"There is a critical need among healthcare providers for an evidence-based, continuously updated, and practical database on complementary and alternative medicine (CAM). With a large percentage of the U.S. population employing CAM therapies, healthcare providers in this country must be able to quickly grasp the clinical significance of these therapies with regard to the overall management of patients' health. Natural Standard provides a credible, rigorously researched, unbiased source of information on an ever-expanding number of complementary and alternative therapies. Boston University School of Medicine Continuing Medical Education has partnered with Natural Standard to sponsor many of the NS modules for AMA PRA Category 1 credit for physicians."

Julie L. White, MS
Administrative Director
Continuing Medical Education
Boston University School of Medicine

"This resource has my highest recommendation."

Jane D. Saxton
Director of Library Services
Bastyr University

"National Standard provides a critical resource for clinicians and researchers, as well as patients and the general public. Using standardized, rigorous research methodology, this multidisciplinary collaboration of experts has set a new standard, literally, for the field. All clinicians and CAM researchers should have access to these evidence-based monographs on complementary and alternative medicine."

Mary Ann Richardson, DrPH
Vice President, Research and Development
National Foundation for Alternative Medicine

"There is a growing popularity for an "evidence-based" approach to CAM. Unfortunately, not everyone takes the time to critically appraise what is out there. As a consequence, some "tomes" regarding natural health product information. Natural Standard's success is due to adopting a rigorous approach to the systematic review of evidence regarding natural health products and its careful selection of leaders in the field to review/edit/collaborate so that well-conducted reviews are paired with clinical experts in the field to assess clinical relevance."

Dr. Sunital Vohra
Director of The Complementary and Alternative
Research and Evaluation (CARE) Program
Stollery Children's Hospital
University of Alberta, Canada

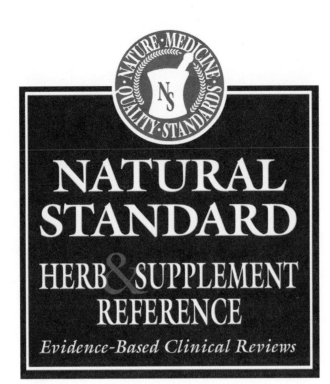

NATURAL STANDARD

HERB & SUPPLEMENT REFERENCE

Evidence-Based Clinical Reviews

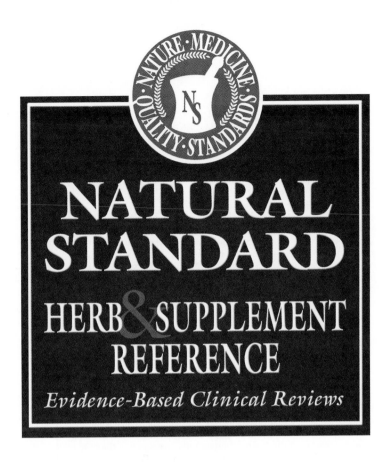

NATURAL STANDARD

HERB & SUPPLEMENT REFERENCE

Evidence-Based Clinical Reviews

Catherine E. Ulbricht, PharmD
Chief Editor

Natural Standard Research Collaboration
Cambridge, Massachusetts
www.naturalstandard.com
Department of Pharmacy
Massachusetts General Hospital
Boston, Massachusetts

Ethan M. Basch, MD, MPhil
Chief Editor

Natural Standard Research Collaboration
Cambridge, Massachusetts
www.naturalstandard.com
Department of Medicine
Memorial Sloan-Kettering Cancer Center
New York, New York

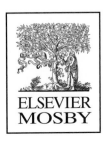

ELSEVIER
MOSBY

ELSEVIER
MOSBY

11830 Westline Industrial Drive
St. Louis, Missouri 63146

NATURAL STANDARD HERB & SUPPLEMENT   ISBN 0-323-02994-9
REFERENCE: EVIDENCE-BASED CLINICAL REVIEWS
Copyright © 2005, Mosby, Inc. All rights reserved.

NOTICE

Pharmacology is an ever-changing field. Standard safety precautions must be followed, but as new research and clinical experience broaden our knowledge, changes in treatment and drug therapy may become necessary or appropriate. Readers are advised to check the most current product information provided by the manufacturer of each drug to be administered to verify the recommended dose, the method and duration of administration, and contraindications. It is the responsibility of the licensed prescriber, relying on experience and knowledge of the patient, to determine dosages and the best treatment for each individual patient. Neither the publisher nor the author assumes any liability for any injury and/or damage to persons or property arising from this publication.

The Publisher

International Standard Book Number 0-323-02994-9

Acquisitions Editor: Kellie White
Senior Developmental Editor: Kim Fons
Publishing Services Manager: Patricia Tannian
Project Manager: John Casey
Book Design Manager: William Drone

Printed in United States of America

Last digit is the print number: 9   8   7   6   5   4   3   2   1

Disclaimer

The content in this book is for general informational purposes only and is not intended as a substitute for medical advice, treatment, or diagnosis. You should consult a physician or other competent medical provider for specific advice applicable to you. If you think you are ill or in need of medical attention, you should seek immediate medical care. Any use of this book or reliance on its content or information is solely at your own risk.

Although some complementary and alternative techniques have been studied scientifically, high-quality data regarding safety, effectiveness, dosage, and mechanism of action are limited or controversial for most therapies. Whenever possible, a practitioner of complementary and alternative techniques should be licensed by a recognized professional organization that adheres to clearly published and generally accepted standards. Before starting any new technique or engaging such a practitioner, an individual should consult with his or her own primary healthcare provider(s). Among other factors, you and your healthcare provider should evaluate the potential risks, benefits, costs, scientific and evidence-based support, and alternatives for the proposed complementary and alternative technique.

As of the date of this publication, the U.S. Food and Drug Administration does not strictly regulate herbs and supplements. There is no guarantee of strength, purity, or safety of unregulated products, and the effects of any such products may vary. Always read product labels fully. If you have a medical condition or are taking a prescription drug or other drugs, herbs, or supplements, you should speak with a qualified healthcare provider about contraindications, interactions, side-effects, and other adverse reactions before starting any new therapy. Immediately consult with a healthcare provider if you experience any unintended side effects or adverse reactions.

In reading and using this book, you agree that the book and its content are provided "as is, where is" and with all faults and that Natural Standard, its shareholders, officers, directors, staff, editors, authors, contributors, and consultants (the "affiliated parties") make no representations or warranties of any kind with respect to the book and its content, including without limitation, as to matters of safety, effectiveness, accuracy, reliability, completeness, timeliness, or results. To the fullest extent allowed by law, Natural Standard and the affiliated parties hereby expressly disclaim any and all representations, guarantees, conditions, and warranties of any and every kind, express or implied or statutory, including without limitation, warranties of title or infringement, and implied warranties of merchantability or fitness for a particular purpose. Readers and users of this book assume full responsibility for the appropriate use of the information it contains and agree to hold Natural Standard and the affiliated parties harmless from and against any and all liabilities, claims, and actions arising from the reader's or user's use of the work or its content. Some jurisdictions do not allow exclusions or limitations of implied warranties, so certain of the above exclusions might not apply.

Because so many individuals contribute to the formation of each Natural Standard monograph, it is not practical to list all who have written, edited, or reviewed each document individually. Therefore a list is provided below of the Natural Standard editors, who are all considered as co-editors of this book.

CHIEF EDITORS

Catherine Ulbricht, PharmD

Dr. Ulbricht serves as senior attending pharmacist, Massachusetts General Hospital and assistant clinical professor at eight universities. She serves on the editorial board of Harvard Health Publications, *Journal of the American Nutraceutical Association, Journal of Integrative Cancer Medicine,* and *Pharmacy Practice News* and is the editor-in-chief of the *Journal of Herbal Pharmacotherapy.* Her background includes experience in the areas of quality improvement, healthcare informatics, and drug therapy decision-support. Dr. Ulbricht has also been trained in physical therapy and chiropractic care.

Ethan Basch, MD, MPhil

Dr. Basch received his medical degree from Harvard Medical School, internal medicine training at Massachusetts General Hospital, and graduate degree in literature from Oxford University. He has held faculty appointments at Harvard Medical School, Northeastern University, University of Rhode Island, University of Missouri, and Massachusetts General Hospital. His background in healthcare decision-support, informatics, and policy includes the design of clinical effectiveness programs and decision-support utilities for multiple healthcare systems. He serves on the editorial board of Harvard Health Publications, the publishing arm of Harvard Medical School, as well as editorial boards of multiple CAM peer-reviewed journals including the *Journal of Herbal Pharmacotherapy, Journal of Cancer Integrative Medicine, Alternative Medicine Research Report,* and *Journal of the American Nutraceutical Association.* He is chief editor of the *Massachusetts General Hospital Primer of Outpatient Medicine* (Lippincott, Williams & Wilkins) and serves as an advisor to the Integrative Medicine Alliance and Cancer Source.

SENIOR EDITORIAL BOARD (ALPHABETICAL ORDER)

Ernie-Paul Barrette, MD, FACP

Dr. Barrette received his medical degree from Harvard Medical School, his MA from Harvard University in Organic Chemistry, and conducted his internal medicine training at Massachusetts General Hospital. He has served as an attending physician and assistant professor at the University of Washington School of Medicine and at Massachusetts General Hospital and is currently on faculty at MetroHealth Medical Center (Ohio) and Case Western Reserve University School of Medicine. He is an expert in complementary and alternative therapies, has contributed to multiple textbooks, and serves as an author and editorial advisor for the newsletter *Alternative Medicine Alert.*

Samuel Basch, MD

Dr. Samuel Basch is an associate clinical professor of psychiatry at Mount Sinai Medical School (NY) and a psychoanalyst. He received his training at Mount Sinai Hospital, where he served as chief resident and at Columbia University Psychoanalytic Clinic. His subspecialties include psychopharmacology and the psychiatric treatment of people with medical illness; he has served as consultant to the cancer unit, the hemodialysis unit, and the organ transplantation unit. His subspecialties also include transcultural psychiatry, and he has worked and taught in Nigeria, Kenya, and Iran, where he studied indigenous treatments and healthcare traditions. Dr. Basch serves on the admissions committee and the board of directors of the Association of Attending Staff at Mount Sinai Hospital and on the Medical Committee of the Riverdale Mental Health Association. He serves on multiple other committees and has published on a wide variety of subjects, including cross-cultural psychiatry, the psychiatric aspects of hemodialysis, and organ transplantation.

William Benda, MD, FACEP, FAAEM

Dr. Benda received his professional training at Duke University, University of Miami School of Medicine, Harbor-UCLA Medical Center, and the Program in Integrative Medicine at the University of Arizona under Dr. Andrew Weil. He has served as director of emergency medical services and assistant clinical professor of medicine at UCLA, as the sole physician in Eastern Rwanda during the 1994 genocide and subsequent cholera epidemic, and as medical director of the Big Sur Health Center. His research and clinical work has focused on patients with breast cancer, animal-assisted therapy, and physician health and well-being. Dr. Benda is a co-founder of the National Integrative Medicine Council, a nonprofit organization for which he has served as Director of Medical and Public Affairs. He is an editor, contributor, and medical advisory board member for several conventional and alternative medicine journals, and he lectures extensively on a variety of topics in the integrative arena.

Stephen Bent, MD

Graduate of Duke University and Vanderbilt University School of Medicine, residency in internal medicine, and fellowship in general internal medicine/clinical epidemiology at the University of California, San Francisco (UCSF), Dr. Bent is an assistant professor of medicine and attending physician at UCSF, where he conducts research evaluating the safety and effectiveness of alternative therapies. He is the project director of an NIH-funded, randomized controlled trial of the herb saw palmetto and the principal investigator of a study evaluating a commonly used Chinese herbal remedy. Dr. Bent is a co-author of textbooks in evidence-based medicine and internal medicine, and he is an expert in the systematic evaluation of alternative therapies.

Heather Boon, BSc Phm, PhD

As an author and researcher, Dr. Boon has gained an international reputation, evidenced by her membership on the prestigious international editorial board of the British journal, *Focus on Alternative and Complementary Therapies* (FACT). She founded and chairs the Toronto CAM Research Network and is an advisor to multiple government and private organizations. In addition, she chaired the Canadian Society for Hospital Pharmacists (CSHP) Task Force to Develop Guidelines for Handling Alternative Medication/Therapy. Dr. Boon has been the principal investigator for myriad large studies focusing on CAM therapies used to treat cancer and on emerging CAM practice patterns. She is widely published as the author of primary research and reviews and maintains a faculty position at the University of Toronto.

Stefan Bughi, MD

Dr. Bughi is president of the Southern California Society of Clinical Hypnosis and a fellow of the American Institute of Stress. He is board certified in internal medicine and endocrinology and serves as assistant professor of clinical medicine at the Keck School of Medicine, University of Southern California in Los Angeles. Presently he works as a physician specialist in the endocrine/diabetes service at Rancho Los Amigos National Rehabilitation Center and at the University of Southern California. Dr. Bughi received his medical degree from the University of Bucharest School of Medicine, Romania, internal medicine training at NE Pennsylvania Affiliated Programs, and endocrinology fellowship at the University of Southern California. His research interests include stress and psychosomatic disorders. He has organized and presented seminars on stress to health professionals and at national and international scientific meetings.

Richard Philip Cohan, DDS, MS, MBA

After Dr. Cohan received an AB in bacteriology from University of California, Berkeley, he engaged in molecular genetic research at Stanford Medical School and Syntex Laboratories. Subsequently, he completed a master's degree in (oral) biology at Southern Methodist University and a DDS at Case Western Reserve University. He joined the faculty of the University of the Pacific (UOP) School of Dentistry in San Francisco in 1972 and became section head of oral diagnosis and treatment planning in 1984. Dr. Cohan has attained both a master's degree in educational psychology and an MBA from UOP during his tenure there. Since 1989, his research, new course development, publishing, editing, and consulting activities have focused primarily on integrative medicine in dentistry. Most recently, he co-authored and submitted for publication a chapter on complementary and alternative medicine for the leading dental pharmacology textbook. He maintains a private dental practice at the California Pacific Medical Center in San Francisco.

William Collinge, MPH, PhD

Dr. Collinge received his MPH and PhD from the University of California, Berkeley, and clinical training at Harvard's Mind/Body Medical Institute. He has served as a peer-review panelist at the National Institutes of Health, National Center for Complementary and Alternative Medicine (NCCAM) and has taught at the UC Berkeley School of Public Health and several other universities. He has conducted research in integrative programs for cancer, HIV, and chronic fatigue syndrome and has extensive clinical background in behavioral, mind/body, and energy medicine. He consults in patient-centered approaches to program development in integrative medicine. He is on the editorial boards of *Subtle Energies & Energy Medicine* and *The International Journal of Healing and Caring*. His books include *Subtle Energy* and *The American Holistic Health Association Complete Guide to Alternative Medicine*.

Cathi Dennehy, PharmD

Dr. Dennehy is an assistant clinical professor in the department of clinical pharmacy in the School of Pharmacy at the University of California, San Francisco (UCSF). Her areas of specialty are herbal medicine and anticoagulation. Dr. Dennehy co-coordinates an evidence-based course in herbal remedies and dietary supplements at UCSF. She has co-authored book chapters on herbs and dietary supplements in various medical and pharmacy textbooks. Dr. Dennehy serves as a consultant to various organizations and journal publications in the area of herbal medicine. In addition, she has coordinated various continuing education programs for state and national pharmacy societies on herbs and dietary supplements and speaks statewide and nationally on this subject.

J. Donald Dishman, DC, MSc

Dr. Dishman is an associate professor in the departments of anatomy and research at the New York Chiropractic College (NYCC) in Seneca Falls, NY. He serves as director of the chiropractic clinic of Monroe Community Hospital in Rochester, NY. In addition to his DC, he was awarded a master of science degree in neurophysiology from the Institute for Sensory Research at Syracuse University. His research has focused on the neurophysiology of spinal manipulative therapy. He maintains a full-time research laboratory at NYCC in which neurophysiological techniques (e.g., H-reflexes, transcranial magnetic stimulation, electromyography) are employed in the investigation of the effects of spinal manipulation on the nervous system. Dr. Dishman also maintains an appointment as adjunct associate professor of bioengineering and neuroscience at the Institute for Sensory Research of Syracuse University. He has published numerous manuscripts in the field of neurophysiology of spinal manipulation, including in the international journal, *Spine*. He also serves as a reviewer for the *Journal of Manipulative and Physiological Therapeutics* and the *Journal of the Neuromusculoskeletal System*.

Joan Engebretson, DrPH, RN

Dr. Engebretson is an associate professor at the University of Texas Health Science Center at Houston, School of Nursing and the School of Public Health. Her background is in maternal child health and community health. She has taught in maternal/child health, women's health, and community health. She is co-editor of the *Maternal, Neonatal and Women's Health Nursing* textbook. Dr. Engebretson has conducted and supervised ethnographic studies examining cultural issues and approaches to healing, as well as clinical research with traditional healers and recipients of touch therapies. She has published numerous articles and book chapters on complementary and alternative therapies, serves on several advisory boards, and consults with many organizations regarding the use of complementary therapies. She teaches a course on culture and complementary therapies at the University of Texas.

Edzard Ernst, MD, PhD, FRCP

Dr. Ernst is one of the best-known worldwide figures in complementary and alternative medicine research, and he has published over 500 major articles and books in this area. His work has focused on the systematic production of rigorous and trustworthy information. He is currently director of the department of complementary medicine at Exeter University, England, which is a premier global center for scientific research in this field.

Mitchell A. Fleisher, MD, DHt, FAAFP, DcABCT

Dr. Fleisher is a board-certified family physician specializing in classical homeopathy, nutritional and botanical medicine, and chelation therapy with over 20 years of clinical experience in integrative medicine. He serves as an active member of the clinical faculty of the National Center for Homeopathy and is clinical instructor for the University of Virginia Health Sciences Center and at the Medical College of Virginia, where he teaches homeopathy in the complementary medicine program. He has lectured throughout the United States and internationally on classical homeopathy and nutritional therapy and regularly contributes as an author and editor to medical journals and popular magazines. Dr. Fleisher attended Stanford University School of Medicine. He has served on the faculty of the New England School of Homeopathy, is currently a clinical preceptor at the Hahnemann College of Homeopathy, and is a graduate of both of these institutions. He is a former assistant clinical professor of family medicine at the Medical College of Virginia and former associate medical director of the MCV/Blackstone Family Practice Residency Training Program, of which he is a graduate. Dr. Fleisher is a fellow of the American Academy of Family Physicians, a diplomate of the American Board of Family Practice and American Board of Homeotherapeutics, and a diplomate candidate of the American Board of Chelation Therapy.

Harley Goldberg, DO

Dr. Goldberg is the director of complementary and alternative medicine for Kaiser Permanente Northern California Medical Care Program and the chief of complementary medicine at Santa Teresa Medical Center in San Jose, California. A graduate of the University of Osteopathic Medicine and Health Sciences, he completed a family medicine residency at Oregon Health Sciences University, Portland, Oregon. He is board certified in family medicine, a fellow of the American Academy of Family Practice, and board certified in neuromusculoskeletal and osteopathic manipulative medicine. Dr. Goldberg has written or edited over 20 systematic reviews of CAM modalities, which are widely used in the Kaiser Permanente system, and he serves on the editorial board of *FACT: Focus on Alternative and Complementary Therapies,* and *Alternative Therapies in Health and Medicine.*

Joerg Gruenwald, PhD

Dr. Gruenwald is primary author of the *PDR for Herbal Medicines* and is a leading European expert in the field of botanicals/phytomedicines. He is the president of Phytopharm Consulting, a unit of analyze & realize ag, Berlin, Germany, a specialized consulting company for natural medicine and dietary supplements. His activities range from market analysis, product development, to R&D, licensing, and medical writing. His main focus is the international exchange of information with an emphasis on Europe and the United States, based on his long experience as medical director of Lichtwer Pharma and on several years as president of Phytopharm Consulting. Dr. Gruenwald has published over 180 scientific articles, five books, and the CD-ROM "Herbal Remedies." He is a regular chairman of international conferences.

Paul Hammerness, MD

Dr. Hammerness is a graduate of Dartmouth Medical School, with postgraduate training in psychiatry and child and adolescent psychiatry at Massachusetts General Hospital and McLean Hospital. He has clinical, administrative, and editorial experience within numerous evidence-based research groups. Dr. Hammerness is committed to continuous quality improvement, particularly when applied to the evaluation of CAM and psychiatric therapies. He is the author of multiple CAM review articles and serves on the editorial board for Harvard Health Publications, the publishing arm of Harvard Medical School.

Charles Holmes, MD, MPH

Dr. Holmes trained in internal medicine at Massachusetts General Hospital and is presently a fellow in infectious disease at Massachusetts General Hospital/Brigham and Women's Hospital and a clinical fellow at Harvard Medical School. Following a graduate degree in epidemiology and international health from the University of Michigan, Dr. Holmes practiced infectious disease epidemiology at the World Health Organization in Geneva, Switzerland. He is currently engaged in HIV research in Boston and sub-Saharan Africa.

Courtney Jarvis, PharmD

Dr. Jarvis serves as an assistant professor in the department of pharmacy practice, Massachusetts College of Pharmacy and Health Sciences (MCPHS), where she teaches graduate level courses involving traditional and complementary medicine. In particular, Dr. Jarvis co-coordinates the therapeutics sequence and an evidence-based course in women's health, which incorporates herbs and dietary supplements into the curriculum. Dr. Jarvis practices clinical pharmacy at UMASS/Memorial Health Care Medical Center with the family medicine residency program.

Karta Purkh Singh Khalsa, CDN, RH (AHG)

KP Khalsa teaches Ayurvedic and botanical medicine in the naturopathic doctoral program and the herbal sciences bachelor's program at Bastyr University, the foremost naturopathic medicine educational institution in the United States. He is a leading member of The American Herbalists Guild, having served two terms on the board of directors. He continues to act as a national association officer. He is a certified dietitian-nutritionist and one of the first registered herbalists in the United States. Author or editor of over a dozen books, he recently co-authored *Herbal Defense* (Warner Books). He is a frequent contributor to mainstream and professional publications in the natural healing field. KP Khalsa is on the faculty of several professional training programs and is the founder of The Professional Herbalist Certificate Course, a 2-year postsecondary curriculum that trains professional herbalists, now being offered at several colleges in Washington and New Mexico. He is a frequent lecturer and presenter to professional healthcare organizations throughout the United States.

Catherine DeFranco Kirkwood, MPH, CCCJS-MAC

Catherine Kirkwood serves as program education coordinator for the Complementary/Integrative Medicine Education Resources (CIMER) Program of the Office of Educational Programs at MD Anderson Cancer Center. She previously served as the director of clinical education and training for the AIDS Education and Training Center for Texas and Oklahoma, a program of the University of Texas School of Public Health. Ms. Kirkwood received her master's degree in public health from the University of Texas. She has more than 20 years of experience in education of healthcare professionals at the Texas Medical Center. She is an appointed member of the Ryan

White Planning Council and serves as a senior member of the Advances in Medications and Treatment subcommittee.

David J. Kroll, PhD

Former research director of the Duke University Center for Integrative Medicine, Dr. Kroll is nationally recognized for his work in alternative medicine education and research. He recently joined the Natural Products Program of Research Triangle Institute where the anticancer drug Taxol was first isolated. He was recently named a president's teaching scholar of the University of Colorado. He has co-authored reference books for clinical and lay audiences on evidence-based evaluation of phytomedicinals and has served as series co-editor for 16 consumer books on alternative medicine. He is a graduate of the Philadelphia College of Pharmacy and Science and of the University of Florida College of Medicine, department of pharmacology and therapeutics, with a post-doctoral fellowship in molecular oncology at the University of Colorado School of Medicine, divisions of endocrinology and medical oncology. Dr. Kroll has spent most of his academic career as an associate professor of pharmacology and toxicology at the University of Colorado School of Pharmacy, where he has conducted NIH-funded research on the molecular pharmacology of natural product drugs that target DNA topoisomerases, herbal remedies that interact with these anti-tumor drugs, and the molecular mechanisms of cytochrome P-450 induction by botanicals.

Richard Liebowitz, MD

Dr. Liebowitz is the director of clinical services for the Duke University Center for Integrative Medicine. Before his current position, he served as director of education for Dr. Andrew Weil's program in integrative medicine, as well as general medicine section chief at the University of Arizona. He has received multiple honors and awards for excellence in teaching at these institutions. Dr. Liebowitz is a graduate of Robert Wood Johnson (Rutgers) Medical School and of the internal medicine residency program at the University of Massachusetts. In addition to his other responsibilities, he currently directs a community-based program in Durham, NC, to improve health in an underserved population. He serves on the editorial board of *Archives of Internal Medicine*.

Ann M. Lynch, RPh, AE-C

Ann Lynch serves as a clinical instructor in the department of pharmacy practice, Massachusetts College of Pharmacy and Health Sciences (MCPHS). She received her BS in pharmacy from Northeastern University and graduate level training at MCPHS. Her professional focus is in the area of herbal medicine and interactions, as well as in community practice with specialty interests in asthma, diabetes, and women's health. Ms. Lynch coordinates on-site screenings and community educational clinics regarding conventional and complementary medicine practices at Fallon Clinic Pharmacies and co-coordinates courses in drug interactions and pharmaceutical care at MCPHS.

Ed Mills DPH, MSc (Oxon)

Dr. Mills is director of research at the Canadian College of Naturopathic Medicine. He is the author of numerous publications, reviews, and original research related to evidence-based complementary and alternative medicine. He has also authored original research articles on issues surrounding risk and risk perception in complementary and alternative medicine. His academic interests and clinical trial work focus on improving the methodology of herb-drug interaction studies. He is the chair of the Evidence-Based Complementary and Alternative Medicine (EBCAM) Working Group.

Shri Kant Mishra, ABMS (BHU), MD, MS, FAAN, FIAA

Dr. Mishra is professor of neurology and coordinator of the integrative medicine program at the Keck School of Medicine, University of Southern California, and staff neurologist at the VA Greater Los Angeles Healthcare System and Olive View UCLA Medical Center. He graduated Ayurveda Charya, bachelor of medicine and surgery (ABMS) from Banaras Hindu University in Varanasi India, and received his master's of science (anatomy) from Queens University, Kingston, Ontario, Canada, his medical degree from the University of Toronto, and his master's degree in administrative medicine from the University of Wisconsin. He is a member of numerous neuroscience and integrative medicine societies and editorial boards, and is president of the American Academy of Ayurvedic Medicine (AAAM). He has been chair of an NCCAM (NIH) study section. He is a practicing neurologist, Ayurvedist, and yoga teacher. He has served as president and chair of the Indian Medical Association of Southern California, FIA of Southern California, and as regional director of AAPI.

Howard Moffet, MS, MPH

Howard Moffet serves as a research program manager at the Kaiser Permanente (KP) Division of Research in Oakland, California, and is a member of the KP Complementary and Alternative Medicine Research Group. He currently teaches in the Department of Health Education, Institute for Holistic Healing Studies, San Francisco State University, and was appointed by former governor Gray Davis to the California Acupuncture Board. He received his graduate degrees from the Harvard School of Public Health and the American College of Traditional Chinese Medicine. He is a licensed acupuncturist, and his research interest is in the physiological mechanisms of acupuncture.

Adrianne Rogers, MD

Dr. Rogers received her medical degree from Harvard Medical School and pathology training at the Mallory Institute of Pathology (Boston City Hospital) and the Peter Bent Brigham Hospital. She is professor and associate chair of pathology and laboratory medicine and director of the Office of Medical Education at Boston University School of Medicine and is on the pathology staff at Boston Medical Center. She is the author of numerous articles on experimental studies of dietary and nutritional effects on chemical carcinogenesis, is a diplomate and member of the American Board of Toxicology, on which she just completed a term as chair of the examination committee, and is a member of the editorial boards of the *Journal of Nutritional Biochemistry, Toxicology,* and *Nutrition and Cancer.* She is a member of the expert panel of the Research Institute for Fragrance Materials (RIFM), which reviews publications and data related to safety of materials used in fragrances, and of the Beryllium Industries Scientific Advisory Committee (BISAC), which reviews basic science and clinical studies of beryllium toxicity. For many years she served on and chaired the grants review panel for the American Institute for Cancer Research (AICR), which supports research in diet and cancer.

Aviva Romm, BSc, RH (AHG), CPM

Aviva Romm has been in clinical practice as an herbalist and midwife since 1986. She is currently president of the American Herbalists Guild (AHG). The author of six books on botanical medicine, Aviva is also the executive editor of the peer-reviewed *Journal of the American Herbalists Guild.* She serves as primary editor for the *Textbook of Botanical Medicine for Women,* to be published by Churchill/Elsevier in 2004. Her policy work has focused on developing national standards for botanical medicine education and practice in the United States. She regularly writes for national health magazines and peer-reviewed publications, is on the advisory board for Bastyr University's bachelor of science program in botanical medicine, and regularly presents at national conferences.

Michael Rotblatt, MD, PharmD

Dr. Rotblatt began his career as a pharmacist, receiving his PharmD from UC San Francisco, and worked as a drug information and clinical pharmacist at Stanford University Hospital. He received his medical degree from UC Irvine and completed internal medicine residency training at a UCLA program. He is currently an associate professor of medicine at UCLA and an attending physician at the Sepulveda VA Ambulatory Care Center and the Olive View–UCLA Medical Center. His area of interest is evaluating herbal medicines and other dietary supplements and educating health care professionals in this field. He is co-author of the book, *Evidence-Based Herbal Medicine,* has lectured nationally to health professional groups, and serves on the editorial board for *Focus on Alternative and Complementary Therapies* (FACT).

Andrew L. Rubman, ND

Dr. Rubman received his naturopathic medical degree from National College of Naturopathic Medicine in Portland, Oregon. A founder and lifetime member of the American Association of Naturopathic Physicians, he has been active in national media and organizations advocating the evolution of a responsible medical continuum among all licensed physicians. He has served as an advisor and lecturer for the White House Commission for Complementary and Alternative Medical Policy and medical schools across the United States. An adjunct associate professor of clinical medicine at the College of Naturopathic Medicine, University of Bridgeport, and an adjunct professor of medicine at the Florida College of Integrative Medicine, he is widely published. Dr. Rubman serves as the content provider in naturopathic medicine for the North American Menopause Society and is an editorial advisor to numerous publications.

Kenneth Sancier, PhD

Dr. Sancier is the founder and chairman of the board of directors of the Qigong Institute. He is a professor at the American College of Traditional Medicine, San Francisco. He received a doctorate from Johns Hopkins University, and his research has focused on basic and applied chemistry. Dr. Sancier developed the computerized Qigong Research Database, has written multiple reviews of qigong scientific investigations, and has published numerous qigong clinical studies. He has participated in international qigong conferences in China, Japan, Canada, and the United States. He is an editor of the *Journal of the International Society of Life Information Science* (JISLIS), director of the California Information Center of ISLIS, on the advisory board of the *Journal Of Alternative Therapies,* and is on the Council of the World Academic Society of Medical Qigong.

Elad Schiff, MD

Dr. Schiff received his internal medicine training at B'nai Zion Medical Center in Israel. He has served as chairman of the Committee for Regulation of Complementary Medicine Studies, Ministries of Education and Health, Israel. He has published multiple articles in the areas of acupuncture and pain medicine and is currently a residential fellow at the Program in Integrative Medicine at the University of Arizona under Dr. Andrew Weil. In addition to practicing internal medicine, he teaches in leading schools of complementary medicine in Israel and is involved with a complementary medicine clinic that provides reflexology, shiatsu, and acupuncture services.

Robb Scholten, MSLIS

Robb Scholten serves as the information officer at the Division for Research and Education on Complementary and Integrative Medical Therapies, Harvard Medical School. Before that he worked as an academic representative at PaperChase, a pioneer organization in consumer-accessible database interfaces. He conducted his graduate work in information science at the University of Tennessee, where he helped design one of the first web-controlled online remote access database services in the state. Robb is also the secretary for the division's three major continuing education courses, which focus on integrative medical therapies.

Michael Smith, MRPharmS, ND

Dr. Smith serves as associate dean for research at the Canadian College of Naturopathic Medicine. He is the author of numerous review articles and texts on the safety and uses of natural products, including *Herbs to Homeopathy,* published by Prentice Hall Canada in 2002. He has served as principal investigator for multiple studies, including a prospective controlled study of echinacea published in the *Archives of Internal Medicine* (2000), studies of alternative therapies in cancer, and studies of alternative therapies in pregnancy. As a recognized authority in Canada, he serves on multiple national and international panels, including the National Advisory Group on Complementary and Alternative Medicine and HIV/AIDS, and the International Editorial Board for Focus on Alternative and Complementary Therapies (FACT).

David Sollars, MAc, HMC

David Sollars holds a master's degree in oriental medicine from the New England School of Acupuncture (NESA). He is currently an adjunct professor of biology at Merrimack College, where he lectures on integrated approaches to sports medicine. He is a diplomat of the National Commission for the Certification of Acupuncturists, NESA's Chinese Herbal Medical Program, the North American Homeopathic Master's Clinician Course, and the International Federation of Homeopathy. He is certified in Japanese Shiatsu, Sotai, and Chinese Tui-Na massage. He has been practicing in the Boston area for over 16 years, has authored books on acupuncture, fitness, and homeopathy, and is a frequent lecturer and consultant for colleges, hospitals, insurance companies, and patient support groups.

Philippe Szapary, MD

Dr. Szapary is a graduate of Brown University and the University of Chicago Pritzker School of Medicine. He conducted his internship and residency in primary care internal medicine at the University of California, San Francisco. Dr. Szapary is an assistant professor of medicine in the division of general internal medicine at the University of Pennsylvania, where he conducts clinical trials in complementary and alternative therapies in cardiovascular disease. He is the principal investigator of a randomized clinical trial of gugulipid in hypercholesterolemia and has participated in several industry-sponsored trials of plant stanol esters in hyperlipidemia. Dr. Szapary has also recently been awarded a career development award from the NIH to study the effects of Ayurvedic botanicals in atherosclerosis. He has authored several chapters in ambulatory medicine, evidence-based medicine, and CAM therapies in cardiovascular disease. Dr. Szapary is also a regular contributor to the publication *Alternative Medicine Alert.*

Candy Tsourounis, PharmD

Dr. Tsourounis is the acting director of the Drug Information Analysis Service at the University of California, San Francisco (UCSF). She also serves as an assistant clinical professor in the department of clinical pharmacy at UCSF. Dr. Tsourounis co-coordinates an evidence-based course in herbal remedies and dietary supplements, sponsored by the Osher Center for Integrative Medicine. She has co-authored multiple book chapters on herbs and dietary supplements in medical and pharmacy textbooks. Dr. Tsourounis serves as a clinical consultant and editor for several drug information publications and computer software programs, particularly in the areas of herbal remedies and dietary supplements. She has coordinated continuing education programs for national pharmacy societies on herbs and dietary supplements and lectures nationally.

Andrew Weil, MD

Andrew Weil is an internationally recognized expert on medicinal plants, alternative medicine, and the reform of medical education. Dr. Weil received his undergraduate degree in biology (botany) from Harvard University, medical degree from Harvard Medical School, and completed a medical internship at Mt. Zion Hospital in San Francisco. In the 1970s, as a fellow of the Institute of Current World Affairs, Dr. Weil traveled widely in North and South America and Africa collecting information on drug use in other cultures, medicinal plants, and alternative methods of treating disease. He subsequently conducted research on medicinal and psychoactive plants at the Harvard Botanical Museum. Dr. Weil currently serves as director of the Program in Integrative Medicine of the College of Medicine, University of Arizona, where he holds appointments as clinical professor of medicine and clinical assistant professor of family and community medicine. The Program in Integrative Medicine aims to change U.S. medical education by including information on alternative therapies, mind-body interactions, healing, and other subjects not currently emphasized in the training of physicians. Dr. Weil is the author of numerous scientific and popular articles, as well as seven books, including the international best sellers *Spontaneous Healing* and *Eight Weeks to Optimum Health.* His most recent books include *Eating Well for Optimum Health: The Essential Guide to Food, Diet, and Nutrition* and *The Healthy Kitchen: Recipes for a Better Body, Life, and Spirit* (with Rosie Daley).

Roger Wood, LMT, Dipl. ABT (NCCAOM)

Roger Wood is a shiatsu practitioner. He received his training at the Boston Shiatsu School and 2 years of advanced training in North Yorkshire, England. He is the founder and president of the American Organization for Bodywork Therapies of Asia (MA), a professional organization for shiatsu and other Asian bodywork therapists. He is a diplomate of the National Certification Commission for Acupuncture and Oriental Medicine. In addition to his clinical practice, he supervises students at the Boston Shiatsu School Student Clinic and participates in NIH-sponsored research on low back pain at the Beth Israel Deaconess Medical Center, Harvard Medical School.

Robert Zori, MD

Dr. Zori is an associate professor, chief of the division of genetics, and director of cytogenetics in the department of pediatrics at the University of Florida. He is a graduate of Odense University Medical School in Denmark and the Baystate Medical Center Residency Program in Massachusetts. He has practiced medicine in both Denmark and the United States.

AUTHORS/CONTRIBUTORS

Acknowledgments

Many individuals have contributed significantly to the content and effort underlying this book and the Natural Standard Research Collaboration in general.

We are grateful to John Martinson, without whose support this project would not have been possible. Our close colleague and friend Paul Hammerness has shouldered significant editorial responsibility, as has Charles Holmes, a fellow co-founder of Natural Standard. Early contributors to Natural Standard provided the solid methodological and editorial foundation that has distinguished the organization, in particular, Michael Smith, Heather Boon, David Sollars, Philippe Szapary, E-P Barrette, and Steve Bent. We would also like to thank several individuals—Adrianne Rogers, Candy Tsourounis, and Cathi Dennehy—who have continued to contribute significantly to the collaboration, including materials in this book.

Invaluable has been the contribution of Chris Wisdo, whose technical aptitude has facilitated the functionality of the Natural Standard database. Members of the Research Team over the past years have fostered a productive and collegial work environment, and we are particularly grateful for the commitment of Regina Gorenshteyn and Michelle Nhuch.

There are several trailblazers in the field of evidence-based/academic CAM who have defined an environment in which the work of Natural Standard is valued. We are thankful to David Eisenberg, who has continued to provide us with valuable guidance and enthusiasm, as has his Information Officer, our friend Robb Scholten. Edzard Ernst has given insights as an editor for Natural Standard and continues to push this field ahead through publishing. Ellen Hughes has persistently provided guidance and support. Harley Goldberg remains a champion of this field, as well as a friend.

We would especially like to thank Kellie White, Kim Fons, Inta Ozols, and Linda Duncan at Elsevier, who have shared our enthusiasm for Natural Standard print projects and have been a pleasure as colleagues. All of the editors and authors of Natural Standard have helped forge this unique multidisciplinary collaboration, yielding a unique consensus and center in an otherwise fractured field. We look forward to our continued work together. Finally, we would like to thank our families and friends, who have supported us through this and other arduous projects.

Kate and Ethan

Contents

INTRODUCTION

Since its establishment in 1999, the Natural Standard Research Collaboration has become one of the world's premier sources of scientifically based information on complementary and alternative medicine (CAM). This international collaborative effort has involved more than 300 contributors from multiple healthcare disciplines across numerous countries. Editors and reviewers range from the most well-known researchers and clinicians in this field to private practitioners.

Natural Standard maintains an online database of evidence-based CAM reviews, including coverage of herbs, supplements, modalities (such as chiropractic or massage), daily news briefings, continuing education, and conditions-based cross-referencing. Subscriptions to this database are available for individuals or institutions at www.naturalstandard.com. In addition, Natural Standard provides CAM information for hospitals, healthcare institutions, HMOs, research organizations, manufacturers, journals, magazines, and textbooks worldwide. Millions of clinicians and patients have relied on Natural Standard content.

This book includes comprehensive systematic reviews of selected herbs and supplements, designed for use by clinicians and researchers. A "Bottom-Line" companion text with abbreviated versions of this content is also available or can be accessed online. The topics covered in this first volume have been selected based on utilization data, sales trends, frequency of information requests by institutional/individual users of Natural Standard, and safety concerns. Tremendous time, labor, and cost are involved with the creation of each piece, involving numerous individuals via an extensive methodology (described below). We are constantly adding new topics and expanding this database. In the interest of saving space and including more topics, in some cases monographs from the companion handbook to this text have been included.

These pieces demonstrate the growing body of literature regarding the efficacy and safety of CAM therapies, although research for many of these therapies is still in its early phases. It is our hope that this information will serve as a helpful guide to these selected agents.

NATURAL STANDARD BACKGROUND

Natural Standard aims to provide high-quality, reliable information about CAM therapies to clinicians, patients, and healthcare institutions. Through systematic aggregation and analysis of scientific data (see below), incorporation of historic and folkloric perspectives, consultation with multidisciplinary editorial experts, use of validated grading scales (see Table 1), and blinded peer-review processes, Natural Standard builds evidence-based and consensus-based content. This content is designed to support safer and more informed therapeutic decisions.

As the volume of CAM safety concerns and scientific research increases, clinicians and patients are faced with progressively complex therapeutic decisions. These issues, coupled with a growing consciousness among practitioners that many patients use CAM therapies, has created a need for high-quality information services and decision support utilities.

However, rigorous, peer-reviewed, evidence-based resources in this area are scarce. Sources of CAM information are often not updated with appropriate frequency, rely on anecdotal evidence rather than an evidence-based approach, are not rooted in academic health centers, are not scientifically rigorous, and do not encompass a multidisciplinary approach.

In response to this need, the Natural Standard Research Collaboration was formed as a multidisciplinary, multi-institution initiative in 1999. Natural Standard content and rigorous methodology are designed to address issues of safety and efficacy that directly pertain to the questions raised by clinicians, patients, and healthcare institutions.

CAM is one part of a larger healthcare context that is becoming progressively integrated. Natural Standard aspires to raise the standards for CAM information, toward improving the quality of healthcare delivery overall.

MONOGRAPH METHODOLOGY: SYSTEMATIC AGGREGATION, ANALYSIS, AND REVIEW OF THE LITERATURE
Search Strategy

To prepare each Natural Standard monograph, electronic searches are conducted in 10 databases, including AMED, CANCERLIT, CINAHL, CISCOM, the Cochrane Library, EMBASE, HerbMed, International Pharmaceutical Abstracts, Medline, and NAPRALERT. Search terms include the common name(s), scientific name(s), and all listed synonyms for each topic. Hand searches are conducted of 20 additional journals (not indexed in common databases) and of bibliographies from 50 selected secondary references. No restrictions are placed on language or quality of publications. Researchers in the CAM field are consulted for access to additional references or ongoing research.

Selection Criteria

All literature is collected pertaining to efficacy in humans (regardless of study design, quality, or language), dosing, precautions, adverse effects, use in pregnancy/lactation, interactions, alteration of laboratory assays, and mechanism of action (*in vitro*, animal research, human data). Standardized inclusion/exclusion criteria are used selection.

Data Analysis

Data extraction and analysis are performed by healthcare professionals conducting clinical work and research at academic centers, using standardized instruments that pertain to each monograph section (defining inclusion and exclusion criteria and analytic techniques, including validated measures of study quality). Data are verified by a second reviewer.

Review Process

Blinded review of monographs is conducted by multidisciplinary research-clinical faculty at major academic centers with expertise in epidemiology and biostatistics, pharmacology, toxicology, CAM research, and clinical practice. In cases of editorial disagreement, a three-member panel of the editorial board addresses conflicts and consults experts when applicable. Authors of studies are contacted when clarification is required.

Update Process

Natural Standard regularly monitors scientific literature and industry warnings. When clinically relevant new data emerge, best efforts are made to update content immediately. In addition, regular updates with renewed searches occur every 3 to 18 months, varying by topic.

NATURAL STANDARD EVIDENCE-BASED VALIDATED GRADING RATIONALE

Multiple grading scales have been developed over the past decade to evaluate the level of available scientific evidence supporting the efficacy of medical interventions. Based on existing grading scales, as well as unique challenges involved in the evaluation of CAM therapies, the Natural Standard grading scale was developed through a multidisciplinary consensus group, widely reviewed, then piloted and validated. This scale

has been found to have a high level of inter-rater reliability, has been used in numerous publications, and has been presented for discussion at the Agency for Healthcare Research and Quality (AHRQ).

These grades are used in all Natural Standard reviews (monographs). Specific grades reflect the level of available scientific evidence in support of the efficacy of a given therapy for a specific indication. Expert opinion and folkloric precedent are not included in this assessment and are reflected in a separate section of each monograph. Evidence of harm is considered separately, and the grades apply only to evidence of benefit (Table 1).

Table 1
Natural Standard Evidence-Based Validated Grading Rationale

Level of Evidence Grade	Criteria
A (Strong scientific evidence)	Statistically significant evidence of benefit from more than two properly randomized controlled trials (RCTs), *or* evidence from one properly conducted RCT *and* one properly conducted meta-analysis, or evidence from multiple RCTs with a clear majority of the properly conducted trials showing statistically significant evidence of benefit *and* with supporting evidence in basic science, animal studies, or theory.
B (Good scientific evidence)	Statistically significant evidence of benefit from one or two properly randomized trials, *or* evidence of benefit from one or more properly conducted meta-analysis *or* evidence of benefit from more than one cohort/case-control/non-randomized trials *and* with supporting evidence in basic science, animal studies, or theory.
C (Unclear or conflicting scientific evidence)	Evidence of benefit from one or more small RCT(s) without adequate size, power, statistical significance, or quality of design by objective criteria,* *or* conflicting evidence from multiple RCTs without a clear majority of the properly conducted trials showing evidence of benefit or ineffectiveness, *or* evidence of benefit from more than one cohort/case-control/non-randomized trials *and* without supporting evidence in basic science, animal studies, or theory, *or* evidence of efficacy only from basic science, animal studies, or theory.
D (Fair negative scientific evidence)	Statistically significant negative evidence (i.e., lack of evidence of benefit) from cohort/case-control/non-randomized trials, and evidence in basic science, animal studies, or theory suggesting a lack of benefit.
F (Strong negative scientific evidence)	Statistically significant negative evidence (i.e. lack of evidence of benefit) from one or more properly randomized adequately powered trial(s) of high-quality design by objective criteria.*
Lack of evidence[†]	Unable to evaluate efficacy due to lack of adequate or available human data.

* Objective criteria are derived from validated instruments for evaluating study quality, including the 5-point scale developed by Jadad et al., in which a score below 4 is considered to indicate lesser quality methodologically (Jadad AR, Moore RA, Carroll D, et al. Assessing the quality of reports of randomized clinical trials: is blinding necessary? *Controlled Clinical Trials* 1996; 17[1]:1-12).

[†]Listed separately in monographs in the section, "Historical or Theoretical Uses That Lack Sufficient Evidence."

CAM IN THE UNITED STATES: A BRIEF BACKGROUND

Various definitions have been assigned to the term "complementary and alternative medicine (CAM)," but it is generally regarded as encompassing a broad group of healing philosophies, diagnostic approaches, and therapeutic interventions that do not belong to the politically dominant (conventional) health system of a particular society.[1,2] Some authors separately define *alternative* therapies as those used in place of conventional practices, whereas *complementary* or *integrative* medicine can be combined with mainstream approaches.[2,3] Other terms

used to refer to CAM include folkloric, holistic, irregular, non-conventional, non-Western, traditional, unconventional, unorthodox, and unproven medicine.

In the United States and other Western countries, CAM therapies are often defined functionally as interventions neither taught in medical schools nor available in hospital-based practices.[4] Examples include dietary supplements (amino acids, herbal products/botanicals, minerals, vitamins, and substances that increase total dietary intake),[5] modalities (manipulative therapies, mind-body medicine, and energy/bioelectromagnetic-based approaches), spiritual healing, and nutritional/dietary alteration. Boundaries between CAM and conventional therapies are not always clear and often change over time. Scientific evidence has led to broader mainstream acceptance of some CAM therapies and rejection of others.

CAM Research

The safety and efficacy of many CAM approaches are not well studied, although the body of research is growing. In 1992, the U.S. Congress established the Office of Alternative Medicine (OAM) within the National Institutes of Health (NIH), with a budget of $2 million to "investigate and evaluate promising unconventional medical practices." In 1998, Congress elevated the status of the OAM to a NIH Center, becoming the National Center for Complementary and Alternative Medicine (NCCAM).

The budget of NCCAM has progressively increased, from $50 million in fiscal year 1999 to $114 million in 2003, toward its mission to "support rigorous research on CAM, to train researchers in CAM, and to disseminate information to the public and professionals on which CAM modalities work, which do not, and why."

Prevalence

In the United States, an estimated 44% of the population used at least one CAM therapy in 1997.[4,6-8] Utilization in specific chronic diseases appears to be even higher. For example, surveys published since 1999 suggest that between 25% to 83% of U.S. cancer patients have used CAM therapies at some point after diagnosis, with variations in use rates depending on geographic area and type of cancer.[9-24] These reports suggest use of high-dose vitamins among cancer patients to be 21% to 81%, herbs and supplements 9% to 60%, combination herbal teas (such as Essiac) 7% to 25%, and lifestyle diets (such as vegan or macrobiotic) 9% to 24%.

Earlier studies generally report lower overall prevalence of CAM use (9% to 54%), possibly due to increasing rates of utilization or to broadening of the definition of CAM in survey questionnaires and in the views of respondents.[25,26]

CAM use appears to be more common among those with higher educational level, higher income, female sex, younger age, use of chemotherapy or surgery, or history of CAM use before diagnosis.[12,15,18] Overall, surveys vary in terms of definitions of CAM and of specific types of therapy included in questionnaires, complicating assessment of overall prevalence.

Safety Concerns

Significant potential morbidity and cost have been indirectly associated with herb/supplement-drug interactions, including increased emergency room visits, outpatient clinic visits, and perioperative complications.[27-29] However, the true direct and indirect costs, morbidity, and mortality associated with CAM-related interactions or adverse effects are not known or well studied.

Systematic study or published data regarding potential interactions between specific herbs and vitamins and prescription drugs is limited.[30-38] (See Appendix A for a list of agents with potentially concerning properties, such as bleeding risk, sedation, hepatotoxicity, estrogenic effects, P450 inhibition or induction, or hypoglycemic effects.)

Standardization

Preparation of herbs and supplements may vary from manufacturer to manufacturer and from batch to batch within one manufacturer. Because it is often not clear what are the active components of a product, standardization may not be possible, and the clinical effects of different brands may not be comparable.

Patient-Clinician Communication

Some research reports that neither adult[23] nor pediatric[39] patients receive sufficient information or discuss CAM therapies with a physician, pharmacist, nurse, or CAM practitioner, whereas other studies find more than 60% of patients discuss CAM with their physician.[20] These discrepancies likely reflect an overall heterogeneity in clinicians' styles of managing patients who use CAM.

Most physicians do not receive formal training regarding the safety and effectiveness of CAM and have limited knowledge in this area.[40] There appears to be significant concern among practitioners about potential safety risks and patient out-of-pocket expenses associated with CAM use.[41,42] Surveys suggest a desire by clinicians for access to quality CAM information, both to improve quality of care and to enhance communication with patients.[43,44] Due to potential adverse effects and interactions associated with CAM use, clinicians are often encouraged to ask patients about CAM use, although it is not known if beneficial outcomes result from this practice. Recommended approaches for clinicians to patients who use CAM have been published[45,46] and generally include suggestions to encourage patients to discuss their reasons for seeking CAM, to provide patients with evidence-based information about specific CAM therapies (or explain when available evidence is insufficient), to explain known safety concerns and note that "natural" does not always equate with safety, to support patients emotionally and psychologically even if they choose a CAM therapy with which the clinician does not agree, and to provide close clinical follow-up of patients using CAM therapies. Several evidence-based CAM informational resources are available online for clinicians and patients and can be used as a starting point for discussions in this area (Table 2).

Table 2
Evidence-Based Online CAM Resources (For Clinicians and Patients)

Natural Standard Collaboration (www.naturalstandard.com)	The online counterpart to this book, containing hundreds of reviews of herbs, supplements, modalities (chiropractic, massage, etc), patient information, and monthly news briefs.
M.D. Anderson CIMER (www.mdanderson.org/departments/CIMER)	An informational site maintained by M.D. Anderson Cancer Center with information on CAM therapies relevant to cancer patients and access to other resources.
National Center for Complementary and Alternative Medicine (NCCAM) (http://nccam.nih.gov)	A site maintained by NCCAM, the NIH Center dedicated to primary CAM research.
Office of Dietary Supplements (http://ods.od.nih.gov/index.aspx)	A federal agency that supports research and disseminates research results in the area of dietary supplements.
Cochrane Collaboration (www.cochrane.org)	An international collaboration which prepares systematic reviews of numerous medical therapies, including many CAM approaches.
ConsumerLab (www.consumerlab.com)	An organization that evaluates commercially available products for constituents and adulterants, and publishes online lists of these test results.

EVIDENCE TABLES

Evidence tables in *Natural Standard* monographs summarize the available evidence around efficacy. Categories in the evidence tables are explained below and are summarized in Table 3.

Condition Treated

Refers to the medical condition or disease targeted by a therapy.

Study Design

Common types include the following:

- **Randomized controlled trial (RCT):** An experimental trial in which participants are assigned randomly to receive either an intervention being tested or placebo. Note that Natural Standard defines RCTs as being placebo-controlled, while studies using active controls are classified as equivalence trials (see below). In RCTs, participants and researchers are often blinded (i.e., unaware of group assignments), although unblinded and quasi-blinded RCTs are also often performed. True random allocation to trial arms, proper blinding, and sufficient sample size are the basis for an adequate RCT.
- **Equivalence trial:** An RCT that compares two active agents. Equivalence trials often compare new treatments to usual (standard) care and may not include a placebo arm.
- **Before and after comparison:** A study that reports only the change in outcome in each group of a study, and does not report between-group comparisons. This is a common error in studies that claim to be RCTs.
- **Case series:** A description of a group of patients with a condition, treatment, or outcome (e.g., 20 patients with migraine headache underwent acupuncture and 17 reported feeling better afterwards). Case series are considered weak evidence of efficacy.
- **Case-control study:** A study in which patients with a certain outcome are selected and compared to similar patients (without the outcome) to see if certain risk factors/ predictors are more common in patients with that outcome. This study design is not common in the complementary and alternative medicine literature.
- **Cohort study:** A study that assembles a group of patients with certain baseline characteristics (for example, use of a drug) and follows them forward in time for outcomes. This study design is not common in the complementary and alternative medicine literature.
- **Meta-analysis:** A pooling of multiple trials to increase statistical power (often used to pool data from a number of RCTs with small sample sizes, none which demonstrates significance alone but in aggregate can achieve significance). Multiple difficulties are encountered when designing/ reviewing these analyses; in particular, outcomes measures or therapies may differ from study to study, hindering direct comparison.
- **Review:** An author's description of his or her opinion based on personal, non-systematic review of the evidence.
- **Systematic review:** A review conducted according to pre-specified criteria in an attempt to limit bias from the investigators. Systematic reviews often include a meta-analysis of data from the included studies.

AUTHOR, YEAR

Identifies the study being described in a row of the table.

N

The total number of subjects included in a study (treatment group plus placebo group). Some studies recruit a larger number of subjects initially but do not use them all because they do not meet the study's entry criteria. In this case, it is the second, smaller number that qualifies as N. N includes all subjects that are part of a study at the start date, even if they drop out, are lost to follow-up, or are deemed unsuitable for analysis by the authors. Trials with a large number of drop-outs that are not included in the analysis are considered to be weaker evidence for efficacy. (For systematic reviews the

Table 3
Explanation of Columns in Natural Standard Evidence Tables

1	2	3	4	5	6	7	8	9	10
Condition Treated	Study Design	Author, Year	N	Statistically Significant?	Quality of study 0-2 = poor 3-4 = good 5 = excellent	Magnitude of Benefit	Absolute Risk Reduction	Number Needed to Treat	Comments

number of studies included is reported. For meta-analyses, the number of total subjects included in the analysis or the number of studies may be reported.)

Statistically Significant?

Results are noted as being statistically significant if a study's authors report statistical significance or if quantitative evidence of significance is present (such as *p* values).

Quality of Study

A numerical score between 0 and 5 is assigned as a rough measure of study design/reporting quality (0 being weakest and 5 being strongest). This number is based on a well-established, validated scale developed by Jadad et al. (Jadad AR, Moore RA, Carroll D, et al. Assessing the quality of reports of randomized clinical trials: is blinding necessary? Controlled Clinical Trials

1996;17[1]:1-12). This calculation does not account for all study elements that may be used to assess quality (other aspects of study design/reporting are addressed in the "Evidence Discussion" sections of monographs).

- A Jadad score is calculated using the seven items in the table below. The first five items are indications of good quality, and each counts as one point towards an overall quality score. The final two items indicate poor quality, and a point is subtracted for each if its criteria are met. The range of possible scores is 0 to 5.

Magnitude of Benefit

This summarizes how strong a benefit is: small, medium, large, or none. If results are not statistically significant, "NA" for "not applicable" is entered. In order to be consistent in defining small, medium, and large benefits across different studies and monographs, Natural Standard defines the magnitude of benefit in terms of the standard deviation (SD) of the outcome measure. Specifically, the benefit is considered:

- **Large:** if >1 SD
- **Medium:** if 0.5 to 0.9 SD
- **Small:** if 0.2 to 0.4 SD

In many cases, studies do not report the standard deviation of change of the outcome measure. However, the change in the standard deviation of the outcome measure (also known as effect size) can be calculated and is derived by subtracting the mean (or mean difference) in the placebo/control group from the mean (or mean difference) in the treatment group, and dividing that quantity by the pooled standard deviation (Effect size=[Mean treatment − Mean placebo]/SDp).

Absolute Risk Reduction

This describes the difference between the percentage of people in the control/placebo group experiencing a specific outcome (control event rate) and the percentage of people in the experimental/therapy group experiencing that same outcome (experimental event rate). Mathematically, absolute risk reduction (ARR) equals experimental event rate minus control event rate. ARR is better able to discriminate between large and small treatment effects than relative risk reduction (RRR), a calculation that is often cited in studies ([Control event rate − Experimental event rate]/Control event rate). Many studies do not include adequate data to calculate the ARR, in which cases "NA" is entered into this column.

Number Needed to Treat

This is the number of patients who would need to use the therapy under investigation, for the period of time described in the study, in order for one person to experience the specified benefit. It is calculated by dividing the Absolute Risk Reduction into 1 (1/ARR).

Jadad Score Calculation	
Item	*Score*
Was the study described as randomized (this includes words such as randomly, random, and randomization)?	0/1
Was the method used to generate the sequence of randomization described and appropriate (table of random numbers, computer-generated, etc)?	0/1
Was the study described as double-blind?	0/1
Was the method of double-blinding described and appropriate (identical placebo, active placebo, dummy, etc)?	0/1
Was there a description of withdrawals and dropouts?	0/1
Deduct one point if the method used to the sequence of randomization was described and it was inappropriate (patients were allocated alternately, or according to date of birth, hospital number, etc).	0/-1
Deduct one point if the study was described as double-blind but the method of blinding was inappropriate (e.g., comparison of tablet vs. injection with no double dummy).	0/-1

Comments

When appropriate, this brief section may comment on design flaws (inadequately described subjects, lack of blinding, brief follow-up, not intention-to-treat, etc.), notable study design elements (crossover, etc.), dosing, and/or specifics of study group/sub-groups (age, gender, etc). More detailed description of studies is found in the "Evidence Discussion" section that follows the "Evidence Table" in Natural Standard monographs.

References

1. Panel on Definition and Description, Office of Alternative Medicine, National Institutes of Health, CAM Research Methodology Conference, Bethesda, MD, April 1995.
2. Zollman C, Vickers A. ABC of complementary medicine: What is complementary medicine? Br Med J 1999;319:693-696.
3. Cassileth BR. "Complementary" or "alternative"? It makes a difference in cancer care. Complement Ther Med 1999;44:22.
4. Eisenberg DM, Davis, RB, Ettner SL, et al. Trends in alternative medicine use in the United States, 1990-1997. Results of a follow-up national survey. JAMA 1998;280(18):1569-1575.
5. Dietary Supplement Health and Education Act of 1994 (DSHEA), Public Law 103-417, October 25, 1994 (103rd Congress).
6. Wolsko PM, Eisenberg DM, Davis RB, et al. Insurance coverage, medical conditions, and visits to alternative medicine providers. Results of a national survey. Arch Intern Med 2002;162:281-287.
7. Astin JA. Why patients use alternative medicine: results of a national survey. JAMA 1998;279:1548-1553.
8. Druss B. Association between use of unconventional therapies and conventional medical services. JAMA 1999;282:651-656.
9. White JD. The National Cancer Institute's perspective and agenda for promoting awareness and research on alternative therapies for cancer (keynote address). J Altern Complement Med 2002;8(5):545-550.
10. Adler SR, Fosket JR. Disclosing complementary and alternative medicine use in the medical encounter: A qualitative study in women with breast cancer. J Fam Pract 1999;48:453-458.
11. Bernstein BJ, Grasso T. Prevalence of complementary and alternative medicine use in cancer patients. Oncology (Huntington) 2001;15(10):1267-1272.
12. Burstein HJ, Gelber S, Guadagnoli E, at al. Use of alternative medicine by women with early-stage breast cancer. N Engl J Med 1999;340(22):1733-1739.
13. Gotay CC, Hara W, Issel BF, et al. Use of complementary and alternative medicine in Hawaii cancer patients. Hawaii Med J 1999;58(4):94-98.
14. Kao GD, Devine P. Use of complementary health practices by prostate carcinoma patients undergoing radiation therapy. Cancer 2000;88(3):615-619.
15. Lee MM, Chang JS, Jacobs B, et al. Complementary and alternative medicine use among men with prostate cancer in four ethnic populations. Am J Public Health 2002;92(10):1606-1609.
16. Lippert MC, McClain R, Boyd JC, et al. Alternative medicine use in patients with localized prostate carcinoma treated with curative intent. Cancer 1999;86(12):2642-2648.
17. Maskarinec G, Shumay DM, Kakai H, et al. Ethnic differences in complementary and alternative medicine use among cancer patients. J Altern Complement Med 2000;6(6):531-538.
18. Morris KT, Johnson N, Homer L, et al. A comparison of complementary therapy use between breast cancer patients and patients with other primary tumor sites (abstract). Am J Surg 2000;179:407-411.
19. Patterson RE, Neuhouser ML, Hedderson MM, et al. Types of alternative medicine used by patients with breast, colon, or prostate cancer: predictors, motives, and costs. J Altern Complement Med 2002;8(4):477-485.
20. Richardson MA, Sanders T, Palmer JL, et al. Complementary/alternative medicine use in a comprehensive cancer center and the implications for oncology. J Clin Oncol 2000;18(13):2505-2514.
21. Shumay DM, Maskarinec G, Gotay CC, et al. Determinants of the degree of complementary and alternative medicine use among patients with cancer. J Altern Complement Med 2002;8(5):661-671.
22. Sparber A, Bauer L, Curt G, et al. Use of complementary medicine by adult patients participating in cancer clinical trials. Oncol Nurs Forum 2000;27(4):623-630.
23. Swisher EM, Cohn DE, Goff BA, et al. Use of complementary and alternative medicine among women with gynecologic cancers. Gynecol Oncol 2002;84:363-367.
24. VandeCreek L, Rogers E, Lester J. Use of alternative therapies among breast cancer outpatients compared with the general population. Altern Ther Health Med 1999;5(1):71-76.
25. Ernst E, Cassileth BR. The prevalence of complementary/alternative medicine in cancer. A systematic review. Cancer 1998;83(4):777-782.
26. Sparber A, Wooten JC. Surveys of complementary and alternative medicine. II. Use of alternative and complementary cancer therapies. J Altern Complement Med 2001;7(3):281-287.
27. Rogers EA, Gough JE, Brewer KL. Are emergency department patients at risk for herb-drug interactions? Acad Emerg Med 2001;8(9):932-934.
28. Farah MH, Edwards R, Lindquist M, et al. International monitoring of adverse health effects associated with herbal medicines. Pharmacoepidemiol Drug Safety 2000;9:105-112.
29. Ang-Lee MK, Moss J, Yuan CS. Herbal medicines and perioperative care. JAMA 2001;286:208-216.
30. Palmer ME, Haller C, McKinney PE, et al. Adverse events associated with dietary supplements: an observational study. Lancet 2003;361(9352):101-106.
31. Fugh-Berman A. Herb-drug interactions. Lancet 2000;355(9198):134-138.
32. Abebe W. Herbal medication: potential for adverse interactions with analgesic drugs. J Clin Pharm Ther 2002;27(6):391-401.
33. Ernst E. Possible interactions between synthetic and herbal medicinal products. 1. A systematic review of the indirect evidence. Perfusion 2000;13:4-15.
34. Ernst E. Interactions between synthetic and herbal medicinal products. 2. A systematic review of the direct evidence. Perfusion 2000;13:60-70.
35. Piscitelli SC, Burstein AH. Herb-drug interactions and confounding in clinical trials. J Herbal Pharmacother 2002;2(1):23-26.
36. Izzo AA, Ernst E. Interactions between herbal medicines and prescribed drugs: a systematic review. Drugs 2001;61(15):2163-2175.
37. Hardy ML. Herb-drug interactions: An evidence-based table. Alternative Medicine Alert 2000;June:64-69.
38. Lambrecht J, Hamilton W, Rabinovich A. A review of herb-drug interactions: documented and theoretical. U S Pharmacist 2000;25(8):1-12.
39. Friedman T, Slayton WB, Allen LS, et al. Use of alternative therapies for children with cancer. Pediatrics 1997;100(6):E1(2-6).
40. Jonas WB. Alternative medicine—learning from the past, examining the present, advancing to the future. JAMA 1998;280:1616-1618.
41. Angell M. Alternative medicine—the risks of untested and unregulated remedies. N Engl J Med 1998;339(123):839-841.
42. Studdert DM. Medical malpractice implications of alternative medicine. JAMA 1998;280(18):1610-1615.
43. Winslow LC, Shapiro H. Physicians want education about complementary and alternative medicine to enhance communication with their patients. Arch Intern Med 2002;162(10):1176-1181.
44. Kroll DJ. Concerns and needs for research in herbal supplement pharmacotherapy and safety. J Herbal Pharmacother 2001;1(2):3-23.
45. Weiger WA, Smith M, Boon H, et al. Advising patients who seek complementary and alternative medical therapies for cancer. Ann Intern Med 2002;137(11):889-903.
46. Eisenberg DM. Advising patients who seek alternative medical therapies. Ann Intern Med 1997;127:61.

Acidophilus (Lactobacillus)
(*Lactobacillus acidophilus*)

SYNONYMS/COMMON NAMES/RELATED SUBSTANCES

- Acidophilus, Acidophilus Extra Strength, acidophilus milk, Actimel, Bacid, DDS-Acidophilus, Enpac, Fermalac, Florajen, Gynoflor, Kala, Kyo-Dophilus, *L. acidophilus* milk, *L. acidophilus* yogurt, Lacteol Fort, Lactinex, Lactobacillaceae, lactobacillus (lactobacilli), Lacto Bacillus, MoreDophilus, Narine, Probiata, Pro-Bionate, probiotic, Superdophilus, yogurt.

CLINICAL BOTTOM LINE
Background

- Lactobacilli are bacteria that normally live in the human small intestine and vagina. *Lactobacillus acidophilus* is considered to be beneficial because it produces vitamin K, lactase, and antimicrobial substances such as acidolin, acidolphilin, lactocidin, and bacteriocin. Multiple trials in humans report the benefits of acidophilus for bacterial vaginosis. Other medicinal uses of acidophilus have not been sufficiently studied to form clear conclusions.
- The term *probiotic* is used to describe organisms that are used medicinally, including bacteria such as *L. acidophilus* and yeast such as *Saccharomyces boulardii*.
- Although it is generally believed to be safe with few side effects, oral *L. acidophilus* should be avoided in people with intestinal damage, a weakened immune system, or overgrowth of intestinal bacteria.

Uses Based on Scientific Evidence	Grade*
Bacterial vaginosis Multiple studies in humans report that *L. acidophilus* vaginal suppositories are effective in the treatment of bacterial vaginosis. A small number of studies suggest that eating yogurt enriched with *Lactobacillus acidophilus* may be similarly beneficial. Additional research is necessary before a firm conclusion can be reached. Persons with persistent vaginal discomfort are advised to seek medical attention.	B
Asthma There is limited research in this area, with unclear results.	C
Diarrhea prevention Limited research studies in humans suggest that *L. acidophilus* may not be effective when used to prevent diarrhea in travelers or in people taking antibiotics. Several studies reported that the related species *Lactobacillus GG* was helpful in the prevention of diarrhea in children and travelers. Additional study is needed in these areas before a firm conclusion can be drawn.	C
Diarrhea treatment (in children) A small amount of studies in children, using different forms of acidophilus, report no improvement in diarrhea. Future studies should use a viable *L. acidophilus* culture to assess its effects. Multiple studies in humans using *Lactobacillus GG*, a different species, suggest that this species may be a safe and effective treatment for diarrhea in otherwise healthy infants and children. *L. acidophilus* may be helpful in the management of chronic or persistent diarrhea and bacterial-overgrowth related diarrhea. Further research is needed to determine potential safe and effective dosing.	C
Hepatic encephalopathy There have been limited studies of *L. acidophilus* as therapy for hepatic encephalopathy, a liver disorder with symptoms including confused thinking. Results were inconclusive.	C
High cholesterol There is conflicting information from several studies in humans regarding the effect of *L. acidophilus*–enriched dairy products on decreasing blood levels of total cholesterol or low-density lipoprotein ("bad cholesterol").	C
Irritable bowel syndrome Studies in humans report mixed results in the improvement of bowel symptoms in patients taking *L. acidophilus* by mouth.	C
Lactose intolerance Several studies in humans examined whether *L. acidophilus* given by mouth improves digestion of lactose. Results were inconclusive, and more research is needed in this area.	C
Necrotizing enterocolitis prevention One study using *L. acidophilus* in combination with another bacterium (*Bifidobacterium infantis*) in infants reported fewer cases of necrotizing enterocolitis (severe inflammation of the gut), and no complications related to treatment. Additional research is necessary in this area before conclusions can be drawn.	C
Vaginal candidiasis (yeast infection) In some studies, *L. acidophilus* has been taken by mouth or as a vaginal suppository for the prevention or treatment of vaginal yeast infections. The results have not been adequately assessed, and more research is needed in this area before a conclusion can be drawn.	C

*Key to grades: *A:* Strong scientific evidence for this use; *B:* Good scientific evidence for this use; *C:* Unclear scientific evidence for this use; *D:* Fair scientific evidence against this use (it may not work); *F:* Strong scientific evidence against this use (it likely does not work). For a more detailed explanation of efficacy criteria, see "Natural Standard Evidence-Based Validated Grading Rationale" in the Introduction.

Uses Based on Tradition, Theory, or Limited Scientific Evidence

Acne, AIDS, allergies, cancer, canker sores, colitis, colon cancer prevention, constipation, Crohn's disease, diaper rash, diverticulitis, *Escherichia coli* infection in cancer patients, fever blisters, heart disease, heartburn, hives, immune enhancer, indigestion, infection, overgrowth of bacteria in the small bowel, preoperative prevention of infections or gut bacteria loss, stomach ulcer, thrush, ulcerative colitis, urinary tract infection.

DOSING/TOXICOLOGY

The following doses are based on scientific research, publications, traditional use, or expert opinion. Many herbs and supplements have not been thoroughly tested, and their safety and effectiveness may not be proven. Brands may be made differently, with variable ingredients even within the same brand. The doses shown may not apply to all products. It is important to always read product labels and discuss doses with a qualified healthcare provider before therapy is started.

Standardization

- Standardization involves measuring the amount of certain chemicals in products to try to make different preparations similar to each other. It is not always known if the chemicals being measured are the "active" ingredients. *L. acidophilus* is commercially prepared as a concentrate, in a freeze-dried form, or as viable cultures. For all formulations, the dose is based on the number of living organisms. Standardization of *L. acidophilus* has been a challenge because it is difficult to assess which products contain live bacteria and are free from contaminants. Significant variations in effectiveness and shelf life have been observed. Storage conditions and the length of time that the product is stored can alter the effectiveness, and refrigeration is recommended for *L. acidophilus* products. Pasteurization kills *L. acidophilus*.

Adults (18 Years and Older)

- **Tablets/capsules/liquid/yogurt:** A dose between 1 billion and 10 billion viable (live) *L. acidophilus* bacteria taken daily in divided doses is considered sufficient for most people. Higher doses may cause mild abdominal discomfort, and smaller doses may not establish a stable population in the gut. For vaginal bacterial infections, a dose that has been used is 8 ounces of yogurt containing *L. acidophilus* in a concentration of 100 million colony-forming units (10^8 CFU) in each milliliter. In one study, capsules containing 1.5 g of *L. acidophilus* were used.
- **Vaginal suppository:** Doses used for vaginal infections include 1 to 2 tablets (containing 10 million to 1 billion CFU in each tablet), inserted into the vagina once or twice daily.

Children (Younger Than 18 Years)

- **Tablets/capsules/liquid:** Some natural medicine textbooks and experts suggest that one-quarter teaspoon or one-quarter capsule of commercially available *L. acidophilus* may be safe for use in children for the replacement of gut bacteria destroyed by antibiotics. Up to 12 billion lyophilized heat-killed *L. acidophilus* has been given every 12 hours for up to 5 days. It is often recommended that *L. acidophilus* supplements be taken at least 2 hours after antibiotic doses, because antibiotics may kill *L. acidophilus* if they are taken at the same time. A qualified healthcare practitioner should be consulted before *L. acidophilus* is given to children. Special caution should be used in children younger than 3 years of age.
- **Topical (applied to the skin):** Acidophilus liquid preparations have been used on the diaper area to treat yeast infections; however, safety and effectiveness have not been well studied. A qualified healthcare practitioner should be consulted before using *L. acidophilus* in children. Special caution should be used in children younger than three years of age.

SAFETY

The U.S. Food and Drug Administration does not strictly regulate herbs and supplements. There is no guarantee of the strength, purity, or safety of products, and effects may vary. It is important to always read product labels. People who have a medical condition, or are taking other drugs, herbs, or supplements, should consult a qualified healthcare provider before starting a new therapy. A healthcare provider should be contacted immediately about any side effects.

Allergies

- Lactose-sensitive people may experience abdominal discomfort from dairy products containing *L. acidophilus*.

Side Effects and Warnings

- Studies report few side effects from *L. acidophilus* when it is used at recommended doses. The most common complaint is abdominal discomfort (gas), which usually resolves with continued use. To reduce the risk of abdominal discomfort, some experts recommend limiting the daily dose to fewer than 10 billion live *L. acidophilus* organisms. Some women have reported a burning sensation in the vagina after using *L. acidophilus* vaginal tablets.
- There have been rare reports of *L. acidophilus* infection of heart valves, and the risk may be greater in people with artificial heart valves. People with severely weakened immune systems (due to disease, cancer chemotherapy drugs, or organ transplant immunosuppressants) may develop serious infections or bacteremia (bacteria in the blood) after taking *L. acidophilus*. Therefore, *L. acidophilus* should be avoided in such individuals. People with intestinal damage or recent bowel surgery also should avoid taking lactobacilli.

Pregnancy and Breastfeeding

- There are not enough scientific studies available to establish safety during pregnancy. Pregnant women should use *L. acidophilus* cautiously and under medical supervision, if at all. A small number of pregnant women have taken part in studies investigating the use of *L. acidophilus* vaginal tablets and a culture of *L. acidophilus*; no negative effects were reported, but further research is needed in this area.

INTERACTIONS

Most herbs and supplements have not been thoroughly tested for interactions with other herbs, supplements, drugs, or foods. The interactions listed here are based on reports in scientific publications, laboratory experiments, or traditional use. It is important to always read product labels. People who have a medical condition, or are taking other drugs, herbs, or supplements, should consult a qualified healthcare provider before starting a new therapy.

Interactions with Drugs

- Some experts believe that *L. acidophilus* taken by mouth should be used 2 to 3 hours after antibiotic doses to prevent killing the acidophilus organisms. It has also been suggested that lactobacilli are damaged by alcohol, and therefore alcohol should be avoided when taking acidophilus products. Scientific research is limited in these areas.
- In theory, *L. acidophilus* taken by mouth may not survive the acidic environment of the stomach. Some experts suggest that antacids should be taken 30 to 60 minutes before taking lactobacilli. However, this has not been well studied in humans.
- In theory, *L. acidophilus* may prolong the effects of some drugs, including birth control pills and benzodiazepines such as diazepam (Valium). Based on laboratory experiments, *L. acidophilus* may reduce the effectiveness of sulfasalazine (Azulfidine), a drug used for inflammatory bowel disease.

Interactions with Herbs and Dietary Supplements

- Fructo-oligosaccharides (FOS, also called *probiotics*) are non-digestible sugar chains that are nutrients for lactobacilli. FOS, taken by mouth at a dose of 2000 to 3000 mg, may stimulate the growth of lactobacilli. Natural food sources of FOS include bananas, Jerusalem artichokes, onions, asparagus, and garlic.
- *Lactobacillus casei, Saccharomyces boulardii,* and other probiotics may add to the effects of *L. acidophilus.*

Selected References

Natural Standard developed the preceding evidence-based information based on a systematic review of more than 200 scientific articles. For comprehensive information about alternative and complementary therapies on the professional level, go to www.naturalstandard.com. Selected references are listed here.

Agerholm-Larsen L, Raben A, Haulrik N, et al. Effect of 8 week intake of probiotic milk products on risk factors for cardiovascular diseases. Eur J Clin Nutr 2000;54(4):288-297.

Alm L. [Acidophilus milk for therapy in gastrointestinal disorders.] Nahrung 1984;28(6-7):683-684.

Anderson JW, Gilliland SE. Effect of fermented milk (yogurt) containing Lactobacillus acidophilus L1 on serum cholesterol in hypercholesterolemic humans. J Am Coll Nutr 1999;18(1):43-50.

Arvola T, Laiho K, Torkkeli S, et al. Prophylactic Lactobacillus GG reduces antibiotic-associated diarrhea in children with respiratory infections: a randomized study. Pediatrics 1999;104(5):e64.

Bayer AS, Chow AW, Betts D, et al. Lactobacillemia—report of nine cases. Important clinical and therapeutic considerations. Am J Med 1978;64(5):808-813.

Berman S, Spicer D. Safety and reliability of lactobacillus dietary supplements in Seattle, Washington. American Public Health Association 130th Annual Meeting, November 9-13 2002; A37244.

Boulloche J, Mouterde O, Mallet E. Management of acute diarrhea in infants and young children: controlled study of the antidiarrheal efficacy of killed L. acidophilus (LB strain) versus a placebo and a reference drug (loperamide). Ann Pediatr 1994;41(7):457-463.

Chomarat M, Espinouse D. Lactobacillus rhamnosus septicemia in patients with prolonged aplasia receiving ceftazidime-vancomycin. Eur J Clin Microbiol Infect Dis 1991;10(1):44.

Clements ML, Levine MM, Ristaino PA, et al. Exogenous lactobacilli fed to man—their fate and ability to prevent diarrheal disease. Prog Food Nutr Sci 1983;7(3-4):29-37.

D'Souza AL, Rajkumar C, Cooke J, et al. Probiotics in prevention of antibiotic associated diarrhoea: meta-analysis. BMJ 2002;324(7350):1361.

Davies AJ, James PA, Hawkey PM. Lactobacillus endocarditis. J Infect 1986;12(2):169-174.

de Roos NM, Schouten G, Katan MB. Yoghurt enriched with Lactobacillus acidophilus does not lower blood lipids in healthy men and women with normal to borderline high serum cholesterol levels. Eur J Clin Nutr 1999;53(4):277-280.

Dehkordi N, Rao DR, Warren AP, et al. Lactose malabsorption as influenced by chocolate milk, skim milk, sucrose, whole milk, and lactic cultures. J Am Diet Assoc 1995;95(4):484-486.

dios Pozo-Olano J, Warram JH Jr, Gomez RG, et al. Effect of a lactobacilli preparation on traveler's diarrhea. A randomized, double blind clinical trial. Gastroenterology 1978;74(5 Pt 1):829-830.

Friedlander A, Druker MM, Schachter A. Lactobacillus acidophilus and vitamin B complex in the treatment of vaginal infection. Panminerva Med 1986;28(1):51-53.

Gaon D, Garcia H, Winter L, et al. Effect of Lactobacillus strains and Saccharomyces boulardii on persistent diarrhea in children. Medicina (B Aires) 2003;63(4):293-298.

Gaon D, Garmendia C, Murrielo NO, et al. Effect of Lactobacillus strains (L. casei and L. Acidophillus strains cerela) on bacterial overgrowth–related chronic diarrhea. Medicina (B Aires) 2002;62(2):159-163.

Gotz V, Romankiewicz JA, Moss J, et al. Prophylaxis against ampicillin-associated diarrhea with a lactobacillus preparation. Am J Hosp Pharm 1979;36(6):754-757.

Griffiths JK, Daly JS, Dodge RA. Two cases of endocarditis due to Lactobacillus species: antimicrobial susceptibility, review, and discussion of therapy. Clin Infect Dis 1992;15(2):250-255.

Hallen A, Jarstrand C, Pahlson C. Treatment of bacterial vaginosis with lactobacilli. Sex Transm Dis 1992;19(3):146-148.

Halpern GM, Prindiville T, Blankenburg M, et al. Treatment of irritable bowel syndrome with Lacteol Fort: a randomized, double-blind, cross-over trial. Am J Gastroenterol 1996;91(8):1579-1585.

Hilton E, Isenberg HD, Alperstein P, et al. Ingestion of yogurt containing Lactobacillus acidophilus as prophylaxis for candidal vaginitis. Ann Intern Med 1992;116(5):353-357.

Hoyos AB. Reduced incidence of necrotizing enterocolitis associated with enteral administration of Lactobacillus acidophilus and Bifidobacterium infantis to neonates in an intensive care unit. Int J Infect Dis 1999;3(4):197-202.

Kim HS, Gilliland SE. Lactobacillus acidophilus as a dietary adjunct for milk to aid lactose digestion in humans. J Dairy Sci 1983;66(5):959-966.

Kostiuk OP, Chernyshova LI, Slukvin II. [Protective effect of Lactobacillus acidophilus on development of infection, caused by Klebsiella pneumoniae.] Fiziol Zh 1993;39(4):62-68.

Larvol L, Monier A, Besnier P, et al. [Liver abscess caused by Lactobacillus acidophilus.] Gastroenterol Clin Biol 1996;20(2):193-195.

Lidbeck A, Nord CE, Gustafsson JA, et al. Lactobacilli, anticarcinogenic activities and human intestinal microflora. Eur J Cancer Prev 1992;1(5):341-353.

Lin SY, Ayres JW, Winkler W Jr, et al. Lactobacillus effects on cholesterol: in vitro and in vivo results. J Dairy Sci 1989;72(11):2885-2899.

Macbeth WA, Kass EH, McDermott WV. Treatment of hepatic encephalopathy by alteration of intestinal flora with lactobacillus acidophilus. Lancet 1965;191:399-403.

Michielutti F, Bertini M, Presciuttini B, et al. [Clinical assessment of a new oral bacterial treatment for children with acute diarrhea.] Minerva Med 1996;87(11):545-550.

Neri A, Sabah G, Samra Z. Bacterial vaginosis in pregnancy treated with yoghurt. Acta Obstet Gynecol Scand 1993;72(1):17-19.

Newcomer AD, Park HS, O'Brien PC, et al. Response of patients with irritable bowel syndrome and lactase deficiency using unfermented acidophilus milk. Am J Clin Nutr 1983;38(2):257-263.

Ozmen S, Turhan NO, Seckin NC. Gardnerella-associated vaginitis: comparison of three treatment modalities. Turkish J Med Sci 1998;28(2):171-173.

Parent D, Bossens M, Bayot D, et al. Therapy of bacterial vaginosis using exogenously-applied Lactobacilli acidophili and a low dose of estriol: a placebo-controlled multicentric clinical trial. Arzneimittelforschung 1996;46(1):68-73.

Patel R, Cockerill FR, Porayko MK, et al. Lactobacillemia in liver transplant patients. Clin Infect Dis 1994;18(2):207-212.

Read AE, McCarthy CF, Heaton KW, et al. Lactobacillus acidophilus (enpac) in treatment of hepatic encephalopathy. BMJ 1966;5498:1267-1269.

Reuman PD, Duckworth DH, Smith KL, et al. Lack of effect of Lactobacillus on gastrointestinal bacterial colonization in premature infants. Pediatr Infect Dis 1986;5(6):663-668.

Saltzman JR, Russell RM, Golner B, et al. A randomized trial of Lactobacillus acidophilus BG2FO4 to treat lactose intolerance. Am J Clin Nutr 1999;69(1):140-146.

Satta A, Delplano A, Cossu P, et al. [Treatment of enterocolitis and other intestinal disorders with a Bifidobacterium bifidum and Lactobacillus acidophilus combination.] Clin Ter 1980;94(2):173-184.

Schaafsma G, Meuling WJ, van Dokkum W, et al. Effects of a milk product, fermented by Lactobacillus acidophilus and with fructo-oligosaccharides added, on blood lipids in male volunteers. Eur J Clin Nutr 1998;52(6):436-440.

Shalev E, Battino S, Weiner E, et al. Ingestion of yogurt containing Lactobacillus acidophilus compared with pasteurized yogurt as prophylaxis for recurrent candidal vaginitis and bacterial vaginosis. Arch Fam Med 1996;5(10):593-596.

Siboulet A. [Vaccination against nonspecific bacterial vaginosis. Double-blind study of Gynatren.] Gynakol Rundsch 1991;31(3):153-160.

Simakachorn N, Pichaipat V, Rithipornpaisarn P, et al. Clinical evaluation of the addition of lyophilized, heat-killed Lactobacillus acidophilus LB to oral rehydration therapy in the treatment of acute diarrhea in children. J Pediatr Gastroenterol Nutr 2000;30(1):68-72.

Sussman JI, Baron EJ, Goldberg SM, et al. Clinical manifestations and therapy of Lactobacillus endocarditis: report of a case and review of the literature. Rev Infect Dis 1986;8(5):771-776.

Tankanow RM, Ross MB, Ertel IJ, et al. A double-blind, placebo-controlled study of the efficacy of Lactinex in the prophylaxis of amoxicillin-induced diarrhea. DICP 1990;24(4):382-384.

Unoki T, Nakamura I, Fujisawa T, et al. [Infective endocarditis due to Lactobacillus acidophilus group. Report of a case and review of the literature.] Kansenshogaku Zasshi 1988;62(9):835-840.

Van Niel CW, Feudtner C, Garrison MM, et al. Lactobacillus therapy for acute infectious diarrhea in children: a meta-analysis. Pediatrics 2002;109(4):678-684.

Wheeler JG, Shema SJ, Bogle ML, et al. Immune and clinical impact of Lactobacillus acidophilus on asthma. Ann Allergy Asthma Immunol 1997;79(3):229-233.

Witsell DL, Garrett CG, Yarbrough WG, et al. Effect of Lactobacillus acidophilus on antibiotic-associated gastrointestinal morbidity: a prospective randomized trial. J Otolaryngol 1995;24(4):230-233.

Alfalfa
(*Medicago sativa* L.)

SYNONYMS/COMMON NAMES/RELATED SUBSTANCES

- Al-fac-facah, arc, buffalo herb, California clover, Chilean clover, Fabaceae, feuille de luzerne, isoflavone, jatt, kaba yonca, Leguminosae, lucerne, medicago, mielga, mu su, phytoestrogen, purple medic, purple medick, purple medicle, sai pi li ka, saranac, Spanish clover, team, weevelchek, yonja.

CLINICAL BOTTOM LINE
Background

- Alfalfa has a long history of medicinal and nutritional use. Basic science, animal research, and preliminary human studies of alfalfa have demonstrated reductions in cholesterol and atherosclerotic plaque formation. Early evidence suggests that alfalfa may also possess hypoglycemic or antifungal properties. However, there is currently insufficient information from clinical trials to adequately evaluate the safety or efficacy of alfalfa for any indication.
- Alfalfa appears to be generally well tolerated. There are several reports of the development of a lupus-like syndrome, or exacerbations of systemic lupus erythematosus (SLE) in patients with known SLE, associated with the ingestion of alfalfa tablets. These reactions may be associated with the amino acid L-canavanine, which appears to be present in alfalfa seeds and sprouts, but not in the leaves. There are also rare cases of pancytopenia, dermatitis, and gastrointestinal symptoms.

Scientific Evidence for Common/Studied Uses	Grade*
Atherosclerosis	C
Diabetes	C
Hyperlipidemia	C

*Key to grades: *A:* Strong scientific evidence for this use; *B:* Good scientific evidence for this use; *C:* Unclear scientific evidence for this use; *D:* Fair scientific evidence against this use (it may not work); *F:* Strong scientific evidence against this use (it likely does not work). For a more detailed explanation of efficacy criteria, see "Natural Standard Evidence-Based Validated Grading Rationale" in the Introduction.

Historical or Theoretical Indications That Lack Sufficient Evidence

- Allergies,[1] antifungal,[2,3] appetite stimulant, asthma, bladder disorders, boils, coagulation disorders, convalescence, coughs, diuresis, gastrointestinal tract disorders, gum healing after orthodontic procedures, hay fever, indigestion, inflammation, insect bites, jaundice, kidney disorders, lactation induction, menopausal symptoms, nutritional support, peptic ulcer disease, prostate disorders, radiotherapy-induced skin damage, rheumatoid arthritis, scurvy, thrombocytopenic purpura, uterine stimulant, vitamin supplementation (vitamins A, C, E, and K).

Expert Opinion and Folkloric Precedent

- Alfalfa has been used medicinally for centuries. Traditionally, alfalfa has been used for the treatment of arthritis, menstrual

irregularities, kidney and bladder disorders, and stomach upset. Alfalfa has been used in Chinese medicine to treat coughs and digestive problems, and in India to treat boils. Native Americans used alfalfa to alleviate jaundice and to promote blood clotting. Reportedly, cattle fed alfalfa were believed to grow stronger, which may have prompted its use in humans.
- Currently, alfalfa is widely used as a food. In the United States, alfalfa is included in the U.S. Food and Drug Administration (FDA) GRAS (generally regarded as safe) category. The Council of Europe lists alfalfa as a source of natural food flavoring.

Safety Summary

- **Likely safe:** When above-ground parts are eaten as a food in moderate quantities, in salads or other food preparations, in otherwise healthy adults without a history of autoimmune disorders.
- **Possibly safe:** When taken in recommended doses in otherwise healthy adults without a history of autoimmune disorders. Human safety trials are lacking.
- **Likely unsafe:** When consumed in large quantities or used by people who have a history of systemic lupus erythematosus (SLE) or other autoimmune diseases, based on reports that link alfalfa consumption to the development of a lupus-like syndrome or exacerbations in individuals with known SLE.[4-7] The amino acid that has been associated with SLE, L-canavanine,[8] appears to be present in alfalfa seeds and sprouts, but not in the leaves, and therefore theoretically should not be present in alfalfa tablets manufactured from the leaves.[4] However, case reports have included a patient taking tablets.[8] Pancytopenia has been reported when large amounts of seeds are consumed.[5] Human safety trials are lacking.

DOSING/TOXICOLOGY
General

- Recommended doses are based on traditional health practice patterns and expert opinion. There are no reliable human trials demonstrating safety or efficacy for any particular dose of alfalfa. In general, with natural products, the optimal doses needed to balance efficacy and safety often have not been determined. Formulations and preparation methods. may vary from manufacturer to manufacturer, and from batch to batch of a specific product made by a single manufacturer. Because often the active components of a product are not known, standardization may not be possible, and the clinical effects of different brands may not be comparable.

Standardization

- Literature review reveals no well-established standardization for alfalfa products.

Dosing: Adult (18 Years and Older)
Oral

- **Tablets:** Cholestaid (esterin-processed alfalfa), 2 tablets (1 g each) orally three times daily for up to 2 months. Decrease to 1 tablet three times daily thereafter (dosing per manufacturer's recommendations).

- **Dried herb:** 5 to 10 g of dried herb three times daily has been used.
- **Liquid extract:** 5 to 10 mL of a liquid extract (1:1 in 25% alcohol) three times daily has been used.
- **Seeds:** For hyperlipidemia, 40 g of heated, prepared seeds three times a day with food has been used.[10]

Dosing: Pediatric (Younger Than 18 Years)

- There is insufficient evidence to recommend for or against the use of alfalfa in children. Safety and efficacy data are not available.

Toxicology

- Alfalfa has been associated with pancytopenia in one case report.[9] Consumption of alfalfa may induce a lupus-like syndrome or exacerbate systemic lupus erythematosus (SLE)[4,6] L-Canavanine is believed to play a role in causing and/or reactivating SLE.[4] This agent appears to exist in the seeds and sprouts of alfalfa, but not in the leaves of mature alfalfa plants. Alfalfa tablets typically are composed of the leaves of mature alfalfa plants, but not the seeds or sprouts.[8]
- In a 6-week study of alfalfa use in six persons consuming 160 g of alfalfa daily for 3 weeks, followed by 80 g of alfalfa daily for 3 weeks, no signs of toxicity were observed.[11] However, reported adverse effects included increased intestinal gas and bulky feces. No signs of toxicity were found in an 18-month study comparing monkeys fed diets consisting of cholesterol plus alfalfa saponins and monkeys fed diets consisting of cholesterol alone.[12] In another study, no signs of toxicity were found in monkeys fed alfalfa saponins for 6 to 8 weeks.[13] Toxicity was defined as no change in general appearance, body weight, food consumption, blood test results, or intestinal biopsy findings. Safety studies of a protein isolated from alfalfa found no toxic effects when the protein was administered to white rats[14]; a 30-day toxicity study found that a solution of 500 μg/mL (0.1% weight/volume polyethylene glycol in 2 mM of sodium hydroxide) of the alfalfa component G2 was nontoxic when injected intraperitoneally in mice. No hemolytic activity was observed in mouse erythrocytes.[2]

ADVERSE EFFECTS/PRECAUTIONS/CONTRAINDICATIONS
Allergy

- Known allergy or hypersensitivity to alfalfa or other members of the Fabaceae or Leguminosae plant family.
- Use alfalfa cautiously in patients with allergies to grass. There are conflicting reports claiming cross-sensitivity between alfalfa and members of the grass family. One article mentions that cross-sensitivity reactions should be unlikely because alfalfa is classified as a legume and is not related to the grass family. However, it is possible that alfalfa may be contaminated by grass pollen and thereby elicit an allergic reaction.[15]

Adverse Effects

- **General:** There has been long-standing historical use of alfalfa, with few adverse effects noted anecdotally or in the available scientific literature. In the few human case reports available, alfalfa appears to be generally well tolerated but has been linked to a few serious adverse effects, including the development of a lupus-like syndrome or exacerbations of systemic lupus erythematosus (SLE), possibly associated with the constituent L-canavanine. Contamination of alfalfa with *Escherichia coli*, *Salmonella*, and *Listeria* has resulted in infections.

- **Dermatologic:** Dermatitis associated with alfalfa use has been reported. In a 1954 publication, dermatitis was noted in a 61-year-old woman consuming 4 to 6 cups of tea made with 2 tablespoons of alfalfa seeds for approximately 2 months before onset.[16] Examination revealed diffuse, confluent edema and erythema on the face, eyelids, ears, hands, forearms, and distal humeral regions. Her dermatitis resolved with topical application of "Shamberg" lotion (ingredients include resorcin, boric acid, glycerin, zinc oxide, witch hazel and distilled water), intravenous calcium gluconate, and oral bromisovalum. Re-exposure to alfalfa resulted in a similar reaction in this patient.
- **Gastrointestinal:** Flatulence and bulkier feces were noted during the first week of a small prospective case series involving three subjects ingesting alfalfa.[11] Increased fecal volume and increased frequency of stools were seen in most patients in a case series of 15 subjects ingesting alfalfa.[10] Additional adverse effects reported included abdominal discomfort in 2 patients, looser than normal stools in 6 patients, diarrhea in 2 patients, and intestinal gas in 13 patients.
- **Endocrine (hypoglycemia):** Alfalfa has been associated with reductions in serum glucose levels in rats.[17,18] Evidence in humans is limited. A 1962 case report documents hypoglycemia in a diabetic man taking alfalfa.[19] After being unresponsive to conventional hypoglycemic agents, his blood glucose reached 648 mg/100 mL. Physicians allowed the patient to prepare an alfalfa extract he had used in the past. Two hours after the patient consumed the extract, he exhibited clinical signs of hypoglycemia with a blood sugar of 68 mg/100 mL. The extract was consumed 12 additional times when the patient had blood glucose levels ranging between 190 and 580 mg per 100 mL, each time resulting in a reduction of blood glucose concentrations.
- **Endocrine (estrogenic):** Constituents of alfalfa include coumestrol, with reported estrogenic activity.[20-22] Effects in humans are not known.
- **Endocrine (hypokalemia):** A case report documents hypokalemia (2.9 mMol/L) in a woman who had been drinking a "cleansing tea" containing alfalfa, licorice, and nettles.[23] Her potassium blood level returned to normal after she stopped drinking the tea and took potassium supplements. The specific cause of the hypokalemia was not clear. Notably, both of the other constituents have been associated with hypokalemia (nettles may exert a diuretic effect, and licorice may decrease potassium levels via an aldosterone-like effect).
- **Endocrine (thyroid):** An immunoreactive thyrotropin-releasing hormone–like material has been found in alfalfa, but its biological action is unknown.[24]
- **Hematologic:** Pancytopenia and splenomegaly were reported in a 59-year-old man who had been taking 80 to 160 g of ground alfalfa seeds for up to 6 weeks at a time, for a 5-month period.[9] His hematologic values and spleen size returned to normal when the alfalfa was discontinued. Alfalfa may contain vitamin K and theoretically could interact with vitamin K–dependent anticoagulants.
- **Rheumatologic (systemic lupus erythematosus [SLE]):** Alfalfa ingestion has been associated with the development of a lupus-like syndrome in animals and humans,[4-7] as well as with possible exacerbations of lupus in patients with known SLE. These reactions may be associated with the amino acid L-canavanine,[4] which appears to be present in alfalfa seeds and sprouts, but not in the leaves, and therefore theoretically should not be present in alfalfa tablets manufactured from

the leaves.[8] However, case reports have included individuals ingesting tablets. A lupus-like syndrome was described in four patients taking 12 to 24 alfalfa tablets daily.[5] Symptoms included arthralgias, myalgias, and rash; positive antinuclear antibodies (ANAs) arose anywhere from 3 weeks to 7 months after initiating alfalfa therapy. Upon discontinuation of alfalfa tablets, all four patients became asymptomatic. In two patients, ANA levels returned to normal. Two additional reports have documented possible exacerbation or induction of SLE associated with alfalfa use.[6] One case involved a woman with a 26-year history of SLE who had been taking 15 tablets of alfalfa daily for 9 months before an exacerbation of SLE. The episode was characterized by a rise in ANA levels, depression, arthralgias, malaise, proteinuria, hypocomplementemia, increased cryoglobulins, and lethargy. Because of the delay in onset of the exacerbation from the initiation of alfalfa therapy, causation cannot be clearly established. In a different report, SLE and arthritis were found in multiple family members who had been taking a combination of vitamin E and alfalfa tablets for 7 years.[7] Again, it is not known what other environmental or genetic factors may have affected these individuals, and the association with alfalfa is not clear. Nonetheless, caution is warranted in patients with SLE or other autoimmune diseases until more reliable or systematic data are available.

- **Rheumatologic (gout):** Alfalfa may increase serum urate levels[10] and could theoretically exacerbate or cause gout.
- **Infectious disease (contaminants):** Bacterial infections have been reported in a number of cases involving alfalfa sprouts, alfalfa seeds, and alfalfa tablets contaminated with *Escherichia coli* (including 0157:H7), *Salmonella*, or *Listeria monocytogenes*.[25-33] In one case report, a 55-year-old man developed *L. monocytogenes* meningitis, bacteremia, and multi-organ failure.[34] Analysis of his prior medications included vitamins, cod liver oil, garlic pills, and alfalfa tablets (650 mg). The alfalfa tablets were found to be contaminated with the same strain of *L. monocytogenes*, and no other products were contaminated. The patient subsequently died as a result of this infection. Several methods of decontamination of commercial alfalfa projects have been evaluated, including irradiation.[35-38]

Precautions/Warnings/Contraindications

- Avoid in patients with grass allergies, due to a possibility of cross-reactivity.
- Avoid in patients with systemic lupus erythematosus (SLE), due to a possible risk of disease exacerbation.[4,6] Use cautiously in patients with other autoimmune disorders.
- Avoid in patients with hormone-sensitive conditions such as breast, uterine, or ovarian cancer, endometriosis, and fibroids; alfalfa contains constituents, including coumestrol, with possible with estrogenic activity .[20-22]
- Use cautiously in patients taking warfarin or other vitamin K–dependent anticoagulants; alfalfa may contain vitamin K.
- Use cautiously in patients with gout; alfalfa may increase serum urate levels.[10]
- Use cautiously in patients with diabetes; alfalfa may reduce blood glucose levels.[19]

Pregnancy and Lactation

- Alfalfa may contain a uterine stimulant, stachydrine, found in *Medicago sativa* var. *italica*.[39] Although teratogenicity caused by alfalfa has not been proven, its use should be avoided during pregnancy because of a lack of safety data. Based on traditional use, alfalfa may be safe in amounts normally found in food.
- Coumestrol, which is present in alfalfa, may possess estrogenic properties,[21] with unclear effects on pregnancy and lactation.
- Alfalfa seeds are traditionally reputed to be lactogenic and to affect the menstrual cycle.[39]

INTERACTIONS

Alfalfa/Drug Interactions

- **Warfarin (Coumadin):** Alfalfa is reported to contain vitamin K, and therefore may reduce the effects of vitamin K–dependent anticoagulant medications.
- **Hypoglycemic drugs:** Based on limited case report data[19] and animal research,[18] alfalfa may lower blood glucose levels, and may have additive effects when used with other hypoglycemic agents.[17]
- **Cholesterol-lowering medications:** Alfalfa may lower total cholesterol, low-density lipoprotein (LDL), and triglyceride concentrations, based on two human case series and animal data[10,11,40,41]; alfalfa may therefore have additive effects when used with other cholesterol-lowering medications.
- **Chlorpromazine (Thorazine):** Chlorpromazine has been reported to have increased drug-induced photosensitivity when taken in combination with alfalfa.
- **Hormone replacement therapy (HRT), oral contraceptives (OCPs):** Alfalfa has been reported to contain coumestrol and other constituents that may possess estrogenic properties.[21,22] Interactions with other hormonal therapies are not known.
- **Thyroid agents:** Immunoreactive thyrotropin-releasing hormone-like material has been found in alfalfa, although its biological action is unknown.[24]

Alfalfa/Herb/Supplement Interactions

- **Anticoagulant herbs and supplements:** Alfalfa has been reported to contain vitamin K, and therefore may reduce the effects of anticoagulant agents that rely on depletion of vitamin K.
- **Hypoglycemic herbs and supplements:** Based on limited case report data[19] and animal research,[18] alfalfa may lower blood glucose levels, and may have additive effects when used with other hypoglycemic agents.[17]
- **Cholesterol-lowering herbs:** Alfalfa may lower total cholesterol, low-density lipoprotein (LDL), and triglyceride concentrations, based on two human case series and animal data[10,11,40,41]; alfalfa may therefore have additive effects when used with other cholesterol-lowering agents.
- **Estrogenic herbs and supplements:** Alfalfa has been reported to contain coumestrol and other constituents that have estrogenic properties.[21,22]
- **Iron:** Alfalfa and other fibers have been shown *in vitro* to bind iron, therefore reducing its absorption.[42]
- **Vitamin E:** Alfalfa contains saponins, which may interfere with absorption or activity of vitamin E. In addition, it has been postulated that vitamin E may potentiate the effects of L-canavanine, a component of alfalfa associated with the development of lupus-like syndrome, or exacerbation of lupus.[7] Data are limited in this area.
- **Vitamin K:** Alfalfa contains vitamin K, and when taken with other sources of vitamin K may additively reduce the efficacy of anticoagulants such as warfarin.

Alfalfa/Food Interactions

- **Vitamin K–containing foods:** Foods containing vitamin K, such as green leafy vegetables, may have additive effects with alfalfa (which also contains vitamin K) in reducing the efficacy of anticoagulants such as warfarin.

Alfalfa/Lab Interactions

- **Serum glucose:** Based on limited case report data and animal research, alfalfa may lower blood glucose levels.[17-19]
- **Plasma lipids:** Alfalfa may lower total cholesterol, low-density lipoprotein (LDL) and triglyceride concentrations.[10,11,40,41]
- **Serum potassium:** Alfalfa may lower serum potassium concentrations, based on a human case report.[23]
- **Uric acid:** Alfalfa may increase serum urate levels.[23]
- **Serum calcium:** Mean serum calcium levels decreased significantly in a case series of 15 patients taking 40 g of heat-prepared alfalfa seed three times daily for 8 weeks.[10] Alfalfa may increase intracellular Ca^{2+} levels, based on an *in vitro* study of the alfalfa constituent L-canavanine.[43]

MECHANISM OF ACTION
Pharmacology

- **Constituents:** Vitamins A, C, E, and K, minerals, and trace elements are present in alfalfa. The amounts of each are unclear, and any benefits or toxicities due to these constituents remain unknown. Alfalfa contains coumestrol, a phytoestrogen has been isolated from three commercially available alfalfa products,[10] and *in vitro* may have a role as a low-density lipoprotein (LDL) antioxidant.[44] Alfalfa saponins rather than alfalfa fiber appear to be responsible for the reduction of cholesterol absorption.[45] Flavonoids have also been isolated from alfalfa.[46] Manganese, found in relatively high concentrations in alfalfa, has been proposed as a possible cause of hypoglycemia in one case-report.[19] Immunoreactive thyrotropin-releasing hormone-like material has been found in alfalfa in significant amounts, although its biological action is unknown.[24] 1,2-dimethylhydrazine, a carcinogen, binds to alfalfa when colon pH is between 10.5-12, and alfalfa has been proposed as possessing protective properties against chemically-induced colon cancer.[47]
- **Antimicrobial effects:** Alfalfa may possess anti-microbial properties.[48] G2, 2-beta-hydroxy-3-beta-O- (beta-D-gluco-pyranosyl)-delta 12-oleanene-23, 28-dionic acid has been isolated from alfalfa roots and has been shown *in vitro* to possess a high degree of activity against *Cryptococcus neoformans* (MIC 2 µg/mL).[49] G2 exhibits activity against a wide range of yeast strains and appears to induce lethal ion leakage from yeast cells.[50] Medicagenic acid, hederagenin glycosides, and soyasapogenols may contribute to the anti-fungal actions of alfalfa, including against *Aspergillus niger*, *Candida albicans*, and *Candida tropicalis*.[3]
- **Cholesterol-lowering effects:** A study in monkeys found that monkeys fed alfalfa saponins had decreased cholesterolemia without changes in high-density lipoprotein (HDL) when compared to monkeys not fed alfalfa saponins.[12] It was also noted that alfalfa saponins decrease intestinal absorption and increase fecal excretion of cholesterol, a finding also reported in rats.[51] Alfalfa has been shown to prevent the expected rise in cholesterol associated with intake of a high cholesterol diet in monkeys.[52] Alfalfa reduces lipid levels in plasma and tissues more effectively than D-thyroxine and pyrimidine, but not as effectively as cholestyramine or diets completely void of cholesterol.[53] Similar cholesterol-lowering effects have been observed in rabbits.[54-56] Rabbits with an ileal bypass required less alfalfa to prevent hyper-cholesterolemia than rabbits with normal gut length[55]; alfalfa was an effective adjuvant to partial ileal bypass in the treat-

ment of hypercholesterolemia in rabbits.[56] Following oral administration of cholesterol to rabbits, elevations in serum cholesterol were prevented when feedings included alfalfa.[54] Hyperlipidemia-induced rabbits fed alfalfa were found to have lower total cholesterol, specifically triglycerides and non-esterified fatty acids, when compared to rabbits not fed alfalfa.[40] A study in 72 monkeys showed that diets consisting of alfalfa and cholesterol reduced cholesterol levels and atherosclerotic plaque formation when compared with diets containing cholesterol alone.[57,58]
- **Hypoglycemic effects:** Alfalfa has been found to significantly lower basal plasma glucose concentrations in streptozotocin diabetic mice.[17] In a different study, streptozotocin diabetic mice fed alfalfa (62.5 g/kg in the diet and 2.5 g/L in drinking water) experienced reduced hyperglycemia when compared with normal mice.[18] The hypoglycemic actions of alfalfa have been postulated to be due to the potentiation of insulin secretion and improvement of insulin action, although human data in this area are limited.
- **Immunologic effects:** The alfalfa constituent L-canavanine, an amino acid, has been associated in animals and humans with the development of a lupus-like syndrome or exacerbation of systemic lupus erythematosus (SLE).[4,59,60] *In vitro*, alfalfa appears to act on CD8 (−) Leu8 (+) T cells to regulate antibody synthesis and proliferation.[43] L-Canavanine may exert an inhibitory effect on CD8 T cells,[60] and may also exert effects on mononuclear cells.[59] The mechanism of action remains unknown. An unsaponifiable substance extracted from alfalfa appeared to be beneficial in treating skin damage secondary to radiotherapy and healing gums after orthodontist operations. The substance contained cycloartenol, sitosterol, campestrol, and stigonosterol.[61]

Pharmacodynamics/Kinetics

- In a rat toxicity study, alfalfa was shown to significantly increase the activity of the hepatic enzyme, aminopyrine *N*-demethylase.[62] It did not affect glutathione *S*-transferase or epoxide hydrolase activities.

HISTORY

- The name alfalfa comes from the Arabian word *al-fac-facah*, meaning "father of all foods." It was used historically by Arabs to feed horses and was believed to make horses stronger.
- Medicinally, alfalfa has been used for a wide range of indications. In traditional Chinese medicine, alfalfa has been used to treat gastrointestinal tract problems and coughs. In India, Ayurvedic priests used alfalfa for poor digestion, treatment of boils, water retention, and arthritis. North American Indians used alfalfa to treat jaundice and to promote blood clotting. Alfalfa has also been used traditionally for arthritis, bladder and kidney problems, prostate problems, menstrual irregularities, diabetes, asthma, and dyspepsia.

REVIEW OF THE EVIDENCE: DISCUSSION
Hyperlipidemia
Summary

- Multiple animal studies have demonstrated cholesterol-lowering and triglyceride-lowering effects of alfalfa, possibly without effects on high-density lipoprotein (HDL).[13,40,52,54-56] Saponins in alfalfa may decrease intestinal absorption and increase fecal excretion of cholesterol.[13,51] However, there is limited human evidence in this area. Two small case-series have reported alfalfa to decrease total cholesterol and low-

Review of the Evidence: Alfalfa

Condition Treated*	Study Design	Author, Year	N[†]	SS[†]	Study Quality[‡]	Magnitude of Benefit	ARR[†]	NNT[†]	Comments
Hyperlipidemia	Case series	Malinow[11] 1980	3	Yes	NA	Small	NA	NA	Small study, short duration, no control group or placebo.
Hyperlipidemia	Case series	Molgaard[10] 1987	15	Yes	NA	Small	NA	NA	Small study, short duration, no control group or placebo.

*Primary or secondary outcome.
[†]N, Number of patients; SS, statistically significant; ARR, absolute risk reduction; NNT, the number of patients who need to undergo a specific intervention in order to observe an outcome in one individual.
[‡]0-2 = poor; 3-4 = good; 5 = excellent.
NA, Not applicable.
For an explanation of each category in this table, please see Table 3 in the Introduction.

density lipoprotein (LDL) levels. Further data from controlled trials are necessary before alfalfa can be recommended for this indication.

Evidence

- Molgaard et al. conducted a case series in 15 patients: 8 with type IIa hyperlipoproteinemia (HLP), 3 with type IIb HLP, and 4 with type IV HLP.[10] Patients were given 40 g of heat-prepared alfalfa seeds three times daily at mealtimes for 8 weeks, followed by a post-treatment period of 8 weeks without any lipid-lowering agents. Patients maintained an American Heart Association phase 1 diet during both phases of the study. In patients with type II HLP, median values of total plasma cholesterol decreased by 17% from 9.58 to 8.00 mmol/L ($p < 0.001$), and low-density lipoprotein (LDL) values decreased by 18% from 7.69 to 6.33 mmol/L ($p < 0.01$). In 2 patients, LDL cholesterol decreased by less than 5%. Apolipoprotein B decreased by 34% from 2.17 to 1.43 g/L ($p < 0.05$) in patients with type II HLP, whereas apolipoprotein A-I did not change. Patients with type IV HLP experienced an increase in LDL cholesterol, but the statistical significance of this increase was not evaluated due to the small group size. Body weight increased significantly during the first 4 weeks. During the post-treatment phase, plasma cholesterol levels returned to baseline. These compelling preliminary results are limited by the lack of control group and small sample size.
- In a small case series, Malinow et al. demonstrated decreased plasma cholesterol levels in three volunteers following alfalfa ingestion.[11] Subjects were given 160 g of alfalfa daily for 3 weeks, followed by 80 g daily for an additional 3 weeks. Blood was drawn for baseline high-density lipoprotein (HDL) and plasma cholesterol values prior to alfalfa administration, and then weekly thereafter. Plasma cholesterol levels were reported to be lowered without changing HDL in all three men. These results are similarly limited by the lack of a control group, as well as by short duration, small study population, and poor reporting of results.

Atherosclerosis
Summary

- There is insufficient human data available to recommend for or against the use of alfalfa in the treatment of atherosclerosis. Current available evidence is limited to animal studies. Regression of atherosclerotic plaque has been demonstrated in animals, associated with the ingestion of alfalfa.[57,58,63] Human data are lacking.

Diabetes
Summary

- Alfalfa has been associated with reductions in serum glucose levels in rat studies[17,18] and in a 1962 human case report. However, there are insufficient human data available to recommend for or against the use of alfalfa in the treatment of diabetes.

Evidence

- A 1962 case report documents hypoglycemia in a diabetic man taking alfalfa.[19] After being unresponsive to conventional hypoglycemic agents, his blood glucose reached 648 mg/100 mL. Physicians allowed the patient to prepare an alfalfa extract he had used in the past. Two hours after the patient consumed the extract, he exhibited clinical signs of hypoglycemia with a blood sugar of 68 mg/100 mL. The extract was consumed 12 additional times when the patient had blood glucose levels ranging between 190 to 580 mg per 100 mL, each time resulting in a reduction of blood glucose concentrations. More recent data are not available.

FORMULARY: BRANDS USED IN CLINICAL TRIALS
Brands Used in Statistically Significant Clinical Trials

- Cholestaid (Nx Nutraceuticals, Sparks, Maryland).

REFERENCES

1. Polk IJ. Alfalfa pill treatment of allergy may be hazardous. JAMA 1982; 247(10):1493.
2. Polacheck I, Zehavi U, Naim M, et al. Activity of compound G2 isolated from alfalfa roots against medically important yeasts. Antimicrob Agents Chemother 1986;30(2):290-294.
3. Jurzysta M, Waller GR. Antifungal and hemolytic activity of aerial parts of alfalfa (Medicago) species in relation to saponin composition. Adv Exp Med Biol 1996;404:565-574.
4. Malinow MR, Bardana EJ, Jr., Pirofsky B, et al. Systemic lupus erythematosus-like syndrome in monkeys fed alfalfa sprouts: role of a nonprotein amino acid. Science 1982;216(4544):415-417.
5. Prete PE. The mechanism of action of L-canavanine in inducing autoimmune phenomena. Arthritis Rheum 1985;28(10):1198-1200.
6. Roberts JL, Hayashi JA. Exacerbation of SLE associated with alfalfa ingestion. N Engl J Med 1983;308(22):1361.
7. Herbert V, Kasdan TS. Alfalfa, vitamin E, and autoimmune disorders. Am J Clin Nutr 1994;60(4):639-640.
8. Farnsworth NR. Alfalfa pills and autoimmune diseases. Am J Clin Nutr 1995;62(5):1026-1028.
9. Malinow MR, Bardana EJ Jr, Goodnight SH Jr. Pancytopenia during ingestion of alfalfa seeds. Lancet 1981;1(8220 Pt 1):615.
10. Molgaard J, von Schenck H, Olsson AG. Alfalfa seeds lower low density lipoprotein cholesterol and apolipoprotein B concentrations in patients with type II hyperlipoproteinemia. Atherosclerosis 1987;65(1-2):173-179.
11. Malinow MR, McLaughlin P, Stafford C. Alfalfa seeds: effects on cholesterol metabolism. Experientia 1980;36(5):562-564.

12. Malinow MR, McNulty WP, Houghton DC, et al. Lack of toxicity of alfalfa saponins in cynomolgus macaques. J Med Primatol 1982;11(2):106-118.

13. Malinow MR, Connor WE, McLaughlin P, et al. Cholesterol and bile acid balance in *Macaca fascicularis*. Effects of alfalfa saponins. J Clin Invest 1981;67(1):156-162.

14. Grigorashvili GZ, Proidak NI. [Analysis of safety and nutritive value of protein isolated from alfalfa]. Vopr Pitan 1982;5:33-37.

15. Brandenburg DM. Alfalfa of the family Leguminosae. JAMA 1983; 249(24):3303.

16. Kaufman W. Alfalfa seed dermatitis. JAMA 1954;155(12):1058-1059.

17. Swanston-Flatt SK, Day C, Bailey CJ, et al. Traditional plant treatments for diabetes. Studies in normal and streptozotocin diabetic mice. Diabetologia 1990;33(8):462-464.

18. Gray AM, Flatt PR. Pancreatic and extra-pancreatic effects of the traditional anti- diabetic plant, *Medicago sativa* (lucerne). Br J Nutr 1997;78(2): 325-334.

19. Rubenstein AH, Levin NW, Elliott GA. Manganese-induced hypoglycemia. Lancet 1962;1348-1351.

20. Shemesh M, Lindner HR, Ayalon N. Affinity of rabbit uterine oestradiol receptor for phyto-oestrogens and its use in a competitive protein-binding radioassay for plasma coumestrol. J Reprod Fertil 1972;29(1):1-9.

21. Elakovich SD, Hampton JM. Analysis of coumestrol, a phytoestrogen, in alfalfa tablets sold for human consumption. J Agric Food Chem 1984;32(1): 173-175.

22. Kurzer MS, Xu X. Dietary phytoestrogens. Annu Rev Nutr 1997;17:353-381.

23. Feingold RM. Should we fear "health foods"? Arch Intern Med 1999; 159(13):1502.

24. Jackson IM. Abundance of immunoreactive thyrotropin-releasing hormone-like material in the alfalfa plant. Endocrinology 1981;108(1):344-346.

25. Mohle-Boetani J, Werner B, Polumbo M, et al. From the Centers for Disease Control and Prevention. Alfalfa sprouts—Arizona, California, Colorado, and New Mexico, February-April, 2001. JAMA 2002;287(5):581-582.

26. Howard MB, Hutcheson SW. Growth dynamics of *Salmonella enterica* strains on alfalfa sprouts and in waste seed irrigation water. Appl Environ Microbiol 2003;69(1):548-553.

27. Strapp CM, Shearer AE, Joerger RD. Survey of retail alfalfa sprouts and mushrooms for the presence of *Escherichia coli* O157:H7, *Salmonella*, and *Listeria* with BAX, and evaluation of this polymerase chain reaction-based system with experimentally contaminated samples. J Food Prot 2003;66(2): 182-187.

28. Winthrop KL, Palumbo MS, Farrar JA, et al. Alfalfa sprouts and *Salmonella* Kottbus infection: a multistate outbreak following inadequate seed disinfection with heat and chlorine. J Food Prot 2003;66(1):13-17.

29. Backer HD, Mohle-Boetani JC, Werner SB, et al. High incidence of extraintestinal infections in a *Salmonella* Havana outbreak associated with alfalfa sprouts. Public Health Rep 2000;115(4): 339-345.

30. Mahon BE, Ponka A, Hall WN, et al. An international outbreak of *Salmonella* infections caused by alfalfa sprouts grown from contaminated seeds. J Infect Dis 1997;175(4):876-882.

31. Ponka A, Andersson Y, Siitonen A, et al. Salmonella in alfalfa sprouts. Lancet 1995;345:462-463.

32. Taormina PJ, Beuchat LR, Slutsker L. Infections associated with eating seed sprouts: an international concern. Emerg Infect Dis 1999;5(5):626-634.

33. Van Beneden CA, Keene WE, Strang RA, et al. Multinational outbreak of *Salmonella enterica* serotype Newport infections due to contaminated alfalfa sprouts. JAMA 1999;281(2):158-162.

34. Farber JM, Carter AO, Varughese PV, et al. Listeriosis traced to the consumption of alfalfa tablets and soft cheese. N Engl J Med 1990;322(5):338.

35. Thayer DW, Rajkowski KT, Boyd G, et al. Inactivation of *Escherichia coli* O157:H7 and *Salmonella* by gamma irradiation of alfalfa seed intended for production of food sprouts. J Food Prot 2003;66(2):175-181.

36. Kim C, Hung YC, Brackett RE, et al. Efficacy of electrolyzed oxidizing water in inactivating *Salmonella* on alfalfa seeds and sprouts. J Food Prot 2003;66(2):208-214.

37. Liao CH, Fett WF. Isolation of *Salmonella* from alfalfa seed and demonstration of impaired growth of heat-injured cells in seed homogenates. Int J Food Microbiol 2003;82(3):245-253.

38. Gill CJ, Keene WE, Mohle-Boetani JC, et al. Alfalfa seed decontamination in a *Salmonella* outbreak. Emerg Infect Dis 2003;9(4):474-479.

39. Farnsworth NR, Bingel AS, Cordell GA, et al. Potential value of plants as sources of new antifertility agents I. J Pharm Sci 1975;64(4):535-598.

40. Yanaura S, Sakamoto M. [Effect of alfalfa meal on experimental hyperlipidemia]. Nippon Yakurigaku Zasshi 1975;71(5):387-393.

41. Kritchevsky D, Story JA. Fiber, hypercholesteremia, and atherosclerosis. Lipids 1978;13(5):366-369.

42. Mackler BP, Herbert V. The effect of raw wheat bran, alfalfa meal and alpha-cellulose on iron ascorbate chelate and ferric chloride in three binding solutions. Am J Clin Nutr 1985;42(4):618-628.

43. Morimoto I. A study on immunological effects of L-canavanine. Kobe J Med Sci 1989;35(5-6):287-298.

44. Hwang J, Hodis HN, Sevanian A. Soy and alfalfa phytoestrogen extracts become potent low-density lipoprotein antioxidants in the presence of acerola cherry extract. J Agric Food Chem 2001;49(1):308-314.

45. Malinow MR, McLaughlin P, Stafford C, et al. Comparative effects of alfalfa saponins and alfalfa fiber on cholesterol absorption in rats. Am J Clin Nutr 1979;32(9):1810-1812.

46. Stochmal A, Piacente S, Pizza C, et al. Alfalfa (*Medicago sativa* L.) flavonoids. 1. Apigenin and luteolin glycosides from aerial parts. J Agric Food Chem 2001;49(2):753-758.

47. Smith-Barbaro P, Hanson D, Reddy BS. Carcinogen binding to various types of dietary fiber. J Natl Cancer Inst 1981;67(2):495-497.

48. Rosenthal GA. The biological effects and mode of action of L-canavanine, a structural analogue of L-arginine. Q Rev Biol 1977;52(2):155-178.

49. Polacheck I, Zehavi U, Naim M, et al. The susceptibility of *Cryptococcus neoformans* to an antimycotic agent (G2) from alfalfa. Zentralbl Bakteriol Mikrobiol Hyg [A] 1986;261(4):481-486.

50. Polacheck I, Levy M, Guizie M, et al. Mode of action of the antimycotic agent G2 isolated from alfalfa roots. Zentralbl Bakteriol 1991;275(4): 504-512.

51. Malinow MR, McLaughlin P, Papworth L, et al. Effect of alfalfa saponins on intestinal cholesterol absorption in rats. Am J Clin Nutr 1977;30(12): 2061-2067.

52. Malinow MR, McLaughlin P, Kohler GO, et al. Prevention of elevated cholesterolemia in monkeys. Steroids 1977;29(1):105-110.

53. Srinivasan SR, Patton D, Radhakrishnamurthy B, et al. Lipid changes in atherosclerotic aortas of *Macaca fascicularis* after various regression regimens. Atherosclerosis 1980;37(4):591-601.

54. Cookson FB, Fedoroff S. Quantitative relationships between administered cholesterol and alfalfa required to prevent hypercholesterolaemia in rabbits. Br J Exp Pathol 1968;49(4):348-355.

55. Barichello AW, Fedoroff S. Effect of ileal bypass and alfalfa on hypercholesterolaemia. Br J Exp Pathol 1971;52(1):81-87.

56. Esper E, Barichello AW, Chan EK, et al. Synergistic lipid-lowering effects of alfalfa meal as an adjuvant to the partial ileal bypass operation. Surgery 1987;102(1):39-51.

57. Malinow MR, McLaughlin P, Naito HK, et al. Effect of alfalfa meal on shrinkage (regression) of atherosclerotic plaques during cholesterol feeding in monkeys. Atherosclerosis 1978;30(1):27-43.

58. Malinow MR, McLaughlin P, Naito HK, et al. Regression of atherosclerosis during cholesterol feeding in *Macaca fascicularis*. Am J Cardiol 1978;41:396.

59. Morimoto I, Shiozawa S, Tanaka Y, et al. L-canavanine acts on suppressor-inducer T cells to regulate antibody synthesis: lymphocytes of systemic lupus erythematosus patients are specifically unresponsive to L-canavanine. Clin Immunol Immunopathol 1990;55(1):97-108.

60. Alcocer-Varela J, Iglesias A, Llorente L, et al. Effects of L-canavanine on T cells may explain the induction of systemic lupus erythematosus by alfalfa. Arthritis Rheum 1985;28(1):52-57.

61. Mac Lean JA. Unsaponifiable substance from alfalfa for pharmaceutical and cosmetic use. Pharmaceuticals 1974;81:339.

62. Garrett BJ, Cheeke PR, Miranda CL, et al. Consumption of poisonous plants (*Senecio jacobaea, Symphytum officinale, Pteridium aquilinum, Hypericum perforatum*) by rats: chronic toxicity, mineral metabolism, and hepatic drug-metabolizing enzymes. Toxicol Lett 1982;10(2-3):183-188.

63. Malinow MR. Experimental models of atherosclerosis regression. Atherosclerosis 1983;48(2):105-118.

Aloe
(Aloe vera)

SYNONYMS/COMMON NAMES/RELATED SUBSTANCES

Acemannan, *Aloe africana*, *Aloe arborescens* Miller, *Aloe barbadesis*, *Aloe capensis*, *Aloe ferox*, aloe latex, aloe mucilage, *Aloe perfoliata*, *Aloe perryi* Baker, *Aloe spicata*, *Aloe vulgari*, Barbados aloe, bitter aloe, burn plant, Cape aloe, carrisyn, hirukattali, Curaçao aloe, elephant's gall, first-aid plant, ghai kunwar, ghikumar, hsiang-dan, jelly leek, kumari, lahoi, laloi, lily of the desert, lu-hui, medicine plant, Mediterranean aloe, miracle plant, mocha aloes, musabbar, natal aloes, nohwa, plant of immortality, plant of life, rokai, sabilla, savila, socotrine aloe, subr, true aloe, Venezuela aloe, za'bila, Zanzibar aloe.

CLINICAL BOTTOM LINE
Background

- Transparent gel from the pulp of the meaty leaves of *Aloe vera* has been used topically for thousands of years to treat wounds, skin infections, burns, and numerous other dermatologic conditions. Dried latex from the inner lining of the leaf has traditionally been used as an oral laxative.
- There is strong scientific evidence in support of the laxative properties of aloe latex, based on the well-established cathartic properties of anthraquinone glycosides (found in aloe latex). However, aloe's therapeutic value compared with other approaches to constipation remains unclear.
- There is promising preliminary support from *in vitro*, animal, and human studies that topical aloe gel has immunomodulatory properties that may improve wound healing and skin inflammation.

Scientific Evidence for Common/Studied Uses	Grade*
Constipation (laxative)	A
Genital herpes	B
Psoriasis vulgaris	B
Seborrheic dermatitis	B
Aphthous stomatitis	C
Cancer prevention	C
Diabetes (type 2)	C
HIV infection	C
Skin burns	C
Infected surgical wounds	D
Pressure ulcers	D
Radiation dermatitis	D

*Key to grades: *A:* Strong scientific evidence for this use; *B:* Good scientific evidence for this use; *C:* Unclear scientific evidence for this use; *D:* Fair scientific evidence against this use (it may not work); *F:* Strong scientific evidence against this use (it likely does not work). For a more detailed explanation of efficacy criteria, see "Natural Standard Evidence-Based Validated Grading Rationale" in the Introduction.

Historical or Theoretical Indications That Lack Sufficient Evidence

- Alopecia (hair loss), antioxidant,[1-3] arthritis (osteoarthritis, rheumatoid arthritis), asthma,[4] bacterial skin infections,[5] candidal skin infections,[6] chronic fatigue syndrome, chronic leg ulcers,[7] congestive heart failure,[8] corneal abrasions/ulcers,[9] coronary artery disease prevention,[10] dry skin (aloe gel gloves),[11] frostbite,[12,13] functional bowel disorders, helminthic infections, hepatitis,[14] hyperlipidemia, inflammatory bowel disease, lichen planus,[15] peptic ulcer,[16] periodontal surgical rinse,[17] post-dermabrasion wound healing,[18] radioprotection,[19] sunburn,[20] systemic lupus erythematosus, tic douloureux,[21] untreatable advanced solid neoplasms,[22] urolithiasis (bladder stones), vaginal contraceptive.[23]

Expert Opinion and Historic Precedent

- Topical aloe first gained popularity in the United States in the 1930s with reports of its success in treating x-ray burns.[24-28] Today, *Aloe vera* gel is an ingredient in hundreds of skin lotions and sun blocks,[29] and the gel's use in cosmetics has been boosted by claims that it possesses similar anti-aging effects to vitamin A derivatives.[30]
- Aloe is popular in traditional Chinese and Ayurvedic medicine. The Chinese literature describes the skin and the inner lining of aloe leaves as a "cold, bitter remedy" which can be "downward draining" and used to clear constipation due to accumulation of "heat" (fire). The gel is considered "cool and moist." In Ayurvedic medicine (the traditional medicine of India), aloe is used internally as a laxative, anthelminthic, hemorrhoid remedy, and uterine stimulant (menstrual regulator); it is also used topically, often in combination with licorice root, to treat eczema or psoriasis. In Arabian medicine, the fresh gel is rubbed on the forehead as a headache remedy, is rubbed on the body to cool fevers, and is also used for wound healing, conjunctivitis, infection, and constipation.
- Some naturopaths promote aloe juice as a way to prevent and treat renal stones.[31] Recently, aloe extracts have gained popularity as a treatment for canker sores, peptic ulcers, and HIV infection. The inner leaf lining is used orally as a natural laxative.
- Many individuals keep a plant in the home (thrives in bright sunlight with little care), and when faced with a minor burn, gel from a fresh leaf is applied directly to the affected skin area.
- Aloe has been cautiously approved by the expert panel, the German Commission E, for use in constipation as a second-line agent. A monograph issued by the World Health Organization has also endorsed this use. Aloe is approved by the U.S. Food and Drug Administration (FDA) as a food flavoring agent (*A. ferox*, *A. perryi*, *A. vera*). The laxative component of aloe is regulated by the FDA as a drug, but its topical applications are not regulated or endorsed.

Safety Summary

- **Likely safe:** When *Aloe vera* gel or extract is used topically to reduce pain and inflammation, to enhance healing of skin wounds (abrasions, cuts, ulcers), or to treat psoriasis, frostbite injury, burns, and HPV I infections (cold sores). Medical attention should be sought for severe burns, wounds, or frostbite.

- **Possibly safe:** When *Aloe vera* is taken orally (potential hypoglycemic properties), or when oral aloe latex is used short-term as a laxative.[32,33]
- **Likely unsafe:** When oral aloe latex is used for prolonged periods as a laxative, because of theoretical risk of dehydration and electrolyte imbalance. Topical aloe gel should be avoided for postoperative wounds, because of findings of delayed healing in one trial.[34]

DOSING/TOXICOLOGY
General

- Recommended doses are based on those most commonly used in available trials or on historical practice. However, with natural products, the optimal doses needed to balance efficacy and safety often have not been determined. Formulations and preparation methods may vary from manufacturer to manufacturer, and from batch to batch of a specific product made by a single manufacturer. Because often the active components of a product are not known, standardization may not be possible, and the clinical effects of different brands may not be comparable.

Standardization

- Standardized products are not widely available. Although this is likely not problematic for topical aloe gel, it may pose dangers with oral aloe (because of potential hypoglycemic properties). Oral aloe preparations often contain 10 to 30 mg of hydroxyanthracene derivatives per daily dose, calculated as anhydrous aloin.[35]
- Penalties have been enforced for illegal marketing of *Aloe vera* products in the United States.[36]

Dosing: Adult (18 Years and Older)
Topical

- **General use:** Pure *Aloe vera* gel is often used liberally on the skin. There are no available reports of systemic absorption leading to clinically relevant events. Commercial preparations combined with or without other active ingredients are available.
- **Psoriasis vulgaris:** Hydrophilic cream of 0.5% (by weight) of a 50% ethanol extract of aloe, combined with mineral and castor oils, three times daily for 5 consecutive days per week, for up to 4 weeks.[37]
- **Genital herpes:** Hydrophilic cream of 0.5% (by weight) of a 50% ethanol extract, combined with liquid paraffin and castor oil, three times daily on lesions for 5 consecutive days per week, for up to 2 weeks.[38]

Oral

- **Constipation:** The dose often recommended is the minimum amount to maintain a soft stool, typically 0.04 to 0.17 g of dried juice (corresponds to 10 to 30 mg of hydroxyanthraquinones). As an alternative, in combination with celandine (300 mg) and psyllium (50 mg), 150 mg of the dried juice daily of aloe has been found effective as a laxative.[39]
- **Diabetes (type 2):** 5 to 15 mL of aloe juice twice daily.[32,33,40] Inconclusive efficacy or safety.
- **HIV infection:** 1000 to 1600 mg of acemannan orally in four equal doses.[41-43] Inconclusive efficacy or safety.

Intravenous/Intramuscular

- No recommended dosage for injectable acemannan exists to date because safety has not been sufficiently evaluated. Cases of death have been associated with *Aloe vera* injections under unclear circumstances.[35,,44]

Dosing: Pediatric (Younger Than 18 Years)
Topical

- Topical use in children is common and appears to be well tolerated.

Oral/Parenteral

- Not recommended internally because of lack of safety data.

Toxicology

- Subchronic oral use of acemannan has been well tolerated in animals.[45] Systemic toxicity of injectable acemannan has not occurred in mice, rats or dogs.[46]
- Although anthraquinones are believed to be genotoxic,[47] the anthraquinones in aloe, including aloe-emodin, do not appear to be well absorbed, and no detectable levels result from ingestion.[48] A low molecular weight fraction from aloe gel has been shown to be cytotoxic *in vitro*.[49]
- Most adverse effects appear to be mediated by potassium depletion after prolonged oral use, for which supportive care with oral or intravenous fluid/electrolyte replacement have been anecdotally reported as effective.
- The U.S. Food and Drug Administration has approved *A. ferox, A. perryi, A. vera,* and certain hybrids for use as natural food flavorings.

ADVERSE EFFECTS/PRECAUTIONS/CONTRAINDICATIONS
Allergy

- Avoid if known allergy to plants of the Liliaceae family (garlic, onions, tulips).
- After prolonged use of topical aloe gel, urticaria,[50] contact dermatitis,[51-53] and widespread dermatitis[54] have been reported.

Adverse Effects

- **Dermatologic:** One randomized trial reported delayed wound healing with topical aloe gel, applied following complicated gynecological surgeries.[34] Thus, topical aloe may not be advisable for the promotion of postoperative incision healing. Photodermatitis has also been reported.[55] In one case report, a 65–year-old woman who was 2 weeks post-dermabrasion applied *Aloe vera* leaf juice to her skin, which produced stinging, induration, and erythema.[56] The patient was prescribed hydrocortisone and diphenhydramine ointment, and the dermatitis subsided over time.[56]
- **Cardiovascular:** Theoretically, a risk of arrhythmia may increase with prolonged use of oral aloe latex, based on anecdotal reports of potassium depletion and based on aloe's laxative properties.
- **Gastrointestinal:** Occasional abdominal cramping and diarrhea with oral use have been reported anecdotally by practitioners. Using laxatives such as aloe latex for more than 7 consecutive days may aggravate constipation or cause dependency. Chronic use or abuse of anthranoid-containing laxatives for longer than 1 year has been associated with increased risk of colorectal cancer, with a relative risk of 3.04 vs. non-anthranoid abusers (triple the risk).[57]
- **Endocrine:** Hypoglycemic effects of oral aloe have been reported in two methodologically weak human trials, with

purported equivalence to a sulfonylurea anti-hyperglycemic oral agent (glibenclamide).[32,33] Laboratory studies have documented beta-cell stimulation and subsequent drops in blood glucose in mice (thus, there may be no effect in type 1 diabetics, in whom beta cells have been destroyed).[58] In contrast, a small randomized trial, published only as a conference abstract, found no evidence of hypoglycemia in 16 type 2 diabetics given aloe juice (15 mL twice daily).[40] The effects of aloe on human blood glucose levels thus remain inconclusive, although caution is warranted in patients taking anti-hyperglycemic agents.

- **Musculoskeletal:** A risk of muscle weakness may increase with prolonged use of aloe latex, based on anecdotal reports of potassium depletion and based on aloe's laxative properties.
- **Renal:** Based on the laxative properties of oral aloe latex, prolonged use may cause potassium depletion; there are anecdotal reports of low potassium, although scant literature exists in this area.

Precautions/Warnings/Contraindications

- Oral aloe products should be used cautiously in patients with diabetes or glucose intolerance, and in patients using glucose-lowering agents. Blood glucose levels should be monitored.
- Avoid oral aloe latex in patients with renal insufficiency, cardiac disease, or electrolyte abnormalities, because of theoretical risk/anecdotal reports of hypokalemia.
- Avoid use of oral aloe latex in patients with ileus, acute surgical abdomen, bowel obstruction, fecal impaction, or appendicitis.
- Avoid *Aloe vera* injections, which have been associated with four cases of death under unclear circumstances.[35,44]

Pregnancy and Lactation

- Although topical application is unlikely to be harmful during pregnancy or lactation,[59] internal use is not recommended because of theoretical stimulation of uterine contractility by anthraquinones. It is not known whether pharmacologically active constituents of aloe may be excreted with breast milk. Consumption of the dried juice from the pericyclic region of aloe leaves is contraindicated during lactation.

INTERACTIONS
Aloe/Drug Interactions

- **Oral hypoglycemic agents:** Concomitant use of glucose-lowering agents with oral forms of aloe may increase hypoglycemic effects. Hypoglycemic properties of aloe have been reported in two methodologically weak human trials, with purported equivalence to an oral hypoglycemic sulfonylurea agent (glibenclamide).[32,33] Laboratory studies have documented beta-cell stimulation and subsequent drops in blood glucose in mice.[58,60] In contrast, a small randomized trial, published as a conference abstract, found no evidence of hypoglycemia in 16 type 2 diabetics given aloe juice (15 mL twice daily).[40]
- **Insulin:** Based on the laxative properties of oral aloe latex, prolonged use may cause potassium depletion and act additively with insulin to reduce serum potassium levels. Concomitant use of insulin with oral forms of aloe may increase hypoglycemic effects, based on preliminary human data.[32,33] One animal study suggests that stimulation of beta cells is responsible for this effect of aloe, and thus the interaction might not apply to type 1 diabetics, in whom beta cells have been destroyed.

- **Digoxin, digitoxin:** Low levels of serum potassium (due to aloe latex laxative overuse) theoretically could interfere with cardiac glycosides or other antiarrhythmic agents.
- **Non–potassium sparing diuretics (loop diuretics, thiazide diuretics):** Based on the laxative properties of oral aloe latex, prolonged use may cause potassium depletion. Hypokalemia may be exacerbated by simultaneous applications of thiazide diuretics.
- **Laxatives:** Theoretically, concomitant use of oral aloe latex and other laxatives may exacerbate hypokalemia, dehydration, metabolic alkalosis, or other electrolyte abnormalities.
- **Oral corticosteroids, oral hydrocortisone:** Based on the laxative properties of oral aloe latex, prolonged use may cause potassium depletion. Hypokalemia may be exacerbated by simultaneous application of steroids.
- **Topical hydrocortisone:** Concomitant topical use of topical aloe may enhance absorption of hydrocortisone, although there is limited evidence in this area.[61]
- **Zidovudine (AZT):** Preliminary reports suggest that AZT levels may be boosted by aloe ingestion, although data remain scant in this area.[62]

Aloe/Herb/Supplement Interactions

- **Licorice root (*Glycyrrhiza glabra* L.):** Based on the laxative properties of oral aloe latex, prolonged use may result in potassium depletion. Hypokalemia may be exacerbated by simultaneous applications of licorice root.
- **Laxative herbs:** Theoretically, concomitant use of oral aloe latex and other laxatives may exacerbate hypokalemia, dehydration, metabolic alkalosis, or other electrolyte abnormalities.
- **Hypoglycemic agents:** Concomitant use of glucose-lowering agents with oral forms of aloe may increase hypoglycemic effects, based on preliminary human data.[32,33]

Aloe/Food Interactions

- **Absorption:** The high mucilage content in aloe taken orally may interfere with absorption of foods and orally administered drugs. Malabsorption may occur after prolonged oral use of aloe.

Aloe/Lab Interactions

- **Serum potassium levels:** Based on the laxative properties of oral aloe latex, prolonged HIV/AIDS use may cause potassium depletion, metabolic alkalosis, and dehydration.
- **Serum glucose levels:** Preliminary evidence from two poorly conducted human trials and from animal data suggests that oral forms of aloe may lower blood sugar levels.[32,33,58]

MECHANISM OF ACTION
Pharmacology

- **Aloe gel:** The gel or mucilage obtained from the flesh of the leaf is 99% water at pH 4.5. The constituent polysaccharide glucomannan is an effective human skin moisturizer, which accounts for its use in many cosmetics. Acemannan, the major carbohydrate fraction in the gel, is a water-soluble long-chain mannose polymer that has been found *in vitro* and in animal studies to modulate immune function (particularly macrophage activation and cytokine production) and to accelerate wound healing. The macrophage-stimulating principle of acemannan appears to reside in the high molecular weight polysaccharide aloeride.[63] Acemannan has also been reported to exhibit antineoplastic and antiviral effects *in vitro*.

- Other constituents include bradykininase, which possesses anti-inflammatory properties, and magnesium lactate, which has antipruritic effects.[8] A mannose-rich polysaccharide fraction of aloe gel has been shown in mice to enhance antibody production.[64] Salicylic acid and other antiprostaglandin compounds may be responsible for aloe's local anti-inflammatory activity, possibly due to an inhibitory effect on the arachidonic acid pathway via cyclooxygenase.[65]
- Antioxidant properties have been attributed to aloesin derived from *Aloe vera*.[1-3]
- Topical aloe's anti-inflammatory properties do not appear to interfere with wound healing, but rather increase wound tensile strength,[66] possibly because of the fibroblast-stimulating activity of mannose-6-phosphate.[67]
- Anti-leukemic and anti-mutagenic effects of aloe *in vitro* have been attributed to di-(2-ethylhexyl) phthalate (DEHP).[68] Promotion of apoptosis has been reported *in vitro* as a possible antineoplastic mechanism.[69] Aloe appears to affect favorably detoxification of reactive metabolites by liver and other organs.[2]
- Calcium isocitrate, isolated from *Aloe sponaria*, has been shown to be inotropic in rat and rabbit hearts.[8]
- Constituents of kitachi aloe leaf pulp and skin have been found to stimulate beta cells in diabetic mice, thereby lowering blood glucose levels.[58]
- **Aloe latex:** Aloe latex contains anthraquinone glycosides (aloin, aloe-emodin and barbaloin) that act as potent stimulant laxatives.[48,70-75] These water-soluble glycosides are split by intestinal bacteria into aglycones, which are believed to exert a more powerful laxative effect than other herbs, including senna, cascara, and rhubarb root. One of these compounds, aloe-emodin-9-anthrone, has been shown to increase the water content in rat large intestine.[76] This appears to be a more important cathartic mechanism than increased intestinal motility (which has also been proposed).[71,72]

Pharmacodynamics/Kinetics

- Anthraquinone glycosides, which are absorbed well only after digestion by intestinal bacteria, are eliminated in the urine, bile, feces, and breast milk.
- The half-life of aloe-emodin is approximately 48 to 50 hours.[77]

HISTORY

- Aloe is depicted as the "plant of immortality" in 6000-year-old Egyptian stone carvings and was a traditional funerary gift to the pharaohs. The ancient Egyptian Book of Remedies notes the use of aloe to cure infections, treat the skin, and prepare laxatives. The New Testament (John 19:39-40) refers to a mixture of myrrh and aloes for the preparation of Jesus' body. Alexander the Great is said to have conquered Socotra to secure control of aloe. The Greek physician Dioscorides recorded its use in 74 AD for wounds, hair loss, genital ulcers, and hemorrhoids. Arab traders found willing buyers for aloe transported to Asia in the 6th century AD, and the Spanish brought aloe to the Americas in the 16th century. In the 1930s, topical aloe gel was hailed as a treatment of roentgen (radiation) dermatitis and has since been widely used in cosmetic and dermatologic preparations.
- Penalties have been enforced for illegal marketing of *Aloe vera* products in the United States.[36]

Review of the Evidence: Aloe

Condition Treated*	Study Design	Author, Year	N[†]	SS[†]	Study Quality[‡]	Magnitude of Benefit	ARR[†]	NNT[†]	Comments
Constipation	RCT, double-blind	Odes[39] 1991	35	Yes	3	Large	NA	NA	Efficacy for treatment of constipation in herbal combination.
Seborrheic dermatitis	RCT, double-blind	Vardy[80] 1999	46	Yes	3	Large	43%	3	Impressive efficacy of aloe lotion; only known study for this indication.
Psoriasis vulgaris	RCT, double-blind	Syed[37] 1996	60	Yes	3	Large	77%	2	Impressive efficacy of aloe lotion; methodologically suspicious.
Genital herpes	RCT, double-blind	Syed[38] 1997	60	Yes	3	Large	60%	2	Impressive efficacy of aloe lotion in first episode of herpes; methodologically suspicious.
Genital herpes	RCT, double-blind	Syed[81] 1996	120	Yes	2	Large	62.5%	2	Brief report in Letter to the Editor format. Found aloe hydrophilic cream superior to placebo or aloe gel.
Skin burns	Equivalence trial	Heck[82] 1981	18	NA	1	Medium	NA	NA	Faster healing with aloe vs. Silvadene.
Skin burns	Non-blinded, not controlled	Visuthikosol[83] 1995	27	Yes	2	Large	NA	NA	Study used "within subject" controls.
Radiation induced dermatitis	Equivalence trial	Bosely[92] 2003	45	Yes	0	None	NA	NA	Aloe gel less effective than 1% APP cream in prevention and treatment of radiation dermatitis in children
Radiation induced dermatitis	RCT, double-blind	Williams[90] 1996	194	No	4	None	NA	NA	No prevention of radiation dermatitis by aloe gel.

Continued

Review of the Evidence: Aloe—cont'd

Condition Treated*	Study Design	Author, Year	N[†]	SS[†]	Study Quality[‡]	Magnitude of Benefit	ARR[†]	NNT[†]	Comments
Radiation induced dermatitis	RCT, double-blind	Heggie[91] 2002	225	Yes	3	None	NA	NA	Aloe gel less effective than aqueous cream for prevention of pain or desquamation from radiation therapy for breast cancer.
Radiation induced dermatitis	RCT, partially blinded	Olsen[89] 2001	70	Yes	1	Medium	NA	NA	Delay in development of radiation-associated skin changes.
Aphthous stomatitis	RCT, double-blind, modified crossover	Garnick[85] 1998	40	Yes	2	Medium	NA	NA	Combination of aloe, allantoin, and silicon dioxide vs. silicon dioxide alone.
Aphthous stomatitis	Equivalence trial, double-blind	Plemons[86] 1994	83	Yes	2	Large	NA	NA	Acemannan (topical) accelerated oral ulcer healing vs. Orabase Plain.
Type 2 diabetes	Placebo-controlled, single-blind	Yongchaiyudha[32] 1996	72	Yes	1	Large	NA	NA	Poor-quality design and reporting.
Type 2 diabetes	Placebo-controlled, single-blind	Bunyapraphatsara[33] 1996	72	Yes	1	Large	NA	NA	Poor-quality design and reporting.
Type 2 diabetes	RCT, double-blind, crossover	Chalaprawat[40] 1997	16	No	2	None	NA	NA	Conference abstract. No effect of aloe juice on mean plasma glucose levels.
Advanced HIV infections	RCT, double-blind	Montaner[41] 1996	63	No	5	None	NA	NA	Acemannan ineffective against HIV.
Pressure ulcers	RCT	Thomas[88] 1998	30	No	2	None	NA	NA	No effect of acemannan on pressure ulcers.
Infected surgical wounds	RCT, non-blinded	Schmidt[34] 1991	21	Yes	4	Negative	NA	NA	Significant delay in wound healing by second intention after gynecologic or obstetric laparotomy.
Multiple indications	Systematic review	Vogler[78] 1999	10	NA	NA	NA	NA	NA	10 studies of various indications analyzed.

*Primary or secondary outcome.
[†]N, Number of patients; SS, statistically significant; ARR, absolute risk reduction; NNT, the number of patients who need to undergo a specific intervention in order to observe an outcome in one individual.
[‡]0-2 = poor; 3-4 = good; 5 = excellent.
APP, Anionic phospholipid-based; NA, not applicable; RCT, randomized, controlled trial.
For an explanation of each category in this table, please see Table 3 in the Introduction.

REVIEW OF THE EVIDENCE: DISCUSSION
Constipation
Summary

- Few clinical studies have been conducted to evaluate the laxative effect of aloe latex in humans. However, the laxative effect of anthraquinone glycosides found in aloe, such as aloin, aloe-emodin and barbaloin, is well established scientifically.[48,70-75] The question of whether aloe latex may offer a reasonable approach to treating constipation remains to be answered. Further study is warranted to establish dosing and to compare efficacy and safety with commonly used laxative agents.

Evidence

- Chapman and Pitelli compared the laxative effect of aloin (1 grain [= 0.0648 g] once) with phenolphthalein (2 grains once), phenolphthalein plus aloin (1 grain and 0.5 grain, respectively), and placebo in 28 healthy adults.[79] Study subjects were randomly allocated to different treatment sequences; stool frequency and transit time were compared for all treatments. Aloin had a laxative effect (compared to placebo), which was reported as stronger than that of phenolphthalein and slightly weaker than the combination. However, no statistical analysis was presented in the paper.
- A randomized double-blind placebo-controlled study found that aloe (in combination with celandine and psyllium) was

an effective laxative in patients suffering from chronic constipation.[39] Thirty-five such patients were randomly allocated to either celandine plus aloe plus psyllium (starting with 1 500-mg capsule per day containing these ingredients in ratios of 6:3:1 and increasing up to three capsules per day as required) or placebo. Three subjects in the placebo group dropped out because of lack of effect, and all subjects in the celandine plus aloe plus psyllium group remained in the study. All indicators of constipation improved in the experimental group vs. placebo, with statistical significance. The mean number of stools increased to 7.9 in the aloe group vs. 4.3 in the placebo group. Stool consistency scores (1 = soft/liquid, 2 = normal, 3 = hard) improved to 1.6 and 2.4, respectively. The number of capsules taken was a third lower in the experimental group vs. placebo (10.1 and 15.8, respectively). Pain scores remained unchanged in both groups. Although this study demonstrated the efficacy of an herbal combination containing aloe as a laxative, the effect of aloe cannot be separated from that of the other ingredients.

Seborrheic Dermatitis
Summary

- Preliminary evidence from one randomized trial supports aloe's efficacy in the treatment of seborrheic dermatitis. Corroboration by studies from independent groups is warranted before a strong recommendation can be made.

Evidence

- Vardy et al. examined the efficacy of aloe emulsion for the treatment of seborrheic dermatitis.[80] Forty-six patients were randomly allocated to treatment with 30% *Aloe vera* emulsion topically twice per day or to placebo for 4 to 6 weeks. At the end of the treatment period, global improvement was seen in the aloe group (58% and 62% according to dermatologist and patient ratings scales, respectively) vs. placebo (15% and 25%, respectively). This study was well designed and reported, and the dramatic results are unlikely due to bias. However, because this is an isolated study, further evaluation is warranted to provide additional support.

Psoriasis Vulgaris
Summary

- Evidence from one randomized trial suggests that 0.5% extract from *Aloe vera* in a hydrophilic cream is an effective treatment of psoriasis vulgaris. Although this study was well designed and reported, the high degree of efficacy is suspicious from a methodological standpoint. Additional research is warranted in this area.

Evidence

- Syed et al. randomized 60 patients with long-standing psoriasis to receive aloe treatment or placebo.[37] Aloe treatments consisted of three daily topical applications of a 0.5% cream for 4 weeks vs. applications of a cream without active ingredients. Patients were followed over 8 months and compared in terms of proportion cured and proportion of plaques cured. More than 80% of plaques and patients were cured in the treatment group vs. <10% in the placebo group (for both comparisons, $p < 0.001$). It is unlikely that such a strong effect is attributable to flawed randomization or blinding. The high degrees of efficacy and compliance reported in this study, and lack of reporting of blinding or randomization, raise questions about the accuracy of these results. However, no firm conclusion can be made without further study.

Genital Herpes
Summary

- Limited evidence suggests that 0.5% extract from *Aloe vera* in a hydrophilic cream is an effective treatment of genital herpes in men (superior to both aloe gel and placebo). The best available study,[38] although seemingly well designed and reported, reports a high degree of efficacy that is suspicious from a methodological standpoint. Additional research is warranted in this area.

Evidence

- Syed et al. randomized 60 men with a first episode of genital herpes to receive topical aloe or placebo.[38] Aloe treatments consisted of three daily applications of a 0.5% cream for 5 days vs. applications of a cream without active ingredients. Two thirds were cured of lesions in the aloe group after 1 week compared to only 2/30 in the placebo group ($p < 0.001$). It is unlikely that this strong effect was accounted for by flawed randomization or blinding procedures (both of which were not disclosed in the paper). From methodological and clinical perspectives, such highly effective results in an isolated study are suspicious. However, without further evaluation in a follow-up randomized trial, a firm conclusion cannot be made.
- In a prior published Letter to the Editor, Syed et al. described a randomized, double-blind controlled trial in 120 men in Pakistan, in which 0.5% topical aloe extract gel or cream, or placebo, was applied to male patients with first episodes of genital herpes.[81] Treatment was administered three times daily for 5 consecutive days/week, for 2 weeks. Aloe in hydrophilic cream was noted to significantly shorten the duration of lesions vs. gel or placebo (4.8 days, 7.0 days, and 14.0 days, respectively). With cream, 70% of patients were cured, vs. 7.5% with placebo. Although promising, the abbreviated format of this publication did not describe blinding, randomization, method of statistical analysis, or measurement criteria for classifying lesions. Therefore, the evidence remains inconclusive.

Skin Burns
Summary

- Preliminary evidence suggests that aloe may be effective in promoting healing of partial-thickness skin burns. However, the existing studies are small and poor in quality, and therefore no clear conclusion can be drawn. Further study is warranted in this area.

Evidence

- Heck et al. topically treated 18 patients with second-degree burns (2% to 12% of total body surface area) with either aloe extract or with Silvadene.[82] The average wound healing time was 13 days with aloe vs. 16 days with Silvadene. No statistical analysis was presented and results were not stratified by burn severity. Therefore, a definitive conclusion cannot be made.
- Visukitosol et al. examined the effect of a topical aloe gel preparation on skin burns in comparison to Vaseline gauze.[83] They found that in 27 patients with partial-thickness skin burns the mean healing time was 12 days with aloe gel treatment vs. 18 days with Vaseline gauze. Although the findings from this trial are suggestive, the lack of true controls (only the distal part of each wound was treated with aloe) or blinding prohibits firm conclusions.
- In a poorly described study, silver sulfadiazine cream was found to be more effective than aloe in the treatment of experimental second-degree burns, with a suggestion that aloe may in fact disrupt the healing process.[84] These conflicting results cannot be considered conclusive but must be considered.

Aphthous Stomatitis
Summary

- There is equivocal evidence from two studies that treatment of recurrent aphthous ulcers with aloe gel reduces pain and prolongs ulcer-free intervals. Further study is warranted.

Evidence

- Garnick at al. examined the effectiveness of a gel containing aloe, in addition to silicon dioxide and allantoin, on the healing of recurrent aphthous ulcers.[85] First, a gel containing aloe, allantoin, and silicon dioxide was compared to a gel containing only silicon dioxide in 40 patients. The mean duration of lesion-free intervals was 5 days in the experimental group vs. 18 days in the silicon dioxide group. However, this trend was not statistically significant. When comparing the experimental treatment to a control gel (n = 18), mean intervals were 9 vs. 2 days ($p = 0.0335$). Because of the multiple agents involved in this study, it is not possible to draw conclusions about the efficacy of aloe itself.
- Plemons et al. randomized 53 patients suffering from recurrent oral ulcers to topical treatment with either the aloe

constituent acemannan (Carrisyn Gel Wound Dressing, modified for oral lesion use) or Orabase-Plain (oral analgesic) four times daily.[86] A third group was treated with freeze-dried acemannan (Carrisyn Gel Wound Dressing cut into small pieces). The average healing time was shorter in the acemannan groups (5.7 days) than in the control group (7.8 days; $p = 0.0031$), whereas other parameters (erythema, discomfort) were only marginally affected. These results suggest that topical acemannan accelerates the healing of ulcers in aphthous stomatitis, but interpretation of the results must take methodological weaknesses into account (randomization inadequately reported, blinding methods inappropriate).

Diabetes (Type 2)
Summary
- Laboratory studies have documented beta-cell stimulation by aloe, as well as drops in blood glucose in mice.[58] Results from two poorly conducted human trials suggest that oral aloe gel may be effective in lowering blood glucose levels, although a third, smaller study has found no effect. More definitive studies are needed to explore efficacy and safety of aloe in diabetics.

Evidence
- Two non-randomized studies conducted by the same group concluded that aloe gel may be similarly effective as glibenclamide (a sulfonylurea antihyperglycemic oral agent) to lower blood glucose in type 2 diabetes mellitus.[32,33] However, methodology, statistics, and results were incompletely described. Thus, firm conclusions cannot be drawn.
- In a randomized double-blind placebo-controlled crossover study published only as a conference abstract, Chalprawat found no hypoglycemic effect of aloe juice (15 mL twice daily) in 16 type 2 diabetics.[40] Although the statistical power of this study was low, a large hypoglycemic effect is unlikely given the results.
- Oral dried aloe gel was studied in five patients with type 2 diabetes.[85] Half a teaspoon of aloe was administered daily over 4 to weeks, after which time fasting glucose was noted to have fallen from a mean of 273 to 151 ($p < 0.05$). In a simultaneous mouse study, both glibenclamide (10 mg/kg twice daily) and aloe (500 mg/kg twice daily) were found to induce hypoglycemia after 5 days (blood sugar reduced by 40%). However, only glibenclamide was effective after 3 days. Although compelling, this study is too preliminary and methodologically weak (small, no controls, poor description of methods) to be of direct relevance to clinical practice.

HIV Infection
Summary
- Acemannan, the major carbohydrate fraction in aloe gel, has been shown *in vitro* to possess immunostimulant and anti-retroviral activities. Preliminary data from human trials are equivocal; because of methodological weaknesses of available studies, firm conclusions are not possible. Without further human trials, the evidence cannot be considered compelling either in favor or against this use of aloe.

Evidence
- Montaner et al. conducted a randomized double-blind study to evaluate the efficacy of acemannan as an adjuvant anti-retroviral agent for HIV.[41] In this trial, 63 patients were randomized to receive either 400 mg of oral acemannan four times daily or placebo. No difference in CD4 counts, CD4/ CD8 ratios, P24 antigen, β_2-microglobulin concentration, or viral load was found between the two treatment groups. Although these results are discouraging, because no power calculation was performed, it is not clear that the sample size was adequate to properly measure differences between groups. Descriptions of blinding and randomization are limited.
- Two non-randomized studies evaluating the efficacy of oral acemannan in the treatment of HIV infection have been published as conference abstracts.[42,43] Both studies found clinical improvement and large increases in circulating monocytes/macrophages. The observational character of these reports provides compelling, albeit preliminary, support.
- In a case report, McDaniel and McAnalley found improvement in several serologic and clinical indicators of HIV infection in eight patients treated with acemannan (Carrisyn) for 90 days (unclear if subjects received four doses of 250 mg or 250 mg in four divided doses).[42] Benefits included decline in HIV core antigen, elimination of diarrhea, fever, diaphoresis, and "loss of culturability."
- In a non-randomized controlled study, McDaniel et al. found circulating monocytes/macrophages to be significantly more numerous in 14 HIV patients treated with 800 mg of acemannan per day (365 per smear) than in 35 patients not receiving acemannan (68 per smear, $p = 0.00027$).[43] These surrogate serologic endpoints require clinical correlation.

Cancer Prevention
Summary
- There is preliminary evidence from a small case-control study that aloe consumption may reduce the risk of developing lung cancer. Further evidence is warranted in this area to clarify if it is aloe itself or other factors that mediate this benefit.

Evidence
- In a multi-center Japanese case-control study of 192 subjects (1 case per 2 controls), a questionnaire was administered to determine the potential correlations between lung cancer incidence, smoking, and consumption of 17 different types of plants.[87] Odds ratios were calculated via an established method (Mantel-Haenszel analysis). A subgroup of 132 subjects (44 "pairs") was analyzed specifically for plant food intake, and it was determined that the odds ratio for the aloe species *Aloe arborescens* Miller was 0.5 ($p < 0.1$), suggesting half the incidence of cancer in regular consumers of aloe vs. non-aloe consumers. Although compelling, the methodological difficulties of case-control studies apply to this report. The possible effect of confounders not detected by the study questionnaire is prominent. For example, aloe/plant eaters may be more likely to exercise than non-plant eaters, which may exert an independent effect on outcome. In addition, it is not clear if this effect is generalizable to other species of aloe.

Infected Surgical Wounds
Summary
- In one study, topical aloe gel was found to prolong wound-healing time following gynecological or obstetrical laparotomy. Further study is warranted, because wound healing is a popular use of topical aloe.

Evidence
- Schmidt et al. examined the effect of aloe gel on the healing of complicated surgical wounds (healing by second intention).[34] In this study, 21 women with complicated wounds

after gynecologic or obstetric surgery were stratified according to incision type and randomized to standard treatment (debridement, irrigation) or standard treatment plus aloe gel. Wounds in the experimental group healed in 83 days on average vs. 53 days in the group with standard treatment (p = 0.003). Due to the clearly prolonged healing in the group treated with aloe, patient recruitment was terminated before the desired sample size (n = 114) was reached. This otherwise well-designed trial was not placebo controlled. However, the size of the effect was unlikely due to a placebo effect. Further study of aloe's role in the healing of wounds of varying severity may be warranted before this traditional use can be strongly discouraged, although use in complicated surgical wounds may not be advisable in light of these results.

- *Aloe vera* rinses have also been used on periodontal surgical sites.[17]

Pressure Ulcers
Summary

- One well-designed randomized trial found no benefit of topical acemannan hydrogel (the major carbohydrate fraction in aloe gel) in the treatment of pressure ulcers.

Evidence

- Thomas et al. conducted a randomized controlled trial in which 30 patients with pressure ulcers were randomly allocated to receive either acemannan hydrogel (daily dressings with 0.25-inch layer) or saline dressing.[88] Ulcers were evaluated weekly for 10 weeks or until ulcers healed. Both the proportion of healed ulcers (63% vs. 64%) and the mean time to healing (5.3 vs. 5.2 weeks) were similar in the two groups. This study had sufficient (80%) power to detect a 25% difference between treatment arms. These results suggest that acemannan hydrogel may not be effective in the treatment of pressure ulcers.

Radiation Dermatitis
Summary

- Reports during the 1930s of topical aloe's beneficial effect on post-radiation dermatitis triggered widespread use in dermatologic and cosmetic products.[24-28] Aloe gel is currently recommended by some practitioners for radiation-induced dermatitis. However, preliminary scientific evaluation suggests that topical aloe may not significantly improve pain or desquamation related to radiotherapy and may be inferior to topical aqueous gel. Additional well-designed studies are necessary before a firm conclusion can be drawn.

Evidence

- Olsen et al. prospectively studied 70 cancer patients receiving radiation doses greater than 2000 cGy.[89] Patients were randomized to either pure *Aloe vera* gel (applied liberally to the irradiated skin area throughout the day) or no specific topical treatment. All patients were instructed to wash the irradiated skin area with mild soap. Skin changes were evaluated by a clinician, blinded to the treatment, at weekly intervals. The only statistically significant difference found between treatment arms was skin texture, which at a cumulative dose below 2700 cGy was rarer in the non-treated group than in the aloe group (p<0.012). No significant differences were seen for erythema, itching, or tanning. However, in a subgroup receiving higher cumulative radiation doses, onset of skin changes was significantly delayed in the aloe group. Although this study found some beneficial

effects of aloe on radiation-associated skin changes, lack of patient blinding or placebo weakens the results.

- Williams et al. conducted a randomized trial addressing the efficacy of aloe gel for radiation-induced dermatitis.[90] In this study, 184 women undergoing treatment for breast cancer were stratified according to age, planned target radiation dose, dose fraction, and skin complexion. Subjects were randomized in a double-blind manner to topical aloe (applied twice/day on the treatment field) vs. placebo (inert gel). No difference was found between groups or within strata. Although this was a fair-sized trial, no power calculation was performed at the onset, and description of methodology was limited. Nonetheless, these results are discouraging.

- Heggie et al. conducted a randomized controlled trial (phase III) in 225 women undergoing radiation therapy for breast cancer.[91] Subjects received either topical aloe vera gel or aqueous cream three times per day throughout radiotherapy and for 2 weeks following therapy. Assessments were made by nursing staff at weekly visits. The authors report that patients receiving aqueous cream experienced significantly less pain and desquamation compared to aloe patients. These results suggest that aqueous gel may be a superior choice in such patients, although because of lack of use of validated evaluation instruments and incomplete reporting of analysis, these results cannot be considered definitive. Comparison of aloe to a non-active intervention would provide additional information about the efficacy of aloe.

- Bosley et al. conducted a randomized controlled trial (phase III) comparing a 1% anionic phospholipid-based (APP) cream with an *Aloe vera*–based gel in the prevention and treatment of radiation dermatitis in 45 pediatric patients treated with radiation therapy.[92] The mean age of subjects was 11 years, with Hodgkin's disease being the most common diagnosis and the thorax being the most common treatment field. Chemotherapy was used before or during radiation treatment. Patients were excluded if they had received prior irradiation for their disease or had coincident dermatological conditions or if there was planned use of other topical products. Treatments were applied topically, symmetrically and adjacent within the field of irradiation once daily after radiation treatment. Skin comfort was evaluated by a questionnaire, and dermatological assessments were made using a 15-item score on a 4-level scale before and weekly during treatment, and up to 6 weeks after radiation. The authors reported statistically significant results favoring the cream on skin assessment variables such as dryness (p = 0.002), comfort (p = 0.002), erythema (p = 0.002), and peeling (p = 0.008). Limitations of the study include a lack of description of randomization, lack of blinding, and lack of reported mean duration of treatment between the two treatment groups. In addition, the skin comfort assessment was based on subjective data.

FORMULARY: BRANDS USED IN CLINICAL TRIALS
Brands Used in Statistically Significant Clinical Trials

- Carrisyn Gel Wound Dressing (preparation of acemannan, the major carbohydrate fraction of aloe gel, found efficacious for oral aphthous ulcers/stomatitis); Carrisyn (internal preparations have been used in HIV with unproven efficacy).

REFERENCES

1. Yagi A, Kabash A, Mizuno K, et al. Radical scavenging glycoprotein inhibiting cyclooxygenase-2 and thromboxane A2 synthase from *Aloe vera* gel. Planta Med 2003;69(3):269-271.
2. Singh RP, Dhanalakshmi S, Rao AR. Chemomodulatory action of *Aloe vera*

on the profiles of enzymes associated with carcinogen metabolism and antioxidant status regulation in mice. Phytomedicine 2000;7(3):209-219.

3. Yagi A, Kabash A, Okamura N, et al. Antioxidant, free radical scavenging and anti-inflammatory effects of aloesin derivatives in *Aloe vera*. Planta Med 2002;68(11):957-960.

4. Shida T, Yagi A, Nishimura H, et al. Effect of Aloe extract on peripheral phagocytosis in adult bronchial asthma. Planta Med 1985;51(3):273-275.

5. Lorenzetti LJ, Salisbury R, Beal JL, et al. Bacteriostatic property of *Aloe vera*. J Pharm Sci 1964;53:1287.

6. Ali MI, Shalaby NM, Elgamal MH, et al. Antifungal effects of different plant extracts and their major components of selected aloe species. Phytother Res 1999;13(5):401-407.

7. Zawahry ME, Hegazy MR, Helal M. Use of aloe in treating leg ulcers and dermatoses. Int J Dermatol 1973;12(1):68-73.

8. Yagi A, Shibata S, Nishioka I, et al. Cardiac stimulant action of constituents of *Aloe saponaria*. J Pharm Sci 1982;71(7):739-741.

9. Green K, Tasi J, Luxenberg M. Effect of aloe vera on corneal epithelial wound healing. J Toxicol Cutan Ocular Toxicol 1996;15(4):301-304.

10. Agarwal OP. Prevention of atheromatous heart disease. Angiology 1985;36(8):485-492.

11. West DP, Zhu YF. Evaluation of aloe vera gel gloves in the treatment of dry skin associated with occupational exposure. Am J Infect Control 2003; 31(1):40-42.

12. Heggers JP, Phillips LG, McCauley RL, et al. Frostbite: experimental and clinical evaluations of treatment. J Wilderness Med 1990;1:27-32.

13. Miller MB, Koltai PJ. Treatment of experimental frostbite with pentoxifylline and aloe vera cream. Arch Otolaryngol Head Neck Surg 1995;121(6): 678-680.

14. Fan YJ, Li M, Yang WL, et al. [Protective effect of extracts from *Aloe vera* L. var. chinensis (Haw.) Berg. on experimental hepatic lesions and a primary clinical study on the injection of in patients with hepatitis.] Zhongguo Zhong Yao Za Zhi 1989;14(12):746-748.

15. Hayes SM. Lichen planusreport of successful treatment with aloe vera. Gen Dent 1999;47(3):268-272.

16. Blitz JJ, Smith JW, Gerard JR. *Aloe vera* gel in peptic ulcer therapy: preliminary report. J Amer Osteopath Assoc 1963;62:731-735.

17. Rieger L, Carson RE. The clinical effects of saline and aloe vera rinses on periodontal surgical sites. J Okla Dent Assoc 2002;92(3):40-43.

18. Fulton JE, Jr. The stimulation of postdermabrasion wound healing with stabilized aloe vera gel-polyethylene oxide dressing. J Dermatol Surg Oncol 1990;16(5):460-467.

19. Pande S, Kumar M, Kumar A. Radioprotective efficacy of Aloe vera leaf extract. Pharmaceut Biol 1998;36(3):227-232.

20. Crowell J, Hilsenbeck S, Penneys N. Aloe vera does not affect cutaneous erythema and blood flow following ultraviolet B exposure. Photodermatol 1989;6(5):237-239.

21. Hayes SM. Tic douloureux: report of successful treatment. Gen Dent 1984;32(5):441-442.

22. Lissoni P, Giani L, Zerbini S, et al. Biotherapy with the pineal immuno-modulating hormone melatonin versus melatonin plus aloe vera in untreatable advanced solid neoplasms. Nat Immun 1998;16(1):27-33.

23. Fahim MS, Wang M. Zinc acetate and lyophilized aloe barbadensis as vaginal contraceptive. Contraception 1996;53(4):231-236.

24. Collins EE, Collins C. Roentgen dermatitis treated with fresh whole leaf of aloe vera. Am J Roentgenol 1935;33(3):396-397.

25. Collins CE. Alvagel as a therapeutic agent in the treatment of roentgen and radium burns. Radiol Rev Chicago Med Recorder 1935;57(6):137-138.

26. Mandeville FB. Aloe vera in the treatment of radiation ulcers of mucous membranes. Radiology 1939;32:598-599.

27. Wright CS. Aloe vera in the treatment of roentgen ulcers and telangiectasis. J Amer Med Assoc 1935;106(16):1363-1364.

28. Rowe TD, Lovell BK, Parks LM. Further observations on the use of *Aloe vera* leaf in the treatment of third degree x-ray reactions. J Amer Pharmaceut Assoc 1941;30:266-269.

29. Grindlay D, Reynolds T. The *Aloe vera* phenomenon: a review of the properties and modern uses of the leaf parenchyma gel. J Ethnopharmacol 1986;16(2-3):117-151.

30. Danhof I. Potential benefits from orally-ingested internal *Aloe vera* gel. International Aloe Science Council Tenth Annual Aloe Scientific Seminar, Irving, Texas, 1991;

31. McGuffin M, Hobbs C, Upton R, et al. American Herbal Products Association's Botanical Safety Handbook. Boca Raton: CRC Press, 1997:

32. Yongchaiyudha S, Rungpitarangsi V, Bunyapraphatsara N, et al. Antidiabetic activity of *Aloe vera* L. juice. I Clinical trial in new cases of diabetes mellitus. Phytomedicine 1996;3(3):241-243.

33. Bunyapraphatsara N, Yongchaiyudha S, Rungpitarangsi V, et al. Antidiabetic activity of *Aloe vera* L. juice. II. Clinical trial in diabetes mellitus patients in combination with glibenclamide. Phytomed 1996;3(3):245-248.

34. Schmidt JM, Greenspoon JS. *Aloe vera* dermal wound gel is associated with a delay in wound healing. Obstet Gynecol 1991;78(1):115-117.

35. Anonymous. MD loses license after injecting aloe kills 3. National Council Against Health Fraud 1997;20:4.

36. Meadows M. Maryland man, Virginia physician sentenced for illegally marketing aloe vera "treatments." FDA Consum 2002;36(3):34-35.

37. Syed TA, Ahmad SA, Holt AH, et al. Management of psoriasis with Aloe vera extract in a hydrophilic cream: a placebo-controlled, double-blind study. Trop Med Int Health 1996;1(4):505-509.

38. Syed TA, Afzal M, Ashfaq AS. Management of genital herpes in men with 0.5% *Aloe vera* extract in a hydrophilic cream. A placebo-controlled double-blind study. J Derm Treatment 1997;8(2):99-102.

39. Odes HS, Madar Z. A double-blind trial of a celandin, aloe vera and psyllium laxative preparation in adult patients with constipation. Digestion 1991; 49(2):65-71.

40. Chalaprawat M. The hypoglycemic effects of *Aloe vera* in Thai diabetic patients. J Clin Epidemiol 1997;50(Suppl 1):3S.

41. Montaner JS, Gill J, Singer J, et al. Double-blind placebo-controlled pilot trial of acemannan in advanced human immunodeficiency virus disease. J Acquir Immune Defic Syn Hum Retrovirol 1996;12:153-157.

42. McDaniel HR, McAnalley BH. Evaluation of polymannoacetate (carrisyn) in the treatment of AIDS. Clin Research 1987;35(3):483a.

43. McDaniel HR, Combs C, McDaniel HR, et al. An increase in circulating monocyte/macrophages (M/M) is induced by oral acemannan (ACE-M) in HIV-1 patients. Amer J Clin Pathol a990;94(4):516-517.

44. Anonymous. License revoked for *Aloe vera* use. Mat Med Law 1998;1:1-2.

45. Fogleman RW, Shellenberger TE, Balmer MF, et al. Subchronic oral administration of acemannan in the rat and dog. Vet Hum Toxicol 1992;34(2): 144-147.

46. Fogleman RW, Chapdelaine JM, Carpenter RH, et al. Toxicologic evaluation of injectable acemannan in the mouse, rat and dog. Vet Hum Toxicol 1992;34(3):201-205.

47. Muller SO, Eckert I, Lutz WK, et al. Genotoxicity of the laxative drug components emodin, aloe-emodin and danthron in mammalian cells: topoisomerase II mediated? Mutat Res 1996;371(3-4):165-173.

48. Krumbiegel G, Schulz HU. Rhein and aloe-emodin kinetics from senna laxatives in man. Pharmacology 1993;47(suppl 1):120-124.

49. Avila H, Rivero J, Herrera F, et al. Cytotoxicity of a low molecular weight fraction from Aloe vera (Aloe barbadensis Miller) gel. Toxicon 1997;35(9): 1423-1430.

50. Morrow DM, Rapaport MJ, Strick RA. Hypersensitivity to aloe. Arch Dermatol 1980;116(9):1064-1065.

51. Shoji A. Contact dermatitis to *Aloe arborescens*. Contact Dermatitis 1982; 8(3):164-167.

52. Nakamura T, Kotajima S. Contact dermatitis from *Aloe arborescens*. Contact Dermatitis 1984;11(1):51.

53. Sauchak U. Acute bullous allergic dermatitis due to local application of aloe leaves. Vestnik Dermatologii i Venerologii 1977;12:44-45.

54. Hogan DJ. Widespread dermatitis after topical treatment of chronic leg ulcers and stasis dermatitis. CMAJ 1988;138(4):336-338.

55. Dominguez-Soto L. Photodermatitis to aloe vera. Int J Dermatol 1992; 31(5):372.

56. Hunter D, Frumkin A. Adverse reactions to vitamin E and aloe vera preparations after dermabrasion and chemical peel. Cutis 1991;47(3): 193-196.

57. Siegers CP, Hertzberg-Lottin E, Otte M, et al. Anthranoid laxative abuse—a risk for colorectal cancer? Gut 1993;34(8):1099-1101.

58. Beppu H, Nagamura Y, Fujita K. Hypoglycemic and antidiabetic effects in mice of aloe-arborescens miller var natalensis berger. Phytother Res 1993;7:S37-S42.

59. Lepik K. Safety in herbal medications in pregnancy. Canadian Pharmaceut J 1997;130:29-33.

60. Okyar A, Can A, Akev N, et al. Effect of *Aloe vera* leaves on blood glucose level in type I and type II diabetic rat models. Phytother Res 2001;15(2): 157-161.

61. Davis RH, Parker WL, Murdoch DP. *Aloe vera* as a biologically active vehicle for hydrocortisone acetate. J Am Podiatr Med Assoc 1991;81(1):1-9.

62. Anonymous. Aloe vera may boost AZT. Med Tribune 1991;22:4.

63. Pugh N, Ross SA, ElSohly MA, et al. Characterization of Aloeride, a new high-molecular-weight polysaccharide from Aloe vera with potent immunostimulatory activity. J Agric Food Chem 2001;49(2):1030-1034.

64. 't Hart LA, van den Berg AJ, Kuis L, et al. An anti-complementary polysaccharide with immunological adjuvant activity from the leaf parenchyma gel of *Aloe vera*. Planta Med 1989;55(6):509-512.

65. Vazquez B, Avila G, Segura D, et al. Antiinflammatory activity of extracts from *Aloe vera* gel. J Ethnopharmacol 1996;55(1):69-75.

66. Davis RH, DiDonato JJ, Johnson RW, et al. *Aloe vera*, hydrocortisone, and sterol influence on wound tensile strength and anti-inflammation. J Am Podiatr Med Assoc 1994;84(12):614-621.

67. Davis RH, Donato JJ, Hartman GM, et al. Anti-inflammatory and wound healing activity of a growth substance in *Aloe vera*. J Am Podiatr Med Assoc 1994;84(2):77-81.

68. Lee KH, Kim JH, Lim DS, et al. Anti-leukaemic and anti-mutagenic effects of di(2-ethylhexyl)phthalate isolated from *Aloe vera* Linne. J Pharm Pharmacol 2000; 52(5):593-598.

69. Pecere T, Sarinella F, Salata C, et al. Involvement of p53 in specific antineuroectodermal tumor activity of aloe-emodin. Int J Cancer 2003;106(6): 836-847.

70. de Witte P, Lemli L. The metabolism of anthranoid laxatives. Hepatogastroenterology1990;37(6):601-605.

71. Ishii Y, Tanizawa H, Takino Y. Studies of aloe. IV. Mechanism of cathartic effect. (3). Biol Pharm Bull 1994;17(4):495-497.
72. Ishii Y, Tanizawa H, Takino Y. Studies of aloe. V. Mechanism of cathartic effect. (4). Biol Pharm Bull 1994;17(5):651-653.
73. Honig J, Geck P, Rauwald HW. Inhibition of Cl– channels as a possible base of laxative action of certain anthraquinones and anthrones. Planta Med 1992;58(Suppl 1):A586-A587.
74. Koch A. Investigations of the laxative action of aloin in the human colon. Planta Med 1993;59:A689.
75. Nelemans FA. Clinical and toxicological aspects of anthraquinone laxatives. Pharmacology 1976;14(Suppl 1):73-77.
76. Ishii Y, Tanizawa H, Takino Y. Studies of aloe. III. Mechanism of cathartic effect. (2). Chem Pharm Bull (Tokyo) 1990;38(1):197-200.
77. Lang W. Pharmacokinetic-metabolic studies with 14C– aloe emodin after oral administration to male and female rats. Pharmacology 1993;47(Suppl 1):110-119.
78. Vogler BK, Ernst E. *Aloe vera*: a systematic review of its clinical effectiveness. Br J Gen Pract 1999;49(447):823-828.
79. Chapman DD, Pittelli JJ. Double-blind comparison of alophen with its components for cathartic effects. Curr Ther Res Clin Exp 1974;16(8):817-820.
80. Vardy AD, Cohen AD, Tchetov T. A double-blind, placebo-controlled trial of *Aloe vera* (*A. barbadensis*) emulsion in the treatment of seborrheic dermatitis. J Derm Treat 1999;10(1):7-11.
81. Syed TA, Cheema KM, Ahmad SA, et al. *Aloe vera* extract 0.5% in hydrophilic cream versus *Aloe vera* gel for the measurement of genital herpes in males. A placebo-controlled, double-blind, comparative study. J Eur Acad Dermatol Venerol 1996;7(3):294-295.
82. Heck E, Head M. *Aloe vera* gel cream as a topical treatment for outpatient burns. Burns 1981;7(4):291-294.
83. Visuthikosol V, Sukwanarat Y, Chowchuen B, et al. Effect of *Aloe vera* gel to healing of burn wounds: a clinical and histologic study. J Med Assoc Thai 1995;78(8):403-409.
84. Kaufman T, Kalderon N, Ullmann Y, et al. *Aloe vera* gel hindered wound healing of experimental second-degree burns: a quantitative controlled study. J Burn Care Rehabil 1988;9(2):156-159.
85. Garnick JJ, Singh B, Winkley G. Effectiveness of a medicament containing silicon dioxide, aloe, and allantoin on aphthous stomatitis. Oral Surg Oral Med Oral Pathol Oral Radiol Endod 1998;86(5):550-556.
86. Plemons JM, Reps PD, Binnie WH, et al. Evaluation of acemannan in the treatment of recurrent aphthous stomatitis, Wounds 1994;6(2):40-45.
87. Sakai R. Epidemiologic survey on lung cancer with respect to cigarette smoking and plant diet. Jpn J Cancer Res 1989;80(6):513-520.
88. Thomas DR, Goode PS, LaMaster K, et al. Acemannan hydrogel dressing versus saline dressing for pressure ulcers. A randomized, controlled trial. Adv Wound Care 1998;11(6):273-276.
89. Olsen DL, Raub W, Jr., Bradley C, et al. The effect of aloe vera gel/mild soap versus mild soap alone in preventing skin reactions in patients undergoing radiation therapy. Oncol Nurs Forum 2001;28(3):543-547.
90. Williams MS, Burk M, Loprinzi CL, et al. Phase III double-blind evaluation of an *Aloe vera* gel as a prophylactic agent for radiation-induced skin toxicity. Int J Radiation Oncol Biol Phys 1996;36(2):345-349.
91. Heggie S, Bryant GP, Tripcony L, et al. A Phase III study on the efficacy of topical aloe vera gel on irradiated breast tissue. Cancer Nurs 2002;25(6):442-451.
92. Bosley C, Smith J, Baratti P, et al. A phase III trial comparing an anionic phospholipid-based (APP) cream and aloe vera-based gel in the prevention and treatment of radiation dermatitis. Int J Radiat Oncol Biol Phys 2003;57(2 Suppl):S438.

Antineoplastons
(Phenylacetate)

SYNONYMS/COMMON NAMES/RELATED SUBSTANCES

- A1, A2, A3, A4, A5, A10, A10-1, AS2-1, AS2-5, AS5, antineoplaston A, antineoplaston H, antineoplaston L, antineoplaston O, antineoplaston F, antineoplaston Ch, antineoplaston K, 3-*N*-phenylacetylaminopiperidine-2,6 dione, phenylacetylglutamine (PAG), phenylacetylisoglutamine (PAIG), phenylacetic acid (PAA), 3-phenylacetylamino-2,6-piperidinedione, sodium phenylacetate.

CLINICAL BOTTOM LINE

Background

- Antineoplastons are a group of naturally occurring peptide fractions that were observed by Stanislaw Burzynski in the late 1970s to be absent in the urine of cancer patients. It was hypothesized that these substances might have anti-tumor properties. In the 1980s, Burzynski identified chemical structures for several of these antineoplastons and developed a process to prepare them synthetically. Antineoplaston A10, identified as 3-phenylacetylamino-2,6-piperidinedione, was the first to be synthesized.
- The use of antineoplastons for the treatment of various types of cancer has been studied in the laboratory, in animals, and in limited preliminary human research. In 1991, the Cancer Therapy Evaluation Program of the National Cancer Institute (NCI) examined records of seven patients with brain tumors treated at the Burzynski Clinic in Texas. Based on their findings, the NCI sponsored a brain tumor clinical trial. However, because of difficulty recruiting patients and disagreement over study design, this research was canceled. The results in nine patients who were included prior to cancellation were reported but were not conclusive. In 1997, Dr. Burzynski encountered legal problems because of permitting antineoplastons to be shipped out of Texas.
- Evidence from randomized, controlled trials is lacking in support of antineoplastons as a cancer treatment, and antineoplaston therapy is not approved by the U.S. Food and Drug Administration. Antineoplastons are not widely available in the United States, and their safety and efficacy has not been proven, although multiple studies of antineoplastons in treatment for various cancers have been sponsored by the Burzynski Research Institute. In recent years, antineoplastons have been suggested as therapy for other conditions such as Parkinson's disease, sickle cell anemia, and thalassemia.

Uses Based on Scientific Evidence	Grade*
Cancer Scientific evidence regarding the effectiveness of antineoplastons in cancer therapy is inconclusive. Several preliminary studies in humans (case series, phase I/II trials) have examined antineoplaston types A2, A5, A10, AS2-1, and AS2-5 as treatment for a variety of cancer types. It remains unclear whether antineoplastons are effective, or what doses may be safe. Until better research is available, no clear conclusion can be drawn.	C
HIV infection A small preliminary study published by Burzynski and colleagues in 1992 reported increased energy and weight in patients with HIV infection, a decreased number of opportunistic infections, and increased CD4+ counts overall. These patients were treated with antineoplaston AS2-1. However, this evidence cannot be considered conclusive. Currently, drug therapy regimens are available for HIV infections with clearly demonstrated effects (HAART, or highly active anti-retroviral therapy), and patients with HIV infection should consult a physician about treatment options.	C
Sickle cell anemia/thalassemia A small preliminary study of the use of antineoplastons as therapy for sickle cell anemia/thalassemia reported positive findings, but there is currently insufficient evidence to make a clear recommendation in this area.	C

*Key to grades: *A:* Strong scientific evidence for this use; *B:* Good scientific evidence for this use; *C:* Unclear scientific evidence for this use; *D:* Fair scientific evidence against this use (it may not work); *F:* Strong scientific evidence against this use (it likely does not work). For a more detailed explanation of efficacy criteria, see "Natural Standard Evidence-Based Validated Grading Rationale" in the Introduction.

Historical or Theoretical Indications That Lack Sufficient Evidence
Acute lymphocytic leukemia, adenocarcinoma, aging, astrocytoma, basal cell epithelioma, bladder cancer, brain/central nervous system tumors, cholesterol/triglyceride abnormalities, chronic lymphocytic leukemia, colon cancer, encephalitis, glioblastoma, hepatocellular carcinoma, leukocytosis, malignant melanoma, medulloblastoma, metastatic synovial sarcoma, Parkinson's disease, promyelocytic leukemia, prostate cancer, rectal cancer, skin cancer, thrombocytosis.

DOSING/TOXICOLOGY

The following doses are based on scientific research, publications, traditional use, and expert opinion. Many herbs and supplements have not been thoroughly tested, and safety and effectiveness may not be proven. Brands may be made differently, with variable ingredients even within the same brand. The doses shown may not apply to all products. It is important to always read product labels and discuss doses with a qualified healthcare provider before therapy is started.

Adults (18 Years and Older)

- Various doses of antineoplastons have been used in preliminary studies. Safety and effectiveness have not been established for any specific dose or use. In studies, oral doses of antineoplaston A10 range from 10 to 40 g, or 100 to 288 mg per kg of body weight, daily. Duration of use has varied. Antineoplaston AS2-1 has been studied at doses of 12 to 30 g, or 97 to 130 mg per kg of body weight, daily. Antineoplastons also have been studied applied to the skin and administered by intravenous (IV) or intramuscular (IM) routes.

A

Children (Younger Than 18 Years)
- There are insufficient data available to recommend the use of antineoplastons in children.

SAFETY

The U.S. Food and Drug Administration does not strictly regulate herbs and supplements. There is no guarantee of strength, purity, or safety of products, and effects may vary. It is important to always read product labels. People who have a medical condition, or are taking other drugs, herbs, or supplements, should consult a qualified healthcare provider before starting a new therapy. A healthcare provider should be contacted immediately about any side effects.

Allergies
- Allergic skin rash has been reported after injection of antineoplaston AS2-1. Persons who have reacted to antineoplaston in the past should avoid this therapy.

Side Effects and Warnings
- Adverse effects have been reported in several preliminary studies. It is not clear how common these reactions are, or if they occur more frequently than with placebo. Because many patients taking antineoplastons have been diagnosed with serious illnesses such as advanced cancer, it is not clear whether these effects may be caused by the illnesses themselves or by the antineoplastons.
- Antineoplaston therapy has been associated with drowsiness, headache, fatigue, mild dizziness/vertigo, and confusion. Antineoplaston A10 is retained in the brain tissue of animals; the importance of this in humans is not known. Weakness, nausea, vomiting, upset stomach, abdominal pain, and increased flatulence (gas) have been reported.
- Various types of antineoplastons administered for a period of weeks to years have been associated with sore throat, fever, chills, reduced blood albumin levels, liver function test abnormalities, low blood sugar levels (hypoglycemia), low potassium levels, and a strong body odor similar to that of urine.
- Palpitations, high blood pressure (hypertension), and mild peripheral edema (water retention) have been noted. Chest pressure and irregular or fast heart beat have also been observed. Joint swelling, muscle/joint pain, muscle contractions in the throat, weakness, and finger rigidity have been reported in clinical trials.
- Decreases in blood platelets, red blood cells, and white blood cells have been observed. Other serious reported effects include slow or abnormal breathing, metabolic/electrolyte abnormalities, cerebral edema (brain swelling), dangerously low blood pressure (hypotension), and death.

Pregnancy and Breastfeeding
- The safety of antineoplastons during pregnancy or breastfeeding is not known, and therefore antineoplastons are not recommended.

INTERACTIONS

Most herbs and supplements have not been thoroughly tested for interactions with other herbs, supplements, drugs, and foods. The interactions listed here are based on reports in scientific publications, laboratory experiments, and traditional use. It is important to always read product labels. People who have a medical condition, or are taking other drugs, herbs, or supplements, should consult a qualified healthcare provider before starting a new therapy.

Interactions with Drugs, Herbs, and Dietary Supplements
- Limited information is available about interactions with antineoplastons. Agents with adverse effects similar to antineoplastons may have additive effects, such as lowering blood potassium and glucose levels and causing liver abnormalities. It is not known whether antineoplastons add to the effects of chemotherapeutic drugs.

Selected References

Natural Standard developed the preceding evidence-based information based on a systematic review of more than 100 scientific articles. For comprehensive information about alternative and complementary therapies on the professional level, go to www.naturalstandard.com. Selected references are listed here.

Badria F, Mabed M, El Awadi M, et al. Immune modulatory potentials of antineoplaston A-10 in breast cancer patients. Cancer Lett 2000;157(1):57-63.

Badria F, Mabed M, Khafagy W, et al. Potential utility of antineoplaston A-10 levels in breast cancer. Cancer Lett 2000;157(1):67-70.

Buckner JC, Malkin MG, Reed E, et al. Phase II study of antineoplastons A10 (NSC 648539) and AS2-1 (NSC 620261) in patients with recurrent glioma. Mayo Clin Proc 1999;74(2):137-145.

Burzynski R. Treatment of bladder cancer with antineoplaston formulations. Adv Exp Clin Chemother 1988;2:37-46.

Burzynski SR, Conde AB, Peters A, et al. Retrospective study of antineoplastons A10 and AS2-1 in primary brain tumors. Clin Drug Invest 1999;18:1-10.

Burzynski SR, Kubove E, Burzynski B. Phase I clinical studies of antineoplaston A5 injections. Drugs Exp Clin Res 1987;13 Suppl 1:37-43.

Burzynski SR, Kubove E, Burzynski B. Phase II clinical trials of antineoplaston A10 and AS2-1 infusion in astrocytoma. In: Adam D, Buchner T, Rubinstein E, editors. Recent Advances in Chemotherapy. Munich, Futuramed Publishers, 1991:2506-2507.

Burzynski SR, Kubove E, Burzynski B. Treatment of hormonally refractory cancer of the prostate with antineoplaston AS2-1. Drugs Exp Clin Res 1990; 16(7):361-369.

Burzynski SR, Kubove E, Szymkowski B, et al. Phase II clinical trials of novel differentiation inducer—antineoplaston AS2-1 in AIDS and asymptomatic HIV infection [abstract]. Int Conf AIDS 1992;8(3):61 (abstract no. Pub 7074).

Burzynski SR, Kubove E. Initial clinical study with antineoplaston A2 injections in cancer patients with five years' follow-up. Drugs Exp Clin Res 1987; 13(Suppl 1):1-11.

Burzynski SR, Kubove E. Phase I clinical studies of antineoplaston A3 injections. Drugs Exp Clin Res 1987;13(Suppl 1):17-29.

Burzynski SR, Kubove E. Toxicology studies on antineoplaston A10 injections in cancer patients. Drugs Exp Clin Res 1986;12(Suppl 10):47-55.

Burzynski SR. Potential of antineoplastons in diseases of old age. Drugs Aging 1995;7(3):157-167.

Burzynski SR. Toxicology studies on antineoplaston AS2-5 injections in cancer patients. Drugs Exp Clin Res 1986;12(Suppl 1):17-24.

Burzynski R. Isolation, purification, and synthesis of antineoplastons. Int J Exper Clin Chemother 1989;2:63-69.

Choi BG. Synthesis of antineoplaston A10 as potential antitumor agents. Arch Pharm Res 1998;21(2):157-163.

Green S. "Antineoplastons." An unproved cancer therapy. JAMA 1992;267(21): 2924-2928.

Juszkiewicz M, Chodkowska A, Burzynski SR, et al. The influence of antineoplaston A5 on particular subtypes of central dopaminergic receptors. Drugs Exp Clin Res 1995;21(4):153-156.

Kumabe T. Antineoplaston treatment for advanced hepatocellular carcinoma. Oncology Rep 1998;5(6):1363-1367.

Liau MC, Szopa M, Burzynski B, et al. Quantitative assay of plasma and urinary peptides as an aid for the evaluation of cancer patients undergoing antineoplaston therapy. Drugs Exp Clin Res 1987;13(Suppl 1):61-70.

Soltysiak-Pawluczuk D, Burzynski SR. Cellular accumulation of antineoplaston AS21 in human hepatoma cells. Cancer Lett 1995;88(1):107-112.

Sugita Y, Tsuda H, Maruiwa H, et al. The effect of Antineoplaston, a new antitumor agent on malignant brain tumors. Kurume Med J 1995;42(3):133-140.

Tsuda H, Hara H, Eriguchi N, et al. Toxicological study on antineoplastons A-10 and AS2-1 in cancer patients. Kurume Med J 1995;42(4):241-249.

Tsuda H, Iemura A, Sata M, et al. Inhibitory effect of antineoplaston A10 and AS2-1 on human hepatocellular carcinoma. Kurume Med J 1996;43(2): 137-147.

Tsuda H, Sata M, Kumabe T, et al. Quick response of advanced cancer to chemoradiation therapy with antineoplastons. Oncol Rep 1998;5(3):597-600.

Tsuda H, Sata M, Saitsu H, et al. Antineoplaston AS2-1 for maintenance therapy in liver cancer. Oncol Rep 1997;4:1213-1216.

Tweddle S, James N. Lessons from antineoplaston. Lancet 1997;349(9054):741.

Arginine
(L-Arginine)

SYNONYMS/COMMON NAMES/RELATED SUBSTANCES

- Arg, arginine hydrochloride (intravenous formulation), ibuprofen-arginate (Spedifen), L-arginine, 2-amino-5-guanidinopentanoic acid.
- *Note:* Arginine vasopressin has an entirely different mechanism than arginine/L-arginine. NG-monomethyl-L-arginine also is different from arginine/L-arginine and functions as an inhibitor of nitric oxide synthesis.
- **Dietary sources of arginine:** Almonds, barley, Brazil nuts, brown rice, buckwheat, cashews, cereals, chicken, chocolate, coconut, corn, dairy products, filberts, gelatin, meats, oats, peanuts, pecans, raisins, sesame and sunflower seeds, walnuts.

CLINICAL BOTTOM LINE

Background

- L-Arginine was first isolated in 1886. In 1932, L-arginine was found to be required for the generation of urea, which is necessary for the removal of toxic ammonia from the body. In 1939, L-arginine was also shown to be required for the synthesis of creatine. Creatine degrades to creatinine at a constant rate and is cleared from the body by the kidney.
- Arginine is considered a semi-essential amino acid, because although it is normally synthesized in sufficient amounts by the body, supplementation is sometimes required (for example, because of inborn errors of urea synthesis, protein malnutrition, excess ammonia production, excessive lysine intake, burns, infection, peritoneal dialysis, rapid growth, and sepsis). Symptoms of arginine deficiency include poor wound healing, hair loss, skin rash, constipation, and fatty liver.
- Arginine is a precursor of nitric oxide, which causes blood vessel relaxation (vasodilation). Preliminary evidence suggests that arginine may be useful in the treatment of medical conditions that are improved by vasodilation, such as angina, atherosclerosis, coronary artery disease, erectile dysfunction, heart failure, intermittent claudication/peripheral vascular disease, and vascular headache. Arginine also stimulates protein synthesis and its role has been studied in wound healing, bodybuilding, enhancement of sperm production (spermatogenesis), and prevention of wasting in people with critical illness.
- Arginine hydrochloride has a high chloride content and has been used for the treatment of metabolic alkalosis. This use should be under the supervision of a qualified healthcare professional.
- Most people likely do not need to take arginine supplements because the body usually makes sufficient amounts.

Uses Based on Scientific Evidence	Grade*
Growth hormone reserve test/pituitary disorder diagnosis Intravenously administered arginine can be used to evaluate growth hormone reserve in individuals with suspected growth hormone deficiency (for example, in patients with suspected panhypopituitarism, growth/stature abnormalities, gigantism/acromegaly, or pituitary adenoma). This is a U.S. Food and Drug Administration (FDA)–labeled indication for arginine.	A
Inborn errors of urea synthesis In patients with inborn errors of urea synthesis, high blood ammonia levels and metabolic alkalosis may occur, particularly in patients with ornithine carbamoyl transferase (OCT) deficiency or carbamoyl phosphate synthetase (CPS) deficiency. Arginine can be helpful by shifting the way that the body processes nitrogen but should be avoided in patients with hyperargininemia (high arginine blood levels). Other drugs, such as citrulline, sodium benzoate, and sodium phenylbutyrate, may have similar benefits, although dialysis may be necessary initially. This use of arginine should be supervised by a qualified healthcare professional.	A
Adrenoleukodystrophy (ALD) Adrenoleukodystrophy (ALD) is a rare inherited metabolic disorder characterized by the loss of fatty coverings (myelin sheaths) on nerve fibers in the brain, and progressive destruction of the adrenal glands. ALD is inherited as an X-linked genetic trait that results in dementia and adrenal failure. Injections of arginine have been proposed to help manage this disorder, although most study results are inconclusive. Further research is needed to evaluate the use of arginine in ALD.	C
Burns A randomized, controlled clinical trial designed to evaluate immune function of patients given 15 mg of arginine orally suggests that arginine may aid in the recovery of immune function and protein function in partial-thickness burn patients. Further research is necessary to confirm these findings.	C
Coronary artery disease / angina Initial evidence from several studies suggests that arginine administered orally or by injection improves exercise tolerance and blood flow in arteries of the heart. Benefits have been shown in some patients with coronary artery disease and angina. A small, randomized, controlled clinical trial studied the effects of a nutritional bar enriched with L-arginine and a combination of other nutrients in the management of chronic stable angina. The authors found that this arginine-rich medical food, when used with traditional therapy, improved vascular function, exercise capacity, and other aspects of quality of life in these patients. However, further research is needed to confirm these findings and to establish safe and effective doses.	C
Critical illness Some studies suggest that arginine may provide benefits when added to nutritional supplements during critical illnesses (for example, in patients being treated in intensive care units [ICUs]). However, the specific role of arginine in improving recovery is unclear. A randomized, controlled clinical trial was designed to study the effects of a high-protein formula enriched with arginine, fiber, and antioxidants in early nutrition	C

Continued

therapy of critically ill patients. The study measured infections in the ICU, length of hospital stay, and death rates. Patients fed the high-protein formula–enriched diet developed fewer hospital infections than patients fed a standard high-protein diet. There was no difference in length of ICU hospital stay or death rate.

Dental pain (ibuprofen arginate)	C

A well-designed multicenter, randomized controlled clinical trial found that ibuprofen arginate (Spedifen) reduced pain faster after dental surgery compared with conventional ibuprofen alone. The study included 498 patients who were given ibuprofen arginate, ibuprofen, or placebo after dental surgery. The degree of the relief of pain, onset of action, and tolerability of both ibuprofen arginate and ibuprofen were compared. It was found that ibuprofen arginate relieved pain faster, and adverse events with ibuprofen arginate were similar to those seen with ibuprofen alone. Another, similar trial concluded that patients treated with ibuprofen arginate rated its overall effectiveness higher than those treated with ibuprofen alone. Adverse event profiles were similar across all treatment groups. Further research is merited in this area.

Erectile dysfunction	C

Early studies suggested that arginine supplements are useful for managing erectile dysfunction (ED) in men with low levels of nitrates in blood or urine. A randomized, controlled clinical trial reported improvements in patients with mild-to-moderate ED following use of a combination of L-arginine, glutamate, and yohimbine hydrochloride. Notably, yohimbine hydrochloride is an FDA-approved therapy for this condition, and the effects caused by arginine alone in this combination therapy are difficult to determine. It is not clear what doses of arginine may be safe or effective in treating this condition, and comparisons have not been made with other agents used for ED.

Gastrointestinal cancer surgery	C

Supplementation with an oral combination of arginine and omega-3 fatty acids may reduce length of hospital stay and infections after surgery in gastrointestinal cancer patients. There is conflicting evidence about whether to give the combination before or after surgery. Both strategies have been reported as superior to conventional treatment (no artificial nutrition) in reducing infections after surgery and hospital stay. In a large, randomized, controlled clinical trial, malnourished cancer patients were given oral enteral nutrition supplemented by arginine, omega-3 fatty acids, and RNA before surgery. It was found that supplementation with the combination given before surgery reduced complications after surgery and hospital stay. Another randomized, controlled clinical trial in patients with gastrointestinal cancer studied the effects of an enteral diet supplemented with arginine, omega-3 fatty acids, and glutamine (administered after surgery) on immune function and inflammatory response. This study reported the supplement to be well tolerated with positive effects on immune and

inflammatory response. Further research is needed to determine the effects of arginine alone.

Congestive heart failure (CHF)	C

Studies of arginine in patients with CHF have shown mixed results. Some studies reported improved exercise tolerance. Additional studies are needed to confirm these findings.

Heart protection during coronary artery bypass grafting (CABG)	C

Arginine-supplemented "blood cardioplegic solution" is proposed to have protective properties. A randomized, controlled clinical trial using this solution in patients undergoing heart surgery (CABG) reported improved heart protection. Further research is needed before a firm conclusion can be drawn.

High blood pressure	C

A small study suggested that arginine taken by mouth may help to dilate the arteries and temporarily reduce blood pressure in hypertensive patients with type 2 diabetes. Larger, high-quality studies are needed before a recommendation can be made.

Migraine headache	C

Preliminary studies suggest that adding arginine to ibuprofen therapy may decrease migraine headache pain.

Peripheral vascular disease/claudication	C

Intermittent claudication is a condition characterized by leg pain and fatigue due to buildup of cholesterol plaques or clots in leg arteries. A small number of studies reported that arginine therapy may improve walking distance in patients with claudication. Further research is needed before a firm conclusion can be drawn.

Recovery after surgery	C

One study suggests that arginine provides benefits when used as a supplement after surgery. It is not clear what the specific role of arginine may be in improving immune function, and safe and effective doses have not been determined.

Wound healing	C

Arginine has been suggested to improve the rate of wound healing in elderly individuals. A randomized, controlled clinical trial reported improved wound healing after surgery in patients with head and neck cancer, following the use of an enteral diet supplemented with arginine and fiber. Arginine has also been used topically (on the skin) to improve wound healing. Further research is necessary in this area before a firm conclusion can be drawn.

Cyclosporine toxicity	D

Studies in animals showed that arginine blocked the toxic effects of cyclosporine, a drug used to prevent organ transplant rejection. However, results from studies in humans did not show that arginine offered any protection from cyclosporine-induced toxicity.

Infertility	D

Although there have been several studies in this area, it is not clear what effects arginine has on improving

Continued

the likelihood of getting pregnant. Early evidence does not support the finding that arginine has any benefits in women who are undergoing *in vitro* fertilization or in men with abnormal sperm.

Interstitial cystitis Arginine has been proposed as a treatment for interstitial cystitis (inflammation of the bladder). However, most well-designed studies in humans have not found that arginine offers any benefit in treating symptoms such as urinary frequency or urgency.	D
Kidney disease It has been suggested that arginine may be a useful supplement in people diagnosed with kidney failure. However, results from available studies do not support this claim. A small, randomized, controlled clinical trial studied the ability of L-arginine to improve dilation of blood vessels in children with chronic renal failure. Results showed that blood vessel dilation (endothelial function) was not improved with oral L-arginine, suggesting that dietary supplementation is not a beneficial or useful clinical approach in children with chronic renal failure.	D
Kidney protection during angiography The contrast media or dye used during angiography to map a patient's arteries (or during some CT scans) can be toxic to the kidneys, especially in people with pre-existing kidney disease. A randomized, parallel, double-blind clinical trial studied the use of L-arginine to protect kidneys in patients with chronic renal failure undergoing angiography. The authors found no evidence that injections of L-arginine protect the kidney from damage due to contrast media. Other therapies, such as *N*-acetylcysteine (NAC), have been found beneficial in protecting the kidneys from contrast-induced damage, particularly in patients at high risk, such as those with diabetes.	D
Asthma Although arginine has been suggested as a treatment for asthma, studies in humans have found that arginine actually *worsens* inflammation in the lungs and *contributes* to asthma symptoms. Therefore, taking arginine by mouth or by inhalation is not recommended for people with asthma.	F

*Key to grades: *A:* Strong scientific evidence for this use; *B:* Good scientific evidence for this use; *C:* Unclear scientific evidence for this use; *D:* Fair scientific evidence against this use (it may not work); *F:* Strong scientific evidence against this use (it likely does not work). For a more detailed explanation of efficacy criteria, see "Natural Standard Evidence-Based Validated Grading Rationale" in the Introduction.

Historical or Theoretical Indications That Lack Sufficient Evidence
AIDS/HIV, ammonia toxicity, anti-aging, beta-hemoglobinopathies, cancer, cardiac syndrome X, cold prevention, cystic fibrosis, dementia, diabetes, enhanced athletic performance, enhanced immune function, glaucoma, growth hormone stimulation, heart

attack, hemolytic uremic syndrome (HUS), hepatic encephalopathy, immunomodulation, infection, pulmonary hypertension (high blood pressure in the lungs), high cholesterol, increased muscle mass, infantile necrotizing enterocolitis, inflammatory bowel disease, ischemic stroke, liver disease, lower esophageal sphincter relaxation, low sperm count, metabolic acidosis, obesity, osteoporosis, pain, peritonitis, preeclampsia, pre-term labor contractions, Raynaud's phenomenon, sepsis, sickle cell anemia, stomach motility disorders, stomach ulcer, stroke, supplementation to a low protein diet, thrombotic thrombocytopenic purpura (TTP).

DOSING/TOXICOLOGY

The following doses are based on scientific research, publications, traditional use, and expert opinion. Many herbs and supplements have not been thoroughly tested, and safety and effectiveness may not be proven. Brands may be made differently, with variable ingredients even within the same brand. The doses shown may not apply to all products. It is important to always read product labels and discuss doses with a qualified healthcare provider before therapy is started.

Standardization

- Intravenous arginine hydrochloride is available as a 10% solution (950 mOsm/L), with 47.5 mEq chloride ion per 100 mL. There is no established standardization for oral arginine products.
- *Note:* Most people likely do not need to take arginine supplements because the body usually makes sufficient amounts.

Adults (18 Years and Older)

- **Tablets/capsules:** There are no standard or well-established doses for arginine, and many different doses have been used and studied. A dose studied for treating coronary artery disease is 2 to 3 g taken by mouth three times daily for 3 to 6 months. A dose studied for treatment of heart failure is 5.6 to 12.6 g, divided into two or three equal doses, taken by mouth daily for 6 weeks. For erectile dysfunction, 1.6 g taken by mouth three times daily for 6 weeks has been studied. For low sperm count, 4 g daily taken by mouth for 3 months has been used. For women undergoing in vitro (test tube) fertilization, an oral dose of 16 g per day has been used; however, this therapy should be discussed with the healthcare provider coordinating the *in vitro* program. For interstitial cystitis, 500 mg taken by mouth three times daily for six weeks has been used. For the long-term management of inborn disorders of the urea cycle, oral doses of 0.5 to 2 g daily have been used.
- **Intravenous:** Intravenous administration of arginine depends on specific institutional dosing guidelines and should be given under the supervision of a qualified healthcare provider.

Children (Younger Than 18 Years)

- Arginine supplements are not recommended for children because scientific information is lacking about this therapy in children and because of potential side effects.

SAFETY

The U.S. Food and Drug Administration does not strictly regulate herbs and supplements. There is no guarantee of strength, purity, or safety of products, and effects may vary. It is important to always read product labels. People who have a medical condition, or are taking other drugs, herbs, or supplements, should consult a qualified healthcare provider before starting a new therapy. A healthcare provider should be contacted immediately about any side effects.

Allergies

- Anaphylaxis (severe allergic reaction) has occurred after arginine injections. People with a known allergy should avoid arginine. Signs of allergy include rash, itching, and shortness of breath.

Side Effects and Warnings

- Arginine has been well tolerated by most people in studies lasting up to 6 months; however, there is the possibility of serious adverse effects in some individuals.
- Stomach discomfort, including nausea, stomach cramps, and an increased number of stools, may occur. People with asthma may experience a worsening of symptoms if arginine is inhaled, which may be related to allergy.
- Other potential side effects include low blood pressure and changes in numerous chemicals and electrolytes in the blood. Examples are high potassium, high chloride, low sodium, low phosphate, high blood urea nitrogen, and high creatinine levels. People with liver or kidney disease may be especially susceptible to these complications and should avoid using arginine except under medical supervision. After injections of arginine, low back pain, flushing, headache, numbness, restless legs, venous irritation, and death of surrounding tissues have been reported.
- In theory, arginine may increase the risk of bleeding. Persons using anticoagulants (blood thinners) or antiplatelet drugs, and those with underlying bleeding disorders, should consult a qualified healthcare provider before using arginine and should be monitored.
- Arginine may increase blood sugar levels. Caution is advised in patients taking prescription drugs to control sugar levels.

Pregnancy and Breastfeeding

- Arginine cannot be recommended as a supplement during pregnancy and breast-feeding because insufficient scientific information is available.

INTERACTIONS

Most herbs and supplements have not been thoroughly tested for interactions with other herbs, supplements, drugs, and foods. The interactions listed here are based on reports in scientific publications, laboratory experiments, and traditional use. It is important to always read product labels. People who have a medical condition, or are taking other drugs, herbs, or supplements, should consult a qualified healthcare provider before starting a new therapy.

Interactions with Drugs

- Because arginine increases the activity of some hormones in the body, many possible drug interactions may occur. The prescription drug aminophylline and the sweetening agent xylitol can decrease the effects of arginine on glucagon.
- Estrogens (found in birth control pills and hormone replacement therapies) may increase the effects of arginine on growth hormone, glucagon and insulin. In contrast, progestins (also found in birth control pills and some hormone replacement therapies) may decrease the responsiveness of growth hormone to arginine.
- When used with arginine, some diuretics such as spironolactone (Aldactone) and ACE-inhibitor blood pressure drugs such as enalapril (Vasotec) may cause elevated potassium levels in the blood. Monitoring of blood potassium levels may be required.

- Arginine should be used carefully with drugs such as nitroglycerin and sildenafil (Viagra) because blood pressure may fall too low. Other adverse effects such as headache and flushing may occur when arginine is used with these drugs.
- Because arginine can cause the stomach to make more acid, it may reduce the effectiveness of drugs that block stomach acid, such as ranitidine (Zantac) and esomeprazole (Nexium).
- In theory, arginine may increase the risk of bleeding when used with anticoagulants (blood thinners) or antiplatelet drugs. Examples are warfarin (Coumadin), heparin, and clopidogrel (Plavix). Some pain relievers may also increase the risk of bleeding if used with arginine. Examples include aspirin, ibuprofen (Motrin, Advil) and naproxen (Naprosyn, Aleve, Anaprox).
- Arginine may raise blood sugar levels. People using arginine and also taking oral drugs for diabetes or using insulin should be monitored closely by a qualified healthcare provider. Dosing adjustments may be necessary.
- Studies suggest that a combination of ibuprofen and arginine (ibuprofen-arginate [Spedifen]) has a faster onset of pain relief than ibuprofen alone. Use of other ibuprofen-based pain relievers such as Motrin or Advil with ibuprofen-arginate may increase the risk of toxic effects. People should consult their healthcare provider before combining these medications.

Interactions with Herbs and Dietary Supplements

- Arginine may block the benefits of lysine in treating cold sores.
- Arginine may increase the activity of growth hormone if used with ornithine.
- In theory, arginine may further increase the risk of bleeding when taken with herbs and supplements that are believed to increase the risk of bleeding. Multiple cases of bleeding have been reported with the use of *Ginkgo biloba*, and fewer cases have been reported with the use of garlic and saw palmetto. Numerous other agents may theoretically increase the risk of bleeding, although this has not been proven in most cases. Examples are alfalfa, American ginseng, angelica, anise, *Arnica montana*, asafetida, aspen bark, bilberry, birch, black cohosh, bladderwrack, bogbean, boldo, borage seed oil, bromelain, capsicum, cat's claw, celery, chamomile, chaparral, clove, coleus, cordyceps, danshen, devil's claw, dong quai, EPA (eicosapentaenoic acid, found in fish oils), evening primrose oil, fenugreek, feverfew, fish oil, flaxseed/ flax powder (not a concern with flaxseed oil), ginger, grapefruit juice, grapeseed, green tea, guggul, gymnestra, horse chestnut, horseradish, licorice root, lovage root, male fern, meadowsweet, nordihydroguaiaretic acid (NDGA), omega-3 fatty acids, onion, papain, *Panax ginseng*, parsley, passion flower, poplar, prickly ash, propolis, quassia, red clover, reishi, Siberian ginseng, sweet clover, rue, sweet birch, sweet clover, turmeric, vitamin E, white willow, wild carrot, wild lettuce, willow, wintergreen, and yucca.
- Because arginine may raise blood sugar level, people taking arginine and also using other herbs or supplements that may raise blood sugar levels (for example, cocoa, dehydroepiandrosterone [DHEA], ephedra [when combined with caffeine], and melatonin) should be monitored closely by their healthcare provider. Dosing adjustments may be necessary.

Selected References

Natural Standard developed the above evidence-based information based on a systematic review of more than 550 articles. For comprehensive information about alternative and complementary therapies on the professional level, go to www.naturalstandard.com. Selected references are listed below.

Bath PM, Willmot M Leonardi-Bee J, et al. Nitric oxide donors (nitrates), L-arginine, or nitric oxide synthase inhibitors for acute stroke. Cochrane Database Syst Rev 2002;(4): CD000398.

Beale RJ, Bryg DJ, Bihari DJ. Immunonutrition in the critically ill: a systematic review of clinical outcome. Crit Care Med 1999;27(12):2799-2805.

Bennett-Richards KJ, Kattenhorn M, Donald AE, et al. Oral L-arginine does not improve endothelial dysfunction in children with chronic renal failure. Kidney Int 2002;62(4): 1372-1378.

Black P, Max MB' Desjardins P, Norwood T, et al. A randomized, double-blind, placebo-controlled comparison of the analgesic efficacy, onset of action, and tolerability of ibuprofen arginate and ibuprofen in postoperative dental pain. Clin Ther 2002;24(7): 1072-1089.

Boger RH, Bode-Boger SM, Thiele W, et al. Restoring vascular nitric oxide formation by L-arginine improves the symptoms of intermittent claudication in patients with peripheral arterial occlusive disease. J Am Coll Cardiol 1998; 32(5):1336-1344.

Braga M, Gianotti L, Nespoli L, Radaelli G, et al. Nutritional approach in malnourished surgical patients: a prospective randomized study. Arch Surg 2002;137(2): 174-180.

Caparros T, Lopez J, Grau T. Early enteral nutrition in critically ill patients with a high-protein diet enriched with arginine, fiber, and antioxidants compared with a standard high-protein diet. The effect on nosocomial infections and outcome. JPEN J Parenter Enteral Nutr 2001;25(6):299-308; discussion 308-309.

Carrier M, Pellerin M, Perrault LP, et al. Cardioplegic arrest with L-arginine improves myocardial protection: results of a prospective randomized clinical trial. Ann Thorac Surg 2002; 73(3): 837-841; discussion 842.

Cartledge JJ, Davies AM, Eardley I. A randomized double-blind placebo-controlled crossover trial of the efficacy of L-arginine in the treatment of interstitial cystitis. BJU Int 2000;85(4):421-426.

Cen Y, Luo XS, Liu XX. Effect of L-arginine supplementation on partial-thickness burned patients. Zhongguo Xiu Fu Chong Jian Wai Ke Za Zhi 1999; 13(4):227-231.

Chen J, Wollman Y, Chernichovsky T, et al. Effect of oral administration of high-dose nitric oxide donor L-arginine in men with organic erectile dysfunction: results of a double- blind, randomized, placebo-controlled study. BJU Int 1999;83(3):269-273.

Chuntrasakul C, Siltharm S, Sarasombath S, et al. Metabolic and immune effects of dietary arginine, glutamine and omega-3 fatty acids supplementation in immunocompromised patients. J Med Assoc Thai 1998;81(5):334-343.

de Luis DA, Aller R, Izaola O, et al. Postsurgery enteral nutrition in head and neck cancer patients. Eur J Clin Nutr 2002;56(11):1126-1129.

de Luis DA, Izaola O, Cuellar L, et al. Effects of c-reactive protein and inter-leukins blood levels in postsurgery arginine-enhanced enteral nutrition in head and neck cancer patients. Eur J Clin Nutr 2003;57(1):96-99.

Desjardins P, Black P, Papageorge M, et al. Ibuprofen arginate provides effective relief from postoperative dental pain with a more rapid onset of action than ibuprofen. Eur J Clin Pharmacol 2002;58(6):387-394.

Gianotti L, Braga M, Nespoli L, et al. A randomized controlled trial of preoperative oral supplementation with a specialized diet in patients with gastrointestinal cancer. Evid Based Nurs 2003;6(2):47.

Huynh NT, Tayek JA. Oral arginine reduces systemic blood pressure in type 2 diabetes: its potential role in nitric oxide generation. J Am Coll Nutr 2002; 21(5):422-427.

Klotz T, Mathers MJ, Braun M, et al. Effectiveness of oral L-arginine in first-line treatment of erectile dysfunction in a controlled crossover study. Urol Int 1999;63(4):220-223.

Korting G, Smith S, Wheeler M, et al. A randomized double-blind trial of oral L-arginine for treatment of interstitial cystitis. J Urol 1999;161(2):558-565.

Lebret T, Herve JM, Gorny P, et al. Efficacy and safety of a novel combination of L-arginine, glutamate, and yohimbine hydrochloride: a new oral therapy for erectile dysfunction. Eur Urol 2002;41(6):608-613.

Lekakis JP, Papathanassiou S, Papioannou TG, et al. Oral L-arginine improves endothelial dysfunction in patients with essential hypertension. Int J Cardiol 2002;86(2-3):317-323.

Maxwell AJ, Zapien MP, Pearce GL, et al. Randomized trial of a medical food for the dietary management of chronic, stable angina. J Am Coll Cardiol 2002; 39(1):37-45.

McGovern MM, Wasserstein MP, Aron A, et al. Biochemical effect of intravenous arginine butyrate in X-linked adrenoleukodystrophy. J Pediatr. 2003;142(6): 709-713.

Mehlisch DR, Ardia A, Pallotta T. A controlled comparative study of ibuprofen arginate versus conventional ibuprofen in the treatment of postoperative dental pain. J Clin Pharmacol 2002;42(8):904-911.

Miller HI, Dascalu A, Rassin TA, et al. Effects of an acute dose of L-arginine during coronary angiography in patients with chronic renal failure: a randomized, parallel, double-blind clinical trial. Am J Nephrol 2003;23(2):91-95.

Sandrini G, Franchini S, Lanfranchi S, et al. Effectiveness of ibuprofen-arginine in the treatment of acute migraine attacks. Int J Clin Pharmacol Res 1998; 18(3):145-150.

Wu GH, Zhang YW, Wu ZH. Modulation of postoperative immune and inflammatory response by immune-enhancing enteral diet in gastrointestinal cancer patients. World J Gastroenterol 2001;7(3): 357-362.

Artichoke
(Cynara scolymus L.)

SYNONYMS/COMMON NAMES/RELATED SUBSTANCES

- Alcachofa, alcaucil, artichaut, artichiocco, artichoke, artischocke, artiskok, carciofo, cardo, cardo de comer, cardon d'Espagne, cardoon, Cynara, *Cynara cardunculus, Cynarae folium, Cynara scolymus* L., French artichoke, garden artichoke, gemuseartischocke, golden artichoke, kardone, tyosen-azami.
- *Note:* Globe artichoke should not be mistaken for Jerusalem artichoke, which is the tuber of *Helianthus tuberosa* L. (a species of sunflower).

CLINICAL BOTTOM LINE
Background

- Globe artichoke is a popular phytomedicine in Europe. It is purported to possess diuretic, choleretic, anti-dyspeptic, lipid-lowering, and antioxidant properties.
- Cynarin, luteolin, cynardoside (luteolin-7-O-glycoside), scolymoside, and chlorogenic acid are believed to be artichoke's active constituents. The most studied component, cynarin, is concentrated in the leaves, and most studies have investigated leaf extract.
- There is preliminary evidence that globe artichoke extract may increase choleresis (secretion of bile) and that components of artichoke (cynarin and luteolin) may lower serum lipids.

Scientific Evidence for Common/Studied Uses	Grade*
Alcohol-induced hangover	C
Antioxidant	C
Choleretic (bile-secretion stimulant)	C
Irritable bowel syndrome (IBS)	C
Lipid-lowering (cholesterol and triglycerides)	C
Non-ulcer dyspepsia	C

*Key to grades: *A:* Strong scientific evidence for this use; *B:* Good scientific evidence for this use; *C:* Unclear scientific evidence for this use; *D:* Fair scientific evidence against this use (it may not work); *F:* Strong scientific evidence against this use (it likely does not work). For a more detailed explanation of efficacy criteria, see "Natural Standard Evidence-Based Validated Grading Rationale" in the Introduction.

Historical or Theoretical Indications That Lack Sufficient Evidence

- Allergies, arthritis, anemia, atherosclerosis, bitter tonic, cholegogue, cholelithiasis, constipation, cystitis, digestion disorders, diuretic,[1] eczema, emesis, hepatoprotection,[2,3] gout, jaundice, nausea,[4] nephrolithiasis, nephrosclerosis, peripheral edema, pruritis, rheumatoid arthritis, snakebite, urolithiasis, vomiting.

Expert Opinion and Folkloric Precedent

- Globe artichoke has a long-standing folkloric tradition, notably in France. Historically, it has been used most commonly as a diuretic and for nausea, jaundice, dyspepsia, rheumatic diseases, gout, pruritis, and urinary stones.

Safety Summary

- **Likely Safe:** When taken orally for short periods of time, globe artichoke has been reported in one study to be safe in 17 patients in doses of up to 750 mg of the artichoke constituent cynarin.[5] Doses up to 1500 mg of cynarin have been reported in studies assessing effects on cholesterol levels. It is unclear if these doses are safe in the long term.[5]

DOSING/TOXICOLOGY
General

- Recommended doses are based on those most commonly used in available trials, or in historical practice. However, with natural products, the optimal doses needed to balance efficacy and safety often have not been determined. Formulation and preparation methods may vary from batch to batch of a specific product made by a single manufacturer. Because often the active components of a product are not known, standardization may not be possible, and the clinical effects of different brands may not be comparable.
- *Note:* Globe artichoke should not be mistaken for Jerusalem artichoke, which is the tuber of *Helianthus tuberosa* L.

Standardization

- There are no uniform standards for artichoke extracts. Some products are standardized to 15% cholorogenic acid, 2% to 5% cynarin per dose, or 1% caffeoyl acid derivatives.[6]

Dosing: Adult (18 Years and Older)
Oral

- **Tablets/Capsules:** Doses of globe artichoke containing 250 to 750 mg of cynarin daily, or dried artichoke extract, 1800 to 1900 mg daily, have been used in clinical trials. However, it is not clear that these are optimal doses.[5,7,8] For dyspepsia, doses of 320 mg vs. 640 mg of daily artichoke leaf extract have been compared, with equal efficacy reported.[9]
- **Liquid/Fluid:** 3 to 8 mL of 1:2 liquid extract per day is often recommended in clinical practice, and up to 10 mL of pressed juice from fresh leaves and flower buds of the artichoke has been used in clinical trials.[10] The expert panel German Commission E has recommended 6 mL of tincture (1:5 g/mL) given three times daily. For lipid-lowering effects, an adult dose of artichoke standardized leaf extract (320 mg) four to six times daily for a minimum of 6 weeks has been suggested.[11-15]
- **Dried Leaves:** A crude dose of artichoke leaves (1 to 4 g) three times daily has been recommended anecdotally.[16] Doses in the range of 4 to 9 g of dried leaves daily are often recommended in clinical practice.
- **Dry extract:** The German Commission E has recommended 0.5 g of a 12:1 (w/w) dried extract given as a single daily dose.

Dosing: Pediatric (Younger Than 18 Years)

- Insufficient evidence to recommend.

Toxicology

- Although contact dermatitis, urticaria, and asthma may be caused by topical globe artichoke exposure,[17-19] there are no known published cases following oral consumption.

- LD$_{50}$ values have been determined to be greater than 265 mg/kg of purified extract in rats.[20]

ADVERSE EFFECTS/PRECAUTIONS/CONTRAINDICATIONS
Allergy

- Artichoke should be used with caution in patients with demonstrated allergy to members of the *Asteraceae* or *Compositae* family (e.g., chrysanthemums, daisies, marigolds, ragweed, arnica), because of possible cross-reactivity.
- A case of severe allergic reaction complicated by asthma exacerbation following topical exposure to artichoke has been reported.[21] Other cases of dermatitis,[17] as well as rhinitis and bronchial asthma,[19] have been reported among workers handling artichokes.

Adverse Effects/Postmarket Surveillance

- **Dermatologic:** Both contact dermatitis and contact urticaria have been noted following topical exposure to artichoke in individual case reports, with symptoms spontaneously subsiding hours or days after exposure.[17,21] Skin testing on four patients with allergic rhinitis and asthma have yielded positive results for artichoke.[18]
- **Gastrointestinal:** Mild flatulence, diarrhea, hunger, and nausea have been reported.[6,11,15,22] Artichoke is purported to increase bile flow, although there is limited scientific evidence in this area. Animal data and historical accounts suggest that globe artichoke may increase bile secretion,[4,23] although human data are limited.[8]
- **Pulmonary:** Dyspnea, cough, chest tightness and a severe asthma exacerbation were described in a case report of a patient who also developed contact urticaria after topical exposure to artichokes, likely the result of a hypersensitivity reaction.[21] Emergency beta-mimetic, oxygen, and corticosteroid treatment were required for the asthmatic attack 24 hours after cessation of exposure, despite the use of antihistamines. Another case of asthma after contact has also been reported.[19]
- **Hematologic:** Significantly reduced platelet aggregation (both spontaneous and ADP-induced) was noted in 62 men taking an artichoke extract (Cynarex) for 2 years (dose not reported), who were also chronically exposed to carbon disulfide.[24] The independent contribution of artichoke is not clear.[18]
- **Endocrine/Renal:** Nephrotoxicity has been reported with artichoke mixtures.[25] There have been reports of kidney failure and/or toxicity from the use of artichoke leaves.[26]

Precautions/Warnings/Contraindications

- Use cautiously in patients with cholelithiasis or biliary/bile duct obstruction, based on historical accounts that globe artichoke may increase bile flow.[4,23]
- Use cautiously in patients with demonstrated allergy to members of the Asteraceae or Compositae family (e.g., chrysanthemums, daisies, marigolds, ragweed, arnica) due to the possibility of cross-sensitivity.
- Use cautiously in patients with kidney disease, based on limited reports of nephrotoxicity.[25,26]

Pregnancy and Lactation

- Not recommended, because of lack of sufficient data.

INTERACTIONS
Artichoke/Drug Interactions

- **Anticoagulant or anti-platelet agents:** Artichoke may increase the risk of bleeding, based on a report of significantly reduced platelet aggregation (both spontaneous and ADP-induced) in 62 men taking an artichoke extract (Cynarex) for 2 years (dose not reported), who were also chronically exposed to carbon disulfide.[24] The independent contribution of artichoke is not clear.
- **Cholesterol-lowering agents:** *Additive effect*: There are multiple published reports of cholesterol-lowering effects of artichoke,[5,7,10,27-37] although the quality of most studies is not sufficient to form a clear conclusion in this area. There is a report that cholesterol synthesis may be inhibited by the artichoke constituent luteolin via inhibition of HMG-CoA reductase, the same action as statin drugs such as atorvastatin (Lipitor).[36] Therefore, artichoke may add to the cholesterol-lowering effects of other agents.

Artichoke/Herb Interactions

- **Anticoagulant or anti-platelet herbs/supplements:** Artichoke may increase the risk of bleeding, based on a report of significantly reduced platelet aggregation (both spontaneous and ADP-induced) in 62 men taking an artichoke extract (Cynarex) for 2 years (dose not reported), who were also chronically exposed to carbon disulfide.[24] The independent contribution of artichoke is not clear.
- **Cholesterol-lowering herbs/supplements:** *Additive effect*: There are multiple published reports of cholesterol-lowering effects of artichoke[5,7,10,27-37] although the quality of most studies is not sufficient to form a clear conclusion in this area. There is a report that cholesterol synthesis may be inhibited by the artichoke constituent luteolin via inhibition of HMG-CoA reductase.[36] Therefore, artichoke may add to the lipid-lowering effects of other agents such as fish oil, garlic, and niacin.

MECHANISM OF ACTION
Pharmacology

- **Constituents:** Cynarin, luteolin, cynardoside (luteolin-7-O-glycoside), scolymoside, and chlorogenic acid are believed to be artichoke's active constituents. The most studied component, cynarin, is most concentrated in the leaves, and most studies have investigated leaf extract. Luteolin is reported to be responsible for inhibition of cholesterol synthesis, whereas cynarin may have no effects.[36]
- **Choleretic effects (stimulation of bile secretion):** Globe artichoke leaf extract has been found to increase bile secretion in perfused rat liver and liver cell cultures.[4,23] It has been suggested that reduction of intrahepatic cholesterol concentration is responsible for globe artichoke extract's ability to treat dyspepsia.[4]
- **Cholesterol-lowering effects:** Cynarin and artichoke extracts have been reported to reduce plasma cholesterol and triglyceride levels in animal studies.[20,38,39] Other animal research has noted that artichoke extracts may prevent the development of atherosclerotic plaques.[40-42] This anti-atherosclerotic action is thought to be the product of two mechanisms of action: an antioxidant effect that reduces low-density lipoprotein (LDL) oxidation,[37] and inhibition of cholesterol synthesis.[34] Gebhardt reported that globe artichoke extract decreased cholesterol synthesis by inhibiting the action of HMG-CoA reductase, which is required to convert HMG-CoA to mevalonate, the same action as statin drugs.[36] In the synthesis of cholesterol, acetyl-CoA is converted to HMG-CoA, then to mevalonate, and ultimately to cholesterol. In this study, luteolin was the compound found to be responsible for inhibition of cholesterol synthesis, whereas cynarin had no effect on cholesterol synthesis.

- **Antioxidant effects:** Antioxidant properties of artichoke have been noted in multiple pre-clinical studies,[2,3,15,37,43-49] although long-term clinical effects in humans are not known.
- **Hepatoprotection:** Several *in vitro* studies report that cynarin and artichoke extracts provide protection against a variety of toxins.[2,3,48-52]

Pharmacodynamics/Kinetics

- Insufficient available evidence.

HISTORY

- The artichoke has been used for centuries for multiple purposes, including as a diuretic, choleretic, or to lessen body odor. Other historical uses include the treatment of edema ("dropsy"), gout, joint pains ("rheumatism"), jaundice, nausea, dyspepsia, urinary stones, and flatulence. Its history of known medicinal use dates to the 4th century BC.

Review of the Evidence: Artichoke

Condition Treated*	Study Design	Author, Year	N[†]	SS[†]	Study Quality[‡]	Magnitude of Benefit	ARR[†]	NNT[†]	Comments
Bile secretion stimulation	Randomized, crossover, placebo-controlled	Kirchhoff[8] 1994	20	Yes	4	Medium	NA	NA	Not clear if the increases in bile secretion reported are clinically significant. Mean increase 127.3% after 30 minutes and 151.5% after 90 minutes.
Gastrointestinal complaints	Case series	Wegener[34] 1995	500	NA	NA	Medium	NA	NA	Included patients diagnosed with non-ulcer dyspepsia, constipation. and functional bile duct obstruction.
Bile duct dyskinesias	Case series	Held[6] 1992	403	NA	NA	NA	NA	NA	375 mg of artichoke standardized to 1% caffeoyl acid derivatives; treatment period not specified.
Cholesterol reduction	Meta-analysis (Cochrane)	Pittler[32] 2002	167 (2 studies)	Yes	NA	NA	NA	NA	Authors concluded evidence is compelling but not definitive.
Cholesterol reduction	Placebo controlled, double-blind	Petrowicz[33] 1997	44	No	NA	NA	NA	NA	Evaluated in healthy volunteers aged 20-49 years; received artichoke leaf extract (ALE; Hepar-SL forte).
Cholesterol reduction	Randomized placebo controlled	Englisch[7] 2000	143	Yes					Mean 18.5% decrease in total cholesterol; also decrease in LDL, but not triglycerides.
Lipid lowering	Open-label, uncontrolled. Case series	Fintelmann[12] 1996	553	Mixed	4	Moderate	NA	NA	3-6 x 320 mg capsules daily for 6 weeks; cholesterol level was a secondary outcome measure and was significantly improved.
Lipid lowering	Case series	Dorn[10] 1995	84	No	NA	Small	NA	NA	Non-significant trend toward decreased LDL and triglycerides.
Cholesterol reduction	Case series	Wegener[34] 1995	500	Yes	NA	Medium	NA	NA	Included patients diagnosed with non-ulcer dyspepsia, constipation, and functional bile duct obstruction.
Familial hyper-lipoproteinemia	Case series	Heckers[5] 1977	17	No	NA	NA	NA	NA	Small study with no placebo control.
Hyperlipidemia; hyper-cholesterolemia	Case series	Von Weiland[35] 1973	142	NA	NA	NA	NA	NA	Assessed cynarin (constituent of artichoke).
Irritable bowel syndrome	Open-label, uncontrolled	Walker[22] 2001	279	Yes	NA	NA	NA	NA	Post-marketing surveillance; all patients also had dyspeptic syndrome.
Dyspepsia	Randomized, controlled	Holtmann[56] 2003	247	Yes	4	Moderate	NA	NA	Overall well designed, suggestive results.
Dyspepsia	Randomized, controlled	Kupke[57] 1991	60	Yes	2	Small	18%	6	Used a combination herbal product containing artichoke.
Dyspepsia	Open-label, uncontrolled	Fintelmann[12] 1996	553	No	NA	NA	NA	NA	3-6 × 320-mg capsules daily for 6 weeks.

*Primary or secondary outcome.
[†]*N*, Number of patients; *SS*, statistically significant; *ARR,* absolute risk reduction; *NNT,* the number of patients who need to undergo a specific intervention in order to observe an outcome in one individual.
[‡]0-2 = poor; 3-4 = good; 5 = excellent.
NA, Not applicable; *LDL,* low-density lipoprotein.
For an explanation of each category in this table, please see Table 3 in the Introduction.

REVIEW OF THE EVIDENCE: DISCUSSION
Choleretic
Summary

- Globe artichoke leaf extract has been found to increase bile secretion in perfused rat liver and liver cell cultures[4,23] and has been reported in one small double-blind, placebo-controlled trial and several case series to increase choleresis (secretion of bile). However, better-quality clinical research is necessary before a firm conclusion can be drawn in this area.

Controlled Trial Evidence

- Kirchhoff et al. conducted a double-blind, placebo-controlled, crossover study in which 20 male patients each received intra-duodenal administration of either placebo or 1.92 g of globe artichoke extract.[8] Intra-duodenal bile secretion was measured using a probe. After an 8-day washout period, the patients were crossed over to receive either placebo or active extract. There was a significant increase in bile secretion in the treatment group as compared to placebo at 30, 60, and 90 minutes ($p < 0.05$). At 30 minutes, 0.93 mL of bile had been secreted in the treatment group as compared to 0.71 mL in the placebo group. At 60 minutes, 0.95 mL vs. 0.64 mL were secreted in the respective groups. At 90 minutes, 0.78 mL vs. 0.55 mL were secreted in the respective groups. No side effects were noted. Whether these findings are clinically significant is unclear, and further study with clinical correlation is necessary before a firm conclusion can be drawn.

Studies of Lesser Design Strength

- A number of additional studies have been conducted of lesser methodological quality, including several case series. The majority of these studies report positive results, although due to methodological weaknesses, their conclusions are of limited clinical relevance. Wegner collected data on a series of patients with abdominal complaints including non-ulcer dyspepsia (16%), constipation (22%), functional bile duct obstruction (21%), dyspepsia (34%), and others (7%) who were treated with artichoke (Heplar SL forte; mean dose, 4.75 capsules daily).[34] After 6 weeks of treatment, interim analysis of 170 cases indicated that 45% to 95% of symptoms had resolved. For example, nausea and vomiting had improved in 95% of patients and abdominal pain had improved in 75% of patients. In addition, a statistically significant decrease in serum cholesterol levels (−14.5%) was noted.
- Held reported a case series in 403 patients treated with bile duct dyskinesias with 375 mg of artichoke extract (Hekbilin A, standardized to 1% caffeoyl acid derivatives; treatment length not specified).[6] The treatment was judged "good" or "very good" by 84.3% of patients and 87.2% of physicians. Mild gastrointestinal adverse effects were noted in 12 cases. Significant reductions of transaminases and total bilirubin were noted. Limited information was provided about selection criteria, and standardized rating scales were not used.
- In an early (1957) open clinical study of 198 patients with biliary fistula, the artichoke constituent cynara extract was reported to possess choleretic and cholagogic effects, and to elicit clinical improvement.[53] However, adequate details regarding patients and outcome measures was not provided.

Lipid-Lowering (Cholesterol/Triglycerides)
Summary

- Several pre-clinical[36,37,54] and human studies report artichoke extract or its constituents cynarin or luteolin to moderately decrease total cholesterol and triglyceride levels. However, the overall quality of available research is not high, and without better-quality research, a firm conclusion cannot be drawn. Reliable comparisons with other lipid-lowering agents have not been conducted, and dosing is not clearly established. Effects on high-density lipoprotein (HDL/"good cholesterol") or low-density lipoprotein (LDL/"bad cholesterol") levels are not clear.

Systematic Review

- Pittler et al. authored a Cochrane systematic review of artichoke leaf extract in the treatment of hypercholesterolemia, including two controlled trials (n = 167 total participants).[32] In one study, cholesterol levels were significantly reduced from 7.74 mmol/L to 6.31 mmol/L after 42 ± 3 days compared to placebo, which reduced cholesterol from 7.69 mmol/ L to 7.03 mmol/L ($p = 0.000001$). A second trial reported significantly reduced cholesterol levels compared to placebo in patients with a baseline total cholesterol greater than 230 mg/dL. The authors concluded that although the lipid-lowering effects of artichoke extract are supported by *in vitro* and animal studies, and small to moderate beneficial effects are reported, the evidence is not compelling enough to form a clear conclusion. Additional trials with larger sample sizes are needed to establish whether artichoke is effective and safe for treatment of patients with hypercholesterolemia.

Controlled Trials

- In an early (1975) controlled trial conducted by Montini et al., two groups of 30 patients presenting with various dislipidemias were treated for 50 days with either cynarin (Listrocol) or placebo.[29] The authors reported that cynarin induced a significant reduction in mean cholesterol levels by 20% compared to placebo ($p < 0.001$), as well as reductions in pre-beta-lipoproteins, beta/alpha-lipoprotein ratio, and patient body weight (by approximately 5 kg). In another early study (1974), Mars et al. conducted a double-blind, placebo-controlled trial, reporting that 500 mg of cynarin taken daily significantly lowered triglyceride levels in elderly patients with hypertriglyceridemia.[30] Neither of these studies clearly described design or methods.
- Petrowicz et al. conducted a placebo-controlled double-blind study in 44 healthy volunteers aged 20 to 49 years.[33] Patients received 640 mg of artichoke leaf extract (ALE; Hepar-SL forte) three times daily or placebo over a 12-week period. Initial mean group values of total cholesterol were relatively low in both groups (203.0 mg/dL in the placebo group, 204.2 mg/dL in the artichoke group). Results overall were not impressive, although sub-group analysis suggested that lipid-lowering effects of artichoke are detectable when baseline total cholesterol levels are greater than 200 mg/dL but are less pronounced with lower values. High-density lipoprotein (HDL/"good cholesterol") levels tended to decrease with artichoke therapy. No major adverse reactions were reported in either group.
- Englisch et al. randomized 143 adults with total cholesterol levels greater than 280 mg/dL to receive either 1800 mg of artichoke dry extract or placebo daily for 6 weeks.[7] In this double-blind clinical trial, mean total cholesterol levels decreased by 18.5% in the treatment group compared to 8.6% in the placebo group ($p = 0.0001$). Low-density lipoprotein (LDL/"bad cholesterol") levels decreased by 22.9% in the treatment group vs. 6.3% in the placebo group ($p = 0.0001$).

There was no difference between groups in HDL levels, but the LDL-to-HDL ratio decreased by 20.2% and 7.2%, respectively. Triglyceride levels were not significantly affected.

Studies of Lesser Design Strength

- Data from uncontrolled or lesser-quality studies is suggestive but cannot be considered clinically conclusive. For example, cynara extract was reported to moderately decrease total cholesterol and triglyceride levels in 132 patients.[31] Other studies report cynarin in oral doses of 750 to 1500 mg per day to significantly reduce levels of total serum cholesterol,[27,28] by up to 15% at a dose of 1000 mg per day over 4 weeks.[55] Fintelmann et al. conducted a 6-week open-label, uncontrolled multicenter clinical trial in order to investigate the activity and tolerability of artichoke leaf extract (3 to 6 capsules daily of Hepar SL forte; each capsule contained 320 mg of artichoke extract) in patients with dyspepsia.[11-15] A significant decrease in serum lipids was observed with a decline in total cholesterol of 11.5% and a 12.5% decline in triglyceride levels.

- Dorn conducted an uncontrolled continuation trial using juice extracted from globe artichoke leaves and flower buds.[10] In the initial phase, 60 patients with hyperlipidemia were given 10 mL of juice three times a day for 6 weeks. In a continuation phase, 30 patients received an additional 6 weeks of therapy. The target end point was a decrease in total cholesterol by 30 mg/dL and was not reached in either study. However, there was a trend toward lowered total cholesterol, lowered LDL, lowered triglycerides, and elevated HDL in the continuation phase. A third trial using the same therapy was conducted over 12 weeks in 24 patients with total cholesterol above 299 mg/dL and/or triglycerides above 449. Mean LDL did not significantly decrease (from 188 mg/dL to 186 mg/dL), and total cholesterol decreased only slightly from 290 to 282, whereas HDL levels did not change. Triglycerides decreased from 481 mg/dL to 460 mg/dL (4.4%). Because of the lack of controls and unclear use of other therapies or lifestyle changes by subjects, a clear conclusion cannot be drawn based on these results.

- Wegner collected data on a series of patients with abdominal complaints including non-ulcer dyspepsia (16%), constipation (22%), functional bile duct obstruction (21%), dyspepsia (34%), and others (7%) who were treated with artichoke (Heplar SL forte; mean dose was 4.75 capsules daily).[34] After six weeks of treatment, a statistically significant decrease in serum cholesterol levels (−14.5%) was noted.

- Heckers et al. studied the ability of cynarin to lower total cholesterol or triglyceride concentrations in 17 patients with familial type IIa or type IIb hyperlipoproteinemia.[5] This open-label, uncontrolled study found no effect of cynarin on serum cholesterol or triglyceride levels after 3 months (at doses of 250 mg or 750 mg per day). Four patients were given cynarin at a dose of 1500 mg daily for an additional 3 months. However, even this high dose was not associated with any change in cholesterol levels.

- Von Weiland et al. assessed the effect of cynarin in two samples: 10 healthy men (a single dose of 20 mg of cynarin followed by another dose of 60 mg of cynarin 3 to 5 days later); and 132 patients diagnosed with hypercholesterolemia and/or hypertriglyceridemia (three doses of cynarin of 20 mg daily for a mean of 7 months).[35] The authors reported that lipolysis was inhibited by a dose of 60 mg of cynarin in group 1. In group 2, total cholesterol was decreased by 31% and triglycerides were reduced by an average of 24%.

Non-Ulcer Dyspepsia
Summary

- One proposed etiology of non-ulcer dyspepsia is bile duct dyskinesia. Because globe artichoke extract has been studied as a choloretic (bile secretion stimulant), it has been hypothesized that it may also function as an anti-dyspeptic agent. Although this hypothesis has been supported by early clinical evidence, available studies are small, with a variety of design flaws. A recommendation for the use of artichoke in the management of non-ulcer dyspepsia cannot be made in the absence of better-designed, adequately powered randomized controlled trials. It should also be noted that patients with chronic or recurrent dyspepsia might require medical evaluation to rule out ulcer or neoplasm; non-ulcer dyspepsia is a diagnosis of exclusion.

Controlled Trials

- In 2003, Holtmann et al. published a double-blind, randomized controlled trial in 247 patients with functional dyspepsia, who were treated with either a commercial artichoke leaf extract preparation (2 320-mg plant extract three times daily) or placebo.[56] The primary outcome measure was patient weekly rating of overall dyspeptic symptom score using a four-point scale. Secondary outcomes were scores for individual dyspeptic symptoms and quality of life as assessed by the validated Nepean Dyspepsia Index (NDI). Data from 244 patients (129 artichoke, 115 placebo) were suitable for analysis, on an intention-to-treat basis. The overall symptom improvement over a 6-week period was significantly greater with artichoke than with placebo (8.3 ± 4.6 vs. 6.7 ± 4.8, $p < 0.01$). In addition, patients treated with artichoke demonstrated significantly greater improvement in global quality-of-life scores compared to placebo, although ranges crossed each other (−41.1 ± 47.6 vs. −24.8 ± 35.6, $p < 0.01$). Although these results are promising, better-quality evidence is necessary before a clear conclusion can be reached.

- Kupke et al. conducted a randomized, controlled trial of a combination herbal product (Cynarzym) containing 50 mg of artichoke in 60 patients with non-ulcer dyspepsia.[57] Length of treatment was not specified. Patients ingested three capsules of either Cynarzym or placebo daily. The study reported a small benefit in terms of bile excretion and amelioration of symptoms of patients in the Cynarzym group. However, because this study assessed a combination herbal product, it is difficult to determine the isolated role of artichoke in the results reported. In addition, design, methods, and statistical analysis were not well described.

Uncontrolled Studies

- In a 2003 open, dose-ranging post-marketing study, 516 healthy patients with self-reported dyspepsia were administered 320 mg or 640 mg of daily artichoke leaf extract.[9] After 2 months, 454 completed the study. In both dosage groups, compared with baseline, there was a significant reduction of all dyspeptic symptoms, with an average reduction of 40% in global dyspepsia score (Nepean Dyspepsia Index). There were no differences in the primary outcome measures between the two groups, although relief of states of anxiety, a secondary outcome, was greater with the higher dose ($p = 0.03$).

- Fintelmann et al. conducted a 6-week open-label, uncontrolled multicenter clinical trial in order to investigate the activity and tolerability of artichoke leaf extract (3 to 6 320-mg capsules daily) in patients with dyspepsia.[11-15] Variations in the symptoms of 533 patients (whose complaints of dyspepsia averaged 155 weeks in duration) were examined. Documented symptoms regressed after 6 weeks of treatment by a mean of 70.5% with a notable decline in vomiting, nausea, lack of appetite, and constipation. The treating doctors for 85% of patients rated the therapeutic efficacy of artichoke leaf extract as "good." This was mirrored by patient responses. The lack of controls or use of a standardized assessment instrument limits the clinical value of these results.

- Wegner collected data on a series of patients with abdominal complaints including non-ulcer dyspepsia (16%), constipation (22%), functional bile duct obstruction (21%), dyspepsia (34%), and others (7%) who were treated with artichoke (Heplar SL forte; mean dose, 4.75 capsules daily).[34] After six weeks of treatment, interim analysis of 170 cases indicated that 45% to 95% of symptoms had resolved. For example, nausea and vomiting improved in 95% of patients and abdominal pain improved in 75% of patients.

Irritable Bowel Syndrome (IBS)
Summary

- The symptom overlap between dyspeptic syndrome and irritable bowel syndrome (IBS) has given rise to the notion that artichoke leaf extract may have potential for treating IBS as well. However, there is insufficient available evidence to form a clear conclusion in this area.

Evidence

- In a 6-week open-label, uncontrolled post-marketing surveillance study, Walker et al. administered Hepar-SL forte, a standardized, high-dose, aqueous-alcohol extract of artichoke leaf (400-mg capsules containing 320 mg of artichoke leaf extract) to 553 patients with dyspeptic syndrome or non-specific gastrointestinal complaints.[22] Patients took six capsules per day on average, consistent with the manufacturer's recommended dose of two capsules three times daily with meals. A sub-group of 279 patients reported having at least three of five irritable bowel syndrome symptoms (abdominal pain, bloating, flatulence, right-sided abdominal cramps, constipation). In this sub-group, mean scores for all five IBS symptoms were significantly reduced ($p < 0.05$), with reductions ranging from 65% to 77% compared to baseline. Patients noted improvement in symptoms after an average of 10.4 days of treatment. On an analog scale of 1 (excellent) to 5 (insufficient), the overall efficacy of treatment was rated as 1.95 by physicians and as 1.99 by patients. Eighty-four percent of both patients and physicians rated the overall effectiveness of ALE as good or excellent. Eighty-six percent of patients rated artichoke therapy as substantially or slightly more effective than previous treatments used. Reported adverse effects included hunger in one patient and transient increased flatulence in two patients. Limitations of this study include a lack of control group and the possible influence of patient expectations. The subset of patients with IBS was defined on the basis of five symptoms that overlap with symptoms of dyspepsia; other IBS symptoms were not considered in defining the subset.

Antioxidant
Summary

- Antioxidant properties of artichoke have been noted in multiple pre-clinical studies,[2,3,15,37,43-49] although long-term clinical effects in humans are not known.

Alcohol-Induced Hangover
Summary

- Artichoke extract has been used as a hangover remedy. However, there is insufficient available evidence to form a clear conclusion in this area.

Evidence

- In a small 2002 randomized, double-blind crossover trial, 15 volunteers received either three capsules of commercially available standardized artichoke extract or placebo before and after alcohol exposure. After a 1-week washout period, volunteers received the opposite treatment. The primary outcome measure was difference in hangover severity scores. Secondary outcome measures included mood profile and cognitive performance test scores administered 1 hour before and 10 hours after alcohol exposure. The authors reported that none of the outcome measures differed significantly between interventions. Adverse events were rare and were mild/transient. Although these results suggest a lack of benefit, this small study may have been underpowered to detect significant between-group differences. Therefore, a clear conclusion cannot be reached based on these results.

FORMULARY: BRANDS USED IN CLINICAL TRIALS

- Hepar SL forte.[8,11-15]
- Valverde Artischoke bei Verdauungsbeschwerden (Artichoke dry extract) as coated tablets containing 450 mg of extract.[7]

References

1. Beggi D, Dettori L. Ricerche sperimentali sull'allzione diuretica della *Cynara scolymus*. Il Policlinico Sez Prat 1931;XLI:489-490.
2. Gebhardt R, Fausel M. Antioxidant and hepatoprotective effects of artichoke extracts and constituents in cultured rat hepatocytes. Toxicol in Vitro 1997; 11:669-672.
3. Gebhardt R. Antioxidative and protective properties of extracts from leaves of the artichoke (*Cynara scolymus* L.) against hydroperoxide-induced oxidative stress in cultured rat hepatocytes. Toxicol Appl Pharmacol 1997; 144(2):279-286.
4. Kraft K. Artichoke leaf extract—Recent findings reflecting effects on lipid metabolism, liver and gastrointestinal tracts. Phytomedicine 1997;4(4): 369-378.
5. Heckers H, Dittmar K, Schmahl FW, et al. Inefficiency of cynarin as therapeutic regimen in familial type II hyperlipoproteinaemia. Atherosclerosis 1977;26(2):249-253.
6. Held C. Von der 1. Deutsche-Ungarischen Phytopharmakon-Konferenz, Budapest, 20. November 1991. Z Klin Med 1992;47:92-93.
7. Englisch W, Beckers C, Unkauf M, et al. Efficacy of Artichoke dry extract in patients with hyperlipoproteinemia. Arzneimittelforschung 2000;50(3): 260-265.
8. Kirchhoff R, Beckers CH, Kirchhoff GM, et al. Increase in choleresis by means of artichoke extract. Phytomedicine 1994;1:107-115.
9. Marakis G, Walker AF, Middleton RW, et al. Artichoke leaf extract reduces mild dyspepsia in an open study. Phytomedicine 2002;9(8):694-699.
10. Dorn M. Improvement in raised lipid levels with artichoke juice (*Cynara scolymus* L.). British J Phytother 1995;4(1):21-26.
11. Fintelmann V. [Antidyspeptic and lipid lowering activity of artichoke extract]. Z Allg Med 1996;72:48-57.
12. Fintelmann V. Antidyspeptic and lipid-lowering effects of artichoke leaf extract—results of clinical studies into the efficacy and tolerance of Hepar-SL forte involving 553 patients. J Gen Med 1996;2:3-19.
13. Fintelmann V, Menssen HG. Artichoke leaf extract: current knowledge concerning its efficacy as a lipid-reducer and antidyspeptic agent. Dtsch Apoth Ztg 1996;136:1405-1414.
14. Fintelmann V, Menssen HG. Artischokenblatterextrakt. Deutsche Apotheker Zeitung 1996;136(17):63-74.
15. Fintelmann V. Therapeutic profile and mechanism of action of artichoke leaf extract: hypolipemic, antioxidant, hepatoprotective and choleretic properties. Phytomedicine 1996;suppl 1:50.
16. Newall CA, Anderson LA, Phillipson JD. Herbal medicines: A guide for health-care professionals. London: The Pharmaceutical Press, 1996: 36.
17. Meding B. Allergic contact dermatitis from artichoke, *Cynara scolymus*. Contact Dermatitis 1983;9(4):314.
18. Romano C, Ferrara A, Falagiani P. A case of allergy to globe artichoke and other clinical cases of rare food allergy. J Invest Allergol Clin Immunol 2000;10(2):102-104.

19. Miralles JC, Garcia-Sells J, Bartolome B, et al. Occupational rhinitis and bronchial asthma due to artichoke (*Cynara scolymus*). Ann Allergy Asthma Immunol 2003;91(1):92-95.
20. Lietti A. Choleretic and cholesterol lowering properties of artichoke extracts. Fitoterapia 1977;48:153-158.
21. Quirce S, Tabar AI, Olaguibel JM, et al. Occupational contact urticaria syndrome caused by globe artichoke (*Cynara scolymus*). J Allergy Clin Immunol 1996;97(2):710-711.
22. Walker AF, Middleton RW, Petrowicz O. Artichoke leaf extract reduces symptoms of irritable bowel syndrome in a post-marketing surveillance study. Phytother Res 2001;15(1):58-61.
23. Matuschowski P. Testing of *Cynara scolymus* in the isolated perfused rat liver. 43rd Ann Congr Soc Med Plant Res 1996;3-7.
24. Woyke M, Cwajda H, Wojcicki J, et al. Platelet aggregation in workers chronically exposed to carbon disulfide and subjected to prophylactic treatment with Cynarex] [in Polish]. Medycyna Pracy 1981;32(4):261-264.
25. Violon C. Belgian (Chinese herb) nephropathy: why? Farmaceutisch Tijdschrift voor Belgie 1997;74:11-36.
26. Farrell J, Campbell E, Walshe JJ. Renal failure associated with alternative medical therapies. Ren Fail 1995;17(6):759-764.
27. Cima G, Bonora R. Artichoke. Minerva Med 1959;50:2288-2291.
28. Mancini M, Oriente P, D'Andrea L. Artichoke. Minerva Med 1960; 51:2460-2463.
29. Montini M, Levoni P, Ongaro A, et al. [Controlled application of cynarin in the treatment of hyperlipemic syndrome. Observations in 60 cases.] Arzneimittelforschung 1975;25(8):1311-1314.
30. Mars G, Brambilla G. [Effect of 1,5-dicafleylquinic acid (cynarine) on hypertriglyceridemia in aged patients]. Med Welt 1974;25(39):1572-1574.
31. Hammerl H, Kindler K, Kranzl C, et al. [Effect of Cynarin on hyperlipidemia with special reference to type II (hypercholesterinemia)]. Wien Med Wochenschr 1973;123(41):601-605.
32. Pittler MH, Thompson CO, Ernst E. Artichoke leaf extract for treating hypercholesterolaemia. Cochrane Database Syst Rev 2002;(3):CD003335.
33. Petrowicz O, Gebhardt R, Donner M, et al. Effects of artichoke leaf extract (ALE) on lipoprotein metabolism in vitro and in vivo. Atherosclerosis 1997;129:147.
34. Wegener T. [About the therapeutic activity of the artichoke.] Pflanzliche Gallentherapeutika 1995;16:81.
35. von Weiland HH, Kindler K, Kranzl Ch, et al. Uber den Einfluss von Cynarin auf Hyperlipidamien unter besonderer Berucksichtigung des Typs II (Hyper-cholesterinamie). Wiener Medizinische Wochenschrift 1973;41: 601-605.
36. Gebhardt R. Inhibition of cholesterol biosynthesis in primary cultured rat hepatocytes by artichoke (*Cynara scolymus* L.) extracts. J Pharmacol Exp Ther 1998;286(3):1122-1128.
37. Brown JE, Rice-Evans CA. Luteolin-rich artichoke extract protects low density lipoprotein from oxidation in vitro. Free Radic Res 1998;29(3): 247-255.
38. Wojcicki J. Effect of 1,5-dicaffeylquinic acid (cynarine) on cholesterol levels in serum and liver of acute ethanol-treated rats. Drug Alcohol Depend 1978;3(2):143-145.
39. Wojcicki J. Effect of 1,5-dicaffeoylquinic acid on ethanol-induced hypertriglyceridemia. Arzneim-Forsch 1976;26(11):2047-2048.
40. Samochowiec L. Artichoke. Diss Pharm 1959;11:99-112.
41. Samochowiec L. The action of herbs and roots of artichokes (*Cynara scolymnus*) and cardoon (*Cynara cardunculus*) on the development of experimental atherosclerosis in white rats. Diss Pharm 1962;14:115.
42. Samochowiec L. The effect of artichokes (*Cynara scolymus* L.) and cardoons (*Cynara cardunculus* L.) on developed atherosclerotic changes in white rats. Fol Biol 1962;10;75-83.
43. Wang M, Simon JE, Aviles IF, et al. Analysis of antioxidative phenolic compounds in artichoke (*Cynara scolymus* L.). J Agric Food Chem 2003; 51(3):601-608.
44. Llorach R, Espin JC, Tomas-Barberan FA, et al. Artichoke (*Cynara scolymus* L.) byproducts as a potential source of health-promoting antioxidant phenolics. J Agric Food Chem 2002;50(12):3458-3464.
45. Jimenez-Escrig A, Dragsted LO, Daneshvar B, et al. In vitro antioxidant activities of edible artichoke (*Cynara scolymus* L.) and effect on biomarkers of antioxidants in rats. J Agric Food Chem 2003;51(18):5540-5545.
46. Zapolska-Downar D, Zapolski-Downar A, Naruszewicz M, et al. Protective properties of artichoke (*Cynara scolymus*) against oxidative stress induced in cultured endothelial cells and monocytes. Life Sci 2002;71(24):2897-08.
47. Betancor-Fernandez A, Perez-Galvez A, Sies H, et al. Screening pharmaceutical preparations containing extracts of turmeric rhizome, artichoke leaf, devil's claw root and garlic or salmon oil for antioxidant capacity. J Pharm Pharmacol 2003;55(7):981-986.
48. Adzet T. Action of an artichoke extract against carbon tetrachloride-induced hepatotoxicity in rats. Acts Pharm Jugosl 1987;37:183-188.
49. Adzet T, Camarasa J, Laguna JC. Hepatoprotective activity of polyphenolic compounds from *Cynara scolymus* against CCl4 toxicity in isolated rat hepatocytes. J Nat Prod 1987;50(4):612-617.
50. Kiso Y, Tohkin M, Hikino H. Antihepatotoxic principles of *Atractylodes* rhizomes. J Nat Prod 1983;46(5):651-654.
51. Kiso Y, et al. Assay method for antihepatotoxic activity using carbon tetrachloride induced cytotoxicity in primary cultured hepatocytes. Planta Medica 1983;49(4):222-225.
52. Camarasa J, Laguna JC, Gaspar A. Biochemical and histological pattern of cyanarin and caffeic acid treatment in CCl4-induced hepatoxicity. Med Sci Res 1987;15:91-92.
53. Hammerl H, Pichler O. Uber eine moglichkeit der kausalen Behandlung von Erkrankungen der Gallenwege mit einem Artischockenpreparat. Wiener Med Wschr 1957;107(25/26):545-546.
54. Panizzi L, Scarpati ML. Constitution of cynarine, the active principle of the artichoke. Nature 1954;174:1062.
55. Adam G, Kluthe R. Cholesterinsenkender Effect von Cynarin. Therapiewoche 1979;29:5673-5640.
56. Holtmann G, Adam B, Haag S, et al. Efficacy of artichoke leaf extract in the treatment of patients with functional dyspepsia: a six-week placebo-controlled, double-blind, multicentre trial. Aliment Pharmacol Ther 2003;18(11-12):1099-1105.
57. Kupke D, Sanden HV, Trinczek-Gartner H, et al. Prüfung der choleretischen Aktivitat eines pflanzlichen Cholagogums. Z Allg Med 1991;67:1046-1058.

Astragalus
(*Astragalus membranaceus*)

SYNONYMS/COMMON NAMES/RELATED SUBSTANCES

- *Astragalus trigonus, Astragalus gummifera, Astragalus mollissimus, Astragalus lentiginosus,* astragel, baak kei (beg kei, bei qi, buck qi), Fabaceae, goat's horn (goat's thorn), green dragon, gum dragon, gum tragacanthae (gummi tragacanthae), hoang ky, hog gum, huang-chi (huang qi, huangoi, huangqi, hwanggi), ji cao, Leguminosae, locoweed, membranous milk vetch, milk vetch, mongolian milk, mongolian milk vetch, neimeng huangqi, ogi (ougi), radix astragali, spino santo, Syrian tragacanth, tai shen, tragacanth, wong kei, yellow vetch, zhongfengnaomitong.
- **Selected combination products that include this agent:** Astragalus-Power, Baoyuan Dahuang, Biomune OSF Plus, Bu Zhong Yi Qi Tang, CH-100, Chi Power, Chinese Thermo-Chi, Deep Defense, Energy Boost Tincture, Equilizer Fast Start, Excel Energy, Fast Start, Fit America Natural Weight Control Aid, Formula One, Formula 3, Formula 3 Cell Activator, Fu-Zheng, Han-Dan-Gan-Le, Herbal Balance, Intra, Jian Yan Ling (JYL), Jiangtangjia, Magic Herb Diet Plus Formula + Chromium Picolinate, Man-Shen-Ling (MSL), Master Herb with Chromium Picolinate, Megawatt, Nature's Nutrition Formula One, Nature's Power Trim Super Fat Burner, New Image, New Image Plus, Sanhuang, Shengxue Mixture (SXM), Shen-Qi, Shi-quan-da-bu-tang (SQT), Thermojetics Beige, Tri-Chromaleane, Ultra Energy Now, Vita Chromaleane, Yi-qi Huo-xue Injection (YHI), Yogi Herbal Tea.

CLINICAL BOTTOM LINE
Background

- Astragalus products are derived from the roots of *Astragalus membranaceus* or related species, which are native to China. In traditional Chinese medicine, astragalus is commonly found in mixtures with other herbs and is used in the treatment of numerous ailments, including heart, liver, and kidney diseases, as well as cancer, viral infections, and immune system disorders. Western herbalists began using astragalus in the 1800s as an ingredient in various tonics. The use of astragalus became popular in the 1980s based on theories about anti-cancer properties, although these proposed effects have not been clearly demonstrated in studies in humans.
- Some medicinal uses of astragalus are based on its proposed immunostimulatory properties, reported in preliminary laboratory and animal experiments, but not conclusively demonstrated in humans. Most astragalus research has been conducted in China and has not been well designed or reported.
- The gummy sap (tragacanth) from astragalus is used as a thickener (ice cream), emulsifier, denture adhesive, and anti-diarrheal agent.

Uses Based on Scientific Evidence	Grade*
Antiviral activity Antiviral activity has been reported with the use of astragalus in laboratory and animal studies. Limited	C

human research has examined the use of astragalus for viral infections in the lung, heart (pericarditis), liver (hepatitis B and C), cervix (papillomavirus), and for HIV infection. Studies have included combinations of astragalus with the drug interferon and astragalus as a component of herbal mixtures. However, most studies have been small and poorly designed. Because of a lack of well-designed research studies, no firm conclusions can be drawn.

Cancer Although early laboratory and animal studies reported increased immune cell function and reduced cancer cell growth associated with the use of astragalus, there is no reliable human evidence in these areas. Because of a lack of well-designed research studies, a firm conclusion cannot be drawn.	C
Chemotherapy side effects In Chinese medicine, astragalus-containing herbal mixtures are sometimes used to reduce the side effects of cancer treatments. Because of the lack of well-designed research studies, a firm conclusion cannot be drawn.	C
Coronary artery disease In Chinese medicine, herbal mixtures containing astragalus have been used to treat coronary artery disease. Several studies in humans report reduced symptoms and improved heart function, although these are not well described. High-quality research studies in humans are necessary before a conclusion can be drawn.	C
Heart failure In Chinese medicine, herbal mixtures containing astragalus have been used to treat various heart diseases. There are several human case reports of reduced symptoms, improved heart function, and diuretic ("water pill") effects, although these are not well described. High-quality research studies in humans are necessary before conclusions can be drawn.	C
Immunostimulation Astragalus has been suggested as an immunostimulant in preliminary laboratory and animal research, and in traditional accounts. Published studies from China report increases in white blood cell counts with the use of astragalus preparations, but details are limited. High-quality research studies in humans are necessary before a firm conclusion can be drawn.	C
Liver protection Several animal and human studies report that astragalus may protect the liver from damage related to toxins or hepatitis B and C. Overall, this research has been poorly designed and reported. Astragalus alone has not been well evaluated. Better-quality research studies are necessary before a conclusion can be drawn.	C

Continued

Myocarditis/endocarditis (heart infections) Antiviral activity has been reported in laboratory studies and animal models of myocarditis/endocarditis. Research studies in humans are limited in this area, and further research is necessary before a conclusion can be drawn.	C
Renal failure Several animal and human studies report that kidney damage from toxins and kidney failure may be improved with the use of astragalus-containing herbal mixtures. Overall, this research has been poorly designed and reported. Astragalus alone has not been well evaluated. Better quality research is necessary before a conclusion can be drawn.	C
Upper respiratory tract infection Astragalus is often used in Chinese medicine as a part of herbal mixtures to prevent or treat upper respiratory tract infections. Antiviral activity has been reported in laboratory and animal studies and in limited reports of studies in humans. However, most studies have been small and poorly designed. Because of a lack of well-designed research studies, no firm conclusions can be drawn.	C

*Key to grades: *A:* Strong scientific evidence for this use; *B:* Good scientific evidence for this use; *C:* Unclear scientific evidence for this use; *D:* Fair scientific evidence against this use (it may not work); *F:* Strong scientific evidence against this use (it likely does not work). For a more detailed explanation of efficacy criteria, see "Natural Standard Evidence-Based Validated Grading Rationale" in the Introduction.

Historical or Theoretical Indications That Lack Sufficient Evidence

Adrenal insufficiency (Addison's disease), aging, AIDS/HIV, allergies, Alzheimer's disease, anemia, angina, ankylosing spondylitis, anorexia, antifungal, antimicrobial, antioxidant, asthma, blood thinner, bone-marrow suppression from cancer or HIV, bronchitis, cervicitis, "chi deficiency" (fatigue, weakness, loss of appetite), chronic fatigue syndrome, chronic hepatitis, cleanser, cyclosporine-induced immunosuppression, dementia, demulcent, denture adhesive (astragalus sap), diabetes, diabetic foot ulcers, diabetic neuropathy, diarrhea, digestion enhancement, diuretic (urination stimulant), edema, fatigue, fever, gangrene, gastrointestinal disorders, genital herpes, graft-versus-host disease, hearing damage from toxins/gentamicin, heart attack, hemorrhage (bleeding), hemorrhoids, high cholesterol, high blood pressure, hyperthyroidism, insomnia, joint pain, laxative, leprosy, leukemia, liver disease, low blood-platelet levels, lung cancer, memory, menstrual disorders, metabolic disorders, minimal brain dysfunction, myalgia (muscle pain), myasthenia gravis, nephritis, night sweats, palpitations, pelvic congestion syndrome, postpartum fever, postpartum urinary retention, prostatitis, rectal prolapse, rotavirus enterocolitis (in infants), shortness of breath, sperm motility, stamina/endurance enhancement, stomach ulcer, stroke, sweating (excessive), systemic lupus erythematosus (SLE), tissue oxygenation, uterine prolapse, uterine bleeding, weight loss, wound healing.

DOSING/TOXICOLOGY

The listed doses are based on scientific research, publications, traditional use, and expert opinion. Many herbs and supplements have not been thoroughly tested, and safety and effectiveness may not be proven. Brands may be made differently, with variable ingredients even within the same brand. The doses shown may not apply to all products. It is important to always read product labels, and discuss doses with a qualified healthcare provider before therapy is started.

Standardization

- Standardization involves measuring the amount of certain chemicals in products when attempting to make different preparations similar to each other. It is not always known if the chemicals being measured are the "active" ingredients.
- Anecdotal reports have recommended the standardization of astragalus to a minimum of 0.4% 4-hydroxy-3-methoxy-isoflavone-7-glycoside per dose. However, because astragalus is often added to herbal mixtures with unclear amounts of astragalus used, standardization is not always possible.

Adults (18 Years and Older)

- **General use by mouth:** In Chinese medicine, astragalus is used in soups, teas, extracts, and pill form. In practice and in most scientific studies, astragalus is one component of multi-herb mixtures. Therefore, precise dosing of astragalus alone is unclear. Safety and effectiveness are not clearly established for any particular dose. Various doses of astragalus that have been used or studied include 250 to 500 mg of extract taken four times daily, 1 to 30 g of dried root taken daily (doses as high as 60 g have been reported), and 500 to 1000 mg of root capsules taken 3 times daily. Dosing of tinctures and fluid extracts depends on the strength of preparations.
- *Note:* In theory, tragacanth (the gummy sap derived from astragalus) may reduce absorption of drugs taken by mouth and thus should not be taken at the same time.

Children (Younger Than 18 Years)

- There is insufficient scientific data to recommend astragalus for use in children.

SAFETY

The U.S. Food and Drug Administration does not strictly regulate herbs and supplements. There is no guarantee of strength, purity, or safety of products, and effects may vary. It is important to always read product labels. People who have a medical condition, or are taking other drugs, herbs, or supplements, should consult a qualified healthcare provider before starting a new therapy. A healthcare provider should be contacted immediately about any side effects.

Allergies

- In theory, patients with allergies to members of the Leguminosae family may react to astragalus. Cross-reactivity with Quillaja bark (soap bark) has been reported for astragalus gum tragacanth.

Side Effects and Warnings

- Some species of astragalus cause poisoning in livestock, although these species are not usually present in human preparations (which primarily include *Astragalus membranaceus*). Livestock toxicity, referred to as "locoweed" poisoning, has occurred with species that contain swainsonine (*Astragalus lentiginosus, Astragalus mollissimus, Astragalus nothrosys, Astragalus pubentissimus, Astragalus thuseri, Astragalus wootoni*) and in species that accumulate selenium

(*Astragalus bisulcatus*, *Astragalus flavus*, *Astragalus praelongus*, *Astragalus saurinus*, *Astragalus tenellus*).

- Overall, it is difficult to determine the side effects or toxicity of astragalus, because it is most commonly used in combination with other herbs. There are numerous reports of side effects, ranging from mild to deadly, in the U.S. Food and Drug Administration computer database, although most of these occur with multi-ingredient products and cannot be attributed to astragalus specifically. Astragalus used alone and in recommended doses is traditionally considered to be safe, although this herb's safety has not been well studied. The most common side effects appear to be mild stomach upset and allergic reactions. In the United States, tragacanth (astragalus gummy sap) has been classified as GRAS (generally recognized as safe) for food use, but astragalus itself does not have GRAS status.
- Based on preliminary animal studies and limited human research, astragalus may decrease blood sugar levels. Caution is advised in patients with diabetes or hypoglycemia and in those taking drugs, herbs, or supplements that affect blood sugar levels. Serum glucose levels may need to be monitored by a healthcare professional, and dosing adjustments may be necessary.
- Based on anecdotal reports and preliminary laboratory research, astragalus may increase the risk of bleeding. Caution is advised in patients with bleeding disorders and in people taking drugs that may increase the risk of bleeding. Dosing adjustments may be necessary.
- Preliminary reports of use in China have noted decreased blood pressure at doses of less than 15 g and increased blood pressure at doses above 30 g. Animal research suggests possible blood pressure–lowering effects. Because of a lack of well-designed studies, no firm conclusions can be drawn. Nonetheless, people with abnormal blood pressure or taking blood pressure medications should use caution when taking astragalus and should be monitored by a qualified healthcare professional. Palpitations have been noted in human reports in China.
- Based on studies of animals, astragalus may act as a diuretic and increase urination. In theory, this may lead to dehydration or metabolic abnormalities. There is one report of pneumonia in an infant who had "breathed in" (inhaled) a combination herbal medicine powder that included *Astragalus sarcocolla*.
- Astragalus may increase growth hormone levels.

Pregnancy and Breastfeeding

- There is insufficient scientific evidence to recommend the use of *Astragalus membranaceus* during pregnancy or breastfeeding. Studies of toxic astragalus species, such as *Astragalus lentiginosus* and *Astragalus mollissimus* (locoweed) have reported harmful effects in pregnant animals, leading to abortions or abnormal heart development.

INTERACTIONS

Most herbs and supplements have not been thoroughly tested for interactions with other herbs, supplements, drugs, and foods. The interactions listed here are based on reports in scientific publications, laboratory experiments, and traditional use. It is important to always read product labels. People who have a medical condition, or are taking other drugs, herbs, or supplements, should consult a qualified healthcare provider before starting a new therapy.

Interactions with Drugs

- Based on preliminary animal studies and limited human research, astragalus may decrease blood sugar levels. Caution is advised in patients with diabetes or hypoglycemia and in people taking drugs that affect blood sugar levels. Serum glucose levels may need to be monitored by a healthcare provider, and dosing adjustments may be necessary.
- Preliminary reports of use in China have noted decreased blood pressure at doses of less than 15 g and increased blood pressure at doses above 30 g. Research in animals suggests possible blood pressure–lowering effects. Although well-designed studies are not available, people taking drugs that affect blood pressure should use caution when taking astragalus and should be monitored by a qualified healthcare professional. It has been suggested that beta-blocker drugs such as propranolol (Inderal) and atenolol (Tenormin) may reduce the effects of astragalus on the heart, although this has not been well studied.
- Based on anecdotal reports, astragalus may further increase the risk of bleeding when taken with drugs that increase the risk of bleeding. Examples are aspirin, anticoagulants ("blood thinners") such as warfarin (Coumadin) and heparin, anti-platelet drugs such as clopidogrel (Plavix), and non-steroidal anti-inflammatory drugs such as ibuprofen (Motrin, Advil) and naproxen (Naprosyn, Aleve).
- Based on animal research and traditional use, astragalus may act as a diuretic and increase urination. In theory, this may lead to dehydration or metabolic abnormalities (low blood levels of sodium or potassium), particularly when used in combination with diuretic drugs such as furosemide (Lasix), chlorothiazide (Diuril), and spironolactone (Aldactone).
- Based on laboratory and animal studies, astragalus may possess immunostimulating properties, although research in humans is not conclusive. Some research suggests that astragalus may interfere with the effects of drugs that suppress the immune system, such as steroids and agents used in organ transplants. Better research is necessary before a firm conclusion can be reached.
- Although there is no reliable scientific evidence in this area, some sources suggest other potential drug interactions. These include reduced effects of astragalus when used with sedative drugs (e.g., phenobarbital) and hypnotic agents (e.g., chloral hydrate), increased effects of astragalus when taken with colchicine, increased effects of paralytics such as pancuronium or succinylcholine when used with astragalus, increased effects of stimulants such as ephedrine or epinephrine, increased side effects of dopamine antagonists such as haloperidol (Haldol), and increased side effects of the cancer drug procarbazine.
- In theory, tragacanth (the gummy sap derived from astragalus) may reduce absorption of drugs taken by mouth and thus should be taken at a different time.

Interactions with Herbs and Dietary Supplements

- Based on preliminary animal studies and limited human research, astragalus may decrease blood sugar levels. Caution is advised in patients with diabetes or hypoglycemia and in people taking herbs or supplements that affect blood sugar levels. Examples are *Aloe vera*, American ginseng, bilberry, bitter melon, burdock, fenugreek, fish oil, gymnema, horse chestnut seed extract (HCSE), marshmallow, milk thistle, *Panax ginseng*, rosemary, Siberian ginseng, stinging nettle and white horehound. Serum glucose levels may need to be monitored by a healthcare provider, and dosing adjustments may be necessary.
- Preliminary reports of human use in China have noted decreased blood pressure at doses of less than 15 g and increased blood pressure at doses above 30 g. Animal research suggests possible blood pressure–lowering effects. Although

well-designed studies are not available, people taking herbs or supplements that affect blood pressure should use caution when taking astragalus and should be monitored by a qualified healthcare professional. Herbs that may lower blood pressure include aconite/monkshood, arnica, baneberry, betel nut, bilberry, black cohosh, bryony, calendula, California poppy, coleus, curcumin, eucalyptol, eucalyptus oil, ginger, goldenseal, green hellebore, hawthorn, Indian tobacco, jaborandi, mistletoe, night blooming cereus, oleander, pasque flower, periwinkle, pleurisy root, shepherd's purse, Texas milkweed, turmeric, and wild cherry.

- Based on anecdotal reports, astragalus may further increase the risk of bleeding when taken with herbs or supplements that increase the risk of bleeding. Multiple cases of bleeding have been reported with the use of *Ginkgo biloba*, and fewer cases have been reported with the use of garlic and saw palmetto. Theoretically, numerous other agents may increase the risk of bleeding, although this has not been proven in most cases. Examples are alfalfa, American ginseng, angelica, anise, *Arnica montana*, asafetida, aspen bark, bilberry, birch, black cohosh, bladderwrack, bogbean, boldo, borage seed oil, bromelain, capsicum, cat's claw, celery, chamomile, chaparral, clove, coleus, cordyceps, danshen, devil's claw, dong quai, evening primrose, fenugreek, feverfew, flaxseed/flax powder (not a concern with flaxseed oil), ginger, grapefruit juice, grapeseed, green tea, guggul, gymnestra, horse chestnut, horseradish, licorice root, lovage root, male fern, meadowsweet, nordihydroguaiaretic acid (NDGA), onion, papain, *Panax ginseng*, parsley, passion flower, poplar, prickly ash, propolis, quassia, red clover, reishi, rue, Siberian ginseng, sweet birch, sweet clover, turmeric, vitamin E, white willow, wild carrot, wild lettuce, willow, wintergreen, and yucca.
- Based on animal research and traditional use, astragalus may act as a diuretic and increase urination. In theory, this may lead to dehydration or metabolic abnormalities (low blood levels of sodium or potassium), particularly when used in combination with other herbs or supplements that may possess diuretic properties. Examples are artichoke, celery, corn silk, couch grass, dandelion, elder flower, horsetail, juniper berry, kava, shepherd's purse, uva ursi, and yarrow.
- Based on laboratory and animal studies, astragalus may possess immunostimulating properties, although research in humans is not conclusive. It is not known if astragalus interacts with other agents proposed to affect the immune system. Examples are bromelain, calendula, coenzyme Q10, echinacea, ginger, ginseng, goldenseal, gotu kola, lycopene, maitake mushroom, marshmallow, polypodium, propolis, and tea tree oil.
- In theory, tragacanth (the gummy sap derived from astragalus) may reduce absorption of other herbs or supplements taken by mouth and thus should be taken at a different time.

Selected References

Natural Standard developed the preceding evidence-based information based on a systematic review of more than 200 publications. For comprehensive information about alternative and complementary therapies on the professional level, go to www.naturalstandard.com. Selected references are listed here.

Al-Fakhri SA. Herbal medicine: possible cause of aspiration pneumonia: a case report. Saudi Pharm J 1998;6(1):88-91.
Batey RG, Bensoussan A, Fan YY, et al. Preliminary report of a randomized, double-blind placebo-controlled trial of a Chinese herbal medicine preparation CH-100 in the treatment of chronic hepatitis C. J Gastroenterol Hepatol 1998;13(3):244-247.
Bedir E, Pugh N, Calis I, et al. Immunostimulatory effects of cycloartane-type triterpene glycosides from astragalus species. Biol Pharm Bull 2000;23(7):834-837.
Bisignano G, Iauk L, Kirjavainen S, et al. Anti-inflammatory, analgesic, anti-pyretic and antibacterial activity of Astragalus siculus biv. Int J Pharm 1994;32(4):400-405.
Burack JH, Cohen MR, Hahn JA, et al. Pilot randomized controlled trial of Chinese herbal treatment for HIV-associated symptoms. J Acquir Immune Defic Syndr Hum Retrovirol 1996;12(4):386-393.
Chen KT, Su CH, Hsin LH, et al. Reducing fatigue of athletes following oral administration of huangqi jianzhong tang. Acta Pharmacol Sin 2002 Aug;23(8):757-761.
Chen LX, Liao JZ, Guo WQ. [Effects of Astragalus membranaceus on left ventricular function and oxygen free radical in acute myocardial infarction patients and mechanism of its cardiotonic action.] Zhonghuo Zhong Xi Yi Jie He Za Zhi 1995;15(3):141-143.
Chu DT, Lepe-Zuniga J, Wong WL, et al. Fractionated extract of Astragalus membranaceus, a Chinese medicinal herb, potentiates LAK cell cytotoxicity generated by a low dose of recombinant interleukin-2. J Clin Lab Immunol 1988;26(4):183-187.
Chu DT, Lin JR, Wong W. [The in vitro potentiation of LAK cell cytotoxicity in cancer and AIDS patients induced by F3—a fractionated extract of Astragalus membranaceus.] Zhonghua Zhong Liu Za Zhi 1994;16(3):167-171.
Chu DT, Sun Y, Lin JR. [Immune restoration of local xenogeneic graft-versus-host reaction in cancer patients in vitro and reversal of cyclophosphamide-induced immune suppression in the rat in vivo by fractionated Astragalus membranaceus.] Zhong Xi Yi Jie He Za Zhi 1989;9(6):351-354, 326.
Chu DT, Wong WL, Mavligit GM. Immunotherapy with Chinese medicinal herbs. II. Reversal of cyclophosphamide-induced immune suppression by administration of fractionated Astragalus membranaceus in vivo. J Clin Lab Immunol 1988;25(3):125-129.
Coppes MJ, Anderson RA, Egeler RM, et al. Alternative therapies for the treatment of childhood cancer. N Engl J Med 1998;339(12):846-847.
Cuellar M, Giner RM, Recio MC, et al. Screening of antiinflammatory medicinal plants used in traditional medicine against skin diseases. Phytother Res 1998;12:18-23.
Cui R, He J, Wang B, Zhang F, et al. Suppressive effect of Astragalus membranaceus Bunge on chemical hepatocarcinogenesis in rats. Cancer Chemother Pharmacol. 2003;51(1):75-80. Epub 2002 Nov 26.
Dai CF, Zhang ZZ, Qi XL, et al. [Clinical and experimental study of treatment of nanmiqing capsule for chronic prostatitis.] Zhonghua Nan Ke Xue 2002;8(5):379-382.
Duan P, Wang ZM. [Clinical study on effect of Astragalus in efficacy enhancing and toxicity reducing of chemotherapy in patients of malignant tumor.] Zhongguo Zhong Xi Yi Jie He Za Zhi 2002;22(7):515-517.
el Sebakhy NA, Asaad AM, Abdallah RM, et al. Antimicrobial isoflavans from Astragalus species. Phytochemistry 1994;36(6):1387-1389.
Fu QL. [Experimental study on Yiqi-huoxue therapy of liver fibrosis.] Zhongguo Zhong Xi Yi Jie He Za Zhi 1992;12(4):228-229, 198.
Gariboldi P, Pelizzoni F, Tato M, et al. Cycloartane triterpene glycosides from Astragalus trigonus. Phytochem 1995;40(6):1755-1760.
Gu W, Yang YZ, He MX. [A study on combination therapy of Western and traditional Chinese medicine of acute viral myocarditis.] Zhongguo Zhong Xi Yi Jie He Za Zhi 1996;16(12):713-716.
Guo SK, Chen KJ, Yu FR, et al. Treatment of acute myocardial infarction with AMI-mixture combined with Western medicine. Planta Med 1983;48(1):63-64.
He Z, Findlay JA. Constituents of Astragalus membranaceus. J Natural Prod 1991;54(3):810-815.
Hikino H, Funayama S, Endo K. Hypotensive principle of Astragalus and Hedysarum roots. Planta Med 1976;30:297-302.
Hirotani M, Zhou Y, Rui H, et al. Cycloartane triterpene glycosides from the hairy root cultures of Astragalus membranaceus. Phytochem 1994;37(5):1403-1407.
Hong CY, Lo YC, Tan FC, et al. Astragalus membranaceus and Polygonum multiflorum protect rat heart mitochondria against lipid peroxidation. Am J Chinese Med 1994;22(1):63-70.
Hong GX, Qin WC, Huang LS. [Memory-improving effect of aqueous extract of Astragalus membranaceus (Fisch.) Bge.] Zhongguo Zhong Yao Za Zhi 1994;19(11):687-688, 704.
Hou YD, Ma GL, Wu SH, et al. Effect of Radix Astragali seu Hedysari on the interferon system. Chin Med J (Engl) 1981;94(1):35-40.
Huang WM, Yan J, Xu J. [Clinical and experimental study on inhibitory effect of Sanhuang mixture on platelet aggregation.] Zhongguo Zhong Xi Yi Jie He Za Zhi 1995;15(8):465-467.
Huang ZQ, Qin NP, Ye W. [Effects of Astragalus membranaceus on T-lymphocyte subsets in patients with viral myocarditis.] Zhongguo Zhong Xi Yi Jie He Za Zhi 1995;15(6):328-330.
Jin R, Wan LL, Mitsuishi T, et al. [Immunomodulative effects of Chinese herbs in mice treated with anti-tumor agent cyclophosphamide.] Yakugaku Zasshi 1994;114(7):533-538.
Kajimura K, Takagi Y, Ueba N, et al. Protective effect of astragali radix by oral administration against Japanese encephalitis virus infection in mice. Biol Pharm Bull 1996;19(9):1166-1169.
Khoo KS, Ang PT. Extract of Astragalus membranaceus and Ligustrum lucidum does not prevent cyclophosphamide-induced myelosuppression. Singapore Med J 1995;36(4):387-390.
Kim C, Ha H, Kim JS, Kim YT, et al. Induction of growth hormone by the roots of Astragalus membranaceus in pituitary cell culture. Arch Pharm Res 2003;26(1):34-39.

Lau BH, Ruckle HC, Botolazzo T, et al. Chinese medicinal herbs inhibit growth of murine renal cell carcinoma. Cancer Biother 1994;9(2):153-161.

Lei ZY, Qin H, Liao JZ. [Action of *Astragalus membranaceus* on left ventricular function of angina pectoris.] Zhongguo Zhong Xi Yi Jie He Za Zhi 1994; 14(4):199-202.

Li C, Luo J, Li L, et al. The collagenolytic effects of the traditional Chinese medicine preparation, Han-Dan-Gan-Le, contribute to reversal of chemical-induced liver fibrosis in rats. Life Sci 2003;72(14):1563-1571.

Li CX, Li L, Lou J, et al. The protective effects of traditional Chinese medicine prescription, Han-dan-gan-le, on CCl4-induced liver fibrosis in rats. Am J Chin Med 1998;26(3-4):325-332.

Li L, Wang H, Zhu S. [Hepatic albumin's mRNA in nephrotic syndrome rats treated with Chinese herbs.] Zhonghua Yi Xue Za Zhi 1995;75(5):276-279.

Li NQ. [Clinical and experimental study on shen-qo injection with chemotherapy in the treatment of malignant tumor of digestive tract.] Zhongguo Zhong Xi Yi Jie He Za Zhi 1992;12(10):579, 588-592.

Li X, et al. Pharmacological study of APS-G: Part 1—effect on reaction to stress. Zhong Cheng Yao 1989;11(3):27-29.

Li X, et al. Pharmacological study of APS-G: Part 3—effect on blood glucose and glycogen content in liver. Zhong Cheng Yao 1989;11(9):32-33.

Liu ZG, Xiong ZM, Yu XY. [Effect of astragalus injection on immune function in patients with congestive heart failure.] Zhongguo Zhong Xi Yi Jie He Za Zhi 2003;23(5):351-353.

Luo HM, Dai RH, Li Y. [Nuclear cardiology study on effective ingredients of *Astragalus membranaceus* in treating heart failure.] Zhongguo Zhong Xi Yi Jie He Za Zhi 1995;15(12):707-709.

Ma J, Peng A, Lin S. Mechanisms of the therapeutic effect of *Astragalus membranaceus* on sodium and water retention in experimental heart failure. Chin Med J 1998;111(1):17-23.

Ma Y, Tian Z, Kuang H, et al. Studies of the constituents of *Astragalus membranaceus* Bunge. III. Structures of triterpenoidal glycosides, huangqiyenins A and B, from the leaves. Chem Pharm Bull 1997;45(2):359-361.

Ning L, Chen CX, Jin RM, et al. [Effect of components of dang-gui-bu-xue decoction on hematopenia.] Zhongguo Zhong Yao Za Zhi. 2002 Jan;27(1): 50-53.

Pan SY. [Pharmacological action of *Astragalus membranaceus* on the central nervous system in mice.] Zhong Yao Tong Bao 1986;11(9):47-49.

Qian ZW, Li YY. [Synergism of *Astragalus membranaceus* with interferon in the treatment of cervical erosion and their antiviral activities.] Zhong Xi Yi Jie He Za Zhi 1987;7(5):268-269, 287, 259.

Raghuprasad PK, Brooks SM, Litwin A, et al. Quillaja bark (soap bark)–induced asthma. J Allergy Clin Immunol 1980;65(4):285-287.

Rios JL, Waterman PG. A review of the pharmacology and toxicology of astragalus. Phytother Res 1997;11:411-418.

Rittenhouse JR, Lui PD, Lau BH. Chinese medicinal herbs reverse macrophage suppression induced by urological tumors. J Urol 1991;146(2):486-490.

Sheng ZL, Li NY, Ge XP. [Clinical study of baoyuan dahuang decoction in the treatment of chronic renal failure.] Zhongguo Zhong Xi Yi Jie He Za Zhi 1994;14(5):268-270, 259.

Shirataki Y, Takao M, Yoshida S, et al. Antioxidative components isolated from the roots of *Astragalus membranaceus* Bunge (Astragali Radix). Phytother Res 1997;11:603-605.

Su ZZ, He YY, Chen G. [Clinical and experimental study on effects of Man-shen-ling oral liquid in the treatment of 100 cases of chronic nephritis.] Zhongguo Zhong Xi Yi Jie He Za Zhi 1993;13(5):269-260.

Sun Y, Hersh EM, Lee S, et al. Preliminary observations on the effects of the Chinese medicinal herbs *Astragalus membranaceus* and *Ligustrum lucidum* on lymphocyte blastogenic responses. J Biol Response Mod 1983;2(3):227-237.

Sun Y, Hersh EM, Talpax M, et al. Immune restoration and/or augmentation of local graft versus host reaction by traditional Chinese medicinal herbs. Cancer 1983;52(1):70-73.

Sun Y. The role of traditional Chinese medicine in supportive care of cancer patients. Recent Results Cancer Res 1988;108:327-334.

Tianqing P, Yingzhen Y, Riesemann H, et al. The inhibitory effect of *Astragalus membranaceus* on Coxsackie B-3 virus RNA replication. Chin Med Sci J 1995; 10(3):146-150.

Wang D, Shen W, Tian Y, et al. [Protective effect of total flavonoids of radix Astragali on mammalian cell damage caused by hydroxyl radical.] Zhongguo Zhong Yao Za Zhi 1995;20(4):240-242.

Wang F. Twenty-eight cases of diabetic foot ulcer and gangrene treated with the Chinese herbal medicine combined with injection of ahylsantinfarctase. J Tradit Chin Med 2002;22(1):3-4.

Wang Q. [Inotropic action of *Astragalus membranaceus* Bge. saponins and its possible mechanism.] Zhongguo Zhong Yao Za Zhi 1992;17(9):557-559.

Wei H, Sun R, Xiao W, et al. Traditional Chinese medicine Astragalus reverses predominance of Th2 cytokines and their up-stream transcript factors in lung cancer patients. Oncol Rep 2003;10(5):1507-1512.

Weng XS. [Treatment of leucopenia with pure Astragalus preparation—an analysis of 115 leucopenic cases.] Zhongguo Zhong Xi Yi Jie He Za Zhi 1995;15(8):462-464.

Wu XS, Chen HY, Li M. [Clinical observation on effect of combined use of Astragalus and compound salviae injection in treating acute cerebral infarction.] Zhongguo Zhong Xi Yi Jie He Za Zhi. 2003;23(5):380-381.

Xiangzhe J. A clinical investigation on 30 cases of senile benign renal arteriosclerosis treated by Huang qi gu jing yin. J Tradit Chin Med 2001;21(3): 177-180.

Xu XY, Li LH, Wu LS, Zhao CL, Lin HY. [Adjustment effect of Dadix Astragalus and Dadix Angelicae sinensis on TNF-alpha and bFGF on renal injury induced by ischemia reperfusion in rabbit.] Zhongguo Zhong Yao Za Zhi. 2002; 27(10):771-773.

Xuan W, Dong M, Dong M. Effects of compound injection of *Pyrola rotundifolia* L. and *Astragalus membranaceus* Bge on experimental guinea pigs' gentamicin ototoxicity. Ann Otol Rhinol Laryngol 1995;104(5):374-380.

Yan HJ. [Clinical and experimental study of the effect of kang er xin-I on viral myocarditis.] Zhong Xi Yi Jie He Za Zhi 1991;11(8):468-470, 452.

Yang Y, Jin P, Guo Q, et al. Effect of *Astragalus membranaceus* on natural killer cell activity and induction of alpha- and gamma-interferon in patients with Coxsackie B viral myocarditis. Chin Med J 1990;103(4):304-307.

Yang Y, Jin P, Guo Q, et al. Treatment of experimental Coxsackie B-3 viral myocarditis with *Astragalus membranaceus* in mice. Chin Med J 1990;103(1): 14-18.

Yin X, Zhang S, Kong Y, et al. Observation on efficiency of Jiangtang capsule in treating diabetes mellitus type 2 with hyperlipidemia. Chin J Integ Tradit West Med 2001;7(3):214-216.

Yu L, Lu Y, Li J, Wang H. Identification of a gene associated with astragalus and angelica's renal protective effects by silver staining mRNA differential display. Chin Med J (Engl) 2002 Jun;115(6):923-927.

Yuan WL, Chen HZ, Yang YZ, et al. Effect of *Astragalus membranaceus* on electric activities of cultured rat beating heart cells infected with Coxsackie B-2 virus. Chin Med J 1990;103(3):177-182.

Zee-Cheng RK. Shi-quan-da-bu-tang (ten significant tonic decoction), SQT. A potent Chinese biological response modifier in cancer immunotherapy, potentiation and detoxification of anticancer drugs. Methods Find Exp Clin Pharmacol 1992;14(9):725-736.

Zhang BZ, Ding F, Tan LW. [Clinical and experimental study on Yi-gan-ning granule in treating chronic hepatitis B.] Zhongguo Zhong Xi Yi Jie He Za Zhi 1993;13(10):597-599, 580.

Zhang H, Huang J. [Preliminary study of traditional Chinese medicine treatment of minimal brain dysfunction: analysis of 100 cases.] Zhong Xi Yi Jie He Za Zhi 1990;10(5):278-279, 260.

Zhang HE, et al. Treatment of adult diabetes with Jiangtangjia tablet. J Tradit Chin Med 1986;27(4):37-39.

Zhang JG, Gao DS, Wei GH. [Clinical study on effect of Astragalus injection on left ventricular remodeling and left ventricular function in patients with acute myocardial infarction.] Zhongguo Zhong Xi Yi Jie He Za Zhi. 2002; 22(5):346-348.

Zhang WJ, Wojta J, Binder BR. Regulation of the fibrinolytic potential of cultured human umbilical vein endothelial cells: Astragaloside IV downregulates plasminogen activator inhibitor-1 and upregulates tissue-type plasminogen activator expression. J Vasc Res 1997;34:273-280.

Zhang YD, Shen JP, Zhu SH, et al. [Effects of astragalus (ASI, SK) on experimental liver injury.] Yao Xue Xue Bao 1992;27(6):401-406.

Zhang ZL, Wen QZ, Liu CX. Hepatoprotective effects of astragalus root. J Ethnopharmacol 1990;30(2):145-149.

Zhao KS, Mancini C, Doria G. Enhancement of the immune response in mice by *Astragalus membranaceus* extracts. Immunopharmacol 1990;20(3):225-233.

Zhao KW, Kong HY. [Effect of Astragalan on secretion of tumor necrosis factors in human peripheral blood mononuclear cells.] Zhongguo Zhong Xi Yi Jie He Za Zhi 1993;13(5):263-265, 259.

Zhao XZ. [Effects of *Astragalus membranaceus* and *Tripterygium hypoglancum* on natural killer cell activity of peripheral blood mononuclear in systemic lupus erythematosus.] Zhongguo Zhong Xi Yi Jie He Za Zhi 1992;12(11):669-671, 645.

Zhou Y, Hirotani M, Rui H, et al. Two triglycosidic triterpene astragalosides from hairy root cultures of *Astragalus membranaceus*. Phytochemistry 1995; 38(6):1407-1410.

Zhou Y, Huang Z, Huang T, et al. Clinical study of Shengxue Mixture in treating aplastic anemia. Chin J Integ Trad West 2001;7(3):186-189.

Zong PP, Yan TY, Gong MM. [Clinical and experimental studies of effects of Huayu decoction on scavenging free radicals.] Zhongguo Zhong Xi Yi Jie He Za Zhi 1993;13(10):591-593, 579.

Zuo L, Guo H. [Quantitative study on synergistic effect of radix astragali A6 and acyclovir against herpes simplex virus type I by polymerase chain reaction.] Zhongguo Zhong Xi Yi Jie He Za Zhi 1998;18(4):233-235.

Barley

(Hordeum vulgare L.), Germinated Barley Foodstuff (GBF)

SYNONYMS/COMMON NAMES/RELATED SUBSTANCES

- Barley malt, barley oil, brewers spent grain, dietary fiber, germinated barley, high-protein barley flour (HPBF), Gramineae, high-fiber barley, hordeum, *Hordeum distychum, Hordeum dislichon, Hordeum murinum,* mai ya, pearl barley, Poaceae, pot barley, scotch barley, wild barley grass.

CLINICAL BOTTOM LINE
Background

- Barley is a cereal used as a staple food in many countries. It is commonly used as an ingredient in baked products and soup in Europe and the United States. Barley malt is used to make beer, and as a natural sweetener called malt sugar or barley jelly sugar.
- Recent data suggest that barley may be promising in reducing total cholesterol and low-density lipoprotein (LDL) in mildly hyperlipidemic patients.[1-6] Barley has a high fiber content; a modest inverse association has been observed between dietary fiber intake and cardiovascular disease in a recent large prospective cohort study, although results were not statistically significant.[7,8]
- Germinated barley foodstuff (GBF) is derived from the aleurone and scutellum fractions of germinated barley. GBF may play a role in the management of ulcerative colitis,[9,10] although further controlled studies are warranted. GBF has also been suggested as a treatment for mild constipation.[11] Barley bran flour accelerates gastrointestinal transit and increases fecal weight.[12] High fiber barley may be useful in the diets of patients with diabetes, because of a low glycemic index and ability to reduce postprandial glucose.[13,14]

Scientific Evidence for Common/Studied Uses	Grade*
Hyperlipidemia	B
Constipation	C
Hyperglycemia	C
Ulcerative colitis	C

*Key to grades: *A:* Strong scientific evidence for this use; *B:* Good scientific evidence for this use; *C:* Unclear scientific evidence for this use; *D:* Fair scientific evidence against this use (it may not work); *F:* Strong scientific evidence against this use (it likely does not work). For a more detailed explanation of efficacy criteria, see "Natural Standard Evidence-Based Validated Grading Rationale" in the Introduction.

Historical or Theoretical Uses That Lack Sufficient Evidence

- Antioxidant[15,16] appetite suppressant, boils, blood circulation, bronchitis, bronchodilation, cancer, colon cancer, diarrhea, gastritis, gastrointestinal inflammation, hair growth stimulant,[17] inflammatory bowel disorders, immunomodulator,[18] stamina enhancer, strength enhancer, sweetener, weight loss.

Expert Opinion and Folkloric Precedent

- Barley was historically used by the Romans to treat boils, and by the Greeks to treat gastrointestinal inflammation.
- In China, barley along with hung gue (red fruit) has been used to treat patients with galactorrhea and high prolactin levels.

Safety Summary

- **Likely safe:** When used orally in recommended doses, or as a food in otherwise healthy adults. No studies of long-term safety are available, but unfermented barley has been used as a staple food in many parts of the world without reported serious adverse effects.
- **Possibly safe:** When used in children in recommended doses, because of insufficient evidence.
- **Possibly unsafe:** When used in large amounts in pregnancy or lactation, based on anecdotal reports. Severe anaphylactic reactions and contact dermatitis have been associated with beer consumption.[19-21]
- **Likely unsafe:** When used in patients with celiac disease.

DOSING/TOXICOLOGY
General

- Recommended doses are based on those most commonly used in available trials, or on historical practice. However, with natural products the optimal doses needed to balance efficacy and safety often have not been determined. Formulations and preparation methods may vary from manufacturer to manufacturer, and from batch to batch of a specific product made by a single manufacturer. Because often the active components of a product are not known, standardization may not be possible, and the clinical effects of different brands may not be comparable.

Dosing: Adult (18 Years and Older)
Oral

- **Mild to moderate ulcerative colitis:** Germinated barley foodstuff (GBF). 10 g three times daily.[22] Doses up to 30 g daily have been reported as tolerated.[10,22]
- **Hypercholesterolemia:** Barley oil, 3 mL daily in two divided doses, or 30 g of barley bran flour daily.[3]
- **Constipation:** Limited research has used 9 g of germinated barley foodstuff (GBF) daily for up to 20 days.[11]
- *Note:* Most trials have used foods containing barley rather than barley oil or other forms.

Dosing: Pediatric (Younger Than 18 Years)

- Insufficient evidence to recommend.

Toxicology

- In rats, a 10% germinated barley foodstuff (GBF) diet administered for 28 days did not elicit signs of toxicity when compared to rats fed a control diet.[23] No deaths, hematological changes, chemistry value changes, behavior changes, growth changes, organ weight changes or histologic differences were found.[24]
- Consumption of concentrated barley beta-glucan (7%) did not cause treatment-related inflammatory or other adverse effects in mice after 28 days.[18,24]

ADVERSE EFFECTS/PRECAUTIONS/CONTRAINDICATIONS
Allergy

- Known allergy/hypersensitivity to barley flour or beer made with barley. Severe anaphylactic reactions and contact dermatitis have been reported from beer.[19-21] Malted barley is a basic ingredient found in beer.
- Numerous cases of type-1 hypersensitivity have been reported following beer ingestion, with confirmation via a positive challenge to beer, and positive skin tests and RAST for barley.[19,20,25,26] In one patient, cooked barley ingestion did not produce any symptoms. Some patients reported previous hypersensitivity to grass pollens and various other allergens, although cross-sensitivity was not determined. Patients with wheat allergy may experience symptoms with barley because of cross-reaction of gamma-3 hordein in barley with omega-5 gliadin in wheat.[27]
- Urticarial rash from beer has been reported in atopic subjects as a type-1 IgE-mediated hypersensitivity reaction.[28] Occupational contact urticaria was reported in a 20-year-old waitress, although drinking beer did not elicit a reaction.[29] Drinking beer has been associated with acute allergic reactions in three reported cases.[25] Symptoms experienced by a 34-year-old woman included tingling in the face, lip angioedema, chest tightness, dyspnea, and rhinoconjunctivitis; tongue angioedema, cough, wheezing, generalized urticaria, and fainting were experienced in a 20-year-old man after drinking beer; a 22-year-old woman experienced generalized urticaria immediately after drinking beer.
- "Bakers' asthma" is an allergic response resulting from the inhalation of cereal flours among workers of the baking and milling industries, and can occur due to barley flour exposure.[30,31] Cross-antigenicity has been shown to exist between different cereals.[32]

ADVERSE EFFECTS/POST-MARKET SURVEILLANCE

- **General:** Barley appears to be generally well tolerated in healthy adults in recommended doses for short periods of time, or as a cereal or in beer. Multiple cases of allergy have been reported, and cross-reactivity may occur with allergy to grass or wheat. Germinated barley foodstuff (GBF) in doses as high as 30 g was tolerated in 10 patients with mild to moderate active ulcerative colitis over a four-week period.[22]
- **Dermatologic:** Contact dermatitis associated with malt in beer has been documented in a case report.[21] Contact dermatitis of the eyelids and extremities has been reported in dock workers and silo operators.[33,34] Skin rash may occur on exposure to barley dust. Urticarial rash from beer has been reported in atopic subjects as a type-1 IgE-mediated hypersensitivity reaction.[28] Occupational contact urticaria was reported in a 20-year-old waitress, although drinking beer did not elicit a reaction.[29] Drinking beer has been associated with acute allergic reactions in three reported cases.[25] Symptoms experienced by a 34-year-old woman included tingling in the face, lip angioedema, chest tightness, dyspnea, and rhinoconjunctivitis; tongue angioedema, cough, wheezing, generalized urticaria, and fainting were experienced in a 20-year-old man after drinking beer; a 22-year-old woman experienced generalized urticaria immediately after drinking beer.
- **Neurologic:** Hordenine, an aminophenol in the root of germinating barley, is a sympathomimetic. In theory, effects may occur in the sympathetic nervous system, although human data in this area are lacking.
- **Ocular/otic:** Eye, nasal, and sinus irritation can occur on exposure to grain dust.

- **Pulmonary/respiratory:** Barley flours can be a source of inhalant allergens in asthma[35,36] and are a source of potential occupational exposure.[37,38] Sixty-nine of 80 dockworkers handling grains experienced "chest symptoms" when exposed to barley dust, and 13 others experienced evening "feverish episodes" after handling barley.[38] "Bakers' asthma" is an allergic response resulting from the inhalation of cereal flours among workers of the baking and milling industries, and can occur due to barley flour exposure.[30,31] Cross-antigenicity has been shown to exist between different cereals.[32] Inhalation of wild barley grass may result in bronchial irritation or pneumonitis.[39,40]
- **Gastrointestinal:** Six out of 10 patients with biopsy-proven celiac disease developed gastrointestinal upset and impairment of xylose excretion when challenged with barley.[41] In these patients, bowel function returned to normal and symptoms abated within 72 hours of stopping barley. A similar effect was noticed in one patient who ingested beer. Barley contains prolamine hordein, which may be responsible for these effects, similar to gliadins in wheat and rye.[45] Five infants fed a formula containing barley water, whole milk, and corn syrup developed malnutrition and microcytic hypochromic anemia, possibly due to deficiencies of iron, vitamin A, and vitamin C.[43] A paper was presented at the "Experimental Biology 2000" meeting suggesting that beta-glucan in barley and oatmeal can help to control appetite by increasing the feeling of fullness.[44]
- **Endocrine:** Barley contains more fermentable carbohydrate than other cereals such as rice. Fermentation of undigested carbohydrate produces short-chain fatty acids, some which may reduce hepatic glucose production and affect postprandial glycemia.[45]
- **Musculoskeletal:** Fungal contamination of barley by *Trichothecium roseum*, *Dreschelera ito*, and *Alternaria nees* has been associated with Kashin-Beck disease (KBD), which is an endemic degenerative osteochondropathy estimated to affect 1 million to 3 million people in rural China and Tibet.[46]

Precautions/Warnings/Contraindications

- Avoid use in patients with celiac disease; gluten found in barley may exacerbate this condition.
- Use cautiously in patients taking hypoglycemic agents, due to possible additive properties.

Pregnancy and Lactation

- Anecdotally, excessive consumption of barley sprouts is not advised during pregnancy.
- Infants fed a formula containing barley water, whole milk, and corn syrup have developed malnutrition and microcytic hypochromic anemia, possibly due to deficiencies of iron, vitamin A, and vitamin C.[43]

INTERACTIONS
Barley/Drug Interactions

- **Oral medications:** Fiber in barley may affect the absorption of oral agents by reducing gastrointestinal transit time.
- **Sympathomimetics:** Hordenine, an aminophenol in the root of germinating barley, is a sympathomimetic, and combination use may theoretically result in additive effects. Human data are lacking in this area.
- **Hypoglycemic drugs:** Barley contains more fermentable carbohydrate than other cereals such as rice. Fermentation of undigested carbohydrate produces short chain fatty acids, some which may reduce hepatic glucose production and

affect postprandial glycemia.[45] Barley use may result in lowered blood glucose concentrations, and when taken with hypoglycemic agents, theoretically may result in lower-than-expected blood glucose values.

- **Hyperlipidemic agents:** Barley use has been associated with decreased total cholesterol and low-density lipoprotein (LDL) concentrations, and may act additively with other cholesterol-lowering agents.[3,4,47,48]

Barley/Herb/Supplement Interactions

- **Oral herbs/supplements:** Fiber in barley may affect the absorption of oral agents by reducing gastrointestinal transit time.
- **Sympathomimetic agents:** Hordenine, an aminophenol in the root of germinating barley, is a sympathomimetic, and theoretically combination use may result in additive effects. Human data are lacking in this area.
- **Hypoglycemic herbs and supplements:** Barley contains more fermentable carbohydrate than other cereals such as rice. Fermentation of undigested carbohydrate produces short-chain fatty acids, some of which may reduce hepatic glucose production and affect postprandial glycemia.[45] Barley may result in lowered blood glucose concentrations, and when taken with hypoglycemic agents, theoretically may result in lower-than-expected blood glucose values.
- **Antihyperlipidemic herbs and supplements:** Barley use has been associated with decreased total cholesterol and low-density lipoprotein (LDL) concentrations, and may act additively with other cholesterol-lowering agents, such as niacin, garlic, guggul, and fish oil.[3,4,47,48]

Barley/Food Interactions

- Insufficient available data.

Barley/Lab Interactions

- **Serum glucose:** Barley contains more fermentable carbohydrate than other cereals such as rice. Fermentation of undigested carbohydrate produces short-chain fatty acids, some of which may reduce hepatic glucose production and affect postprandial glycemia.[45]
- **Lipid panel:** Barley use has been associated with decreased total cholesterol and low-density lipoprotein (LDL) concentrations.[3,4,47,48]

MECHANISM OF ACTION
Pharmacology

- **Glycemic effects:** Barley contains more fermentable carbohydrate than other cereals such as rice. Fermentation of undigested carbohydrate produces short-chain fatty acids, some of which may reduce hepatic glucose production and affect postprandial glycemia.[45] Because of viscous properties of beta-glucans, boiled flours appear to produce higher glucose and insulin responses compared to milled kernels.[49]
- **Metabolic effects:** Barley products composed of boiled intact (rice extender) and milled kernels (porridge) with different amylose-amylopectin ratios (7% to 44% amylose) have been reported to lower metabolic responses and raise satiety scores compared to white/wheat bread.[49]
- **Cholesterol effects:** Plasma lipid–lowering effects of barley have been attributed to rich amounts of beta-glucan, a water-soluble fiber.[4,50] The beta-glucan component of barley is believed to slow gastric emptying time, prolong the feeling of fullness, and stabilize blood sugars. Other contributory factors may be d-alpha–tocotrienol.[51] In chicks, high-protein barley flour (HPBF)–based diets increase body weight (18%),

suppress HMG-CoA reductase (−36%), impair fatty acid synthetase (−40%), and decrease serum triglyceride (−9%) and cholesterol levels (−23%).[48]

- **Sympathomimetic effects:** Hordenine, an aminophenol in the root of germinating barley, is a sympathomimetic. Human effects in this area have not been studied.
- **Gastrointestinal effects:** Germinated barley foodstuff (GBF) is derived from the aleurone and scutellum fractions of germinated barley. GBF appears to induce proliferation of intestinal epithelial cells and facilitate defecation through bacterial production of short-chain fatty acids, especially butyrate. GBF is believed to facilitate epithelial repair and suppress epithelial NFkB-DNA binding activity through butyrate (by the microflora bifidobacterium and eubacterium). GBF has been associated with increased growth of these microflora in the intestinal tract.[22,52]

Pharmacodynamics/Kinetics

- Barley contains greater amounts of soluble and non-soluble starches compared to other cereals, and approximately 17% of the carbohydrate in barley is not absorbed. This leads to fermentation in the colon by microflora, measurable by the hydrogen breath test.[45]
- Barley was historically used by the Romans to treat boils, and by the Greeks to treat gastrointestinal inflammation. The Roman physician Pliny reported that if a person affected with a boil took nine grains of barley, traced a circle around the boil three times with each grain, and then threw the barley into a fire with his left hand, the boil would be cured. Gladiators ate barley for strength and stamina and were called "hordearii" from the Latin word for barley, "hordeum."

REVIEW OF THE EVIDENCE: DISCUSSION
Hyperlipidemia
Summary

- Several small, randomized studies suggest that high-fiber barley, barley bran flour, and barley oil elicit small reductions in serum cholesterol levels by increasing cholesterol excretion. There is good evidence from existing research to support the use of barley along with a cholesterol-lowering diet in mild cases of hypercholesterolemia. Larger and longer studies are warranted to more rigorously confirm lasting benefits.

Controlled Trials

- McIntosh et al. compared the effects of barley and wheat in 21 men (aged 30-59 years) with hyperlipidemia (210-270 mg/dL) in a randomized, crossover trial.[4] No subjects were taking lipid-lowering drugs, none had a prior history of cardiovascular disease, and all appeared to be free of any overt liver, kidney, or thyroid disease. All patients were placed on a baseline diet for 3 weeks before entering two 4-week treatment periods of consuming barley or wheat foods. The authors reported that subjects in the barley group experienced a mean decrease in total cholesterol by 6% ($p < 0.05$), and in low-density lipoprotein (LDL) by 7% ($p < 0.02$). Triglycerides and glucose did not change significantly. Although this study appears to have been properly randomized, methods and statistical analysis were poorly described.
- Newman et al. examined the effects of barley or wheat in 14 healthy volunteers without chronic illnesses and not taking lipid-lowering drugs.[53] Volunteers were randomly assigned to receive barley or a 75% wheat/25% wheat bran diet for 6 weeks. Results showed an increase of serum cholesterol

Review of the Evidence: Barley

Condition Treated*	Study Design	Author, Year	N[†]	SS[†]	Study Quality[‡]	Magnitude of Benefit	ARR[†]	NNT[†]	Comments
Hyperlipidemia	Randomized, controlled, crossover trial	McIntosh[4] 1991	21	Yes	3	Small	NA	NA	Significant reductions in total cholesterol levels, no changes in triglycerides
Hyperlipidemia	Randomized, controlled, single-blind trial	Lupton[3] 1994	79	Yes	3	Small	NA	NA	Significant reductions in total cholesterol and LDL-C values.
Hyperlipidemia	Randomized, controlled, single-blind trial	Newman[53] 1989	14	No	2	None	NA	NA	No significant differences between diets with barley vs. barley/wheat (75%/25%) combination. Sample size may have been too small to detect between-group differences.
Hyperlipidemia	Randomized, controlled, single-blind, crossover trial	Keogh[8] 2003	18	No	1	None	NA	NA	No significant difference in serum cholesterol levels between diets with beta-glucan enriched barley and isoenergetic doses of glucose. Study likely underpowered.

*Primary or secondary outcome.
[†]N, Number of patients; SS, statistically significant; ARR, absolute risk reduction; NNT, the number of patients who need to undergo a specific intervention in order to observe an outcome in one individual.
[‡]0-2 = poor; 3-4 = good; 5 = excellent.
NA, Not applicable; LDL-C, low-density lipoprotein C.
For an explanation of each category in this table, please see Table 3 in the Introduction.

and low-density lipoprotein C (LDL-C) in the wheat group. Subjects with average pretreatment cholesterol concentrations did not experience any significant difference after receiving barley. However, those volunteers with higher pretreatment cholesterol concentrations experienced decreases in total cholesterol and LDL-C after receiving barley. Limiting factors of this trial were a lack of a placebo group, and a sample size that was potentially too small to adequately detect between-group differences.

- In a randomized, controlled trial, Lupton et al. studied the effects of barley oil, barley extract, and cellulose in 79 men and women with hyperlipidemia (230 mg/dL or higher).[3] Subjects were included who were not taking lipid-lowering therapy, were within 30% of ideal body weight, and had no significant history of diabetes mellitus, hypothyroidism, hyperthyroidism, alcohol or drug abuse, or liver or kidney disease. All subjects were instructed to follow the National Cholesterol Education Program Step I diet and were randomly assigned to one of three treatment arms during a 30-day study period: 30 g of added cellulose, 3 g of added barley oil extract, or 30 g of added barley bran flour. There was no placebo arm. Outcome measures included serologic cholesterol levels. The authors reported that barley bran flour decreased mean total cholesterol levels by 0.60 mmol/L (23.2 mg/dL) ($p = 0.0001$), and decreased LDL-C by 6.5% ($p = 0.036$). Barley oil was noted to decrease total cholesterol by 0.50 mmol/L (19.3 mg/dL) ($p = 0.002$) and LDL-C by 9.2% ($p = 0.003$). Total serum cholesterol or LDL-C of the cellulose control group did not decrease significantly over the same period. The lack of a placebo control or active control (such as an established drug therapy) limits the value of these results, as the reported data were compared with baseline values and may have been attributable to dietary changes only. In addition, the single-blind design may have allowed for the introduction of bias.
- An unpublished study presented at the "Experimental Biology 2000" meeting examined the effects of barley vs. wheat in mildly overweight individuals.[44] Sixty subjects

received muffins with either barley endosperm (containing 7 g of beta-glucan) in an easily absorbable form, barley (5 g of beta-glucan) in a form less easily absorbable, or refined wheat flour. All groups followed the National Cholesterol Education Program's Step I diet. Subjects were asked to rank their feelings of fullness, hunger, and satiety throughout the study. Results showed that those who ate barley muffins felt "fuller" and "more satisfied" throughout the study than those who ate wheat muffins. Other results revealed a weight loss of an average of 0.5 pound per week in those who ate barley compared to a weight gain of 0.5 pound in those who ate wheat muffins. The barley group demonstrated significant reductions in total cholesterol (11%) and LDL (12%). Although these results are suggestive, as unpublished results, they cannot be analyzed in detail.

- In a small randomized, controlled, single-blind crossover trial, Keogh et al. studied the effects of beta-glucan–enriched barley on serum cholesterol levels in 18 mildly hyperlipidemic men.[8] Subjects included were mildly hyperlipidemic men (4.0 +/− 0.6 mmol LDL cholesterol/L) with a body mass index of 27.4 ± 4.6 kg/m. All subjects were randomly assigned either to a treatment arm (8.1 to 11.9 g of beta-glucan per day scaled to body weight) or to a control arm (6.5 to 9.2 g of isoenergetic glucose per day), for 4 weeks. Then, after a 4-week washout period, the regimens were crossed over. At the study's end, the authors reported no statistically significant differences between groups in the primary outcomes of total serum cholesterol, low-density lipoprotein (LDL), or high-density lipoprotein (HDL). However, the small sample size and lack of power calculation allow for the possibility that absence of between-group differences was due to inadequate sample size rather than to a true lack of difference. In addition, aside from cholesterol levels, other specific inclusion/exclusion criteria were not specified, and baseline characteristics of subjects were not detailed. Therefore, some degree of heterogeneity may have characterized the cohort, and the two groups may have been dissimilar despite randomization. The single-blind design may have allowed for the introduction of bias. Notably, the effect of beta-glucan–enriched barley on lipid profiles was highly variable among subjects, suggesting that certain subgroups may be more sensitive to this intervention (although this study would not be able to detect such distinctions).

Case Series

- Lia et al. reported a case series of nine subjects who had undergone proctocolectomy 1 to 23 years earlier for ulcerative colitis, and had well-functioning ileostomies.[2] Subjects were administered one of four possible diets containing oat bran (OB), oat bran with beta-gluconase (OBE), barley (B), or wheat flour (W) for two consecutive days in random order, with 5 days between diet periods. The 24-hour excretion of bile acids and cholesterol was measured from samples collected every 2 hours by changing ileostomy bags. Results showed that mean total bile acid excretion was 53% higher in the OB diet period than in the OBE diet period. The excretion of beta-sitosetol and campesterol was significantly higher in the B diet period than in the OBE and W diet periods. Net cholesterol excretion was significantly higher in the B diet period than in the OBE and W diet periods. Median fatty acid excretion was 5.6%, 4.8%, 2.3%, and 0.9% in the OB, OBE, B, and W diet periods, respectively, with no significant differences found. This study was limited by a lack of control group and small sample size.

- Ikegami et al. conducted a case series to assess the effects of a rice-barley preparation on the lipid profiles of normolipidemic subjects (n = 5), hyperlipidemic men (n = 20), and mildly hyperlipidemic women (n = 7).[47] In place of rice, subjects received a boiled barley/rice (1:1 by weight) supplement twice a day for 2 to 4 weeks. Normolipidemic patients experienced no significant changes in their lipid profiles after 4 weeks of barley administration. Hypercholesterolemic men and women experienced a significant 10% mean decrease in total cholesterol levels and a 13% reduction in LDL values. Although these results are promising, limitations of the study include lack of a control group and small sample size.

Ulcerative Colitis
Summary

- Germinated barley foodstuff (GBF), derived from the aleurone and scutellum fractions of germinated barley, has been shown to increase short-chain fatty acids (especially butyrate) in the bowel, as well as fecal bifidobacterium and eubacterium.[52] Beneficial effects of GBF in ulcerative colitis have been proposed to result from maintenance of intestinal epithelial cells, and facilitation of colonic epithelial repair. Oral butyrate is completely absorbed in the small bowel and does not reach the colon, hence the potential utility of bacterial butyrate produced from GBF, which does appear to reach the large bowel.[22] Evidence of clinical benefit in this area is preliminary.

Evidence

- Kanauchi et al. published an open case series in 21 patients with mild to moderate active ulcerative colitis given 20 to 30 g of GBF daily for 24 weeks, in conjunction with baseline treatments of 5-ASA and/or steroids.[10] The authors noted a significant mean decrease in clinical activity index compared to baseline, particularly in the degree of visible blood in stools and nocturnal diarrhea. No clinically relevant side effects were detected. In a previous non-randomized controlled study, the same research group reported decreases in clinical index activity without adverse effects in a similar patient population (n = 18) administered 20 to 30 g of GBF over 4 weeks.[54] GBF was associated with increased fecal concentrations of bifidobacterium and eubacterium. The same research group (Kanauchi et al.) published a prior case series of 10 healthy volunteers given 30 g daily of GBF, and reported increased production of short-chain fatty acids, particularly butyrate, and increased fecal weight and water content.[55] Subsequently, 10 patients with mild to moderate active ulcerative colitis who had failed standard treatment were given 30 g of GBF in a non-randomized open-label fashion for 4 weeks.[22] Clinical and endoscopic improvement independent of disease extent was noted in these patients. Although these results are suggestive, the lack of use of standardized outcome measures, blinding, randomization, or parallel controls limits the clinical value of this research.

- In a similar case series reported by Mitsuyama et al., 10 patients with mild to moderate active ulcerative colitis who failed standard treatment were given 30 g of GBF in an open-label fashion for 4 weeks.[9] Results revealed a significant 59% decrease in mean clinical activity index score and 63% decrease in mean endoscopic index score. A significant increase in stool butyrate concentrations was also noted following GBF treatment ($p < 0.05$).

Hyperglycemia
Summary

- Preliminary evidence suggests that barley meal may improve glucose tolerance. This is believed to be due to fermentation of undigested carbohydrates in barley that decrease hepatic glucose production by up to 30%. Barley products have been shown to have a lower glycemic index compared to wheat or rice.

Evidence

- In a study by Thorburn et al., 10 healthy volunteers received 90 g of carbohydrates in the form of brown rice or barley in random order 1 week apart.[45] All subjects were found to have normal glucose tolerance. Outcomes were measured via an oral glucose tolerance test. Peak plasma glucose at 170 minutes in the barley meal group was found to be 0.7 mmol/L (~27 mg/dL) lower than in the rice group, and hepatic glucose production was significantly reduced following the barley meal. Plasma insulin concentrations were not significantly different after either the barley or rice meals. Breath test results demonstrated a greater amount of fermentable carbohydrate associated with barley than with rice. Notably, barley contains greater amount of soluble fiber and resistant starch than rice. No placebo group was evaluated.

- Liljeberg et al. examined the effects of two different diets in nine healthy volunteers with normal body mass indices.[13] Subjects were administered a diet containing high-fiber barley, white bread, whole meal oats, or whole meal barley porridge. Outcomes were measured via an oral glucose tolerance test. The authors reported a statistically significant decrease in the post-prandial glucose rise and insulin response in patients given high-fiber barley as a carbohydrate load vs. white bread, whole meal oats, or barley porridges. Although compelling, the small size and lack of placebo group limit the clinical applicability of this study.

Constipation
Summary

- Barley has been used traditionally as a treatment for constipation because of its high fiber content. However, there is limited clinical evidence in this area.

Evidence

- In a case series, Kanauchi et al. reported the effects of germinated barley foodstuff (GBF) on healthy and constipated patients.[11] Nine healthy volunteers received 9 g of GBF daily for 10 days, after which the dose was increased to 18 g for an additional 10 days. Outcome parameters included fecal weight and short-chain fatty acid content, which were compared to baseline values. Results indicated that GBF at both doses resulted in significant increases in fecal butyrate content and fecal weight compared to baseline. Following this study, a second investigation was conducted in 16 chronically constipated volunteers. These subjects were administered 9 g of GBF daily for 14 days. Measured outcome parameters included frequency and volume of stool and were assessed by a subjective questionnaire survey. The authors reported that GBF significantly improved these measures compared to baseline. However, a standardized measurement instrument was not used, long-term outcomes were not assessed, and the results were not compared to a control group. Due to these methodological weaknesses, this study can only be considered preliminary.

FORMULARY: BRANDS USED IN CLINICAL TRIALS

Forms of Barley Used in Statistically Significant Clinical Trials

- Barley bran flour, barley oil, germinated barley foodstuff (GBF), high-fiber barley.

References

1. Bourdon I, Yokoyama W, Davis P, et al. Postprandial lipid, glucose, insulin, and cholecystokinin responses in men fed barley pasta enriched with beta-glucan. Am J Clin Nutr 1999;69(1):55-63.
2. Lia A, Hallmans G, Sandberg AS, et al. Oat beta-glucan increases bile acid excretion and a fiber-rich barley fraction increases cholesterol excretion in ileostomy subjects. Am J Clin Nutr 1995;62(6):1245-1251.
3. Lupton JR, Robinson MC, Morin JL. Cholesterol-lowering effect of barley bran flour and oil. J Am Diet Assoc 1994;94(1):65-70.
4. McIntosh GH, Whyte J, McArthur R, et al. Barley and wheat foods: influence on plasma cholesterol concentrations in hypercholesterolemic men. Am J Clin Nutr 1991;53(5):1205-1209.
5. Newman RK, Newman CW, Graham H. The hypocholesterolemic function of barley beta-glucans. Cereal Foods World 1989;34:883-886.
6. Roberts DC, Truswell AS, Bencke A, et al. The cholesterol-lowering effect of a breakfast cereal containing psyllium fibre. Med J Aust 1994;161(11-12):660-664.
7. Liu S, Buring JE, Sesso HD, et al. A prospective study of dietary fiber intake and risk of cardiovascular disease among women. J Am Coll Cardiol 2002;39(1):49-56.
8. Keogh GF, Cooper GJ, Mulvey TB, et al. Randomized controlled crossover study of the effect of a highly beta-glucan-enriched barley on cardiovascular disease risk factors in mildly hypercholesterolemic men. Am J Clin Nutr 2003;78(4):711-718.
9. Mitsuyama K, Saiki T, Kanauchi O, et al. Treatment of ulcerative colitis with germinated barley foodstuff feeding: a pilot study. Aliment Pharmacol Ther 1998;12(12):1225-1230.
10. Kanauchi O, Mitsuyama K, Homma T, et al. Treatment of ulcerative colitis patients by long-term administration of germinated barley foodstuff: Multi-center open trial. Int J Mol Med 2003;12(5):701-704.
11. Kanauchi O, Mitsuyama K, Saiki T, et al. Germinated barley foodstuff increases fecal volume and butyrate production at relatively low doses and relieves constipation in humans. Int J Mol Med 1998;2(4):445-450.
12. Lupton JR, Morin JL, Robinson MC. Barley bran flour accelerates gastrointestinal transit time. J Am Diet Assoc 1993;93(8):881-885.
13. Liljeberg HG, Granfeldt YE, Bjorck IM. Products based on a high fiber barley genotype, but not on common barley or oats, lower postprandial glucose and insulin responses in healthy humans. J Nutr 1996;126(2):458-466.
14. Ostman EM, Liljeberg Elmstahl HG, Bjorck IM. Barley bread containing lactic acid improves glucose tolerance at a subsequent meal in healthy men and women. J Nutr 2002;132(6):1173-1175.
15. Yu YM, Wu CH, Tseng YH, et al. Antioxidative and hypolipidemic effects of barley leaf essence in a rabbit model of atherosclerosis. Jpn J Pharmacol 2002;89(2):142-148.
16. Yu YM, Chang WC, Chang CT, et al. Effects of young barley leaf extract and antioxidative vitamins on LDL oxidation and free radical scavenging activities in type 2 diabetes. Diabetes Metab 2002;28(2):107-114.
17. Kamimura A, Takahashi T. Procyanidin B-3, isolated from barley and identified as a hair-growth stimulant, has the potential to counteract inhibitory regulation by TGF-beta1. Exp Dermatol 2002;11(6):532-541.
18. Delaney B, Carlson T, Zheng GH, et al. Repeated dose oral toxicological evaluation of concentrated barley beta-glucan in CD-1 mice including a recovery phase. Food Chem Toxicol 2003;41(8):1089-1102.
19. Bonadonna P, Crivellaro M, Dama A, et al. Beer-induced anaphylaxis due to barley sensitization: two case reports. J Investig Allergol Clin Immunol 1999;9(4):268-270.
20. Santucci B, Cristaudo A, Cannistraci C, et al. Urticaria from beer in 3 patients. Contact Dermatitis 1996;34(5):368.
21. van Ketel WG. Immediate type allergy to malt in beer. Contact Dermatitis 1980;6(4):297-298.
22. Kanauchi O, Iwanaga T, Mitsuyama K. Germinated barley foodstuff feeding. A novel neutraceutical therapeutic strategy for ulcerative colitis. Digestion 2001;63 Suppl 1:60-67.
23. Nakamura T, Kanauchi O, Koike T. Toxic study of germinated barley foodstuff by 28 days continuous administration in rats. Pharmacometrics 1997;54(4):201-207.
24. Delaney B, Carlson T, Frazer S, et al. Evaluation of the toxicity of concentrated barley beta-glucan in a 28-day feeding study in Wistar rats. Food Chem Toxicol 2003;41(4):477-487.
25. Fernandez-Anaya S, Crespo JF, Rodriguez JR, et al. Beer anaphylaxis. J Allergy Clin Immunol 1999;103(5 Pt 1):959-960.
26. Keller K, Schwanitz HJ. Type I hypersensitivity to beer. Contact Dermatitis 1994;30(1):44-45.
27. Palosuo K, Alenius H, Varjonen E, et al. Rye gamma-70 and gamma-35 secalins and barley gamma-3 hordein cross-react with omega-5 gliadin, a major allergen in wheat-dependent, exercise-induced anaphylaxis. Clin Exp Allergy 2001;31(3):466-471.
28. Curioni A, Santucci B, Cristaudo A, et al. Urticaria from beer: an immediate hypersensitivity reaction due to a 10-kDa protein derived from barley. Clin Exp Allergy 1999;29(3):407-413.
29. Gutgesell C, Fuchs T. Contact urticaria from beer. Contact Dermatitis 1995;33(6):436-437.
30. Weiss W, Huber G, Engel KH, et al. Identification and characterization of wheat grain albumin/globulin allergens. Electrophoresis 1997;18(5):826-833.
31. Barber D, Sanchez-Monge R, Gomez L, et al. A barley flour inhibitor of insect alpha-amylase is a major allergen associated with baker's asthma disease. FEBS Lett 1989;248(1-2):119-122.
32. Block G, Tse KS, Kijek K, et al. Baker's asthma. Studies of the cross-antigenicity between different cereal grains. Clin Allergy 1984;14(2):177-185.
33. Cronin E. Contact dermatitis from barley dust. Contact Dermatitis 1979;5(3):196.
34. Pereira F, Rafael M, Lacerda MH. Contact dermatitis from barley. Contact Dermatitis 1998;39(5):261-262.
35. Nakase M, Usui Y, Alvarez-Nakase AM, et al. Cereal allergens: rice-seed allergens with structural similarity to wheat and barley allergens. Allergy 1998;53(46 Suppl):55-57.
36. Vidal C, Gonzalez-Quintela A. Food-induced and occupational asthma due to barley flour. Ann Allergy Asthma Immunol 1995;75(2):121-124.
37. Yap JC, Chan CC, Wang YT, et al. A case of occupational asthma due to barley grain dust. Ann Acad Med Singapore 1994;23(5):734-736.
38. Cockcroft AE, McDermott M, Edwards JH, et al. Grain exposure—symptoms and lung function. Eur J Respir Dis 1983;64(3):189-196.
39. Ammari FF, Faris KT, Mahafza TM. Inhalation of wild barley into the airways: two different outcomes. Saudi Med J 2000;21(5):468-470.
40. Dutau G. [Pneumopleurocutaneous fistula after inhalation of an ear of barley (Hordeum murinum)]. Ann Pediatr (Paris) 1990;37(6):367-370.
41. Baker PG, Read AE. Oats and barley toxicity in coeliac patients. Postgrad Med J 1976;52(607):264-268.
42. Ellis HJ, Doyle AP, Day P, et al. Demonstration of the presence of coeliac-activating gliadin-like epitopes in malted barley. Int Arch Allergy Immunol 1994;104(3):308-310.
43. Fabius RJ, Merritt RJ, Fleiss PM, et al. Malnutrition associated with a formula of barley water, corn syrup, and whole milk. Am J Dis Child 1981;135(7):615-617.
44. Keenan JM. Whole grains, refined grains. Paper presented at "Experimental Biology 2000" meeting, April 17, 2000, San Diego, California.
45. Thorburn A, Muir J, Proietto J. Carbohydrate fermentation decreases hepatic glucose output in healthy subjects. Metabolism 1993;42(6):780-785.
46. Chasseur C, Suetens C, Nolard N, et al. Fungal contamination in barley and Kashin-Beck disease in Tibet. Lancet 1997;350(9084):1074.
47. Ikegami S, Tomita M, Honda S, et al. Effect of boiled barley-rice-feeding in hypercholesterolemic and normolipemic subjects. Plant Foods Hum Nutr 1996;49(4):317-328.
48. Burger WC, Qureshi AA, Din ZZ, et al. Suppression of cholesterol biosynthesis by constituents of barley kernel. Atherosclerosis 1984;51(1):75-87.
49. Granfeldt Y, Liljeberg H, Drews A, et al. Glucose and insulin responses to barley products: influence of food structure and amylose-amylopectin ratio. Am J Clin Nutr 1994;59(5):1075-1082.
50. Delaney B, Nicolosi RJ, Wilson TA, et al. Beta-glucan fractions from barley

and oats are similarly antiatherogenic in hypercholesterolemic Syrian golden hamsters. J Nutr 2003;133(2):468-475.

51. Qureshi AA, Burger WC, Peterson DM, et al. The structure of an inhibitor of cholesterol biosynthesis isolated from barley. J Biol Chem 1986;261(23): 10544-10550.

52. Kanauchi O, Fujiyama Y, Mitsuyama K, et al. Increased growth of *Bifidobacterium* and *Eubacterium* by germinated barley foodstuff, accompanied by enhanced butyrate production in healthy volunteers. Int J Mol Med 1999;3(2):175-179.

53. Newman RK, Lewis SE, Newman CW, et al. Hypocholesterolemic effect of barley foods on healthy men. Nutr Rep Int 1989;39:749-760.

54. Kanauchi O, Suga T, Tochihara M, et al. Treatment of ulcerative colitis by feeding with germinated barley foodstuff: first report of a multicenter open control trial. J Gastroenterol 2002;37 Suppl 14:67-72.

55. Kanauchi O, Mitsuyama K, Saiki T, et al. Germinated barley foodstuff increases fecal volume and butyrate production in humans. Int J Mol Med 1998;1(6):937-941.

B

Belladonna
(*Atropa belladonna* L. or var. acuminata Royle ex Lindl)

SYNONYMS/COMMON NAMES/RELATED SUBSTANCES

- Beladona, belladone, belladonnae herbae pulvis standardisatus, belladonna herbum, belladonna leaf, belladonna pulvis normatus, belladonnae folium, belladonna radix, belladonne, deadly nightshade, deadly nightshade leaf, devil's cherries, devil's herb, die belladonna, die tollkirsche, divale, dwale, dwayberry, galnebaer, great morel, herba belladonna, hoja de belladonna, naughty man's cherries, poison black cherries, powdered belladonna, Solanaceae, solanum mortale, solanum somniferum, stryshon, strygium, tollekirsche, tollkirschenblatter.
- **Selected combination products:** Bellergal, Bellergal-S, Bellergil, Bel-Phen-Ergot S, B&O Supprettes, Cafergot-PB, Distovagal, Phenerbel-S, PMS-Opium & Beladonna.

CLINICAL BOTTOM LINE
Background

- Belladonna is an herb that has been used for centuries for a variety of indications, including headache, menstrual symptoms, peptic ulcer disease, inflammation, and motion sickness. Belladonna is known to contain active agents with anticholinergic properties, such as the tropane alkaloids atropine, hyoscine (scopolamine) and hyoscyamine.
- There are few available studies of belladonna monotherapy for any indication. Most research has evaluated belladonna in combination with other agents such as ergot alkaloids or barbiturates, or in homeopathic (diluted) preparations. Preliminary evidence suggests possible efficacy in combination with barbiturates for the management of symptoms associated with irritable bowel syndrome. However, there is currently insufficient scientific evidence regarding the use of belladonna for this or any other indication.
- There is extensive literature on the adverse effects and toxicity of belladonna, related principally to its known anticholinergic actions. Common adverse effects include dry mouth, urinary retention, flushing, papillary dilation, constipation, confusion, and delirium. Many of these effects may occur at therapeutic doses.

Scientific Evidence for Common/Studied Uses	Grade
Airway obstruction	C
Autonomic nervous system disturbances	C
Headache	C
Irritable bowel syndrome	C
Otitis media	C
Premenstrual syndrome	C
Radiodermatitis	C
Menopausal symptoms	D

*Key to grades: *A:* Strong scientific evidence for this use; *B:* Good scientific evidence for this use; *C:* Unclear scientific evidence for this use; *D:* Fair scientific evidence against this use (it may not work); *F:* Strong scientific evidence against this use (it likely does not work). For a more detailed explanation of efficacy criteria, see "Natural Standard Evidence-Based Validated Grading Rationale" in the Introduction.

Historical or Theoretical Uses That Lack Sufficient Evidence

- Abnormal menstrual bleeding, acute inflammation, anesthetic, antispasmodic, anxiety,[1,2] arthritis, asthma, chickenpox, colds, colitis, conjunctivitis, diarrhea, diuresis, diverticulitis, earache, encephalitis, fever, flu, gout, hay fever, hemorrhoids, hyperemesis gravidarum, hyperkinesis (excessive motor function), hyperhidrosis (excessive sweating), measles, menstrual irregularities,[3] motion sickness, mumps, muscle and joint pain, mydriasis, nausea and vomiting during pregnancy, neuralgia, nocturnal enuresis, organophosphate poisoning, Parkinson's disease, pancreatitis, peptic ulcer disease,[4] rash, scarlet fever, sciatica, sedative, sore throat, teething, toothache, ulcerative colitis, urolithiasis, urinary retention,[5] warts, whooping cough.

Expert Opinion and Historic Precedent

- Belladonna was used during ancient times as a poison, and likely a medicinal, although knowledge of its therapeutic action dates to the 19th century.[6] A prominent 19th century London physician, Charles Williams, studied belladonna as part of his investigations into the pathophysiology of asthma.[7] In the same era in Paris, belladonna was introduced in the treatment of Parkinson's disease by Ordenstein, a pupil of Charcot.[8]
- Belladonna was also prescribed by the founder of homeopathy, the German physician Samuel Hahnemann. By the principle of homeopathy, that "like cures like," belladonna in homeopathic dilutions is said to be a remedy for inflammation characterized by the triad of redness, swelling, and pain. It is believed to act during the night and to have an affinity for the head, throat, and ears.[9]
- While studies in the late 1970s examined the effects of belladonna on irritable bowel syndrome, more recent placebo-controlled trials have examined homeopathic prophylaxis for migraine,[10] homeopathic treatment of radiodermatitis,[11] and the treatment of airway obstruction in infants.[12]

Safety Summary

- **Possibly safe:** When taken by healthy individuals in recommended doses for a short duration, or when taken in homeopathic dilutions. Notably, there are numerous available preparations of belladonna alkaloids, the majority of which have not been evaluated for safety in controlled trials.
- **Possibly unsafe:** When taken by individuals with medical conditions such as congestive heart failure, hypertension, coronary artery disease, cardiac arrhythmias, constipation, partial or complete bowel obstruction, narrow-angle glaucoma, prostatic obstruction, myasthenia gravis, and urinary retention.
- **Likely unsafe:** When taken in large doses by children or adults. When taken by breastfeeding or pregnant women. When taken concurrently with other agents that possess anticholinergic properties.

DOSING/TOXICOLOGY
General

- Recommended doses are based on those most commonly used in available trials, or on historical practice. However, with natural products, the optimal doses needed to balance efficacy and safety often have not been determined. Formulations and preparation methods may vary from manufacturer to manufacturer, and from batch to batch of a specific product made by a single manufacturer. Non-homeopathic dilutions of belladonna should clearly state the quantity of tropane alkaloids contained.

Standardization

- There is no current widely used standardized preparation of belladonna.
- Doses of belladonna are generally calculated by milligrams of total alkaloids. *Atropa belladonna* contains up to 20 different tropane alkaloid compounds. Those present in the largest concentration in leaves include hyoscyamine (68.7%), apoatropine (17.9%), 3α-phenylacetoxytropane (2.8%), cuscohygrine (2.5%), and scopolamine (0.8%). Those present in the largest concentration in roots include hyoscyamine (36.7%), cuscohygrine (31.5%), 6-hydroxyhyoscyamine (8.9%), hygrine (6%), 6-hydroxyapoatropoine (3.6%), scopolamine (2.9%), and apoatropine (1.7%).[13]
- The commercial preparation Bellergal contains 40 mg of phenobarbital, 0.6 mg of ergotamine tartrate, and 0.2 mg of levorotatory alkaloids of belladonna.[14-16]
- The commercial preparation Donnatal contains 0.1037 mg of hyoscyamine sulfate, 0.0194 mg of atropine sulfate, 0.0065 mg of hyoscine hydrobromide, and 16.2 mg of phenobarbital.[17]

Dosing: Adult (18 Years and Older)
Oral

- **Traditional dosing:** Traditional doses have included belladonna leaf powder, 50 to 100 mL per dose, with a maximum single dose of 200 mg (0.6 mg of total alkaloids, calculated as hyoscyamine) and a maximum daily dose of 600 mg (equivalent to 1.8 mg of total alkaloids calculated as hyoscyamine); belladonna root, 50 mg per dose, with a maximum single dose of 100 mg (0.5 mg of total alkaloids, calculated as hyoscyamine) and a maximum daily dose of 300 mg (equivalent to 1.5 mL of total alkaloids calculated as hyoscyamine); or belladonna extract, 10 mg per dose, with a maximum single dose of 100 mg (0.5 mg of total alkaloids, calculated as hyoscyamine) and a maximum daily dose of 150 mL (equivalent to 2.2 mL of total alkaloids calculated as hyoscyamine). These doses have been noted by the expert German panel, the Commission E, principally for the treatment of "gastrointestinal spasm." Other anecdotal reports have suggested a tincture of belladonna (27 to 33 mg of belladonna leaf alkaloids per 100 mL), at 1.5 mg per day, divided into three doses per day with a double dose at bedtime, or 0.6 to 1 mL (0.18 to 0.3 mg of belladonna leaf alkaloids) three to four times daily.
- **Irritable bowel syndrome:** Placebo-controlled trials during the 1960s and 1970s examined several doses and preparations of belladonna for irritable bowel, including Hyoscine butylbromide, 10 mg taken four times daily, or a combination preparation containing 0.25 mg of levorotatory alkaloids of belladonna plus 50 mg of phenobarbital.[18,19] Donnatal tablets (0.1037 mg of hyoscyamine sulfate, 0.0194 mg of atropine sulfate, 0.0065 mg of hyoscine hydrobromide, 16.2 mg of phenobarbital) have also been used.[17] A higher daily dose was used in one study, including 8 mg of belladonna and 30 mg of phenobarbital, although because of the known toxicity of belladonna, that dose may not be advisable.[20] Traditional doses are listed above.

- **Autonomic nervous system disturbances:** Limited data are available in this area. One small clinical trial administered a combination formula, including 15 mg of belladonna, 60 mg of ergot alkaloids, 15 mg of propranolol, and 25 mg of amobarbital, taken three times a day for 2 weeks, and noted improvements in 72% of subjects with autonomic dysfunction (diseases poorly described).[21]
- **Headache:** Studies in the 1960s and 1970s reported unimpressive effects on headache with the combination product Bellergal (40 mg of phenobarbital, 0.6 mg of ergotamine tartrate, 0.2 mg of levorotatory alkaloids of belladonna, taken twice daily).[14-16]
- **Premenstrual syndrome:** Bellergal (40 mg of phenobarbital, 0.6 mg of ergotamine tartrate, 0.2 mg of levorotatory alkaloids of belladonna) taken twice daily for 10 days prior to menses was evaluated in one poorly reported 1970s trial.[22]
- **Menopausal symptoms:** A placebo-controlled trial found no effects on menopausal symptoms with 4 weeks of Bellergal Retard (total daily dose: 80 mg of phenobarbital, 1.2 mg of ergotamine tartrate, 0.4 mg of levorotatory alkaloids of belladonna).[23]
- **Homeopathic dosing:** (*Note:* Homeopathic dosing is often dependent on the indication, presentation, and philosophy of the practitioner, and dosing standards may range widely.) In general, homeopathic preparations are initially diluted 1:10 or 1:100. Serial dilutions are continued until desired concentrations are achieved. When a 1:10 dilution is diluted 30 times, it is said to be a 30X or 30D potency. When a 1:100 dilution is diluted 30 times, it is referred to as a 30C potency. "Proving studies" have been conducted to investigate the effects of homeopathic belladonna in healthy volunteers and have used preparations of Belladonna 30CH (Deutsche Homöopathie-Union Karlsruhe, Germany)[9] and Belladonna C30 (Ainsworth's Homeopathic Pharmacy, UK), 1 tablet twice daily.[24]
- **Radiodermatitis:** Belladonna 7CH (Laboratoires Boiron, France), 3 granules sublingually taken twice daily, has been used in a controlled trial in patients with breast cancer.[11]

Topical

- **Musculoskeletal:** The topical use of a belladonna plaster produced by Cuxson Gerrard (England) containing 0.25% belladonna alkaloids (hysoscine 2%, atropine 1%) has been described in a case report and may be associated with contact dermatitis after prolonged use.[25]

Dosing: Pediatric (Younger Than 18 Years)
Oral

- **Traditional dosing:** Anecdotal use suggests a typical pediatric dose to be 0.03 mL/kg three times daily or 0.8mL/m^2 three times daily (27 to 33 mg of belladonna leaf alkaloids per 100 mL). Maximum dose has been reported as 3.5 mL per day. Safety and efficacy have not been clearly demonstrated.
- **Airway obstruction:** A poorly reported controlled trial administered a tincture of belladonna, in a dose equivalent to 0.01 mg/kg of atropine, at bedtime to infants.[12]
- *Note:* Death in children may occur at 0.2 mg/kg of atropine.[26] Thus, two fruits may be lethal for a small child (2 mg of atropine are often found in a fruit).[27]
- **Homeopathic dosing:** (*Note:* Homeopathic dosing is often dependent on the indication, presentation, and philosophy of the practitioner, and dosing standards may range widely.) In general, homeopathic preparations are initially diluted 1:10 or 1:100. Serial dilutions are continued until desired concentrations are achieved. When a 1:10 dilution is diluted

30 times, it is said to be a 30X or 30D potency. When a 1:100 dilution is diluted 30 times, it is referred to as a 30C potency.

- **Otitis media:** An observational study comparing homeopathic with conventional treatment for children with otitis media utilized Belladonna 30X globules (brand and dose not specified).[28] Favorable results were reported, although the study was poorly designed and described.

Toxicology

- At a dose of up to 1.5 mg per day, belladonna is traditionally considered to be safe, although many people will experience anticholinergic side effects. The most common manifestations of belladonna overdose include anticholinergic symptoms such as dilated pupils, flushing, dry mouth, tachycardia, confusion, agitation, and hallucinations.[6,29] The anticholinergic effects of belladonna can be dangerous at high doses and may result in severe side effects or death. Death in children may occur at 0.2 mg/kg atropine.[26] Thus, two fruits may be lethal for a small child (2 mg of atropine are often found in a fruit).[27]
- Cases of belladonna poisoning with plant ingestions have long been reported in the literature, including an early (1921) report of belladonna poisoning from eating rabbits that had been feeding on belladonna.[30] Case reports include anticholinergic poisoning symptoms in children and adults after ingestion of deadly nightshade berries.[27,31,32] Several case reports exist of belladonna poisoning after ingestion of tomatoes grown from a plant grafted to jimson weed (*Datura stramonium*).[33] A case report describes a 68-year-old Italian man who presented with agitation, hallucinations, slurred speech, tachycardia, dilated pupils, hypertonia, and myoclonic jerks after ingestion of berries from deadly nightshade (*Atropa belladonna*).[34] A study of plant intoxications in Switzerland over a period of 29 years revealed 152 severe cases, of which 62 were caused by *Atropa belladonna, Datura stramonium,* and *Hyoscyamus niger.*[29]
- A case report from Chicago describes a 4-year-old girl with symptoms consistent with anticholinergic poisoning after ingestion of woody nightshade (*Solanum dulcamara*), a relative of belladonna that contains solanine, not generally thought to have anticholinergic effects. She was administered 0.2 mg (0.02 mg/kg) of physostigmine three times in an hour with complete resolution of symptoms. Despite the unusual plant exposure, this report serves as evidence of the efficacy of physostigmine as an antidote for anticholinergic poisoning.[35] However, a recent case report of two adults with belladonna poisoning reports supportive therapy, not physostigmine, to be efficacious.[27]
- Belladonna toxicity has been reported with various routes of administration, including topical plaster.[36] There are several case series of ingestion of approximately 0.5 to 1.5 teaspoons of Asthmadore powder (belladonna and stramonium alkaloids, 0.23% to 0.31%; R. Schiffman Co., Los Angeles) for the purpose of experiencing hallucinatory effects that resulted in hallucinations, agitation, tachycardia, tachypnea, dilated pupils, blurred vision, and unsteady gait. After 7 to 24 hours of observation, the subjects in these case series fully recovered.[37-39]
- Belladonna overdose should be considered serious and should be treated by qualified medical professionals. Due to the anticholinergic inhibitory effects on gastric emptying, delayed ingestion with resultant prolonged toxicity may occur.[26]

ADVERSE EFFECTS/PRECAUTIONS/CONTRAINDICATIONS
Allergy

- Known allergy/hypersensitivity to belladonna and anticholinergic drugs.
- Known allergy to other members of the Solanaceae (nightshade) family, such as bell peppers, potatoes, and eggplants.
- Allergic contact dermatitis may develop with prolonged use of topical belladonna preparations, even at low concentrations.[25]

Adverse Effects

- **General:** Adverse reactions are common with belladonna alkaloid use. Doses of 0.5 mg or greater may cause anticholinergic side effects of varying severity. Anticholinergic effects may include dry mouth, urinary retention, flushing, pupillary dilation, constipation, and confusion. There is some evidence that in homeopathic (dilute) concentrations, oral belladonna may not elicit clinically relevant anticholinergic signs or symptoms.[40]
- **Dermatologic:** Case reports of toxicity have described redness of the skin, flushing, and dry skin. Allergic contact dermatitis has been reported with use of topical belladonna plaster, even at dilute concentrations.[25] Two incidences of rash and hives were noted with belladonna-phenobarbital-ergotamine treatment.[16] Anecdotal reports have mentioned such other adverse effects as fixed drug eruptions, Stevens-Johnson syndrome, and photosensitivity.
- **Neurologic/CNS:** Case reports have described headache, excitement, agitation, dizziness, lightheadedness, drowsiness, unsteadiness, confusion, hallucinations, slurred speech, sedation, hyperreflexia, convulsions, vertigo and coma.[29,30,33,34,37-39,41]
- **Ocular/Otic:** Ocular effects may include mydriasis, photophobia, blurred vision, and dilation of pupils.[30,35,37-39,41,42] Belladonna splinters placed in the eye have been associated with fixed mydriasis.[43]
- **Psychiatric:** Hallucinations and acute psychosis have been documented in cases of toxicity.[26,27,29,34,37-39]
- **Respiratory:** Rapid respiration has been reported in cases of toxicity,[37] as well as coma with respiratory arrest requiring mechanical ventilation.[26]
- **Cardiovascular:** Tachycardia has been reported in cases of toxicity.[26,30,37,38,41,44] Belladonna contains atropine, which is commonly used in hospitals to increase heart rate. In one report, infants who received hyoscyamine sulfate developed heart rates of 155 to 220 beats per minute when given 2 to 4 mL of hyoscyamine.[42] Severe hypertension has been documented,[45] as have ventricular premature beats, in patients with belladonna poisoning.[46]
- **Gastrointestinal:** Case reports have noted dry mouth resulting from belladonna use or toxicity.[30,33,37-39,41,44] Other anecdotal or theoretical effects include abdominal distention and reduction in salivary flow.[33]
- **Genitourinary:** Urinary retention has been documented.[38,44]
- **Endocrine:** Case reports have documented decreased perspiration.[35] Anecdotal references note a possibility of decreased flow of breast milk.
- **Musculoskeletal:** Anecdotal reports have noted muscle tremor, rigidity, and crampy leg pains.[27,33,36]

Precautions/Warnings/Contraindications

- Avoid in elderly patients and in children, based on numerous case reports of serious effects of belladonna poisoning in these age groups.

- Avoid in patients using other anticholinergic agents.
- Use cautiously in patients with cardiac disease, including coronary heart disease, congestive heart failure, hypertension, cardiac arrhythmias, or unstable cardiovascular status, because of case reports of cardiac effects (hypertension, tachycardia, arrhythmias) with belladonna poisoning.
- Use cautiously in patients with gastrointestinal tract disease such as ulcers, esophageal reflux, hiatal hernia, obstructive gastrointestinal disease, constipation, ileus or atony, colitis, ileostomy, and colostomy. Belladonna's anticholinergic effects may delay gastric emptying and decrease esophageal pressure.
- Use cautiously in patients with urinary retention, prostatic hypertrophy or obstruction, or obstructive uropathy. Due to belladonna's anticholinergic effects, these conditions may be aggravated.
- Use cautiously in patients with narrow-angle glaucoma, because of a theoretical increase in ocular tension.
- Use cautiously in patients with Sjögren's syndrome, xerostomia, or lachrymal problems, because of belladonna's anticholinergic effects.
- Use cautiously in patients with neuromuscular disorders such as myasthenia gravis, as belladonna may cause neuromuscular blockade resulting in weakness or paralysis.
- Use cautiously in patients with fever.
- Use cautiously in patients with Down syndrome, as they may be particularly sensitive to anticholinergic effects of belladonna.

Pregnancy and Lactation

- Not recommended because of the potential for toxicity and adverse outcomes.
- Belladonna is listed under category C according to the U.S. Food and Drug Administration. Belladonna alkaloids are excreted in breast milk, thereby exposing infants to potential toxicity.
- One small, case-control study of neonatal death and congenital malformations showed no increase in these outcomes in mothers ingesting belladonna alkaloids.[47] In another study, there was an increase in birth defects in the offspring of mothers who had taken belladonna, although no relationship between first trimester use of atropine and birth defects was found.[48]
- There have been anecdotal reports that use of belladonna during pregnancy may increase risk of respiratory abnormalities, hypospadias (penile urethral anomalies in males), and eye/ear malformations.

INTERACTIONS
Belladonna/Drug Interactions

- **Oral medications:** Belladonna may delay gastrointestinal transit time and thereby affect absorption of some medications.
- **Drugs that interact with anticholinergic agents:** Numerous drugs and drug classes may interact with anticholinergic agents. Examples include acetophenenazine, amantadine, amitriptyline, atropine, benztropine, bethanechol, biperiden, brompheniramine, carbinoxamine, chlorpromazine, clemastine, clindinium, clozapine, cyclopentolate, cyproheptadine, dicyclomine, diphenhydramine, dixyrazine, ethopropazine, fenoterol, fluphenazine, haloperidol, homatropine, hyoscyamine, ipratropium, loxapine, mesoridazine, methdilazine, methotrimeprazine, olanzapine, oxybutynin, perazine, periciazine, perphenazine, pimozide, pipotiazine, prochlorperazine, procyclidine, promazine, promethazine, propiomazine, quinidine, scopolamine, thiethylperazine, thioridazine, thiothixene, trifluoperazine, triflupromazine, trihexyphenidyl, trimeprazine, and triprolidine.
- **Drugs that interact with atropine:** Atropine is a constituent of belladonna. Theoretically, drugs that interact with atropine may also interact with belladonna. Examples include ambenonium, arbutamine, belladonna, cisapride, cromolyn, halothane, methacholine, and procainamide.
- **Tricyclic antidepressant drugs:** Because of the anticholinergic properties of belladonna, interactions may occur with tricyclic antidepressant drugs.
- **Cisapride:** Atropine, a constituent of belladonna, has been reported to block the effects of cisapride on peristaltic contractions.[49] When atropine was administered before cisapride, the effects of cisapride on lower esophageal sphincter pressure were antagonized. The effect did not occur when atropine was administered after cisapride.
- **Antiarrhythmic drugs:** Administering belladonna with procainamide may result in additive anti-vagal effects on atrioventricular nodal conduction.
- **Alcohol:** Concomitant use of alcohol with belladonna may theoretically result in additive CNS depression.
- **Tacrine (Cognex):** In mice, cognitive deficits associated with belladonna alkaloid administration are attenuated by tacrine.[50]

Belladonna/Herb/Supplement Interactions

- **Oral agents:** Belladonna may delay gastrointestinal transit time and thereby affect absorption of some agents.
- **Anticholinergic herbs and supplements:** Combination use of belladonna with anticholinergic agents may potentiate its therapeutic and adverse effects. Examples of anticholinergic herbs include bittersweet (*Solanum dulcamara*), henbane (*Hyoscyamus niger*), and jimsonweed (*Datura stramonium*).

Belladonna/Food Interactions

- Insufficient available evidence.

Belladonna/Lab Interactions

- Insufficient available evidence.

MECHANISM OF ACTION
Pharmacology

- Belladonna alkaloids are competitive inhibitors of the muscarinic actions of acetylcholine, acting at receptors located in exocrine glands, smooth and cardiac muscle, and intramural neurons.
- The belladonna constituent scopolamine exerts greater effects on the CNS, eye, and secretory glands than the constituents atropine and hyoscyamine. Atropine exerts more activity on the heart, intestine, and bronchial muscle, and exhibits a more prolonged duration of action compared to scopolamine. Hyoscyamine exerts similar actions to atropine but has more potent central and peripheral nervous system effects.
- A single-blind placebo-controlled study was conducted to investigate the cardiorespiratory effects of belladonna, as a surrogate measure of vagal activity.[51] Single doses of an oral belladonna tincture containing 0.1 mg/mL alkaloid concentration were administered, with a proportion of atropine to scopolamine of 20:1. In eight healthy young subjects, heart rate and noninvasive arterial finger blood pressure were recorded for 4 hours following oral application of 1 mL,

2 mL, or 5 mL of this belladonna tincture or placebo. The authors reported that 1 hour after administration of 5 mL, mean respiratory rate, heart rate, and baroreflex sensitivity decreased significantly in six of eight subjects. In contrast, following administration of 1 to 2 mL, mean respiratory rate and heart rate increased compared to placebo.

Pharmacodynamics/Kinetics

- The belladonna constituent atropine has a reported half-life of several hours and is rarely detectable in the plasma after 24 hours. Elimination half-life of atropine from raw or cooked belladonna berries was reported to be approximately 120 to 140 minutes in a case report of toxic ingestion.[26]
- Atropine is primarily renally excreted. Renal clearance of atropine following ingestion of raw or cooked belladonna berries is variable, depending on the form ingested, but may be as high as 3.6 mg/24 hours.[26]

HISTORY

- The name belladonna means "beautiful woman" in Italian, and is derived from the use of this herb by 16th-century Venetian women to self-induce dilated pupils and flushed cheeks in order to make them appear more attractive.
- Possible references to the intoxicating properties of belladonna alkaloids appear throughout historical literature, including Homer's *Iliad* and *Odyssey*. The poison used by Friar Lawrence to put Juliet to sleep in Shakespeare's *Romeo and Juliet* may have been belladonna.
- Belladonna has been used for centuries in the religious rites of Native North and South Americans, including the Algonquians and Incas. It was reported to be the agent in a poisoning of soldiers in Jamestown, Virginia in 1676, where *Datura stramonium* (a relative of *Atropa belladonna*) was known as "Jamestown weed."[6]
- In the late 1960s, there were several reports that Asthmador, a compound of belladonna and stramonium alkaloids, was being used in a number of different communities in the United States as a hallucinogen. There are case reports in the medical literature describing overdoses of Asthmador taken for this effect.[52]

REVIEW OF THE EVIDENCE: DISCUSSION
Irritable Bowel Syndrome
Summary

- Anticholinergic medications have been used for years in the treatment of irritable bowel syndrome. Patients with this disorder are thought to have abnormal colonic motility, and their symptoms may be replicated with a cholinergic agonist. Although the mechanism of action provides a compelling case for the use of belladonna, there have only been limited controlled trials of belladonna in combination with phenobarbital in heterogeneous samples, and one study that showed a trend toward improved symptoms in patients treated with the belladonna constituent hyoscine (scopolamine). Therefore, there is currently insufficient evidence to recommend belladonna as a monotherapy for the treatment of irritable bowel syndrome.

Evidence

- An early (1959) contribution to the literature was a 15-month double-blind trial of 75 patients with "irritable colon," treated with Belladenal spacetabs (0.25 mg of levorotatory alkaloids of belladonna plus 50 mg of phenobarbital), placebo, or both.[18] The percentage of patients that improved

was 70% with Belladenal treatment, compared to a 24% placebo response. The study provides limited detail, and methods, outcome measurement techniques, and statistical analysis were not adequately described.

- A 1966 double-blind, crossover trial of 140 patients with gastrointestinal spasm compared Donnatal tablets (belladonna [0.1037 mg of hyoscyamine sulfate, 0.0194 mg of atropine sulfate, 0.0065 mg of hyoscine hydrobromide] plus 16.2 mg of phenobarbital) with Valpin (anisotropine, with or without phenobarbital).[17] Baseline diagnoses of subjects were heterogeneous, including spastic colon and peptic ulcer disease. The authors reported "excellent" or "good" results in 96% of subjects treated with anisotropine plus phenobarbital, 86% of subjects treated with anisotropine alone, and 70% of subjects treated with belladonna plus phenobarbital. However, inconsistent results were noted depending on the order of crossover, suggesting a possible lack of adequate washout period. In addition, greater variability was observed in the results for belladonna than for the other medications. This study was poorly designed and reported, and evaluated outcomes subjectively. It is therefore of limited clinical value.
- In a randomized, double-blind trial, Rhodes et al. compared five different sedative-anticholinergic medications with placebo in 22 patients with irritable bowel syndrome.[20] Treatments were administered serially, and effects were measured via a patient questionnaire. Each treatment was given four times daily for 1 month. The dose of belladonna administered was 8 mg, combined with 30 mg phenobarbital. The symptom index questionnaire revealed no significant effect of any of the treatments vs. placebo. However, a significant number of patients (7/15) "preferred" the belladonna/phenobarbital combination to the other treatments. This study was limited by a small sample size, lack of use of a validated outcomes measure, inadequate descriptions of blinding, randomization, or statistical analysis, and a high dropout rate (27%).
- The effects of hyoscine butylbromide (10 mg four times a day), lorazepam, and ispaghula husk were studied in a sample of 96 patients with irritable bowel syndrome.[19] Eight groups of 12 patients were randomized to all possible combinations of these three therapies and placebo. Each therapy demonstrated a trend toward improved symptoms over the 3-month trial, although results were only significant for ispaghula husk. Methods and statistical analysis were not well described.

Prevention of Airway Obstruction
Summary

- Anticholinergic agents such as belladonna cause relaxation of smooth muscles of the airway and a reduction in production of mucus. Although the known mechanism of belladonna is compelling for this use, there is only limited human research in this area. One study looking at treatment of airway obstruction during sleep in infants demonstrated a beneficial effect of belladonna. However, because of a lack of other controlled trials, there is currently insufficient evidence to recommend belladonna for the prevention of airway obstruction.

Evidence

- Kahn et al. studied obstructed breathing in the sleep of 20 infants (average age, 12 weeks) with a history of breath-holding spells.[12] This randomized, double-blind, crossover trial lasted for 14 days, with each infant spending one night

Review of the Evidence: Belladonna

Condition Treated*	Study Design	Author, Year	N[†]	SS[†]	Study Quality[‡]	Magnitude of Benefit	ARR[†]	NNT[†]	Comments
Irritable bowel syndrome	Randomized controlled trial	Lichstein[18] 1959	75	Unclear	3	46%	2	NA	Combination formula Belladenal spacetabs studied (0.25 mg of belladonna alkaloids and 50 mg of phenobarbital).
Gastrointestinal spasm	Randomized controlled trial	King[17] 1966	140	No	3	NA	NA	NA	Combination formula Donnatal studied (hyoscyamine, atropine, hyoscine, + phenobarbital) vs. Valpin (anisotropine ± phenobarbital). Crossover design.
Irritable bowel	Randomized controlled trial	Rhodes[20] 1978	16	Mixed	3	Small	NA	NA	No improvement in symptom index compared to placebo. 27% dropout.
Irritable bowel	Randomized controlled trial	Ritchie[19] 1979	96	No	3	NA	NA	NA	Of three therapies, only ispaghula husk significantly improved symptoms.
Airway obstruction prevention	Randomized controlled trial	Kahn[12] 1991	20	Yes	4	Medium	30%	3.3	Tincture of belladonna studied (contained ethanol) in infants with breath-holding spells.
Autonomic nervous system dysfunction	Equivalence trial, non-randomized.	Dobrescu[21] 1970	36	Yes	0	Medium	36%	2.8	Two combination formulas containing barbiturates compared; superior results with formula containing higher concentration of belladonna and propranolol. No placebo control.
Vagal response	Randomized controlled dosing study	Bettermann[52] 2001	8	Unclear	3	Medium	NA	NA	Belladonna tincture higher dose associated with respiratory and heart rate. Tinctures contain ethanol.
Headache prophylaxis (homeopathic treatment)	Randomized controlled trial	Whitmarsh[10] 1997	63	No	4	None	NA	NA	Homeopathic migraine prophylaxis administered for 4 months.
Headache	Randomized controlled trial	Stieg[16] 1977	76	Mixed	3	Variable	NA	NA	Combination formula BEP (belladonna, ergotamine, phenobarbital) associated with benefits in one study arm but not another. 28% dropout.
Headache	Randomized controlled trial	Lance[14] 1965	110	No	0	None	NA	NA	Combination formula Bellergal compared to other therapies or placebo. Poorly described study.
Otitis media (homeopathic treatment)	Observational study	Friese[28] 1997	131	Yes	0	Medium	14.2%	7	Various homeopathic remedies studied, including belladonna preparation. Benefits reported vs. antibiotics.
Pre-menstrual syndrome	Randomized controlled trial	Robinson[22] 1977	32	Yes	4	Medium	NA	NA	Combination formula Bellergal studied over 3 menstrual cycles. Reduced symptoms reported. 23% dropout.
Radiodermatitis (homeopathic treatment)	Randomized controlled trial	Balzarini[11] 2000	66	Yes	5	Small	NA	NA	Homeopathic belladonna dilution studied for 8 weeks. Significant effects in total severity score only.
Menopausal symptoms	Randomized controlled trial	Bergmans[23] 1987	71	No	4	None	None	NA	Combination formula including belladonna studied. Trend toward improvement at 2-4 weeks, but no effect at 8 weeks.

*Primary or secondary outcome.
[†] N, Number of patients; SS, statistically significant; ARR, absolute risk reduction; NNT, the number of patients who need to undergo a specific intervention in order to observe an outcome in one individual.
[‡] 0-2 = poor; 3-4 = good; 5 = excellent.
NA, Not applicable.
For an explanation of each category in this table, please see Table 3 in the Introduction.

undergoing polysomnography with each treatment (placebo or belladonna). Tincture of belladonna was administered in a dose equivalent to 0.01 mg/kg of atropine at bedtime. The authors reported a significant reduction in obstructed breathing events, with response noted in 50% (10/20) of infants receiving belladonna and in 20% (4/20) of infants in the placebo group. Differences between groups were statistically significant. No significant adverse effects were observed, although decreased "water evaporation rates" were noted in the belladonna-treated patients. It is unclear if a history of breath-holding spells correlates clearly with physiologic airway obstruction. The authors recognized that belladonna overdose in infants and children can be deadly, and that the long-term effects of belladonna treatment are unknown. In addition, tinctures contain ethanol, which may have elicited effects in subjects.

Autonomic Nervous System Disturbances
Summary

- Literature review reveals limited evidence regarding the use of belladonna for treatment of symptoms associated with autonomic nervous system dysfunction. Therefore, there is currently insufficient evidence to support the use of belladonna for symptoms of autonomic nervous system dysfunction.

Evidence

- In a 1970 trial, Dobrescu compared two different combination formulas, each taken three times daily by patients with disturbances of the autonomic nervous system[21]: "Formula I" contained a low concentration of belladonna (0.25 mg of belladonna, 0.3 mg of alkaloids of ergot, 30 mg of phenobarbital); "Formula II" contained a higher concentration of belladonna (15 mg of belladonna extract, 60 mg of ergot extract, 15 mg of propranolol, 25 mg of amobarbital). A total of 36 subjects were enrolled in this single-blind, crossover trial and received treatment for 1 week, followed by crossover to the alternate therapy for 1 week. "Very good" results were noted in 72% of subjects receiving Formula II (higher belladonna concentration), compared with 36% treated with Formula I. Limitations of this study include the small sample size, lack of adequate randomization, use of subjective outcome measures, and failure to report the dropout rate. In addition, because of multiple variations between the two formulas, it is not clear which constituent(s) might be responsible for the differing effects.

- A single-blind placebo-controlled study was conducted to investigate the cardiorespiratory effects of belladonna, as a surrogate measure of vagal activity.[51] Single doses of an oral belladonna tincture containing 0.1 mg/mL of alkaloid concentration were administered, with a proportion of atropine to scopolamine of 20:1. In eight healthy young subjects, heart rate and noninvasive arterial finger blood pressure were recorded for 4 hours following oral application of 1 mL, 2 mL, or 5 mL of this belladonna tincture, or placebo. The authors reported that 1 hour after administration of 5 mL, mean respiratory rate, heart rate, and baroreflex sensitivity decreased significantly in six of eight subjects. In contrast, following administration of 1 or 2 mL, mean respiratory rate and heart rate increased compared to placebo.

Headache
Summary

- Studies comparing belladonna-containing compounds with placebo have been small and have reported limited or

no benefits. However, this research has been of poor quality and has examined combination products containing other agents such as ergotamine or phenobarbital (which may be efficacious in the absence of belladonna), or used homeopathic (dilute) belladonna preparations. There is currently insufficient evidence to support the use of belladonna for the treatment or prophylaxis of headache.

Evidence

- A study conducted by Stieg compared a combination formula belladonna-ergotamine-phenobarbital (BEP) to placebo in a randomized crossover and parallel group design trial.[16] BEP is equivalent to the commercially available product Bellergal-S, which contains 40 mg of phenobarbital, 0.6 mg of ergotamine tartrate, and 0.2 mg of levorotatory alkaloids of belladonna. The trial enrolled 76 patients with recurrent throbbing headaches at least once a week. No other prophylactic headache medication was allowed, but the use of medications for symptomatic relief was allowed during the study period. BEP or placebo was administered twice daily to subjects during the trial. The authors reported that over a 4-week period, there was no difference in drug effectiveness or headache severity between groups. A modest, significant decrease in headache severity and increase in days without headache medication was noted in a crossover substudy. Problems with this trial include the use of subjective measures of effect, small sample size, and 28% dropout, with no intention-to-treat analysis, and lack of description of randomization.

- In a poorly described 1965 study by Lance et al., Bellergal was compared to methysergide, cyproheptadine, and placebo in the treatment of 110 subjects with migraine headache.[14] Compared to placebo, Bellergal was reported to elicit no significant effect. No randomization or blinding was described, no dropout rate was reported, and the methods of the study were not described.

- Whitmarsh et al. conducted a randomized, placebo-controlled study in 63 outpatients with migraine headache diagnosed by International Headache Society criteria.[10] Subjects received either a belladonna-containing homeopathic remedy or placebo for 4 months. No significant differences were detected between groups, and overall, headache frequency was 19% in the homeopathy group and 16% with placebo. The sample size may have been too small to detect significant between-group differences, and the groups were dissimilar at baseline.

- A 1965 placebo-controlled trial compared methysergide, cyproheptadine, and Bellergal (40 mg phenobarbital). Uncontrolled studies have been reported, reporting small benefits from belladonna-containing compounds. Steele et al. reported a 1954 case series in which administration of Bellergal for headache yielded "satisfactory results" in 73.3% of patients.[15]

Otitis Media
Summary

- There is currently insufficient evidence to support the use of belladonna for the treatment of otitis media.

Evidence

- A German homeopath and four otolaryngologists performed an observational study comparing homeopathic with conventional treatment for children with otitis media.[28] The homeopathic practitioner chose from among 12 remedies for otitis, including belladonna 30X globules (brand not specified). The homeopathic treatment group was reported to experience significantly fewer recurrences of otitis (29.3% vs. 43.5%), a shorter treatment duration, and a shorter duration of symptoms than the otolaryngologist-treated group (which received antibiotics). However, the frequency with which belladonna was used from among the 12 remedies was not specified, and there was no randomization or blinding in this trial (allowing for the possible introduction of bias or confounding). Therefore, although these results are compelling, they cannot be considered conclusive.

Premenstrual Syndrome
Summary
- Bellergal, a combination formula containing 40 mg of phenobarbital, 0.6 mg of ergotamine tartrate, and 0.2 mg of levorotatory alkaloids of belladonna, has been reported in one controlled human trial to decrease symptoms associated with premenstrual syndrome, including fatigue, breast tenderness, and irritability. Further study is warranted before an evidence-based recommendation can be made.

Evidence
- Robinson et al. performed a randomized, double-blind, placebo-controlled trial in 32 patients experiencing symptoms associated with premenstrual syndrome.[22] Patients were administered oral Bellergal or placebo three times daily, beginning 10 days prior to menses. The primary outcome assessed was presence of any of nine "typical symptoms" of premenstrual syndrome over three menstrual cycles. The authors reported significantly less fatigue, breast tenderness, and lethargy in the treatment group vs. placebo. Although these results are suggestive, limitations of this study included its short duration, small sample size, 23% dropout, and unclear reporting of results or statistical analysis. The use of a combination formula leaves open the question of belladonna's efficacy.

Radiodermatitis
Summary
- Homeopathic application of belladonna for the management of radiodermatitis has been proposed based on the observed similarities between symptoms of radiodermatitis and the effects of belladonna (based on the dictum that "like cures like"). One randomized trial has reported modest benefits of a homeopathic (dilute) oral belladonna preparation for this indication, although there is no known biochemical basis for this use. There is currently insufficient evidence to support the use of belladonna for the management of radiodermatitis.

Evidence
- A randomized, double-blind, placebo controlled trial was conducted in 66 patients undergoing radiation therapy following surgery for breast cancer.[11] Subjects were assigned to receive either the homeopathic dilution Belladonna 7CH (3 granules sublingually twice daily), the homeopathic preparation X-ray 15CH (3 granules sublingually once daily), or placebo. The authors reported that after 8 weeks, there was a small significant improvement measured by a subjective index of severity in the two treated groups vs. placebo. This study was properly randomized and blinded, although dosing regimens varied by therapy, which may have revealed group assignments. The study was limited by the use of a non-standard outcomes measurement scale. Further study may be warranted in this area.

Menopausal Symptoms
Summary
- Bellergal, a combination formula containing 40 mg of phenobarbital, 0.6 mg of ergotamine tartrate, and 0.2 mg of levorotatory alkaloids of belladonna, has been used historically and reported anecdotally to reduce the incidence of hot flashes. One randomized control trial has reported negative results. There is currently insufficient evidence to recommend for or against the use of belladonna for the alleviation of menopausal symptoms.

Evidence
- Bergmans et al. conducted a randomized, double-blind, placebo-controlled trial in 71 patients experiencing menopausal symptoms.[23] After 8 weeks of follow-up, no benefit of Bellergal was observed vs. placebo. Notably, a trend towards improved symptoms was seen at 2-4 weeks. These results cannot be considered conclusive due to limitations, including a 46% dropout rate.

FORMULARY: BRANDS USED IN CLINICAL TRIALS
Brands Used in Statistically Significant Clinical Trials
- Bellergal (40 mg of phenobarbital, 0.6 mg of ergotamine tartrate, and 0.2 mg of levorotatory alkaloids of belladonna).[14-16] Also available: Bellergal-R, Bellergal-S.

International Brand Names
- Astrobel, Belladonnysat Burger, Bellafolin, Bellafolina, Bellanorm, Tremoforat.

References
1. Samet CM. The evaluation of Bellergal Tablets compared to librium and placebo in the treatment of symptoms of anxiety tension states associated with functional gastrointestinal disorders. Psychosomatics 1976;17(4):202-209.
2. Steadman HE. Treatment of psychosomatic disorders with Bellergal. J Med Assoc Ga 1968;57(8):384-386.
3. Reichenberg-Ullman J. Homeopathy for women: menstrual discomfort and abnormal bleeding; relieved with Belladonna. Resonance (Magazine Internat Foundation Homeop) 1991;13(2):12-13.
4. Sodeman WA, Augur NA, Pollard HM. Physiology and pharmacology of belladonna therapy in acid-peptic disease. Med Clin North Am 1969;53(6):1379-1388.
5. Tita B, Bolle P, Martinoli L, et al. A comparative study of Atropa belladonna and atropine on an animal model of urinary retention. Pharmacol Res Commun 1988;20 Suppl 5:55-58.
6. Shader RI, Greenblatt DJ. Uses and toxicity of belladonna alkaloids and synthetic anticholinergics. Semin Psychiatry 1971;3(4):449-476.
7. Lotvall J. Contractility of lungs and air-tubes: experiments performed in 1840 by Charles J.B. Williams. Eur Respir J 1994;7(3):592-595.
8. Kapp W. The history of drugs for the treatment of Parkinson's disease. J Neural Transm Suppl 1992;38(Suppl):1-6.
9. Walach H. Does a highly diluted homeopathic drug act as a placebo in healthy volunteers? Experimental study of belladonna 30C in double-blind crossover design—a pilot study. J Psychosom Res 1993;37(8):851-860.
10. Whitmarsh TE, Coleston-Shields DM, Steiner TJ. Double-blind randomized placebo-controlled study of homeopathic prophylaxis of migraine. Cephalalgia 1997;17(5):600-604.
11. Balzarini A, Felisi E., Martini A., et al. Efficacy of homeopathic treatment of skin reactions during radiotherapy for breast cancer: a randomised, double-blind clinical trial. Br Homeopath J 2000;89(1):8-12.
12. Kahn A., Rebuffat E, Sottiaux M, et al. Prevention of airway obstructions during sleep in infants with breath-holding spells by means of oral belladonna: a prospective double-blind crossover evaluation. Sleep 1991;14(5):432-438.
13. Hartmann T, Witte L, Oprach F, et al. Reinvestigation of the alkaloid composition of Atropa belladonna plants, root cultures, and cell suspension cultures. Planta Med 1986;5:390-395.
14. Lance JW, Curran DA, Anthony M. Investigations into the mechanism and treatment of chronic headache. Med J Aust 1965;2(22):909-914.
15. Steele CH. The use of Bellergal in the prophylactic treatment of some types of headaches. Ann Allergy 1954;42-46.
16. Stieg RL. Double-blind study of belladonna-ergotamine-phenobarbital for interval treatment of recurrent throbbing headache. Headache 1977;17(3):120-124.

17. King JC. Anisotropine methylbromide for relief of gastrointestinal spasm: double- blind crossover comparison study with belladonna alkaloids and phenobarbital. Curr Ther Res Clin Exp 1966;8(11):535-541.

18. Lichstein J, Mayer JD. Drug therapy in the unstable bowel (irritable colon). A 15-month double-blind clinical study in 75 cases of response to a prolonged-acting belladonna alkaloid-phenobarbital mixture or placebo. J Chron Dis 1959;9(4):394-404.

19. Ritchie JA, Truelove SC. Treatment of irritable bowel syndrome with lorazepam, hyoscine butylbromide, and ispaghula husk. Br Med J 1979; 1(6160):376-378.

20. Rhodes JB, Abrams JH, Manning RT. Controlled clinical trial of sedative-anticholinergic drugs in patients with the irritable bowel syndrome. J Clin Pharmacol 1978;18(7):340-345.

21. Dobrescu DI. Propranolol in the treatment of disturbances of the autonomic nervous system. Curr Ther Res Clin Exp 1971;13(1):69-73.

22. Robinson K, Huntington KM, Wallace MG. Treatment of the premenstrual syndrome. Br J Obstet Gynaecol 1977;84(10):784-788.

23. Bergmans M, Merkus J, Corbey R, et al. Effect of Bellergal Retard on climacteric complaints: a double-blind, placebo-controlled study. Maturitas 1987;9:227-234.

24. Goodyear K., Lewith G., Low JL. Randomized double-blind placebo-controlled trial of homeopathic 'proving' for Belladonna C30. J R Soc Med 1998;91(11):579-582.

25. Williams HC, du Vivier A. Belladonna plaster—not as bella as it seems. Contact Dermatitis 1990;23(2):119-120.

26. Schneider F, Lutun P, Kintz P, et al. Plasma and urine concentrations of atropine after the ingestion of cooked deadly nightshade berries. J Toxicol Clin Toxicol 1996;34(1):113-117.

27. Southgate HJ, Egerton M, Dauncey EA. Lessons to be learned: a case study approach. Unseasonal severe poisoning of two adults by deadly nightside (*Atropa belladonna*). Journal of the Royal Society of Health 2000;120(2): 127-130.

28. Friese KH, Kruse S, Ludtke R, et al. The homeopathic treatment of otitis media in children—comparisons with conventional therapy. Int J Clin Pharmacol Ther 1997;35(7):296-301.

29. Jaspersen-Schib R, Theus L, Guirguis-Oeschger M, et al. [Serious plant poisonings in Switzerland 1966-1994. Case analysis from the Swiss Toxicology Information Center.] Schweiz Med Wochenschr 1996;126(25): 1085-1098.

30. Firth D, Bentley JR. Belladonna poisoning from eating rabbit. Lancet 1921;2:901.

31. Joll ME. Three cases of belladonna poisoning. Lancet 1916;2:647.

32. Minors EH. Five cases of belladonna poisoning. Br Med J 1948;2:518-519.

33. Eichner ER, Gunsolus JM, Powers JF. "Belladonna" poisoning confused with botulism. JAMA 1967;201(9):695-696.

34. Trabattoni G, Visintini D, Terzano GM, et al. Accidental poisoning with deadly nightshade berries: a case report. Human Toxicol 1984;3(6):513-516.

35. Ceha LJ, Presperin C, Young E, et al. Anticholinergic toxicity from nightshade berry poisoning responsive to physostigmine. The Journal of Emergency Medicine 1997;15(1):65-69.

36. Sims SR. Poisoning due to belladonna plasters. Br Med J 1954;1531.

37. Gabel MC. Purposeful ingestion of belladonna for hallucinatory effects. J Pediatr 1968;72(6):864-866.

38. Goldsmith SR, Frank I, Ungerleider JT. Poisoning from ingestion of a stramonium-belladonna mixture: flower power gone sour. JAMA 1968; 204(2):169-170.

39. Cummins BM, Obetz SW, Wilson MR, et al. Belladonna poisoning as a facet of psychodelia. Jama 1968;204(11):153.

40. Walach H, Koster H, Hennig T, et al. The effects of homeopathic belladonna 30CH in healthy volunteers—a randomized, double-blind experiment. J Psychosom Res 2001;50(3):155-160.

41. Hamilton M, Sclare AB. Belladonna poisoning. Br Med J 1947;611-612.

42. Myers JH, Moro-Sutherland D, Shook JE. Anticholinergic poisoning in colicky infants treated with hyoscyamine sulfate. Am J Emerg Med 1997; 15(5):532-535.

43. Berney C, Wolfensberger TJ. [Mydriasis induced by splinter from belladonna bush.] Klin Monatsbl Augenheilkd 2000;216(5):346-347.

44. Heindl S, Binder C, Desel H, et al. [Etiology of initially unexplained confusion of excitability in deadly nightshade poisoning with suicidal intent. Symptoms, differential diagnosis, toxicology and physostigmine therapy of anticholinergic syndrome.] Dtsch Med Wochenschr 2000;125(45): 1361-1365.

45. Pentel P, Mikell F. Reaction to phenylpropalamine/chlorpheniramine/ belladonna compound in a women with unrecognised autonomic dysfunction. Lancet 1982;2(8292):274.

46. Golwalla A. Multiple extrasystoles: an unusual manifestation of belladonna poisoning. Dis Chest 1965;48:83-84.

47. Mellin GW. Drugs in the first trimester of pregnancy and the fetal life of Homo sapiens. Am J Obst Gynec 1964;90(7):1169-1180.

48. Diaz DM, Diaz SF, Marx GF. Cardiovascular effects of glycopyrrolate and belladonna derivatives in obstetric patients. Bull N Y Acad Med 1980;56(2):245-248.

49. Corazziari E, Bontempo I, Anzini F. Effects of cisapride on distal esophageal motility in humans. Dig Dis Sci 1989;34(10):1600-1605.

50. Pan SY, Han YF. Learning deficits induced by 4 belladonna alkaloids are preferentially attenuated by tacrine. Acta Pharmacol Sin 2000;21(2):124-130.

51. Bettermann H, Cysarz D, Portsteffen A, et al. Bimodal dose-dependent effect on autonomic, cardiac control after oral administration of Atropa belladonna. Auton Neurosci 2001;90(1-2):132-137.

52. Jacobs KW. Asthmador: a legal hallucinogen. Int J Addict 1974;9(4):503-512.

Betel Nut
(Areca catechu L.)

SYNONYMS/COMMON NAMES/RELATED SUBSTANCES
- Amaska, areca nut, arecoline, arequier, betal, betelnusspalme, betel quid, chavica etal, gutkha, hmarg, maag, marg, mava, mawa, paan, Palmaceae, pan, pan masala, pan parag, pinang, pinlang, Piper betel L. (leaf of vine used to wrap betel nuts), pugua, quid, Sting, supai, ugam.

CLINICAL BOTTOM LINE
Background
- Betel nut use refers to a combination of three ingredients: the nut of the betel palm (*Areca catechu*), part of the *Piper betel* vine, and lime. Anecdotal reports have indicated that small doses generally lead to euphoria and increased flow of energy, whereas large doses often result in sedation. Although all three ingredients may contribute to these effects, most experts attribute the psychoactive effects to the alkaloids found in betel nuts.
- Betel nut is reportedly used by a substantial portion of the world's population as a recreational drug, due to its central nervous system (CNS) stimulant activity. Found originally in tropical southern Asia, betel nut has been introduced to the communities of east Africa, Madagascar, and the West Indies. There is little evidence from adequately controlled studies to support clinical use of betel, but the constituents have demonstrated pharmacologic actions. The main active component, the alkaloid arecoline, has potent cholinergic activity.
- Constituents of areca are potentially carcinogenic. Long-term use has been associated with oral submucous fibrosis (OSF), pre-cancerous oral lesions, and squamous cell carcinoma. Acute effects of betel chewing include asthma.

Scientific Evidence for Common/Studied Uses	Grade*
Anemia	C
CNS stimulant	C
Dental caries	C
Salivary stimulant	C
Schizophrenia	C
Stroke recovery	C
Ulcerative colitis	C

*Key to grades: *A:* Strong scientific evidence for this use; *B:* Good scientific evidence for this use; *C:* Unclear scientific evidence for this use; *D:* Fair scientific evidence against this use (it may not work); *F:* Strong scientific evidence against this use (it likely does not work). For a more detailed explanation of efficacy criteria, see "Natural Standard Evidence-Based Validated Grading Rationale" in the Introduction.

Historical or Theoretical Indications That Lack Sufficient Evidence
- Alcoholism, anthelmintic, aphrodisiac, appetite stimulant, asthma, cough, dermatitis (topical), digestive aid, diphtheria, diuretic, gas, glaucoma, impotence, joint pain (rheumatism), leprosy, menorrhagia, methanol-induced blindness,[1] otitis media, polydipsia/excessive thirst, respiratory stimulant, syncope, toothache, veterinary cathartic/anthelminthic.

Expert Opinion and Folkloric Precedent
- In traditional Indian medicine, betel nut is recommended for its laxative and carminative (anti-flatus) effects and as a household and veterinary anthelminthic. Betel nut is not frequently recommended medically because of its toxicity profile. Toothpaste containing areca nut was once used due to the belief that areca nut could protect against tooth decay while strengthening gums, but its use has now been discontinued.[2] Presently, the majority of betel use is recreational.

Safety Summary
- **Likely unsafe:** Despite widespread recreational use, because of documented toxicity associated with acute or chronic chewing/oral consumption, betel nut cannot be considered safe for human use (particularly when used chronically or in high doses).

DOSING/TOXICOLOGY
General
- Recommended doses are based on those most commonly used in available trials, or on historical practice. However, with natural products, the optimal doses needed to balance efficacy and safety often have not been determined. Formulations and preparation methods may vary from manufacturer to manufacturer, and from batch to batch of a specific product made by a single manufacturer. Because often the active components of a product are not known, standardization may not be possible, and the clinical effects of different brands may not be comparable.

Standardization
- There is inadequate information available regarding standardization of betel nut.

Dosing: Adult (18 Years and Older)
Oral
- Betel nut can be chewed alone but is more often chewed as a quid, or a combination of ingredients. Ingredients other than betel nut may include calcium hydroxide, water, catechu gum, cardamom, cloves, anise seeds, cinnamon, tobacco, nutmeg, and gold or silver metal. These ingredients are often wrapped in a betel leaf, which is sucked in the lateral gingival pocket.
- Anecdotal reports have indicated that ingestion of 8 to 30 g of areca nut may be lethal.

Dosing: Pediatric (Younger Than 18 Years)
- Not recommended, due to risk of carcinogenesis, exacerbation of asthma, and cardiovascular effects.

Toxicology
- **Convulsions:** Anecdotal reports have noted that chewing areca nut in high doses may lead to convulsions and death.

- **Carcinogenicity:** A retrospective study of betel nut users demonstrated an association between chewing betel nut and oral squamous cell carcinoma involving the cheek and tongue.[3] Epithelial cells isolated from the mouths of betel nut chewers were significantly more likely to undergo cell proliferation than cells from non-chewers. The use of tobacco as part of the chewed material may be a contributing factor in the oral carcinogenicity seen with betel.[4] Esophageal and liver cancer have also been reported in limited numbers of betel users.[5-11]
- **Lead toxicity:** A 36-year-old patient experienced lead toxicity from betel nut ingestion. The patient was admitted for generalized abdominal pain lasting for 3 months. Other symptoms included nausea, vomiting, weakness, and muscle aches. Urine lead concentrations were above normal, which resolved after treatment with EDTA (ethylenediamine-tetraacetic acid) infusions.[12] A follow-up Chinese study found no correlation between lead and betel nut use.[13]
- **Aflatoxin contamination:** Betel nut samples have been found contaminated with aflatoxin.[14]

ADVERSE EFFECTS/PRECAUTIONS/CONTRAINDICATIONS
Allergy

- Acute bronchoconstriction has been reported, although no hypersensitivity reactions are found in the available literature.[15] In theory, cross-reactivity may occur with other members of the Palmaceae family.

Adverse Effects

- **General:** Despite widespread recreational use, because of documented toxicity associated with acute or chronic chewing or oral ingestion, betel nut cannot be considered safe for human use (particularly when used chronically or in high doses).
- **Dermatologic:** Chemicals in betel leaves has been associated with inducing contact leukomelanosis, believed to occur via inhibition of melanin synthesis or melanocytotoxicity.[16]
- **Ocular:** Pupil dilation, miosis, and blurred vision have been noted anecdotally.
- **Neurologic (extrapyramidal effects):** Extrapyramidal symptoms (EPS) such as tremor and stiffness have been reported in patients who chewed betel while receiving antipsychotic drugs.[17,18] In one case-report, a 51-year-old man with chronic schizophrenia maintained on depot fluphenazine and procyclidine developed pronounced rigidity, bradykinesia. and deterioration in orofacial dyskinesia after consumption of betel nut over a 2-week period. The patient had no prior symptoms of extrapyramidal symptoms other than orofacial dyskinesia. One week after discontinuation of betel nut, the patient's symptoms were reported to have resolved.[18] Another patient with schizoaffective disorder maintained on flupenthixol developed stiffness, tremor, and akathisia after 2 weeks of betel nut use. Procyclidine was given but did not resolve the patient's symptoms. Four days following discontinuation of betel nut, the patient's symptoms resolved.[18] The betel constituent, arecoline, at a dose of 20 mg, has been found to worsen chorea in patients with Huntington's disease.[19] Seizure activity has also been reported.[20]
- **Neurologic (cholinergic effects):** Cholinergic toxicity (salivation, lacrimation, urinary incontinence, sweating, diarrhea, emesis, facial flushing, and fever) may be seen with the use of betel,[21,22] likely due to the cholinergic alkaloid constituent of betel, arecoline, which appears to possess muscarinic properties as well as nicotinic properties at higher doses. Anecdotally, the betel constituent arecaine has been noted to cause dizziness and tetanic convulsions. Betel chewing may cause electroencephalographic changes associated with arousal and relaxation.[23] Chewing betel nut was shown to reduce performance reaction times with statistical significance.[24] In one study of 15 male subjects, betel quid ingestion lengthened reaction time latencies.[25] Another study found that reaction time and short-term memory did not appear to be impeded by betel use.[26]
- **Neurologic (anti-thiamine effects):** Betel nut has been shown to have anti-thiamine effects,[27] which theoretically may result in neurologic damage, including Wernicke-Korsakoff syndrome. Wernicke's encephalopathy is characterized by confusion, ataxia, nystagmus, and ophthalmoplegia (weakness of the lateral rectus muscle and conjugate gaze palsies), whereas Korsakoff's psychosis involves confabulation, anterograde amnesia, and retrograde amnesia.
- **Psychiatric:** Constituents of betel have been shown to possess psychoactive and euphoric effects.[28] Habituation has been reported in long-term users, with dependency in up to 20% of users,[28-30] and signs of withdrawal (anxiety, despondency, memory lapses) have been reported in limited studies of regular users of betel.[31]
- **Cardiovascular:** Patients chewing betel nuts have reported acute chest pain, ventricular arrhythmias, tachycardia, palpitations, and hemodynamic instability (hypotension/hypertension),[30,32-36] which may be attributed to the cholinergic betel nut constituent arecoline.[19] Pan masala (mixture of betel nut, lime and calcium hydroxide, water, catechu gum, cardamom, cloves, anise seeds, cinnamon, tobacco, nutmeg, and gold or silver metal) has been associated with acute elevations in blood pressure and pulse rate.[37] Cardiovascular effects of betel nut were studied in 47 healthy male subjects who were divided into groups of chronic, occasional, and new chewers. Following betel chewing, all groups showed a significant increase in heart rate lasting an average of 16.8 minutes. Only the new chewers showed an increase in systolic blood pressure, which suggests that habitual users may develop tolerance to the pressor effects of betel nut.[38] Betel nut was also shown to produce a sympathetic response, with an increase in concentrations of circulating norepinephrine and epinephrine.[33] Myocardial infarction has been documented in a 47-year-old man who experienced severe anterior chest pain instantly after chewing betel nut. The patient was a smoker for several years but had never tried betel nut prior to this incident. He had a negative medical history but a positive family history of coronary artery disease. The patient experienced dizziness, shortness of breath, cold sweats, and ventricular premature beats, and cardiac enzymes revealed myocardial necrosis.[36]
- **Gastrointestinal (GI discomfort):** There are anecdotal reports of nausea, vomiting, diarrhea, and abdominal cramps after betel nut ingestion.
- **Oral (oral health):** Betel quid chewing was shown to impair gingival fibroblast functions and thereby have a harmful effect on gingival tissues.[39] Betel chewers have been shown to have higher rates of periodontal disease than non-chewers.[40] Although betel chewing has been believed to cause or exacerbate temporomandibular joint (TMJ) pain dysfunction syndrome, one study found no correlation between betel chewing and incidence and TMJ pain dysfunction syndrome.[41] Betel nut chewing may also cause a gradual absorption of calcium by the lime constituent, as well as gingivitis, periodontitis, and chronic osteomyelitis.[42] Chewing areca nut may result in red-stained teeth, mouth, lips and feces.

- **Oral (oral submucous fibrosis):** Oral submucous fibrosis (OSF), characterized by deposition of fibrous tissue in the oral tissue and esophagus, has been associated with betel use in Asian populations.[3,43-47] OSF appears to be related to the frequency and duration of betel chewing.[48-51] However, one study found that frequency and duration of betel chewing were not accurate predictors of when mucosal changes occur, or to what extent.[52] Another study found that frequency of chewing rather than total duration directly correlate to OSF.[53] Babu et al. showed that pan masala/gutkha chewers (perfumed, sweetened mixtures of betel quid and tobacco) developed oral fibrosis after an average of 2.7 ± 0.6 years of use, whereas chewers of betel quid developed oral fibrosis after an average of 8.6 ± 2.3 years of use.[4] Clinical symptoms of blanching of mucosa, fibrous bands, burning and dryness of mouth were present in ex–betel nut chewers, who had discontinued betel anywhere from 1 to 13 years (mean cessation duration = 6.4 years).[54]
- **Oral (oral leukoplakia/cancer):** Betel use has been associated with leukoplakia,[55,56] as has the combination of pan chewing and tobacco.[57] Chronic oral inflammation may be seen in the absence of fibrosis,[52] with oral and esophageal carcinoma as a further consequence.[5,7,11,30] However, the contribution of tobacco and/or the corrosive effects of lime, which are often combined with betel in the chewed material, are confounders.[58,59] Slaked lime has been shown to increase pH to levels at which reactive oxygen species occur, which may thereby contribute to oral cancer.[60] Tobacco habits have been found to be more common in patients with OSF and carcinoma.[61] However, one study did not show an increased risk of OSF with tobacco use in those who chewed betel quid or pan masala.[53]
- **Gastrointestinal (hepatocellular carcinoma):** Amount and duration of betel nut consumption have been found to increase the risk of developing hepatocellular carcinoma (HCC), in a case-controlled study and a case report.[6,10] The risk of HCC appears to be increased in patients with hepatitis B or C who chew betel nuts.
- **Pulmonary:** Wheezing, bronchoconstriction, dyspnea, and pulmonary edema have been noted anecdotally in users of betel nuts. Acute toxicity of betel nut has resulted in tachypnea and dyspnea.[34] Aggravation of asthma with a decrease in forced expiratory volume has been reported in patients who chew betel nuts.[15,62,63]
- **Endocrine:** Betel nut extract may induce glucose intolerance in mice,[64] whereas the arecoline fraction from betel nuts reduces blood sugar in diabetic rabbits.[65] Consumption of betel nut has been associated with obesity, which may be a confounder in epidemiologic research that suggests an association between betel nut use and diabetes.[66] Other epidemiologic evidence has failed to demonstrate an association between betel chewing and diabetes.[67] Betel nut has exhibited both stimulatory and inhibitory effects on thyroid function in male mice.[68] Betel chewing has been shown to increase skin temperature among healthy volunteers who were occasional or habitual betel nut chewers.[69]
- **Genitourinary:** A retrospective study found women with a habit of betel nut chewing to have a 50.9% incidence of cervical dysplasia vs. 4.1% in women who did not chew betel nut.[70]
- **Renal:** Two patients who chewed large quantities of betel nuts developed milk-alkali syndrome, characterized by hypercalcemia, metabolic alkalosis, and renal insufficiency.[71] The betel nut preparation contained a paste composed of calcium carbonate. Metabolic abnormalities resolved after discontinuation of betel nut chewing and administration of saline.
- **Oncologic:** Chaudhry reviewed human and animal data and findings suggest that pan masala–containing tobacco is likely to be carcinogenic.[72] A two-year study in mice reported the development of liver, stomach, prostate, sebaceous gland, and lung carcinomas, with lung adenocarcinoma being the most frequent malignant tumor type.[73] A retrospective study found women with a habit of betel nut chewing to have a 50.9% incidence of cervical dysplasia vs. 4.1% in women who did not chew betel nut.[70] A study of 195 cases of oral squamous cell carcinoma found 73.85% (n = 144) of patients to be regular betel nut chewers. The mean age of betel chewers was significantly lower than that of non-chewers who developed oral squamous cell carcinoma.[74] Oral lichen planus–like lesions were found in 35 betel-tobacco chewers. Lesions were described as white, wavy, parallel, and non-elevated lines that could not be scraped off.[75] This has also been noted in a case report.[76]

Precautions/Warnings/Contraindications

- Betel nut chewing and oral ingestion have been associated with acute and chronic toxicity, and may result in adverse effects to users (particularly when used chronically or in high doses).
- Avoid in patients with asthma.
- Avoid in patients with hepatitis B or C, due to an increased risk of hepatocellular carcinoma.
- Use cautiously in patients taking anticholinergic or cholinergic drugs because of the cholinergic properties of betel nut (arecoline constituent).
- Use cautiously in patients with coronary artery disease, hypertension, diabetes, extrapyramidal disorders (Huntington's chorea, Parkinson's disease, etc.), or drugs that may cause extrapyramidal effects (neuroleptics, etc.).

Pregnancy and Lactation

- Avoid use in pregnant or lactating women because of potential carcinogenic or fetotoxic effects. Betel nut also has CNS stimulant and cholinergic effects that may adversely affect fetuses or breast-fed babies. A mouse study found betel nut ingestion to result in fetal death, reduction in fetal weight, and delay in skeletal maturity.[77] In a human study of adverse effects of betel nut on pregnancy in Aboriginal women in Taiwan, it was found that prevalence of adverse pregnancy outcomes were 2.8-fold greater among women who chewed betel nut.[78] In an earlier study, however, no adverse effects on fetuses was found when betel nut was administered to pregnant women.[79]

INTERACTIONS
Betel Nut/Drug Interactions

- **Anticholinergic agents:** Anticholinergic effects may be reduced when used in combination with betel nut, due to the cholinergic properties of the betel constituent arecoline.[17] The skin temperature–elevating effects of betel in humans has been found to be completely inhibited by atropine.[69] However, anecdotal reports have noted that atropine may enhance the CNS stimulatory effects of the arecoline constituent of betel.
- **Cholinergic agents:** Cholinergic toxicity (salivation, lacrimation, urinary incontinence, sweating, diarrhea, emesis, facial flushing, and fever) may be seen with the use of betel,[21,22] and has been attributed to the cholinergic properties of

the betel constituent arecoline.[17] Betel may lead to additive effects when used with other cholinergic agents.

- **Insulin, hypoglycemic agents:** The arecoline fraction from betel nuts has been found to reduce blood sugar in diabetic rabbits.[65] Use of betel may have additive effects with hypoglycemic agents.
- **Phenothiazines:** Extrapyramidal symptoms (EPS) such as tremor and stiffness may result when used concomitantly with betel nut.[17,18]
- **Monoamine oxidase inhibitors (MAOIs):** The dichloromethane fraction of betel nut has been shown to inhibit monoamine oxidase in a rat model[80] and therefore may potentiate the effects of MAOIs.
- **Angiotensin-converting enzyme (ACE) inhibitors:** Areca II-5-C, a fraction isolated from betel nut (*Areca catechu* L.), showed ACE inhibitory activity *in vitro*.[81] Use of betel nut with ACE inhibitors may result in additive effects.
- **CNS stimulants:** Constituents of betel have been shown to possess psychoactive and euphoric effects.[28] Theoretically, betel use may result in additive effects with other CNS stimulants.
- **Lipid-lowering agents:** Betel nut extracts lowered concentrations of cholesterol and triglycerides significantly in rats fed a diet containing cholesteryl oleate.[82] Use of betel with hyperlipidemic agents may result in additive effects.
- **Glaucoma agents:** Anecdotal reports have noted that betel may either increase or decrease effects of antiglaucoma medications. Review of the scientific literature reveals no reliable human data in this area.
- **Beta blockers, calcium channel blockers, cardiac glycosides:** The betel nut constituent arecoline possesses cholinergic properties and may cause bradycardia. Concomitant use with beta blockers, calcium channel blockers, digoxin, or other agents that reduce heart rate may increase the risk of bradycardia. In a human study, the skin temperature–elevating effects of betel were found to be partially inhibited by the beta adrenergic antagonist propranolol,[69] which is of unclear clinical significance.

Betel Nut/Herb/Supplement Interactions

- **Cholinergic herbs:** Cholinergic toxicity (salivation, lacrimation, urinary incontinence, sweating, diarrhea, emesis, facial flushing, and fever) may be seen with the use of betel[21,22] and has been attributed to the cholinergic properties of the betel constituent arecoline.[17] Betel may lead to additive effects when used with other agents with cholinergic properties, such as American hellebore (*Veratrum viride*), jaborandi (*Pilocarpus jaborandi*), lobelia (*Lobelia inflata*), pulsatilla (*Anemone pulsatilla* L.), and snakeroot (*Rauwolfia serpentina*).
- **Anticholinergic herbs:** Cholinergic toxicity (salivation, lacrimation, urinary incontinence, sweating, diarrhea, emesis, facial flushing, and fever) may be seen with the use of betel[21,22] and has been attributed to the cholinergic properties of the betel constituent arecoline.[17] Betel may reduce the effects of agents with possible anticholinergic properties, such as belladonna, henbane (*Hyoscyamus niger*), hyoscyamine, and *Swertia japonica* Makino (Gentianaceae).
- **Hypoglycemic herbs and supplements:** The arecoline fraction from betel nuts has been found to reduce blood sugar in diabetic rabbits.[65] Use of betel may have additive effects with hypoglycemic agents.
- **Monoamine oxidase inhibitor (MAOI) herbs:** The dichloromethane fraction of betel nut has been shown to inhibit monoamine oxidase in a rat model[80] and therefore may potentiate the effects of agents with MAOI effects.

- **Lipid-lowering agents:** Betel nut extracts lowered concentrations of cholesterol and triglycerides significantly in rats fed a diet containing cholesteryl oleate.[82] Use of betel with hyperlipidemic agents may result in additive effects.
- **CNS stimulants:** Constituents of betel have been shown to possess psychoactive and euphoric effects.[28] Theoretically, betel use may result in additive effects with other CNS stimulants, such as caffeine, guarana, or ephedra (ma huang).
- **Cardiac glycoside herbs:** The betel nut constituent arecoline possesses cholinergic properties and may cause bradycardia. Concomitant use with cardiac glycoside herbs, or other agents that reduce heart rate, may increase the risk of bradycardia.
- **Thiamine (Vitamin B$_1$):** Betel has been reported to possess anti-thiamine effects[27] and theoretically may precipitate neurologic damage, including Wernicke-Korsakoff syndrome. Wernicke's encephalopathy is characterized by confusion, ataxia, nystagmus, and ophthalmoplegia (weakness of the lateral rectus muscle and conjugate gaze palsies), whereas Korsakoff's psychosis involves confusion and amnesia.
- **Alcohol:** Theoretically, concomitant chronic use of betel and alcohol may lead to an increased risk of oral cancer.

Betel Nut/Lab Interactions

- **Thyroid stimulating hormone (TSH), thyroxine (T$_4$), triiodothyronine (T$_3$):** Betel nut has exhibited both stimulatory and inhibitory effects on thyroid function in male mice[68] and may have unpredictable effects on serum levels of thyroid hormones.
- **Glucose:** The arecoline fraction from betel nuts has been found to reduce blood sugar in diabetic rabbits.[65] Systematic study in humans is lacking.
- **Total cholesterol, triglycerides:** Betel nut extracts lowered concentrations of cholesterol and triglycerides significantly in rats fed a diet containing cholesteryl oleate.[82] Systematic study in humans is lacking.
- **Fecal occult blood test/stool guaiac:** Anecdotal reports have noted that chewing areca nuts can stain feces red and may interfere with fecal lab tests.

MECHANISM OF ACTION
Pharmacology

- **Constituents:** Betel nut contains a number of related pyridine alkaloids, notably arecoline, which may range in concentration from 0.1% to 0.9%. Other alkaloids include arecaidine, arecaine, arecolidine, betel-phenol, chavicol, guvacine, and isoguvacine. Anecdotal reports have indicated that chavicol and betel-phenol are counterirritants and salivary stimulants. Tannins are also found.[83] The concentration of betel constituents in the mouth after chewing a single nut has been approximated to be 50 µg/mL of arecoline, 80 µg/mL of catechin, and 1.8 mg/mL of tannic acid.[84] The betel component arecoline is hydrolyzed to arecaidine *in vitro*.[85]
- **Neurotransmitter effects:** The betel nut constituent arecoline possesses muscarinic agonist properties,[86] which may account for the central and autonomic effects produced by betel (as well as nicotinic properties at higher doses). The betel nut constituents arecaidine and guvacine inhibit gamma-aminobutyric acid (GABA) uptake in rat brain slices with potency similar to that of nipecotic acid.[87,88] Arecadine has been found to inhibit the uptake of GABA and enhance the effects of GABA on firing of cerebellar Purkinje cells in a cat.[89] The dichloromethane fraction of betel has been shown to inhibit monoamine oxidase.[80]
- **Gastrointestinal effects:** Incubation of isolated brush border membrane with betel nut extracts decreased activity

of alkaline phosphatase, sucrase, and calcium/magnesium adenosine triphosphatase (ATPase),[90] which may result in interference with intestinal nutrient absorption.

- **Effects on inflammation:** Arecoline, in high concentrations, had an inhibitory effect on neutrophil functions.[91] Betel nut extracts stimulate the production of prostaglandin E_2 and induce COX-2 mRNA in human gingival keratinocytes *in vitro*, providing a potential explanation for the oral inflammation seen in betel nut users. However, cytotoxicity appears to occur independently from prostaglandin alterations.[92]

- **Antimicrobial effects:** De Miranda et al. investigated the growth of salivary and oral microorganisms exposed to extracts of betel or to the saliva after chewing betel nut.[84] The extract of baked or boiled nuts (10%) inhibited the growth of *Staphylococcus aureus*, *Fusobacterium nucleatum*, and *Streptococcus salivarius*, but not *Candida albicans*. Growth was measured as CFUs of inoculated cultures grown in blood agar for 24 to 48 hours. Growth suppression was also produced by tannic acid (>0.45 mg/mL), but not by arecoline or catechin. Incubation of saliva from subjects chewing betel for more than an hour also suppressed the growth of oral microorganisms compared to saliva from controls.

- **Mutagenic effects:** Chewing betel nuts increases the generation of hydroxyl free radicals in the saliva.[93] Betel quid chewing may increase mitochondrial DNA mutations in oral tissues and thereby contribute to oral cancer.[94] Betel nut extracts *in vitro* increase the rate of cell division, reduce cell cycle time, induce DNA strand breaks, induce DNA synthesis, and induce the expression of proto-oncogenes.[95-99] Areca nut, *Piper betel* L. and arecoline appear to contribute to the pathogenesis of oral mucosal lesions via genotoxic and nongenotoxic mechanisms.[100-103] Areca nut appears to impair growth of oral mucosal fibroblasts[104] and thereby may aid in the development of oral submucous fibrosis (OSF) and oral cancer.[105] The betel component arecaidine has been implicated as a carcinogenic component of betel nut.[106] Arecoline also appears to be cytotoxic to human gingival fibroblast function.[39,107,108] Arecoline and arecaidine may enhance cell proliferation and affect fibroblasts to synthesize interleukin-6, which may contribute to OSF.[109] Betel nut alkaloids stimulate collagen synthesis and proliferation of human buccal mucosal fibroblasts *in vitro*; the constituent arecaidine appears to be more potent than arecoline.[85] Copper content found in areca nuts may be associated with the development of OSF.[110] Those who chewed soaked or boiled nuts demonstrated a lower incidence of mucosal changes than those who chewed raw, sundried, or roasted nuts.[111] In studies with mice, processed areca nuts were found to have lower carcinogenicity than unprocessed areca nuts.[112] Incorporation of lime and tobacco to betel nut appears to increase the incidence of mucosal changes. The lime component of betel quid may be responsible for free radical production rather than betel itself.[113] Use of lime results in increased pH and thereby may enhance the extent of absorption of arecoline and arecadine across oral mucous membranes.[114] Pan (*Piper betel* leaf preparation), lime, and tobacco were found to contain uranium, which may correlate with an increased incidence of oral cancers.[115] Betel leaf was not found to be tumorigenic in mice study, whereas betel quid was associated with tumorigenicity.[116]

- **Other effects:** Areca II-5-C, a fraction isolated from betel, showed angiotensin-converting enzyme inhibitory activity *in vitro*.[81] Areca nut extracts lowered concentrations of cholesterol and triglycerides significantly in rats fed a diet containing cholesteryl oleate.[82] Pan masala has been shown to cause sperm abnormalities in mice.[117]

Pharmacodynamics/Kinetics

- Areca nut has been found to decrease mace-induced elevations in hepatic glutathione s-transferase and increase elevations in levels of cytochrome b5 and cytochrome P450.[118]
- Minutes after mastication of betel, the onset of effects occurs and may last for a mean period of 17 minutes.[21]

HISTORY

- *Areca catechu* resembles a thin coconut palm tree. Seeds of this tree are referred to as betel nuts. Betel nuts mixed with lime and other spices/herbs are often wrapped in leaves of a vine plant, *Piper betel* L. Betel nut is chewed for its mild CNS stimulating effects by a large number of people throughout the world, especially in southern Asia and the Pacific basin. It is believed to be the oldest known masticatory agent and has been described in Chinese and Indian medicine for over 2000 years.
- The betel nut (fruit) may be chewed alone or in a combination with other ingredients known as a quid. The quid is often mixed with slaked lime, which hydrolyzes some of the alkaloids to other active components. The quid may also include the leaves of the unrelated *Piper betel* L. ("betel vine" or "betel pepper") and tobacco. Chewing is prohibited in public places in some countries because when spit, the red saliva produces stains on floors or sidewalks.[21,119] Betel nut reddens saliva and blackens teeth.

REVIEW OF THE EVIDENCE: DISCUSSION
Stroke Recovery/Cerebrovascular Accident (CVA)
Summary

- A small number of poor-quality studies have been conducted in patients recovering from thromboembolic CVAs (stroke). Recovery of various measures of functional status have been reported to improve statistically significantly faster in subjects ingesting an aqueous extract of betel nut vs. patients not using betel nut. It is not clear if these results may be due to CNS stimulant or cholinergic activity. Because of methodological weaknesses with the available data, and the known risks associated with betel use, it is not clear that the potential benefits outweigh the risks.

Evidence

- Mannan et al. conducted a double-blind, placebo-controlled study in 60 hospitalized stroke patients.[120] Hemorrhagic CVA patients were excluded from the study. Subjects were randomized to receive an aqueous solution containing 2.125 g of betel nut extract or placebo. Outcomes measured included speech function, muscle power, and bladder function, although the methods of measurement were not described. The authors reported a statistically significant improvement in speech patterns in 30% of betel nut patients vs. 0% of the placebo group; improved strength in 70% of betel patients vs. 23% of placebo; and improved bladder function in 40% of betel patients vs. 12% of placebo. Although these results are suggestive, this was a poorly described study, with no details provided of baseline patient characteristics, measurement instruments, or statistical methods. The data cannot therefore be analyzed, and the study is of limited value.
- In a brief published abstract by the same principal author, a study of betel nut administration in 100 patients was described.[121] It is not clear if this is a report of the same study

Review of the Evidence: Betel Nut

Condition Treated*	Study Design	Author, Year	N†	SS†	Study Quality‡	Magnitude of Benefit	ARR†	NNT†	Comments
Stroke recovery	RCT	Mannan[120] 1988	60	Yes	2	Small	30%	3	Improved speech, muscle strength, and bladder function in stroke patients using betel; outcomes measures not described.
Stroke recovery	Controlled study	Mannan[121] 1987	100	Yes	0	Unclear	NA	NA	Published abstract; details of study design, dosing, duration of administration, control group regimen, measurement instruments, and specific baseline patient characteristics not described.
Schizophrenia	Cohort	Sullivan[122] 2000	70	Yes	NA	Small	NA	NA	Data not prospective; self-medicated patients studied; higher levels of betel nut use associated with fewer schizophrenia symptoms.
Anemia	Case series	Taufa[79] 1988	453	Yes	NA	Small	NA	NA	Pregnant, self-reported betel users had lower frequency of anemia than non-users.
Ulcerative colitis	Prospective cohort, matched controls	Lee 1996	195	Yes	NA	Small	NA	NA	Lower incidence of ulcerative colitis found in betel chewers and smokers.

*Primary or secondary outcome.
†N, Number of patients; SS, statistically significant; ARR, absolute risk reduction; NNT, the number of patients who need to undergo a specific intervention in order to observe an outcome in one individual.
‡0-2 = poor; 3-4 = good; 5 = excellent.
NA, Not applicable; RCT, randomized, controlled trial.
For an explanation of each category in this table, please see Table 3 in the Introduction.

as described above, with a larger initial patient cohort. Subjects with cerebrovascular disease (CVD) and "various disabilities" were studied. Although not stated explicitly in the abstract, the patients appear to be individuals with recent CVAs, whose courses of recovery were followed in this study. Outcome parameters of consciousness, dysphagia, bladder function, and activity of daily living were reported as improving or recovering significantly earlier than in a control group ($p = 0.01$). However, details of study design, dosing, duration of administration, control group regimen, measurement instruments, and specific baseline patient characteristics were not described. Therefore, this report may serve as an anecdote but cannot be adequately evaluated as a study.

Schizophrenia
Summary

- Preliminary studies have reported improvements in positive and negative symptoms of schizophrenia in betel nut chewers. However, there are no high-quality, prospective studies in this area. The arecoline constituent of betel nut has been found to possess cholinergic properties, and extrapyramidal side effects have been observed with betel use. Until further data are available, the risks associated with short- and long-term chewing or ingestion of betel nut may outweigh the benefits.

Evidence

- Sullivan et al. studied 70 hospitalized patients in Micronesia with a diagnosis of schizophrenia or schizoaffective disorder.[122,123] Self-reports were used to divide patients into two groups, based on levels of betel nut utilization: "serious" betel nut chewers (>2 betel nuts per day; n = 40), and "casual"/non-users (n = 30). A standardized measurement instrument was then used to assess the severity of schizophrenia positive

and negative symptoms, the PANSS (positive and negative syndrome scale). The authors reported that the "casual"/non-user group had significantly higher scores on the PANSS, correlated with more severe disease, than the "serious" users. A sub-group analysis found that the differences between groups were present both in patients who were taking antipsychotic medications, and in those who were not medicated (although improvements in positive symptoms were not observed in the unmedicated group). Limitations of this study include the lack of controls or use of a prospective cohort, and self-reporting by patients as a means of group separation. In addition, it is not clear if betel nut chewing was the cause of improved symptoms or if patients who already might have had higher baseline scores on the PANSS were more highly functioning, and therefore capable of participating in activities such as betel nut chewing. Prospective data would address this issue.

- A case report documents betel use in a Micronesian woman diagnosed with chronic paranoid schizophrenia.[124] She stopped betel nut use prior to her diagnosis and treatment. Despite two months of therapy with fluphenazine, the patient continued to experience psychotic symptoms. When the patient resumed betel nut use, she was observed to experience an improvement in her symptoms. However, it is not clear if betel chewing was the cause of her improvement or if an improvement in her symptoms for other reasons may have affected her level of functioning, such that she could resume betel nut chewing.

Anemia
Summary

- An observational study reports a small statistically significant decrease in the incidence of anemia in pregnant betel nut chewers vs. non-chewers. Until further data are available, the risks of betel use likely outweigh any potential benefits.

Evidence

- Taufa studied the frequency of anemia among non-smoking women in New Guinea at the time of delivery.[79] All women (n = 453) admitted to a labor ward were interviewed for betel nut utilization. Betel use, defined as any amount of use during the course of pregnancy, was found in 315 subjects, while 138 women were defined as non-users. Hemoglobin levels were measured in antenatal blood at the time of labor. The incidence of anemia, defined as hemoglobin <10 g/dL, was found in 59% of non-users and in 48% of betel users, with statistical significance. Notably, there were no significant differences between the two groups in terms of socio-economic status or method of delivery, and two subjects in each group were diagnosed with malaria. Only one measurement of hemoglobin was made per subject, which, due to potential variability in results of the assay, may have reduced the reliability of the overall results. The lack of controls or prospective design allows for the possible introduction of confounding factors; although no differences were detected in socioeconomic status or malaria status, there may be other fundamental differences between individuals who choose to chew betel nuts or to abstain that might affect levels of hemoglobin.

Dental Caries
Summary

- Toothpaste containing areca nut was once used due to the belief that areca nut could protect against tooth decay while strengthening gums, but its use has now has been discontinued.[2] Results from poorly described retrospective analyses suggest that betel nut chewing may serve a protective role against the development of dental caries. *In vitro* data suggest antimicrobial effects of betel nut, which may play a role. However, because of the known toxicity associated with acute or chronic betel use, and the availability of other therapies with demonstrated efficacy against the development of dental caries, the risks of betel nut use likely outweigh the potential benefits.

Evidence

- Howden assessed the effects of betel nut chewing on dental health in a retrospective analysis.[125] Subjects who were non-chewers were compared to regular betel nut chewers. The prevalence of dental caries was found to be 23% for betel chewers vs. 49% for non-chewers, with statistical significance. In a retrospective analysis of 982 subjects, an inverse relationship was noted between the incidence of dental caries and frequency of betel nut chewing.[126] In a similar study of 301 subjects in New Guinea, the prevalence of dental caries was also found to be inversely proportional to the frequency of betel nut chewing.[127]

Ulcerative Colitis
Summary

- Currently there is a lack of sufficient evidence to recommend the use of betel nut as a protective agent for ulcerative colitis. Based on the known toxicities associated with acute or chronic betel use, the risks likely outweigh any potential benefits.

Evidence

- In a prospective cohort study with matched controls, 116 Asian patients with inflammatory bowel disease were compared to 79 healthy controls.[128] All subjects were given questionnaires regarding their betel nut chewing and smoking habits. It was found that the prevalence of ulcerative colitis was 13% in betel nut chewers vs. 20% in non-chewers ($p < 0.05$). Smokers were also found to have a decreased incidence of developing ulcerative colitis. This preliminary finding suggests that betel nut chewing may reduce the risk of developing ulcerative colitis.

Central Nervous System (CNS) Stimulation
Summary

- Constituents of betel have been shown to possess psychoactive and euphoric effects.[28] Although not systematically evaluated in humans, betel nut is often used recreationally for its reported stimulant effects. Other substances that may be combined with betel nut when chewing, such as tobacco, may serve as confounders. Based on the known toxicities associated with acute or chronic betel use, the risks likely outweigh any potential benefits.

Salivary Stimulation
Summary

- Although not systematically evaluated in humans, betel nut chewing has been noted to produce copious salivation in users, possibly due to the muscarinic agonist activity of betel components. However, based on the known toxicities associated with acute or chronic betel use, the risks likely outweigh any potential benefits.

References

1. Scrimgeour EM, Dethlefs RF, Kevau I. Delayed recovery of vision after blindness caused by methanol poisoning. Med J Aust 1982;2(10):481-483.
2. Schullian D. Notes and Events. J Hist Med 1984;39:65-68.
3. van Wyk CW, Stander I, Padayachee A, et al. The areca nut chewing habit and oral squamous cell carcinoma in South African Indians. A retrospective study. S Afr Med J 1993;83(6):425-429.
4. Babu S, Bhat RV, Kumar PU, et al. A comparative clinico-pathological study of oral submucous fibrosis in habitual chewers of pan masala and betelquid. J Toxicol Clin Toxicol 1996;34(3):317-322.
5. Fendell LD, Smith JR. Betel-nut-associated cancer: report of case. J Oral Surg 1970;28(6):455-456.
6. Liu CJ, Chen CL, Chang KW, et al. Safrole in betel quid may be a risk factor for hepatocellular carcinoma: case report. CMAJ 2000;162(3):359-360.
7. Phukan RK, Ali MS, Chetia CK, et al. Betel nut and tobacco chewing; potential risk factors of cancer of oesophagus in Assam, India. Br J Cancer 2001;85(5):661-667.
8. Sheikh MY, Rizvi IH, Ahmed I. Oesophageal carcinoma caused by betel nut. J Pak Med Assoc 1992;42(6):145-146.
9. Srivatanakul P, Parkin DM, Khlat M, et al. Liver cancer in Thailand. II. A case-control study of hepatocellular carcinoma. Int J Cancer 1991;48(3):329-332.
10. Tsai JF, Chuang LY, Jeng JE, et al. Betel quid chewing as a risk factor for hepatocellular carcinoma: a case-control study. Br J Cancer 2001;84(5):709-713.
11. Wu MT, Lee YC, Chen CJ, et al. Risk of betel chewing for oesophageal cancer in Taiwan. Br J Cancer 2001;85(5):658-660.
12. Cunningham L, Worrel T, Leflore J. Acute lead poisoning from the betel nut. A case report. J Tenn Med Assoc 1985;78(8):491-492.
13. Liou SH, Wu TN, Chiang HC, et al. Blood lead levels in the general population of Taiwan, Republic of China. Int Arch Occup Environ Health 1994;66(4):255-260.
14. Raisuddin S, Misra JK. Aflatoxin in betel nut and its control by use of food preservatives. Food Addit.Contam 1991;8(6):707-712.
15. Taylor RF, al-Jarad N, John LM, et al. Betel-nut chewing and asthma. Lancet 1992;339(8802):1134-1136.
16. Liao YL, Chiang YC, Tsai TF, et al. Contact leukomelanosis induced by the leaves of *Piper betel* L. (Piperaceae): a clinical and histopathologic survey. J Am Acad Dermatol 1999;40(4):583-589.
17. Deahl M. Betel nut-induced extrapyramidal syndrome: an unusual drug interaction. Mov Disord 1989;4(4):330-332.
18. Deahl MP. Psychostimulant properties of betel nuts. BMJ 1987;294:841.
19. Nutt JG, Rosin A, Chase TN. Treatment of Huntington disease with a cholinergic agonist. Neurology 1978;28(10):1061-1064.
20. Huang Z, Xiao B, Wang X, et al. Betel nut indulgence as a cause of epilepsy. Seizure 2003;12(6):406-408.

21. Nelson BS, Heischober B. Betel nut: a common drug used by naturalized citizens from India, Far East Asia, and the South Pacific Islands. Ann Emerg Med 1999;34(2):238-243.
22. Chu NS. Effect of betel chewing on RR interval variation. J Formos Med Assoc 1995;94(3):106-110.
23. Chu NS. Effects of betel chewing on electroencephalographic activity: spectral analysis and topographic mapping. J Formos Med Assoc 1994; 93(2):167-169.
24. Chu NS. Effect of betel chewing on performance reaction time. J Formos Med Assoc 1994;93(4):343-345.
25. Stricherz ME, Pratt P. Betel quid and reaction time. Pharmacol Biochem Behav 1976;4(5):627-628.
26. Wyatt TA. Betel nut chewing and selected psychophysiological variables. Psychol Rep 1996;79(2):451-463.
27. Vimokesant SL, Hilker DM, Nakornchai S, et al. Effects of betel nut and fermented fish on the thiamin status of northeastern Thais. Am J Clin Nutr 1975;28(12):1458-1463.
28. Talonu NT. Observations on betel-nut use, habituation, addiction and carcinogenesis in Papua New Guineans. P N G Med J 1989;32(3):195-197.
29. Pickwell SM, Schimelpfening S, Palinkas LA. 'Betelmania'. Betel quid chewing by Cambodian women in the United States and its potential health effects. West J Med 1994;160(4):326-330.
30. Chu NS. Effects of Betel chewing on the central and autonomic nervous systems. J Biomed Sci 2001;8(3):229-236.
31. Wiesner DM. Betel-nut withdrawal. Med J Aust 1987;146(8):453.
32. Chiang WT, Yang CC, Deng JF, et al. Cardiac arrhythmia and betel nut chewing—is there a causal effect? Vet Hum Toxicol 1998;40(5):287-289.
33. Chu NS. Sympathetic response to betel chewing. J Psychoactive Drugs 1995;27(2):183-186.
34. Deng JF, Ger J, Tsai WJ, et al. Acute toxicities of betel nut: rare but probably overlooked events. J Toxicol Clin Toxicol 2001;39(4):355-360.
35. Frewer LJ. The effect of betel nut on human performance. P N G Med J 1990;33(2):143-145.
36. Hung DZ, Deng JF. Acute myocardial infarction temporally related to betel nut chewing. Vet Hum Toxicol 1998;40(1):25-28.
37. Sharma AK, Gupta R, Gupta HP, et al. Haemodynamic effects of pan masala in healthy volunteers. J Assoc Physicians India 2000;48(4):400-401.
38. Chu NS. Cardiovascular responses to betel chewing. J Formos Med Assoc 1993;92(9):835-837.
39. Chang MC, Kuo MY, Hahn LJ, et al. Areca nut extract inhibits the growth, attachment, and matrix protein synthesis of cultured human gingival fibroblasts. J Periodontol 1998;69(10):1092-1097.
40. Metha FS, et al. Relation of betel leaf chewing to periodontal disease. JADA 1955;50(5):531-536.
41. Rao MB, Rao CB. Incidence of temporomandibular joint pain dysfunction syndrome in rural population. Int J Oral Surg 1981;10(4):261-265.
42. Westermeyer J. Betel Nut Chewing. JAMA 1982;248(15):1835.
43. Gupta PC, Sinor PN, Bhonsle RB, et al. Oral submucous fibrosis in India: a new epidemic? Natl Med J India 1998;11(3):113-116.
44. Murlidhar V, Upmanyu G. Tobacco chewing, oral submucous fibrosis, and anaesthetic risk. Lancet 1996;347:1840.
45. Seedat HA, van Wyk CW. Betel-nut chewing and submucous fibrosis in Durban. S Afr Med J 1988;74(11):568-571.
46. Seedat HA, van Wyk CW. Betel chewing and dietary habits of chewers without and with submucous fibrosis and with concomitant oral cancer. S.Afr.Med J 1988;74(11):572-575.
47. Tang JG, Jian XF, Gao ML, et al. Epidemiological survey of oral sub-mucous fibrosis in Xiangtan City, Hunan Province, China. Community Dent Oral Epidemiol 1997;25(2):177-180.
48. Anil S, Beena VT. Oral submucous fibrosis in a 12-year-old girl: case report. Pediatr Dent 1993;15(2):120-122.
49. Cox SC, Walker DM. Oral submucous fibrosis. A review. Aust Dent J 1996;41(5):294-299.
50. Hazare VK, Goel RR, Gupta PC. Oral submucous fibrosis, areca nut and pan masala use: a case-control study. Natl Med J India 1998;11(6):299.
51. Sinor PN, Gupta PC, Murti PR, et al. A case-control study of oral sub-mucous fibrosis with special reference to the etiologic role of areca nut. J Oral Pathol Med 1990;19(2):94-98.
52. Seedat HA, van Wyk CW. The oral features of betel nut chewers without submucous fibrosis. J Biol Buccale 1988;16(3):123-128.
53. Shah N, Sharma PP. Role of chewing and smoking habits in the etiology of oral submucous fibrosis (OSF): a case-control study. J Oral Pathol Med 1998;27(10):475-479.
54. Seedat HA, van Wyk CW. Submucous fibrosis (SF) in ex-betel nut chewers: a report of 14 cases. J Oral Pathol Med 1988;17(5):226-229.
55. Shiu MN, Chen TH, Chang SH, et al. Risk factors for leukoplakia and malignant transformation to oral carcinoma: a leukoplakia cohort in Taiwan. Br J Cancer 2000;82(11):1871-1874.
56. Yang YH, Lee HY, Tung S, et al. Epidemiological survey of oral submucous fibrosis and leukoplakia in aborigines of Taiwan. J Oral Pathol Med 2001; 30(4):213-219.
57. Pearson N, Croucher R, Marcenes W, et al. Prevalence of oral lesions among a sample of Bangladeshi medical users aged 40 years and over living in Tower Hamlets, UK. Int Dent J 2001;51(1):30-34.
58. Chin CT, Lee KW. The effects of betel-nut chewing on the buccal mucosa of 296 Indians and Malays in West Malaysia. A clinical study. Br J Cancer 1970;24(3):427-432.
59. Tennekoon GE, Bartlett GC. Effect of betel chewing on the oral mucosa. Br J Cancer 1969;23(1):39-43.
60. Thomas SJ, MacLennan R. Slaked lime and betel nut cancer in Papua New Guinea. Lancet 1992;340(8819):577-578.
61. Maher R, Lee AJ, Warnakulasuriya KA, et al. Role of areca nut in the causation of oral submucous fibrosis: a case-control study in Pakistan. J Oral Pathol Med 1994;23(2):65-69.
62. Kiyingi KS. Betel-nut chewing may aggravate asthma. PNG Med J 1991; 34(2):117-121.
63. Kiyingi KS, Saweri A. Betelnut chewing causes bronchoconstriction in some asthma patients. PNG Med J 1994;37(2):90-99.
64. Boucher BJ, Ewen SW, Stowers JM. Betel nut (Areca catechu) consumption and the induction of glucose intolerance in adult CD1 mice and in their F1 and F2 offspring. Diabetologia 1994;37(1):49-55.
65. Chempakam B. Hypoglycaemic activity of arecoline in betel nut Areca catechu L. Indian J Exp Biol 1993;31(5):474-475.
66. Mannan N, Boucher BJ, Evans SJ. Increased waist size and weight in relation to consumption of Areca catechu (betel-nut); a risk factor for increased glycaemia in Asians in east London. Br J Nutr 2000;83(3): 267-273.
67. Dowse GK. Betel-nut chewing and diabetes in Papua New Guinea and elsewhere. Diabetologia 1994;37(10):1062-1064.
68. Panda S, Kar A. Dual role of betel leaf extract on thyroid function in male mice. Pharmacol Res 1998;38(6):493-496.
69. Chu NS. Betel chewing increases the skin temperature: effects of atropine and propranolol. Neurosci Lett 1995;194(1-2):130-132.
70. Chakrabarti RN, Dutta K, Ghosh K, et al. Uterine cervical dysplasia with reference to the betel quid chewing habit. Eur J Gynaecol Oncol 1990; 11(1):57-59.
71. Wu KD, Chuang RB, Wu FL, et al. The milk-alkali syndrome caused by betelnuts in oyster shell paste. J Toxicol Clin Toxicol 1996;34(6):741-745.
72. Chaudhry K. Is pan masala-containing tobacco carcinogenic? Natl Med J India 1999;12(1):21-27.
73. Bhisey RA, Ramchandani AG, D'Souza AV, et al. Long-term carcinogenicity of pan masala in Swiss mice. Int J Cancer 1999;83(5):679-684.
74. Chen GS, Chen CH. [A statistical analysis of oral squamous cell carcinoma]. Gaoxiong.Yi Xue Ke Xue Za Zhi 1995;11(10):582-588.
75. Daftary DK, Bhonsle RB, Murti RB, et al. An oral lichen planus–like lesion in Indian betel-tobacco chewers. Scand J Dent Res 1980;88(3):244-249.
76. Stoopler ET, Parisi E, Sollecito TP. Betel quid–induced oral lichen planus: a case report. Cutis 2003;71(4):307-311.
77. Sinha A, Rao AR. Embryotoxicity of betel nuts in mice. Toxicology 1985; 37(3-4):315-326.
78. Yang MS, Chang FT, Chen SS, et al. Betel quid chewing and risk of adverse pregnancy outcomes among aborigines in southern Taiwan. Public Health 1999;113(4):189-192.
79. Taufa T. Betel-nut chewing and pregnancy. Papua New Guinea Med J 1988;31:229-234.
80. Dar A, Khatoon S. Behavioral and biochemical studies of dichloromethane fraction from the Areca catechu nut. Pharmacol Biochem Behav 2000; 65(1):1-6.
81. Inokuchi J, Okabe H, Yamauchi T, et al. Antihypertensive substance in seeds of Areca catechu L. Life Sci 1986;38(15):1375-1382.
82. Jeon SM, Kim HS, Lee TG, et al. Lower absorption of cholesteryl oleate in rats supplemented with Areca catechu L. extract. Ann Nutr Metab 2000; 44(4):170-176.
83. Raghavan V, Baruah HK. Areca nut: India's popular masticatory—history, chemistry and utilization. Economic Botany 1958;12:315-345.
84. de Miranda CM, van Wyk CW, van der BP, et al. The effect of areca nut on salivary and selected oral microorganisms. Int Dent J 1996;46(4):350-356.
85. Harvey W, Scutt A, Meghji S, et al. Stimulation of human buccal mucosa fibroblasts in vitro by betel-nut alkaloids. Arch Oral Biol 1986;31(1):45-49.
86. Hanley MR, Iversen LL. Muscarinic cholinergic receptors in rat corpus striatum and regulation of guanosine cyclic 3',5'-monophosphate. Mol Pharmacol 1978;14(2):246-255.
87. Johnston GA, Krogsgaard-Larsen P, Stephanson A. Betel nut constituents as inhibitors of gamma-aminobutyric acid uptake. Nature 1975; 258(5536):627-628.
88. Smythies JR. Betel nut as a GABA blocker. Am J Psychiatry 1977; 134(7):822.
89. Lodge D, Johnston GA, Curtis DR, et al. Effects of the Areca nut constituents arecaidine and guvacine on the action of GABA in the cat central nervous system. Brain Res 1977;136(3):513-522.
90. Kumar M, Kannan A, Upreti RK. Effect of betel/areca nut (Areca catechu) extracts on intestinal epithelial cell lining. Vet Hum Toxicol 2000;42(5): 257-260.
91. Hung SL, Chen YL, Wan HC, et al. Effects of areca nut extracts on the functions of human neutrophils in vitro. J Periodontal Res 2000;35(4): 186-193.
92. Jeng JH, Ho YS, Chan CP, et al. Areca nut extract up-regulates prostaglandin production, cyclooxygenase-mRNA and protein expression of human oral keratinocytes. Carcinogenesis 2000;21(7):1365-1370.
93. Nair UJ, Nair J, Friesen MD, et al. Ortho- and meta-tyrosine formation

from phenylalanine in human saliva as a marker of hydroxyl radical generation during betel quid chewing. Carcinogenesis 1995;16(5):1195-1198.

94. Lee HC, Yin PH, Yu TN, et al. Accumulation of mitochondrial DNA deletions in human oral tissues—effects of betel quid chewing and oral cancer. Mutat Res 2001;493(1-2):67-74.

95. Dave BJ, Trivedi AH, Adhvaryu SG. Role of areca nut consumption in the cause of oral cancers. A cytogenetic assessment. Cancer 1992;70(5): 1017-1023.

96. Ho TJ, Chiang CP, Hong CY, et al. Induction of the c-jun protooncogene expression by areca nut extract and arecoline on oral mucosal fibroblasts. Oral Oncol 2000;36(5):432-436.

97. Sundqvist K, Grafstrom RC. Effects of areca nut on growth, differentiation and formation of DNA damage in cultured human buccal epithelial cells. Int J Cancer 1992;52(2):305-310.

98. Liu TY, Chen CL, Chi CW. Oxidative damage to DNA induced by areca nut extract. Mutat Res 1996;367(1):25-31.

99. Lin MH, Chou FP, Huang HP, et al. The tumor promoting effect of lime–piper betel quid in JB6 cells. Food Chem Toxicol 2003;41(11): 1463-1471.

100. Dave BJ, Trivedi AH, Adhvaryu SG. *In vitro* genotoxic effects of areca nut extract and arecoline. J Cancer Res Clin Oncol 1992;118(4):283-288.

101. Jeng JH, Hahn LJ, Lin BR, et al. Effects of areca nut, inflorescence piper betel extracts and arecoline on cytotoxicity, total and unscheduled DNA synthesis in cultured gingival keratinocytes. J Oral Pathol Med 1999; 2(28):64-71.

102. Jeng JH, Kuo ML, Hahn LJ, et al. Genotoxic and non-genotoxic effects of betel quid ingredients on oral mucosal fibroblasts *in vitro*. J Dent Res 1994;73(5):1043-1049.

103. Jeng JH, Chang MC, Hahn LJ. Role of areca nut in betel quid–associated chemical carcinogenesis: current awareness and future perspectives. Oral Oncol 2001;37(6):477-492.

104. Van Wyck CW, Olivier A, De Miranda CM, et al. Observations on the effect of areca nut exracts on oral fibroblast proliferation. J Oral Pathol Med 1994;23(4):145-148.

105. Chang MC, Ho YS, Lee PH, et al. Areca nut extract and arecoline induced the cell cycle arrest but not apoptosis of cultured oral KB epithelial cells: association of glutathione, reactive oxygen species and mitochondrial membrane potential. Carcinogenesis 2001;22(9):1527-1535.

106. Ashby J, Styles JA, Boyland E. Betel nuts, arecaidine, and oral cancer. Lancet 1979;1(8107):112.

107. Chang YC, Tai KW, Lii CK, et al. Cytopathologic effects of arecoline on human gingival fibroblasts *in vitro*. Clin Oral Investig. 1999;3(1):25-29.

108. Chang YC, Hu CC, Lii CK, et al. Cytotoxicity and arecoline mechanisms in human gingival fibroblasts *in vitro*. Clin Oral Investig 2001;5(1):51-56.

109. Chen CC, Huang JF, Tsai CC. *In vitro* production of interleukin-6 by human gingival, normal buccal mucosa, and oral submucous fibrosis fibroblasts treated with betel-nut alkaloids. Gaoxiong Yi Xue Ke Xue Za Zhi 1995;11(11):604-614.

110. Trivedy C, Baldwin D, Warnakulasuriya S, et al. Copper content in Areca *catechu* (betel nut) products and oral submucous fibrosis. Lancet 1997; 349(9063):1447.

111. Awang MN. Fate of betel nut chemical constituents following nut treatment prior to chewing and its relation to oral precancerous & cancerous lesion. Dent J Malays. 1988;10(1):33-37.

112. Rao AR, Das P. Evaluation of the carcinogenicity of different preparations of areca nut in mice. Int J Cancer 1989;43(4):728-732.

113. Nair UJ, Friesen M, Richard I, et al. Effect of lime composition on the formation of reactive oxygen species from areca nut extract in vitro. Carcinogenesis 1990;11(12):2145-2148.

114. Kiyingi KS. Slaked lime and betel nut cancer in Papua New Guinea. Lancet 1992;340(8831):1357-1358.

115. Chakarvarti SK, Dhiman J, Nagpaul KK. Uranium trace analysis of a chewable betel-leaf preparation and tea-leaves. Health Physics 1981;40: 78-81.

116. Shirname LP, Menon MM, Nair J, et al. Correlation of mutagenicity and tumorigenicity of betel quid and its ingredients. Nutr Cancer 1983; 5(2):87-91.

117. Mukherjee A, Chakrabarti J, Chakrabarti A, et al. Effect of 'Pan Masala' on the germ cells of male mice. Cancer Lett 1991;58(3):161-165.

118. Singh A, Rao AR. Modulatory effect of Areca nut on the action of mace (*Myristica fragrans*, Houtt) on the hepatic detoxification system in mice. Food Chem Toxicol 1993;31(7):517-521.

119. Norton SA. Betel: consumption and consequences. J Am Acad Dermatol 1998;38(1):81-88.

120. Mannan MA, Mohammad QD, Haqua A, et al. Role of areca-catechu (betel-nut) in cerebrovascular disease: a double blind clinical trial. Bangladesh J Neuro 1988;4(2):46-51.

121. Mannan MA. *Areca catechu* for treatment of cerebrovascular disease (CVD). Neuroscience 1987;22(Suppl):S539.

122. Sullivan RJ, Allen JS, Otto C, et al. Effects of chewing betel nut (*Areca catechu*) on the symptoms of people with schizophrenia in Palau, Micronesia. Br J Psychiatry 2000;177:174-178.

123. Kuruppuarachchi KA, Williams SS. Betel use and schizophrenia. Br J Psychiatry 2003;182:455.

124. Wilson LG. Cross-cultural differences in indicators of improvement from psychosis: the case of betel nut chewing. J Nerv Ment Dis 1979;167(4): 250-251.

125. Howden GF. The cariostatic effect of betel nut chewing. P N G Med J 1984;27(3-4):123-131.

126. Moller IJ, Pindborg JJ, Effendi I. The relation between betel chewing and dental caries. Scand J Dent Res 1977;85(1):64-70.

127. Schamschula RG, Adkins BL, Barmes DE, et al. Betal chewing and caries experience in New Guinea. Community Dent Oral Epidemiol 1977;5(6): 284-286.

128. Lee CN, Jayanthi V, McDonald B, et al. Betel nut and smoking. Are they both protective in ulcerative colitis? A pilot study. Arq Gastroenterol 1996;33(1):3-5.

Bilberry
(*Vaccinium myrtillus*)

SYNONYMS/COMMON NAMES/RELATED SUBSTANCES

- Airelle, bickbeere, black whortle, blaubeere, blaubessen, bleaberry, blueberry, burren myrtle, dwarf bilberry, dyeberry, European blueberry, heidelbeere, heidelberry, hurtleberry, huckleberry, mirtillo nero, myrtilli fructus, trackleberry, *Vaccinium myrtillus* anthocyanoside (VMA) extract, *Vaccinium myrtillus* extract (VME), whortleberry, wineberry.

CLINICAL BOTTOM LINE
Background

- Bilberry, a close relative of blueberry, has a long history of medicinal use. The dried fruit has been popular for the symptomatic treatment of diarrhea, for topical relief of minor mucous membrane inflammation, and for a variety of eye disorders, including poor night vision, eyestrain, and myopia.
- Bilberry fruit and its extracts contain a number of biologically active components, including a class of compounds called anthocyanosides. These have been the focus of recent research in Europe.
- Bilberry extract has been evaluated for efficacy as an antioxidant, mucostimulant, hypoglycemic, anti-inflammatory, "vasoprotectant," and lipid-lowering agent. Although preclinical studies have been promising, human data are limited and largely of poor quality. At this time, there is not sufficient evidence in support of or against the use of bilberry for most indications. Notably, the evidence suggests a lack of benefit of bilberry for the improvement of night vision.
- Bilberry is commonly used to make jams, pies, cobblers, syrups, and alcoholic/non-alcoholic beverages. Fruit extracts are used as a coloring agent in wines.

Scientific Evidence for Common/Studied Uses	Grade*
Atherosclerosis and peripheral vascular disease	C
Cataracts	C
Chronic venous insufficiency	C
Diabetes mellitus	C
Diarrhea	C
Dysmenorrhea	C
Fibrocystic breast disease	C
Peptic ulcer disease (PUD)	C
Retinopathy (diabetic, vascular)	C
Night vision	D

*Key to grades: *A:* Strong scientific evidence for this use; *B:* Good scientific evidence for this use; *C:* Unclear scientific evidence for this use; *D:* Fair scientific evidence against this use (it may not work); *F:* Strong scientific evidence against this use (it likely does not work). For a more detailed explanation of efficacy criteria, see "Natural Standard Evidence-Based Validated Grading Rationale" in the Introduction.

Historical or Theoretical Uses That Lack Sufficient Evidence

- Angina, antioxidant,[1-4] arthritis, bleeding gums, cancer,[5,6] common cold, cough, dermatitis, dysentery, dyspepsia, fevers, functional heart disease, glaucoma,[7] gout, hematuria, hemorrhoids,[8-10] hyperlipidemia,[4,11-13] hypertension, infantile dyspepsia, kidney disease, myopia,[7,14,15] liver disease, oral ulcers, pharyngitis, poor circulation, prevention/stopping of lactation,[16] retinitis pigmentosa,[7,17,18] scurvy, skin infections, urinary tract infections, varicose veins of pregnancy.[19]

Expert Opinion and Historic Precedent

- Currently, bilberry products are used in Europe as vasoprotective agents and as prevention or treatment of various disorders of the eye, especially night blindness. In addition, bilberry has been used to treat eye conditions such as cataracts, diabetic retinopathy, retinitis pigmentosa, glaucoma, and macular degeneration.
- Herbalists have commonly used the berries to treat diarrhea. Some surgeons in Europe recommend bilberry for enhanced wound healing. Many herbalists have used an extract made from the leaves to treat urinary tract infections. Some believe that bilberry's tannin content accounts for its historical use as a treatment for diarrhea, oral ulcers, and sore throat, but there are no confirmatory studies.
- Use of bilberry leaf extracts in high doses is often regarded as unsafe owing to potential toxic side effects.

Safety Summary

- **Likely safe:** When taken as fruit in amounts typically found in foods, or as fruit extract in recommended doses by otherwise healthy individuals for brief periods of time.
- **Possibly unsafe:** When used in patients with disorders of platelet function, with bleeding disorders, or taking oral anticoagulant therapy, because of increased risk of bleeding (theoretical); or in combination with hypoglycemic medications, because of increased risk of hypoglycemia (theoretical).
- **Likely unsafe:** In large quantities, acute toxicity may occur in the form of hydroquinone poisoning, anticoagulation, or gastrointestinal distress.[20]

DOSING/TOXICOLOGY
General

- Recommended doses are based on those most commonly used in available trials, or on historical practice. However, with natural products, the optimal doses needed to balance efficacy and safety often have not been determined. Formulations and preparation methods may vary from manufacturer to manufacturer, and from batch to batch of a specific product made by a single manufacturer. Because often the active components of a product are not known, standardization may not be possible, and the clinical effects of different brands may not be comparable.

Standardization

- Bilberry VMA (*Vaccinium myrtillus* anthocyanoside, the anthocyanoside component of the extract) standardized to contain 25% anthocyanidin has been used in most European studies. However, the strength and dosing of preparations available in the United States may differ from those used in European studies. Patients may be advised to follow specific dosing instructions for each formulation.

Dosing: Adult (18 Years and Older)
Oral

- **Circulatory and ophthalmologic uses:** Bilberry VMA extract doses range from 80 to 480 mg daily in 2 to 3 divided doses. A common recommended dose is 80 mg of extract twice daily (standardized to contain 25% anthocyanidin).[21-31]
- **Acute diarrhea:** No reliable scientific data exist to support the use of bilberry for diarrhea. Experts, however, recommend dried fruit 4 to 8 g orally with water two times/day, or a decoction of dried fruit orally three times/day (made by boiling 5 to 10 g of crushed dried fruit in 150 mL of water for 10 minutes and straining while hot), or cold macerate of dried fruit orally three times/day (made by soaking dried crushed fruit in 150 mL water for several hours). Experts caution that for the treatment of diarrhea, only preparations of dried bilberry should be used, as the fresh fruit may actually exert a laxative effect.
- **Ulcer prevention:** There are no human studies on ulcer prevention using bilberry. However, in rats, a natural flavonoid, IdB1027 (VMA extract from bilberry), has demonstrated promising anti-ulcer effects.[16,32,33] Despite the lack of human trials, experts recommend half a cup of fresh bilberries (difficult to acquire in the United States) or 20 to 40 mg of standardized anthocyanidin extract three times/day.[34]
- **Dysmenorrhea:** 160 mg of bilberry VMA extract taken orally twice daily for 8 days, started three days before menses, has been used in a small trial.[34]
- **General:** Doses recommended by some experts based on traditional use include 55 to 115 g of fresh berries three times daily, or 80 to 160 mg of aqueous extract three times daily (standardized to 25% anthocyanosides).

Topical

- **Mucous membrane inflammation:** Experts recommend gargle mouthwash of 10% dried fruit decoction as needed.

Dosing: Pediatric (Younger Than 18 Years)
- Insufficient available evidence.

Toxicology
- Safety of bilberry fruit is often presumed based on food exposure history. Literature review reveals neither animal nor human studies that report toxicity. In large quantities, acute toxicity may occur in the form of hydroquinone poisoning, anticoagulation, or gastrointestinal distress.[20]

ADVERSE EFFECTS/PRECAUTIONS/CONTRAINDICATIONS
Allergy

- Avoid in patients with allergy to bilberry or any of its constituents. Literature review reveals no reports of clinically significant allergic reactions. Herbal products carry the potential for contamination with other herbal products, pesticides, herbicides, heavy metals, and pharmaceuticals.

Adverse Effects/Postmarket Surveillance

- **General:** The long-term safety and side effects of bilberry have not been extensively studied. Safety is often presumed based on bilberry's history as a food source. Morazzoni and Bombardelli reported the results of French postmarketing

surveillance data from 2295 individuals using the bilberry extract Tegens before 1987.[8] Adverse effects were experienced by 4% of patients overall, with 1% complaining of gastrointestinal discomfort, and <1% experiencing nausea or "heartburn."

- **Gastrointestinal:** Theoretically, bilberry fresh fruit may exert a laxative effect. For this reason, only dried bilberry or preparations of the dried bilberry are usually recommended for the treatment of diarrhea. One postmarket surveillance report of patients using bilberry extract (Tegens) found 1% of patients complaining of gastrointestinal discomfort, and <1% experiencing nausea or "heartburn."
- **Endocrine:** Hypoglycemia has been demonstrated in animal studies, even in the setting of intravenous glucose administration.[13] Human data are limited.
- **Cardiovascular:** Bilberry has been theorized to potentially decrease blood pressure, based on pre-clinical evidence of vascular smooth muscle–relaxing properties.[35-37] Bilberry products are sometimes marketed for the treatment of hypertension. However, literature review reveals no human data to support these assertions.
- **Hematologic:** With the use of bilberry leaf extract, there is a theoretical bleeding risk, based on the antiplatelet and potential anticoagulant actions of bilberry extract, although there have been no human reports of bleeding in the available literature.[38]

Precautions/Warnings/Contraindications

- Long-term side effects and safety of bilberry remain unknown.
- Use cautiously in doses higher than recommended. European studies have used 25% anthocyanoside extract dosed at 80 to 160 mg three times/day.[21,38] Toxicity may theoretically occur at higher doses.
- Use bilberry cautiously in patients with bleeding disorders or using anticoagulant/antiplatelet medications, because of a theoretical increased risk of bleeding.
- Use bilberry cautiously in patients with diabetes or on hypoglycemic medications, because of the theoretical risk of hypoglycemia.
- Safety in pregnancy and during lactation has not been established but is presumed by many to be safe, based on the use of bilberry as a food product.
- Avoid ingesting bilberry leaves: experts suggest possible toxicity.

Pregnancy and Lactation

- Safety of bilberry in pregnancy has not been established or studied systematically. However, one study used bilberry extract to treat pregnancy-induced lower extremity edema, and no adverse effects were reported.[19] Bilberry fruit is presumed to be safe on the basis of the use of bilberry as a food product.

INTERACTIONS
Bilberry/Drug Interactions

- **Non-steroidal anti-inflammatory drugs (NSAIDs), anticoagulants, antiplatelet agents:** There is a theoretical bleeding risk based on the antiplatelet and potential anticoagulant actions of bilberry extract, although there have been no human reports of bleeding in the available literature.[38]
- **Insulin, oral hypoglycemic drugs:** When treated with bilberry leaf extract, diabetic rats developed hypoglycemia,

even in the setting of intravenous glucose administration.[13] Therefore, there is a theoretical risk of additive or synergistic effects when taken with anti-hyperglycemic agents. However, literature review reveals no controlled trials evaluating the effects of bilberry fruits or leaves on blood sugar levels in humans, or any trials evaluating bilberry's potential interaction with standard diabetic medications.

Bilberry/Herb Interactions

- **Anticoagulant/antiplatelet agents:** There is a theoretical bleeding risk, based on the antiplatelet and potential anticoagulant actions of bilberry extract, although there have been no human reports of bleeding in the available literature.[38]
- **Hypoglycemic agents:** Hypoglycemia has been demonstrated in animal studies. An extract was made from bilberry leaves and given to diabetic rats, which then developed hypoglycemia, even in the setting of intravenous glucose administration.[13] In the absence of human data, there exists a theoretical risk of additive or synergistic effects when bilberry products are taken concomitantly with hypoglycemic agents.

Bilberry/Food Interactions

- Insufficient data available.

Bilberry/Lab Interactions

- **Serum glucose:** Hypoglycemia has been demonstrated in animal studies. Rats given an extract made from bilberry developed hypoglycemia, even in the setting of intravenous glucose administration.[13] Human data are lacking.
- **Coagulation panel:** Bilberry extract has been shown to have potential anticoagulant and antiplatelet actions, although there have been no human reports of bleeding in the available literature.[38]

MECHANISM OF ACTION
Pharmacology

- Bilberry contains several compounds with demonstrated biological activity. The main chemicals contained in the extract are anthocyanins, flavonoids, hydroquinone, loeanolic acid, neomyrtillin, sodium, tannins, and ursolic acid.[20,33,39] The anthocyanosides, tannins, and flavonoids have been of particular scientific interest. Tannins are used medicinally as astringents and to treat diarrhea.
- Flavonoids have been shown *in vitro* to possess a number of biological properties, including inhibition of prostacyclin synthesis, reduction of capillary permeability and fragility, free radical scavenging, inhibition of a wide range of enzymes, impairment of coagulation and platelet aggregation, and anti-carcinogenicity.[5]
- Bilberry contains anthocyanosides that are flavonoid derivatives of anthocyanins (the blue, red, or violet pigments found in many berry varieties). These are closely related in structure and activity to flavonoids[20] and possess free radical scavenging/antioxidant properties. An *in vitro* study has suggested that anthocyanosides appear to stabilize connective tissue by enhancing collagen synthesis, inhibiting collagen degradation, and enhancing collagen cross-linking.[40] In contrast, Boniface and Robert. found a significant decrease in connective tissue synthesis (collagen and glycoproteins) in gingival tissue samples of 12 adult diabetics treated with 600 mg of anthocyanosides per day for 2 months.[41]
- Anthocyanosides have been shown to inhibit cyclic adenosine monophosphate (AMP) phosphodiesterase, which is involved in intracellular signal transduction pathways.[16] Anthocyanoside

extract has been shown to have smooth muscle–relaxing activity, which may account for its purported effects in one series of women with dysmenorrhea.[34] Anthocyanosides have also been shown to exert direct effects on the retina, including the alteration of local enzymatic reactions and enhancement of the recovery of rhodopsin.[17]
- Antioxidant properties have been attributed to bilberry based on *in vitro* study,[1-4] although study in humans is not available.

Pharmacodynamics/Kinetics

- There are limited data regarding the pharmacodynamics and kinetics of *Vaccinium myrtillus* (bilberry) anthocyanosides (VMA). In one animal study, bilberry anthocyanosides were rapidly distributed after intraperitoneal injection and intravenous administration.[42] In another animal study, bilberry anthocyanosides were found to be eliminated via the bile and urine, with a modest level of liver extraction.[39]
- Bioavailability in animals is low. Following oral doses in rats, plasma levels of VMA reached a peak at 15 minutes and declined rapidly within 2 hours, and the absolute bioavailability was 1.2% of the administered dose. The gastrointestinal absorption of VMA was 5% of the administered dose.[42] Another study found a differential affinity of VMA for certain tissues (especially skin and kidney). This suggests that different tissues may have more persistent local concentrations.[33]

HISTORY

- The bilberry plant is a deciduous, leafy, freely branched perennial shrub that is native to Northern Europe, Northern America, and Canada. It is found in heaths, moors, and woods in most of Europe, in northern Asia, and in mountain/sub-alpine western North America. Bilberry grows to 35 to 60 cm in height and flowers from April through June. It produces a fruit similar to that of the American blueberry, and the ripe fruits can be collected July through September. The name bilberry is derived from the Danish *bollebar*, which means "dark berry." The berries are purple-black and coarsely wrinkled and contain many small, shiny, brownish-red seeds.
- Bilberry's medicinal use was described by the 12th century German herbalist Hildegard von Bingen (1098-1179), who recommended it for the induction of menses. Herbalists in the 1700s reported its use as well. Decoctions of the dried fruit have a long history of oral use to treat diarrhea, and of topical use to treat mild inflammation of the mouth and mucous membranes. Bilberry preparations have also been used traditionally to help stop the flow of breast milk, and as a treatment for urinary complaints, including nephrolithiasis and urinary tract infections. Tea made from bilberry plant leaves has a long history of use in the management of diabetes mellitus. Bilberry has also been traditionally used as a nutritional supplement in the treatment or prevention of scurvy, because of its vitamin C content.
- The modern use of bilberry in the treatment of various visual disorders dates back to World War II. British Royal Air Force pilots reported that the ingestion of bilberry jam just before missions seemed to improve their vision. Poor-quality studies during the 1960s and 1970s supported these claims. Recently, there have been several open trials and some randomized trials in the European literature investigating the use of bilberry in treating and preventing various visual disorders. Today, bilberry and VMA extracts are used as prophylaxis against cataracts, diabetic retinopathy, glaucoma, macular degeneration, and impaired night vision. Some European

B

surgeons use VMA extract to promote surgical wound healing.

REVIEW OF THE EVIDENCE: DISCUSSION
Chronic Venous Insufficiency
Summary

- Chronic venous insufficiency (CVI) is a syndrome characterized by lower extremity edema, varicosities, pain, pruritis, atrophic skin changes, and ulcerations. *Vaccinium myrtillus*

anthocyanoside (VMA), an extract of bilberry standardized to 25% anthocyanin, is often used in Europe for the treatment of CVI. Literature review reveals several human case series and a single-blind trial that have reported significant improvements in edema and lower extremity discomfort related to CVI. However, due to methodological weaknesses with the available data, there is not sufficient evidence to recommend either for or against the use of bilberry extract for CVI.

Review of the Evidence: Bilberry

Condition Treated*	Study Design	Author, Year	N[†]	SS[†]	Study Quality[‡]	Magnitude of Benefit	ARR[†]	NNT[†]	Comments
Chronic venous insufficiency	Single-blind, placebo-controlled	Gatta[43] 1988	60	Yes	2	Small	NA	NA	30-day trial showing significant improvement, but poor methodological quality.
Diabetic microangiopathy	Case series	Lagrue[49] 1979	54	Unclear	NA	Small	NA	NA	Examined polymeric collagen and structural glycoprotein levels.
Vascular retinopathy (diabetic or hypertensive)	Before and after	Perossini[25] 1987	40	Yes	2	NA	NA	NA	Ophthalmoscopic improvement in 77%-90% of treated patients; poor hypertensive).
Diabetic retinopathy	Controlled trial	Repossi[50] 1987	NA	Yes	1	NA	NA	NA	Ophthalmoscopic end points.
Diabetic retinopathy	Case series	Mosci[26] 1988	30	Yes	NA	Medium	NA	NA	Subjects with and without retinopathy given procyanidolic anthocyanosides; positive ophthalmoscopic end points, but statistical significance not calculated.
Diabetic retinopathy	Case series	Scharrer[51] 1981	31	No	NA	Small	NA	NA	Small study; included small numbers of other eye disorders (macular degeneration, anticoagulant-related hemorrhage).
Cataracts	Double-blind, placebo-controlled	Bravetti[52] 1989	50	Unclear	NA	Large	NA	NA	Combined treatment with vitamin E.
Dysmenorrhea	Randomized, double-blind	Colombo[34] 1985	30	Yes	2	NA	NA	NA	Treatments three days before and during menses reduced nausea, vomiting, headache in treatment group vs. placebo.
Fibrocystic disease of the breast	Case series	Leonardi[57] 1993	257	N/A	NA	Medium	NA	NA	Open trial measuring improvements from baseline.
Night vision	Placebo-controlled	Jayle[31] 1965	60	Yes	3	Medium	NA	NA	Limited description of blinding, randomization, or measurement technique.
Night vision	Placebo-controlled	Jayle[30] 1964	40	Yes	2	N/A	NA	NA	Crossover design; limited description of blinding, randomization, or measurement technique.
Night vision	Double-blind, placebo-controlled, crossover	Zadok[24] 1997	18	Yes	3	None	NA	NA	Early negative study with ophthalmoscopic end points; power calculation performed, but small study nonetheless.
Night vision	Double-blind, placebo-controlled, crossover	Levy[23] 1998	16	Yes	3	None	NA	NA	Negative study, but no power calculation done; examined single-dose VMA effect on 3 tests of night vision.
Night vision	Double-blind, placebo-controlled, crossover	Muth[21] 2000	15	Yes	3	None	NA	NA	3 weeks of high-dose VMA failed to show effect on night vision.

*Primary or secondary outcome.
[†]*N*, Number of patients; *SS*, statistically significant; *ARR*, absolute risk reduction; *NNT*, the number of patients who need to undergo a specific intervention in order to observe an outcome in one individual.
[‡]0-2 = poor; 3-4 = good; 5 = excellent.
NA, Not applicable; *RCT*, randomized, controlled trial. *VMA*, vaccinium myrtillus anthocyanoside.
For an explanation of each category in this table, please see Table 3 in the Introduction.

Evidence

- Bilberry extract has been shown to exert potent effects on vascular permeability and fragility in animal and *in vitro* models. VMA extracts have been widely used in Europe for arterial, venous, and capillary disorders.
- A single-blind placebo-controlled study in 60 patients with chronic venous insufficiency showed significant reduction in symptom severity after 30 days of bilberry therapy.[43] Subjects were given bilberry extract equivalent to 173 mg of anthrocyanins each day or placebo. Reporting of blinding technique and randomization was limited, thus weakening the conclusions of this trial.
- A number of case series of poor methodological quality conducted between 1968 and 1985 reported positive findings. These results can only be considered preliminary because of lack of statistical analysis in some cases, inconsistent classification of subjects, and the use of non-validated measurement instruments to measure outcomes. Since the signs and symptoms of CVI may wax and wane over time, the lack of controls makes it impossible to discern whether improvements were due to bilberry or to the natural history of the disease. Coget and Merlin administered 100 to 150 mg of bilberry anthocyanins daily for 2 weeks per month over 2 months to 27 subjects with varicosities or other lower extremity venous malformations.[44] Subjective improvements in edema, pain, and bruising were reported, with no statistical analysis provided. In a French case series, a heterogeneous group of patients with "lowered capillary resistance" was treated with VMA extract (Difrarel 100, 4 tablets/day) for 12 to 69 days (mean, 28 days).[45] The authors reported a mean increase in capillary resistance over baseline. However, the study enrolled 40 patients with diverse conditions, including atherosclerosis, hypertension, and venous insufficiency of the lower limbs, thus limiting generalization. Ghiringhelli et al. studied 480 mg of bilberry anthocyanins daily (Tegens) for 1 month in 47 subjects with CVI.[46] Statistically significant improvements in lower extremity edema and subjective pain and burning were reported. However, it was not reported if concomitant therapies were used during the trial period. In a 6-month study, Tori and D'Errico administered 480 mg of bilberry anthocyanins daily (Tegens) to 97 patients with lower extremity varicosities.[47] Statistically significant improvements were reported in measurements of edema and discomfort, although it is not clear that the measurements used would be reproducible. Based on these studies, no definitive conclusions can be drawn regarding the use of bilberry in CVI.

Retinopathy (Diabetic, Vascular)
Summary

- Although the efficacy of bilberry in the treatment of retinal and microvascular disease of diabetes has yet to be firmly established, many animal studies and a few small placebo-controlled trials have reported promising results in this area. Clinical trials in the European literature, mostly from Italy, have reported effects on parameters of retinopathy and microangiopathy in humans.

Preclinical Evidence

- Numerous animal experiments have documented protective effects of *Vaccinium myrtillus* anthocyanoside (VMA), an extract of bilberry standardized to 25% anthocyanin, on blood vessels.[33,35,39,48] VMA has been shown to improve microvascular oxygen delivery, and to function as an antioxidant and anti-inflammatory agent. Lagrue et al. demon-

strated improvements in levels of "pathologic proteins" (collagen and structural lipoprotein levels) in diabetic microangiopathy.[49] These early data have made bilberry an attractive candidate for use in diabetic retinopathy and microangiopathy, both of which involve vascular damage at the level of the small blood vessels.

Human Evidence

- A double-blind, placebo-controlled study was conducted in 40 patients with vascular retinopathy (diabetic or hypertensive).[25] Bilberry extract (Tegens) was administered at a dose of 160 mg twice/day for 1 month. Placebo patients were then given bilberry for a month (although bilberry patients were not crossed over to placebo). Moderate mean improvements in ophthalmoscopic and fluoroangiographic findings were found following bilberry treatment, as measured by a multi-item clinician questionnaire. According to the authors, a 77% to 90% improvement was seen in bilberry-treated patients. The clinical validity of these results is limited by the lack of adequate description of blinding or randomization, and by the lack of crossover of the placebo group (preventing true between-group comparisons).
- In a case series, Mosci et al. dosed 30 subjects (10 with diabetic retinopathy, 10 with nondiabetic retinopathy, and 10 normal "controls") with procyanidolic anthocyanosides.[26] A statistically significant improvement in microangiopathic measures was noted for patients with retinopathy, although details of measurement instrument and method of analysis were not reported.
- Similar effects have been demonstrated in additional small studies of poor methodological quality by Repossi et al.[50] and Scharrer and Ober.[51]

Diabetes Mellitus (Hyperglycemia)
Summary

- Bilberry is a traditional therapy used in the treatment of diabetes. Tea made from the leaves of bilberry is often used for this indication. Limited animal data suggest that bilberry leaf extract possesses hypoglycemic and lipid-lowering properties that may be beneficial in diabetes.[13] However, literature review reveals no human studies. Since there are no available human trials evaluating the safety or efficacy of the use of bilberry leaf extract as a hypoglycemic agent, or evaluating interaction of bilberry leaf extract with oral hypoglycemic medications, bilberry cannot be recommended for the treatment of diabetic patients.

Cataracts
Summary

- Bilberry extract has been used and recommended clinically for a number of eye disorders, including the prevention of cataract progression. It has been hypothesized that the bioflavonoids in bilberry may benefit cataracts. At this time, there are limited data available in support of this use of bilberry or quercetin (also a source of bioflavonoids).[29]

Evidence

- In one case series of 50 elderly Italians with early-stage cataracts (62 eyes studied), a combination of vitamin E and anthocyanosides (extracted from bilberry) was found to slow the progression of lens opacities in 97% of cases.[52] However, without controls, the progression rate in the absence of bilberry cannot be assessed. In addition, the effects of bilberry cannot be separated from those of vitamin E.

Dysmenorrhea
Summary
- Limited evidence suggests that bilberry extract may improve symptoms associated with dysmenorrhea, such as headache, nausea, vomiting, and pelvic pain. However, at this time, the data are not sufficient to recommend either for or against this use of bilberry.

Evidence
- Bioflavonoids and extracts of anthocyanosides (such as those present in bilberry) have been shown to relax vascular smooth muscle in experimental models, possibly via stimulation of prostaglandins.[35-37] It has been hypothesized that such smooth muscle–relaxing effects might improve the symptoms of dysmenorrhea.
- Colombo and Vescovini performed a small (n = 30) placebo-controlled double-blind study that examined treatment of dysmenorrhea.[34] A dose of 160 mg twice daily of bilberry *Vaccinium myrtillus* anthocyanoside (Tegens) was started 3 days before menses and continued for 8 days, and repeated for two consecutive menstrual cycles. This treatment was found to statistically significantly reduce pelvic pain, lumbosacral pain, breast pain, nausea, vomiting, and headache vs. placebo. However, there was limited description of blinding, randomization, measurement instruments used, patient baseline characteristics, and statistical analysis. Therefore, this trial can only be considered suggestive, and not definitive.

Atherosclerosis and Peripheral Vascular Disease
Summary
- Bilberry has been used traditionally to treat symptoms of vascular disease (including coronary artery disease). However, there is limited human study in this area. Preliminary evidence from numerous *in vitro* and animal studies have suggested that bilberry extracts may be useful in the prevention of vascular disease[35,48,53] and may reduce oxidation of low-density lipoproteins (LDL).[4,11-13] Without additional human data, a recommendation cannot be made either in favor or against this use of bilberry.

Evidence
- Bilberry extracts have been shown to decrease platelet aggregation and LDL oxidation in animal models.[4,54] In an animal experiment looking at ischemia-reperfusion injury in hamster cheek microcirculation, *Vaccinium myrtillus* (bilberry) anthocyanoside (VMA) extract was shown to reduce microvascular impairment after reperfusion.[55] In another animal study, VMA extract was shown to reduce vascular permeability in the setting of hypertension.[53] Decreases in lipid deposition and intimal proliferation have also been demonstrated in VMA-treated animals.[56] These studies suggest there may be a vasoprotective role for VMA in the prevention of vascular disease.

Fibrocystic Breast Disease
Summary
- There is preliminary evidence suggesting possible benefit of bilberry in the treatment of fibrocystic disease of the breast.

Evidence
- A case series examining bilberry extract in the treatment of fibrocystic mastopathy reported encouraging early results. Marked improvement was seen in 33% of patients, reduction in symptoms was reported in 27%, and complete resolution was reported in 6% of patients. However, no effect was seen in 32% of patients.[57] Without a control group, it is not clear to what extent improvements would not have occurred spontaneously. Therefore, results can only be considered preliminary.

Diarrhea
Summary
- Treatment of diarrhea is a popular use of bilberry products. However, literature review reveals no laboratory, animal or human studies investigating this role for bilberry products. A recommendation for this indication can therefore not be based on scientific merit.

Peptic Ulcer Disease
Summary
- Bilberry extract has been suggested as a promoter of gastric ulcer healing, with support from animal data.[58] In rats, a natural flavonoid IdB1027 (VMA extract from bilberry) has demonstrated promising anti-ulcer effects.[16,32,33,39] At this time, however, there is not adequate human evidence to recommend for or against this use of bilberry. It should be noted that the bacterium *Helicobacter pylori* has been implicated in many cases of gastric and duodenal ulcers, and testing and/or treatment for *H. pylori* should be considered in patients with known or suspected peptic ulcer disease.

Night Vision
Summary
- Uncontrolled studies during the 1960s and 1970s, and anecdotal reports, suggested a beneficial effect of bilberry on night vision. However, more recent controlled human trials with well-defined outcomes have failed to demonstrate any effect. Although these trials have been methodologically flawed, the balance of available evidence suggests lack of efficacy. It is possible that the doses used have not been adequate to elicit a measurable effect. Nonetheless, without additional positive evidence from well-designed trials, the use of bilberry products for night vision cannot be considered scientifically supported.

Early Positive Evidence
- Jayle and Aubert conducted an early randomized, crossover trial in 40 healthy subjects.[30] Individuals were administered anthrocyanosides from bilberry and were found to have a statistically significant small improvement in night vision. However, details of blinding, randomization, and the measurement instrument were limited, thus reducing the clinical applicability of these results. In a follow-up randomized, placebo-controlled trial by Jayle et al., 1000 g of anthrocyanosides from bilberry were administered to 60 healthy individuals.[31] Again, a moderate statistically significant improvement was documented, although blinding and randomization were not adequately reported.

Negative Evidence
- Levy and Glovinsky performed a double-blind, placebo-controlled, crossover study to examine the effect of a single oral dose of bilberry extract (VMA) on night vision in normal individuals.[23] The researchers evaluated three parameters of night vision (scotopic retinal threshold, dark adaptation rate, and mesopic contrast sensitivity). Sixteen normal volunteers were tested and no significant effect was noted. The study was more carefully controlled than the studies

from the 1960s; patients were normal individuals with no report of visual impairments. The study population was small, and with a sample size of 16 and no power calculation conducted, a positive result could have been missed. It is also possible that the duration of therapy was insufficient, and that more than one dose of VMA is needed in order to elicit an improvement in night vision.

- A double-blind, placebo-controlled, crossover study examined the effects of high-dose bilberry extract over a 3-week period. Bilberry extract at a dose of 160 mg or placebo was given three times daily to 15 subjects. At the end of 21 days, patients were crossed to the other treatment arm. Results failed to demonstrate any effect on night visual acuity or night contrast sensitivity. Subjects were healthy young males. The authors reported that two had "below-average" night vision parameters, and that "subset analysis" did not show any improvement in these two.[21] This small study with no power calculation does not allow for definitive conclusions.

- In the late 1990s, Israeli investigators reported similar negative results in a trial using bilberry.[22,24] This double-blind, placebo-controlled crossover study in 18 subjects used a lower dose of bilberry (12 to 24 mg of anthrocyanosides) given twice daily for 4 weeks. No statistically significant improvement in night vision was observed, as measured by full-field absolute scotopic retinal threshold (SRT), dark absorption rate (DAR), or mesopic contrast sensitivity (MCS). Although this trial was small, a power calculation found the sample to be adequate to measure the stated outcomes. Nonetheless, with a sample size of 18, the adequacy of the sample size must come into question. The power was calculated to 80%, which is a standard approach, although this leaves a 20% chance that there are true benefits of therapy.

FORMULARY: BRANDS USED IN CLINICAL TRIALS
Brands Used In Human Studies

- Tegens (Europe).

References

1. Martin-Aragon S, Basabe B, Benedi JM, et al. In vitro and in vivo antioxidant properties of Vaccinium myrtillus. Pharmaceutical Biology 1999;37(2):109-113.
2. Prior R, Cao G, Martin A, et al. Antioxidant capacity as influence by total phenolic and anthocyanin content, maturity, and variety of Vaccinium species. J Agricult Food Chem 1998;46:2686-2693.
3. Martin-Aragon S, Basabe B, Benedi J, et al. Antioxidant action of Vaccinium myrtillus L. Phytotherapy 1998;46:S104-S106.
4. Laplaud PM, Lelubre A, Chapman MJ. Antioxidant action of Vaccinium myrtillus extract on human low density lipoproteins in vitro: initial observations. Fundam Clin Pharmacol 1997;11(1):35-40.
5. Bomser J, Madhavi DL, Singletary K, et al. In vitro anticancer activity of fruit extracts from Vaccinium species. Planta Med 1996;62(3):212-216.
6. Katsube N, Iwashita K, Tsushida T, et al. Induction of apoptosis in cancer cells by Bilberry (Vaccinium myrtillus) and the anthocyanins. J Agric Food Chem 2003;51(1):68-75.
7. Caselli L. [Clinical and electroretinographic study on activity of anthocyanosides]. Arch Med Interna 1985;37:29-35.
8. Morazzoni P, Magistretti MJ. Effects of Vaccinium myrtillus anthocyanosides on prostacyclin-like activity in rat arterial issue. Fitoterapia 1986;57:11-14.
9. Pezzangora V, Barina R, de Stefani R, et al. La terapia medica con antocianosidi del mirtillo nei pazienti operati di emorroidectomia. Gaz Med It 1984;143:405-409.
10. Oliva E, Nicastro A, Sorcini A, et al. Gli anticianosidi del mirtillo nel trattamento postoperatorio delle emorroidi. Aggior Med Chir 1990;8(1):1-6.
11. Rasetti FRM, Caruso D, Galli G, et al. Extracts of Ginkgo biloba L. leaves and Vaccinium myrtillus L. fruits prevent photo induced oxidation of low density lipoprotein cholesterol. Phytomedicine 1997;3:335-338.
12. Viana M, Barbas C, Bonet B, et al. In vitro effects of a flavonoid-rich extract on LDL oxidation. Atherosclerosis 1996;123(1-2):83-91.
13. Cignarella A, Nastasi M, Cavalli E, et al. Novel lipid-lowering properties of Vaccinium myrtillus L. leaves, a traditional antidiabetic treatment, in several models of rat dyslipidaemia: a comparison with ciprofibrate. Thromb Res 1996;84(5):311-322.
14. Grosse-Ruyken FJ. [The drug treatment of "myopia syndrome" (author's transl)]. Klin Monatsbl Augenheilkd 1977;171(4):623-627.
15. Politzer M. [Experiences in the medical treatment of progressive myopia (author's transl)]. Klin Monatsbl Augenheilkd 1977;171(4):616-619.
16. Magistretti MJ, Conti M, Cristoni A. Antiulcer activity of an anthocyanidin from Vaccinium myrtillus. Arzneimittelforschung 1988;38(5):686-690.
17. Cluzel C, Bastide P, Wegman R, et al. [Enzymatic activities of retina and anthocyanoside extracts of Vaccinium myrtillus (lactate dehydrogenase, alpha-hydroxybutyrate dehydrogenase, 6-phosphogluconate dehydrogenase, glucose-6-phosphate dehydrogenase, alpha-glycerophosphate dehydrogenase, 5-nucleotidase, phosphoglucose isomerase)]. Biochem Pharmacol 1970;19(7):2295-2302.
18. Fiorini G, Biancacci A, Graziano FM. [Perimetric and adaptometric modifications after ingestion of myrtillin associated with betacarotene]. Ann Ottalmol Clin Ocul 1965;91(6):371-386.
19. Grismondi GL. [Treatment of phlebopathies caused by stasis in pregnancy]. Minerva Ginecol 1981;33(2-3):221-230.
20. Havsteen B. Flavonoids, a class of natural products of high pharmacological potency. Biochem Pharmacol 1983;32(7):1141-1148.
21. Muth ER, Laurent JM, Jasper P. The effect of bilberry nutritional supplementation on night visual acuity and contrast sensitivity. Altern Med Rev 2000;5(2):164-173.
22. Zadok D, Levy Y, Glovinsky Y. The effect of anthocyanosides in a multiple oral dose on night vision. Eye 1999;13(Pt 6):734-736.
23. Levy Y, Glovinsky Y. The effect of anthocyanosides on night vision. Eye 1998;12(Pt 6):967-969.
24. Zadok D, Levy Y, Glovinskly Y, et al. The effect of anthocyanosides on night vision tests. Investigative Ophthalmology and Visual Science 1997; 38(4):S633.
25. Perossini M, et al. Diabetic and hypertensive retinopathy therapy with Vaccinium myrtillus anthocyanosides (Tegens): Double blind placebo controlled clinical trial. Annali di Ottalmaologia e Clinica Oculistica 1987; 113:1173-1190.
26. Mosci C, Fioretto M, Polizzi A, et al. The influence of procyanidolic anthocyanosides on macular recovery time and oscillatory potentials in the diabetic subject. Annli di Ottalmologi e Clinica Oculistica 1988;114:473-479.
27. Pautler EL, Maga JA, Tengerdy C. A pharmacologically potent natural product in the bovine retina. Exp Eye Res 1986;42(3):285-288.
28. Spinella G. Natural anthocyanosides in treatment of peripheral venous insufficiency. Arch Med Int 1985;37:219.
29. Varma SD, Mizuno A, Kinoshita JH. Diabetic cataracts and flavonoids. Science 1977;195(4274):205-206.
30. Jayle GE, Aubert L. Action des glucosides d'anthocyanes sur la vision scotopique et mésopique du sujet normal. Therapie 1964;19:171-185.
31. Jayle GE, Aubry M, Gavini H, et al. [Study concerning the action of anthocyanoside extracts of Vaccinium Myrtillus on night vision]. Ann Ocul (Paris) 1965;198(6):556-562.
32. Mertz-Nielsen A, Munck LK, Bukhave K, et al. A natural flavonoid, IdB 1027, increases gastric luminal release of prostaglandin E_2 in healthy subjects. Ital J Gastroenterol. 1990;22(5):288-290.
33. Lietti A, Cristoni A, Picci M. Studies on Vaccinium myrtillus anthocyanosides. I. Vasoprotective and antiinflammatory activity. Arzneimittelforschung 1976;26(5):829-832.
34. Colombo D, Vescovini R. Controlled clinical trial of anthocyanosides from Vaccinium myrtillus in primary dysmenorrhea. G Ital Obstet Ginecol 1985; 7:1033-1038.
35. Colantuoni A, Bertuglia S, Magistretti MJ, et al. Effects of Vaccinium myrtillus anthocyanosides on arterial vasomotion. Arzneimittelforschung 1991;41(9):905-909.
36. Bettini V. Effects of Vaccinium myrtillus anthocyanosides on vascular smooth muscle. Fitoterapia 1984;55(5):265-272.
37. Bettini V, Mayellaro F, Ton P, et al. Interactions between Vaccinium myrtillus anthocyanosides and serotonin on splenic artery smooth muscle. Fitoterapia 1984;55(4):201-208.
38. Pulliero G, Montin S, Bettini V, et al. Ex vivo study of the inhibitory effects of Vaccinium myrtillus anthocyanosides on human platelet aggregation. Fitoterapia 1989;60:69-75.
39. Lietti A, Forni G. Studies on Vaccinium myrtillus anthocyanosides. II. Aspects of anthocyanins pharmacokinetics in the rat. Arzneimittelforschung 1976;26(5):832-835.
40. Jonadet M, Meunier MT, Bastide J, et al. [Anthocyanosides extracted from Vitis vinifera, Vaccinium myrtillus and Pinus maritimus. I. Elastase-inhibiting activities in vitro. Compared angioprotective activities in vivo]. J Pharm Belg 1983;38(1):41-46.
41. Boniface R, Robert AM. [Effect of anthocyanins on human connective tissue metabolism in the human]. Klin Monatsbl Augenheilkd 1996;209(6):368-372.
42. Morazzoni P, Livio S, Scilingo A, et al. Vaccinium myrtillus anthocyanosides pharmacokinetics in rats. Arzneimittelforschung 1991;41(2):128-131.
43. Gatta L. Experimental single-blind study: 60 pts with venous insufficiency received Bilberry extract equivalent to 173 mg anthocyanins daily or placebo for 30 days. Fitoterapia 1988;59(suppl 1):19.

44. Coget J, Merlen JF. [Clinical study of a new chemical agent for vascular protection, Difrarel 20, composed of anthocyanosides extracted from *Vaccinium myrtillus*]. Phlebologie 1968;21(2):221-228.

45. Amouretti M. [Therapeutic value of *Vaccinium myrtillus* anthocyanosides in an internal medicine department]. Therapeutique 1972;48(9):579-581.

46. Ghiringhelli C, Gregoratti L, Marastoni F. [Capillarotropic action of anthocyanosides in high dosage in phlebopathic statis]. Minerva Cardio-angiol 1978;26(4):255-276.

47. Tori A, D'Errico F. [*Vaccinium myrtillus* anthocyanosides in the treatment of stasis venous diseases of the lower limbs.]. Gazz Med Ital 1980;139: 217-224.

48. Gabor M. Pharmacologic effects of flavonoids on blood vessels. Angiologica 1972;9(3-6):355-374.

49. Lagrue G, Robert AM, Miskulin M, et al. Pathology of the microcirculation in diabetes and alterations of the biosynthesis of intercellular matrix macromolecules. Front Matrix Biol 1979;7:324-335.

50. Repossi P, Malagola R, De Cadilhac C. The role of anthocyanosides on vascular permeability in diabetic retinopathy. Ann Ottalmol Clin Ocul 1987; 113:357-361.

51. Scharrer A, Ober M. [Anthocyanosides in the treatment of retinopathies (author's transl)]. Klin Monatsbl Augenheilkd 1981;178(5):386-389.

52. Bravetti GO, Fraboni E, Maccolini E. Preventive medical treatment of senile cataract with vitamin E and *Vaccinium myrtillus* anthocyanosides: Clinical evaluation. Ann Ottalmol Clin Ocul 1989;115:109-116.

53. Detre Z, Jellinek H, Miskulin M, et al. Studies on vascular permeability in hypertension: action of anthocyanosides. Clin Physiol Biochem 1986;4(2): 143-149.

54. Buliero G. The inhibitory effects of anthocyanosides on human platelet aggregation. Fitoterapia 1989;60:69.

55. Bertuglia S, Malandrino S, Colantuoni A. Effect of *Vaccinium myrtillus* anthocyanosides on ischaemia reperfusion injury in hamster cheek pouch microcirculation. Pharmacol Res 1995;31(3-4):183-187.

56. Kadar A, Robert L, Miskulin M, et al. Influence of anthocyanoside treatment on the cholesterol-induced atherosclerosis in the rabbit. Paroi Arterielle 1979;5(4):187-205.

57. Leonardi M. [Treatment of fibrocystic disease of the breast with myrtillus anthocyanins. Our experience]. Minerva Ginecol 1993;45(12):617-621.

58. Cristoni A, Magistretti MJ. Antiulcer and healing activity of *Vaccinium myrtillus* anthocyanosides. Farmaco [Prat] 1987;42(2):29-43.

Bitter Almond

(Prunus amygdalus Batch var. amara [DC.] Focke; Laetrile)

SYNONYMS/COMMON NAMES/RELATED SUBSTANCES:

- Aci badem, almendra amara, amande amere, amendoa amarga, amygdala amara, amygdalis dulcis amara, bitter almond oil, bittere amandel, bittermandel, gorkiy mindal, karvasmanteli, keseru mandula, ku wei bian tao, ku xing ren, lawz murr, mandorla amara, *Prunus communis amara*, *Prunus dulcis* (Mill.) D.A. Webb var. *amara* (DC.) H.E. Moore, *Prunus amygalus amara*, Rosaceae, volatile almond oil.

- *Note:* Bitter almond should not be confused with sweet almond. Sweet almond seeds do not contain amygdalin and can be eaten, whereas bitter almonds are toxic.

CLINICAL BOTTOM LINE
Brief Background

- The almond is closely related to the peach, apricot, and cherry (all classified as drupes). Unlike the others, however, the outer layer of the almond is not edible. The edible portion of the almond is the seed. A compound called amygdalin differentiates the bitter almond from the sweet almond. In the presence of water (hydrolysis), amygdalin yields glucose as well as benzaldehyde and hydrocyanic acid (HCN). HCN, the salts of which are known as cyanide, is poisonous. To be used in food or as a flavoring agent, the HCN must be removed from the bitter almond oil. Once it is removed, the oil is called volatile almond oil and is considered to be almost pure benzaldehyde. Volatile almond oil can still be toxic in large amounts.

- Historically, bitter almond oil was once used as a cough suppressant and as an antipruritic. It is also said to possess anti–peptic ulcer, local anesthetic, and antispasmodic properties. HCN-free bitter almond oil is used in very small amounts as a flavoring agent in products such as marzipan.

- "Laetrile," an alternative cancer drug marketed in Mexico and other countries outside of the U.S., is derived from amygdalin. Based on a phase II trial in 1982, the U.S. National Cancer Institute concluded that laetrile is not an effective chemotherapeutic agent. Nonetheless, many people still travel to use this therapy outside the United States. Multiple cases of cyanide poisoning, including deaths, have been associated with laetrile therapy.

Scientific Evidence for Common/Studied Uses	Grade*
Cancer (Laetrile)	D

*Key to grades: *A:* Strong scientific evidence for this use; *B:* Good scientific evidence for this use; *C:* Unclear scientific evidence for this use; *D:* Fair scientific evidence against this use (it may not work); *F:* Strong scientific evidence against this use (it likely does not work). For a more detailed explanation of efficacy criteria, see "Natural Standard Evidence-Based Validated Grading Rationale" in the Introduction.

Historical or Theoretical Indications That Lack Sufficient Evidence

- Analgesic, antibacterial, anti-inflammatory, antipruritic, antispasmodic, cough suppressant, local anesthetic, narcotic.

Expert Opinion and Historic/Folkloric Precedent

- There is little historical precedent for therapeutic use of bitter almond in the literature.

Brief Safety Summary

- **Possibly safe:** When small amounts of HCN-free bitter almond oil are used.
- **Likely unsafe:** When large amounts of HCN-free bitter almond oil are used or when bitter almonds are ingested as food. When bitter almond volatile oil containing HCN is used orally, benzaldehyde can cause fatal CNS depression and respiratory failure. Laetrile in oral or intravenous formulations has been associated with multiple cases of cyanide poisoning.

DOSING/TOXICOLOGY
Standardization

- Hydrocyanic acid (HCN), also known as cyanide, is poisonous. To be used in food or as a flavoring agent, the HCN must be removed from the bitter almond oil. Once it is removed, the oil is called volatile almond oil and is considered to be almost pure benzaldehyde. Volatile almond oil can still be toxic in large amounts.

- Mexico supplies the majority of laetrile to the United States, and standardization has been problematic. Laetrile samples produced in Mexico were randomly selected and analyzed for potency and contamination. Results showed laetrile samples to include lower concentrations of the compound than labeled and to be contaminated with amygdalinamide, amygdalin acid, and 2-propanol.[1]

Dosing: Adult (18 Years And Older)

- There is no standard dose for bitter almond.

Dosing: Pediatric (Younger Than 18 Years)

- Because of potential toxicity, bitter almond products should be avoided in children.

Toxicology

- Laetrile, a purported chemotherapeutic agent, is derived from amygdalin, found in the pits of fruits and nuts such as bitter almond. Use of laetrile is associated with a significant risk of cyanide poisoning, which appears to be more severe with oral administration than with intravenous or intramuscular dosing. Multiple cases of cyanide poisonings have been reported in the literature.[2-6]

- A 32-year-old woman, with suicidal intent, swallowed nine grams of the intravenous formulation of laetrile. The patient was treated with lavage, amyl nitrite, sodium nitrite, and sodium thiosulfate. The patient recovered with a decrease in her cyanide level from 143 μmol/L to 12 μmol/L the following day.[4]

- After 3 weeks of laetrile therapy, a patient developed a diffuse, nonpruritic, erythematous macular rash. Within two days of discontinuation of laetrile and treatment with prednisone, the patient's rash subsided.[7]

ADVERSE EFFECTS/PRECAUTIONS/CONTRAINDICATIONS
Allergy

- Allergies to almonds are common and have led to severe reactions, including oral allergic syndrome (OAS), angioedema, and laryngeal edema.[8]
- After 3 weeks of laetrile therapy, a patient developed a diffuse, nonpruritic, erythematous macular rash. Within 2 days of discontinuation of laetrile and treatment with prednisone, the patient's rash subsided.[7]

Adverse Effects

- **General:** Laetrile, derived from the amygdalin found in bitter almonds, is considered unsafe in any form due to its potential for causing cyanide toxicity. Reactions appear to be more severe with oral administration than with intravenous or intramuscular dosing.
- **Neurologic/CNS:** High doses of bitter almond or laetrile may lead to CNS and respiratory depression. A patient taking laetrile, 500 mg daily for approximately 6 months, was admitted for bilateral eyelid ptosis and bilateral upper and lower extremity proximal muscle weakness. The patient was also taking phenytoin since the previous year. Upon discontinuation of laetrile, the ptosis and muscle weakness completely resolved within 6 days.[7] Headache, dizziness, and obtundation have also been reported with laetrile therapy.[9]
- **Hematologic:** Agranulocytosis occurred in a 61-year-old woman who had been consuming laetrile for 5 years. Upon discontinuation of laetrile, agranulocytosis resolved. Approximately 3 months later, the patient resumed taking laetrile and was readmitted for agranulocytosis, which again resolved upon discontinuation of laetrile.[10]
- **Gastrointestinal:** Nausea and vomiting have been reported with laetrile therapy.[9]
- **Cyanide Poisoning:** Multiple cases of cyanide poisonings, some of which were fatal, have been associated with the use of laetrile.[2-6,11-14]
  - In order to make up for missed doses, a 22-year-old male took 12 to 18 laetrile tablets at once. The patient developed acute onset of grand mal seizures and was admitted for cyanide poisoning. During admission, the patient was noted to have an odor similar to that of almonds. The patient recovered full neurologic function after supportive measures and treatment with naloxone, amyl nitrite, sodium nitrite, sodium bicarbonate, and sodium thiosulfate.[6]
  - An 11-month-old girl swallowed 1 to 5 of the 500-mg laetrile tablets. Approximately 30 minutes following ingestion, the child developed lethargy. The patient was brought to a hospital in a comatose state, had symptoms of shock, irregular respiration, and metabolic acidosis. Despite endotracheal intubation, gastric lavage, and intravenous bicarbonate administration, the patient died 71 hours post laetrile ingestion.[2,12]
  - A 32-year-old woman with suicidal intent swallowed 9 g of intravenous (IV) laetrile. The patient was treated with lavage, amyl nitrite, sodium nitrite, and sodium thiosulfate. The patient recovered with a decrease in her cyanide level from 143 μmol/L to 13 μmol/L the following day.[4]
  - A 2-year-old patient was administered laetrile, 500 mg orally and 3.5 g intravenously, on a daily basis. Due to eventual difficulty of IV administration, the patient's normal IV dose was administered as an enema. Following the second rectal dose, the patient was diagnosed with cyanide poisoning, with symptoms of vomiting, diarrhea, lethargy, tachypnea, and cyanosis. Following oxygen therapy and hydration, the patient recovered.[3]
  - A 17-year-old girl with mild, asymptomatic pulmonary stenosis had a radical excision of a right frontal astrocytoma. Two months later, the patient started IV laetrile therapy at a dose of 12 g daily for four weeks. Approximately 1 month later, the patient was unable to take the medication intravenously and therefore swallowed 3.5 ampuls (3 g each). Shortly after ingestion, the patient developed dizziness, a severe headache, tetanic contractures of her hands, generalized convulsions, difficulty breathing, and dilated pupils. She then became comatose and despite lavage and respiratory assistance, died 1 day later.[14]
  - A 67-year-old woman taking oral laetrile tablets at erratic doses was admitted for acute cyanide poisoning after ingesting 12 bitter almonds. She developed abdominal pain, collapsed, and was brought to a hospital. The patient was noted to have an odor of almonds. Her condition was complicated by lactic acidosis and pulmonary edema. The patient responded to supportive care and treatment with sodium nitrite and sodium thiosulfate.[5]

Precautions/Warnings/Contraindications

- Use bitter almond products cautiously because of the potential for cyanide toxicity.

Pregnancy and Lactation

- Not recommended because of insufficient available data. Oral laetrile administered to pregnant hamsters resulted in skeletal malformations in offspring. However, intravenous laetrile did not result in any malformations. It was reported that oral laetrile increased *in situ* cyanide concentration significantly, whereas intravenous laetrile in these animals did not.[15]

INTERACTIONS
Bitter Almond/Drug Interactions

- **Sedatives, CNS depressants:** Theoretically, depressant effects caused by bitter almond may be potentiated when administered with CNS depressants.
- **Alcohol:** Almond oil was shown in mice to be an inducer of hepatic alcohol dehydrogenase. This finding suggests a possible adverse interaction between almond oil and alcohol. Bitter almond may result in a disulfiram-like flushing reaction with concomitant alcohol use.[16]

Bitter Almond/Herb/Supplement Interactions

- **Sedative herbs and supplements, CNS depressants:** Theoretically, depressant effects caused by bitter almond may be potentiated when administered with CNS depressants.
- **Alcohol:** Some herbal extracts or tinctures contain high concentrations of alcohol. Almond oil was shown in mice to be an inducer of hepatic alcohol dehydrogenase. This finding suggests a possible adverse interaction between almond oil and alcohol. Bitter almond may result in a disulfiram-like flushing reaction with concomitant alcohol use.[16]

Bitter Almond/Food Interactions

- **Alcohol:** Some foods may contain alcohol (e.g., salad dressing, sauces). Almond oil was shown in mice to be an inducer of hepatic alcohol dehydrogenase. This finding suggests a possible adverse interaction between almond oil and alcohol.

Bitter almond may result in a disulfiram-like flushing reaction with concomitant alcohol use.[16]

- **Laetrile and raw almonds:** When using bitter almond products or laetrile, concomitant ingestion of raw almonds has been reported in several cases to increase the incidence of cyanide poisoning.[5,17]

Bitter Almond/Lab Interactions

- Insufficient available evidence.

MECHANISM OF ACTION
Pharmacology

- Analysis of almonds has revealed the following components: protein, emulsin, prunasin, daucosterol and other sterols, as well as trace amounts of vitamin A. Other substances found include B complex, vitamin E, and amino acids such as glutamic acid, aspartic acid, and arginine. Amygdalin is present in the bitter almond at a level of 3% to 4%.
- Almond oil was shown in mice to be an inducer of hepatic alcohol dehydrogenase and a non-competitive inhibitor of cytoplasmic and mitochondrial liver aldehyde dehydrogenase. It did not affect heart lactate dehydrogenase.[16]
- Amygdalin was shown to have an analgesic effect in mice without inducing tolerance. It did not show evidence of anti-inflammatory activity.[18]

Pharmacodynamics/Kinetics

- After intravenous laetrile, amygdalin has been shown to be excreted primarily unchanged, with urinary recoveries as high as 100%. Peak plasma levels following a 6-g intramuscular dose of laetrile were 180 µg/mL.[19]
- Prunasin, a metabolite of amygdalin, has a bioavailability of approximately 50%. Prunasin's volume of distribution and clearance are larger than those of amygdalin.[20]

HISTORY

- References to almonds are found throughout history, as far back as the Old Testament.
- The almond tree is native to Western Asia, but it has been extensively cultivated in modern times. Large amounts of almonds are produced in California and in Spain.

REVIEW OF THE EVIDENCE: DISCUSSION
Cancer
Summary

- Laetrile is an alternative cancer drug marketed in Mexico and other countries outside of the U.S. Laetrile is derived from amygdalin, which is found in the pits of fruits and nuts such as bitter almond. There are multiple animal studies and initial human evidence to suggest that laetrile is not beneficial in the treatment of cancer. Based on a phase II trial in 1982, the U.S. National Cancer Institute concluded that laetrile is not an effective chemotherapeutic agent. Nonetheless, many people still travel to use this therapy outside the U.S. Multiple cases of cyanide poisoning, including deaths, have been associated with laetrile therapy.

Evidence

- Although initially promising results were reported from a small number of *in vitro*[21-23] and animal studies,[24] multiple studies have demonstrated a lack of effect of laetrile or amygdalin in animal models of cancer, including lung carcinoma, sarcoma, melanoma, and leukemia.[25-32] Several poorly described human case reports have provided inadequate evidence of efficacy.[33-36] A case series of 10 patients with several types of metastatic cancer reported use of various doses of intravenous laetrile (9 to 133 g total), with short-term subjective improvements in lymphadenopathy and tumor size, but no statistical analysis or long-term follow-up.[37] An earlier case series of 44 patients reported use of laetrile concurrently with other therapies, but mixed results were reported, and it is unclear what effects laetrile may have had.[38]
- The U.S. National Cancer Institute sponsored a phase II study of laetrile for cancer in 1982 based on a prior phase I (dosing) study in 6 patients.[17] The phase II study was conducted in 178 patients with various cancer types, including colon, breast, and lung.[9] All subjects were considered to be in "good condition," as none were disabled or in a preterminal state. One third of these patients had not received any prior chemotherapy. For 21 days, intravenous laetrile therapy was administered, combined with "metabolic therapy" (including diet, pancreatic enzymes, and vitamins). Of the 175 patients who could be evaluated, only one subject was felt to have improved, based on diminished gastric carcinoma tumor mass. However, 95 patients experienced tumor progression, and all evaluable subjects experienced disease progression seven months after completing treatment. Adverse effects included nausea, vomiting, headache, dizziness, mental obtundation, dermatitis, and cyanide toxicity. Although this study had several methodological weaknesses, including a mixed patient population, based on these results the National Cancer Institute concluded that laetrile is not a beneficial chemotherapeutic agent and should not be approved for use in the United States. Although laetrile is still used by individuals outside of the United States, based on the available research and known significant toxicity, the evidence does not support use of this treatment.

Review of the Evidence: Bitter Almond

Condition Treated*	Study Design	Author, Year	N[†]	SS[†]	Study Quality[‡]	Magnitude of Benefit	ARR[†]	NNT[†]	Comments
Cancer	Phase II trial	Moertel[9] 1982	178	No	2	None	NA	NA	Combination of laetrile with "metabolic" therapy in patients with various tumor types.

*Primary or secondary outcome.
[†] *N*, Number of patients; *SS*, statistically significant; *ARR*, absolute risk reduction; *NNT*, the number of patients who need to undergo a specific intervention in order to observe an outcome in one individual.
[‡] 0-2 = poor; 3-4 = good; 5 = excellent.
NA, Not applicable.
For an explanation of each category in this table, please see Table 3 in the Introduction.

References

1. Jee J, Yoshikawa F, Pont L, et al. Assay of amygdalin dosage forms from Mexico. J Pharm Sci 1978;67(3):438-440.
2. Humbert JR, Tress JH, Braico KT. Fatal cyanide poisoning: accidental ingestion of amygdalin. JAMA 1977;238(6):482.
3. Ortega JA, Creek JE. Acute cyanide poisoning following administration of Laetrile enemas. J Pediatr 1978;93(6):1059.
4. Moss M, Khalil N, Gray J. Deliberate self-poisoning with Laetrile. Can Med Assoc J 1981;125(10):1126, 1128.
5. Shragg TA, Albertson TE, Fisher CJ, Jr. Cyanide poisoning after bitter almond ingestion. West J Med 1982;136(1):65-69.
6. Beamer WC, Shealy RM, Prough DS. Acute cyanide poisoning from laetrile ingestion. Ann Emerg Med 1983;12(7):449-451.
7. Smith FP, Butler TP, Cohan S, et al. Laetrile toxicity: a report of two patients. Cancer Treat Rep 1978;62(1):169-171.
8. Pasini G, Simonato B, Giannattasio M, et al. IgE binding to almond proteins in two CAP-FEIA-negative patients with allergic symptoms to almond as compared to three CAP-FEIA-false-positive subjects. Allergy 2000;55(10):955-958.
9. Moertel CG, Fleming TR, Rubin J, et al. A clinical trial of amygdalin (Laetrile) in the treatment of human cancer. N Engl J Med 1982;306(4):201-206.
10. Liegner KB, Beck EM, Rosenberg A. Laetrile-induced agranulocytosis. JAMA 1981;246(24):2841-2842.
11. Anonymous. Toxicity of Laetrile. FDA Drug Bull 1977;7:26-32.
12. Braico KT, Humbert JR, Terplan KL, et al. Laetrile intoxication. Report of a fatal case. N Engl J Med 1979;300(5):238-240.
13. Pack WK, Raudonat HW, Schmidt K. [Lethal poisoning with hydrocyanic acid after ingestion of bitter almonds (*Prunus amygdalus*).] Z Rechtsmed 1972;70(1):53-54.
14. Sadoff L, Fuchs K, Hollander J. Rapid death associated with laetrile ingestion. JAMA 1978;239(15):1532.
15. Willhite CC. Congenital malformations induced by laetrile. Science 1982;215(4539):1513-1515.
16. Messiha FS. Effect of almond and anis oils on mouse liver alcohol dehydrogenase, aldehyde dehydrogenase and heart lactate dehydrogenase isoenzymes. Toxicol Lett 1990;54(2-3):183-188.
17. Moertel CG, Ames MM, Kovach JS, et al. A pharmacologic and toxicological study of amygdalin. JAMA 1981;245(6):591-594.
18. Zhu YP, Su ZW, Li CH. [Analgesic effect and no physical dependence of amygdalin.] Zhongguo Zhong.Yao Za Zhi. 1994;19(2):105-107, 128.
19. Ames MM, Kovach JS, Flora KP. Initial pharmacologic studies of amygdalin (laetrile) in man. Res Commun Chem Pathol Pharmacol 1978;22(1):175-185.
20. Rauws AG, Olling M, Timmerman A. The pharmacokinetics of prunasin, a metabolite of amygdalin. J Toxicol Clin Toxicol 1982;19(8):851-856.
21. Biaglow JE, Durand RE. The enhanced radiation response of an in vitro tumour model by cyanide released from hydrolysed amygdalin. Int J Radiat Biol Relat Stud Phys Chem Med 1978;33(4):397-401.
22. Bhatti RA, Ablin RJ, Guinan PD. Tumour-associated directed immunity in prostatic cancer: effect of amygdalin. IRCS Med Sci 1981;9(1):19.
23. Syrigos KN, Rowlinson-Busza G, Epenetos AA. *In vitro* cytotoxicity following specific activation of amygdalin by beta-glucosidase conjugated to a bladder cancer-associated monoclonal antibody. Int J Cancer 1998;78(6):712-719.
24. Manner HW, DiSanti SJ, Maggio MI, et al. Amygdalin, vitamin A and enzyme induced regression of murine mammary adenocarcinomas. J Manip Physiol Ther 1978;1(4):246-248.
25. Gostomski FE. The effects of amygdalin on the Krebs-2 carcinoma in adult and fetal DUB (ICR) mice. Disseration Abstracts International 1978;39(5):2075-B.
26. Wodinsky I, Swiniarski JK. Antitumor activity of amygdalin MF (NSC-15780) as a single agent and with beta-glucosidase (NSC-128056) on a spectrum of transplantable rodent tumors. Cancer Chemother Rep 1975;59(5):939-950.
27. Laster WR, Jr., Schabel FM, Jr. Experimental studies of the antitumor activity of amygdalin MF (NSC- 15780) alone and in combination with beta-glucosidase (NSC-128056). Cancer Chemother Rep 1975;59(5):951-965.
28. Stock CC, Tarnowski GS, Schmid FA, et al. Antitumor tests of amygdalin in transplantable animal tumor systems. J Surg Oncol 1978;10(2):81-88.
29. Hill GJ, Shine TE, Hill HZ, et al. Failure of amygdalin to arrest B16 melanoma and BW5147 AKR leukemia. Cancer Res 1976;36(6):2102-2107.
30. Lea MA, Koch MR. Effects of cyanate, thiocyanate, and amygdalin on metabolite uptake in normal and neoplastic tissues of the rat. J Natl Cancer Inst 1979;63(5):1279-1283.
31. Khandekar JD, Edelman H. Studies of amygdalin (laetrile) toxicity in rodents. JAMA 1979;242(2):169-171.
32. Ovejera AA, Houchens DP, Barker AD, et al. Inactivity of DL-amygdalin against human breast and colon tumor xenografts in athymic (nude) mice. Cancer Treat Rep 1978;62(4):576-578.
33. Ross WE. Unconventional cancer therapy. Compr Ther 1985;11(9):37-43.
34. Navarro MD. The Philippine experience in the early detection and chemotherapy of cancer. Santo Tomas J Med 1970;25(3):125-133.
35. Morrone JA. Chemotherapy of inoperable cancer: preliminary report of 10 cases treated with laetrile. J Exper Med Surg 1962;20:299-308.
36. Brown WE, Wood CD, Smith AN. Sodium cyanide as a cancer chemotherapeutic agent: laboratory and clinical studies. Amer J Obstet Gyn 1960;80(5):907-918.
37. Navarro MD. Five years experience with laetrile therapy in advanced cancer. Acta Unio Internat Contra Cancrum 1959;15(Suppl 1):209-221.
38. Anonymous. Report by the cancer commission of the California Medical Association: the treatment of cancer with "laetrile." California Med 1953;78(4):320-326.

Bitter Melon
(*Momordica charantia* L. Cucurbitaceae) and MAP30

SYNONYMS/COMMON NAMES/RELATED SUBSTANCES

- African cucumber, balsam-apple, balsambirne, balsam pear, balsamo, beta-momorcharin, bitter apple, bitter cucumber, bitter gourd, bittergurke, carilla gourd, charantin, chinli-chih, cundeamor, kakara, karela, kuguazi, k'u-kua, lai margose, MAP30, *Mormodica angustipala*, momordique, pavakkachedi, pepino montero, p'u-t'ao, sorosi, sushavi, vegetable insulin, wild cucumber.

CLINICAL BOTTOM LINE
Background

- Bitter melon (*Momordica charantia* L. Cucurbitaceae) has traditionally been used as a remedy for lowering blood glucose levels in patients with diabetes mellitus. Extracts and powdered formulations of the fruit are most frequently used, although teas made from the stems and leaves are sometimes recommended.
- Data from *in vitro*, animal, and several poorly designed human studies suggest a moderate hypoglycemic effect of bitter melon and some of its crude extracts. The available human investigations have principally tested bitter melon juice in type 2 diabetics. However, dosage, toxicity, standardization, adverse effects, and long-term outcomes have not been systematically assessed.[1] Further study is warranted in this area.
- Constituents of bitter melon have been isolated that possess antiviral and antineoplastic activities *in vitro*. In particular, a protein called MAP30 has shown some promise, although no human trials have been conducted.[2-9]
- Bitter melon is also consumed as a foodstuff and is found as an ingredient in some South Asian curries. The raw fruit is available in specialty Asian markets, where it is known as *karela*.

Scientific Evidence for Common/Studied Uses	Grade*
Diabetes mellitus (hypoglycemic agent)	B
Cancer	C
Human immunodeficiency virus (HIV)	C

*Key to grades: *A*: Strong scientific evidence for this use; *B*: Good scientific evidence for this use; *C*: Unclear scientific evidence for this use; *D*: Fair scientific evidence against this use (it may not work); *F*: Strong scientific evidence against this use (it likely does not work). For a more detailed explanation of efficacy criteria, see "Natural Standard Evidence-Based Validated Grading Rationale" in the Introduction.

Historical or Theoretical Uses That Lack Sufficient Evidence

- Abortifacient,[10-12] analgesia,[13] gastrointestinal cramps, glaucoma,[14] hemorrhoids, hyperlipidemia,[15] infertility, psoriasis, retinopathy.[16]

Expert Opinion and Folkloric Precedent

- Bitter melon has a long history of use as a hypoglycemic agent in Asia, Africa, and Latin America. The plant extract is sometimes called "vegetable insulin." More recently, bitter melon has been proposed as an antiviral or antineoplastic agent. However, despite some encouraging *in vitro* studies, there is no reliable human trial evidence for these effects. Folkloric uses have included myriad other indications, including psoriasis, infertility, gastrointestinal cramps, infections, cancer, and as a traditional abortifacient.

Safety Summary

- **Possibly safe:** When used as an oral hypoglycemic agent under close medical supervision, with regular blood glucose monitoring.[17,18]
- **Possibly unsafe:** When used in patients taking other oral hypoglycemic agents, or without close supervision of blood sugars.[17]
- **Likely unsafe:** Bitter melon should not be taken by pregnant women, as it may cause spontaneous abortion, based on animal data.[10,11] Use should be avoided in children, based on two case reports of hypoglycemic coma in children following ingestion of bitter melon tea.[19,20]

DOSING/TOXICOLOGY
General

- Recommended doses are based on those most commonly used in available trials, or on historical practice. However, with natural products, the optimal doses needed to balance efficacy and safety often have not been determined. Formulations and preparation methods may vary from manufacturer to manufacturer, and from batch to batch of a specific product made by a single manufacturer. Because often the active components of a product are not known, standardization may not be possible, and the clinical effects of different brands may not be comparable.

Standardization

- Insufficient data available.

Dosing: Adult (18 Years and Older)
Oral

- Because of the wide variations in preparation techniques of bitter melon, the proper dosing cannot be determined at the present time. In the available studies, bitter melon has sometimes been administered as a fruit juice in doses of 50 mL[17] or 100 mL.[21] Juice formulations have been reported to have more potent effects on blood sugar and glycosylated hemoglobin (HbA1c) than the powder of the sun-dried fruit.[22] However, safety and efficacy have not been established for any specific dose(s) of bitter melon.

Subcutaneous

- Subcutaneous administration of bitter melon has been studied in humans,[18] although safety, efficacy, and dosing have not been clearly established.

Dosing: Pediatric (Younger Than 18 Years)

- Insufficient data are available. Caution is warranted, based on two case reports of hypoglycemic coma in children following ingestion of bitter melon tea.[19,20]

Toxicology

- The seeds and outer rind of bitter melon fruit contain a toxic lectin, which inhibits protein synthesis in the intestinal wall (the clinical significance of this is not clear).[23]
- There have been two case reports of hypoglycemic coma in children following ingestion of bitter melon tea.[19,20]

ADVERSE EFFECTS/PRECAUTIONS/CONTRAINDICATIONS
Allergy

- Known allergy/hypersensitivity to bitter melon or members of the Cucurbitaceae (gourd or melon) family, including Persian melon, honeydew, casaba, muskmelon, and cantaloupe.

Adverse Effects

- **Neurologic/CNS:** Headaches have been reported after the ingestion of bitter melon seeds.[20] However, details regarding severity and duration of headaches are limited.
- **Gastrointestinal:** Significant rises in gamma-glutamyl transferase (GGT) and alkaline phosphatase have been observed in animals following oral administration of bitter melon fruit juice and seed extract. These rises, however, have not been associated with significant histopathologic changes in the liver.[24] The clinical relevance in humans has not been studied, and caution is warranted, particularly in patients with underlying liver disease. The seeds and outer rind of bitter melon contain a toxic lectin that inhibits protein synthesis in the intestinal wall. However, this has not been correlated with clinical signs or symptoms in humans.[23]
- **Endocrine:** Bitter melon has been found to lower blood glucose levels in animal studies[25-29] and in several methodologically weak human trials.[17,18,20-22] Proposed mechanisms include insulin-like effects,[18,30] stimulation of pancreatic insulin secretion,[31] decreased hepatic gluconeogenesis, increased hepatic glycogen synthesis, and increased peripheral glucose oxidation.[32] Two case reports have documented hypoglycemic coma and convulsions in children after administration of a bitter melon tea.[19,20]
- **Hematologic:** Individuals with glucose-6-phosphate dehydrogenase deficiency are at risk of developing "favism" following ingestion of bitter melon seeds. Favism is defined by the onset of hemolytic anemia with symptoms including headache, fever, stomach pain, and coma.[20] The glycosidic compound vicine, a favism-inducing chemical, has been isolated from bitter melon.[33] Glucose-6-phosphate dehydrogenase deficiency and favism are most common in persons of Mediterranean and Middle Eastern lineage.
- **Genitourinary:** The fertility rate of mice fed daily bitter melon juice dropped from 90% to 20% in one study.[34] Spermatogenesis was inhibited in dogs fed a bitter melon fruit extract for 60 days.[35] However, studies of a protein isolated from bitter melon seeds called MAP30 (under investigation as a potential therapy for cancer or HIV) has been found not to affect sperm motility *in vitro*.[4]

Precautions/Warnings/Contraindications

- Avoid ingestion of bitter melon seeds or outer rind, due to toxic lectins.[23]
- Avoid bitter melon in patients with glucose-6-phosphate dehydrogenase deficiency, due to the risk of hemolytic reaction and "favism."
- Use with caution in patients with diabetes, glucose intolerance, or taking hypoglycemic agents, due to the risk of hypoglycemia.[17,18,20,21]

Pregnancy and Lactation

- Bitter melon is not recommended during pregnancy because two proteins isolated from the raw fruit possess abortifacient properties in animals.[10-12] The fertility rate of mice fed daily bitter melon juice dropped from 90% to 20% in one study.[34] Spermatogenesis was inhibited in dogs fed a bitter melon fruit extract for 60 days.[35]

INTERACTIONS
Bitter Melon/Drug Interactions

- **Insulin, oral hypoglycemic agents:** Bitter melon has been found to lower blood glucose levels in animal experiments[25-29] and in several methodologically weak human studies.[17,18,20-22] Bitter melon may have additive effects when taken concomitantly with other blood glucose-lowering agents. A poorly described case series (n = 9) reported additive glucose-lowering effects of bitter melon juice or fried fruit when taken concomitantly with sulfonylurea drugs in 8 subjects (measured via glucose tolerance tests).[17] In a poorly described case report, a 40-year-old woman with type 2 diabetes experienced additive glucose-lowering effects when ingesting both the sulfonylurea drug chlorpropamide (Diabinese) and a curry containing bitter melon and garlic.[36] (Notably, garlic has been said anecdotally to possess hypoglycemic properties, although there is limited human evidence in this area.) In rats, oral bitter melon juice has been found to potentiate the glucose-lowering effects of the sulfonylurea tolbutamide (Orinase).[37]

Bitter Melon/Herb/Supplement Interactions

- **Hypoglycemic herbs and supplements:** Bitter melon has been found to lower blood glucose levels in animal studies[25-29] and in several methodologically weak human trials.[17,18,20-22] Bitter melon may have additive effects when taken concomitantly with other blood glucose-lowering agents.[36]

Bitter Melon/Food Interactions

- Insufficient data available.

Bitter Melon/Lab Interactions

- **Gamma-glutamyl transferase (GGT), alkaline phosphatase, liver function tests:** Rises in GGT and alkaline phosphatase have been observed in animals following oral administration of bitter melon fruit juice and seed extract. These rises have not been associated with significant histopathologic changes in the liver.[24] However, the potential for hepatotoxicity has not been systematically studied in humans.

MECHANISM OF ACTION
Pharmacology

- **Hypoglycemic effect:** Multiple mechanisms have been proposed as the cause of bitter melon's hypoglycemic properties. Components of bitter melon extract appear to have structural similarities to animal insulin, as measured by electrophoresis and infrared spectrum analysis.[18] Preliminary investigation has reported some insulin-like properties of bitter melon.[30,38,39] Other evidence suggests that bitter melon may decrease hepatic gluconeogenesis, increase hepatic glycogen synthesis, and increase peripheral glucose oxidation in erythrocytes and adipocytes.[32] One study reported that bitter melon increases pancreatic insulin secretion,[31] but this was not confirmed by subsequent studies.[40,41] Although several constituents of bitter melon have been found to possess hypoglycemic properties,[25-29] most interest has focused on a polypeptide isolated from the seeds called "polypeptide p," and a mixture of two steroid glycosides referred to as "charantin."[23,42]

- **Antiviral activity:** Antiviral activity observed *in vitro* has been attributed to a 30 kD protein called MAP30, which has been isolated from bitter melon seeds.[2] This protein has been reported to inhibit HIV viral integrase and cause irreversible relaxation of supercoiled viral nucleic acids.[5] These changes render viruses unable to integrate into host cell genomes. Reduced rates of T lymphocyte infection with HIV-1 and reduced rates of viral replication in infected cells have also been reported *in vitro*.[8,9] The *MAP30* gene has been cloned and expressed, and the recombinant protein re-MAP30 possesses similar properties *in vitro* to native MAP30. However, the antiviral activity of MAP30 (or bitter melon) has not been studied in humans.

- **Cancer:** MAP30, a protein isolated from bitter melon extract, has been reported to possess antineoplastic effects *in vitro*.[2,3,5] These effects have been attributed to the reduced expression of growth factor receptors such as the transmembrane tyrosine kinase receptor HER2 (also known as *neu* or *c-erb*-2), which has been implicated in breast cancer.[3] MAP30 was originally identified as a single-chain ribosome inactivating protein (SCRIP), but its *in vitro* activities appear to be unrelated to its effect on ribosomes. Bitter melon has been suggested to potentiate the function of natural killer cells in cancer patients.[43,44]

HISTORY

- Bitter melon has been used for centuries as a therapeutic agent in Asia, Africa, and Latin America. Folkloric uses include treatment of diabetes, psoriasis, infertility, gastrointestinal cramps, infections, and cancer. Bitter melon has also been used as a traditional abortifacient.

- Bitter melon is also consumed as a foodstuff and is found as an ingredient in some South Asian curries. The raw fruit is available in specialty Asian markets, where it is known as *karela*.

REVIEW OF THE EVIDENCE: DISCUSSION
Diabetes Mellitus (Hypoglycemic Agent)
Summary

- Bitter melon has been demonstrated to decrease serum glucose levels in animal experiments and in a small number of methodologically weak human studies. None of these investigations has been randomized or controlled. Dosage, toxicity, and adverse effects have not been systematically assessed. Preparation techniques have varied in the literature, and potency and chemical constituents may have varied accordingly. Nonetheless, the human, animal, and *in vitro* evidence collectively suggests a moderate hypoglycemic effect of bitter melon and some of its crude extracts. Reductions in serum blood sugars may occur as soon as 30 minutes after dosing, peak at 4 hours, and persist for at least 12 hours. Since neither safety nor efficacy have been established, bitter melon should be avoided by diabetics except under the strict supervision of a licensed healthcare professional, with careful monitoring of serum blood sugars. Properly designed randomized, controlled trials are warranted in order to further establish the clinical role of bitter melon for diabetes.

Evidence

- In 1977, Baldwa et al. conducted a controlled, nonrandomized, nonblinded trial examining the hypoglycemic effects of bitter melon on patients with diabetes.[18] Nineteen subjects were enrolled, including five healthy volunteers and 14 patients with either type 1 or type 2 diabetes. An extraction method was performed to isolate "vegetable insulin" from bitter melon, which was suspended in sterile water and

Review of the Evidence: Bitter Melon

Condition Treated*	Study Design	Author, Year	N[†]	SS[†]	Study Quality[‡]	Magnitude of Benefit	ARR[†]	NNT[†]	Comments
Diabetes types 1 and 2	Controlled trial, non-randomized, non-blinded	Baldwa[18] 1977	19	No	1	Large	NA	NA	Subcutaneous bitter melon extract lowered mean blood glucose after 30 minutes (21% drop), with peak effects at 4 hours (49% drop), and lasting effects at 12 hours (28% drop); methodologically weak study.
Diabetes type 2	Case series	Leatherdale[17] 1981	9	Yes	NA	Medium	NA	NA	Statistically significant 12% improvement in GTT after bitter melon juice; methodologically weak study.
Diabetes type 2	Case series	Welihinda[21] 1986	18	Yes	NA	Medium	NA	NA	Improved GTT in 13 subjects with bitter melon juice; poorly described study.
Diabetes type 2	Case series	Srivastava[22] 1993	12	NA	NA	Large	NA	NA	Bitter melon juice superior to dried fruit powder for reduction of mean serum glucose levels; methodologically weak study.

*Primary or secondary outcome.
[†]*N*, Number of patients; *SS*, statistically significant; *ARR*, absolute risk reduction; *NNT*, the number of patients who need to undergo a specific intervention in order to observe an outcome in one individual.
[‡]0-2 = poor; 3-4 = good; 5 = excellent.
NA, Not applicable; *GTT*, glucose tolerance test.
For an explanation of each category in this table, please see Table 3 in the Introduction.

available in a subcutaneous form with a concentration of 1.8 mg of vegetable insulin per 40-unit dose. Nine diabetic patients were placed on a sliding scale to receive 10 units of this suspension for a fasting blood sugar below 180, 20 units for 180 to 250, and 30 units for >250. Five diabetics and five nondiabetics received placebo. The primary end point measured was a decrease in fasting blood glucose, measured at multiple points over 12 hours. The authors reported a mean decrease in serum glucose levels for the diabetics receiving bitter melon, with effects noted as early as 30 minutes (21.5% drop from a mean baseline glucose level of 295), a maximum reduction at 4 hours (49.2% drop), and persistent effects after 12 hours (28% drop). In contrast, in both the diabetic and nondiabetic controls, a mean decrease in serum glucose of approximately 5% was seen throughout the study period. Although these results appear promising, multiple methodological weaknesses reduce their usefulness. No statistical analysis was performed (although with such dramatic differences between groups, it is likely that the differences would have been significant). Blinding was not performed, potentially introducing bias. Randomization was not performed, potentially introducing confounders. The diabetics receiving bitter melon had quite different mean baseline serum glucose values from the placebo group (295 vs. 210). Therefore, it is not clear that these groups were comparable. Furthermore, this study mixed type 1 and type 2 diabetics and diseases with different etiologies and mechanisms. As a result of these weaknesses, these results can only be considered preliminary.

- In 1981, Leatherdale et al. conducted a case series involving nine type 2 diabetics, of whom eight were taking concomitant sulfonylurea drugs.[17] Subjects underwent a baseline glucose tolerance test (GTT), a GTT following ingestion of 50 mL of bitter melon juice (obtained from approximately 200 g of fresh bitter melon fruit), and then a GTT after 8 to 11 weeks of daily ingestion of fried bitter melon (0.23 g daily). The GTT following fried fruit intake revealed a mean drop in glucose levels of approximately 6% after 1 hour. This result does not appear to have been statistically significant. In the juice group GTT, a statistically significant mean drop of approximately 12% was observed after 1 hour. A secondary end point was the effect of 8 to 11 weeks of fried bitter melon on glycosylated hemoglobin (HbA1c). Mean HbA1c values were found to have fallen by 8% from baseline. The results of this brief, poorly reported study are suggestive, but due to methodological weaknesses, including lack of controls, description of baseline patient characteristics, and adequate explanation of statistical methods, firm conclusions cannot be drawn.

- In 1986, Welihinda et al. reported a case series in 18 patients with newly diagnosed type 2 diabetes (average age 38 years).[21] Subjects were each given 100 mL of bitter melon fruit juice 30 minutes prior to glucose loading for a glucose tolerance test (GTT). Results were compared to the subjects' own responses to a GTT on a prior day, when water was administered as a control. Thirteen of the patients (73%) showed statistically significant moderate improvements in their GTT after taking bitter melon. Five patients did not improve. It is not clear what baseline differences might have existed in these 5 non-responders. Although suggestive, these results cannot be considered conclusive, due to methodological weaknesses. Even with patients serving as their own controls, the lack of true controls or randomization increases

the possibility of confounding. Without blinding, bias is more likely to be introduced. Baseline characteristics of patients were not clearly defined.

- In 1993, Srivastava et al. conducted a case series study involving 12 type 2 diabetic patients over 21 days.[22] Patients were not using other treatments, aside from "diabetic diets." Each subject was given one of two possible bitter melon preparations: (1) an aqueous extract prepared by boiling 100 g of chopped bitter melon in 200 mL of water until the volume was reduced to 100 mL, given daily as a single morning dose; or (2) 5 g of dried fruit powder given three times daily. After 3 weeks of therapy, patients in the powder group (n = 5) experienced a nonsignificant 25% reduction in mean blood sugar levels. In the aqueous extract group (n = 7), a statistically significant 54% reduction in mean blood sugars was observed, and mean glycosylated hemoglobin levels fell from 8.37 to 6.95 ($p < 0.01$). Although these results are promising, this was not a well-described or well-designed study. Statistical analysis was not clearly described. The lack of controls, description of baseline patient characteristics, and measurement of fasting glucose levels makes these conclusions difficult to interpret.

- The hypoglycemic effects of bitter melon powder dosed at 50 mg/kg have been observed to persist for as long as 7 days in one poorly described human case series.[45] These results cannot be considered conclusive, due to lack of controls, blinding, randomization, and clear statistical analysis. Nonetheless, these results are suggestive and add to the weight of other conducted studies.

Human Immunodeficiency Virus (HIV)
Summary

- Antiviral activity observed *in vitro* has been attributed to a 30kD protein called MAP30, which has been isolated from bitter melon seeds.[2,3,8,9] This protein has been reported to inhibit HIV viral integrase and cause irreversible relaxation of supercoiled viral nucleic acids.[5] These changes render viruses unable to integrate into host cell genomes. Reduced rates of T lymphocyte infection with HIV-1 and reduced rates of viral replication in infected cells have also been reported *in vitro*.[8,9] The *MAP30* gene has been cloned and expressed, and the recombinant protein re-MAP30 possesses similar properties *in vitro* as native MAP30. However, the antiviral activity of MAP30 (or bitter melon) has not been studied in humans.

Cancer
Summary

- MAP30, a protein isolated from bitter melon extract, has been reported to possess antineoplastic effects *in vitro*.[3,6] These effects have been attributed to the reduced expression of growth factor receptors such as the transmembrane tyrosine kinase receptor HER2 (also known as *neu* or *c-erb-2*), which has been implicated in breast cancer.[3] MAP30 was originally identified as a single-chain ribosome inactivating protein (SCRIP), but its *in vitro* antineoplastic activities appear to be unrelated to its effect on ribosomes. The *MAP30* gene has been cloned and expressed, and the recombinant protein re-MAP30 possesses similar properties *in vitro* as native MAP30. However, the antineoplastic effects of MAP30 (or bitter melon) have not been studied in humans.

- Bitter melon has been suggested to potentiate the function of natural killer cells in cancer patients.[43,44]

References

1. Basch E, Gabardi S, Ulbricht C. Bitter melon (*Momordica charantia*): a review of efficacy and safety. Am J Health Syst Pharm 2003;60(4):356-359.
2. Wang YX, Jacob J, Wingfield PT, et al. Anti-HIV and anti-tumor protein MAP30, a 30 kDa single-strand type-I RIP, shares similar secondary structure and beta-sheet topology with the A chain of ricin, a type-II RIP. Protein Sci 2000;9(1):138-144.
3. Lee-Huang S, Huang PL, Sun Y, et al. Inhibition of MDA-MB-231 human breast tumor xenografts and HER2 expression by anti-tumor agents GAP31 and MAP30. Anticancer Res 2000;20(2A):653-659.
4. Schreiber CA, Wan L, Sun Y, et al. The antiviral agents, MAP30 and GAP31, are not toxic to human spermatozoa and may be useful in preventing the sexual transmission of human immunodeficiency virus type 1. Fertil Steril 1999;72(4):686-690.
5. Wang YX, Neamati N, Jacob J, et al. Solution structure of anti-HIV-1 and anti-tumor protein MAP30: structural insights into its multiple functions. Cell 1999;99(4):433-442.
6. Bourinbaiar AS, Lee-Huang S. The activity of plant-derived antiretroviral proteins MAP30 and GAP31 against herpes simplex virus in vitro. Biochem Biophys Res Commun 1996;219(3):923-929.
7. Bourinbaiar AS, Lee-Huang S. Potentiation of anti-HIV activity of anti-inflammatory drugs, dexamethasone and indomethacin, by MAP30, the antiviral agent from bitter melon. Biochem Biophys Res Commun 1995;208(2):779-785.
8. Lee-Huang S, Huang PL, Chen HC, et al. Anti-HIV and anti-tumor activities of recombinant MAP30 from bitter melon. Gene 1995;161(2):151-156.
9. Lee-Huang S, Huang PL, Huang PL, et al. Inhibition of the integrase of human immunodeficiency virus (HIV) type 1 by anti-HIV plant proteins MAP30 and GAP31. Proc Natl Acad Sci U S A 1995;92(19):8818-8822.
10. Aguwa CN, Mittal GC. Abortifacient effects of the roots of *Momordica angustisepala*. J Ethnopharmacol 1983;7(2):169-173.
11. Chan WY, Tam PP, Yeung HW. The termination of early pregnancy in the mouse by beta-momorcharin. Contraception 1984;29(1):91-100.
12. Leung SO, Yeung HW, Leung KN. The immunosuppressive activities of two abortifacient proteins isolated from the seeds of bitter melon (*Momordica charantia*). Immunopharmacology 1987;13(3):159-171.
13. Biswas AR, Ramaswamy S, Bapna JS. Analgesic effect of *Momordica charantia* seed extract in mice and rats. J Ethnopharmacol 1991;31(1):115-118.
14. Mistry PP, Patel V. Ayurvedic herbal preparation in the treatment of high intraocular pressure. Clin Res 1991;39(2):420A.
15. Ng TB, Wong CM, Li WW, et al. A steryl glycoside fraction from *Momordica charantia* seeds with an inhibitory action on lipid metabolism *in vitro*. Biochem Cell Biol 1986;64(8):766-771.
16. Srivastava Y, Venkatakrishna-Bhatt H, Verma Y, et al. Retardation of retinopathy by *Momordica charantia* L. (bitter gourd) fruit extract in alloxan diabetic rats. Indian J Exp Biol 1987;25(8):571-572.
17. Leatherdale BA, Panesar RK, Singh G, et al. Improvement in glucose tolerance due to *Momordica charantia* (karela). Br Med J (Clin Res Ed) 1981;282(6279):1823-1824.
18. Baldwa VS, Bhandara CM, Pangaria A, et al. Clinical trials in patients with diabetes mellitus of an insulin-like compound obtained from plant source. Upsala J Med Sci 1977;82:39-41.
19. Hulin et al. Intoxication aigue pour *Momordica charantica* (Sorrossi). A proposdeux cas. Semaine Hospitaux 1988;64:2847-2848.
20. Raman A, Lau C. Anti-diabetic properties and phytochemistry of *Momordica charantia* L. (Cucurbitaceae). Phytomedicine 1996;2(4):349-362.
21. Welihinda J, Karunanayake EH, Sheriff MH, et al. Effect of *Momordica charantia* on the glucose tolerance in maturity onset diabetes. J Ethnopharmacol 1986;17(3):277-282.
22. Srivastava Y. Antidiabetic and adaptogenic properties of *Momordica charantia* extract: an experimental and clinical evaluation. Phytother Res 1993;7:285-289.
23. Marles R, Farnsworth N. Antidiabetic plants and their active constituents: an update. Phytomedicine 1997;2(2):137-189.
24. Tennekoon KH, Jeevathayaparan S, Angunawala P, et al. Effect of *Momordica charantia* on key hepatic enzymes. J Ethnopharmacol 1994;44(2):93-97.
25. Chen Q, Chan LL, Li ET. Bitter melon (*Momordica charantia*) reduces adiposity, lowers serum insulin and normalizes glucose tolerance in rats fed a high fat diet. J Nutr 2003;133(4):1088-1093.
26. Virdi J, Sivakami S, Shahani S, et al. Antihyperglycemic effects of three extracts from *Momordica charantia*. J Ethnopharmacol 2003;88(1):107-111.
27. Rathi SS, Grover JK, Vats V. The effect of *Momordica charantia* and *Mucuna pruriens* in experimental diabetes and their effect on key metabolic enzymes involved in carbohydrate metabolism. Phytother Res 2002;16(3):236-243.
28. Miura T, Itoh C, Iwamoto N, et al. Hypoglycemic activity of the fruit of the *Momordica charantia* in type 2 diabetic mice. J Nutr Sci Vitaminol (Tokyo) 2001;47(5):340-344.
29. Vikrant V, Grover JK, Tandon N, et al. Treatment with extracts of *Momordica charantia* and *Eugenia jambolana* prevents hyperglycemia and hyperinsulinemia in fructose fed rats. J Ethnopharmacol 2001;76(2):139-143.
30. Wong CM, Yeung HW, Ng TB. Screening of *Trichosanthes kirilowii*, *Momordica charantia* and *Cucurbita maxima* (family Cucurbitaceae) for compounds with antilipolytic activity. J Ethnopharmacol 1985;13(3):313-321.
31. Welihinda J, Arvidson G, Gylfe E, et al. The insulin-releasing activity of the tropical plant *Momordica charantia*. Acta Biol Med Ger 1982;41(12):1229-1240.
32. Shibib BA, Khan LA, Rahman R. Hypoglycaemic activity of *Coccinia indica* and *Momordica charantia* in diabetic rats: depression of the hepatic gluconeogenic enzymes glucose-6-phosphatase and fructose-1,6-bisphosphatase and elevation of both liver and red-cell shunt enzyme glucose-6-phosphate dehydrogenase. Biochem J 1993;292 (Pt 1):267-270.
33. Dutta PK, Chakravarty AK, Chowdhury US, et al. Vicine, a favism-inducing toxin from *Momordica charantia* Linn. seeds. Indian J Chem 1981;20B(August):669-671.
34. Stepka W, Wilson KE, Madge GE. Antifertility investigation on *Momordica*. Lloydia 1974;37(4):645.
35. Dixit VP, Khanna P, Bhargava SK. Effects of *Momordica charantia* L. fruit extract on the testicular function of dog. Planta Med 1978;34(3):280-286.
36. Aslam M, Stockley IH. Interaction between curry ingredient (karela) and drug (chlorpropamide). Lancet 1979;1:607.
37. Kulkarni RD, Gaitonde BB. Potentiation of tolbutamide action by jasad bhasma and karela (*Momordica charantia*). Indian J Med Res 1962;50(5):715-719.
38. Ng TB, Wong CM, Li WW, et al. Isolation and characterization of a galactose binding lectin with insulinomimetic activities. From the seeds of the bitter gourd *Momordica charantia* (Family Cucurbitaceae). Int J Peptide Protein Res 1986;28(2):163-172.
39. Ng TB, Wong CM, Li WW, et al. Insulin-like molecules in *Momordica charantia* seeds. J Ethnopharmacol 1986;15(1):107-117.
40. Day C, Cartwright T, Provost J, et al. Hypoglycaemic effect of *Momordica charantia* extracts. Planta Med 1990;56(5):426-429.
41. Sarkar S, Pranava M, Marita R. Demonstration of the hypoglycemic action of *Momordica charantia* in a validated animal model of diabetes. Pharmacol Res 1996;33(1):1-4.
42. Khanna P, Jain SC, Panagariya A, et al. Hypoglycemic activity of polypeptide-p from a plant source. J Nat Prod 1981;44(6):648-655.
43. Pongnikorn S, Fongmoon D, Kasinrerk W, et al. Effect of bitter melon (*Momordica charantia* Linn) on level and function of natural killer cells in cervical cancer patients with radiotherapy. J Med Assoc Thai 2003;86(1):61-68.
44. Cunnick JE, Sakamoto K, Chapes SK, et al. Induction of tumor cytotoxic immune cells using a protein from the bitter melon (*Momordica charantia*). Cell Immunol 1990;126(2):278-289.
45. Akhtar MS. Trial of *Momordica charantia* Linn (Karela) powder in patients with maturity-onset diabetes. J Pak Med Assoc 1982;32(4):106-107.

Black Cohosh
(*Cimicifuga racemosa* [L.] Nutt.)

SYNONYMS/COMMON NAMES/RELATED SUBSTANCES

- *Actaea macrotys, Actaea racemosa* L., actée à grappes, Amerikanisches wanzenkraut, baneberry, black snakeroot, botrophis serpentaria, bugwort, cohosh bugbane, cimicifuga, *Cimicifugae racemosae* rhizoma, cimicifugawurzelstock, herbe au punaise, macrotys, *Macrotys actaeoides*, rattle root, rattle snakeroot, rattle top, rattle weed, rich weed, schwarze schlangenwurzel, solvlys, squaw root, *Thalictrodes racemosa*, traubensilberkerze, wanzwnkraut.
- *Note:* Do not confuse black cohosh with blue cohosh (*Caulophyllum thalictroides*), which contains potentially cardiotoxic/vasoconstrictive chemicals. Do not confuse black cohosh (*Cimicifuga racemosa*) with *Cimicifuga foetida*, bugbane, fairy candles, or sheng ma; these are species from the same family (Ranunculaceae) with different therapeutic effects.

CLINICAL BOTTOM LINE
Background

- Black cohosh is popular as an alternative to hormonal therapy in the treatment of menopausal (climacteric) symptoms such as hot flashes, mood disturbances, diaphoresis, palpitations, and vaginal dryness. Several controlled trials and case series have reported black cohosh to improve menopausal symptoms for up to 6 months. Although these initial studies are suggestive, they have been few in number and have universally suffered from methodological weaknesses.
- The mechanism of action of black cohosh remains unclear, and the effects on estrogen receptors or hormonal levels (if any) have not been fully elucidated. Recent publications suggest that there may be no direct effects on estrogen receptors, although this is an area of active controversy.[1-8] Safety and efficacy data beyond 6 months are not available, although recent reports suggest safety of short-term use, including in women experiencing menopausal symptoms for whom estrogen replacement therapy is contraindicated.[9,10] Nonetheless, due to a lack of long-term follow-up, caution is advisable until better-quality safety data are available. Use of black cohosh in high-risk populations (such as in women with a history of breast cancer) should be under the supervision of a licensed healthcare professional.

Scientific Evidence for Common/Studied Uses	Grade*
Menopausal symptoms	B
Arthritis pain (rheumatoid arthritis, osteoarthritis)	C

*Key to grades: *A:* Strong scientific evidence for this use; *B:* Good scientific evidence for this use; *C:* Unclear scientific evidence for this use; *D:* Fair scientific evidence against this use (it may not work); *F:* Strong scientific evidence against this use (it likely does not work). For a more detailed explanation of efficacy criteria, see "Natural Standard Evidence-Based Validated Grading Rationale" in the Introduction.

Historical or Theoretical Uses That Lack Sufficient Evidence

- Amenorrhea, antitussive, anxiety, aphrodisiac, appetite stimulant, asthma, astringent, back pain, bronchitis, cardiac diseases, cervical dysplasia, chorea, depression, diarrhea, diaphoretic, dysmenorrhea, edema, endocarditis, endometriosis, fever, fibrocystic disease, gall bladder disorders, headache, hypertension,[11] infertility, inflammation, insect repellent, labor induction, leukorrhea, liver disease, malaise, malaria, mastitis, miscarriage, myalgia, nephritis, neurovegetative complaints, osteoporosis, palpitations, pancreatitis, parturition, pertussis (whooping cough), polycystic breast disease, polycystic ovarian syndrome, polymenorrhea, premenstrual syndrome (PMS), pruritis, sleep disorders, snakebites, sore throat, tinnitus, thrombocytopenia, uterine bleeding, uterine fibroids, uterine prolapse,[12] vertigo, yellow fever.[13]

Expert Opinion and Folkloric Precedent

- Black cohosh has been approved by the German expert panel, the Commission E, for premenstrual discomfort (weight gain, swelling, mood fluctuations, breast tenderness), dysmenorrhea, and perimenopausal symptoms and is a popular therapy in Europe for these uses.
- Native North Americans used the roots of black cohosh primarily for gynecologic conditions, joint pains, and labor pain relief. Other members of the genus *Cimicifuga* have been used within traditional Asian healing models as anti-inflammatory and analgesic agents. Black cohosh has been studied primarily in Germany over the past 40 years, with a standardized extract (Remifemin) available since the 1950s.
- In a survey of 500 nurse-midwives in the United States, out of 172 respondents, 33% indicated that they use black cohosh to stimulate labor.[14]
- Members of the genus *Cimicifuga*, notably *C. dahurica* (Turcz. Ex Fish. and C.A. Mey.) and *C. japonica* (Thunb.) Spreng, are frequently used within many traditional Asian healing models.

Safety Summary

- **Likely safe:** When used for up to 6 months in otherwise healthy, non-pregnant, non-lactating individuals. Long-term safety data are not available.
- **Possibly safe:** When taken by individuals with a history of hormone-sensitive conditions, such as breast cancer, uterine cancer, or endometriosis due to possible estrogenic effects and unknown risks,[15,16] although there is recent evidence that estrogenic properties may not be clinically relevant.[1-8] Black cohosh has been found to inhibit the growth of breast cancer cells *in vitro*,[17,18] and has been well tolerated in breast cancer patients for 6 weeks taken concomitantly with tamoxifen[19] and in breast cancer survivors with hot flashes.[10]
- **Possibly unsafe:** When taken as a labor-inducing agent concomitantly with blue cohosh (*Caulophyllum thalictroides*). There is a report of severe multi-organ hypoxic injury in a child delivered naturally (at home) with the aid of blue and black cohosh, who was not breathing at the time of birth.[14,20,21]
- **Likely unsafe:** When taken during pregnancy due to possible emmenagogic (menstrual flow–stimulating) effects (particularly during the first two trimesters).

DOSING/TOXICOLOGY
General

- Recommended doses are based on those most commonly used in available trials, or on historical practice. However, with natural products, the optimal doses needed to balance efficacy and safety often have not been determined. Formulations and preparation methods may vary from manufacturer to manufacturer, and from batch to batch of a specific product made by a single manufacturer. Because often the active components of a product are not known, standardization may not be possible, and the clinical effects of different brands may not be comparable.

Standardization

- The dosage of black cohosh is often based on its content of triterpenes, calculated as 27-deoxyactein. The German product Remifemin, used in the majority of clinical studies, contains an alcoholic extract of black cohosh rhizoma standardized to contain 1 mg of 27-deoxyactein per 20-mg tablet.[22] The manufacturing process and dosing recommendations for Remifemin have changed over the past 20 years, and doses used in different studies may not be comparable. A standardized liquid formulation of Remifemin was used in some studies.

Dosing: Adult (18 Years and Older)
Oral

- **Tablets:** For perimenopausal symptoms, studies have used 20 and 40 mg Remifemin tablets (corresponding to 1 to 2 mg of 27-deoxyactein) twice daily or 40 drops of a liquid ethanolic extract. The manufacturing process and dosing recommendations for Remifemin have changed over the past 20 years, and doses used in different studies may not be comparable. The dosing regimen currently recommended is 20 mg twice daily. A study of 40 mg per day vs. 127 mg per day of an isopropanolic extract of black cohosh for 6 months reported similar effects on menopausal symptoms.[23]
- **Dried rhizome (root):** The British Herbal Compendium has recommended 40 to 200 mg of dried rhizome daily in divided doses, although traditional doses have been as high as 1 g three times daily.
- **Tincture/liquid:** The British Herbal Compendium has recommended 0.4 to 2 mL of a (1:10) 60% ethanol tincture daily.
- **Other:** Powdered root or tea, 1 to 2 g three times daily, has been used.

Dosing: Pediatric (Younger Than 18 Years)

- Insufficient evidence to recommend.

Toxicology

- Anecdotally, overdose of black cohosh may cause headache, nausea, vomiting, dizziness, bradycardia, visual disturbances, and perspiration. A review of the literature reveals no reports of toxicity in humans.[24] In animals, administration of high doses of black cohosh for up to 6 months did not result in toxicity,[25] and no specific organ toxicity was seen in rats fed high doses (up to 5 g of extract/kg) for 26 weeks.[26] In an *in vitro* study, no evidence of mutagenicity from an isopropanolic extract of black cohosh was noted.[27]

ADVERSE EFFECTS/PRECAUTIONS/CONTRAINDICATIONS
Allergy

- Avoid if allergic to black cohosh or other members of the Ranunculaceae (buttercup or crowfoot) family.

- Native black cohosh contains small amounts of salicylic acid, but it is not clear how much (if any) is present in commercially available or standardized extracts. Caution is warranted in patients allergic to aspirin or other salicylates.

Adverse Effects/Postmarket Surveillance

- **General:** Reviews of the literature have reported black cohosh to be generally well tolerated in recommended doses for up to 6 months.[7,9,12,23,28,29] The potential effects of black cohosh on estrogen-sensitive conditions such as breast cancer, uterine cancer, and endometriosis are not known.
- **Neurologic/CNS:** Tonic-clonic seizures were reported in a 45-year-old woman who had been taking black cohosh, chaste tree berries/seeds (*Vitex agnus-castus*), and evening primrose oil (*Oenothera biennis*) for 4 months, who also consumed alcohol.[30] The relative contribution of each agent is not clear. Anecdotally, high doses of black cohosh may cause frontal headaches, dizziness, diaphoresis, and visual disturbances.
- **Cardiovascular:** Arrhythmia of unspecified type was reported in one patient in a 2-month placebo-controlled trial of black cohosh (n = 85).[19] Anecdotally, high doses of black cohosh may cause bradycardia. In a 1962 study, acteina, a constituent of black cohosh, was found to cause peripheral vasodilation in humans and was noted to elicit hypotension in animals.[31] Additional supporting data in humans is lacking.
- **Gastrointestinal (hepatitis):** There are three reported cases in Australia of hepatitis in patients taking herbal combinations containing black cohosh, including two cases of fulminant hepatic failure requiring transplantation.[32,33] The specific role of black cohosh in these cases is not clear. In 2003, a case report was published of acute liver failure in a 52-year-old woman using an herbal combination for 3 months (for tinnitus), including black cohosh and several other herbs (200-mL bottle containing fluid extracts of black cohosh, 20 mL; *Nepeta hederacea* [ground ivy], 80 mL; *Hydrastis canadensis* [goldenseal], 20 mL; *Ginkgo biloba*, 40 mL; *Avena sativa* [oat seed], 40 mL; concentration: 1 g of each herb per mL of extract, except goldenseal [0.5 g per mL]). The patient ingested 7.5 mL twice daily as needed, with an estimated total of 600 mL taken over 3 months. Liver transplantation was required. Laboratory analysis revealed no undeclared drugs in the preparation (which had been prepared by the patient's pharmacist). Notably, ground ivy contains very low concentrations of pulegone, a known hepatotoxin. Some authors feel that these cases have not been adequately substantiated, and given the widespread use of black cohosh and paucity of other such reports, merit further investigation.[34]
- **Gastrointestinal (gastrointestinal symptoms):** Mild gastrointestinal discomfort was found in 7% of a clinical sample of 629 women taking black cohosh.[35] Constipation was noted in one subject, and indigestion in another subject taking both black cohosh and tamoxifen in a placebo controlled trial.[19] Anecdotally, high doses of black cohosh may cause nausea and vomiting.
- **Endocrine (estrogenic effects):** The estrogenic activity of black cohosh remains debated, and specific estrogenic constituents have not been identified. It is not clear if black cohosh is safe in individuals with hormone-sensitive conditions such as breast cancer, uterine cancer, and endometriosis. Recent publications suggest that there may be no direct effects on estrogen receptors, although this is an area of active controversy.[1-8] Safety and efficacy data beyond

6 months are not available, although recent reports suggest safety of short-term use, including in women experiencing menopausal symptoms for whom estrogen replacement therapy is contraindicated.[9,10] In a 2-month trial in breast cancer survivors, endometrial hyperplasia was noted in one patient taking both black cohosh and tamoxifen (out of 42 subjects receiving black cohosh), and one instance each was noted of vaginal bleeding, weight gain, dilation and curettage, hysterectomy, and breast cancer recurrence.[19] The influence of black cohosh alone or in combination with tamoxifen is not clear in these cases, although these complications were not reported among 43 non–black cohosh subjects. Black cohosh was administered for 12 months in combination with tamoxifen to 136 breast cancer survivors for the prevention of hot flashes, and was well tolerated, although long-term safety data are not available.[10] In animals and *in vitro*, initial reports of estrogen receptor–binding activity[36] stand in contrast to more recent data suggesting no significant estrogen receptor–binding activity or estrogenic activities.[16,37-39] One *in vitro* study found no effects of black cohosh alone on estrogen receptors, but reported that black cohosh antagonized proliferative effects on cells induced by estradiol.[40] Several studies have aimed to assess estrogenic activity by measuring luteinizing hormone (LH), follicle-stimulating hormone (FSH), or prolactin levels.[41,42] One study reported lower FSH levels (but not LH) in patients treated with black cohosh vs. placebo (n = 110), although the results are not clear, because of lack of known baseline hormone levels in either group.[41] Results from other trials have found no effects on these hormone levels after up to 6 months of black cohosh therapy[19,29,43] Premature onset of estrus could not be precipitated in female infantile mice by administration of black cohosh.[44] Estrogenic effects on vaginal epithelium were noted in one 3-month trial of black cohosh,[45] whereas a more recent 6-month trial reported no effects on vaginal cytology.[23] Nonetheless, because of lack of long-term follow-up safety data, caution is advisable until better-quality safety data are available. Use of black cohosh in high-risk populations (such as in women with a history of breast cancer) should be under the supervision of a licensed healthcare professional.

- **Oncologic:** It remains unclear if black cohosh possesses estrogenic activity that may affect hormone-sensitive cancers, such as some types of breast or uterine cancer. Initial *in vitro* studies have reported black cohosh to possess inhibitory effects on estrogen-responsive cancer cell lines/breast cancer cells.[17,18,46] In a 2-month trial in breast cancer survivors, endometrial hyperplasia was noted in one patient taking both black cohosh and tamoxifen (out of 42 subjects receiving black cohosh), and one instance each was noted of vaginal bleeding, weight gain, dilation and curettage, hysterectomy, and breast cancer recurrence.[19] The influence of black cohosh alone or in combination with tamoxifen is not clear in these cases, although these complications were not reported among 43 non–black cohosh subjects. Black cohosh was administered for 12 months in combination with tamoxifen to 136 breast-cancer survivors for the prevention of hot flashes, and was well tolerated, although long-term safety data are not available.[10]

- **Hematologic:** It is not clear if black cohosh increases the risk of blood clots or stroke, and there have been no reports of these complications from the small number of existing case studies and trials. It is not clear if black cohosh possesses a similar mechanism of action as estrogen and raloxifene, which have been associated with these complications.

- **Musculoskeletal:** It has been hypothesized that black cohosh may exert negative effects on bone resorption, and that black cohosh, as potential substitute for estrogen therapy, may not possess the beneficial effects that estrogen may have on bone mass. However, there are no supporting human data in this area.

Precautions/Warnings/Contraindications

- Use cautiously in patients with known allergy to aspirin, other salicylates, or members of the Ranunculaceae (buttercup or crowfoot) family.
- Use cautiously in patients with known estrogen-sensitive conditions, such as breast cancer, uterine cancer, and endometriosis. Effects are not known.
- Use cautiously in patients on hormone replacement therapy, including tamoxifen and raloxifene. Effects of black cohosh are not known.
- Use cautiously in patients with known seizure disorder, based on one case report.
- Use cautiously in patients on antihypertensive medications, because of a theoretical risk of hypotension.
- Use cautiously in patients with history of thromboembolic disease or stroke. Although there are no reports of these complications in the available literature, there may be a theoretical risk.
- Use cautiously in patients with liver disease, because of three case reports of liver damage.
- If black cohosh is used as an alternative to prescription hormone replacement therapy, follow bone mass and be aware that beneficial effects on bone mass may not occur.

Pregnancy and Lactation

- Safety during pregnancy has not been established, and use of black cohosh may be inadvisable because of purported effects on the uterus ("uterotonic" effects), and possible estrogenic properties.
- In a survey of 500 nurse-midwives in the United States, out of 172 respondents, 33% indicated that they use black cohosh to stimulate labor.[14] There is one report of severe multi-organ hypoxic injury in a child delivered "naturally" with the aid of both blue and black cohosh (*Caulophyllum thalictroides*) who was not breathing at the time of birth.[21] The child survived with permanent central nervous system damage. Notably, blue cohosh possesses a vasoconstrictive glycoside that may have been responsible for the adverse effects.
- There is insufficient evidence regarding use of black cohosh during lactation, and it is therefore not recommended.
- Tinctures may be ill-advised during pregnancy because of their high alcohol content, although the absolute quantity of alcohol ingested from tinctures at recommended doses is likely to be relatively small.

INTERACTIONS
Black Cohosh/Drug Interactions

- **Hormone replacement therapy (HRT), oral contraceptives (OCPs):** The estrogenic activity of black cohosh remains debated. Specific estrogenic constituents have not been identified, and it is not clear how (or if) black cohosh interacts with estrogens/estrogen receptors and/or progestins. Recent publications suggest that there may be no direct effects on estrogen receptors, although this is an area of active controversy.[1-8] Therefore, caution is warranted in individuals taking both black cohosh and estrogens because of unknown effects, and interaction data in this area are lacking. In animals and *in vitro*, initial reports of estrogen receptor–binding activity[36] stand in contrast to more recent data suggesting no significant estrogen receptor–binding activity or estrogenic activities.[16,37-39] One *in vitro* study found no effects of black cohosh alone on estrogen receptors but reported that black cohosh antagonized proliferative effects on cells induced by estradiol.[40] Several studies have aimed to assess estrogenic activity by measuring luteinizing hormone (LH), follicle-stimulating hormone (FSH), or prolactin levels.[41,42] One study reported lower FSH levels (but not LH) in patients treated with black cohosh vs. placebo (n = 110), although baseline hormone levels were not known in either group.[41] Results from other trials have found no effects on these hormone levels after up to 6 months of black cohosh therapy.[19,29,43] Premature onset of estrus in female infantile mice could not be precipitated by administration of black cohosh.[44] Estrogenic effects on vaginal epithelium were noted in one 3-month trial of black cohosh,[45] whereas a more recent 6-month trial reported no effects on vaginal cytology.[23]

- **Tamoxifen, raloxifene:** Controversy surrounds the use of black cohosh in combination with tamoxifen. In a 2003 randomized, open-label controlled trial of black cohosh for the prevention of hot flashes in women survivors of breast cancer taking tamoxifen, 136 women, ages 36 to 52 years, received either black cohosh (CR BNO 1055, Menofem/Klimadynon, 20 mg daily) with their tamoxifen, or tamoxifen alone.[10] After 12 months, 24.4% of black cohosh subjects experienced hot flashes, compared to 73.9% in the tamoxifen-only group ($p < 0.01$). These results are promising, although the introduction of bias due to the open-label design is possible. Long-term follow-up of disease-free interval was not conducted, and therefore the safety of black cohosh in breast cancer patients was not established. In a 2001 trial of 85 breast cancer survivors, endometrial hyperplasia was noted in one patient taking both black cohosh and tamoxifen (out of 42 subjects receiving black cohosh), and one instance each was noted of vaginal bleeding, weight gain, dilation and curettage, hysterectomy, and breast cancer recurrence.[19] The influence of black cohosh alone or in combination with tamoxifen is not clear in these cases, although these complications were not reported among 43 non–black cohosh subjects. In this study, no improvements in hot flashes, other menopausal symptoms, or overall well-being were noted over a 2-month period (in contrast to other preliminary research suggesting efficacy of black cohosh for menopausal symptoms). It is not clear if tamoxifen antagonized the effects of black cohosh, or if hot flashes induced by tamoxifen are refractory to black cohosh therapy. Although this trial suggests that black cohosh may not be useful in the short-term treatment of tamoxifen-related hot flashes, because of methodological weaknesses further study is warranted. Also in this trial, constipation was noted in one subject, and indigestion in one subject.[19] Recent *in vitro* study suggests possible additive anti-proliferative effects of black cohosh and tamoxifen.[47]

- **Hypotensive drugs:** Because of theoretical hypotensive effects, black cohosh should be used cautiously with other hypotensive agents.[11,13] There have been reports of hypotension in animals, although human data are limited in this area; increased peripheral blood flow was associated with black cohosh administration in a 1962 study.[31]

- **Antiplatelet drugs, anticoagulants:** Native black cohosh contains small amounts of salicylic acid and may potentiate the antiplatelet effects of other agents. This is a theoretical concern, as it is not clear if therapeutic amounts of salicylates are present in commercial or processed black cohosh products.

- **Disulfiram (Antabuse):** Tinctures may contain high alcohol content and theoretically may elicit a disulfiram reaction.

- **Metronidazole (Flagyl):** A disulfiram reaction can occur when metronidazole and alcohol are used concomitantly. Because of the high alcohol content in some tinctures, this combination theoretically may cause such a reaction.

Black Cohosh/Herb/Supplement Interactions

- **Antiplatelet/anticoagulant herbs and supplements:** Native black cohosh contains small amounts of salicylic acid and may potentiate the antiplatelet effects of other agents. This is a theoretical concern, as it is not clear if therapeutic amounts of salicylates are present in commercial or processed black cohosh products.

- **Herbs and supplements containing phytoestrogens:** The estrogenic activity of black cohosh remains debated. Specific estrogenic constituents have not been identified, and it is not clear if black cohosh interacts with other estrogenic compounds. Recent publications suggest that there may be no direct effects on estrogen receptors, although this is an area of active controversy.[1-8] Therefore, caution is warranted in subjects taking both black cohosh and herbs containing phytoestrogens, because of unknown effects, and interaction data in this area are lacking. In animals and *in vitro*, initial reports of estrogen receptor–binding activity[36] stand in contrast to more recent data suggesting no significant estrogen receptor–binding activity or estrogenic activities.[16,37-39] Several studies have aimed to assess estrogenic activity by measuring luteinizing hormone (LH), follicle-stimulating hormone (FSH), or prolactin levels.[41,42] One study reported lower FSH levels (but not LH) in patients treated with black cohosh vs. placebo (n = 110), although baseline hormone levels were not known in either group.[41] Results from other trials have found no effects on these hormone levels after up to 6 months of black cohosh therapy.[19,29,34] Premature onset of estrus in female infantile mice could not be precipitated by administration of black cohosh.[44] Estrogenic effects on vaginal epithelium were noted in one 3-month trial of black cohosh,[45] whereas a more recent 6-month trial reported no effects on vaginal cytology.[23]

- **Evening primrose oil, chasteberry:** Tonic-clonic seizures have been reported in a 45-year-old woman who had been taking black cohosh, chaste tree (berries and seeds), and primrose oil for 4 months, who also consumed alcohol.[30] The relative contribution of each agent or risk of combination is not clear.

- **Blue cohosh:** Both black cohosh and blue cohosh (*Caulophyllum thalictroides*) are commonly used by nurse-midwives in the United States to assist birth.[14] There is a report of severe multi-organ hypoxic injury in a child delivered "naturally" with the aid of both blue and black cohosh, who was not breathing at the time of birth.[14,20,21] The child survived with permanent central nervous system damage. Notably, blue cohosh possesses a vasoconstrictive glycoside that may have been responsible for the adverse effects.

- **American pennyroyal:** Pennyroyal (*Hedeoma pulegioides* L.) and black cohosh are sometimes taken together to induce abortion, although the use of these herbs together cannot be recommended because of the possibility of increased toxicity and death. There is a case report of a 24-year-old woman who took 48% to 56% of pennyroyal herb in an alcohol base and an unknown amount of black cohosh root for 2 weeks in an attempt to induce abortion.[48] Following a single subsequent dose of this combination, the patient died within 48 hours.

MECHANISM OF ACTION
Pharmacology

- **Constituents:** Constituents of black cohosh with proposed or demonstrated pharmacological activity include triterpene glycosides (actein, 27-deoxyactein, cimicifugoside),[17] cyclolanostanol xylosides,[49] formononetin, and organic acids (isoferulic, salicylic acid).
- **Estrogenic effects:** It is not clear what constituent(s) of black cohosh, if any, possesses estrogenic properties. In animals and *in vitro,* initial reports of estrogen receptor–binding activity[36] stand in contrast to more recent data suggesting no significant estrogen receptor–binding activity or estrogenic activities.[1,2,16,37-39] One *in vitro* study found no effects of black cohosh alone on estrogen receptors but reported that black cohosh antagonized proliferative effects on cells induced by estradiol.[40] Several studies have aimed to assess estrogen activity by measuring luteinizing hormone (LH), follicle-stimulating hormone (FSH), or prolactin levels.[41,42] One study reported lower FSH levels (but not LH) in patients treated with black cohosh vs. placebo (n = 110), although baseline hormone levels were not known in either group.[41] Results from other trials have found no effects on these hormone levels after up to 6 months of black cohosh therapy.[19,29,43] Premature onset of estrus in female infantile mice could not be precipitated by administration of black cohosh.[44] Estrogenic effects on vaginal epithelium were noted in one 3-month trial of black cohosh,[45] whereas a more recent 6-month trial reported no effects on vaginal cytology.[23]
- **CNS effects:** Recent studies suggest that the mechanism of action of black cohosh may be centrally mediated, with possible action at the level of serotonin or dopamine receptors.[6,8]
- **Cancer cell lines:** *In vitro* studies have reported black cohosh to possess inhibitory effects on estrogen-responsive cancer cell lines/breast cancer cells.[17,18,46]
- **Vascular effects:** In a 1962 study, acteina, a constituent of black cohosh, was found to cause peripheral vasodilation and has been noted to elicit hypotension in animals.[31] Additional supporting data in humans are lacking.
- **Other:** Cimicifugoside from *Cimicifuga simplex* has been found to inhibit cellular thymidine-3H uptake and to act as a selective inhibitor of nucleoside transport into mammalian cells.[13,50,51]

HISTORY

- Native American and Chinese herbalists have traditionally used black cohosh for a variety of ailments, and as an insect repellent.
- In the 19th century, black cohosh was used by medical practitioners for a variety of rheumatic disorders, dysmenorrhea, and to induce labor. An eclectic physician of obstetrics and gynecology in the 1800s, John King was a strong proponent of medicinal use of this herb. A popular product sold in the United States in the late 1800s for menstrual cramps was Lydia E. Pinkham's Vegetable Compound, which contained black cohosh and alcohol.
- Black cohosh has been widely used in Germany since the 1950s, principally for disorders associated with menopause and menstruation.

REVIEW OF THE EVIDENCE: DISCUSSION
Menopausal/Perimenopausal Symptoms
Summary

- Black cohosh is popular as an alternative to prescription hormonal therapy in the treatment of menopausal (climacteric) symptoms such as hot flashes, mood disturbances, diaphoresis, palpitations, and vaginal dryness. Several controlled trials and case series have reported black cohosh to improve menopausal symptoms for up to 6 months. Although these initial studies are suggestive, they have been small in number and have universally suffered from methodological weaknesses. Most trials have utilized a standardized measurement scale to assess menopausal symptoms called the Kupperman Index, which does not measure vaginal dryness/atrophy but does measure paresthesias and vertigo (which are not classically associated with menopause). The mechanism of action of black cohosh remains unclear, and effects on estrogen receptors or hormonal levels have not been demonstrated. Safety and efficacy data beyond 6 months are not available. Therefore, while the available evidence does suggest possible efficacy of black cohosh for the short-term treatment of menopausal symptoms, this is an area where a well-designed, long-term, three-arm (black cohosh vs. standard therapy vs. placebo) evaluation of efficacy and safety is warranted.

Randomized Controlled Trials

- In a randomized, double-blind trial, Stoll et al. compared 4 mg of black cohosh extract (Remifemin) taken twice daily vs. 0.625 mg of conjugated estrogens vs. placebo in 80 women with menopausal symptoms.[45] Outcomes measures included the Kupperman Index, anxiety as measured by the Hamilton anxiety scale (HAM-A), and proliferation of vaginal epithelium. After 12 weeks, all measures were significantly improved in the black cohosh group vs. placebo, with reported equivalence to conjugated estrogens. In a separate measure of and frequency of hot flashes, improvement in the black cohosh group was superior to estrogens or placebo, with a mean reduction in the black cohosh group from 4.9 to 0.7 hot flashes per day vs. 5.2 to 3.2 in the estrogen group (which was similar to placebo). Despite methodological weaknesses of this study, including incomplete descriptions of baseline patient characteristics, blinding, or randomization, the three-arm design and use of multiple outcomes measures add strength to the results.
- Jacobson et al. conducted a randomized, double-blind study in 85 breast cancer survivors who had completed their primary breast cancer treatment and were experiencing hot flashes.[19] In this group, 69% were taking tamoxifen. Subjects were randomized to receive either an unidentified black cohosh preparation or placebo for 2 months, after which time both groups were reported to experience significant reductions in hot flashes, with no advantage of black cohosh over placebo in the 81% of subjects that completed the study. No between-group differences were detected on visual analog scales of well-being, global health, or menopausal symptoms (diaphoresis, palpitations, sleep quality, depression, anxiety, headache). The weaknesses of this study include the short duration, which may not be adequate to assess menopausal symptoms, concomitant use of tamoxifen, which induces hot flashes that may require a different treatment approach than menopausal hot flashes, unclear black cohosh product used, and large dropout (19%) without adequate analysis of dropouts. Nonetheless, these negative

Review of the Evidence: Black Cohosh

Condition Treated*	Study Design	Author, Year	N[†]	SS[†]	Study Quality[‡]	Magnitude of Benefit	ARR[†]	NNT[†]	Comments
Menopausal symptoms	Randomized, double-blind, placebo-controlled, equivalence study	Stoll[45] 1987	80	Yes	4	Medium	NA	NA	8 mg of Remifemin (black cohosh) vs. conjugated estrogens or placebo for 12 weeks. Black cohosh superior to placebo and equal to estrogens on Kupperman Index, HAM-A, and vaginal epithelial proliferation; hot flashes reduced more than estrogens.
Menopausal symptoms (breast cancer survivors)	Randomized, double-blind, placebo-controlled	Jacobson[19] 2001	85	NA	3	None	NA	NA	No improvement in hot flashes in breast cancer survivors from black cohosh vs. placebo. 69% of subjects taking tamoxifen. 19% dropout.
Menopausal symptoms	Dosing trial (randomized, double-blind)	Liske and Wüstenberg[23] 1998	152	NA	3	Large	NA	NA	Published conference abstract. 40 mg vs. 127 mg per day of black cohosh extract for 6 months. No differences found in Kupperman Index, LH, FSH, or vaginal epithelium. No placebo group.
Menopausal symptoms	Randomized, double-blind, placebo-controlled	Boblitz[55] 2000	179	Yes	2	Medium	NA	NA	Published conference abstract. Fixed combination of black cohosh and St. John's wort improved Kupperman Index after 6 weeks.
Menopausal symptoms	Equivalence trial, randomized, non-blinded, no placebo	Lehmann-Willenbrock[29] 1988	60	NA	1	Medium	NA	NA	Black cohosh vs. 3 hormone replacement therapies for 6 months in hysterectomy patients. Equal improvements in all groups on Kupperman Index. Sample size may have been inadequate.
Menopausal symptoms	Equivalence trial, non-blinded, no placebo	Warnecke[52] 1985	60	Yes	1	Medium	NA	NA	Black cohosh vs. conjugated estrogens vs. diazepam. Equal improvement on Kupperman Index and HAM-A.
Hot flashes in breast cancer survivors using tamoxifen	Randomized, controlled, open-label trial	Hernandez[10] 2003	139	Yes	4	Medium	49.5%	2	Tamoxifen plus black cohosh vs. tamoxifen alone reported to reduce hot flash incidence. Open-label design allows for bias.

*Primary or secondary outcome.
[†] N, Number of patients; SS, statistically significant; ARR, absolute risk reduction; NNT, the number of patients who need to undergo a specific intervention in order to observe an outcome in one individual.
[‡] 0-2 = poor; 3-4 = good; 5 = excellent.
FSH, Follicle-stimulating hormone; HAM-A, Hamilton anxiety scale; LH, luteinizing hormone; NA, not applicable.
For an explanation of each category in this table, please see Table 3 in the Introduction.

results warrant further evaluation, particularly in the setting of tamoxifen use, which may be common in women who seek black cohosh as an alternative to estrogen therapy (or in women with breast cancer history or risk).

• In a six-month randomized, non-blinded study, Lehmann-Willenbrock and Riedel randomized 60 women younger than 40 years of age who had undergone hysterectomy (but were left with at least one ovary) to receive either black cohosh (2 20-mg tablets of Remifemin twice daily), estriol (1 mg once daily), conjugated estrogens (1.25 mg once daily), or estrogen/progestin combination (1 tablet of unclear dosage daily).[29] Notably, these were not cancer patients and had undergone hysterectomy for non-malignant conditions. Subjects were all experiencing menopausal symptoms prior to the study. Outcomes measures included a modified Kupperman Index (a sum score of menopausal symptoms), as well as serum LH and FSH levels. Assessment at 1, 2, 3, and 6 months found improvements on the Kupperman Index to be comparable in all groups. The Kupperman Index

score was noted to decrease in all groups by at least 50% vs. baseline (more in the conjugated estrogen and estrogen-gestagen groups, without statistical significance). FSH and LH levels decreased in all hormonal replacement groups, but not in the black cohosh group. These results are compromised by the lack of placebo group, poor description of baseline patient characteristics, and unclear procedures for blinding or randomization. The small sample size despite multiple subgroups, without a power calculation to determine adequate sample size, leaves open the possibility that results are due to lack of statistical power, rather than true equivalence of therapies.

• In a non-blinded study of 60 women with menopausal symptoms, Warnecke compared black cohosh (40 drops of daily Remifemin liquid twice daily, standardized to 27-deoxyactein) vs. 0.625 mg of conjugated estrogens daily vs. 2 mg of the benzodiazepine diazepam daily.[52] Outcomes measures included the Kupperman Index of menopausal symptoms, Hamilton anxiety scale (HAM-A), Clinical

Global Impressions (CGI) scale, and a patient self-assessment scale for depression. After 12 weeks, statistically significant improvements were noted in both groups in Kupperman, HAM-A, and self-assessment scores, without differences between groups. Non-significant improvements were noted in CGI scores in both groups. Although suggestive, the lack of placebo group or blinding allows for the influence of bias and confounders. The results may reflect the natural history of menopausal symptoms rather than the benefits of therapy.

- Hernandez et al. investigated the use of black cohosh for the prevention of hot flashes in women survivors of breast cancer taking tamoxifen.[10] In this randomized, open-label controlled trial, 136 women, ages 36 to 52 years, received either black cohosh (CR BNO 1055, Menofem/Klimadynon, 20 mg daily) with their tamoxifen, or tamoxifen alone. After 12 months, 24.4% of black cohosh subjects experienced hot flashes, compared to 73.9% in the tamoxifen-only group ($p < 0.01$). These results are promising, although the introduction of bias due to the open-label design is possible. Long-term follow-up of disease-free interval was not conducted, and therefore the safety of black cohosh in breast cancer patients was not established.

Case Series

- In a case series, 40 drops of daily Remifemin (standardized to 27-deoxyactein) was administered for 6 to 8 weeks to 629 women with menopausal symptoms.[35] Primary outcomes measures included diaphoresis, hot flashes, headache, palpitations, and anxiety. After 4 weeks, 80% of subjects were reported to have experienced symptomatic relief. Although suggestive, this study is limited by the lack of a control group. The observed improvements may therefore reflect the natural history of menopausal symptoms to wax and wane, or confounding by a "placebo effect" (rather than effects of black cohosh).
- Two poor-quality case series with similar designs have been reported from gynecology practices.[53,54] In combination, 86 cases were presented of women treated with Remifemin liquid, 40 drops twice daily for approximately 3 months. Improvements were reported in Kupperman Index scores for menopausal symptoms, and in Clinical Global Impressions (CGI) score. Although suggestive, the short duration and lack of controls weakens these results.

Dosing Study

- In a published abstract, Liske and Wüstenberg reported a comparison of two doses of an iso-propanolic extract of black cohosh.[23] Menopausal women (n = 152, ages 43 to 60 years) were randomized to receive either 40 mg or 127 mg of black cohosh daily for 6 months. Improvements on the Kupperman Index were reported after 2 weeks in both groups. After 6 months, the groups were found to have similar results on the Kupperman Index (90% of subjects in both groups improving), without changes in either group in levels of LH, FSH, or prolactin, and without changes in vaginal epithelial proliferation. Although this report suggests equal efficacy of the two doses of black cohosh, the lack of placebo arm weakens the results; benefits over time due to the natural history of menopausal symptoms to wax and wane cannot be ruled out as causative. In addition, as a published abstract, descriptions of methodology were limited. Although no power calculation was conducted, the sample size was likely adequate to detect between-group differences.

Combination Product

- Boblitz et al. conducted a double-blind, randomized, placebo-controlled trial of Remifemin Plus, which contains a fixed combination of St. John's wort (*Hypericum perforatum*) and black cohosh.[55] In this study, 179 patients with complaints associated with menopause were treated with 2 capsules given together once daily of either Remifemin Plus or placebo. The Kupperman Index of those ingesting Remifemin Plus decreased from 31.4 to 18.7, compared with a decrease in the placebo group from 30.3 to 22.3 ($p < 0.001$). Psychological parameters were also significantly improved in the Remifemin Plus group. However, it is not possible to separate the possible effects of black cohosh from those of St. John's wort, which has been found to improve symptoms of mild to moderate depression and may exert influence on Kupperman measures. As a published abstract, this report included only limited descriptions of baseline patient characteristics and methods.

Arthritis Pain (Rheumatoid Arthritis, Osteoarthritis)
Summary

- Literature review reveals no high-quality studies of black cohosh monotherapy for symptoms of rheumatoid arthritis or osteoarthritis. Native black cohosh does contain small amounts of salicylates, although it is not clear if these are present in therapeutic amounts in commercial preparations. One study of a combination product containing black cohosh and several other salicylate-containing herbs for rheumatoid arthritis or osteoarthritis found small improvements in pain scores, but no improvement in joint function or decrease in self-medication with analgesics.

Evidence

- A randomized, double-blind, placebo-controlled trial administered a fixed combination product (Reumalex) to 82 male and female patients with rheumatoid arthritis or osteoarthritis.[56] Each Reumalex tablet contains 35 mg of black cohosh, 100 mg of white willow bark, 25 mg of sarsaparilla (4:1), 17 mg of poplar bark (7:1), and 40 mg of guaiacum resin. Notably, several constituents contain salicylates, and it has been estimated that each Reumalex tablet may include up to 10 to 20 mg of salicylates. Two Reumalex tablets or placebo were administered to subjects over a 2-month period. Outcomes measures included scores on the validated Arthritis Impact Measurement Scales Health Status Questionnaire (AIMS-2). Small significant improvements in pain were noted in the Reumalex group vs. placebo, although there were no other significant differences between groups, including measures of joint function and use of over-the-counter analgesics. These results cannot be extrapolated to any of the constituents alone.

FORMULARY: BRANDS USED IN CLINICAL TRIALS/ THIRD-PARTY TESTING
Brands Used In Clinical Trials

- Remifemin (originally manufactured by Schaper & Brümmer; now manufactured and distributed by GlaxoSmithKline).
- CR BNO 1055 (Menofem/Klimadynon).
- **Other trade names:** Biophylin, Black Cohosh Liquid Extract (Bio-pro), Black Cohosh Root Powder (Global Botanical), Cimisan, Femilla N, Klimadyon, Ligvites, Vegetex.
- **Combination products:** Black Cohosh CX, Cimicifuga-Amyda-Shell Decoction, Estroven, FC with Dong Quai, GNC Menopause Formula, Natrol, Nature's Herbs, Qingwei san,

Remifemin Plus (black cohosh plus St. John's wort), Reumalex (35 mg of black cohosh, 100 mg of white willow bark, 25 mg of sarsaparilla [4:1], 17 mg of poplar bark [7:1], and 40 mg of guaiacum resin).

Brands Shown to Contain Claimed Ingredients Through Third-Party Testing

• Remifemin

References

1. Borrelli F, Izzo AA, Ernst E. Pharmacological effects of *Cimicifuga racemosa*. Life Sci 2003;73(10):1215-1229.
2. Lupu R, Mehmi I, Atlas E, et al. Black cohosh, a menopausal remedy, does not have estrogenic activity and does not promote breast cancer cell growth. Int J Oncol 2003;23(5):1407-1412.
3. Mahady GB. Is black cohosh estrogenic? Nutr Rev 2003;61(5 Pt 1):183-186.
4. Seidlova-Wuttke D, Jarry H, Becker T, et al. Pharmacology of *Cimicifuga racemosa* extract BNO 1055 in rats: bone, fat and uterus. Maturitas 2003; 44 Suppl 1:S39-S50.
5. Seidlova-Wuttke D, Hesse O, Jarry H, et al. Evidence for selective estrogen receptor modulator activity in a black cohosh (*Cimicifuga racemosa*) extract: comparison with estradiol-17beta. Eur J Endocrinol 2003;149(4):351-362.
6. Jarry H, Metten M, Spengler B, et al. In vitro effects of the *Cimicifuga racemosa* extract BNO 1055. Maturitas 2003;44 Suppl 1:S31-S38.
7. Huntley A, Ernst E. A systematic review of the safety of black cohosh. Menopause 2003;10(1):58-64.
8. Burdette JE, Liu J, Chen SN, et al. Black cohosh acts as a mixed competitive ligand and partial agonist of the serotonin receptor. J Agric Food Chem 2003;51(19):5661-5670.
9. Dog TL, Powell KL, Weisman SM. Critical evaluation of the safety of *Cimicifuga racemosa* in menopause symptom relief. Menopause 2003;10(4):299-313.
10. Hernandez MG, Pluchino S. *Cimicifuga racemosa* for the treatment of hot flushes in women surviving breast cancer. Maturitas 2003;44 Suppl 1:S59-S65.
11. Hailemeskel B, Lee HJ, Thomhe H. Incidence of potential herb-drug interactions among herbal users. ASHP Midyear Clinical Meeting 2000; 35:p-267e.
12. Hunter A. *Cimicifuga racemosa*: pharmacology, clinical trials and clinical use. Eur J Herbal Med 1999;5(1):19-25.
13. Takahira M, Kusano A, Shibano M, et al. Antimalarial activity and nucleoside transport inhibitory activity of the triterpenic constituents of *Cimicifuga* spp. Biol Pharm Bull 1998;21(8):823-828.
14. McFarlin BL, Gibson MH, O'Rear J, et al. A national survey of herbal preparation use by nurse-midwives for labor stimulation. Review of the literature and recommendations for practice. J Nurse Midwifery 1999; 44(3):205-216.
15. Liske E, Wustenberg P. Efficacy and safety of phytomedicines with particular references to *Cimicifuga racemosa*. J Med Assoc Thai 1998;Jan:s108.
16. Einer-Jensen N, Zhao J, Andersen KP, et al. *Cimicifuga* and *Melbrosia* lack oestrogenic effects in mice and rats. Maturitas 1996;25(2):149-153.
17. Struck D, Tegtmeier M, Harnischfeger G. Flavones in extracts of *Cimicifuga racemosa*. Planta Med 1997;63:289-290.
18. Nesselhut T, Schellhase C, Dietrich R, et al. [Investigations into the growth-inhibitive efficacy of phytopharmacopia with estrogen-like influences on mammary gland carcinoma cells] (translated from German). Arch Gynecol Obstet 1993;254:817-818.
19. Jacobson JS, Troxel AB, Evans J, et al. Randomized trial of black cohosh for the treatment of hot flashes among women with a history of breast cancer. J Clin Oncol 2001;19(10):2739-2745.
20. Baillie N, Rasmussen P. Black and blue cohosh in labour. N Z Med J 1997;110(1036):20-21.
21. Gunn TR, Wright IM. The use of black and blue cohosh in labour. N Z Med J 1996;109(1032):410-411.
22. Pepping J. Black cohosh: *Cimicifuga racemosa*. Am J Health Syst Pharm 1999;56(14):1400-1402.
23. Liske E, Wüstenberg P. Therapy of climacteric complaints with *Cimicifuga racemosa*: herbal medicine with clinically proven evidence [poster presentation]. Menopause 1998;5(4):250.
24. McKenna DJ, Jones K, Humphrey S, et al. Black cohosh: efficacy, safety, and use in clinical and preclinical applications. Altern Ther Health Med 2001; 7(3):93-100.
25. Beuscher N, Reichert R. *Cimicifuga racemosa* L.—black cohosh. Zeit Phytother 1995;16:301-310.
26. Korn WD. Six month oral toxicity study with remifemin-granulate in rats followed by an 8-week recovery period. International Bioresearch, Hannover, Germany 1991;1.
27. Liske E. Therapeutic efficacy and safety of *Cimicifuga racemosa* for gynecologic disorders. Adv Ther 1998;15(1):45-53.
28. Lieberman S. A review of the effectiveness of *Cimicifuga racemosa* (black cohosh) for the symptoms of menopause. J Womens Health 1998;7(5): 525-529.
29. Lehmann-Willenbrock E, Riedel HH. [Clinical and endocrinologic studies of the treatment of ovarian insufficiency manifestations following hysterectomy with intact adnexa.] Zentralbl Gynakol 1988;110(10):611-618.
30. Shuster J. Heparin and thrombocytopenia. Black Cohosh root? Chasteberry tree? Seizures! Hosp Pharm 1996;31:1553-1554.
31. Genazzani E, Sorrentino L. Vascular action of acteina: active constituent of *Actaea racemosa* L. Nature 1962;194(4828):544-545.
32. Whiting PW, Clouston A, Kerlin P. Black cohosh and other herbal remedies associated with acute hepatitis. Med J Aust 2002;177(8):440-443.
33. Lontos S, Jones RM, Angus PW, et al. Acute liver failure associated with the use of herbal preparations containing black cohosh. Med J Aust 2003; 179(7):390-391.
34. Thomsen M, Schmidt M. Hepatotoxicity from *Cimicifuga racemosa*? Recent Australian Case Report not sufficiently substantiated. J Altern Complement Med 2003;9(3):337-340.
35. Stolze H. [An alternative to treat menopausal complaints.] Gynecologie 1982;1:14-16.
36. Jarry H, Harnischfeger G, Duker E. [The endocrine effects of constituents of *Cimicifuga racemosa*. 2. *In vitro* binding of constituents to estrogen receptors.] Planta Med 1985;51(4):316-319.
37. Zava DT, Dollbaum CM, Blen M. Estrogen and progestin bioactivity of foods, herbs, and spices. Proc Soc Exp Biol Med 1998;217(3):369-378.
38. Liu J, Burdette JE, Xu H, et al. Evaluation of estrogenic activity of plant extracts for the potential treatment of menopausal symptoms. J Agric Food Chem 2001;49(5):2472-2479.
39. Liu Z, Yang Z, Zhu M, et al. [Estrogenicity of black cohosh (*Cimicifuga racemosa*) and its effect on estrogen receptor level in human breast cancer MCF-7 cells.] Wei Sheng Yan Jiu 2001;30(2):77-80.
40. Zierau O, Bodinet C, Kolba S, et al. Antiestrogenic activities of *Cimicifuga racemosa* extracts. J Steroid Biochem Mol Biol 2002;80(1):125-130.
41. Duker EM, Kopanski L, Jarry H, et al. Effects of extracts from *Cimicifuga racemosa* on gonadotropin release in menopausal women and ovariectomized rats. Planta Med 1991;57(5):420-424.
42. Jarry H, Harnischfeger G. [Endocrine effects of constituents of *Cimicifuga racemosa*. 1. The effect on serum levels of pituitary hormones in ovariectomized rats.] Planta Med 1985;51(1):46-49.
43. Liske E, Wüstenberg P, Boblitz N. Human-pharmacological investigations during treatment of climacteric complaints with *Cimicifuga racemosa* (Remifemin): No estrogen-like effects. ESCOP 2001;1:1.
44. Siess VM, Seybold G. [Studies on the effects of *Pulsatilla pratensis*, *Cimicifuga racemosa* and *Aristolochia clematitis* on the estrus in infantile and castrated white mice.] Arzneimittelforschung 1960;10:514-520.
45. Stoll W. Phytotherapeutikum beeinflusst atrophisches Vaginal epithel. Doppelblindversuch *Cimicifuga* vs. Oestrogenpraeparat [Phytopharmaceutical influences on atrophic vaginal epithelium. Double-blind study on *Cimicifuga* vs. an estrogen preparation]. Therapeuticon 1987;1:23-32.
46. Dixon-Shanies D, Shaikh N. Growth inhibition of human breast cancer cells by herbs and phytoestrogens. Oncol Rep 1999;6(6):1383-1387.
47. Freudenstein J, Bodinet C. Influence of an isopropanolic aqueous extract of *Cimicifuga racemosae* rhizoma on the proliferation of MCF-7 cells. 23rd International LOF-Symposium on Phytoestrogens, University of Ghent, Belgium (January 15, 1999).
48. Anderson IB, Mullen WH, Meeker JE, et al. Pennyroyal toxicity: measurement of toxic metabolite levels in two cases and review of the literature. Ann Intern Med 1996;124(8):726-734.
49. Koeda M, Aoki Y, Sakurai N, et al. Studies on the Chinese crude drug "shoma." IX. Three novel cyclolanostanol xylosides, cimicifugosides H-1, H-2 and H-5, from cimicifuga rhizome. Chem Pharm Bull (Tokyo) 1995; 43(5):771-776.
50. Hemmi H, Kusano G, Ishida N. Selective inhibition of nucleoside transport into mouse lymphoma L-5178Y cells by cimicifugoside. J Pharmacobiodyn 1980;3(12):636-642.
51. Hemmi H, Kitame F, Ishida N, et al. Inhibition of thymidine transport into phytohemagglutinin-stimulated lymphocytes by triterpenoids from *Cimicifuga* species. J Pharm Dyn 1979;2:339-349.
52. Warnecke G. Using phyto-treatment to influence menopause symptoms. Med Welt 1985;36:871-874.
53. Daiber W. Menopause symptoms: success without hormones. Arztl Praxis 1983;35:1946-1947.
54. Vorberg G. Treatment of menopause symptoms. ZFA 1984;60:626-629.
55. Boblitz N, Schrader E, Henneicke-von Zepelin HH, et al. Benefit of a fixed drug combination containing St. John's wort and black cohosh for climacteric patients—results of a randomised clinical trial (poster presentaion from 6th Annual Symposium on Complementary Health Care, Exeter, England, December 2-4, 1999). Focus Alt Comp Ther (FACT) 2000;5(1): 85-86.
56. Mills SY, Jacoby RK, Chacksfield M, et al. Effect of a proprietary herbal medicine on the relief of chronic arthritic pain: a double-blind study. Br J Rheumatol 1996;35(9):874-878.

Black Tea
(Camellia sinensis)

SYNONYMS/COMMON NAMES/RELATED SUBSTANCES

- *Camellia assamica*, camellia tea, camellia, *Camellia sinensis*, catechin, Chinese tea, tea for America, theifers, *Thea sinensis, Thea bohea, Thea viridis*.
- *Note:* Also see the chapter on green tea.

CLINICAL BOTTOM LINE

Background

- Black tea is made from the dried leaves of *Camellia sinensis*, a perennial evergreen shrub. Black tea has a long history of use, dating back to China approximately 5000 years ago. Green tea, black tea, and oolong tea are all derived from the same plant.
- Black tea is a source of caffeine, a methylxanthine which stimulates the central nervous system, relaxes smooth muscle in the airways to the lungs (bronchioles), stimulates the heart, and acts on the kidney as a diuretic (increasing urine flow). One cup of tea contains approximately 50 mg of caffeine, depending on the strength and size of cup (compare with coffee, which contains 65 to 175 mg of caffeine per cup). Tea also contains polyphenols (catechins, anthocyanins, and phenolic acids), tannin, trace elements, and vitamins.
- The tea plant is native to Southeast Asia and can grow to a height of 40 feet but is usually maintained at a height of 2 to 3 feet by regular pruning. The first spring leaf buds, called the *first flush*, are considered the highest-quality leaves. When the first flush leaf bud is picked, another one grows, which is called the *second flush*; this sequence continues until an *autumn flush*. The older leaves picked farther down the stems are considered to be of poorer quality.
- Tea varieties reflect the growing region (e.g., Ceylon or Assam), the district (e.g., Darjeeling), the form (e.g., pekoe is cut, gunpowder is rolled), and the processing method (e.g., black, green, and oolong). India and Sri Lanka are the major producers of black tea.
- Historically, tea has been served as a part of various ceremonies, and people have used tea to stay alert during long meditations. A legend in India describes the story of Prince Siddhartha Gautama, the founder of Buddhism, who tore off his eyelids in frustration at his inability to stay awake during meditation while journeying through China. A tea plant is said to have sprouted from the spot where his eyelids fell, providing him with the ability to stay awake, meditate, and reach enlightenment.
- Turkish traders reportedly introduced tea to Western cultures in the 6th century. By the 18th century, tea was commonly consumed in England, where it became customary to drink tea at 5 o'clock in the afternoon.
- Black tea reached the Americas with the first European settlers in 1492. Black tea gained notoriety in America in 1773 when American colonists, protesting unfair taxation, tossed a shipload of black tea overboard during what is now known as the *Boston Tea Party*.

Uses Based on Scientific Evidence	Grade*
Asthma Research has shown that caffeine causes improvements in airflow to the lungs (bronchodilation). However, it is unclear whether caffeine or tea use has significant clinical benefits in people with asthma. Better research is needed in this area before a conclusion can be drawn.	C
Cancer prevention Several studies have explored a possible association between regular consumption of black tea and rates of cancer in populations. This research has yielded conflicting results, with some studies suggesting benefits, and others reporting no effects. Laboratory studies have shown that components of tea such as polyphenols have antioxidant properties and effects against tumors. However, effects in humans remain unclear, and these components may be more common in green tea than in black tea. Some laboratory research and studies in animals suggest that components of black tea may be carcinogenic, although effects in humans are unclear. Overall, the relationship of black tea consumption and cancer in humans remains undetermined.	C
Dental cavity prevention There are limited studies of black tea as a mouthwash for the prevention of dental cavities (caries). It is not clear if this is a beneficial therapy.	C

	Grade*
Heart attack prevention/cardiovascular risk There is conflicting evidence from a small number of studies examining the relationship of tea intake and the risk of heart attack. Tea may reduce the risk of platelet aggregation or endothelial dysfunction and is proposed to be beneficial against blockage of arteries in the heart. The long-term effects of tea consumption on cardiovascular risk factors such as cholesterol levels, blood pressure, and atherosclerosis are unknown. One study reports that drinking black tea regularly does not alter plasma homocysteine concentrations.	C
Memory enhancement Several preliminary studies have examined the effects of caffeine, tea, or coffee use on short- and long-term memory. It remains unclear whether tea is beneficial for this use.	C
Mental performance/alertness Limited, poor-quality research studies have reported that the use of black tea may improve cognition and sense of alertness (black tea contains caffeine, which is a stimulant).	C
Methicillin-resistant *Staphylococcus aureus* (MRSA) infection In one small study, inhaled tea catechin was reported to be temporarily effective in the reduction of MRSA infection and shortening of hospital stay in elderly	C

Continued

patients with MRSA-infected sputum. Additional research is needed to further explore these results.	
Osteoporosis prevention Preliminary research suggests that regular use of black tea may improve bone mineral density in older women. Better research is needed in this area before a conclusion can be drawn.	C

*Key to grades: *A:* Strong scientific evidence for this use; *B:* Good scientific evidence for this use; *C:* Unclear scientific evidence for this use; *D:* Fair scientific evidence against this use (it may not work); *F:* Strong scientific evidence against this use (it likely does not work). For a more detailed explanation of efficacy criteria, see "Natural Standard Evidence-Based Validated Grading Rationale" in the Introduction.

Historical or Theoretical Indications That Lack Sufficient Evidence

Acute pharyngitis, antioxidant, anxiety, cancer multidrug resistance, circulatory/blood flow disorders, "cleansing" colorectal cancer, Crohn's disease, diabetes, diarrhea, diuretic (increasing urine flow), energy metabolism, gum disease, headache, hyperactivity (in children), immune enhancement/improving resistance to disease, influenza, joint pain, kidney stone prevention, melanoma, obesity, osteoarthritis, pain, prostate cancer, stomach disorders, toxin/alcohol elimination from the body, trigeminal neuralgia, vomiting, weight loss.

DOSING/TOXICOLOGY

The following doses are based on scientific research, publications, traditional use, or expert opinion. Many herbs and supplements have not been thoroughly tested, and their safety and effectiveness may not be proven. Brands may be made differently, with variable ingredients even within the same brand. The doses shown may not apply to all products. It is important to always read product labels and discuss doses with a qualified healthcare provider before therapy is started.

Adults (18 Years and Older)

- Black tea has not been proven as an effective therapy for any condition, and benefits of specific doses are not established. Studies of the use of tea for heart disease prevention evaluated 250 to 900 ml of tea consumed daily for up to 4 weeks. In research studies of the effect of tea on cognitive performance, an example dose is 400 ml of black tea taken three times daily. In studies of the effect of tea on dental cavity prevention, 20 ml of black tea gargled for 60 seconds daily has been used.
- One cup of tea contains approximately 50 mg of caffeine, depending on tea strength and cup size.

SAFETY

The U.S. Food and Drug Administration does not strictly regulate herbs and supplements. There is no guarantee of the strength, purity, or safety of products, and effects may vary. It is important to always read product labels. People who have a medical condition, or are taking other drugs, herbs, or supplements, should consult a qualified healthcare provider before starting a new therapy. A healthcare provider should be contacted immediately if there are any side effects.

Allergies

- People with known allergy/hypersensitivity to caffeine or tannin should avoid black tea. Skin rash and hives have been reported following caffeine ingestion.

Side Effects and Warnings

- Studies of the side effects of black tea specifically are limited. However, black tea contains caffeine, from which multiple reactions have been reported.
- Caffeine is a stimulant of the central nervous system and may cause insomnia in adults, children, and infants (including nursing infants of mothers who take caffeine). Caffeine acts on the kidneys as a diuretic (increasing urine flow and urine sodium/potassium levels and potentially decreasing blood sodium/potassium levels) and may worsen urge incontinence. Caffeine-containing beverages may increase the production of stomach acid, and may worsen ulcer symptoms. Tannin in tea can cause constipation. Caffeine in doses of 250 to 350 mg can increase heart rate and blood pressure, although people who consume caffeine regularly do not seem to experience these effects over the long term.
- An increase in blood sugar levels may occur after drinking black tea containing the equivalent of 200 mg of caffeine (4 to 5 cups, depending on tea strength and cup size). Caffeine-containing beverages such as black tea should be used cautiously in persons with diabetes. People with severe liver disease should use caffeine cautiously, as levels of caffeine in the blood may accumulate and be long-lasting. Skin rashes have been associated with caffeine ingestion. In laboratory research studies and studies in animals, caffeine has been found to affect blood clotting, but effects in humans are unknown.
- **Caffeine toxicity/high doses:** When 500 mg of caffeine are consumed (usually more than 8 to 10 cups per day, depending on tea strength and cup size), symptoms of anxiety, delirium, agitation, psychosis, and detrusor instability (unstable bladder) may occur. Conception may be delayed in women who consume large amounts of caffeine. Seizures, muscle spasms, life-threatening muscle breakdown (rhabdomyolysis), and life-threatening abnormal heart rhythms have been reported with caffeine overdose. Doses greater than 1000 mg may be fatal.
- **Caffeine withdrawal:** Chronic use can result in tolerance and psychological dependence. Abrupt discontinuation may result in withdrawal symptoms such as headache, irritation, nervousness, anxiety, tremors, and dizziness. In people with psychiatric disorders such as affective disorder and schizoaffective disorder, caffeine withdrawal may worsen symptoms or cause confusion, disorientation, excitement, restlessness, violent behavior, or mania.
- **Chronic effects:** Several population studies initially suggested a possible association between caffeine use and fibrocystic breast disease, but more recent research has not confirmed this connection. Limited research studies have reported a possible relationship between caffeine use and multiple sclerosis, although evidence is not definitive in this area. Studies in animals reported that tannin fractions from tea plants may increase the risk of cancer, although it is not clear that the tannin present in black tea has significant carcinogenic effects in humans.
- Drinking tannin-containing beverages such as tea may contribute to iron deficiency, and, in infants, tea has been associated with impaired iron metabolism and microcytic anemia.

Pregnancy and Breastfeeding

- Large amounts of black tea should be used cautiously in pregnant women, as caffeine crosses the placenta and has been associated with spontaneous abortion, intrauterine growth retardation, and low birth weight. Heavy caffeine intake (400 mg per day or greater) during pregnancy may increase the risk of later developing SIDS (sudden infant death syndrome). Very high doses of caffeine (greater than or equal to 1100 mg daily) have been associated with birth defects, including limb and palate malformations.

- Caffeine is readily transferred in breast milk. Caffeine ingestion by infants can lead to sleep disturbances/insomnia. Infants nursing from mothers consuming greater than 500 mg of caffeine daily have been reported to experience tremors and heart rhythm abnormalities. Components present in breast milk may reduce an infant's ability to metabolize caffeine, resulting in higher than expected blood levels. Tea consumption by mothers of breastfeeding infants has been associated with anemia, reductions in iron metabolism, and irritability in these infants.

INTERACTIONS

Most herbs and supplements have not been thoroughly tested for interactions with other herbs, supplements, drugs, or foods. The interactions listed here are based on reports in scientific publications, laboratory experiments, or traditional use. It is important to always read product labels. People who have a medical condition, or are taking other drugs, herbs, or supplements, should consult a qualified healthcare provider before starting a new therapy.

Interactions with Drugs

Studies of the interactions of black tea with drugs are limited. However, black tea is an important source of caffeine, from which multiple interactions have been documented.

- The combination of caffeine with ephedrine, an ephedra alkaloid, has been implicated in numerous severe and life-threatening cardiovascular events such as abnormally high blood pressure, stroke, and heart attack. This combination is commonly used in over-the-counter weight loss products and may also be associated with other adverse effects, including abnormal heart rhythms, insomnia, anxiety, headache, irritability, poor concentration, blurred vision, and dizziness. Stroke has been reported after the nasal ingestion of caffeine with amphetamine.
- Caffeine may add to the effects of other stimulants, including nicotine, beta-adrenergic agonists such as albuterol (Ventolin), and other methylxanthines such as theophylline. Caffeine can counteract drowsy effects and mental slowness caused by benzodiazepines such as lorazepam (Ativan) and diazepam (Valium). Phenylpropanolamine and caffeine should not be used together because of reports of numerous, potentially serious adverse effects; oral phenylpropanolamine formulations have been removed from the United States market because of reports of bleeding into the head.
- When taken with caffeine, a number of drugs may increase caffeine blood levels or the length of time that caffeine acts on the body. Examples are disulfiram (Antabuse), oral contraceptives, hormone replacement therapy, ciprofloxacin (Cipro), norfloxacin, fluvoxamine (Luvox), cimetidine (Tagamet), verapamil, and mexiletine. Caffeine levels may be lowered by taking dexamethasone (Decadron). The metabolism of caffeine by the liver (cytochrome P-450 isoenzyme 1A2) may be affected by multiple drugs, although the effects in humans are not clear.
- Caffeine may lengthen the effects of carbamazepine (Tegretol) and increase the effects of clozapine (Clozaril) and dipyridamole (Persantine, Aggrenox). Caffeine may affect serum lithium levels, and abrupt discontinuation of caffeine use by regular caffeine users taking lithium may result in high levels of lithium or lithium toxicity. Levels of aspirin or phenobarbital may be lowered in the blood, although clinical effects in humans are not clear.
- Although caffeine by itself does not appear to have pain-relieving properties, it is used in combination with ergotamine tartrate in the treatment of migraine or cluster headaches (e.g., Cafergot). It has been shown to increase the headache-relieving effects of other pain relievers such as acetaminophen and aspirin (e.g., Excedrin). Caffeine may also increase the pain-relieving effects of codeine and ibuprofen (Advil, Motrin).
- As a diuretic, caffeine increases urine and sodium losses through the kidneys and may add to the effects of other diuretics such as furosemide (Lasix).

Interactions with Herbs and Dietary Supplements

- Studies of black tea interactions with herbs and supplements are limited. However, black tea is a source of caffeine, from which multiple interactions have been documented.
- Caffeine may add to the effects and side effects of other stimulants. The combination of caffeine with ephedrine, which is present in ephedra (ma huang), has been implicated in numerous severe or life-threatening cardiovascular events such as abnormally high blood pressure, stroke, and heart attack. This combination is commonly used in over-the-counter weight loss products, and may also be associated with other adverse effects, including abnormal heart rhythms, insomnia, anxiety, headache, irritability, poor concentration, blurred vision, and dizziness.
- Cola nut, guarana (*Paullina cupana*), and yerba mate (*Ilex paraguariensis*) are also sources of caffeine, and may add to the effects and side effects of caffeine in black tea. A combination product containing caffeine, yerba mate, and damania (*Turnera difussa*) has been reported to cause weight loss, slowing of gastrointestinal tract motility, and a feeling of stomach fullness.
- As a diuretic, caffeine increases urine and sodium losses through the kidneys, and may add to the effects of other diuretic agents such as artichoke, celery, corn silk, couchgrass, dandelion, elder flower, horsetail, juniper berry, kava, shepherd's purse, uva ursi, and yarrow.

Selected References

Natural Standard developed the preceding evidence-based information based on a systematic review of more than 575 articles. For comprehensive information about alternative and complementary therapies on the professional level, go to www.naturalstandard.com. Selected references are listed here.

Arab L, Il'yasova D. The epidemiology of tea consumption and colorectal cancer incidence. J Nutr 2003;133(10):3310S-3318S.
Arts IC, Hollman PC, Feskens EJ, et al. Catechin intake might explain the inverse relation between tea consumption and ischemic heart disease: the Zutphen Elderly Study. Am J Clin Nutr 2001;74(2):227-232.
Birkett NJ, Logan AG. Caffeine-containing beverages and the prevalence of hypertension. J Hypertens Suppl 1988;6(4):S620-S622.
Blot WJ, Chow WH, McLaughlin JK. Tea and cancer: a review of the epidemiological evidence. Eur J Cancer Prev 1996;5(6):425-438.
Blot WJ, McLaughlin JK, Chow WH. Cancer rates among drinkers of black tea. Crit Rev Food Sci Nutr 1997;37(8):739-760.
Brinckmann J, Sigwart H, van Houten Taylor L. Safety and efficacy of a traditional herbal medicine (Throat Coat) in symptomatic temporary relief of pain in patients with acute pharyngitis: a multicenter, prospective, randomized, double-blinded, placebo-controlled study. J Altern Complement Med 2003;9(2):285-298.
Brown CA, Bolton-Smith C, Woodward M, et al. Coffee and tea consumption and the prevalence of coronary heart disease in men and women: results from the Scottish Heart Health Study. J Epidemiol Community Health 1993; 47(3):171-175.
Brown SL, Salive ME, Pahor M, et al. Occult caffeine as a source of sleep problems in an older population. J Am Geriatr Soc 1995;43(8):860-864.

Cerhan JR, Putnam SD, Bianchi GD, et al. Tea consumption and risk of cancer of the colon and rectum. Nutr Cancer 2001;41(1-2):33-40.

Chow WH, Blot WJ, McLaughlin JK. Tea drinking and cancer risk: epidemiologic evidence. Proc Soc Exp Biol Med 1999;220(4):197.

Chow WH, Swanson CA, Lissowska J, et al. Risk of stomach cancer in relation to consumption of cigarettes, alcohol, tea and coffee in Warsaw, Poland. Int J Cancer 1999;81(6):871-876.

Clausson B, Granath F, Ekbom A, et al. Effect of caffeine exposure during pregnancy on birth weight and gestational age. Am J Epidemiol 2002;155(5):429-436.

Cnattingius S, Signorello LB, Anneren G, et al. Caffeine intake and the risk of first-trimester spontaneous abortion. N Engl J Med 2000;343(25):1839-1845.

Davies MJ, Judd JT, Baer DJ, et al. Black tea consumption reduces total and LDL cholesterol in mildly hypercholesterolemic adults. J Nutr 2003;133(10):3298S-3302S.

Dlugosz L, Belanger K, Hellenbrand K, et al. Maternal caffeine consumption and spontaneous abortion: a prospective cohort study. Epidemiology 1996;7(3):250-255.

Dora I, Arab L, Martinchik A, et al. Black tea consumption and risk of rectal cancer in Moscow population. Ann Epidemiol 2003;13(6):405-411.

Duffy SJ, Keaney JF, Jr., Holbrook M, et al. Short- and long-term black tea consumption reverses endothelial dysfunction in patients with coronary artery disease. Circulation 2001;104(2):151-156.

Esimone CO, Adikwu MU, Nwafor SV, et al. Potential use of tea extract as a complementary mouthwash: comparative evaluation of two commercial samples. J Altern Complement Med 2001;7(5):523-527.

Fernandes O, Sabharwal M, Smiley T, et al. Moderate to heavy caffeine consumption during pregnancy and relationship to spontaneous abortion and abnormal fetal growth: a meta-analysis. Reprod Toxicol 1998;12(4):435-444.

Ford RP, Schluter PJ, Mitchell EA, et al. Heavy caffeine intake in pregnancy and sudden infant death syndrome. New Zealand Cot Death Study Group. Arch Dis Child 1998;78(1):9-13.

Geleijnse JM, Launer LJ, Van der Kuip DA, et al. Inverse association of tea and flavonoid intakes with incident myocardial infarction: the Rotterdam Study. Am J Clin Nutr 2002;75(5):880-886.

Goldbohm RA, Hertog MG, Brants HA, et al. Consumption of black tea and cancer risk: a prospective cohort study. J Natl Cancer Inst 1996;88(2):93-100.

Grosso LM, Rosenberg KD, Belanger K, et al. Maternal caffeine intake and intrauterine growth retardation. Epidemiology 2001;12(4):447-455.

Hadeed A, Siegel S. Newborn cardiac arrhythmias associated with maternal caffeine use during pregnancy. Clin Pediatr (Phila) 1993;32(1):45-47.

Hakim IA, Harris RB, Brown S, et al. Effect of increased tea consumption on oxidative DNA damage among smokers: a randomized controlled study. J Nutr 2003;133(10):3303S-3309S.

Hodgson JM, Burke V, Beilin LJ, et al. Can black tea influence plasma total homocysteine concentrations? Am J Clin Nutr 2003;77(4):907-911.

Hodgson JM, Devine A, Puddey IB, et al. Tea intake is inversely related to blood pressure in older women. J Nutr 2003;133(9):2883-2886.

Jatoi A, Ellison N, Burch PA, et al. A phase II trial of green tea in the treatment of patients with androgen independent metastatic prostate carcinoma. Cancer 2003;97(6):1442-1446.

Lambert JD, Yang CS. Mechanisms of cancer prevention by tea constituents. J Nutr 2003;133(10):3262S-3267S.

Lambert JD, Yang CS. Cancer chemopreventive activity and bioavailability of tea and tea polyphenols. Mutat Res 2003;523-524:201-208.

Mameleers PA, Van Boxtel MP, Hogervorst E. Habitual caffeine consumption and its relation to memory, attention, planning capacity and psychomotor performance across multiple age groups. Hum Psychopharmacol 2000;15(8):573-581.

Mei Y, Wei D, Liu J. Reversal of cancer multidrug resistance by tea polyphenol in KB cells. J Chemother 2003;15(3):260-265.

Hegarty VM, May HM, Khaw KT. Tea drinking and bone mineral density in older women. Am J Clin Nutr 2000;71(4):1003-1007.

Heilbrun LK, Nomura A, Stemmermann GN. Black tea consumption and cancer risk: a prospective study. Br J Cancer 1986;54(4):677-683.

Hindmarch I, Quinlan PT, Moore KL, et al. The effects of black tea and other beverages on aspects of cognition and psychomotor performance. Psychopharmacology (Berl) 1998;139(3):230-238.

Hodgson JM, Puddey IB, Burke V, et al. Effects on blood pressure of drinking green and black tea. J Hypertens 1999;17(4):457-463.

Infante-Rivard C, Fernandez A, Gauthier R, et al. Fetal loss associated with caffeine intake before and during pregnancy. JAMA 1993;270(24):2940-2943.

James JE. Chronic effects of habitual caffeine consumption on laboratory and ambulatory blood pressure levels. J Cardiovasc Risk 1994;1(2):159-164.

Kinlen LJ, McPherson K. Pancreas cancer and coffee and tea consumption: a case-control study. Br J Cancer 1984;49(1):93-96.

Kinlen LJ, Willows AN, Goldblatt P, et al. Tea consumption and cancer. Br J Cancer 1988;58(3):397-401.

Klatsky AL, Armstrong MA, Friedman GD. Coffee, tea, and mortality. Ann Epidemiol 1993;3(4):375-381.

Kohlmeier L, Weterings KG, Steck S, et al. Tea and cancer prevention: an evaluation of the epidemiologic literature. Nutr Cancer 1997;27(1):1-13.

Lawson DH, Jick H, Rothman KJ. Coffee and tea consumption and breast disease. Surgery 1981;90(5):801-803.

Nakagawa K, Ninomiya M, Okubo T, et al. Tea catechin supplementation increases antioxidant capacity and prevents phospholipid hydroperoxidation in plasma of humans. J Agric Food Chem 1999;47(10):3967-3973.

Ohno Y, Wakai K, Genka K, et al. Tea consumption and lung cancer risk: a case-control study in Okinawa, Japan. Jpn J Cancer Res 1995;86(11):1027-1034.

Rechner AR, Wagner E, Van Buren L, et al. Black tea represents a major source of dietary phenolics among regular tea drinkers. Free Radic Res 2002;36(10):1127-1135.

Santos IS, Victora CG, Huttly S, et al. Caffeine intake and pregnancy outcomes: a meta-analytic review. Cad Saude Publica 1998;14(3):523-530.

Sesso HD, Gaziano JM, Buring JE, et al. Coffee and tea intake and the risk of myocardial infarction. Am J Epidemiol 1999;149(2):162-167.

Shirlow MJ, Mathers CD. A study of caffeine consumption and symptoms; indigestion, palpitations, tremor, headache and insomnia. Int J Epidemiol 1985;14(2):239-248.

Stavchansky S, Combs A, Sagraves R, et al. Pharmacokinetics of caffeine in breast milk and plasma after single oral administration of caffeine to lactating mothers. Biopharm Drug Dispos 1988;9(4):285-299.

Stoner GD, Mukhtar H. Polyphenols as cancer chemopreventive agents. J Cell Biochem Suppl 1995;22:169-180.

Wrenn KD, Oschner I. Rhabdomyolysis induced by a caffeine overdose. Ann Emerg Med 1989;18(1):94-97.

Yamada H, Ohashi K, Atsumi T, et al. Effects of tea catechin inhalation on methicillin-resistant *Staphylococcus aureus* in elderly patients in a hospital ward. Hosp Infect 2003;53(3):229-231.

Yang CS, Wang ZY. Tea and cancer. J Natl Cancer Inst 1993;85(13):1038-1049.

Bladderwrack/Seaweed/Kelp
(*Fucus vesiculosus*)

SYNONYMS/COMMON NAMES/RELATED SUBSTANCES

- Black-tang, bladder, bladder fucus, blasen-tang, common seawrack, cut weed, Dyers fucus, Fucus, hai-ts'ao, kelp, kelpware, knotted wrack, meereiche, *Quercus marina*, popping wrack, red fucus, rockrack, rockweed, schweintang, sea kelp, sea oak, seetang, seaware, seaweed, sea wrack, swine tang, tang, Varech vesiculeux, vraic, wrack.

CLINICAL BOTTOM LINE
Background

- *Fucus vesiculosus* is a brown seaweed of the family Fucaceae that grows on the northern coasts of the Atlantic and Pacific oceans and the North and Baltic seas. Its name is sometimes used to refer to *Ascophyllum nodosum,* another brown seaweed that grows alongside *F. vesiculosus.* These species are often components of kelp preparations along with other types of seaweed.
- *F. vesiculosus*, also commonly referred to as bladderwrack, has traditionally been used to treat disorders of the thyroid gland and as a component of weight loss formulas. It has also been shown in pre-clinical studies to possess anticoagulant and hypoglycemic properties. However, review of the literature reveals no clinical trial evidence in support of (or against) the efficacy of bladderwrack for any use in humans.
- The active ingredients of bladderwrack have not been fully identified, and little research exists on its components. Therefore, most pharmacologic activities attributed to *F. vesiculosus* are generally recognized for brown seaweed species and are not specific to *F. vesiculosus.*

Scientific Evidence for Common/Studied Uses	Grade*
Anorectic (weight loss)	C
Antibacterial	C
Anticoagulant	C
Antifungal	C
Antioxidant	C
Cancer	C
Goiter, thyroid disease	C
Hyperglycemia (diabetes)	C

*Key to grades: *A:* Strong scientific evidence for this use; *B:* Good scientific evidence for this use; *C:* Unclear scientific evidence for this use; *D:* Fair scientific evidence against this use (it may not work); *F:* Strong scientific evidence against this use (it likely does not work). For a more detailed explanation of efficacy criteria, see "Natural Standard Evidence-Based Validated Grading Rationale" in the Introduction.

Historical or Theoretical Indications That Lack Sufficient Evidence

- Anti-parasitic, arthritis, atherosclerosis, benign prostatic hypertrophy (BPH), bladder inflammatory disease, bulk laxative, desquamative nephritis, dyspepsia, eczema, edema, enlarged glands, exophthalmos, fatigue, fatty heart, goiter, hair loss, heartburn, hyperlipemia, laxative, lymphadenoid goiter, malnutrition, menstrual irregularities (menorrhagia), myxedema, obesity, orchitis (swollen or painful testes), psoriasis, radiation protection, rheumatism, sore throat, stool softener, ulcer, urinary tract tonic.

Expert Opinion and Folkloric Precedent

- Seaweed has been used medicinally in China for over 5000 years. Bladderwrack was used in the 18th century as a major dietary source of iodine and has been used traditionally to treat goiter.
- In the 1860s, it was discovered that some seaweeds serve as hypermetabolic thyroid stimulants. They have since been included as a component of numerous weight loss formulas.

Safety Summary

- **Possibly unsafe:** Bladderwrack contains varying amounts of iodine (up to 600 μg per gram, and regular use may elicit hyperthyroidism, hypothyroidism, goiter, or myxedema, although many individuals remain euthyroid (normal human iodine intake is 100 to 200 μg/day).[1-4] Bladderwrack also concentrates heavy metals found in the ocean, including arsenic, cadmium and lead, and ingestion carries with it the risk of heavy metal poisoning. Bladderwrack may act additively with CNS stimulants, anticoagulants, laxatives, hypoglycemic agents, nephrotoxic agents, amiodarone (source of iodine), and lithium carbonate (potential induction of hypothyroidism with concomitant use). At high doses of iodine, a brassy taste, increased salivation, gastric irritation, and acneiform skin lesions may occur.
- **Likely unsafe:** Bladderwrack is likely unsafe when taken by children or pregnant/lactating women, because of high iodine content and potential disruption of thyroid function. Prolonged therapy may be inadvisable for these reasons and also because of possible contamination with toxic heavy metals. Bladderwrack should be avoided in patients with heart failure or renal insufficiency because of its potentially high sodium content, and in hyperthyroid patients because of its iodine content.

DOSING/TOXICOLOGY
General

- No data are available from high-quality human trials that demonstrate safety or efficacy for any specific dose of bladderwrack. The following doses are based on those most commonly suggested by historical practice, expert opinion, and/or anecdote. Because of the potential contamination of bladderwrack with heavy metals, its consumption should always been considered potentially unsafe.

Standardization

- Some bladderwrack products are beginning to list iodine content, although there is no widely accepted standard at this time.

Dosing: Adult (18 Years and Older)
Oral

- **Tablets/capsules:** Soft capsules (alcohol extract) in a dosage of 200 to 600 mg daily has been recommended; or tablets taken initially 3 times/day and gradually increased to 24 tablets/day.
- **Liquid/fluid:** 16 g of bruised plant mixed with one pint of water, administered in 2 fluid ounce doses three times/day; or alcoholic liquid extract in a dose of 4 to 8 mL before meals.

Topical

- **Patch:** Bladderwrack and seaweed patches are sold commercially as weight loss products, although there are no commonly accepted or tested doses.

Dosing: Pediatric (Younger Than 18 Years)

- Administration of bladderwrack to children is not recommended because of potential toxicity.

Toxicology

- Most toxicities associated with bladderwrack are likely due to high concentrations of iodine or heavy metals. A case report of nephrotoxicity in an 18-year-old girl taking *F. vesiculosus* as part of a weight loss formulation was attributed to the high arsenic content of the seaweed.[5] The high iodine content of kelp tablets was found to be the most likely cause of two case reports of acneiform eruption of the skin.[6] A 74-year-old woman who had been taking kelp supplements for several months presented to a hospital with peripheral neuropathy of unknown etiology. She was found to have an elevated 24-hour urinary excretion of arsenic.[7] Ninety days after discontinuation of the kelp supplement, her urine arsenic level returned to normal.

ADVERSE EFFECTS/PRECAUTIONS/CONTRAINDICATIONS
Allergy

- Known allergy/hypersensitivity to *Fucus vesiculosus* or any of its components, or known iodine sensitivity.

Adverse Effects

- **General:** Most adverse effects appear related to high iodine content or heavy metal contamination of bladderwrack preparations rather than to the seaweed itself.
- **Dermatologic:** High doses of iodine are known to potentially cause acneiform lesions. Two case reports have documented exacerbation of severe acne in a 24-year-old and a 29-year-old female following the commencement of a health-food diet including kelp tablets.[6]
- **Neurologic/CNS:** There is a case report of arsenic-induced peripheral neuropathy in a 74-year-old woman taking kelp tablets.[7]
- **Renal:** There is a case report of nephrotoxicity in an 18-year-old female taking 400-mg *Fucus vesiculosus* tablets orally three times/day for weight loss. The toxicity appears to have been caused by high levels of arsenic found within the *F. vesiculosis* preparation.
- **Endocrine:** Based on the known sequelae of iodine toxicity, the high iodine content in bladderwrack may lead to hyperthyroidism, hypothyroidism, goiter, or myedema.[1-4] There are human case reports of hyperthyroidism from ingestion

of kelp products: A report of transient hyperthyroidism in a 27-year-old female taking the dietary supplement Energy-V and a multivitamin, both containing kelp, for approximately 1 month has been documented.[2] Thyroid function returned to normal upon discontinuation of the kelp-containing products. A second case report details the induction of hyperthyroidism, as confirmed clinically and with laboratory tests, in a 72-year-old female with no preexisting thyroid condition after ingestion of Vitalia (sea-kelp tablets).[4] All signs and symptoms of hyperthyroidism dissipated 6 months after discontinuing the sea-kelp tablets, and her condition was determined to be iodine-induced. Extracts of *Fucus vesiculosus* have been found to cause significant hypoglycemia in laboratory animals and may have additive effects with hypoglycemic agents in humans.[8] Bladderwrack may contain vitamins and minerals, calcium, magnesium, potassium, and sodium, thereby increasing serum levels.
- **Hematologic:** A 54-year-old woman taking a vitamin and kelp tablets presented to her physician with abnormal bleeding and petechiae.[9] She was diagnosed with autoimmune thrombocytopenic purpura with dyserythropoiesis, attributed to "contaminants" in the kelp preparation. Three months after withdrawal of the kelp supplement and treatment with immunoglobulin, prednisolone and azathioprine, her dyserythropoiesis was reversed. Bladderwrack exhibits *in vitro* anticoagulant properties.[10,11]
- **Gastrointestinal:** Laxative properties have traditionally been attributed to chronic use of bladderwrack and other brown seaweeds, and mechanistically may be due to the component alginic acid, a hydrophilic colloidal polysaccharide present in many laxative agents. Iodine toxicity, which may occur with chronic bladderwrack use, may cause a brassy taste, increased salivation, and/or gastric irritation.

Precautions/Warnings/Contraindications

- Avoid in patients with hyperthyroidism, hypothyroidism, or autoimmune thyroid disease, based on potentially high levels of iodine in seaweed preparations.
- Avoid in patients taking thyroid hormone supplements, lithium carbonate, or amiodarone, due to potentially high iodine levels in bladderwrack.
- Use cautiously in patients with known iron deficiency due to theoretical reduction of iron absorption after prolonged use.
- Use cautiously in patients with heart failure, renal insufficiency, or taking diuretics, due to potentially high sodium content of bladderwrack.
- Use cautiously in diabetic patients, based on reports of hypoglycemia in animal studies.
- Use cautiously in patients taking aspirin or anticoagulants, based on *in vitro* evidence of anticoagulant properties and on a case report of autoimmune thrombocytopenic purpura (likely due to contaminants in a product).
- Use cautiously in patients with diarrhea, due to possible laxative effects of bladderwrack.

Pregnancy and Lactation

- Bladderwrack is often not recommended during pregnancy and lactation, because of potentially high iodine concentrations and frequent contamination with heavy metals.[12]

INTERACTIONS
Bladderwrack/Drug Interactions

- **Amiodarone:** In theory, concomitant use of bladderwrack and amiodarone may alter thyroid function because of high iodine levels in both agents.

- **CNS stimulant drugs (amphetamines, methylphenidate):** Stimulants may act synergistically with bladderwrack, due to its purported hypermetabolic thyroid stimulant properties.
- **Anticoagulants, aspirin, NSAIDs, antiplatelet agents:** Bladderwrack may increase the risk of bleeding if taken concomitantly with anticoagulants, because of its *in vitro* exhibition of anticoagulant properties.[10,11]
- **Diuretics:** In theory, bladderwrack may decrease the effectiveness of diuretics, because of its high sodium content. Bladderwrack may contain vitamins and minerals, calcium, magnesium, potassium, and sodium, thereby increasing serum levels.
- **Insulin, oral hypoglycemics:** Extracts of *Fucus vesiculosus* have been found to cause significant hypoglycemia in laboratory animals and may have additive effects with hypoglycemic agents in humans.[8]
- **Laxatives:** Laxative properties have traditionally been attributed to chronic use of bladderwrack and other brown seaweeds. Mechanistically, this may be due to the component alginic acid, a hydrophilic colloidal polysaccharide present in some laxative agents as well as in bladderwrack.
- **Lithium carbonate:** Concomitant use of iodine-containing agents, such as bladderwrack and kelp, may alter thyroid function when used with lithium.
- **Nephrotoxic drugs:** The presence of heavy metal contaminants in bladderwrack preparations, including arsenic, cadmium, chromium, and lead, may potentiate renal damage if taken with known nephrotoxic agents.
- **Thyroxine (T_4), liothyroxine (T_3), propylthiouracil (PTU), methimazole:** In theory, the high iodine content of bladderwrack may interfere with the function of drugs that act on the thyroid. There are case reports of transient hyperthyroidism associated with kelp products taken alone.
- **Calcium, magnesium, potassium, sodium:** Bladderwrack preparations contain variable levels of calcium, magnesium, potassium, sodium, vitamins, and minerals and may therefore increase serum levels.

Bladderwrack/Herb/Supplement Interactions

- **CNS stimulant herbs (ma huang, ephedra):** A theoretical interaction exists if stimulants and bladderwrack are ingested simultaneously, based on possible potentiation of hypermetabolic effects.
- **Hypoglycemic agents:** Extracts of *Fucus vesiculosus* have been found to cause significant hypoglycemia in laboratory animals and may have additive effects with hypoglycemic agents in humans.[8]
- **Diuretic agents:** In theory, bladderwrack may decrease the effectiveness of diuretics due to its high sodium content. Bladderwrack may also contain potassium, increasing serum potassium levels.
- **Anticoagulants, antiplatelet agents:** Bladderwrack may increase the risk of bleeding if taken concomitantly with anticoagulants because of its *in vitro* exhibition of anticoagulant properties.
- **Agents with thyroid activity:** In theory, the high iodine content of bladderwrack may interfere with the function of agents that act on the thyroid. There are case reports of transient hyperthyroidism associated with kelp products taken alone.
- **Nephrotoxic agents:** The presence of heavy metals in bladderwrack preparations, including arsenic, cadmium, chromium, and lead, may potentiate renal damage if taken with known nephrotoxic agents.[5,10,11]

- **Iron:** In theory, bladderwrack may decrease iron absorption, especially if ingested for a prolonged period of time.
- **Calcium, magnesium, potassium, sodium:** Bladderwrack preparations contain variable levels of calcium, magnesium, potassium, sodium, vitamins, and minerals and may therefore increase serum levels.

Bladderwrack/Food Interactions

- Insufficient data available.

Bladderwrack/Lab Interactions

- **Activated partial thromboplastin time (aPTT):** Bladderwrack may increase aPTT test results because of the heparin-like activity of its fucoidan component.[10,11]
- **Thyroid-stimulating hormone (TSH):** In theory, bladderwrack may increase serum TSH levels because of its iodine-induced alteration of thyroid function.
- **Thyroxine (T_4) levels:** In theory, bladderwrack may increase serum T_4 levels because of its iodine-induced alteration of thyroid function.
- **Radioactive iodine uptake:** In theory, bladderwrack may interfere with radioactive iodine uptake and thyroid function tests because of its iodine-induced alteration of thyroid function.
- **Electrolytes:** Bladderwrack preparations contain variable levels of calcium, magnesium, potassium, sodium, vitamins, and minerals and may therefore increase serum levels.

MECHANISM OF ACTION
Pharmacology

- **Anticoagulant:** Fucoidan, a high-molecular-weight sulfated polysaccharide isolated from *Fucus vesiculosus,* has been found *in vitro* to enhance the heparin-cofactor II-thrombin reaction through the formation of a ternary complex with both heparin-cofactor II and thrombin.[10,11,13] An additional *ex vivo* analysis using human plasma has demonstrated the ability of fucoidan to prolong the activated partial thromboplastin time.[10] Fucoidans isolated from *F. vesiculosus* have stronger anticoagulant properties than fucans isolated from other brown algae species, including *Sargassum muticum* and *Laminaria digitata*, because of higher contents of fucose and sulfate.[14]
- **Antifungal:** A lectin-like mucopolysaccharide isolated from *Fucus vesiculosus* has been found to be specific for complex carbohydrates. This mucopolysaccharide causes agglutination of the yeast *Candida guilliermondii,* and inhibits the growth of *C. guilliermondii* by 99.2%.[15] *In vivo* studies are lacking.
- **Antioxidant:** *In vitro* analysis has demonstrated that *F. vesiculosus* inhibits oxidation of methyl linoleate with a shortened induction period similar to results seen with Vitamin E, but without the oxygen uptake suppression at t_0.[15]
- **Antibacterial:** A lectin-like mucopolysaccharide found *in vitro* to have activity against *Candida guilliermondii* also inhibits growth of multiple *Neisseria meningitidis* and *Escherichia coli* strains.[16]
- **Laxative:** Laxative properties of bladderwrack and other brown seaweeds (Phaeophyceae) have been attributed to the component alginic acid, a hydrophilic colloidal polysaccharide.
- **Thyroid activity:** Kelp and bladderwrack products are frequently high in iodine content and have been used traditionally for thyroid diseases. In humans, there are case reports of transient hyperthyroidism as a result of bladderwrack ingestion.[2,4] Bladderwrack products contain up to 600 µg per gram of iodine, whereas normal human iodine intake is

on the order of 100 to 200 µg/day. Individuals ingesting bladderwrack or kelp products as food or supplements may ingest up to 30 times this amount. Chronic iodine toxicity may result in hypothyroidism, hyperthyroidism, goiter, or myxedema, although many individuals remain euthyroid. Systematic study of the effects of bladderwrack in humans is lacking, and there may be other active constituents. In terms of iodine content, there is no widely accepted standardization of iodine content in bladderwrack, although some products may list iodine content on the label.

Pharmacodynamics/Kinetics

- Insufficient data available.

HISTORY

- Kelp has traditionally been used to preserve shellfish in packing, and as a fertilizer. It has also long been included in the diets of people in Japan and the Polynesian islands. Seaweed has historically been ingested as a dietary source of iodine and used in the treatment of goiter and other thyroid disorders.

REVIEW OF THE EVIDENCE

- No studies qualify for inclusion in the evidence table.

REVIEW OF THE EVIDENCE: DISCUSSION

Goiter, Thyroid Disease

Summary

- Bladderwrack contains variable levels of iodine (up to 600 µg per gram). As a result, it has been used to treat thyroid disorders such as goiter. Although there are case reports of kelp products inducing hyperthyroidism, there have not been systematic studies of dosing, safety, or efficacy, and there is no widely accepted standardization of iodine content for these products. Although the evidence does suggest thyroid activity, there are inadequate studies to strongly support this use of bladderwrack.

Evidence

- There have been case reports of hyperthyroidism resulting from sea kelp ingestion: Transient hyperthyroidism occurred in a 27-year-old female taking the dietary supplement Energy-V and a multivitamin, both containing kelp, for approximately 1 month.[2] Thyroid function returned to normal upon discontinuation of the kelp-containing products. A second report details the induction of hyperthyroidism, as confirmed clinically and with laboratory tests, in a 72-year-old female with no preexisting thyroid condition, after ingestion of Vitalia (sea-kelp tablets).[4] All signs and symptoms of hyperthyroidism dissipated 6 months after discontinuing the sea-kelp tablets, and her condition was determined to be iodine-induced.
- Due to the lack of standardization of seaweed products, it may be difficult to accurately control thyroid function via this method. Clearly, there are drug therapies such as thyroxine or liothyroxine that act directly via known mechanisms. For patients who lack sufficient dietary iodine, such as in some cases of goiter, bladderwrack or kelp may offer a dietary source when other sources (such as iodized salt) are not available.

Obesity

Summary

- Bladderwrack and other seaweed products are often marketed for weight loss. Theoretically, the thyroid stimulatory properties of bladderwrack may cause hypermetabolic weight loss. However, its anorectic properties and safety for this purpose have not been adequately evaluated in humans.

Anticoagulant

Summary

- Fucans or fucoidans found in brown algae such as bladderwrack appear *in vitro* to have anticoagulant properties, but their use as anticoagulants has not been evaluated adequately in humans.

Evidence

- Springer et al. first demonstrated the anticoagulant properties of fucoidans isolated from *Fucus vesiculosus in vitro* and in rabbits.[17] More recent studies have confirmed the anticoagulant properties of fucoidans from *F. vesiculosus* and other brown seaweeds, including *Ascophyllum nodosum*, *Laminaria religiosa*, and *Pelvitia caniculata*.[10,14,18,19]
- Soeda et al. found that fucoidan derivatives isolated from *F. vesiculosus* stimulate tissue plasminogen activator (tPA)–induced clot lysis through the activation of plasminogen, and slow the rate of fibrin polymerization *in vitro*.[19] They have also found that intravenous fucoidan administered weekly to hyperlipidemic rats decreases the size of hepatic vein thrombi induced by endotoxin.
- Maruyama et al. reported that the fucoidan extract from *Laminaria religiosa* possesses greater antithrombin activity than does heparin and activated plasminogen.[18] Grauffel et al. found that fucans with higher fucose and sulfate levels, like those isolated from *Fucus vesiculosus*, had more potent anticoagulant properties than the fucans with low sulfate and fucose concentrations.[14] Church et al. found that fucoidan from *F. vesiculosus* increases the rate of heparin cofactor II-thrombin inhibition, resulting in *in vitro* anticoagulant effects.[10]

Antifungal/Antibacterial

Summary

- A lectin-like mucopolysaccharide found in *Fucus vesiculosus* (bladderwrack) appears to possess antifungal and antibacterial activity *in vitro*. Literature review reveals no human evidence.

Evidence

- Criado and Ferreiros reported that a lectin-like mucopolysaccharide isolated from *Fucus vesiculosus* agglutinates *Candida guilliermondii* cells. It also inhibited the growth of *C. guilliermondii in vitro*, while other species of *Candida* were not found to be susceptible to that mucopolysaccharide.[15] The mucopolysaccharide inhibited the growth of many *Neisseria meningitidis* strains at a concentration of 5 µg/mL and was bactericidal at concentrations above 10 µg/mL.[16] The growth of select *Escherichia coli* strains was also inhibited by this mucopolysaccharide at concentrations over 10 µg/mL.

Antioxidant

Summary

- Fucoidans from some brown algae, including bladderwrack (*Fucus vesiculosus*), exhibit some antioxidant activity *in vitro*. Human data are lacking.

Evidence

- Le Tutour et al. found that extracts from various brown seaweed species, including *Fucus vesiculosus* and *Ascophyllum nodosum,* extended the induction period of oxidation of methyl linoleate but were ineffective at suppressing the rate of oxygen uptake at time zero (as does Vitamin E, a known antioxidant).[20]

Cancer
Summary

- Several brown algae, including *Fucus vesiculosus,* appear to suppress the growth of various neoplastic cells in animals and *in vitro.* Human data are lacking.

Evidence

- Yamamoto et al. found the extract of *Sargassum fulvellum* to possess antitumor activity against human sarcoma-180 ascitic cells both *in vitro* and in mice and attributed these effects to a sulfated polysaccharide.[21] These components have since been isolated from *Ascophyllum nodosum* and *Fucus vesiculosus,* as well as from other brown seaweed species. A fucan isolated from *A. nodosum* was shown to suppress human sarcoma-180 ascitic cells both *in vitro* and in mice.[22,23] The mechanism of this anti-neoplastic effect is unknown.
- These fucans were also found to suppress growth of non-small-cell human bronchopulmonary carcinoma (NSCLC-N6) cells *in vitro* and *in vivo.*[23]
- Furthermore, a low-molecular-weight fucan isolated from the brown seaweed *Ascophyllum nodosum* seems to suppress the growth of CCL39 fibroblasts and COLO320DM human colon adenocarcinoma cells *in vitro.*[22]

Hyperglycemia (Diabetes)
Summary

- *Fucus vesiculosus* exhibits some hypoglycemic properties in animals. Human data are lacking.

Evidence

- Lamela et al. demonstrated that an extract of *Fucus vesiculosus* lowers the blood glucose in normoglycemic rabbits after oral administration of 10 mg/kg (9.6% reduction after 4 hours), but not after higher doses of the extract.[8] The mechanism of action has not been clearly elucidated.

References

1. Clark CD, Bassett B, Burge MR. Effects of kelp supplementation on thyroid function in euthyroid subjects. Endocr Pract 2003;9(5):363-369.
2. Eliason BC. Transient hyperthyroidism in a patient taking dietary supplements containing kelp. J Am Board Fam Pract 1998;11(6):478-480.
3. Hartman AA. [Hyperthyroidism during administration of kelp tablets,] Ned Tijdschr Geneeskd 1990;134(28):1373.
4. Shilo S, Hirsch HJ. Iodine-induced hyperthyroidism in a patient with a normal thyroid gland. Postgrad Med J 1986;62(729):661-662.
5. Conz PA, La Greca G, Benedetti P, et al. *Fucus vesiculosus*: a nephrotoxic alga? Nephrol Dial Transplant 1998;13(2):526-527.
6. Harrell BL, Rudolph AH. Letter: kelp diet: a cause of acneiform eruption. Arch Dermatol 1976;112(4):560.
7. Walkiw O, Douglas DE. Health food supplements prepared from kelp—a source of elevated urinary arsenic. Clin Toxicol 1975;8(3):325-331.
8. Lamela M, Anca J, Villar R, et al. Hypoglycemic activity of several seaweed extracts. J Ethnopharmacol 1989;27(1-2):35-43.
9. Pye KG, Kelsey SM, House IM, et al. Severe dyserythropoiesis and auto-immune thrombocytopenia associated with ingestion of kelp supplements. Lancet 1992;339(8808):1540.
10. Church FC, Meade JB, Treanor RE, et al. Antithrombin activity of fucoidan. The interaction of fucoidan with heparin cofactor II, antithrombin III, and thrombin. J Biol Chem 1989;264(6):3618-3623.
11. Durig J, Bruhn T, Zurborn KH, et al. Anticoagulant fucoidan fractions from *Fucus vesiculosus* induce platelet activation *in vitro.* Thromb Res 1997;85(6):479-491.
12. Norman JA, Pickford CJ, Sanders TW, et al. Human intake of arsenic and iodine from seaweed-based food supplements and health foods available in the UK. Food Addit Contam 1987;5(1):103-109.
13. Colliec S, Fischer AM, Tapon-Bretaudiere J, et al. Anticoagulant properties of a fucoidan fraction. Thromb Res 1991;64(2):143-154.
14. Grauffel V, Kloareg B, Mabeau S, et al. New natural polysaccharides with potent antithrombic activity: fucans from brown algae. Biomaterials 1989;10(6):363-368.
15. Criado MT, Ferreiros CM. Selective interaction of a *Fucus vesiculosus* lectin-like mucopolysaccharide with several Candida species. Ann Microbiol (Paris) 1983;134A(2):149-154.
16. Criado MT, Ferreiros CM. Toxicity of an algal mucopolysaccharide for *Escherichia coli* and *Neisseria meningitidis* strains. Rev Esp Fisiol 1984;40(2):227-230.
17. Springer GF, Wurzel HA, McNeal GM, et al. Isolation of anticoagulant fractions from crude fucoidin. Proc Soc Exp Biol Med 1957;94:404-409.
18. Maruyama H, Nakajima J, Yamamoto I. A study on the anticoagulant and fibrinolytic activities of a crude fucoidan from the edible brown seaweed *Laminaria religiosa,* with special reference to its inhibitory effect on the growth of sarcoma-180 ascites cells subcutaneously implanted into mice. Kitasato Arch Exp Med 1987;60(3):105-121.
19. Soeda S, Sakaguchi S, Shimeno H, et al. Fibrinolytic and anticoagulant activities of highly sulfated fucoidan. Biochem Pharmacol 1992;43(8):1853-1858.
20. Le Tutour B, Benslimane F, Gouleau MP, et al. Antioxidant and pro-oxidant activities of the brown algae, *Laminaria digitata, Himanthalia elongata, Fucus vesiculosus, Fucus serratus* and *Ascophyllum nodosum.* J Applied Phycology 1998;10(2):121-129.
21. Yamamoto I, Nagumo T, Fujihara M, et al. Antitumor effect of seaweeds. II. Fractionation and partial characterization of the polysaccharide with antitumor activity from Sargassum fulvellum. Jpn J Exp Med 1977;47(3): 133-140.
22. Ellouali M, Boisson-Vidal C, Durand P, et al. Antitumor activity of low molecular weight fucans extracted from brown seaweed *Ascophyllum nodosum.* Anticancer Res 1993;13(6A):2011-2020.
23. Riou D, Colliec-Jouault S, Pinczon du Sel D, et al. Antitumor and anti-proliferative effects of a fucan extracted from ascophyllum nodosum against a non-small-cell bronchopulmonary carcinoma line. Anticancer Res 1996;16(3A):1213-1218.

Blessed Thistle
(*Cnicus Benedictus* L.)

SYNONYMS/COMMON NAMES/RELATED SUBSTANCES

- Bitter thistle, cardin, carbenia benedicta, chardon Benit, cardo santo, carduus benedictus, *Cnici benedicti herba*, cnicus, holy thistle, kardo-benedictenkraut, St. Benedict thistle, spotted thistle.
- *Note:* Blessed thistle should not be mistaken for milk thistle (*Silybum marianus*) or other members of the thistle family.

CLINICAL BOTTOM LINE
Background

- Blessed thistle leaves, stems, and flowers have traditionally been used in "bitter" tonic drinks and in other oral preparations to enhance appetite and digestion. Blessed thistle may also be included in the unproven anti-cancer herbal remedy Essiac. The herb has been tested *in vitro* for its antimicrobial, anticancer, and anti-inflammatory effects, with some positive results. However, no controlled trials have documented clinical benefits in humans.

Scientific Evidence for Common/Studied Uses	Grade*
Abortifacient	C
Dyspepsia/indigestion/flatulence	C
Viral infections	C

*Key to grades: *A:* Strong scientific evidence for this use; *B:* Good scientific evidence for this use; *C:* Unclear scientific evidence for this use; *D:* Fair scientific evidence against this use (it may not work); *F:* Strong scientific evidence against this use (it likely does not work). For a more detailed explanation of efficacy criteria, see "Natural Standard Evidence-Based Validated Grading Rationale" in the Introduction.

Historical or Theoretical Indications That Lack Sufficient Evidence

- Anorexia, antibiotic, antimicrobial, antipyretic, appetite stimulant, astringent, blood purifier, boils, bubonic plague, cervical dysplasia, colds, contraceptive,[1] choleretic, diaphoretic, diarrhea, digestive tonic, diuretic, dysmenorrhea,[2] emmenagogue,[3] expectorant, fever, galactagogue, gallbladder disease, hemorrhage, hepatic disorders, inflammation, jaundice, malaria, memory improvement, menstrual disorders, pneumonitis, rabies, salivary stimulant, skin ulcers, wound healing.

Expert Opinion and Folkloric Precedent

- Traditionally, blessed thistle leaves, stems, and flowers have been used in "bitter" tonics to stimulate appetite and digestion. Preparations of blessed thistle have been used medicinally in Europe and India for multiple conditions, including anorexia, dyspepsia, flatulence, indigestion, and loss of appetite. The German expert panel, the Commission E, has approved the internal use of blessed thistle for loss of appetite and dyspepsia. The British Herbal Compendium indicates its use for loss of appetite, anorexia, and "flatulent dyspepsia."

- Anecdotally, blessed thistle has also been recommended for cervical dysplasia, diarrhea, hemorrhage, wound healing, stimulation of lactation, and dysmenorrhea.

Safety Summary

- **Likely safe:** When blessed thistle is used as flavoring agent, it is generally considered to be safe. In the United States it is an allowable flavoring for alcoholic beverages such as Benedictine liqueur.
- **Possibly safe:** The above-ground parts of blessed thistle may be safe when taken orally in recommended doses; allergic reactions have been reported.
- **Possibly unsafe:** Oral use of blessed thistle is possibly unsafe during pregnancy, because of potential emmenagogue (menstruation stimulant) and abortifacient properties. Gastric toxicity may occur with high doses.

DOSING/TOXICOLOGY

General

- Recommended doses are based on historical practice. With natural products, the optimal doses needed to balance efficacy and safety often have not been determined. Formulations and preparation methods may vary from manufacturer to manufacturer, and from batch to batch of a specific product made by a single manufacturer. Because often the active components of a product are not known, standardization may not be possible, and the clinical effects of different brands may not be comparable.

Standardization

- There is no widely accepted standardization for blessed thistle, although there are assays available to determine the presence of the "bitter" constituent cnicin.[4] Pharmacopeial-grade blessed thistle herb is reported to require a "bitterness value" that is ≥800.
- Blessed thistle herbal preparations are often obtained from the leaves and flowers of the plant.

Dosing: Adult (18 Years and Older)
Oral

- **Tincture:** 7.5 to 10 mL (1.5 g/L of blessed thistle) three times daily.
- **Liquid extract (1:1 g/mL in 25% alcohol):** 1.5 to 3.0 mL three times daily.
- **Infusion:** 1.5 to 2 g of blessed thistle in 150 mL of water three times daily.
- **Tea:** 1.5-3 g of dried blessed thistle flowering tops steeped in boiling water and taken as tea three times daily, or 1-3 teaspoons of dried blessed thistle herb steeped in 1 cup of boiling water for 5 to 15 minutes; 1 cup may be taken three times daily; recommended by some to be used 30 minutes before meals. It may be bitter in taste.

Dosing: Pediatric (Younger Than 18 Years)

- Safety and efficacy data for children are lacking, and blessed thistle is generally not recommended in infancy or early childhood.

Toxicology

- **Acute toxicity:** Gastric irritation and vomiting have been reported from high doses of blessed thistle (>5 g per cup of tea).
- Water extracts of blessed thistle have exhibited no mutagenicity at concentrations up to 200 μL/disc in the standard Ames test,[5] although alcoholic extracts in concentrations of 400 μL/disc possess mild mutagenic effects (in combination with other herbs, which reduces the clarity of this finding).[6] The LD_{50} of cnicin, a constituent of blessed thistle, has been reported as 1.6 to 3.2 mmol/kg in mice.
- In theory, tannins in blessed thistle may be hepatotoxic or nephrotoxic if ingested chronically.

ADVERSE EFFECTS/PRECAUTIONS/CONTRAINDICATIONS
Allergy

- Allergy/hypersensitivity to blessed thistle has been reported, as well as cross-reactivity to mugwort and echinacea. In theory, cross-reactivity may occur to other plants in the Asteraceae/Compositae family. Cross-reactivity may occur with bitter weed, blanket flower, chrysanthemum, coltsfoot, daisy, dandelion, dwarf sunflower, goldenrod, marigold, prairie sage, and ragweed.[7]
- Sesquiterpene lactones are the elements of Asteraceae/Compositae plants believed to be responsible for allergic cross-sensitivity. A study in guinea pigs using 20 different species of Compositae plants demonstrated blessed thistle to possess relatively strong sensitizing properties.[7]

Adverse Effects/Postmarket Surveillance

- **General:** Blessed thistle is generally considered to be safe when used in recommended doses for short periods of time, with few reported adverse effects. Allergic cross-sensitivity may occur with other members of the Compositae family.
- **Dermatologic:** Blessed thistle may cause contact dermatitis. Cross-reactivity may occur with other members of the Compositae family.
- **Ocular/Otic:** Direct exposure to growing blessed thistle plants may result in irritation of the eyes.
- **Gastrointestinal:** Anecdotally, blessed thistle taken in high doses (greater than 5 g per cup of tea) may cause stomach irritation and vomiting. Blessed thistle contains approximately 8% tannins; notably, chronic ingestion of plants that contain ≥10% tannins may cause gastrointestinal upset, hepatic necrosis, or increased risk of developing esophageal or nasal cancer. Traditionally, blessed thistle is believed to stimulate gastric acid secretion, and use may be inadvisable in patients with peptic ulcer disease.
- **Hematologic:** Blessed thistle has been shown to possess platelet-activating factor (PAF) antagonist properties, which in theory may reduce PAF-stimulated platelet aggregation, increasing bleeding risk.[8]
- **Renal:** Blessed thistle contains approximately 8% tannins; notably, chronic ingestion of plants that contain ≥10% tannins may result in nephrotoxicity.

Precautions/Warnings/Contraindications

- Use blessed thistle cautiously in patients with peptic ulcer disease, based on the traditional belief that blessed thistle stimulates gastric acid secretion.

Pregnancy and Lactation

- Blessed thistle has been used traditionally to stimulate menstruation or induce abortion, and therefore should be avoided during pregnancy.
- Although blessed thistle has been used traditionally to stimulate lactation, it is not recommended during lactation because of insufficient available safety information.

INTERACTIONS
Blessed Thistle/Drug Interactions

- **Antacids, H2-receptor antagonists, proton pump inhibitors, sucralfate:** Traditionally, blessed thistle is believed to stimulate gastric acid secretion and may reduce the efficacy of antacids.
- **Anticoagulant drugs, anti-platelet agents, NSAIDS:** Blessed thistle has been shown to possess platelet-activating factor (PAF) antagonist properties, which in theory may reduce PAF-stimulated platelet aggregation, increasing bleeding risk.[8] Clinical effects in humans have not been assessed.

Blessed Thistle/Herb/Supplement Interactions

- **Anticoagulant Herbs and Supplements:** Blessed thistle has been shown to possess platelet-activating factor (PAF) antagonist properties, which in theory may reduce PAF-stimulated platelet aggregation, increasing bleeding risk.[8] Clinical effects in humans have not been assessed.

Blessed Thistle/Lab Interactions

- Insufficient available evidence.

Blessed Thistle/Food Interactions

- Insufficient available evidence.

MECHANISM OF ACTION
Pharmacology

- **Constituents:** The chemical constituents of blessed thistle include sesquiterpene lactone glycosides such as cnicin (0.2 to 0.7%), polyacetylen,[9] and absinthin[10]; triterpenoids such as a-amyrenone, a-amyrin acetate, a-amyrine, and multiflorenol acetate[10,11]; lignans such as trachelogenin, arctigenin, and nortracheloside[12]; flavonoids; polyenes; tannins (8%); and essential/volatile oils (0.3%) such as p-cymene, fenchon, citral and cinnamaldehyde.[13] Lignans such as trachelogenin may contribute to the bitter characteristics of blessed thistle. Cnicin has also been identified as a principal bitter ingredient in blessed thistle.[14]
- **Antimicrobial effects:** Antimicrobial activity of blessed thistle has been attributed to cnicin and polyacetylene constituents.[13,15,16] Antibacterial activity of cnicin and the essential oil of blessed thistle herb have been observed *in vitro* against *Bacillus subtilis*, *Brucella* species, *Escherichia coli*, *Proteus* species, *Pseudomonas aeruginosa*, *Staphylococcus aureus*, and *Streptococcus faecalis*.[13,15,16] Other studies have demonstrated no activity against *Klebsiella*, *Pseudomonas*, *S. aureus*, *Salmonella typhi*, or yeast.[17-19] Several lignans have also been under investigation as antiviral (particularly anti-HIV) and anticancer agents.[20-23]
- **Anti-inflammatory effects:** In the standard rat paw model of inflammation, cnicin had mild anti-inflammatory effects.[24] Lignans such as arctigenin and trachelogenin appear to exert inhibitory effects on cyclic adenosine monophosphate (AMP), phosphodiesterase, and histamine release in rat mast cells.[8] Antagonist activities against calcium ions and platelet-activation factor have also been observed.[8]
- **Antiproliferative effects:** Cnicin and arctigenin have exhibited cytotoxic activity against some tumor cell lines, including leukemia (HL-60), hepatomas, and sarcomas via inhibition

of cellular DNA, RNA or protein synthesis.[16,20,21,25-28] Arctigenin has been noted to induce differentiation in mouse myeloid leukemia cell lines.[29] Blessed thistle is included in some brands of the unproven anti-cancer herbal remedy Essiac.

Pharmacodynamics/Kinetics

- Following oral ingestion of blessed thistle by rats, the lignans arctiin and tracheloside are metabolized to their genins, arctigenin and trachelogein. Peak serum levels are reached at 4 hours for arctigenin and at 8 hours for trachelogenin.[8]

HISTORY

- The blessed thistle plant grows 30-50 cm high. The stems are heavily branched, fuzzy, and sticky; the leaves are thorny and dentate, and the upper leaves form a cup around the flower (which is pale yellow and daisy-like). The leaves, flowering tops, and seeds have been used medicinally. Blessed thistle is native to the Mediterranean region of Europe, and has been naturalized throughout the United States and Europe.
- Blessed or "holy" thistle has been used for more than 2000 years as a "bitter" to stimulate appetite, enhance bile secretion, strengthen the liver, diminish jaundice, decrease flatulence, and aid digestion. Preparations of blessed thistle have also been used historically as a diuretic, diaphoretic, emmenagogue, contraceptive, and antipyretic; as a cure for bubonic plague sores and malaria; and as a general tonic/cure-all. Currently, blessed thistle is most often recommended as a bitter tonic to treat dyspepsia, flatulence, and indigestion. It is also sometimes used as a treatment for diarrhea or hemorrhage, wound healing, lactation stimulation, or dysmenorrhea. Blessed thistle is sometimes added as a fifth ingredient to the unproven anti-cancer herbal remedy Essiac.
- Blessed thistle is also used as a flavoring agent in Benedictine liqueur.

REVIEW OF THE EVIDENCE: TABLE

- No studies qualify for inclusion in the evidence table.

REVIEW OF THE EVIDENCE: DISCUSSION

Viral Infections
Summary

- *In vitro* studies suggest a broad spectrum of antimicrobial activity of blessed thistle. Lignans in blessed thistle have been investigated as anti-HIV agents.[30] However, blessed thistle has exhibited no antiviral activity against herpes, influenza, or polioviruses.[31] There are no reliable human trials of blessed thistle as a treatment for viral infections. There is insufficient scientific evidence to recommend for or against the use of blessed thistle for this indication.

Evidence

- There is one case report of an HIV-infected woman who used an herbal mixture including blessed thistle.[32] Although she reportedly felt symptomatic improvement with the use of this preparation, she subsequently died of pneumonia. Additional details, such as viral load or CD4+ counts, are not available. The potential effects of other herbs in the preparation are not known.

Dyspepsia, Indigestion, Flatulence
Summary

- Blessed thistle is sometimes recommended as a treatment for dyspepsia, indigestion, and flatulence (although historically,

blessed thistle is believed to stimulate gastric acid secretion). There is limited scientific study in this area, and the extent of these gastrointestinal effects remains unclear.
- Abortifacient

Evidence

- Blessed thistle has sometimes been used traditionally as an abortifacient. There is limited human study in this area. Safety and efficacy have not been established.

FORMULARY: BRANDS USED IN CLINICAL TRIALS

European Trade Names (Herbal Mixtures Containing Blessed Thistle)

- Asgocholan, Bilisan forte, Bomgall forte S, Carvomin, Cheiranthol, Chola-Dolan, Digestivum Hetterich, Esberigal, Frisoman, Gallexier, Gallitophen, Gastritol, Gastrosan, Gladlax, Hepaticum-Divinal, Hevert-Gall S, Losapan, Mag Kottas, Leber-Gallentee, Mariazeller, Rasyana, Tisane Anti-biliaire et Stomachique, Tisane pour le coeur et la circulation H, Ventrodigest.

References

1. Krag K. Plants used as contraceptives by the North American Indians: an ethnobotanical study. Cambridge, MA: Harvard University, 1976: 1177.
2. Novitch M, Schweiker R. Orally administered menstrual drug products for over-the-counter human use. Federal Register 1982;47:55076-55101.
3. de Laszlo H, Henshaw P. Plant materials used by primitive peoples to affect fertility. Science 1954;119:626-631.
4. Anon. In: Bradley PR, editor. British Herbal Compendium. Bournemouth, Dorset, UK: British Herbal Medicine Association, 1992:
5. Schimmer O, Kruger A, Paulini H, et al. An evaluation of 55 commercial plant extracts in the Ames mutagenicity test. Pharmazie 1994;49(6): 448-451.
6. Goggelmann W, Schimmer O. Mutagenicity testing of beta-asarone and commercial calamus drugs with *Salmonella typhimurium*. Mutat Res 1983; 121(3-4):191-194.
7. Zeller W, de Gols M, Hausen BM. The sensitizing capacity of Compositae plants. VI. Guinea pig sensitization experiments with ornamental plants and weeds using different methods. Arch Dermatol Res 1985;277(1):28-35.
8. Nose M, Fujimoto T, Nishibe S, et al. Structural transformation of lignan compounds in rat gastrointestinal tract; II. Serum concentration of lignans and their metabolites. Planta Med 1993;59(2):131-134.
9. Vanhaelen-Fastre R. [Polyacetylen compounds from Cnicus benedictus.] Planta Medica 1974;25:47-59.
10. Kataria H. Phytochemical investigation of medicinal plant *Cnicus wallichii* and *Cnicus benedictus* L. Asian J Chem 1995;7:227-228.
11. Ulbelen A, Berkan T. Triterpenic and steroidal compounds of *Cnicus benedictus*. Planta Medica 1977;31:375-377.
12. Vanhaelen M, Vanhaelen-Fastre R. Lactonic lignans from *Cnicus benedictus*. Phytochemistry 1975;14:2709.
13. Vanhaelen-Fastre R. [Constitution and antibiotical properties of the essential oil of *Cnicus benedictus* (author's transl).] Planta Med 1973;24(2): 165-175.
14. Schneider G, Lachner I. [Analysis and action of cnicin]. Planta Med 1987; 53(3):247-251.
15. Vanhaelen-Fastre R. [Antibiotic and cytotoxic activity of cnicin isolated from *Cnicus benedictus* L.] J Pharm Belg 1972;27(6):683-688.
16. Vanhaelen-Fastre R, Vanhaelen M. [Antibiotic and cytotoxic activity of cnicin and of its hydrolysis products. Chemical structure—biological activity relationship (author's transl).] Planta Med 1976;29(2):179-189.
17. Perez C, Anesini C. Inhibition of *Pseudomonas aeruginosa* by Argentinean medicinal plants. Fitoterapia 1994;65(2):169-172.
18. Perez C, Anesini C. *In vitro* antibacterial activity of Argentine folk medicinal plants against *Salmonella typhi*. J Ethnopharmacol 1994;44(1):41-46.
19. Recio M, Rios J, Villar A. Antimicrobial activity of selected plants employed in the Spanish Mediterranean area. Part II. Phytother Res 1989;3:77-80.
20. Eich E, Pertz H, Kaloga M, et al. (-)-Arctigenin as a lead structure for inhibitors of human immunodeficiency virus type-1 integrase. J Med Chem 1996;39(1):86-95.
21. Hirano T, Gotoh M, Oka K. Natural flavonoids and lignans are potent cytostatic agents against human leukemic HL-60 cells. Life Sci 1994;55(13): 1061-1069.
22. Maeda Y, Mitsuya H. Antiretroviral chemotherapy against AIDS. Med Biol Environ 1995;23:267-278.
23. Yang L, Lin S, Yang T, et al. Synthesis of anti-HIV activity of dibenzylbutyrolactone lignans. Bioorg Med Chem Lett 1996;6(8):941-944.
24. Mascolo N, Autore G, Caspasso F, et al. Biological screening of Italian medicinal plants for antiinflammatory activity. Phytother Res 1987;1:28-31.

25. Barrero AF, Oltra JE, Morales V, et al. Biomimetic cyclization of cnicin to malacitanolide, a cytotoxic eudesmanolide from *Centaurea malacitana*. J Nat Prod 1997;60(10):1034-1035.
26. Cobb E. Antineoplastic agent from *Cnicus benedictus*. Patent Brit 1973; 335:181.
27. Moritani S, Nomura M, Takeda Y, et al. Cytotoxic components of *Bardanae fructus* (Goboshi). Biol Pharm Bull 1996;19:1515-1517.
28. Ryu SY, Ahn JW, Kang YH, et al. Antiproliferative effect of arctigenin and arctiin. Arch Pharm Res 1995;18(6):462-463.

29. Umehara K, Sugawa A, Kuroyanagi M, et al. Studies on the differentiation-inducers from *Arctium fructus*. Chem Pharm Bull 1993;41:1774-1779.
30. Pfeiffer K, Trumm S, Eich E, et al. HIV-1 integrase as a target for anti-HIV drugs. Arch STD/HIV Res 1999;6:27-33.
31. May G, Willuhn G. [Antiviral effect of aqueous plant extracts in tissue culture.] Arzneimittelforschung 1978;28(1):1-7.
32. Duke JA. Green Pharmacy. Emmaus: Rodale Press, 1997, p 507.

B

Boron

SYNONYMS/COMMON NAMES/RELATED SUBSTANCES

- Atomic number 5, B, Borax, boric acid, boric anhydride, boron aspartate, boron citrate, boron glycinate, boron oxide, boron sesquioxide, Dobill's solution, magnesium perborate, sodium biborate, sodium borate, sodium metaborate, sodium perborate, sodium pyroborate, sodium tetraborate, Tincal.

CLINICAL BOTTOM LINE
Background

- Boron is a trace element that is found throughout the global environment. The inorganic compound of boron (boric acid, borax) has been used for many decades as an antiseptic and food preservative.
- In the 1980s, boron was discovered to play a role in regulating mineral metabolism (such as calcium and magnesium) and enhancing the vitamin D activation process in humans. These discoveries led to the hypothesis of using boron both in the prevention of osteoporosis and the treatment of osteoarthritis. Although studies assessing these purposes are in preliminary stages, reports are promising.
- There is conflicting evidence to support the use of boron in hormonal regulation and cognitive function. Several ongoing studies are examining the use of boron neutron capture technology in radiation therapy for the treatment of brain tumors.
- Excessive use of boron has led to fatal poisonings. Boron is easily absorbed and subsequently eliminated primarily through the kidney; it should be used cautiously in patients with renal insufficiency.

Scientific Evidence for Common/Studied Uses	Grade*
Improving cognitive function	C
Osteoarthritis	C
Osteoporosis	C
Vaginitis (topical)	C
Bodybuilding aid (increasing testosterone)	D
Menopausal symptoms	D
Prevention of blood clotting (coagulation effects)	D
Psoriasis (boric acid ointment)	D

*Key to grades: A: Strong scientific evidence for this use; B: Good scientific evidence for this use; C: Unclear scientific evidence for this use; D: Fair scientific evidence against this use (it may not work); F: Strong scientific evidence against this use (it likely does not work). For a more detailed explanation of efficacy criteria, see "Natural Standard Evidence-Based Validated Grading Rationale" in the Introduction.

Historical or Theoretical Indications That Lack Sufficient Evidence

- Antiseptic, breast cancer, boron deficiency, diaper rash (avoid because of case reports of death in infants from absorbing boron through skin or when taken by mouth), cancer, eye cleansing, high cholesterol, increasing lifespan, leukemia, rheumatoid arthritis, vitamin D deficiency, wound care.

Expert Opinion and Historic/Folkloric Precedent

- Boron historically has been viewed as a poison but more recently has been used therapeutically in humans. Oral boron supplements have been used to treat osteoarthritis or to prevent bone loss. The topical preparation is used for vaginitis and psoriasis. Other uses of boron are under study.

Safety Summary

- **Likely safe:** When taken by otherwise healthy individual in trace amounts similar to amounts found in foods. A recommended daily allowance for boron is not established.
- **Likely unsafe:** Poisoning has occurred with the ingestion of the equivalent of 0.2 g/kg of boron,[1] or with exposure to boron oxide and boric acid dust at 4.1 mg/m^3. Safety concerns have also been raised when boron has been taken in excessive amounts for more than 3 or 4 days, when it has been used in patients with renal function impairment, or when it has been used in infants and young adults. Most toxicity is due to exposure to excessive amounts of inorganic boron. The available nutritional products are boron citrate, boron aspartate, boron glycinate chelates, and sodium borax.

DOSING/TOXICOLOGY
General

- Recommended doses are based on those most commonly used in available trials or on historical practice. However, with natural products, the optimal doses needed to balance efficacy and safety often have not been determined. Formulations and preparation methods may vary from manufacturer to manufacturer, and from batch to batch of a specific product made by a single manufacturer. Because often the active components of a product are not known, standardization may not be possible, and the clinical effects of different brands may not be comparable.

Standardization

- Most of the nutritional boron products available commercially are either sodium borax or a boron-chelated agent combined with aspartate, glycinate, or citrate. Boron (as boric acid or borax) can be easily absorbed by mouth, through the skin, or by breathing.

Dosing: Adult (18 Years and Older)
Oral

- **Dietary intake:** The average reported daily boron intake in the American diet is 1.17 mg for men, 0.96 mg for women and 1.29 to 1.47 mg for vegetarians. High–boron content foods include peanut butter, wine, grapes, beans, and peaches.[3]
- **Osteoarthritis:** 3 to 6 mg of elemental boron (as sodium tetraborate decahydrate) taken by mouth daily for up to 8 weeks has been used.[4,5]
- **Osteoporosis prevention:** 3 mg of boron taken by mouth per day for individuals with low-boron diet (low vegetable, fruit diet) has been studied.

- **Improvement of cognitive function:** 3 mg of elemental boron taken by mouth daily has been studied.[6]
- **Menopausal symptoms:** 2.5 to 3 mg of elemental boron taken by mouth daily has been studied.[7,8]

Topical

- **Psoriasis:** 1.5% boric acid with 3% zinc oxide applied to the skin as needed has been studied.[9]

Vaginal Application

- **Vaginitis:** Boric acid powder capsules administered vaginally daily have been studied. Safety and effectiveness are not established.[10-12]

Dosing: Pediatric (Younger Than 18 Years)

- There is not enough scientific data to recommend the safe use of boron in children. Case reports exist of death in infants following use of boron (taken by mouth or placed on the skin).

Toxicology

- Although boron, as boric acid and borax, is potentially toxic to all organisms, higher animals usually do not accumulate boron due to their ability to rapidly excrete it. However, because boron can be easily absorbed by mouth, through skin and inhalation, incidental exposure to excessive boron may cause potentially fatal toxic reactions. The most common reactions include skin rash, desquamation, nausea, vomiting (blue-green emesis), diarrhea (in blue-green color), abdominal pain, and headache.[1,13-16] Hypotension and metabolic acidosis have also been reported.[17] Chronic exposure may cause convulsions, anemia, and dehydration, as well as renal and hepatic damage.[15,18-20] Exposure to boric acid or boron oxide dust can cause eye irritation, dryness of the mouth and nose, sore throat, and productive cough.[2] Excessive amounts of boron ingestion have been shown to cause testicular toxicity, decreased sperm motility, and reduced fertility in male rats.[20-23] Alopecia totalis has also been reported anecdotally with boron poisoning.
- The toxic effects of boron appear to be more severe in infants. There are fatal case reports of infants who have been exposed to boron by either oral or topical route. Historically, a honey and borax solution was used to clean infant pacifiers, and topical boric acid powder was used to prevent diaper rash. However, these practices were associated with several infant deaths due to boron toxicity.[24,25]
- **Management:** Boron can be dialyzed, which shortens its half-life. In addition to charcoal and gastric lavage, hemodialysis and peritoneal dialysis have been used to treat acute boron poisoning.[13] N-acetylcysteine is effective in increasing boron excretion and shortens its half-life in rats.[26] It has been recommended that patients with acidosis, renal impairment, or ingestion (greater than 6 g in adults or greater than 200 mg/kg in children) be admitted to a hospital for management.

ADVERSE EFFECTS/PRECAUTIONS/CONTRAINDICATIONS
Allergy

- Known allergy/hypersensitivity to boron, boric acid, borax, citrate, aspartate, and glycinate.

Adverse Effects/Postmarket Surveillance

- **General:** Adverse reactions in doses below 10 mg per day are believed to be unlikely. Large doses can result in acute poisoning. There are fatal case reports of infants who have been exposed to boron by either oral or topical route. Boron toxicity may cause skin rash, nausea, vomiting (may be blue-green color), diarrhea (may be blue-green color), abdominal pain, headache, hypotension, or metabolic acidosis.
- **Dermatologic:** Dermatologic reactions such as skin erythema, desquamation and exfoliation have been reported in the literature.[24] Alopecia totalis has also been reported anecdotally with boron poisoning.
- **Neurologic/CNS:** Both CNS stimulation as well as CNS depression have been reported anecdotally. Specific symptoms may include hyperexcitability, irritability, tremors, seizure disorder, weakness, lethargy, headache, and depression.[18] Fever and hyperthermia have been reported anecdotally.
- **Ocular/Otic:** Exposure to boric acid or boron oxide dust has been reported to cause eye irritation.[2]
- **Pulmonary/Respiratory:** Exposure to boric acid and boron oxide dust has been reported to cause mouth and nasal passage irritation, sore throat and productive cough.[2]
- **Gastrointestinal:** Boron has been noted to cause diarrhea.[24]
- **Endocrine:** Boron has been reported to increase serum levels of 17β-estradiol and testosterone.[27] Clinical effects are not clear. Boron may be associated with reduced serum calcitonin, insulin, or phosphorus, and with increased levels of vitamin D_2, calcium, copper, magnesium, or thyroxine.
- **Genitourinary:** Ingesting large amounts of boron has been associated with infertility in male rats.[21] There are no reports of boron-induced human infertility in the available literature.

Precautions/Warnings/Contraindications

- Avoid use in infants and children, because of case reports of fatalities.
- Avoid use in renal failure patients who are not on dialysis, as boron is eliminated primarily via the kidneys. For patients on dialysis, however, boron supplementation may be needed because dialysis removes boron from the bloodstream. This should be discussed with the patient's nephrologist.
- Use cautiously in patients with estrogen-sensitive cancers (breast, ovarian), based on anecdotal reports of increased serum estrogen concentrations.

Pregnancy and Lactation

- There is not enough scientific evidence to recommend the safe use of boron during pregnancy or breastfeeding. There is a trace amount of boron distributed to human milk.

INTERACTIONS
Boron/Drug Interactions

- **Magnesium, Antacids:** Magnesium may interfere with the normal physiologic effects of boron in the body.[27-29] Sources of magnesium may include antacids containing magnesium oxide or magnesium sulfate (milk of magnesia, Maalox).
- **Estrogens, Testosterone:** In theory, use of boron with estrogen-active drugs such as birth control pills or hormone replacement therapy may result in increased estrogen effects.[27] Use of boron with testosterone-active drugs such as Testoderm may result in increased testosterone effects.

Boron/Herb/Supplement Interactions

- **Calcium, Vitamin D:** Boron supplementation may result in increased calcium levels in the blood and may add to the effects of calcium or vitamin D supplementation.
- **Phytoestrogens:** In theory, use of boron with estrogen-active herbs or supplements may result in increased estrogen

effects.[27] Possible examples include alfalfa, black cohosh, bloodroot, burdock, hops, kudzu, licorice, pomegranate, red clover, soy, thyme, white horehound, and yucca.

Boron/Lab Interactions

- **Phosphorus:** Supplemental doses of boron may reduce serum phosphorus concentrations.[30]
- **Plasma vitamin D_2:** Supplementation of boron may result in increased plasma concentrations of vitamin D_2 in men and women with low magnesium and copper diets.[30,32]
- **Plasma ionized and total calcium:** Boron supplementation may result in increased concentrations of plasma ionized and total calcium as well as reduced serum calcitonin concentration and urinary excretion of calcium.[31,32]
- **Plasma copper:** Boron supplementation may result in higher serum concentrations of plasma copper.[31,32]
- **Plasma magnesium:** Boron supplementation may result in increased plasma magnesium concentrations.[32]
- **Plasma insulin:** According to anecdotal reports, boron may decrease plasma insulin levels.
- **Plasma thyroxine (T_4):** According to anecdotal reports, boron may increase plasma thyroxine.
- **Estrogen:** Use of boron may result in increased endogenous estrogen.[27]
- **Total testosterone:** Boron supplementation may increase concentrations of serum testosterone.[34]

MECHANISM OF ACTION
Pharmacodynamics/Kinetics

- Both inorganic boron (i.e., borate or borax) and organic boron (i.e., boron amino acid chelate) are well absorbed orally by humans. Dermal absorption of boron is insignificant through intact skin, although boron has been demonstrated to penetrate damaged or abraded skin.[35]
- Boron distributes to all tissues with the highest concentration in bone and lowest in adipose tissue. Boron levels generally achieve a steady state in 3 to 4 days.[35]
- Boric acid and borates are not well metabolized by humans. Greater than 90% of the administered dose is excreted unchanged primarily via the urine (50% within 12 hours and 80% to 100% over 5 to 7 days). More than 50% of the oral dose is reported to be eliminated during the first 24 hours in healthy volunteers.[36] The half-life of boron is between 13 hours[13] and 23 hours.[36] Peak CNS concentrations may occur within 3 hours (faster in other tissues); volume of distribution is reported as 0.17 to 0.5 L/kg.

HISTORY

- The Babylonians used borax as a flux for working gold 4000 years ago. The Egyptians then used boron as a mummifying and medicinal agent. In the 8th century, Arabs traded borax between Medina and China. The use of borax flux by European goldsmiths dates to the 12th century.[37] In

Review of the Evidence: Boron

Condition Treated*	Study Design	Author, Year	N[†]	SS[†]	Study Quality[‡]	Magnitude of Benefit	ARR[†]	NNT[†]	Comments
Osteoarthritis	Randomized, placebo-controlled, double blind	Travers[4,5] 1990	20	Yes	3	Small	40%	3	8-week study.
Bone mineral and hormone metabolism	Randomized, placebo-controlled, single-blind	Volpe[48] 1993	28	No	1	Small	NA	NA	Female college students.
Bone mineral and hormone metabolism	Cohort	Nielsen 1987[27]	13	NA	NA	Small	NA	NA	Postmenopausal women; healthy volunteers.
Bone mineral and hormone metabolism	Cohort	Hunt[33] 1997	11	NA	NA	Small	NA	NA	Postmenopausal women; healthy volunteers.
Bone marrow density	Randomized, placebo-controlled	Biquet[42] 1996	87	No	1	Small	NA	NA	12 months follow-up.
Perimenopausal discomfort	Double-blind, Crossover	Nielsen[7] 1999	43	No	1	Small	NA	NA	More women experienced exacerbations than symptom relief.
Vaginitis	Comparison trial	Van Slyke[10,11] 1981	112	Yes	2	Small	28%	4	Boric acid compared with nystatin.
Ergogenic aid	Randomized, placebo-controlled, double-blind	Green[47] 1994	19	No	3	None	NA	NA	Weight training 4 times a week in both groups; 7-week trial.
Psoriasis	Randomized, placebo-controlled, double blind	Limaye[9] 1997	30	No	3	Small	NA	NA	Dropout rate, 46%.
Cognitive function	Cohort	Penland[6] 1994	28	Yes	NA	NA	NA	NA	Cohort study.

*Primary or secondary outcome.
[†]N, Number of patients; SS, statistically significant; ARR, absolute risk reduction; NNT, the number of patients who need to undergo a specific intervention in order to observe an outcome in one individual.
[‡]0-2 = poor; 3-4 = good; 5 = excellent.
NA, Not applicable.
For an explanation of each category in this table, please see Table 3 in the Introduction.

1702, William Homberg introduced borax into medical practice. It was purported to be a sedative, anodyne and antispasmodic.[24]

- Boron exists in nature in a hydrated form, which can be found in soil, water, vegetables, and fruits. Most boron that enters the human body comes from the ingestion of leafy vegetables, fruit, nuts, and legumes.

REVIEW OF THE EVIDENCE: DISCUSSION

Osteoarthritis

Summary

- Based on human population research, in a boron rich environment, people appear to have fewer joint disorders.[38,39] It has also been proposed that boron deficiency may contribute to the development of osteoarthritis. However, there is no clear human evidence that supplementation with boron is beneficial as prevention against or as a treatment for osteoarthritis.

Evidence

- Travers et al. conducted a double-blind study to examine the effect of boron supplements for the treatment of osteoarthritis. Twenty patients were assigned to take either 6 mg of elemental boron orally (as sodium tetraborate decahydrate) or placebo.[4,5] To evaluate the improvement of joint conditions, patients were examined at weeks 0, 3, and 8. The authors reported "slight" improvements in 50% of patients taking boron supplementation vs. 10% of patients in the placebo group. However, the small number of patients included in this study, high dropout rate (25%), and lack of use of validated measures make the results difficult to interpret.

Osteoporosis

Summary

- Animal and preliminary human studies report boron to play a role in mineral metabolism, with effects on calcium, phosphorus, and vitamin D.[27,40,41] However, research of bone mineral density in women taking boron supplements does not clearly demonstrate benefits in osteoporosis. Additional study is needed before a firm conclusion can be drawn.
- **Evidence:** Nielsen et al. examined the effects of boron in 13 postmenopausal women by comparing urinary calcium excretion before and after boron supplementation in the setting of a low boron diet (<1 mg of boron per day).[27] The authors reported that boron reduced calcium loss in the urine. In a study by Hunt et al., the authors reported similar results in 11 postmenopausal women.[33] In both of these reports, it was found that a low magnesium diet in addition to boron supplementation enhances calcium preservation. Beattie also reported positive calcium balance with boron supplementation in 6 postmenopausal women selected from 200 volunteers.[8] Although these studies may shed some light onto the physiology of boron in human body, they are limited by design, and comparisons were made between a very low boron diet (less than 0.25 mg/day while average boron intake in the United States is 1 to 1.5 mg/day) and a high boron intake (3.25 mg/day), and bone marrow density and risk of fracture were not examined. Therefore, the clinical implications of these studies are limited.
- Biquet et al. reported the results of a randomized, placebo-controlled trial comparing bone mineral density of the lumbar spine, hip, and femoral neck regions in a group of

healthy postmenopausal women taking boron supplementation (3 mg/day) versus placebo.[42] After 1 year of follow-up, no significant difference in bone marrow density between the two groups was observed, further clouding the evidence supporting the use of boron in the prevention of bone loss.

Vaginitis

Summary

- Inorganic boron (boric acid, borax) has been used as an antiseptic based on proposed antibacterial and antifungal properties. It is proposed that boric acid may have effects against candidal and non-candidal vulvovaginitis.[43] A limited amount of poor-quality research reports that boric acid capsules used in the vagina may be effective for vaginitis. Further evidence is needed before a recommendation can be made.

Evidence

- Van Slyke et al. compared a 600-mg boric acid capsule to a nystatin vaginal capsule in the treatment of vulvovaginitis in 112 patients.[10,11] After 7 to 10 days of therapy, the authors reported a 92% cure rate in the boric acid group and a 64% cure rate in the nystatin group. However, this study has been criticized for using a low dose of nystatin in the comparison group.[42]
- In a case series,[12] 21 out of 26 patients with *Torulopsis* (*Candida*) *glabrata* vaginitis were reported as being cured or experiencing improved symptom control with boric acid therapy.
- In a case report,[45] boric acid was successfully used to treat azole-refractory candidal vaginitis in a woman with AIDS.

Improving Cognitive Function

Summary

- Preliminary human study reports better performance on tasks of eye-hand coordination, attention, perception, short-term memory and long-term memory with boron supplementation. However, additional research is needed before a firm conclusion can be drawn.

Evidence

- Penland examined the effect of boron on cognitive function in older men and women.[6] The author compared boron supplementation (3 mg) to a low boron diet, and reported that a low boron diet results in significantly poorer cognitive performance. The boron-supplemented group experienced increased rates of "higher-frequency activity," as well as significantly greater performance on tasks emphasizing manual dexterity, eye-hand coordination, attention, perception, encoding, short-term memory, and long-term memory. It is not clear if boron supplements are beneficial in those with a normal (non–boron-depleted) diet.

Prevention of Blood Clotting (Coagulation Effects)

Summary

- It has been proposed that boron may affect the activity of certain blood clotting factors. There is not enough evidence in this area to form a clear conclusion.
- A small (15 healthy men aged 45 to 65 years), randomized, placebo-controlled, double-blind, crossover study concluded that there is no evidence of boron lowering clotting factor VIIa, and therefore it should not alter bleeding risk.[46] Notably, a manufacturer of boron funded this study.

Bodybuilding Aid (Increasing Testosterone)

Summary

- There is preliminary negative evidence for the use of boron for improving performance in bodybuilding by increasing testosterone. Although boron is suggested to raise testosterone levels, in early human research, total lean body mass has not been affected by boron supplementation in bodybuilders. Additional research is necessary before a firm conclusion can be drawn.

Evidence

- The effect of boron supplementation (2.5 mg) was investigated in 19 male bodybuilders, using a randomized, double-blind, placebo-controlled design.[47] Subjects in both the boron-supplemented group and the placebo group underwent 7 weeks of weight training. The authors reported that testosterone levels and total lean body mass were increased from baseline in both groups but were unaffected by boron supplementation.

Menopausal Symptoms

Summary

- It has been proposed that boron affects estrogen levels in postmenopausal women. However, preliminary studies have found no changes in menopausal symptoms.

Evidence

- In two studies, serum 17β-estradiol levels were raised when postmenopausal women ingested boron supplements.[8,27] It appears that boron, magnesium and other factors may play a complex role in estrogen regulation, and it is not clear that boron directly interferes with serum estrogen levels. In a follow-up study, Nielsen and Penland conducted a double-blind crossover study to examine the effects of boron in women with menopausal discomfort.[7] The authors reported that more women receiving boron supplements experienced exacerbation of symptoms (46%) rather than relief (22%). As in previous investigations, estrogen levels were found to increase during the period of boron supplementation.
- In a randomized, placebo-controlled trial, Volpe et al. investigated the effects of boron supplementation on hormonal levels in two groups of young women: college female athletes and sedentary women.[48] After a 10-month follow-up, the authors found no significant differences in serum 17β estradiol and testosterone levels between the boron and placebo arms. However, the athlete group did show a significant increase in 17β-estradiol and testosterone levels compared to baseline. Nonetheless, the authors concluded that boron does not affect sex steroid levels in young women.

Psoriasis (Topical)

Summary

- Preliminary human study of an ointment including boric acid does not report significant benefits in psoriasis.
- An ointment consisting of boric acid and zinc oxide was compared to placebo in treating plaque-type psoriasis in 30 subjects.[9] Although use of the boron ointment demonstrated a trend toward better performance vs. placebo, this result did not reach statistical significance. A high dropout rate (14 subjects) hinders this result.

References

1. Linden CH, Hall AH, Kulig KW, et al. Acute ingestions of boric acid. J Toxicol Clin Toxicol 1986;24(4):269-279.
2. Garabrant DH, Bernstein L, Peters JM, et al. Respiratory and eye irritation from boron oxide and boric acid dusts. J Occup Med 1984;26(8):584-586.
3. Rainey CJ, Nyquist LA, Christensen RE, et al. Daily boron intake from the American diet. J Am Diet Assoc 1999;99(3):335-340.
4. Travers RL, Rennie GC, Newnham RE. Boron and arthritis: the results of a double-blind pilot study. J Nutritional Med 1990;1:127-132.
5. Travers RL, Rennie GC. Clinical trial: boron and arthritis. The results of a double blind pilot study. Townsend Lett Doctors 1990;360-362.
6. Penland JG. Dietary boron, brain function, and cognitive performance. Environ Health Perspect 1994;102 Suppl 7:65-72.
7. Nielsen FH, Penland JG. Boron supplementation of peri-menopausal women affects boron metabolism and indices associated with macromineral metabolism, hormonal status and immune function. J Trace Elem Exp Med 1999;12(3):251-261.
8. Beattie JH, Peace HS. The influence of a low-boron diet and boron supplementation on bone, major mineral and sex steroid metabolism in postmenopausal women. Br J Nutr 1993;69(3):871-884.
9. Limaye S, Weightman W. Effect of an ointment containing boric acid, zinc oxide, starch and petrolatum on psoriasis. Australas J Dermatol 1997;38(4):185-186.
10. Van Slyke KK, Michel VP, Rein MF. The boric acid powder treatment of vulvovaginal candidiasis. J Am Coll Health Assoc 1981;30(3):107-109.
11. Van Slyke KK, Michel VP, Rein MF. Treatment of vulvovaginal candidiasis with boric acid powder. Am J Obstet Gynecol 1981;141(2):145-148.
12. Sobel JD, Chaim W. Treatment of Torulopsis glabrata: retrospective review of boric acid therapy. Clin Infect Dis 1997;24(4):649-652.
13. Litovitz TL, Klein-Schwartz W, Oderda GM, et al. Clinical manifestations of toxicity in a series of 784 boric acid ingestions. Am J Emerg Med 1988;6(3):209-213.
14. Tangermann RH, Etzel RA, Mortimer L, et al. An outbreak of a food-related illness resembling boric acid poisoning. Arch Environ Contam Toxicol 1992;23(1):142-144.
15. Chao TC, Maxwell SM, Wong SY. An outbreak of aflatoxicosis and boric acid poisoning in Malaysia: a clinicopathological study. J Pathol 1991; 164(3):225-233.
16. Schillinger Pediatric BM, Berstein M, Goldberg LA, et al. Boric acid poisoning. J Am Acad Dermatol 1982;7(5):667-673.
17. Restuccio A, Mortensen ME, Kelley MT. Fatal ingestion of boric acid in an adult. Am J Emerg Med 1992;10(6):545-547.
18. Gordon AS, Prichard JS, Freedman MH. Seizure disorders and anemia associated with chronic borax intoxication. Can Med Assoc J 1973;108(6): 719-721.
19. O'Sullivan K, Taylor M. Chronic boric acid poisoning in infants. Arch Dis Child 1983;58(9):737-739.
20. Ishii Y, Fujizuka N, Takahashi T, et al. A fatal case of acute boric acid poisoning. J Toxicol Clin Toxicol 1993;31(2):345-352.
21. Fukuda R, Hirode M, Mori I, et al. Collaborative work to evaluate toxicity on male reproductive organs by repeated dose studies in rats. Testicular toxicity of boric acid after 2- and 4-week administration periods. J Toxicol Sci 2000;25 Spec No:233-239.
22. Lee IP, Sherins RJ, Dixon RL. Evidence for induction of germinal aplasia in male rats by environmental exposure to boron. Toxicol Appl Pharmacol 1978;45(2):577-590.
23. Chapin RE, Ku WW. The reproductive toxicity of boric acid. Environ Health Perspect 1994;102(Suppl 7):87-91.
24. Valdes-Dapena MA, Arey JB. Boric acid poisoning. J Pediatr 1962;61: 531-546.
25. Goldbloom RB, Goldbloom A. Boron acid poisoning: report of four cases and a review of 109 cases from the world literature. J Pediatr 1953; 43(6): 631-643.
26. Banner W, Jr., Koch M, Capin DM, et al. Experimental chelation therapy in chromium, lead, and boron intoxication with N-acetylcysteine and other compounds. Toxicol Appl Pharmacol 1986;83(1):142-147.
27. Nielsen FH, Hunt CD, Mullen LM, et al. Effect of dietary boron on mineral, estrogen, and testosterone metabolism in postmenopausal women. FASEB J 1987;1(5):394-397.
28. Nielsen FH, Hunt CD, Mullen LM, et al. Effect of dietary boron on mineral, estrogen, and testosterone metabolism in postmenopausal women. FASEB J 1987;1(5):394-397.
29. Nielsen FH, Gallagher SK, Johnson LK, et al. Boron enhances and mimics some effects of estrogen therapy in postmenopausal women. J Trace Elem Exp Med 1992;5(4):237-246.
30. Meacham SL, Taper LJ, Volpe SL. Effects of boron supplementation on bone mineral density and dietary, blood, and urinary calcium, phosphorus, magnesium, and boron in female athletes. Environ Health Perspect 1994;102(Suppl 7):79-82.
31. Nielsen FH. Studies on the relationship between boron and magnesium which possibly affects the formation and maintenance of bones. Magnes Trace Elem 1990;9(2):61-69.
32. Nielsen FH, Mullen LM, Gallagher SK. Effect of boron depletion and repletion on blood indicators of calcium status in humans fed a magnesium-low diet. J Trace Elem Exp Med 1990;3:45-54.
33. Hunt CD, Herbel JL, Nielsen FH. Metabolic responses of postmenopausal women to supplemental dietary boron and aluminum during usual and low magnesium intake: boron, calcium, and magnesium absorption and retention and blood mineral concentrations. Am J Clin Nutr 1997;65(3): 803-813.
34. Ferrando AA, Green NR. The effect of boron supplementation on lean body

mass, plasma testosterone levels, and strength in male bodybuilders. Int J Sport Nutr 1993;3(2):140-149.

35. Murray FJ. A human health risk assessment of boron (boric acid and borax) in drinking water. Regul Toxicol Pharmacol 1995;22(3):221-230.

36. Jansen JA, Andersen J, Schou JS. Boric acid single dose pharmacokinetics after intravenous administration to man. Arch Toxicol 1984;55(1):64-67.

37. Woods WG. An introduction to boron: history, sources, uses, and chemistry. Environ Health Perspect 1994;102(Suppl 7):5-11.

38. Newnham RE. Essentiality of boron for healthy bones and joints. Environ Health Perspect 1994;102 Suppl 7:83-85.

39. Newnham RE. The role of boron in human nutrition. J Applied Nutrition 1994;46(3):81-85.

40. Hunt CD. The biochemical effects of physiologic amounts of dietary boron in animal nutrition models. Environ Health Perspect 1994;102 Suppl 7: 35-43.

41. Hunt CD, Herbel JL, Idso JP. Dietary boron modifies the effects of vitamin D3 nutrition on indices of energy substrate utilization and mineral metabolism in the chick. J Bone Miner Res 1994;9(2):171-182.

42. Biquet I, Collette J, Dauphin JF, et al. Prevention of postmenopausal bone loss by administration of boron. Osteoporos Int 1996;6(Suppl 1):249.

43. Prutting SM, Cerveny JD. Boric acid vaginal suppositories: a brief review. Infect Dis Obstet Gynecol 1998;6(4):191-194.

44. Orley J. Nystatin versus boric acid powder in vulvovaginal candidiasis. Am J Obstet Gynecol 1982;144(8):992-993.

45. Shinohara YT, Tasker SA. Successful use of boric acid to control azole-refractory Candida vaginitis in a woman with AIDS. J Acquir Immune Defic Syndr Hum Retrovirol 1997;16(3):219-220.

46. Wallace JM, Hannon-Fletcher MP, Robson PJ, et al. Boron supplementation and activated factor VII in healthy men. Eur J Clin Nutr 2002;56(11): 1102-1107.

47. Green NR, Ferrando AA. Plasma boron and the effects of boron supplementation in males. Environ Health Perspect 1994;102(Suppl 7):73-77.

48. Volpe SL, Taper LJ, Meacham S. The relationship between boron and magnesium status and bone mineral density in the human: a review. Magnes Res 1993;6(3):291-296.

Boswellia

(Boswellia serrata Roxb.)/Frankincense

SYNONYMS/COMMON NAMES/RELATED SUBSTANCES

- African elemi *(Boswellia frereana)*, Bibal incense *(Boswellia carterii)*, Burseraveae, carterii, dhup, guggals, H15, indish incense, olibanum, S-compound, sacra, salai guggal, sallai guggul, Sallaki.
- **Selected combination products that include boswellia:** Articulin-F *(Withania somnifera* [ashwagandha], *Boswellia serrata, Curcuma longai* [turmeric], zinc complex); RA-1 *(Withania somnifera* [ashwagandha], *Boswellia serrata, Zingiber officinale* [ginger], *Curcma longa* [turmeric]).

CLINICAL BOTTOM LINE

Background

- Resin extracts from the *Boswellia serrata* tree have been found to inhibit the synthesis of pro-inflammatory mediators, including leukotrienes. Animal and *in vitro* studies suggest possible efficacy for inflammatory conditions such as inflammatory bowel disease, rheumatoid arthritis, and osteoarthritis, although high-quality human data are lacking. Initial human evidence from one well-designed trial suggests the efficacy of boswellia as a chronic therapy for asthma (but *not* for the relief of acute asthma exacerbations). Further studies are warranted in this area.
- As opposed to nonsteroidal anti-inflammatory drugs (NSAIDs), long-term use of boswellia has not been shown to cause gastrointestinal irritation or ulceration, although adverse effects have not been systematically studied in humans.

Scientific Evidence for Common/Studied Uses	Grade*
Asthma (chronic therapy)	B
Crohn's disease	C
Osteoarthritis	C
Rheumatoid arthritis	C
Ulcerative colitis	C

*Key to grades: *A:* Strong scientific evidence for this use; *B:* Good scientific evidence for this use; *C:* Unclear scientific evidence for this use; *D:* Fair scientific evidence against this use (it may not work); *F:* Strong scientific evidence against this use (it likely does not work). For a more detailed explanation of efficacy criteria, see "Natural Standard Evidence-Based Validated Grading Rationale" in the Introduction.

Historical or Theoretical Uses That Lack Sufficient Evidence

- Acne, amenorrhea, analgesic,[1] antifungal,[2] anti-inflammatory,[3,4] antiseptic, astringent, belching, blood "purification," breast cysts, bursitis, cancer,[5] carminative, cervical spondylosis,[6] chronic obstructive pulmonary disease (COPD), cicatrizant (scar formation), cystitis, digestive, diuretic, dyspepsia, emmenagogue (induces menstruation), expectorant, genital area infections, hyperlipidemia,[7] multiple sclerosis, nephritis, peptic ulcer disease, pimples, sedative,[1] sexually transmitted diseases (STDs), skin ulcers/sores, syphilis, tendonitis, toxin-induced liver damage,[4] uterine infections, wound healing.

Expert Opinion and Historic Precedent

- Boswellia has traditionally been used for a number of topical applications, including treatment of acne, bacterial and fungal infections, boils, wound healing, scars, and varicose veins. It is used cosmetically as a facial toner and to smooth wrinkles.
- Chinese herbalists use boswellia in powder form and in teas for rheumatism and menstrual pain and as an external wash for sores and bruises.
- Historically, boswellia has been utilized to improve emotional well-being and as part of religious rituals. It has been reported that it has the ability to enhance spirituality, mental perception, meditation, prayer, and consciousness when burned (burning is said to produce a psychoactive substance, trans-hydrocannabinole).[6]
- "Olibanum" oil from boswellia is used in food products, alcoholic and non-alcoholic beverages, frozen dairy desserts, baked goods, pudding, and gelatins. The level often found in these meat products is 0.001%. Olibanum oil and extracts are used as fixative and/or fragrance components in soaps, detergents, creams, lotions, and perfumes (commonly 0.8%).

Safety Summary

- **Likely safe:** When consumed in amounts found in foods (maximum levels 0.001% in meat products).
- **Possibly safe:** When used in recommended doses as an oral agent to treat arthritis, inflammatory bowel disease, and asthma.[8-13]
- **Likely unsafe:** When used in pregnant women, based on reports in the Indian literature that resin from boswellia may be an emmenagogue and induce abortion.[14]

DOSING/TOXICOLOGY

General

- Recommended doses are based on those most commonly used in available trials, or on historical practice. However, with natural products, the optimal doses needed to balance efficacy and safety often have not been determined. Formulations and preparation methods may vary from manufacturer to manufacturer, and from batch to batch of a specific product made by a single manufacturer. Because often the active components of a product are not known, standardization may not be possible, and the clinical effects of different brands may not be comparable.

Standardization

- The gum resin typically contains 30% boswellic acids, whereas ethanol extracts contain 43% boswellic acids.[15] Some commercial sources contain up to 65% boswellic acids. Oral doses of 200 to 400 mg are often standardized to contain 37.5% boswellic acids per dose.[8]
- The standardized boswellia products Sallaki (India) and H15 (Switzerland) contain 11-keto-β-boswellic acid (1.8%), acetyl-11-keto-β-boswellic acid (1.4%), and acetyl-β-boswellic acid/β-boswellic acid (2%).[12]
- The standardized boswellia product S-compound contains 11-keto-β-boswellic acid (0.63%), acetyl-11-keto-β-boswellic acid (0.7%), and acetyl-β-boswellic acid/β-boswellic acid (1.5%).[13]

Dosing: Adult (18 Years and Older)
Oral Tablets/Capsules

- **Asthma:** 300 mg three times a day of boswellia powdered gum resin capsules (S-compound was used in one trial),[13] or 400 mg three times daily (extract standardized to 37.5% boswellic acids per dose) (anecdotal).
- **Crohn's disease:** 1200 mg three times daily of standardized *Boswellia serrata* gum resin H15, for up to 8 weeks.[16]
- **Osteoarthritis:** Two capsules, 3 times daily of Aticulin-F (combination formula containing 100 mg of *Boswellia serrata*, 450 mg of *Withania somnifera* [ashwagandha], 50 mg of *Curcuma longa* [turmeric], and 50 mg of zinc complex).[10]
- **Rheumatoid arthritis:** 400 mg three times daily of standardized *Boswellia serrata* gum resin H15,[8] or 2 capsules, three times daily of Aticulin-F (combination formula containing 100 mg of *Boswellia serrata*, 450 mg of *Withania somnifera* [ashwagandha], 50 mg of *Curcuma longa* [turmeric], and 50 mg of zinc complex).[11]
- **Ulcerative colitis:** 350 to 400 mg three times daily (extract standardized to 37.5% boswellic acids per dose).[12]

Dosing: Pediatric (Younger Than 18 Years)

- Review of the literature reveals no adverse events specifically related to the use of boswellia in children. However, safety, efficacy, and dosing have not been systematically studied. Some experts believe that regular use of boswellia may mask the symptoms of asthma in children and may delay diagnosis. Use in children should be supervised by an appropriately licensed healthcare professional.

Toxicology

- The LD_{50} of boswellic acids is >2 g/kg in rats and mice; doses of 2 g/kg in mice, rats, and monkeys have not caused death; high doses have reportedly not yielded significant effects on behavior or clinical, hematologic, biochemical and pathologic data.[15,17]

ADVERSE EFFECTS/PRECAUTIONS/CONTRAINDICATIONS
Allergy

- No allergic or hypersensitivity reactions to boswellia have been reported in the available literature, although this area lacks systematic study.

Adverse Effects

- **General:** Boswellia is generally believed to be safe when used as directed, although safety and toxicity have not been systematically studied in humans. The most common complaints in trials have been nausea and acid reflux. A licensed healthcare provider should be consulted prior to use.
- **Dermatologic:** Dermatitis was reported in 4 of 62 patients (6%) in two clinical trials using Articulin-F, a combination product containing gum resin from *Boswellia serrata* as well as *Withania somnifera* (ashwagandha), *Curcuma longa* (turmeric), and zinc complex.[10,11] The independent effects of boswellia are not clear.
- **Gastrointestinal:** Boswellia extract has been associated with mild gastrointestinal upset in a randomized controlled trial in patients with osteoarthritis.[18] In a study of patients with ulcerative colitis, abdominal fullness, epigastric pain, gastroesophageal reflux symptoms, diarrhea, and nausea were reported by 6 of 34 patients (18%) receiving 350 mg three times daily of boswellia for 6 weeks.[12] It is not clear to what extent these symptoms were related to the patients' under-

lying colitis. Two of 80 patients (3%) receiving the boswellia powdered gum resin formulation S-compound complained of epigastric pain, hyperacidity, and nausea.[13] Nausea was reported in 3 of 62 patients (5%), and abdominal fullness in 7 of 62 patients (11%) in two clinical trials using Articulin-F (combination product containing *Boswellia serrata*, *Withania somnifera* [ashwagandha], *Curcuma longa* [turmeric], and zinc complex).[10,11] However, the independent effects of boswellia could not be determined.

Precautions/Warnings/Contraindications

- Use cautiously in patients with pre-existing gastritis or gastroesophageal reflux disease (GERD), as reflux and epigastric pain have been associated with the use of boswellia.
- Use cautiously in patients taking lipid-soluble medications, as the gum resin of boswellia has been reported to lower cholesterol and triglyceride levels,[7] and may bind to/impair absorption of these medications.

Pregnancy and Lactation

- Reports in the Indian literature suggest that resin from boswellia is an emmenagogue and may induce abortion.[14] Safety of boswellia during pregnancy has not been systematically studied and therefore cannot be recommended.

INTERACTIONS
Boswellia/Drug Interactions

- **Leukotriene inhibitors:** Boswellia has been found in animal and *in vitro* studies to inhibit 5-lipoxygenase, thereby reducing the production of leukotrienes.[3,4,6,19] Boswellia therefore may potentiate the actions of pharmaceutical leukotriene inhibitors such as zafirlukast (Accolate) and montelukast (Singulair), which are used in the treatment of asthma.
- **Antineoplastic agents:** Boswellic acids have been found *in vitro* to inhibit protein synthesis via effects on nucleic acids, and to inhibit proliferation of human leukemic HL-60 cells.[5,20] Theoretically, concomitant use with other antiproliferative agents may potentiate effects or toxicity.
- **Lipid-lowering agents:** The gum of boswellia has been reported to lower cholesterol and triglyceride levels in rats[7] and may potentiate the effects of lipid-lowering agents.
- **Fat-soluble medications:** The gum resin of boswellia has been reported to lower cholesterol and triglyceride levels[7] and may bind to/impair absorption of lipid-soluble agents.
- **Nonsteroidal anti-inflammatory agents (NSAIDs), COX-2 inhibitors:** In the treatment of arthritic conditions, the purported mechanism of boswellia's activity is reduction of glycosaminoglycan (GAG) degradation, based on rat studies.[21] This potentially beneficial mechanism may theoretically be disrupted by concomitant use of NSAIDs.
- **Antifungal agents (potential positive interaction):** The essential oil from *Boswellia serrata* has been reported to possess antifungal activity, with weak activity against human fungal pathogens *in vitro* (but greater effect against plant fungal pathogens).[2]

Boswellia/Herb/Supplement Interactions

- **Glycosaminoglycans (GAGs), chondroitin sulfate, glucosamine:** Boswellia has been reported to reduce the degradation of glycosaminoglycans in rats[21] and may act additively or synergistically with agents shown to be efficacious in the treatment of osteoarthritis, such as glucosamine and chondroitin.

- **Antiproliferative agents:** Boswellic acids have been found *in vitro* to inhibit protein synthesis via effects on nucleic acids and to inhibit proliferation of human leukemic HL-60 cells.[5,20] Theoretically, concomitant use with other antiproliferative agents may potentiate effects or toxicity.
- **Antifungal agents (potential positive interaction):** The essential oil from *Boswellia serrata* has been reported to possess antifungal activity, with weak activity against human fungal pathogens *in vitro* (but greater effect against plant fungal pathogens).[2]
- **Lipid-lowering agents:** The gum of boswellia has been reported to lower cholesterol and triglyceride levels in rats[7] and may potentiate the effects of lipid-lowering agents such as garlic.

Boswellia/Food Interactions

- Literature review reveals no reported interactions.

Boswellia/Lab Interactions

- **Serum lipids:** The gum of boswellia has been reported to lower cholesterol and triglyceride levels in rats,[7] although human studies are lacking.
- **Liver function tests (transaminases):** Toxin-induced transaminitis in mice was reduced by administration of boswellia, although effects on normal liver or on humans are not clear.[4]

MECHANISM OF ACTION
Pharmacology

- *Boswellia serrata* is a branching tree found in India, North Africa, and the Middle East. A gummy oleoresin is found under the bark, which contains oil, resins, and gum. Extracts of this gummy exudate have been used medicinally and scientifically evaluated.
- *In vitro* and rat studies have reported that acetyl-11-keto-β-boswellic acid from boswellia inhibits the enzyme 5-lipoxygenase, which produces 5-hydroxyeicosatetraenoic (5-HETE) and leukotriene B4 (LTB4).[3,6,22,23] These products are involved with the induction of bronchoconstriction, chemotaxis, and vascular permeability.[3,4,6,19] Additional studies have found that boswellia inhibits human leukocyte elastase (HLE), which is involved in the pathogenesis of emphysema, cystic fibrosis, chronic bronchitis, and acute respiratory distress syndrome.[3,6] Multiple pentacyclic triterpenic acids have been isolated from boswellia.[24-26]
- Anti-inflammatory effects of boswellic acids have been reported in animal studies.[22,27] Doses of 50 to 200 mg/kg given orally to mice, after intrapleural injection of carrageenan, inhibited polymorphonuclear leukocyte (PMN) infiltration into the pleural cavity. This response was similar to that of indomethacin (1.25 to 5 mg/kg). Alcoholic extracts of boswellia in oral doses of 50 to 200 mg/kg inhibited carrageenan-induced paw edema in rats, similar to phenylbutazone (50 to 100 mg/kg), and improved blood supply to joint tissues.[17] Mixed acetylboswellic acids extracted from the gum resin of *Boswellia serrata* significantly inhibited ionophone-stimulated release of leukotrienes B4 and C4 from intact human PMNs.[28] Boswellic acids have demonstrated anti-inflammatory and anti-arthritic activity in chronic models of adjuvant-induced polyarthritis and formaldehyde arthritis in rats[17] and in BSA-induced arthritis in rabbits.[29] Boswellic acids produced a protective effect in sodium urate gouty arthritis in dogs, reduced exudate volume and inhibited leukocyte migration in carrageenan-induced pleurisy in rats, and was antipyretic in rats and rabbits.[27]
- In animals, ingestion of defatted alcoholic extracts of boswellia decreases PMN infiltration and migration, decreases primary antibody synthesis, and inhibits the classical complement pathway.[26,29,30] Humoral responses are also inhibited by oral boswellia extract, 25 to 200 mg/kg in mice (similar to the effect of azathioprine, 100 mg/kg orally).[17] Prolonged administration of boswellic acids (25 to 100 mg/kg for 21 days) increases body weight and total leukocyte counts in rats.[30,31]
- The non-phenolic ration of *Boswellia serrata* gum resin (20 to 300 mg/kg) exhibits an analgesic effect in rats similar to that of morphine (4.5 mg/kg), and a sedative effect (55 to 300 mg/kg) comparable to that of chlorpromazine (7.5 mg/kg).[1]
- In biochemical studies, boswellic acids have acted to reduce arthritis-associated elevated enzymes such as glutamic pyruvic transaminase, glycohydrolase, and β-glucuronidase.[32,33] Inhibition of glycosaminoglycan (GAG) synthesis and urinary excretion of connective tissue metabolites by boswellic acids have been proposed as support for the purported beneficial effects of boswellia in preventing the degradation of connective tissue in inflammatory arthritic conditions.[21]
- In anti-hyperlipidemic studies performed in rats, boswellic acids have been found to reduce serum cholesterol and triglycerides.[7]
- Boswellic acids have not been found to act as antioxidants.[4]

Pharmacodynamics/Kinetics

- The LD_{50} of boswellic acid is >2 g/kg in rats and mice when administered orally or intraperitoneally. Subacute toxicity studies in rabbits over 3 months, and chronic toxicity studies in rats and monkeys over 6 months, have found no toxic effects of boswellic acids at high doses.[27,34] Pentacylic triterpene boswellic acids from *Boswellia serrata* Roxb. inhibited leukotriene B4 and C4 biosynthesis in intact PMNs.[28] Acetyl-11-keto-β-boswellic acid induced inhibition of 5-lipoxygenase product formation noncompetitively and reversibly.
- 1200 mg of boswellia resulted in plasma concentrations of 10-32 μM of 11-keto-β-boswellia acid and 18-20 μM acetyl-11-keto-β-boswellia acid, measured 2-3 hours following administration.[12]

HISTORY

- Boswellia traditionally has been used for numerous medicinal purposes, including skin disorders, infections, wound healing, and varicosities. In traditional Chinese medicine, powders and teas from boswellia were used to treat rheumatic diseases, menstrual disorders, and bruises. Cosmetically, it has been recommended as a facial toner and to smooth wrinkles.
- The use of boswellia dates back to ancient Egypt, where "olibanum" was used as an ingredient in embalming liquids for mummification. Boswellia historically has been utilized to improve emotional well-being and as a part of religious rituals. It has been reported to enhance spirituality, mental perception, meditation, prayer, and consciousness when burned (burning is said to produce a psychoactive substance, trans-hydrocannabinole).[6]
- Recent interest in the use of boswellia for inflammatory diseases such as arthritis, inflammatory bowel disease, and

asthma stems from scientific reports that boswellia inhibits leukotriene synthesis.

REVIEW OF THE EVIDENCE: DISCUSSION
Asthma (Chronic Therapy)
Summary

- Boswellia has been proposed as a potential asthma chronic therapy, based on its known properties as an inhibitor of leukotriene biosynthesis (a mechanism known to be involved with the progression of asthmatic bronchoconstriction). One randomized, controlled trial of good-quality in 80 subjects has demonstrated improvements in FEV_1 (forced expiratory volume in 1 second), FVC (forced vital capacity), number of asthma exacerbations, and wheezing, following 41 days of boswellia therapy.[13] However, baseline characteristics between patients in this study may not have been comparable. Nonetheless, the existing data provide good initial evidence

in favor of this use of boswellia. Future studies are warranted to assess the long-term efficacy and safety of boswellia, the temporality of effects, and the efficacy of boswellia vs. standard therapies. Boswellia should not be used for the relief of acute asthma exacerbations.

Evidence

- In a 6-week double-blind, placebo-controlled study, Gupta et al. examined the use of boswellia gum resin in 80 patients with bronchial asthma.[13] Subjects were randomized to receive either 300 mg of boswellia powdered gum resin capsules (S-compound) or 300 mg of lactose (as placebo), orally three times daily. Baseline patient characteristics were compared between groups. Overall, the boswellia group was older than the placebo group (mean age 37.7 years vs. 33.0 years), although this difference was not statistically significant. However, there were significant differences in

Review of the Evidence: Boswellia

Condition Treated*	Study Design	Author, Year	N[†]	SS[†]	Study Quality[‡]	Magnitude of Benefit	ARR[†]	NNT[†]	Comments
Asthma	Randomized, controlled	Gupta[13] 1998	80	Yes	4	Medium	NA	NA	70% showed improvement.
Crohn's disease	Randomized equivalence study, double-blind	Gerhardt[16] 2001	102	No	3	None	NA	NA	19% dropout; no difference between boswellia (H15) and mesalazine; unclear if equivalent, or inadequately powered to detect differences.
Osteoarthritis	Randomized controlled, crossover	Kulkarni[10] 1991	42	Yes	4	Large	NA	NA	Combination product used (Articulin-F); effects of boswellia alone not clear.
Osteoarthritis (knee)	Randomized, placebo-controlled, crossover	Kimmatkar[18] 2003	30	Yes	2	Medium	NA	NA	*Boswellia serrata* extract (BSE) associated with improved pain, flexion, walking distance after 8 weeks.
Rheumatoid arthritis	Randomized, controlled	Chopra[35] 2000	182	Yes	5	Small	NA	NA	Combination product used (RA-1); strong effect seen in placebo group.
Rheumatoid arthritis	Before and after comparison	Sander[9] 1998	37	No	3	NA	NA	NA	No improvement in pain with boswellia product H15, but no power calculation done.
Rheumatoid arthritis	Review of 11 unpublished studies	Etzel[8] 1996	>260	NA	NA	NA	NA	NA	Poorly described review with no numeric or statistical data; inclusion and exclusion criteria not noted.
Rheumatoid arthritis	Randomized, controlled, crossover	Kulkarni[11] 1992	20	Yes	3	Large	NA	NA	Combination product used (Articulin F); effects of boswellia alone not clear.
Ulcerative colitis	Non-randomized, open, equivalence study	Gupta[36] 2001	30	No	0	NA	NA	NA	Improved signs and symptoms with boswellia vs. baseline, but no difference from control (sulfasalazine); no placebo; methodologically weak.
Ulcerative colitis	Non-randomized, open, equivalence study	Gupta[12] 1997	42	No	0	NA	NA	NA	Improved signs and symptoms with boswellia vs. baseline, but no difference from control (sulfasalazine); no placebo; methodologically weak.

*Primary or secondary outcome.
[†] N, Number of patients; SS, statistically significant; ARR, absolute risk reduction; NNT, the number of patients who need to undergo a specific intervention in order to observe an outcome in one individual.
[‡] 0-2 = poor; 3-4 = good; 5 = excellent.
NA, Not applicable.
For an explanation of each category in this table, please see Table 3 in the Introduction.

quantitative baseline characteristics in the boswellia subjects vs. placebo, including a lower mean FEV_1 (1.6 L vs. 2.0 L), a lower FVC (1.9 L vs. 2.3 L), and a lower PEFR (peak expiratory flow rate) (244 L/minute vs. 306 L/ minute). Clinical and laboratory assessments were performed on days 1 and 42, and a log of asthma exacerbations was documented. Mean improvements were seen in both groups for multiple parameters, and improvements in the boswellia group were greater. The median improvement in FEV_1 was 25% in the boswellia group vs. 5% in placebo, the difference being statistically significant. However, it should be noted that the mean FEV_1 in the boswellia group was 20% lower than in the control group at baseline, and therefore at the study's end, the values for the two groups were nearly equivalent. The mean FVC improved by 21% in the boswellia group vs. 9% in the control group, with statistical significance. Again, however, there were significant differences in baseline values. Secondary effects such as reduced dyspnea and eosinophilia and absence of rhonchi after treatment, were also apparent in the boswellia group vs. placebo. In addition, the number of asthma exacerbations was significantly reduced in the boswellia group ($p < 0.0001$). Overall, these results are promising and have a basis in basic science studies that demonstrate boswellia to inhibit leukotriene biosynthesis (a mechanism known to be involved in the biochemical progression of asthmatic bronchoconstriction). The principal weakness of this study is the significant difference in baseline characteristics between groups, raising questions about appropriate randomization, and about whether the groups were comparable. Future studies should assess the long-term efficacy and safety of boswellia and the temporality of boswellia's effects and compare boswellia with standard therapies.

Crohn's Disease
Summary
• Boswellia has been noted in animal and *in vitro* studies to possess anti-inflammatory properties. Based on these observations, boswellia has been suggested as a potential treatment for Crohn's disease. However, limited human data exist, and there is inadequate evidence in favor of or against this use of boswellia.

Evidence
• Gerhardt et al. conducted an 8-week randomized, double-blind equivalence study using the *Boswellia serrata* standardized extract H15 or mesalazine in 102 patients with active Crohn's disease.[16] Three times daily, subjects were administered either 1200 mg of H15 or 1.5 g of mesalazine. The primary outcome measure used was the validated Crohn's Disease Activity Index (CDAI) which takes into account multiple signs and symptoms. At the end of 8 weeks, moderate improvements in CDAI scores were seen in both groups, with greater improvements in the H15 group. However, the difference in mean scores between groups was not statistically significant. Since no power calculation was conducted, it remains unclear if the lack of significance of results between groups is due to actual equivalence between therapies or to an inadequate sample size (although a sample size of 102 may have been adequate). Because there was no placebo group, the improvements in the H15 group vs. baseline cannot be discerned from the natural history of the disease. The procedures for blinding and randomization

were not described. Nineteen subjects (19%) dropped out of the study (6 in the boswellia group and 13 in the mesalazine group), and it is not clear that there was an intent-to-treat analysis. Although the improvements observed in the H15 group appear promising, due to the methodological weaknesses of this study the results cannot be considered clinically relevant. Further investigation is warranted in this area.

Osteoarthritis
Summary
• Boswellia has been noted in animal and *in vitro* studies to possess anti-inflammatory properties. Based on these observations, boswellia has been suggested as a potential treatment for osteoarthritis. To date, there is limited clinical evaluation of boswellia for this indication. Although promising results are reported, due to methodological problems with available data, no clear conclusion can be drawn.

Evidence
• Kulkarni et al. conducted a randomized, double-blind, placebo-controlled, crossover study in 42 patients with osteoarthritis.[10] Patients were randomized to receive either the combination product Articulin-F (2 capsules 3 times daily) or placebo for 3 months. Each tablet of Articulin-F contains extracts of 100 mg of *Boswellia serrata*, 450 mg of *Withania somnifera* (ashwagandha), 50 mg of *Curcuma longa* (turmeric), and 50 mg of zinc complex. Pain severity and disability scores were tabulated using validated instruments (Ritchie articular index, American Rheumatism Association joint score). At the study's end, treatment with Articulin-F was found to have significantly improved the mean pain severity score ($p < 0.001$) and mean disability score ($p < 0.05$). Other parameters such as morning stiffness, grip strength, and joint score also showed improvement, but without statistical significance. The lack of significance of these results may reflect an absence of true benefit or inadequate sample size to detect true benefits. Weaknesses of this study also include poor description of randomization and blinding methods and unclear diagnostic criteria by which patients were judged to have osteoarthritis (unclear inclusion criteria). As a result, the patient population may not have been uniform. The mixed statistical significance of results and the isolated nature of this study leave open the question of the efficacy of Articulin-F for osteoarthritis. Because Articulin-F is a combination product, no firm conclusions can be drawn regarding boswellia specifically.
• Kimmatkar et al. conducted a randomized, double-blind, placebo-controlled, crossover trial in 30 patients with osteoarthritis of the knee.[18] Subjects were administered either placebo or a formulation of *Boswellia serrata* extract (BSE) for 8 weeks, followed by a washout period and crossover for an additional 8 weeks. The authors reported statistically significant mean improvements in the BSE group compared to placebo in terms of pain, flexion, and walking distance. Although these results are promising, the descriptions of blinding, randomization, and statistical analysis were not well delineated, diminishing the quality of this publication overall. Better-quality study is necessary to confirm these findings.

Rheumatoid Arthritis
Summary
• Boswellia has been noted in animal and *in vitro* studies to possess anti-inflammatory properties. Based on these

observations, boswellia has been suggested as a potential treatment for rheumatoid arthritis (RA). Two methodologically weak publications have reported conflicting results for boswellia monotherapy. Two positive studies of combination products containing boswellia (RA-1 and Articulin-F) have not provided adequate data regarding the effects of boswellia alone. Therefore, there is currently insufficient evidence to recommend for or against the use of boswellia for rheumatoid arthritis.

Evidence (Boswellia Monotherapy)

- In a German double-blind, placebo-controlled, pilot study, a 37-patient single-center subset of 78 rheumatoid arthritis patients recruited for a multi-center trial were treated with the standardized boswellia extract H15.[9] For 12 weeks, a daily dose of 3600 mg of H15 or placebo was given to subjects, in addition to their baseline medications (NSAIDs and/or steroids). At the study's conclusion, a small, non–statistically significant reduction in the use of NSAIDs was observed in the boswellia group vs. placebo (5.8% vs. 3.1%). H15 was not found to be effective in reducing pain or improving function as measured by validated scales, and no differences in C-reactive protein were observed between groups. Because no power calculation was performed, it is not clear that the sample size of this study was adequate to discern true benefits. In addition, methods of randomization and blinding were not well described. Therefore, the results cannot be considered definitive.
- Etzel reported the cumulative findings of 11 unpublished studies conducted between 1985 and 1990, ranging from 1 to 6 months in duration, in which >260 patients with rheumatoid arthritis were treated with the standardized boswellia extract H15.[8] Results were tabulated for a total of 375 subjects, but apparently some of the described patients were the same individuals, assessed in different investigations. Study designs varied from direct observation (most common) to placebo-controlled and double-blind (although methodological details of each study were not provided in detail). The authors concluded that across investigations, H15 was not efficacious for the relief of acute pain but may improve chronic symptoms such as joint swelling and stiffness and may reduce NSAID intake. However, no numeric or statistical data were provided to support these assertions. Benefits were reported to be additive to other therapies, such as NSAIDs. Adverse effects were reported as being minimal. No statistical analysis was reported in this review. The primary data are not available for analysis, and the majority of evidence was derived from non-controlled studies. Therefore, no evidence-based conclusions can be drawn from this report.

Evidence (Combination Products That Include Boswellia)

- Equivocal results from a well-designed study were reported by Chopra et al.[35] The authors conducted a 16-week randomized, double-blind, placebo-controlled trial to assess the efficacy of the standardized combination product RA-1 in 182 patients with rheumatoid arthritis (RA). RA-1 is an herbal mixture of *Boswellia serrata*, *Withania somnifera* (Ashwagandha), *Zingiber officinale* (ginger), and *Curcuma longa* (turmeric). Subjects received 2 tablets three times daily (444 mg/day), and discontinued other RA therapies. Signs and symptoms associated with RA were assessed by validated instruments, taking into account joint tenderness, pain, swelling, stiffness, rheumatoid factor, C-reactive protein, and interleukin 6 (IL-6). Baseline patient characteristics in the two groups were comparable. An initial calculation was performed to assure at least 80% power (required total n ≥130), and result tabulation was designed as an intent-to-treat analysis. Seventeen patients withdrew, but none due to drug toxicity. Significant improvements over baseline were observed in both the RA-1 and placebo groups ($p < 0.001$). Although results for the RA-1 group were numerically superior to placebo across outcomes, these differences were not statistically significant except for three measures: (1) a slightly increased proportion of subjects with a 50% reduction in the number of swollen joints/swollen joint score; (2) reduced rheumatoid factor (30% reduction vs. 0%); and (3) a relative improvement in the ACR 20 (American College of Rheumatism) assessment score (39% vs. 30%). Although suggestive, these results cannot be applied to clinical practice because of their mixed statistical significance. It is not clear if the lack of significance for most results reflects a lack of benefit of RA-1 vs. placebo, or if the study was not adequately powered to detect differences. Although a power calculation was performed, because of large improvements in multiple parameters in the placebo group, true differences across categories may not have been detected with statistical significance. Notably, rheumatoid factor, a serologic marker which is less subject to a "placebo effect", did improve in the RA-1 group over placebo, although C-reactive protein did not. In addition, because this study examined a combination product, the relative contributions of each constituent are not clear, and the amounts of each may have been lower than in common monotherapy doses. The results remain equivocal, and may merit confirmation by additional studies.
- In a randomized, double-blind, placebo-controlled, crossover study, Kulkarni et al. studied the combination product Articulin-F in 20 patients with RA.[11] Each tablet of Articulin-F contains extracts of 100 mg of *Boswellia serrata*, 450 mg of *Withania somnifera* (ashwagandha), 50 mg of *Curcuma longa* (turmeric), and 50 mg of zinc complex. Treatment included Articulin-F (2 capsules, 3 times a day) or placebo for 3 months. All previous drugs were withdrawn 1 month prior to the study. Inclusion criteria for subjects included morning stiffness, joint swelling, pain severity, disability/loss of function, spells of remission, and serologically positive rheumatoid factor. Assessment was based on measures of stiffness and pain (by both validated [Ritchie articular index, American Rheumatism Association joint score] and non-validated scales), erythrocyte sedimentation rate (ESR), and rheumatoid factor. Treatment with Articulin-F was reported to moderately improve all measurements of pain, morning stiffness duration, grip strength, and disability score vs. placebo ($p < 0.001$). Benefits were noted after 2 weeks of therapy and persisted throughout the study. After 3 months, rheumatoid factor seroconversion (to seronegativity) occurred in 9 patients taking Articulin-F® and in none taking placebo. Nonsteroidal anti-inflammatory drugs were required to control symptoms in 3 patients taking Articulin-F vs. 18 taking placebo ($p < 0.05$). Overall, these results are promising, although procedures for randomization and blinding were not reported. As a result, bias and confounders may have been introduced that affected outcomes. To some extent, the crossover design would reduce the potential effects of confounders. Since a combination product was used, the isolated effects of boswellia cannot be assessed.

Ulcerative Colitis
Summary

- Boswellia has been noted in animal and *in vitro* studies to possess anti-inflammatory properties. Based on these observations, boswellia has been suggested as a potential treatment for ulcerative colitis. At this time, however, only a limited number of poor-quality human trials have evaluated this use of boswellia, with inconclusive results. Therefore, there is inadequate evidence for or against this use of boswellia.

- Gupta et al. conducted a poor-quality, open, non-randomized equivalence study in 30 patients with chronic colitis, in which subjects were administered either *Boswellia serrata* gum resin (S compound, manufactured in India) or sulfasalazine.[36] Subjects between the ages of 18 and 48 years were treated for 6 weeks with either boswellia, 900 mg daily in three divided doses (n = 20), or sulfasalazine, 3 g daily in three divided doses (n = 10). Measured outcomes included sigmoidoscopic examination, rectal biopsy histopathology, stool characteristics, and serum values (hemoglobin, iron, calcium, phosphorus, proteins, total leukocytes and eosinophils). These values were entered into a formula to determine a "remission rate," although the specifics of the formula and calculation were not adequately described. The authors noted that 18 of 20 boswellia patients entered "remission," vs. 6 of 10 in the sulfasalazine group, but the difference between groups was not statistically significant. Histologic improvement of biopsies was noted in 75% of boswellia subjects vs. 40% of sulfasalazine subjects, but, again, no statistically significant difference between groups was found. These results cannot be clinically interpreted. Although the authors report statistically significant improvements in the "remission rate" and biopsy histopathology of boswellia subjects vs. baseline, comparisons with controls were not statistically significant. Since no power calculation was conducted, it remains unclear if the lack of significance is due to actual equivalence between therapies or to an inadequate sample size. Because there was no placebo group, the improvements in the boswellia group vs. baseline cannot be discerned from the natural history of the disease. The lack of blinding introduces the possibility of bias, and lack of randomization affords an opportunity for confounding.

- In an earlier open, non-randomized trial, the same group of authors administered encapsulated powdered *Boswellia serrata* gum resin (350 mg three times daily) or sulfasalazine (1 g three times daily) for 6 weeks to 42 patients with ulcerative colitis.[12] Patients were allowed to select their choice of therapy: 34 chose boswellia and 8 chose sulfasalazine. Measured outcomes included symptoms improvement (abdominal pain, diarrhea), sigmoidoscopic examination, rectal biopsy histopathology, stool characteristics, and serum values (hemoglobin, iron, calcium, phosphorus, proteins, total leukocytes and eosinophils). These values were entered into a formula together to determine a "remission rate," although the specifics of the formula and calculation were not adequately described. The authors reported improved abdominal pain and diarrhea in all sulfasalazine patients, and in approximately 90% of boswellia patients, without statistical significance between groups. Histopathologic improvements were observed in approximately 75% of both boswellia and sulfasalazine patients, again without significant differences between groups. "Remission" occurred in 82.4% of boswellia patients and 75% of sulfasalazine patients with no significant differences between groups. Since no power calculation was

conducted, it remains unclear if the lack of significance of results between groups is due to actual equivalence between therapies or to an inadequate sample size. Because there was no placebo group, the improvements in the boswellia group vs. baseline cannot be discerned from the natural history of the disease. The lack of blinding or randomization, as well as allowing patients to choose their own therapies, increases the risk of bias or confounding. No firm conclusions can be drawn because of the methodological weaknesses of this study.

FORMULARY: BRANDS USED IN CLINICAL TRIALS

- Sallaki (India) and H15 (Switzerland) are standardized extracts of *Boswellia serrata*, marketed by M/S Gufic Ltd., India. This compound contains 11-keto-β-boswellic acid (1.8%), acetyl-11-keto-β-boswellic acid (1.4%), and acetyl-β-boswellic acid/β-boswellic acid (2 %).[12]
- S-compound is manufactured by Rahul Pharma, Jammu Tawi, India. This compound contains 11-keto-β-boswellic acid (0.63%), acetyl-11-keto-β-boswellic acid (0.7%), acetyl-β-boswellic acid/β-boswellic acid (1.5%).[13]
- RA-1 is a herbal mixture of *Boswellia serrata*, *Withania somnifera* (ashwagandha), *Zingiber officinale* (ginger), and *Curcuma longa* (turmeric).[35]
- Articulin-F is a herbomineral combination containing 100 mg of *Boswellia serrata*, 450 mg of *Withania somnifera* [ashwagandha], 50 mg of *Curcuma longa* [turmeric], and 50 mg of zinc complex.[10]

References

1. Menon MK, Kar A. Analgesic and psychopharmacological effects of the gum resin of *Boswellia serrata*. Planta Med 1971;19(4):333-341.
2. Gangwal ML, Vardhan DK. Antifungal studies of volatile constituents of *Boswellia serrata*. Asian J Chem 1995;7:675-676.
3. Ammon HP, Mack T, Singh GB, et al. Inhibition of leukotriene B4 formation in rat peritoneal neutrophils by an ethanolic extract of the gum resin exudate of *Boswellia serrata*. Planta Med 1991;57(3):203-207.
4. Safayhi H, Mack T, Sabieraj J, et al. Boswellic acids: novel, specific, nonredox inhibitors of 5-lipoxygenase. J Pharm Exper Ther 1992;261(3): 1143-1146.
5. Shao Y, Ho CT, Chin CK, et al. Inhibitory activity of boswellic acids from *Boswellia serrata* against human leukemia HL-60 cells in culture. Planta Med 1998;64(4):328-331.
6. Ammon HP. Salai Guggal—*Boswellia serrata*: from a herbal medicine to a non-redox inhibitor of leukotriene biosynthesis. Eur J Med Res 1996; 1(8):369-370.
7. Atal CK, Gupta OP, Singh GB. Salai guggal: a promising anti-arthritic and anti-hyperlipidemic agent. Proc BPS 1981;203P-204P.
8. Etzel R. Special extract of *Boswellia serrata* (H15) in the treatment of rheumatoid arthritis. Phytomed 1996;3(1):91-94.
9. Sander O, Herborn G, Rau R. [Is H15 (resin extract of *Boswellia serrata*, "incense") a useful supplement to established drug therapy of chronic polyarthritis? Results of a double-blind pilot study.] Z Rheumatol 1998; 57(1):11-16.
10. Kulkarni RR, Patki PS, Jog VP, et al. Treatment of osteoarthritis with a herbomineral formulation: a double-blind, placebo-controlled, cross-over study. J Ethnopharm 1991;33(1-2):91-95.
11. Kulkarni RR, Patki PS, Jog VP, et al. Efficacy of an Ayurvedic formulation in rheumatoid arthritis: a double-blind, placebo-controlled, cross-over study. Indian J Pharm 1992;24:98-101.
12. Gupta I, Parihar A, Malhotra P, et al. Effects of *Boswellia serrata* gum resin in patients with ulcerative colitis. Eur J Med Res 1997;2(1):37-43.
13. Gupta I, Gupta V, Parihar A, et al. Effects of *Boswellia serrata* gum resin in patients with bronchial asthma: results of a double-blind, placebo-controlled, 6-week clinical study. Eur J Med Res 1998;3(11):511-514.
14. Kamboj VP. A review of Indian medicinal plants with interceptive activity. Indian J Med Res 1988;87:336-355.
15. Singh GB, Bani S, Singh S. Toxicity and safety evaluation of boswellic acids. Phytomed 1996;3(1):87-90.
16. Gerhardt H, Seifert F, Buvari P, et al. [Therapy of active Crohn disease with *Boswellia serrata* extract H 15]. Z Gastroenterol 2001;39(1):11-17.
17. Singh GB, Atal CK. Pharmacology of an extract of salai guggal ex-*Boswellia serrata*, a new non-steroidal anti-inflammatory agent. Agents Actions 1986;18(3-4):407-412.
18. Kimmatkar N, Thawani V, Hingorani L, et al. Efficacy and tolerability of

Boswellia serrata extract in treatment of osteoarthritis of knee—A randomized double blind placebo controlled trial. Phytomedicine 2003;10(1):3-7.

19. Safayhi H, Sailer ER, Amnon HP. 5-lipoxygenase inhibition by acetyl-11-keto-beta-boswellic acid (AKBA) by a novel mechanism. Phytomed 1996; 3(1):71-72.

20. Jing Y, Nakajo S, Xia L, et al. Boswellic acid acetate induces differentiation and apoptosis in leukemia cell lines. Leuk.Res 1999;23(1):43-50.

21. Reddy GK, Chandrakasan G, Dhar SC. Studies on the metabolism of glycosaminoglycans under the influence of new herbal anti-inflammatory agents. Biochem Pharmacol 1989;38(20):3527-3534.

22. Ammon HP. [Boswellic acids (components of frankincense) as the active principle in treatment of chronic inflammatory diseases.] Wien Med Wochenschr 2002;152(15-16):373-378.

23. Ammon HP, Safayhi H, Mack T, et al. Mechanism of antiinflammatory actions of curcumine and boswellic acids. J Ethnopharmacol. 1993;38(2-3): 113-119.

24. Buchele B, Simmet T. Analysis of 12 different pentacyclic triterpenic acids from frankincense in human plasma by high-performance liquid chromatography and photodiode array detection. J Chromatogr B Analyt Technol Biomed Life Sci 2003;795(2):355-362.

25. Buchele B, Zugmaier W, Simmet T. Analysis of pentacyclic triterpenic acids from frankincense gum resins and related phytopharmaceuticals by high-performance liquid chromatography. Identification of lupeolic acid, a novel pentacyclic triterpene. J Chromatogr B Analyt Technol Biomed Life Sci 2003;791(1-2):21-30.

26. Knaus U, Wagner H. Effects of Boswellic acid of *Boswellia serrata* and other triterpenic acids on the Complement System. Phytomedicine 1996;3(1): 77-80.

27. Singh GB, Singh S, Bani S. Anti-inflammatory actions of boswellic acids. Phytomed 1996;3(1):81-85.

28. Wildfeuer A, Neu IS, Safayhi H, et al. Effects of boswellic acids extracted from a herbal medicine on the biosynthesis of leukotrienes and the course of experimental autoimmune encephalomyelitis. Arzneimittelforschung 1998; 48(6):668-674.

29. Sharma ML, Bani S, Singh GB. Anti-arthritic activity of boswellic acids in bovine serum albumin (BSA)-induced arthritis. Int J Immunopharmacol. 1989;11(6):647-652.

30. Sharma ML, Khajuria A, Kaul A, et al. Effect of salai guggal ex-*Boswellia serrata* on cellular and humoral immune responses and leucocyte migration. Agents Actions 1988;24(1-2):161-164.

31. Sharma ML, Kaul A, Khajuria A, et al. Immunomodulatory activity of Boswellic acids (pentacyclic triterpene acids) from Boswellia serrata. Phytother Res 1996;10:107-112.

32. Kesava RG, Dhar SC. Effect of a new non-steroidal anti-inflammatory agent on lysosomal stability in adjuvant induced arthritis. Ital J Biochem 1987; 36(4):205-217.

33. Kesava RG, Dhar SC, Singh GB. Urinary excretion of connective tissue metabolites under the influence of a new non-steroidal anti-inflammatory agent in adjuvant induced arthritis. Agents Actions 1987;22(1-2):99-105.

34. Singh GB, Singh S, Bani S. Alcoholic extract of salai-guggal ex-*Boswellia serrata*, a new natural source NSAID. Drugs Today 1996;32(2):109-112.

35. Chopra A, Lavin P, Patwardhan B, et al. Randomized double blind trial of an ayurvedic plant derived formulation for treatment of rheumatoid arthritis. J Rheumatol 2000;27(6):1365-1372.

36. Gupta I, Parihar A, Malhotra P, et al. Effects of gum resin of *Boswellia serrata* in patients with chronic colitis. Planta Med 2001;67(5):391-395.

Bromelain
(Ananas comosus)

SYNONYMS/COMMON NAMES/RELATED SUBSTANCES

- *Ananas sativus*, Ananase, bromeline, bromelainum, Bromeliaceae bromelin, pineapple extract, plant protease concentrate, Traumanase.

CLINICAL BOTTOM LINE

Background

- Bromelain is a digestive enzyme that is extracted from the stem and fruit of the pineapple.

Uses Based on Scientific Evidence	Grade*
Inflammation Several preliminary studies suggest that bromelain, when taken by mouth, can reduce inflammation or pain caused by inflammation. Better-quality studies are needed to confirm these results.	B
Sinusitis It has been proposed that bromelain may be a useful addition to other therapies used for sinusitis (such as antibiotics) because of its ability to reduce inflammation and swelling. Studies report mixed results, although overall bromelain appears to be beneficial for reducing swelling and improving breathing. Better-quality studies are needed before a strong recommendation can be made.	B
Cancer Scientific evidence is insufficient to recommend for or against the use of bromelain in the treatment of cancer, whether it is used alone or in addition to other therapies.	C
Chronic obstructive pulmonary disease (COPD) There is not enough information to recommend for or against the use of bromelain in COPD.	C
Digestive enzyme/pancreatic insufficiency Bromelain is an enzyme with the ability to digest proteins. However, there have been few reliable research studies on whether bromelain is helpful as a digestive aid. Better-quality and more extensive studies are needed before a firm conclusion can be made.	C
Nutrition supplementation Scientific evidence is insufficient to recommend for or against the use of bromelain as a nutritional supplement.	C
Rheumatoid arthritis (RA) There is not enough information to recommend for or against the use of bromelain in rheumatoid arthritis (RA). Notably, most studies and case reports in this area have been published by the same authors.	C
Steatorrhea (fatty stools due to poor digestion) There is not enough information to recommend for or against the use of bromelain in the treatment of steatorrhea.	C
Urinary tract infection (UTI) There is not enough information to recommend for or against the use of bromelain in urinary tract infections.	C

*Key to grades: *A:* Strong scientific evidence for this use; *B:* Good scientific evidence for this use; *C:* Unclear scientific evidence for this use; *D:* Fair scientific evidence against this use (it may not work); *F:* Strong scientific evidence against this use (it likely does not work). For a more detailed explanation of efficacy criteria, see "Natural Standard Evidence-Based Validated Grading Rationale" in the Introduction.

Historical or Theoretical Indications That Lack Sufficient Evidence
Acquired immunodeficiency syndrome (AIDS), allergic rhinitis (hay fever), amyloidosis, angina, antibiotic absorption problems in the gut, appetite suppressant, atherosclerosis ("hardening of the arteries"), autoimmune disorders, back pain, blood clot treatment, bronchitis, bruises, burn and wound care, bursitis, cancer prevention, carpal tunnel syndrome, cellulitis/skin infections, colitis, common cold, cough, diarrhea, epididymitis, episiotomy pain (after childbirth), food allergies, food lodged in the esophagus, frostbite, gout, heart disease, hemorrhoids, immune system regulation, indigestion, infections, injuries, joint disease, "leaky gut" syndrome, menstrual pain, pain (general), pancreatic problems with food digestion, Peyronie's disease (abnormal curvature, pain, and scar tissue in the penis), platelet inhibition (blood thinner), pneumonia, poor absorption of digested food, poor blood circulation in the legs, upper respiratory tract infection, sciatica, scleroderma, shingles pain/postherpetic neuralgia, shortening of labor, smooth muscle relaxation, sports-related or other physical injuries, staphylococcal bacterial infections, stimulation of muscle contractions, stomach ulcer prevention, swelling after surgery or injury, tendonitis, thick mucus, thrombophlebitis, treatment of scar tissue, ulcerative colitis, varicose veins, wound healing.

DOSING/TOXICOLOGY

The following doses are based on scientific research, publications, traditional use, or expert opinion. Many herbs and supplements have not been thoroughly tested, and their safety and effectiveness may not be proven. Brands may be made differently, with variable ingredients even within the same brand. The doses shown may not apply to all products. It is important to always read product labels and discuss doses with a qualified healthcare provider before therapy is started.

Standardization

- Standardization involves measuring the amounts of certain chemicals in products to try to make different preparations similar to each other. It is not always known if the chemicals being measured are the "active" ingredients. Bromelain may be standardized to milk clotting units (MCU), gelatin digesting units (GDU), FIP units, or Rorer units (RU) per gram. The MCU is officially recognized by the Food Chemistry Codex. Some experts recommend using bromelain standardized to contain at least 2000 MCU per gram, whereas other sources recommend a range of 1200 to 1800 MCU per gram.

Adults (18 Years and Older)

- **Oral (by mouth):** A variety of doses have been used and studied. Research studies in the 1960s and 1970s used 120 to 240 mg of bromelain concentrate tablets daily (Traumanase or Ananase; 2500 RU per mg) in three or four divided doses for up to 1 week to treat inflammation. The German expert panel (Commission E) has recommended 80 to 320 mg (200 to 800 FIP units) taken two to three times daily. Some authors recommend 500 to 1000 mg of bromelain to be taken three times daily, and many manufacturers sell products standardized to 2000 GDU in 500-mg tablets. The effects of bromelain may occur at lower doses, and treatment may be started at a low dose and increased as needed.
- **Topical (applied to the skin):** Cream containing 35% bromelain in an oil-containing base has been used to clean wounds.

Children (Younger Than 18 Years)

- Scientific research evidence is insufficient to recommend the safe use of bromelain in children.

SAFETY

The U.S. Food and Drug Administration does not strictly regulate herbs and supplements. There is no guarantee of the strength, purity, or safety of products, and effects may vary. It is important to always read product labels. People who have a medical condition, or are taking other drugs, herbs, or supplements, should consult a qualified healthcare provider before starting a new therapy. A healthcare provider should be contacted immediately about any side effects.

Allergies

- There have been multiple reports of allergic and asthmatic reactions to bromelain products, including throat swelling and difficulty breathing. Allergic reactions to bromelain may occur in people who are allergic to pineapples or other members of the Bromeliaceae family, and in those who are sensitive or allergic to birch pollen, carrot, celery, cypress pollen, fennel, grass pollen, honeybee venom, latex, papain, rye flour, or wheat flour.

Side Effects and Warnings

- Few serious side effects have been reported with the use of bromelain at daily doses up to 10 g for each kilogram (2.2 pounds) of body weight. The most common side effects reported are stomach upset and diarrhea. Other reactions include increased heart rate, nausea, vomiting, irritation of mucous membranes, and menstrual problems.
- In theory, bromelain may increase the risk of bleeding. Caution is advised in people who have bleeding disorders or are taking drugs that increase the risk of bleeding. Dosing adjustments may be necessary. Bromelain should be used with caution in people with stomach ulcers, active bleeding, or a history of bleeding, in those who are taking medications that thin the blood or who are going to have certain dental or surgical procedures.
- Higher doses of bromelain may increase the heart rate, and it should be used cautiously in people with heart disease. Some experts warn against bromelain use by people with liver or kidney disease, although there is limited scientific information in this area. Bromelain may cause abnormal uterine bleeding or heavy/prolonged menstruation.

Pregnancy and Breastfeeding

- Bromelain is not recommended during pregnancy or when a woman is breastfeeding because information about its safety is limited.

INTERACTIONS

Most herbs and supplements have not been thoroughly tested for interactions with other herbs, supplements, drugs, or foods. The interactions listed here are based on reports in scientific publications, laboratory experiments, or traditional use. It is important to always read product labels. People who have a medical condition, or are taking other drugs, herbs, or supplements, should consult a qualified healthcare provider before starting a new therapy.

Interactions with Drugs

- In theory, bromelain may increase the risk of bleeding when taken with drugs that increase the risk of bleeding. Examples are anticoagulants (blood thinners) such as warfarin (Coumadin) and heparin, antiplatelet drugs such as clopidogrel (Plavix), aspirin, and nonsteroidal anti-inflammatory drugs (NSAIDs) such as ibuprofen (Motrin, Advil) and naproxen (Naprosyn, Aleve). In addition, bromelain theoretically may add to the anti-inflammatory effects of NSAIDs.
- Studies in humans suggest that bromelain may increase the absorption of some antibiotics, notably amoxicillin and tetracycline, and increase levels of these drugs in the body. Bromelain may increase the actions of the chemotherapy (anti-cancer) drugs 5-fluorouracil and vincristine, although reliable scientific research in this area is lacking. In theory, the use of bromelain with blood pressure medications in the "ACE inhibitor" class, such as captopril (Capoten) and lisinopril (Zestril), may cause larger decreases in blood pressure than expected.
- Some experts suggest that bromelain may cause drowsiness or sedation and may increase the amount of drowsiness caused by some drugs. Examples are alcohol, some antidepressants, barbiturates such as phenobarbital, benzodiazepines such as lorazepam (Ativan) and diazepam (Valium), and narcotics such as codeine. Caution is advised in people who are driving or operating machinery.

Interactions with Herbs and Dietary Supplements

- In theory, bromelain may increase the risk of bleeding when taken with herbs and supplements that are believed to increase the risk of bleeding. Multiple cases of bleeding have been reported with the use of *Ginkgo biloba*, and fewer cases with garlic and with saw palmetto. Numerous other agents may theoretically increase the risk of bleeding, although this has not been proven in most cases. Examples are alfalfa, American ginseng, angelica, anise, *Arnica montana*, asafetida, aspen bark, bilberry, birch, black cohosh, bladderwrack, bogbean, boldo, borage seed oil, capsicum, cat's claw, celery, chamomile, chaparral, clove, coleus, cordyceps, danshen, devil's claw, dong quai, eicosapentaenoic acid (EPA), evening primrose, fenugreek, feverfew, fish oil, flaxseed/flax powder (not a concern with flaxseed oil), ginger, grapefruit juice, grapeseed, green tea, guggul, gymnestra, horse chestnut, horseradish, licorice root, lovage root, male fern, meadowsweet, nordihydroguaiaretic acid (NDGA), onion, *Panax ginseng*, papain, parsley, passion flower, poplar, prickly ash, propolis, quassia, red clover, reishi, rue, Siberian ginseng, sweet birch, sweet clover, turmeric, vitamin E, white willow, wild carrot, wild lettuce, willow, wintergreen, and yucca.

- Based on preliminary studies in animals, bromelain and the enzyme trypsin may have stronger anti-inflammatory effects when combined. It has been suggested that zinc may block the effects of bromelain in the body, whereas magnesium may increase the effects, although scientific research in this area is lacking.

Interactions with Foods

- Some studies suggest that potato protein and soybeans may reduce the effects of bromelain in the body. Some experts recommend taking bromelain on an empty stomach.

Selected References

Natural Standard developed the preceding evidence-based information based on a systematic review of more than 250 scientific articles. For comprehensive information about alternative and complementary therapies on the professional level, go to www.naturalstandard.com. Selected references are listed here.

Balakrishnan V, Hareendran A, Nair CS. Double-blind cross-over trial of an enzyme preparation in pancreatic steatorrhoea. J Assoc Phys India 1981; 29(3):207-209.

Cirelli MG. Five years of clinical experience with bromelains in therapy of edema and inflammation in postoperative tissue reaction, skin infections and trauma. Clin Med 1967;74(6):55-59.

Cohen A, Goldman J. Bromelains therapy in rheumatoid arthritis. Penn Med J 1964;67:27-30.

Cowie DH, Fairweather DV, Newell DJ. A double-blind trial of bromelains as an adjunct to vaginal plastic repair operations. J Obstet Gynaecol Br Commonw 1970;77(4):365-368.

Gerard G. [Anticancer treatment and bromelains.] Agressologie 1972;13(4): 261-274.

Glade MJ, Kendra D, Kaminski MV. Improvement in protein utilization in nursing-home patients on tube feeding supplemented with an enzyme product derived from *Aspergillus niger* and Bromelain. Nutrition 2001;17(4):348-350.

Gylling U, Rintala A, Taipale S, et al. The effect of a proteolytic enzyme combinate (bromelain) on the postoperative oedema by oral application. A clinical and experimental study. Acta Chir Scand 1966;131(3):193-196.

Hotz G, Frank T, Zoller J, et al. [Antiphlogistic effect of bromelaine following third molar removal.] Dtsch Zahnärztl Z 1989;44(11):830-832.

Howat RC, Lewis GD. The effect of bromelain therapy on episiotomy wounds—a double blind controlled clinical trial. J Obstet Gynaecol Br Commonw 1972; 79(10):951-953.

Hunter RG, Henry GW, Civin WH. The action of papain and bromelain on the uterus. Part III. The physiologically incompetent internal cervical os. Am J Obst Gynec 1957;73(4):875-880.

Korlof B, Ponten B, Ugland O. Bromelain—a proteolytic enzyme. Scand J Plast Reconstr Surg 1969;3(1):27-29.

Kugener H, Bergmann D, Beck K. [Efficacy of bromelain in pancreatogenic digestive insufficiency.] Zeitschrift fur Gastroenterologie 1968;6:430-433.

Mader H. [Comparative studies on the effect of bromelin and oxyphenbutazone in episiotomy pains.] Schweiz Rundsch Med Prax 1973;62(35):1064-1068.

Masson M. [Bromelain in blunt injuries of the locomotor system. A study of observed applications in general practice.] Fortschr Med 1995;113(19): 303-306.

Miller JM, Ginsberg M, McElfatrick GC, et al. The administration of bromelain orally in the treatment of inflammation and edema. Exper Med Surg 1964;22: 293-299.

Mori S, Ojima Y, Hirose T, et al. The clinical effect of proteolytic enzyme containing bromelain and trypsin on urinary tract infection evaluated by double blind method. Acta Obstet Gynaecol Jpn 1972;19(3):147-153.

Morrison AW, Morrison MC. Bromelain—a clinical assessment in the postoperative treatment of arthrotomies of the knee and facial injuries. Brit J Clin Pract 1965;19(4):207-210.

Mudrak J, Bobak L, Sebova I. Adjuvant therapy with hydrolytic enzymes in recurrent laryngeal papillomatosis. Acta Otolaryngol Suppl 1997;527: 128-130.

Ryan RE. A double-blind clinical evaluation of bromelains in the treatment of acute sinusitis. Headache 1967;7(1):13-17.

Seligman B. Bromelain: an anti-inflammatory agent. Angiology 1962;13:508-510.

Seligman B. Oral bromelains as adjuncts in the treatment of acute thrombophlebitis. Angiology 1969;20(1):22-26.

Seltzer AP. Adjunctive use of bromelains in sinusitis: a controlled study. Eye Ear Nose Throat Mon 1967;46(10):1281, 1284, 1286-1288.

Spaeth GL. The effect of bromelains on the inflammatory response caused by cataract extraction: a double-blind study. Eye Ear Nose Throat Mon 1968; 47(12):634-639.

Stange R, Schneider R, Maurer R, et al. Proteolytic enzyme bromelaine enhances zytotoxicity in patients with breast cancer [abstract]. Nat Scien Conf Compl Altern Integ Med Res, Boston, April 12-14, 2002.

Tassman GC, Zafran JN, Zayon GM. A double-blind crossover study of a plant proteolytic enzyme in oral surgery. J Dent Med 1965;20(2):51-54.

Tassman GC, Zafran JN, Zayon GM. Evaluation of a plant proteolytic enzyme for the control of inflammation and pain. J Dental Med 1964;19(2):73-77.

Taub SJ. The use of bromelains in sinusitis: a double-blind clinical evaluation. Eye Ear Nose Throat Mon 1967;46(3):361.

Weiss S, Scherrer M. [Crossed double-blind trial of potassium iodide and bromelain (Traumanase) in chronic bronchitis.] Schweiz Rundsch Med Prax 1972;61(43):1331-1333.

Zatuchni GI, Colombi DJ. Bromelains therapy for the prevention of episiotomy pain. Obstet Gynecol 1967;29(2):275-278.

Burdock
(Arctium lappa)

SYNONYMS/COMMON NAMES/RELATED SUBSTANCES

- Akujitsu, anthraxivore, arctii, *Arctium minus*, *Arctium tomentosa*, bardana, bardanae radix, bardane, bardane grande, beggar's buttons, burdock root, burr, burr seed, chin, clotburr, clotbur, cocklebur, cockle button, cocklebuttons, cuckold, daiki kishi, edible burdock, fox's clote, grass burdock, great bur, great burdock, great burdocks, gobo (Japanese), grosse klette (German), happy major, hardock, hare burr, hurrburr, kletterwurzel (German), lampazo (Spanish), lappola, love leaves, niu bang zi, oil of lappa, personata, Philanthropium, thorny burr, turkey burrseed, woo-bang-ja, wild gobo.

CLINICAL BOTTOM LINE
Background

- Burdock historically has been used to treat a wide variety of ailments, including arthritis, diabetes, and hair loss. It is a principal herbal ingredient in the popular cancer remedies Essiac (rhubarb, sorrel, slippery elm) and Hoxsey formula (red clover, poke, prickly ash, bloodroot, barberry).
- Burdock fruit has been found to cause hypoglycemia in animals, and preliminary human studies have examined the efficacy of burdock root in diabetes. *In vitro* and animal studies have explored the use of burdock for bacterial infections, cancer, HIV, and nephrolithiasis. However, there is currently insufficient human evidence regarding the efficacy of burdock for any indication.

Scientific Evidence for Common/Studied Uses	Grade*
Diabetes	C

*Key to grades: A: Strong scientific evidence for this use; B: Good scientific evidence for this use; C: Unclear scientific evidence for this use; D: Fair scientific evidence against this use (it may not work); F: Strong scientific evidence against this use (it likely does not work). For a more detailed explanation of efficacy criteria, see "Natural Standard Evidence-Based Validated Grading Rationale" in the Introduction.

Historical or Theoretical Indications That Lack Sufficient Evidence

- Abscesses, acne, analgesia, anorexia nervosa, aphrodisiac, arthritis, bacterial infections, bladder disorders, boils, burns, cancer, canker sores, catarrh, common cold, cosmetic uses, cough, cystitis, dandruff, detoxification, diaphoretic, diuretic, eczema, fever, fluid retention, fungal infections, gout, gonorrhea, hair loss (baldness), hair tonic, headache, hemorrhoids, hepatoprotection,[1,2] hives, HIV infection,[3,4] impotence, inflammation, ichthyosis, kidney disease, laxative, lice, lumbar pain, measles, nephrolithiasis, pimples, pleurisy, pneumonia, psoriasis, respiratory infections, rheumatoid arthritis, ringworm, sciatica, scurvy, scrapes, seborrhea (sebaceous gland overactivity), skin disorders, skin moisturizer, sores, sterility, syphilis, tonsillitis, upper respiratory tract infections, urinary tract infections, urolithiasis, venereal diseases, warts, wound healing.

Expert Opinion and Folkloric Precedent

- Burdock is believed to exhibit a range of healing properties when used orally or topically. There is no consensus on what are the active constituents. Burdock has been used to treat diabetes and is an ingredient of two anticancer combination therapies: Essiac (also contains rhubarb, sorrel, slippery elm), and Hoxsey formula (also contains red clover, poke, prickly ash, bloodroot, barberry).

Safety Summary

- **Likely safe:** Burdock is generally regarded as safe for oral or topical use in recommended amounts. It is consumed as a vegetable in Japan and is used in sukiyaki, with no reports of toxicity found in literature review. Toxicity has not been systematically studied.
- **Possibly unsafe:** There are rare reports of contact dermatitis associated with burdock.[5] Burdock is considered unsafe in pregnancy/lactation, based on its oxytocic and uterine stimulatory effects in animals. There is insufficient pediatric safety information. Reports of hypoglycemia in rats may warrant caution in diabetics.
- **Likely unsafe:** Burdock root tea has been associated with atropine poisoning as a result of adulteration with belladonna root or deadly nightshade.[6,7] The roots of these plants closely resemble each other, and confusion occasionally occurs during harvesting. Eye trauma has occurred from the plant's needles becoming embedded in palpebral conjunctiva and causing linear corneal scratch marks.[8]

DOSING/TOXICOLOGY
General

- Recommended doses are based on historical practice and published reports. However, with natural products, the optimal doses needed to balance efficacy and safety often have not been determined. Formulations and preparation methods may vary from manufacturer to manufacturer, and from batch to batch of a specific product made by a single manufacturer. Because often the active components of a product are not known, standardization may not be possible, and the clinical effects of different brands may not be comparable.

Standardization

- There is no widely accepted standardization for burdock products.

Dosing: Adult (18 Years and Older)
Oral

- **Dried root:** 2 to 6 g of pure dried root daily, or 2 to 6 g of dried root in the form of a decoction three times daily.
- **Tablets/capsules:** Burdock is available as 425- to 475-mg capsules.
- **Decoction (1:20):** 500 mL daily.
- **Tincture:** 8 to 12 mL (1:5) three times daily, or 2 to 8 mL (1:10 in 25% alcohol) three times daily, or 0.25 to 1 teaspoon (1:10 in 45% alcohol) up to three times daily. (*Note:* 1 teaspoon = 4 to 5 mL.)
- **Fluid extract (1:1 in 25% alcohol):** 2 to 8 mL three times daily. (*Note:* 1 teaspoon = 4 to 5 mL.)

- **Root tea:** 2 to 6 g of dried burdock root in 500 mL of water three times daily, or 1 cup three or four times daily, or 1 teaspoon of dried burdock root boiled in 3 cups of water for 30 minutes, up to 3 cups daily.
- **Seeds:** Burdock has been used as a diuretic, with preparations made from powdered burdock seeds yielding a yellow, bland fixed product called oil of lappa. Human studies are lacking.

Topical

- Burdock is used topically for eczema, psoriasis, baldness, and warts and may be used as a compress or plaster.

Dosing: Pediatric (Younger Than 18 Years)

- Insufficient available data.

Toxicology

- Burdock, like other herbal products, carries the potential for contamination with other herbs, pesticides, heavy metals, and pharmaceuticals. This is particularly concerning with imports from developing countries. There have been reports of acute anticholinergic reactions following consumption of burdock products.[6-9] These cases are believed to be due to contamination with belladonna alkaloids, which resemble burdock during harvesting. Burdock itself has not been found to contain atropine or other constituents that would be responsible for these reactions.
- A rat study found no toxicity or carcinogenicity following 120 days of a diet containing burdock and other plants.[10]
- Tannins present in burdock are potentially toxic. Tannins are phenolic compounds that can induce stomach upset, and in high concentrations they may cause nephrotoxicity or hepatic necrosis. Long-term use may increase the risk of nasopharyngeal or esophageal cancer. Literature review reveals no documented human cases.

ADVERSE EFFECTS/PRECAUTIONS/CONTRAINDICATIONS
Allergy

- Anaphylaxis after consuming burdock has been reported in a 53-year-old Japanese man, with a history of urticaria that occurred multiple times after consuming boiled burdock with carrot, curry, and rice.[11] The patient presented with all-over body erythema, dyspnea, hypotension, and stridor 1 hour after eating boiled burdock. He recovered following subcutaneous injection of epinephrine and intravenous steroids. A skin prick evaluation was subsequently performed (Prick-Lancetter, Sweden), revealing hypersensitivity to raw and boiled burdock and carrot.
- Contact dermatitis associated with burdock has also been reported.[5]
- Sensitivity to burdock may occur in individuals with allergy to members of the Asteraceae/Compositae family, including ragweed, chrysanthemums, marigolds, and daisies.

Adverse Effects

- **General:** Oral use of burdock is generally believed to be safe, although reports of hypoglycemia in rats may warrant caution in diabetics. Handling the plant or using topical preparations has occasionally been associated with contact dermatitis.
- **Dermatologic:** Allergic dermatitis has been associated with the use of burdock plasters in several case reports.[5] Two men and a 14-year-old girl developed erythematous, vesicular,

pruritic, exudative reactions in areas corresponding to the application of burdock root plasters.[5] Reactions occurred up to 7 days after initial use. Patch testing was positive for burdock sensitivity in all three patients, and was nonreactive in matched controls.

- **Neurologic/CNS:** Anticholinergic effects have been observed in HIV patients taking burdock root and are believed to be due to contamination with belladonna alkaloids.[3] Multiple other reports of anticholinergic reactions have been reported following consumption of burdock products.[6-9] Contamination with belladonna may occur during harvesting, because of its close resemblance to burdock. Burdock itself has not been found to contain atropine or other constituents that would be responsible for these reactions.
- **Cardiovascular:** Atropine-like (anticholinergic) reactions such as bradycardia have been reported following consumption of burdock products.[6-9] These cases are believed to be due to contamination with belladonna alkaloids, which resemble burdock during harvesting. Burdock itself has not been found to contain atropine or other constituents that would be responsible for these reactions.
- **Ocular/otic:** Exposure to common burdock in nature carries a risk of eye trauma from the plant's needles, which have been reported to become embedded in the palpebral conjunctiva and produce characteristic random linear corneal scratch marks.[8]
- **Renal:** Diuretic effects have been associated with oral burdock use in HIV patients.[3] Additional supporting data are lacking.
- **Endocrine:** Estrogenic effects have been associated with oral burdock use in HIV patients.[3] Burdock fruit extracts have demonstrated hypoglycemic activity in rats[12] and may lower blood glucose levels in humans.[13-15] Although mice with streptozotocin-induced diabetes given burdock paradoxically experienced hyperglycemia,[16] the mechanism of burdock's effects on serum glucose is not clear, and the clinical relevance of this conflicting report is uncertain.

Precautions/Warnings/Contraindications

- Avoid in pregnancy, especially during the first trimester, because of the presence of anthraquinone glycosides in burdock root, and oxytocic and uterine stimulant activities observed in animals.[17]
- Use cautiously in patients with diabetes or glucose intolerance, because of reports of hypoglycemia in animal studies.
- Use cautiously in patients taking diuretics, with electrolyte imbalances, or with dehydration, because of diuretic effects of burdock observed in one study.
- Monitor patients for anticholinergic effects, because of possible contamination of burdock preparations with belladonna alkaloids.

Pregnancy and Lactation

- Traditionally, burdock has been avoided during pregnancy and lactation, especially during the first trimester, because of the presence of anthraquinone glycosides in burdock root, and oxytocic and uterine stimulant activities observed in animals.[17]

INTERACTIONS
Burdock/Drug Interactions

- **Insulin and oral hypoglycemic agents:** Burdock fruit extracts have demonstrated hypoglycemic activity in rats[12] and may lower blood glucose levels in humans.[13-15] Concomitant use with insulin or oral hypoglycemic agents may additively reduce blood glucose levels, and doses may require adjustment.

- **Diuretic agents:** Oral burdock use has been associated with diuretic effects in HIV patients[13] and may act additively when used concomitantly with diuretic agents. Evidence is limited.
- **Estrogens:** Oral burdock use has been associated with estrogenic effects in HIV patients[13] and may act additively with estrogens. Evidence is limited.
- **Antiplatelet agents:** Lignans in burdock have been found to inhibit binding of platelet-activating factor (PAF) to platelets in rabbits[18] and theoretically may act additively with other anti-platelet agents. Human data are limited.
- **General:** Some tinctures contain high concentrations of ethanol, and may lead to vomiting if used concomitantly with disulfiram (Antabuse) or metronidazole (Flagyl).

Burdock/Herb/Supplement Interactions

- **Hypoglycemic agents:** Burdock fruit extracts have demonstrated hypoglycemic activity in rats,[12] and may lower blood glucose levels in humans.[13-15] Concomitant use with other hypoglycemic agents may additively reduce blood glucose levels, and doses may require adjustment.
- **Diuretic agents:** Oral burdock use has been associated with diuretic effects in HIV patients[3] and may act additively when used concomitantly with diuretic agents. Evidence is limited.
- **Phytoestrogens:** Oral burdock use has been associated with estrogenic effects in HIV patients[3] and may act additively with estrogenic herbs or supplements. Evidence is limited.
- **Antiplatelet agents:** Lignans in burdock have been found to inhibit binding of platelet-activating factor (PAF) to platelets in rabbits[18] and theoretically may act additively with other anti-platelet agents. Human data are limited.

Burdock/Food Interactions

- Insufficient available data.

Burdock/Lab Interactions

- **Serum glucose:** Burdock fruit extracts have demonstrated hypoglycemic activity in rats[12] and may lower blood glucose levels in humans.[13-15] Although mice with streptozotocin-induced diabetes given burdock paradoxically experienced hyperglycemia, the mechanism of burdock's effects on serum glucose is not clear,[16] and the clinical relevance of this conflicting report is uncertain.

MECHANISM OF ACTION
Pharmacology

- **Constituents:** Burdock (*Arctium lappa*) contains sterols, tannins, sulfur-containing polyacetylenes (<0.1%),[19,20] volatile and fatty oils, and polysaccharides/mucilages (xyloglucan).[21] Six compounds have been isolated from the seeds of *Arctium lappa*, including a lignan (neoarctin), daucosterol, arctigenin, arctiin, mataresinol, and lappaol.[22] Burdock leaves contain arctiol, fukinone, fukinanolide, and petastilone. The active constituents of burdock are believed to be sequisterpene lactones and carbohydrate inulin (50%).[23]
- **Antiviral/antibacterial:** Inhibition of HIV-1 infection has been demonstrated *in vitro*.[4] Several lignans are now under investigation as antiviral agents (particularly anti-HIV).[24] The antibacterial activity of burdock has been attributed

to the presence of polyacetylonenes[19]; burdock has been reported to exhibit *in vitro* activity against gram-negative bacteria, including *E. coli*, *Shigella flexneri*, and *Shigella sonnei*.
- **Antineoplastic:** Burdock exhibits *in vitro* cytostatic activity against experimental cancer cell lines and has been found to inhibit the tumor-promoting activity of Epstein-Barr virus in Swiss mice (resulting in inhibition, hemorrhagic necrosis, and liquefaction of tumors).[25,26] *In vitro* data have found dismutagenic activity of burdock against 4-NO2-1, 2-DAB, ethidium bromide, and other mutagens,[27] which has been attributed to the burdock constituent arctigenin.[22] *In vitro* studies suggest that fresh burdock juice inhibits DMBA-induced chromosomal abnormalities.[23,28]
- **Antioxidant/anti-inflammatory:** In an animal model, subcutaneous administration of *Arctium lappa* crude extract exhibits free radical scavenging activity and has been found to reduce rat paw edema.[29] Burdock exhibits hepatoprotective properties in mice injected with acetaminophen or carbon tetrachloride, which has been attributed to antioxidant properties.[2] Lignans in burdock exhibit antagonism of platelet-activating factor (PAF) binding to platelets in rabbits.[18]
- **Renal:** Oral burdock use has been associated with diuretic effects in humans,[3] and with inhibition of kidney stone formation in Wistar rats.[30]

Pharmacodynamics

- The burdock constituent arctiin remains stable in gastric juice and is rapidly transformed into arctigenin metabolite 1 in rat intestinal flora, followed by conversion into its metabolite 2 through C-3 methylation.[31]
- Following an oral dose of 200 mg/kg in rats, the arctiin metabolite 1 reaches its peak serum level after four hours.[31]

HISTORY

- Burdock's formal name "*Arctium lappa*" is derived from the Greek words *arktos* or "bear" and *lappa* meaning "to seize." *Arctium minus* is the American source of root.
- In medieval Germany, Hildegard of Bingen used burdock to treat cancerous tumors. In 14th century Europe, a combination of burdock and wine was used to treat leprosy. Later European herbalists used burdock for fevers, a variety of dermatological conditions (baldness, scrapes, burns), syphilis, and gonorrhea. In Chinese medicine, burdock has been used to treat upper respiratory tract infections and pneumonia arising from a "hot wind"; the seeds, known as *niu-bang-zi*, are the main parts used. Burdock has also been used in Indian Ayurvedic medicine for upper respiratory infections and pneumonia.
- Native Americans included burdock root in herbal preparations used by women in labor. American herbalists have used burdock for arthritis, urinary tract infections, lice, ringworm, and eczema. It has also been used as a diuretic, with preparations made from powdered burdock seeds yielding a yellow bland fixed product called "oil of lappa." Burdock has also traditionally been used as a liver tonic, diaphoretic, diuretic, blood purifier, laxative, antipyretic, and antimicrobial. In the 1930s, Harry Hoxsey included burdock in an herbal cancer treatment which gained some popularity. Burdock is also an ingredient in the widely used Canadian cancer remedy Essiac.
- Burdock roots and leaves are eaten as vegetables in Japan and are sold in specialty groceries in the United States.

REVIEW OF THE EVIDENCE: TABLE

• No studies qualify for inclusion in the evidence table.

REVIEW OF THE EVIDENCE: DISCUSSION
Diabetes
Summary

• Burdock has been used traditionally to treat diabetes. Preliminary animal data and poor-quality human data suggest possible hypoglycemic effects of burdock root or fruit, although reliable data are lacking. Further study is warranted in this area before a firm conclusion can be drawn.

Evidence

• Burdock fruit extracts have demonstrated hypoglycemic activity in rats[12] and have been speculated to lower blood glucose levels in humans.[13-15] Although mice with streptozotocin-induced diabetes given burdock paradoxically experienced hyperglycemia, the mechanism of burdock's effects on serum glucose is not clear,[16] and the clinical relevance of this conflicting animal report is uncertain.

• In a human case series from the 1930s, the effects of dried burdock root on diabetic patients were observed.[13] Subjects were fed a batter prepared from 90 g of burdock powder (exposed to low heat), 36 g of butter, water, salt, saccharin, and several drops of ginger fluid extract. Baseline serum sugar levels were recorded and were compared to levels following burdock administration after 30 minutes, 90 minutes, 165 minutes, and 225 minutes. Subjects served as their own controls, and on a different day received 100 g of carbohydrate in the form of oatmeal, corn, wheat bread, and bananas, with similar serum measurements. The authors reported that burdock inhibited the expected hyperglycemia caused by administration of common polysaccharides at the measured time intervals. In "mild diabetic" subjects, normal blood sugar levels were maintained by the administration of burdock in the form of crackers.[13] Although the results are compelling, the methodological weaknesses and unclear reporting in this early study make the clinical application of these results impossible. Further study is warranted in this area in order to establish the safety and efficacy of burdock in diabetes therapy.

References

1. Lin SC, Lin CH, Lin CC, et al. Hepatoprotective effects of *Arctium lappa* Linne on liver injuries induced by chronic ethanol consumption and potentiated by carbon tetrachloride. J Biomed Sci 2002;9(5):401-409.
2. Lin SC, Chung TC, Lin CC, et al. Hepatoprotective effects of *Arctium lappa* on carbon tetrachloride- and acetaminophen-induced liver damage. Am J Chin Med 2000;28(2):163-173.
3. Kassler WJ, Blanc P, Greenblatt R. The use of medicinal herbs by human immunodeficiency virus-infected patients. Arch Intern Med 1991;151(11):2281-2288.
4. Yao XJ, Wainberg MA, Parniak MA. Mechanism of inhibition of HIV-1 infection in vitro by purified extract of *Prunella vulgaris*. Virology 1992;187(1):56-62.
5. Rodriguez P, Blanco J, Juste S, et al. Allergic contact dermatitis due to burdock (*Arctium lappa*). Contact Dermatitis 1995;33(2):134-135.
6. Bryson PD, Watanabe AS, Rumack BH, et al. Burdock root tea poisoning. Case report involving a commercial preparation. JAMA 1978;239(20):2157.
7. Bryson PD. Burdock root tea poisoning. JAMA 1978;240(15):1586.
8. Breed FB, Kuwabara T. Burdock ophthalmia. Arch Ophthalmol 1966;75(1):16-20.
9. Rhoads PM, Tong TG, Banner W, Jr., et al. Anticholinergic poisonings associated with commercial burdock root tea. J Toxicol Clin Toxicol 1984;22(6):581-584.
10. Hirono I, Mori H, Kato K, et al. Safety examination of some edible plants, Part 2. J Environ Pathol Toxicol 1978;1(1):71-74.
11. Sasaki Y, Kimura Y, Tsunoda T, et al. Anaphylaxis due to burdock. Int J Dermatol 2003;42(6):472-473.
12. Lapinina L, Sisoeva T. Investigation of some plants to determine their sugar lowering action. Farmatsevtichnyi Zhurnal 1964;19:52-58.
13. Silver AA, Krantz JC. The effect of the ingestion of burdock root on normal and diabetic individuals: A preliminary report. Ann Int Med 1931;5:274-284.
14. Bever BO, Zahnd GR. Plants with oral hypoglycaemic action. Q J Crude Drug Res 1979;17:139-196.
15. Farnsworth NR, Segelman AB. Hypoglycemic plants. Tile Till 1971;57:52-56.
16. Swanston-Flatt SK, Day C, Flatt PR, et al. Glycaemic effects of traditional European plant treatments for diabetes. Studies in normal and streptozotocin diabetic mice. Diabetes Res 1989;10(2):69-73.
17. Farnsworth NR, Bingel AS, Cordell GA, et al. Potential value of plants as sources of new antifertility agents I. J Pharm Sci 1975;64(4):535-598.
18. Iwakami S, Wu JB, Ebizuka Y, et al. Platelet activating factor (PAF) antagonists contained in medicinal plants: lignans and sesquiterpenes. Chem Pharm Bull (Tokyo) 1992;40(5):1196-1198.
19. Schulte KE, Rucker G, Boehme R. [Polyacetylenes as components of the roots of bur.] Arzneimittelforschung 1967;17(7):829-833.
20. Washino T. New sulfur-containing acetylenic compounds from *Arctium lappa*. Agric Biol Chem 1986;50(263):269.
21. Kato Y, Watanabe T. Isolation and characterization of a xyloglucan from gobo (*Arctium lappa* L.). Biosci Biotechnol Biochem 1993;57(9):1591-1592.
22. Wang HY, Yang JS. [Studies on the chemical constituents of *Arctium lappa* L.] Yao Xue Xue Bao [Acta Pharmaceutica Sinica] 1993;28(12):911-917.
23. Ichihara A. New sesquilignans from *Arctium lappa* L. The structure of lappaol C, D and E. Agric Biol Chem 1977;41:1813-1814.
24. Yang L, Lin S, Yang T, et al. Synthesis of anti-HIV activity of dibenzylbutyrolactone lignans. Bioorganic Medicinal Chem Lett 1996;6:941-944.
25. Dombradi CA, Foldeak S. Screening report on the antitumor activity of purified *Arctium lappa* extracts. Tumori 1966;52(3):173-175.
26. Sato A. [Studies on anti-tumor activity of crude drugs. I. The effects of aqueous extracts of some crude drugs in shortterm screening test. (1).] Yakugaku Zasshi 1989;109(6):407-423.
27. Morita K, Kada T, Namiki M. A desmutagenic factor isolated from burdock (*Arctium lappa* Linne). Mutat Res 1984;129(1):25-31.
28. Morita K. Chemical nature of a desmutagenic factor isolated from burdock (*Arctium lappa* Linne). Agric Biol Chem 1985;49:925-932.
29. Lin CC, Lu JM, Yang JJ, et al. Anti-inflammatory and radical scavenge effects of *Arctium lappa*. Am J Chin Med 1996;24(2):127-137.
30. Grases F, Melero G, Costa-Bauza A, et al. Urolithiasis and phytotherapy. Int Urol Nephrol 1994;26(5):507-511.
31. Nose M, Fujimoto T, Nishibe S, et al. Structural transformation of lignan compounds in rat gastrointestinal tract; II. Serum concentration of lignans and their metabolites. Planta Med 1993;59(2):131-134.

Calendula

(Calendula officinalis L.) , Marigold

SYNONYMS/COMMON NAMES/RELATED SUBSTANCES

- Asteraceae, bride of the sun, bull flower, butterwort, *Caltha officinalis, Calendula arvensis* L., calendula flower, calendula herb, calendulae flos, calendulae herba, claveton (Spanish), Compositae, cowbloom, death-flower, drunkard gold, fior d'ogni (Italian), flaminquillo (Spanish), fleurs de tous les mois (French), gauche-fer (French), gold bloom, goldblume (German), golden flower of Mary, goulans, gouls, holligold, holygold, husband's dial, kingscup, maravilla, marigold, marybud, marygold, mejorana (Spanish), poet's marigold, pot marigold, publican and sinner, ringelblume (German), ruddles, Scotch marigold, shining herb, solsequia, souci (French), souci des champs (French), souci des jardins (French), summer's bride, sun's bride, water dragon, yolk of egg.
- *Note:* Not to be confused with the common garden or French marigold (*Tagetes* spp), African marigold (*Tagetes erecta*), or Inca marigold (*Tagetes minuta*).
- **Combination products:** Traumeel.

CLINICAL BOTTOM LINE
Background

- Calendula (*Calendula officinalis*), also known as marigold, has been widely used topically to treat minor skin wounds, skin infections, burns, bee stings, sunburn, warts and cancer. Most scientific evidence regarding its efficacy as a wound-healing agent is based on animal and *in vitro* studies, whereas human evidence is virtually lacking.

Scientific Evidence for Common/Studied Uses	Grade*
Otitis media	C
Skin inflammation	C
Wound healing	C

*Key to grades: *A:* Strong scientific evidence for this use; *B:* Good scientific evidence for this use; *C:* Unclear scientific evidence for this use; *D:* Fair scientific evidence against this use (it may not work); *F:* Strong scientific evidence against this use (it likely does not work). For a more detailed explanation of efficacy criteria, see "Natural Standard Evidence-Based Validated Grading Rationale" in the Introduction.

Historical or Theoretical Indications That Lack Sufficient Evidence

- Abscesses, acne, amenorrhea, analgesia, anemia, antibacterial, antifungal, antiviral, anxiety, appetite stimulant, atherosclerosis, athlete's foot, benign prostatic hypertrophy, bladder irritation, blood purification, bruises, burns, cardiac disease, cholera, circulation, colitis,[1,2] conjunctivitis,[3,4] constipation, cosmetic, cough, cramps, diaper rash, dizziness, diuresis, dystrophic nervous disturbances, eczema, edema, epididymitis, epistaxis, fatigue, fever, frostbite, gastrointestinal tract disorders, gastritis, gout, headache, hemorrhoids, herpes simplex,[5] herpes keratitis,[6] HIV, indigestion, immunostimulant, influenza,[5] insomnia, jaundice, liver-gallbladder function stimulator, metabolic disorders, mouth and throat infections, muscular atrophy, nausea, peptic ulcer disease,[7] proctitis, prostatitis, purging agent, skin cancer, sore throat, spasms, spleen disorders, stones, syphilis, thrombophlebitis, tinnitus, toothache, tuberculosis, ulcerative colitis, urinary retention, uterine tonic, varicose ulcers,[8] warts, yeast infections.

Expert Opinion and Folkloric Precedent

- Traditionally, calendula has been used topically for treating minor wounds, burns and other skin problems. Multiple references are made to calendula as a wound healing aid and topical anti-infective agent. However, no strong scientific evidence supports these properties.
- Powder from the plant's petals is occasionally used as an inexpensive alternative to saffron for coloring and flavoring foods.

Safety Summary

- Insufficient data are available to support the safety of these ingredients in medicinal or cosmetic formulations.[9]

DOSING/TOXICOLOGY
General

- Recommended doses are based on those most commonly used in available trials, or on historical practice. However, with natural products, the optimal doses needed to balance efficacy and safety often have not been determined. Formulations and preparation methods may vary from manufacturer to manufacturer, and from batch to batch of a specific product made by a single manufacturer. Because often the active components of a product are not known, standardization may not be possible, and the clinical effects of different brands may not be comparable.

Standardization

- Insufficient evidence available.

Dosing: Adult (18 Years and Older)
Topical

- According to expert panels, the German Commission E and the European Scientific Cooperative on Phytotherapy, 2% to 5% ointment is often used. Topical preparations may be applied three or four times daily as needed. According to these sources, a 1:1 tincture in 40% alcohol or 1:5 in 90% alcohol may be diluted at least 1:3 with freshly boiled water for compresses.

Otic (Ear Drops)

- 5 drops of Otikon Otic Solution, instilled into the affected ear three times a day, has been used.[10]

Dosing: Pediatric (Younger Than 18 Years)

- Insufficient evidence to recommend.

Toxicology

- *In vitro*, some calendula saponins have cytotoxic properties.[11] Genotoxicity has been described from calendula extract.[12] The relevance of these findings is unclear.

- An LD_{50} of 375 mg/kg and an LD_{100} of 580 mg/kg has been determined in mice by intravenous and intraperitoneal administration of aqueous extracts. In hydroalcoholic extracts an LD_{50} of 45 mg/mouse (subcutaneous) and an LD_{50} of 526 mg/100 g in rats (intravenous) has been reported.
- *Calendula officinalis* extract is reported to be used in almost 200 cosmetic formulations, over a wide range of product categories.[9] Acute toxicity studies in rats and mice suggest that the extract is relatively nontoxic. Animal tests have demonstrated minimal skin irritation, and no sensitization or phototoxicity. Minimal ocular irritation was seen with one formulation and no irritation with others. Six saponins isolated from *C. officinalis* flowers were not mutagenic in an Ames test, and a tea derived from *C. officinalis* was not genotoxic in *Drosophila melanogaster*. Clinical testing of cosmetic formulations containing the extract elicited little irritation or sensitization. Published accounts assert that until more data are available, there is insufficient evidence to support the safety of these ingredients in cosmetic formulations.[9]

ADVERSE EFFECTS/PRECAUTIONS/CONTRAINDICATIONS
Allergy

- Known allergy/hypersensitivity to members of the Aster/Compositae family, such as ragweed, chrysanthemums, marigolds and daisies.[13] Anaphylactic shock after gargling with a calendula infusion has been reported, and one patient had a positive skin patch test to calendula 10% tincture.[14]
- Reider et al. tested 443 consecutive patients with Compositae mix, sesquiterpene lactone mix, arnica, calendula, and propolis.[15] Five subjects (1.13%) reacted to arnica, and 9 (2.03%) to calendula. The *Compositae* mix elicited a reaction in 18 cases (approximately 4.06%). Sensitization to arnica and calendula was often accompanied by reactions to nickel, *Myroxylon pereirae* resin, propolis, and colophonium.

Adverse Effects/Postmarket Surveillance

- There is limited evidence other than reports of hypersensitivity reactions.

Precautions/Warnings/Contraindications

- Use cautiously in patients with allergy/hypersensitivity to members of the Aster/Compositae family.

Pregnancy and Lactation

- *In vitro*, calendula has exhibited moderate "uterotonic" effects in isolated rabbit and guinea pig uterine tissues.[16] Anecdotal reports indicate that calendula may possess spermatocide and abortifacient effects.[17] Use during pregnancy and lactation has not been shown to be safe, and systemic effects from topical use are not clear.

INTERACTIONS
Calendula/Drug Interactions

- **Sedative drugs:** In early animal studies, high doses of ingested calendula preparations were reported to act as sedatives.[18] Therefore, combination use with sedative agents may lead to additive effects. In rats, calendula was shown to increase hexobarbital sleeping time.[19] Systemic effects after topical use of calendula in humans are not clear.
- **Antihypertensive drugs:** In early animal studies, high doses of calendula preparations were reported to possess hypotensive effects.[18] Therefore, combination use with hypotensive agents may lead to additive effects. Systemic effects after topical use of calendula in humans are not clear.

Calendula/Herb/Supplement Interactions

- **Sedative herbs and supplements:** In early animal studies, high doses of ingested calendula preparations were reported to act as sedatives.[18] Therefore, combination use with sedative agents may lead to additive effects. In rats, calendula was shown to increase hexobarbital sleeping time.[19] Systemic effects after topical use of calendula in humans are not clear.
- **Hypotensive herbs:** In early animal studies, high doses of calendula preparations were reported to possess hypotensive effects.[18] Therefore, combination use with hypotensive agents may lead to additive effects. Systemic effects after topical use of calendula in humans are not clear.

Calendula/Food Interactions

- Insufficient available evidence.

Calendula/Lab Interactions

- Insufficient available evidence.

MECHANISM OF ACTION
Pharmacology

- **Constituents:** The principal identified constituents of calendula are triterpenoids and flavonoids,[20,21] which have numerous alleged pharmacological properties, including anti-inflammatory, immunostimulating, antibacterial, antiviral, antiprotozoal, and antineoplastic. The mechanisms underlying these possible effects are poorly understood. Hypoglycemic, gastric emptying inhibitory, and gastroprotective properties have been attributed to calendasaponins A, B, C, and D; two additional ionone glucosides (officinosides A and B), and two sesquiterpene oligoglycosides (officinosides C and D), have been isolated from the flowers of Egyptian *Calendula officinalis*.[22] Two homologous cDNAs, CoFad2 and CoFac2, were isolated from a *Calendula officinalis* developing seed by polymerase chain reaction.[23] Both sequences share similarity to FAD2 desaturases and FAD2-related enzymes. In *C. officinalis* plants, CoFad2 was expressed in all tissues tested, whereas CoFac2 expression was specific to developing seeds. Expression of CoFad2 cDNA in yeast (*Saccharomyces cerevisiae*) indicated it encodes a delta 12 desaturase that introduces a double bond at the 12 position of 16:1(9Z) and 18:1(9Z). Expression of CoFac2 in yeast revealed that the encoded enzyme acts as a fatty acid conjugase converting 18:2(9Z, 12Z) to calendic acid 18:3(8E, 10E, 12Z). The enzyme also has weak activity on the mono-unsaturates 16:1(9Z) and 18:1(9Z) producing compounds with the properties of 8,10 conjugated dienes.
- **Anti-inflammatory effects:** The active components of calendula's anti-inflammatory activity are thought to be the triterpenoids, particularly faradiol monoester. Free ester faradiol is the most active and exhibits the same effects as an equimolar dose of indomethacin.[23-26] Calendula's glycosides also have inhibited lipoxygenase activity *in vitro*.[27]
- **Wound-healing effects:** Rao et al. observed a reduction of epithelization time, an increase in wound strength, and improvement of wound contraction in rats with experimental incision wounds that were topically treated with calendula.[28] Effects may also be mediated by stimulation of phagocytosis and increased granulation,[13] and via effects on metabolism of glycoproteins, nucleoproteins and collagen proteins in tissue regeneration.[29]
- **Antiviral effects:** Anti-HIV activity of calendula has been demonstrated *in vitro*,[30] specifically involving inhibition of HIV-1 (IIIB)-induced cytopathogenicity in CD4+

lymphocytic Molt-4 clone 8 cells. Triterpenoid saponins from *Calendula arvensis* have inhibited multiplication of vesicular stomatitis virus and rhinovirus *in vitro*.[31]

- **Antibacterial effects:** Hydroacetonic extract from fresh plants inhibits the growth of *Staphylococcus aureus* at a concentration of 1 mg/mL *in vitro*.[32] Calendula extract was tested on biofilms of infant dentifrices and did not demonstrate antimicrobial effects against *A. viscosus*, *Candida albicans*, *Lactobacillus casei*, *Streptococcus mitis*, *S. mutans*, *S. oralis*, *S. sanguis*, and *S. sobrinus*.[33]
- **Antiprotozoal effects:** Oxygenated terpene alcohols and terpene lactones from calendula have been observed to possess trichomonacidal activity.[34]
- **Antiproliferative effects:** In a mouse model, dietary lutein derived from calendula extract has been found to suppress mammary tumor growth, increase tumor latency, and enhance lymphocyte proliferation.[35] Saponins isolated from calendula express *in vitro* antimutagenic and tumor cell cytotoxic activity.[11,36] *C. officinalis* does not exert a direct mitogenic effect on human lymphocytes *in vitro* and exhibits inhibitory effects on lymphocyte proliferation.[37] A preparation of several herbs (*Calendula officinalis*, *Echinacea purpurea*, *Scorzonera humilis*, *Aconitum moldavicum*) has been associated with "normalization" of pathologic enzyme activity by rat hepatocytes affected by carcinoma.[38]
- **Other effects:** *In vitro*, calendula exhibited moderate "uterotonic" effects in isolated rabbit and guinea pig uterine tissues.[16] In early (1964) animal studies, high doses of calendula preparations were reported to act as sedatives and hypotensive agents.[18]

Pharmacodynamics/Kinetics

- Insufficient available evidence.

HISTORY

- Calendula (*Calendula officinalis* L.), commonly known as marigold, is an annual flower in the daisy family that grows to a height of 12 to 18 inches and is native to Asia and southern Europe. Calendula has been cultivated for centuries in ornamental gardens, where it readily grows in poor soils.
- Calendula has been used medicinally since the 12th century throughout central Europe and the Mediterranean area. The name calendula is derived from the Latin word *kalends*, meaning the first day of each month, when the flowers bloom. Calendula has also been called the "herb of the sun," because its flowers bloom in the morning and close in

the evening. According to Greek mythology, calendula was named after four wood nymphs who fell in love with Apollo.

REVIEW OF THE EVIDENCE: DISCUSSION
Wound Healing
Summary

- Although minor skin wounds are a common indication for topical treatment with calendula, few scientific studies have been conducted in this area. Limited evidence from animal and *in vitro* studies lend support to the use of calendula to promote wound healing; these studies have noted a reduction in epithelization time, an increase in wound strength, and an improvement in wound contraction of experimental incisions treated with topical calendula.[28] However, high-quality human evidence is lacking.

Evidence

- In a poorly described case series, Neto el al. studied calendula's effects on promoting burn healing.[8] Calendula and a combination of calendula and barbatimao (derived from *Stryphnodendron barbadetiman*) were studied in 15 patients with burns, varicose ulcers, abrasions, or dermatitis. All patients had been "unresponsive" to conventional therapy. The authors reported that all subjects with burns experienced complete healing in 2 to 6 days, 8 of 12 patients with varicose ulcers experienced complete healing within 30 days, and 7 of 11 patients with abrasions or chronic dermatitis were healed within 10 days. The method of evaluating wound healing was not described in detail, and statistical analysis was not provided.
- In a poorly designed and described comparison study, a group of patients with second- or third-degree burns was treated topically with calendula, pure Vaseline, or a commercial "proteolytic ointment."[39] A successful outcome was defined as the absence of eschar or local infection, as evaluated by subjective criteria. After 12 days of therapy, the authors reported that 70% of the calendula group was considered a "success," compared to 66% of the proteolytic ointment group ($p > 0.05$) and 54% of the Vaseline group ($p = 0.05$). Analgesia was reported by 60% of calendula patients vs. 21% receiving the proteolytic ointment. This study was not randomized or blinded, allowing for the possible introduction of confounders or bias. The lack of placebo arm leaves open the question of whether improvements were due to the natural course of wound healing rather than to therapeutic intervention(s).

Review of the Evidence: Calendula

Condition Treated*	Study Design	Author, Year	N[†]	SS[†]	Study Quality[‡]	Magnitude of Benefit	ARR[†]	NNT[†]	Comments
Otitis media	Randomized controlled trial	Sarrell[10] 2001	110	Yes	1	Small	NA	NA	Comparison of Otikon Otic solution[§] with anesthetic eardrops as a symptomatic treatment of otalgia in children with acute otitis media.

*Primary or secondary outcome.
†*N*, Number of patients; *SS*, statistically significant; *ARR*, absolute risk reduction; *NNT*, the number of patients who need to undergo a specific intervention in order to observe an outcome in one individual.
‡0-2 = poor; 3-4 = good; 5 = excellent.
§Composed of *Allium sativum*, *Verbascum thapsus*, *Calendula flores*, and *Hypericum perforatum*.
NA, Not applicable.
For an explanation of each category in this table, please see Table 3 in the Introduction.

Skin Inflammation

Summary

- Limited animal research suggests that calendula extracts may possess anti-inflammatory properties when applied topically to the skin. Human studies are lacking in this area.

Evidence

- Della Loggia et al. reported that hydroalcoholic extracts of calendula exhibit mild anti-inflammatory activity with dose-dependent effects in mice with experimental inflammation of the ear canal.[24] A carbon dioxide extract appeared to be more active with a dose-dependent effect. In a subsequent study, the most active anti-inflammatory component of the carbon dioxide extract was found to be free faradiol, which demonstrated a dose-dependent effect equal to that of indomethacin.[25] The authors suggested that esterified faradiol may be the main active constituent, based on its quantitative prevalence.

Otitis Media

Summary

- There is insufficient human evidence to recommend calendula for the treatment of otitis media or for pain associated with otitis media.

Evidence

- Sarrell et al. compared Otikon Otic solution (a naturopathic herbal solution containing *Allium sativum*, *Verbascum thapsus*, *Calendula flores*, and *Hypericum perforatum*) with anesthetic eardrops as a symptomatic treatment of otalgia in 110 children with acute otitis media.[10] Subjects were randomized to receive 5 drops of either Otikon Otic or anesthetic ear drops in the affected ear three times daily. Pain was measured using a subjective pain scale (1-10). Throughout the study, mean pain levels remained lower in the Otikon Otic group, although this difference was only statistically significant during the first day, 30 minutes after application. Although this study is suggestive, the lack of placebo group limits the distinction between pain relief due to the natural history of otitis pain vs. analgesia due to therapeutic intervention. In addition, inadequate blinding may have allowed for the introduction of bias. The simple 1-10 pain scale may not have been sensitive enough to detect between-group differences. The effects of *Calendula flores* monotherapy cannot be extrapolated from this study of a combination product.
- A 1979 study assessing the efficacy of multiple herbal products in the treatment of chronic otitis media found calendula to be "minimally effective."[40] Additional details are limited.

FORMULARY: BRANDS USED IN CLINICAL TRIALS

Brands Used in Statistically Significant Clinical Trials

- Otikon Otic solution (combination product).[10]

References

1. Chakurski I, Matev M, Stefanov G, et al. [Treatment of duodenal ulcers and gastroduodenitis with a herbal combination of *Symphitum officinalis* and *Calendula officinalis* with and without antacids.] Vutr Boles 1981; 20(6):44-47.
2. Chakurski I, Matev M, Koichev A, et al. [Treatment of chronic colitis with an herbal combination of *Taraxacum* officinale, *Hipericum perforatum*, *Melissa officinaliss*, *Calendula officinalis* and *Foeniculum vulgare*.] Vutr Boles 1981;20(6):51-54.
3. Marinchev VN, Bychkova LN, Balvanovich NV, et al. [Use of calendula for therapy of chronic inflammatory diseases of eyelids and conjunctiva.] Oftal'mologicheskii Zhurnal 1971;26(3):196-198.
4. Mozherenkov VP, Shubina LF. [Treatment of chronic conjunctivitis with Calendula.] Med Sestra 1976;35(4):33-34.
5. Bogdanova NS, Nikolaeva IS, Shcherbakova LI, et al. [Study of antiviral properties of Calendula officinalis.] Farmakol Toksikol 1970;33(3):349-355.
6. Corina P, Dimitris S, Emanuil T, et al. [Treatment with acyclovir combined with a new Romanian product from plants.] Oftalmologia 1999;46(1):55-57.
7. Matev M, Chakurski I, Stefanov G, et al. [Use of an herbal combination with laxative action on duodenal peptic ulcer and gastroduodenitis patients with a concomitant obstipation syndrome.] Vutr Boles 1981;20(6):48-51.
8. Neto JJ, Fracasso JF, Neves MDCLC, et al. Treatment of varicose ulcer and skin lesions with calendula. Revista de Ciencias Farm Sao Paulo 1996;17:181-186.
9. Anonymous. Final report on the safety assessment of *Calendula officinalis* extract and *Calendula officinalis*. Int J Toxicol 2001;20(Suppl 2):13-20.
10. Sarrell EM, Mandelberg A, Cohen HA. Efficacy of naturopathic extracts in the management of ear pain associated with acute otitis media. Arch Pediatr Adolesc Med 2001;155(7):796-799.
11. Quetin-Leclercq J, Elias R, Balansard G, et al. Cytotoxic activity of some triterpenoid saponins. Planta Med 1992;58(3):279-281.
12. Ramos A, Edreira A, Vizoso A, et al. Genotoxicity of an extract of *Calendula officinalis* L. J Ethnopharmacol 1998;61(1):49-55.
13. Dietz V. Calendula preparations to treat cutaneous infections. Alt Med Alert 1998;1(12):140-142.
14. Bruynzeel DP, van Ketel WG, Young E, et al. Contact sensitization by alternative topical medicaments containing plant extracts. The Dutch Contact Dermatoses Group. Contact Dermatitis 1992;27(4):278-279.
15. Reider N, Komericki P, Hausen BM, et al. The seamy side of natural medicines: contact sensitization to arnica (*Arnica montana* L.) and marigold (*Calendula officinalis* L.). Contact Dermatitis 2001;45(5):269-272.
16. Shipochliev T. [Uterotonic action of extracts from a group of medicinal plants.] Vet Med Nauki 1981;18(4):94-98.
17. Brinker F. Herb Contraindications and Drug Interactions. Sandy: Eclectic Medical Publications, 1998, p 46.
18. Bojadjiev C. On the sedative and hypotensive effect of preparations from the plant *Calendula officinalis*. Nauch Trud Visshi Med Inst Sof 1964;43: 15-20.
19. Samochowiec L. Pharmacological study of saponosides from *Aralia mandshurica* Rupr. et Maxim and *Calendula officinalis* L. Herba Pol 1983; 29:151-155.
20. Yoshikawa M, Murakami T, Kishi A, et al. Medicinal flowers. III. Marigold. (1): hypoglycemic, gastric emptying inhibitory, and gastroprotective principles and new oleanane-type triterpene oligoglycosides, calendasaponins A, B, C, and D, from Egyptian *Calendula officinalis*. Chem Pharm Bull (Tokyo) 2001;49(7):863-870.
21. Vidal-Ollivier E, Elias R, Faure F, et al. Flavonol glycosides from *Calendula officinalis* flowers. Planta Med 1989;55:73-74.
22. Marukami T, Kishi A, Yoshikawa M. Medicinal flowers. IV. Marigold. (2): Structures of new ionone and sesquiterpene glycosides from Egyptian *Calendula officinalis*. Chem Pharm Bull (Tokyo) 2001;49(8):974-978.
23. Qiu X, Reed DW, Hong H, et al. Identification and analysis of a gene from *Calendula officinalis* encoding a fatty acid conjugase. Plant Physiol 2001; 125(2):847-855.
24. Della Loggia R., et al. Topical anti-inflammatory activity of *Calendula officinalis* extracts. Planta Med 1990;56:658.
25. Della LR, Tubaro A, Sosa S, et al. The role of triterpenoids in the topical anti-inflammatory activity of *Calendula officinalis* flowers. Planta Med 1994;60(5):516-520.
26. Zitterl-Eglseer K, Sosa S, Jurenitsch J, et al. Anti-oedematous activities of the main triterpendiol esters of marigold (*Calendula officinalis* L.). J Ethnopharmacol 1997;57(2):139-144.
27. Bezakova L, Masterova I, Paulikova I, et al. Inhibitory activity of isorhamnetin glycosides from *Calendula officinalis* L. on the activity of lipoxygenase. Pharmazie 1996;51(2):126-127.
28. Rao S, Udupa A, Udupa SL, et al. Calendula and Hypericum: Two homeopathic drugs promoting wound healing in rats. Fitoterapia 1991; 62(6): 508-510.
29. Klouchek-Popova E, Popov A, Pavlova N, et al. Influence of the physiological regeneration and epithelialization using fractions isolated from *Calendula officinalis*. Acta Physiol Pharmacol Bulg. 1982;8(4):63-67.
30. Kalvatchev Z, Walder R, Garzaro D. Anti-HIV activity of extracts from *Calendula officinalis* flowers. Biomed Pharmacother 1997;51(4):176-180.
31. De Tommasi N, Conti C, Stein ML, et al. Structure and in vitro antiviral activity of triterpenoid saponins from *Calendula arvensis*. Planta Med 1991; 57(3):250-253.
32. Dumenil G, Chemli R, Balansard C, et al. [Evaluation of antibacterial properties of marigold flowers (*Calendula officinalis* L.) and other homeopathic tinctures of C. *officinalis* L. and C. *arvensis* L. (author's transl).] Ann Pharm Fr 1980;38(6):493-499.
33. Modesto A, Lima KC, de Uzeda M. Effects of three different infant dentifrices on biofilms and oral microorganisms. J Clin Pediatr Dent 2000; 24(3):237-243.

34. Gracza L. Oxygen-containing terpene derivatives from *Calendula officinalis.* Planta Med 1987;53:227.

35. Chew BP, Wong MW, Wong TS. Effects of lutein from marigold extract on immunity and growth of mammary tumors in mice. Anticancer Res 1996;16(6B):3689-3694.

36. Elias R, De Meo M, Vidal-Ollivier E, et al. Antimutagenic activity of some saponins isolated from *Calendula officinalis* L., *C. arvensis* L. and *Hedera helix* L. Mutagenesis 1990;5(4):327-331.

37. Amirghofran Z, Azadbakht M, Karimi MH. Evaluation of the immuno-modulatory effects of five herbal plants. J Ethnopharmacol 2000;72(1-2): 167-172.

38. Marchenko MM, Kopyl'chuk HP, Hrygor'ieva OV. [Activity of cytoplasmic proteinases from rat liver in Heren's carcinoma during tumor growth and treatment with medicinal herbs.] Ukr Biokhim Zh 2000;72(3):91-94.

39. Lievre M, Marichy J, Baux S, et al. Controlled study of three ointments for the local management of 2nd and 3rd degree burns. Clin Trials Meta-analysis 1992;28:9-12.

40. Shaparenko BA, Slivko AB, Bazarova OV, et al. On use of medicinal plants for treatment of patients with chronic suppurative otitis. Zh Ushn Gorl Bolezn 1979;39:48-51.

Chamomile
(Matricaria recutita, Chamaemelum nobile)

SYNONYMS/COMMON NAMES/RELATED SUBSTANCES

- *Anthemis arvensis, Anthemis cotula, Anthemis nobile, Anthemis nobilis*, Asteraceae/Compositae, baboonig, babuna, babunah camomile, babunj, bunga kamil, camamila, camomile, camomile sauvage, camomilla, camomille allemande, Campomilla, *Chamaemelum nobile* L., Chamomilla, chamomilla recutita, chamomillae ramane flos, chamomille commune, classic chamomile, common chamomile, double chamomile, echte kamille, English chamomile, feldkamille, fleur de camomile, fleurs de petite camomille, flores anthemidis, flos chamomillae, garden chamomile, German chamomile, grosse kamille, grote kamille, ground apple, Hungarian chamomile, kamille, kamillen, Kamillosan, kamitsure, kamiture, kleine, kleme kamille, lawn chamomile, low chamomile, manzanilla, manzanilla chiquita, manzanilla comun, manzanilla dulce, *Matricaria chamomilla, Matricaria recutita, Matricaria suaveolens*, matricariae flos, matricariae flowers, matricaire, may-then, nervine, pin heads, rauschert, romaine, romaine manzanilla, Roman chamomile, romische kamille, single chamomile, sweet chamomile, sweet false chamomile, sweet feverfew, true chamomile, whig-plant, wild chamomile.

CLINICAL BOTTOM LINE

Background

- Chamomile has been used medicinally for thousands of years and is widely used in Europe. It is a popular treatment for numerous ailments, including sleep disorders, anxiety, diaper rash, digestion/intestinal conditions, infantile colic, skin infections/inflammation (including eczema), teething pains, and wound healing. In the United States, chamomile is best known as an ingredient in herbal tea preparations proposed to have mild sedating effects.
- German chamomile (*Matricaria recutita*) and Roman chamomile (*Chamaemelum nobile*) are the two major types of chamomile used for health conditions. They are believed to have similar effects on the body, although German chamomile may be slightly stronger. Most research has focused on German chamomile, which is more commonly used everywhere except in England, where Roman chamomile is more common.
- Although chamomile is widely used, there is not enough reliable research in humans to support its use for any condition. Despite its reputation as a GENTLE medicinal plant, there have been many reports of allergic reactions (including life-threatening anaphylaxis) in people after eating or coming into contact with chamomile preparations.

Uses Based on Scientific Evidence	Grade*
Common cold One study reported that inhaling steam with chamomile extract improved common cold symptoms. More extensive and better-quality research is needed before a recommendation can be made.	C
Diarrhea in children One study reported that chamomile with apple pectin may reduce the length of time that children experience diarrhea. However, neither the design nor the results were well reported, and it is unclear whether the benefits reported were owing to the effects of chamomile or of the apple pectin.	C
Gastrointestinal conditions Chamomile is used traditionally for numerous gastrointestinal conditions, including digestion disorders, "spasm" or colic, upset stomach, flatulence (gas), ulcers, and gastrointestinal irritation. However, there have been no reliable studies in humans in these areas. In large doses, chamomile may cause vomiting.	C
Hemorrhagic cystitis (bladder irritation with bleeding) One poor-quality study reported that the combination of chamomile baths, chamomile bladder washes, and antibiotics was superior to antibiotics alone as therapy for hemorrhagic cystitis. Additional research is necessary before a conclusion can be reached. Hemorrhagic cystitis is a potentially serious condition for which medical attention should be sought.	C
Hemorrhoids One poor-quality study reported that chamomile ointment may improve hemorrhoids. Better evidence is needed before a recommendation can be made.	C
Mucositis from cancer treatment (mouth ulcers/irritation) Poor-quality studies have used chamomile mouthwash for the prevention or treatment of mouth mucositis caused by radiation therapy or cancer chemotherapy. Results are conflicting, and it remains unclear whether chamomile is helpful in this situation.	C
Quality of life in cancer patients A small amount of research suggests that massage using chamomile essential oil may improve anxiety and quality of life in patients with cancer. However, this evidence is not of high quality, and it is unclear whether this approach is superior to massage alone without essential oils. Additional study is needed before a firm conclusion can be reached.	C
Skin conditions (eczema/radiation damage/wound healing) Laboratory research and studies in animals have reported that chamomile has anti-inflammatory properties. Studies in humans suggest that chamomile ointment may work as well as hydrocortisone cream for eczema and that it may improve wound healing, but that chamomile cream may not work as well as almond oil for treating skin damage after radiation	C

Continued

therapy. Relief of inflammation and itching has been observed in clinical trials. These studies were not well designed or reported, and better-quality research is needed before a firm conclusion can be reached.

Sleep aid/sedation Traditionally, chamomile preparations such as tea and essential oil aromatherapy have been used for insomnia and sedation (calming effects). Small, poor-quality studies have reported mild hypnotic effects of chamomile aromatherapy and possible sedative properties of tea. However, there are no well-designed trials in humans in these areas. Better-quality research is needed before a recommendation can be made.	C
Vaginitis (inflammation of the vagina) Symptoms of vaginitis include itching, discharge, and pain with urination. A small study reported that chamomile douche improved symptoms of vaginitis with few side effects. Because vaginitis can be caused by infection (including sexually transmitted diseases), poor hygiene, or nutritional deficiencies. People with this condition should consult a qualified healthcare provider. More extensive and better-quality research studies are needed before a conclusion can be drawn regarding the role of chamomile in the management of vaginitis.	C
Postoperative sore throat/hoarseness due to intubation A trial in humans compared chamomile extract spray with normal saline spray (control), administered before placement of a breathing (endotracheal) tube, to determine effects on postoperative sore throat and hoarseness. Results did not show that chamomile prevented postoperative sore throat and hoarseness any more effectively than normal saline.	D

*Key to grades: A: Strong scientific evidence for this use; B: Good scientific evidence for this use; C: Unclear scientific evidence for this use; D: Fair scientific evidence against this use (it may not work); F: Strong scientific evidence against this use (it likely does not work). For a more detailed explanation of efficacy criteria, see "Natural Standard Evidence-Based Validated Grading Rationale" in the Introduction.

Historical or Theoretical Indications That Lack Sufficient Evidence
Abdominal bloating, abrasions, abscesses, acne, anorexia, antibacterial, antifungal, anti-inflammatory, antioxidant, anxiety, arthritis, back pain, bedsores, blocked tear ducts, burns, cancer, carpal tunnel syndrome, chickenpox, constipation, contact dermatitis, convulsions, delirium tremens (DTs), diaper rash, diaphoretic, diuretic (increasing urination), dysmenorrhea, ear infections, eye infections, fever, fistula healing, flatulence (gas), frostbite, fungal infections, gingivitis, gum irritation, hay fever, heartburn, heat rash, hives, impetigo, infantile colic, insect bites, irritable bowel syndrome, liver disorders, malaria, mastitis (breast inflammation), menstrual disorders, morning sickness, motion sickness, neuralgia (nerve pain), nausea, parasites/worms, poison ivy, psoriasis, restlessness, sciatica, sea sickness, seizure disorder, sinusitis, skin infections, teething pain (mouth rinse), uterine disorders.

DOSING/TOXICOLOGY

The following doses are based on scientific research, publications, traditional use, or expert opinion. Many herbs and supplements have not been thoroughly tested, and their safety and effectiveness may not be proven. Brands may be made differently, with variable ingredients even within the same brand. The doses shown may not apply to all products. It is important to always read product labels and discuss doses with a qualified healthcare provider before therapy is started.

Standardization

- Standardization involves measuring the amounts of certain chemicals in products to try to make different preparations similar to each other. It is not always known if the chemicals being measured are the "active" ingredients.
- Most American chamomile products are not standardized to any particular constituent. Many German chamomile products, such as Kamillosan, which contains 20 mg chamomile essential oil per 100 g of cream, are standardized to a minimum value of chamazulene and alpha-bisobolol. Tablets and capsules of chamomile may be standardized to contain 1.2% apigenin and 0.5% essential oil per dose. Examples of standardized chamomile preparations are Nutritional Dynamics German Chamomile (400 mg of chamomile flower per capsule, standardized to 1.25% apigenin and 0.5% essential oil), Nature's Way German chamomile (125 mg of extract standardized to 1.25% apigenin, and 350 mg of chamomile flower per capsule).

Adults (18 Years and Older)

- **Tea/infusion:** Traditional doses include tea made from 150 ml of boiling water poured over 2 to 4 g of fresh flower heads and steeped for 10 minutes, taken by mouth three times daily. One to 4 cups of chamomile tea (made from tea bags) taken daily has also been used.
- **Liquid extract/tincture:** As a liquid extract (1:1 in 45% alcohol), 1 to 4 ml taken by mouth three times daily has been used. As a tincture (1:5 in alcohol), 15 ml taken three or four times daily has been used.
- **Capsules/tablets:** 400 to 1600 mg taken by mouth daily in divided doses has been used.
- **Skin use:** There are no standard doses for chamomile used on the skin. Some natural medicine publications have recommended paste, plaster, or ointment containing 3% to 10% chamomile flower heads.
- **Douche:** There is no standard or well-studied dose for chamomile used as a douche. Some natural medicine publications have recommended a preparation containing 3% to 10% chamomile.
- **Mouth-rinse/gargle:** 1% fluid extract or 5% tincture has been used.
- **Bath:** 5 g of chamomile or 0.8 g of alcoholic extract per liter of water has been used.

Children (Younger Than 18 Years)

- Reliable scientific data are insufficient to recommend the safe use of chamomile products in children. Some natural medicine publications recommend that the dose of chamomile tea for children should be half of the adult dose.

SAFETY

The U.S. Food and Drug Administration does not strictly regulate herbs and supplements. There is no guarantee of the strength, purity, or safety of products, and effects may vary. It is important to always read product labels. People who have a medical condition, or are taking other drugs, herbs, or supplements, should consult a qualified healthcare provider before starting a new therapy. A healthcare provider should be contacted immediately about any side effects.

Allergies

- There have been multiple reports of serious allergic reactions (including anaphylaxis, throat swelling, and shortness of breath) to chamomile taken by mouth or used as an enema. Skin allergic reactions have been reported frequently, including dermatitis and eczema. Chamomile eyewash can cause allergic conjunctivitis (pink eye).
- People with allergies to other plants in the Asteraceae/Compositae family should avoid chamomile. Examples are aster, chrysanthemum, mugwort, ragweed, and ragwort. Cross-reactions may occur with birch pollen, celery, chrysanthemum, feverfew, and tansy. Individuals with allergies to these plants should avoid chamomile.

Side Effects and Warnings

- Impurities (adulterants) in chamomile products are common and may cause adverse effects.
- Chamomile in various forms may cause drowsiness or sedation. Caution should be used in people who are driving or operating heavy machinery. In large doses, chamomile can cause vomiting.
- Because of its coumarin content, chamomile may theoretically increase the risk of bleeding. Caution is advised in people who have bleeding disorders or are taking drugs that may increase the risk of bleeding. Dosing adjustments may be necessary.
- One poor-quality study reported slight increases in blood pressure from chamomile, but the evidence is insufficient to make a firm conclusion.

Pregnancy and Breastfeeding

- In theory, chamomile may act as a uterine stimulant or lead to abortion. Therefore, its use should be avoided during pregnancy. There are insufficient scientific data to recommend the safe use of chamomile by women who are breastfeeding.

INTERACTIONS

Most herbs and supplements have not been thoroughly tested for interactions with other herbs, supplements, drugs, or foods. The interactions listed here are based on reports in scientific publications, laboratory experiments, or traditional use. It is important to always read product labels. People who have a medical condition, or are taking other drugs, herbs, or supplements, should consult a qualified healthcare provider before starting a new therapy.

Interactions with Drugs

- Interactions of chamomile with drugs have not been well studied.
- Chamomile may increase the level of drowsiness caused by some drugs. Examples are alcohol, some antidepressants, barbiturates such as phenobarbital, benzodiazepines such as lorazepam (Ativan) and diazepam (Valium), and narcotics such as codeine. Caution is advised in people who are driving or operating machinery.
- In theory, chamomile may increase the risk of bleeding when used with anticoagulants or antiplatelet drugs. Examples are anticoagulants (blood thinners) such as warfarin (Coumadin) and heparin, antiplatelet drugs such as clopidogrel (Plavix), aspirin, and nonsteroidal anti-inflammatory drugs (NSAIDs) such as ibuprofen (Motrin, Advil) and naproxen (Naprosyn, Aleve).

- Limited laboratory research and studies in animals suggest that chamomile may interfere with how the body uses the liver's cytochrome P450 enzyme system to process components of some drugs. As a result, blood levels of these components may be elevated and may cause increased effects or potentially serious adverse reactions. People who are using any medications should always read the package insert and consult with their healthcare provider or pharmacist about possible interactions. This effect of chamomile has not been reliably tested in humans.
- *Note*: Many tinctures contain high levels of alcohol and may cause vomiting when taken with metronidazole (Flagyl) and disulfiram (Antabuse).

Interactions with Herbs and Dietary Supplements

- Chamomile may increase the level of drowsiness caused by some herbs or supplements. Examples are calamus, calendula, California poppy, capsicum, catnip, celery, couchgrass, dogwood, elecampane, goldenseal, gotu kola, hops, kava (may help sleep without drowsiness), lavender aromatherapy, lemon balm, sage, sassafras, scullcap, shepherd's purse, Siberian ginseng, stinging nettle, St. John's wort, valerian, wild carrot, wild lettuce, withania root, and yerba mansa. Caution is advised in people who are driving or operating machinery.
- In theory, chamomile may increase the risk of bleeding when taken with other products that are believed to increase the risk of bleeding. Multiple cases of bleeding have been reported with the use of *Ginkgo biloba*, and fewer cases with garlic and saw palmetto. Numerous other agents may theoretically increase the risk of bleeding, although this has not been proven in most cases. Examples are alfalfa, American ginseng, angelica, anise, *Arnica montana*, asafetida, aspen bark, bilberry, birch, black cohosh, bladderwrack, bogbean, boldo, borage seed oil, bromelain, capsicum, cat's claw, celery, chaparral, clove, coleus, cordyceps, danshen, devil's claw, dong quai, evening primrose, fenugreek, feverfew, flaxseed/flax powder (not a concern with flaxseed oil), ginger, grapefruit juice, grape seed, green tea, guggul, gymnestra, horseradish, licorice root, lovage root, male fern, meadowsweet, nordihydroguaiaretic acid (NDGA), onion, *Panax ginseng*, papain, parsley, passion flower, poplar, prickly ash, propolis, quassia, red clover, reishi, rue, Siberian ginseng, sweet birch, sweet clover, turmeric, vitamin E, white willow, wild carrot, wild lettuce, willow, wintergreen, and yucca.
- Limited laboratory research and studies in animals suggest that chamomile may interfere with how the body uses the liver's cytochrome P450 enzyme system to process components of other herbs and supplements. As a result, blood levels of these components may be elevated. Chamomile may alter the effects of other herbs on the cytochrome P450 system. Examples of such herbs are bloodroot, cat's claw, chaparral, chasteberry, damiana, *Echinacea angustifolia*, goldenseal, grapefruit juice, licorice, oregano, red clover, St. John's wort, wild cherry, and yucca. People who are using any medications should always read the package insert and consult their healthcare provider or pharmacist about possible interactions.

Selected References

Natural Standard developed the preceding evidence-based information based on a systematic review of more than 160 articles. For comprehensive information about alternative and complementary therapies on the professional level, go to www.naturalstandard.com. Selected references are listed here.

C

Aertgeerts P, Albring M, Klaschka F, et al. [Comparative testing of Kamillosan cream and steroidal (0.25% hydrocortisone, 0.75% fluocortin butyl ester) and non-steroidal (5% bufexamac) dermatologic agents in maintenance therapy of eczematous diseases.] Z Hautkr 1985;60(3):270-277.

Balslev T, Moller AB. [Burns in children caused by camomile tea.] Ugeskr Laeger 1990;152(19):1384.

Benetti C, Manganelli F. [Clinical experiences in the pharmacological treatment of vaginitis with a camomile-extract vaginal douche.] Minerva Ginecol 1985; 37(12):799-801.

Benner MH, Lee HJ. Anaphylactic reaction to chamomile tea. J Allergy Clin Immunol 1973;52(5):307-308.

Carl W, Emrich LS. Management of oral mucositis during local radiation and systemic chemotherapy: a study of 98 patients. J Prosthet Dent 1991;66(3): 361-369.

Casterline CL. Allergy to chamomile tea. JAMA 1980;244(4):330-331.

de la Motte S, Bose-O'Reilly S, Heinisch M, et al. [Double-blind comparison of an apple pectin-chamomile extract preparation with placebo in children with diarrhea.] Arzneimittelforschung 1997;47(11):1247-1249.

de la Torre orin F, Sanchez Machin I, Garcia Robaina JC, et al. Clinical cross-reactivity between *Artemisia vulgaris* and *Matricaria chamomilla* (chamomile). J Investig Allergol Clin Immunol 2001;11(2):118-122.

Fidler P, Loprinzi CL, O'Fallon JR, et al. Prospective evaluation of a chamomile mouthwash for prevention of 5-FU-induced oral mucositis. Cancer 1996; 77(3):522-525.

Foti C, Nettis E, Panebianco R, et al. Contact urticaria from *Matricaria chamomilla*. Contact Dermatitis 2000;42(6):360-361.

Giordano-Labadie F, Schwarze HP, Bazex J. Allergic contact dermatitis from camomile used in phytotherapy. Contact Dermatitis 2000;42(4):247.

Gowania HJ, Raulin C, Swoboda M. [Effect of chamomile on wound healing— a clinical double-blind study.] Z Hautkr 1987;62(17):1262, 1267-1271.

Gould L, Reddy CV, Gomprecht RF. Cardiac effects of chamomile tea. J Clin Pharmacol 1973;13(11):475-479.

Jensen-Jarolim E, Reider N, Fritsch R, et al. Fatal outcome of anaphylaxis to camomile-containing enema during labor: a case study. J Allergy Clin Immunol 1998;102(6 Pt 1):1041-1042.

Kagawa D, Jokura H, Ochiai R, Tokimitsu I, Tsubone H. The sedative effects and mechanism of action of cedrol inhalation with behavioral pharmacological evaluation. Planta Med 2003;69(7):637-641.

Kyokong O, Charuluxananan S, Muangmingsuk V, et al. Efficacy of chamomile-extract spray for prevention of post-operative sore throat. J Med Assoc Thai 2002;85(Suppl 1):S180-S185.

Maiche A, Grohn P, Maki-Hokkonen H. Effect of chamomile cream and almond ointment on acute radiation skin reaction. Acta Oncol 1991;30:395-397.

Maiche A, Maki-Hokkonen H, Grohn P. [Comparative trial of chamomile cream in radiotherapy.] Suomen Laakarilehti 1991;46(24):2206-2208.

Maliakal PP, Wanwimolruk S. Effect of herbal teas on hepatic drug metabolizing enzymes in rats. J Pharm Pharmacol 2001;53(10):1323-1329.

McGeorge BC, Steele MC. Allergic contact dermatitis of the nipple from Roman chamomile ointment. Contact Dermatitis 1991;24(2):139-140.

Patzelt-Wenczler R, Ponce-Poschl E. Proof of efficacy of Kamillosan cream in atopic eczema. Eur J Med Res 2000;5:171-175.

Paulsen E. Contact sensitization from Compositae-containing herbal remedies and cosmetics. Contact Dermatitis 2002;47(4):189-198.

Pereira F, Santos R, Pereira A. Contact dermatitis from chamomile tea. Contact Dermatitis 1997;36(6):307.

Reider N, Sepp N, Fritsch P, et al. Anaphylaxis to camomile: clinical features and allergen cross-reactivity. Clin Exp Allergy 2000;30(10):1436-1443.

Rodriguez B, Rodriguez A, de Barrio M, et al. Asthma induced by canary food mix. Allergy Asthma Proc 2003;24(4):265-268.

Ross SM. An integrative approach to eczema (atopic dermatitis). Holist Nurs Pract 2003;17(1):56-62.

Rycroft RJ. Recurrent facial dermatitis from chamomile tea. Contact Dermatitis. 2003;48(4):229.

Saller R, Beschomer M, Hellenbrecht D, et al. Dose dependency of symptomatic relief of complaints by chamomile steam inhalation in patients with common cold. Eur J Pharmacol 1990;183:728-729.

Seidler-Lozykowska K. Determination of the ploidy level in chamomile (*Chamomilla recutita* [L.] Rausch.) strains rich in alpha-bisabolol. J Appl Genet 2003;44(2):151-155.

Smolinski AT, Pestka JJ. Modulation of lipopolysaccharide-induced pro-inflammatory cytokine production *in vitro* and *in vivo* by the herbal constituents apigenin (chamomile), ginsenoside Rb(1) (ginseng) and parthenolide (feverfew). Food Chem Toxicol 2003;41(10):1381-1390.

Subiza J, Subiza JL, Alonso M, et al. Allergic conjunctivitis to chamomile tea. Ann Allergy 1990;65(2):127-132.

Subiza J, Subiza JL, Hinojosa M, et al. Anaphylactic reaction after the ingestion of chamomile tea: a study of cross-reactivity with other composite pollens. J Allergy Clin Immunol 1989;84(3):353-358.

Thien FC. Chamomile tea enema anaphylaxis. Med J Aust 2001;175(1):54.

van Ketel WG. Allergy to *Matricaria chamomilla*. Contact Dermatitis 1987; 16(1):50-51.

Weizman Z, Alkrinawi S, Goldfarb D, et al. Efficacy of herbal tea preparation in infantile colic. J Pediatr 1993;122(4):650-652

Wilkinson S, Aldridge J, Salmon I, et al. An evaluation of aromatherapy massage in palliative care. Palliat Med 1999;13(5):409-417.

Chaparral

(Larrea tridentata [DC] Coville, *Larrea divaricata* Cav)

SYNONYMS/COMMON NAMES/RELATED SUBSTANCES

- Chaparro, creosote bush, dwarf evergreen oak, el gobernadora, falsa alcaparra, geroop, gobernadora, greasewood, guamis, gumis, hediondilla, hideonodo, jarillo, kovanau, kreosotstrauch, *Larrea divaricata, Larrea tridentate, Larrea glutiosa, Larrea mexicana* Moric, nordihydroguaiaretic acid (NDGA), palo ondo, shoegoi, sonora covillea, tasago, ya-tmep, yah-temp, Zygophyllaceae.

CLINICAL BOTTOM LINE
Background

- Chaparral and its constituent nordihydroguaiaretic acid (NDGA) have been reported to possess antioxidant/free-radical scavenging properties. Although proposed as a treatment for cancer, effectiveness has not been demonstrated in clinical trials. Chaparral and NDGA have been associated with cases of hepatitis, cirrhosis, liver failure, renal cysts, and renal cell carcinoma. In response to these reports, the U.S. Food and Drug Administration removed chaparral from its "generally recognized as safe" (GRAS) list in 1970. Chaparral and NDGA are generally considered unsafe and are not recommended for use.

Scientific Evidence for Common/Studied Uses	Grade*
Cancer	C

*Key to grades: *A:* Strong scientific evidence for this use; *B:* Good scientific evidence for this use; *C:* Unclear scientific evidence for this use; *D:* Fair scientific evidence against this use (it may not work); *F:* Strong scientific evidence against this use (it likely does not work). For a more detailed explanation of efficacy criteria, see "Natural Standard Evidence-Based Validated Grading Rationale" in the Introduction.

Historical or Theoretical Uses That Lack Supportive Evidence:

- Allergies, analgesia, antibacterial, anti-flatulent, anti-inflammatory, antiparasitic, antiviral, arthritis, autoimmune disorders, "blood purifier," bowel cramps, bruises, chickenpox (varicella), CNS disorders, colds, chronic cutaneous disorders, diabetes, diarrhea, diuretic, dysmenorrhea, dyspepsia, emesis, expectorant, gastrointestinal cramps, gastrointestinal disorders, genitourinary infections, hair tonic, hallucinations (including those due to lysergic acid diethylamide (LSD) ingestion), heartburn, indigestion, influenza, menstrual cramps, pain, peptic ulcer disease, respiratory tract infections, rheumatic diseases, skin disorders, snakebite pain, tuberculosis, venereal disease, wound healing.

Expert Opinion and Folkloric Precedent

- Because of chaparral's adverse effect profile, many natural medicine experts discourage its use.

Safety Summary

- **Likely unsafe:** The U.S. Food and Drug Administration removed chaparral from the "generally recognized as safe" (GRAS) list in 1970. Capsule and tablet forms of chaparral have been associated with more toxicity reports than steeped teas. Because of the adverse effects of hepatic and renal toxicity, chaparral is not recommended for use. Chaparral is unsafe in pregnancy and lactation based on *in vitro* uteroactivity as well as toxicity. The chaparral constituent nordihydroguaiaretic acid (NGDA) inhibits RNA protein and lipid syntheses by mammary glands following prolactin stimulation *in vitro* and theoretically should be avoided during lactation.[1]
- **Possibly unsafe:** A supplement called Herp-Eeze (formerly called Larreastat) made with *Larrea tridentate* (chaparral), has been claimed to be nontoxic. Supportive data are limited.

DOSING/TOXICOLOGY
General

- Chaparral is generally considered unsafe and is not recommended for use. The doses listed are based on those most commonly used in historical practice. In general, with natural products, the optimal doses needed to balance safety and efficacy often have not been determined. Formulations and preparation methods may vary from manufacturer to manufacturer, and from batch to batch of a specific product made by a single manufacturer. Because often the active components of a product are not known, standardization may not be possible, and the clinical effects of different brands may not be comparable.

Standardization

- There is no widely accepted standardization for chaparral.

Dosing: Adult (18 Years and Older)
Oral:

- **General:** Capsules or tablets may deliver large doses, leading to toxicity. Small doses of tea or tincture have been associated with less toxicity and possibly contain fewer allergenic compounds than found in capsules or tablets. Exposure to lignans, which may yield toxicity, appears to be greater from capsules or tablets than from decoctions of chaparral tea.[2]
- **Tablets/Capsules:** Not recommended due to potential toxicity.
- **Tea:** 1 teaspoon of chaparral leaves and flowers steeped in 1 pint of water for 15 minutes; 1 to 3 cups daily up to a maximum of several days. May be toxic.
- **Tincture:** 20 drops up to 3 times daily. May be toxic.
- **Topical:** Apply oil or powdered form of chaparral over affected area several times daily.

Dosing: Pediatric (Younger Than 18 Years)

- Chaparral is not recommended for use because of potential toxicity.

Toxicology

- Rats fed the chaparral constituent nordihydroguaiaretic acid (NDGA) titrated to a total of 3% in their diet over 4 weeks developed multiple cortical and medullary renal cysts.[3] In a 1947 study, Cranston et al. conducted chronic toxicity studies assessing oral and intraperitoneal administration of 0.25%

C

to 0.5% NDGA over a period of 2 years in rats and mice.[4] The authors noted no significant pathology of the liver, spleen or kidneys, although instances of liver necrosis were noted in both the control and the NDGA groups. In one NDGA group, hemorrhage into the cecum was noted in half of the rats, but this was not reproduced in a larger sample. Several rats administered a higher concentration of NDGA developed mesenteric cysts.

- Anecdotally, decontamination with ipecac or activated charcoal with lavage and supportive therapy are recommended for overdose treatment.

ADVERSE EFFECTS/PRECAUTIONS/CONTRAINDICATIONS
Allergy

- Avoid if there is known allergy/hypersensitivity to chaparral or any of its constituents including nordihydroguaiaretic acid (NDGA), nor-isoguaiasin, dihydroguaiaretic acid, partially demethylated dihydroguaiaretic acid, and demethoxyisoguaiasin.[2]
- There have been human case reports of allergic hypersensitivity (contact dermatitis) to chaparral or its resin.[5,6]

Adverse Effects

- **General:** Chaparral has been associated with multiple serious and potentially fatal adverse effects. The U.S. Food and Drug Administration removed chaparral from the "generally recognized as safe" (GRAS) list in 1970 and now considers chaparral to be unsafe. Exposure to lignans, which may yield toxicity, appears to be greater from capsule or tablets than from decoctions of chaparral tea.[2]
- **Dermatologic:** In a case series of 59 patients, adverse effects included rash and stomatitis; however, frequency and severity were not noted.[7] Six men with acute contact dermatitis had positive patch tests to various species of the genus *Larrea*.[5] Dermatitis was reported on the face, neck, arms, legs, and scrotum (most chemical constituents including nordihydroguaiaretic acid [NDGA] are found in all species of *Larrea*, and therefore these reactions may be pertinent to chaparral). There have been human case reports of allergic hypersensitivity (contact dermatitis) to the plant or its resin.[5,6]
- **Neurologic/CNS:** Fever has been reported in case reports,[7,8] but it is unclear if this was due to chaparral ingestion.
- **Renal:** Chaparral has been reported to induce kidney failure.[8] Renal cystic disease, renal insufficiency, and renal cell carcinoma were reported in a patient who consumed 3 to 4 cups of chaparral tea daily for 3 months.[9] The patient presented with mild hypertension, a creatinine of 1.5 mg/dL, and had a history of pyelonephritis. The patient was followed for 2 years and subsequently was noted to have a creatinine of 1.7 mg/dL. It is not clear that chaparral was the causative agent in this case. Chaparral has been noted to cause renal cysts in rats, theorized to be due to renal accumulation of the o-quinone metabolite of the chaparral component nordihydroguaiaretic acid (NDGA).[3] Rat feedings including 2% NDGA have been associated with cystic changes to the kidney.[10] Partial nephron obstruction was noted and was believed to be a contributor to cyst formation.
- **Hepatic:** Multiple case-reports linking chaparral to liver toxicity are available in the literature.[8,11-17] The most serious outcomes of liver toxicity documented include four case reports of cirrhosis, and two of fulminant liver failure requiring transplantation. In most cases, symptoms arose 3 to 52 weeks after initiating chaparral and resolved in 1 to 17 weeks after

discontinuation.[8] Symptoms reported include fatigue, right upper quadrant abdominal pain, dark urine, light stools, nausea, diarrhea, anorexia, weight loss, icterus, fatigue, pedal edema, and increased abdominal girth. Also noted were elevations in alkaline phosphatase, alanine aminotransferase (ALT) and aspartate aminotransferase (AST), total bilirubin, and gamma-glutamyltranspeptidase (GGT).

Precautions/Warnings/Contraindications

- Chaparral and its constituent nordihydroguaiaretic acid (NDGA) are potentially toxic or fatal, and are not recommended for general use.
- Avoid in patients with renal dysfunction: Chaparral has been linked to renal cysts and carcinoma.[9] Patients with renal dysfunction may be more susceptible to accumulation and toxicity of chaparral.
- Avoid in patients with hepatic disease: Patients with hepatic dysfunction may be more likely to develop chaparral-induced hepatitis, cirrhosis or liver failure.

Pregnancy and Lactation

- Chaparral is not recommended for use. Anecdotally it has been reported that chaparral induced uterine contractions in animals. The chaparral component nordihydroguaiaretic acid (NDGA) was shown to inhibit prolactin effects on RNA, lipid, and casein biosynthesis in cultured mouse mammary gland explants.[1] The clinical significance of this finding is unclear.

INTERACTIONS
Chaparral/Drug Interactions

- **Anticoagulants, antiplatelet agents, NSAIDs:** In theory, there may be an increased risk of bleeding with concurrent use of chaparral and other agents. The chaparral component nordihydroguaiaretic acid (NDGA) diminishes platelet aggregation evoked by collagen or adenosine diphosphate and delays its onset.[18]
- **Nephrotoxic medications:** Theoretically, use of chaparral with other agents known to induce renal toxicity should be avoided. Chaparral has been reported to induce kidney failure.[8] Renal cell carcinoma and renal cystic disease have also been reported with chaparral.[9]
- **Hepatotoxic medications:** Chaparral has been reported to induce liver injury.[8,13,15-17] Theoretically, use of chaparral with other agents known to induce liver toxicity should be avoided, such as amiodarone, carmustine, danazol, fluoxymesterone, isoniazid, ketoconazole, mercaptopurine, methotrexate, methyltestosterone, oxandrolone, oxymetholone, plicamycin, stanozolol, tacrine, testosterone, and valproic acid.
- **Hypoglycemic agents, insulin:** In theory, chaparral may have additive effects when taken concurrently with hypoglycemic agents. In mouse models of type 2 diabetes, the chaparral component nordihydroguaiaretic acid (NDGA) was shown to decrease plasma glucose concentrations, without any change in insulin concentration.[19] NDGA improved glucose tolerance and ability of insulin to decrease glucose concentrations.
- **Agents metabolized by cytochrome P450:** The chaparral component nordihydroguaiaretic acid (NDGA) inhibits cytochrome P450-mediated monoxygenase activity in rat hepatic microsomes.[20] In theory, chaparral, which contains NDGA, may interact with other agents metabolized by the cytochrome P450 pathway and raise the levels of P450 substrates.

- **Monoamine oxidase inhibitors (MAOIs):** Chaparral has been reported anecdotally to pose a risk of reacting with MAOIs. There are limited data in this area.

Chaparral/Herb/Supplement Interactions

- **Anticoagulant/antiplatelet herbs and supplements:** In theory, there may be an increased risk of bleeding with concurrent use of chaparral and other agents. The chaparral component nordihydroguaiaretic acid (NDGA) diminishes platelet aggregation evoked by collagen or adenosine-diphosphate, and delays its onset.[18]
- **Nephrotoxic agents:** Theoretically, use of chaparral with other agents known to induce renal toxicity should be avoided. Chaparral has been reported to induce kidney failure.[18] Renal cell carcinoma and renal cystic disease have also been reported with chaparral.[9]
- **Hepatotoxic agents:** Chaparral has been reported to induce liver injury.[8,13,15-17] Theoretically, use of chaparral with other agents known to induce liver toxicity should be avoided. Hepatotoxicity has often been reported following ingestion of chaparral over weeks to months, and case reports have noted elevated liver enzymes.[11]
- **Hypoglycemic herbs and supplements:** In theory, chaparral may have additive effects when taken concurrently with hypoglycemic agents. In mouse models of type 2 diabetes, the chaparral component nordihydroguaiaretic acid (NDGA) was shown to decrease plasma glucose concentrations, without any change in insulin concentration. NDGA improved glucose tolerance and ability of insulin to decrease glucose concentrations.[19]
- **Agents metabolized by cytochrome P450:** The chaparral component nordihydroguaiaretic acid (NDGA) inhibits cytochrome P450-mediated monoxygenase activity in rat hepatic microsomes.[20] Theoretically chaparral, which contains NDGA, may interact with other agents metabolized by the cytochrome P450 pathway.
- **Monoamine oxidase inhibitor herbs and supplements:** Chaparral has been reported anecdotally to pose a risk of reacting with monoamine oxidase inhibitors. There are limited data in this area.

Chaparral/Food Interactions

- Insufficient available evidence.

Chaparral/Lab Interactions

- **Alanine aminotransferase (ALT), aspartate aminotransferase (AST), gamma-glutamyltransferase (GGT), lactate dehydrogenase (LDH), alkaline phosphatase, total bilirubin:** Hepatotoxicity has often been reported following ingestion of chaparral over weeks to months, and case reports have noted elevated liver enzymes.[11]

- **Plasma glucose:** Chaparral may lower serum glucose levels. In mouse models of type 2 diabetes, the chaparral component nordihydroguaiaretic acid (NDGA) was shown to decrease plasma glucose concentrations, without any change in insulin concentration. NDGA improved glucose tolerance and ability of insulin to decrease glucose concentrations.[19]
- **Serum creatinine:** Chaparral has been reported to induce kidney failure[8] and has been associated with elevations of creatinine to 1.5 mg/dL (without subsequent improvement of renal function despite cessation of chaparral therapy).[9]

MECHANISM OF ACTION
Pharmacology

- The chaparral constituent nordihydroguaiaretic acid (NDGA) has been theorized to block cellular respiration and exert antioxidant effects, although pharmacologic studies are limited. NDGA has been shown to inhibit induction of ornithine decarboxylase, a lipoxygenase inhibitor in mice,[21] and in vitro.[22] NDGA diminishes platelet aggregation evoked by collagen or adenosine diphosphate and delays its onset.[18] Hydroxyl groups of NDGA may play a role in inhibiting cytochrome P450 monoxygenase activity.[20]
- In mouse models of type 2 diabetes, NDGA was shown to decrease plasma glucose concentrations, without any change in insulin concentration. NDGA improved glucose tolerance and ability of insulin to decrease glucose concentrations.[19]

Pharmacodynamics/Kinetics

- In rats, the chaparral component nordihydroguaiaretic acid (NDGA) is metabolized to an o-quinone metabolite in the ileum and is absorbed in the bloodstream, filtered by the glomeruli, and retained by the proximal tubule where it accumulates.[3,23] Free NDGA is not found in the rat kidney, but is found in the feces.[3]

HISTORY

- Chaparral is a shrub found in the desert regions of southwestern United States and Mexico. It was used by Native American populations for indications including chickenpox (varicella), colds, diarrhea, menstrual cramps, pain, rheumatic diseases, skin disorders, and snake bites and as an emetic. Chaparral tea was also used for purported effects of removing lysergic acid diethylamide (LSD) residue and thereby preventing recurrent hallucinations. Chaparral leaves also have been used externally for bruises, scratches, wounds, and hair growth. The chaparral component nordihydroguaiaretic acid (NDGA) has been evaluated as a treatment for cancer.
- Before 1967, NDGA was used as a food additive to prevent fermentation and decomposition, possibly due to its antioxidant properties.

Review of the Evidence: Chaparral

Condition Treated*	Study Design	Author, Year	N[†]	SS[†]	Study Quality[‡]	Magnitude of Benefit	ARR[†]	NNT[†]	Comments
Cancer (tumor regression)	Case series	Smart[7] 1970	59	No	NA	None	NA	NA	Heterogeneous tumor types studied, short duration; improvements seen in 4 patients.

*Primary or secondary outcome.
[†]N, Number of patients; SS, statistically significant; ARR, absolute risk reduction; NNT, the number of patients who need to undergo a specific intervention in order to observe an outcome in one individual.
[‡]0-2 = poor; 3-4 = good; 5 = excellent.
NA, Not applicable.
For an explanation of each category in this table, please see Table 3 in the Introduction.

REVIEW OF THE EVIDENCE: DISCUSSION
Cancer
Summary

- Possible anticancer effects of chaparral or its component nordihydroguaiaretic acid (NDGA) were initially suggested by animal research and a human case report. However, a subsequent small case series did not observe impressive benefits.[7] Without further controlled trial evidence, the data must be considered inconclusive. Because of the known toxicity of chaparral, the risks of this therapy may outweigh the potential benefits.

Evidence

- In a 1970 case series of 59 patients with advanced malignancies (types not documented), subjects were treated with either 16 to 24 oz. of chaparral tea or 250 to 3000 mg of nordihydroguaiaretic acid (NDGA) daily for 4 weeks.[7] Patients were considered to have a benefit if tumor size decreased by 25% or greater. Although four patients experienced significant tumor regression, other patients experienced no change or growth in tumor size. Adverse effects included nausea, vomiting, diarrhea, abdominal cramps, rash, stomatitis, and fever. Details pertaining to the four subjects who benefited are limited.

- In a 1969 published case report, a patient 85 years of age with metastatic malignant melanoma ingested chaparral tea equivalent to approximately 3.5 to 6 g daily. The patient refused all other medical treatment. Within a year, the lesion on his face was reportedly reduced from 3 to 4 cm to a diameter of 2 to 3 cm. A submandibular lesion, which was 5 to 7 cm in diameter, completely resolved.[24]

- Rats were given the carcinogen methylazoxymethanol to induce bowel tumors in order to evaluate the effect of NDGA on carcinogenesis.[25] Results indicated that 13 out of 14 rats in the control group developed tumors, whereas only 5 out of 14 rats in the NDGA treatment group developed tumors.

References

1. Rillema JA. Effect of NDGA, a lipoxygenase inhibitor, on prolactin actions in mouse mammary gland explants. Prostaglandins Leukot.Med 1984; 16(1): 89-94.
2. Obermeyer WR, Musser SM, Betz JM, et al. Chemical studies of phytoestrogens and related compounds in dietary supplements: flax and chaparral. Proc Soc Exp Biol Med 1995;208(1):6-12.
3. Goodman T, Grice HC, Becking GC, et al. A cystic nephropathy induced by nordihydroguaiaretic acid in the rat. Light and electron microscopic investigations. Lab Invest 1970;23(1):93-107.
4. Cranston EM, Jensen MJ, Moren MJ, et al. The acute and chronic toxicity of nordihydroguaiaretic acid. Fed Proc 1947;6:318-319.
5. Leonforte JF. Contact dermatitis from *Larrea* (creosote bush). J Am Acad Dermatol 1986;14(2 Pt 1):202-207.
6. Shasky DR. Contact dermatitis from *Larrea tridentata* (creosote bush). J Am Acad Dermatol 1986;15(2 Pt 1):302.
7. Smart CR, Hogle HH, Vogel H, et al. Clinical experience with nordihydroguaiaretic acid—"chaparral tea" in the treatment of cancer. Rocky Mt Med J 1970;67(11):39-43.
8. Sheikh NM, Philen RM, Love LA. Chaparral-associated hepatotoxicity. Arch Intern Med 1997;157(8):913-919.
9. Smith AY, Feddersen RM, Gardner KD, Jr., et al. Cystic renal cell carcinoma and acquired renal cystic disease associated with consumption of chaparral tea: a case report. J Urol 1994;152(6 Pt 1):2089-2091.
10. Evan AP, Gardner KD, Jr. Nephron obstruction in nordihydroguaiaretic acid-induced renal cystic disease. Kidney Int 1979;15(1):7-19.
11. Alderman S, Kailas S, Goldfarb S, et al. Cholestatic hepatitis after ingestion of chaparral leaf: confirmation by endoscopic retrograde cholangio-pancreatography and liver biopsy. J Clin Gastroenterol 1994;19(3):242-247.
12. Anonymous. Chaparral-induced toxic hepatitis—California and Texas, 1992. MMWR Morb Mortal Wkly Rep 1992;41(43):812-814.
13. Batchelor WB, Heathcote J, Wanless IR. Chaparral-induced hepatic injury. Am J Gastroenterol 1995;90(5):831-833.
14. Clark F. Chaparral-induced toxic hepatitis: California and Texas, 1992. MMWR Morb Mortal Wkly Rep 1992;41:812-814.
15. Gordon DW, Rosenthal G, Hart J, et al. Chaparral ingestion. The broadening spectrum of liver injury caused by herbal medications. JAMA 1995;273(6):489-490.
16. Katz M, Saibil F. Herbal hepatitis: subacute hepatic necrosis secondary to chaparral leaf. J Clin Gastroenterol 1990;12(2):203-206.
17. Smith BC, Desmond PV. Acute hepatitis induced by ingestion of the herbal medication chaparral. Aust N Z J Med 1993;23(5):526.
18. Gimeno MF, Shattner MA, Borda E, et al. Lipoxygenase inhibitors alter aggregation and adhesiveness of human blood platelets from aspirin-treated patients. Prostaglandins Leukot Med 1983;11(1):109-119.
19. Luo J, Chuang T, Cheung J, et al. Masoprocol (nordihydroguaiaretic acid): a new antihyperglycemic agent isolated from the creosote bush (*Larrea tridentata*). Eur J Pharmacol 1998;346(1):77-79.
20. Agarwal R, Wang ZY, Bik DP, et al. Nordihydroguaiaretic acid, an inhibitor of lipoxygenase, also inhibits cytochrome P-450-mediated monooxygenase activity in rat epidermal and hepatic microsomes. Drug Metab Dispos 1991; 19(3):620-624.
21. Nakadate T, Yamamoto S, Aizu E, et al. Inhibition of 12-O-tetra-decanoylphorbol-13-acetate-induced increase in vascular permeability in mouse skin by lipoxygenase inhibitors. Jpn J Pharmacol 1985;38(2):161-168.
22. Salari H, Braquet P, Borgeat P. Comparative effects of indomethacin, acetylenic acids, 15-HETE, nordihydroguaiaretic acid and BW755C on the metabolism of arachidonic acid in human leukocytes and platelets. Prostaglandins Leukot Med 1984;13(1):53-60.
23. Grice HC, Becking G, Goodman T. Toxic properties of nordihydroguaiaretic acid. Food Cosmet Toxicol 1968;6(2):155-161.
24. Smart CR, Hogle HH, Robins RK, et al. An interesting observation on nordihydroguaiaretic acid (NSC-4291; NDGA) and a patient with malignant melanoma—a preliminary report. Cancer Chemother Rep 1969;53(2):147-151.
25. Birkenfeld S, Zaltsman YA, Krispin M, et al. Antitumor effects of inhibitors of arachidonic acid cascade on experimentally induced intestinal tumors. Dis Colon Rectum 1987;30(1):43-46.

Chasteberry
(Vitex agnus-castus)

SYNONYMS/COMMON NAMES/RELATED SUBSTANCES

- Abraham's balm, Abrahams-strauch, agneau chaste (French), agni casti fructus, agnocasto, agnus castus, chaste berry, chaste tree, chaste tree berry, chastetree, gattilier (French), hemp tree, keuschlammfruchte (German), kyskhedstrae (Danish), monk's pepper, moenchspfeffer (German), petit poivre (French), Verbenaceae, vitex.

CLINICAL BOTTOM LINE
Background

- The chaste tree is native to the Mediterranean and Central Asia. Its berries have long been used for a variety of abnormalities including "corpus luteum deficiency," mastalgia, and menstrual abnormalities.
- Chasteberry has been shown to inhibit prolactin secretion by competitively binding to dopamine receptors. Available evidence suggests that chasteberry may be an effective treatment option for hyperprolactinemic conditions and premenstrual syndrome. Chasteberry does not appear to affect levels of luteinizing hormone or follicle-stimulating hormone.
- To date, clinical trials have found that treatment with chasteberry has been well tolerated with minimal side effects.

Scientific Evidence for Common/Studied Uses	Grade*
Hyperprolactinemia	B
Corpus luteum deficiency/luteal phase deficiency	C
Cyclic mastalgia	C
Irregular menstrual cycles	C
Premenstrual dysphoric disorder (PMDD)	C
Premenstrual syndrome (PMS)	C

*Key to grades: *A:* Strong scientific evidence for this use; *B:* Good scientific evidence for this use; *C:* Unclear scientific evidence for this use; *D:* Fair scientific evidence against this use (it may not work); *F:* Strong scientific evidence against this use (it likely does not work). For a more detailed explanation of efficacy criteria, see "Natural Standard Evidence-Based Validated Grading Rationale" in the Introduction.

Historical or Theoretical Uses That Lack Supportive Evidence

- Acne,[1] amenorrhea, antifungal,[2] anti-inflammatory, anxiety, benign prostatic hypertrophy (BPH), chastity, constipation, cystic endometrial hyperplasia, dementia, depression due to menopause,[3] diarrhea, dysmenorrhea, dyspepsia, endometriosis, epilepsy, female infertility,[4] fevers, fibrocystic breasts, flatulence, fluid retention, follicular ovarian cysts, hangovers, hot flashes, hypogonadism, impotence, inflammation, lactation, menopause, menorrhagia (heavy menstruation), menstrual dermatoses, "menstrual neuroses," metrorrhagia (from functional causes), mouth ulcers, nervousness, oligomenorrhea (lengthened cycle),[5] orofacial herpes simplex, overactive libido, placenta expulsion, polymenorrhea (shortened cycle),[5] postpartum bleeding, premenstrual aphthous ulcerative stomatitis,[6] prevention of miscarriage in patients with progesterone insufficiency, reducing sexual desire, rheumatic conditions, secondary amenorrhea, snake bite, upper respiratory tract infections, vaginal dryness.

Expert Opinion and Folkloric Precedent

- The dried fruit of chasteberry plants has been used for thousands of years as a means of treating various ailments ranging from impotence to breast pain. It was popular in ancient Greece and Rome to help promote celibacy. More recently, chasteberry has gained recognition for its success in alleviating some signs and symptoms of hyperprolactinemia and premenstrual syndrome.[7,8] It is thought to have a normalizing effect on the menstrual cycle and has been used successfully to treat both amenorrhea and menorrhagia.[9]
- A preparation of chasteberry has been available in Germany since the 1950s and is used in the treatment of menstrual cycle irregularities, premenstrual complaints, and mastalgia.

Safety Summary

- **Likely safe:** When used orally in otherwise healthy adults taken in appropriate doses for the short-term alleviation of signs and symptoms associated with premenstrual syndrome or hyperprolactinemia.[7,8,10-12]
- **Likely safe:** When used concomitantly with oral contraceptives or hormone replacement therapy.[13,14] There are no studies evaluating the long-term effects of chasteberry, and safety is not established.
- **Possibly unsafe:** When used concomitantly with dopamine agonists/antagonists, because of the binding of chasteberry to dopamine-2 receptors in the pituitary.[15,16]
- **Likely unsafe:** When used in patients during pregnancy or lactation.[7]

DOSING/TOXICOLOGY
General

- Recommended doses are based on those most commonly used in available trials, or on historical practice. However, with natural products, the optimal doses needed to balance efficacy and safety often have not been determined. Formulations and preparation methods may vary from manufacturer to manufacturer, and from batch to batch of a specific product made by a single manufacturer. Because often the active components of a product are not known, standardization may not be possible, and the clinical effects of different brands may not be comparable.

Standardization

- Although there is no universal standardization for chasteberry products, many extracts are standardized to contain 0.5% agnuside or 0.6% aucubin, and may be standardized to casticin content.
- Various formulations have been used, including Femicur (Schaper & Brummer GmbH & Co. KG, Salzgitter, Germany), which contains 1.6 to 3.0 mg of dried extract per capsule; Agnolyt (Madaus AG, Cologne, Germany) liquid or

capsules, standardized to 3.5 to 4.2 mg of dried chasteberry extract; *Vitex agnus castus* L extract Ze 440, in which each 20-mg tablet is standardized for casticin; Agnucaston/BNO 1095 (a 70% ethanol, 30% water extract, Bionorica, Neumarkt, Germany) liquid or tablets, Mastodynon (53% v/v ethanol, Bionorica, Neumarkt, Germany) liquid or tablets, daily dose of 60 drops is equivalent to 32.4 mg of the extract.

Dosing: Adult (18 Years and Older)
Oral

- *Note:* Some experts recommend taking chasteberry on an empty stomach in the morning for maximal benefits. However, no studies have confirmed this finding.
- Various doses of chasteberry have been used in studies and practice. For example, for premenstrual syndrome, 20 mg of chasteberry extract ZE 440 has been used (standardized to 60% ethanol m/m, extract ratio 6 to 12:1; standardized for casticin),[13,14] 40 mg daily of Femicur (corresponding to 3.2 to 6.0 mg of dried chasteberry fruit).[11] Traditional doses have ranged from 3.5 to 4.5 mg per day of dried extract to 600 mg three times per day of dried fruit. There is no standard dosing recommendation for hyperprolactinemia, although studies have used 20 mg of Strotan capsules daily in women,[7] and 40 to 160 mg of a chasteberry extract up to three times daily in men.[12] For cyclic mastalgia, 1.8 mL per day (60 drops) of Mastodynon chasteberry extract has been given daily,[17,18] or 1 Mastodynon tablet daily.[8]
- Other traditional dosing includes an aqueous alcoholic extract derived from 30 to 40 mg of dried fruit daily in 50% to 70% alcohol (v/v); 0.03 to 0.04 mL daily of fluid extract (1:1 g/mL), 0.15 to 0.2 mL daily of tincture (1:5 g/mL); 2.6 to 4.2 mg daily of a dried extract (9.5 to 11.5:1 w/w); or 0.5 to 1.0 g of dried fruit taken three times daily.

Dosing: Pediatric (Younger Than 18 Years)

- Insufficient evidence to recommend.

Toxicology

- Although rare, there has been one case report of multiple follicular development after taking an herbal supplement containing chasteberry.[19] The patient had symptoms of a mild ovarian hyperstimulation syndrome with an observed luteinizing hormone surge. Hormone levels returned to normal following cessation of the supplement.

ADVERSE EFFECTS/PRECAUTIONS/CONTRAINDICATIONS
Allergy

- Known allergy/hypersensitivity to members of the Vitex (Verbenaceae) family or any chasteberry components.
- Mild skin reactions have been reported in clinical trials, including eczema, itching, rash, skin eruptions, urticaria,[10,11,13,14,18] and allergic exanthema.[20]

Adverse Effects

- **General:** When taken in recommended doses, chasteberry appears to be generally well tolerated, with few adverse events reported.[11,13,14] In an observational trial of 551 patients, approximately 5% experienced side effects, which were primarily mild.[21]
- **Dermatologic:** Acne, alopecia, eczema, itching, rash, skin eruptions, and urticaria have been noted in clinical trials.[10,11,13,14] In an open trial, seven patients were noted to develop acne.[22] One patient developed allergic exanthema in a randomized trial.[20]

- **Neurologic/CNS:** Headache,[21,22] vertigo,[12] and seizure[23] have been reported, although causality is not clear. Anecdotal reports have noted drowsiness, agitation, fatigue, sweating, and dry mouth. One patient developed depressed mood during a randomized trial.[20]
- **Otic:** Increased intraocular pressure has been reported anecdotally, although this has not been studied.
- **Cardiovascular:** Although there are anecdotal reports of tachycardia, palpitations, circulatory disorders, and pulmonary edema with the use of chasteberry, no changes in heart rate or blood pressure were noted in a controlled trial comparing chasteberry to placebo at dose escalations of 120 mg/day, 240 mg/day, and 480 mg/day.[12]
- **Gastrointestinal:** Diarrhea, nausea, gas (flatulence), heartburn, and vomiting have been reported rarely in clinical studies.[10-12,22]
- **Endocrine:** There is a case report of altered gonadotropin and ovarian hormone levels with chasteberry, in which a patient experienced symptoms suggestive of mild ovarian hyperstimulation in the luteal phase.[19] Mastodynia was reported in one patient in a randomized trial.[20] Hot flashes, mastalgia, cycle changes, fibroid growth, and weight gain have also rarely been reported.
- **Renal:** Polyuria has been reported anecdotally.
- **Genitourinary:** Menstrual bleeding has rarely been reported in clinical trials.[11,13,14,22] Vaginitis and pelvic disease have been reported anecdotally.
- **Hematologic:** One subject in a large, uncontrolled clinical trial reported that after treatment with chasteberry she experienced a nosebleed.[11]

Precautions/Warnings/Contraindications

- Use cautiously in patients taking oral contraceptives or hormone replacement therapy.
- Use cautiously in patients taking dopamine agonists or antagonists.
- Avoid using in patients with hormone-sensitive cancers or conditions.
- Avoid using in women who are pregnant or breastfeeding.
- Avoid using in women undergoing *in vitro* fertilization.[19]

Pregnancy and Lactation

- Except under strict medical supervision, chasteberry should not be used in pregnancy because of potential uterine stimulatory properties. Some clinicians have used chasteberry in progesterone-deficient women during their first trimester to prevent miscarriage,[24] but it is not known if chasteberry is helpful or safe for this indication.
- Theoretically, chasteberry should be avoided during lactation. Chasteberry competitively binds to dopamine receptors and has been shown to affect prolactin secretion,[15,16] possibly resulting in decreased breast milk production. However, some clinicians actually use low doses to stimulate milk production, with some reported benefits.

INTERACTIONS
Chasteberry/Drug Interactions

- **Dopamine antagonists:** Chasteberry has been shown to bind to dopamine-2 receptors and therefore may negate the action of dopamine antagonists.
- **Dopamine agonists:** Chasteberry competitively binds to dopamine-2 receptors, and may result in increased serum levels of dopamine, thereby exacerbating dopaminergic effects.

- **Oral contraceptives/hormone replacement therapy:** Chasteberry may increase plasma levels of estrogens and progesterone.

Chasteberry/Herb/Supplement Interactions

- **Estrogenic or progestational herbs:** Chasteberry may increase plasma levels of estrogens and progesterone and may add to the effects of estrogenic or progestational herbs.

Chasteberry/Food Interactions

- Insufficient data.

Chasteberry/Lab Interactions

- **Prolactin:** Low doses of chasteberry have been observed to increase serum prolactin levels,[7,12] and higher doses of chasteberry have resulted in inhibition of prolactin secretion and lower serum levels of prolactin.

MECHANISM OF ACTION
Pharmacology

- **Constituents:** The dried fruit of chasteberry is used to prepare commercial products. The fruit contains essential oils (limonene, cineole, and sabinene), iridoid glycosides (aucubin and agnoside), flavonoids (primarily castican, orientin, and isovitexin), and essential fatty acids (oleic acid, linolenic acid, palmitic acid, stearic acid).
- **Hormonal effects:** *In vitro*, constituents in chasteberry bind selectively to estrogen receptor beta.[25,26] Apigenin, a flavonoid, has been identified as an active phytoestrogen in chasteberry. It has been debated whether chasteberry alters the secretion of follicle-stimulating hormone (FSH) or luteinizing hormone (LH). Most clinical trials have found that levels remain unaffected.[8,16] The reported effects of chasteberry on prolactin levels in humans are variable and not well characterized. *In vitro* and animal studies report that constituents of chasteberry bind to dopamine-2 receptors in the pituitary, thereby inhibiting prolactin secretion.[15,16] Haloperidol, a dopamine agonist, was able to counteract the prolactin-lowering effect of chasteberry.[27] One animal study suggests that chasteberry possesses antiandrogenic effects,[28] noting that a flavonoid-rich fraction of chasteberry administered to male dogs resulted in disruption of the latter stages of spermatogenesis. Reduced androgen production was reflected in low levels of sialic acid in the testes.
- **Antimicrobial effects:** Ethanolic and etheric extracts of chaste tree demonstrate *in vitro* antimicrobial activity against *Staphylococcus aureus, Streptococcus faecalis* (6.5% to 20% extracts), *Salmonella, Escherichia coli* (10% to 20%), *Candida albicans, C. tropicalis, C. pseudotropicalis* and *C. krusei* (10% to 40%). Chasteberry extracts have also demonstrated high levels of toxicity against the mycelial growth of *Trichophyton mentagrophytes, Epidermophyton floccosum, Microsporum canis, M. gypseum* (1.5% to 12%) and *Penicillium viridicatum* (9% to 23%).[29] Essential oil from chasteberry has shown greater activity against *E. coli* and *C. albicans* than against *S. aureus* or *Bacillus anthracoides*.[30] Five flavonoids and two iridoids extracted from *Vitex agnus-castus* possess inhibitory action against *Bacillus cereus, B. megaterium,* and *Staphylococcus aureus*.[31]

Pharmacodynamics/Kinetics

- The effects of dosing on clinical effects from chasteberry are not well understood. In one small study among men with normal prolactin levels, acute administration of low doses of chasteberry resulted in a small increase in prolactin secretion, whereas high doses resulted in a small decrease in prolactin secretion.[12]

HISTORY

- Chasteberry's name originates from the Latin words *castitas*, meaning chastity, and *agnus*, meaning lamb. It has long been a belief that the plant inspires chastity. The dried fruits of the plant, which have a peppery taste and smell, were used in monasteries instead of pepper to help monks remain celibate, hence the historical name "monk's pepper." Chasteberry was also used in ancient Greece and Rome as a means to diminish sexual desire. Although preparations of chasteberry are not regulated in the United States, a standardized preparation of chasteberry has been available in Germany since the 1950s.

REVIEW OF THE EVIDENCE: DISCUSSION
Hyperprolactinemia
Summary

- Several controlled trials and pre-clinical studies report the ability of chasteberry to inhibit prolactin secretion.[8,15,16,27,32] Chasteberry has thus been suggested as a potential therapy in hyperprolactinemia, a condition characterized by elevated serum prolactin levels. Prolactin is an amino acid protein produced in the anterior pituitary gland, and its primary action in the body is to enhance breast development during pregnancy and to induce milk production. Prolactin binds to receptors in the gonads, lymphoid cells, and liver. Estrogen stimulates pituitary lactotroph cells that produce prolactin, although lactation is inhibited by high levels of estrogen and progesterone during pregnancy. When estrogen and progesterone levels rapidly decline during the postpartum period, lactation occurs. During this period, ovulation is often suppressed by the suppression of gonadotropins due to prolactin. Dopamine is the principal regulator of prolactin secretion, acting via dopamine-2 receptors on lactotrophs. Prolactin production is also stimulated by thyrotropin-releasing hormone (TRH), hypothalamic peptides, and vasoactive intestinal peptide (VIP).

Evidence

- Merz et al. conducted an open, intra-individual comparison in 20 healthy men to determine the effect of a chasteberry extract on prolactin (PRL) secretion, as well as to elucidate tolerable, effective doses of chasteberry in humans.[12] The study included four 2-week phases in which subjects received placebo and 120, 240, and 480 mg doses of the extract, divided three times daily. Each phase was followed by a 1-week washout period. Blood pressure, heart rate, basal PRL level, and testosterone, follicle-stimulating hormone (FSH), luteinizing hormone (LH), and clinical chemistry laboratory assays (including complete blood counts) were recorded. Compliance was based on pill counts and patient affirmation. The trial reported that at the 120-mg dose, PRL levels rose approximately 16% from baseline; using the 480-mg dose, PRL levels fell approximately 10% from baseline. Based on the limited number of subjects and the inter-individual cyclic variation of PRL, the significance of the findings is unclear. Overall, 26 adverse events were reported: 7 reports on the lowest dose, 3 reports at the middle dose, and 8 reports at the highest dose. Reports were mainly of "slight feelings of ill-health." Limitations of this trial include lack of blinding and small changes in PRL levels.

Review of the Evidence: Chasteberry

Condition Treated*	Study Design	Author, Year	N[†]	SS[†]	Study Quality[‡]	Magnitude of Benefit	ARR[†]	NNT[†]	Comments
Prolactin secretion	Observational, case series	Merz[12] 1996	20	No	0	NA	NA	NA	Small study group and inter-individual variations in prolactin may have confounded results.
"Corpus luteum deficiency" due to latent hyper-prolactinemia	Randomized, controlled, double-blind	Milewicz[7] 1993	89	Yes	5	Large	NA	NA	Treatment was effective as measured by biochemical markers.
Premenstrual dysphoric disorder	Randomized, controlled, single-blind comparison trial	Atmaca[33] 2003	42	Yes	3	Large	NA	NA	Reported as equal to fluoxetine, but no placebo control; may be underpowered for adequate comparison.
Premenstrual syndrome (PMS)	Randomized, controlled, double-blind	Schellenberg[13] 2001	178	Yes	5	Large	NA	NA	Demonstrated beneficial effect on symptom relief.
PMS	Randomized, double-blind, equivalence trial	Lauritzen[10] 1997	175	Yes	4	Small	NA	NA	Differences in baseline characteristics underscore true benefit; no placebo control but equal response to pyridoxine. May be underpowered for adequate comparison.
PMS	Randomized, controlled, double-blind	Turner[34] 1993	600	No	4	None	NA	NA	Only 217 patients completed study.
Amenorrhea, infertility, corpus luteum deficiency	Randomized, controlled, double-blind	Gerhard[24] 1998	96	Unclear	2	Medium	22	5	38 women with secondary amenorrhea, 31 with luteal insufficiency, 27 with idiopathic infertility treated over 3 months; variable outcomes measured in each group; published once with non-significant results, then groups re-organized and re-published, claiming significance.
Cyclic mastalgia	Randomized, double-blind comparison trial	Kubista[18] 1987	160	Yes	4	Large	38	3	Mastodynon and Gestagene were equally effective and superior to placebo.
Cyclic mastalgia	Randomized, controlled double-blind	Halaska[17] 1999	97	Yes	3	Medium	NA	NA	Significant benefits observed with 1 or 2 treatment cycles but not with 3.
Cyclic mastalgia	Randomized, controlled, double-blind	Wuttke[8] 1997	104	Yes	2	Medium	NA	NA	Improved symptoms and altered prolactin levels observed. No changes in FSH or LH.

*Primary or secondary outcome.
[†]N, Number of patients; SS, statistically significant; ARR, absolute risk reduction; NNT, the number of patients who need to undergo a specific intervention in order to observe an outcome in one individual.
[‡]0-2 = poor; 3-4 = good; 5 = excellent.
NA, Not applicable.
FSH, Follicle-stimulating hormone; LH, luteinizing hormone.
For an explanation of each category in this table, please see Table 3 in the Introduction.

• Milewicz et al. conducted a randomized, controlled, double-blind trial in 52 women with luteal phase defects due to latent hyperprolactinemia.[7] The women were given either Strotan capsules, standardized to 20 mg of chasteberry, or placebo daily. Blood for hormonal analysis was taken on days 5 through 8 and on day 20 of the menstrual cycle before and after 3 months of therapy. Latent hyperprolactinemia was assessed by monitoring prolactin release 15 and 30 minutes after injection of 200 µg of thyrotropin-releasing hormone. After 3 months of therapy, PRL release was reduced, luteal phase normalized, and deficits in progesterone synthesis eliminated. Long-term use of chasteberry has not been systematically investigated.

Premenstrual Dysphoric Disorder (PMDD)
Summary
• There is limited controlled trial evidence suggesting possible benefits of chasteberry in the alleviation of symptoms of PMDD.[33] Further evidence is necessary before a firm conclusion can be drawn.

Evidence
• Atmaca et al. enrolled 41 patients with PMDD, diagnosed according to *Diagnostic and Statistical Manual of Mental Disorders*, third edition, revised (DSM IV) criteria, in a 2-month trial comparing a daily dose of 20 to 40 mg of fluoxetine vs. chasteberry extract.[33] The trial was randomized

and single-blinded (rater-blinded), and the specific chasteberry extract used was not described. Outcome measures included the Penn Daily Symptom Report (DSR), the Hamilton Depression Rating scale (HAM-D), and the Clinical Global Impression–Severity of Illness and Improvement scales (CGI-SI and CGI-I scales). At the trial endpoint, all markers were significantly improved from baseline and not significantly different between groups. However, because of the small sample size, the typically large placebo effect observed in trials of anti-depressants, and lack of a placebo group, it is likely that this study was not adequately powered to detect differences between groups. Therefore, results cannot be considered conclusive.

Premenstrual Syndrome (PMS)
Summary

- Most studies evaluating chasteberry in PMS have been of poor study design, although one recent trial demonstrating benefit is of high quality. Further evidence is necessary before a firm conclusion can be drawn.

Controlled Trials

- Schellenberg et al. conducted a multi-center, randomized, controlled, double-blind study evaluating the effects of chasteberry for PMS symptoms over the course of 3 menstrual cycles in 178 women.[13,14] Premenstrual syndrome was diagnosed according to *Diagnostic and Statistical Manual of Mental Disorders*, third edition, revised (DSM III-R) criteria. Subjects received either a 20-mg tablet of chasteberry extract ZE 440 (standardized to 60% ethanol m/m, extract ratio 6 to 12:1; standardized for casticin) or placebo. Prior to and post-treatment, all patients were asked to self-assess irritability, mood, anger, headache, bloating, and breast fullness, undergo clinical global evaluation by a trained clinician, and undergo various laboratory tests (hematology, biochemistry, pregnancy). Self-assessment was rated according to a validated visual analog scale. Final analysis reported that in the chasteberry group, scores evaluating irritability, mood, anger, headache, and breast fullness all significantly improved compared to the placebo group. More than half the women had at least a 50% reduction in symptoms. Water retention was unaffected by treatment. Self-assessment scores were corroborated by physicians. Treatment was well tolerated. Overall, this was a reasonably well-conducted trial suggesting short-term benefits of chasteberry for the relief of PMS symptoms. Further study using established outcome measures is merited.
- Turner and Mills conducted a randomized, double-blind, placebo-controlled trial assessing the efficacy of chasteberry in the treatment of 600 patients with PMS.[34] Patients were randomized to receive a soy-based placebo or chasteberry at a dose of 600 mg three times daily for 3 months. Outcome measures included evaluations from a questionnaire based on the validated Menstrual Distress Questionnaire. A total of 217 women completed the study, with 105 patients in the chasteberry group and 112 in the placebo group. Results did not reveal any significant differences between the chasteberry and placebo groups. A difference in water retention was seen, although it did not reach statistical significance ($p = 0.09$). The high drop-out rate is a significant limitation of this trial, as is the use of soy as a placebo, given the purported estrogenic effects of soy that theoretically may have affected patient symptoms.
- Lauritzen et al. conducted a randomized, double-blind, equivalence trial in 175 women with "premenstrual tension syndrome" (PMTS).[10] Women were administered either 1 capsule of Agnolyt (standardized to 3.5 to 4.2 mg of dried chasteberry extract) and 1 capsule of placebo daily, or 2 capsules of placebo on days 1 through 15 followed by 2 capsules of pyridoxine, 100 mg each, on days 16 through 35 over the course of three menstrual cycles. Therapeutic response was assessed using the PMTS scale, consisting of 36 items specific for the symptoms of PMTS, and the NIH Clinical Global Impression (CGI) scale. Secondary endpoints were the rating of six characteristic common PMTS complaints and efficacy and tolerability of treatment, assessed by both patient and physician. The authors reported a small but significant difference between the chasteberry and pyridoxine groups in PMTS scores (10.1 points and 6.8 points, respectively). CGI scores improved in 77.1% of the chasteberry group compared to 60.6% of the pyridoxine group, and chasteberry was found to be twice as effective, as assessed by the investigator (24.4% and 12.1% respectively). Withdrawal due to adverse events was minimal (5 in the chasteberry group), and treatment was reportedly "very well tolerated." Although these results are promising, this was not an intention-to-treat analysis: of the 175 women initially randomized, only 105 were included in the final treatment analysis (46, chasteberry; 59, pyridoxine). Secondary endpoints were not analyzed for statistical significance.

Uncontrolled Studies

- Berger et al. conducted a multi-center, open-label study to investigate the efficacy of *Vitex agnus-castus* extract Ze 440 in 50 patients suffering from PMS.[22] Subjects were treated daily with 1 tablet (20 mg of native extract) during three menstrual cycles. The main effect parameter was the validated Moor menstrual distress self-assessment questionnaire (MMDQ), and secondary outcomes included a visual analog scale (VAS, self-assessment) and a global impression scale (GI, self-assessment). Questionnaires were administered to subjects at baseline, at the end of three cycles of treatment, and at the end of three cycles after the treatment phase. The MMDQ score was significantly reduced (42.5%, $p < 0.001$), but symptoms gradually returned after treatment cessation. However, a difference from baseline remained (20%, $p < 0.001$) up to three cycles later. Twenty of the 43 subjects were considered "responders," with a 50% reduction in MMDQ score relative to baseline. The VAS score during the luteal phase was reduced progressively by treatment (47.2%, $p < 0.001$), and at the end of the post-treatment observation period the score was still 21.7% below baseline ($p < 0.001$). GI was considered moderate to excellent by 38 patients; 5 patients indicated no GI. The number of days with PMS symptoms was reduced slightly from 7.5 to 6 days ($p < 0.001$). Six subjects withdrew from the study for reasons unrelated to the medication, and one subject complained of fatigue and headache related to the medication 4 days after starting treatment. Although this trial is promising, the lack of control group and open study design are limitations.
- Loch et al. conducted an open, uncontrolled trial to investigate the efficacy and tolerance of Femicur capsules, a chasteberry preparation, in 1698 patients suffering from PMS.[11] A standard questionnaire was developed to evaluate four commonly seen traits in PMS, including depression, anxiety, craving, and water retention. Questionnaires were administered to subjects prior to and after three cycles of treatment. Ninety-six percent of the questionnaires were completed, with a self-reported compliance rate of 98%. Ninety-three percent of subjects reported a decrease in

number of symptoms, of which more than 40% reported complete symptom resolution. Anxiety was significantly alleviated after treatment with chasteberry (71.3% versus 18.8%). Water retention and mastodynia were still reported in greater than 30% of subjects; however, most reported that symptoms had waned. Ninety-four percent of patients rated their tolerance of *Vitex* treatment as good or very good. These results are promising, but as this was an uncontrolled study, they can only be considered suggestive.

- In a case series, Peters-Welte and Albrecht. assessed the efficacy of chasteberry in 551 patients with menstrual disorders, including PMS, uterine fibroids, mastodynia, corpus luteum insufficiency, hypermenorrhea, polymenorrhea, menorrhagia, metrorrhagia, infertility, anovulation, acyclic permanent bleeding, and secondary amenorrhea.[21] Improvements of symptoms occurred within the first 4 weeks in 31.9% of patients and in 83.5% of patients within 12 weeks. According to patient evaluations, 29% became symptom free, 52% observed improvements, and 11% experienced no change. According to physician observations, 69% were symptom free, 19% observed improvement, and 9% experienced no change. Approximately 5% experienced mild side effects, but one patient did experience "heavy headaches."
- Dittmar conducted a study using Agnolyt in the treatment of 1542 women diagnosed with PMS.[35] Patients received an average dose of 42 drops daily (range of 20 to 120 drops). Results reported an improvement in symptoms after a mean of 25.3 days (range of 1 to 365 days) with treatment being discontinued in 3.8% of cases because of "inadequate effects." Both patients and physicians rated treatment as satisfactory or better in 95% of cases. Although adverse effects were reported in 32 women, only 17 withdrew from the study.
- Other studies of lesser-quality design have also been conducted in this area, with inconclusive results.[36-38]

Corpus Luteum Deficiency / Luteal Phase Deficiency
Summary

- Corpus luteum deficiency (CLD) is a term more commonly used in Europe than in the United States and refers to irregular development of the corpus luteum following ovulation, resulting in abnormal progesterone secretion and incomplete endometrial differentiation. The term luteal phase deficiency (LPD) has also been used in this setting and has been implicated both in infertility and recurrent pregnancy loss. This condition is still not fully characterized and appears to be multifactorial in its causes. As many as 20% of patients who are infertile and 60% of women with recurrent pregnancy loss have been diagnosed with LPD, although up to 10% of women who are fertile appear to have an inadequate luteal phase, raising questions about the nature of CLD/LPD. The use of chasteberry for this condition remains controversial.

Controlled Trials

- Gerhard et al. conducted a randomized, placebo-controlled, double-blind study in 38 women with secondary amenorrhea, 31 women with luteal insufficiency, and 27 women with idiopathic sterility.[24] Ninety-six subjects received 30 drops of Mastodynon or placebo twice daily over a period of 3 months. Outcome measures included pregnancy or menstrual bleeding in women with amenorrhea, and pregnancy or improved concentrations of luteal hormones in both other groups. Blinding, randomization, and drop-out rates were not described. The target criterion was achieved in 31 out of 66 women who were suitable for evaluation. Although

improvements were greater in the group receiving Mastodynon compared to placebo (57.6% vs. 36.0%, $p = 0.069$), the results did not reach statistical significance. Seven subjects with amenorrhea, four with idiopathic sterility, and four with luteal insufficiency conceived during the observation period. Notably, this study was re-published and reported statistically significant data, stating that 30 out of 66 women were suitable for evaluation and that the target criterion was achieved statistically more frequently with Mastodynon than with placebo (54.5% vs. 36.4%, $p = 0.049$). The unclear description of results, pooling of diverse conditions and outcomes, and variable significance reported in publications raises questions about the quality of this study, and its results cannot be considered conclusive.

Uncontrolled Studies

- Feldmann et al. studied the effects of chasteberry on 1571 women with menstrual disturbances and diagnoses of corpus luteum insufficiency or ovarian dysfunction.[39] Patients received Agnolyt at an average daily dose of 40 drops taken on an empty stomach for an average of 135 days. The reported response rate was 90%. Adverse effects were noted in 1.9% of patients and included malaise, gastrointestinal complaints, nausea, and diarrhea. Single cases of heavy menses, dizziness, weight gain, allergy and heartburn were also noted.
- Propping conducted a study in 1592 women with secondary amenorrhea (n = 202), dysmenorrhea (n = 186), PMS anovulation (n = 175), perimenopausal symptoms or sterility (n = 145), oligomenorrhea or menorrhagia (n = 66), disturbed menstruation (n = 32), hypermenorrhea (n = 418), polymenorrhea (n = 369), or primary amenorrhea (n = 1).[40] Subjects received 40 drops of chasteberry daily for 6 months. A total of 173 patients received some form of concurrent therapy. As rated by physicians, 33% were free of complaints and another 51% had satisfactory results. A total of 6.5% of subjects had unsatisfactory results, and in 9% of patients, data were missing. As rated by patients, 61% had good results, 29% had satisfactory results, 6% had unsatisfactory results, and 4% had missing data. Approximately 4.5% of patients became pregnant, and 3.9% of patients started oral contraceptives. In terms of withdrawals, 5.5% discontinued use because of inadequate effects, and 1% discontinued use because of side effects.
- Probst and Roth reported a case series examining the effects of chasteberry on 57 women with secondary amenorrhea, oligomenorrhea, cystic glandular hyperplasia, or anovular cycles.[41] Patients were treated with 15 drops three times daily for 6 weeks. There was an increase in temperature in the secretory phase detected in the endometrium. Results showed that 87.7% of subjects demonstrated normalization of menstrual bleeding, whereas 12% of patients failed to respond. No side effects were noted.
- Bubenzer assessed the effects of chasteberry in 120 women with polymenorrhea (n = 25), oligomenorrhea (n = 44), or corpus luteum insufficiency (n = 44).[5] As many as 60% of women had sought treatment to help them conceive. All patients were treated with Strotan for 6 months. The authors reported that average serum progesterone increased from 6.5 to 9.3 ng/mL, that 29% of the women became pregnant, and that 63% had their cycle normalized. The temperatures of the women with disturbed temperatures during the menstrual cycle normalized. Women with very low progesterone levels appeared to derive the most benefit. Adverse effects were reported in 5% to 10% of patients and included headache, "sickness," and bloating.

- Propping et al. conducted an experimental study in 45 young women diagnosed with CLD.[42] Baseline levels of progesterone, prolactin, and thyroid-stimulating hormone were measured on the 21st day of the menstrual cycle. The authors reported an 87% "therapeutic success" rate; 15% of the women became pregnant.

Cyclic Mastalgia

Summary

- More than 60% of women with chronic breast pain have a condition called cyclic mastalgia. In this condition, pain is usually worse during the premenstrual phase of the menstrual cycle and is relieved with menstruation. The pain may also occur throughout the menstrual cycle. It is believed to be caused by hormonal changes and is most common in younger women or older women who are taking hormone replacement therapy. Despite preliminary promising results, due to methodological problems with available studies, it remains unclear if chasteberry is an effective treatment in the management of cyclic mastalgia.

Evidence

- Kubista et al. conducted a randomized, double-blind comparison study of chasteberry (Mastodynon), lynestrenol (Gestagene, a progestational agent), and placebo in the treatment of 160 cases of severe mastopathy with cyclic mastalgia.[18] Subjects in the Mastogynon group received 30 drops twice daily. The authors reported that the percentages of patients reporting "good relief" were 74.5% among those receiving chasteberry, 82.1% in the lynestrenol group, and 36.8% in the placebo group. Differences compared to placebo were statistically significant. A significant increase in prolactin levels and a significant decrease in progesterone levels were also noted. In terms of adverse effects, one patient developed nausea and weight gain that prompted cessation of therapy. Three other cases of weight gain, indigestion, and rash on the neck and face were also reported. Limitations include poor description of randomization.
- Wuttke et al. evaluated the efficacy of Mastodynon in a randomized, double-blind, placebo-controlled trial including 104 patients with mastalgia.[8] Subjects that had experienced mastalgia for at least three cycles and who complained of breast pain on at least 3 days in the cycle before treatment were included. All subjects were randomized to receive either a solution or tablet containing chasteberry (Mastodynon) or placebo for three cycles. Patients were required to report the intensity of breast pain on a validated visual analogue scale (VAS). Estradiol, progesterone, basal prolactin, follicle-stimulating hormone (FSH), and luteinizing hormone (LH) levels were also measured during premenstrual weeks 0, 1, 2, and 3. At the end of treatment, the two groups treated with chasteberry solution and tablets were found to have significantly lower VAS scores compared to placebo ($p = 0.0067$ and $p = 0.0076$, respectively). When compared with placebo, basal prolactin levels fell significantly by a mean of 4.35 ng/mL (= 0.039) with chasteberry solution and by 3.7 ng/mL ($p = 0.015$) with chasteberry tablets. Chasteberry did not have any significant effects on LH and FSH.
- Halaska et al. conducted a randomized, controlled, double-blind trial in 100 women complaining of cyclic mastalgia over the course of three menstrual cycles.[17] Subjects received either 1.8 mL of a chasteberry extract or placebo daily. Symptoms were assessed using a validated visual analogue scale (VAS). Ninety-seven women were analyzed. Breast pain was reportedly lower in the treatment group. Intensity of breast pain diminished at a quicker rate in the chasteberry group. Tolerability was reported as satisfactory. Results and statistical analysis were not well described.
- Other studies of lesser-quality design have also been conducted in this area, with inconclusive results.[43-50]

Irregular Menstrual Cycles

Summary

- It remains unclear if chasteberry is an effective therapy in the management of irregular menses.
- Bleier conducted an observational study in 126 women with menstrual disorders.[9] Women were administered 15 drops of a chasteberry extract three times daily over several cycles. In 33 women suffering from polymenorrhea, the duration between menstrual cycles lengthened from a mean of 20.1 days to 26.3 days. In 58 women with menorrhagia, cycles were significantly shortened. Three women with primary infertility and two women with secondary infertility became pregnant. Due to a lack of control group and limited discussion of methods or statistical analysis, further evidence is necessary before reaching a firm conclusion.
- Other studies of lesser quality design have also been conducted in this area, with inconclusive results.[51-54]

FORMULARY: BRANDS USED IN CLINICAL TRIALS

Brands Used in Statistically Significant Clinical Trials

- Strotan caps.[7]
- Femicur caps (Schaper & Brummer, Germany); 1 cap = 1.6 to 3.0 mg of dried extract, corresponding to 20 mg of drug.[11]
- Mastodynon solution or tablets (Binorica Laboratories, France).[8,18]
- Agnolyt.[10,42]

U.S. Equivalents of Most Commonly Recommended European Brands

- Agnolyt is available in the United States as Femaprin, manufactured by Natures Way.

References

1. Amann W. [Improvement of acne vulgaris following therapy with agnus castus (Agnolyt)]. Ther Ggw 1967;106(1):124-126.
2. Amayanti M, Susheela K, Sharma GJ. Effect of plant extracts and systemic fungicide on the pineapple fruit- rotting fungus, *Ceratocystis paradoxa*. Cytobios 1996;86(346):155-165.
3. Dantas SM. Menopausal symptoms and alternative medicine. Prim Care Update Ob/Gyns 1998;unlisted:212-220.
4. Farnsworth NR, Bingel AS, Cordell GA, et al. Potential value of plants as sources of new antifertility agents I. J Pharm Sci 1975;64(4):535-598.
5. Bubenzer RH. Therapy with *Agnus castus* extract (Strotan). Therapiewoche 1993;43(32-3):1705-1706.
6. Hillebrand H. [The treatment of premenstrual aphthous ulcerative stomatitis with Agnolyt]. Z Allgemeinmed 1964;40(36):1577.
7. Milewicz A, Gejdel E, Sworen H, et al. [*Vitex agnus castus* extract in the treatment of luteal phase defects due to latent hyperprolactinemia: results of a randomized placebo- controlled double-blind study]. Arzneimittelforschung 1993;43(7):752-756.
8. Wuttke W, Splitt G, Gorkow C, et al. Behandlung zyklusabhangiger brustschmerzen mit einem *Agnus castus*-haltigen arzneimittel. Geburtsh Frauenheilk 1997;57:569-574.
9. Bleier W. Therapie von Zyklus- und Blutungsstorungen und weiteren endokrin bedingten Erkrankungen der Frau mit pflanzlichen Wirkstoffen. Zbl Gynakol 1959;81:701-709.
10. Lauritzen C, Reuter HD, Repges R, et al. Treatment of premenstrual tension syndrome with *Vitex angus castus*. Controlled, double-blind study versus pyridoxine. Phytomedicine 1997;4(3):183-189.
11. Loch EG, Selle H, Boblitz N. Treatment of premenstrual syndrome with a phytopharmaceutical formulation containing *Vitex agnus castus*. J Womens Health Gend Based Med 2000;9(3):315-320.
12. Merz PG, Gorkow C, Schrodter A, et al. The effects of a special *Agnus castus* extract (BP1095E1) on prolactin secretion in healthy male subjects. Exp Clin Endocrinol Diabetes 1996;104(6):447-453.

C

13. Schellenberg R. Treatment for the premenstrual syndrome with *agnus castus* fruit extract: prospective, randomised, placebo controlled study. BMJ 2001;322(7279):134-137.

14. Schellenberg R, Schrader E, Brattström A. Vitex agnus castus extrakt Ze440 bei pramenstruellem syndrom: ergebnisse einer RCT im vergleich mit plazebo bei 170 patientinnen. Abstracts Book—Symposium Phytopharmaka VII.Forschung und klinische anwendung, October 12-13 2001;

15. Sliutz G, Speiser P, Schultz AM, et al. Agnus castus extracts inhibit prolactin secretion of rat pituitary cells. Horm Metab Res 1993;25(5):253-255.

16. Jarry H, Leonhardt S, Gorkow C, et al. *In vitro* prolactin but not LH and FSH release is inhibited by compounds in extracts of Agnus castus: direct evidence for a dopaminergic principle by the dopamine receptor assay. Exp Clin Endocrinol 1994;102(6):448-454.

17. Halaska M, Raus K, Beles P, et al. [Treatment of cyclical mastodynia using an extract of *Vitex agnus castus*: results of a double-blind comparison with a placebo]. Ceska Gynekol 1998;63(5):388-392.

18. Kubista E, Muller G, Spona J. [Treatment of mastopathies with cyclic mastodynia. Clinical results and hormonal profiles]. Rev Fr Gynecol Obstet 1987;82(4):221-227.

19. Cahill DJ, Fox R, Wardle PG, et al. Multiple follicular development associated with herbal medicine. Hum Reprod 1994;9(8):1469-1470.

20. Blank A, Gerhard I. *Agnus castus* containing preparation on female sterility. Fact: Focus Altern Compl Therap 1998;3(4):182.

21. Peters-Welte C, Albrecht M. [Menstrual abnormalities and PMS. *Vitex agnus-castus* in a study of application]. Therapiewoche Gynakologie 1994;7(1):49-52.

22. Berger D, Schaffner W, Schrader E, et al. Efficacy of *Vitex agnus castus* L. extract Ze 440 in patients with pre- menstrual syndrome (PMS). Arch Gynecol Obstet 2000;264(3):150-153.

23. Shuster J. Heparin and thrombocytopenia: Black Cohosh root? Chastberry tree? Seizures! Hosp Pharm 1996;31:1553-1554.

24. Gerhard I, I, Patek A, Monga B, et al. Mastodynon®) bei weiblicher Sterilitat.Randomisierte, plazebokontrollierte klinische Doppelblindstudie. Forsch Komplementarmed 1998;5(6):272-278.

25. Jarry H, Spengler B, Porzel A, et al. Evidence for estrogen receptor beta-selective activity of *Vitex agnus-castus* and isolated flavones. Planta Med 2003;69(10):945-947.

26. Wuttke W, Jarry H, Christoffel V, et al. Chaste tree (*Vitex agnus-castus*) pharmacology and clinical indications. Phytomedicine 2003;10(4):348-357.

27. Winterhoff H, Gorkow C, Behr B. Die Hemmung der Laktation bei Ratten als indirekter Beweis fur die Senkung von Prolaktin durch Agnus castus. Zeitschrift fur Phytotherapie 1991;12:175-179.

28. Bhargava SK. Antiandrogenic effects of a flavonoid-rich fraction of Vitex negundo seeds: a histological and biochemical study in dogs. J Ethnopharmacol 1989;27(3):327-339.

29. Pepeljnjak S, Antolic A, Kustrak D. Antibacterial and antifungal activities of the *Vitex agnus-castus* L. extracts. Acta Pharmaceutica Zagreb 1996;46(3):201-206.

30. Mishurova SS. Essential oil in *Vitex agnus astus* L., its component composition and antimicrobial activity. Rastitel 'nye Resursy 1986;22(4):526-530.

31. Gomaa CS. Flavonoids and iridoids from *Vitex agnus-castus*. Planta Medica 1978;33:277.

32. Jarry H, Leonhardt S, Wuttke W, et al. [*Agnus castus* as a dopaminergic active constituent in Mastodynon N]. Zeitschrift fur Phytotherapie 1991; 12:77-82.

33. Atmaca M, Kumru S, Tezcan E. Fluoxetine versus *Vitex agnus castus* extract in the treatment of premenstrual dysphoric disorder. Hum Psychopharmacol 2003;18(3):191-195.

34. Turner S, Mills S. A double-blind clinical trial on a herbal remedy for premenstrual syndrome: a case study. Compl Therap Med 1993;1(2):73-77.

35. Dittmar FW. Premenstrual syndrome: treatment with a phytopharmaceutical [in German]. TW Gynakologie 1992;5(1):60-68.

36. Liebel H. Behandlung des prämenstruellen Syndromes. *Agnus castus*-haltige Kombinationsarzneimittel im Test. Therapiewoche Gynakol 1992;5:2-12.

37. Meyl C. Therapie des prämenstruellen syndroms. Therapie einer kombinierten behandlung von mastodynon und vitamin E mit der vitamin E-monotherapie. Therapeutikon 1991;5(10):518-525.

38. Coeugniet E. Premenstrual syndrome and its treatment. Arztezeitchr Naturheilverf 1986;27:619-622.

39. Feldmann HU, Albrecht M, Lamertz M, et al. The treatment of corpus luteum insufficiency and premenstrual syndrome. Experience in a multi-center study under clinical practice conditions. [in German]. Gyne 1990; 11(12):421-425.

40. Propping D. *Vitex agnus-castus*: treatment of gynecological syndromes. [in German]. Therapeutikon 1991;5:581-585.

41. Probst V, Roth OA. On a plant extract with a hormone-like effects. Deutsch Medizin Zeitschrift 1954;35:1271-1274.

42. Propping D, Katzorke T, Belkien L. Diagnostik und therapie der gelbkorperschwache in der praxis. Therapiewoche 1988;38:2992-3001.

43. Fikentscher H. [Aetiology, diagnosis and therapy of mastopathy and mastodynia. Experiences of treatment with mastodynon (author's transl)]. Med Klin 1977;72(34):1327-1330.

44. Schwalbe E. [Treatment of mastodynia]. ZFA (Stuttgart)1979;55(22): 1239-1242.

45. Opitz G, Liebl A. [Conservative treatment of mastopathy with Mastodynon]. Ther Ggw 1980;119(7):804-809.

46. Göbel R. Results of the clinical evaluations of Danazol in benign breast disease compared with local treatment, gestagens, and bromocriptine. *In* Baum M, George WD, Hughes LE (eds): Benign Breast Diseases. London, Roy Soc Med Int, 1985, pp 115-120.

47. Gregl A. Klinik und therapie der mastodynie. Med Welt 1985;36:242-246.

48. Fournier D, Grumbrecht C. Behandlung der mastopathie, mastodynie und des prämenstruellen syndroms. Verleich medikamentöser behandlung zu unbehandelten kontrollen. Therapiewoche 1987;37(5):430-434.

49. Fersizoglou NE. Hormonale und thermographische veränderungen unter konservativer therapie der mastophathie. Vergleich von danazol, tamoxifen, lisurid, lynesterenol und einem phytopharmakon. Dissertation, 1989.

50. Krapfl E. Prospektiv randomisierte klinische thrapiestudie zum wirksamkeitsvergleich von Orgametril®, einem 19 nor-testosteron-derivat, versus Mastodynon®, agnus castus-haltigen alkoholischen pflanzenextrakt, bei schmerzhafter mastopathie. Dissertation, 1988.

51. Halder R. Über die anwendungsmoglichkeiten von vitex agnus-castus L. in der frauenheilkunde unter besonderer berücksichtigung der blutungsstörungen. Dissertation 1957.

52. Roth OA. Zur therapie der gelbkörperinsuffizienz in der praxis. Med Klin1956;51:1263-1265.

53. Mergner R. Zyklusstörungen: therapie mit einem vitex-agnus-castus-haltigen kombinationsarzneimittel. Der Kassenarzt 1992;7:51-60.

54. Kayser HW, Istanbulluoglu S. *Vitex agnus castus*. Hippokrates 1954;25: 717-719.

Chondroitin Sulfate

SYNONYMS/COMMON NAMES/RELATED SUBSTANCES

- ACS4-ACS6, CDS, chondroitin sulfate A, chondroitin sulfate C, chondroitin sulphate A sodium, chondroitin-4-sulfate, chondroitin-6-sulfate, chondroitin sulfuric acid, chondro-protective agents, chonsurid, condroitin, Condrosulf CS, CSA, CSC, disease-modifying osteoarthritis drugs (DMOADs), GAG, galacotosaminoglucuronoglycan sulfate (Matrix), mesoglycan (heparan sulfate-52%, dermatan sulfate-35%, heparin-8%, chondroitin sulfate-5%), symptomatic slow-acting drug in osteoarthritis (SYSADOA).

CLINICAL BOTTOM LINE

Background

- Chondroitin was first extracted and purified in the 1960s. It is currently manufactured from natural sources (shark/beef cartilage or bovine trachea) or by synthetic means. The consensus of expert and industry opinions support the use of chondroitin and its common partner agent, glucosamine, for improving symptoms and arresting (or possibly reversing) the degenerative process of osteoarthritis.

Uses Based on Scientific Evidence	Grade*
Osteoarthritis Multiple controlled clinical trials since the 1980s have examined the use of oral chondroitin in patients with osteoarthritis of the knee and other locations (spine, hips, finger joints). Most of these studies have reported significant benefits in terms of symptoms (such as pain), function (such as mobility), and reduced medication requirements (such as anti-inflammatories). However, most studies have been brief (6 months' duration) with methodological weaknesses: a wide variety of patient classifications and outcome variables have been used, resulting in heterogeneity between trials; most analyses were not on an intention-to-treat basis; relationships between investigators and manufacturers were often not clarified; and blinding and randomization were frequently not well described. Despite these weaknesses and potential for bias in the available results, the weight of scientific evidence points to a beneficial effect when chondroitin is used for 6 to 24 months. Longer term effects are not clear. Preliminary studies of topical chondroitin have also been conducted. Chondroitin is frequently used with glucosamine. Glucosamine has independently been demonstrated to benefit patients with osteoarthritis (particularly of the knee). It remains unclear whether there is added benefit of using these two agents together compared to using either alone.	A
Ophthalmologic uses Chondroitin is sometimes used as a component of eye drop solutions, including prescription-only preparations such as Viscoat. These solutions should be used only under the supervision of an ophthalmologist.	B
Coronary artery disease (secondary prevention) Several studies in the early 1970s assessed the use of oral chondroitin for the prevention of subsequent coronary events in patients with a history of heart disease or myocardial infarction. Although favorable results were reported, because of methodological weaknesses in this research and the widespread current availability of more proven drug therapies for patients in this setting, a recommendation cannot be made in this area.	C
Interstitial cystitis There is preliminary research administering intravesicular chondroitin in patients diagnosed with interstitial cystitis. Additional evidence is necessary before a firm conclusion can be drawn.	C

*Key to grades: *A:* Strong scientific evidence for this use; *B:* Good scientific evidence for this use; *C:* Unclear scientific evidence for this use; *D:* Fair scientific evidence against this use (it may not work); *F:* Strong scientific evidence against this use (it likely does not work). For a more detailed explanation of efficacy criteria, see "Natural Standard Evidence-Based Validated Grading Rationale" in the Introduction.

Historical or Theoretical Indications That Lack Sufficient Evidence
Angina, anti-inflammatory, chronic venous ulcers, gonarthrosis, hyperlipidemia, iron deficiency anemia, kidney stones, leukemia, malaria, myocardial infarction, osteoporosis, premature labor prevention.

DOSING/TOXICOLOGY

The following doses are based on scientific research, publications, traditional use, or expert opinion. Many herbs and supplements have not been thoroughly tested, and their safety and effectiveness may not be proven. Brands may be made differently, with variable ingredients even within the same brand. The doses shown may not apply to all products. It is important to always read product labels and discuss doses with a qualified healthcare provider before therapy is started.

Standardization

- Standardization involves measuring the amounts of certain chemicals in products to try to make different preparations similar to each other. It is not always known if the chemicals being measured are the "active" ingredients.

Adult (18 Years and Older)

Oral (by Mouth)

- **Monotherapy:** Doses of 200 to 400 mg twice to three times daily, or 800 to 1200 mg once daily have been used. Higher doses (up to 2000 mg) appear to have similar efficacy. In the treatment of osteoarthritis, full effects may take several weeks to occur.
- **Combination with glucosamine:** It is not clear what dose is optimal when chondroitin is used in combination with glucosamine or whether the combination is as effective as or more effective than either agent alone.

Intravenous/Intramuscular

- For osteoarthritis, 50 to 100 mg as a single daily injection or divided into two daily injections has been used. Medical supervision is recommended.

Children (Younger Than 18 Years)

- Because of insufficient scientific evidence, chondroitin is not recommended for use in children.

SAFETY

The U.S. Food and Drug Administration does not strictly regulate herbs and supplements. There is no guarantee of the strength, purity, or safety of products, and effects may vary. It is important to always read product labels. People who have a medical condition, or are taking other drugs, herbs, or supplements, should consult a qualified healthcare provider before starting a new therapy. A healthcare provider should be contacted immediately about any side effects.

Allergies

- Use cautiously if allergic or hypersensitive to chondroitin sulfate products.

Side Effects and Warnings

- There are limited data about the long-term safety of chondroitin, although it appears to be well tolerated in most trials.
- Adverse effects that have been rarely reported or are theoretical include bone marrow suppression, breathing difficulties, chest pain, constipation, diarrhea, elevated blood pressure, euphoria, exacerbation of previously well-controlled asthma, eyelid edema, gastrointestinal pain/dyspepsia, hair loss, headache, hives, increased risk of bleeding, lower extremity edema, motor uneasiness, nausea, photosensitivity, rash, subjective tightness in the throat or chest, and transaminitis.
- Chondroitin should be used with caution in people who have bleeding disorders or are taking anticoagulant medications.

Pregnancy and Breastfeeding

- The use of chondroitin should be avoided in pregnant or breastfeeding women because effects are unknown, and chondroitin is structurally similar to heparin, which is contraindicated during pregnancy.

INTERACTIONS

Most herbs and supplements have not been thoroughly tested for interactions with other herbs, supplements, drugs, or foods. The interactions listed here are based on reports in scientific publications, laboratory experiments, or traditional use. It is important to always read product labels. People who have a medical condition, or are taking other drugs, herbs, or supplements, should consult a qualified healthcare provider before starting a new therapy.

Interactions with Drugs

- In theory, chondroitin may increase the risk of bleeding when taken with other agents that may increase the risk of bleeding. Examples of such agents are anticoagulants (blood thinners) such as warfarin (Coumadin) and heparin, antiplatelet drugs such as clopidogrel (Plavix), aspirin, and non-steroidal anti-inflammatory drugs such as ibuprofen (Motrin, Advil) and naproxen (Naprosyn, Aleve).

Interactions with Herbs and Dietary Supplements

- In theory, chondroitin may increase the risk of bleeding when taken with herbs and supplements that may also increase the risk of bleeding. Multiple cases of bleeding have been reported with the use of *Ginkgo biloba*, and fewer cases with garlic and saw palmetto. Numerous other agents may theoretically increase the risk of bleeding, although this has not been proven in most cases. Examples of such agents are alfalfa, American ginseng, angelica, anise, *Arnica montana*, asafetida, aspen bark, bilberry, birch, black cohosh, bladderwrack, bogbean, boldo, borage seed oil, bromelain, capsicum, cat's claw, celery, chamomile, chaparral, clove, coleus, cordyceps, dandelion, danshen, devil's claw, dong quai, eicosapentaenoic acid (EPA), evening primrose oil, fenugreek, feverfew, fish oil, flaxseed/flax powder (not a concern with flaxseed oil), ginger, grapefruit juice, grape seed, green tea, guggul, gymnestra, horse chestnut, horseradish, licorice root, lovage root, male fern, meadowsweet, melatonin, nordihydroguaiaretic acid (NDGA), omega-3 fatty acids, onion, *Panax ginseng*, papain, parsley, passion flower, poplar, prickly ash, propolis, quassia, red clover, reishi, rue, Siberian ginseng, sweet birch, sweet clover, turmeric, vitamin E, white willow, wild carrot, wild lettuce, willow, wintergreen, and yucca.

Selected References

Natural Standard developed the preceding evidence-based information based on a systematic review of more than 175 articles. For comprehensive information about alternative and complementary therapies on the professional level, go to www.naturalstandard.com. Selected references are listed here.

Blotman F, Loyau G. Clinical trial with chondroitin sulfate in gonarthrosis [abstract]. Osteoarthritis Cartilage 1993;1:68.

Bourgeois P, Chales G, Dehais J, et al. Efficacy and tolerability of chondroitin sulfate 1200 mg/day vs chondroitin sulfate 3 x 400 mg/day vs placebo. Osteoarthritis Cartilage 1998;6(Suppl A):25-30.

Bucsi L, Poor G. Efficacy and tolerability of oral chondroitin sulfate as a symptomatic slow-acting drug for osteoarthritis (SYSADOA) in the treatment of knee osteoarthritis. Osteoarthritis Cartilage 1998;6(Suppl A)31-36.

Cohen M, Wolfe R, Mai T, et al. A randomized, double blind, placebo controlled trial of a topical cream containing glucosamine sulfate, chondroitin sulfate, and camphor for osteoarthritis of the knee. J Rheumatol 2003;30(3):523-528.

Conrozier T. [Anti-arthrosis treatments: efficacy and tolerance of chondroitin sulfates (CS 4 & 6).] Presse Med 1998;27(36):1862-1865.

Danao-Camara T. Potential side effects of treatment with glucosamine and chondroitin. Arthritis Rheum 2000;43(12):2853.

Das A Jr, Hammad TA. Efficacy of a combination of FCHG49 glucosamine hydrochloride, TRH122 low molecular weight sodium chondroitin sulfate and manganese ascorbate in the management of knee osteoarthritis. Osteoarthritis Cartilage 2000;8(5):343-350.

Du J, White N, Eddington ND. The bioavailability and pharmacokinetics of glucosamine hydrochloride and chondroitin sulfate after oral and intravenous single dose administration in the horse. Biopharm Drug Dispos 2004;25(3):109-116.

Fleish AM, Merlin C, Imhoff A, et al. A one-year randomized, double-blind, placebo-controlled study with oral chondroitin sulfate in patients with knee osteoarthritis. Osteoarthritis Cartilage 1997;5:70.

L'Hirondel JL. [Clinical double blind study with oral application of chondroitin sulfate vs. placebo for treatment of tibio femoral gonarthrosis in 125 patients.] Litera Rheumatologica 1992;14:77-84.

Leeb BF, Petera P, Neumann K. [Results of a multicenter study of chondroitin sulfate (Condrosulf) use in arthroses of the finger, knee and hip joints.] Wien Med Wochenschr 1996;146(24):609-614.

Leeb BF, Schweitzer H, Montag K, et al. A metaanalysis of chondroitin sulfate in the treatment of osteoarthritis. J Rheumatol 2000;27(1):205-211.

Leffler CT, Philippi AF, Leffler SG, et al. Glucosamine, chondroitin, and manganese ascorbate for degenerative joint disease of the knee or low back: a randomized, double-blind, placebo-controlled pilot study. Mil Med 1999;164(2):85-91.

Limberg MB, McCaa C, Kissling GE, et al. Topical application of hyaluronic acid and chondroitin sulfate in the treatment of dry eyes. Am J Ophthalmol 1987;103(2):194-197.

Malaise M, et al. Efficacy and tolerability of 800 mg oral chondroitin sulfate in the treatment of knee osteoarthritis: a randomized double-blind multicentre study versus placebo. Litera Rheumatologica 1999;24:31-42.

Mazieres B, Loyau G, Menkes CJ, et al. [Chondroitin sulfate in the treatment of gonarthrosis and coxarthrosis. 5-months result of a multicenter double-blind controlled prospective study using placebo.] Rev Rhum Mal Osteoartic 1992;59(7-8):466-472.

McAlindon TE, LaValley MP, Gulin JP, et al. Glucosamine and chondroitin for treatment of osteoarthritis: a systematic quality assessment and meta-analysis. JAMA 2000;283(11):1469-1475.

McGee M, Wagner WD. Chondroitin sulfate anticoagulant activity is linked to water transfer: relevance to proteoglycan structure in atherosclerosis. Arterioscler Thromb Vasc Biol 2003;23(10):1921-1927.

Morreale P, Manopulo R, Galati M, et al. Comparison of the antiinflammatory efficacy of chondroitin sulfate and diclofenac sodium in patients with knee osteoarthritis. J Rheumatol 1996;23(8):1385-1391.

Morrison LM, Branwood AW, Ershoff BH, et al. The prevention of coronary arteriosclerotic heart disease with chondroitin sulfate A: preliminary report. Exp Med Surg 1969;27(3):278-289.

Morrison LM. Reduction of ischemic coronary heart disease by chondroitin sulfate A. Angiology 1971;22(3):165-174.

Obara M, Hirano H, Ogawa M, et al. Does chondroitin sulfate defend the human uterine cervix against ripening in threatened premature labor? Am J Obstet Gynecol 2000;182(2):334-339.

Richy F, Bruyere O, Ethgen O, et al. Structural and symptomatic efficacy of glucosamine and chondroitin in knee osteoarthritis: a comprehensive meta-analysis. Arch Intern Med 2003;163(13):1514-1522.

Rozenfeld V, Crain JL, Callahan AK. Possible augmentation of warfarin effect by glucosamine-chondroitin. Am J Health Syst Pharm 2004;61(3):306-307.

Shankland WE. The effects of glucosamine and chondroitin sulfate on osteoarthritis of the TMJ: a preliminary report of 50 patients. Cranio 1998;16(4):230-235.

Steinhoff G, Ittah B, Rowan S. The efficacy of chondroitin sulfate 0.2% in treating interstitial cystitis. Can J Urol 2002;9(1):1454-1458.

Tallia AF, Cardone DA. Asthma exacerbation associated with glucosamine-chondroitin supplement. J Am Board Fam Pract 2002;15(6):481-484.

Towheed TE, Anastassiades TP. Glucosamine and chondroitin for treating symptoms of osteoarthritis: evidence is widely touted but incomplete. JAMA 2000;283(11):1483-1484.

Uebelhart D, Chantraine A. Efficacite clinique du sulfate de chondroitine dans la gonarthrose: Etude randomisee en double-insu versus placebo [abstract]. Rev Rhumatisme 1994;10:692.

Uebelhart D, Knüssel O, Theiler R. Efficacy and tolerability of oral avian chondroitin sulfate in painful knee osteoarthritis [abstract]. Schweiz Med Wochenschr 1999;129(33):1174.

Uebelhart D, Thonar EJ, Zhang J, et al. Protective effect of exogenous chondroitin 4,6-sulfate in the acute degradation of articular cartilage in the rabbit. Osteoarthritis Cartilage 1998;6(Suppl A):6-13.

Uebelhart D, Malaise M, Marcolongo R, et al. Intermittent treatment of knee osteoarthritis with oral chondroitin sulfate: a one-year, randomized, double-blind, multicenter study versus placebo. Osteoarthritis Cartilage 2004;12(4):269-276.

Van Blitterswijk WJ, Van De Nes JC, Wuisman PI. Glucosamine and chondroitin sulfate supplementation to treat symptomatic disc degeneration: Biochemical rationale and case report. BMC Complement Altern Med 2003;3(1):2.

Verbruggen G, Goemaere S, Veys EM. Chondroitin sulfate: S/DMOAD (structure/disease modifying anti-osteoarthritis drug) in the treatment of finger joint OA. Osteoarthritis Cartilage 1998;6 Suppl A:37-38.

Volpi N. Oral bioavailability of chondroitin sulfate (Condrosulf) and its constituents in healthy male volunteers. Osteoarthritis Cartilage 2002;10(10):768-777.

Clay

SYNONYMS/COMMON NAMES/RELATED SUBSTANCES

- Akipula, aluminium silicate, anhydrous aluminum silicates, askipula, beidellitic montmorillonite, benditos, bioelectrical minerals, cipula, chalk, clay dust, clay lozenges, clay suspension products, clay tablets, colloidal minerals, colloidal trace minerals, fossil farina, humic shale, Indian healing clay, kipula, mountain meal, panito del senor, plant-derived liquid minerals, tirra santa, terra sigillata, white clay, white mud.

CLINICAL BOTTOM LINE
Background

- Clay has been used medicinally for centuries in Africa, India, and China, and by Native American groups. Uses have included gastrointestinal disorders and as an antidote for poisoning.
- The practice of eating dirt, clay, or other non-nutritious substances is referred to as "pica" or "geophagia" and is common in young children and in mentally handicapped or psychotic patients. There is some evidence that mineral deficiencies such as iron deficiency may lead to pica, and prevalence is higher in developing countries and in poor communities. Chronic clay ingestion may lead to iron malabsorption and further precipitate this condition.
- There is insufficient scientific evidence to recommend for or against the use of clay for any medical condition. The potential for adverse effects with chronic oral ingestion of clay may outweigh any potential benefits.

Scientific Evidence for Common/Studied Uses	Grade*
Encopresis (fecal incontinence associated with psychiatric disorders): clay modeling therapy in children	C
Functional gastrointestinal disorders	C
Mercuric chloride poisoning	C
Protection from aflatoxins	C

Historical or Theoretical Uses That Lack Sufficient Evidence

- Animal bites, cardiovascular disorders, constipation, diarrhea, dysentery, gastric disorders, hyperemesis gravidarum, malignant fevers, menstruation difficulties, nutrition, ophthalmologic disorders, plague, poisoning, skin fairness, smoking, syphilis, vomiting, water purification,[1] weight loss.

Expert Opinion and Folkloric Precedent

- Currently, clay is not often recommended medicinally because of potential toxicities that may occur with ingestion. It has been reported that traditionally some African ethnic groups have practiced clay eating during pregnancy.

Safety Summary

- **Possibly unsafe:** Clay products used orally may contain varying amounts of aluminum, arsenic, barium, lead, nickel, and titanium. Colloidal mineral supplements may also contain unsafe concentrations of radioactive metals. Possibly unsafe when used in patients during pregnancy or lactation, or when used in children. Clay possesses potassium-binding capacity, and chronic ingestion has been associated with severe hypokalemia, particularly in patients with renal insufficiency.[2-4] Habitual clay eating (pica or geophagia) may lead to iron malabsorption and severe deficiency and has been associated with anemia.[3,5]

DOSING/TOXICOLOGY
General

- Recommended doses are based on those most commonly used in available trials, or on historical practice. However, with natural products, optimal doses needed to balance efficacy and safety often have not been determined. Formulations and preparation methods may vary from manufacturer to manufacturer, and from batch to batch of a specific product made by a single manufacturer. Because often the active components of a product are not known, standardization may not be possible, and the clinical effects of different brands may not be comparable.

Dosing: Adult (18 Years and Older)

- Insufficient evidence to recommend. May cause adverse effects.

Dosing: Pediatric (Younger Than 18 Years)

- Insufficient evidence to recommend. May cause adverse effects.

Toxicology

- Clay or dirt eating has been associated with lead poisoning in infants and children.[6] Clay products may contain varying amounts of aluminum, arsenic, barium, lead, nickel, and titanium.
- Because of its ion-exchange property, clay may absorb toxic heavy metals such as mercuric chloride, making them unavailable for absorption.[7]

ADVERSE EFFECTS/PRECAUTIONS/CONTRAINDICATIONS
Allergy

- Known allergy/hypersensitivity to clay, clay products, or constituents of clay.

Adverse Effects/Post-Market Surveillance

- **General:** The practice of eating dirt, clay, or other non-nutritious substances is referred to as "pica" or "geophagia" and is common in early childhood and in mentally handicapped or psychotic patients. There is some evidence that mineral deficiencies such as iron deficiency may lead to pica.[8-10] Clay ingestion may lead to iron malabsorption and further precipitate this condition.[3,5,11] Habitual clay eating has been associated with electrolyte imbalances and may carry a risk of lead toxicity. In the 19th century, a syndrome was described as associated with chronic pica called "Cachexia Africana," characterized by an edematous appearance, dilated cardiomyopathy, polyuria, and death.[12]

- **Dermatologic:** Descriptions of individuals who chronically ate clay in the 19th century noted skin that was initially dry and shiny; in late stages of disease, especially in children, skin ulcerations were noted over the upper and lower extremities.[12]
- **Neurologic/CNS:** Pica has been associated with the development of lead poisoning in children and may carry a risk of CNS damage.[6] In one case report, a 6-year-old girl died from complications of lead poisoning and encephalopathy after ingesting lemonade from a glazed clay pitcher.[13]
- **Psychiatric:** Habitual clay eating (pica or geophagia) may occur in patients with mental illness, including psychotic disorders.
- **Pulmonary/Respiratory:** In the 1960s, it was reported that children with a history of pica were predisposed to develop more frequent and severe respiratory infections than healthy children.[14] Chronic bronchitis, dyspnea, and pneumoconiosis have been associated with dust exposure in the heavy clay industry.[15]
- **Cardiovascular:** Chronic clay eating (pica or geophagia) was reported in the 19th century to be associated with dilated cardiomyopathy and death.[12]
- **Gastrointestinal:** Clay eating may precipitate constipation or diarrhea. Heartburn, flatulence, loss of appetite, and vomiting after meals have been reported. Clay eating has also been associated with intestinal obstruction and necrotizing enteritis, leading to bowel perforation.[16-18] Colonic stones have been reported in two children with pica.[19] Geophagia has been associated with hepatosplenomegaly.[20]
- **Renal:** Clay possesses potassium-binding capacity, and chronic clay ingestion has been associated with severe hypokalemia,[2-4] particularly in patients with renal insufficiency,[2] but not in those receiving hemodialysis.[21]
- **Genitourinary:** Chronic clay eating has been associated with polyuria and urge incontinence, as well as hypogonadism.
- **Hematologic:** Habitual clay eating (pica or geophagia) may lead to iron malabsorption and severe deficiency and has been associated with anemia.[3,5]
- **Musculoskeletal:** Myositis has been associated with chronic clay ingestion.
- **Infectious Disease:** Hookworm infections have been associated with ingestion of clay. Tetanus contracted from clay has been described in an infant who ate clay, and in a newborn whose umbilical cord was wrapped in clay.[22]
- **Other:** Clay pots containing candy (Jarritos brand Tamarindo candy) have been recalled in the United States by the U.S. Food and Drug Administration because of high levels of lead in the candy, absorbed from the clay pots. Clay products may contain varying amounts of aluminum, arsenic, barium, lead, nickel, and titanium. Elevated levels of 2,3,7,8-tetra-cholorodibenzo-*p*-dioxin have been found in farm-raised catfish and in eggs from chickens fed a diet including ball clay from a mine in Mississippi.[23] Chronic clay eating may be associated with trace element deficiency.[3]

Precautions/Warnings/Contraindications

- Avoid use in patients during pregnancy or lactation. Clay ingestion during pregnancy may be associated with an increased incidence of toxemia.[24]
- Avoid use in patients with Wilson's disease.
- Avoid use in patients with renal insufficiency.
- Use cautiously in infants and children.

Pregnancy and Lactation

- Not recommended. Clay ingestion during pregnancy may be associated with an increased incidence of toxemia.[24] In a 1964 report of 62 infants delivered to patients with clay- or cornstarch- eating habits, 24% of infants in the clay group and 33% in the cornstarch group were rated by clinicians as being in "poor" or "very poor" condition at birth, associated with increased mortality, vs. 11% in a control group.[25] This was not a clearly described study.

INTERACTIONS
Clay/Drug Interactions

- **Cimetidine:** When administered simultaneously, clay has been found to inhibit the absorption of cimetidine (Tagamet).[26]

Clay/Herb/Supplement Interactions

- **Iron:** Clay has been demonstrated to interfere with iron absorption.[3]

Clay/Food Interactions

- Insufficient data available.

Clay/Lab Interactions

- **Iron, Calcium, Magnesium:** Clay may act as a cation exchange resin. Calcium and magnesium in clay are replaced by iron, making iron unabsorbable because of formation of insoluble iron complexes.[5] Iron deficiency may result, and levels of calcium or magnesium may increase.
- **Potassium:** Clay possesses potassium-binding capacity and has been associated with hypokalemia.[2-4]

MECHANISM OF ACTION
Pharmacology

- The constituents vary in different types of clay. Aluminum and silicon compounds may constitute >90%. Iron and calcium compounds may constitute 2% to 3%. Clay often contains organic matter as humus and fossils, and may contain small amounts of other minerals, including zinc, bismuth, lead, copper, nickel, and manganese.[16,27]
- The pH of clay ranges from 4.6 to 10.2.[5]
- Some clay preparations have been found to be similar to Kaolin and Kaopectate, which are used to treat gastrointestinal disturbances including diarrhea.
- Clay material has been reported to remove 81% of microcystin-LR hepatotoxins from water and may offer an effective method of stripping these toxins from drinking water supplies.[1]

Pharmacodynamics/Kinetics

- Clay may act as a cation exchange resin. Calcium and magnesium in clay are replaced by iron, making iron unabsorbable because of formation of insoluble iron complexes.[5]
- Clay possesses potassium-binding capacity, and chronic clay ingestion has been associated with severe hypokalemia.[2-4]
- Because of its ion-exchange property, clay may absorb toxic heavy metals such as mercuric chloride, making them unavailable for absorption.[7]

HISTORY

- Clay eating has been noted in diverse cultural groups and geographical regions throughout history. The practice of habitually eating dirt, clay, or other non-nutritious substances is referred to as "pica" or "geophagia" and is common in early childhood and in mentally handicapped or psychotic patients. There is some evidence that mineral deficiencies such as iron deficiency may lead to pica. Clay ingestion may lead to iron malabsorption and further precipitate the condition. Treatment with iron supplements has been found to stop pica.

- Records dating to 40 BC indicate that clay dug on a single day of the year from caves on the island of Lemnos in the Northern Aegean sea were used to make medicinal lozenges. This clay was mixed with goat's blood, dried and formed into lozenges, and stamped with the seal of a goat's figure. These lozenges may have been used to treat cases of poisoning and conditions including fever, diarrhea, and bubonic plague. These lozenges have been found throughout southern Europe, including in Portugal, Italy, Turkey, and Armenia.[7]
- Small tablets of sacred earth called "tierra santa" are sold at the shrine of Esquipulas in Guatemala. These white clay tablets, blessed by the Roman Catholic Church before sale, are said to possess health-giving properties. They are also known as "benditos" or "blessed ones," and have been used in diseases of the stomach, heart, and eyes and for menstrual difficulties.[28]
- There is a historical account that in 1581, a prisoner in Langenburg, Baden, Germany was condemned to death and requested that clay lozenges ("terra sigillata") be administered to him concomitantly with the assigned poison, mercuric chloride (approximately 6 grams).[7] The prisoner survived, and it was hypothesized that the clay lozenges were protective.

REVIEW OF THE EVIDENCE: DISCUSSION
Functional Gastrointestinal Disorders
Summary

- There is insufficient scientific evidence to recommend for or against the medicinal use of clay in patients with gastrointestinal disorders. Some clay preparations have been found to be similar to Kaolin and Kaopectate, which are used to treat gastrointestinal disturbances including diarrhea.

Evidence

- Pariente and De La Garoullaye conducted a randomized, single-blind trial comparing the effects of clay vs. a mucilage product containing Karaya gum plus polyvinyl polypyrrolidone (Polykaraya, Synthelabo, France) in the treatment of 289 ambulatory patients with functional gastrointestinal disorders.[29] Inclusion criteria and specific symptoms or diagnoses of subjects were not clearly described. Patients were assigned to receive a daily oral dose of 3 sachets

of Karaya gum plus polyvinyl polypyrrolidone or clay for 8 weeks. The authors reported that mean chronic pain was reduced in both groups by >50% at week 4 and >80% at week 8, without the difference being statistically significant between groups. A significant decrease in the use of analgesics and antispasmodics was noted in the mucilage group at week 4 vs. clay, and intestinal transit time was also significantly improved in the mucilage group vs. clay at week 4. Compliance was reported as "good" in both groups, without any observed adverse effects. The methods, outcome measures, and statistical analysis of this study were not well described, and no placebo arm was included.

Encopresis (Fecal Incontinence Associated with Psychiatric Disorders): Clay Modeling Therapy in Children
Summary

- It is not clear if play with modeling clay is an effective therapeutic intervention in children with constipation and encopresis.

Evidence

- In a case series, Feldman et al. assessed the effects of play with modeling clay in the treatment of children with intractable encopresis.[30] Six children (ages 4 to 12 years) affected with constipation with encopresis for 2 to 8 years (mean, 5.4 years) were included. Play with modeling clay was hypothesized by the authors to be potentially therapeutic, because of the physical resemblance of brown clay to feces. It was felt that clay modeling might allow children to express frustrations with their condition. The authors noted that four children experienced resolution of encopresis during the 2-month study without relapse during 1 year of follow-up. A fifth child showed improvement and the sixth child failed to respond. Because this was an uncontrolled study, confounding factors (such as increased attention to children enrolled in a study) may have contributed to the observed outcome. In addition, it is not clear if these children might have improved without intervention.

Mercuric Chloride Poisoning
Summary

- Clay lozenges have been used historically in the treatment of mercuric chloride poisoning, and were officially mentioned

Review of the Evidence: Clay

Condition Treated*	Study Design	Author, Year	N[†]	SS[†]	Study Quality[‡]	Magnitude of Benefit	ARR[†]	NNT[†]	Comments
Functional gastrointestinal disorders	Randomized, single-blind comparison trial	Pariente and De La Garoullaye, 1994[29]	289	Mixed	2	Medium	NA	NA	Clay vs. Karaya gum plus polyvinyl polypyrrolidone for 8 weeks; equal pain reduction in both groups; decreased use of analgesics and improved gastrointestinal transit time with Karaya gum compared with clay.
Encopresis (fecal incontinence associated with psychiatric disorders)	Case series	Feldman, 1993[30]	6	NA	NA	NA	NA	NA	Play with modeling clay associated with improvement in 5 of 6 children, but study limited by lack of control group.

*Primary or secondary outcome.
[†]N, Number of patients; SS, statistically significant; ARR, absolute risk reduction; NNT, the number of patients who need to undergo a specific intervention in order to observe an outcome in one individual.
[‡]0-2 = poor; 3-4 = good; 5 = excellent.
NA, Not applicable.
For an explanation of each category in this table, please see Table 3 in the Introduction.

in several European pharmacopeias, including the Royal College, until the mid 19th century. There is limited evidence of efficacy in this area. There is a historical account that in 1581, a prisoner in Langenburg, Baden, Germany was condemned to death and requested that clay lozenges ("terra sigillata") be administered to him concomitantly with the assigned poison, mercuric chloride (approximately 6 grams).[7] The prisoner survived, and it was hypothesized that the clay lozenges were protective.

Protection from Aflatoxins

Summary

- Aflatoxins are toxic substances from the spores of the fungus *Aspergillus flavus*. This fungus infects peanuts, and ingestion of aflatoxins from peanuts and cereals (primarily in warm and humid regions) has been associated with the development of liver cancers in humans and multiple cancer types in animals. Phyllosilicate clay has been shown to tightly bind aflatoxins in aqueous solutions,[31] and HSACS clay in animal diets may diminish or block exposure to aflatoxins.[32] However, the risks of chronic clay exposure may not justify the proposed beneficial effects, and other preventive measures may carry less risk. Evidence of benefits in humans is lacking.

References

1. Morri RJ, Williams DE, Luu HA, et al. The adsorption of microcystin-LR by natural clay particles. Toxicon 2000;38(2):303-308.
2. Gonzalez JJ, Owens W, Ungaro PC, et al. Clay ingestion: a rare cause of hypokalemia. Ann Intern Med 1982;97(1):65-66.
3. Mengel CE, Carter WA, Horton ES. Geophagia with iron deficiency and hypokalemia. Arch Intern Med 1964;114:470-474.
4. Severance HW, Jr., Holt T, Patrone NA, et al. Profound muscle weakness and hypokalemia due to clay ingestion. South Med J 1988;81(2):272-274.
5. Minnich V, Okcuoglu A, Tarcon Y, et al. Pica in Turkey. II. Effect of clay upon iron absorption. Am J Clin Nutr 1968;21(1):78-86.
6. Guinee VF. Pica and lead poisoning. Nutr Rev 1971;29(12):267-269.
7. Halsted JA. Geophagia in man: its nature and nutritional effects. Am J Clin Nutr 1968;21(12):1384-1393.
8. Beron R, Valero A. Pica and hypochromic anemia: a survey of 14 cases seen in Israel. Harefuah 1961;61(2):35-39.
9. Crosby WH. Food pica and iron deficiency. Arch Intern Med 1971;127(5):960-961.
10. McDonald R, Marshall SR. The value of iron therapy in pica. Pediatrics 1964;34:558-562.
11. Blum M, Orton C, Rose L. The effect of starch ingestion on excessive iron association, abstracted. Ann Intern Med 1968;68:1165.
12. Carpenter WM. Observations on Cachexia Africana, on habits and effects of dirt eating in negro race. New Orleans Med Surg J 1844;1:146-168.
13. Montoya-Cabrera MA, Hernandex-Zamora A, Portilla-Aguilar J, et al. [Fatal lead poisoning caused by the ingestion of lemonade from glazed clay chinaware]. Gac Med Mex 1981;117(4):154-158.
14. Gutelius MF, Millican FK, Layman EM, et al. Nutritional studies of children with pica: I. Controlled study evaluating nutritional states. Pediatrics 1962;29:1012-1017.
15. Love RG, Waclawski ER, Maclaren WM, et al. Risks of respiratory disease in the heavy clay industry. Occup Environ Med 1999;56(2):124-133.
16. Bateson EM, Lebroy T. Clay eating by Aboriginals of the Northern Territory. Med J Aust 1978;1(Suppl 1):1-3.
17. Delaitre B, Lemaigre G, Acar JF, et al. [Necrotizing enteritis and geophagia]. Nouv Presse Med 1976;5(28):1743-1746.
18. Sanchez JE. Perforation of the colon due to clay ball. Arch Surg 1978;113(7):906.
19. Murty TV, Rao NN, Bopardikar KV. "Geophagia with mechanical obstructive symptoms." Indian Pediatr 1976;13(7):575-576.
20. Prasad AS, Halsted JA, Nadimi M. Syndrome of iron deficiency anemia, hepatospelenomegaly, hypogonadism, dwarfism and geophagia. Am J Med 1961;31:532-546.
21. Obialo CI, Crowell AK, Wen XJ, et al. Clay pica has no hematologic or metabolic correlate in chronic hemodialysis patients. J Ren Nutr 2001;11(1):32-36.
22. Booth EM. A case of tetanus of intestinal origin. Irish J Med Sci 1934;6:670-674.
23. Hayward DG, Nortrup D, Gardner A, et al. Elevated TCDD in chicken eggs and farm-raised catfish fed a diet with ball clay from a Southern United States mine. Environ Res 1999;81(3):248-256.
24. O'Rourke DE, Quinn JG, Nicholson JO, et al. Geophagia during pregnancy. Obstet Gynecol 1967;29(4):581-584.
25. Edwards CE, McDonald S, Mitchell JK, et al. Effect of clay and cornstarch intake on women and their infants. J Amer Diet Assoc 1964;44:109-115.
26. Fredj G, Farinotti R, Salvadori C, et al. [Topical digestive drugs with a clay base. Influence on the absorption of cimetidine]. Therapie 1986;41(1):23-25.
27. Edwards CH, McDonald S, Mitchell J. Clay- and cornstarch-eating women. J Amer Diet Assoc 1959;35:810-815.
28. Hunter JM, DeKleine R. Geophagy in Central America. Geogr Rev 1984;74(2):157-169.
29. Pariente EA, De La Garoullaye G. [A multicenter comparative study of a mucilage (Karaya gum + PVPP) versus clay in functional intestinal disorders]. Med Chir Dig 1994;23(3):193-199.
30. Feldman PC, Villanueva S, Lanne V, et al. Use of play with clay to treat children with intractable encopresis. J Pediatr 1993;122(3):483-488.
31. Phillips TD, Sarr AB, Grant PG. Selective chemisorption and detoxification of aflatoxins by phyllosilicate clay. Nat Toxins 1995;3(4):204-213.
32. Phillips TD. Dietary clay in the chemoprevention of aflatoxin-induced disease. Toxicol Sci 1999;52(2 Suppl):118-126.

Clove and Clove Oil (Eugenol)
(Eugenia aromatica)

SYNONYMS/COMMON NAMES/RELATED SUBSTANCES

- 2-methoxy-4-(2-propenyl)-phenol, caryophylli, *Caryophylli atheroleum*, caryophyllum, caryophyllus, *Caryophyllus aromaticus*, chiodo di garofano, clavos, clous de girolfe, clove cigarettes, clove oil, *Eugenia caryophyllata*, *Eugenia caryophyllus*, *Flores caryophylli*, gewurznelken nagelein, kreteks, Myrtaceae, oil of clove, oleum caryophylli, pentogen, *Syzigium aromaticum*, tropical myrtle.
- **Combination products:** Dent-Zel-Ite toothache relief drops, Red Cross Toothache Medication.

CLINICAL BOTTOM LINE
Background

- Clove is widely cultivated in Indonesia, Sri-Lanka, Madagascar, Tanzania, and Brazil. It is used in limited amounts in food products as a fragrant, flavoring agent, and antiseptic.
- Clinical trials assessing clove monotherapy are limited, although the expert panel German Commission E has approved the use of clove as a topical antiseptic and anesthetic. Other uses for clove, such as treatment for premature ejaculation, inflammation after tooth extraction (dry socket), and fever reduction, lack reliable human clinical evidence.
- Clove is sometimes added to tobacco in cigarettes. Clove cigarettes (kreteks) typically contain 60% tobacco and 40% ground cloves.

Uses Based on Scientific Evidence	Grade*
Fever reduction Studies in animals suggest that clove can lower fever, but no reliable studies in humans are available.	C
Inflammation after tooth extraction (dry socket) Preliminary studies have reported that oil of clove combined with zinc oxide paste is effective for treatment of dry socket. The benefits of clove alone need to be studied before a recommendation can be made.	C
Premature ejaculation A small amount of human research reports that a combination cream with clove and other herbs may be helpful in the treatment of premature ejaculation. However, well-designed studies of the effectiveness of clove alone are needed before a conclusion can be drawn.	C

*Key to grades: *A:* Strong scientific evidence for this use; *B:* Good scientific evidence for this use; *C:* Unclear scientific evidence for this use; *D:* Fair scientific evidence against this use (it may not work); *F:* Strong scientific evidence against this use (it likely does not work). For a more detailed explanation of efficacy criteria, see "Natural Standard Evidence-Based Validated Grading Rationale" in the Introduction.

Historical or Theoretical Indications That Lack Sufficient Evidence

Abdominal pain, antifungal, antihistamine, antioxidant, antiseptic, antiviral, asthma, athlete's foot, bad breath, blood purifier, blood thinner (antiplatelet agent), cancer, dental cavities, colic, cough, counterirritant, decreased gastric transit time, diabetes, diarrhea, dust mites, expectorant, flatulence (gas), flavoring for food and cigarettes, gout, hernia, herpes simplex virus, hiccups, high blood pressure, inflammation, mouth and throat inflammation, mouthwash, muscle spasm, nausea and vomiting, pain, parasites, smooth muscle relaxant, tooth or gum pain, vasorelaxant.

DOSING/TOXICOLOGY

The following doses are based on scientific research, publications, traditional use, or expert opinion. Many herbs and supplements have not been thoroughly tested, and their safety and effectiveness may not be proven. Brands may be made differently, with variable ingredients even within the same brand. The doses shown may not apply to all products. It is important to always read product labels and discuss doses with a qualified healthcare provider before therapy is started.

Standardization

- Standardization involves measuring the amounts of certain chemicals in products to try to make different preparations similar to each other. It is not always known if the chemicals being measured are the "active" ingredients. Some sources recommend that clove oil should not be used in concentrations higher than 0.06%, and that the daily dose of eugenol, a component of clove, should not be higher than 2.5 milligrams for each kilogram of body weight.

Adults (18 Years and Older)

- There is insufficient scientific evidence available to recommend a specific dose of clove by mouth, on the skin, or by any other route.

Children (Younger Than 18 Years)

- There is insufficient scientific evidence available to recommend a specific dose of clove by mouth, on the skin, or by any other route.

SAFETY

The U.S. Food and Drug Administration does not strictly regulate herbs and supplements. There is no guarantee of the strength, purity, or safety of products, and effects may vary. It is important to always read product labels. People who have a medical condition, or are taking other drugs, herbs, or supplements, should consult a qualified healthcare provider before starting a new therapy. A healthcare provider should be contacted immediately about any side effects.

Allergies

- Allergic reactions to clove and its component eugenol have been reported, including severe reactions (anaphylaxis). Eugenol or clove can cause allergic rashes when applied to the skin or inside the mouth. Hives have been reported in clove cigarette smokers. People who are allergic to balsam of Peru may also be allergic to clove. Persons with known allergy to clove, its component eugenol, or to balsam of Peru should avoid the use of clove by mouth, inhaled from cigarettes, or applied to the skin.

Side Effects and Warnings

- Clove is generally regarded as safe for food use in the United States. However, when clove is taken by mouth in large doses, in its undiluted oil form, or used in clove cigarettes, side effects may occur, including vomiting, sore throat, seizure, sedation, difficulty breathing, fluid in the lungs, vomiting of blood, blood disorders, kidney failure, and liver damage. People with kidney or liver disorders or who have had seizures should avoid clove. Serious side effects are reported more often in young children. It is recommended to avoid the use of clove supplements in children and pregnant or nursing women.
- Laboratory research studies suggest that clove or clove oil may cause an increased risk of bleeding. Caution is advised in people with bleeding disorders or those taking drugs that may increase the risk of bleeding. Dosing adjustments may be necessary. It is unclear what doses or methods of using clove may contribute to this risk. One case of disseminated intravascular coagulation (DIC) (a severe reaction including bleeding and liver damage) was reported in a person taking clove by mouth.
- When applied to the skin or the inside of the mouth, clove can cause burning, loss of sensation, local tissue damage, dental pulp damage, and lip sores and can increase the risk of cavities. There is a high risk of contact dermatitis (rash) and even burns if undiluted, full-strength clove oil is applied to the skin. The application of clove combination herbal creams to the penis has been reported to cause episodes of difficulty with erection or ejaculation.
- Based on an infant case report, clove oil taken by mouth may lower blood sugar levels. Caution is advised in patients with diabetes or hypoglycemia, and in those taking drugs, herbs, or supplements that affect blood sugar levels. Serum glucose levels may need to be monitored by a healthcare provider, and medication adjustments may be necessary.
- Contamination of clove can occur if the herb is improperly stored. Fungi and aflatoxins are among the most common contaminants. Ingesting contaminated clove can result in health problems in humans as well as in animals.

Pregnancy and Breastfeeding

- Insufficient information about safety is available to recommend the use of clove supplements in pregnant or breastfeeding women.

INTERACTIONS

Most herbs and supplements have not been thoroughly tested for interactions with other herbs, supplements, drugs, or foods. The interactions listed here are based on reports in scientific publications, laboratory experiments, or traditional use. It is important to always read product labels. People who have a medical condition, or are taking other drugs, herbs, or supplements, should consult a qualified healthcare provider before starting a new therapy.

Interactions with Drugs

- Based on laboratory research, clove theoretically may increase the risk of bleeding when taken with drugs that increase the risk of bleeding. It is unclear what doses or methods of using clove may increase this risk. Examples of such drugs are anticoagulants (blood thinners) such as warfarin (Coumadin) and heparin, antiplatelet drugs such as clopidogrel (Plavix), aspirin, and nonsteroidal anti-inflammatory drugs such as ibuprofen (Motrin, Advil) and naproxen (Naprosyn, Aleve).
- Based on an infant case report, clove oil taken by mouth may lower blood sugar levels. Caution is advised when using medications that may also lower blood sugar levels. People taking drugs for diabetes by mouth or insulin should be monitored closely by a qualified healthcare provider. Medication adjustments may be necessary.
- When applied to the skin, eugenol, a component of clove, may reduce the ability to feel and react to painful stimulation. Therefore, use of clove products on the skin with other numbing or pain-reducing products such as lidocaine/prilocaine cream (Emla) theoretically may increase effects.

Interactions with Herbs and Dietary Supplements

- Based on laboratory research studies, clove may increase the risk of bleeding when taken with herbs and supplements that may also increase the risk of bleeding. It is unclear what doses or methods of using clove may increase this risk. Multiple cases of bleeding have been reported with the use of *Ginkgo biloba*, some cases with garlic, and fewer cases with saw palmetto. Numerous other agents may theoretically increase the risk of bleeding, although this has not been proven in most cases. Examples of such agents are alfalfa, American ginseng, angelica, anise, *Arnica montana*, asafetida, aspen bark, bilberry, birch, black cohosh, bladderwrack, bogbean, boldo, borage seed oil, bromelain, capsicum, cat's claw, celery, chamomile, chaparral, coleus, cordyceps, danshen, devil's claw, dong quai, eicosapentaenoic acid (EPA), evening primrose, fenugreek, feverfew, fish oil, flaxseed/flax powder (not a concern with flaxseed oil), ginger, grapefruit juice, grape seed, green tea, guggul, gymnestra, horse chestnut, horseradish, licorice root, lovage root, male fern, meadowsweet, nordihydroguaiaretic acid (NDGA), onion, *Panax ginseng*, papain, parsley, passion flower, poplar, prickly ash, propolis, quassia, red clover, reishi, rue, Siberian ginseng, sweet birch, sweet clover, turmeric, vitamin E, white willow, wild carrot, wild lettuce, willow, wintergreen, and yucca.
- Based on an infant case report, clove may lower blood sugar levels. Caution is advised when using herbs or supplements that may also lower blood sugar levels. Blood glucose levels may require monitoring, and doses may need adjustment. Examples of such herbs are *Aloe vera*, American ginseng, bilberry, bitter melon, burdock, fenugreek, fish oil, gymnema, horse chestnut seed extract (HCSE), maitake mushroom, marshmallow, milk thistle, *Panax ginseng*, rosemary, Siberian ginseng, stinging nettle, and white horehound.
- When applied to the skin, eugenol, a component of clove, may reduce the ability to feel and react to painful stimulation. Therefore, use with other numbing or pain-reducing products such as capsaicin cream (Zostrix) may in theory cause exaggerated effects.

Selected References

Natural Standard developed the preceding evidence-based information based on a systematic review of more than 220 scientific articles. For comprehensive information about alternative and complementary therapies on the professional level, go to www.naturalstandard.com. Selected references are listed here.

Burt SA, Reinders RD. Antibacterial activity of selected plant essential oils against *Escherichia coli* O157:H7. Lett Appl Microbiol 2003;36(3):162-167.

Choi HK, Jung GW, Moon KH, et al. Clinical study of SS-cream in patients with lifelong premature ejaculation. Urology 2000;55(2):257-261.

Consolini AE, Sarubbio MG. Pharmacological effects of *Eugenia uniflora* (Myrtaceae) aqueous crude extract on rat's heart. J Ethnopharmacol 2002; 81(1):57-63.

Damiani CE, Rossoni LV, Vassallo DV. Vasorelaxant effects of eugenol on rat thoracic aorta. Vascul Pharmacol 2003;40(1):59-66.

Dragland S, Senoo H, Wake K, et al. Several culinary and medicinal herbs are important sources of dietary antioxidants. J Nutr 2003;133(5):1286-1290.

Elshafie AE, Al-Rashdi TA, Al-Bahry SN, et al. Fungi and aflatoxins associated with spices in the Sultanate of Oman. Mycopathologia 2002;155(3):155-160.

Friedman M, Henika PR, Mandrell RE. Bactericidal activities of plant essential oils and some of their isolated constituents against *Campylobacter jejuni*, *Escherichia coli*, *Listeria monocytogenes*, and *Salmonella enterica*. J Food Prot 2002;65(10):1545-1560.

Grover JK, Rathi SS, Vats V. Amelioration of experimental diabetic neuropathy and gastropathy in rats following oral administration of plant (*Eugenia jambolana*, *Mucuna pruriens* and *Tinospora cordifolia*) extracts. Indian J Exp Biol 2002;40(3):273-276.

Guynot ME, Ramos AJ, Seto L, et al. Antifungal activity of volatile compounds generated by essential oils against fungi commonly causing deterioration of bakery products. J Appl Microbiol 2003;94(5):893-899.

Huss U, Ringbom T, Perera P, et al. Screening of ubiquitous plant constituents for COX-2 inhibition with a scintillation proximity based assay. J Nat Prod 2002;65(11):1517-1521.

Juglal S, Govinden R, Odhav B. Spice oils for the control of co-occurring mycotoxin-producing fungi. J Food Prot 2002;65(4):683-687.

Kalemba D, Kunicka A. Antibacterial and antifungal properties of essential oils. Curr Med Chem 2003;10(10):813-829.

Kim EH, Kim HK, Ahn YJ. Acaricidal activity of clove bud oil compounds against *Dermatophagoides farinae* and *Dermatophagoides pteronyssinus* (Acari: Pyroglyphidae). J Agric Food Chem 2003;51(4):885-889.

Pallares DE. Link between clove cigarettes and urticaria? Postgrad Med 1999;106(4):153.

Sanchez-Perez J, Garcia-Diez A. Occupational allergic contact dermatitis from eugenol, oil of cinnamon and oil of cloves in a physiotherapist. Contact Dermatitis 1999;41(6):346-347.

Soetiarto F. The relationship between habitual clove cigarette smoking and a specific pattern of dental decay in male bus drivers in Jakarta, Indonesia. Caries Res 1999;33(3):248-250.

Coenzyme Q10
(Ubiquinone)

SYNONYMS/COMMON NAMES/RELATED SUBSTANCES

- Adelir, coenzymeQ, co-enzyme Q10, coenzyme Q (50), coQ, coQ10, coQ(50), co-Q10, CoQ-10, 2,3-dimethoxy-5-methyl-6-decaprenyl benzoquinone, Heartcin, idebenone (synthetic analogue), mitoquinone, Neuquinone, Q10, Taidecanone, ubidecarenone, ubiquinone, ubiquinone-10, ubiquinone-Q10, Udekinon, vitamin q10, vitamin Q10.

CLINICAL BOTTOM LINE

Background

- Coenzyme Q10 (CoQ10) is produced by the human body and is necessary for the basic functioning of cells. CoQ10 levels are reported to decrease with age and to be low in people with chronic diseases such as heart conditions, muscular dystrophy, Parkinson's disease, cancer, diabetes, and HIV/AIDS. Some prescription drugs may also decrease CoQ10 levels. Levels of CoQ10 in the body can be increased by taking CoQ10 supplements, although it is not clear whether this is beneficial. CoQ10 has been used, recommended, or studied for numerous conditions and remains controversial as a treatment in many areas.

Uses Based on Scientific Evidence	Grade*
High blood pressure (hypertension) Preliminary research suggests that CoQ10 causes small decreases in blood pressure (systolic and possibly diastolic). Low blood levels of CoQ10 have been found in people with hypertension, although it is not clear if CoQ10 "deficiency" is a cause of high blood pressure. It is not known what dose is safe or effective. CoQ10 is less commonly used to treat hypertension than it is for other heart conditions such as congestive heart failure. Well-designed long-term research is needed to strengthen this recommendation.	B
Alzheimer's disease Promising preliminary evidence from human research suggests that CoQ10 supplements may slow down, but not cure, dementia in people with Alzheimer's disease. Additional well-designed studies are needed to confirm this result before a firm recommendation can be made.	C
Angina (chest pain from clogged heart arteries) Preliminary small human studies suggest that CoQ10 may reduce angina and improve exercise tolerance in people with clogged heart arteries. Better studies are needed before a firm recommendation can be made.	C
Anthracycline chemotherapy heart toxicity Anthracycline chemotherapy drugs, such as doxorubicin (Adriamycin), are commonly used to treat cancers such as breast cancer or lymphoma. Heart damage (cardiomyopathy) is a major concern with the use of anthracyclines, and CoQ10 has been suggested to protect the heart. However, studies in this area are small and not high quality, and the effects of CoQ10 remain unclear.	
Breast cancer Several studies in women with breast cancer report reduced levels of CoQ10 in diseased breast tissue or blood. It has been suggested by some researchers that raising CoQ10 levels with supplements might be helpful. However, it is not clear if CoQ10 is beneficial in these patients or if the low levels of CoQ10 may actually be a part of the body's natural response to cancer, helping to fight disease. Supplementation with CoQ10 has not been proven to reduce cancer and has not been compared with other forms of treatment for breast cancer.	C
Cardiomyopathy (dilated, hypertrophic) There is conflicting evidence from research on the use of CoQ10 in patients with dilated or hypertrophic cardiomyopathy. Different levels of disease severity have been studied (New York Heart Association heart failure classes I through IV). Some studies report improved heart function (ejection fraction, stroke volume, cardiac index, exercise tolerance), while others find no improvements. Most trials are small or not well designed. Better research is needed in this area before a recommendation can be made.	C
Exercise performance The effects of CoQ10 on exercise performance have been tested in athletes, normal healthy individuals, and people with chronic lung disease. Results are variable; some studies reported benefits, and others showed no effects. Most trials have not been well designed. Better research is necessary before a firm conclusion can be drawn.	C
Friedreich's ataxia Preliminary research reports promising evidence for the use of CoQ10 in the treatment of Friedreich's ataxia. Further evidence is necessary before a firm conclusion can be drawn.	C
Gum disease (periodontitis) Preliminary studies in humans suggest possible benefits of CoQ10 taken by mouth or placed on the skin or gums in the treatment of periodontitis. Improvement in bleeding, swelling, and pain were reported. However, the available studies are small and of poor quality. Better research is needed before a conclusion can be drawn.	C
Heart attack (acute myocardial infarction) There is preliminary human study of CoQ10 given to patients within 3 days after a heart attack. Reductions in deaths, abnormal heart rhythms, and second heart	C

Continued

attacks are reported, although better research is needed before a firm conclusion can be drawn.	
Heart failure The evidence for CoQ10 in the treatment of heart failure is controversial and remains unclear. Different levels of disease severity have been studied (New York Heart Association classes I through IV). Some studies report improved heart function (ejection fraction, stroke volume, cardiac index, exercise tolerance), while others find no improvements. Most trials are small or not well designed. In some parts of Europe, Russia, and Japan, CoQ10 is considered a part of standard therapy for congestive heart failure patients. Better research is needed in this area, studying effects on quality of life, hospitalization, and death rates, before a recommendation can be made.	C
Heart protection during surgery Several studies suggest that cardiac function may be improved following major heart surgery such as coronary artery bypass graft (CABG) or valve replacement when CoQ10 is given to patients before or during surgery. Better-designed studies that measure effects on long-term cardiac function and survival are necessary before a recommendation can be made.	C
HIV/AIDS Limited evidence suggests that natural levels of CoQ10 in the body may be reduced in people with HIV/AIDS. There is no reliable scientific research showing that CoQ10 supplements have any effect on this disease.	C
Mitochondrial diseases and Kearns-Sayre syndrome CoQ10 is often recommended for people with mitochondrial diseases such as myopathies, encephalomyopathies, and Kearns-Sayre syndrome. Several early studies reported improvement in metabolism and physical endurance in people with these conditions after treatment with CoQ10, although most available research is not of high quality or definitive. Better studies are needed before a strong recommendation can be made.	C
Muscular dystrophy Preliminary studies in people with muscular dystrophy who were given CoQ10 supplements reported improvement in exercise capacity, heart function, and overall quality of life. Additional research is needed in this area.	C
Diabetes Evidence from preliminary studies suggests that CoQ10 does not affect blood sugar levels in people with type 1 or type 2 diabetes and does not alter the need for diabetes medications.	D

*Key to grades: A: Strong scientific evidence for this use; B: Good scientific evidence for this use; C: Unclear scientific evidence for this use; D: Fair scientific evidence against this use (it may not work); F: Strong scientific evidence against this use (it likely does not work). For a more detailed explanation of efficacy criteria, see "Natural Standard Evidence-Based Validated Grading Rationale" in the Introduction.

Historical or Theoretical Indications That Lack Sufficient Evidence

Amyotrophic lateral sclerosis (ALS), antioxidant, asthma, Bell's palsy, breathing difficulties, cancer, cerebellar ataxia, chronic fatigue syndrome, chronic obstructive pulmonary disease (COPD), deafness, decreased sperm motility (idiopathic asthenozoospermia), gingivitis, hair loss (and hair loss from chemotherapy), hepatitis B, high cholesterol, Huntington's chorea/disease, immune system diseases, infertility, insomnia, irregular heart beat, kidney failure, leg swelling (edema), life extension, liver enlargement/disease, lung cancer/disease, macular degeneration, maternally inherited diabetes mellitus and deafness (MIDD), MELAS syndrome, mitral valve prolapse, obesity, Papillon-Lefevre syndrome, Parkinson's disease, physical performance enhancement, prevention of muscle damage from statin cholesterol-lowering drugs, psychiatric disorders, QT-interval shortening; reduction of phenothiazine side effects, reduction of tricyclic antidepressant (TCA) side effects, stomach ulcers.

DOSING/TOXICOLOGY

The following doses are based on scientific research, publications, traditional use, or expert opinion. Many herbs and supplements have not been thoroughly tested, and their safety and effectiveness may not be proven. Brands may be made differently, with variable ingredients even within the same brand. The doses shown may not apply to all products. It is important to always read product labels and discuss doses with a qualified healthcare provider before therapy is started.

Standardization

- Standardization involves measuring the amounts of certain chemicals in products to try to make different preparations similar to each other. It is not always known if the chemicals being measured are the "active" ingredients. CoQ10 products sold in stores have been found to contain variable amounts of claimed ingredients. Early studies used low doses, while more recent research suggests that higher doses may be safe and have greater effects.

Adults (18 Years and Older)
Oral Use (by Mouth)

- **High blood pressure:** 30 to 360 mg of CoQ10 per day have been used. The ideal starting dose is not established. The reason why some people seem to respond better than others is unclear.
- **Congestive heart failure/cardiomyopathy:** Studies have used 100 to 200 mg of CoQ10 per day, or 2 mg per kilogram (2.2 pounds) of body weight per day. Limited research suggests that up to 600 mg per day may be tolerated. CoQ10 has been tested alone or as an addition to prescription drugs for these conditions. People with congestive heart failure or cardiomyopathy should consult a qualified healthcare provider before starting a new therapy.
- **Heart attack:** 120 mg of CoQ10 per day started 3 days after a heart attack has been studied, but the safety and effectiveness of this therapy are not established. People should consult a qualified healthcare provider before starting a new therapy.
- **Breast cancer:** 90 mg of CoQ10 per day in combination with multivitamin/multi-mineral supplementation has been studied.

- **Alzheimer's disease:** Doses of CoQ10 ranging from 60 mg once daily to 120 mg three times a day have been used. A preliminary study reported that higher doses may be more beneficial, although this has not been proven.
- **Anthracycline chemotherapy heart toxicity:** Preliminary research studies have used 50 to 100 mg of CoQ10 per day in children and adults receiving doxorubicin (Adriamycin) chemotherapy.
- **Angina:** 60 mg of CoQ10 per day for up to 4 weeks has been studied.
- **Heart protection during surgery:** Several studies in the 1980s and early 1990s used 30 to 150 mg of CoQ10 per day, starting 1 to 2 weeks prior to surgery and continuing for up to 1 month after surgery. Patients should consult their surgeon before starting a new therapy.
- **Exercise performance:** 90 to 150 mg per day of CoQ10 has been studied.
- **HIV/AIDS:** A dose of CoQ10 per day has been studied, but effectiveness has not been proved.
- **Muscular dystrophy:** In one study, 100 mg of CoQ10 per day divided into three doses was used.
- **Mitochondrial diseases:** 120 to 160 mg per day, or 2 mg per kilogram of body weight, has been used.
- **Gum disease (periodontitis):** In one study, 5 ml (1 teaspoonful) per day, concentrated to 200 mg of CoQ10 per ml of corn oil, taken by mouth in divided doses has been used.

Topical (on the skin)

- **Gum disease (periodontitis):** In one study, 85 mg of CoQ10 per ml of soybean oil suspension was applied to the surface of affected areas once weekly using a plastic syringe.

Intravenous (through the veins)

- **Heart protection during surgery:** Most studies of the use of CoQ10 for heart protection during bypass surgery have used CoQ10 taken by mouth. However, one study used intravenous CoQ10, 5 mg per kilogram of body weight, given 2 hours prior to surgery. Safety was not proved. People who are planning to use any therapies close to the time of surgery should discuss this with their surgeon.

Children (Younger Than 18 Years)

- There is not enough scientific information to recommend the safe use of CoQ10 in children. A qualified healthcare provider should be consulted before considering use. One small study in children used 100 mg of CoQ10 by mouth twice daily to reduce the heart toxicity of anthracycline (doxorubicin) chemotherapy. Another study used 3 to 3.4 mg per kilogram of body weight daily in children with mitral valve prolapse.

SAFETY

The U.S. Food and Drug Administration does not strictly regulate herbs and supplements. There is no guarantee of the strength, purity, or safety of products, and effects may vary. It is important to always read product labels. People who have a medical condition, or are taking other drugs, herbs, or supplements, should consult a qualified healthcare provider before starting a new therapy. A healthcare provider should be contacted immediately about any side effects.

Allergies

- In theory, allergic reactions to supplements containing CoQ10 may occur.

Side Effects and Warnings

- Few serious side effects of CoQ10 have been reported. Side effects typically are mild and brief, stopping without any treatment needed. Reactions may include diarrhea, dizziness, fatigue, flu-like symptoms, headache, heartburn, increased sensitivity to light, insomnia, irritability, itching, loss of appetite, nausea and vomiting, rash, and stomach upset.
- CoQ10 may decrease blood sugar levels. Caution is advised in people with diabetes or hypoglycemia, and in those taking drugs, herbs, or supplements that affect blood sugar levels. Serum glucose levels may need to be monitored by a healthcare provider, and medication adjustments may be necessary.
- Low blood platelet numbers were reported in one person taking CoQ10. However, other factors (viral infection, other medications) may have been responsible. A decrease in platelets may increase the risk of bruising or bleeding, although there are no known reports of bleeding caused by CoQ10. Caution is advised in people who have bleeding disorders or who are taking drugs that increase the risk of bleeding. Dosing adjustments may be necessary.
- CoQ10 may decrease blood pressure, and caution is advised in patients with low blood pressure or taking blood pressure medications. Elevations of liver enzymes have been reported rarely, and caution is advised in people with liver disease or taking medications that may harm the liver. CoQ10 may lower blood levels of cholesterol or triglycerides. In one study, thyroid hormone levels were altered.
- Organ damage due to lack of oxygen/blood flow during intense exercise was reported in a study of people with heart disease, although the specific role of CoQ10 was not clear. Vigorous exercise is often discouraged in people using CoQ10 supplements.

Pregnancy and Breastfeeding

- Scientific evidence is insufficient to recommend the safe use of CoQ10 during pregnancy or breastfeeding.

INTERACTIONS

Most herbs and supplements have not been thoroughly tested for interactions with other herbs, supplements, drugs, or foods. The interactions listed here are based on reports in scientific publications, laboratory experiments, or traditional use. It is important to always read product labels. People who have a medical condition, or are taking other drugs, herbs, or supplements, should consult a qualified healthcare provider before starting a new therapy.

Interactions with Drugs

- In theory and based on a single case report, coenzyme Q10 may reduce the effectiveness of warfarin (Coumadin), and may limit or prevent effective anticoagulation (blood thinning). CoQ10 may reduce blood pressure and may add to the effects of other blood pressure–lowering agents. In theory, CoQ10 may affect thyroid hormone levels and alter the effects of thyroid drugs such as levothyroxine (Synthroid), although this has not been proved in humans.
- In theory and based on research studies in humans, a number of drugs may deplete natural levels of CoQ10 in the body. It has not been shown that there are benefits of CoQ10 supplements in people using these agents. Examples of such agents are antipsychotic medications such as chlorpromazine, fluphenazine, haloperidol, mesoridazine, prochlorperazine, promethazine, thioridazine, trifluoperazine, and trimipramine; beta-blocker drugs such as acebutolol, atenolol, betaxolol, bisoprolol, carvedilol, esmolol, labetalol, metoprolol,

nadolol, penbutolol, pindolol, propranolol, sotalol, and timolol; clonidine; diabetes drugs such as acetohexamide, chlorpropamide, glimepiride, glipizide, glyburide, metformin, tolazamide, and tolbutamide; diuretic drugs ("water pills") such as benzthiazide, chlorothiazide, hydralazine, hydrochlorothiazide, indapamide, methyclothiazide, metolazone, and polythiazide; gemfibrozil; HMG-CoA reductase inhibitors ("statins") such as atorvastatin, cerivastatin (no longer available in U.S.), fluvastatin, lovastatin, pravastatin, and simvastatin; methyldopa; and tricyclic antidepressant drugs such as amitriptyline, clomipramine, doxepin, imipramine, and trimipramine.

Interactions with Herbs and Dietary Supplements

- CoQ10 may reduce blood pressure and may result in additive effects when taken with other herbs or supplements that also lower blood pressure. Herbs that may lower blood pressure include aconite/monkshood, arnica, baneberry, betel nut, bilberry, black cohosh, bryony, calendula, California poppy, coleus, curcumin, eucalyptol, eucalyptus oil, ginger, goldenseal, green hellebore, hawthorn, horsetail, Indian tobacco, jaborandi, licorice, mistletoe, night blooming cereus, oleander, pasque flower, periwinkle, pleurisy root, shepherd's purse, Texas milkweed, turmeric, and wild cherry.
- Based on results of studies in humans, vitamin E may reduce CoQ10 blood levels. In theory, red rice yeast may decrease CoQ10 levels. CoQ10 may add to the effects or side effects of L-carnitine.

Selected References

Natural Standard developed the preceding evidence-based information based on a systematic review of more than 600 scientific articles. For comprehensive information about alternative and complementary therapies on the professional level, go to www.naturalstandard.com. Selected references are listed here.

Albano CB, Muralikrishnan D, Ebadi M. Distribution of coenzyme Q homologues in brain. Neurochem Res 2002;27(5):359-368.

Baggio E, Gandini R, Plancher AC, et al. Italian multicenter study on the safety and efficacy of coenzyme Q10 as adjunctive therapy in heart failure. CoQ10 Drug Surveillance Investigators. Mol Aspects Med 1994;15(Suppl): s287-s294.

Baker SK, Tarnopolsky MA. Targeting cellular energy production in neurological disorders. Expert Opin Investig Drugs 2003;12(10):1655-1679.

Balercia G, Arnaldi G, Lucarelli G, et al. Effects of exogenous CoQ10 administration in patients with idiopathic asthenozoospermia. Int J Andrology 2000; 23(Suppl):43.

Batino M, Ferreiro MS, Quiles JL, et al. Alterations in the oxidation products, antioxidant markers, antioxidant capacity and lipid patterns in plasma of patients affected by Papillon-Lefevre syndrome. Free Radic Res 2003;37(6): 603-609.

Blasi MA, Bovina C, Carella G, et al. Does coenzyme Q10 play a role in opposing oxidative stress in patients with age-related macular degeneration? Ophthalmologica 2001;215(1):51-54.

Bleske B, Willis R, Anthony M, et al. The effect of pravastatin and atorvastatin on coenzyme Q10. Am Heart J 2001;142(2):e2.

Bonetti A, Solito F, Carmosino G, et al. Effect of ubidecarenone oral treatment on aerobic power in middle-aged trained subjects. J Sports Med Phys Fitness 2000;40(1):51-57.

Braun B, Clarkson PM, Freedson PS, et al. Effects of coenzyme Q10 supplementation on exercise performance, VO_{2max}, and lipid peroxidation in trained cyclists. Int J Sport Nutr 1991;1(4):353-365.

Bresolin N, Doriguzzi C, Ponzetto C, et al. Ubidecarenone in the treatment of mitochondrial myopathies: a multi-center double-blind trial. J Neurol Sci 1990;100(1-2):70-78.

Burke BE, Neuenschwander R, Olson RD. Randomized, double-blind, placebo-controlled trial of coenzyme Q10 in isolated systolic hypertension. South Med J 2001;94(11):1112-1117.

Chello M, Mastroroberto P, Romano R, et al. Protection by coenzyme Q10 from myocardial reperfusion injury during coronary artery bypass grafting. Ann Thorac Surg 1994;58(5):1427-1432.

Chen RS, Huang CC, Chu NS. Coenzyme Q10 treatment in mitochondrial encephalomyopathies. Short-term double-blind, crossover study. Eur Neurol 1997;37(4):212-218.

Chen YF, Lin YT, Wu SC. Effectiveness of coenzyme Q10 on myocardial preservation during hypothermic cardioplegic arrest. J Thorac Cardiovasc Surg 1994;107(1):242-247.

de Bustos F, Jimenez-Jimenez FJ, Molina JA, et al. Serum levels of coenzyme Q10 in patients with multiple sclerosis. Acta Neurol Scand 2000;101(3): 209-211.

Digiesi V, Cantini F, Brodbeck B. Effect of coenzyme Q10 on essential arterial hypertension. Curr Ther Res 1990;47(5):841-845.

Eaton S, Skinner R, Hale JP, et al. Plasma coenzyme Q(10) in children and adolescents undergoing doxorubicin therapy. Clin Chim Acta 2000;302(1-2): 1-9.

Eriksson JG, Forsen TJ, Mortensen SA, et al. The effect of coenzyme Q10 administration on metabolic control in patients with type 2 diabetes mellitus. Biofactors 1999;9(2-4):315-318.

Folkers K, Langsjoen P, Willis R, et al. Lovastatin decreases coenzyme Q levels in humans. Proc Natl Acad Sci U S A 1990;87(22):8931-8934.

Folkers K, Vadhanavikit S, Mortensen SA. Biochemical rationale and myocardial tissue data on the effective therapy of cardiomyopathy with coenzyme Q10. Proc Natl Acad Sci U S A 1985;82(3):901-904.

Fujimoto S, Kurihara N, Hirata K, et al. Effects of coenzyme Q10 administration on pulmonary function and exercise performance in patients with chronic lung diseases. Clin Investig 1993;71(Suppl 8):S162-S166.

Gazdikova K, Gvozdjakova A, Kucharska J, et al. Effect of coenzyme Q10 in patients with kidney diseases. Cas Lek Cesk 2000;140:307-310.

Ghirlanda G, Oradei A, Manto A, et al. Evidence of plasma CoQ10-lowering effect by HMG-CoA reductase inhibitors: a double-blind, placebo-controlled study. J Clin Pharmacol 1993;33(3):226-229.

Gutzmann H, Hadler D. Sustained efficacy and safety of idebenone in the treatment of Alzheimer's disease: update on a 2-year double-blind multicentre study. J Neural Transm Suppl 1998;54:301-310.

Hanioka T, Tanaka M, Ojima M, et al. Effect of topical application of coenzyme Q10 on adult periodontitis. Mol Aspects Med 1994;15(Suppl):s241-s248.

Henriksen JE, Andersen CB, Hother-Nielsen O, et al. Impact of ubiquinone (coenzyme Q10) treatment on glycaemic control, insulin requirement and well-being in patients with Type 1 diabetes mellitus. Diabet Med 1999; 16(4):312-318.

Ishiyama T, Morita Y, Toyama S, et al. A clinical study of the effect of coenzyme Q on congestive heart failure. Jpn Heart J 1976;17(1):32-42.

Jimenez-Jimenez FJ, Molina JA, de Bustos F, et al. Serum levels of coenzyme Q10 in patients with Parkinson's disease. J Neural Transm 2000;107(2): 177-181.

Judy WV, Stogsdill WW, Folkers K. Myocardial preservation by therapy with coenzyme Q10 during heart surgery. Clin Investig 1993;71(Suppl 8): S155-S161.

Kamikawa T, Kobayashi A, Yamashita T, et al. Effects of coenzyme Q10 on exercise tolerance in chronic stable angina pectoris. Am J Cardiol 1985;56(4): 247-251.

Khatta M, Alexander BS, Krichten CM, et al. The effect of coenzyme Q10 in patients with congestive heart failure. Ann Intern Med 2000;132(8):636-640.

Lampertico M, Comis S. Italian multicenter study on the efficacy and safety of coenzyme Q10 as adjuvant therapy in heart failure. Clin Investig 1993; 71(8 Suppl):S129-S133.

Landbo C, Almdal TP. [Interaction between warfarin and coenzyme Q10.] Ugeskr Laeger 1998;160(22):3226-3227.

Langsjoen H, Langsjoen P, Langsjoen P, et al. Usefulness of coenzyme Q10 in clinical cardiology: a long-term study. Mol Aspects Med 1994;15(Suppl): s165-s175.

Langsjoen P, Langsjoen P, Willis R, et al. Treatment of essential hypertension with coenzyme Q10. Mol Aspects Med 1994;15(Suppl):s265-s272.

Langsjoen PH, Folkers K, Lyson K, et al. Pronounced increase of survival of patients with cardiomyopathy when treated with coenzyme Q10 and conventional therapy. Int J Tissue React 1990;12(3):163-168.

Langsjoen PH, Langsjoen PH, Folkers K. A six-year clinical study of therapy of cardiomyopathy with coenzyme Q10. Int J Tissue React 1990;12(3):169-171.

Langsjoen PH, Langsjoen PH, Folkers K. Long-term efficacy and safety of coenzyme Q10 therapy for idiopathic dilated cardiomyopathy. Am J Cardiol 1990;65(7):521-523.

Lerman-Sagie T, Rustin P, Lev D, et al. Dramatic improvement in mitochondrial cardiomyopathy following treatment with idebenone. J Inherit Metab Dis 2001;24(1):28-34.

Lockwood K, Moesgaard S, Folkers K. Partial and complete regression of breast cancer in relation to dosage of coenzyme Q10. Biochem Biophys Res Commun 1994;199(3):1504-1508.

Lockwood K, Moesgaard S, Hanioka T, et al. Apparent partial remission of breast cancer in "high risk" patients supplemented with nutritional antioxidants, essential fatty acids and coenzyme Q10. Mol Aspects Med 1994;15(Suppl): s231-s240.

Lockwood K, Moesgard S, Yamamoto T, et al. Progress on therapy of breast cancer with vitamin Q10 and the regression of metastases. Biochem Biophys Res Commun 1995;212(1):172-177.

Matsumura T, Saji S, Nakamura R, et al. Evidence for enhanced treatment of periodontal disease by therapy with coenzyme Q. Int J Vitam Nutr Res 1973; 43(4):537-548.

Mazzola C, Guffanti EE, Vaccarella A, et al. Noninvasive assessment of coenzyme Q10 in patients with chronic stable effort angina and moderate heart failure. Curr Ther Res 1987;41(6):923-932.

Miyake Y, Shouzu A, Nishikawa M, et al. Effect of treatment with 3-hydroxy-3-methylglutaryl coenzyme A reductase inhibitors on serum coenzyme Q10 in diabetic patients. Arzneimittelforschung 1999;49(4):324-329.

Morisco C, Trimarco B, Condorelli M. Effect of coenzyme Q10 therapy in patients with congestive heart failure: a long-term multicenter randomized study. Clin Investig 1993;71(Suppl 8):S134-S136.

Mortensen SA. Coenzyme Q10 as an adjunctive therapy in patients with congestive heart failure. J Am Coll Cardiol 2000;36(1):304-305.

Mortensen SA, Leth A, Agner E, et al. Dose-related decrease of serum coenzyme Q10 during treatment with HMG-CoA reductase inhibitors. Mol Aspects Med 1997;18(Suppl):s137-s144.

Mortensen SA, Vadhanavikit S, Muratsu K, et al. Coenzyme Q10: clinical benefits with biochemical correlates suggesting a scientific breakthrough in the management of chronic heart failure. Int J Tissue React 1990;12(3):155-162.

Munkholm H, Hansen HH, Rasmussen K. Coenzyme Q10 treatment in serious heart failure. Biofactors 1999;9(2-4):285-289.

Musumeci O, Naini A, Slonim AE, et al. Familial cerebellar ataxia with muscle coenzyme Q10 deficiency. Neurology 2001;56(7):849-855.

Nielsen AN, Mizuno M, Ratkevicius A, et al. No effect of antioxidant supplementation in triathletes on maximal oxygen uptake, 31P-NMRS detected muscle energy metabolism and muscle fatigue. Int J Sports Med 1999;20(3):154-158.

Ogasahara S, Nishikawa Y, Yorifuji S, et al. Treatment of Kearns-Sayre syndrome with coenzyme Q10. Neurology 1986;36(1):45-53.

Permanetter B, Rossy W, Klein G, et al. Ubiquinone (coenzyme Q10) in the long-term treatment of idiopathic dilated cardiomyopathy. Eur Heart J 1992;13(11):1528-1533.

Pogessi L, Galanti G, Corneglio M, et al. Effect of coenzyme Q10 on left ventricular function in patients with dilative cardiomyopathy. Curr Ther Res 1991;49:878-886.

Porter DA, Costill DL, Zachwieja JJ, et al. The effect of oral coenzyme Q10 on the exercise tolerance of middle-aged, untrained men. Int J Sports Med 1995;16(7):421-427.

Shults CW, Beal MF, Fontaine D, et al. Absorption, tolerability, and effects on mitochondrial activity of oral coenzyme Q10 in parkinsonian patients. Neurology 1998;50(3):793-795.

Singh RB, Khanna HK, Niaz MA. Randomized, double-blind placebo-controlled trial of coenzyme Q10 in chronic renal failure: discovery of a new role. J Nutr Environ Med 2000;10:281-288.

Singh RB, Niaz MA, Rastogi SS, et al. Effect of hydrosoluble coenzyme Q10 on blood pressures and insulin resistance in hypertensive patients with coronary artery disease. J Hum Hypertens 1999;13(3):203-208.

Singh RB, Wander GS, Rastogi A, et al. Randomized, double-blind placebo-controlled trial of coenzyme Q10 in patients with acute myocardial infarction. Cardiovasc Drugs Ther 1998;12(4):347-353.

Soja AM, Mortensen SA. [Treatment of chronic cardiac insufficiency with coenzyme Q10, results of meta-analysis in controlled clinical trials.] Ugeskr Laeger 1997;159(49):7302-7308.

Sunamori M, Tanaka H, Maruyama T, et al. Clinical experience of coenzyme Q10 to enhance intraoperative myocardial protection in coronary artery revascularization. Cardiovasc Drugs Ther 1991;5 Suppl 2:297-300.

Tanaka J, Tominaga R, Yoshitoshi M, et al. Coenzyme Q10: the prophylactic effect on low cardiac output following cardiac valve replacement. Ann Thorac Surg 1982;33(2):145-151.

The Huntington Study Group. A randomized, placebo-controlled trial of coenzyme Q10 and remacemide in Huntington's disease. Neurology 2001;57(3):397-404.

Tran MT, Mitchell TM, Kennedy DT, et al. Role of coenzyme Q10 in chronic heart failure, angina, and hypertension. Pharmacotherapy 2001;21(7):797-806.

Watson PS, Scalia GM, Galbraith A, et al. Lack of effect of coenzyme Q on left ventricular function in patients with congestive heart failure. J Am Coll Cardiol 1999;33(6):1549-1552.

Weston SB, Zhou S, Weatherby RP, et al. Does exogenous coenzyme Q10 affect aerobic capacity in endurance athletes? Int J Sport Nutr 1997;7(3):197-206.

Yamagami T, Takagi M, Akagami H, et al. Effect of coenzyme Q10 on essential hypertension: a double-blind controlled study. In Folkers K, Yamamura Y (eds): Biomedical and Clinical Aspects of Coenzyme Q. Amsterdam, Elsevier, 1986, pp 337-343.

Yikoski T, Piirainen J, Hanninen O, et al. The effect of coenzyme Q10 on the exercise performance of cross-country skiers. Molec Aspects Med 1997;18(Suppl):s283-s290.

Zhou M, Zhi Q, Tang Y, et al. Effects of coenzyme Q10 on myocardial protection during cardiac valve replacement and scavenging free radical activity in vitro. J Cardiovasc Surg (Torino) 1999;40(3):355-361.

Cranberry
(Vaccinium macrocarpon)

SYNONYMS/COMMON NAMES/RELATED SUBSTANCES

- American cranberry, arandano Americano, arandano trepador, bear berry, black cranberry, bog cranberry, Ericaceae, European cranberry, grosse moosebeere, isokarpalo, kranbeere, kronsbeere, large cranberry, low cranberry, marsh apple, mountain cranberry, moosebeere, mossberry, *Oxycoccus hagerupii*, *Oxycoccus microcarpus*, *Oxycoccus macrocarpus*, *Oxycoccus palustris*, *Oxycoccus quadripetalus*, pikkukarpalo, preisselbeere, ronce d'Amerique, trailing swamp cranberry, tsuru-kokemomo, *Vaccinium edule*, *Vaccinium erythrocarpum*, *Vaccinium hageruppi*, *Vaccinium microcarpum*, *Vaccinium occycoccus*, *Vaccinium plaustre*, *Vaccinium vitis*.
- **Similar Berries:** Blueberry (*Vaccinium angustifolium*), bilberry (*Vaccinium myrtilis*), bear berry (*uva ursi*), alpine cranberry (*Vaccinium vitis-idaea*).

CLINICAL BOTTOM LINE
Background

- Cranberry is widely used to prevent urinary tract infection (UTI). It was initially believed to function by acidifying urine. However, the mechanism is now thought to be inhibition of adhesion of bacteria to uroepithelial cells by proanthocyanadin, a compound present in cranberry.
- There is preliminary clinical evidence in support of the use of cranberry juice and cranberry supplements to *prevent* UTI, although most available studies are of poor methodological quality. Most evidence has focused on effects against *E. coli*, although *in vitro* research suggests activity against *Proteus*, *Pseudomonas* and other bacteria. There are no clear dosing guidelines, but given the safety of cranberry, it may be reasonable to recommend the use of moderate amounts of cranberry juice cocktail to prevent UTI in non-chronically ill individuals.
- Cranberry has not been shown effective as a *treatment* for documented UTI. Although cranberry may be a viable adjunct therapy in a time when antimicrobial resistance is of concern, given the proven efficacy of antibiotics, cranberry should not be considered a first-line agent.
- Cranberry has been investigated for numerous other medicinal uses, and promising areas of investigation include prevention of *H. pylori* infection and dental plaque.

Scientific Evidence for Common/Studied Uses	Grade*
Urinary tract infection *prophylaxis*	B
Achlorhydria and B12 absorption	C
Antioxidant	C
Antiviral and antifungal	C
Cancer prevention	C
Dental (oral) plaque	C
Helicobacter pylori gastric infection	C
Nephrolithiasis	C
Reduction of odor associated with incontinence/bladder catheterization	C
Urinary tract infection *treatment*	C
Urine acidification	C
Urostomy care	C
Chronic urinary tract infection *prophylaxis*: children with neurogenic bladder	D

*Key to grades: *A:* Strong scientific evidence for this use; *B:* Good scientific evidence for this use; *C:* Unclear scientific evidence for this use; *D:* Fair scientific evidence against this use (it may not work); *F:* Strong scientific evidence against this use (it likely does not work). For a more detailed explanation of efficacy criteria, see "Natural Standard Evidence-Based Validated Grading Rationale" in the Introduction.

Historical or Theoretical Uses That Lack Sufficient Evidence

- Anorexia, atherosclerosis,[1] blood disorders, cancer treatment, cholecystitis, diabetes,[2] diuresis, liver disorders, nephrolithiasis prevention, radiation-induced urinary symptoms,[3] scurvy, stomach ailments, urostomy site care, vomiting, wound care (poultice).

Expert Opinion and Historic Precedent

- There is an almost universal consensus among complementary medicine practitioners, and among many physicians, that cranberry is safe and effective for use in preventing urinary tract infections.
- Cranberry has also been used to treat scurvy. Although there are no studies regarding this use, cranberry is notably high in vitamin C content.

Safety Summary

- **Likely safe:** Commercially available cranberry juice products are likely safe when taken orally in amounts as high as 4 L/day in healthy individuals. Commercially available cranberry capsules are likely safe when used at recommended doses. Literature review has revealed no reported toxic events. In children (2 to 18 years old), 300 mL/day for 3 months has been tolerated, as reported in one study.[4]

DOSING/TOXICOLOGY
General

- Recommended doses are based on those most commonly used in available trials, or on historical practice. However, with natural products, the optimal doses needed to balance efficacy and safety often have not been determined. Formulations and preparation methods may vary from manufacturer to manufacturer, and from batch to batch of a specific product made by a single manufacturer. Because often the active components of a product are not known, standardization may not be possible, and the clinical effects of different brands may not be comparable.

Standardization

- There is no widely accepted standardization for cranberry juice products. In general, cranberry juice contains glucose, fructose, ascorbic acid, benzoic acid, citric acid, quinic acid, malic acid, proanthocyanidins, triterpenoids, catechins, lectins, and 90% water.
- Some cranberry preparations are standardized to 11% to 12% quinic acid per dose.

Dosing: Adult (18 Years and Older)
Oral (Prevention of Urinary Tract Infection)

- *Note:* Studied doses are for preventing, not treating urinary tract infection (UTI). There is no widely accepted dosing standard.
- **Juice:** 300 mL/day (10 oz) of commercially available cranberry cocktail (Ocean Spray) was studied in the best-designed available trial.[5,6] Recommended doses range from 90 to 480 mL (3 to 16 oz) of cranberry cocktail twice daily, or 1 to 30 mL of unsweetened 100% cranberry juice daily.
- **Capsules (encapsulated cranberry juice powder):** Many experts recommend between 1 and 6 300- to 400-mg capsules of hard gelatin concentrated cranberry juice extract, taken twice a day, with water 1 hour before meals or 2 hours after meals. Soft gelatin capsules contain vegetable oil and less of the cranberry compound.[7]
- **Concentrate:** 1.5 ounces of frozen juice concentrate twice/day has been used. Concentrate has almost 30 times the "unit strength" of juice cocktail.[8]
- **Tincture:** 4 to 5 mL of cranberry tincture can be given three times/day (anecdotal).

Oral (Prevention of Urinary Stones)

- **Juice:** 1 quart of cranberry juice cocktail daily,[9] 8 oz of cranberry juice 4 times daily for several days, then 8 oz 2 times daily.[10] Efficacy is not proven.

Other Forms

- Cranberry is available in other forms that have not been studied specifically. These include cranberry sauce (half the "unit strength" of juice cocktail); fresh/frozen cranberries (half the "unit strength" of juice cocktail); dried cranberry press cake (used as a fiber source, four times the "unit strength" of cranberry).[8]

Dosing: Pediatric (Younger Than 18 Years)

- Insufficient evidence to recommend, but has been used safely in doses of 15 mL/kg in one study. In children (2 to 18 years old), 300 mL/day of cranberry juice for 3 months was tolerated.[4] High doses may cause toxicity.[11]

Toxicology

- Cranberry juice consumed in quantities of up to 4 L/day has been shown not to be toxic in normal individuals.[12] High doses (>3L/day) may cause gastrointestinal distress and diarrhea, or toxicity in infants or young children.[11]

ADVERSE EFFECTS/PRECAUTIONS/CONTRAINDICATIONS
Allergy

- Known allergy or hypersensitivity to *Vaccinium* species (cranberries and blueberries).

Adverse Effects

- **Gastrointestinal:** Doses greater than 3 L/day may cause gastrointestinal distress and diarrhea. Some commercially available products are high in calories, although on average,

6 ounces of cranberry juice contain approximately 100 calories.
- **Renal:** Patients with a history of oxalate stones may wish to limit intake to 1 L/day, based on anecdotal/expert opinion.
- **Endocrine:** Diabetic patients should drink sugar-free cranberry juice to avoid high glycemic excursion.

Precautions/Warnings/Contraindications

- Cranberry juice should not be considered a substitute for antibiotics in cases of acute documented urinary tract infections.
- Use with caution in patients with diabetes or glucose intolerance, because of the risk of hyperglycemia. Some commercially available cranberry juice products contain large amounts of sugar. Sugar-free cranberry juice products are also available.

Pregnancy and Lactation

- Safety has not been determined in pregnancy and lactation, although cranberry juice is believed by many experts to be safe in recommended amounts based on historical use.

INTERACTIONS
Cranberry/Drug Interactions

- **Proton pump inhibitors (PPIs):** Cranberry juice has been noted to increase absorption of vitamin B_{12} in patients using proton pump inhibitors.[3]
- **Antacid drugs:** Theoretically, cranberry juice may counteract antacids, due to its acidic pH.
- **Antibiotics:** Theoretically, cranberry juice could increase the effects of antibiotics in the urinary tract.
- **Renally eliminated drugs:** Theoretically, cranberry juice could enhance the elimination of drugs excreted in the urine.
- **Warfarin (Coumadin):** A preliminary report suggests a possible interaction between cranberry and warfarin, although further data are necessary before a clear conclusion can be reached.[14]

Cranberry/Herb/Supplement Interactions

- **Renally eliminated agents:** Theoretically, cranberry juice may enhance the elimination of agents excreted in the urine.

MECHANISM OF ACTION
Pharmacology

- **UTI prophylaxis:** Cranberry was long thought to prevent urinary tract infection (UTI) by means of urinary acidification. However, it has now been demonstrated that cranberry juice inhibits bacterial adherence to uroepithelial cells by 75% for 60 of 77 *E. coli* clinical isolates *in vitro* when controlling for pH.[15-19] Uropathogenic *Escherichia coli* adhere to urinary bladder cells because they have substances that mediate adhesion on the hair-like fimbriae or pili on their surfaces. Cranberry juice contains two compounds that have been found to block *E. coli* adhesion.[20] One is fructose (present in most fruit juices). It has been found that fructose in guava, pineapple, mango, grapefruit, blueberry and cranberry juice inhibits the mannose-sensitive type-1 fimbrial adhesin in yeast aggregation assays. The second inhibitor is a high molecular weight compound called proanthocyanidin, found in cranberry and blueberry juices (genus *Ericaceae*), which acts on the mannose-resistant P fimbriae or pili expressed by uropathogenic *E. coli*.[16,21,22] *In vitro*, this inhibition is irreversible.
- **Spectrum of activity:** Although *E. coli* is the best-studied organism, *in vitro* examinations of bacterial adherence to

urinary epithelial cells have shown that pre-incubation of *Proteus, Pseudomonas,* and *E. coli* with cranberry juice cocktail results in decreased adhesion to epithelial cells.[23] This effect has been more pronounced *in vitro* than *in vivo*, and cranberry juice has not been found to eradicate the most adherent bacteria. Cranberry supplements (Cranactin tablets, 400 mg three times daily for 2 days) and ascorbic acid (500 mg twice daily for 2 days) each have decreased deposition rates and numbers of adherent *E. coli* and *Entero-coccus faecalis in vitro*, but not *Pseudomonas aeruginosa, Staphylococcus epidermidis,* or *Candida albicans.*[24] Recently, investigators used a fivefold concentrated preparation of cranberry juice adjusted to a pH of 7.0 and incubated bacterial strains in broth with cranberry and plain controls. At 24 hours, the cranberry-inoculated broth showed no growth of *E. coli, Staphylococcus aureus, Pseudomonas, Klebsiella,* and *Proteus* and decreased growth of *Enterococcus faecalis* and *Salmonella.*[25] Cranberry has not been shown to be bactericidal.

- **Urinary acidification:** With consumption of cranberry juice of up to 4 L/day, hippuric acid excretion increases, as does urine volume, leading to no changes in urine pH and minimal increases in hippuric acid concentration (to a level that is insufficient for bacteriostasis).[12] One study showed only transient decreases in urinary pH in three of four subjects.[26] A study in 40 normal subjects found urinary pH to decrease by 0.5, to a minimum of 5.4, with consumption of 250 mL of 80% cranberry juice three times daily for 12 days.[27] A limitation of this study was that the beverage contained 80% cranberry juice, as opposed to commercially available cocktails that are 25% to 33% juice. Notably, bacteriostasis has been achieved at pH levels of 5.5.

- **Constituents:** Six ounces of cranberry juice cocktail (Ocean Spray) on average contain 96 calories, 24 g of carbohydrates, 0.17 g of crude fiber, 0.02 g of benzoic acid, 0.28 g of citric acid, 0.30 g of malic acid, and 0.45 g of quinic acid.[7] In 94.5 g of fresh frozen cranberries, on average there are 35 calories, 7.8 g of carbohydrates, 2.1 g of crude fiber, 0.01 g of benzoic acid, 0.52 g of citric acid, 0.48 g of malic acid, and 0.53 g of quinic acid.[7] Cranberry powder hard gelatin capsules (6.9 g in 12 capsules, tested brand manufactured by Murdock Pharmaceuticals) contains 24 calories, 5 g of carbohydrates, 0.97 g of crude fiber, 0.001 g of benzoic acid, 0.46 g of citric acid, 0.53 g of malic acid, and 0.50 g of quinic acid.[7]

Pharmacodynamics/Kinetics

- Human studies have not adequately addressed the precise absorption, bioavailability, volume of distribution, metabolism, elimination half-life, onset of action, time to peak, or duration of activity of cranberry.

- In multiple studies of urinary acidification, urine samples were obtained 2 to 4 hours after ingestion of cranberry juice, although some trials collected 24-hour urine samples (others do not report the time of collection). One study of plasma antioxidant capacity of cranberry juice determined that plasma phenol levels peaked at 1 hour and that vitamin C concentrations plateaued at 2 hours.[28] Since neither of these are the putative active agents for preventing urinary tract infection, the influence of these findings on dosing is not clear.

HISTORY

- Native Americans traditionally used cranberries medicinally and as food. *Pemmican*, a combination of crushed cranberries, fat, and dried meat, was prepared as a meal. Cranberries were

used for prevention of kidney stones, and were believed to remove toxins from the blood. Upon arrival in North America, European settlers were introduced to the nutritional and medicinal uses of cranberries. German scientists researched the connection between cranberries and incidence of urinary tract infection in the 1840s, after noting that cranberry ingestion increased hippuric acid secretion, which is bacteriostatic in high concentration. It has subsequently been demonstrated that the acidification of urine is not antibacterial,[15] and other mechanisms have been suggested.

- In modern times, cranberry is popular as a food and is often consumed as relish, sauce, jam, juice, or dried berries.

REVIEW OF THE EVIDENCE: DISCUSSION
Chronic Urinary Tract Infection (UTI) Prophylaxis
Summary

- There is highly suggestive but not definitive evidence to support the use of cranberry for prophylaxis of urinary tract infections (UTIs). No single study convincingly demonstrates the ability of cranberry to prevent UTIs. However, the aggregation of favorable evidence combined with a plausible biological mechanism does tend to support this use, despite the poor methodological quality of nearly all available studies. Notably, many of the positive and negative studies have been sponsored by the manufacturer Ocean Spray. The effective dose and duration of treatment has not been determined. A properly randomized, double-blind, placebo-controlled trial with adequate follow-up or intention-to-treat analysis, using several doses of cranberry juice or cranberry supplement to determine effective dose, and with hard outcomes such as symptomatic UTI rather than asymptomatic bacteriuria, would assist in settling this question.

Systematic Review

- Five of the available published randomized controlled trials of cranberry for UTI were reviewed by Jepson et al.,[29] including studies by Avorn et al.,[5,6] Haverkorn and Mandigers,[30] Foda et al.,[31] Walker et al.,[32] and Schlager et al.[4] (each is discussed below in detail). Based on this evidence, the authors concluded that there is no definitive evidence to recommend cranberry juice for the prevention of UTI, given the lack of clear effect, large dropout rates, and uncertainty regarding appropriate dose. This review did not incorporate a study by Kontiokari et al.,[33] which did not adequately blind to treatment but showed a significant decrease in symptomatic UTI (discussed below). Nor did it include a well-conducted positive case-control study by Foxman et al.,[34] which suggests a role for further study of cranberry (discussed below).

Human Trials (Nursing Home Residents)

- A widely cited trial, published in the *Journal of the American Medical Association* (*JAMA*), was performed in 153 elderly female nursing home residents (mean age 78.5) with a high rate of asymptomatic bacteriuria.[5,6] This randomized, double-blind, placebo-controlled study was designed to determine the effect of regular intake of cranberry juice on bacteriuria and pyuria. Commercially available cranberry cocktail sweetened with saccharin was used along with an identically appearing placebo beverage. Subjects drank 300 mL/day of either cranberry juice or placebo for 6 months. At study completion, the treated group was found to have an odds ratio of 0.42 for bacteriuria with pyuria in relation to controls ($p = 0.004$) (no significant effect on urinary pH). Although the results are suggestive, several

Review of the Evidence: Cranberry

Condition Treated*	Study Design	Author, Year	N[†]	SS[†]	Study Quality[‡]	Magnitude of Benefit	ARR[†]	NNT[†]	Comments
Prevention of UTI	Systematic review	Jepson[29] 2000	5 studies	No	NA	None	NA	NA	Review of studies by Avorn,[5,6] Haverkorn,[30] Foda,[31] Schlager,[4] and Walker.[32]
Prevention of bacteriuria with pyuria	Randomized, controlled	Avorn[5,6] 1994	153	Yes	4	Small	13%	8	Reduced rate of asymptomatic bacteriuria and pyuria; significance unclear.
Prevention of bacteriuria	Controlled, crossover	Schlager[4] 1999	15	No	4	None	NA	NA	Study in 15 children with neurogenic bladder.
Prevention of UTI	Randomized controlled, crossover	Walker[32] 1997	10	Yes	3	Moderate	NA	NA	10 women completers, mean age 37, using cranberry capsules; UTI incidence of 6/person-year decreased to 2.4/person-year.
Prevention of UTI	Randomized controlled, single-blind	Kontiokari[33] 2001	150	Yes	2	Moderate	20%	5	Three arms included cranberry, lactobacillus, and nothing; participants were female.
Prevention of UTI	Randomized controlled, crossover	Foda[31] 1995	40	No	2	None	NA	NA	Results not statistically significant; small numbers.
Prevention of bacteriura	Randomized controlled, crossover	Haverkorn[30] 1994	7	Yes	1	Small	NA	NA	High dropout rate precludes interpretation.
Prevention of UTI	Case-control	Foxman[34] 1995	374	No	NA	Moderate	13%	8	Study of young women showed near-significant risk reduction with sporadic juice use.
Prevention of UTI	Case series	Dignam[37] 1997	538	Yes	NA	Small	NA	NA	Apparent decrease in symptomatic UTI when institutionalized elderly subjects were given cranberry.
Prevention of UTI (nursing home)	Case series	Gibson[38] 1991	28	No	NA	Unclear	NA	NA	Methodologically weak study.
Treatment of UTI	Case series	Papas[40] 1966	60	No	NA	Unclear	NA	NA	Methodologically weak study.
Urine acidification	Case series	Tsukada[56] 1994	13	No	NA	None	NA	NA	Methodologically weak study.

*Primary or secondary outcome.
[†] N, Number of patients; SS, statistically significant; ARR, absolute risk reduction; NNT, the number of patients who need to undergo a specific intervention in order to observe an outcome in one individual.
[‡] 0-2 = poor; 3-4 = good; 5 = excellent.
NA, Not applicable. UTI, urinary tract infection.
For an explanation of each category in this table, please see Table 3 in the Introduction.

problems with this study limit the utility of its results: The placebo group experienced twice as many urinary tract infections by history (33% vs. 17%), and was treated with antibiotics twice as often after randomization (16% vs. 8%). One fifth of specimens contained mixed flora, suggesting the absence of a UTI (or inadequate collection). Eighty-three percent of subjects in the treatment group completed the study, vs. 75% of controls. The study was sponsored by the manufacturer of Ocean Spray, which may have biased results. The clinical significance of asymptomatic pyuria and bacteriuria determined by non-catheterized specimens in elderly women is unclear. Even if the outcomes measures are considered reliable, the study has limited generalizability to younger populations: E. coli was isolated from only 43% of specimens, compared with 80% incidence in younger women. Since cranberry juice likely exerts its strongest effect on E. coli, different populations may benefit to different

degrees. The conclusions of this study have also been questioned because of the uncertainty of clean urine specimens[35] and because of lack of equivalency of the groups with regard to history of previous urinary tract infections.[36]

- In a poorly designed study, the rate of symptomatic UTIs was followed in a 538-bed nursing home when subjects were given cranberry capsules (6/day of Azo-cranberry) or 4 oz of cranberry juice daily.[37] There was no concurrent placebo control. The authors found that the rate in their study was 20.7 per month compared to 27.7 per month in historical controls. Problems of this study include the lack of randomization, lack of data regarding the number of patients in the treatment group and historical control group, and the absence of a case definition of UTI.
- In a poorly described study of 28 nursing home patients with a history of recurrent UTI, subjects were given 4 to 6 oz of cranberry juice/day for 7 weeks.[38] Notably, 19 had

no further urinary tract infections during the 7-week follow-up period, although it is not clear what the rate would have been in the absence of cranberry juice. These results are of limited clinical utility. Similarly, in a nursing home population, 4 to 6 oz/day of cranberry juice was reported to significantly prevent UTIs, although details are limited.[38]

- A 6-month study by Fleet suggests that bacterial infections (bacteriuria) and associated influx of white blood cells into the urine (pyuria) can be reduced by nearly 50% in elderly women who drink 300 mL of cranberry juice cocktail/day.[39] Along with earlier reports on the ability of cranberry juice to inhibit bacterial adherence to urinary epithelial cells in cell culture, this work suggests that drinking cranberry juice each day may be clinically useful.

Human Trials (Healthy Women)

- Haverkorn and Mandigers studied 38 normal women in a randomized, crossover study, in which 15 mL of cranberry juice twice/day was given vs. water (control) for 1 month, and then the reverse treatment was administered the following month.[30] Twenty-one did not complete the study (55%), and 3 patients with constant bacteriuria and 7 without any bacteriuria were excluded from analysis (not intention-to-treat). Of the 7 patients analyzed, the authors reported "fewer occurrences of bacteriuria during the period when cranberry juice was being taken." Given the small numbers, high dropout rate, and lack of specific data, the significance of these findings is unclear.

- A well-conducted examination of this topic was a case-control study of sexually active college women, designed to determine the risk of various exposures on first-time urinary tract infection.[34] In the 374 subjects, 86 cases of UTI were diagnosed, of which 86% were caused by *E. coli*. After adjusting for frequency of vaginal intercourse, which was a significant risk factor for UTI, they found that "habitual cranberry juice use" had an odds ratio for UTI of 0.48 with 95% confidence intervals slightly crossing 1 (0.19 to 1.02). These data suggest that individuals with a high rate of *E. coli* infection are most likely to benefit from cranberry. "Habitual cranberry juice use" was not clearly defined and was not monitored and is unlikely to have been daily. However, this would bias results against statistical significance, rather than in favor of positive results. Further study of regular use is warranted.

- One letter describes a randomized, double-blind, crossover trial among healthy women using cranberry capsules containing 400 mg of cranberry solids and an identical placebo capsule given daily, each for 3 months.[32] Unfortunately, only ten subjects completed the study. Six UTIs in total occurred during the cranberry months, and 15 occurred during the placebo months. The authors did not note whether few or many subjects were responsible for the majority of infections. Although the study was described as being well designed, the investigators do not provide their data, making it difficult to evaluate their calculation of effect. The authors did note $p < 0.05$ for reducing the incidence of UTI.

- A well-designed study of a cranberry-lingonberry combination[33] was not included in Jepson's Cochrane review.[29] This trial, conducted in Finland, randomized (method not described) 150 women with *E. coli* UTI into three groups: 50 mL of cranberry-lingonberry juice concentrate (7.5 g of cranberry concentrate and 1.5 g of lingonberry concentrate) daily for 6 months; 100 mL of *Lactobacillus* GG drink

(4×10^{10} CFU/100 mL) 5 days per week for 1 year; or an open control. When patients developed symptoms, their urine was cultured, and 100,000 CFU was the criterion for infection. Women taking antimicrobial prophylaxis were excluded. The groups were well matched for age (mean age 30), frequency of intercourse, use of birth control, history of UTI, proportion of *E. coli* UTI (80%), and daily fluid intake. Over the first 6 months of the study, 8 women in the cranberry-lingonberry group, 19 in the lactobacillus group, and 18 in the control group developed at least one UTI. An absolute risk reduction of 20% in the treatment group at 6 months was sustained at 1 year. This study demonstrated the benefits of a cranberry-lingonberry juice combination in preventing UTI. Problems include lack of blinding to treatment, use of a combination product, which makes evaluation of cranberry's individual effect impossible, and the curious fact that the effect was sustained over 12 months when the treatment was only given for 6 months (unclear if baseline differences existed between groups, long-term protection was mediated, or cranberry-lingonberry juice subjects elected to continue ingesting juice by choice).

Pediatrics

- In a 6-month trial, Foda et al. treated 40 pediatric neuropathic bladder patients, mean age 9 years, with 15 mL/kg of 30% cranberry cocktail, divided into 3 or 4 doses vs. water (control).[31] Subjects then crossed over to the opposite treatment. Specimens were obtained by clean catheterization. Patients who were previously on antibiotic prophylaxis remained on that treatment. Twenty-one patients completed the study (52%), including 12 that remained on prophylactic antibiotics. Monthly cultures and symptoms were recorded. No significant difference between groups was found. Thirty percent dropped out due to taste, cost, or caloric content of the cranberry juice. Strengths of this study include clean catheterization of specimens and strict definition of infection. Weaknesses include poor generalizability, lack of intention-to-treat analysis, and small numbers.

Urinary Tract Infection (UTI) Treatment
Summary

- Literature review reveals no reliable evidence to support the use of cranberry in the treatment of documented urinary tract infection (UTI). One reason for this may be that cranberry fails to eradicate the most adherent bacteria *in vitro*.[23] Without explicit study in this area, a recommendation cannot be made.

- In a poorly described 1962 study of 60 patients (44 female, 16 male) with acute UTI, subjects received 480 mL (16 oz) of cranberry juice for 21 days.[40] Half were noted to experience a positive clinical response, and an additional 20% had moderate improvement. Six weeks after the juice was discontinued, 27 patients had persistent or recurrent infection (asymptomatic in 8), and 17 patients had negative urine cultures. These results can only be considered preliminary.

- In a 1962 brief report, 6 oz of cranberry juice twice/day was reported to improve chronic pyelonephritis in a 66-year-old woman.[41] The author noted personal clinical experience in which this dose of cranberry juice relieved symptoms of UTI in multiple patients.

- Nahata et al. conducted a randomized, controlled, crossover trial of 27 subjects with bacteriuria, comparing methenamine madelate alone, ascorbic acid, and ascorbic acid plus cranberry juice.[42,43] Each patient was randomized to 5 days of each therapy. However, the primary purpose of the study was to access the effect of methenamine on formaldehyde concentrations and had no outcomes specific to UTI treatment with cranberry juice.

Antiviral and Antifungal
Summary

- Literature review reveals no human studies to support the use of cranberry as an antiviral or antifungal agent.

Evidence

- In a study of the ability of 19 juices to inactivate poliovirus type 1 *in vitro*, less than 1% of the virus survived after incubation with cranberry juice for 2 hours at pH 7.0. The clinical significance of this finding is unclear.[44]
- Cranberry juice at 40% concentration inhibits the growth *in vitro* of *Microsporum* spp., some *Trichophyton* spp., and one *Epidermophyton* spp.[45] *Candida albicans* growth has not been inhibited. The clinical significance of these findings is unclear.

Antioxidant
Summary

- Cranberry may possess antioxidant properties *in vitro*, but no studies with hard clinical outcomes have been published to support a benefit of cranberry as an antioxidant in humans. Antioxidant properties may be due to ascorbic acid present in cranberry, although further study is warranted.

Evidence

- Nine healthy female volunteers consumed 500 mL of cranberry juice and blueberry juice.[28] After 60 to 120 minutes, a functional assay of antioxidant capacity of the plasma revealed a significant increase after ingestion of cranberry but not blueberry juice. This effect was attributed to an increase in ascorbic acid, which cranberry juice contains but blueberry juice does not. The clinical significance of this finding is unclear.
- *In vitro*, polyphenolic compounds from cranberry have been found to possess antioxidant properties,[46] and LDL oxidation appears to be inhibited by cranberry extracts,[47] although clinical effect has not been studied.

Dental (Oral) Plaque
Summary

- Based on results of *in vitro* research, Weiss et al. suggest that reducing the bacterial flora of dental plaque with cranberry may decrease gingival irritation and periodontal disease.[48] However, there are no available clinical data to support this. The authors note that commercially available cranberry juice with its high fructose and dextrose content may not be suitable for this purpose, because of the known ability of those substances to *cause* plaque accumulation.

Nephrolithiasis
Summary

- Although cranberry consumption may increase urinary excretion of oxalate, possibly predisposing to calcium oxalate stone formation, it also increases magnesium and potassium excretion, which can decrease the rate of stone formation.[49,50] Cranberry juice of unspecified amounts has been found to decrease urinary calcium by 50% in patients with renal stones.[51] The clinical significance and net outcome of these findings in various subgroups has not been elucidated.

Cancer Prevention
Summary

- Although cranberry's potential antioxidant properties are supported by preliminary pre-clinical data, the use of cranberry for cancer prevention (other than as part of a healthy diet) requires further study.

Evidence

- One study assayed four *Vaccinium* species (lowbush blueberry, bilberry, cranberry, lingonberry) for anticarcinogenic activity. *In vitro*, the proanthocyanidin fraction inhibited a tumor promoter enzyme.[52] Further investigation is required before a conclusion can be drawn.

Achlorhydria and B₁₂ Absorption

Achlorhydria and B_{12} Absorption
Summary

- Cranberry juice consumption promotes vitamin B_{12} absorption in elderly patients taking proton pump inhibitors, but this effect appears to be related to the acidity of the juice rather than the cranberry itself.

Evidence

- In a study of elderly patients taking omeprazole, ingestion of protein-bound vitamin B_{12} along with cranberry juice (120 mL with a pH to 2.5-2.6, unspecified brand and concentration) doubled absorption of vitamin B_{12}, but ingestion with 0.1 N hydrochloric acid (pH 1.2) increased vitamin B_{12} absorption by a factor of 8.[13] The study showed that ingestion of an acidic drink improved protein-bound vitamin B_{12} absorption in patients taking proton pump inhibitors. The specific contribution of cranberry as opposed to other acidic drinks is not clear.

Helicobacter Pylori Gastric Infection
Summary

- *In vitro*, cranberry inhibits adhesion of *H. pylori* to gastric mucus. Literature search reveals no reliable human clinical data.

Evidence

- A research group that demonstrated the anti-adhesin properties of cranberry in *E. coli* turned its attention to *Helicobacter pylori*, the bacteria associated with peptic ulcer disease and gastric cancer.[53] A high-molecular-weight compound in cranberry juice that irreversibly inhibits the P fimbriae of *E. coli* was incubated with three strains of *H. pylori*. *In vitro*, this compound inhibited the sialic acid–specific adhesion of *H. pylori* to human gastric mucus and to human erythrocytes. The authors suggest that consumption of cranberry may find a therapeutic use in prevention or treatment of *H. pylori* infection, but this has yet to be studied *in vivo*.

Urine Acidification
Summary

- In large quantities, cranberry juice may lower urine pH, although the clinical significance is not clear. Contrary to prior opinion, urine acidification does not appear to be the mechanism of action by which cranberry prevents urinary tract infections.

Evidence

- In early case series, adults who consumed large amounts of cranberries were noted to have acidic urine.[54] In normal subjects in one study, drinking cranberry juice with meals significantly reduced urinary pH for several hours after meals.[27] Urinary acidification effects appear to be transient,[26] and patients would need to drink a quart or more (1500 mL) of cranberry juice daily to cause a significant long-term impact on urinary acidity.[55]
- In 13 patients with urostomies, 160 to 320 mL of cranberry juice/day for 6 months did not significantly alter urine pH.[56]

Urostomy Care
Summary

- It has been proposed that skin irritation at urostomy sites is related to alkaline pH. Therefore, cranberry juice, purported to lower urine pH, has been suggested as a possible therapy for this indication.[57] However, cranberry juice does not clearly significantly lower urine pH. Although preliminary evidence from one case series suggests possible improvement of skin irritation at urostomy sites, the mechanism of action is not clear. Increased volume of urine may be causative.

Evidence

- In a case series of 13 urostomy patients, 160 to 320 mL of cranberry juice was administered daily for 6 months.[56] Four of six patients with peristomal skin irritation noted significant improvement, although urine pH was unchanged. No other patients developed peristomal skin problems during treatment with cranberry. Without controls, the clinical relevance of these results is unclear.

Reduction of Odor Associated with Incontinence/Bladder Catheterization
Summary

- There is preliminary evidence that cranberry juice may reduce urine odor associated with incontinence or intermittent bladder catheterization. Without objective outcomes or controlled trial evidence, the results can only be considered preliminary. Nonetheless, given the low toxicity of cranberry juice, incontinent or catheterized patients may choose to try cranberry for this purpose.

Evidence

- In a case series of incontinent adults, and studies of children who require intermittent catheterization, there have been significant subjective reductions in urinary odors in those given daily cranberry juice.[57,58] It has been suggested that this effect is secondary to reductions in rates of subclinical cystitis, although data are scant in this area.

Chronic Urinary Tract Infection (UTI) Prophylaxis: Children with Neurogenic Bladder
Summary

- There is preliminary evidence that cranberry is not effective as urinary tract infection (UTI) prophylaxis for children with neurogenic bladder.

Evidence

- Schlager et al. studied 15 children (ages 2-18) with neurogenic bladder, receiving clean intermittent catheterization.[4] Subjects were given cranberry juice concentrate equivalent to 300 mL of cranberry juice cocktail or identical placebo

for 3 months, and then crossed over. Rates of bacteriuria were equal (75% in both groups), and rates of UTI were also similar. *E. coli* constituted 48% of isolates from the placebo group and 43% of isolates from the cranberry group. This study suggests that cranberry has little role in the prevention of bacteriuria and UTI in this population. However, this trial may not have been adequately powered to detect significant effect.

FORMULARY: BRANDS USED IN CLINICAL TRIALS/ THIRD-PARTY TESTING
Brands Used in Statistically Significant Clinical Trials

- Ocean Spray cranberry juice cocktail (sponsor of multiple trials).
- Many studies do not list the brand of juice or capsule used.

Brands Shown to Contain Claimed Ingredients Through Third-Party Testing

- **Capsules:** Nature's Resource (405 mg of standardized cranberry juice extract/capsule); Spring Valley (475 mg of cranberry fruit/capsule); Cranberry Fruit Sundown Herbals (425 mg of cranberry fruit/capsule); Celestial Seasonings Cranberry (400 mg of cranberry extract standardized to >35% organic acid).
- **Juice:** Ocean Spray Cranberry Juice Cocktail: 27% cranberry juice, water, high fructose corn syrup, cranberry juice concentrate, ascorbic acid.

References

1. Reed J. Cranberry flavonoids, atherosclerosis and cardiovascular health. Crit Rev Food Sci Nutr 2002;42(3 Suppl):301-316.
2. Chambers BK, Camire ME. Can cranberry supplementation benefit adults with type 2 diabetes? Diabetes Care 2003;26(9):2695-2696.
3. Campbell G, Pickles T, D'yachkova Y. A randomised trial of cranberry versus apple juice in the management of urinary symptoms during external beam radiation therapy for prostate cancer. Clin Oncol (R Coll Radiol) 2003;15(6):322-328.
4. Schlager TA, Anderson S, Trudell J, et al. Effect of cranberry juice on bacteriuria in children with neurogenic bladder receiving intermittent catheterization. J Pediatr 1999;135(6):698-702.
5. Avorn J, Monane M, Gurwitz JH, et al. Reduction of bacteriuria and pyuria after ingestion of cranberry juice. JAMA 1994;271(10):751-754.
6. Avorn J, Monane M, Gurwitz J, et al. Reduction of bacteriuria and pyuria using cranberry juice. JAMA 1994;272(8):588-590.
7. Hughes BG, Lawson LD. Nutritional content of cranberry products. Am J Hosp Pharm 1989;46(6):1129.
8. Siciliano AA. Cranberry. Herbalgram 1996;38:51-54.
9. Zinsser HH, Seneca H, Light I, et al. Management of infected stones with acidifying agents. N Y State J Med 1968;68:3001-3009.
10. Sternlieb P. Cranberry juice in renal disease [letter]. New Engl J Med 1963;268(1):57.
11. Garcia-Calatayud S, Larreina Cordoba JJ, Lozano De La Torre MJ. [Severe cranberry juice poisoning]. An Esp Pediatr 2002;56(1):72-73.
12. Bodel P, Cotran R, Kass E. Cranberry juice and the antibacterial action of hippuric acid. J Lab Clin Med 1959;54(6):881-888.
13. Saltzman JR, Kemp JA, Golner BB, et al. Effect of hypochlorhydria due to omeprazole treatment or atrophic gastritis on protein-bound vitamin B$_{12}$ absorption. J Am Coll Nutr 1994;13(6):584-591.
14. Suvarna R, Pirmohamed M, Henderson L. Possible interaction between warfarin and cranberry juice. BMJ 2003;327(7429):1454.
15. Sobota AE. Inhibition of bacterial adherence by cranberry juice: potential use for the treatment of urinary tract infections. J Urol 1984;131(5):1013-1016.
16. Howell AB, Vorsa N, Der MA, et al. Inhibition of the adherence of P-fimbriated Escherichia coli to uroepithelial-cell surfaces by proanthocyanidin extracts from cranberries. N Engl J Med 1998;339(15):1085-1086.
17. Howell AB, Foxman B. Cranberry juice and adhesion of antibiotic-resistant uropathogens. JAMA 2002;287(23):3082-3083.
18. Ahuja S, Kaack B, Roberts J. Loss of fimbrial adhesion with the addition of Vaccinum macrocarpon to the growth medium of P-fimbriated Escherichia coli. J Urol 1998;159(2):559-562.
19. Allison DG, Cronin MA, Hawker J, et al. Influence of cranberry juice on attachment of Escherichia coli to glass. J Basic Microbiol 2000;40(1):3-6.

20. Zafriri D, Ofek I, Adar R, et al. Inhibitory activity of cranberry juice on adherence of type 1 and type P fimbriated *Escherichia coli* to eucaryotic cells. Antimicrob Agents Chemother 1989;33(1):92-98.
21. Ofek I, Goldhar J, Zafriri D, et al. Anti-*Escherichia coli* adhesin activity of cranberry and blueberry juices. N Engl J Med 1991;324(22):1599.
22. Ofek I, Goldhar J, Sharon N. Anti-*Escherichia coli* adhesin activity of cranberry and blueberry juices. Adv Exp Med Biol 1996;408:179-183.
23. Schmidt DR, Sobota AE. An examination of the anti-adherence activity of cranberry juice on urinary and nonurinary bacterial isolates. Microbios 1988;55(224-225):173-181.
24. Habash MB, Van der Mei HC, Busscher HJ, et al. The effect of water, ascorbic acid, and cranberry derived supplementation on human urine and uropathogen adhesion to silicone rubber. Can J Microbiol 1999; 45(8):691-694.
25. Lee YL, Owens J, Thrupp L, et al. Does cranberry juice have antibacterial activity? JAMA 2000;283(13):1691.
26. Kahn HD, Panariello VA, Saeli J, et al. Effect of cranberry juice on urine. J Am Diet Assoc 1967;51(3):251-254.
27. Kinney AB, Blount M. Effect of cranberry juice on urinary pH. Nurs Res 1979;28(5):287-290.
28. Pedersen CB, Kyle J, Jenkinson AM, et al. Effects of blueberry and cranberry juice consumption on the plasma antioxidant capacity of healthy female volunteers. Eur J Clin Nutr 2000;54(5):405-408.
29. Jepson RG, Mihaljevic L, Craig J. Cranberries for preventing urinary tract infections. Cochrane Database Syst Rev 2000;(2):CD001321.
30. Haverkorn MJ, Mandigers J. Reduction of bacteriuria and pyuria using cranberry juice. JAMA 1994;272(8):590.
31. Foda M, Middlebrook PF, Gatfield CT, et al. Efficacy of cranberry in prevention of urinary tract infection in a susceptible pediatric population. Canadian J Urology 1995;2(1):98-102.
32. Walker EB, Barney DP, Mickelsen JN, et al. Cranberry concentrate: UTI prophylaxis. J Fam Pract 1997;45(2):167-168.
33. Kontiokari T, Sundqvist K, Nuutinen M, et al. Randomised trial of cranberry-lingonberry juice and *Lactobacillus* GG drink for the prevention of urinary tract infections in women. BMJ 2001;322(7302):1571-1573.
34. Foxman B, Geiger AM, Palin K, et al. First-time urinary tract infection and sexual behavior. Epidemiology 1995;6(2):162-168.
35. Goodfriend R. Reduction of bacteriuria and pyuria using cranberry juice. JAMA 1994;272(8):588-590.
36. Hopkins WJ, Heisey DM, Jonler M, et al. Reduction of bacteriuria and pyuria using cranberry juice. JAMA 1994;272(8):588-589.
37. Dignam R, Ahmed M, Denman S, et al. The effect of cranberry juice on UTI rates in a long-term care facility. J Amer Geriat Soc 1997;45(9):S53.
38. Gibson L, Pike L, Kilbourne J. Effectiveness of cranberry juice in preventing urinary tract infections in long-term care facility patients. J Naturopath Med 1991;2(1):45-47.
39. Fleet JC. New support for a folk remedy: cranberry juice reduces bacteriuria and pyuria in elderly women. Nutr Rev 1994;52(5):168-170.
40. Papas PN, Brusch CA, Ceresia GC. Cranberry juice in the treatment of urinary tract infections. Southwest Med 1966;47(1):17-20.
41. Moen DV. Observations on the effectiveness of cranberry juice in urinary infections. Wisconsin Med J 1962;61:282-283.
42. Nahata MC, Cummins BA, McLeod DC, et al. Predictability of methenamine efficacy based on type of urinary pathogen and pH. J Am Geriatr Soc 1981;29(5):236-239.
43. Nahata MC, Cummins BA, McLeod DC, et al. Effect of urinary acidifiers on formaldehyde concentration and efficacy with methenamine therapy. Eur J Clin Pharmacol 1982;22(3):281-284.
44. Konowalchuk J, Speirs JI. Antiviral effect of commercial juices and beverages. Appl Environ Microbiol 1978;35(6):1219-1220.
45. Swartz JH, Medrek TF. Antifungal properties of cranberry juice. Appl Microbiol 1968;16(10):1524-1527.
46. Yan X, Murphy BT, Hammond GB, et al. Antioxidant activities and anti-tumor screening of extracts from cranberry fruit (*Vaccinium macrocarpon*). J Agric Food Chem 2002;50(21):5844-5849.
47. Wilson T, Porcari JP, Harbin D. Cranberry extract inhibits low density lipoprotein oxidation. Life Sci 1998;62(24):L381-L386.
48. Weiss EI, Lev-Dor R, Kashamn Y, et al. Inhibiting interspecies coaggregation of plaque bacteria with a cranberry juice constituent [published errata appear in J Am Dent Assoc 1999 Jan;130(1):36 and 1999 Mar;130(3):332]. J Am Dent Assoc 1998;129(12):1719-1723.
49. Terris MK, Issa MM, Tacker JR. Dietary supplementation with cranberry concentrate tablets may increase the risk of nephrolithiasis. Urology 2001; 57(1):26-29.
50. McHarg T, Rodgers A, Charlton K. Influence of cranberry juice on the urinary risk factors for calcium oxalate kidney stone formation. BJU Int 2003;92(7):765-768.
51. Light I, Gursel E, Zinnser HH. Urinary ionized calcium in urolithiasis. Effect of cranberry juice. Urology 1973;1(1):67-70.
52. Bomser J, Madhavi DL, Singletary K, et al. *In vitro* anticancer activity of fruit extracts from Vaccinium species. Planta Med 1996;62(3):212-216.
53. Burger O, Ofek I, Tabak M, et al. A high molecular mass constituent of cranberry juice inhibits Helicobacter pylori adhesion to human gastric mucus. FEMS Immunol Med Microbiol 2000;29(4):295-301.
54. Blatherwick NR, Long ML. Studies of urinary acidity II: The increased acidity produced by eating prunes and cranberries. J Biol Chem 1923; 57:815.
55. Leaver RB. Cranberry juice. Prof Nurse 1996;11(8):525-526.
56. Tsukada K, Tokunaga K, Iwama T, et al. Cranberry juice and its impact on peri-stomal skin conditions for urostomy patients. Ostomy Wound Manage 1994;40(9):60-68.
57. Walsh BA. Urostomy and urinary pH. J ET Nurs 1992;19(4):110-113.
58. DuGan C, Cardaciotto P. Reduction of ammoniacal urinary odors by the sustained feeding of cranberry juice. J Psych Nurs 1966;4:467-470.

Creatine

SYNONYMS/COMMON NAMES/RELATED SUBSTANCES

- N-amidinosarcosine, N-(aminoiminomethyl)-N methyl glycine, Athletic Series Creatine, beta-GPA, Challenge Creatine Monohydrate, Creapure, Creatine Booster, creatine citrate, creatine monohydrate powder, creatine phosphate, Creatine Powder Drink Mix, Creatine Xtreme Lemonade, Creatine Xtreme Punch, Creavescent, cyclocreatine, EAS Phospagen HP, Hardcore Formula Creatine Powder, HPCE pure creatine monohydrate, methyl guanidine–acetic acid, Neoton, Performance Enhancer Creatine Fuel, Phosphagen, Power Creatine, Total Creatine Transport.
- **Selected combination products that contain creatine:** Creatine Xtreme Punch (6 g creatine monohydrate, 1000 mg taurine, 500 mg L-glutamine, 500 mg L-glutamicacid, 200 mg hydroxycitrate, 15 mg vanadyl nicotinate, 120 g chromium); Met-Rx Anabolic Drive Series (12.4 g micronized creatine, 400 mg alpha-lipoic acid, 10 g glutamine peptide); Muscle Link/Effervescent Creatine Elite (5 g 99.5% pure creatine monohydrate, 20 g dextrose); Optimum Nutrition Creatine Liquid Energy Tropical Punch (6 g 99% pure pharmaceutical grade creatine monohydrate, 500 mg methylsulfonylmethane); Phosphagain (64 g daily carbohydrate, 67 g daily protein, 5 g daily fat, 20 g daily creatine, yeast-derived RNA, taurine).

CLINICAL BOTTOM LINE
Background

- Creatine is naturally synthesized in the human body from amino acids, primarily in the kidney and liver, and transported in the blood to the muscles. Approximately 95% of the body's total creatine content is located in skeletal muscle. Creatine is found in meat and fish; on average, most adults in the United States consume 1-2 g of creatine daily from dietary sources.
- Creatine was discovered in the 1800s as an organic constituent of meat. In the 1970s, Soviet scientists reported that oral creatine supplements improved athletic performance during brief, intense activities such as sprints. Creatine gained popularity in the 1990s as a "natural" way to enhance athletic performance and build lean body mass. It was reported that skeletal muscle total creatine content increased with oral creatine supplementation, although response was variable. Factors that may account for this variation are carbohydrate intake, physical activity, training status, and muscle fiber type. The finding that carbohydrate enhanced muscle creatine uptake increased the market for creatine multi-ingredient sports drinks.
- Annual consumption of creatine products is estimated to exceed four million kilograms. The use of creatine is especially popular among adolescent athletes, who are reported to take doses that are not consistent with scientific evidence and that frequently exceed recommended loading and maintenance doses.
- Published reports suggest that approximately 25% of professional baseball players and up to 50% of professional football players consume creatine supplements. According to a survey of high school athletes, creatine use is common among football players, wrestlers, hockey players, gymnasts, and lacrosse players. In 1998, the creatine market in the United States. was estimated at $200 million. Most athletic associations (including the International Olympic Committee, the International Amateur Athletic Federation, and the National Collegiate Athletic Association) have not banned this supplement.
- Creatinine excreted in urine is derived from creatine stored in muscle.

Uses Based on Scientific Evidence	Grade*
Congestive heart failure (chronic) It has been reported that cardiac creatine levels lowered in people with chronic heart failure. Several studies reported that creatine supplementation was associated with improved heart muscle strength and endurance in patients with heart failure. However, standards for a safe and effective dose have not been established. Creatine supplementation has also been reported to increase creatine levels in skeletal muscle in these patients, helping to increase strength and endurance. Comparisons with drugs used to treat heart failure have not been conducted. People who have symptoms of heart failure should consult a qualified healthcare provider.	C
Enhanced athletic endurance It has been suggested that creatine may help improve athletic endurance by increasing time to fatigue (possibly by shortening muscle recovery periods). However, the results of research evaluating this claim are mixed. Findings from different studies disagree with each other, and most studies do not support the use of creatine to enhance sustained aerobic activities.	C
Enhanced athletic sprinting Creatine has been suggested to enhance athletic performance and to delay onset of fatigue during short sprints. Effects have been attributed to increased creatine concentrations in muscle. Although results from different studies disagree with each other, most research reports some improvement when creatine is used as a supplement. Creatine may enhance performance when used during brief bursts of aerobic activities and when there are short recovery times between bouts of activity. Better research is necessary before a firm conclusion can be reached.	C
Enhanced muscle mass/strength Multiple studies suggest that creatine may improve muscle mass and strength in men and women, particularly when accompanied by increased physical activity. However, studies of creatine in athletes have disagreed with each other. Although many experts believe that creatine may be useful for high-intensity, short-duration exercise, it has not been demonstrated effective in endurance sports. Benefit may be greatest	C

Continued

when levels of creatine before supplementation are low, and in specific sub-populations such as older men. Of the approximately 300 studies that have evaluated the potential ergogenic value of creatine supplementation, about 70% report statistically significant results while the remaining studies generally report non-significant gains in performance. Because of methodological problems with available studies, a firm conclusion cannot be reached.

GAMT deficiency   C
Some individuals are born with a genetic disorder in which there is a deficiency of the enzyme guanidinoacetate methyltransferase (GAMT). A lack of this enzyme causes severe developmental delays and abnormal movement disorders. The condition is diagnosed by a lack of creatine in the brain. Although there is only limited research in this area, significant improvements were noted in two individuals who were given supplemental creatine, suggesting that this supplement may be an effective treatment for disorders caused by a lack of creatine.

Heart muscle protection during heart surgery   C
There is early evidence that heart muscle may recover better and more rapidly after open-heart surgery if intravenous creatinine is administered during the operation. Further study is needed before a recommendation can be made.

High cholesterol   C
There is limited research in this area, and results from different studies disagree with each other (with some trials noting reductions in total cholesterol and triglyceride levels). It remains unclear what effect creatine has on lipids. Additional studies are needed before a clear conclusion can be drawn.

Hyperornithinemia (high levels of ornithine in the blood)   C
Ornithine is a by-product formed in the liver. Some persons are born with a genetic disorder that prevents the breakdown of ornithine, resulting in excessively high levels of ornithine in the blood. This imbalance can result in muscle weakness, reduced storage of creatine in the muscles and brain, and blindness. Although research in this area is limited, early evidence suggests that long-term, daily creatine supplements may replace the deficient creatine and may slow vision loss.

McArdle's disease   C
McArdle's disease is characterized by a deficiency of energy compounds stored in muscle, resulting in muscle fatigue, exercise intolerance, and pain when exercising. Creatine has been proposed as a possible therapy for this condition. However, research in this area has been limited, and the results of existing studies disagree. It is unclear whether creatine offers any benefits to patients with McArdle's disease.

Muscular dystrophy   C
Creatine loss is suspected to cause muscle weakness and breakdown in Duchenne muscular dystrophy. Studies in animals report increased muscle formation

and survival with creatine. Studies in humans have been small, although early evidence suggests that creatine may be beneficial in treating muscular dystrophies. Further research is needed.

Myocardial infarction (heart attack)   C
There is early evidence that intravenous creatine following a heart attack may be beneficial to heart muscle function and may prevent ventricular arrhythmias. Further study is needed before a recommendation can be made in this area.
It has been reported that use of creatine phosphate may have a favorable effect on mental deterioration in "cardio-cerebral syndrome" following heart attacks in the elderly.

Neuromuscular disorders   C
Numerous studies suggest that creatine may be helpful in the treatment of various neuromuscular diseases, such as amyotrophic lateral sclerosis (ALS) and myasthenia gravis, and may delay onset of symptoms when used as an adjunct to conventional treatment. However, creatine ingestion does not appear to have a significant effect on muscle creatine stores or high-intensity exercise capacity in individuals with multiple sclerosis.
Although early studies were encouraging, recent research reports no beneficial effects on survival or disease progression. Additional studies are needed to provide clearer answers.

*Key to grades: A: Strong scientific evidence for this use; B: Good scientific evidence for this use; C: Unclear scientific evidence for this use; D: Fair scientific evidence against this use (it may not work); F: Strong scientific evidence against this use (it likely does not work). For a more detailed explanation of efficacy criteria, see "Natural Standard Evidence-Based Validated Grading Rationale" in the Introduction.

Historical or Theoretical Indications That Lack Sufficient Evidence

Alzheimer's disease, anti-arrhythmic, anti-convulsant, anti-inflammatory, antioxidant, arginine:glycine amidinotransferase (AGAT) deficiency, breast cancer, cervical cancer, circadian clock acceleration, colon cancer, diabetes and diabetic complications, disuse muscle atrophy, fibromyalgia, growth stimulation, herpes, , Huntington's disease, hyperhomocysteinemia, hypoxic seizures, mitochondrial diseases, neuroprotection, Parkinson's disease, rheumatoid arthritis, wasting of brain regions.

DOSING/TOXICOLOGY
The following doses are based on scientific research, publications, traditional use, or expert opinion. Many herbs and supplements have not been thoroughly tested, and their safety and effectiveness may not be proven. Brands may be made differently, with variable ingredients even within the same brand. The doses shown may not apply to all products. It is important to always read product labels and discuss doses with a qualified healthcare provider before therapy is started.

Standardization
- Standardization involves measuring the amounts of certain chemicals in products to try to make different preparations similar to each other. It is not always known if the chemicals

being measured are the "active" ingredients. Products contain different forms of creatine (e.g., creatine monohydrate, creatine monophosphate) in varying concentrations and may be combined with other supplements. There are no standard doses of creatine, and many different doses are used.

Adults (18 Years and Older)

- *Note*: Creatine appears to be absorbed best as a solution, although it is also readily absorbed when natural sources such as meat and fish are ingested. Elevation of muscle creatine levels may best be achieved by taking creatine with carbohydrates. Experts often recommend maintaining good hydration during creatine use.
- **Oral (powder):** A wide range of dosing has been used or studied. To enhance athletic performance, 9 to 20 g daily in divided doses for 4 to 7 days has been used, with maintenance doses of 2 to 5 g, or 0.3 mg per kilogram of body weight, daily. For cholesterol reduction, 20 to 25 g daily for 5 days, followed by 5 to 10 g thereafter, has been used. To treat hyperornithinemia, 1.5 g daily has been used. For neuromuscular diseases, including muscular dystrophy, 10 g daily has been suggested, although lower doses (5 g) and higher doses (20 g) have also been used. A dose of 400 to 670 mg per kilogram of body weight daily has been used to treat GAMT deficiency. For congestive heart failure, 20 g per day has been studied. For symptomatic therapy of ALS, 20 g daily for 7 days, and then 3 g daily for 3 to 6 months has been used. A dose of 150 mg per kilogram of body weight has been used daily for 5 days, followed by 60 mg per kilogram daily for 5 weeks, for McArdle's disease.
- **Intravenous/intramuscular (IV/IM):** Numerous dosing regimens have been used in studies in humans. IV/IM dosing should be administered only under strict medical supervision.

Children (Younger Than 18 Years)

- Dosing in children should be carried out under medical supervision because of potential adverse effects. A dose of 5 g daily has been used in children with muscular dystrophy, and various doses have been used in children with GAMT deficiency, including 2 g per kilogram of body weight, 4-8 g daily in an infant, and 400-670 mg per kilogram of body weight.

SAFETY

The U.S. Food and Drug Administration does not strictly regulate herbs and supplements. There is no guarantee of the strength, purity, or safety of products, and effects may vary. It is important to always read product labels. People who have a medical condition, or are taking other drugs, herbs, or supplements, should consult a qualified healthcare provider before starting a new therapy. A healthcare provider should be contacted immediately about any side effects.

Allergies

- Creatine has been associated with asthmatic symptoms. People should not take creatine if they have a known allergy to this supplement.

Side Effects and Warnings

- Systematic studies of the safety, pharmacology, and toxicology of creatine are limited. People using creatine, including athletes, should be monitored by a qualified healthcare provider.
- Some individuals may experience gastrointestinal symptoms, including loss of appetite, stomach discomfort, diarrhea, or nausea.

- Creatine may cause muscle cramps or muscle breakdown, leading to discomfort and possibly muscle tears. Weight gain and increased body mass may occur. Heat intolerance, fever, dehydration, reduced blood volume, and electrolyte imbalances (and resulting seizures) may occur.
- There is less concern today than formerly about possible kidney damage from creatine, although there have been reports of kidney damage, such as interstitial nephritis. People with kidney disease should avoid the use of creatine. Similarly, because liver function may be affected by creatine supplements, caution is advised in people with underlying liver disease.
- In theory, creatine may alter the activities of insulin. Caution is advised in people with diabetes or hypoglycemia, and in those taking drugs, herbs, or supplements that affect blood sugar levels. Serum glucose levels may need to be monitored by a healthcare provider, and medication adjustments may be necessary.
- Chronic administration of a large quantity of creatine is reported to increase the production of formaldehyde, which may cause serious side effects.
- Based on a case report, creatine may increase the risk of compartment syndrome of the lower leg, a condition characterized by pain in the lower leg associated with inflammation and ischemia (diminished blood flow), which is a potential surgical emergency.

Pregnancy and Breastfeeding

- Creatine cannot be recommended during pregnancy or breastfeeding because of the lack of scientific information in these areas.
- Pasteurized cow's milk appears to contain higher levels of creatine than human milk. The clinical significance of this is unclear.

INTERACTIONS

Most herbs and supplements have not been thoroughly tested for interactions with other herbs, supplements, drugs, or foods. The interactions listed here are based on reports in scientific publications, laboratory experiments, or traditional use. It is important to always read product labels. People who have a medical condition, or are taking other drugs, herbs, or supplements, should consult a qualified healthcare provider before starting a new therapy.

Interactions with Drugs

- In theory, creatine may alter the activities of insulin, particularly when it is taken with carbohydrates. Caution is advised in people who are using medications that may also alter blood sugar levels. People taking drugs for diabetes by mouth or insulin should be monitored closely by a qualified healthcare provider. Medication adjustments may be necessary.
- Use of creatine with probenecid may increase levels of creatine in the body, leading to increased side effects.
- Use of creatine with diuretics such as hydrochlorothiazide and furosemide (Lasix) should be avoided because of the risks of dehydration and electrolyte disturbances. The likelihood of kidney damage may be greater when creatine is used with drugs that may damage the kidneys, including amikacin, anti-inflammatory drugs such as ibuprofen (Advil, Motrin), cimetidine (Tagamet), cyclosporine (Neoral, Sandimmune), gentamicin, tobramycin, and trimethoprim.
- Creatine may increase the cholesterol-lowering effects of other drugs used to lower cholesterol levels, such as lovastatin (Mevacor).

- Studies in animals reported that the combination of creatine and nonsteroidal anti-inflammatory drugs was more effective in reducing inflammation than either agent used alone.
- Creatine and nifedipine, when used together, may enhance heart function, although research in this area is limited.

Interactions with Herbs and Dietary Supplements

- Creatine may increase the risk of adverse effects, including stroke, when used with caffeine and ephedra. In addition, caffeine may reduce the beneficial effects of creatine during intense intermittent exercise.
- Because creatine theoretically may alter the activities of insulin, caution is advised when using herbs or supplements that may also alter blood sugar levels. Blood glucose levels may require monitoring, and doses may need adjustment. Examples of herbs and supplements that may cause hypoglycemia (low blood sugar levels) are *Aloe vera*, American ginseng, bilberry, bitter melon, burdock, fenugreek, fish oil, gymnema, horse chestnut seed extract (HCSE), maitake mushroom, marshmallow, milk thistle, *Panax ginseng*, rosemary, shark cartilage, Siberian ginseng, stinging nettle, and white horehound. Agents that may raise blood sugar levels (hyperglycemia) include arginine, cocoa, and ephedra (when combined with caffeine).
- Creatine may reduce the effectiveness of vitamins A, D, E, and K.
- Creatine may affect liver function, and should be used cautiously with potentially hepatotoxic (liver-damaging) herbs and supplements. Examples are ackee, bee pollen, birch oil, blessed thistle, borage, bush tea, butterbur, chaparral, coltsfoot, comfrey, DHEA, *Echinacea purpurea*, *Echium* spp., germander, *Heliotropium* spp., horse chestnut (parenteral preparations), jin-bu-huan (*Lycopodium serratum*), kava, lobelia, mate, niacin (vitamin B$_3$), niacinamide, Paraguay tea, periwinkle, *Plantago lanceolata*, pride of Madeira, rue, sassafras, scullcap, *Senecio* spp./groundsel, tansy ragwort, L-tetrahydropalmatine (THP), turmeric/curcumin, tu-san-chi (*Gynura segetum*), uva ursi, valerian, and white chameleon.
- Use of creatine with diuretics should be avoided because of the risk of dehydration and electrolyte disturbances. Herbs with possible diuretic effects include artichoke, celery, corn silk, couchgrass, dandelion, elder flower, horsetail, juniper berry, kava, shepherd's purse, uva ursi, and yarrow.
- It is possible that creatine may increase the cholesterol-lowering effects of herbs and supplements that lower cholesterol levels, such as red yeast (*Monascus purpureus*).

Selected References

Natural Standard developed the preceding evidence-based information based on a systematic review of more than 3000 articles. For comprehensive information about alternative and complementary therapies on the professional level, go to www.naturalstandard.com. Selected references are listed here.

Aaserud R, Gramvik P, Olsen SR, Jensen J. Creatine supplementation delays onset of fatigue during repeated bouts of sprint running. Scand J Med Sci Sports 1998;8(5 Pt 1):247-251.

Andrews R, Greenhaff P, Curtis S, et al. The effect of dietary creatine supplementation on skeletal muscle metabolism in congestive heart failure. Eur Heart J 1998;19(4):617-622.

Balestrino M, Lensman M, Parodi M, et al. Role of creatine and phosphocreatine in neuronal protection from anoxic and ischemic damage. Amino Acids 2002; 23(1-3):221-229.

Batley MA, Walton T, Scott DL, et al. Creatine supplementation in fibromyalgia. ULAR 2002 European Congress of Rheumatology, June 12-15, 2002, Stockholm.

Battini R, Leuzzi V, Carducci C, et al. Creatine depletion in a new case with AGAT deficiency: clinical and genetic study in a large pedigree. Mol Genet Metab 2002;77(4):326-331.

Becque MD, Lochmann JD, Melrose DR. Effects of oral creatine supplementation on muscular strength and body composition. Med Sci Sports Exerc 2000;32(3):654-658.

Bemben MG, Bemben DA, Loftiss DD, et al. Creatine supplementation during resistance training in college football athletes. Med Sci Sports Exerc 2001;33(10):1667-1673.

Biwer CJ, Jensen RL, Schmidt WD, Watts PB. The effect of creatine on treadmill running with high-intensity intervals. J Strength Cond Res 2003;17(3): 439-445.

Branch JD. Effect of creatine supplementation on body composition and performance: a meta-analysis. Int J Sport Nutr Exerc Metab 2003;13(2):198-226.

Brose A, Parise G, Tarnopolsky MA. Creatine supplementation enhances isometric strength and body composition improvements following strength exercise training in older adults. J Gerontol A Biol Sci Med Sci 2003;58(1): 11-19.

Chwalbinska-Moneta J. Effect of creatine supplementation on aerobic performance and anaerobic capacity in elite rowers in the course of endurance training. Int J Sport Nutr Exerc Metab 2003;13(2):173-183.

Delecluse C, Diels R, Goris M. Effect of creatine supplementation on intermittent sprint running performance in highly trained athletes. J Strength Cond Res 2003;17(3):446-454.

Eijnde BO, Van Leemputte M, Goris M, et al. Effects of creatine supplementation and exercise training on fitness in men 55-75 yr old. J Appl Physiol 2003; 95(2):818-828.

Fagbemi O, Kane KA, Parratt JR. Creatine phosphate suppresses ventricular arrhythmias resulting from coronary artery ligation. J Cardiovasc Pharmacol 1982;4(1):53-58.

Farquhar WB, Zambraski EJ. Effects of creatine use on the athlete's kidney. Curr Sports Med Rep 2002;1(2):103-106.

Ferraro S, Codella C, Palumbo F, et al. Hemodynamic effects of creatine phosphate in patients with congestive heart failure: a double-blind comparison trial versus placebo. Clin Cardiol 1996;19(9):699-703.

Gordon A, Hultman E, Kaijser L, et al. Creatine supplementation in chronic heart failure increases skeletal muscle creatine phosphate and muscle performance. Cardiovasc Res 1995;30(3):413-418.

Gotshalk LA, Volek JS, Staron RS, et al. Creatine supplementation improves muscular performance in older men. Med Sci Sports Exerc 2002;34(3):537-543.

Green AL, Hultman E, Macdonald IA, et al. Carbohydrate ingestion augments skeletal muscle creatine accumulation during creatine supplementation in humans. Am J Physiol 1996;271(5 Pt 1):E821-E826.

Green AL, Simpson EJ, Littlewood JJ, et al. Carbohydrate ingestion augments creatine retention during creatine feeding in humans. Acta Physiol Scand 1996;158(2):195-202.

Greenwood M, Kreider RB, Melton C, et al. Creatine supplementation during college football training does not increase the incidence of cramping or injury. Mol Cell Biochem 2003;244(1-2):83-88.

Grindstaff PD, Kreider R, Bishop R, et al. Effects of creatine supplementation on repetitive sprint performance and body composition in competitive swimmers. Int J Sport Nutr 1997;7(4):330-346.

Groeneveld GJ, Veldink JH, van der Tweel I, et al. A randomized sequential trial of creatine in amyotrophic lateral sclerosis. Ann Neurol 2003;53(4):437-445.

Hespel P, Op't Eijnde B, Van Leemputte M. Opposite actions of caffeine and creatine on muscle relaxation time in humans. J Appl Physiol 2002;92(2): 513-518.

Hulsemann J, Manz F, Wember T, Schoch G. [Administration of creatine and creatinine with breast milk and infant milk preparations.] Klin Padiatr 1987; 199(4):292-295.

Izquierdo M, Ibanez J, Gonzalez-Badillo JJ, Gorostiaga EM. Effects of creatine supplementation on muscle power, endurance, and sprint performance. Med Sci Sports Exerc 2002;34(2):332-343.

Jacobstein MD, Gerken TA, Bhat AM, Carlier PG. Myocardial protection during ischemia by prior feeding with the creatine analog: cyclocreatine. J Am Coll Cardiol 1989;14(1):246-251.

Jones AM, Atter T, Georg KP. Oral creatine supplementation improves multiple sprint performance in elite ice-hockey players. J Sports Med Phys Fitness 1999; 39(3):189-196.

Kilduff LP, Vidakovic P, Cooney G, et al. Effects of creatine on isometric bench-press performance in resistance-trained humans. Med Sci Sports Exerc 2002; 34(7):1176-1183.

Klopstock T, Querner V, Schmidt F, et al. A placebo-controlled crossover trial of creatine in mitochondrial diseases. Neurology 2000;55(11):1748-1751.

Komura K, Hobbiebrunken E, Wilichowski EK, Hanefeld FA. Effectiveness of creatine monohydrate in mitochondrial encephalomyopathies. Pediatr Neurol 2003;28(1):53-58.

Koshy KM, Griswold E, Schneeberger EE. Interstitial nephritis in a patient taking creatine. N Engl J Med 1999;340(10):814-815.

Kreider RB, Ferreira M, Wilson M, et al. Effects of creatine supplementation on body composition, strength, and sprint performance. Med Sci Sports Exerc 1998;30(1):73-82.

Kreider RB, Melton C, Rasmussen CJ, et al. Long-term creatine supplementation does not significantly affect clinical markers of health in athletes. Mol Cell Biochem 2003;244(1-2):95-104.

Kuehl K, Goldberg L, Elliot D. Long-term oral creatine supplementation does not impair renal function in healthy athletes. Med Sci Sports Exerc 2000; 32(1):248-249.

Lawler JM, Barnes WS, Wu G, et al. Direct antioxidant properties of creatine. Biochem Biophys Res Commun 2002;290(1):47-52.

Lehmkuhl M, Malone M, Justice B, et al. The effects of 8 weeks of creatine monohydrate and glutamine supplementation on body composition and performance measures. J Strength Cond Res 2003;17(3):425-438.

Mayhew DL, Mayhew JL, Ware JS. Effects of long-term creatine supplementation on liver and kidney functions in American college football players. Int J Sport Nutr Exerc Metab 2002;12(4):453-460.

Mazzini L, Balzarini C, Colombo R, et al. Effects of creatine supplementation on exercise performance and muscular strength in amyotrophic lateral sclerosis: preliminary results. J Neurol Sci 2001;191(1-2):139-144.

McNaughton LR, Dalton B, Tarr J. The effects of creatine supplementation on high-intensity exercise performance in elite performers. Eur J Appl Physiol Occup Physiol 1998;78(3):236-240.

Mujika I, Chatard JC, Lacoste L, et al. Creatine supplementation does not improve sprint performance in competitive swimmers. Med Sci Sports Exerc 1996;28(11):1435-1441.

Mujika I, Padilla S, Ibanez J, et al. Creatine supplementation and sprint performance in soccer players. Med Sci Sports Exerc 2000;32(2):518-525.

Newman JE, Hargreaves M, Garnham A, Snow RJ. Effect of creatine ingestion on glucose tolerance and insulin sensitivity in men. Med Sci Sports Exerc 2003;35(1):69-74.

O'Reilly DS, Carter R, Bell E, et al. Exercise to exhaustion in the second-wind phase of exercise in a case of McArdle's disease with and without creatine supplementation. Scott Med J 2003;48(2):46-48.

Peyrebrune MC, Nevill ME, Donaldson FJ, Cosford DJ. The effects of oral creatine supplementation on performance in single and repeated sprint swimming. J Sports Sci 1998;16(3):271-279.

Potteiger JA, Randall JC, Schroeder C, et al. Elevated anterior compartment pressure in the leg after creatine supplementation: A controlled case report. J Athl Train 2001;36(1):85-88.

Preen D, Dawson B, Goodman C, et al. Effect of creatine loading on long-term sprint exercise performance and metabolism. Med Sci Sports Exerc 2001; 33(5):814-821.

Robinson TM, Sewell DA, Casey A, et al. Dietary creatine supplementation does not affect some haematological indices, or indices of muscle damage and hepatic and renal function. Br J Sports Med 2000;34(4):284-288.

Romer LM, Barrington JP, Jeukendrup AE. Effects of oral creatine supplementation on high intensity, intermittent exercise performance in competitive squash players. Int J Sports Med 2001;22(8):546-552.

Rooney KB, Bryson JM, Digney AL, et al. Creatine supplementation affects glucose homeostasis but not insulin secretion in humans. Ann Nutr Metab 2003;47(1):11-15.

Schneider-Gold C, Beck M, Wessig C, et al. Creatine monohydrate in DM2/PROMM: a double-blind placebo-controlled clinical study. Proximal myotonic myopathy. Neurology 2003;60(3):500-502.

Schroeder C, Potteiger J, Randall J, et al. The effects of creatine dietary supplementation on anterior compartment pressure in the lower leg during rest and following exercise. Clin J Sport Med 2001;11(2):87-95.

Skare OC, Skadberg, Wisnes AR. Creatine supplementation improves sprint performance in male sprinters. Scand J Med Sci Sports 2001;11(2):96-102.

Tarnopolsky MA, MacLennan DP. Creatine monohydrate supplementation enhances high-intensity exercise performance in males and females. Int J Sport Nutr Exerc Metab 2000;10(4):452-463.

Vandenberghe K, Gillis N, Van Leemputte M, et al. Caffeine counteracts the ergogenic action of muscle creatine loading. J Appl Physiol 1996;80(2): 452-457.

Vorgerd M, Zange J, Kley R, et al. Effect of high-dose creatine therapy on symptoms of exercise intolerance in McArdle disease: double-blind, placebo-controlled crossover study. Arch Neurol 2002;59(1):97-101.

Dandelion
(*Taraxacum officinale*)

SYNONYMS/COMMON NAMES/RELATED SUBSTANCES

- Asteraceae (family), blowball, cankerwort, clock flower, common dandelion, Cichoroideae, Compositae, dandelion herb, dent de lion, diente de lion, dudhal, dumble-dor, fairy clock, fortune teller, huang hua di ding (yellow flower earth nail), hokouei-kon, irish daisy, *Leontodon taraxacum*, lion's teeth, lion's tooth, lowenzahn, lowenzahnwurzel, maelkebotte, milk gowan, min-deul-rre, monk's head, mongoloid dandelion, pee in the bed, pissenlit, piss-in-bed, pries' crown, priest's crown, puffball, pu gong ying, pu kung ying, radix taraxaci, swine snout, taraxaci herba, taraxacum, *Taraxacum mongolicum*, *Taraxacum palustre*, *Taraxacum vulgare*, telltime, white endive, wild endive, witch gowan, witches' milk, yellow flower earth nail.

CLINICAL BOTTOM LINE
Background

- Dandelion is a member of the Asteraceae/Compositae family and is closely related to chicory. It is a perennial herb, native throughout the Northern Hemisphere, found growing wild in meadows, pastures, and waste grounds of temperate zones.
- Dandelion root and leaf are used widely in Europe for gastrointestinal ailments. The European Scientific Cooperative on Phytotherapy (ESCOP) recommends dandelion root for "restoration of hepatic and biliary function, dyspepsia [indigestion], and loss of appetite." The German Commission E authorizes the use of combination products containing dandelion root and herb for biliary abnormalities, appetite loss, dyspepsia, and stimulation of diuresis (urine flow). Some modern naturopathic physicians assert that dandelion can detoxify the liver and gallbladder, reduce side effects of medications metabolized (processed) by the liver, and relieve symptoms associated with liver disease.
- Dandelion leaves are a source of vitamin A, containing up to 1400 IU per 100 g.
- Dandelion is generally regarded as safe, with rare side effects including contact dermatitis, diarrhea, and gastrointestinal upset. Traditionally, the herb is not recommended in patients with liver or gallbladder disease, based on the belief that dandelion stimulates bile secretion (an assertion not demonstrated in animal or human studies).
- Dandelion is used as a salad ingredient, and the roasted root and its extracts are sometimes used as a coffee substitute.

Scientific Evidence for Common/Studied Uses	Grade*
Anti-inflammatory	C
Antioxidant	C
Cancer	C
Colitis	C
Diabetes	C
Diuretic	C
Hepatitis B	C

*Key to grades: *A:* Strong scientific evidence for this use; *B:* Good scientific evidence for this use; *C:* Unclear scientific evidence for this use; *D:* Fair scientific evidence against this use (it may not work); *F:* Strong scientific evidence against this use (it likely does not work). For a more detailed explanation of efficacy criteria, see "Natural Standard Evidence-Based Validated Grading Rationale" in the Introduction.

Historical or Theoretical Uses That Lack Sufficient Evidence

- Abscess, acne, age spots, AIDS, alcohol withdrawal, allergies, analgesia, anemia, antibacterial, antifungal, antioxidant, antiviral, aphthous ulcers, appendicitis, appetite stimulant, arthritis, benign prostate hypertrophy, bile flow stimulation, bladder irritation, blood purifier, boils, breast augmentation, breast cancer, breast infection, breast inflammation, breast milk stimulation, bruises, cardiovascular disorders, chronic fatigue syndrome, circulation, clogged arteries, coffee substitute, congestive heart failure, dandruff, diarrhea, dropsy, eye problems, fertility, fever reduction, food uses, frequent urination, gallbladder disease, gallstones, gas, gout, headache, heartburn, high blood pressure, high cholesterol, immune stimulation, increased sweating, jaundice, kidney disease, kidney stones,[1] leukemia, liver disease, liver cleansing, menopause, menstrual period stimulation, muscle aches, nutrition, osteoarthritis, postpartum support, pregnancy, premenstrual syndrome, psoriasis, rheumatoid arthritis, skin conditions, skin toner, smoking cessation, stiff joints, stimulant, stomachache, urinary stimulant, urinary tract inflammation, warts, weight loss.

Expert Opinion and Folkloric Precedent

- Dandelion root has been used like other bitter herbs, to improve appetite and treat minor digestive disorders. Modern naturopathic physicians consider dandelion to have the ability to detoxify the liver and gallbladder, reduce the side effects of medications processed by the liver, and relieve symptoms of diseases in which impaired liver function plays a role. *In vitro* data and human studies do not support the belief that dandelion stimulates bile secretion.

Safety Summary

- **Likely safe:** When taken orally in amounts naturally found in foods and when taken orally in recommended doses by otherwise healthy adults for medicinal purposes. Dandelion is Generally Recognized as Safe (GRAS) in the United States for food use, with a maximum level of 0.014% for the fluid extract and 0.003% for the solid extract.
- **Possibly unsafe:** When used in amounts greater than recommended doses or when used for a long duration. When used in doses greater than that found in food in patients during pregnancy or lactation. When used in doses greater than that found in food in pediatric patients.

- **Likely unsafe:** When used in patients with hypersensitivity to dandelion or other members of the Asteraceae/Compositae family (e.g. ragweed, chrysanthemums, marigolds, and daises).

DOSING/TOXICOLOGY
General

- Recommended doses are based on those most commonly used in available trials, or on historical practice. However, with natural products, the optimal doses needed to balance efficacy and safety often have not been determined. Formulations and preparation methods may vary from manufacturer to manufacturer, and from batch to batch of a specific product made by a single manufacturer. Because often the active components of a product are not known, standardization may not be possible, and the clinical effects of different brands may not be comparable.

Standardization

- There are no standard or well-studied doses of dandelion, and many different doses are used traditionally. Safety of use beyond 4 months has not been evaluated.
- Dandelion leaves are a source of vitamin A, containing up to 1400 IU per 100 g.

Dosing: Adults (18 Years and Older)

- **Dried root:** Doses of 2 to 8 g taken by infusion or decoction have been used.
- **Leaf fluid extract:** Doses of 4 to 8 mL of a 1:1 extract in 25% alcohol have been used.
- **Root tincture:** Doses of 1 or 2 teaspoons of a 1:5 tincture in 45% alcohol have been used.

Dosing: Pediatric (Younger Than 18 Years)

- There is not enough scientific research to recommend dandelion for use in children in amounts greater than found in food.

Toxicology

- The acute toxicity of dandelion (mice intraperitoneal injection) is low, with an LD_{50} value estimated at 36.8 g/kg for the root and 28.8 g/kg for the herb. Tita et al. administered up to 10 g/kg orally and 4 g/kg intraperitoneally in rats and mice and observed a "low toxicity."[2]
- Twenty rats were fed a diet composed of 32% dandelion rhizomes to evaluate carcinogenic activity.[3] One rat died 20 days after the experiment began and 6 rats died >200 days after the start of the experiment. No tumors were observed in this group.
- Rabbits administered dandelion at doses up to 6 g/kg body weight for 7 days did not demonstrate visible toxicity.[4]

ADVERSE EFFECTS/PRECAUTIONS/CONTRAINDICATIONS
Allergies

- Dandelion should be avoided by individuals with known allergy to dandelion,[5,6] honey,[7] chamomile, chrysanthemums, yarrow, feverfew or any members of the Asteraceae/Compositae plant families (ragweed, sunflower, daisies).[8]
- The most common type of allergy to dandelion is dermatitis following direct skin contact,[9-12] which may include itching, rash, or red/swollen or eczematous areas on the skin.[12] Skin reactions are also reported in dogs.[14] The main chemicals in dandelion responsible for allergic reactions are believed to

be sesquiterpene lactones. Patch tests have been developed to assess for dandelion allergy.[15-17]
- Rhinoconjunctivitis and asthma have been reported after handling products such as birdfeed containing dandelion and other herbs, with reported positive skin tests for dandelion hypersensitivity.[18]

Side Effects and Warnings

- **General:** Dandelion has been well tolerated in a small number of available human studies. Safety of use beyond 4 months has not been evaluated.
- **Dermatologic:** The most common reported adverse effects are skin allergy, eczema, and increased sun sensitivity following direct contact.[9-13]
- **Gastrointestinal:** According to traditional accounts, gastrointestinal symptoms may occur, including stomach discomfort, diarrhea and heartburn. There is a 1966 case of a patient who developed intestinal blockage from ingesting a large amount of dandelion greens 3 weeks after undergoing a stomach operation.[19]
- **Infectious (contamination):** Parasitic infection due to ingestion of contaminated dandelion has been reported, affecting the liver and bile ducts and characterized by fever, stomach upset, vomiting, loss of appetite, coughing, and liver damage.[20]
- **Endocrine:** Dandelion may lower blood sugar levels, based on one animal study,[4] although another study notes no changes.[21] Effects in humans are not known. Caution is advised in patients with diabetes or hypoglycemia and in those taking drugs, herbs, or supplements that affect blood sugar levels. Serum glucose levels may need to be monitored by a healthcare provider, and medication adjustments may be necessary.
- **Hematologic:** In theory, because of coumarins found in dandelion leaf extracts, dandelion may increase the risk of bleeding when taken with drugs that increase the risk of bleeding. Platelet aggregation may also be inhibited.
- **Renal:** Historically, dandelion is believed to possess diuretic (increased urination) properties and to lower blood potassium levels.
- **Neurologic:** Dandelion may be prepared as a tincture containing high levels of alcohol. Tinctures should therefore be avoided during pregnancy or when driving or operating heavy machinery.

Precautions/Warnings/Contraindications

- Avoid use in patients with hypersensitivity/allergy to dandelion or other members of the Asteraceae/Compositae family.
- Use cautiously in patients with bile duct and intestinal obstruction, acute cholecystitis, empyema, or acute gallbladder inflammation (theoretical).
- Use cautiously in patients with digestive disorders, stomach inflammation, or irritable bowel syndrome.
- Use cautiously in patients with diabetes.
- Use cautiously in patients with renal failure.

Pregnancy and Lactation

- Dandelion cannot be recommended during pregnancy and lactation in amounts greater than found in foods, because of a lack of scientific information. Many tinctures contain high levels of alcohol and should be avoided during pregnancy.

INTERACTIONS
Interactions with Drugs

- **General:** Drug interactions with dandelion have rarely been identified, although there is limited study in this area.
- **Ciprofloxacin (Cipro):** Based on animal research, dandelion may reduce the effects of the antibiotic ciprofloxacin (Cipro) because of reduced absorption of the drug.[23] In theory, dandelion may reduce the absorption of other drugs taken at the same time.
- **Hypoglycemic drugs:** Based on an animal study, dandelion may lower blood sugar levels,[4] although another study notes no changes.[21] Although effects in humans are not known, caution is advised in patients taking prescription drugs that may also lower blood sugar levels. Those using oral drugs for diabetes or insulin should be monitored closely by a healthcare provider while using dandelion. Dosing adjustments may be necessary.
- **Diuretics:** Historically, dandelion is believed to possess diuretic (increased urination) properties and to lower blood potassium levels. In theory, the effects or side effects of other drugs may be increased, including other diuretics, lithium, digoxin (Lanoxin), and corticosteroids such as prednisone.
- **Niacin/nicotinic acid:** The effects or side effects of niacin or nicotinic acid may be increased (such as flushing and gastrointestinal upset), because of small amounts of nicotinic acid present in dandelion.
- **Anticoagulants:** In theory, because of coumarins found in dandelion leaf extracts, dandelion may increase the risk of bleeding when used with anticoagulants or antiplatelet drugs. Platelet aggregation may also be inhibited.[22]
- **Antacids:** It is possible that dandelion may reduce the effectiveness of antacids or drugs commonly used to treat peptic ulcer disease, such as famotidine (Pepcid) and esomeprazole (Nexium).
- **P450 1A2 and 2E metabolized drugs:** There is animal evidence that dandelion may interfere with the way the liver breaks down certain drugs (using the P450 1A2 and 2E enzyme systems). As a result, the levels of these drugs may be raised in the blood, and increase the intended effects or side effects. Patients using medications should check the package insert and speak with a healthcare provider or pharmacist about possible interactions.
- **Flagyl:** Be aware that many tinctures contain high levels of alcohol and may cause nausea or vomiting when taken with metronidazole (Flagyl).
- **Disulfiram (Antabuse):** Be aware that many tinctures contain high levels of alcohol and may cause nausea or vomiting when taken with disulfiram (Antabuse).

Interactions with Herbs and Dietary Supplements

- **General:** Interactions of dietary supplements with dandelion have rarely been published, although there is limited study in this area.
- **Hypoglycemic agents:** Based on an animal study, dandelion may lower blood sugar levels,[4] although another study notes no changes.[21] Although effects in humans are not known, caution is advised when using herbs or supplements that may also lower blood sugar levels. Blood glucose levels may require monitoring, and doses may need adjustment.
- **Diuretic agents:** Historically, dandelion is believed to possess diuretic (increased urination) properties and may increase the effects of other herbs with potential diuretic effects.
- **Anticoagulant agents:** In theory, because of coumarins found in dandelion leaf extracts, dandelion may increase the risk of bleeding when taken with herbs and supplements that are believed to increase the risk of bleeding. Platelet aggregation may also be inhibited.[22]
- **P450 1A2 and 2E metabolized agents:** There is animal evidence that dandelion may interfere with the way the liver breaks down certain drugs (using the P450 1A2 and 2E enzyme systems). As a result, the levels of other herbs or supplements to be too high in the blood. In theory, dandelion may also alter the effects that other herbs or supplements possibly have on the P450 system, such as bloodroot, cat's claw, chamomile, chaparral, chasteberry, damiana, *Echinacea angustifolia*, goldenseal, grapefruit juice, licorice, oregano, red clover, St. John's wort, wild cherry, and yucca.
- **Vitamin A, lutein, beta-carotene:** Dandelion leaves contain vitamin A, lutein, and beta-carotene, and supplemental doses of these agents may have additive effects or toxicity. Vitamin A is fat-soluble and can accumulate in tissues.

Dandelion/Lab Interactions

- **Urine drug screens:** Dandelion has been used historically by substance abusers with the intention of masking illicit substances in urine drug screens (anecdotal). However, there is no reliable study in this area.
- **Glucose:** Because of potential hypoglycemic effects, serum glucose concentration may be reduced by dandelion.
- **Electrolytes:** Because of diuretic effects, plasma sodium or potassium concentrations may decrease with dandelion use. However, no such effects have been found in the available literature.

MECHANISM OF ACTION
Pharmacology

- Dandelion's therapeutic effects historically have been attributed to the bitter constituents found in the roots and leaves.[24] Research in laboratory animals suggests that dandelion root may possess anti-inflammatory properties.[25] Sesquiterpene lactones are responsible for diuretic effects and may contribute to dandelion's mild anti-inflammatory activity.[25] Lactones may increase gastric acid secretion.
- Dandelion is suggested to increase bile production and flow to the gallbladder (choleretic), and exert a direct effect on the gallbladder, causing contraction and release of stored bile (cholagogue).[26] Dandelion leaves contain appetite-stimulating substances, eudesmanolides, previously known as taraxacum.
- Inulin, a constituent of dandelion, may act to buffer blood glucose levels and has experimental hypoglycemic activity in animals.[27]
- Several laboratory studies report antioxidant properties of dandelion flower extract.[28-31]
- Potassium is present in dandelion leaves at a concentration of 297 mg per 100 g.[32] The leaves are a source of vitamin A (1400 IU per 100 g), as well as lutein and beta-carotene. Dandelion is also a source of fiber, potassium, iron, calcium, magnesium, phosphorus, thiamine and riboflavin. Dandelion contains sodium, vitamin C, and vitamin D in lesser concentrations.

Pharmacodynamics/Kinetics

- **Effects on phase 1 metabolism:** Activity of hepatic enzyme CYP1A2 in the liver microsomes of rats receiving dandelion in a green tea extract solution was decreased to 15% of that in a control group (which received water).[33] In the same study, CYP2E activity was decreased to 48% of that in the control group.

- **Effects on phase 2 metabolism:** Following the ingestion of dandelion in a green tea extract solution, detoxifying enzyme UDP-glucoronosyl transferase activity increased to 244% of the control group enzyme activity.[33]

HISTORY

- Dandelion was commonly used in Native American medicine. The Iroquois, Ojibwe, and Rappahannock prepared infusions and decoctions of the root and herb to treat kidney disease, dyspepsia, and heartburn. In traditional Arabian medicine, dandelion has been used to treat liver and spleen ailments. In traditional Chinese medicine (TCM), dandelion is combined with other herbs to treat hepatitis, to enhance immune response to upper respiratory tract infections, bronchitis, or pneumonia, and as a topical compress for mastitis (breast inflammation).
- Dandelion is a perennial herb native throughout the Northern Hemisphere, found growing wild in meadows, pastures, and waste grounds in temperate zones. Dandelion is very adaptable but prefers moist nitrogen-rich soils and altitudes less than 6000 feet. Most commercial dandelion is cultivated in Bulgaria, Hungary, Poland, Romania, and the United Kingdom.

REVIEW OF EVIDENCE: TABLE

- No studies qualify for inclusion in the evidence table.

REVIEW OF THE EVIDENCE: DISCUSSION

Anti-inflammatory
Evidence

- Research in laboratory animals suggests that dandelion root may possess anti-inflammatory properties.[25] There are no well-conducted human studies in this area.

Antioxidant
Evidence

- Several laboratory studies report antioxidant properties of dandelion flower extract,[28-31] although this research is preliminary and effects in humans are not known.

Cancer
Evidence

- Limited animal research does not provide a clear assessment of the effects of dandelion on tumor growth.[34,35] There are no well-conducted human studies in this area.

Colitis
Evidence

- There is a report in several patients that a combination herbal preparation containing dandelion improved chronic pain associated with colitis.[36] Because multiple herbs were used, and this study is not well designed or reported, the effects of dandelion are not clear.

Diabetes
Evidence

- There is limited animal research on the effects of dandelion on blood sugar levels in animals. One study reports decreases in glucose levels in non-diabetic rabbits,[4] whereas another notes no changes in mice.[21] Effects in humans are not known.

Diuretic
Evidence

- Dandelion leaves have traditionally been used to increase urine production and excretion. Animal studies report mixed

results, and there is no reliable human research in this area.[2,32,37]

Hepatitis B
Evidence

- One human study reports improved liver function in people with hepatitis B after taking a combination herbal preparation containing dandelion root, called jiedu yanggan gao (also including *Artemisia capillaris, Taraxacum mongolicum*, plantago seed, cephalanoplos segetum, hedyotis diffusa, flos chrysanthemi indici, smilax glabra, astragalus membranaceus, salviae miltiorrhizae, fructus polygonii orientalis, radix paeoniae alba, and polygonatum sibiricum).[38] Because multiple herbs were used, and this study is not well designed or reported, the effects of dandelion are not clear.

References

1. Grases F, Melero G, Costa-Bauza A, et al. Urolithiasis and phytotherapy. Int Urol Nephrol 1994;26(5):507-511.
2. Tita B, Bello U, Faccendini P, et al. Taraxacum officinale W.: pharmacological effect of ethanol extract. Pharmacological Res 1993;27(Suppl 1):23-24.
3. Hirono I, Mori H, Kato K, et al. Safety examination of some edible plants, Part 2. J Environ Pathol Toxicol 1978;1(1):71-74.
4. Akhtar MS, Khan QM, Khaliq T. Effects of *Portulaca oleracae* (Kulfa) and *Taraxacum officinale* (Dhudhal) in normoglycaemic and alloxan-treated hyperglycaemic rabbits. J Pak Med Assoc 1985;35(7):207-210.
5. Cohen SH, Yunginger JW, Rosenberg N, Fink JN. Acute allergic reaction after composite pollen ingestion. J Allergy Clin Immunol 1979;64(4):270-274.
6. Jovanovic M, Mimica-Dukic N, Poljacki M, Boza P. Erythema multiforme due to contact with weeds: a recurrence after patch testing. Contact Dermatitis 2003;48(1):17-25.
7. Helbling A, Peter C, Berchtold E,et al. Allergy to honey: relation to pollen and honey bee allergy. Allergy 1992;47(1):41-49.
8. Fernandez C, Martin-Esteban M, Fiandor A, et al. Analysis of cross-reactivity between sunflower pollen and other pollens of the Compositae family. J Allergy Clin Immunol 1993;92(5):660-667.
9. Ingber A. Seasonal allergic contact dermatitis from *Taraxacum officinale* (dandelion) in an Israeli florist. Contact Dermatitis 2000;43(1):49.
10. Dawe RS, Green CM, MacLeod TM, Ferguson J. Daisy, dandelion and thistle contact allergy in the photosensitivity dermatitis and actinic reticuloid syndrome. Contact Dermatitis 1996;35(2):109-110.
11. Wakelin SH, Marren P, Young E, Shaw S. Compositae sensitivity and chronic hand dermatitis in a seven-year-old boy. Br J Dermatol 1997;137(2):289-291.
12. Guin JD, Skidmore G. Compositae dermatitis in childhood. Arch Dermatol 1987;123(4):500-502.
13. Davies MG, Kersey PJ. Contact allergy to yarrow and dandelion. Contact Dermatitis 1986;14(4):256-257.
14. Youn HY, Kang HS, Bhang DH, et al. Allergens causing atopic diseases in canine. J Vet Sci 2002;3(4):335-341.
15. Lovell CR, Rowan M. Dandelion dermatitis. Contact Derm 1991;25(3):185-188.
16. Goulden V, Wilkinson SM. Patch testing for Compositae allergy. Br J Dermatol 1998;138(6):1018-1021.
17. Mark KA, Brancaccio RR, Soter NA, Cohen DE. Allergic contact and photoallergic contact dermatitis to plant and pesticide allergens. Arch Dermatol 1999;135(1):67-70.
18. Rodriguez B, Rodriguez A, de Barrio M, et al. Asthma induced by canary food mix. Allergy Asthma Proc 2003;24(4):265-268.
19. Collins JM, Miller DR. Dandelion green bezoar following antrectomy and vagotomy—case report. J Kansas Med Soc 1966;67(6):303-304.
20. Merino AJ, Amerigo Garcia MJ, Alvarez RL, Erdozain R. I. [Human fascioliasis with atypical severe presentation. Treatment with triclabendazole]. Enferm Infecc Microbiol Clin 1998;16(1):28-30.
21. Swanston-Flatt SK, Day C, Flatt PR, et al. Glycaemic effects of traditional European plant treatments for diabetes. Studies in normal and streptozotocin diabetic mice. Diabetes Res 1989;10(2):69-73.
22. Neef H, Cilli F, Declerck PJ, et al. Platelet anti-aggregating activity of *Taraxacum officinale* Weber. Phytotherapy Research 1996;10:s138-s140.
23. Zhu M, Wong PY, Li RC. Effects of *Taraxacum mongolicum* on the bioavailability and disposition of ciprofloxacin in rats. J Pharm Sci 1999;88(6):632-634.
24. Kuusi T, Pyylaso H, Autio K. The bitterness properties of dandelion. II. Chemical investigations. Lebensm-Wiss Technol 1985;18:347-349.
25. Mascolo N, Autore G, Capasso F, et al. Biological screening of Italian medicinal plants for anti-inflammatory activity. Phytotherapy Res 1987;1(1):28-31.
26. Bohm K. Studies on the choleretic action of some drugs. Azneim-Forsh 1959;9:376-378.

27. Rutherford PP, Deacon AC. The mode of action of dandelion root fructofuranosidases on inulin. Biochem J 1972;129(2):511-512.

28. Hu C, Kitts DD. Antioxidant, prooxidant, and cytotoxic activities of solvent-fractionated dandelion (*Taraxacum officinale*) flower extracts in vitro. J Agric Food Chem 2003;51(1):301-310.

29. Hagymasi K, Blazovics A, Feher J, et al. The *in vitro* effect of dandelions antioxidants on microsomal lipid peroxidation. Phytother Res 2000;14(1): 43-44.

30. Kim HM, Oh CH, Chung CK. Activation of inducible nitric oxide synthase by *Taraxacum officinale* in mouse peritoneal macrophages. Gen Pharmacol 1999;32(6):683-688.

31. Kim HM, Lee EH, Shin TY, et al. *Taraxacum officinale* restores inhibition of nitric oxide production by cadmium in mouse peritoneal macrophages. Immunopharmacol Immunotoxicol 1998;20(2):283-297.

32. Hook I, McGee A, Henman M, et al. Evaluation of dandelion for diuretic activity and variation in potassium content. Int J Pharmacog 1993;31(1): 29-34.

33. Maliakal PP, Wanwimolruk S. Effect of herbal teas on hepatic drug metabolizing enzymes in rats. J Pharm Pharmacol 2001;53(10):1323-1329.

34. Baba K, Abe S, Mizuno D. [Antitumor activity of hot water extract of dandelion, *Taraxacum officinale*—correlation between antitumor activity and timing of administration (author's transl)]. Yakugaku Zasshi 1981; 101(6):538-543.

35. Hata K, Ishikawa K, Hori K, Konishi T. Differentiation-inducing activity of lupeol, a lupane-type triterpene from Chinese dandelion root (Hokouei-kon), on a mouse melanoma cell line. Biol Pharm Bull 2000;23(8):962-967.

36. Chakurski I, Matev M, Koichev A, et al. [Treatment of chronic colitis with an herbal combination of *Taraxacum officinale*, *Hipericum perforatum*, *Melissa officinalis*, *Calendula officinalis* and *Foeniculum vulgare*]. Vutreshni bolesti 1981;20(6):51-54.

37. Racz-Kotilla E, Racz G, Solomon A. The action of *Taraxacum officinale* extracts on the body weight and diuresis of laboratory animals. Planta Med 1974;26(3):212-217.

38. Chen Z. [Clinical study of 96 cases with chronic hepatitis B treated with jiedu yanggan gao by a double-blind method]. Zhong Xi Yi Jie He Za Zhi 1990;10(2):71-4, 67.

Danshen
(*Salvia miltiorrhiza*)

D

SYNONYMS/COMMON NAMES/RELATED SUBSTANCES

- Bunge, Ch'ih shen, dan-shen, dan shen, danshen root, hang ken, hung ken, pin-ma ts'ao (horse-racing grass), radix salvia miltiorrhiza, red-rooted sage, red sage root, red sage root, red roots, *Salvia bowelyana*, *Salviae miltiorrhizae*, *Salvia przewalskii*, *Salvia przewalskii* mandarinorum, *Salvia yunnanensis*, salvia root, scarlet sage, sh'ih shen, shu-wei ts'ao (rat-tail grass), tan seng, tan-shen, tzu tan-ken (roots of purple sage).

CLINICAL BOTTOM LINE
Background

- Danshen (*Salvia miltiorrhiza*) is widely used in traditional Chinese medicine (TCM), often in combination with other herbs. Remedies containing danshen are used traditionally to treat a diversity of ailments, particularly cardiac (heart) and vascular (blood vessel) disorders such as atherosclerosis (hardening of the arteries with cholesterol plaques) and blood clotting abnormalities.
- The ability of danshen to thin the blood and reduce blood clotting is well documented, although the herb's purported ability to "invigorate" the blood or improve circulation has not been demonstrated in high-quality trials in humans. Constituents of the danshen root, particularly proto-catechualdehyde and 3,4-dihydroxyphenyl-lactic acid, are believed to be responsible for its vascular effects. Because danshen can inhibit platelet aggregation and has been reported to potentiate (increase) the blood-thinning effects of warfarin, it should be avoided in persons with bleeding disorders, prior to some surgical procedures, or in those taking anticoagulant (blood-thinning) drugs, herbs, or supplements.
- In the mid-1980s, scientific interest was shown in danshen's possible cardiovascular benefits, particularly in patients with ischemic stroke or coronary artery disease/angina. More recent studies have focused on danshen's possible role in the treatment of liver disease (hepatitis and cirrhosis), and as an antioxidant. However, most research in these areas has been in studies in animals and small trials of poor methodological quality in humans. Therefore, firm evidence-based conclusions are not possible at this time about the effects of danshen for any medical condition.

Uses Based on Scientific Evidence	Grade*
Asthmatic bronchitis A small amount of research studies in humans suggest that danshen may improve breathing and lessen cough and wheeze in persons with chronic asthmatic bronchitis. Better studies are needed that compare danshen with established treatments for this condition before a clear conclusion can be drawn.	C
Burn healing Although studies in animals suggest that danshen may speed healing of burns and wounds, there are no reliable studies in humans available that evaluate this claim.	C
Cardiovascular disease/angina A small number of poor-quality studies in animals and humans report that danshen may provide benefits for treating disorders of the heart and blood vessels, including heart attacks, cardiac chest pain (angina), or myocarditis. Traditionally, danshen is most frequently used for these problems in combination with other herbs. Because most studies have been small and brief with flaws in their designs, and the results of different trials have disagreed with each other, it is not clear whether there is any benefit from danshen for these conditions. No specific dose or standardized preparation is widely accepted for these disorders. Danshen may have effects on blood clotting and therefore may be unsafe when combined with other drugs used in patients with cardiovascular disease. Patients should check with a physician and pharmacist before combining danshen with prescription drugs.	C
Glaucoma Danshen has been proposed as a possible glaucoma therapy, but further studies are needed in humans before a clear conclusion can be drawn. Danshen should not be used in place of established therapies, and patients with glaucoma should be evaluated by a qualified eye care specialist.	C
Increased rate of peritoneal dialysis One study suggested that danshen may speed peritoneal dialysis and ultrafiltration rates when added to dialysate solution. Although this evidence is promising, it is not known whether danshen is safe for this use.	C
Ischemic stroke In limited research from the 1970s, danshen was administered intravenously (through the veins) for up to 4 weeks in patients with ischemic stroke. Due to poor quality of this evidence, unclear safety, and the existence of more proven treatments for ischemic stroke, this use of danshen cannot be recommended.	C
Liver disease (cirrhosis / chronic hepatitis B) Some studies suggest that danshen may provide benefits for treating liver diseases such as cirrhosis and chronic hepatitis B. Traditionally, danshen is most frequently used for these problems in combination with other herbs. Although early research in humans suggests a possible reduction in liver fibrosis in people with cirrhosis, as well as some improvements in liver function in chronic hepatitis, these studies have been small with flaws in their designs. Therefore it is unclear whether there are any clinically significant effects of danshen in patients with liver disease.	C

*Key to grades: A: Strong scientific evidence for this use; B: Good scientific evidence for this use; C: Unclear scientific evidence for this use; D: Fair scientific evidence against this use (it may not work); F: Strong scientific evidence against this use (it likely does not work). For a more detailed explanation of efficacy criteria, see "Natural Standard Evidence-Based Validated Grading Rationale" in the Introduction.

177

Historical or Theoretical Indications That Lack Sufficient Evidence

Acne, anoxic brain injury, antioxidant, antiphospholipid syndrome, anxiety, bleomycin-induced lung fibrosis, blood-clotting disorders, bruising, cancer, cataracts, circulation, clogged arteries, diabetic nerve pain, ectopic pregnancy, eczema, gastric ulcers, gentamicin toxicity, hearing loss, heart palpitations, high cholesterol, HIV, hypercoagulability, intrauterine growth retardation, kidney failure, left ventricular hypertrophy, leukemia, liver cancer, lung fibrosis, menstrual problems, preeclampsia, psoriasis, pulmonary hypertension, radiation-induced lung damage, restlessness, sleep difficulties, stimulation of gamma-aminobutyric acid (GABA) release, stomach ulcers, wound healing.

DOSING/TOXICOLOGY

The following doses are based on scientific research, publications, traditional use, or expert opinion. Many herbs and supplements have not been thoroughly tested, and their safety and effectiveness may not be proven. Brands may be made differently, with variable ingredients even within the same brand. The doses shown may not apply to all products. It is important to always read product labels and discuss doses with a qualified healthcare provider before therapy is started.

Standardization

- Standardization involves measuring the amounts of certain chemicals in products to try to make different preparations similar to each other. It is not always known if the chemicals being measured are the "active" ingredients. There is no widely accepted standardization or well-studied dosing of danshen, and many different doses are used traditionally. Danshen is frequently used in combination with other herbs.

Adults (18 Years and Older)

- **By mouth:** Oral dosing has not been studied in well-conducted trials in humans, and therefore no specific dose can be recommended.
- **By intravenous injection:** In research from the 1970s, an 8-ml injection of danshen (16 g of the herb) was given intravenously (diluted in 500 ml of a 10% glucose solution) for up to 4 weeks for ischemic stroke. Safety and effectiveness have not been established for this route of administration and it cannot be recommended at his time.

Children (Younger Than 18 Years)

- There is insufficient scientific evidence to recommend the safe use of danshen in children, and its use should be avoided because of potentially serious side effects.

SAFETY

The U.S. Food and Drug Administration does not strictly regulate herbs and supplements. There is no guarantee of the strength, purity, or safety of products, and effects may vary. It is important to always read product labels. People who have a medical condition, or are taking other drugs, herbs, or supplements, should consult a qualified healthcare provider before starting a new therapy. A healthcare provider should be contacted immediately about any side effects.

Allergies

- People with known allergy to danshen or its constituents (i.e., protocatechualdehyde, 3,4-dihydroxyphenyl-lactic acid, tanshinone I, dihydrotanshinone, cryptotanshione, miltirone, salvianolic acid B) should avoid this herb. Danshen is often found in combination with other herbs in various formulations, and patients should read product labels carefully and consult their healthcare provider and pharmacist about possible interactions.

Side Effects and Warnings

- Although danshen has been well tolerated in most studies, there is limited research using preparations consisting of danshen only for extended periods of time, and safety has not been studied systematically.
- Danshen may increase the risk of bleeding. This herb has been reported to inhibit platelet aggregation and increase the blood-thinning effects of warfarin in humans. Caution is advised in people with bleeding disorders who are taking drugs that may increase the risk of bleeding, or prior to some surgical procedures. Dosing adjustments may be necessary.
- Some people may experience stomach discomfort, reduced appetite, or itching.
- In theory, danshen may lower blood pressure and therefore it should be used cautiously by patients with blood pressure abnormalities or taking drugs that alter blood pressure.
- In theory, the chemical miltirone, which is present in danshen, may increase drowsiness. Caution is advised in people who are driving or operating machinery.

Pregnancy and Breastfeeding

- Danshen should be avoided during pregnancy and breastfeeding. In theory, the blood-thinning properties of danshen may increase the risk of miscarriage, and effects on the fetus or nursing infants are unknown.

INTERACTIONS

Most herbs and supplements have not been thoroughly tested for interactions with other herbs, supplements, drugs, or foods. The interactions listed here are based on reports in scientific publications, laboratory experiments, or traditional use. It is important to always read product labels. People who have a medical condition, or are taking other drugs, herbs, or supplements, should consult a qualified healthcare provider before starting a new therapy.

Interactions with Drugs

- Danshen may increase the risk of bleeding when it is taken with drugs that increase the risk of bleeding. This herb has been reported to inhibit platelet aggregation and to cause excessive anticoagulation (blood-thinning effects) in persons taking the blood thinner warfarin (Coumadin). Examples of drugs that increase the risk of bleeding are anticoagulants such as warfarin (Coumadin) and heparin, antiplatelet drugs such as clopidogrel (Plavix), aspirin, and nonsteroidal anti-inflammatory drugs such as ibuprofen (Motrin, Advil) and naproxen (Naprosyn, Aleve).
- In theory, the risk of side effects or toxicity from digoxin (Lanoxin) may be increased if this agent is taken with danshen. In addition, danshen may cause inaccurate (too high or too low) laboratory measurements of digoxin blood levels.
- Danshen may cause hypotension (dangerously low blood pressure) if it is taken with drugs that also lower blood pressure. Examples of such drugs are ACE-inhibitors such as captopril (Capoten) and lisinopril (Prinivil) and beta-blockers such as atenolol (Tenormin) and propranolol (Inderal). In addition, the use of danshen with beta-blockers may cause bradycardia (dangerously slow heart rate).
- In theory, the chemical miltirone, which is present in danshen, may increase sleepiness or other side effects associated with some drugs taken for anxiety or insomnia, such as lorazepam

(Ativan), alprazolam (Xanax), and diazepam (Valium), and alcohol. In addition, based on studies in animals, danshen may affect the absorption of alcohol in the blood.

Interactions with Herbs and Dietary Supplements

- Danshen may increase the risk of bleeding when taken with herbs and supplements that may also increase the risk of bleeding. Multiple cases of bleeding have been reported with the use of *Ginkgo biloba*, and fewer cases with garlic and saw palmetto. Numerous other agents may theoretically increase the risk of bleeding, although this has not been proven in most cases. Examples are alfalfa, American ginseng, angelica, anise, *Arnica montana*, asafetida, aspen bark, bilberry, birch, black cohosh, bladderwrack, bogbean, boldo, borage seed oil, bromelain, capsicum, cat's claw, celery, chamomile, chaparral, clove, coleus, cordyceps, devil's claw, dong quai, eicosapentaenoic acid (EPA), evening primrose oil, fenugreek, feverfew, fish oil, flaxseed/flax powder (not a concern with flaxseed oil), ginger, grapefruit juice, grape seed, green tea, guggul, gymnestra, horse chestnut, horseradish, licorice root, lovage root, male fern, meadowsweet, nordihydroguaiaretic acid (NDGA), omega-3 fatty acids, onion, *Panax ginseng*, papain, parsley, passion flower, poplar, prickly ash, propolis, quassia, red clover, reishi, rue, Siberian ginseng, sweet birch, sweet clover, turmeric, vitamin E, white willow, wild carrot, wild lettuce, willow, wintergreen, and yucca.

- In theory, danshen may add to the effects of other herbs with potential cardiac glycoside properties, potentially resulting in slow heart rate or toxicity. Examples of such agents are adonis, balloon cotton, black hellebore root/melampode, black Indian hemp, bushman's poison, cactus grandifloris, convallaria, eyebright, figwort, foxglove/digitalis, frangipani, hedge mustard, hemp root/Canadian hemp root, king's crown, lily-of-the-valley, motherwort, oleander leaf, pheasant's eye plant, plantain leaf, pleurisy root, psyllium husks, redheaded cotton-bush, rhubarb root, rubber vine, seamango, senna fruit, squill, strophanthus, uzara, wallflower, wintersweet, yellow dock root, and yellow oleander. Notably, bufalin/chan suis is a Chinese herbal formula that has been reported as toxic or fatal when taken with cardiac glycosides.

- Danshen should be used cautiously with herbs/supplements that may also lower blood pressure, such as aconite/ monkshood, arnica, baneberry, betel nut, bilberry, black cohosh, bryony, calendula, California poppy, coleus, curcumin, eucalyptol, eucalyptus oil, flaxseed/flaxseed oil, garlic, ginger, ginkgo, goldenseal, green hellebore, hawthorn, Indian tobacco, jaborandi, mistletoe, night-blooming cereus, oleander, pasque flower, periwinkle, pleurisy root, *Polypodium vulgare*, shepherd's purse, Texas milkweed, turmeric, and wild cherry.

- In theory, the chemical miltirone, which is present in danshen, can increase the amount of drowsiness that may be caused by other herbs or supplements, including calamus, calendula, California poppy, capsicum, catnip, celery, couchgrass, dogwood, elecampane, German chamomile, goldenseal, gotu kola, hops, kava (may help sleep without drowsiness), lavender aromatherapy, lemon balm, sage, sassafras, scullcap, shepherd's purse, Siberian ginseng, St. John's wort, stinging nettle, valerian, wild carrot, wild lettuce, withania root, and yerba mansa.

Selected References

Natural Standard developed the preceding evidence-based information based on a systematic review of more than 225 articles. For comprehensive information about alternative and complementary therapies on the professional level, go to www.naturalstandard.com. Selected references are listed here.

Brunetti G, Serra S, Vacca G, et al. IDN 5082, a standardized extract of *Salvia miltiorrhiza*, delays acquisition of alcohol drinking behavior in rats. J Ethnopharmacol 2003;85(1):93-97.

Cao CM, Xia Q, Zhang X, et al. *Salvia miltiorrhiza* attenuates the changes in contraction and intracellular calcium induced by anoxia and reoxygenation in rat cardiomyocytes. Life Sci 2003;72(22):2451-2463.

Chan TY. Interaction between warfarin and danshen (*Salvia miltiorrhiza*). Ann Pharmacother 2001;35(4):501-504.

Chen Y, Ruan Y, Li L, et al. Effects of *Salvia miltiorrhiza* extracts on rat hypoxic pulmonary hypertension, heme oxygenase-1 and nitric oxide synthase. Chin Med J (Engl) 2003;116(5):757-760.

Cheng TO. Warfarin danshen interaction. Ann Thorac Surg 1999;67(3):894.

Ji X, Tan BK, Zhu YC, et al. Comparison of cardioprotective effects using ramipril and DanShen for the treatment of acute myocardial infarction in rats. Life Sci 2003;73(11):1413-1426.

Kang DS, Chung HY, Byun DS, et al. Further isolation of antioxidative (+)-1-hydroxypinoresinol-1-*O*-beta-D-glucoside from the rhizome of *Salvia miltiorrhiza* that acts on peroxynitrite, total ROS and 1,1-diphenyl-2-picrylhydrazyl radical. Arch Pharm Res 2003;26(1):24-27.

Lay IS, Chiu JH, Shiao MS, et al. Crude extract of *Salvia miltiorrhiza* and salvianolic acid B enhance *in vitro* angiogenesis in murine SVR endothelial cell line. Planta Med 2003;69(1):26-32.

Lee TY, Mai LM, Wang GJ, et al. Protective mechanism of *Salvia miltiorrhiza* on carbon tetrachloride–induced acute hepatotoxicity in rats. J Pharmacol Sci 2003;91(3):202-210.

Liu GY. Analysis of effect of composite danshen droplet pills in treatment of chronic stable angina. Hubei J Trad Chin Med 1997;19(2):33-34.

Liu F, Liu Y, Li J. [Effects of danshen on solute transport by peritoneal dialysis.] Hunan Yi Ke Da Xue Xue Bao 1997;22(3):237-239.

Lo CJ, Lin JG, Kuo JS, et al. Effect of *Salvia miltiorrhiza* Bunge on cerebral infarct in ischemia-reperfusion injured rats. Am J Chin Med 2003;31(2):191-200.

Mashour NH, Lin GI, Frishman WH. Herbal medicine for the treatment of cardiovascular disease: clinical considerations. Arch Intern Med 1998;158(20): 2225-2234.

Sha Q, Cheng HZ, Xie XY. *Salviae miltiorrhizae* composita pill for treating 47 cases of active liver cirrhosis. Chin J Integrat Trad West Med Liver Dis 1999;9(6):50.

Vacca G, Colombo G, Brunetti G, et al. Reducing effect of *Salvia miltiorrhiza* extracts on alcohol intake: influence of vehicle. Phytother Res 2003;17(5): 537-541.

Wu CT, Mulabagal V, Nalawade SM, et al. Isolation and quantitative analysis of cryptotanshinone, an active quinoid diterpene formed in callus of *Salvia miltiorrhiza* BUNGE. Biol Pharm Bull 2003;26(6):845-848.

Yagi A, Takeo S. [Anti-inflammatory constituents, aloesin and aloemannan in Aloe species and effects of tanshinon VI in Salvia miltiorrhiza on heart.] Yakugaku Zasshi 2003;123(7):517-532.

Devil's Claw
(*Harpagophytum procumbens*)

SYNONYMS/COMMON NAMES/RELATED SUBSTANCES

- Algophytum, Arthrosetten H, Arthrotabs, Artigel, Artosan, Defencid, Devil's Claw Capsule, Devil's Claw Secondary Root, Devil's Claw Vegicaps, Doloteffin, duiwelsklou, Fitokey Harpagophytum, grapple plant, *griffe du diable*, Harpadol, Hariosen, HarpagoMega, Harpagon, harpagophyti radix, *Harpagophytum zeyheri*, Jucurba N, Pedaliaceae, Rheuma-Sern, Rheuma-Tee, Salus, sengaparile, sudafrikanische, teufelskralle, trampelklette, venustorn, Windhoek's root, wood spider.
- **Multi-ingredient preparations containing devil's claw root:** Arktophytum, Arthritic Pain Herbal Formula, Devil's Claw Plus, Lifesystem Herbal Formula 1 Arthritic Aid, Lifesystem Herbal Formula 12 Willowbark, Prost-1, green-lipped mussel (FM).

CLINICAL BOTTOM LINE
Background

- The medicinal ingredient of devil's claw (*Harpagophytum procumbens*) is extracted from the dried tuberous roots of the plant, which originated in the Kalahari and savannah desert regions of South and Southeast Africa, where it has historically been used to treat a wide range of conditions including fever, malaria, and indigestion.
- Currently, the major clinical uses of devil's claw are as an anti-inflammatory and analgesic (pain reliever) for joint diseases, back pain, and headache. Initial evidence from scientific studies in animals and humans has been popularized and has resulted in widespread use of standardized devil's claw as a mild analgesic for joint pain in Europe. Scientific evaluation is lacking regarding its effectiveness as an appetite stimulant or liver tonic, but it is widely used for these purposes as well.
- Potential side effects include gastrointestinal upset, hypotension (low blood pressure) and arrhythmic (abnormal) heartbeat. Devil's claw may have chronotropic (increased heart rate) and inotropic (increased heart squeezing) effects.
- Traditionally, it has been recommended to avoid using devil's claw in people with gastric or duodenal ulcers and in those using anticoagulants (blood thinners). Clinical data to substantiate these recommendations are insufficient.

Uses Based on Scientific Evidence	Grade*
Osteoarthritis A small amount of research reports that devil's claw may be effective for treating pain and for improving mobility in individuals with osteoarthritis (particularly affecting the hip or knee). These studies suggest that the use of devil's claw may allow the dose of pain medications to be reduced. However, there are problems with the design and reporting of these trials, and better research is needed before a firm conclusion can be drawn.	B

Low back pain The results of several studies in humans of devil's claw for low back pain were conflicting, and additional research is needed to provide clearer answers.	C

*Key to grades: *A:* Strong scientific evidence for this use; *B:* Good scientific evidence for this use; *C:* Unclear scientific evidence for this use; *D:* Fair scientific evidence against this use (it may not work); *F:* Strong scientific evidence against this use (it likely does not work). For a more detailed explanation of efficacy criteria, see "Natural Standard Evidence-Based Validated Grading Rationale" in the Introduction.

Historical or Theoretical Indications That Lack Sufficient Evidence

Allergies, anti-inflammatory, antioxidant, appetite stimulant, arrhythmias, atherosclerosis (clogged arteries), bitter tonic, blood diseases, boils (used topically), childbirth difficulties, choleretic (bile secretion), constipation, diabetes, diarrhea, diuretic, dyspepsia, edema, fever, fibromyalgia, flatulence (gas), gastrointestinal disorders, gout, headache, heartburn, high cholesterol, hip pain, indigestion, irregular heartbeat, knee pain, liver and gallbladder tonic, loss of appetite, malaria, menopausal symptoms, menstrual cramps, migraines, muscle pain, nerve pain, nicotine poisoning, pain, rheumatoid arthritis, sedative, skin cancer (used topically), skin ulcers (used topically), sores (used topically), spasmolytic, tendonitis, urinary tract infections, wound healing for skin injuries (used topically).

DOSING/TOXICOLOGY

The following doses are based on scientific research, publications, traditional use, or expert opinion. Many herbs and supplements have not been thoroughly tested, and their safety and effectiveness may not be proven. Brands may be made differently, with variable ingredients even within the same brand. The doses shown may not apply to all products. It is important to always read product labels and discuss doses with a qualified healthcare provider before therapy is started.

Standardization

- Standardization involves measuring the amounts of certain chemicals in products to try to make different products similar to each other. It is not always known if the chemicals being measured are the "active" ingredients. Devil's claw products may be standardized to contain a specific amount of harpagoside and often contain greater than 1% to 2% harpagoside. Some studies have used a special preparation called WS 1531, which contains 8.5% harpagoside.

Adults (18 Years and Older)

- **Tablets:** A dose of 600 to 1200 mg (standardized to contain 50 to 100 mg of harpagoside) by mouth three times daily has been used in studies of therapy for joint and muscle problems.
- **Dried root:** A dose of 0.5 to 1.5 g by mouth three times daily in an aqueous (water-based) solution has been used traditionally for appetite loss and stomach discomfort.

- **Tincture:** A dose of 0.2 to 1 ml (1:5 in 25% alcohol) by mouth three times daily has been used traditionally. A dose of 3 ml (1:10 in 25% alcohol) by mouth three times daily has also been used traditionally.
- **Fluid extract:** A dose of 0.25 to 1.5 ml (1:1 in 25% alcohol) by mouth three times daily has been used traditionally.

Children (Younger Than 18 Years)
- The dosing and safety of devil's claw have not been studied thoroughly in children, and safety is not established.

SAFETY

The U.S. Food and Drug Administration does not strictly regulate herbs and supplements. There is no guarantee of the strength, purity, or safety of products, and effects may vary. It is important to always read product labels. People who have a medical condition, or are taking other drugs, herbs, or supplements, should consult a qualified healthcare provider before starting a new therapy. A healthcare provider should be contacted immediately about any side effects.

Allergies
- People with allergies to *Harpagophytum procumbens* should avoid devil's claw products.

Side Effects and Warnings
- At recommended doses, devil's claw traditionally is believed to be well tolerated. However, there are published reports of headache, ringing in the ears, loss of taste and appetite, and diarrhea in those taking this herb. Whether the use of devil's claw for longer than 3 to 4 months is safe or effective is unknown.
- Devil's claw may change the rate and force of heartbeats (chronotropic and inotropic effects). People with heart disease or arrhythmias (abnormal heart rhythms) should consult their cardiologist or qualified healthcare provider before taking devil's claw. Devil's claw may affect levels of acid in the gastrointestinal tract and should be avoided by people with gastric (stomach) or duodenal (intestinal) ulcers. Devil's claw should be used cautiously in people with gallstones.
- In theory, devil's claw may lower blood sugar levels. Caution is advised in people with diabetes or hypoglycemia and in those taking drugs, other herbs, or supplements that affect blood sugar levels. Serum glucose levels may need to be monitored by a healthcare provider, and medication adjustments may be necessary.
- In theory, devil's claw may increase the risk of bleeding. Caution is advised in people with bleeding disorders or those taking drugs that may increase the risk of bleeding. Dosing adjustments may be necessary. People may need to stop taking devil's claw before some surgeries and should discuss this with their primary healthcare provider.
- Devil's claw products may be contaminated with other herbs or with pesticides, herbicides, heavy metals, or drugs.

Pregnancy and Breastfeeding
- Devil's claw may stimulate contractions of the uterus and cannot be recommended during pregnancy and breastfeeding. People should be aware that many tinctures contain high levels of alcohol and should be avoided during pregnancy.

INTERACTIONS

Most herbs and supplements have not been thoroughly tested for interactions with other herbs, supplements, drugs, or foods. The interactions listed here are based on reports in scientific publications, laboratory experiments, or traditional use. It is important to always read product labels. People who have a medical condition, or are taking other drugs, herbs, or supplements, should consult a qualified healthcare provider before starting a new therapy.

Interactions with Drugs
- Devil's claw may lower blood sugar levels. Caution is advised in people who are using medications that may also lower blood sugar levels. Persons taking drugs for diabetes by mouth or insulin closely should be monitored by a qualified healthcare provider, and medication adjustments may be necessary.
- In theory, devil's claw may have an additive effect when taken with drugs used for pain, inflammation, high cholesterol, and gout. Devil's claw may add to the effects of drugs that reduce cholesterol levels. Devil's claw may also increase stomach acidity and therefore may affect drugs used to decrease the amount of acid in the stomach, such as antacids, esomeprazole (Nexium), ranitidine (Zantac), and sucralfate. People who are taking any of these drugs should consult their healthcare provider and pharmacist before taking devil's claw.
- Because devil's claw may affect heart rhythm, heart rate, and the force of heartbeats, individuals taking prescription drugs such as antiarrhythmics and digoxin (Lanoxin) should consult their healthcare provider before taking devil's claw.
- In theory, devil's claw may increase the risk of bleeding when taken with drugs that increase the risk of bleeding. Examples are anticoagulants (blood thinners) such as warfarin (Coumadin) and heparin, antiplatelet drugs such as clopidogrel (Plavix), aspirin, and nonsteroidal anti-inflammatory drugs such as ibuprofen (Motrin, Advil) and naproxen (Naprosyn, Aleve).

Interactions with Herbs and Dietary Supplements
- In theory, devil's claw may lower blood sugar levels. Caution is advised in people who are using herbs or supplements that may also lower blood sugar levels. Blood glucose levels may require monitoring, and doses may need adjustment. Examples of herbs that may lower blood sugar levels are *Aloe vera*, American ginseng, bilberry, bitter melon, burdock, fenugreek, fish oil, gymnema, horse chestnut seed extract (HCSE), maitake mushroom, marshmallow, milk thistle, *Panax ginseng*, rosemary, shark cartilage, Siberian ginseng, stinging nettle, and white horehound. Agents that may raise blood sugar levels include arginine, cocoa, and ephedra (when combined with caffeine). In theory, devil's claw may interfere with other herbs and dietary supplements that affect heart rhythm, heart rate, and the force of heartbeats. Potential cardiac glycoside herbs and supplements include adonis, balloon cotton, black hellebore root/melampode, black Indian hemp, bushman's poison, cactus grandifloris, convallaria, eyebright, figwort, foxglove/digitalis, frangipani, hedge mustard, hemp root/Canadian hemp root, king's crown, lily-of-the-valley, motherwort, oleander leaf, pheasant's eye plant, plantain leaf, pleurisy root, psyllium husks, redheaded cotton-bush, rhubarb root, rubber vine, seamango, senna fruit, squill, strophanthus, uzara, wallflower, wintersweet, yellow dock root, and yellow oleander. Notably, bufalin/chan suis is a Chinese herbal formula that has been reported as toxic or fatal when taken with cardiac glycosides.
- Devil's claw may affect herbs and dietary supplements that are used for pain, inflammation, high cholesterol, and gout.

Because devil's claw may increase stomach acidity, it may affect herbs and supplements used to decrease the amount of acid in the stomach.

- Devil's claw may increase the risk of bleeding when taken with herbs and supplements that may also increase the risk of bleeding. Multiple cases of bleeding have been reported with the use of *Ginkgo biloba*, and fewer cases with garlic and saw palmetto. Numerous other agents may theoretically increase the risk of bleeding, although this has not been proven in most cases. Examples are alfalfa, American ginseng, angelica, anise, *Arnica montana*, asafetida, aspen bark, bilberry, birch, black cohosh, bladderwrack, bogbean, boldo, borage seed oil, bromelain, capsicum, cat's claw, celery, chamomile, chaparral, clove, coleus, cordyceps, danshen, dong quai, eicosapentaenoic acid (EPA), evening primrose oil, fenugreek, feverfew, fish oil, flaxseed/flax powder (not a concern with flaxseed oil), ginger, grapefruit juice, grape seed, green tea, guggul, gymnestra, horse chestnut, horseradish, licorice root, lovage root, male fern, meadowsweet, nordihydroguaiaretic acid (NDGA), omega-3 fatty acids, onion, *Panax ginseng*, papain, parsley, passion flower, poplar, prickly ash, propolis, quassia, red clover, reishi, rue, Siberian ginseng, sweet birch, sweet clover, turmeric, vitamin E, white willow, wild carrot, wild lettuce, willow, wintergreen, and yucca.

Selected References

Natural Standard developed the preceding evidence-based information based on a systematic review of more than 75 articles. For comprehensive information about alternative and complementary therapies on the professional level, go to www.naturalstandard.com. Selected references are listed here.

Chantre P, Cappelaere A, Leblan D, et al. Efficacy and tolerance of *Harpagophytum procumbens* versus diacerhein in treatment of osteoarthritis. Phytomedicine 2000;7(3):177-183.

Chrubasik S, Zimpfer C, Schutt U, et al. Effectiveness of *Harpagophytum procumbens* in treatment of acute low back pain. Phytomedicine 1996;3(1):1-10.

Chrubasik S, Junck H, Conradt C, et al. Effectiveness of oral *Harpagophytum* extract WS 1531 in treating low back pain [abstract]. Arthr Rheum 1998; 41(Suppl 9):S261.

Chrubasik S, Junck H, Breitschwerdt H, et al. Effectiveness of *Harpagophytum* extract WS 1531 in the treatment of exacerbation of low back pain: a randomized, placebo-controlled, double-blind study. Eur J Anaesthesiol 1999; 16(2):118-129.

Chrubasik S, Junck H, Breitschwerdt H, et al. Effectiveness of *Harpagophytum* extract WS 1531 in the treatment of exacerbation of low back pain: a randomized, placebo-controlled, double-blind study. Eur J Anaesthesiol 1999; 16(2):118-129.

Chrubasik S, Sporer F, Dillmann-Marschner R, et al. Physicochemical properties of harpagoside and its *in vitro* release from *Harpagophytum procumbens* extract tablets. Phytomedicine 2000;6(6):469-473.

Chrubasik S, Künzel O, Thanner J, et al. A short-term follow-up after a randomised double-blind pilot study comparing Doloteffin vs Rofecoxib for low back pain. 9th Annual Symposium on Complementary Health Care, Exeter, UK, 2002.

Chrubasik S, Model A, Ullmann H, et al. Doloteffin vs Vioxx for low back pain—a randomized, double-blind pilot study. Focus Altern Complement Ther 2002; 7:90.

Chrubasik S, Fiebich B, Black A, et al. Treating low back pain with an extract of *Harpagophytum procumbens* that inhibits cytokine release. Eur J Anaesthesiol 2002;19:209.

Chrubasik S, Pollak S, Black A. Effectiveness of devil's claw for osteoarthritis. Rheumatology (Oxford) 2002;41(11):1332-1333.

Chrubasik S, Thanner J, Kunzel O, et al. Comparison of outcome measures during treatment with the proprietary *Harpagophytum* extract doloteffin in patients with pain in the lower back, knee or hip. Phytomedicine 2002;9(3):181-194.

Chrubasik S, Pollak S. Pain management with herbal antirheumatic drugs. Wien Med Wochenschr 2002; 152(7-8):198-203.

Ernst E, Chrubasik S. Phyto-anti-inflammatories: a systematic review of randomized, placebo-controlled, double-blind trials. Rheum Dis Clin North Am 2000;26(1):13-27.

Grahame R, Robinson BV. Devil's claw (*Harpagophytum procumbens*): pharmacological and clinical studies. Ann Rheum Dis 1981;40(6):632.

Guyader M. Les plantes antirhumatismales. Etude historique et pharmacologique, et etude clinique du nebulisat d'*Harpagophytum procumbens* DC chez 50 patients arthrosiques suivis en service hospitalier [Dissertation]. Paris, Universite Pierre et Marie Curie, 1984.

Leblan D, Chantre P, Fournie B. *Harpagophytum procumbens* in the treatment of knee and hip osteoarthritis: four-month results of a prospective, multicenter, double-blind trial versus diacerhein. Joint Bone Spine 2000;67(5):462-467.

Lecomte A, Costa JP. *Harpagophytum* dans l'arthrose: Etude en double insu contre placebo. Le Magazine 1992;15:27-30.

Munkombwe NM. Acetylated phenolic glycosides from *Harpagophytum procumbens*. Phytochemistry 2003;62(8):1231-1234.

DHEA
(Dehydroepiandrosterone)

SYNONYMS/COMMON NAMES/RELATED SUBSTANCES

- 5-androsten-3-β-ol-17-one Atlantic yam, barbasco, China root, colic root, dehydroepiandrosterone sulfate, devil's bones, DHEA-S, dioscorea, *Dioscorea composita*, *Dioscorea floribunda*, *Dioscorea macrostachya*, *Dioscorea mexicana*, *Dioscorea villosa*, Mexican yam, natural DHEA, phytoestrogen, Prasterone, rheumatism root, wild Mexican yam, yam, yuma.
- **Combination products/trade names:** Born Again's DHEA Eyelift Serum, DHEA Men's Formula, DHEA with Antioxidants 25 mg, DHEA with Bioperine 50 mg.
- *Note*: DHEA can be synthesized in the laboratory using wild yam extract. However, it is believed that wild yam cannot be converted by the body into DHEA. Therefore, information citing wild yam as "natural DHEA" may be inaccurate.

CLINICAL BOTTOM LINE
Background

- DHEA (dehydroepiandrosterone) is an endogenous hormone (made in the human body), and secreted by the adrenal glands. DHEA serves as a precursor to male and female sex hormones (androgens and estrogens). DHEA levels in the body begin to decrease after age 30, and are reported to be low in some people with anorexia, end-stage kidney disease, type 2 diabetes (non-insulin dependent diabetes), AIDS, adrenal insufficiency, and in the critically ill. DHEA levels may also be depleted by a number of drugs, including insulin, corticosteroids, opiates, and danazol.
- No studies of the long-term effects of DHEA have been conducted. DHEA can cause higher than normal levels of androgens and estrogens in the body and theoretically may increase the risk of prostate, breast, ovarian, and other hormone-sensitive cancers. Therefore, it is not recommended for regular use without supervision by a qualified healthcare provider.

Uses Based on Scientific Evidence	Grade*
Adrenal insufficiency Several studies suggest that DHEA may improve well-being, quality of life, exercise capacity, sex drive, and hormone levels in people with insufficient adrenal function (Addison's disease). These studies have been small, and better research is needed to provide more definitive answers. Adrenal insufficiency is a serious medical condition and should be treated under the supervision of a qualified healthcare provider.	C
Atherosclerosis (cholesterol plaques in the arteries) Initial studies report possible benefits of DHEA supplementation in patients with cholesterol plaques in the arteries (hardening of the arteries). However, other, more proven therapies are available, and people with high cholesterol, atherosclerosis, or heart disease should discuss treatment options with their primary healthcare provider.	C
Bone density The ability of DHEA to increase bone density is under investigation. Effects are unclear at this time.	C
Cervical dysplasia Initial research studies suggest that the use of intravaginal DHEA is safe and promotes regression of low-grade cervical lesions. However, further study is necessary in this area before a firm conclusion can be drawn. Patients should not substitute the use of DHEA for better-established therapies, and should discuss management options and follow-up with their primary healthcare provider or a gynecologist.	C
Chronic fatigue syndrome Scientific evidence is unclear regarding the effects of DHEA supplementation in patients with chronic fatigue syndrome. Better-quality research is necessary before a clear conclusion can be drawn.	C
Critical illness Scientific evidence is unclear regarding the safety and effectiveness of DHEA supplementation in critically ill patients. At this time, it is recommended that severe illness in the intensive care unit be treated with better-established therapies.	C
Crohn's disease Initial research studies suggested that DHEA supplements are safe for short-term use in patients with Crohn's disease. Preliminary trials suggest possible beneficial effects, but additional research is necessary before a clear conclusion can be drawn.	C
Depression Results of studies on the use of DHEA supplements for depression are conflicting, with some results suggesting benefits, and others reporting no effects. Better-quality research is necessary before a clear conclusion can be drawn.	C
Heart failure There is conflicting scientific evidence regarding the use of DHEA supplements in patients with heart failure or diminished ejection fraction. Other, more proven therapies are available in this area, and people with heart failure or other types of heart disease should discuss treatment options with their primary healthcare provider or a cardiologist.	C
HIV/AIDS Although some studies suggest that DHEA supplementation may be beneficial in patents with HIV, results from different studies do not agree. Most research in this area was not well designed or reported. There is currently not enough scientific evidence to recommend DHEA for this condition, and other, more proven therapies are available in this area.	C

Continued

Menopausal disorders Many different aspects of menopause have been studied using DHEA as a treatment. When DHEA is applied topically (on the skin) as a cream, it may lessen vaginal pain and discomfort associated with menopause. However, it is not clear whether DHEA cream has any benefits in treating osteoporosis after menopause. Early evidence suggests that DHEA is not an effective treatment for hot flashes or emotional disturbances such as fatigue, irritability, anxiety, depression, insomnia, difficulties with concentration, memory, or decreased sex drive (which may occur at the time of menopause).	C
Muscle mass/body DHEA has been studied for improving body mass index, decreasing body fat, and increasing muscle mass. Early research reports that muscle mass is not increased when adding DHEA supplements to compensate for the natural decrease in dehydroepiandrosterone levels that occurs with aging (in otherwise healthy adults). It is not known if there are medical conditions in which DHEA supplementation might contribute to the preservation or improvement of muscle mass.	C
Myotonic dystrophy There is conflicting scientific evidence regarding the use of DHEA supplements for myotonic dystrophy. Better-quality research is necessary before a clear conclusion can be drawn.	C
Ovulation disorders Low-quality studies suggest that DHEA supplementation may be beneficial in women with ovulation disorders. However, results of research in this area are conflicting, and safety is not established. Currently, there is insufficient scientific evidence to form a clear conclusion about the use of DHEA for this condition.	C
Schizophrenia Initial research studies suggest benefits of DHEA supplementation in the management of negative, depressive, and anxiety symptoms of schizophrenia. Further study is needed to confirm these results before a firm conclusion can be drawn.	C
Septicemia (serious bacterial infections in the blood) Scientific evidence is unclear concerning the safety and effectiveness of DHEA supplementation in patients with septicemia. Other, more proven therapies are available.	C
Sexual function/libido/erectile dysfunction The results of studies vary on the benefits of use of DHEA in erectile dysfunction and sexual function in both men and women. Better-quality research is necessary before a clear conclusion can be drawn.	C
Systemic lupus erythematosus (SLE) Most studies on DHEA supplementation in people with SLE have not been well designed or reported. The results of various studies do not agree, with some	C

results suggesting benefits, and others reporting no effects. Better-quality research is necessary before a clear conclusion can be drawn.	
Alzheimer's disease Initial studies suggest that DHEA does not significantly improve cognitive performance or change symptom severity in people with Alzheimer's disease. Additional research is warranted in this area.	D
Brain function and well-being in the elderly Some textbooks and review articles suggest that DHEA supplements may improve brain function, memory, and overall feelings of well-being in the elderly. However, most studies reported no benefits. Additional study is warranted in this area.	D
Immune system stimulant It is suggested in some textbooks and review articles that DHEA may stimulate the immune system. However, current scientific evidence does not support this claim.	D

*Key to grades: *A:* Strong scientific evidence for this use; *B:* Good scientific evidence for this use; *C:* Unclear scientific evidence for this use; *D:* Fair scientific evidence against this use (it may not work); *F:* Strong scientific evidence against this use (it likely does not work). For a more detailed explanation of efficacy criteria, see "Natural Standard Evidence-Based Validated Grading Rationale" in the Introduction.

Historical or Theoretical Indications That Lack Sufficient Evidence

Aging, allergic disorders, amenorrhea associated with anorexia, andropause/andrenopause, angioedema, anxiety, asthma, bone diseases, bone loss associated with anorexia, bladder cancer, breast cancer, burns, colon cancer, dementia, diabetes, heart attack, high cholesterol, Huntington's disease, influenza, joint diseases, lipodystrophy in HIV, liver protection, malaria, malnutrition, movement disorders, multiple sclerosis, obesity, osteoporosis, pancreatic cancer, Parkinson's disease, performance enhancement, polycystic ovarian syndrome, post-traumatic stress disorder (PTSD), premenstrual syndrome, prostate cancer, psoriasis, Raynaud's phenomenon, rheumatic diseases, skin graft healing, sleep disorders, stress, tetanus, ulcerative colitis, viral encephalitis, weight loss.

DOSING/TOXICOLOGY

The following doses are based on scientific research, publications, traditional use, or expert opinion. Many herbs and supplements have not been thoroughly tested, and their safety and effectiveness may not be proven. Brands may be made differently, with variable ingredients even within the same brand. The doses shown may not apply to all products. It is important to always read product labels and discuss doses with a qualified healthcare provider before therapy is started.

Standardization

- Standardization involves measuring the amounts of certain chemicals in products to try to make different preparations similar to each other. It is not always known if the chemicals being measured are the "active" ingredients.
- *Note:* Some products are micronized and compounded with polyunsaturates. Information on the safety of long-term use of DHEA supplements is not available.

Adults (18 Years and Older)
Oral (Capsules/Tablets)

- **Addison's disease:** A dose of 50 mg taken daily has been used for Addison's disease/adrenal insufficiency. Adrenal insufficiency is a serious medical condition and should be treated under the supervision of a qualified healthcare provider.
- **Depression:** A dose of 30 to 90 mg taken daily has been used for depression. Higher doses of 200 to 500 mg per day have been studied for depression in HIV/AIDS.
- **Crohn's disease/ulcerative colitis:** A dose of 200 mg taken daily has been used in a small pilot study of therapy for Crohn's disease and ulcerative colitis.
- **Systemic lupus erythematosus (SLE):** Doses of 50 to 200 mg taken daily have been used in multiple studies for treatment of SLE.

Intravenous Administration

- **Dementia (multi-infarct):** A dose of 200 mg taken daily has been studied for multi-infarct dementia given intravenously. Safety is not established.

Topical (Cream)

- **Menopausal symptoms:** A cream containing 10% DHEA was applied on an area 20 cm by 20 cm on both thighs once daily for vaginal discomfort associated with menopause.

Children (Younger Than 18 Years)

- The dosing and safety of DHEA have not been well studied in children. In theory, DHEA may interfere with normal hormone balance and growth in children.

SAFETY

The U.S. Food and Drug Administration does not strictly regulate herbs and supplements. There is no guarantee of the strength, purity, or safety of products, and effects may vary. It is important to always read product labels. People who have a medical condition, or are taking other drugs, herbs, or supplements, should consult a qualified healthcare provider before starting a new therapy. A healthcare provider should be contacted immediately about any side effects.

Allergies

- People who are allergic to any DHEA product should avoid the use of all DHEA products.

Side Effects and Warnings

- Few side effects have been reported when DHEA supplements have been taken by mouth in recommended doses. The most common complaints include fatigue, nasal congestion, and headache. Rarely, rapid/irregular heartbeats or palpitations have been reported. People taking DHEA supplements may have a higher risk of developing blood clots or liver damage, although these effects have not been widely studied in humans. Individuals with a history of abnormal heart rhythms, blood clots, or hypercoagulability, and those with a history of liver disease, should avoid DHEA supplements.
- Because DHEA is a hormone related to other male and female hormones, there may be side effects related to its hormonal activities. For example, masculinization may occur in women, including acne, increased facial hair, hair loss, increased sweating, weight gain around the waist, and development of a deeper voice. Likewise, men may develop more prominent breasts (gynecomastia) and breast tenderness. Men may also experience increased blood pressure, testicular wasting, and increased aggressiveness.

- DHEA supplementation may alter the production or balance of various other hormones in the body. Possible hormone-related side effects include increased blood sugar levels, insulin resistance, altered cholesterol levels, altered thyroid hormone levels, and altered adrenal function. Caution is advised in persons with diabetes or hyperglycemia, high cholesterol, thyroid disorders, and other endocrine (hormonal) abnormalities. Serum glucose, cholesterol, and thyroid levels may need to be monitored by a healthcare provider, and medication adjustments may be necessary.
- In theory, DHEA may increase the risk of developing prostate, breast, and ovarian cancer. Based on laboratory research, DHEA may contribute to tamoxifen resistance in persons with breast cancer. Other possible side effects include insomnia, agitation, delusions, mania, nervousness, irritability, and psychosis.
- High DHEA levels have been correlated with Cushing's syndrome, which may be caused by excessive supplementation.

Pregnancy and Breastfeeding

- DHEA is not recommended during pregnancy or breastfeeding. Because DHEA is a hormone, it may be unsafe for the fetus or nursing infant. DHEA has caused abortions in studies of rats.

INTERACTIONS

Most herbs and supplements have not been thoroughly tested for interactions with other herbs, supplements, drugs, or foods. The interactions listed here are based on reports in scientific publications, laboratory experiments, or traditional use. It is important to always read product labels. People who have a medical condition, or are taking other drugs, herbs, or supplements, should consult a qualified healthcare provider before starting a new therapy.

Interactions with Drugs

- Laboratory research and studies in animals suggest that DHEA may interfere with how the body uses the liver's cytochrome P450 enzyme system to process components of some drugs. As a result, blood levels of these components may be elevated and may cause increased effects or potentially serious adverse reactions. Central nervous system agents, including carbamazepine and phenytoin, induce the P450 enzymes that metabolize DHEA and DHEA-S and therefore can decrease circulating concentrations of these hormones. People who are using any medications should always read the package insert and consult their healthcare provider or pharmacist about possible interactions.
- Based on data from studies in humans, DHEA may increase blood sugar levels. Caution is advised in people who are using medications that may also lower blood sugar levels such as metformin (Glucophage). In postmenopausal women, DHEA (1600 mg daily by mouth for 28 days) has been shown to cause insulin resistance. People who are taking drugs for diabetes by mouth or insulin should be closely monitored by a qualified healthcare provider. Medication adjustments may be necessary.
- In theory, DHEA may increase the risk of blood clotting. Persons who are taking anticoagulants (blood thinners) or antiplatelet drugs (such as aspirin) to prevent blood clots should discuss the use of DHEA with their healthcare provider. Examples of blood-thinning drugs are clopidogrel (Plavix), heparin, and warfarin (Coumadin). The risk of blood clots is also increased by smoking and by taking other hormones (such as oral contraceptives or hormone

replacement therapy), and these hormones should not be combined with DHEA except under medical supervision.

- DHEA may alter heart rates or rhythm, and should be used cautiously with heart medications or drugs that may also affect heart rhythm.

- Although studies in this area have been limited, there are some reports that drugs such as amlodipine, nicardipine and other calcium channel blockers (e.g., diltiazem [Cardizem] and alprazolam [Xanax]) may increase DHEA levels in the body, which may lead to increased side effects when taken with DHEA supplements. In theory, increased hormone levels may occur if DHEA is used with estrogen or androgen hormonal therapies. DHEA may interact with psychiatric drugs such as clozapine (Clozaril).

- DHEA may interact with GABA-receptor drugs used for seizures or pain. Studies in animals suggest that DHEA may decrease the effectiveness of methadone and may add to the effects of clofibrate. Laboratory research studies reported that DHEA may contribute to tamoxifen resistance in breast cancer.

- Drugs that reduce the normal levels of DHEA produced by the body include dopamine, insulin, corticosteroids such as dexamethasone, drugs used to treat endometriosis such as danazol, opiate pain-killers, and estrogen-containing drugs. Metopirone and benfluorex may increase blood DHEA levels.

Interactions with Herbs and Dietary Supplements

- Laboratory research and studies in animals suggest that DHEA may interfere with how the body uses the liver's cytochrome P450 enzyme system to process components of other herbs and supplements. As a result, blood levels of these components may be elevated. DHEA may alter the effects that other herbs have on the cytochrome P450 system. Examples of such herbs are bloodroot, cat's claw, chamomile, chaparral, chasteberry, damiana, *Echinacea angustifolia*, goldenseal, grapefruit juice, licorice, oregano, red clover, St. John's wort, wild cherry, and yucca. People who are using any medications should always read the package insert and consult their healthcare provider and pharmacist about possible interactions.

- DHEA may raise blood sugar levels or cause insulin resistance, and may add to the effects of herbs/supplements that may also increase blood sugar levels, such as arginine, cocoa, ephedra (when combined with caffeine), and melatonin. DHEA may work against the effects of herbs/supplements that may decrease blood sugar levels, such as *Aloe vera*, American ginseng, bilberry, bitter melon, burdock, fenugreek, fish oil, gymnema, horse chestnut seed extract (HCSE), maitake mushroom, marshmallow, milk thistle, *Panax ginseng*, rosemary, shark cartilage, Siberian ginseng, stinging nettle, and white horehound. Serum glucose levels in people with diabetes who are using DHEA should be monitored closely by a qualified healthcare provider. Dosing adjustments may be necessary.

- In theory, DHEA may increase the risk of blood clotting and may add to the effects of herbs and supplements that may also increase the risk of clotting, such as coenzyme Q10 and *Panax ginseng*. DHEA may work against the effects of herbs and supplements that may have blood-thinning effects and may reduce the risk of clotting. Examples of such herbs are alfalfa, American ginseng, angelica, anise, *Arnica montana*, asafetida, aspen bark, bilberry, birch, black cohosh, bladderwrack, bogbean, boldo, borage seed oil, bromelain, capsicum, cat's claw, celery, chamomile, chaparral, coleus, clove, cordyceps, danshen, devil's claw, dong quai, eicosapentaenoic acid (EPA), evening primrose oil, fenugreek, feverfew, fish oil, flaxseed/flax powder (not a concern with flaxseed oil), garlic, ginger, *Ginkgo biloba*, grapefruit juice, grape seed, green tea, guggul, gymnestra, horse chestnut, horseradish, licorice root, lovage root, male fern, meadowsweet, nordihydroguaiaretic acid (NDGA), omega-3 fatty acids, onion, *Panax ginseng*, papain, parsley, passion flower, poplar, prickly ash, propolis, quassia, red clover, reishi, rue, saw palmetto, Siberian ginseng, sweet birch, sweet clover, turmeric, vitamin E, white willow, wild carrot, wild lettuce, willow, wintergreen, and yucca.

- It is not known what effects occur when DHEA is used with herbs that may have hormonal effects in the body. Examples of agents with possible estrogen-like (phytoestrogenic) effects in the body are alfalfa, black cohosh, bloodroot, burdock, hops, kudzu, licorice, pomegranate, red clover, soy, thyme, white horehound, and yucca. Agents with possible progestin-like (phytoprogestational) effects in the body include bloodroot, chasteberry, damiana, oregano, and yucca.

- DHEA may alter heart rates and rhythms. Caution is advised in people who are taking herbs or supplements that may alter heart function or that contain cardiac glycosides. Examples are adonis, balloon cotton, black hellebore root/melampode, black Indian hemp, bushman's poison, cactus grandifloris, convallaria, eyebright, figwort, foxglove/digitalis, frangipani, hedge mustard, hemp root/Canadian hemp root, king's crown, lily-of-the-valley, motherwort, oleander leaf, pheasant's eye plant, plantain leaf, pleurisy root; psyllium husks, redheaded cotton-bush, rhubarb root, rubber vine, sea-mango, senna fruit, squill, strophanthus, uzara, wallflower, wintersweet, yellow dock root, and yellow oleander. Notably, bufalin/chan suis is a Chinese herbal formula that has been reported as toxic or fatal when taken with other agents that may alter conduction properties of the heart.

- Chromium picolinate may increase blood DHEA levels. Carnitine combined with DHEA may have additive effects. Studies in animals suggest that DHEA may increase melatonin secretion and prevent breakdown of vitamin E in the body.

Selected References

Natural Standard developed the preceding evidence-based information based on a systematic review of more than 800 articles. For comprehensive information about alternative and complementary therapies on the professional level, go to www.naturalstandard.com. Selected references are listed here.

Achermann JC, Silverman BL. Dehydroepiandrosterone replacement for patients with adrenal insufficiency. Lancet 2001;357(9266):1381-1382.

Andus T, Klebl F, Rogler G, et al. Patients with refractory Crohn's disease or ulcerative colitis respond to dehydroepiandrosterone: a pilot study. Aliment Pharmacol Ther 2003;17(3):409-414.

Angold A. Adolescent depression, cortisol and DHEA. Psychol Med 2003;33(4):573-581.

Arlt W, Callies F, Allolio B. DHEA replacement in women with adrenal insufficiency—pharmacokinetics, bioconversion and clinical effects on well-being, sexuality and cognition. Endocr Res 2000;26(4):505-511.

Arlt W, Callies F, Koehler I, et al. Dehydroepiandrosterone supplementation in healthy men with an age-related decline of dehydroepiandrosterone secretion. J Clin Endocrinol Metab 2001;86(10):4686-4692.

Arlt W, Callies F, van Vlijmen JC, et al. Dehydroepiandrosterone replacement in women with adrenal insufficiency. N Engl J Med 1999;341(14):1013-1020.

Arlt W, Haas J, Callies F, et al. Biotransformation of oral dehydroepiandrosterone in elderly men: significant increase in circulating estrogens. J Clin Endocrinol Metab 1999;84(6):2170-2176.

Arlt W, Justl HG, Callies F, et al. Oral dehydroepiandrosterone for adrenal androgen replacement: pharmacokinetics and peripheral conversion to androgens and estrogens in young healthy females after dexamethasone suppression. J Clin Endocrinol Metab 1998;83(6):1928-1934.

Azuma T, Nagai Y, Saito T, et al. The effect of dehydroepiandrosterone sulfate administration to patients with multi-infarct dementia. J Neurol Sci 1999; 162(1):69-73.

Barry NN, McGuire JL, van Vollenhoven RF. Dehydroepiandrosterone in systemic lupus erythematosus: relationship between dosage, serum levels, and clinical response. J Rheumatol 1998;25(12):2352-2356.

Baulieu EE, Thomas G, Legrain S, et al. Dehydroepiandrosterone (DHEA), DHEA sulfate, and aging: contribution of the DHEAge study to a socio-biomedical issue. Proc Natl Acad Sci U S A 2000;97(8):4279-4284.

Bloch E, Newman E. Comparative placental steroid synthesis. I. Conversion of (7-3-H)-dehydroepiandrosterone to (3-H)-androst-4-ene-3,17-dione. Endocrinology 1966;79(3):524-530.

Bloch M, Schmidt PJ, Danaceau MA, et al. Dehydroepiandrosterone treatment of midlife dysthymia. Biol Psychiatry 1999;45(12):1533-1541.

Brown RC, Han Z, Cascio C, et al. Oxidative stress-mediated DHEA formation in Alzheimer's disease pathology. Neurobiol Aging 2003;24(1):57-65.

Buffington CK, Givens JR, Kitabchi AE. Opposing actions of dehydro-epiandrosterone and testosterone on insulin sensitivity. In vivo and in vitro studies of hyperandrogenic females. Diabetes 1991;40(6):693-700.

Buffington CK, Pourmotabbed G, Kitabchi AE. Case report: amelioration of insulin resistance in diabetes with dehydroepiandrosterone. Am J Med Sci 1993;306(5):320-324.

Calhoun K, Pommier R, Cheek J, et al. The effect of high dehydroepiandrosterone sulfate levels on tamoxifen blockade and breast cancer progression. Am J Surg 2003;185(5):411-415.

Callies F, Fassnacht M, van Vlijmen JC, et al. Dehydroepiandrosterone replace-ment in women with adrenal insufficiency: effects on body composition, serum leptin, bone turnover, and exercise capacity. J Clin Endocrinol Metab 2001; 86(5):1968-1972.

Casson PR, Andersen RN, Herrod HG, et al. Oral dehydroepiandrosterone in physiologic doses modulates immune function in postmenopausal women. Am J Obstet Gynecol 1993;169(6):1536-1539.

Casson PR, Buster JE, Lindsay MS, et al. Dehydroepiandrosterone (DHEA) supplementation augments ovulation induction (OI) in poor responders: a case series [abstract]. Fertil Steril 1998;70(2S)(Suppl 1):475S-476S.

Casson PR, Buster JE. DHEA administration to humans: panacea or palaver? Semin Reprod Endocrinol 1995;13:247-256.

Casson PR, Carson SA, Buster JE, et al. Replacement dehydroepiandrosterone in elderly: rationale and prospects for the future. Endocrinologist 1998;8: 187-194.

Casson PR, et al. Dehydroepiandrosterone (DHEA) replacement in post-menopausal women: present status and future promise. J North Am Meno-pause Soc 1997;4:225.

Casson PR, Faquin LC, Stentz FB, et al. Replacement of dehydroepiandrosterone enhances T-lymphocyte insulin binding in postmenopausal women. Fertil Steril 1995;63(5):1027-1031.

Casson PR, Fisher J, Umstot ES, et al. Vaginal dehydroepiandrosterone (DHEA) bioavailability in a hypopituitary woman with induction of adrenarche [Abstract P17]. Society for Gynecologic Investigation 1994.

Casson PR, Lindsay MS, Pisarska MD, et al. Dehydroepiandrosterone supple-mentation augments ovarian stimulation in poor responders: a case series. Hum Reprod 2000;15(10):2129-2132.

Casson PR, Santoro N, Elkind-Hirsch K, et al. Postmenopausal dehydro-epiandrosterone administration increases free insulin-like growth factor-I and decreases high-density lipoprotein: a six-month trial. Fertil Steril 1998;70(1): 107-110.

Casson PR, Straughn AB, Umstot ES, et al. Delivery of dehydroepiandrosterone to premenopausal women: effects of micronization and nonoral administration. Am J Obstet Gynecol 1996;174(2):649-653.

Centurelli MA, Abate MA. The role of dehydroepiandrosterone in AIDS. Ann Pharmacother 1997;31(5):639-642.

Chang DM, Lan H, Lan HY, et al. GL701 (Prasterone, DHEA) significantly reduces flares in female patients with mild to moderate systemic lupus erythematosus. Arthritis Rheum 2000;43(Suppl):S241.

Chassany O. [Does dehydroepiandrosterone improve well-being?] Presse Med 2000;29(24):1354-1355.

Colker C, Torina G, Swain M, et al. Double-blind, placebo-controlled, randomized clinical trial evaluating the effects of exercise plus 3-acetyl-7-oxo-dehydroepiandrosterone on body composition and the endocrine system in overweight adults [abstract]. J Exercise Physiol 1999;2(4).

Derksen RH. Dehydroepiandrosterone (DHEA) and systemic lupus erythematosus. Semin Arthritis Rheum 1998;27(6):335-347.

Dockhorn R, Wanger J, McKay L, et al. Safety and efficacy of DHEA in asthmatics undergoing a cat room challenge [abstract]. Ann Allergy Asthma Immunol 1999;82(1):111.

Dyner T, Lang W, Geaga JV, et al. Phase I study of dehydroepiandrosterone (EL-10) therapy in symptomatic HIV disease [abstract]. 6th Intl Conf on AIDS 1990;3:208.

Dyner TS, Lang W, Geaga J, et al. An open-label dose-escalation trial of oral dehydroepiandrosterone tolerance and pharmacokinetics in patients with HIV disease. J Acquir Immune Defic Syndr 1993;6(5):459-465.

Fassati P, Fassati M, Sonka J, et al. [New approach to the treatment of angina pectoris by dehydroepiandrosterone-sulfate.] Cas Lek Cesk 1971;110(26): 606-609.

Fassati P, Fassati M, Sonka J, et al. Dehydroepiandrosterone sulphate—a new approach to some cases of angina pectoris therapy. Agressologie 1970;11(5): 445-448.

Forrest AD, Drewery J, Fotherby K, et al. A clinical trial of dehydroepiandrosterone (Diandrone). J Neurol Neurosurg Psychiat 1960;23:52-55.

Furie R. Dehydroepiandrosterone and biologics in the treatment of systemic lupus erythematosus. Curr Rheumatol Rep 2000;2(1):44-50.

Gebre-Medhin G, Husebye ES, Mallmin H, et al. Oral dehydroepiandrosterone (DHEA) replacement therapy in women with Addison's disease. Clin Endocrinol (Oxf) 2000;52(6):775-780.

Giltay EJ, van Schaardenburg D, Gooren LJ, et al. Dehydroepiandrosterone sulfate in patients with rheumatoid arthritis. Ann N Y Acad Sci 1999;876: 152-154.

Giltay EJ, van Schaardenburg D, Gooren LJ, et al. Effects of dehydro-epiandrosterone administration on disease activity in patients with rheumatoid arthritis. Br J Rheumatol 1998;37(6):705-706.

Gordon CM, Grace E, Emans SJ, et al. Changes in bone turnover markers and menstrual function after short-term oral DHEA in young women with anorexia nervosa. J Bone Miner Res 1999;14(1):136-145.

Gordon GB, Bush DE, Weisman HF. Reduction of atherosclerosis by administration of dehydroepiandrosterone. A study in the hypercholesterolemic New Zealand white rabbit with aortic intimal injury. J Clin Invest 1988; 82(2):712-720.

Gordon GB, Bush TL, Helzlsouer KJ, et al. Relationship of serum levels of dehydroepiandrosterone and dehydroepiandrosterone sulfate to the risk of developing postmenopausal breast cancer. Cancer Res 1990;50(13):3859-3862.

Gordon GB, Helzlsouer KJ, Alberg AJ, et al. Serum levels of dehydro-epiandrosterone and dehydroepiandrosterone sulfate and the risk of developing gastric cancer. Cancer Epidemiol Biomarkers Prev 1993;2(1):33-35.

Gordon GB, Helzlsouer KJ, Comstock GW. Serum levels of dehydro-epiandrosterone and its sulfate and the risk of developing bladder cancer. Cancer Res 1991;51(5):1366-1369.

Gordon GB, Shantz LM, Talalay P. Inhibitory effects of dehydroepiandrosterone on cell proliferation, differentiation, and carcinogenesis: role of glucose-6-phosphate dehydrogenase. In Hardy HA, Stratman F (eds): Proceedings of the Eighteenth Steenbock Symposium. Hormones, Thermogenesis, and Obesity. New York, Elsevier Science, 1989, pp 339-354.

Gordon GB, Shantz LM, Talalay P. Modulation of growth, differentiation and carcinogenesis by dehydroepiandrosterone. Adv Enzyme Regul 1987;26: 355-382.

Guay AT. Decreased testosterone in regularly menstruating women with decreased libido: a clinical observation. J Sex Marital Ther 2001;27(5):513-519.

Himmel P, Seligman TM. A pilot study employing dehydroepiandrosterone (DHEA) in the treatment of chronic fatigue syndrome. J Clin Rheumatol 1999;5(2):56-59.

Holzmann H, Krapp R, Morsches B, et al. [Therapy of psoriasis using dehydroepiandrosterone-sulfate.] Arztl Forsch 1971;25(11):345-353.

Holzmann H, Morsches B, Krapp R, et al. [Therapy of psoriasis using dehydroepiandrosterone-enanthate.] Z Haut Geschlechtskr 1972;47(3): 99-110.

Holzmann H, Morsches B, Krapp R, et al. [Therapy of psoriasis with dehydro-epiandrosterone-enanthate. II. Intramuscular depot application of 300 mg weekly (author's transl).] Archiv fur Dermatol Forsch 1973;247(1):23-28.

Hunt PJ, Gurnell EM, Huppert FA, et al. Improvement in mood and fatigue after dehydroepiandrosterone replacement in Addison's disease in a random-ized, double blind trial. J Clin Endocrinol Metab 2000;85(12):4650-4656.

Huppert FA, Van Niekerk JK. Dehydroepiandrosterone (DHEA) supplementa-tion for cognitive function (Cochrane Review). Cochrane Database (Issue 2) 2001;2:CD000304.

Ishikawa M, Shimizu T. Dehydroepiandrosterone sulfate and induction of labor. Am J Perinatol 1989;6(2):173-175.

Johannsson G, Burman P, Wiren L, et al. Low dose dehydroepiandrosterone affects behavior in hypopituitary androgen–deficient women: a placebo-controlled trial. J Clin Endocrinol Metab 2002;87(5):2046-2052.

Jones DL, James VH. Determination of dehydroepiandrosterone and dehydro-epiandrosterone sulphate in blood and tissue. Studies of normal women and women with breast or endometrial cancer. J Steroid Biochem 1987;26(1): 151-159.

Jones JA, Nguyen A, Straub M, et al. Use of DHEA in a patient with advanced prostate cancer: a case report and review. Urology 1997;50(5):784-788.

Kalman DS, Colker CM, Swain MA, et al. A randomized, double-blind, placebo-controlled study of 3-acetyl-7-oxo-dehydroepiandrosterone in healthy overweight adults. Current Therapeutic Research 2000;61(7):435-442.

Kim SS, Brody KH. Dehydroepiandrosterone replacement in Addison's disease. Eur J Obstet Gynecol Reprod Biol 2001;97(1):96-97.

Knopman D, Henderson VW. DHEA for Alzheimer's disease: a modest showing by a superhormone. Neurology 2003;60(7):1060-1061.

Kodama M, Kodama T, Murakami M. The value of the dehydroepiandrosterone-annexed vitamin C infusion treatment in the clinical control of chronic fatigue syndrome (CFS). I. A Pilot study of the new vitamin C infusion treatment with a volunteer CFS patient. In Vivo 1996;10(6):575-584.

Kodama M, Kodama T, Murakami M. The value of the dehydroepiandrosterone-annexed vitamin C infusion treatment in the clinical control of chronic fatigue syndrome (CFS). II. Characterization of CFS patients with special reference to their response to a new vitamin C infusion treatment. In Vivo 1996;10(6):585-596.

Koo E, Feher KG, Feher T, et al. Effect of dehydroepiandrosterone on hereditary angioedema. Klin Wochenschr 1983;61(14):715-717.

Lahita RG. Dehydroepiandrosterone (DHEA) and lupus erythematosus: an update. Lupus 1997;6(6):491-493.

Lahita RG. Dehydroepiandrosterone (DHEA) for serious disease, a possibility? Lupus 1999;8(3):169-170.

Lauritzen C. [Therapeutic attempts with dehydroepiandrosterone sulfate in threatened pregnancies.] Arch Gynakol 1971;211(1):247-249.

Lauritzen C. Conversion of DHEA-sulfate to estrogens as a test of placental function. Horm Metab Res 1969;1(2):96.

Leenstra T, Ter Kuile FO, Kariuki SK, et al. Dehydroepiandrosterone sulfate levels associated with decreased malaria parasite density and increased hemoglobin concentration in pubertal girls from Western Kenya. J Infect Dis 2003;188(2):297-304.

Marcelli C. Can DHEA be used to prevent bone loss and osteoporosis? Joint Bone Spine 2003;70(1):1-2.

Marx C, Petros S, Bornstein SR, et al. Adrenocortical hormones in survivors and nonsurvivors of severe sepsis: diverse time course of dehydroepiandrosterone, dehydroepiandrosterone-sulfate, and cortisol. Crit Care Med 2003;31(5):1382-1388.

Mease PJ, Merrill JT, Lahita R, et al. GL701 (prasterone, dehydroepiandrosterone) improves or stabilizes disease activity in systemic lupus erythematosus. The Endocrine Society's 82nd Annual Meeting, 2000.

Mease PJ, Merrill JT, Lahita RG, et al. GL701 (Prasterone, DHEA) improves systemic lupus erythematosus. Arthritis Rheum 2000;43(Suppl):S271.

Mease PL, Ginzler EM, Gluck OS, et al. Improvement in bone mineral density in steroid-treated patients during treatment with GL701 (Prasterone, DHEA). Arthritis Rheum 2000;43(Suppl):S230.

Munarriz R, Talakoub L, Flaherty E, et al. Androgen replacement therapy with dehydroepiandrosterone for androgen insufficiency and female sexual dysfunction: androgen and questionnaire results. J Sex Marital Ther 2002;28(Suppl 1):165-173.

Munarriz RM, Talakoub L, Flaherty E, et al. Hormone, sexual function and personal sexual distress outcomes following dehydroepiandrosterone (DHEA) treatment for multi-dimensional female sexual dysfunction and androgen deficiency syndrome [abstract]. American Urological Association Annual Meeting, June 2-7, 2001.

Oelkers W. Dehydroepiandrosterone for adrenal insufficiency. N Engl J Med 1999;341(14):1073-1074.

Patavino T, Brady DM. Natural medicine and nutritional therapy as an alternative treatment in systemic lupus erythematosus. Altern Med Rev 2001;6(5):460-471.

Percheron G, Hogrel JY, Denot-Ledunois S, et al. Effect of 1-year oral administration of dehydroepiandrosterone to 60- to 80-year-old individuals on muscle function and cross-sectional area: a double-blind placebo-controlled trial. Arch Intern Med 2003;163(6):720-727.

Petri M, Lahita RG, McGuire J, et al. Results of the GL701 (DHEA) multicenter steroid-sparing SLE study. Arthritis Rheum 1997;40(Suppl):S327.

Rabkin JG, Ferrando SJ, Wagner GJ, et al. DHEA treatment for HIV+ patients: effects on mood, androgenic and anabolic parameters. Psychoneuroendocrinology 2000;25(1):53-68.

Rommler A. [Adrenopause and dehydroepiandrosterone: pharmacological therapy versus replacement therapy.] Gynakol Geburtshilfliche Rundsch 2003;43(2):79-90.

Sasaki K, Nakano R, Kadoya Y, et al. Cervical ripening with dehydroepiandrosterone sulphate. Br J Obstet Gynaecol 1982;89(3):195-198.

Shun YP, Shun LH, Feng YY, et al. [The effect of DHEA on body fat distribution and serum lipids in elderly overweight males.] Pract Geriatr 1999;13(1):31-33.

Stomati M, Monteleone P, Casarosa E, et al. Six-month oral dehydroepiandrosterone supplementation in early and late postmenopause. Gynecol Endocrinol 2000;14(5):342-363.

Strous RD, Maayan R, Lapidus R, et al. Dehydroepiandrosterone augmentation in the management of negative, depressive, and anxiety symptoms in schizophrenia. Arch Gen Psychiatry 2003;60(2):133-141.

Strous RD, Maayan R, Lapidus R, et al. Dehydroepiandrosterone augmentation in the management of negative, depressive, and anxiety symptoms in schizophrenia. Arch Gen Psychiatry 2003;60(2):133-141.

Sugino M, Ohsawa N, Ito T, et al. A pilot study of dehydroepiandrosterone sulfate in myotonic dystrophy. Neurology 1998;51(2):586-589.

Suh-Burgmann E, Sivret J, Duska LR, et al. Long-term administration of intravaginal dehydroepiandrosterone on regression of low-grade cervical dysplasia—a pilot study. Gynecol Obstet Invest 2003;55(1):25-31.

Trichopoulou A, Bamia C, Kalapothaki V, et al. Dehydroepiandrosterone relations to dietary and lifestyle variables in a general population sample. Ann Nutr Metab 2003;47(3-4):158-164.

Usiskin KS, Butterworth S, Clore JN, et al. Lack of effect of dehydroepiandrosterone in obese men. Int J Obes 1990;14(5):457-463.

Vakina TN, Shutov AM, Shalina SV, et al. [Dehydroepiandrosterone and sexual function in men with chronic prostatitis]. Urologiia 2003;Jan-Feb(1):49-52.

Van Vollenhoven RF, Engleman EG, McGuire JL. An open study of dehydroepiandrosterone in systemic lupus erythematosus. Arthritis Rheum 1994;37(9):1305-1310.

Van Vollenhoven RF, Engleman EG, McGuire JL. Dehydroepiandrosterone in systemic lupus erythematosus. Results of a double-blind, placebo-controlled, randomized clinical trial. Arthritis Rheum 1995;38(12):1826-1831.

Van Vollenhoven RF, McDevitt H. Studies of the treatment of nephritis in NZB/NZW mice with dehydroepiandrosterone [abstract]. Arthritis Rheum 1992;35(Suppl):S207.

Van Vollenhoven RF, McGuire JL. Studies of dehydroepiandrosterone (DHEA) as a therapeutic agent in systemic lupus erythematosus. Ann Med Interne (Paris) 1996;147(4):290-296.

Van Vollenhoven RF, Morabito LM, Engleman EG, et al. Treatment of systemic lupus erythematosus with dehydroepiandrosterone. Two-year follow-up from an open-label clinical trial [abstract]. Arthritis Rheum 1994;37:S407.

Van Vollenhoven RF, Morabito LM, Engleman EG, et al. Treatment of systemic lupus erythematosus with dehydroepiandrosterone: 50 patients treated up to 12 months. J Rheumatol 1998;25(2):285-289.

Van Vollenhoven RF, Morales A, Yen S, et al. In patients with systemic lupus erythematosus, treatment with oral dehydroepiandrosterone restores abnormally low in vitro production of IL-2, IL-6 and TNF-alpha [abstract]. Arthritis Rheum 1994;37:S407.

Van Vollenhoven RF, Park JL, Genovese MC, et al. A double-blind, placebo-controlled, clinical trial of dehydroepiandrosterone in severe systemic lupus erythematosus. Lupus 1999;8(3):181-187.

Van Vollenhoven RF. Dehydroepiandrosterone for the treatment of systemic lupus erythematosus. Expert Opin Pharmacother 2002;3(1):23-31.

Van Vollenhoven RF. Dehydroepiandrosterone in systemic lupus erythematosus. Rheum Dis Clin North Am 2000;26(2):349-362.

Van Vollenhoven RF. Dehydroepiandrosterone in the treatment of systemic lupus erythematosus. Rheumatology (Oxford) 2000;39(8):929-930.

Van Weering HG, Gutknecht DR, Schats R. Augmentation of ovarian response by dehydroepiandrosterone. Hum Reprod 2001;16(7):1537-1539.

Villareal DT, Holloszy JO, Kohrt WM. Effects of DHEA replacement on bone mineral density and body composition in elderly women and men. Clin Endocrinol (Oxf) 2000;53(5):561-568.

Wallace D. Current and emerging lupus treatments. Am J Manag Care 2001;7(16 Suppl):S490-S495.

Wallace MB, Lim J, Cutler A, et al. Effects of dehydroepiandrosterone vs androstenedione supplementation in men. Med Sci Sports Exerc 1999;31(12):1788-1792.

Wolkowitz OM, Kramer JH, Reus VI, et al. DHEA treatment of Alzheimer's disease: a randomized, double-blind, placebo-controlled study. Neurology 2003;60(7):1071-1076.

Wolkowitz OM, Reus VI, Keebler A, et al. Double-blind treatment of major depression with dehydroepiandrosterone. Am J Psychiatry 1999;156(4):646-649.

Wolkowitz OM, Reus VI, Roberts E, et al. Antidepressant and cognition-enhancing effects of DHEA in major depression. Ann N Y Acad Sci 1995;774:337-339.

Wolkowitz OM, Reus VI, Roberts E, et al. Dehydroepiandrosterone (DHEA) treatment of depression. Biol Psychiatry 1997;41(3):311-318.

Wren BG, Day RO, McLachlan AJ, et al. Pharmacokinetics of estradiol, progesterone, testosterone and dehydroepiandrosterone after transbuccal administration to postmenopausal women. Climacteric 2003;6(2):104-111.

Zelissen PM, Thijssen JH. [Role of prasterone (dehydroepiandrosterone) in substitution therapy for adrenocortical insufficiency]. Ned Tijdschr Geneeskd 2001;145(42):2018-2022.

Zumoff B, Levin J, Rosenfeld RS, et al. Abnormal 24-hr mean plasma concentrations of dehydroisoandrosterone and dehydroisoandrosterone sulfate in women with primary operable breast cancer. Cancer Res 1981;41(9 Pt 1):3360-3363.

Zumoff B, Troxler RG, O'Connor J, et al. Abnormal hormone levels in men with coronary artery disease. Arteriosclerosis 1982;2(1):58-67.

Zumoff B, Walsh BT, Katz JL, et al. Subnormal plasma dehydroisoandrosterone to cortisol ratio in anorexia nervosa: a second hormonal parameter of ontogenic regression. J Clin Endocrinol Metab 1983;56(4):668-672.

Zumoff BV, Bradlow HL. Sex difference in the metabolism of dehydroisoandrosterone sulfate. J Clin Endocrinol Metab 1980;51(2):334-336.

Dong Quai
(*Angelica sinensis* [Oliv.] Diels)

SYNONYMS/COMMON NAMES/RELATED SUBSTANCES

- American angelica, *Angelica acutiloba* (Japanese), *Angelica archangelica*, *Angelica atropurpurea*, *Angelica dahurica*, *Angelica edulis*, *Angelica gigas*, *Angelica keiskei*, *Angelica koreana*, *Angelica polymorpha* var. sinensis Oliv., *Angelica pubescens*, angelica radix, angelica root, angelica silvestris, angelique, Apiaceae/Umbellifera, *Archangelica officinalis* Moench or Hoff, beta-sitosterol, Chinese angelica, Chinese danggui, danggui, Dang Gui, danggui-nian-tong-tang (DGNTT), dang quai, dong kwai, dong qua, dong quai extract, dong quai root, dong qui, dry-kuei, engelwurzel, European angelica, European dong quai, female ginseng, FP3340010, FP334015, FT334010, garden angelica, heiligenwurzel, Japanese angelica, kinesisk kvan, kinesisk kvanurt, ligusticum glaucescens franch, ligusticum officinale Koch, ligustilides, phytoestrogen, qingui, radix angelica sinensis, root of the holy ghost, tan kue bai zhi, tang kuei, tang kuei root, tang kwei, tanggui (Korean), tanggwi (Korean), tang quai, toki (Japanese), wild angelica, wild chin quai, women's ginseng, yuan nan wild dong quai, yungui.
- **Combination herbal formulations:** Angelica-Alunite Solution, Angelica-Paeonia Powder, Bloussant Breast Enhancement Tablets, Bust Plus, Dong Quai and Royal Jelly, Dong Quai 4, Dong Quai 4, Danggui Buxue Tang, Danggui Huoxue Tang, Female Corrective Combination Containing Dong Quai, Four Things Soup, Shenyan Huayu Tang, Shimotus To, Shou Wu Chih, Sini Decoction, Siwu tang, tokishakuyakusan, Xiao Yao Powder, Yishen Tang.
- *Note:* The related species *Angelica acutiloba* appears to have properties similar to those of dong quai (*Angelica sinensis*) in laboratory experiments.

CLINICAL BOTTOM LINE
Background

- Dong quai (*Angelica sinensis*), also known as Chinese angelica, has been used for thousands of years in traditional Chinese, Korean, and Japanese medicine. It remains one of the most popular plants in Chinese medicine and is used primarily for health conditions in women. Dong quai has been called "female ginseng," based on its use for gynecologic disorders such as painful menstruation (dysmenorrhea), pelvic pain, recovery from childbirth or illness, and fatigue/low vitality. It is also given for strengthening *xue* (loosely translated as "the blood") and for cardiovascular conditions, high blood pressure, inflammation, headache, infections, and neuropathic (nerve) pain.
- In the late 1800s, an extract of dong quai called *Eumenol* became popular in Europe as a treatment for gynecologic complaints. Recently, interest in dong quai has resurged because of its proposed weak estrogen-like properties. However, it remains unclear whether dong quai has the same effects on the body as estrogens, blocks the activity of estrogens, or has no significant hormonal effects. Results of animal studies are conflicting, and one trial in humans found no short-term estrogen-like effects on the body. Additional research is necessary in this area before a firm conclusion can be drawn.
- In Chinese medicine, dong quai is most often used in combination with other herbs. Within the Chinese medical framework, dong quai is used as a component of formulas for liver *qi* stasis and spleen deficiency. It is believed to work best in persons with a *yin* profile and is considered to be a mildly warming herb. Dong quai is thought to return the body to proper order by nourishing the blood and harmonizing vital energy. The name *dong quai* translates as "return to order," based on its alleged restorative properties.
- The part of the plant most often cultivated for medicinal use is the root, which is divided into three parts (head, body, tail). Each section is believed to have different actions within the body. For example, the tail is proposed to be best for promoting blood circulation, while the head is considered the worst.
- Although dong quai has many historical and theoretical uses based on studies in animals, there is little evidence from studies in humans supporting the effects of dong quai for any condition. Clinical studies have been limited, and in general have been either poorly designed or have reported insignificant results. Most of these studies have examined combination formulas containing multiple ingredients, making it difficult to determine which ingredient causes certain effects.

Uses Based on Scientific Evidence	Grade*
Amenorrhea (lack of menstrual period) There have been limited poor-quality studies of dong quai as a component of herbal combinations given for amenorrhea. It is unclear from laboratory studies whether dong quai has the same effects on the body as estrogens or blocks the activity of estrogens (or neither), and how this may affect women with amenorrhea. One study in humans suggested that dong quai may not have significant short-term estrogen-like effects on the body. Additional research is necessary before a firm conclusion can be drawn.	C
Angina pectoris/coronary artery disease There is insufficient evidence to support the use of dong quai for the treatment of heart disease.	C
Arthritis Dong quai is traditionally used in the treatment of arthritis. However, there is insufficient reliable scientific evidence from studies in humans to recommend the use of dong quai alone or in combination with other herbs for osteoarthritis or rheumatoid arthritis.	C
Dysmenorrhea (painful menstruation) Results were inconclusive in preliminary, poor-quality research studies in humans of the use of dong quai in combination with other herbs for dysmenorrhea. Studies in animals reported conflicting results, with both relaxing and stimulatory effects of dong quai on the uterus. Reliable scientific evidence concerning the effects of dong quai alone in women with dysmenorrhea is not available.	C

Continued

It is traditionally believed that therapy should begin on day 14 of the menstrual cycle and continue until menstruation has ceased.

Glomerulonephritis   C
There is insufficient evidence to support the use of dong quai as a treatment for kidney diseases such as glomerulonephritis. Results were unclear in preliminary poor-quality studies of dong quai used in combination with other herbs.

Idiopathic thrombocytopenic purpura (ITP)   C
One poor-quality study reported that dong quai was beneficial in patients diagnosed with ITP. However, these patients were not compared to individuals who were not receiving dong quai, and therefore the results can only be considered preliminary.

Menstrual migraine headache   C
One small study reported a reduced average number of menstruation-associated migraine attacks during prophylactic treatment with a daily combination of 60 mg of soy isoflavones, 100 mg of dong quai, and 50 mg of black cohosh, with each component standardized to its primary alkaloid. Subjects in the study received medication for 24 weeks. The effects of dong quai alone for this condition are unclear, and further research is necessary before a clear conclusion can be reached.

Nerve pain   C
There is insufficient evidence to support the use of dong quai as a treatment for neuropathic pain. High-quality human research is lacking.

Pulmonary hypertension   C
A preliminary controlled trial reports that the combination of dong quai with the drug nifedipine may be better than either agent alone to improve pulmonary hypertension in individuals with chronic obstructive pulmonary disease (COPD). A second study of dong quai alone also noted benefits. These studies were small, not well reported, and cannot be considered conclusive. It remains unclear if dong quai is beneficial for other causes of pulmonary hypertension. Further research is needed before a recommendation can be made.

Menopausal symptoms   D
Dong quai is used in traditional Chinese formulas for menopausal symptoms. It has been proposed that dong quai may contain "phytoestrogens" (chemicals with estrogen-like effects in the body). However, it remains unclear from laboratory studies whether dong quai has the same effects on the body as estrogens, blocks the activity of estrogens, or has no significant effect on estrogens.
A well-designed 24-week human trial compared the effects of dong quai to a placebo in 71 women with menopausal symptoms. This study found no differences in hot flashes or in the Kupperman Index (a commonly used measure of menopausal symptoms) between dong quai and placebo groups. No changes occurred in blood estrogen levels, thickness of the uterus lining, or vaginal dryness. This study suggests that dong quai may not have short-term estrogen-like effects on the body. However, there may have been too few patients enrolled in the study to accurately measure effects. In addition, the dong quai extract used, prepared by East Earth herbs, Inc. (4.5 mg per day, standardized to 0.5 mg per kg of ferulic acid), may not be manufactured in the same way as other dong quai products and may yield different results. Additional research is necessary before a strong recommendation can be made.

*Key to grades: *A:* Strong scientific evidence for this use; *B:* Good scientific evidence for this use; *C:* Unclear scientific evidence for this use; *D:* Fair scientific evidence against this use (it may not work); *F:* Strong scientific evidence against this use (it likely does not work). For a more detailed explanation of efficacy criteria, see "Natural Standard Evidence-Based Validated Grading Rationale" in the Introduction.

Historical or Theoretical Indications That Lack Sufficient Evidence

Abscesses, abdominal pain, abnormal fetal movement, abnormal heart rhythms, age-related nerve damage, allergy, anemia, anorexia nervosa, antibacterial, anti-aging, antifungal, antiseptic, antispasmodic, anti-tumor, antiviral, anxiety, aortitis, asthma, atherosclerosis, back pain, bleeding hemorrhoids, bleomycin-induced lung damage, blood clots, blood flow disorders, blood purifier, blood stagnation, blood vessel disorders, blurred vision, body pain, boils, bone growth, breast enlargement, bronchitis, Buerger's disease, cancer, central nervous system disorders, cervicitis, chilblains, cholagogue, chronic hepatitis, chronic obstructive pulmonary disease (COPD), chronic rhinitis, cirrhosis, colchicine-induced learning impairment, congestive heart failure (CHF), constipation, cough, cramps, dermatitis, diabetes, digestion disorders, diuretic (increasing urine flow), dysentery, eczema, emotional instability, endometritis, expectorant, fatigue, fibrocystic breast disease, fibroids, flatulence (gas), fluid retention, gastric ulcer, glaucoma, hay fever, headache, heartburn, hematopoiesis (stimulation of blood cell production), hemolytic disease of the newborn, hernia, high blood pressure, high cholesterol, hormonal abnormalities, immune cytopenias, immunosuppressant, infections, infertility, irritable bowel syndrome, joint pain, kidney disease, labor aid, laxative, leukorrhea (vaginal discharge), liver protection, lung disease, malaria, menorrhagia (heavy menstrual bleeding), menstrual cramping, migraine, miscarriage prevention, morning sickness, muscle relaxant, osteoporosis, ovulation abnormalities, pain, pain from bruises, palpitations, pelvic congestion syndrome, pelvic inflammatory disease, peritoneal dialysis, pleurisy, postpartum weakness, pregnancy support, premenstrual syndrome (PMS), prolapsed uterus, psoriasis, pulmonary fibrosis, Raynaud's disease, reperfusion injury, respiratory tract infection, retained placenta, Rhesus (Rh) factor incompatibility, rheumatic diseases, sciatica, sedative, sepsis, shingles (herpes zoster), skin pigmentation disorders, skin ulcers, stiffness, stomach cancer, stress, stroke, tinnitus (ringing in the ear), toothache, vaginal atrophy, vitamin E deficiency, wound healing.

DOSING/TOXICOLOGY

The following doses are based on scientific research, publications, traditional use, or expert opinion. Many herbs and supplements have not been thoroughly tested, and their safety and effectiveness may not be proven. Brands may be made differently, with variable ingredients even within the same brand. The doses shown may not apply to all products. It is important to always read product labels and discuss doses with a qualified healthcare provider before therapy is started.

Standardization

- Standardization involves measuring amounts of certain chemicals in products to try to make different preparations similar to each other. It is not always known if the chemicals being measured are the "active" ingredients.
- There are no standard or well-studied doses of dong quai, and many different doses are used traditionally. Some products standardize dong quai to 0.8% to 1.1% ligustilide per dose, or to 0.5 mg per kg of ferulic acid. One gram of 100% dong quai extract has been reported to be equivalent to approximately 4 g of raw dong quai root. Safety and effectiveness are not established for any dose.
- In Asia, dong quai is primarily used medicinally, whereas in the United States and Europe it is more common as a flavoring agent in food products (e.g., in liqueurs, vermouth, ice cream, candy, gelatins, puddings). A related species, *Angelica acutiloba*, appears to have similar properties to dong quai in laboratory experiments.

Adults (18 Years and Older)
Root preparations

- **Combination preparations:** Dong quai is used in numerous herbal combinations, and various doses have been used traditionally and in Chinese research. Because of this variation and lack of high-quality studies, no specific recommendations can be made. Safety and effectiveness are not established for most herbal combinations, and the amounts of dong quai present may vary from batch to batch.
- **Powdered/dried root/root slices:** A dose of 1 to 5 g of root taken by mouth three times daily has been used traditionally, although more common doses range from 1 to 2 g taken three times daily. Weight-based dosing has been proposed, although there is no scientific evidence to support this practice.
- **Fluid extract/tincture:** Doses of 3 to 8 ml of a fluid extract (1:2) or 10 to 40 drops of tincture (1:5 in 50% to 70% alcohol) taken by mouth three times daily have been used.
- **Decoction:** To prepare, 1 teaspoon to 1 tablespoon of cut root is simmered for 2 to 5 minutes in 1 cup of water that has been brought to a boil; it is then removed from the heat and left to stand for 5 to 10 minutes. One to three cups have been consumed by mouth daily.
- **Intravenous injection:** Safety of intravenous use is not established, although it has been reported in research.
- **Topical (on the skin):** Ten to 15 drops of diluted essential oil has been used for skin irritation (anecdotal).

Leaf Preparations (Less Common Than Root Preparations)

- **Dried leaf:** A dose of 2 to 5 g taken by mouth three times daily has been used.
- **Leaf tincture:** A dose of 2 to 5 ml (1:5 in 45% alcohol) taken by mouth three times daily has been used.
- **Leaf fluid extract:** A dose of 0.5 to 2 ml (1:1) taken 3 times daily has been used.

Children (Younger Than 18 Years)

- There are insufficient scientific data to recommend dong quai for use in children, and it is not recommended because of potential side effects.

SAFETY

The U.S. Food and Drug Administration does not strictly regulate herbs and supplements. There is no guarantee of the strength, purity, or safety of products, and effects may vary. It is important to always read product labels. People who have a medical condition, or are taking other drugs, herbs, or supplements, should consult a qualified healthcare provider before starting a new therapy. A healthcare provider should be contacted immediately about any side effects.

Allergies

- People with known allergy/hypersensitivity to *Angelica radix* or members of the Apiaceae/Umbelliferae family (anise, caraway, carrot, celery, dill, parsley) should avoid dong quai products. Skin rash has been reported with the use of dong quai, although it is unclear whether this was an allergic response. An asthma response occurred after a person breathed in dong quai powder.

Side Effects and Warnings

- Although the safety of dong quai is accepted as a food additive in the United States and Europe, its safety in medicinal doses is not known. There are no reliable long-term studies of side effects. Most precautions are based on theory, laboratory research, tradition, or isolated case reports.
- Components of dong quai may increase the risk of bleeding due to anticoagulant and antiplatelet effects, although there are no reliable reports of clinically significant bleeding in humans. Caution is advised in people with bleeding disorders or those who are taking drugs that may increase the risk of bleeding. Dosing adjustments may be necessary. Use of dong quai products should be discontinued in persons who are going to have surgical or major dental procedures.
- It is unclear whether dong quai has the same effects on the body as estrogens, blocks the activity of estrogens, or has no significant hormonal effects. Results of studies in animals are conflicting, and one trial in human subjects reported that there were no short-term estrogen-like effects (including no hormonal changes or increases in uterus-wall thickness after 24 weeks of treatment). It is unclear whether dong quai is safe in individuals with hormone-sensitive conditions such as breast cancer, uterine cancer, ovarian cancer, or endometriosis. It is not known if dong quai possesses the beneficial effects that estrogen is believed to have on bone mass, or the potential harmful effects such as increased risk of stroke or hormone-sensitive cancers.
- Increased sun sensitivity with a risk of severe skin reactions (photosensitivity) may occur because of certain chemicals in dong quai (i.e., furocoumarins, psoralen, and bergapten). Prolonged exposure to sunlight or ultraviolet light should be avoided in people who are using dong quai. It has been reported that steam-distilled oils of the root and seed may not possess these phototoxic chemicals.
- Safrole, a volatile oil in dong quai, may be carcinogenic (cancer-causing). Long-term use should therefore be avoided, and suntan lotions that contain dong quai often limit the amount of dong quai to less than 1%.
- Dong quai has traditionally been associated with gastrointestinal symptoms (particularly with prolonged use), including laxative effects/diarrhea, upset stomach, nausea,

vomiting, loss of appetite, burping, and bloating. Published literature is limited in this area.

- Dong quai preparations may contain high levels of sucrose and should be used cautiously by patients with diabetes or glucose intolerance.

- Various other side effects have rarely been reported with dong quai taken alone or in combination with other herbs, including abnormal heart rhythms, blood pressure abnormalities, fever, gynecomastia (increased male breast size), headache, hot flashes, insomnia, irritability, kidney problems (nephrosis), lightheadedness/dizziness, reduced menstrual flow, sedation/drowsiness, skin rash, sweating, weakness, wheezing/asthma, and worsening premenstrual symptoms. However, side effects have not been evaluated in well-designed studies.

- The safety of dong quai injected into the skin, muscles, or veins is unknown, and this method of administration should be avoided. In one study, dogs stopped breathing after essential oil of dong quai was injected under their skin.

Pregnancy and Breastfeeding

- Dong quai is not recommended during pregnancy because of possible hormonal and anticoagulant/anti-platelet properties. Results of studies in animals of the effects of dong quai on the uterus were conflicting, with reports of both stimulation and relaxation. There is a published report of miscarriage in a woman taking dong quai, although it is not clear whether dong quai was the cause. Dong quai is traditionally viewed as increasing the risk of abortion. Women who are breastfeeding should avoid the use of dong quai because there is insufficient evidence regarding its safety.

INTERACTIONS

Most herbs and supplements have not been thoroughly tested for interactions with other herbs, supplements, drugs, or foods. The interactions listed here are based on reports in scientific publications, laboratory experiments, or traditional use. It is important to always read product labels. People who have a medical condition, or are taking other drugs, herbs, or supplements, should consult a qualified healthcare provider before starting a new therapy.

Interactions with Drugs

- Dong quai when taken alone may increase the risk of bleeding because of its anticoagulant and antiplatelet effects and may increase the risk of bleeding when taken with drugs that increase the risk of bleeding. Examples are anticoagulants (blood thinners) such as warfarin (Coumadin) and heparin, antiplatelet drugs such as clopidogrel (Plavix), aspirin, and nonsteroidal anti-inflammatory drugs such as ibuprofen (Motrin, Advil) and naproxen (Naprosyn, Aleve). In one review, it was reported that the effects of warfarin (Coumadin) were increased in a woman taking 565 mg of dong quai one to two times daily, as measured by 2.5-fold increases in values of blood tests for prothrombin time (PT) and international normalized ratio (INR).

- It remains unclear whether dong quai has the same effects on the body as estrogens, blocks the activity of estrogens, or has no significant hormonal effects. It has not been shown whether taking dong quai increases or decreases the effects of oral contraceptives, of hormone replacement therapies (such as Premarin) that contain estrogen, or of the anti-tumor properties of selective estrogen receptor modulators (SERMs) such as tamoxifen.

- Chemicals in dong quai may cause increased sun sensitivity, with a risk of severe skin reactions (photosensitivity). Dong quai should be avoided in people who are taking other drugs that cause photosensitivity, such as tretinoin (Retin-A, Renova), and some types of antidepressants, cancer drugs, antibiotics, and antipsychotic medications. People who are considering the use of dong quai and who are taking other medications should always read the package insert and consult their healthcare provider or pharmacist about possible interactions.

- Based on laboratory research, dong quai may increase the effects of drugs that affect heart rhythms. Examples of such drugs are beta-blockers such as metoprolol (Lopressor, Toprol), calcium channel blockers such as nifedipine (Procardia), and digoxin. Studies in animals and one report in humans noted reduced blood pressure after administration of dong quai; dong quai should be used cautiously in individuals taking blood pressure–lowering medications.

Interactions with Herbs and Dietary Supplements

- In theory, because of their anticoagulant and antiplatelet effects, components of dong quai may increase the risk of bleeding when taken with herbs and supplements that may increase the risk of bleeding. Multiple cases of bleeding have been reported with the use of *Ginkgo biloba*, and fewer cases with garlic and saw palmetto. Numerous other agents may theoretically increase the risk of bleeding, although this has not been proven in most cases. Examples are alfalfa, American ginseng, angelica, anise, *Arnica montana*, asafetida, aspen bark, bilberry, birch, black cohosh, bladderwrack, bogbean, boldo, borage seed oil, bromelain, capsicum, cat's claw, celery, chamomile, chaparral, clove, coleus, cordyceps, danshen, devil's claw, eicosapentaenoic acid (EPA), evening primrose oil, fenugreek, feverfew, fish oil, flaxseed/flax powder (not a concern with flaxseed oil), ginger, grapefruit juice, grape seed, green tea, guggul, gymnestra, horse chestnut, horseradish, licorice root, lovage root, male fern, meadowsweet, nordihydroguaiaretic acid (NDGA), onion, *Panax ginseng*, papain, parsley, passion flower, poplar, prickly ash, propolis, quassia, red clover, reishi, rue, Siberian ginseng, sweet birch, sweet clover, turmeric, vitamin E, white willow, wild carrot, wild lettuce, willow, wintergreen, and yucca.

- It is unclear whether dong quai has the same effects on the body as estrogens, blocks the activity of estrogens, or has no significant hormonal effects. Dong quai may alter the effects of agents that may have estrogen-like properties, such as alfalfa, black cohosh, bloodroot, burdock, hops, kudzu, licorice, pomegranate, red clover, soy, thyme, white horehound, and yucca.

- Chemicals in dong quai may cause increased sun sensitivity, with a risk of severe skin reactions (photosensitivity). Dong quai should not be taken with products containing *Hypericum perforatum* (St. John's wort) or capsaicin, which are also reported to cause photosensitivity.

Selected References

Natural Standard developed the preceding evidence-based information based on a systematic review of more than 200 articles. For comprehensive information about alternative and complementary therapies on the professional level, go to www.naturalstandard.com. Selected references are listed here.

Abebe W. An overview of herbal supplement utilization with particular emphasis on possible interactions with dental drugs and oral manifestations. J Dent Hyg 2003;77(1):37-46

Bian X, Xu Y, Zhu L, et al. Prevention of maternal-fetal blood group incompatibility with traditional Chinese herbal medicine. Chin Med J (Engl) 1998; 111(7):585-587.

Burke BE, Olson RD, Cusack BJ. Randomized, controlled trial of phytoestrogen in the prophylactic treatment of menstrual migraine. Biomed Pharmacother 2002;56(6):283-288.

Bradley RR, Cunniff PJ, Pereira BJ, et al. Hematopoietic effect of Radix *Angelicae sinensis* in a hemodialysis patient. Am J Kidney Dis 1999;34(2): 349-354.

Chou CT, Kuo SC. The anti-inflammatory and anti-hyperuricemic effects of Chinese herbal formula danggui-nian-tong-tang on acute gouty arthritis: a comparative study with indomethacin and allopurinol. Am J Chin Med 1995; 23(3-4):261-271.

Dai L, Hou J, Cai H. [Using ligustrazini and *Angelica sinensis* to treat the bleomycin-induced pulmonary fibrosis in rats.] Zhonghua Jie He He Hu Xi Za Zhi 1996;19(1):26-28.

Day C, Bailey CJ. Hypoglycaemic agents from traditional plant treatments for diabetes. Internat Industrial Biotech 1998;8(3):5-8.

Deng Y, Yang L. Effect of *Angelica sinensis* (Oliv.) on melanocytic proliferation, melanin synthesis and tyrosinase activity *in vitro*. Di Yi Jun Yi Da Xue Xue Bao 2003;23(3):239-241.

Ding H, Shi GG, Yu X, et al. Modulation of GdCl3 and *Angelica sinensis* polysaccharides on differentially expressed genes in liver of hepatic immunological injury mice by cDNA microarray. World J Gastroenterol 2003;9(5):1072-1076.

Fu YF. Treatment of 34 cases of infertility due to tubal occlusion with compound Danggui injection by irrigation. Jiangsu J Trad Chin Med 1988;9:15-16.

Fugh-Berman A. "Bust enhancing" herbal products. Obstet Gynecol 2003; 101(6):1345-1349.

Goy SY, Loh KC. Gynaecomastia and the herbal tonic "Dong quai." Singapore Med J 2001;42(3):115-116.

Hann SK, Park YK, Im S, et al. Angelica-induced phytophotodermatitis. Photodermatol Photoimmunol Photomed 1991;8(2):84-85.

Harada M, Suzuki M, Ozaki Y. Effect of Japanese Angelica root and peony root on uterine contraction in the rabbit *in situ*. J Pharmacobiodyn 1984;7(5):304-311.

He ZP, Wang DZ, Shi LY, et al. Treating amenorrhea with energy-deficient patients with *angelica sinensis*–astragalus membranaceus menstruation-regulating decoction. J Trad Chin Med 1986;6(3):187-190.

Hirata JD, Swiersz LM, Zell B, et al. Does Dong Quai have estrogenic effects in postmenopausal women? A double-blind, placebo-controlled trial. Fertil Steril 1997;68(6):981-986.

Huang LN, Yang BZ, Wang ZS. Treating 150 cases of postnatal lack of lactation by medicinal extract of "Zeng-Ru-Bao-Yu." Shan Xi J Trad Chin Med (Chiang-Su I Tsa Chih) 1997;18(6):251.

Huang Z, Guo B, Liang K. [Effects of Radix *Angelicae sinensis* on systemic and portal hemodynamics in cirrhotics with portal hypertension.] Zhonghua Nei Ke Za Zhi 1996;35(1):15-18.

Hudson TS, Standish L, Breed C, et al. Clinical and endocrinological effects of a menopausal botanical formula. J Naturopath Med 1998;7(1):73-77.

Huntley AL, Ernst E. A systematic review of herbal medicinal products for the treatment of menopausal symptoms. Menopause 2003;10(5):465-476.

Jujie T, Huaijun H. Effects of Radix Angelicae sinensis on hemorrheology in patients with acute ischemic stroke. J Trad Chin Med 1984;4:225-228.

Kiong HN. Gynaecomastia and the herbal tonic "Dong Quai." Singapore Med J 2001;42(6):286-287.

Kotani N, Oyama T, Sakai I, et al. Analgesic effect of a herbal medicine for treatment of primary dysmenorrhea—a double-blind study. Am J Chin Med 1997;25(2):205-212.

Kronenberg F, Fugh-Berman A. Complementary and alternative medicine for menopausal symptoms: a review of randomized, controlled trials. Ann Intern Med 2002;137(10):805-813.

Lee SK, Cho HK, Cho SH, et al. Occupational asthma and rhinitis caused by multiple herbal agents in a pharmacist. Ann Allergy Asthma Immunol 2001; 86(4):469-474.

Li JC, Yang ZR, Zhang K. [The intervention effects of *Angelica sinensis*, *Salvia miltiorrhiza* and ligustrazine on peritoneal macrophages during peritoneal dialysis.] Zhongguo Zhong Xi Yi Jie He Za Zhi 2002;22(3):190-192.

Li KX, You ZL, Zhang H, et al. Clinical study on "Yi-Qi-Hua-Yu" method in treatment of pelvis congestion syndrome. J Hunan Coll Trad Chin Med 1997; 17(2):11-13, 28.

Li YH. [Local injection of *Angelica sinensis* solution for the treatment of sclerosis and atrophic lichen of the vulva.] Zhonghua Hu Li Za Zhi 1983;18(2):98-99.

Liao JZ, Chen JJ, Wu ZM, et al. Clinical and experimental studies of coronary heart disease treated with yi-qi huo-xue injection. J Tradit Chin Med 1989; 9(3):193-198.

Lo AC, Chan K, Yeung JH, et al. Danggui (*Angelica sinensis*) affects the pharmacodynamics but not the pharmacokinetics of warfarin in rabbits. Eur J Drug Metab Pharmacokinet 1995;20(1):55-60.

Lu MC. Danggui shaoyao can improve colchicine-induced learning acquisition impairment in rats. Acta Pharmacol Sin 2001;22(12):1149-1153.

Mei QB, Tao JY, Cui B. Advances in the pharmacological studies of radix Angelica sinensis (Oliv) Diels (Chinese Danggui). Chin Med J (Engl) 1991; 104(9):776-781.

Nambiar S, Schwartz RH, Constantino A. Hypertension in mother and baby linked to ingestion of Chinese herbal medicine. West J Med 1999;171(3):152.

Oerter Klein K, Janfaza M, Wong JA, et al. Estrogen bioactivity in fo-ti and other herbs used for their estrogen-like effects as determined by a recombinant cell bioassay J Clin Endocrinol Metab 2003;88(9):4077-4079.

Ozaki Y, Ma JP. Inhibitory effects of tetramethylpyrazine and ferulic acid on spontaneous movement of rat uterus *in situ*. Chem Pharm Bull (Tokyo) 1990; 38(6):1620-1623.

Page RL, Lawrence JD. Potentiation of warfarin by Dong quai. Pharmacotherapy 1999;19(7):870-876.

Pan SQ, Zhang ZD, Zhang SX, et al. Clinical observation on 121 cases of primary thrombocytopenic purpura treated by SHEN-XUE-LING powder. Hunan J Chin Trad Med 1997;13(4):3-4.

Seibel MM. Treating hot flushes without hormone replacement therapy. J Fam Pract 2003;52(4):291-296.

Sha H, Chou Y. The modified Dan-Guei-Nein-Tong-Tang to treat gouty arthritis with tophi. J Trad Chinese Med 1987;2:60.

Shang P, Qian AR, Yang TH, et al. Experimental study of anti-tumor effects of polysaccharides from *Angelica sinensis*. World J Gastroenterol 2003;9(9): 1963-1967

Shimuzu M, Matsuzawa T, Suzuki S, et al. Evaluation of *Angelicae radix* (Touki) by the inhibitory effect on platelet aggregation. Chem Pharm Bull 1991; 39(8):2046-2048.

Sun SW, Wang JF. [Efficacy of danggui funing pill in treating 162 cases of abdominal pain.] Zhongguo Zhong Xi Yi Jie He Za Zhi 1992;12(9):531-532, 517.

Tao JY, Ruan YP, Mei QB, et al. [Studies on the antiasthmatic action of ligustilide of dang-gui, Angelica sinensis (Oliv.) Diels.] Yao Xue Xue Bao 1984;19(8): 561-565.

Tu JJ. Effects of radix *Angelicae sinensis* on hemorrheology in patients with acute ischemic stroke. J Tradit Chin Med 1984;4(3):225-228.

Usuki S. Effects of herbal components of Tokishakuyakusan on progesterone secretion by corpus luteum in vitro. Am J Chin Med 1991;19(1):57-60.

Wang CH, Zhang ZH, Wang Q. Therapeutic effect on 106 acute urticaria patients with the added ingredient of radix *Angelicae sinesis*. Journal Shanxi Coll Trad Chin Med 1997;20(3):25.

Wang X, Wei L, Ouyang JP, et al. Effects of an angelica extract on human erythrocyte aggregation, deformation and osmotic fragility. Clin Hemorheol Microcirc 2001;24(3):201-205.

Wang Y, Zhu B. [The effect of angelica polysaccharide on proliferation and differentiation of hematopoietic progenitor cell.] Zhonghua Yi Xue Za Zhi 1996;76(5):363-366.

Wang ZH, Wang XP, Ma L. 103 cases of neonatal hemolytic disease due to ABO blood group incompatibility prevented and treated by Huo Xue Xiao Yu decoction. Forum Trad Chin Med 1997;12(2):26.

Wilasrusmee C, Siddiqui J, Bruch D, et al. *In vitro* immunomodulatory effects of herbal products. Am Surg. 2002;68(10):860-864.

Wilasrusmee C, Kittur S, Siddiqui J, et al. *In vitro* immunomodulatory effects of ten commonly used herbs on murine lymphocytes. J Altern Complement Med 2002;8(4):467-475.

Wu Y, Zhu B. [Effect of danggui buxue decoction on proliferation and expression of intercellular adhesion molecule-1 in human umbilical vein endothelial cells.] Hua Xi Yi Ke Da Xue Xue Bao 2001;32(4):593-595.

Xu JY, Li BX, Cheng SY. [Short-term effects of *Angelica sinensis* and nifedipine on chronic obstructive pulmonary disease in patients with pulmonary hypertension.] Zhongguo Zhong Xi Yi Jie He Za Zhi 1992;12(12):716-718, 707.

Xuan GC, Feng QF, Xue FM. Clinical observation on treating 400 cases of cerebral infarction with traditional Chinese herb powder. Henan J Trad Chin Med Pharmacy 1997;12(4):28-29.

Yan TY, Hou AC, Sun BT. [Injection of *Angelica sinensis* in treating infantile pneumonia and its experimental study in rabbits]. Zhong Xi Yi Jie He Za Zhi 1987;7(3):161-162, 133.

Yang Q, Populo SM, Zhang J, et al. Effect of *Angelica sinensis* on the proliferation of human bone cells. Clin Chim Acta 2002;324(1-2):89-97.

Ye YN, Koo MW, Li Y, et al. *Angelica sinensis* modulates migration and proliferation of gastric epithelial cells. Life Sci 2001;68(8):961-968.

Ye YN, Liu ES, Li Y, et al. Protective effect of polysaccharides-enriched fraction from *Angelica sinensis* on hepatic injury. Life Sci 2001;69(6):637-646.

Ye YN, Liu ES, Shin VY, et al. A mechanistic study of proliferation induced by *Angelica sinensis* in a normal gastric epithelial cell line. Biochem Pharmacol 2001;61(11):1439-1448.

Ye YN, So HL, Liu ES, et al. Effect of polysaccharides from *Angelica sinensis* on gastric ulcer healing. Life Sci 2003;72(8):925-932.

Yim TK, Wu WK, Pak WF, et al. Myocardial protection against ischaemia-reperfusion injury by a *Polygonum multiflorum* extract supplemented 'Dang-Gui decoction for enriching blood', a compound formulation, ex vivo. Phytother Res 2000;14(3):195-199.

Zheng L. [Short-term effect and the mechanism of radix Angelicae on pulmonary hypertension in chronic obstructive pulmonary disease.. Zhonghua Jie He He Hu Xi Za Zhi 1992;15(2):95-97, 127.

Zheng M, Wang YP. Experimental study on effect of Angelica polysaccharide in inhibitory proliferation and inducing differentiation of K562 cells. Zhongguo Zhong Xi Yi Jie He Za Zhi 2002;22(1):54-57.

Zhiping H, Dazeng W, Lingyi S, et al. Treating amenorrhea in vital energy-deficient patients with *Angelica sinensis–Astragalus membranaceus* menstruation-regulating decoction. J Trad Chin Med 2002;6(3):187-190.

Zschocke S, Liu J, Stuppner H, et al. Comparative study of roots of *Angelica sinensis* and related Umbelliferous drugs by thin layer chromatography, high-performance liquid chromatography, and liquid chromatography–mass spectrometry. Phytochem Anal 1998;9(6):283-290.

Echinacea
(*Echinacea angustifolia* DC, *Echinacea pallida*, *Echinacea purpurea*)

SYNONYMS/COMMON NAMES/RELATED SUBSTANCES

- American coneflower, Echinacin, Echinaforce, Echinaguard, black Sampson, black Susan, cock-up-hat, combflower, hedgehog, igelkopf, Indian head, Kansas snake root, kegelblume, narrow-leaved purple coneflower, purple coneflower, red sunflower, rudbeckia, scurvy root, snakeroot, solhat, sun hat.

CLINICAL BOTTOM LINE
Background

- Echinacea species are perennials that belong to the Aster family and originated in eastern North America. Traditionally used for a range of infections and malignancies, the roots and herb (above-ground parts) of echinacea species have attracted recent scientific interest due to purported "immunostimulant" properties. Oral preparations are popular in Europe and the United States for prevention and treatment of upper respiratory tract infections (URIs), and *Echinacea purpurea* herb is believed to be the most potent echinacea species for this indication. In the United States, sales of echinacea are believed to represent approximately 10% of the dietary supplement market.[1]
- For URI *treatment*, numerous human trials have found echinacea to reduce duration and severity, particularly when initiated at the earliest onset of symptoms. However, the majority of trials, largely conducted in Europe, have been small or methodologically flawed. Although highly suggestive, the evidence cannot be considered definitive in favor of this use. Lack of benefit in children ages 2 to 11 years has been reported.[2] There are also recent negative results of a trial in the United States in adults, although this study used a whole-plant echinacea preparation containing both *E. purpurea* and *E. angustifolia*. Additional research is merited in this area.
- For URI *prevention* (prophylaxis), daily echinacea has not been shown effective in human trials.
- Preliminary studies of oral echinacea for genital herpes and radiation-associated toxicity remain inconclusive. Topical *E. purpurea* juice has been suggested for skin and oral wound healing, and oral/injectable echinacea for vaginal *Candida albicans* infections, but evidence is lacking in these areas.
- The German Commission E discourages use of echinacea in patients with autoimmune diseases, but this warning is based on theoretical considerations rather than human data.

Scientific Evidence for Common/Studied Uses	Grade*
Upper respiratory tract infections: treatment	B
Cancer	C
Radiation-associated leukopenia	C
Upper respiratory tract infections: prevention	C
Genital herpes	D

*Key to grades: *A:* Strong scientific evidence for this use; *B:* Good scientific evidence for this use; *C:* Unclear scientific evidence for this use; *D:* Fair scientific evidence against this use (it may not work); *F:* Strong scientific evidence against this use (it likely does not work). For a more detailed explanation of efficacy criteria, see "Natural Standard Evidence-Based Validated Grading Rationale" in the Introduction.

Historical or Theoretical Uses That Lack Sufficient Evidence

- Abscesses, acne, bacterial infections, bee stings, boils, burn wounds,[3] candidiasis, diphtheria, dizziness, dyspepsia, catarrh, eczema,[3] gingivitis, hemorrhoids, herpes labialis,[4] HIV infection,[5] insect bites,[6-8] malaria, migraine headache, nasopharyngeal catarrh, pain, psoriasis, pyorrhea, recurrent vaginal candidiasis,[9] respiratory infections in dogs,[10] rheumatism, septicemia, skin ulcers,[3] skin wounds,[3] snake bites, staphylococcal infections, streptococcal infections, syphilis, tonsillitis, typhoid, urinary tract infection, urinary disorders,[11] whooping cough.[12]

Expert Opinion and Historic/Folkloric Precedent

- Natural medicine experts frequently recommend echinacea species oral extracts for treatment of the common cold and for other conditions requiring "immunostimulation." It is occasionally recommended for topical treatment of wounds. Internal use of *Echinacea pallida* root and *E. purpurea* herb (above ground parts) has been approved by the German Commission E expert panel for supportive therapy of influenza-like infections.
- Despite a paucity of scientific evidence, the German Commission E has approved *E. purpurea* orally for supportive treatment of chronic respiratory infections and lower urinary tract infections and for topical treatment of poorly healing wounds/chronic ulcerations. These indications are also noted in monographs published by the World Health Organization.
- Traditionally, echinacea roots and herbs were used by indigenous Americans for a wide variety of conditions, ranging from snakebites to malignancies.

Safety Summary

- **Likely safe:** Echinacea is considered safe for internal use by most practitioners. Scientific evidence suggests safety when used orally or topically in recommended doses for a maximum of 8 consecutive weeks.
- **Possibly safe:** One small preliminary study suggests safety in pregnant women and in children if taken as directed, although further evidence is warranted in this area.
- **Possibly unsafe:** Echinacea may cause allergic reactions in atopic patients. Some experts discourage use in patients with cancer, tuberculosis, leukocytosis, collagenosis, multiple sclerosis, AIDS, HIV infection, or autoimmune diseases,

although this is based on theory rather than on human data, and there are no case reports of adverse events in such patients.

- **Likely unsafe:** Echinacea may cause allergic reactions in patients with allergies to members of the Asteraceae/Compositae plant family (ragweed, chrysanthemum, marigold, daisy).

DOSING/TOXICOLOGY
General

- Recommended doses are based on those most commonly used in available trials, or on historical practice (not necessarily proven efficacious). However, with natural products, the optimal doses needed to balance efficacy and safety often have not been determined. Formulations and preparation methods may vary from manufacturer to manufacturer, and from batch to batch of a specific product made by a single manufacturer. Because often the active components of a product are not known, standardization may not be possible, and the clinical effects of different brands may not be comparable.
- Combination echinacea products, such as those containing goldenseal, may not be clinically active because of low echinacea concentrations.

Standardization

- Some manufacturers standardize echinacea extracts to 4.0% to 5.0% echinacoside, and others standardize to cichoric acid. Because the active constituent(s) has not been identified, standardization may not be clinically relevant in predicting effectiveness.
- A recent well-conducted study examined the constituents of 59 commercially available echinacea preparations and found that 10% contained no measurable echinacea, and that, of the 21 standardized products, 43% met the quality standards listed on the labels.[1]

Dosing: Adult (18 Years and Older)
Oral

- **Capsules (of powdered herb):** For treatment of upper respiratory tract infections, the dose recommended most often by experts is 500 to 1000 mg three times/day, for 5 to 7 days.[13] A total daily dose of 900 mg/day has been shown superior to 450 mg/day for improvement of cold/flu symptoms.[14]
- **Expressed juice:** The dose recommended most often by experts is 6-9 mL daily in divided doses, for 5 to 7 days.
- **Tincture (1:5):** The dose recommended most often by experts is 0.75 to 1.5 mL, gargled and then swallowed, 2 to 5 times/day, for 5 to 7 days (daily dose should contain equivalent of 900 mg of dried echinacea root). Some herbalists prefer tinctures, because of purported immunostimulation at the level of the tonsillar lymphoid tissues when tinctures are gargled before swallowing.
- **Tea:** The dose recommended most often by experts is 2 teaspoons (4 g of echinacea) of coarsely powdered herb simmered in 1 cup of boiling water for 10 minutes, daily for 5 to 7 days. Echinacea Plus tea, manufactured by Traditional Medicinals (equivalent of 1.275 mg of dried herb and root per tea bag) has been shown to reduce upper respiratory tract infection symptoms when 5 to 6 cups are taken on the first day and titrated down by 1 cup/day for the next 5 days.[15]

Topical

- **Semisolid preparation:** For wound/ulcer healing, the dose often recommended by experts is a semisolid preparation of 15% pressed herb (non-root) juice applied daily.

Parenteral

- Parenteral preparations of echinacea are no longer approved for use in Germany and are generally not available commercially. Severe reactions have been reported following parenteral use.[16]

Dosing: Pediatric (Younger Than 18 Years)

- *Note:* In a study of echinacea for the treatment of cold symptoms in children ages 2 to 11 years, an increased incidence of rash was reported, without significant measured benefits.[2]

Oral

- In general, the dosage recommended for children is weight-based and calculated from the adult dosage (adult dose is based on the weight of a 70-kg male; dose should be reduced proportionately for child's weight).

Intramuscular/Parenteral

- Three studies of 257 subjects total (infants to 14-year-old children) with whooping cough found no adverse effects from 1 to 2 mL of squeezed aqueous extract (0.1 g/2 mL) given intramuscularly twice daily for 3 to 21 days.[12,17-21] Safety of intramuscular preparations has not been established and their use should be approached cautiously. Parenteral preparations of echinacea are no longer approved for use in Germany.

Toxicology

- Symptoms after parenteral administration (not often recommended) have included shivering, fever, and muscle weakness, as documented in one human report of acute toxicity.[22]
- *In vitro* toxic effects have been observed on cells at extremely high echinacea concentrations.[9]
- The LD_{50} of intravenous echinacea juice was found to be 50 mL/kg in one animal study.[23]

ADVERSE EFFECTS/PRECAUTIONS/CONTRAINDICATIONS
Allergy

- **Oral and topical formulations:** Individuals with asthma or atopy may be predisposed to allergic reactions from oral/topical use of echinacea, consistent with IgE-mediated hypersensitivity.[24] Anaphylaxis associated with echinacea has been reported in a 37-year-old woman with a history of atopy.[25] She subsequently was found to have a positive skin prick test, and radioallergosorbent (RAST) testing confirmed IgE binding to echinacea. In a poorly described series of 23 case reports of IgE-mediated hypersensitivity reactions, causality was ascribed to echinacea as "certain" in 2 cases, and "probable" in 10 cases. Adequate details of methodology were not provided.[26] The same authors published a 2002 report from their referral center in Australia that documented four cases of anaphylaxis or bronchospasm following ingestion of echinacea, and one case of maculopapular rash.[24] All five individuals subsequently reacted positively to skin prick and RAST testing for echinacea hypersensitivity. The authors also noted 26 cases reported to the Australian Adverse Drug Reactions Advisory Committee between 1979 and 2000 of urticaria, angioedema, bronchospasm, or anaphylaxis associated with echinacea use. More than six brands and multiple formulations (tea, tablets, liquid) were implicated. No deaths occurred.

- In a study of echinacea use in children ages 2 to 11 years, an increased incidence of rash was reported (7.1% with echinacea vs. 2.7% with placebo; $p = 0.008$).
- To determine the prevalence of echinacea sensitivity in the population at large, 100 atopic patients who had never taken echinacea were tested with skin prick tests, and a positive response was elicited in 20%, with negative controls.[24,26]
- In a study of 1032 subjects who were patch tested topically with various plant extracts, 2 reacted to *Echinacea angustifolia*.[27]
- **Injections:** Five cases of severe reactions following injection of Echinacin have been reported, characterized by angioedema, hypotension, anaphylactic shock, and rash; a 63-year-old patient developed bilateral hand swelling, erythema, and pruritis after oral ingestion of Esberitox.[16] Other cases of allergic reactions have been reported after parenteral use of echinacea products,[28,29] and there is no supportive evidence from human trials to favor parenteral over oral use.
- Theoretically, individuals sensitive to members of the Asteraceae/Compositae plant family (ragweed, chrysanthemums, marigolds, daisies) may be more likely to experience allergic responses.

Adverse Effects

- **General:** Echinacea has been well tolerated in clinical practice and in trials, with few adverse events reported. Three studies of 257 subjects total (infants to 14-year-old children) with whooping cough found no adverse effects from 1 to 2 mL of squeezed aqueous extract (0.1 g/2 ml) given intramuscularly twice daily for 3 to 21 days.[12,17-21]
- **Dermatologic:** Urticaria and allergic rashes have been reported.[24] There is one published case of recurrent erythema nodosum in association with use of echinacea.[30] In a study of children ages 2 to 11 years, rash occurred in 7.1% of children treated with echinacea, vs. 2.7% with placebo ($p = 0.008$).
- **Neurologic/CNS:** Mild drowsiness and headache have been reported in <1% of study subjects.[31] Dizziness has been rarely noted.[24]
- **Cardiovascular:** One case of atrial fibrillation has been reported in association with echinacea use.[24] Specific details are not available.
- **Gastrointestinal:** The most frequently cited adverse events from clinical trials are gastrointestinal, including transient mild nausea or vomiting (<1%), sore throat (<1%), and abdominal pain (<1%).[22] In one study, 13% reported adverse effects that were largely gastrointestinal, although the authors felt that echinacea was the likely cause in only one case (additional details were not provided).[31] Seven cases of hepatitis associated with echinacea use were reported to the Australian Adverse Drug Reactions Advisory Committee between 1979 and 2000.[24] However, specific details of these cases are not available.
- **Genitourinary/Reproductive:** One *in vitro* study of zona free hamster oocytes concluded that high concentrations of echinacea reduce the penetration of hamster sperm. At low concentrations, penetration was comparable to control. *In vitro* incubation of hamster sperm with echinacea for 7 days indicated significant denaturation of sperm DNA and reduced viability.[32]

- **Renal:** One case of acute renal failure has been reported in association with echinacea use.[24] Specific details are not available.
- **Hematologic:** Long-term use of echinacea may be associated with leukopenia,[33] although further data are needed in this area before a firm conclusion can be reached.

Precautions/Warnings/Contraindications

- Use cautiously in patients prone to atopic reactions, because of predisposition toward allergic reactions with oral/topical echinacea.
- Use caution with parenteral preparations of echinacea (no longer approved for use in Germany). Safety is not established, and in diabetics, parenteral administration may worsen glycemic control.
- Use tinctures cautiously in alcoholic patients and in patients taking disulfiram or metronidazole: many tinctures contain significant concentrations of alcohol (range, 15% to 90%).
- The German Commission E warns against use of echinacea in patients with AIDS/HIV infection, collagen vascular diseases, multiple sclerosis, or tuberculosis, due to theoretical adverse effects on immune function, although no specific trial data support this assertion.

Pregnancy and Lactation

- In preliminary studies, oral echinacea has not appeared to pose a teratogenic risk. One controlled, prospective study of 206 pregnant women found no differences in the incidence of birth defects, gestational age, maternal weight gain, birth weight, pregnancy outcome, or fetal distress from echinacea use.[34,35] In this study, different formulations were used by pregnant women: 58% used capsule/tablets (250 to 1000 mg/day) and 38% used tinctures (5 to 30 drops/day) varying in alcoholic content from 25% to 45%. Duration of use varied but typically was continuous for 5 to 7 days. The statistical power of this study, however, was limited, leaving the possibility of undetected adverse gestational effects.
- The German Commission E expert panel considers oral echinacea in recommended doses safe for use in pregnancy and lactation. However, most experts do not recommend parenteral administration during pregnancy. Tinctures may be ill-advised because of their 15% to 90% alcohol content, although the absolute quantity of alcohol ingested from tinctures at recommended doses is likely to be relatively small.
- Further data are warranted in this area.

INTERACTIONS
Echinacea/Drug Interactions

- **Amoxicillin:** There is one poorly described case report of a 19-year-old patient ingesting amoxicillin and an unclear echinacea preparation who developed rhabdomyolysis, shock, and death; further details were not provided.[16]
- **Disulfiram (Antabuse):** Echinacea tinctures often have a high alcohol content (15% to 90%) and theoretically may elicit a disulfiram reaction.
- **Econazole nitrate (Spectazole):** There is preliminary evidence to suggest that use of echinacea with topical Econazole decreases the recurrence rate of vaginal *Candida* infections.[36]
- **Hepatotoxic agents:** Natural medicine practitioners often caution that echinacea may cause hepatotoxicity, and recommend avoiding concomitant use with other potentially

hepatotoxic drugs (anabolic steroids, amiodarone, methotrexate, ketoconazole, etc.). However, there is no clear evidence from basic science or human reports that echinacea causes significant liver toxicity. Some have noted that it lacks the 1,2-unsaturated necrine ring system that causes hepatotoxicity of pyrrolizidine alkaloids.[37]

- **Immunosuppressant drugs, oral corticosteroids:** In theory, echinacea's immunostimulant properties may interfere with immunosuppressant therapy (including azathioprine, cyclosporin, and prednisone). This possibility has not been systematically studied in humans.
- **Metronidazole (Flagyl):** A disulfiram reaction can occur when metronidazole and alcohol are used concomitantly. Because of the high alcohol content in some echinacea tinctures, this combination theoretically may cause such a reaction.

Echinacea/Herb/Supplement Interactions

- **Immunostimulant agents:** *Positive interaction:* Echinacea is sometimes used in combination products that are purported to synergistically stimulate the immune system. For example, Esberitox (PhytoPharmica, Germany) contains *Echinacea purpurea*, *Echinacea pallida*, wild indigo root (*Baptisia tinctoria*), and thuja (white cedar). There is no available human evidence supporting these interactions.
- **Vitamin B:** Although echinacea itself has not been found to interact with vitamin B, many echinacea preparations are coupled with goldenseal (*Hydrastis canadensis*), which is purportedly an antibiotic and may decrease intestinal microflora and absorption of vitamin B. These preparations may have low levels of echinacea and may not be efficacious against virus-induced upper respiratory tract infections.
- **Kava:** Multiple reports of hepatotoxicity associated with kava use have been reported, believed to be most common with heavy or chronic use. Caution should be exercised with concomitant use of echinacea, which some natural medicine practitioners have warned may cause liver toxicity as well. However, there is no clear evidence from basic science or human reports that echinacea causes significant liver toxicity. Some have noted that it lacks the 1,2-unsaturated necrine ring system that causes hepatotoxicity of pyrrolizidine alkaloids.[37] This potential interaction remains theoretical.

Echinacea/Food Interactions

- Insufficient available evidence.

Echinacea/Lab Interactions

- Insufficient available evidence.

MECHANISM OF ACTION
Pharmacology

- Immunostimulatory properties of echinacea appear to target both nonspecific and specific immune function. Nonspecific effects include increases in macrophage proliferation and phagocytosis, as well as secretion of interferon, tumor necrosis factor, and interleukin-1 (*in vitro* and *in vivo*).[38-43] Specific immune responses include activation of alternate complement pathway components, and elevated levels/activity of T lymphocytes and natural killer (NK) cells.[14,44-46] The echinacea species *E. purpurea* is believed to have the strongest potency on the immune system.[47] Immunostimulation may depend on dosage and frequency of administration: Cell-mediated immunity can be stimulated by one therapeutic administration followed by a "free" interval of 1 week, but immunity can be depressed by daily administration of higher doses.[9] Other studies have failed to elicit these responses.
- In animal studies, *Echinacea angustiflora* has exhibited anti-inflammatory[48] and antihyaluronidase activity, a likely function of its polysaccharide fraction,[49] which may stimulate wound healing.[50]
- In rats, an increase of primary and secondary antigen-specific IgG production has been seen with continuous echinacea treatment.[51]
- Echinacea may possess microbiocidal activity against *Candida albicans*, *Listeria monocytogenes*,[52] influenza virus,[53] vesicular stomach virus, and herpes simplex virus (HSV-1 and HSV-2).[54] The relevance of these *in vivo* findings remains unclear.
- Constituents of the root oil of *E. angustiflora* and *Echinacea pallida* have been shown to possess antitumor activity *in vivo*.[55]

Pharmacodynamics/Kinetics

- Insufficient available reliable data.

HISTORY

- Used in traditional medicine by Native Americans of the Great Plains region, there are nine known species of echinacea, all which grow east of the Rocky Mountains.
- Echinacea was adopted by central U.S. settlers in the 1800s. In the 1920s, American Eclectic physicians added echinacea to their pharmacopoeia. However, after the introduction of antibiotics, echinacea use fell out of favor.
- Echinacea's historical use against infections has found renewed interest due to recent rises in antibiotic resistance and the limitations of available antiviral drugs.

Review of the Evidence: Echinacea

Condition Treated*	Study Design	Author, Year	N†	SS†	Study Quality‡	Magnitude of Benefit	ARR†	NNT†	Comments
URI treatment	RCT, double-blind	Brinkeborn[31] 1999	246	Yes	5	Medium	25-35%	3-4	Examined severity but not duration of symptoms; higher concentration more effective.
URI treatment	RCT, double-blind	Barrett[72] 2002	148	No	5	None	NA	NA	No differences in self-reported severity or duration of symptoms; unrefined combination of *E. purpurea* and *E. angustifolia* compared to alfalfa ("placebo"); may not have been adequately powered.

Continued

Review of the Evidence: Echinacea—*cont'd*

Condition Treated*	Study Design	Author, Year	N[†]	SS[†]	Study Quality[‡]	Magnitude of Benefit	ARR[†]	NNT[†]	Comments
URI treatment (children)	RCT, double-blind	Taylor[2] 2003	407	No	4	None	NA	NA	No differences in parent-reported symptom severity or duration; increased risk of rash with echinacea.
URI treatment	RCT, double-blind	Brinkeborn[63] 1998	119	Yes	5	NA	NA	NA	This is a preliminary report of Brinkeborn, 1999 (same trial).
URI treatment	RCT, double-blind	Henneicke-von Zepelin[69] 1999	263	Yes	5	Small	NA	NA	Combination product Esberitox reduced severity and duration.
URI treatment	RCT, double-blind	Hoheisel[64] 1997	120	Yes	4	Medium	20%	5	Decreased duration and severity; subjective outcome.
URI treatment	RCT	Dorn[13] 1997	160	Yes	3	Large	NA	NA	Decreased duration and severity.
URI treatment	RCT	Lindenmuth[15] 2000	95	Yes	3	Small	NA	NA	Decreased duration and severity with early treatment.
URI treatment	RCT, double-blind	Thom[70] 1997	66	Yes	3	Large	NA	NA	Kanjan herbal mixture decreased duration of symptoms.
URI treatment	RCT, dosing trial	Bräunig[14] 1992	180	Yes	2	Large	NA	NA	900 mg/day more effective than 450 mg; methods poorly described.
URI treatment	RCT, dosing trial	Bräunig[58] 1993	160	Yes	2	Large	NA	NA	Use of *Echinacea pallida*; methods poorly described.
URI treatment	RCT, single-blind	Scaglione[71] 1995	32	Yes	1	Medium	NA	NA	Cold-X (combination) reduced the no. of tissues used and duration.
URI prevention	RCT, double-blind	Grimm[67] 1999	109	No	4	Small	9%	11	Level of statistical power questionable; no significant preventive effect; median symptom duration reduced by one third.
URI prevention	Equivalence trial, double-blind	Melchart[66] 1998	302	Yes	4	Small	6%	17	*E. angustifolia* vs. *E. purpurea*; no effect of echinacea vs. placebo on URI incidence, but positive subjective efficacy.
URI prevention	RCT, double-blind	Schoneberger[80] 1992	108	NA	3	Large	7%	14	Reduced incidence, severity, and duration, but methods and statistics insufficiently described.
URI prevention	RCT	Berg[86] 1998	42	Yes	2	Medium	NA	NA	Methodologically weak study in male athletes prior to competition.
URI prevention	Controlled (not randomized or blinded)	Turner[82] 2000	117	No	1	None	13%	8	Poor statistical power; low content of pharmacologically active compounds.
URI prevention	RCT	Forth[81] 1981	95	Yes	1	Large	32%	3	Large preventive effect; methodologically weak.
Radiation-associated leukopenia	RCT	Bendel[87] 1988	50	No	1	None	NA	NA	No power calculation; unclear if sample size is sufficient to sense differences.
Radiation-associated leukopenia	RCT	Sartor[88] 1972	48	Yes	1	Large	NA	NA	Combination product Esberitox reduced no. of days of radiation missed due to leukopenia.
Genital herpes	RCT	Vonau[92] 2001	50	No	4	NA	NA	NA	No effect of 6 months of combination product Esberitox.

*Primary or secondary outcome.
[†]*N*, Number of patients; *SS*, statistically significant; *ARR*, absolute risk reduction; *NNT*, the number of patients who need to undergo a specific intervention in order to observe an outcome in one individual.
[‡]0-2 = poor; 3-4 = good; 5 = excellent.
NA, Not applicable; *RCT*, randomized controlled trial; *URI*, upper respiratory tract infection.
For an explanation of each category in this table, please see Table 3 in the Introduction.

REVIEW OF THE EVIDENCE: DISCUSSION
Upper Respiratory Tract Infection: Treatment
Summary

- Oral echinacea is frequently recommended to reduce the duration and severity of upper respiratory tract infections (URIs). Numerous trials have been conducted in this area but have largely been of limited methodological quality (or they have used combination products). Nonetheless, the sum of existing positive evidence is highly suggestive—albeit not definitive. A sufficiently sized, rigorously blinded study using doses previously found effective (*Echinacea purpurea* extract, 900 mg/day for 6 to 8 days) and using accepted outcome measures is warranted, in order to further characterize optimal timing, dosage, frequency of administration, and magnitude of benefit. Consideration should also be given to the possible differential efficacy of various echinacea species and of their different plant parts (root vs. above-ground herb).

Systematic Reviews

- A systematic review of studies (before 1994) of echinacea for immunomodulatory indications[56] found six randomized, placebo-controlled, double-blind trials examining efficacy in the treatment and prevention of URI.[14,57-61] The authors concluded that, despite some evidence of immunomodulatory action of echinacea, no clear recommendations could be made for the treatment of URI with echinacea. Individual trials are discussed below.
- Barrett et al. published a similar review, but included trials published up to 1998.[62] Nine studies evaluating treatment efficacy,[13,14,58-61,63,64] plus one unpublished trial (Galea, 1996), were identified. Most studies had significant methodological limitations, and often used *ad hoc* symptom scores. The authors nevertheless concluded that the use of echinacea for treatment of early cold symptoms may be "cautiously supported," while long-term or preventive use was not recommended.
- Giles et al. presented a review of studies on echinacea efficacy in prevention and treatment of the common cold published since 1994.[65] Five such trials were included in the analysis.[13,31,64,66,67] The authors concluded that the "efficacy of echinacea for treating common cold symptoms remains unclear, yet it appears a suitable alternative for suitable patients."
- A review of the efficacy of echinacea to prevent or treat the common cold[68] concluded that echinacea may be effective for preventing and treating the common cold, but that more studies are needed to determine which preparations are most effective. All included randomized controlled trials are discussed in detail below.

Randomized Trials (Higher Quality)

- A well-conducted randomized, placebo-controlled double-blind trial of 246 participants found that Echinaforce (6.78 mg of *Echinacea purpurea* crude extract based on 95% herb and 5% root per tablet) and a 7X concentration (48.27 mg) both significantly reduced severity of cold symptoms.[31] Participants took 2 tablets three times daily after onset of symptoms and were advised to continue until they "felt healthy" (7 days maximum). The primary end point was reduction in a 12-symptom complaint-index scale: improvement was documented for subjects who experienced reductions in complaint-index by >60% (physician scale) or >50% (patient scale). This otherwise methodologically

strong study would have benefited from a more established, validated symptom scale. Preliminary results of this trial in 119 patients were reported elsewhere.[63]

- Bräunig et al. conducted a randomized, placebo-controlled, double-blind dosing trial on the efficacy of echinacea extract in the treatment of the common cold.[14] In this study, 180 otherwise healthy patients with symptoms of the common cold were allocated to either placebo (no details provided), *Echinacea purpura* radix 50% ethanolic extract, 450 mg/day or 900 mg/day. Randomization and blinding procedures and treatment plans were not clearly described. At days 0, 3-4, and 8-10, cold symptoms (fatigue, sweats, teary eyes, stinging eyes, sore throat, earache, myalgia, headache) were assessed by a 4-point scale (0 = not present, 1 = mild, 2 = moderate, 3 = severe) and patients were clinically assessed. The two target variables were duration of illness and reduction of symptoms. Only the higher dose of echinacea was superior to placebo in reducing symptoms ($p < 0.0001$). Although this finding is suggestive, the poor description of methods limits the usefulness of this study.
- A randomized, placebo-controlled double-blind trial of 160 patients with symptoms of acute URI found an alcoholic extract of *Echinacea pallidae radix* to significantly reduce both severity and duration of URI symptoms.[13] Neither the method of herb extraction nor a product name was specified. Ninety drops/day were given over 8 to 10 days (unclear whether one or several doses were given). Benefit of echinacea vs. placebo was reported in terms of illness length ($p < 0.0001$), overall symptom score ($p < 0.0004$), and "whole" clinical score ($p < 0.001$). However, limited information was provided regarding statistical analysis or measurement instruments. Although this study is suggestive, without further methodological details, results are difficult to interpret.
- A randomized, double-blind, placebo-controlled study of 120 participants found the duration and severity of common cold symptoms to be significantly decreased with Echinaguard (squeezed sap of *E. purpurea*).[64] The dose given was 20 drops in water every 2 hours for the first day, followed by 3 times daily (up to a total of 10 days). Efficacy was assessed by a short, structured interview which included questions regarding the nature of illness ("real cold?"), fever, severity vs. previous episodes of common cold, onset of improvement, and duration of treatment. Fewer subjects in the Echinaguard group experienced a "real cold" after initiation of treatment vs. placebo (40% vs. 60%, $p = 0.044$). Median time to improvement was significantly shorter in the Echinaguard group than in the placebo group (0 vs. 5 days, $p < 0.0001$). Limitations of this study include unclear standardization of the product used, and incomplete description of randomization, blinding, statistical analysis, dropouts, and validation of the measuring questionnaire.
- Lindenmuth and Lindenmuth conducted a randomized controlled trial of Echinacea Plus tea vs. a placebo for upper respiratory tract symptoms.[15] The tea contained the equivalent of 1.275 mg of dried herb and root per tea bag. Participants were instructed to drink 5 to 6 cups of tea on the first day and titrate down by 1 cup/day for the next 5 days. The experimental group rated the effectiveness of echinacea tea as 4.1 on a 5-point scale (SD, 0.96), while the control group rated their tea 2.8 (SD, 0.095), with a $p < 0.001$. There was also a statistically significant (although small) difference in the number of days symptoms lasted and in the number of days before symptoms diminished in

the treatment group vs. control. Statistical analysis may not have been appropriate (t-test for sum scores), but this methodological weakness would not likely explain the results. Therefore, echinacea tea, when taken at the first onset of symptoms, may be effective in relieving symptoms of the common cold and in abbreviating the course of the illness.

- In a well-conducted randomized, double-blind, placebo-controlled multicenter trial, Henneicke-von Zepelin et al. examined the efficacy of the combination product Esberitox (includes ethanolic-aqueous extracts of 2 mg of herba thujae occidentalis, 7.5 mg of radix echinaceae, 10 mg radix of baptisiae tinctoriae).[69] The study enrolled 263 patients with acute common colds who were not suffering from any chronic condition affecting immune system function. Patients received either Esberitox N, 3 tablets/day, or placebo for 7 to 9 days. Primary outcomes were general well-being (Welzel-Kohnen color scale), physician-evaluated symptom severity (clinical global impression item-1 [CGI-1]), and rhinitis score/bronchitis score (10-point scales). Patient follow-up was on days 0, 4, and 8. The "total efficacy value," a combination of all outcome measures, showed a >20% effect at study completion ($p < 0.05$). The improvement in well-being was most prominent (33.9%, $p = 0.0048$), followed by rhinitis score. Time to response, defined as a 50% decrease in symptom score, was significantly shorter in the treatment group vs. placebo ($p = 0.022$). These findings suggest that an herbal combination containing echinachea significantly reduces the severity and duration of the common cold when given at the early onset of symptoms. However, the question of whether this effect is attributable to the echinacea component of Esberiox cannot be addressed within the framework of this study.

- Thom and Wollan found a significantly faster improvement of cold symptoms with Kanjang, a mixture containing echinacea, Siberian ginseng, and Vasaka.[70] Sixty-six patients with common cold symptoms were randomly assigned to either Kanjang (15 mL three times daily, containing 4.5g/day of Echinacea purpurea radix) or placebo. Improvement of cold symptoms was assessed by a 10-point Visual Analogue Scale (VAS) on days 2, 4, and 10 after onset of treatment. The difference between groups was most pronounced on day 4, when the average global efficacy VAS score was approximately 6 in the Kanjang group vs. 1 in the placebo group ($p = 0.001$). As with other studies using combination products, this study does not permit specific inference regarding the efficacy of echinacea.

Lesser Quality Studies

- Bräunig and Knick report a study evaluating the efficacy of Echinacea pallida for the treatment of URI.[58] In this study, 180 otherwise healthy patients with symptoms of URI were randomly allocated to either E. pallida radix (Pascotox, 900 mg/day) or placebo for 8 to 10 days. Outcome was measured by "overall clinical assessment" and by symptom scores as described for the previous study.[14] Follow-up was at days 0, 3-4, and 8-10. Duration of illness was reduced from 13 to 10 days for bacterial infections and from 13 to 9 days for viral infections (neither the end point of illness nor the basis for diagnosis of viral vs. bacterial infection was clearly defined). Improvement in total symptom score was faster with E. pallida than with placebo ($p < 0.0001$) and faster for viral vs. bacterial infections. The authors concluded that E. pallida is effective in the treatment of URI and

at least as effective as E. purpurea. However, the poor description of methods limits the usefulness of this study.

- Scaglione and Lund evaluated the efficacy of an herbal mixture containing echinacea for the treatment of the common cold in a randomized, placebo-controlled, single-blind trial.[71] Thirty-two patients with cold symptoms, but otherwise healthy, were randomized to receive either 4 effervescent tablets/day of Cold-X, which contains Vitamin C (100 mg), Echinacea purpurea root extract (20.1 mg), eucalyptus leaf extract (2.3 mg), and fennel seed extract (10.3 mg), or placebo (4 glucose tablets/day). Main outcome variables were duration of illness based on rhinorrhea and the number of paper tissues used (measurement method not described). Overall number of tissues used was 882 in the echinacea group vs. 1168 in the control group. Mean duration of cold symptoms was 3.4 and 4.4 days, respectively ($p < 0.01$; the statistical method used was incompletely described and may have been inappropriate). These findings suggest that treatment of the common cold with Cold-X may be effective. However, due to the lack of double-blinding and the use of an herbal combination, no firm conclusions can be drawn.

Negative Studies

- Barrett et al. conducted a randomized, controlled, double-blind study in 148 college students with recent onset of cold symptoms.[72] Enrollees were assigned to receive either alfalfa ("placebo"), or an encapsulated mixture of unrefined Echinacea purpurea herb (25%) and root (25%), plus Echinacea angustifolia root (50%). The dose of echinacea was 1 g taken six times on the first day of symptoms, then three times daily on each additional day of illness, up to 10 days. Measured outcomes included self-reported symptom duration and severity. The authors found no differences between groups: mean duration of symptoms was 5.75 days with placebo, and 6.27 days with echinacea (between-group difference—0.52, 95% CI—1.09 to 0.22 days). No significant treatment effect was found. This study has been criticized for the lack of use of a standardized alcohol extract of echinacea, the choice of a product that contained more than one echinacea species, and the choice of alfalfa as a placebo because it may have some action itself.[73-78] In addition, although there were 148 participants, the sample size may not have been adequate to detect differences in the primary outcome of self-reported symptoms. Therefore, because of methodological weaknesses, this study cannot be considered conclusive.

- Taylor et al. conducted a randomized, double-blind, placebo-controlled study in 407 children (ages 2-11 years), in whom 337 URIs were treated with echinacea, and 370 with placebo.[2] The primary outcome was parent-reported symptom duration and severity. Secondary outcomes included peak severity of symptoms, number of days of fever, and global assessment of symptoms. The median duration of URIs overall was 9 days, and there was no significant difference in duration between groups. Also, no differences in any secondary outcomes were noted. Although there was no significant difference between groups in adverse events overall, there was a significantly greater incidence of rash in the echinacea group than in the placebo group (7.1% with echinacea vs. 2.7% with placebo, $p = 0.008$). This study suggests that echinacea may not alleviate URI symptoms in young children.

Upper Respiratory Tract Infection: Prevention

Summary

- The evidence for echinacea's efficacy in the prevention of upper respiratory tract infections (URIs) is equivocal. The available randomized controlled studies have substantial methodological weaknesses. Lack of statistical power may explain some of the negative results, which are largely based on moderate sample sizes and brief follow-up periods (person–time of observation may be insufficient). Even if there is a preventive effect of echinacea, it is likely small at best. A large, well-designed longitudinal study is warranted in this area.

Systematic Reviews

- A systematic review of studies (before 1994) of echinacea for immunomodulatory indications[56] found three randomized, placebo-controlled and double-blind trials which examined the efficacy of echinacea in the prevention of URI.[79-81] The authors concluded that, despite some evidence of immunomodulatory action of echinacea, no clear recommendations could be made for the prevention of URI with echinacea.

- Barrett et al. published a similar review but included trials published up to 1998.[62] Four trials evaluating prevention efficacy were included.[66,79-81] Most studies had significant methodological limitations, and often used *ad hoc* symptom scores. The authors concluded that the long-term or preventive use of echinacea should not be recommended.

- A review of the efficacy of echinacea to prevent or treat the common cold concluded that echinacea may be effective for preventing and treating the common cold, but more studies are needed to determine which preparations are most effective.[68] All included randomized controlled trials are discussed in detail below.

Randomized Trials (Higher Quality)

- A double-blind, randomized, placebo-controlled trial of 109 participants found that *E. purpurea* (fresh expressed juice of the whole flowering plant harvested without roots), 4 mL twice/day for 8 weeks, did not significantly lower the incidence or severity of common colds.[67] Although no preventive effect of *E. purpurea* juice was found, there was a statistically nonsignificant reduction in the duration of cold symptoms (4.5 days in the echinacea group vs. 6.5 days in the placebo group, $p = 0.45$). The size of this study, considering its prospective nature, may not have been adequate to detect small but significant benefits with sufficient statistical power. It was otherwise well conducted.

- In a placebo-controlled, non-randomized, unblinded experiment, Turner et al. investigated the effect of echinacea vs. placebo in 92 subjects challenged with rhinovirus type 23.[82] Subjects were treated for 2 weeks before and 5 days after inoculation with 300 mg three times/day of echinacea (n = 50) or placebo (n = 42). A clinical diagnosis of a cold was subsequently made in 44% of echinacea subjects and 57% of placebo subjects. Mean symptom scores were lower in the echinacea group vs. placebo throughout the study (overall mean, 13.6 vs. 11.4), and similar differences were observed for individual symptom scores (total rhinorrhea and mean nasal obstruction scales). However, none of the differences was statistically significant. A potential weakness is that almost no echinacosides or alkamides were found by high-pressure liquid chromatography in the echinacea

preparation. In addition, the power of this study to detect a reduction in risk from 50% to 20% was only 75%.

- In a randomized, controlled, open trial, Forth and Beuscher examined the efficacy of two echinacea preparations to prevent URI.[81] Ninety-five healthy subjects were randomly allocated to Esberitox liquid, 25 drops three times daily; Esberitox, three tablets daily; or placebo. Esberitox liquid includes ethanolic-aqueous extracts of herba thujae occidentalis (2 mg), radix echinaceae (7.5 mg), and radix baptisiae tinctoriae (10 mg), whereas Esberitox tablets contain 20 mg of vitamin C/tablet in addition to these ingredients. Treatment duration varied from 3 to 17 weeks, and the main outcome measured was rhinitis. In both echinacea groups combined, two thirds did not suffer from URI, whereas in a placebo group this proportion was only one third ($p < 0.005$). The difference between the two echinacea groups was not statistically significant. Although these results suggest efficacy of echinacea, a proper statistical analysis would have compared the number of events per treatment time rather than the overall risk per group. It is unlikely, however, that this would have substantially changed the results.

- Melchart et al. conducted a randomized, placebo-controlled, double-blind study comparing the efficacy of *E. angustifolia* vs. *E. purpurea*.[66] In this equivalence trial, 302 healthy volunteers without signs of URI were randomly assigned to receive 1 mL of extract from the root of either plant in 30% alcohol (twice daily from Monday through Friday, for 12 weeks) or placebo. There was no difference between the three treatment arms in terms of the main effect measure (time to first URI episode). However, because of low statistical power, the study may have been too small to detect small to medium-sized treatment effects. Notably, 78% in the *Echinacea angustifolia*, 70% in the *E. purpurea* group, and 56% in the placebo group believed subjectively that they benefited from the treatment ($p = 0.04$). Although these findings are suggestive, the use of validated symptom indices might have been advantageous for identifying effects of either treatment.

- Schoneberger evaluated the potential of echinacea to prevent URI in a randomized, placebo-controlled trial.[80] In this study, 108 otherwise healthy patients "at risk for URI" were randomly allocated to receive *E. purpura* juice (4 mL twice daily) or placebo juice for 8 weeks. Randomization and blinding methods were not described. Primary outcome variables were the number and severity of URI episodes. Secondary outcomes included time to first URI and URI duration. In the echinacea group, 23 URIs were observed (78% were mild) vs. 35 in placebo (63% were mild). The average duration of symptoms was 5.3 vs. 7.5 days. The proportion of URI-free patients was 35% vs. 27%. Although no statistical analysis was presented, the difference between the echinacea and placebo groups appeared to be substantial in terms of overall number, duration, and severity of URI.

Lesser Quality Studies

- Several trials of lower methodological quality have examined the effects of echinacea for the prevention of URI symptoms. In a 1974 study of 284 children attending a summer camp, Freyer treated half of the subjects with an herbal combination containing echinacea (Esberitox) and left the other half untreated.[83] In the echinacea group, 30% contracted a cold vs. >50% in the no-treatment group. Although these findings are suggestive, the observational nature renders interpretation difficult. In an earlier (1965) study, children on a pediatric ward were given either oral Esberitox (6 weeks on average) or no treatment.[84] Incidence, prevalence and number of febrile days were substantially lower in the Esberitox group vs. control, but the lack of randomization or blinding limits the value of this study. In a 1961 study, Helbig enrolled 644 children hospitalized for non-URI causes and randomly allocated them to Esberitox or no treatment.[85] Overall, there was no difference between the two groups. A post-study analysis limited to children hospitalized for >14 days found that fewer children treated with Esberitox suffered from new common cold episodes, but no statistical analysis was presented. This method of historical data reshuffling cannot be considered valid. In a randomized, controlled trial in 42 male athletes given echinacea for 28 days prior to competition, subjects receiving echinacea were found to have lower serum and urine levels of soluble interleukin 2 receptors (sIL-2R) and significantly fewer respiratory infections vs. placebo.[86] However, details of methodology and statistical analysis are limited.

Radiation-Associated Leukopenia
Summary
- The evidence from a small number of randomized trials evaluating efficacy of echinacea in the treatment of radiation-induced leukopenia is equivocal. Studies have used the combination product Esberitox, which includes ethanolic-aqueous extracts of *herba thujae occidentalis, radix echinaceae,* and *radix baptisiae tinctoriae.*

Evidence
- Bendel et al. randomly allocated 50 women receiving post-mastectomy radiation therapy to an herbal combination containing echinacea (Esberitox N, 50 drops daily throughout the radiation treatment period) or to placebo.[87] Effects on leukocyte counts and other hematological parameters were assessed before and after radiation. No statistically significant differences were found. Despite the questionable statistical power of the study, the benefit of echinacea is likely to be small at best.
- In contrast, Sartor found a substantial effect of Esberitox on radiation-induced leukopenia.[88] Forty-eight patients undergoing 6 weeks of radiation therapy were assigned randomly to Esberitox or no adjuvant treatment. In the Esberitox group, 46% missed zero days of therapy because of leukocyte counts <3000/mm³, vs. 18% in the untreated group. Although these proportions were not statistically compared, they are highly suggestive. The mean number of missed treatment days did not differ significantly, although these results are not interpretable because of an inadequate t-test.
- In a case series, Pohl found a statistically significant increase in leukocyte counts in 55 patients undergoing radiation therapy after treatment with Esberitox (various doses and routes of administration).[89] This observational study is suggestive mechanistically but of limited clinical value.
- Additional weak evidence is provided by Bendel et al. in a randomized trial of 70 women receiving radiation therapy for breast cancer.[90] No change in incidence of infection was noted, although bone marrow toxicity was reportedly lessened. The methodological and histologic criteria were poorly described, weakening the clinical applicability of results.

Cancer
Summary
- There is insufficient evidence to recommend for or against the use of echinacea for any type of cancer. Only preliminary data from case series are available, without any evidence of benefit.

Evidence
- Cytokine levels were monitored in 35 brain tumor patients who were given 3 mL/day of a 40% *E. angustifolia* herbal therapy. After 4 weeks, no change in white blood cell counts or cytokine production was noted. The clinical significance of these findings is unclear.[91]
- Preliminary studies have been conducted to assess the safety of combination chemotherapy including Echinacin (*E. purpurea*). In one study, 15 patients with advanced, metastatic colon cancer who had already undergone standard treatment with chemotherapy/surgery were given low-dose cyclophosphamide, thymostimulin, and Echinacin.[80] The mean survival time was 4 months. In a case series, five patients with advanced hepatocellular carcinoma were treated with a combination regimen including Echinacin, and mean survival was 10 weeks.[81]

Genital Herpes
Summary
- A small clinical trial assessing the potential benefit of oral echinacea for recurrent herpes genitalis found no effect. Conclusions cannot be considered definitive without further trials.
- Vonau et al. conducted a randomized, placebo-controlled, crossover trial to evaluate the therapeutic use of echinacea for recurrent genital herpes.[92] Fifty patients were randomly allocated to a treatment sequence of either echinacea extract (800 mg orally twice/day) for 6 months followed by placebo for 6 months, or vice versa. Number of recurrences and several indicators of disease status (Visual Analogue Scale of pain, CD4 counts, neutrophil counts) were assessed before and after treatments. No statistically significant differences were found between the groups. Although the sample size was relatively small, a relevant treatment benefit would likely have been detected if present.

FORMULARY: BRANDS USED IN CLINICAL TRIALS
Brands Used in Statistically Significant Clinical Trials
- Echinacin (Madaus AG, Germany), Echinaguard (Nature's Way, USA), Echinaforce (Bioforce), EchinaFresh (Enzymatic Therapy), Esberitox (Enzymatic Therapy), Esberitox N, Pascotox, Resistan, Biracial (Destiny BioMediX Corp).
- Echinacea Plus tea (Traditional Medicinals): equivalent of 1.275 mg of dried herb and root per tea bag.

References
1. Gilroy CM, Steiner JF, Byers T, et al. Echinacea and truth in labeling. Arch Intern Med 2003;163(6):699-704.
2. Taylor JA, Weber W, Standish L, et al. Efficacy and safety of echinacea in treating upper respiratory tract infections in children: a randomized controlled trial. JAMA 2003;290(21):2824-2830.
3. Viehmann P. [Results of treatment with an Echinacea-based ointment]. Erfahrungsheilkunde 1978;27(6):353-358.
4. Bockhorst H, Gollnick N, Guran S, et al. [Therapy of herpes simplex in practice. Report on the treatment of herpes simplex labialis with Esberitox]. ZFA (Stuttgart) 1982;58(32):1795-1798.
5. See D, Berman S, Justis J, et al. A phase I study on the safety of *Echinacea angustifolia* and its effect on viral load in HIV infected individuals. J Amer Nutr Assoc 1998;1(1):14-17.

6. Hill N, van Haselen RA. Clinical trial of a homeopathic insect after-bite treatment. Hom Int R&D Newslet 1993;3/4:4-5.

7. Hill N, Stam C, Tuinder S, et al. A placebo controlled clinical trial investigating the efficacy of a homeopathic after-bite gel in reducing mosquito bite induced erythema. Eur J Clin Pharmacol 1995;49(1-2):103-108.

8. Hill N, Stam C, van Haselen RA. The efficacy of Prrrikweg gel in the treatment of insect bites: a double-blind, placebo-controlled clinical trial. Pharm World Sci 1996;18(1):35-41.

9. Coeugniet EG, Elek E. Immunomodulation with Viscum album and Echinacea purpurea extracts. Onkologie 1987;10(3 Suppl):27-33.

10. Reichling J, Fitzi J, Furst-Jucker J, et al. Echinacea powder: treatment for canine chronic and seasonal upper respiratory tract infections. Schweiz Arch Tierheilkd 2003;145(5):223-231.

11. Timmermans LM, Timmermans LG, Jr. [Determination of the activity of extracts of Echinaceae and Sabal in the treatment of idiopathic megabladder in women]. Acta Urol Belg 1990;58(2):43-59.

12. Baetgen D. Erfolge in der keuchhusten-behandlung mit Echinacin. Therapiewoche 1984;34:5115-5119.

13. Dorn M, Knick E, Lewith G. Placebo-controlled, double-blind study of Echinaceae pallidae radix in upper respiratory tract infections. Complement Ther Med 1997;5:40-42.

14. Bräunig B, Dorn M, Limburg E, et al. Enhancement of resistance in common cold by Echinacea purpurea radix. Zeitschrift fur Phytotherpie 1992;13:7-13.

15. Lindenmuth GF, Lindenmuth EB. The efficacy of echinacea compound herbal tea preparation on the severity and duration of upper respiratory and flu symptoms: a randomized, double-blind placebo-controlled study. J Altern Complement Med 2000;6(4):327-334.

16. Anonymous. Immunallergische reaktionen nach echinacea-extrakten (Echinacin, Exberitox N U.A.). Arznei-telegramm 1991;(April):39.

17. Heesen W. Unspezifische behandlungsmoglichkeiten bei tuberkulosen erkrankungen. Erfahrungsheikunde 1964;13:210-217.

18. Volz G. Zur keuchhustenbehandlung mit Myo-Echinacin. Ther Gegenwart 1957;96:312-313.

19. Zimmermann O. Die therapie des keuchhusten mit Myo-Echinacin. Hippokrates 1969;6:223-235.

20. Barrett B, Vohmann M, Calabrese C. Echinacea for upper respiratory infection. J Fam Pract 1999;48(8):628-635.

21. Ertel G, Manley H, McQueen C, et al. Information on additional Echinacea trials. J Fam Pract 1999;48(12):1001-1002.

22. Parnham MJ. Benefit-risk assessment of the squeezed sap of the purple coneflower (Echinacea purpurea) for long-term oral immunostimulation. Phytomed 1996;3:95-102.

23. Mengs U, Clare CB, Poiley JA. Toxicity of Echinacea purpurea. Acute, subacute and genotoxicity studies. Arzneimittelforschung 1991;41(10):1076-1081.

24. Mullins RJ, Heddle R. Adverse reactions associated with echinacea: the Australian experience. Ann Allergy Asthma Immunol 2002;88(1):42-51.

25. Mullins RJ. Echinacea-associated anaphylaxis. Med J Aust 1998;168(4):170-171.

26. Mullins R. Allergic reactions to echinacea. J Allergy Clin Immunol 2000;105(1 part 2):s268-s269.

27. Bruynzeel DP, van Ketel WG, Young E, et al. Contact sensitization by alternative topical medicaments containing plant extracts. The Dutch Contact Dermatoses Group. Contact Dermatitis 1992;27(4):278-279.

28. Bauer R. [Echinacea drugs—effects and active ingredients]. Z Arztl Fortbild. (Jena) 1996;90(2):111-115.

29. Schonhofer PS, Schulte-Sasse H. [Are botanical immunostimulants effective and harmless?]. Dtsch Med Wochenschr 1989;114(46):1804-1806.

30. Soon SL, Crawford RI. Recurrent erythema nodosum associated with Echinacea herbal therapy. J Am Acad Dermatol 2001;44(2):298-299.

31. Brinkeborn RM, Shah DV, Degenring FH. Echinaforce and other Echinacea fresh plant preparations in the treatment of the common cold: A randomized, placebo controlled, double-blind clinical trial. Phytomedicine 1999;6(1):1 6.

32. Ondrizek RR, Chan PJ, Patton WC, et al. Inhibition of human sperm motility by specific herbs used in alternative medicine. J Assist Reprod Genet 1999;16(2):87-91.

33. Kemp DE, Franco KN. Possible leukopenia associated with long-term use of echinacea. J Am Board Fam Pract 2002;15(5):417-419.

34. Gallo M, Sarkar M, Au W, et al. Pregnancy outcome following gestational exposure to echinacea: a prospective controlled study. Arch Intern Med 2000;160(20):3141-3143.

35. Gallo M, Koren WA, Koren G. The safety of Echinacea use during pregnancy: a prospective controlled cohort study. Proceedings of the 11th International Conference of the Organization of Teratology. Teratology 1998;57:283.

36. Coeugniet E, Kuhnast R. Rezidivierende candidiasis. Therapiewoche 1986;36:3352-3358.

37. Miller LG. Herbal medicinals: selected clinical considerations focusing on known or potential drug-herb interactions. Arch Intern Med 1998;158(20):2200-2211.

38. Bauer R, Wagner H. Echinacea species as potential immunostimulatory drugs. In Wagner H, Farnsworth NR (eds): Economic and Medicinal Plant Research. New York: Academic Press, 1991, pp 253-321.

39. Stimpel M, Proksch A, Wagner H, et al. Macrophage activation and induction of macrophage cytotoxicity by purified polysaccharide fractions from the plant Echinacea purpurea. Infect Immun 1984;46(3):845-849.

40. Mose JR. [Effect of Echinacin on phagocytosis and natural killer cells]. Med Welt 1983;34(51-52):1463-1467.

41. Burger RA, Torres AR, Warren RP, et al. Echinacea-induced cytokine production by human macrophages. Int J Immunopharmacol 1997;19(7):371-379.

42. Burger RA, Torres AR, Warren RP, et al. Echinacea purpurea induced cytokine production in human peripheral blood adherent mononuclear cells (PBAC). J Allergy Clin Immunol 1997;99(1, part 2):283.

43. Luettig B, Steinmuller C, Gifford GE, et al. Macrophage activation by the polysaccharide arabinogalactan isolated from plant cell cultures of Echinacea purpurea. J Natl Cancer Inst 1989;81(9):669-675.

44. Jurcic K, Melchart D, Holzmann M. Two proband studies for the stimulation of granulocyte phagocytosis through echinacea extract containing preparations. Z Phytotherapie 1989;10:67-70.

45. Bany J, Siwicki AK, Zdanowska D, et al. Echinacea purpurea stimulates cellular immunity and anti-bacterial defence independently of the strain of mice. Pol J Vet Sci 2003;6(3 Suppl):3-5.

46. See DM, Broumand N, Sahl L, et al. In vitro effects of echinacea and ginseng on natural killer and antibody-dependent cell cytotoxicity in healthy subjects and chronic fatigue syndrome or acquired immunodeficiency syndrome patients. Immunopharmacology 1997;35(3):229-235.

47. Bodinet C, Willigmann I, Beuscher N. Host-resistance increasing activity of root extracts from Echinacea species. Planta Med 1993;59(Suppl):a672-a673.

48. Tragni E, Tubaro A, Melis S, et al. Evidence from two classic irritation tests for an anti-inflammatory action of a natural extract, Echinacina B. Food Chem Toxicol 1985;23(2):317-319.

49. Tubaro A, Tragni E, Del Negro P, et al. Anti-inflammatory activity of a polysaccharidic fraction of Echinacea angustifolia. J Pharm Pharmacol 1987;39(7):567-569.

50. Tunnerhoff FK, Schwabe HK. Studies in human beings and animals on the influence of echinacea extracts on the formation of connective tissue following the implantation of fibrin. Arzneim Forsch 1956;6:330-334.

51. Rehman J, Dillow JM, Carter SM, et al. Increased production of antigen-specific immunoglobulins G and M following in vivo treatment with the medicinal plants Echinacea angustifolia and Hydrastis canadensis. Immunol Lett 1999;68(2-3):391-395.

52. Steinmuller C, Roesler J, Grottrup E, et al. Polysaccharides isolated from plant cell cultures of Echinacea purpurea enhance the resistance of immunosuppressed mice against systemic infections with Candida albicans and Listeria monocytogenes. Int J Immunopharmacol 1993;15(5):605-614.

53. Wacker A, Hilbig W. [Virus-inhibition by Echinacea purpurea (author's transl)]. Planta Med 1978;33(1):89-102.

54. Thompson KD. Antiviral activity of Viracea against acyclovir susceptible and acyclovir resistant strains of herpes simplex virus. Antiviral Res 1998;39(1):55-61.

55. Voaden DJ, Jacobson M. Tumor inhibitors. 3. Identification and synthesis of an oncolytic hydrocarbon from American coneflower roots. J Med Chem 1972;15(6):619-623.

56. Melchart D, Linde K, Worku F, et al. Immunomodulation with echinacea—a systematic review of controlled clinical trials. Phytomed 1994;1:245-254.

57. Dorn M. Milderung grippaler Infekte durch ein pflanzliches Immunstimulans [Treatment of influenza-like syndromes with a phytotherapeutic immunostimulatory preparation]. Natur-und-Ganzheitsmedizin 1990;2:314-319.

58. Bräunig B, Knick E. [Therapeutic experiences with Echinacea pallida in upper respiratory tract infections]. Naturheilpraxis 1993;1:72-75.

59. Vorberg G, Schneider B. Pflanzliches Immunstimulans verkürzt grippalen Infekt. Doppelblindstudie belegt die Steigerung der unspezifischen Infektabwehr [Phytotherapeutic immunostimulator decreases the duration of influenza-like syndromes. Double-blind trial proves the enhancement of unspecific immune defense]. Ärztliche Forschung 1989;36:3-8.

60. Reitz HD. Immunodulatoren mit pflanzlichen Wirkstoffen: eine wissenschaftliche Studie am Beispiel Esberitox N [Immunomodulation with phytotherapeutic agents: a scientific study on the example of Esberitox]. Notabene Medici 1990;20:362-366.

61. Vorberg G. Bei Erkältung unspezifische Immunabwehr stimulieren. [Stimulation of the immune defense in common colds]. Ärztliche Praxis 1984; 36:97-98.

62. Barrett B, Vohmann M, Calabrese C. Echinacea for upper respiratory tract infection. J Fam Pract 1999;48(8):628-635.

63. Brinkeborn R, Shah D, Geissbuhler S, et al. Echinaforce in the treatment of acute colds. Results of a placebo-controlled double-blind study carried out in Sweden. Schweiz Zschr Ganzheits Medizin 1998;10:26-29.

64. Hoheisel O, Sandberg M, Bertram S, et al. Echinacea treatment shortens the course of the common cold: a double blind, placebo-controlled clinical trial. European J Clin Research 1997;9:261-269.

65. Giles JT, Palat CT, III, Chien SH, et al. Evaluation of echinacea for treatment of the common cold. Pharmacotherapy 2000;20(6):690-697.

66. Melchart D, Walther E, Linde K, et al. Echinacea root extracts for the prevention of upper respiratory tract infections: a double-blind, placebo-controlled randomized trial. Arch Fam Med 1998;7(6):541-545.

67. Grimm W, Muller HH. A randomized controlled trial of the effect of fluid extract of *Echinacea purpurea* on the incidence and severity of colds and respiratory infections. Am J Med 1999;106(2):138-143.

68. Melchart D, Linde K, Fischer P, et al. Echinacea for preventing and treating the common cold. Cochrane Database Syst Rev 2000;(2):CD000530.

69. Henneicke-von Zepelin H, Hentschel C, Schnitker J, et al. Efficacy and safety of a fixed combination phytomedicine in the treatment of the common cold (acute viral respiratory tract infection): results of a randomised, double blind, placebo controlled, multicentre study. Curr Med Res Opin 1999; 15(3):214-227.

70. Thom E, Wollan T. A controlled clinical study of Kanjang mixture in the treatment of uncomplicated upper respiratory tract infections. Phytother Research 1997;11:207-210.

71. Scaglione F, Lund B. Efficacy in the treatment of the common cold of a preparation containing an echinacea extract. IntJ Immunother 1995;11(4): 163-166.

72. Barrett BP, Brown RL, Locken K, et al. Treatment of the common cold with unrefined echinacea. A randomized, double-blind, placebo-controlled trial. Ann Intern Med 2002;137(12):939-946.

73. Millea PJ. Echinacea for the common cold. Ann Intern Med 2003; 139(7):601.

74. Shober S. Echinacea for the common cold. Ann Intern Med 2003;139(7): 600.

75. Mittman P, Wollner D, Kim L. Echinacea for the common cold. Ann Intern Med 2003;139(7):600-601.

76. Russo EB. Echinacea for the common cold. Ann Intern Med 2003; 139(7):599.

77. Applequist WL. Echinacea for the common cold. Ann Intern Med 2003; 139(7):599-600.

78. Abrahams SG. Echinacea for the common cold. Ann Intern Med 2003; 139(7):599.

79. Schmidt U, Albrecht M, Schenk N. Immunstimulas senkt Häufigkeit grippaler Infekte. Plazebokontrollierte Doppelblindstudie mit einem kombinierten Echinacea-Präparat mit 646 Studenten der Kölner Universität. [Immunstimulator decreases the frequency of influenza-like syndromes.

80. Double-blind placebo-controlled trial on 646 students of the University of Cologne]. Natur-und-Ganzheitsmedizin 1990;3:277-281.

Schoneberger D. [The influence of immune-stimulating effects of pressed juice from *Echinacea purpurea* on the course and severity of colds. Results of a double-blind study]. Forum Immunologie 1992;8(18):2-12.

81. Forth H, Beuscher N. [Effect on the frequency of banal cold infections by esberitox]. ZFA (Stuttgart) 1981;57(32):2272-2275.

82. Turner RB, Riker DK, Gangemi JD. Ineffectiveness of echinacea for prevention of experimental rhinovirus colds. Antimicrob Agents Chemother 2000;44(6):1708-1709.

83. Freyer HU. [Incidence of banal infections in childhood and possibilities of their prevention]. Fortschr Med 1974;92(4):165-168.

84. Kleinschmidt H. Versuche zur herabsetzung der infektneigung bei kleinkindern mit esberitox. Therapie ger Gegenwart 1965;104:1258-1262.

85. Helbig G. Unspezifische Reizkörpertherapie zur Infektprophylaxe. Medizinische Klinik 1961;35:1512-1514.

86. Berg A, Northoff H, Konig D, et al. Influence of Echinacin (EC31) treatment on exercise-induced immune response in athletes. J Clin Res 1998; 1:367-380.

87. Bendel R, Bendel V, Renner K, et al. [Supplementary treatment with Esberitox of female patients undergoing curative adjuvant irradiation following breast cancer]. Strahlenther Onkol 1988;164(5):278-283.

88. Sartor KJ. [Efficacy of Esberitox in the treatment of radiation-induced leukopenia]. Ther Ggw 1972;111(8):1147-1150.

89. Pohl P. [Treatment of radiation-induced leukopenia with Esberitox]. Ther Ggw 1970;109(6):902-906.

90. Bendel R, Bendel V, Renner K, et al. [Additional treatment with Esberitox N in patients with chemo-radiotherapy treatment of advanced breast cancer]. Onkologie. 1989;12 Suppl 3:32-38.

91. Elsasser-Beile U, Willenbacher W, Bartsch HH, et al. Cytokine production in leukocyte cultures during therapy with Echinacea extract. J Clin Lab Anal 1996;10(6):441-445.

92. Vonau B, Chard S, Mandalia S, et al. Does the extract of the plant *Echinacea purpurea* influence the clinical course of recurrent genital herpes? Int J STD AIDS 2001;12(3):154-158.

Elderberry and Elder Flower
(*Sambucas nigra* L.)

SYNONYMS/COMMON NAMES/RELATED SUBSTANCES

- Almindelig hyld, baccae, baises de sureau, battree, blackberried alder, black elder, black elderberry, boor tree, bountry, boure tree, busine , Caprifoliaceae, devil's eye, elderberry, ellanwood, ellhorn, European alder, European elder, European elderberry, European elderflower, European elder fruit, frau holloe, German elder, holunderbeeren, holunderblüten, lady elder, old gal, old lady, pipe tree, Rubini (elderberry extract), sambreo, sambuco, *Sambucus sieboldiana*, sambucipunct sambucus, sambuci flos, sauco, schwarzer holunder, stinking elder, sureau noir, sweet elder, tree of doom, yakori bengestro.
- **Selected combination products that include *Sambucus nigra*:** Sinupret (contains *Sambucus nigra* flowers, gentian root, verbena, cowslip flower, and sorrel), Sambucol Active Defense (contains elderberry extract, vitamin C, zinc, *Echinacea angustifolia*, *Echinacea purpurea*, and propolis).
- *Note:* Several species of *Sambucus* produce elderberries. Most scientific literature pertains to *S. nigra*. Other species with similar chemical components include the American elder or common elder (*Sambucus canadensis*), antelope brush (*Sambucus tridentata*), blue elderberry (*Sambucus caerulea*), danewort (*Sambucus ebulus*), dwarf elder (*Sambucus ebulus*), red-fruited elder (*Sambucus pubens, Sambucus racemosa*), and *Sambucus formosana*. American elder (*Sambucus canadensis*) and European elder (*S. nigra*) are often discussed simultaneously in the literature since they have many of the same uses and contain common constituents.

CLINICAL BOTTOM LINE
Background

- Several species of *Sambucus* produce elderberries. Most research and publications refer to *S. nigra*. Other species with similar chemical components include the American elder or common elder (*S. canadensis*), antelope brush (*S. tridentata*), blue elderberry (*S. caerulea*), danewort (*S. ebulus*), dwarf elder (*S. ebulus*), red-fruited elder (*S. pubens, S. racemosa*), and *S. formosana*. American elder (*S. canadensis*) and European Elder (*S. nigra*) are often discussed simultaneously in the literature because they have many of the same uses and contain common constituents.
- European elder grows up to 30 feet tall, is native to Europe, but has been naturalized to the Americas. Historically, the flowers and leaves have been used for pain relief, swelling/inflammation, diuresis (urine production), and as a diaphoretic or expectorant. The leaves have been used externally for sitz baths. The bark, when aged, has been used as a diuretic, laxative, or emetic (to induce vomiting). The berries have been used traditionally in food as flavoring and in the preparation of elderberry wine and pies.
- The flowers and berries (blue/black only) are used most often medicinally. They contain flavonoids, which have been found preclinically to possess a variety of biochemical and pharmacologic actions, including antioxidant and immunologic properties. Although it is hypothesized to be beneficial, there is no definitive evidence from well-conducted human clinical trials regarding the use of elder.
- The bark, leaves, seeds, and raw/unripe fruit contain the cyanogenic glycoside sambunigrin, which is potentially toxic.

Scientific Evidence for Common/Studied Uses	Grade*
Bacterial sinusitis	C
Bronchitis	C
Influenza	C

*Key to grades: *A:* Strong scientific evidence for this use; *B:* Good scientific evidence for this use; *C:* Unclear scientific evidence for this use; *D:* Fair scientific evidence against this use (it may not work); *F:* Strong scientific evidence against this use (it likely does not work). For a more detailed explanation of efficacy criteria, see "Natural Standard Evidence-Based Validated Grading Rationale" in the Introduction.

Historical, Common, or Theoretical Indications That Lack Sufficient Evidence

- Alzheimer's disease, anti-inflammatory,[1] antioxidant,[2,3] antispasmodic, asthma, astringent, blood vessel disorders, burns, cancer,[4,5] chafing, circulatory stimulant, cold sores, colds, colic, cough suppressant, diabetes, diaphoretic,[6] diuretic,[7] edema, epilepsy, fever, flavoring, gut disorders, hair dye, hay fever, headache, herpesvirus infection, HIV infection, immunostimulant,[8] increased sweating, insomnia, joint swelling, kidney disease, laryngitis, laxative, liver disease, measles, migraine, mosquito repellent, nerve pain, psoriasis, respiratory distress, sedative, stress reduction, syphilis, toothache, ulcerative colitis, vomiting, weight loss.

Strength of Expert Opinion and Historic/Folkloric Precedent

- Historically, the leaves have been considered to relieve pain and promote healing when applied as a poultice. Native Americans used elder for infections, coughs, and skin conditions. Elderflower has been used as an insect repellent. When mixed with sage, lemon juice, vinegar, and honey, elder has been used as a gargle for coughs, head colds, laryngitis, flu-like symptoms, and shortness of breath. It has been used on the skin as an astringent in rheumatism and for swelling/inflammation. When mixed with peppermint and honey, hot elder has been used to induce diaphoresis to treat colds. Ancient Egyptians used elder flowers to improve complexion and heal burns.
- Elder extracts are used in foods and beverages as flavoring and in perfumes, hair dyes, scented ointments, skin lotions, and insect repellent. Elder has also been used in wine, pies, and lemonade.

Safety Summary

- **Likely safe:** When cooked berries are consumed in amounts usually found in foods. Short-term use of elder flowers has not been associated with adverse effects in the available literature.
- **Possibly unsafe:** Elderberry products should be used under the direction of a qualified healthcare provider, due to the risk of cyanide toxicity, especially from elder bark, root, leaves, or juice.[9,10] The berries must be cooked sufficiently to avoid the risk of nausea/vomiting or cyanide toxicity. Long-term

or high-dose consumption of elder flowers may exert diuretic properties.

- **Likely unsafe:** When the bark, roots, leaves, and unripe berries of the elder plant are consumed, due to the risk of cyanide poisoning.

DOSING/TOXICOLOGY
General

- Recommended doses are based on those most commonly used in available trials, or on historical practice. However, with natural products, the optimal doses needed to balance efficacy and safety often have not been determined. Formulations and preparation methods may vary from manufacturer to manufacturer, and from batch to batch of a specific product made by a single manufacturer. Because often the active components of a product are not known, standardization may not be possible, and the clinical effects of different brands may not be comparable.

Standardization

- Dried elderflower is often standardized to contain at least 0.8% total flavonoids calculated as isoquercitrin. Dried flower preparations often contain at least 25% water-soluble extract.
- The standardized elderberry product Sambucol is a 38% standardized black elderberry extract containing three flavonoids. The elderberry product formulated for children, Sambucol for Kids, is a 19% standardized black elderberry juice.[6]
- Sambucol Active Defense contains a 38% standardized black elderberry extract, plus vitamin C, zinc, propolis, and a proprietary blend of *Echinacea angustifolia* and *E. purpurea*.
- The standardized elderberry product Sinupret (Quantera Sinus Defense) is an herbal mixture containing 18 mg of flos sambucus nigra elder flower), 18 mg of herba verbenae Off. (shop vervain wort herbs), 6 mg of radix gentianae luteae (gentian root), 18 mg of flos primulae veris cum calycibus (cowslip flowers with calyx) and 18 mg of herba rumicis acetosae (sorrel).[11]

Dosing: Adult (18 Years and Older)
Oral

- **Tea:** A dose of 3 to 5 g of dried elder flowers steeped in one cup of boiling water for 10 to 15 minutes and taken by mouth three times daily has been used. Be aware of possible toxicity.
- **Sinupret tablets:** For bacterial sinusitis, a dose of 2 tablets of Sinupret taken by mouth three times daily with antibiotics has been used. Sinupret is a combination formula containing elder and several other herbs.[11,12]
- **Extract:** For treating influenza or flu-like symptoms, a dose of 4 tablespoons of a standardized elderberry extract syrup (Sambucol) taken daily by mouth for three days has been used.[6]

Topical

- **Hand cream:** Cream has been prepared by mixing several handfuls of fresh elder flowers in liquefied petroleum jelly, simmering for 40 minutes, heating, filtering, and allowing the formula to solidify. This cream has been applied to the hands at bedtime.

Dosing: Pediatric (Younger Than 18 Years)

- For influenza or flu-like symptoms, a dose of 1 teaspoon of elderberry juice containing extract syrup (Sambucol for Kids) taken twice daily has been suggested.[6] However, there is not enough scientific information available to recommend the safe use of elder in children. Toxicity has been reported, and caution is recommended.

Toxicology

- The bark, root, and leaves of *S. nigra* contain the cyanogenic glycoside sambunigrin, which is potentially toxic, and contact can lead to cyanide poisoning. Flowers may be used in food, provided hydrocyanic acid (HCN) levels are below 25 ppm. Purified galactose-specific lectin from *S. nigra* flowers at 2 mg/mL possesses mutagenic activity.[5]
- **Overdose:** Ipecac (within 30 minutes) has been recommended following ingestion of elder leaves, roots, bark, or unripe fruit. Activated charcoal with cathartic may be used, although cathartics may be inadvisable if diarrhea has developed. Emesis and gastric lavage are recommended in cases of cyanide toxicity. Amyl nitrate, sodium nitrate, and sodium thioulfate may also be used.

ADVERSE EFFECTS/PRECAUTIONS/CONTRAINDICATIONS
Allergy

- There are no reports of allergy/hypersensitivity to elderberry or elderflower in the available literature, although this area lacks systematic study. There are anecdotal reports of allergies in children playing with toys made from fresh elder stems. In theory, based on *in vitro* study, lectins from *Sambucus nigra* may have the ability to stimulate cytokine release and induce type I hypersensitivity.[13]
- Elder should be avoided in patients with known allergy to plants in the Caprifoliaceae (honeysuckle) family.

Adverse Effects/Postmarket Surveillance

- **General:** Hydrocyanic acid (HCN), also known as cyanide, is poisonous. Elderberry products should be used under the direction of a qualified healthcare provider, due to the risk of cyanide toxicity, especially from elder bark, root, leaves, and juice.[9,10] The berries must be cooked to prevent nausea or cyanide toxicity.
- **Neurologic/CNS:** Cyanide poisoning from bark, root, leaves, or juice may lead to toxicity,[9,10] including CNS and respiratory depression, and weakness.
- **Gastrointestinal:** There are reports of gastrointestinal distress, diarrhea, vomiting, abdominal cramps, and weakness after drinking elderberry juice made from crushed leaves, stems, and uncooked elderberries.[9,10,14] Elder may also possess laxative effects.
- **Endocrine:** Based on laboratory studies, elder may lower blood sugar levels via stimulation of glucose metabolism and promotion of insulin secretion from beta cells.[15]
- **Renal:** In theory, high-dose or long-term use of elder flowers may have diuretic effects.[7]

Precautions/Warnings/Contraindications

- Elderberry products should be used under the direction of a qualified healthcare provider, because of the risk of cyanide toxicity, including from elder bark, root, leaves, uncooked berries, or juice.[9,10]
- Use cautiously in patients taking diuretics.

Pregnancy and Lactation

- Not recommended, due to insufficient data and risk of toxicity. One study reports gastrointestinal discomfort in pregnant women taking elderberry.[14]

INTERACTIONS
Elder/Drug Interactions

- **Diuretic drugs:** Elder may possess diuretic effects and should be used cautiously with drugs that increase urination.[7]
- **Laxatives:** Elder may possess laxative effects and should be used cautiously with other laxatives.
- **Hypoglycemic drugs:** Based on laboratory studies, elder may lower blood sugar levels.[15] Caution is advised when using medications that may also lower blood sugar levels. A qualified healthcare provider should closely monitor patients taking drugs for diabetes by mouth or insulin. Medication adjustments may be necessary.
- **Methylxanthines (caffeine, theophylline):** The flavonoid quercitin, which is found in elder, has been reported to inhibit xanthine oxidase and may affect caffeine and theophylline levels. Patients using theophylline should consult their healthcare provider before using elder.
- **Cancer chemotherapy drugs:** Preclinical research reports that elder may increase the effects and possible adverse effects of some cancer chemotherapies, including alkylating agents.[4,5]
- **Decongestants:** Based on preliminary research in patients, increased benefits may be seen when elder is used in combination with decongestants such as oxymetazoline (Afrin), and antibiotics.
- **Anti-inflammatory drugs:** Anti-inflammatory properties have been demonstrated in animal studies using elder flowers.[1]

Elder/Herb/Supplement Interactions

- **Antioxidants:** Elder preparations may exert antioxidant activity, and increased effects may be seen when elder is used in combination with other antioxidants.[2,3]
- **Diuretic agents:** Elder may possess diuretic effects and should be used cautiously with other agents that increase urination.[7]
- **Laxative agents:** Elder may possess laxative effects and should be used cautiously with other laxatives.
- **Hypoglycemic agents:** Based on laboratory studies, elder may lower blood sugar levels.[15] Caution is advised when using medications that may also lower blood sugar levels. A qualified healthcare provider should closely monitor patients taking drugs for diabetes by mouth or insulin. Medication adjustments may be necessary.
- **Caffeine:** The flavonoid quercitin, which is found in elder, has been reported to inhibit xanthine oxidase and may affect caffeine levels.
- **Anti-inflammatory agents:** Anti-inflammatory properties have been demonstrated in animal studies using elder flowers.[1]

MECHANISM OF ACTION
Pharmacology

- **Constituents:** There are multiple chemical and biochemical studies of chemical constituents in *Sambuca nigra*. The bark contains α-amyrenone, α-amyrin, betulin, oleanolic acid, beta-sitosterol[16] as well as nigrin b, a lectin similar to ricin, and other type 2 ribosome-inactivating proteins (RIPs) that are less toxic to cells and animals.[17] The flowers/leaves contain flavonoids including quercitin (up to 3%), rutin, and hyperoside,[18] as well as essential oils (responsible for the muscat aroma characteristic of elder flowers),[19] mucilage, tannins (3%), organic acids, glycoside (0.042% by weight), plastocyanin,[20] and sambunigrin (0.042% by weight).
  - The fruit contains the protein *S. nigra* agglutinin Ivf (SNAIVf), which is homologous to type 2 ribosome inactivating protein (RIP),[21] while the bark contains a novel type 2 RIP (SNLRP) consisting of an A chain with *N*-glycosidase activity and a B chain devoid of carbohydrate-binding activity normally present.[22,23] Two additional RIPs were further identified in bark (SNAI and SNAI'),[24] demonstrating the complexity of Type 2 RIP/lectins in *S. nigra*. The lectin isolated from bark is tetrameric with two distinct subunits and is rich in glutamine/glutamic acid, valine, and leucine.[24] The fruit type 2 RIP lectin is 10 amino acids longer than the bark lectin.[25] Elder RIPs with *N*-glycosidase activity are reported to inhibit protein synthesis in rabbits but not in plants.[4]
- **Quercitin,** present in elder, has been shown to be a potent inhibitor of xanthine oxidase.[26] *S. nigra* has been shown to bind heavy metals.[27]
- **Experimental assays:** The lectin of *S. nigra* (*Sambucus nigra* agglutinin, or SNA) has been used in multiple experimental clinical assays because of its carbohydrate-binding properties and its ability to precipitate highly sialylated glycoproteins,[28] including the use of SNA binding to identify pregnant women at risk for pre-term delivery (by detecting fibronectin in cervicovaginal secretions using a glycoprotein lectin immunosorbent assay)[29]; distinguishing normal from stone-forming kidneys (using *N*-acetylneuraminic acid–calcium binding ratios)[30]; examining colorectal carcinoma by examining rates of colonic mucin sialylation (by comparing alpha 2,6–linked sialic acid vs. sialyl-Tn antigen)[31]; evaluating ulcerative colitis by monitoring differences in sialylation in Asian vs. European colitis patients[32]; examining increased beta-galactoside alpha 2,6-sialyltransferase activity (by detection of digoxigenin-conjugated SNA)[33]; evaluating SNA levels in women with breast and ovarian cancer[34]; glycohistochemically identifying microglial cells from Alzheimer's disease samples[35]; measuring decreased sialylation of glycoproteins in nasal glands of patients with sinusitis[36]; monitoring elevated serum sialic acids associated with increase cardiovascular mortality[37]; and enriching stem cell samples/depleting T-cells in bone marrow harvests.[38]
- **Anti-oxidant activity:** Elderberries contain flavonoids (flavone, flavonone, isoflavone derivatives, and anthocyanins), which are reported to possess anti-oxidant activity and to protect against oxidative stressors such as hydrogen peroxide, 2-amidinopropane, and dihydrochloride (AAPH), ferrous sulfate and ascorbic acid.[39-42]
- **Anti-inflammatory activity:** *S. nigra* is reported to modulate the inflammatory cytokines IL-1 and TNF-alpha[1,43]; increased human basophil secretion of Il-4, IL-13, and histamine[13]; and alter the function of human neutrophils.[44]
- **Antiproliferative effects:** SNA has been reported to inhibit nuclear protein transport in neuroblastoma cells, suggesting a functional significance of sialation.[45]
- **Glucose/insulin metabolism:** Recent *in vitro* research[15] refutes earlier study[46] and reports stimulation of glucose metabolism and promotion of insulin secretion from beta cells.
- **Antiviral effects:** A combination product, SHS-174, containing flowers of *S. nigra*, aerial parts of *Hypericum perforatum* L. (St. John's wort), and roots of *Saponaria officinalis* (soap wort) (100 g:70 g:40 g) exhibited antiviral effects and inhibited influenza virus types A and B and herpes simplex virus-1 *in vitro* and in mice.[47] In a different study, *S. nigra* reduced hemagglutination of red blood cells and inhibited replication of several strains of Influenza types A and B *in vitro*.[6]

- **Diuretic effects:** In a rat study, diuretic effects and sodium excretion were associated with an extract of *S. nigra* flowers.[7]

Pharmacodynamics/Kinetics

- The maximum concentration of anthocyanins found in blood after injection of a highly concentrated solution was 35 mg/mL at 1 hour, followed by a quick decay.[40]
- At a dose of 3 g/kg, *S. nigra* extract did not modify the growth rate of rats.[1]
- Elder flowers are believed to be safe for use in food, provided HCN levels are below 25 ppm.

HISTORY

- Legend states that Judas Iscariot was hung from an elder tree, and that the cross on which Jesus was hung was made of elder. Traditionally, elder was used to ward off evil influences, witches, spirits, and death in England and Russia. Knots made from elder twigs were sometimes carried as charms to protect from rheumatism in England. The Serbs considered elder to be good luck.

REVIEW OF THE EVIDENCE: DISCUSSION

Bacterial Sinusitis

Summary

- Elder has been observed to reduce excessive sinus mucus secretion in laboratory studies.[36] There is only limited research specifically using elder to treat sinusitis in humans. Combination products containing elder and other herbs (such as Sinupret) have been reported to have beneficial effects when used with antibiotics to treat sinus infections, although these results require confirmation with additional study.[11,12] Research suggests that herbal preparations containing elder may result in less swelling of mucous membranes, better drainage, milder headache, and decreased nasal congestion. There is no evidence regarding the effects of elder when used alone for treatment of this condition.

Evidence

- Neubauer and Marz conducted a 2-week randomized double-blind, placebo-controlled trial to assess the efficacy of the standardized combination product Sinupret in 160 patients with acute bacterial sinusitis.[11] Sinupret contains 18 mg of flos sambucus nigra (elder flower), 18 mg of herba verbenae off. (shop vervain wort herbs), 6 mg of radix

gentianae luteae (gentian root), 18 mg of flos primulae veris cum calycibus (cowslip flowers with calyx) and 18 mg of herba rumicis acetosae (sorrel). Subjects received 2 tablets three times daily concurrently with the antibiotic doxycycline (Vibramycin) and the decongestant xylometazoline (Otriven). The aim was to determine if the response rate of doxycycline/xylometazoline was improved by adding the herbal combination. The primary outcome measures were x-ray findings and patient assessment. Secondary outcomes were clinical findings (mucosal swelling, obstruction of drainage, headache, discharge, patency of nose). Results were assessed as trichotomous and dichotinous variables, respectively, and evaluated by contingency tables (first visit × follow-up visit) with 95% confidence intervals. All 160 patients were found to have a complete or partially opacified x-ray after 2 weeks, with significant improvement in the treatment group compared to the placebo group in terms of overall response rate and quality of response. No adverse effects were noted in either treatment group. Although 10% of subjects used nose drops during the study (a protocol violation), this noncompliance was distributed equally between groups. Dropouts were not accounted for and 24 observations were lost, with distribution equal among groups. The use of a combination product leaves open the question of elder's activity as a monotherapy. The short follow-up period leaves open the question of longer-term efficacy and safety. Due to limited descriptions of methods and statistical analysis, additional study is needed in this area before a firm conclusion can be drawn.
- Marz et al. published a review of the evidence regarding the use of Sinupret for sinusitis.[48] The authors cited preclinical reports of secretolytic, anti-inflammatory, immunomodulatory, and antiviral effects. They also noted human research suggesting a favorable safety profile and efficacy when added to antibiotics and conventional decongestant drugs.

Influenza Treatment

Summary

- Laboratory studies suggest that elder may reduce mucus production and possess anti-inflammatory and antiviral effects. One study reports that elderberry juice may improve flu-like symptoms, such as fever, fatigue, headache, sore throat, cough, and aches, in less than half the time that it

Review of the Evidence: Elderberry

Condition Treated*	Study Design	Author, Year	N[†]	SS[†]	Study Quality[‡]	Magnitude of Benefit	ARR[†]	NNT[†]	Comments
Sinusitis (bacterial)	RCT	Neubauer[11] 1994	160	Yes	3	Large	28	4	Improved x-rays and symptoms after 2 weeks with herbal combination Sinupret vs. placebo; all subjects received antibiotics and decongestants.
Influenza treatment	RCT	Zakay-Rones[6] 1995	27	Yes	3	Large	53	2	Improved symptoms after 3 days in elderberry group vs. 6 days in controls; Not an intent-to-treat analysis (40 subjects initially randomized).

*Primary or secondary outcome.
[†]*N*, Number of patients; *SS*, statistically significant; *ARR*, absolute risk reduction; *NNT*, the number of patients who need to undergo a specific intervention in order to observe an outcome in one individual.
[‡]0-2 = poor; 3-4 = good; 5 = excellent.
NA, Not applicable; *RCT*, randomized, controlled trial.
For an explanation of each category in this table, please see Table 3 in the Introduction.

normally takes to get over the flu. However, this study was small with design flaws, and it should be noted that the berries must be cooked to prevent nausea or cyanide toxicity. It remains unclear whether there is any benefit from elder for this condition. Additional research is needed in this area before a firm conclusion can be reached. Elder should not be used in the place of other, more proven therapies, and patients are advised to discuss influenza vaccination with their primary healthcare provider.

Evidence

- Zakay-Rones et al. conducted a randomized, double-blind, placebo-controlled study of Sambucol (a syrup containing elderberry juice, raspberry extract, glucose, citric acid, and honey) in the treatment of influenza in otherwise healthy individuals (children and adults) not previously vaccinated against the flu, located in an Israeli agricultural community.[6] Patients were included who had at least three symptoms (fever, myalgia, nasal discharge, cough) of less than 24 hours' duration. Children received 2 tablespoons daily and adults received 4 tablespoons daily for 3 days. Age range and mean age were similar between groups. This was not an intent-to-treat analysis, and out of 40 subjects who were initially enrolled and randomized, 13 were disqualified prior to analysis due to crossover or protocol violations (5 in the treatment group and 8 in the placebo group). In subjects who were analyzed, convalescent phase serologies demonstrated higher antibody titers to Influenza B in the group treated with Sambucol, although these results were not statistically significant and only demonstrated a trend in favor of the treatment group. Follow-up of symptoms was adequately recorded over 6 days, and significant improvement in symptoms was observed in 93.3% of treated patients within 2 days, versus the control group in which it took 6 days to see improvement in 92.7% of patients ($p < 0.001$). A complete cure was seen within 2 to 3 days in Sambucol-treated patients (90%), whereas 6 days were needed in the placebo group. Although randomization and blinding were adequately described, this study is limited by the small sample size, lack of intent-to-treat analysis, and use of influenza-B rather than influenza-A titer measurement. These results are promising. Additional study is needed in this area before a firm conclusion can be drawn.

Bronchitis
Summary

- There is no reliable human evidence evaluating elder monotherapy as a treatment for bronchitis. However, it is an ingredient in the combination herbal product Sinupret. This proprietary formula has been used historically in Europe for the treatment of acute bronchitis and sinusitis. Although no studies have been conducted comparing the combination product to placebo, there is initial evidence from a comparison trial of various expectorants vs. Sinupret in the treatment of acute bronchitis.[12] Additional evidence is necessary before a firm conclusion can be drawn regarding the use of sorrel or Sinupret in the management of bronchitis.

Evidence

- Ernst et al. conducted a comparison trial to evaluate the safety and efficacy of Sinupret vs. 72 commonly prescribed expectorants, chosen freely by physicians at the point of care (for example, products containing acetylcysteine, bromhexine, carbocysteine).[12] The trial was open (non-

blinded, non-randomized) and included 3187 patients with acute, uncomplicated bronchitis, ages 1 to 94 years. The product was administered for 10 days, and the primary outcome was improvement in bronchitis-related symptoms. The authors reported that Sinupret was superior to the mean improvement seen with the reference drugs, both in terms of efficacy and adverse effects. However, Sinupret was not compared to individual expectorants. A sub-group analysis of 535 patients with acute-on-chronic bronchitis demonstrated lower efficacy of both Sinupret and the reference expectorants. Because Sinupret was compared to multiple agents and the study was neither randomized nor blinded, the results can only be considered preliminary.

References

1. Mascolo N, Autore G, Capasso F, et al. Biological screening of Italian medicinal plants for anti-inflammatory activity. Phytotherapy Research 1987;1(1):28-31.
2. Cao G, Prior RL. Anthocyanins are detected in human plasma after oral administration of an elderberry extract. Clin Chem 1999;45(4):574-576.
3. Kaack K, Austed T. Interaction of vitamin C and flavonoids in elderberry (*Sambucus nigra* L.) during juice processing. Plant Foods Hum Nutr 1998; 52(3):187-198.
4. de Benito FM, Iglesias R, Ferreras JM, et al. Constitutive and inducible type 1 ribosome-inactivating proteins (RIPs) in elderberry (*Sambucus nigra* L.). FEBS Lett 1998;428(1-2):75-79.
5. Lukash LL, Karpova IS, Miroshnichenko OS, et al. [The effect of the lectin from *Sambucus nigra* inflorescences on spontaneous and alkylating agent-induced mutagenesis in mammalian somatic cells]. Tsitol Genet 1997; 31(5):52-60.
6. Zakay-Rones Z, Varsano N, Zlotnik M, et al. Inhibition of several strains of influenza virus *in vitro* and reduction of symptoms by an elderberry extract (*Sambucus nigra* L.) during an outbreak of influenza B Panama. J Altern Complement Med 1995;1(4):361-369.
7. Beaux D, Fleurentin J, Mortier F. Effect of extracts of *Orthosiphon stamineus* Benth, *Hieracium pilosella* L., *Sambucus nigra* L. and *Arctostaphylos uva-ursi* (L.) Spreng. in rats. Phytother Res 1999;13(3):222-225.
8. Barak V, Halperin T, Kalickman I. The effect of Sambucol, a black elderberry-based, natural product, on the production of human cytokines: I. Inflammatory cytokines. Eur Cytokine Netw 2001;12(2):290-296.
9. Kunitz S, Melton RJ, Updyke T, et al. Poisoning from elderberry juice. MMWR 1984;33(13):173-174.
10. Anonymous. Leads from the MMWR. Poisoning from elderberry juice. JAMA 1984;251(16):2075.
11. Neubauer N, März RW. Placebo-controlled, randomized double-blind clinical trial with Sinupret® sugar coated tablets on the basis of a therapy with antibiotics and decongestant nasal drops in acute sinusitis. Phytomedicine 1994;1:177-181.
12. Ernst E, Marz RW, Sieder C. [Acute bronchitis: effectiveness of Sinupret. Comparative study with common expectorants in 3,187 patients]. Fortschr Med 1997;115(11):52-53.
13. Haas H, Falcone FH, Schramm G, et al. Dietary lectins can induce in vitro release of IL-4 and IL-13 from human basophils. Eur J Immunol 1999; 29(3):918-927.
14. Tsui B, Dennehy CE, Tsourounis C. A survey of dietary supplement use during pregnancy at an academic medical center. Am J Obstet Gynecol 2001;185(2):433-437.
15. Gray AM, Abdel-Wahab YH, Flatt PR. The traditional plant treatment, *Sambucus nigra* (elder), exhibits insulin-like and insulin-releasing actions in vitro. J Nutr 2000;130(1):15-20.
16. Lawrie W, McLean J, Paton AC. Triterpenoids in the bark of elder (*Sambucus nigra*). Phytochemistry 1964;3:267-268.
17. Battelli MG, Citores L, Buonamici L, et al. Toxicity and cytotoxicity of nigrin b, a two-chain ribosome- inactivating protein from *Sambucus nigra*: comparison with ricin. Arch Toxicol 1997;71(6):360-364.
18. Davidek J. Isolation of chromatographically pure rutin from flowers of elder. Nature 1961;189(4763):487-488.
19. Toulemonde B, Richard HM. Volatile constituents of dry elder (*Sambucus nigra* L.) flowers. J Agric Food Chem 1983;31(2):365-370.
20. Scawen MD, Ramshaw JA, Brown RH, et al. The amino-acid sequence of plastocyanin from *Sambucus nigra* L. (Elder). Eur J Biochem 1974;44(1): 299-303.
21. van Damme EJ, Roy S, Barre A, et al. The major elderberry (*Sambucus nigra*) fruit protein is a lectin derived from a truncated type 2 ribosome-inactivating protein. Plant J 1997;12(6):1251-1260.
22. van Damme EJ, Roy S, Barre A, et al. Elderberry (*Sambucus nigra*) bark contains two structurally different Neu5Ac(alpha2,6)Gal/GalNAc-binding type 2 ribosome-inactivating proteins. Eur J Biochem 1997;245(3): 648-655.

E

23. van Damme EJ, Barre A, Rouge P, et al. Isolation and molecular cloning of a novel type 2 ribosome-inactivating protein with an inactive B chain from elderberry (*Sambucus nigra*) bark. J Biol Chem 1997;272(13):8353-8360.

24. Broekaert WF, Nsimba-Lubaki M, Peeters B, et al. A lectin from elder (*Sambucus nigra* L.) bark. Biochem J 1984;221(1):163-169.

25. Peumans WJ, Roy S, Barre A, et al. Elderberry (*Sambucus nigra*) contains truncated Neu5Ac(alpha- 2,6)Gal/GalNAc-binding type 2 ribosome-inactivating proteins. FEBS Lett 1998;425(1):35-39.

26. Chang WS, Lee YJ, Lu FJ, et al. Inhibitory effects of flavonoids on xanthine oxidase. Anticancer Res 1993;13:2165-2170.

27. Coupe SA, Taylor JE, Roberts JA. Characterisation of an mRNA encoding a metallothionein-like protein that accumulates during ethylene-promoted abscission of *Sambucus nigra* L. leaflets. Planta 1995;197(3):442-447.

28. Shibuya N, Goldstein IJ, Broekaert WF, et al. The elderberry (*Sambucus nigra* L.) bark lectin recognizes the Neu5Ac(alpha 2-6)Gal/GalNAc sequence. J Biol Chem 1987;262(4):1596-1601.

29. Hampel DJ, Kottgen B, Dudenhausen JW, et al. Fetal fibronectin as a marker for an imminent (preterm) delivery. A new technique using the glycoprotein lectin immunosorbent assay. J Immunol Methods 1999;224(1-2):31-42.

30. Hofbauer J, Fang-Kircher S, Steiner G, et al. N-acetylneuraminic acids (nana): a potential key in renal calculogenesis. Urol Res 1998;26(1):49-56.

31. Murayama T, Zuber C, Seelentag WK, et al. Colon carcinoma glycoproteins carrying alpha 2,6-linked sialic acid reactive with *Sambucus nigra* agglutinin are not constitutively expressed in normal human colon mucosa and are distinct from sialyl-Tn antigen. Int J Cancer 1997;70(5):575-581.

32. McMahon RF, Warren BF, Jones CJ, et al. South Asians with ulcerative colitis exhibit altered lectin binding compared with matched European cases. Histochem J 1997;29(6):469-477.

33. Dall'Olio F, Trere D. Expression of alpha 2,6-sialylated sugar chains in normal and neoplastic colon tissues. Detection by digoxigenin-conjugated *Sambucus nigra* agglutinin. Eur J Histochem 1993;37(3):257-265.

34. Goodarzi MT, Turner GA. Decreased branching, increased fucosylation and changed sialylation of alpha-1-proteinase inhibitor in breast and ovarian cancer. Clin Chim Acta 1995;236(2):161-171.

35. Zambenedetti P, Giordano R, Zatta P. Histochemical localization of glycoconjugates on microglial cells in Alzheimer's disease brain samples by using *Abrus precatorius*, *Maackia amurensis*, *Momordica charantia*, and *Sambucus nigra* lectins. Exp Neurol 1998;153(1):167-171.

36. Ueno K, Wang ZH, Hanamure Y, et al. Reduced sialylation of glycoproteins in nasal glands of patients with chronic sinusitis. Acta Otolaryngol 1997;117(3):420-423.

37. Crook JR, Goldman JH, Dalziel M, et al. Increased ventricular sialylation in patients with heart failure secondary to ischemic heart disease. Clin Cardiol 1997;20(5):455-458.

38. Mumcuoglu M, Manor D, Slavin S. Enrichment for GM-CFU from human bone marrow using *Sambucus nigra* agglutinin: potential application to bone marrow transplantation. Exp Hematol 1986;14(10):946-950.

39. Abuja PM, Murkovic M, Pfannhauser W. Antioxidant and prooxidant activities of elderberry (*Sambucus nigra*) extract in low density lipoprotein oxidation. J Agric Food Chem 1998;46:4091-4096.

40. Murkovic M, Adam U, Pfannhauser W. Analysis of anthocyane glycosides in human serum. Fresenius J Anal Chem 2000;366(4):379-381.

41. Youdim KA, Martin A, Joseph JA. Incorporation of the elderberry anthocyanins by endothelial cells increases protection against oxidative stress. Free Radic Biol Med 2000;29(1):51-60.

42. Middleton E Jr, Kandaswami C. Effects of flavonoids on immune and inflammatory cell functions. Biochem Pharmacol 1992;43(6):1167-1179.

43. Yesilada E, Ustun O, Sezik E, et al. Inhibitory effects of Turkish folk remedies on inflammatory cytokines: interleukin-1alpha, interleukin-1beta and tumor necrosis factor alpha. J Ethnopharmacol 1997;58(1):59-73.

44. Timoshenko AV, Cherenkevich SN. [H_2O_2 generation and human neutrophil aggregation as affected by lectins]. Gematol Transfuziol 1995;40(4):32-35.

45. Emig S, Schmalz D, Shakibaei M, et al. The nuclear pore complex protein p62 is one of several sialic acid- containing proteins of the nuclear envelope. J Biol Chem 1995;270(23):13787-13793.

46. Swanston-Flatt SK, Day C, Flatt PR, et al. Glycaemic effects of traditional European plant treatments for diabetes. Studies in normal and streptozotocin diabetic mice. Diabetes Res 1989;10(2):69-73.

47. Serkedjieva J, Manolova N, Zgorniak-Nowosielska I, et al. Antiviral activity of the infusion (SHS-174) from flowers of *Sambucus nigra* L., aerial parts of Hypericum perforatum L., and roots of *Saponaria officinalis* L. against influenza and herpes simplex viruses. Phytotherapy Research 1990;4(3):97-100.

48. Marz RW, Ismail C, Popp MA. [Profile and effectiveness of a phytogenic combination preparation for treatment of sinusitis]. Wien Med Wochenschr 1999;149(8-10):202-208.

Ephedra/Ma Huang
(*Ephedra sinica*)

SYNONYMS/COMMON NAMES/ RELATED SUBSTANCES

- Amsania, Brigham tea, budshur, cao ma huang, chewa, Chinese ephedra, Chinese joint fir, desert herb, *Ephedra altissima, E. americana, E. anti-syphilitica, E. distacha, E. distachya, E. equisetina* (Mongolian ephedra), *E. geradiana, E. helvetica, E. intermedia* (intermediate ephedra), *E. major, E. nevadensis, E. shennungiana, E. trifurca, E. viridis, E. vulgaris,* Ephedraceae, ephedrae herba, epitonin, European ephedra, herba ephedrae, horsetail, hum, huma, Indian joint fir, intermediate ephedra, joint fir, khama, mahoàng, máhuáng, mao, mao-kon, mahuuanggen, Mexican tea, mốc tac ma hoàng, Mongolian ephedra, Mormon tea, mu-tsei-ma-huang, muzei mu huang, natural ecstasy, phok, popotillo, san-ma-huang, sea grape, shrubby, soma, song tuê ma hoàng, squaw tea, teamster's tea, trun aa hoàng, tsao-ma-huang, tutgantha, yellow astringent, yellow horse, zhong ma huang.
- *Note:* There are approximately 40 species of ephedra.

CLINICAL BOTTOM LINE
Background

- *Note:* On February 6, 2004 the U.S. Food and Drug Administration (FDA) issued a final rule prohibiting the sale of dietary supplements containing ephedrine alkaloids (ephedra) because such supplements present an unreasonable risk of illness or injury. The rule became effective 60 days from the date of publication.
- *Ephedra sinica,* a species of ephedra (ma huang), contains the alkaloids ephedrine and pseudoephedrine, which have been found to induce central nervous system stimulation, bronchodilation, and vasoconstriction. In combination with caffeine, ephedrine appears to elicit weight loss (in trials of 1 to 12 months' duration). However, studies of ephedra and ephedrine monotherapy have been equivocal. The majority of human trials of weight loss have been small with methodological weaknesses, including large dropout rates due to adverse effects and incomplete reporting of blinding or randomization. Numerous trials have documented the efficacy of ephedrine in the management of asthmatic bronchoconstriction and hypotension. However, commercial preparations of non-prescription supplements containing ephedra have not been systematically studied for these indications.
- Major safety concerns have been associated with ephedra and ephedrine use, including hypertension, tachycardia, CNS excitation, arrhythmia, myocardial infarction, and stroke. In 1997, due to over 800 U.S. reports of serious toxicity (and many more worldwide) including at least 22 deaths in adolescents and young adults, the FDA adopted a policy that ephedra-containing products must (1) be labeled with all possible adverse effects, including death; (2) contain no more than 8 mg of ephedrine per serving; and (3) be used for no more than 7 days. The FDA also proposed a maximum daily dose of 24 mg, and a ban on ephedra-caffeine combination products (these proposed limits were subsequently withdrawn).
- In 2002, Samenuk et al. identified 926 cases of possible ephedra toxicity reported to the Adverse Reaction Monitoring System of the FDA between 1995 and 1997.[1] In 37 patients, use of ephedra was temporally related to stroke (16 patients), myocardial infarction,[10] or sudden death.[11] Autopsies performed in patients who experienced sudden death showed a normal heart in one, coronary atherosclerosis in three, and cardiomyopathies in three. In 36 of the 37 patients, use of ephedra was reported to be within the manufacturers' dosing guidelines.
- In 2003, a report was prepared by the RAND Southern California Evidence-Based Practice Center for the Agency for Healthcare Research and Quality, U.S. Department of Health and Human Services.[2,3] This study reviewed available clinical trials, as well as more than 1500 adverse event reports to the FDA and adverse event reports to the manufacturer Metabolife. Although most prospective trials were not sufficiently large and most adverse event reports were not sufficiently detailed, the authors identified three deaths, two myocardial infarctions, two cerebrovascular accidents, one seizure, and three psychiatric cases that were considered to be "sentinel events" (i.e., strongly tied to ephedra use within 24 hours without other plausible explanations). In addition, 50 other possible sentinel events were identified.
- A 2003 analysis by Bent et al. in *Annals of Internal Medicine* found that products containing ephedra account for 64% of all adverse reactions to herbs in the United States, but represent only 0.82% of herbal product sales.[4-9] The relative risk for an adverse reaction in a person using ephedra compared with other herbs was extremely high, ranging from 100 (95% CI, 83 to 140) for kava to 720 (95% CI, 520 to 1100) for *Ginkgo biloba*. It was concluded that ephedra use poses a greatly increased risk of adverse reactions compared with other herbs. A 2003 analysis published in *Neurology* also found increased risk of stroke associated with ephedra-containing products.[10,11]
- Despite widely publicized safety concerns[7,12-20] and the highly publicized death of a U.S. major league baseball pitcher thought to be related to ephedra,[21] before the final ban on ephedra, 14% of individuals using non-prescription weight loss products in the U.S. continued to take ephedra or ephedrine-containing products.[22]

Scientific Evidence for Common/Studied Uses	Grade*
Weight loss	A
Asthmatic bronchoconstriction	B
Allergic rhinitis	C
Hypotension	C
Sexual arousal	C

*Key to grades: *A:* Strong scientific evidence for this use; *B:* Good scientific evidence for this use; *C:* Unclear scientific evidence for this use; *D:* Fair scientific evidence against this use (it may not work); *F:* Strong scientific evidence against this use (it likely does not work). For a more detailed explanation of efficacy criteria, see "Natural Standard Evidence-Based Validated Grading Rationale" in the Introduction.

Historical or Theoretical Uses That Lack Sufficient Evidence

- Acute coryza (rhinitis), anaphylaxis,[23] anti-inflammatory, antipyretic, appetite suppressant, athletic performance enhancer,[24,25] bodybuilding, chills, colds, congenital myasthenic syndrome,[26] cough, decongestant, depression, diaphoretic, diuretic, dyspnea, edema, energy-enhancer, enuresis, euphoria, fevers, flu, gonorrhea, gout, hay fever, joint pain, lack of perspiration, metabolic enhancement, myasthenia gravis, narcolepsy,[27] nasal congestion, nephritis, syphilis, stimulant, upper respiratory tract infection, urticaria, uterotonic, water retention.

Expert Opinion and Folkloric Precedent

- Ephedra is native to Asia and has been used in traditional Chinese medicine (TCM) for over 5000 years. It was found in a Middle Eastern Neolithic grave, indicating that it may have been used up to 60,000 years ago. Zen monks used ephedra to improve concentration and to induce calm during meditation.
- The German expert panel, the Commission E, has approved the use of ephedra to treat "diseases of the respiratory tract with mild bronchospasm in adults and children over the age of six," and notes that there are a variety of side effects and potential adverse interactions.
- In TCM, ephedra is used to treat asthma and acute nephritis. It is typically used in conjunction with other herbs.

Safety Summary

- **Possibly safe:** When a product formulation containing a standardized ephedrine content is taken in recommended doses by otherwise healthy adults for a short duration (<7 days) under the strict supervision of a qualified healthcare professional.
- **Likely unsafe:** When used in children, based on numerous cases of heart attack, seizure, and stroke reported to the U.S. Food and Drug Administration. When taken in doses greater than recommended, or when used for longer than 7 days. When used in pregnancy or lactation. When used by patients with anorexia/bulimia, anxiety, benign prostatic hypertrophy, cerebrovascular disease, history of stroke or transient ischemic attack, closed-angle glaucoma, depression, diabetes, heart disease, hypertension, hyperthyroidism, hypovolemia, insomnia, pheochromocytoma, or tremor. When used in combination with other stimulants such as caffeine. There have been over 800 reports of serious toxicity, including at least 22 deaths, in adolescents and young adults using ephedra.

DOSING/TOXICOLOGY
General

- Recommended doses are based on those most commonly used in available trials, or on historical practice. However, with natural products, the optimal doses needed to balance efficacy and safety often have not been determined. Formulations and preparation methods may vary from manufacturer to manufacturer, and from batch to batch of a specific product made by a single manufacturer. Because often the active components of a product are not known, standardization may not be possible, and the clinical effects of different brands may not be comparable.

Standardization

- There is wide variability in the alkaloid content of different preparations of ephedra. A 1998 study examined the pseudo-ephedrine and ephedrine content of nine commercially available nutritional supplements containing *Ephedra sinica*. Significant variations in content were found for pseudoephedrine, ranging from 0.52 to 9.46 mg, and for ephedrine from 1.08 to 13.54 mg per recommended dose.[28] A 1992 study was conducted by collecting 22 different ephedra products from herbal shops throughout Taiwan. A fourfold difference was found in the amounts of the various alkaloids, ranging from 0.536% to 2.308%.[29] Average ephedra supplement content is 1% of the crude plant.
- Different ephedra species, yielding markedly different quantities of active alkaloids, are all sold as ma huang in China, leading to difficulties for consumers trying to find standardized products.[30] *Ephedra sinica* plants grown in northern China often have a different morphology and alkaloid content than the same species grown in southern China.[30]

Dosing: Adult (18 Years and Older)
Oral

- **Controversy regarding dosing:** There is disagreement regarding the optimal form and dose of ephedra. Traditionally, herbalists have recommended a wide range of doses, which are typically higher than U.S. Food and Drug Administration (FDA) recommendations. The FDA has recommended a maximum of 8 mg up to every 6 hours (total daily dose of 24 mg) for up to 7 days. However, doses up to 25 mg of total ephedra alkaloids four times daily have been recommended by some experts, and doses in some studies have been as high as 50 to 100 mg of ephedra three times daily. Over-the-counter drugs containing ephedra generally contain warning labels advising adults to take 12.5 to 25 mg every 4 to 6 hours and not to exceed 150 mg in 24 hours.
- **Weight loss:** The FDA has recommended no greater than 8 mg every 6 hours for up to 7 days. Doses used in some clinical trials have been 25 to 50 mg three times daily.[31-33]

Dosing: Pediatric (Younger Than 18 Years)

- Ephedrine is not recommended in children, due to the risk of toxicity and death. Purified ephedrine has been given to children older than 2 years of age in doses of 2 to 3 mg/kg/day divided into 4 to 6 daily doses.

Toxicology

- Higher than recommended doses, or prolonged use of ephedra (>7 days), can cause anxiety, nausea, cardiac arrhythmias, headache, tremor, hypertension, restlessness, insomnia, gastric mucosal irritation, and diuresis. Due to over 800 reports of serious toxicity, including at least 22 deaths in adolescents and young adults using ephedra, the U.S. Food and Drug Administration (FDA) convened a special advisory committee on "Ephedra-containing Dietary Supplements." In 1997, the FDA adopted a policy that ephedra-containing products must (1) be labeled with all possible adverse effects, including death; (2) contain no more than 8 mg of ephedrine per serving; and (3) be used for no more than 7 days. The FDA also proposed a maximum daily dose of 24 mg, and a ban on ephedra-caffeine combination products. However, the FDA has more recently withdrawn these proposed limits for ephedra consumption. This remains an area of controversy.
- **Acute toxicity:** Ephedrine toxicity has been associated with anxiety, dizziness, insomnia, chest tightness, decreased appetite, hypertension, tachycardia, arrhythmias, stroke, urinary retention, vomiting, psychosis, and death.[34-40] Ooms et al. retrospectively evaluated the clinical signs of toxicity following ingestion of an herbal supplement containing

guarana (a caffeine-containing herb) and ephedra (ma huang) in dogs, using information from the National Animal Poison Control Center database.[41] The authors found that 80% of dogs developed clinical signs of toxicity within 8 hours of ingestion, and these signs persisted for up to 48 hours. Hyperactivity, tremors, seizures, and behavior changes were reported in 83% of animals; other signs included vomiting (47%), tachycardia (30%), and hyperthermia (28%). Estimated ingested doses of guarana and ma huang ranged from 4.4 to 296.2 mg/kg (1.98 to 133.2 mg/lb) and 1.3 to 88.9 mg/kg (0.58 to 40.0 mg/lb) of body weight, respectively. The minimum dose at which death was reported was 19.1 mg of guarana/kg (8.7 mg/lb) and 5.8 mg of ma huang/kg (2.6 mg/lb). Most dogs recovered with supportive treatment, although 17% of the animals died or were euthanized.

- **Chronic toxicity:** Ephedrine can cause weight loss, insomnia, and other amphetamine-like side effects, including hypertension, dry mouth, arrhythmias, palpitations, anxiety, and nervousness. Sustained use may lead to cardiac hypertrophy and focal myocardial necrosis.[42,43] Tea made from the European species, *Ephedra altissima*, exhibited mutagenic effects in the standard Ames test for mutagenicity.[44,45] Lee et al. investigated the relative toxicity of ma huang extracted under different conditions.[46] The toxicities of various extracts were assayed using MTT colorimetry on a battery of cell lines, and ephedrine alkaloids were analyzed with HPLC. The cytotoxicity of all ma huang extracts could not be totally accounted for by their ephedrine contents, suggesting the presence of other toxins. High sensitivity of the Neuro-2a cell line to the toxicity of ma huang extracts suggests activity on neuronal cells.
- Grinding the herb has been found to significantly enhance toxicity, and boiling the whole herb for 2 hours produces an extract with high ephedrine-to-toxins ratio.

ADVERSE EFFECTS/PRECAUTIONS/CONTRAINDICATIONS
Allergy

- Known allergy/hypersensitivity to ephedra or to ephedra constituents such as ephedrine or pseudoephedrine.

Adverse Effects/Postmarket Surveillance

- **General:** The FDA has collected over 1500 reports of serious toxicity (including 22 deaths). Haller et al. conducted a review of 140 reports of adverse events related to the use of dietary supplements containing ephedra alkaloids, submitted to the FDA between 1997 and 1999.[47] A standardized rating system for assessing causation was applied to each adverse event, and 31% of cases were considered to be "definitely" or "probably" related to the use of supplements containing ephedra alkaloids, and an additional 31% were deemed to be "possibly" related. Among these adverse events, 47% involved cardiovascular symptoms and 18% involved the central nervous system. Hypertension was the single most frequent adverse effect (17 reports), followed by palpitations, tachycardia, or both[13]; stroke[14]; and seizures.[7] Ten events resulted in death, and 13 events produced permanent disability.
- In 2003, a report was prepared by the RAND Southern California Evidence-Based Practice Center for the Agency for Healthcare Research and Quality, U.S. Department of Health and Human Services.[2,3] This study reviewed available clinical trials, as well as adverse event reports to the FDA and adverse event reports to the manufacturer, Metabolife. Although most prospective trials were not sufficiently

large and most adverse event reports were not sufficiently detailed, the authors identified three deaths, two myocardial infarctions, two cerebrovascular accidents, one seizure, and three psychiatric cases that were considered to be "sentinel events" (i.e., strongly tied to ephedra use within 24 hours without other plausible explanations). In addition, 50 other possible sentinel events were identified.

- A 2003 analysis by Bent et al. in *Annals of Internal Medicine* found that products containing ephedra account for 64% of all adverse reactions to herbs in the United States, but represent only 0.82% of herbal product sales.[4-9] The relative risk for an adverse reaction in a person using ephedra compared with other herbs was extremely high, ranging from 100 (95% CI, 83 to 140) for kava to 720 (95% CI, 520 to 1100) for *Ginkgo biloba*. It was concluded that ephedra use poses a greatly increased risk of adverse reactions compared with other herbs. A 2003 analysis published in *Neurology* also found increased risk of stroke associated with ephedra-containing products.[10,11]
- **Dermatologic:** Anecdotal reports have noted the occurrence of allergic reactions including contact dermatitis, erythroderma, and exfoliative dermatitis.
- **Neurologic/CNS:** Numerous neurologic adverse effects of ephedra have been noted in the scientific literature. One case-report documents a 38-year-old woman with no history of seizures who experienced new onset of tonic-clonic seizures with complex partial seizures when taking a dietary supplement containing ephedrine.[48] Concomitant use of ma huang and guarana (a caffeine-containing herb) has been linked to cerebral infarction.[49] One case report documents ischemic stroke in a sportsman who consumed ma huang extract and creatine monohydrate for bodybuilding.[39] Another case report of ephedrine-induced stroke resulted in death.[50] Hemorrhagic stroke has also been associated with ephedrine use.[10,11] Other adverse effects mentioned repeatedly in anecdotal reports and in human studies include dizziness, restlessness, anxiety, nervousness, irritability, excitation, euphoria, delirium, confusion, syncope, insomnia, vertigo, and headache (particularly when ephedra/ephedrine is combined with caffeine).[51,52]
- **Psychiatric:** Reports exist of ephedrine-induced mania[53] and psychosis.[54-56] Three patients who habitually used ephedrine developed psychosis with a clinical picture resembling schizophrenia and amphetamine psychosis.[56] Another case report describes a 57-year-old woman who had been taking ephedrine for bronchial asthma (50 mg, three times daily) for more than 30 years. After the death of her husband, she increased her dose of ephedrine to 500 to 1000 mg daily for 6 months and developed paranoid psychosis with delusions of persecution and auditory hallucinations, despite a clear sensorium. The patient recovered after ephedrine was gradually tapered.[57] Other psychiatric adverse effects noted in anecdotal reports include confusion, paranoid psychosis, and auditory/visual hallucinations. There is a case of a suicide attempt and mood disorder associated with use of a diet pill containing ma huang.[58] Psychosis occurred in a 32-year-old male following the consumption of alcohol, caffeine, and Vigueur Fit tablets containing ephedra alkaloids.[59] Fewer than 2 days after the event, a urine sample was found to contain 22 μg/mL of ephedrine and 5 μg/mL of pseudoephedrine. Agitation has been reported in trials in which ephedrine was combined with caffeine.[52]
- **Pulmonary/respiratory:** One case report documents diffuse cardiogenic pulmonary edema in a 25-year-old man after

intravenously injecting himself with ephedrine, believing it to be amphetamine.[60] Anecdotal reports have noted respiratory depression as well as tachypnea and labored breathing to be associated with ephedra.

- **Cardiovascular:** Multiple serious cardiovascular adverse effects have been associated with ephedra or its constituent ephedrine, including myocardial infarction, stroke, cardiac arrhythmia, and hypertension, occurring in individuals with diseased or normal hearts.[1,60] There is a Holter monitor study identifying QT-prolongation with the use of ephedra.[61] In 2003 a report was prepared for the U.S. Department of Health and Human Services.[2,3] A review of available clinical trials, as well as more than 1500 adverse event reports to the FDA and adverse event reports to the manufacturer Metabolife, identified two myocardial infarctions, two cerebrovascular accidents, three deaths, and several other possible adverse cardiovascular events. A case report of coronary artery spasm possibly associated with ephedrine was noted in a 69-year-old man receiving high spinal anesthesia.[62] One case report documents diffuse myocardial injury in a 25-year-old man who presented with pulmonary edema after intravenously injecting himself with ephedrine, believing it to be amphetamine.[60] A 35-year-old woman experienced an acute myocardial infarction secondary to cardiac spasm while taking a dietary supplement containing ephedrine for approximately 30 days.[48] A 44-year-old man who consumed a dietary supplement containing ephedrine for 3 weeks developed acute coronary artery thrombosis and a cardiorespiratory arrest.[48] Ephedra may also elicit arrhythmias, and one case report documented bradycardia/asystole in a patient treated with both atropine and ephedrine (although atropine alone could account for these effects).[63] Ephedra use may lead to hypertension and tachycardia, and in a series of 12 normotensive adults administered an ephedra product in the morning (approximately 20 mg of ephedrine and 5 mg of pseudoephedrine per dose) and again 9 hours later, 50% of patients experienced significant tachycardia, although effects on blood pressure were variable. In contrast, in several trials of ephedrine/caffeine combinations for weight loss, no significant changes in mean heart rate or blood pressure were observed vs. placebo or control.[65-67] Ephedra has been associated with myocarditis,[68,69] although this finding has been disputed.[70] Samenuk et al. evaluated possible cardiovascular toxic effects associated with use of dietary supplements containing ma huang (ephedra).[1] The authors reviewed the Adverse Reaction Monitoring System of the Food and Drug Administration, which included clinical records, investigative reports, and autopsy reports related to ma huang use. From 1995 to 1997, 926 cases of possible ma huang toxicity were reported. In 37 patients, use of ma huang was temporally related to stroke (16 patients), myocardial infarction,[10] or sudden death.[11] Autopsies performed in 7 of the 11 patients who experienced sudden death showed a normal heart in 1, coronary atherosclerosis in 3, and cardiomyopathies in 3. In 36 of the 37 patients, use of ma huang was reported to be within the manufacturers' dosing guidelines. The authors concluded that (1) ma huang use is temporally related to stroke, myocardial infarction, and sudden death; (2) underlying heart or vascular disease is not a prerequisite for ma huang–related adverse events; and (3) the cardiovascular toxic effects associated with ma huang were not limited to massive doses.
- **Gastrointestinal:** Anecdotal reports note gastrointestinal adverse effects including nausea, vomiting, dry mouth, anorexia, constipation, and xerostomia. Increases in aminotransferase levels have been noted anecdotally, although in one study, alanine aminotransferase (ALT) and aspartate aminotransferase (AST) levels were found to decrease significantly from baseline in patients using ephedra/ephedrine and guarana/caffeine.[51] A case of acute hepatitis has been associated with the use of ephedra, possibly due to the presence of a contaminant.[71] A case of fulminant exacerbation of autoimmune hepatitis was associated with use of ephedrine in a 58-year-old woman.[72] Jonderko and Kucio reported that ephedrine inhibits gastric emptying, which may result in a feeling of satiety.[73]
- **Endocrine:** Crude extracts of *Ephedra distachya* have elicited hypoglycemia in normal and diabetic mice.[74] However, hyperglycemia has been reported in human studies of ephedrine used in combination with caffeine. A significant increase in mean glucose levels was associated with an ephedra/guarana (caffeine) combination (70 mg/240 mg daily) in an 8-week double-blind, placebo-controlled study of 67 overweight subjects—although several other constituents were included in this formulation, such as chromium, which may have affected the outcome.[51] In a different double-blind, placebo-controlled study of six healthy and lean subjects, significantly increased mean plasma glucose, insulin, and C-peptide levels were noted in subjects taking a single dose of an ephedrine/caffeine combination (10/200 mg, 20/100 mg, or 20/200 mg) vs. placebo.[75] Anecdotal reports have noted the occurrence of hypokalemia with ephedra use, although potassium levels were not significantly altered in one small human trial.[75] Diaphoresis has been reported anecdotally.
- **Renal:** Ephedra has been associated with nephrolithiasis (kidney stones). One case report describes a 27-year-old body builder who developed nephrolithiasis after taking 60 to 180 mg of ephedrine daily for 10 months.[76] Another case report describes a 24-year-old man who developed kidney stones after chronically ingesting 1 to 3 g of ephedrine daily.[77] Other reported effects include diuresis, urinary retention, and dysuria.
- **Genitourinary:** Anecdotal reports note the occurrence of uterine contractions.
- **Musculoskeletal:** Reported adverse effects include tremors, hyperactive reflexes, weakness, myalgia, rhabdomyolysis, eosinophilia-myalgia syndrome, and parkinsonism.

Precautions/Warnings/Contraindications

- Avoid use in individuals less than 18 years old.
- Avoid use during pregnancy or lactation.
- Avoid use for prolonged periods, due to risk of abuse or toxicity.
- Discontinue use at least 24 hours prior to surgery.
- Use cautiously in patients with cardiovascular disease, including structural heart disease, arrhythmia, coronary artery disease, hypertension, cerebrovascular disease, history of stroke, and transient ischemic attack.
- Use cautiously in patients with depression, anxiety disorders, anorexia/bulimia, or history of suicidal ideation.
- Use cautiously in patients sensitive to stimulants, with insomnia or tremor.
- Use cautiously in patients with urinary retention or benign prostatic hypertrophy.
- Use cautiously in diabetics due to risk of hyperglycemia or hypoglycemia; dosing adjustments of medications may be necessary.

- Use cautiously in patients with previous monoamine oxidase inhibitor (MAOI) use, and discontinue MAOIs at least 2 weeks prior to starting ephedra.
- Use cautiously in patients with kidney disease due to risk of nephrolithiasis.
- Use cautiously in patients with glaucoma.
- Use cautiously in patients with thyroid disease.
- Use cautiously in patients with peptic ulcer disease.

Pregnancy and Lactation
- Ephedra should not be used during pregnancy. Ephedrine crosses the placenta and has been found to increase fetal heart rate.[78,79] Ephedra may induce uterine contractions.
- Ephedra should not be used during breastfeeding. Ephedrine crosses into breast milk and has been associated with irritability, crying, and insomnia in infants.[80]

INTERACTIONS
Ephedra/Drug Interactions
- **Alcohol:** A brief episode of acute psychosis in a 32-year-old male followed the consumption of alcohol, caffeine, and Vigueur Fit tablets containing ephedra alkaloids.[59]
- **Antiadrenergic agents (alpha blockers):** Sympathomimetic effects of ephedrine such as mydriasis and hypertension may be antagonized by antiadrenergic drugs including clonidine, reserpine, and terazosin.
- **Antiarrhythmic agents, antihypertensive drugs, cardiac glycosides (Digoxin, Digitoxin):** Both the ephedrine and pseudoephedrine constituents of ephedra can induce hypertension and chronotropic and inotropic effects in humans.[64,81-83] Ephedra may antagonize the activity of antihypertensive agents such as beta-blockers, diuretics, angiotensin-converting enzyme inhibitors, and calcium-channel blockers. However, in several trials of ephedrine/caffeine combinations taken for weight loss, no significant changes in mean heart rate or blood pressure were observed vs. placebo or control.[65-67]
- **Bronchodilators:** Both ephedrine and pseudoephedrine cause bronchodilation,[81] and use with other bronchodilators or asthma medications may lead to additive effects.
- **CNS stimulants:** Both ephedrine and pseudoephedrine cause central nervous system (CNS) stimulation,[81] and use with other CNS stimulants may lead to additive effects.
- **Diuretics:** The ephedra constituents ephedrine and pseudoephedrine possess diuretic properties and may add to the effects of other diuretics.
- **Ergot alkaloids (bromocriptine, dihydroergotamine, ergotamine):** Ergot alkaloids exert alpha-adrenergic vasoconstrictive effects, and in combination with ephedra may increase hypertensive effects.
- **General anesthetics:** Ephedra may decrease the effectiveness of general anesthetics such as halothane, cyclopropane, and propofol, and increase the risk of arrhythmia.[78,79,84,85]
- **Methylxanthines (theophylline, caffeine):** Use of ephedra with caffeine, theophylline, or other methylxanthines may result in additive neurologic, cardiovascular, and psychiatric adverse effects or toxicity. Fatalities have been associated with simultaneous caffeine and ephedrine use.[86,87] A brief episode of acute psychosis in a 32-year-old male followed the consumption of alcohol, caffeine, and Vigueur Fit tablets containing ephedra alkaloids.[59] Notably, many commercial products contain both ephedra and caffeine. Theophylline combined with ephedrine can induce insomnia, anxiety, and adverse gastrointestinal effects including vomiting.[88]

- **Monoamine oxidase inhibitors (MAOIs):** When ephedra is administered in combination with MAOIs, increased sympathomimetic activity may increase the risk of hypertensive crisis. One case report notes a 28-year-old woman who developed encephalopathy, neuromuscular irritability, hypotension, tachycardia, rhabdomyolysis, and hyperthermia after taking a combination tablet containing ephedrine, caffeine, and theophylline (a "Do-Do") 24 hours after discontinuing phenelzine treatment.[89]
- **Oral hypoglycemic agents, insulin:** Ephedrine has been associated with hyperglycemia in studies combining ephedrine with caffeine. A significant increase in mean glucose levels was associated with an ephedra/guarana (caffeine) combination (70 mg/240 mg daily) in an 8-week double-blind, placebo-controlled study of 67 overweight subjects—although several other constituents were included in this formulation, such as chromium, which may have affected the outcome.[51] In a different double-blind, placebo-controlled study of six healthy and lean subjects, significantly increased mean plasma glucose, insulin, and C-peptide levels were noted in subjects taking a single dose of an ephedrine/caffeine combination (10/200 mg, 20/100 mg, or 20/200 mg) vs. placebo.[75] In contrast, crude extracts of *Ephedra distachya* have elicited hypoglycemia in normal and diabetic mice.[74]
- **Oxytocin (Pitosin), secale alkaloid derivatives:** Concomitant use with ephedra may increase risk of hypertension.
- **Phenothiazine antipsychotics:** Phenothiazines may block the alpha-adrenergic effects of ephedra.
- **Phenylpropanolamine (removed from U.S. market):** Combination use of ephedra and phenylpropanolamine may lead to additive effects.[90]
- **Steroids:** Ephedrine has been reported to increase the clearance and reduce the effectiveness of dexamethasone.[91,92]
- **Thyroid agents:** Ephedra may increase serum levels of thyroid hormones (T_3), and combination use with thyroid hormones may result in additive effects. In one study, the ratio of serum T_3 to T_4 was significantly increased after 4 weeks of treatment with ephedra, although after 12 weeks of treatment the ratio decreased.[93]
- **Tricyclic antidepressants:** In one case report, concomitant use of amitriptyline and ephedrine was associated with hypotension in a 61-year-old woman undergoing ovarian cancer resection.[94]
- **Triglyceride-lowering agents:** In one trial, triglyceride concentrations decreased with ephedra/guarana (caffeine) use—although several other constituents were included in this formulation, such as chromium, which may have affected the outcome.[51]
- **Urine acidifiers/alkalinizers:** Ephedrine and pseudoephedrine are excreted more rapidly with urinary acidifiers (such as ammonium chloride) and more slowly with urinary alkalinizers (such as disodium bicarbonate). Combination use with urinary acidifiers may enhance effects, while urinary alkalinizers may diminish effects.

Ephedra/Herb/Supplement Interactions
- **Caffeine, cola nut, guarana (*Paullina cupana*), yerba mate (*Ilex paraguariensis*):** Cola, guarana, and yerba mate contain caffeine, and combination use may increase the risk of cardiovascular, neurologic, or psychiatric adverse effects. Fatalities have been associated with simultaneous caffeine and ephedrine use.[86,87] Use of concomitant ephedra and guarana has been associated with a case of cerebral

infarction.[49] A brief episode of acute psychosis in a 32-year-old male followed the consumption of alcohol, caffeine, and Vigueur Fit tablets containing ephedra alkaloids.[59] Commercial products are sold that contain both ephedra and guarana. Ephedrine has been associated with hyperglycemia in studies combining ephedrine with caffeine. A significant increase in mean glucose was associated with an ephedrine/caffeine combination (70 mg/240 mg daily) in an 8-week double-blind, placebo-controlled study of 67 overweight subjects.[51] In a different double-blind, placebo-controlled study of six healthy and lean subjects, significantly increased mean plasma glucose, insulin, and C-peptide levels were noted in subjects taking a single dose of an ephedrine/caffeine combination (10/200 mg, 20/100 mg, or 20/200 mg) vs. placebo.[75]

- **CNS stimulant agents:** Both ephedrine and pseudoephedrine cause central nervous system (CNS) stimulation,[81] and use with other CNS stimulants may lead to additive effects.
- **Monoamine oxidase inhibitors (MAOIs):** When ephedra is administered in combination with agents possessing MAOI activity, increased sympathomimetic activity may increase the risk of hypertensive crisis. One case report notes a 28-year-old woman who developed encephalopathy, neuromuscular irritability, hypotension, tachycardia, rhabdomyolysis, and hyperthermia after taking a combination tablet containing ephedrine, caffeine, and theophylline (a "Do-Do") 24 hours after discontinuing phenelzine treatment.[89]
- **Hypotensive herbs and supplements:** Both the ephedrine and pseudoephedrine constituents of ephedra can induce hypertension and chronotropic and inotropic effects in humans.[64,81-83] However, in several trials of ephedrine/caffeine combinations taken for weight loss, no significant changes in mean heart rate or blood pressure were observed vs. placebo or control.[65-67]
- **Cardiac glycosides:** Both the ephedrine and pseudoephedrine constituents of ephedra can induce hypertension and chronotropic and inotropic effects.[64,81] Ephedra may potentiate the inotropic effects of cardiac glycosides and antagonize the negative chronotropic effects.
- **Diuretics:** The ephedra constituents ephedrine and pseudoephedrine possess diuretic properties and may add to the effects of other diuretics.
- **Hypoglycemic agents:** Ephedrine has been associated with hyperglycemia in studies combining ephedrine with caffeine. A significant increase in mean glucose was associated with an ephedra/guarana (caffeine) combination (70 mg/240 mg daily) in an 8-week double-blind, placebo-controlled study of 67 overweight subjects—although several other constituents were included in this formulation, such as chromium, which may have affected the outcome.[51] In a different double-blind, placebo-controlled study of six healthy and lean subjects, significantly increased mean plasma glucose, insulin, and C-peptide levels were noted in subjects taking a single dose of an ephedrine/caffeine combination (10/200 mg, 20/100 mg, or 20/200 mg) vs. placebo.[75] In contrast, crude extracts of *Ephedra distachya* have elicited hypoglycemia in normal and diabetic mice.[74]
- **Hypolipidemic agents:** In one trial, triglyceride concentrations decreased with ephedra/guarana (caffeine) use, although several other constituents were included in this formulation, such as chromium, which may have affected the outcome.[51] Other agents with possible hypolipidemic properties include fish oil, garlic, guggul, and niacin.

Ephedra/Food Interactions

- **Coffee/tea:** Foods containing caffeine taken in combination with ephedra may increase the risk of cardiovascular, neurologic, or psychiatric adverse effects. Fatalities have been associated with simultaneous caffeine and ephedrine use.[86,87] A brief episode of acute psychosis in a 32-year-old male followed the consumption of alcohol, caffeine, and Vigueur Fit tablets containing ephedra alkaloids.[59]

Ephedra/Lab Interactions

- **Triglycerides:** In one trial, triglyceride concentrations decreased with ephedrine/caffeine use.[51]
- **Pulmonary function tests (PFTs):** Due to the bronchodilator effects of ephedra, PFT results may be affected.
- **Thyroid hormones (T_3/T_4 ratio):** In one study, the ratio of serum T3 to T4 was significantly increased after 4 weeks of treatment with ephedra, although after 12 weeks of treatment the ratio decreased.[93]
- **Serum glucose:** Ephedrine has been associated with hyperglycemia in studies combining ephedrine with caffeine. A significant increase in mean glucose was associated with an ephedrine/caffeine combination (70 mg/240 mg daily) in an 8-week double-blind, placebo-controlled study of 67 overweight subjects.[51] In a different double-blind, placebo-controlled study of six healthy and lean subjects, significantly increased mean plasma glucose, insulin, and C-peptide levels were noted in subjects taking a single dose of an ephedrine/caffeine combination (10/200 mg, 20/100 mg, or 20/200 mg) vs. placebo.[75] In contrast, crude extracts of *Ephedra distachya* have elicited hypoglycemia in normal and diabetic mice.[74]
- **Urine amphetamine/methamphetamine:** Ephedra may cause false-positive urine amphetamine or methamphetamine test results.[95]
- **Liver function tests:** Increases in aminotransferase levels have been noted anecdotally, although in one study, alanine aminotransferase (ALT) and aspartate aminotransferase (AST) levels were found to decrease significantly from baseline in patients using ephedrine and caffeine.[51] A case of acute hepatitis has been associated with the use of ephedra, possibly due to the presence of a contaminant.[71] A case of fulminant exacerbation of autoimmune hepatitis was associated with use of ephedrine in a 58-year-old woman.[72]

MECHANISM OF ACTION
Pharmacology

- **Constituents:** Ephedra contains the alkaloids ephedrine, pseudoephedrine (isoephedrine), norpseudoephedrine (cathine), norephedrine, methylephedrine, methylpseudoephedrine,[96] tannins,[97] and other constituents, including quinoline and 6-hydroxykynurenic acid.[98] The stem contains approximately 0.5% to 2.5% alkaloids, with ephedrine accounting for 30% to 90% of the total alkaloid content. The variation in content depends upon the species harvested and the part of the plant used; for example, the woody stems are low in alkaloids and the fruits and roots have practically none, whereas the softer stems contain up to 2.5% active alkaloids. *Ephedra sinica* generally contains substantially greater concentrations of alkaloids than *Ephedra intermedia*.[29,99] The North American species, *Ephedra nevadensis* (Mormon tea, Mexican tea, squaw tea, or desert tea), is apparently devoid of alkaloids altogether. Different extraction methods also yield different quantities of active compounds.[100] In *Ephedra sinica*, pseudoephedrine is typically found as dextro-rotatory (D-pseudoephedrine), and ephedrine is typically levorotatory (L-ephedrine), whereas synthetically manufactured ephedrine is usually a racemic mixture.[101]

- **Alkaloids:** Ephedrine and pseudoephedrine are found in the leaves and stems of ephedra and are structurally related to amphetamines. They increase the availability and action of the endogenous neurotransmitters norepinephrine and epinephrine and stimulate catecholamine receptors in the brain, heart, and blood vessels both directly and indirectly. Both ephedrine and pseudoephedrine elicit central nervous system stimulation, bronchodilation, hypertension, and chronotropic/inotropic effects.[81] The synthetic form of pseudoephedrine is widely used in non-prescription decongestants. Pseudoephedrine is a more potent diuretic than ephedrine. Ephedrine stimulates thermogenesis in adipocytes *in vitro* and in animal studies, an effect which appears to be enhanced by chronic administration.[102] In mice, rats, and monkeys, ephedrine has been associated with significant weight loss, possibly by enhancing thermogenesis or anorexia.[103-108] These effects have been enhanced by combining ephedrine with aspirin and/or methylxanthines (caffeine or theophylline).[109-113] Jonderko and Kucio reported that ephedrine inhibits gastric emptying, which may result in a feeling of satiety and thereby aid in weight loss.[73]
- **Tannins:** Tannins present in ephedra possess astringent effects and have historically been used in topical preparations to reduce oozing and weeping of skin lesions. Ephedra's tannins have been proposed to possess some renal protective properties, based on experimental models of kidney failure in rats.[114]
- **Anti-inflammatory effects:** Ephedra's stems have demonstrated anti-inflammatory activity in a mouse paw model of carageenan-induced inflammation. These effects are thought to be due to pseudoephedrine content.[115] Ephedra extracts have been found to inhibit complement activity *in vitro*.[116]

Pharmacodynamics/Kinetics

- Ephedrine is well absorbed after oral administration, with a reported half-life of 3 to 6 hours. Following oral administration, 88% is excreted in the urine within 24 hours, and 97% is excreted within 48 hours. Ephedrine and pseudoephedrine are excreted more rapidly with urinary acidifiers (such as ammonium chloride) and more slowly with urinary alkalinizers (such as disodium bicarbonate).
- Per anecdotal reports, the onset of bronchodilatory effects with oral ephedrine occurs within 15 to 60 minutes, with a duration of 2 to 4 hours. Oral ephedrine causes pressor and cardiac effects for 4 hours. Intramuscular or subcutaneous administration of ephedrine results in cardiac effects lasting for 1 hour.
- The natural and synthetic forms of ephedrine have similar absorption and pharmacokinetics in adults, but the available natural products contain considerably different concentrations of active alkaloids.[28] Pharmacokinetics have not been extensively studied in children.

HISTORY

- *Ephedra sinica* is an evergreen, shrub-like plant native to arid regions of China and Mongolia. The parts used medicinally are the dried green stems. The plant has horse-shaped yellow flowers, accounting for one of its common names,

"yellow horse." The plants have a strong pine-like odor and an astringent taste. Ephedra plants currently grow in China, northern India, Pakistan, Mongolia and the southwestern United States. A related species indigenous to North America, *Ephedra nevadensis*, appears to be devoid of alkaloid constituents.

- *Ephedra altissima*, a species closely related to modern *Ephedra sinica*, was found along with several other medicinal plants in a Neanderthal gravesite dating back 60,000 years. Juice made from ephedra, known as "soma," was consumed as a longevity-producing beverage in ancient India. Ephedra (ma huang) has been used in traditional Chinese medicine (TCM) for over 5000 years. Its historical uses include the alleviation of fevers, cough, colds, chills, shortness of breath, bone and joint pain, and water retention (edema). It is included in many TCM remedies for asthma.
- Ephedra's principal medicinal constituent, ephedrine, was isolated in 1887 and became popular in the United States as a decongestant and bronchodilator during the 1920s. In the last quarter of the 20th century, ephedrine was used as a therapy for asthma, and to correct hypotension resulting from spinal or epidural anesthesia, including in laboring women. Natural health practitioners sometimes recommend ephedra as an herbal remedy for colds, asthma, allergic rhinitis, cough and bronchitis and as an herbal weight loss agent. It is also used as a CNS stimulant (to enhance alertness) and cardiovascular stimulant.
- In 1998, Blanck investigated the prevalence of non-prescription weight loss product use in Florida, Iowa, Michigan, West Virginia, and Wisconsin.[22] Using the Behavioral Risk Factor Surveillance System and a random-digit telephone survey, a population-based sample of 14,679 non-institutionalized adults 18 years or older was polled. Seven percent of the sample reported non-prescription weight loss product use, which was especially common among young obese women (28.4% of sample). Of those individuals using diet products, 14% used ephedra formulations.
- Ephedrine can also be used as a starting material for the illegal manufacture of "speed," or methamphetamine. Ephedrine itself is known as "natural ecstasy." Some athletes use ephedra to boost their performance naturally; however, in at least one case, an elite athlete was eliminated from competition because the product he used had been spiked with norpseudoephedrine, which is banned by the International Olympic Committee.
- Due to over 800 reports of serious toxicity (including at least 22 deaths) among adolescents and young adults using ephedra (in most cases as a natural stimulant), the U.S. Food and Drug Administration (FDA) convened a special advisory committee on "Ephedra-containing Dietary Supplements." In June 1997, the FDA adopted the policy that ephedra-containing products must (1) be labeled with all possible adverse effects, including death; (2) contain no more than 8 mg of ephedrine per serving; and (3) be used for no more than 7 days. The FDA also proposed a maximum daily dose of 24 mg and a ban on ephedra-caffeine combination products. However, the FDA has more recently withdrawn these proposed limits for ephedra consumption. This remains an area of controversy. In the late 1990s, several states, including Nebraska, Ohio and Texas, banned or severely limited the sale of products containing ephedra. However, products containing more than 10 mg of ephedra are available for purchase on several websites.

- The German expert panel, the Commission E, has approved of the use of ephedra to treat "diseases of the respiratory tract with mild bronchospasm in adults and children over the age of six." The Commission E has also noted a variety of side effects and potential adverse interactions with commonly used medications.

REVIEW OF THE EVIDENCE: DISCUSSION

Weight Loss

Summary

- Up to 7% of the U.S. population uses non-prescription weight loss products, and 14% of those taking such products use an ephedra or ephedrine-containing formulation.[22]

Scientific evidence suggests that the ephedra constituent ephedrine can elicit weight loss when combined with caffeine, as demonstrated in several trials of 1 to 12 months' duration. However, studies of ephedra or ephedrine monotherapy have been equivocal. Overall, the available trials have been small, with methodological weaknesses including large dropout rates due to adverse effects and incomplete reporting of blinding or randomization. Because of the variable concentrations of ephedrine found in commercial preparations, and numerous reports of serious adverse effects (particularly when combined with caffeine), ephedra may not be a safe therapy for this indication. Future studies may determine sub-populations for which this therapy warrants the associated risks.

Review of the Evidence: Ephedra

Condition Treated*	Study Design	Author, Year	N[†]	SS[†]	Study Quality[‡]	Magnitude of Benefit	ARR[†]	NNT[†]	Comments
Weight loss (combination therapy with caffeine)	RCT, double-blind	Daly[66] 1993	24	Yes	4	Medium	NA	NA	Ephedrine + caffeine + aspirin combination superior to placebo over 8-20 weeks.
Weight loss (combination therapy with caffeine)	RCT, double-blind l	Astrup[65] 1992	180	Yes	4	Medium	NA	NA	Ephedrine + caffeine combination superior to ephedrine or caffeine alone, or to placebo, over 24 weeks. All subjects placed on calorie controlled diet.
Weight loss (combination therapy with caffeine)	RCT, double-blind	Molnar[118] 2000	32	Yes	4	Medium	NA	NA	Ephedrine + caffeine combination superior to placebo over 20 weeks. All subjects placed on calorie controlled diet.
Weight loss (combination therapy with caffeine)	RCT, double-blind	Boozer[51] 2001	67	Yes	3	Medium	NA	NA	Ephedrine + caffeine combination superior to placebo over 8 weeks.
Weight loss (combination therapy with caffeine)	Comparison trial, double-blind	Breum[52] 1994	103	Yes	3	Medium	NA	NA	Ephedrine + caffeine combination superior to dexfenfluramine over 15 weeks; all subjects placed on calorie controlled diet.
Weight loss (monotherapy)	RCT, double-blind	Pasquali[33] 1987	10	Yes	3	Medium	NA	NA	Ephedrine superior to placebo over 16 weeks; all subjects placed on calorie controlled diet.
Weight loss (monotherapy)	RCT, double-blind, crossover	Pasquali[31] 1992	10	No	2	None	NA	NA	Ephedrine not superior to placebo over 2 weeks; study may have been underpowered, and low-calorie diet in all subjects may have blunted results.
Weight loss (monotherapy)	RCT, double-blind	Pasquali[32] 1985	62	No	2	None	NA	NA	Ephedrine not superior to placebo over 12 weeks; study may have been underpowered, and low-calorie diet in all subjects may have blunted results.
Allergic rhinitis	RCT, double-blind	Shaikh[142] 1995	118	Yes	3	Medium	NA	NA	Nasally inhaled ephedrine 1% saline solution superior to placebo over 4 weeks.
Sexual arousal in women	Double-blind cross-over controlled	Meston[143] 1998	20	Mixed	2	Medium	NA	NA	Ephedrine superior to placebo, but mixed statistical significance and use of unvalidated measurement scales.

*Primary or secondary outcome.
[†]N, Number of patients; SS, statistically significant; ARR, absolute risk reduction; NNT, the number of patients who need to undergo a specific intervention in order to observe an outcome in one individual.
[‡]0-2 = poor; 3-4 = good; 5 = excellent.
NA, Not applicable; RCT, randomized, controlled trial.
For an explanation of each category in this table, please see Table 3 in the Introduction.

Ephedrine/Caffeine Combination Therapy Trials

- Astrup et al. conducted a randomized, double-blind, placebo-controlled, four-arm trial in 180 obese patients.[65] Subjects were randomized to receive either an ephedrine/caffeine combination (20/200 mg), ephedrine monotherapy (20 mg), caffeine monotherapy (200 mg), or placebo three times daily for 24 weeks. Caloric intake was controlled in all groups (4.2 MJ daily). After weeks 8 and 24, a significant mean weight loss was noted in the combination ephedrine/caffeine group vs. placebo (16.6 kg and 13.2 kg, respectively; a difference of 3.4 kg). However, neither monotherapy yielded significant differences from placebo. These compelling results suggest that combination ephedrine/caffeine therapy may be more effective than either agent alone. As a follow-up, Toubro et al. studied the 99 subjects in the ephedrine/caffeine arm of this trial.[117] An open study was conducted for 25 weeks immediately following the initial trial. At the end of the research period, a statistically significant mean weight loss of 1.1 kg was measured. However, this follow-up was neither blinded nor randomized, allowing for the possible introduction of bias or confounding.
- Boozer et al. conducted a double-blind, placebo-controlled study of a combination of ephedrine from ephedra (72 mg daily) and caffeine from guarana (240 mg daily) in 67 overweight men and women (body mass indices $\geq$29 kg/m^2 and $\leq$35 kg/m^2, respectively).[51] Subjects were randomized to receive either the combination of ephedrine and caffeine or placebo over an 8-week period. The authors reported that subjects in the ephedrine/caffeine group experienced significant weight loss vs. placebo (−4.0 kg and −2.1%, respectively), as well as a significant reduction in fat composition vs. placebo (−0.8 kg and 0.2%, respectively).
- Breum et al. conducted a 15-week double-blind, randomized trial study to compare the efficacy and safety of dexfenfluramine and ephedrine/caffeine therapy in 103 patients who were 20% to 80% overweight.[52] Participants were treated with either 15 mg of dexfenfluramine or 20 mg/200 mg of ephedrine/caffeine three times daily. All subjects received a calorie-controlled diet (5 MJ daily). After 15 weeks of treatment, mean weight reductions in the dexfenfluramine and ephedrine/caffeine groups were 6.9 kg and 8.3 kg, respectively ($p = 0.12$). In a sub-group of patients with a body mass index (BMI) 30 kg/m^2, the mean weight loss was 7.0 kg in the dexfenfluramine group and 9.0 kg in the ephedrine/caffeine group ($p < 0.05$). The lack of a placebo group leaves open the question of how great these weight losses would be compared to dietary control alone.
- Daly et al. conducted a randomized, double-blind, placebo-controlled trial assessing the safety and efficacy of a mixture of ephedrine (75 to 150 mg), caffeine (150 mg), and aspirin (330 mg) in 24 obese individuals.[66] After 8 weeks of therapy, overall mean weight loss was 2.2 kg in the ephedrine/caffeine/aspirin group vs. 0.7 kg in placebo ($p < 0.05$). In a second phase of this study, eight patients in the placebo group were given ephedrine/caffeine/aspirin for an additional 8 weeks, while a different group continued placebo therapy. A mean weight loss of 3.2 kg was found in the ephedrine/caffeine/aspirin group vs. 1.3 kg in placebo ($p = 0.036$). In a third phase of this trial, six patients in the ephedrine/caffeine/aspirin group and five in the placebo group continued therapy for an additional 5 months, after which time a mean weight loss of 5.2 kg was noted in the ephedrine/caffeine/aspirin group compared to a 0.03 kg weight gain in the placebo group. However, one of the placebo patients was discounted from the analysis due to a 66 kg weight loss achieved via self-imposed caloric restriction. The post-analysis disqualification of this outlier patient reveals the weaknesses of small sample sizes and diminished the value of the results. This study was not adequately blinded.
- Molnar et al. conducted a randomized double-blind, placebo-controlled study investigating the efficacy and safety of an ephedrine/caffeine mixture in 32 obese adolescents.[118] Subjects were assigned to receive either ephedrine/caffeine or placebo for 20 weeks in conjunction with a calorie-controlled diet (calculated daily energy requirement minus 500 kcal). Participants whose weight was <80 kg took 1 tablet three times daily (10 mg/100 mg), and participants weighing >80 kg took 2 tablets three times daily (20 mg/200 mg). The authors reported that relative body weight, BMI, and body fat were significantly decreased in the ephedrine/caffeine group (14.4 + 10.5%, 2.9 + 1.9 kg/m^2, and 6.6 + 6.0 kg) vs. placebo (2.2 + 5.8%, 0.5 + 1.6 kg/m^2, 0.5 + 2.7 kg) ($p < 0.05$). Relative body weight decreased by more than 5% occurred in 81% of the ephedrine/caffeine group vs. in 31% of the placebo group.

Ephedrine/Ephedra Monotherapy Trials

- Pasquali et al. conducted a randomized, double-blind, crossover study to determine the effects of ephedrine in 10 obese patients during 6 weeks of a "very-low-calorie diet" (1965 kJ, 60 g of protein, 45 g of carbohydrate).[31] Subjects were randomized to receive either ephedrine hydrochloride (50 mg three times daily) or placebo for two weeks. No difference in weight loss between the two groups was observed. However, the effects of ephedra may have been blunted by concomitant use of the low-calorie diet in both groups. In addition, the small sample size and brief study duration may not have been adequate to detect between-group differences.
- The same principal author conducted a prior double-blind trial in which 10 obese women received either placebo or ephedrine (50 mg) three times daily for 2 months, followed by crossover.[33] Both treatment groups received concomitant diet therapy of 1000 to 1400 kcal/day. The authors reported significant weight loss in the ephedrine group (2.41 ± 0.61 kg) vs. placebo (0.64 ± 0.50 kg).
- The same principal author conducted a prior double-blind, controlled study to assess the effects of ephedrine on weight loss in obese outpatients over a 3-month period.[32] Subjects were assigned to receive either placebo, 25 mg of ephedrine three times daily, or 50 mg of ephedrine three times daily. Dietary intake in all groups was restricted to 1000 kcal/day for women and 1200 kcal/day for men. No significant differences were detected between groups. The group treated with 150 mg of ephedrine experienced more side effects than other groups. The effects of ephedra may have been blunted by concomitant use of the low-calorie diet in both groups. The small sample size and brief study duration may not have been adequate to detect between-group differences.
- Astrup et al. conducted an open trial involving five healthy female volunteers who were 14% overweight.[93] Subjects received 20 mg of ephedrine three times daily for 3 months. After 4 and 12 weeks of treatment, mean body weight was significantly reduced (2.5 kg and 5.5 kg, respectively). However, an average regain of 0.5 kg was experienced 2 months after discontinuation of ephedrine. Limitations of this study include small sample size and lack of blinding or randomization.

E

In Vitro/Animal Data

- Ephedrine stimulates thermogenesis in adipocytes *in vitro* and in animal studies, an effect which appears to be enhanced by chronic administration.[102] In mice, rats and monkeys, ephedrine has been associated with significant weight loss, possibly by enhancing thermogenesis or anorexia.[103-108] These effects have been enhanced by combining ephedrine with aspirin and/or methylxanthines (caffeine or theophylline).[109-113] Jonderko and Kucio reported that ephedrine inhibits gastric emptying, which may result in a feeling of satiety and thereby aid in weight loss.[73]

Asthmatic Bronchoconstriction
Summary

- Ephedra contains both ephedrine and pseudoephedrine and has long been used as a bronchodilator to treat asthma and chronic obstructive pulmonary disease (COPD). The use of ephedrine to treat asthma in children was first reported in Western medicine in 1927[119]; its clinical effectiveness and side effects, including the death of a child from an accidental overdose of an ephedra-containing asthma medication, were subsequently reported in several studies.[120-122] Synthetic forms of ephedrine were used to treat asthma in the United States until the advent of more specific beta-agonist medications. Despite the evidence of efficacy of ephedrine, because of the variable concentrations of ephedrine found in commercial preparations of ephedra and numerous reports of serious adverse effects, the non-prescription dietary supplement ephedra does not appear to be a safe alternative therapy for this indication.

Evidence

- Numerous trials have reported the efficacy of ephedrine as a bronchodilator.[92,123-129] In a double-blind, placebo-controlled study of 16 asthmatic children (13 receiving concomitant aminophylline, and 4 receiving alternate day prednisone), ephedrine sulfate (25 mg every 8 hours) was associated with a significant improvement in pulmonary function tests within 30 minutes of administration, with benefits lasting 3 to 4 hours.[130] This trial was limited by a small sample size and concurrent use of other therapies.
- McLaughlin et al. conducted a double-blind, crossover trial in 16 asthmatic children comparing the effects of ephedrine (24 mg), fenoterol (doses of 2.5 mg, 5 mg, and 7.5 mg), and placebo.[131] Fenoterol and ephedrine were reported to be significantly superior to placebo in the parameters of FEV1 and FEF25-75. Fenoterol, at a dose of 7.5 mg, was shown to be the most effective treatment. These results are limited by small sample size and incomplete descriptions of blinding, randomization, or statistical analysis.
- Weinberger and Bronsky conducted a randomized, double-blind, crossover study examining the bronchodilator effects of oral ephedrine, aminophylline, and the combination of both agents.[132] Twelve asthmatic children were dosed every 6 hours for 1 week in a randomized sequence. Aminophylline in high doses (7.3 mg/kg/dose) appeared to have an effect in relieving signs and symptoms of asthma, and the addition of ephedrine did not produce further benefits, although it increased the frequency of adverse effects.
- In a case series, May et al. studied the effects of ephedrine in promoting bronchodilation acutely and chronically in eight asthmatic patients.[133] No change was reported in the bronchodilator response after receiving a single dose of 22 mg of ephedrine, or following 2 weeks of 11 mg of ephedrine three times daily. No deterioration in pulmonary function was reported during the 2-week treatment period. The small sample size and lack of a control group allowed for the possible introduction of confounders or bias, which may have affected these results.

Hypotension
Summary

- A substantial body of historical evidence, clinical experience, and scientific data supports the potent cardiovascular effects of ephedrine and related sympathomimetic compounds. In published studies, ephedrine has been administered as a pharmaceutical in controlled quantities, generally in the hospital setting. In particular, ephedrine has been used historically to manage the hypotensive effects of epidural and spinal anesthesia during labor and delivery.[78,79,82,134] Ephedrine is a constituent of the non-prescription dietary supplement ephedra. Because of the variable concentrations of ephedrine found in commercial preparations of ephedra, and significant safety concerns, ephedra is likely not a safe alternative therapy for this indication. Notably, in several trials of ephedrine/caffeine combinations taken for weight loss, which may be closer in dose to commercial ephedra products, no significant changes in blood pressure were observed vs. placebo or control.[65-67]

Evidence

- Multiple trials have evaluated ephedrine in the management of hypotension,[85,135-138] particularly for the prevention and treatment of maternal blood pressure decreases during delivery.[82,139,140] Lee et al. conducted a quantitative systematic review of randomized controlled trials studying the efficacy of ephedrine or phenylephrine for the management of maternal hypertension associated with spinal anesthesia during cesarean delivery.[82] Both therapies demonstrated efficacy, with no statistically significant difference between therapies. Notably, maternal bradycardia was more common in the phenylephrine group.
- Prophylactic doses of 12 mg of ephedrine intravenously have been associated with lower incidence of hypotension during spinal anesthesia for cesarean section.[134] Increased uterine artery blood pressure during uterine contractions has been associated with ephedrine use.[141]
- In a case series in 12 normotensive adults given an ephedra product in the morning (approximately 20 mg of ephedrine and 5 mg of pseudoephedrine per dose), and a second dose 9 hours later, 50% of patients experienced significant tachycardia, whereas effects on blood pressure were variable.[64]
- In a double-blind, placebo-controlled study of six healthy and lean subjects, significantly increased mean systolic blood pressure by 5 to 7 mm Hg was noted in subjects taking a single dose of an ephedrine/caffeine combination vs. placebo.[75] Effects were dose-dependent, and were noted at ephedrine/caffeine doses of 10 mg/200 mg, and increased at 20 mg/200 mg. Changes in diastolic blood pressure were variable, and heart rate increases occurred only at the higher doses of ephedrine. Conclusions from this study specific to ephedrine may be confounded by the concomitant use of caffeine.
- In contrast, in several trials of ephedrine/caffeine combinations taken for weight loss, which may be closer in dose to commercial ephedra products, no significant changes in mean heart rate or blood pressure were observed vs. placebo or control.[65-67]

Allergic Rhinitis

Summary

• A randomized, controlled trial has shown promising results of a 1% ephedrine saline nasal wash in the treatment of allergic rhinitis. Results from further randomized, controlled trials are warranted before recommending for or against the use of ephedrine in the treatment of allergic rhinitis. The mechanism of action is not clear, although in theory, local vasoconstriction may play a role. Although effects in this study reportedly lasted for 2 to 4 weeks, there is a theoretical concern that tolerance might develop. Notably, saline nasal washes alone have been demonstrated as efficacious. Further study is warranted in this area, with a long-term comparison to saline monotherapy and nasally inhaled corticosteroids.

Evidence

• Shaikh conducted a randomized, placebo-controlled, crossover trial with 118 patients with perennial allergic rhinitis.[142] Patients were randomized to receive placebo or a 1% ephedrine-saline nasal wash once every 48 hours. After a 4-week interval, patients were crossed over to the opposite treatment. Results indicated that ephedrine-saline significantly improved symptom scores and peak nasal inspiratory flow rates ($p \leq 0.001$). Statistical significance was seen after the second week, and effects lasted for greater than 2 weeks, without notable side effects seen in the majority of patients.

Sexual Arousal

Summary

• One methodologically weak human trial has evaluated the effects of ephedrine on sexual arousal, with inconclusive results.

Evidence

• Meston and Heiman conducted a randomized, double-blind, crossover study to examine the effects of ephedrine sulfate on subjective (self-reported) and physiologic measures of sexual arousal (assessed via vaginal photoplethysmography).[143] Twenty "sexually functional" women received either 50 mg of ephedrine sulfate or placebo prior to exposure to erotic stimuli. The authors reported that ephedrine was associated with a significant mean increase in vaginal pulse amplitude responses to erotic films ($p < 0.01$) but did not have significant effects on subjective ratings ($p < 0.1$)

FORMULARY: BRANDS USED IN CLINICAL TRIALS

Brands Used in Statistically Significant Clinical Trials

• Not applicable.

Multi-Ingredient Preparations Containing Ephedra

• Acceleration, AllerClear, AllerPlus, Andro Heat, Better BodyEnergy for Life, Bio Trim, Biovital Plus, Bladderwrack-Dandelion Virtue, Breathe-Aid Formula, Breath Easy, Cordephrine XC, Diet Fuel, Dymetadrine Xtrem, EPH-833, Ephedra Plus, Thermogen, Guarana-Gotu Kola Virtue, Herba Fuel, Herbal Decongestant Expectorant Capsules, Herbalife—Thermojetics Original Green, Metabolife 356, Metabolift, Metaboloss, MetaboTRIM, Naturafed, Naturally Ripped, Naturatussin 1, Nettle-Reishi Virtue, Power Thin, ProLab Stoked, Pro-Ripped Ephedra, Respa-Herb, Respiratory Support Formula, Ripped Fuel, SinuCheck, SinuClear, SnoreStop, Thermadrene, Thermic Blast, Thermicore, Thermo Cuts, ThermoDiet, Ultra Diet Pep, Xenadrine RFA-1 (discontinued).

References

1. Samenuk D, Link MS, Homoud MK, et al. Adverse cardiovascular events temporally associated with ma huang, an herbal source of ephedrine. Mayo Clin Proc 2002;77(1):12-16.
2. Shekelle P, Morton S, Maglione M, et al. Ephedra and Ephedrine for Weight Loss and Athletic Performance Enhancement: Clinical Efficacy and Side Effects. Evidence Report/Technology Assessment No. 76 (Prepared by Southern California Evidence-based Practice Center, RAND, under Contract No 290-97-0001, Task Order No. 9). Agency for Healthcare Research and Quality. Rockville, MD. February, 2003.
3. Shekelle PG, Hardy ML, Morton SC, et al. Efficacy and safety of ephedra and ephedrine for weight loss and athletic performance: a meta-analysis. JAMA 2003;289(12):1537-1545.
4. Bent S, Tiedt TN, Odden MC, et al. The relative safety of ephedra compared with other herbal products. Ann Intern Med 2003;138(6):468-471.
5. Kingston RL, Borron SW. The relative safety of ephedra compared with other herbal products. Ann Intern Med 2003;139(5 Pt 1):385-387.
6. Dickinson A. The relative safety of ephedra compared with other herbal products. Ann Intern Med 2003;139(5 Pt 1):385-387.
7. Whitaker JM. The relative safety of ephedra compared with other herbal products. Ann Intern Med 2003;139(5 Pt 1):385-387.
8. Kimmel SE. The relative safety of ephedra compared with other herbal products. Ann Intern Med 2003;139(3):234.
9. Kalman DS, Antonio J, Kreider RB. The relative safety of ephedra compared with other herbal products. Ann Intern Med 2003;138(12):1006-1007.
10. Morgenstern LB, Viscoli CM, Kernan WN, et al. Use of Ephedra-containing products and risk for hemorrhagic stroke. Neurology 2003;60(1):132-135.
11. Karch SB. Use of Ephedra-containing products and risk for hemorrhagic stroke. Neurology 2003;61(5):724-725.
12. Anon. Working to get ephedra banned. Consum Rep 2003;68(2):6.
13. Ashar BH, Miller RG, Getz KJ, et al. A critical evaluation of Internet marketing of products that contain ephedra. Mayo Clin Proc 2003;78(8):944-946.
14. Fontanarosa PB, Rennie D, DeAngelis CD. The need for regulation of dietary supplements—lessons from ephedra. JAMA 2003;289(12):1568-1570.
15. Food & Drug Administration. Press Release, February 28, 2003: HHS Acts to Reduce Potential Risks of Dietary Supplements Containing Ephedra.
16. Guharoy R, Noviasky JA. Time to ban ephedra—now. Am J Health Syst Pharm 2003;60(15):1580-1582.
17. Marcus DM, Grollman AP. Ephedra-free is not danger-free. Science 2003;301(5640):1669-1671.
18. Meadows M. Public health officials caution against ephedra use. Health officials caution consumers against using dietary supplements containing ephedra. The stimulant can have dangerous effects on the nervous system and heart. FDA Consum 2003;37(3):8-9.
19. Schulman S. Addressing the potential risks associated with ephedra use: a review of recent efforts. Public Health Rep 2003;118(6):487-492.
20. Worley J, Lindbloom E. Ephedra and ephedrine: modest short-term weight loss, at a price. J Fam Pract 2003;52(7):518-520.
21. Charatan F. Ephedra supplement may have contributed to sportsman's death. BMJ 2003;326(7387):464.
22. Blanck HM, Khan LK, Serdula MK. Use of nonprescription weight loss products: results from a multistate survey. JAMA 2001;286(8):930-935.
23. Wittbrodt ET, Spinler SA. Prevention of anaphylactoid reactions in high-risk patients receiving radiographic contrast media. Ann Pharmacother 1994;28(2):236-241.
24. Bell DG, Jacobs I, Ellerington K. Effect of caffeine and ephedrine ingestion on anaerobic exercise performance. Med Sci Sports Exerc 2001;33(8):1399-1403.
25. Bell DG, McLellan TM, Sabiston CM. Effect of ingesting caffeine and ephedrine on 10-km run performance. Med Sci Sports Exerc 2002;34(2):344-349.
26. Felice KJ, Relva GM. Ephedrine in the treatment of congenital myasthenic syndrome. Muscle Nerve 1996;19(6):799-800.
27. Sonka K. [Treatment of excessive daytime sleepiness]. Ceska Slov Psychiatr 1996;92 Suppl 1:15-22.
28. Gurley BJ, Wang P, Gardner SF. Ephedrine-type alkaloid content of nutritional supplements containing Ephedra sinica (Ma-huang) as determined by high performance liquid chromatography. J Pharm Sci 1998;87(12):1547-1553.
29. Liu YM, Sheu SJ. Determination of Ephedrine alkaloids by capillary electrophoresis. J Chromatog 1992;600:370-372.
30. Zhang JS, Li SH, Lou ZC. [Morphological and histological studies of Chinese Ephedra mahuang. I. Seven species produced in north China]. Yao Xue Xue Bao 1989;24(12):937-948.
31. Pasquali R, Casimirri F, Melchionda N, et al. Effects of chronic administration of ephedrine during very-low-calorie diets on energy expenditure, protein metabolism and hormone levels in obese subjects. Clin Sci (Colch) 1992;82(1):85-92.

32. Pasquali R, Baraldi G, Cesari MP, et al. A controlled trial using ephedrine in the treatment of obesity. Int J Obes 1985;9(2):93-98.

33. Pasquali R, Cesari MP, Melchionda N, et al. Does ephedrine promote weight loss in low-energy-adapted obese women? Int J Obes 1987;11(2): 163-168.

34. Backer R, Tautman D, Lowry S, et al. Fatal ephedrine intoxication. J Forensic Sci 1997;42(1):157-159.

35. Doyle H, Kargin M. Herbal stimulant containing ephedrine has also caused psychosis. BMJ 1996;313(7059):756.

36. Garriott JC, Simmons LM, Poklis A, et al. Five cases of fatal overdose from caffeine-containing "look-alike" drugs. J Anal Toxicol 1985;9(3):141-143.

37. Snook C, Otten M, Hassan M. Massive ephedrine overdose: case report and toxicokinetic analysis. Vet Hum Toxicol 1992;34(4):335.

38. Theoharides TC. Sudden death of a healthy college student related to ephedrine toxicity from a ma huang-containing drink. J Clin Psychopharmacol 1997;17(5):437-439.

39. Vahedi K, Domigo V, Amarenco P, et al. Ischaemic stroke in a sportsman who consumed MaHuang extract and creatine monohydrate for body building. J Neurol Neurosurg Psychiatry 2000;68(1):112-113.

40. Weesner KM, Denison M, Roberts RJ. Cardiac arrhythmias in an adolescent following ingestion of an over-the-counter stimulant. Clin Pediatr (Phila) 1982;21(11):700-701.

41. Ooms TG, Khan SA, Means C. Suspected caffeine and ephedrine toxicosis resulting from ingestion of an herbal supplement containing guarana and ma huang in dogs: 47 cases (1997-1999). J Am Vet Med Assoc 2001; 218(2):225-229.

42. To LB, Sangster JF, Rampling D, et al. Ephedrine-induced cardiomyopathy. Med J Aust 1980;2(1):35-36.

43. Van Mieghem W, Stevens E, Cosemans J. Ephedrine-induced cardiopathy. Br Med J 1978;1(6116):816.

44. Tricker AR, Wacker CD, Preussmann R. 2-(N-nitroso-N-methylamino) propiophenone, a direct acting bacterial mutagen found in nitrosated Ephedra altissima tea. Toxicol Lett 1987;38(1-2):45-50.

45. Tricker AR, Wacker CD, Preussmann R. Nitrosation products from the plant Ephedra altissima and their potential endogenous formation. Cancer Lett 1987;35(2):199-206.

46. Lee MK, Cheng BW, Che CT, et al. Cytotoxicity assessment of Ma-huang (Ephedra) under different conditions of preparation. Toxicol Sci 2000; 56(2):424-430.

47. Haller CA, Benowitz NL. Adverse cardiovascular and central nervous system events associated with dietary supplements containing ephedra alkaloids. N Engl J Med 2000;343(25):1833-1838.

48. Perrotta DM. From the Centers for Disease Control and Prevention. Adverse events associated with ephedrine-containing products—Texas, December 1993-September 1995. JAMA 1996;276(21):1711-1712.

49. du BF, Lannuzel A, Caparros-Lefebvre D, et al. [Cerebral infarction in a patient consuming MaHuang extract and guarana]. Presse Med 2001; 30(4):166-167.

50. Bruno A, Nolte KB, Chapin J. Stroke associated with ephedrine use. Neurology 1993;43(7):1313-1316.

51. Boozer CN, Nasser JA, Heymsfield SB, et al. An herbal supplement containing Ma Huang-Guarana for weight loss: a randomized, double-blind trial. Int J Obes Relat Metab Disord 2001;25(3):316-324.

52. Breum L, Pedersen JK, Ahlstrom F, et al. Comparison of an ephedrine/ caffeine combination and dexfenfluramine in the treatment of obesity. A double-blind multi-centre trial in general practice. Int J Obes Relat Metab Disord 1994;18(2):99-103.

53. Capwell RR. Ephedrine-induced mania from an herbal diet supplement. Am J Psychiatry 1995;152(4):647.

54. Herridge CF, a'Brook MF. Ephedrine psychosis. BMJ 1968;2(598):160.

55. Walton R, Manos GH. Psychosis related to ephedra-containing herbal supplement use. South Med J 2003;96(7):718-720.

56. Roxanas MG, Spalding J. Ephedrine abuse psychosis. Med J Aust 1977; 2(19):639-640.

57. Shufman NE, Witztum E, Vass A. [Ephedrine psychosis]. Harefuah 1994; 127(5-6):166-8, 215.

58. Traboulsi AS, Viswanathan R, Coplan J. Suicide attempt after use of herbal diet pill. Am J Psychiatry 2002;159(2):318-319.

59. Tormey WP, Bruzzi A. Acute psychosis due to the interaction of legal compounds—ephedra alkaloids in 'vigueur fit' tablets, caffeine in 'red bull' and alcohol. Med Sci Law 2001;41(4):331-336.

60. Cockings JG, Brown M. Ephedrine abuse causing acute myocardial infarction. Med J Aust 1997;167(4):199-200.

61. Gardner SF, Franks AM, Gurley BJ, et al. Effect of a multicomponent, ephedra-containing dietary supplement (Metabolife 356) on Holter monitoring and hemostatic parameters in healthy volunteers. Am J Cardiol 2003;91(12):1510-3, A9.

62. Hirabayashi Y, Saitoh K, Fukuda H, et al. Coronary artery spasm after ephedrine in a patient with high spinal anesthesia. Anesthesiology 1996; 84(1):221-224.

63. Lovstad RZ, Granhus G, Hetland S. Bradycardia and asystolic cardiac arrest during spinal anaesthesia: a report of five cases. Acta Anaesthesiol Scand 2000;44(1):48-52.

64. White LM, Gardner SF, Gurley BJ, et al. Pharmacokinetics and cardio-

vascular effects of ma-huang (Ephedra sinica) in normotensive adults. J Clin Pharmacol 1997;37(2):116-122.

65. Astrup A, Breum L, Toubro S, et al. The effect and safety of an ephedrine/ caffeine compound compared to ephedrine, caffeine and placebo in obese subjects on an energy restricted diet. A double blind trial. Int J Obes Relat Metab Disord 1992;16(4):269-277.

66. Daly PA, Krieger DR, Dulloo AG, et al. Ephedrine, caffeine and aspirin: safety and efficacy for treatment of human obesity. Int J Obes Relat Metab Disord 1993;17 Suppl 1:S73-S78.

67. Martinet A, Hostettmann K, Schutz Y. Thermogenic effects of commercially available phytotherapy compounds aimed at treating human obesity. Phytomedicine 1999;6(4):S174.

68. Zaacks SM, Klein L, Tan CD, et al. Hypersensitivity myocarditis associated with ephedra use. J Toxicol Clin Toxicol 1999;37(4):485-489.

69. Leikin JB, Klein L. Ephedra causes myocarditis. J Toxicol Clin Toxicol 2000; 38(3):353-354.

70. Kurt TL. Hypersensitivity myocarditis with ephedra use. J Toxicol Clin Toxicol 2000;38(3):351.

71. Nadir A, Agrawal S, King PD, et al. Acute hepatitis associated with the use of a Chinese herbal product, ma-huang. Am J Gastroenterol 1996; 91(7):1436-1438.

72. Borum ML. Fulminant exacerbation of autoimmune hepatitis after the use of ma huang. Am J Gastroenterol 2001;96(5):1654-1655.

73. Jonderko K, Kucio C. Effect of anti-obesity drugs promoting energy expenditure, yohimbine and ephedrine, on gastric emptying in obese patients. Aliment Pharmacol Ther 1991;5(4):413-418.

74. Konno C, Mizuno T, Hikino H. Isolation and hypoglycemic activity of ephedrans A, B, C, D and E, glycans of Ephedra distachya herbs. Planta Med 1985;(2):162-163.

75. Astrup A, Toubro S, Cannon S, et al. Thermogenic synergism between ephedrine and caffeine in healthy volunteers: a double-blind, placebo-controlled study. Metabolism 1991;40(3):323-329.

76. Powell T, Hsu FF, Turk J, et al. Ma-huang strikes again: ephedrine nephrolithiasis. Am J Kidney Dis 1998;32(1):153-159.

77. Blau JJ. Ephedrine nephrolithiasis associated with chronic ephedrine abuse. J Urol 1998;160(3 Pt 1):825.

78. Hughes SC, Ward MG, Levinson G, et al. Placental transfer of ephedrine does not affect neonatal outcome. Anesthesiology 1985;63(2):217-219.

79. Wright RG, Shnider SM, Levinson G, et al. The effect of maternal administration of ephedrine on fetal heart rate and variability. Obstet Gynecol 1981;57(6):734-738.

80. Mortimer EA, Jr. Drug toxicity from breast milk? Pediatrics 1977; 60(5):780-781.

81. Kalix P. The pharmacology of psychoactive alkaloids from ephedra and catha. J Ethnopharmacol 1991;32(1-3):201-208.

82. Lee A, Ngan Kee WD, Gin T. A quantitative, systematic review of randomized controlled trials of ephedrine versus phenylephrine for the management of hypotension during spinal anesthesia for cesarean delivery. Anesth Analg 2002;94(4):920-6.

83. Meerssschaert K, Brun L, Gourdin M, et al. Terlipressin-ephedrine versus ephedrine to treat hypotension at the induction of anesthesia in patients chronically treated with angiotensin converting-enzyme inhibitors: a prospective, randomized, double-blinded, crossover study. Anesth Analg 2002;94(4):835-40, table.

84. Kanaya N, Satoh H, Seki S, et al. Propofol anesthesia enhances the pressor response to intravenous ephedrine. Anesth Analg 2002;94(5): 1207-1211.

85. Ueda W, Kataoka Y, Takimoto E, et al. Ephedrine-induced increases in arterial blood pressure accelerate regression of epidural block. Anesth Analg 1995;81(4):703-705.

86. Rejent T, Michalek R, Rajewski M. Caffeine fatality with coincident ephedrine. Bull Int Assoc Forensic Toxicol 1981;16:18-19.

87. Ryall JE. Caffeine and ephedrine fatality. Bull Int Assoc Forensic Toxicol 1984;17:13.

88. Weinberger M, Bronsky E. Interaction of ephedrine and theophylline. Clin Pharmacol Ther 1974;15(2):223.

89. Dawson JK, Earnshaw SM, Graham CS. Dangerous monoamine oxidase inhibitor interactions are still occurring in the 1990s. J Accid Emerg Med 1995;12(1):49-51.

90. Kernan WN, Viscoli CM, Brass LM, et al. Phenylpropanolamine and the risk of hemorrhagic stroke. N Engl J Med 2000;343(25):1826-1832.

91. Jubiz W, Meikle AW. Alterations of glucocorticoid actions by other drugs and disease states. Drugs 1979;18(2):113-121.

92. Brooks SM, Sholiton LJ, Werk EE, Jr., et al. The effects of ephedrine and theophylline on dexamethasone metabolism in bronchial asthma. J Clin Pharmacol 1977;17(5-6):308-318.

93. Astrup A, Lundsgaard C, Madsen J, et al. Enhanced thermogenic responsiveness during chronic ephedrine treatment in man. Am J Clin Nutr 1985; 42(1):83-94.

94. Boada S, Solsona B, Papaceit J, et al. [Hypotension refractory to ephedrine after sympathetic blockade in a patient on long-term therapy with tricyclic antidepressants]. Rev Esp Anestesiol Reanim 1999;46(8):364-366.

95. Nishiguchi M, Kinoshita H, Higasa K, et al. [The false positive reaction of the Triage panel drug-of-abuse by herbal drugs ma-huang (Ephedra sinica (Ephedraceae))]. Nippon Hoigaku Zasshi 2001;55(3):331-338.

96. Cui JF, Niu CQ, Zhang JS. [Determination of six Ephedra alkaloids in Chinese Ephedra (Ma Huang) by gas chromatography]. Yao Xue Xue Bao 1991;26(11):852-857.

97. Friedrich H, Wiedemeyer H. [Quantitative determination of the tannin-precursors and the tannins in *Ephedra helvetica* (author's transl)]. Planta Med 1976;30(3):223-231.

98. Caveney S, Starratt A. Glutamatergic signals in Ephedra. Nature 1994; 372:509.

99. Liu YM, Sheu SJ, Chiou SH, et al. A comparative study on commercial samples of Ephedrae herba. Planta Med 1993;59:376-378.

100. Zhang Z, Sun X, Wang L, et al. [Comparison of two extraction methods for maxingshigan decoction]. Chin J Integ Trad West Med 1997;22(7): 413-5, 447.

101. Gurley BJ, Gardner SF, White LM, et al. Ephedrine pharmacokinetics after the ingestion of nutritional supplements containing *Ephedra sinica* (ma huang). Ther Drug Monit 1998;20(4):439-445.

102. Astrup A, Madsen J, Holst JJ, et al. The effect of chronic ephedrine treatment on substrate utilization, the sympathoadrenal activity, and energy expenditure during glucose-induced thermogenesis in man. Metabolism 1986;35(3):260-265.

103. Arch JR, Ainsworth AT, Cawthorne MA. Thermogenic and anorectic effects of ephedrine and congeners in mice and rats. Life Sci 1982; 30(21):1817-1826.

104. Dulloo AG, Miller DS. Thermogenic drugs for the treatment of obesity: sympathetic stimulants in animal models. Br J Nutr 1984;52(2):179-196.

105. Dulloo AG, Seydoux J, Girardier L. Potentiation of the thermogenic antiobesity effects of ephedrine by dietary methylxanthines: adenosine antagonism or phosphodiesterase inhibition? Metabolism 1992;41(11): 1233-1241.

106. Ramsey JJ, Colman RJ, Swick AG, et al. Energy expenditure, body composition, and glucose metabolism in lean and obese rhesus monkeys treated with ephedrine and caffeine. Am J Clin Nutr 1998;68(1):42-51.

107. Yen TT, McKee MM, Bemis KG. Ephedrine reduces weight of viable yellow obese mice (Avy/a). Life Sci 1981;28(2):119-128.

108. Zarrindast MR, Hosseini-Nia T, Farnoodi F. Anorectic effect of ephedrine. Gen Pharmacol 1987;18(5):559-561.

109. Astrup A, Toubro S. Thermogenic, metabolic, and cardiovascular responses to ephedrine and caffeine in man. Int J Obes Relat Metab Disord 1993;17 Suppl 1:S41-S43.

110. Dulloo AG, Miller DS. Aspirin as a promoter of ephedrine-induced thermogenesis: potential use in the treatment of obesity. Am J Clin Nutr 1987;45(3):564-569.

111. Dulloo AG, Miller DS. The thermogenic properties of ephedrine/methylxanthine mixtures: animal studies. Am J Clin Nutr 1986;43(3): 388-394.

112. Dulloo AG, Miller DS. Reversal of obesity in the genetically obese fa/fa Zucker rat with an ephedrine/methylxanthines thermogenic mixture. J Nutr 1987;117(2):383-389.

113. Dulloo AG. Ephedrine, xanthines and prostaglandin-inhibitors: actions and interactions in the stimulation of thermogenesis. Int J Obes Relat Metab Disord 1993;17 Suppl 1:S35-S40.

114. Wang GZ, Hikokichi O. [Experimental study in treating chronic renal failure with dry extract and tannins of herba ephedra]. Chinese J Integ Trad West Med 1994;14(8):485-488.

115. Hikino H, Konno C, Takata H, et al. Antiinflammatory principle of Ephedra Herbs. Chem Pharm Bull (Tokyo) 1980;28(10):2900-2904.

116. Ling M, Piddlesden SJ, Morgan BP. A component of the medicinal herb ephedra blocks activation in the classical and alternative pathways of complement. Clin Exp Immunol 1995;102(3):582-588.

117. Toubro S, Astrup AV, Breum L, et al. Safety and efficacy of long-term treatment with ephedrine, caffeine and an ephedrine/caffeine mixture. Int J Obes Relat Metab Disord 1993;17 Suppl 1:S69-S72.

118. Molnar D, Torok K, Erhardt E, et al. Safety and efficacy of treatment with an ephedrine/caffeine mixture. The first double-blind placebo-controlled pilot study in adolescents. Int J Obes Relat Metab Disord 2000;24(12): 1573-1578.

119. Munns G, Aldrich C. Ephedrine in the treatment of bronchial asthma in children. JAMA 1927;88:1233.

120. Gardner R, Hansen A, Eewing P. Unexpected fatality in a child from accidental consumption of antiasthmatic preparation containing ephedrine, theophylline and phenobarbital. Texas State J Med 1950;46:516-520.

121. Taylor WF, Heimlich EM, Strick L, et al. Ephedrine and theophylline in asthmatic children: quantitive observations on the combination and ephedrine tachyphylaxis. Ann Allergy 1965;23(9):437-440.

122. Weinberger MM. Use of ephedrine in bronchodilator therapy. Pediatr Clin North Am 1975;22(1):121-127.

123. Tashkin DP, Meth R, Simmons DH, et al. Double-blind comparison of acute bronchial and cardiovascular effects of oral terbutaline and ephedrine. Chest 1975;68(2):155-161.

124. Faurschou M, Svendsen UG. [The bronchodilating effect of ephedrine tablets in bronchial asthma]. Ugeskr Laeger 1993;155(46):3784-3785.

125. Pinnas JL, Schachtel BP, Chen TM, et al. Inhaled epinephrine and oral theophylline-ephedrine in the treatment of asthma. J Clin Pharmacol 1991; 31(3):243-247.

126. Direkwattanachai C, Phanichyakarn P, Srianujatra S. Sustained release theophylline and ephedrine therapy in chronic asthma. J Med Assoc Thai 1986;69 Suppl 2:31-37.

127. Lyons HA, Thomas JS, Steen SN. Theophylline and ephedrine in asthma. Curr Ther Res Clin Exp 1975;18(4):573-577.

128. Gotz M. [Long-term out-patient treatment of children with asthma with a theophylline-ephedrine-hydroxyzine combination (author's transl)]. Padiatr Padol 1975;10(4):466-473.

129. Jiang MH, Liu L, Wang QA, et al. [Effects of ephedrine and its analogs on beta-adrenoceptors of rat lung cell membranes]. Zhongguo Yao Li Xue Bao 1987;8(4):318-320.

130. Tinkelman DG, Avner SE. Ephedrine therapy in asthmatic children. Clinical tolerance and absence of side effects. JAMA 1977;237(6):553-557.

131. McLaughlin ET, Bethea LH, Wittig HJ. Comparison of the bronchodilator effect of oral fenoterol and ephedrine in asthmatic children. Ann Allergy 1982;49(4):191-195.

132. Weinberger MM, Bronsky EA. Evaluation of oral bronchodilator therapy in asthmatic children. Bronchodilators in asthmatic children. J Pediatr 1974;84(3):421-427.

133. May CS, Pickup ME, Paterson JW. The acute and chronic bronchodilator effects of ephedrine in asthmatic patients. Br J Clin Pharmacol 1975; 2(6):533-537.

134. Loughrey JP, Walsh F, Gardiner J. Prophylactic intravenous bolus ephedrine for elective Caesarean section under spinal anaesthesia. Eur J Anaesthesiol 2002;19(1):63-68.

135. Saito H. [Mechanism of reversal of the blood pressure by ephedrine. (2)]. Nippon Yakurigaku Zasshi 1977;73(1):83-92.

136. Saito H. [Mechanisms of reversal of the blood pressure by ephedrine. (1)]. Nippon Yakurigaku Zasshi 1977;73(1):73-82.

137. Furukawa T, Kuroda M. [Effects of ephedrine, tyramine and norepinephrine on the blood pressure response to dopamine]. Nippon Yakurigaku Zasshi 1974;70(3):377-384.

138. Unger DL. Blood pressure and pulse rate changes in hypertensive asthmatic patients: effects of an ephedrine compound. Ann Allergy 1968;26(12): 637-638.

139. Ngan Kee WD, Lau TK, Khaw KS, et al. Comparison of metaraminol and ephedrine infusions for maintaining arterial pressure during spinal anesthesia for elective cesarean section. Anesthesiology 2001;95(2):307-313.

140. Kee WD, Khaw KS, Lee BB, et al. A dose-response study of prophylactic intravenous ephedrine for the prevention of hypotension during spinal anesthesia for cesarean delivery. Anesth Analg 2000;90(6):1390-1395.

141. Ducros L, Bonnin P, Cholley BP, et al. Increasing maternal blood pressure with ephedrine increases uterine artery blood flow velocity during uterine contraction. Anesthesiology 2002;96(3):612-616.

142. Shaikh WA. Ephedrine-saline nasal wash in allergic rhinitis. J Allergy Clin Immunol 1995;96(5 Pt 1):597-600.

143. Meston CM, Heiman JR. Ephedrine-activated physiological sexual arousal in women. Arch Gen Psychiatry 1998;55(7):652-656.

Essiac

SYNONYMS/COMMON NAMES/RELATED SUBSTANCES

- **Burdock root (*Arctium lappa*) synonyms/related terms**: Akujitsu, anthraxivore, arctii, *Arctium minus*, *Arctium tomentosa*, bardana, bardanae radix, bardane, bardane grande, beggar's buttons, burr, burr seed, chin, clot-burr, clotbur, cocklebur, cockle button (cocklebutton), cuckold, daiki kishi, edible burdock, fox's clote, grass burdock, great bur, great burdock, gobo, grosse klette, happy major, hardock, hare burr, hurrburr, kletterwurzel, lampazo, lappola, love leaves, niu bang zi, oil of lappa, personata, philanthropium, thorny burr, turkey burrseed, woo-bang-ja, wild gobo.
- **Sheep sorrel (*Rumex acetosella*) synonyms/related terms**: Acedera, acid sorrel, azeda-brava, buckler leaf, cigreto, common sorrel, cuckoo sorrow, cuckoo's meate, dock, dog-eared sorrel, field sorrel, French sorrel, garden sorrel, gowke-meat, greensauce, green sorrel, herba acetosa, kemekulagi, Polygonaceae, red sorrel, red top sorrel, round leaf sorrel, *Rumex scutatus*, *Rumex acetosa* L., sheephead sorrel, sheep's sorrel, sorrel, sorrel dock, sour dock, sour grass, sour sabs, sour suds, sour sauce, wiesensauerampfer, wild sorrel.
- **Slippery elm inner bark (*Ulmus fulva*) synonyms/related terms**: Indian elm, moose elm, red elm, rock elm, slippery elm, sweet elm, Ulmaceae, ulmi rubrae cortex, *Ulmus fulva* Michaux, ulmus rubra, winged elm.
- **Turkish rhubarb (*Rheum palmatum*) synonyms/related terms**: baoshen pill, Canton rhubarb, Chinesischer rhabarber, Chinese rhubarb, chong-gi-huang, common rhubarb, da huang, daio, da huang liujingao, English rhubarb, extractum rhei liquidum, Himalayan rhubarb, Indian rhubarb, Japanese rhubarb, jiang-zhi jian-fel yao (JZJFY), jinghuang tablet, medicinal rhubarb, pie rhubarb, Polygonaceae, pyralvex, pyralvex berna, racine de rhubarbee, RET (rhubarb extract tablet), rhabarber, rhei radix, rhei rhizoma, rheum, rheum australe, *Rheum emodi* Wall., *Rheum officinale* Baill., *Rheum rhabarbarum*, *Rheum rhaponticum* L., *Rheum tanguticum* Maxim., *Rheum tanguticum* Maxim. ex. Balf., *Rheum tanguticum* Maxim. L., Rheum *undulatum*, Rheum x *cultorum*, *Rheum webbianum* (Indian or Himalayan rhubarb), rhizoma, rheirhubarbe de Chine, rhubarb, rubarbo, ruibarbo, shenshi rhubarb, tai huang, Turkey rhubarb.

CLINICAL BOTTOM LINE
Background

- Essiac is a combination of herbs, including burdock root (*Arctium lappa*), sheep sorrel (*Rumex acetosella*), slippery elm inner bark (*Ulmus fulva*), and Turkish rhubarb (*Rheum palmatum*). The original formula was developed by the Canadian nurse Rene Caisse (1888-1978) in the 1920s ("Essiac" is Caisse spelled backward). The recipe is said to be based on a traditional Ojibwa (Native American) remedy, and Caisse administered the formula by mouth and injection to numerous cancer patients during the 1920s and 1930s. The exact ingredients and amounts in the original formulation remain a secret.
- During investigations by the Canadian government and public hearings in the late 1930s, it remained unclear if Essiac was an effective cancer treatment. Amidst controversy, Caisse closed her clinic in 1942. In the 1950s, Caisse provided samples of Essiac to Dr. Charles Brusch, founder of the Brusch Medical Center in Cambridge, Massachusetts, who administered Essiac to patients (it is unclear if Brusch was given access to the secret formula). According to some accounts, additional herbs were added to these later formulations, including blessed thistle (*Cnicus benedictus*), red clover (*Trifolium pratense*), kelp (*Laminaria digitata*), and watercress (*Nasturtium officinale*).
- A laboratory at Memorial Sloan-Kettering Cancer Center tested Essiac samples (provided by Caisse) on mice during the 1970s. This research was never formally published, and there is controversy regarding the results, with some accounts noting no benefits, and others reporting significant effects (including an account by Dr. Brusch). Questions were later raised about improper preparation of the formula. Caisse subsequently refused requests by researchers at Memorial Sloan-Kettering and the U.S. National Cancer Institute for access to the recipe.
- In the 1970s, Caisse provided the formula to Resperin Corporation Ltd., with the understanding that Resperin would coordinate a scientific trial in humans. Although a study was initiated, it was stopped early because of questions about improper preparation of the formula and inadequate study design. This research was never completed. Resperin, which owned the Essiac name, formally went out of business after transferring rights to the Essiac name and selling the secret formula to Essiac Products Ltd., which currently distributes products through Essiac International.
- Despite the lack of available scientific evidence, Essiac and Essiac-like products (with similar ingredients) remain popular, particularly among people with cancer.
- Essiac is most commonly taken as a tea. A survey conducted in 2000 found that almost 15% of Canadian women with breast cancer were using Essiac. Essiac also has become popular in people with HIV and diabetes and in healthy individuals for its purported immune-enhancing properties, although there has been no reliable scientific research in these areas.
- More than 40 Essiac-like products are available in North America, Europe, and Australia. Flor-essence includes the original four herbs (burdock root, sheep sorrel, slippery elm bark, Turkish rhubarb) as well as herbs that were later added as "potentiators" (blessed thistle, red clover, kelp, watercress). Virginias Herbal E contains the four original herbs along with echinacea and black walnut. Other commercial formulations may include additional ingredients, such as cat's claw (*Uncaria tomentosa*).

Uses Based on Scientific Evidence	Grade*
Cancer There are no properly conducted published human studies of Essiac for the treatment of cancer. A laboratory at Memorial Sloan-Kettering Cancer Center tested Essiac on mice during the 1970s, although the results were never formally published and remain	C

Continued

controversial. Questions were raised about improper preparation of the formula. A study in humans was begun in Canada in the late 1970s but was stopped early because of concerns about inconsistent preparation of the formula and inadequate study design. In the 1980s, the Canadian Department of National Health and Welfare collected information about 86 cancer patients treated with Essiac. Results were inconclusive (17 patients had died at the time of the study, inadequate information was available for 8 patients, "no benefits" were found in 47 patients, 5 patients reported reduced need for pain medications, and 1 noted subjective improvement). Most patients had also received other cancer treatments such as chemotherapy, making the effects of Essiac impossible to isolate.

Currently, there is not enough evidence to recommend for or against the use of this herbal mixture as a therapy for cancer. Different brands may contain variable ingredients, and the comparative effectiveness of these formulas is not known. None of the individual herbs used in Essiac has been tested in rigorous human cancer trials (rhubarb has shown some anti-tumor properties in experiments in animals; slippery elm inner bark has not; sheep sorrel and burdock have been used traditionally in other cancer remedies). Numerous individual patient testimonials and reports from manufacturers are available on the Internet, although these cannot be considered scientifically viable as evidence. Individuals with cancer are advised not to delay treatment with more proven therapies.

*Key to grades: A: Strong scientific evidence for this use; B: Good scientific evidence for this use; C: Unclear scientific evidence for this use; D: Fair scientific evidence against this use (it may not work); F: Strong scientific evidence against this use (it likely does not work). For a more detailed explanation of efficacy criteria, see "Natural Standard Evidence-Based Validated Grading Rationale" in the Introduction.

Historical or Theoretical Indications That Lack Sufficient Evidence

AIDS/HIV, appetite stimulant, arthritis, asthma, bladder cancer, blood cleanser, breast cancer, chelating agent (heavy metals), chronic fatigue syndrome, colon cancer, "detoxification," diabetes, endometrial cancer, energy enhancement, head/neck cancers, Hodgkin's disease, immune system enhancement, kidney diseases, leukemia, lip cancer, liver cancer (hepatocellular carcinoma), longevity, lung cancer, Lyme disease, lymphoma, multiple myeloma, non-Hodgkin's lymphoma, nutritional supplement, ovarian cancer, supportive care in advanced cancer patients, pancreatic cancer, paralysis, prostate cancer, reduction of chemotherapy side effects, stomach cancer, systemic lupus erythematosus (SLE), throat cancer, thyroid disorders, tongue cancer, well-being.

DOSING/TOXICOLOGY

The following doses are based on scientific research, publications, traditional use, or expert opinion. Many herbs and supplements have not been thoroughly tested, and their safety and effectiveness may not be proven. Brands may be made differently, with variable ingredients even within the same brand. The doses shown may not apply to all products. It is important to always read product labels and discuss doses with a qualified healthcare provider before therapy is started.

Standardization

- Standardization involves measuring the amounts of certain chemicals in products to try to make different preparations similar to each other. It is not always known if the chemicals being measured are the "active" ingredients. Because the formula for Essiac remains a secret, it is not clear what standards for manufacturing are followed. Some brands of Essiac-like products publish the amounts of herbal constituents, although the basis for standardization of these individual ingredients is not always clear.

Adults (18 Years and Older)

- Historically, Essiac has been administered by mouth or injection. The most common current use is as a tea. There are no reliable published human studies of Essiac or Essiac-like products, and safety or effectiveness has not been established scientifically for any dose. Instructions for tea preparation and dosing vary from product to product. People are advised to read product labels and consult their cancer healthcare provider before starting any new therapy, such as the use of Essiac or Essiac-like products.

Children (Younger Than 18 Years)

- There are insufficient scientific data available to recommend the safe use of Essiac or Essiac-like products in children.

SAFETY

The U.S. Food and Drug Administration does not strictly regulate herbs and supplements. There is no guarantee of the strength, purity, or safety of products, and effects may vary. It is important to always read product labels. People who have a medical condition, or are taking other drugs, herbs, or supplements, should consult a qualified healthcare provider before starting a new therapy. A healthcare provider should be contacted immediately about any side effects.

Allergies

- There are no reports of allergy to Essiac in published scientific literature, although reactions potentially can occur due to any of the included herbs. Anaphylaxis (severe allergic reaction) has been reported after rhubarb leaf ingestion, and allergic reactions to sorrel products taken by mouth have been reported. Contact dermatitis (skin rash after direct contact) has been reported with exposure to burdock, slippery elm bark, and rhubarb leaves. Cross-sensitivity to burdock may occur in individuals with allergy to members of the Asteraceae/Compositae family, such as ragweed, chrysanthemums, marigolds, and daisies.

Side Effects and Warnings

- The safety of Essiac has not been well studied scientifically. Safety concerns are based on theoretical and known reactions associated with herbal components of Essiac: burdock root (*Arctium lappa*), sheep sorrel (*Rumex acetosella*), slippery elm bark (*Ulmus fulva*), and Turkish rhubarb (*Rheum palmatum*). However, the safety and toxicities of these individual herbs also have not been well studied. Essiac-like products may contain different or additional ingredients, and people who plan to use such products should always read the product labels.
- Potentially toxic compounds present in Essiac. include tannins, oxalic acid, and anthraquinones. Tannins, which are

present in burdock, sorrel, rhubarb, and slippery elm, may cause stomach upset and, in high concentrations, may lead to kidney or liver damage. In theory, long-term use of tannins may increase the risk of head and neck cancers, although there are no documented cases in humans.

- Oxalic acid, which is present in rhubarb, slippery elm, and sorrel, can cause serious adverse effects when taken in high doses (particularly in children). Signs and symptoms of oxalic acid toxicity/poisoning include nausea and vomiting, mouth/throat burning, dangerously low blood pressure, blood electrolyte imbalances, seizures, throat swelling that interferes with breathing, and liver and kidney damage. Death from oxalic acid poisoning was reported in an adult man who had eaten soup containing sorrel and in a 4-year-old child who had eaten rhubarb leaves. The lethal dose of oxalic acid for adults has been estimated as 15 to 30 g, although doses as low as 5 g may be fatal. The amount of oxalic acid in Essiac preparations is not known. In cases of suspected oxalic acid poisoning, medical attention should be sought immediately. Regular intake of oxalic acid may increase the risk of kidney stones.
- Anthraquinones in rhubarb root and sheep sorrel may cause diarrhea, intestinal cramping, and loss of fluid and electrolytes (such as potassium). Use of rhubarb may result in discoloration of the urine (bright yellow or red) or of the inner mucosal surface of the intestine (a condition called melanosis coli). Fluoride poisoning has been reported in persons taking rhubarb fruit juice. Rhubarb products manufactured in China have been found to be contaminated with heavy metals. Chronic use of rhubarb products may lead to dependence.
- Based on research in animals and limited studies in humans, burdock may increase or decrease blood sugar levels. Caution is advised in patients with diabetes or hypoglycemia, and in those taking drugs, herbs, or supplements that affect blood sugar levels. Serum glucose levels may need to be monitored by a healthcare provider, and medication adjustments may be necessary. Diuretic effects (increasing urine flow) and estrogen-like effects have been reported in persons with HIV who were taking oral burdock supplements.
- Reports of anticholinergic reactions (such as slow heart rate and dry mouth) with the use of burdock products, reported in studies made in the 1970s, are believed to have been due to contamination with belladonna alkaloids, which resemble burdock and can be introduced during harvesting. Burdock itself has not been found to contain constituents that would be responsible for these reactions.

Pregnancy and Breastfeeding

- There is insufficient scientific evidence to recommend the safe use of Essiac or Essiac-like products in women who are pregnant or are breastfeeding, and there are potential risks from the herbal constituents. Oxalic acid and anthraquinone glycosides, which are present in the included herbs, may be unsafe during pregnancy. Rhubarb and burdock may cause contractions of the uterus; some publications note that whole slippery elm bark can lead to abortion, although there is limited supporting scientific evidence.

INTERACTIONS

Most herbs and supplements have not been thoroughly tested for interactions with other herbs, supplements, drugs, or foods. The interactions listed here are based on reports in scientific publications, laboratory experiments, or traditional use. It is important to always read product labels. People who have a medical condition, or are taking other drugs, herbs, or supplements, should consult a qualified healthcare provider before starting a new therapy.

Interactions with Drugs

- Essiac interactions have not been well studied scientifically. Most potential interactions are based on theoretical and known reactions associated with the herbal components of Essiac: burdock root (*Arctium lappa*), sheep sorrel (*Rumex acetosella*), slippery elm bark (*Ulmus fulva*), and Turkish rhubarb (*Rheum palmatum*). However, the interactions of these individual herbs also have not been well studied. Essiac-like products may contain different or additional ingredients, and people who plan to use such products should always read the product labels.
- Essiac may interfere with how the body uses the liver's cytochrome P450 enzyme system to process components of some drugs. As a result, blood levels of these components may be altered and may cause increased effects or potentially serious adverse reactions. This study reported that a patient who was taking the experimental drug DX-8951f (metabolized by CYP3A4 and CYP1A2) experienced toxic side effects and drug clearance that was 4 to 5 times slower than in other patients. This patient was also taking "Essiac tea"; however, further details are lacking, and it is unclear whether the patient was taking Essiac or an Essiac-like product. People who are using any medications should always read the package insert and consult with their healthcare provider and pharmacist about possible interactions.
- Anthraquinones in rhubarb root and sheep sorrel may lead to diarrhea, dehydration, or loss of electrolytes (such as potassium) and may increase the effects of other laxative agents. In one study in humans, burdock was associated with diuretic effects (increased urine flow), and in theory burdock may cause excess fluid loss (dehydration) and electrolyte imbalances (such as changes in blood potassium or sodium levels). These effects may be increased when burdock is taken at the same time as diuretic drugs such as chlorothiazide (Diuril), furosemide (Lasix), hydrochlorothiazide (HCTZ), and spironolactone (Aldactone). The laxative and diuretic properties of the herbs in Essiac may lead to low potassium blood levels that are potentially dangerous in people taking digoxin or digitoxin.
- Based on animal research and limited human study, burdock may decrease or increase blood sugar levels. Caution is advised in people who are using medications that may also affect blood sugar levels. Persons who are taking drugs for diabetes by mouth or insulin should be monitored closely by a qualified healthcare provider. Medication adjustments may be necessary.
- Based on limited human evidence that is not entirely clear, burdock may have estrogen-like properties, and may act to increase the effects of estrogenic agents, including hormone replacement therapies (e.g., Premarin) and birth control pills.

Interactions with Herbs and Dietary Supplements

- One human report suggests that Essiac may interfere with how the body uses the liver's cytochrome P450 enzyme system to process components of other herbs and supplements. As a result, blood levels of these components may be elevated. Essiac may alter the effects of other herbs on the cytochrome P450 system. Examples of such herbs are bloodroot, cat's claw, chamomile, chaparral, chasteberry, damiana, *Echinacea angustifolia*, goldenseal, grapefruit juice, licorice, oregano, red clover, St. John's wort, wild cherry, and yucca.

- Anthraquinones in rhubarb root and sheep sorrel may cause diarrhea, dehydration, or loss of electrolytes (such as potassium) and may increase the effects of other agents with possible laxative properties, such as alder buckthorn, aloe dried leaf sap, black root, blue flag rhizome, butternut bark, dong quai, European buckthorn, eyebright, cascara bark, castor oil, chasteberry, colocynth fruit pulp, dandelion, gamboges bark, horsetail, jalap root, manna bark, plantain leaf, podophyllum root, psyllium, rhubarb, senna, wild cucumber fruit, and yellow dock root.
- Burdock has been associated with diuretic effects (increased urine flow) in one study in humans and, in theory, may cause excessive fluid loss (dehydration) or electrolyte imbalances (such as changes in blood potassium and sodium levels) when used with other diuretic herbs or supplements, such as artichoke, celery, corn silk, couchgrass, dandelion, elder flower, horsetail, juniper berry, kava, shepherd's purse, uva ursi, and yarrow.
- The laxative and diuretic properties of herbs in Essiac may result in low potassium blood levels that are potentially dangerous in people taking cardiac glycoside-containing herbs such as adonis, balloon cotton, black hellebore root/melampode, black Indian hemp, bushman's poison, cactus grandifloris, convallaria, eyebright, figwort, foxglove/digitalis, frangipani, hedge mustard, hemp root/Canadian hemp root, king's crown, lily-of-the-valley, motherwort, oleander leaf, pheasant's eye plant, plantain leaf, pleurisy root; psyllium husks, redheaded cotton-bush, rhubarb root, rubber vine, sea-mango, senna fruit, squill, strophanthus, uzara, wallflower, wintersweet, yellow dock root, and yellow oleander.
- Based on research in animals and limited studies in humans, burdock may decrease or increase blood sugar levels. Caution is advised in people who are using other herbs or supplements that may also alter blood sugar levels. Blood glucose levels may require monitoring, and doses may need adjustment. Examples of herbs that may lower blood sugar levels are *Aloe vera*, American ginseng, bilberry, bitter melon, fenugreek, fish oil, gymnema, horse chestnut seed extract (HCSE), marshmallow, milk thistle, *Panax ginseng*, rosemary, Siberian ginseng, stinging nettle, and white horehound.
- Because burdock may contain estrogen-like chemicals, the effects of other agents believed to have estrogen-like properties may be altered. Examples of such agents are alfalfa, black cohosh, bloodroot, hops, kudzu, licorice, pomegranate, red clover, soy, thyme, white horehound, and yucca. These possible interactions are based on initial and unclear evidence.
- In theory, use of rhubarb and sheep sorrel may decrease the absorption of minerals such as calcium, iron, and zinc.

Selected References

Natural Standard developed the preceding evidence-based information based on a systematic review of more than 75 articles. For comprehensive information about alternative and complementary therapies on the professional level, go to www.naturalstandard.com. Selected references are listed here.

Bever BO, Zahnd GR. Plants with oral hypoglycaemic action. Quart J Crude Drug Res 1979;17:139-196.

Boon H, Stewart M, Kennard MA, et al. Use of complementary/alternative medicine by breast cancer survivors in Ontario: prevalence and perceptions. J Clin Oncol 2000;18(13):2515-2521.

Bryson PD, Watanabe AS, Rumack BH, et al. Burdock root tea poisoning. Case report involving a commercial preparation. JAMA 1978;239(20):2157.

Bryson PD. Burdock root tea poisoning. JAMA 1978;240(15):1586.

De Jager R, Cheverton P, Tamanoi K, et al. (DX-8931f Investigators). DX-8951f: summary of phase I clinical trials. Ann N Y Acad Sci 2000;922:260-273.

Dog TL. Author of CME article offers clarification about Essiac. Altern Ther Health Med 2001;7(4):20.

Fraser SS, Allen C. Could Essiac halt cancer? Homemaker's 1977 (August issue).

Geyer C, Hammond L, Johnson T, et al. Dose-schedule optimization of the hexacyclic camptothecin (CPT) analog DX-8951f: a phase I and pharmacokinetic study with escalation of both treatment duration and dose [meeting abstract]. Proc Ann Meet Amer Soc Clin Oncol 1999:A813.

Kaegi E. Unconventional therapies for cancer: 1. Essiac. The Task Force on Alternative Therapies of the Canadian Breast Cancer Research Initiative. CMAJ 1998;158(7):897-902.

Karn H, Moore MJ. The use of the herbal remedy Essiac in an outpatient cancer population [meeting abstract]. Proc Ann Meet Amer Soc Clin Oncol 1997:A245.

LeMoine L. Essiac: an historical perspective. Can Oncol Nurs J 1997;7(4):216-221.

Rhoads PM, Tong TG, Banner W, Jr., et al. Anticholinergic poisonings associated with commercial burdock root. J Toxicol Clin Toxicol 1984;22(6):581-584.

Silver AA, Krantz JC. The effect of the ingestion of burdock root on normal and diabetic individuals: a preliminary report. Ann Int Med 1931;5:274-284.

Tamayo C, Richardson MA, Diamond S, et al. The chemistry and biological activity of herbs used in Flor-Essence herbal tonic and Essiac. Phytother Res 2000;14(1):1-14.

Thomas R. The Essiac report: the true story of a Canadian herbal cancer remedy and of the thousands of lives it continues to save. Los Angeles: Altern Treat Inform Network, 1993.

U.S. Congressional Office of Technology Assessment. Essiac. Washington, DC: U.S. Government Printing Office, 1990.

Zarembski PM, Hodgkinson A. Plasma oxalic acid and calcium levels in oxalate poisoning. J Clin Path 1967;20:283-285.

Eucalyptus Oil

(Eucalyptus globulus Labillardiere, *Eucalyptus fructicetorum* F. Von Mueller, *Eucalyptus smithii* R.T. Baker)

SYNONYMS/COMMON NAMES/RELATED SUBSTANCES

- Australian fever tree leaf, blauer gommibaum, blue gum, catheter oil, cineole, 1,8-cineole, essence of eucalyptus rectifiee, essencia de eucalipto, eucalypti aetheroleum, eucalypti folium, eucalyptol, *Eucalyptus polybractea*, eucalytpo setma ag, fevertree, gommier bleu, gum tree, kafur ag, malee, myrtaceae, oleum eucalypti, schonmutz, southern blue gum, Tasmanian blue gum.

CLINICAL BOTTOM LINE

Background

- Eucalyptus oil is used commonly as a decongestant and expectorant for upper respiratory tract infections or inflammations, as well as for various musculoskeletal conditions. The oil is found in numerous over-the-counter cough and cold lozenges as well as in inhalation vapors and topical ointments. Veterinarians use the oil topically for its reported antimicrobial activity, which is supported by *in vitro* and *in vivo* study. Numerous applications are suggested in the sparse literature on this topic; however, there is not sufficient controlled support for any human indication at this time. Other applications include as an aromatic in soaps or perfumes, as flavoring in foodstuffs and beverages, and as a dental and industrial solvent.
- Eucalyptus oil contains 70% to 85% 1,8-cineole (eucalyptol), which is also present in other plant oils. Eucalyptol is used as an ingredient in some mouthwash and dental preparations and as an endodontic solvent and may possess antimicrobial properties. Listerine mouthrinse is a combination of essential oils (eucalyptol, menthol, thymol, methyl salicylate) that has been shown to be efficacious for the reduction of dental plaque and gingivitis.
- Topical use or inhalation use of eucalyptus oil at low concentrations may be safe, although significant and potentially lethal toxicity has been consistently reported with oral use and may occur with inhalation use as well. All routes of administration should be avoided in children.

Scientific Evidence for Common/Studied Uses	Grade*
Asthma	C
Decongestant-expectorant/upper respiratory tract infection (oral/inhalation)	C
Dental plaque/gingivitis (mouthwash)	C
Headache (topical)	C

*Key to grades: A: Strong scientific evidence for this use; B: Good scientific evidence for this use; C: Unclear scientific evidence for this use; D: Fair scientific evidence against this use (it may not work); F: Strong scientific evidence against this use (it likely does not work). For a more detailed explanation of efficacy criteria, see "Natural Standard Evidence-Based Validated Grading Rationale" in the Introduction.

Historical or Theoretical Uses That Lack Sufficient Evidence

- Alertness,[1] AIDS,[2] analgesia,[3] antibacterial, antifungal, antipyretic, antispasmodic, antiviral, aromatherapy, arthritis, astringent, back pain, bronchitis, burns, cancer prevention,[4,5] chronic obstructive pulmonary disease (COPD), chronic suppurative otitis,[6] cleaning solvent, colds,[7] cough, croup, deodorant, diabetes,[8] dysentery, emphysema, fever, flavoring, fragrance, hepatoprotection,[9] herpes, hookworm, inflammation, inflammatory bowel disease,[10] influenza, insect repellant,[11,12] muscle/joint pain (topical), muscle spasm, nerve pain, parasitic infection, rheumatoid arthritis (topical), rhinitis, ringworm, shingles, sinusitis,[13] skin infections in children,[14] skin ulcers, snoring,[15] stimulant, strains/sprains (topical), tinnea, tuberculosis, urinary retention,[16] urinary tract infection,[16] whooping cough, wound healing.

Expert Opinion and Folkloric Precedent

- Eucalyptus is licensed in Germany as a medicinal tea for bronchitis or throat inflammation and has been approved by the German expert panel, the Commission E, for "catarrh" (mucous membrane inflammation) of the respiratory tract. The oil is also approved for topical use for rheumatic complaints. Eucalyptus is known as the "oil of respiration" in holistic aromatherapy practice, due to its suggested anti-inflammatory, antiseptic, expectorant, and anti-spasmodic properties. Eucalyptol (1,8-cineole), which is present in eucalyptus oil, has a long history of use in endodontics as a solvent, and to soften gutta percha (a thermoplastic root canal filling material) and various sealers.[17] The oil is also used as an industrial degreasing solvent.

Safety Summary

- **Likely safe:** When the oil is consumed in amounts commonly found in foods. In the United States, eucalyptus is approved for food use.
- **Possibly safe:** When used topically by healthy adults for a short duration.
- **Likely unsafe:** When used in infants and children, or when used in large amounts orally or in nondiluted form by anyone, regardless of age.

DOSING/TOXICOLOGY

General

- The following doses are based on traditional health practice patterns, expert opinion, and anecdote. No available reliable human trials demonstrate safety or efficacy of a particular dose of eucalyptus. In general, with natural products, the optimal doses needed to balance efficacy and safety often have not been determined. Formulations and preparation methods may vary from manufacturer to manufacturer, and from batch to batch of specific product made by a single manufacturer. Because often the active components of a product are not known, standardization may not be possible, and the clinical effects of different brands may not be comparable.

Standardization

- Standardization data are lacking. It has been suggested that in order to be effective medicinally, eucalyptus leaf oil must contain 70% to 85% 1,8-cineole (eucalyptol).

Dosing: Adult (18 Years and Older)

Topical

- External application of 5% to 20% in oil-based formulation or 5% to 10% in alcohol-based formulation. Although likely less toxic than oral ingestion, topical use may lead to toxicity.[18]

Inhalation

- Tincture with 5% to 10% oil or a few drops placed into a vaporizer as an inhalant. Adverse events associated with inadvertent ingestion of vaporizer solutions containing eucalyptus have been reported.[19]

Oral

- *Note:* Eucalyptus oil should be taken with caution because small amounts of oil taken internally have resulted in toxic and fatal reactions.[18,20]
- **Eucalyptus oil:** 0.05 to 0.2 mL or 0.3 to 0.6 g daily has been used traditionally, but may result in toxicity.
- **Infusion prepared with eucalyptus leaf:** 2 to 3 g of leaf in 150 mL of water, three times a day, has been used traditionally, but may result in toxicity.
- **Small gut–soluble capsules:** 200 mg of 1,8-cineol was taken three times daily by mouth for asthma in one trial.[21]
- **Mouthwash:** Eucalyptol (1,8-cineole) is a principal constituent of eucalyptus oil and is present in some mouthwash products. In low concentrations, eucalyptol appears to be well tolerated.

Dosing: Pediatric (Younger Than 18 Years)

- Due to toxicity data involving small doses of eucalyptus through topical[18] or oral[19] administration, eucalyptus is not recommended for use by infants and young children. Adverse events associated with inadvertent ingestion of vaporizer solutions containing eucalyptus have been reported.[19]

Toxicology

- Toxicity can lead to central nervous system depression; subsequent aspiration of stomach contents may be a risk. Multiple cases of toxicity have been reported in the literature beginning in the early 1900s, including coma, seizure, and death.[20] Anecdotally, toxicity has been suggested to follow as little as ingestion of 1 teaspoon, and toxicity may occur following topical[18] or inhalation-vaporizer exposure.[19]
- Toxicity has been reported in both children and adults. In a review of 109 pediatric admissions following ingestion, 59% had clinical effects. The authors suggested that significant central nervous system (CNS) depression is likely to occur following ingestion of 5 mL or greater of 100% oil[22]; however, another review did not find a relationship between amount ingested and symptom severity.[23] In an example of a pediatric case, Hindle[24] reported the accidental ingestion of eucalyptus oil in an 11-month-old infant. The infant developed lethargy, pallor, with difficulty breathing, coarse pulmonary crackles and a brief generalized seizure following ingestion of 10 to 15 mL of oil. Recovery was over 2 to 3 days following intubation and instillation of gastric charcoal. In an adult case with greater ingestion, a 73-year-old woman was found unconscious, hypotensive, hypothermic, and

hypoventilating following intentional ingestion of approximately 200 to 250 mL of oil. She developed aspiration pneumonitis and died 3 months later of pneumonia.[25]

- An LD_{50} of 2480 mg/kg has been reported in rats.

ADVERSE EFFECTS/PRECAUTIONS/CONTRAINDICATIONS

Allergy

- Multiple case reports of allergic reactions have been reported in the literature. Contact allergy to eucalyptus and other oils was demonstrated in patch-testing of a 53-year-old man using aromatherapy.[26] IgE-mediated contact urticaria from eucalyptus pollen has been reported in a 55-year-old woman after contact with eucalyptus leaves.[27] IgE activity has also been found in asthmatic children.[28] A maculopapular rash was described in a 3-year-old girl following ingestion of 15 mL of oil.[23] Allergic contact dermatitis was reported due to application of a topical cream containing the eucalyptus constituent 1,8-cineole (eucalyptol).[29]

Adverse Effects/Postmarket Surveillance

- **General:** Significant and potentially lethal toxicity has been consistently reported with internal (oral) use of eucalyptus oil in children and adults. In adults, topical and inhalation use are likely safer than oral use but may also carry a risk of toxicity[18,19] In children, topical use or inhalation have caused severe toxicity and death and should be avoided. It may be safe for adults to consume small amounts of diluted eucalyptus oil or to use topical or inhaled eucalyptus for brief periods of time, although caution is warranted. The signs and symptoms of eucalyptus toxicity may include epigastric burning, nausea, vomiting, dizziness, muscular weakness, constricted pupils, a feeling of suffocation, cyanosis, delirium, and convulsions.
- **Dermatologic:** Transient local redness, burning, and irritation have been reported following topical (bath) exposure.[30] A systemic, fine maculopapular rash was described in a 3-year-old girl following ingestion of 15 mL of oil.[23] Allergic contact dermatitis has been reported due to application of a topical cream containing the eucalyptus constituent 1,8-cineole (eucalyptol).[29]
- **Neurologic/CNS:** Central nervous system (CNS) depression with drowsiness and loss of consciousness as well as CNS excitation, ataxia, slurred speech, vertigo, hyperreflexia. and headache have been described in case reports.[20,23,31] Fever and headache are reported in a case involving a heavy consumer of eucalyptus extract.[32] In a review of 109 pediatric admissions following ingestion, 28% had CNS depression and 15% experienced ataxia.[22] Convulsions have been reported in case reports of oral ingestion,[24] and in exposure in bath water.[33] In the latter case, a 12-month-old girl was given five prolonged baths with eucalyptus oil, pine, and thyme, and developed multiple convulsions (133 in 24 hours), which continued over the following 4 years, necessitating anticonvulsant medication. Because of the chronic nature of the seizure disorder, it is not clear if the baths were the cause. Other effects mentioned in anecdotal reports include muscle weakness, paresis. and absence of deep tendon reflexes. Fever has been reported in a case of a heavy consumer of eucalyptus extract.[32]
- **Ocular/otic:** Pupillary constriction has been reported.[20,23]
- **Pulmonary/respiratory:** Respiratory effects, including hypoventilation, dyspnea, tachypnea, bronchospasm, pneumonitis, and aspiration pneumonia have been described in

reviews.[20,22] Apnea has also been reported.[30] Other effects per anecdotal reports include cough and tachypnea.

- **Cardiovascular:** Cardiovascular collapse with severe intoxication has been cited in case reports.[20,23] Premature ventricular contractions (PVCs) and trigeminy were described in a previously well 29-year-old man who ingested approximately 1 ounce of eucalyptus oil.[30] Anecdotal reports have also indicated the occurrence of hypotension and tachycardia. Cardiac asystole was reported in an alcoholic patient who ingested a large volume of Listerine mouthrinse, a combination product containing the eucalyptus constituent eucalyptol (1,8-cineole) as well as menthol, thymol, and methyl salicylate.[34]

- **Hematological:** There has been one case report documenting epistaxis following eucalyptus ingestion.[30] There are anecdotal reports that eucalyptus oil may induce adverse reactions ("attacks") in patients with acute intermittent porphyria and therefore should be avoided in these individuals.

- **Gastrointestinal:** In a review of 109 pediatric admissions following ingestion, 37% experienced vomiting.[22] This adverse effect has been reported elsewhere.[23,30] Abdominal pain has been reported in a trial of the eucalyptus constituent 1,8-cineol (eucalyptol) for inflammatory bowel disease.[10] Anecdotal reports have indicated that nausea and diarrhea have also occurred following eucalyptus ingestion.

- **Endocrine:** Eucalyptus has been found to lower blood glucose concentrations in diabetic animals.[8] Human data are lacking.

Precautions/Warnings/Contraindications

- Avoid if known allergy/hypersensitivity to eucalyptus oil.
- Avoid in infants and young children, due to case reports of significant toxicity following oral and topical exposure.
- Use cautiously in patients with asthma or other pulmonary disease, due to reports of dyspnea, tachypnea, bronchospasm, and pneumonitis.
- Use cautiously in patients with seizure disorder, due to case reports of seizures in children following ingestion and bath exposure.
- Use cautiously in patients with hypotension, because cardiovascular collapse with severe intoxication has been cited in case reports.
- Use cautiously in patients with severe liver disease, because anecdotal reports have indicated that eucalyptus oil may activate liver enzymes as well as interact with medications metabolized by the liver.
- Use cautiously in patients with kidney disease. Anecdotal reports have indicated that eucalyptol, a volatile component of eucalyptus, may cause irritation during urinary excretion.
- Use cautiously in patients with inflammation of the bile duct and gastrointestinal tract. Volatile constituents may cause mucosal irritation and possible choleretic activity.

Pregnancy and Lactation

- Because of the known toxicity of eucalyptus and unknown effects during pregnancy and lactation, eucalyptus should be avoided by patients who are pregnant or breastfeeding.

INTERACTIONS
Eucalyptus/Drug Interactions

- **CNS depressants/sedatives:** In multiple case reports, oral ingestion of eucalyptus oil has been associated with central nervous system (CNS) depression, characterized by drowsiness, loss of consciousness, ataxia, slurred speech, vertigo,

hyperreflexia, and headache.[20,23,31] Animal study has revealed sedative effects that are not mediated by a mu-receptor mechanism.[3] Additive effects may occur when eucalyptus is taken with other sedative agents.

- **Oral hypoglycemic agents, insulin:** Eucalyptus has been shown to lower blood glucose concentrations in diabetic animals.[8] Use with hypoglycemic agents may result in additive effects.

- **Drugs metabolized by cytochrome P450:** The terpine 1,8-cineole (eucalyptol), a principal component of eucalyptus, has been found to possess cytochrome P450–inducing activity in animals[35] and *in vitro*, specifically affecting levels of aminopyrine, amphetamine, zoxazolamine, and phenylbutazone.[36] Initial evidence suggests that 1,8-cineole is a substrate (metabolite) of CYP 3A specifically, with levels affected by that enzyme.[37] Other research has isolated the metabolite of eucalyptol, 2-exo-hydroxy-1,8-cineole, as a substrate of cytochrome P450.[37,38]

- **Pentobarbital:** *In vivo* and *in vitro* studies have demonstrated reductions in pentobarbital levels when used with eucalyptol, a component of eucalyptus.[36] Human data are lacking.

- **Amphetamine:** *In vivo* and *in vitro* studies have demonstrated reductions in amphetamine levels when used with eucalyptol, a component of eucalyptus.[36] Human data are lacking.

- **5-Fluorouracil (5-FU):** Eucalyptus has been found to enhance permeation of topical 5-FU through rat skin.[39] Using topical 5-FU and eucalyptus concomitantly may potentiate the effects of 5-FU.

Eucalyptus/Herb/Supplement Interactions

- **Sedating herbs and supplements:** In multiple case reports, oral ingestion of eucalyptus oil has been associated with central nervous system (CNS) depression, characterized by drowsiness, loss of consciousness, ataxia, slurred speech, vertigo, hyperreflexia, and headache.[20,23,31] Animal study has revealed sedative effects that are not mediated by a mu-receptor mechanism.[3] Additive effects may occur when eucalyptus is taken with other sedative agents.

- **Hypoglycemic herbs and supplements, insulin:** Eucalyptus has been shown to lower blood glucose concentrations in diabetic animals.[8] Eucalyptus used with hypoglycemic agents may result in additive effects.

- **Herbs and supplements metabolized by cytochrome P450:** The terpine 1,8-cineole (eucalyptol), a principal component of eucalyptus, has been found to possess cytochrome P450–inducing activity in animals[35] and *in vitro*, specifically affecting levels of aminopyrine, amphetamine, zoxazolamine, and phenylbutazone.[36] Initial evidence suggests that 1,8-cineole is a substrate (metabolite) of CYP 3A specifically, with levels affected by that enzyme.[37] Other research has isolated the metabolite of eucalyptol, 2-exo-hydroxy-1,8-cineole, as a substrate of cytochrome P450.[37,38]

- **Pyrrolizidine alkaloid-containing plants:** Based on anecdote, eucalyptus may potentiate the toxicity of borage, coltsfoot, comfrey, hound's tooth, and *Senecio* species.

Eucalyptus/Food Interactions

- **Milk and lipids:** In theory, the absorption of eucalyptus may be increased in the presence of milk or lipids.

Eucalyptus/Lab Interactions

- **Plasma glucose concentration:** Eucalyptus has been shown to lower blood glucose concentrations in diabetic animals.[8] Human data are lacking.

MECHANISM OF ACTION
Pharmacology

- **Constituents:** There are over 500 species of eucalyptus, ranging from shrubs to several 100-foot-tall trees. Eucalyptus leaves and oil are utilized for medicinal and other uses, such as fragrance in perfumes. Volatile oils are derived principally from species that are rich in 1,8-cineol (eucalyptol), such as *Eucalyptus globulus* Labillardiere (blue gum), *E. smithii*, and *E. fructicetorum*. *E.s globulus* Labillardiere is the most common medicinal species. Eucalyptus oil preparations may contain up to 80% 1,8-cineole.[40] 1,8-Cineol is present in the oils of other plants as well, such as tea tree oil. Other compounds present include macrocarpals (phloroglucinol-sesquiterpenes), other monoterpenes (D-limonene, α-pinene, β-pinene), alkaloids, phenols, and tannins.[41-44] The exact mechanism of action of eucalyptus oil is unknown at this time but may involve antimicrobial and anti-inflammatory effects.

- **Antimicrobial effects:** Antimicrobial activity has been studied in animal and basic science research. It has been suggested that the Australian koala's ingestion and skin surface excretion of eucalyptus may serve an antiparasitic function (and may also serve a homeostatic/thermal regulatory function).[45] *In vitro* antifungal properties have been reported in multiple eucalyptus species.[46,47] Antiviral activity against herpes simplex virus (HSV-1, HSV-2) has been demonstrated in cell cultures.[40] Eucalyptus oil in laboratory and laundry testing has shown significant reduction in live mites[48] and repellent activity against four biting arthropods.[12] Studies of medicinal plant extracts have demonstrated broad antimicrobial activity of eucalyptus against *Escherichia coli*, *Staphylococcus aureus*, and *Candida albicans* isolates,[41] as well as against gram-positive and gram-negative oral cariogenic and periodontopathic bacteria.[44] This research supports earlier studies demonstrating antibacterial activity.[49,50]

- **Anti-inflammatory and pulmonary effects:** An *in vitro* study of human blood monocytes reported dose-dependent, significant inhibition of multiple cytokines, with suggested application in the treatment of airway inflammation.[51,52] Anti-inflammatory activity and antinociceptive effect have been demonstrated elsewhere in animal models[3,53] may be related to antioxidant activity.[54] In addition, expectorant activity,[45] anti-oxidant effects,[55] and effects on surface tension in respiratory distress syndrome[56] have been studied. Burrow et al. reported stimulation of nasal cold receptors without effects on nasal resistance to airflow,[57] thus hypothesizing that the oil may simply act as a counter-irritant. Acknowledging possible slight symptomatic benefit and antimicrobial activity in respiratory conditions, Riechelmann et al. demonstrated that the *in vitro* function of human ciliary respiratory cells is impaired at higher concentrations of eucalyptus oil.[58]

- **Vascular effects:** Hong and Shellock. conducted a study of topical Eucalyptamint (eucalyptus oil, lanolin, and 15% menthol) on cutaneous blood flow and temperature.[59] Ten healthy subjects served as their own controls and consecutively received either the active agent or placebo. Subjective ratings, blood flow, and skin and muscle temperature were monitored for 60 minutes following application. Subjective perceptions were not significantly different, although blood flow, skin, and muscle temperatures were significantly altered for 45 minutes compared to placebo or to baseline measurements.

- **Other effects:** Other research into eucalyptus' mechanism of action has included demonstration of antitumor promoting effects with *in vitro* and *in vivo* studies of euglobal compounds isolated from eucalyptus plants[4,5]; inhibition of human plasminogen activator inhibitor[60]; examination of a serotonergic (5HT3) mechanism; appetite suppressant effects in animal feeding studies[61]; stimulation of insulin secretion; and enhancement of muscle glucose uptake and metabolism in diabetic animal models.[8] An *in vitro* study demonstrated that high concentrations of essential oils may reduce human nasal respiratory cell ciliary activity.[58]

Pharmacodynamics/Kinetics

- There is limited available human pharmacodynamic/kinetic information on eucalyptus at this time. Lipophilic monoterpenes appear to be readily orally absorbed, with a primarily oxidative metabolism that may require induction of the cytochrome P450 enzyme system, and subsequent urinary excretion.[43] Gastrointestinal absorption of eucalyptus is rapid and is likely enhanced by lipids and milk. Eucalyptus is believed to be eliminated via the gastrointestinal tract and the lungs.

- Eucalyptol (1,8-cineole), which is present in eucalyptus oil, is well absorbed via inhalation, with a reported peak plasma level at 18 minutes.[62]

- Eucalyptol (1,8-cineole) has been found *in vitro* and in animals to possess cytochrome P450–inducing activity.[35-37]

HISTORY

- Eucalyptus is native to Australia and serves as a primary food and water source for the koala. Australian Aborigines traditionally utilized the leaves as a source of water and to treat fevers. Marshes in which the trees took root dried, thereby reducing the habitat for mosquitoes carrying malaria. The eucalyptus was thus aptly named the "Australian fever tree."

- European explorers believed that the trees possessed antimicrobial activity, and brought saplings back to their homelands. Later uses included the treatment of various pulmonary conditions and as an antiseptic for urinary catheters.

- Eucalyptus trees were introduced into California and Hawaii in the mid-1800s. The initial small groves grew rapidly over the years, eventually dominating habitats and posing a significant fire hazard, as witnessed in the Oakland fire of 1991. Therefore, the state of California performed a eucalyptus tree removal and restoration project from 1990 to 1996, removing tens of thousands of tons of logs. Conversely, in Western Australia over the past 20 years there has been a project to replant trees in an effort to rehabilitate land, with a concurrent initiative by commercial industry to market the oil as an industrial solvent.

- Eucalyptus plants and trees are utilized in floral arrangements, planted as roadway wind or sound breaks, used as landscaping, and burned as a source of fuel.

REVIEW OF THE EVIDENCE: DISCUSSION
Asthma
Summary

- Initial research reports that long-term systemic therapy with 1,8-cineol may decrease the amount of oral corticosteroids required in steroid-dependent asthma. Further research is needed to confirm anti-inflammatory and mucolytic activity before this agent can be recommended in upper and lower airway diseases. In addition, comparison would be required with other agents used in asthma (such as leukotriene inhibitors, salmeterol, and inhaled corticosteroids) before a firm conclusion could be reached.

Review of the Evidence: Eucalyptus

Condition Treated*	Study Design	Author, Year	N†	SS†	Study Quality‡	Magnitude of Benefit	ARR†	NNT†	Comments
Asthma	RCT	Juergens[21] 2003	32	Yes	3	Small	NA	NA	Study to establish oral glucocorticoid-sparing capacity of 1,8-cineol (eucalyptol).

*Primary or secondary outcome.
†N, Number of patients; SS, statistically significant; ARR, absolute risk reduction; NNT, the number of patients who need to undergo a specific intervention in order to observe an outcome in one individual.
‡0-2 = poor; 3-4 = good; 5 = excellent.
NA, Not applicable; RCT, randomized, controlled trial.
For an explanation of each category in this table, please see Table 3 in the Introduction.

Evidence

- 1,8-cineol (eucalyptol), the major monoterpene of eucalyptus oil, suppresses arachidonic acid metabolism and cytokine production in human monocytes. A randomized controlled trial was conducted to evaluate the anti-inflammatory efficacy of 1,8-cineol by determining its prednisolone equivalent potency in patients with severe asthma.[21] Thirty-two patients with steroid-dependent bronchial asthma were enrolled in a double-blind, placebo-controlled trial. After determining the effective oral steroid dose during a 2-month run-in phase, subjects were randomly allocated to receive either 200 mg of 1,8-cineol three times daily or placebo, taken as small gut soluble capsules for 12 weeks. Oral glucocorticosteroids were reduced by 2.5-mg increments every 3 weeks. The primary end point of this investigation was to establish the oral glucocorticosteroid-sparing capacity of 1,8-cineol in severe asthma. Reductions were seen in daily prednisolone dosage of 36% with 1,8-cineol treatment (range, 2.5 to 10 mg; mean, 3.75 mg) vs. a decrease of 7% (2.5 to 5 mg; mean, 0.91 mg) in the placebo group ($p = 0.006$). Twelve of 16 cineol vs. 4 of 16 placebo patients achieved a reduction of oral steroids ($p = 0.012$). Further research is needed in this area before a firm conclusion can be drawn.

Decongestant-Expectorant/Upper Respiratory Tract Infection
Summary

- Despite eucalyptus oil's widespread use in multiple over-the-counter agents and inhalation vapors, there is insufficient available evidence to recommend either for or against eucalyptus oil as a decongestant-expectorant (in oral or inhaled form), due to a lack of controlled clinical trials. The available studies have been poor quality and largely used combination therapies or other sources of 1,8-cineole (eucalyptol), which is a principal constituent of eucalyptus.

Evidence

- A combination inhalation mixture of eucalyptus, menthol, and camphor was compared to placebo (tap water inhalation) in 24 healthy non-smoking adults with "common colds."[7] Following nasal spraying with phenylephrine, inhalation was conducted for 20 or 60 minutes. The authors noted significant improvements in forced vital capacity (FVC) and forced expiratory volume after 3 seconds (FEV_3) with the aromatic therapy vs. control (for both exposure time periods). However, there were no clear descriptions of baseline patient characteristics or differences, and this study was not properly randomized or blinded. In addition, the effects of eucalyptus cannot be separated from the possible benefits of the other included agents.

- A combination therapy which contains eucalyptus oil (Kanjang mixture) was compared to placebo in a double-blind study of 66 healthy adults with uncomplicated upper respiratory tract infections.[63] A visual analog scale was used to assess affects on coughing, sleep quality, and mucus production. All parameters significantly improved after 2 to 4 days vs. placebo, but after 10 days there were no differences between groups. It is not clear if this was due to the temporality of the infections. Although this study is promising, the incomplete reporting of baseline patient characteristics, origin of the scale used, and blinding or randomization procedures reduces the clinical utility of these results.

- A fixed combination therapy containing eucalyptus oil, juniper oil, and cajeput oil (Olbas drops) was compared to placebo in the treatment of 40 patients with upper respiratory tract infections.[64] Inhalation and topical treatments were administered, and after 7 days, the authors reported that the Olbas drops group experienced a shorter mean duration of symptoms, without statistical significance. This trial was poorly described and the effects of eucalyptus cannot be separated from the possible benefits of the other agents.

- A poor-quality case series reported improvement of maxillary sinus inflammation and peri-tonsillar abscesses in children with chronic sinusitis following the use of the eucalyptus product Eucalymine. Methods and results were not clearly reported.[13]

- Additional studies have been conducted on Myrtol, which contains the constituent 1,8-cineole (eucalyptol), which is also present in eucalyptus oil.[65-71] Efficacy has been reported in the treatment of respiratory infections, bronchitis, and chronic obstructive pulmonary disease (COPD), although these studies have generally been of low methodological quality. It is not clear that these results can be directly extrapolated to eucalyptus oil.

Dental (Supragingival) Plaque/Gingivitis
Summary

- Studies of medicinal plant extracts have demonstrated broad antimicrobial activity of eucalyptus against *Escherichia coli*, *Staphylococcus aureus* and *Candida albicans* isolates,[41] as well as gram-positive and gram-negative oral cariogenic and periodontopathic bacteria.[44] This research supports earlier studies demonstrating antibacterial activity.[49,50] Eucalyptol (1,8-cineole), a principal constituent of eucalyptus oil, has a long history of use in endodontics as a solvent, and to soften gutta percha (a thermoplastic root canal filling material) and various sealers.[17] Several studies have assessed the effects of eucalyptus extract or eucalyptol for the treatment of mouth flora associated with plaque or gingivitis. There are promising early results, although the evidence remains equivocal. Several well-conducted human trials have demonstrated the efficacy of Listerine antiseptic mouthrinse (Pfizer) against dental (supragingival) plaque and gingivitis. Listerine is a broad-spectrum antibacterial mouthrinse that contains a combination of essential oils (eucalyptol, menthol, thymol, methyl salicylate). Although promising, these results cannot be extrapolated to eucalyptol or eucalyptus oil as a monotherapy.

Evidence

- Sato et al. performed a double-blind crossover study to assess the effects on plaque formation of a chewing gum containing a 0.3% eucalyptus extract (*E. globulus*), a gum containing 0.3% funoran (a galactan present in red algae containing 3,6-anhydro-L-galactose and D-galactose), or a control gum.[72] Subjects received gum to chew after meals for 4 days. Plaque evaluation was performed at baseline and following treatment. Both treatments were noted to significantly lower plaque scores vs. placebo using a validated plaque-measurement scale (Quigley & Hein Index), with no significant differences between treatments. Although this preliminary trial was not adequately randomized or blinded, the results are promising for both therapies.
- The effects of a teeth-cleaning solution (dentifrice) containing fluoride and a fixed combination of several essential oils (thymol, menthol, methyl salicylate, and eucalyptol), or a control product containing fluoride only, was assessed in a 66-member subpopulation of a larger study of 361 individuals.[73] Effects were assessed after 3 and 6 months, and it was found that there was no difference in the concentrations of the most important pathogenic oral microbial flora in the essential oil-plus-fluoride group vs. the fluoride-only group. Because this trial did not specifically study eucalyptus oil, there is limited relevance. In terms of the use of eucalyptol (1,8-cineole) for this indication, the study may not have been adequately powered to detect true differences between groups. A subsequent rat study of a similar fixed essential oil combination containing fluoride was found to be more effective in preventing dental caries, although it appears that there was no fluoride present in the control dentifrice, which would likely have confounded the results.[74]

Listerine

- Listerine antiseptic mouthrinse contains a combination of essential oils, including eucalyptol, menthol, thymol, and methyl salicylate. Broad-spectrum antibiotic properties have been demonstrated for Listerine,[75] including against *Streptococcus mutans*,[76] herpes simplex virus, and influenza A virus.[77] Listerine has been demonstrated in several randomized, double-blind trials to be efficacious in the treatment of supragingival plaque and gingivitis for up to 6 months.
- Lamster conducted a 6-month randomized trial in 129 healthy adults with plaque and gingivitis, but no periodontitis.[78] Subjects were randomized to Listerine, sterile water, or a "vehicle control" with Listerine components minus the active ingredients. Subjects rinsed twice daily, intermittently supervised, in addition to their "normal" oral hygiene. After 6 months, mean plaque scores on the standardized Quigley-Hein Plaque Index (Turesky modification) were significantly reduced by 20.8% vs. vehicle (1.93 vs. 2.44) control and 22.2% vs. sterile water (1.93 vs. 2.48), whereas mean scores on the Modified Gingival Index were significantly reduced by 27.7% vs. vehicle control (1.20 vs. 1.66) and 28.2% vs. sterile water (1.20 vs. 1.67). Although this study was well

designed, randomization, blinding, and statistical analysis were not thoroughly described. Nonetheless, these are promising results.

- Gordon et al. conducted a randomized, double-blind study with similar design in 85 healthy adults.[79] All subjects received several weekly professional dental prophylaxis treatments, followed by 9 months of twice-daily mouth rinses with either Listerine, sterile water, or "vehicle control." Notably, after 9 months, plaque and gingival scores increased in the non-Listerine groups. In the Listerine group, mean Quigley-Hein Plaque Index scores were 13.8% better than vehicle control (1.93 vs. 2.36) and 19.5% better than sterile water (1.93 vs. 2.49), whereas scores on the Modified Gingival Index were 19.5% better than vehicle control (1.13 vs. 1.43) and 21.3% better than sterile water (1.13 vs. 1.49). All values had reported statistical significance. This study was also well designed, but the results are weakened by lack of description of randomization, blinding, or statistical analysis. In addition, the use by subjects of professional dental prophylaxis treatments may limit generalizability to patient populations that do not receive these prophylactic treatments.
- DePaola et al. conducted a randomized, double-blind trial in 108 individuals with gingivitis and plaque, but without periodontitis.[80] Plaque samples were taken at baseline to assess the presence of bacterial species. Over the following 6 months, subjects rinsed daily with either Listerine or a 5% hydroalcoholic placebo that appeared and tasted like Listerine. During this time, subjects continued routine oral hygiene and received professional dental prophylaxis treatments every 6 months. After 6 months, a significant 34% mean reduction in Quigley-Hein Plaque Index scores was noted vs. control (1.15 vs. 1.75), and a significant 34.4% reduction was noted on the Modified Gingival Index (0.92 vs. 1.39). Microbiological samples after 6 months compared to baseline samples revealed no significant differences between groups or vs. baseline. No opportunistic organisms were noted, a result confirmed in a subsequent 6-month study.[81] Notably, the plaque index that is more commonly used currently is the Turesky-modified Plaque Index, not the Quigley-Hein Plaque Index.
- Listerine mouthrinse has been reported to significantly reduce gingivitis and plaque in several additional human studies[82-84] and to be less efficacious than Peridex (chlorhexidine) against plaque,[85-87] but less likely than Peridex to cause tongue, dental, or restoration stains or supragingival calculus,[88] an effect shown to be due to Peridex binding to bacterial surfaces. A 2001 human trial conducted by Pfizer (the manufacturer of Listerine), reported Listerine mouthrinse plus a fluoride toothpaste to be superior to Colgate Total dentifrice (toothpaste) for the reduction of plaque and gingivitis in 316 individuals with plaque after 6 months.[89] There is early evidence that Listerine is able to penetrate dental plaque biofilm and kill gram-positive organisms interproximally (in the area most associated with periodontitis and dental caries, previously thought to be cleansed primarily only via flossing).[90,91] Adverse effects of Listerine have included case reports of allergic contact dermatitis[92] attributed to thymol, and cardiac asystole in an alcoholic patient who ingested a large volume of Listerine.[34] Listerine should be avoided in patients taking metronidazole or disulfiram. Other uses of Listerine include the removal of orally inhaled corticosteroids following inhalation[93] and wound-dressing following periodontal surgery.[94]

Headache (Topical)

Summary

- Eucalyptus has been associated with analgesia in animal studies.[3] The effects of topical eucalyptus oil on mechanisms associated with the pathophysiology of headache have been assessed in one study, in combination with peppermint oil. No effects were found on pain sensitivity. Additional trials with clinical outcomes are necessary before topical eucalyptus oil can be recommended for the treatment of headache.

Evidence

- A double-blind, randomized, placebo-controlled, crossover trial was conducted in healthy subjects (n = 32) to assess the effects of topical treatment with a combination peppermint oil/eucalyptus oil preparation on neurophysiologic, psychological, and experimental analgesic parameters.[95,96] Four treatment measures were compared: peppermint/eucalyptus/ethanol vs. peppermint/ethanol/trace eucalyptus vs. eucalyptus/ethanol/trace peppermint vs. placebo/ethanol/trace peppermint/trace eucalyptus. The combination of peppermint oil, eucalyptus oil, and ethanol was reported to increase cognitive performance and to possess muscle-relaxing and "mental relaxing" effects. It did not, however, have a significant effect on pain sensitivity. A significant analgesic effect with a reduction in sensitivity to headache was produced by a combination of peppermint oil/ethanol/trace eucalyptus, but not with the combination eucalyptus/ethanol/trace peppermint. This was a poor-quality study, with incomplete descriptions of methodology, blinding, and randomization. Nonetheless, it suggests that peppermint oil may be efficacious as a topical therapy for headache, whereas eucalyptus is not.

FORMULARY: BRANDS USED IN CLINICAL TRIALS

Brands Used in Clinical Trials

- Eucalyptamint (Naturopathic Laboratories, Florida); Enelbin-Rheuma (Germany).

Other Brand Names

- Bosisto's Eucalyptus Spray; Gelodurat.

References

1. Ilmberger J, Heuberger E, Mahrhofer C, et al. The influence of essential oils on human attention. I: alertness. Chem Senses 2001;26(3):239-245.
2. Nishizawa M, Emura M, Kan Y, et al. Macrocarpals: HIV-RTase inhibitors of *Eucalyptus globulus*. Tetrahedron Lett 1992;33:2983-2986.
3. Santos FA, Rao VS. Antiinflammatory and antinociceptive effects of 1,8-cineole a terpenoid oxide present in many plant essential oils. Phytother Res 2000;14(4):240-244.
4. Takasaki M, Konoshima T, Fujitani K, et al. Inhibitors of skin-tumor promotion. VIII. Inhibitory effects of euglobals and their related compounds on Epstein-Barr virus activation. (1). Chem Pharm Bull (Tokyo) 1990;38(10):2737-2739.
5. Takasaki M, Konoshima T, Kozuka M, et al. Anti-tumor-promoting activities of euglobals from Eucalyptus plants. Biol Pharm Bul. 1995;18(3):435-438.
6. Shaparenko BA, Slivko AB, Bazarova OV, et al. On use of medicinal plants for treatment of patients with chronic suppurative otitis. Zh Ushn Gorl Bolezn 1979;39:48-51.
7. Cohen BM, Dressler WE. Acute aromatics inhalation modifies the airways. Effects of the common cold. Respiration 1982;43(4):285-293.
8. Gray AM, Flatt PR. Antihyperglycemic actions of *Eucalyptus globulus* (Eucalyptus) are associated with pancreatic and extra-pancreatic effects in mice. J Nutr 1998;128(12):2319-2323.
9. Santos FA, Silva RM, Tome AR, et al. 1,8-cineole protects against liver failure in an *in-vivo* murine model of endotoxemic shock. J Pharm Pharmacol 2001;53(4):505-511.
10. Juergens UR. [Reducing the need for cortisone. Does eucalyptus oil work in asthma? (interview by Brigitte Moreano)]. MMW Fortschr Med 2001; 143(13):14.
11. Trigg JK. Evaluation of a eucalyptus-based repellent against *Anopheles* spp. in Tanzania. J Am Mosq Control Assoc 1996;12(2 Pt 1):243-246.
12. Trigg JK, Hill N. Laboratory evaluation of a eucalyptus-based repellent against four biting arthropods. Phytother Res 1996;10:313-316.
13. Tarasova GD, Krutikova NM, Pekli FF, et al. [Experience in the use of eucalymine in acute inflammatory ENT diseases in children]. Vestn Otorinolaringol 1998;(6):48-50.
14. Kriazheva SS, Khamaganova IV. [External use of eucalimine in pediatric patients]. Pediatriia 1989;8:97-98.
15. Ishizuka Y, Imamura Y, Tereshima K, et al. Effects of nasal inhalation capsule. Oto-Rhino-Laryngology Tokyo 1997;40:9-13.
16. Belzner S. [Eucalyptus oil dressings in urinary retention]. Pflege Aktuell 1997;51(6):386-387.
17. Morse DR, Wilcko JM. Gutta percha-eucapercha: a pilot clinical study. Gen Dent 1980;28(3):24-9, 32.
18. Darben T, Cominos B, Lee CT. Topical eucalyptus oil poisoning. Australas J Dermatol 1998;39(4):265-267.
19. Day LM, Ozanne-Smith J, Parsons BJ, et al. Eucalyptus oil poisoning among young children: mechanisms of access and the potential for prevention. Aust N Z J Public Health 1997;21(3):297-302.
20. Gurr RW, Scroogie JG. Eucalyptus oil poisoning treated by dialysis and mannitol infusion with an appendix on the analysis of biological fluids for alcohol and eucalyptol. Aust Ann Med 1965;4:238-249.
21. Juergens UR, Dethlefsen U, Steinkamp G, et al. Anti-inflammatory activity of 1.8-cineol (eucalyptol) in bronchial asthma: a double-blind placebo-controlled trial. Respir Med 2003;97(3):250-256.
22. Tibballs J. Clinical effects and management of eucalyptus oil ingestion in infants and young children. Med J Aust 1995;163(4):177-180.
23. Webb NJ, Pitt WR. Eucalyptus oil poisoning in childhood: 41 cases in south-east Queensland. J Paediatr Child Health 1993;29(5):368-371.
24. Hindle RC. Eucalyptus oil ingestion. N Z Med J 1994;107(977):185-186.
25. Anpalahan M, Le Couteur DG. Deliberate self-poisoning with eucalyptus oil in an elderly woman. Aust N Z J Med 1998;28(1):58.
26. Schaller M, Korting HC. Allergic airborne contact dermatitis from essential oils used in aromatherapy. Clin Exp Dermatol 1995;20(2):143-145.
27. Vidal C, Cabeza N. Contact urticaria due to eucalyptus pollen. Contact Dermatitis 1992;26(4):265.
28. Wang JY, Chen WY. Inhalant allergens in asthmatic children in Taiwan: comparison evaluation of skin testing, radioallergosorbent test and multiple allergosorbent chemiluminescent assay for specific IgE. J Formos Med Assoc 1992;91(12):1127-1132.
29. Vilaplana J, Romaguera C. Allergic contact dermatitis due to eucalyptol in an anti-inflammatory cream. Contact Dermatitis 2000;43(2):118.
30. Spoerke DG, Vandenberg SA, Smolinske SC, et al. Eucalyptus oil: 14 cases of exposure. Vet Hum Toxicol 1989;31(2):166-168.
31. Patel S, Wiggins J. Eucalyptus oil poisoning. Arch Dis Child 1980;55: 405-406.
32. Tascini C, Ferranti S, Gemignani G, et al. Clinical microbiological case: fever and headache in a heavy consumer of eucalyptus extract. Clin Microbiol Infect 2002;8(7):437, 445-437, 446.
33. Burkhard PR, Burkhardt K, Haenggeli CA, et al. Plant-induced seizures: reappearance of an old problem. J Neurol 1999;246(8):667-670.
34. Westermeyer RR, Terpolilli RN. Cardiac asystole after mouthwash ingestion: a case report and review of the contents. Mil Med 2001;166(9):833-835.
35. Pass GJ, McLean S, Stupans I, et al. Microsomal metabolism of the terpene 1,8-cineole in the common brushtail possum (*Trichosurus vulpecula*), koala (*Phascolarctos cinereus*), rat and human. Xenobiotica 2001;31(4):205-221.
36. Jori A, Bianchetti A, Prestini PE, et al. Effect of eucalyptol (1,8-cineole) on the metabolism of other drugs in rats and in man. Eur J Pharmacol 1970; 9(3):362-366.
37. Miyazawa M, Shindo M, Shimada T. Oxidation of 1,8-cineole, the mono-terpene cyclic ether originated from eucalyptus polybractea, by cytochrome P450 3A enzymes in rat and human liver microsomes. Drug Metab Dispos 2001;29(2):200-205.
38. Miyazawa M, Shindo M. Biotransformation of 1,8-cineole by human liver microsomes. Nat Prod Lett 2001;15(1):49-53.
39. Abdullah D, Ping QN, Liu GJ. Enhancing effect of essential oils on the penetration of 5-fluorouracil through rat skin. Yao Xue Xue Bao 1996; 31(3):214-221.
40. Schnitzler P, Schon K, Reichling J. Antiviral activity of Australian tea tree oil and eucalyptus oil against herpes simplex virus in cell culture. Pharmazie 2001;56(4):343-347.
41. Ahmad I, Beg AZ. Antimicrobial and phytochemical studies on 45 Indian medicinal plants against multi-drug resistant human pathogens. J Ethnopharmacol 2001;74(2):113-123.
42. Hou AJ, Liu YZ, Yang H, et al. Hydrolyzable tannins and related polyphenols from *Eucalyptus globulus*. J Asian Nat Prod Res 2000;2(3):205-212.
43. McLean S, Foley WJ. Metabolism of Eucalyptus terpenes by herbivorous marsupials. Drug Metab Rev 1997;29(1-2):213-218.
44. Osawa K, Yasuda H, Morita H, et al. Macrocarpals H, I, and J from the leaves of *Eucalyptus globulus*. J Nat Prod 1996;59(9):823-827.
45. Whitman BW, Ghazizadeh H. Eucalyptus oil: therapeutic and toxic aspects of pharmacology in humans and animals. J Paediatr Child Health 1994; 30(2):190-191.
46. Egawa H, Tsutsui O, Tatsuyama K, et al. Antifungal substances found in leaves of Eucalyptus species. Experientia (Specialia) 1977;33(7):889-890.

47. Shahi SK, Shukla AC, Bajaj AK, et al. Broad spectrum herbal therapy against superficial fungal infections. Skin Pharmacol Appl Skin Physiol 2000;13(1): 60-64.

48. Tovey ER, McDonald LG. A simple washing procedure with eucalyptus oil for controlling house dust mites and their allergens in clothing and bedding. J Allergy Clin Immunol 1997;100(4):464-466.

49. Kumar A, Sharma VD, Sing AK, et al. Antibacterial properties of different Eucalyptus oils. Fitoterapia 1988;59(2):141-144.

50. Pizsolitto AC, Mancini B, Fracalanzza L, et al. Determination of antibacterial activity of essential oils officialized by the Brazilian pharmacopeia, 2nd edition. Chem Abstr 1977;86:12226s.

51. Juergens UR, Stober M, Vetter H. Inhibition of cytokine production and arachidonic acid metabolism by eucalyptol (1.8-cineole) in human blood monocytes in vitro. Eur J Med Res 1998;3(11):508-510.

52. Juergens UR, Stober M, Schmidt-Schilling L, et al. Antiinflammatory effects of eucalyptol (1.8-cineole) in bronchial asthma: inhibition of arachidonic acid metabolism in human blood monocytes ex vivo. Eur J Med Res 1998; 3(9):407-412.

53. Atta AH, Alkofahi A. Anti-nociceptive and anti-inflammatory effects of some Jordanian medicinal plant extracts. J Ethnopharmacol. 1998;60(2): 117-124.

54. Grassmann J, Hippeli S, Dornisch K, et al. Antioxidant properties of essential oils. Possible explanations for their anti-inflammatory effects. Arzneimittelforschung 2000;50(2):135-139.

55. Siurin SA. [Effects of essential oil on lipid peroxidation and lipid metabolism in patients with chronic bronchitis]. Klin Med (Mosk) 1997;75(10):43-45.

56. Banerjee R, Bellare JR. In vitro evaluation of surfactants with eucalyptus oil for respiratory distress syndrome. Respir Physiol 2001;126(2):141-151.

57. Burrow A, Eccles R, Jones AS. The effects of camphor, eucalyptus and menthol vapour on nasal resistance to airflow and nasal sensation. Acta Otolaryngol. 1983;96(1-2):157-161.

58. Riechelmann H, Brommer C, Hinni M, et al. Response of human ciliated respiratory cells to a mixture of menthol, eucalyptus oil and pine needle oil. Arzneimittelforschung 1997;47(9):1035-1039.

59. Hong CZ, Shellock FG. Effects of a topically applied counterirritant (Eucalyptamint) on cutaneous blood flow and on skin and muscle temperatures. A placebo-controlled study. Am J Phys Med Rehabil 1991; 70(1):29-33.

60. Neve J, Leone PA, Carroll AR, et al. Sideroxylonal C, a new inhibitor of human plasminogen activator inhibitor type-1, from the flowers of Eucalyptus albens. J Nat Prod 1999;62(2):324-326.

61. Lawler IR, Foley WJ, Pass GJ, et al. Administration of a 5HT3 receptor antagonist increases the intake of diets containing Eucalyptus secondary metabolites by marsupials. J Comp Physiol [B] 1998;168(8):611-618.

62. Jager W, Nasel B, Nasel C, et al. Pharmacokinetic studies of the fragrance compound 1,8-cineol in humans during inhalation. Chem Senses 1996; 21(4):477-480.

63. Thom E, Wollan T. A controlled clinical study of Kanjang mixture in the treatment of uncomplicated upper respiratory tract infections. Phytother Res 1997;11(3):207-210.

64. Hansen B, Babiak G, Schilling M, et al. A mixture of volatile oils in treatment of the common cold. Therapiewoche 1984;34(13):2015-2019.

65. Federspil P, Wulkow R, Zimmermann T. [Effects of standardized Myrtol in therapy of acute sinusitis—results of a double-blind, randomized multicenter study compared with placebo]. Laryngorhinootologie 1997;76(1):23-27.

66. Sengespeik HC, Zimmermann T, Peiske C, et al. [Myrtol standardized in the treatment of acute and chronic respiratory infections in children. A multicenter post-marketing surveillance study]. Arzneimittelforschung 1998;48(10):990-994.

67. Matthys H, de Mey C, Carls C, et al. Efficacy and tolerability of myrtol standardized in acute bronchitis. A multi-centre, randomised, double-blind, placebo-controlled parallel group clinical trial vs. cefuroxime and ambroxol. Arzneimittelforschung 2000;50(8):700-711.

68. Dorow P, Weiss T, Felix R, et al. [Effect of a secretolytic and a combination of pinene, limonene and cineole on mucociliary clearance in patients with chronic obstructive pulmonary disease]. Arzneimittelforschung 1987; 37(12):1378-1381.

69. Meister R, Wittig T, Beuscher N, et al. Efficacy and tolerability of myrtol standardized in long-term treatment of chronic bronchitis. A double-blind, placebo-controlled study. Study Group Investigators. Arzneimittelforschung 1999;49(4):351-358.

70. Behrbohm H, Kaschke O, Sydow K. [Effect of the phytogenic secretolytic drug Gelomyrtol forte on mucociliary clearance of the maxillary sinus]. Laryngorhinootologie 1995;74(12):733-737.

71. Ulmer WT, Schott D. [Chronic obstructive bronchitis. Effect of Gelomyrtol forte in a placebo-controlled double-blind study]. Fortschr Med 1991; 109(27):547-550.

72. Sato S, Yoshinuma N, Ito K, et al. The inhibitory effect of funoran and eucalyptus extract-containing chewing gum on plaque formation. J Oral Sci 1998;40(3):115-117.

73. Charles CH, Vincent JW, Borycheski L, et al. Effect of an essential oil-containing dentifrice on dental plaque microbial composition. Am J Dent 2000;13(Spec No):26C-30C.

74. Yu D, Pearson SK, Bowen WH, et al. Caries inhibition efficacy of an antiplaque/antigingivitis dentifrice. Am J Dent 2000;13(Spec No):14C-17C.

75. Ross NM, Charles CH, Dills SS. Long-term effects of Listerine antiseptic on dental plaque and gingivitis. J Clin Dentistry 1988;1(4):92-95.

76. Fine DH, Furgang D, Barnett ML, et al. Effect of an essential oil-containing antiseptic mouthrinse on plaque and salivary Streptococcus mutans levels. J Clin Periodontol 2000;27(3):157-161.

77. Dennison DK, Meredith GM, Shillitoe EJ, et al. The antiviral spectrum of Listerine antiseptic. Oral Surg Oral Med Oral Pathol Oral Radiol Endod 1995;79(4):442-448.

78. Lamster IB. The effect of Listerine antiseptic on reduction of existing plaque and gingivitis. Clin Prev Dent 1983;5:12-16.

79. Gordon JM, Lamster IB, Seiger MC. Efficacy of Listerine antiseptic in inhibiting the development of plaque and gingivitis. J Clin Periodontol 1985;12(8):697-704.

80. DePaola LG, Overholser CD, Meiller TF, et al. Chemotherapeutic inhibition of supragingival dental plaque and gingivitis development. J Clin Periodontol 1989;16(5):311-315.

81. Minah GE, DePaola LG, Overholser CD, et al. Effects of 6 months use of an antiseptic mouthrinse on supragingival dental plaque microflora. J Clin Periodontol 1989;16(6):347-352.

82. Brecx M, Brownstone E, MacDonald L, et al. Efficacy of Listerine, Meridol and chlorhexidine mouthrinses as supplements to regular tooth cleaning measures. J Clin Periodontol 1992;19(3):202-207.

83. Nelson RF, Rodasti PC, Tichnor A, et al. Comparative study of four over-the-counter mouthrinses claiming antiplaque and/or antigingivitis benefits. Clin Prev Dent 1991;13(6):30-33.

84. Pitts G, Brogdon C, Hu L, et al. Mechanism of action of an antiseptic, anti-odor mouthwash. J Dent Res 1983;62(6):738-742.

85. Maruniak J, Clark WB, Walker CB, et al. The effect of 3 mouthrinses on plaque and gingivitis development. J Clin Periodontol 1992;19(1):19-23.

86. McKenzie WT, Forgas L, Vernino AR, et al. Comparison of a 0.12% chlorhexidine mouthrinse and an essential oil mouthrinse on oral health in institutionalized, mentally handicapped adults: one-year results. J Periodontol 1992;63(3):187-193.

87. Brecx M, Netuschil L, Reichert B, et al. Efficacy of Listerine, Meridol and chlorhexidine mouthrinses on plaque, gingivitis and plaque bacteria vitality. J Clin Periodontol 1990;17(5):292-297.

88. Overholser CD, Meiller TF, DePaola LG, et al. Comparative effects of 2 chemotherapeutic mouthrinses on the development of supragingival dental plaque and gingivitis. J Clin Periodontol 1990;17(8):575-579.

89. Charles CH, Sharma NC, Galustians HJ, et al. Comparative efficacy of an antiseptic mouthrinse and an antiplaque/antigingivitis dentifrice. A six-month clinical trial. J Am Dent Assoc 2001;132(5):670-675.

90. Pan P, Barnett ML, Coelho J, et al. Determination of the in situ bactericidal activity of an essential oil mouthrinse using a vital stain method. J Clin Periodontol 2000;27(4):256-261.

91. Fine DH, Furgang D, Barnett ML. Comparative antimicrobial activities of antiseptic mouthrinses against isogenic planktonic and biofilm forms of Actinobacillus actinomycetemcomitans. J Clin Periodontol 2001;28(7): 697-700.

92. Fisher AA. Allergic contact dermatitis due to thymol in Listerine for treatment of paronychia. Cutis 1989;43(6):531-532.

93. Kelloway JS, Wyatt NN, Adlis S, et al. Does using a mouthwash instead of water improve the oropharyngeal removal of inhaled flovent (fluticasone propionate)? Allergy Asthma Proc 2001;22(6):367-371.

94. Yukna RA, Broxson AW, Mayer ET, et al. Comparison of Listerine mouthwash and periodontal dressing following periodontal flap surgery. I. Initial findings. Clin Prev Dent 1986;8(4):14-19.

95. Gobel H, Schmidt G, Soyka D. Effect of peppermint and eucalyptus oil preparations on neurophysiological and experimental algesimetric headache parameters. Cephalalgia 1994;14(3):228-234.

96. Gobel H, Schmidt G. Effect of peppermint and eucalyptus oil preparations on headache parameters. Zeitschrift Fur Phytotherapie 1995;16(1):23, 29-26, 33.

Evening Primrose Oil
(*Oenothera biennis* L.)

SYNONYMS/COMMON NAMES/RELATED SUBSTANCES

- Echte nachtkerze, EPO, fever plant, gamma-linolenic acid (GLA), herbe aux anes, huile d'onagre, kaempe natlys, king's cureall, la belle de nuit, nachtkerzenol, night willow-herb, *Oenothera communis* Leveill, *Oenothera graveolens* Gilib, omega-6 essential fatty acid, *Onagra biennis* Scop, *Onogra vulgaris*, onagre bisannuelle, scabish, spach, stella di sera, sun drop, teunisbloem.

CLINICAL BOTTOM LINE
Background

- Evening primrose oil (EPO) contains an omega-6 essential fatty acid, gamma-linolenic acid (GLA), which is felt to be the active ingredient. EPO has been studied in a wide variety of disorders, particularly those affected by metabolic products of essential fatty acids. However, high-quality evidence for its use in most indications is still lacking. GLA has been officially licensed for the treatment of noncyclical breast pain (mastalgia) in England, and for the treatment of eczema in numerous countries, including England, Germany, Ireland, South Africa and Italy.[1]
- Preliminary evidence suggests efficacy of EPO for atopic dermatitis and eczema, although further trials are warranted before the data can be considered definitive.

Scientific Evidence for Common/Studied Uses Grade*	
Atopic dermatitis (children and adults)	B
Eczema (children and adults)	B
Breast cancer	C
Breast cysts	C
Breast pain (mastalgia)	C
Diabetes	C
Diabetic peripheral neuropathy	C
Ichthyosis vulgaris	C
Multiple sclerosis	C
Obesity/weight loss	C
Pre-eclampsia/pregnancy-induced hypertension	C
Postviral/chronic fatigue syndrome	C
Raynaud's phenomenon	C
Rheumatoid arthritis	C
Asthma	D
Attention deficit hyperactivity disorder (ADHD)	D
Menopause (flushing/bone metabolism)	D
Premenstrual syndrome (PMS)	D
Psoriasis	D
Schizophrenia	D

*Key to grades: *A:* Strong scientific evidence for this use; *B:* Good scientific evidence for this use; *C:* Unclear scientific evidence for this use; *D:* Fair scientific evidence against this use (it may not work); *F:* Strong scientific evidence against this use (it likely does not work). For a more detailed explanation of efficacy criteria, see "Natural Standard Evidence-Based Validated Grading Rationale" in the Introduction.

Historical or Theoretical Uses That Lack Sufficient Evidence

- Alcoholism, antioxidant,[2] atherosclerosis,[3] bruises (topical), cancer,[4,5] cancer prevention, cardiovascular disease, Crohn's disease, cystic fibrosis, fibrocystic breast disease, gastrointestinal disorders, hangover remedy, hepatitis B (chronic), hypercholesterolemia,[6] inflammation,[2] irritable bowel syndrome, melanoma, multiple sclerosis, pain, Sjogren's syndrome,[7] systemic lupus erythematosus (SLE), ulcerative colitis,[8] uremic skin conditions in dialysis patient,[9] urolithiasis,[10,11] weight loss, whooping cough, wound healing (poultice).

Expert Opinion and Folkloric Precedent

- Medicinal use of evening primrose oil (EPO) is a recent phenomenon. Native Americans traditionally considered the seeds a food and used poultices (of the whole plant) to treat bruises and root decoctions for the management of hemorrhoids. The leaves were thought to be helpful to treat minor wounds, gastrointestinal complaints and sore throats.
- Despite the theoretical benefits of supplementing with EPO to obtain the essential fatty acid gamma-linolenic acid (GLA), and its wide use for a variety of conditions, well-controlled, randomized studies to date have been either lacking or unable to demonstrate a consistent and clear benefit.

Safety Summary

- **Likely safe:** When evening primrose oil (EPO) is used orally in recommended doses for up to one year, for premenstrual syndrome, cyclical mastalgia, or atopic dermatitis.
- **Possibly unsafe:** When EPO is used in patients with seizure disorders or patients currently taking phenothiazine neuroleptics (e.g., chlorpromazine, thioridazine, trifluoperazine, fluphenazine).[12,13] The effects of long-term use (>1 year) are unknown. Therefore, long-term use of EPO without supervision by a licensed healthcare professional often is not recommended.

DOSING/TOXICOLOGY
General

- Recommended doses are based on those most commonly used in available trials, or on historical practice. However, with natural products, the optimal doses needed to balance efficacy and safety often have not been determined. Formulations and preparation methods may vary from manufacturer to manufacturer, and from batch to batch of a specific product made by a single manufacturer. Because often the active components of a product are not known, standardization may not be possible, and the clinical effects of different brands may not be comparable.

Standardization

- Standardized capsules of evening primrose oil (EPO) contain approximately 320 mg of linoleic acid (LA), 40 mg of gamma-linolenic acid (GLA), and 10 IU of vitamin E.[14] Preparations may also be identified according to percent content (70% LA, 9% GLA).[15] Dietary conversion of LA provides approximately 250 to 1000 mg/day of GLA.[1]

Dosing: Adult (18 Years and Older)
Oral

- **Atopic dermatitis:** 4 to 8 g of evening primrose oil (EPO)/day in divided doses have been used in trials.
- **Cyclical mastalgia:** 3 g of EPO/day in divided doses have been used in trials.[16]

Dosing: Pediatric (Younger Than 18 Years)
Oral

- **Atopic dermatitis:** 3 g of EPO/day in divided doses (to a maximum of 0.5 g/kg/day) have been used in trials.[16]

Toxicology

- Insufficient evidence at this time. Although no significant toxicity was reported in a 1992 review of animal trials and of approximately 500,000 users of EPO in the United Kingdom,[1] adverse effects including seizures and gastrointestinal discomfort are found in the literature.

ADVERSE EFFECTS/PRECAUTIONS/CONTRAINDICATIONS
Allergy

- Allergy or hypersensitivity to evening primrose oil (EPO) has not been widely reported. Individuals with allergy to plants in the Onagraceae family, gamma-linolenic acid, or other ingredients in EPO l should avoid its use.

Adverse Effects

- **General:** Evening primrose oil (EPO) has been well tolerated when taken in doses up to 3 g daily for up to 1 year.[17] A 1992 review found no significant toxicity in a review of animal trials and of approximately 500,000 users of EPO in the United Kingdom.[1] In 241 patients treated with EPO for cyclic mastalgia, 4% reported adverse events, vs. 30% of 295 treated with danazol and 35% of 216 treated with bromocriptine.[18,19]
- **Neurologic:** There have been several case reports of seizures associated with the use of EPO in patients with/without known seizure disorders,[12,13] and possibly with the combination of EPO and anesthetics. Headache has been reported in reviews.[15]
- **Cardiovascular:** In several rat studies by Engler et al., gamma-linolenic acid, an active constituent of EPO, has been found to decrease central venous blood pressure in both normotensive and hypertensive animals.[20-22] This is potentially due to angiotensin II receptor inhibition.[23,24] Preliminary human evidence is equivocal, with some data suggesting a blood pressure–lowering effect in humans[25] and other data showing no effect on blood pressure.[6]
- **Gastrointestinal:** Abdominal pain, nausea, and loose stools have been reported in studies and clinical reviews.[15,26]

Precautions/Warnings/Contraindications

- Use cautiously in patients with known seizure disorders, based on case reports of seizure.
- Use cautiously in patients currently taking phenothiazine neuroleptics such as chlorpromazine (Thorazine), thioridazine (Mellaril), trifluoperazine (Stelazine), or fluphenazine (Prolixin), due to reports of seizure.
- Use cautiously in patients undergoing anesthesia, based on the possibility of seizure.

Pregnancy and Lactation

- Cannot be recommended, due to insufficient available data.

INTERACTIONS
EPO/Drug Interactions

- **Phenothiazine neuroleptics:** There are multiple case reports of seizures occurring in patients taking both evening primrose oil (EPO) and phenothiazine neuroleptics such as chlorpromazine (Thorazine), thioridazine (Mellaril), trifluoperazine (Stelazine), or fluphenazine (Prolixin).[12,13]
- **Anesthetics:** Based on case reports of seizures, it has been hypothesized that EPO may increase risk of seizure when used concomitantly with general anesthetics.
- **Anticonvulsants:** Based on case reports of seizures, it has been hypothesized that EPO may lower seizure threshold.
- **Antihypertensive agents, pressors:** In several rat studies by Engler et al., gamma-linolenic acid, an active constituent of EPO, has been found to decrease central venous blood pressure in both normotensive and hypertensive animals.[20-22,27] This is potentially due to angiotensin II *receptor* inhibition.[23,24] Preliminary human evidence is equivocal, with some data suggesting a blood pressure-lowering effect in humans[25] and other data showing no effect on blood pressure.[6]

EPO/Herb/Supplement Interactions

- **Hypotensive agents:** In several rat studies by Engler et al., gamma-linolenic acid, an active constituent of evening primrose oil (EPO), has been found to decrease central venous blood pressure in both normotensive and hypertensive animals.[20-22,27] This is potentially due to angiotensin II receptor inhibition.[23,24] Preliminary human evidence is equivocal, with some data suggesting a blood pressure–lowering effect in humans[25] and other data showing no effect on blood pressure.[6]

EPO/Food Interactions

- Insufficient data available.

EPO/Lab Interactions

- Insufficient data available.

MECHANISM OF ACTION
Pharmacology

- The seed of the evening primrose plant (*Oenothera biennis* L.) is processed to extract evening primrose oil (EPO). The oil is usually packaged in capsules, and a small amount of vitamin E is added to help prevent oxidation. The active ingredient in EPO is thought to be gamma-linolenic acid (GLA), one of the omega-6 essential fatty acids. The amount of GLA in EPO varies but is approximately 9%.[15] EPO also contains linoleic acid (LA), which may be found in a variety of other vegetable oils. LA is metabolized to GLA, which is further metabolized to dihomo-gamma-linolenic acid (DGLA) and to arachidonic acid (AA).

- Omega-6 and omega-3 fatty acids are termed essential fatty acids because humans must obtain them from the diet (i.e., cannot make them from other fats). Essential fatty acids are building blocks for a number of molecules in the body and are essential in the creation of leukotrienes and prostaglandins (an array of signaling molecules important in biological processes, including inflammation). Some evidence suggests that disease may result from deficiencies in certain essential fatty acids and may be due to a defect in conversion. It has been suggested that a defect in conversion of LA to GLA may occur in patients with atopic eczema and in alcoholics.[1]
- GLA is also found in borage and black currant oils, although EPO is the simplest oil, containing few other components.[1]
- In several rat studies by Engler et al., GLA has been found to decrease central venous blood pressure in both normotensive and hypertensive animals.[20-22,27] This is potentially due to angiotensin II receptor inhibition.[23,24]

Pharmacodynamics/Kinetics
- The time course by which linoleic acid and gamma-linolenic acid affect metabolism of prostaglandins and leukotrienes has not been firmly established. After administration of EPO, t_{max} of linoleic acid is approximately 3 to 5 hours.[28] Metabolic effects may occur within hours of ingestion and may persist for months.
- A recent study of healthy volunteers given EPO found small changes in serum fatty acid levels, with only GLA demonstrating an absorption-elimination pattern.[28]

HISTORY
- The dermatologic use of linolenic acid may have been the first medical application of the essential fatty acids (EFAs). Researchers in the 1930s studied EFA-deficient animals and associated dermatitis, which appeared similar to clinical cases of atopic eczema. For many years following that work, high-dose linolenic acid was used for this condition, its use declining only after topical steroids were introduced in the 1950s. Horrobin, who works with a manufacturer, began extensive studies of evening primrose oil in the late 1970s.[1]

REVIEW OF THE EVIDENCE: DISCUSSION
Atopic Dermatitis and Eczema (Children and Adults)
Summary
- Several small trials with methodological flaws have examined oral evening primrose oil (EPO) for dermatitis and eczema (including premenstrual worsening of eczema). Overall, the weight of the evidence points to a moderate improvement of these conditions with EPO (6 to 8 g/day in divided doses). There is early evidence that the combination of EPO and fish oil may be less effective for eczema than EPO alone. Despite the fact that a large, well-conducted randomized trial is needed to provide definitive evidence, EPO has been approved for atopic dermatitis and eczema in several countries outside the United States.

Meta-analysis
- A meta-analysis of nine controlled trials by Morse et al. investigated the efficacy of one proprietary brand of EPO (Epogam) for atopic eczema.[29] All trials were conducted prior to 1989, including seven studies not published in the peer-reviewed literature, and two published studies.[26,30] The analysis concluded that EPO administration is associated with significant symptom improvements in studies with parallel designs. However, studies with crossover designs failed to note a significant effect from EPO treatment. The authors argued that these findings indicate a significant carry-over effect of EPO treatment. The analysis also documented that change in clinical condition was correlated with changes in plasma levels of dihomo-gamma-linolenic acid (DGLA) and arachidonic acid (AA). All patients in the trials continued topical treatment for eczema throughout the study periods. The quality of the seven unpublished trials cannot be assessed objectively. One negative trial by Bamford et al. was excluded from the analysis by the authors[26] because the placebo and treatment groups both experienced elevations in DGLA and AA (a phenomenon they noted had never previously occurred in their 20 unpublished studies, which they felt suggested that some patients "assigned to receive placebo actually received active treatment or vice versa"). Since these previous trials have not been published, it is impossible to access the validity of this assertion. Nonetheless, even if the results from the negative study were included in the meta-analysis, the meta-analysis results would indicate that Epogam produces a significant improvement in symptoms compared to baseline, and that this effect is better than placebo in 2 out of 3 parameters (patient global score was not significant). Finally, it should be noted that several of the authors of the meta-analysis (including the first author) have direct affiliations with Scotia Pharmaceuticals (the manufacturer of multiple EPO products).

Positive Trials
- Wright and Burton completed a double-blind crossover study of 99 patients (adults and children) with moderate to severe atopic eczema.[30] This was the only published trial considered but not excluded in the Morse meta-analysis.[29] Subjects received 12 weeks of EPO or placebo in random order. Four doses of EPO were studied, ranging from 1 capsule (equivalent to 360 mg of linoleic acid and 45 mg of gamma-linolenic acid [GLA]) twice daily to 6 capsules twice daily. All patients continued their normal treatment (mild topical steroids, emollients, and oral antihistamines) throughout the study period. In subjects on low-dose EPO, itching was the only symptom that significantly improved, whereas in the high-dose group, itching, scaling, and overall severity were all significantly reduced compared to placebo. However, only 80 subjects completed the study. Randomization was not well described and may have been inappropriate.
- Schalin-Karrila et al. conducted a double-blind placebo-controlled trial in which patients (n = 25) with atopic eczema received either EPO (4 capsules twice daily, each capsule containing 360 mg of linoleic acid and 45 mg of GLA) or placebo for 12 weeks.[31] The authors reported that the patients receiving EPO showed a significantly greater reduction in inflammation than those in the placebo group. However, subjects were taking concomitant medications with unclear effects on results. Blinding was not adequately described.
- Bordoni et al. completed a randomized, placebo-controlled, double-blind trial in 24 children suffering from atopic eczema.[32] Subjects were allowed to continue using emollients and weak topical steroids as needed throughout the trial. EPO-treated children improved significantly when compared with those ingesting placebo. Blinding, randomization, compliance, and method of analysis were incompletely described.
- Additional evidence of the benefit associated with EPO in treating children with atopic dermatitis has been provided

Review of the Evidence: Evening Primrose Oil

Condition Treated*	Study Design	Author, Year	N[†]	SS[†]	Study Quality[‡]	Magnitude of Benefit	ARR[†]	NNT[†]	Comments
Atopic dermatitis	Meta-analysis	Morse[29] 1989	311	Yes	NA	Medium	NA	NA	9 trials included (7 unpublished), with heterogeneous methodology; concomitant medications; possible author bias.
Atopic dermatitis	RCT	Berth-Jones[36] 1993	123	No	4	NA	NA	NA	Parallel design.
Atopic eczema	RCT	Humphreys[33] 1994	58	Yes	5	Medium	37%	3	Well conducted, in setting of premenstrual exacerbation.
Atopic eczema	RCT	Biagi[16] 1994	51	Yes	4	Medium	NA	NA	Study in children; concomitant medications.
Atopic eczema	RCT	Schalin-Karrila[31] 1987	25	Yes	4	Small	NA	NA	Concomitant medications.
Atopic eczema	RCT	Bamford[26] 1985	154	No	4	NA	NA	NA	Adults and children; varying doses.
Atopic eczema	RCT, dose comparison	Wright[30] 1982	99	Yes	4	Medium	NA	NA	30% decrease in symptoms with low dose EPO; 43% with high dose; adults and children; varying doses.
Atopic eczema	RCT	Bordoni[32] 1988	24	Yes	3	Medium	59%	2	Study in children; concomitant medications.
Atopic eczema	Open, uncontrolled	Biagi[34] 1988	12	Yes	NA	Medium	NA	NA	Study in children; concomitant medications.
Chronic dermatitis	RCT	Whitaker[35] 1996	39	No	4	NA	NA	NA	Small sample size; no power calculation performed.
Diabetic peripheral neuropathy	RCT	Keen[45] 1993	111	Yes	4	Medium	NA	NA	Multicenter trial for 1 year.
Rheumatoid arthritis	Review	Joe[46] 1993	129	No	NA	NA	NA	NA	4 trials reviewed; poor quality noted.
Rheumatoid arthritis	RCT	Brzeski[49] 1991	40	No	4	NA	NA	NA	Evaluated NSAID use.
Rheumatoid arthritis	RCT	Belch[50] 1988	49	Yes	4	Medium	40%	2.5	Outcome measured; stopped or reduced NSAID intake.
Rheumatoid arthritis	RCT	Jantti[48] 1988	20	Yes	2	NA	NA	NA	Assessed changes in serum lipids, but not symptom relief.
Psoriatic arthritis	RCT	Veale[51] 1994	38	No	4	Negative	−9%	NA	Placebo group did better; no effect in skin or arthritis symptoms.
Pre-eclampsia	RCT	Moodley[54] 1989	47	NA	4	Negative	−19%	NA	Placebo group did better.
Pre-eclampsia	RCT	D'Almeida[55] 1992	150	Yes	2	Small	18%	6	Possibly under-powered trial.
Mastalgia	RCT, double-blind	Blommers[56] 2002	120	No	3	None	NA	NA	Neither evening primrose oil nor fish oil offered clear benefit vs. control oils in the treatment of mastalgia.
Mastalgia	"Before and after" study	Pashby[57] 1981	73	Yes	2	Small	NA	NA	Statistical analysis not adequately described.
Mastalgia	RCT, single-blind	Gateley[18,19] 1992	36	No	2	Small	NA	NA	Some improvement in essential fatty acid profile, but no clear clinical correlate.
Mastalgia	Open, uncontrolled	Gateley[59] 1990	126	NA	NA	NA	NA	NA	Response rate of patients who failed first line therapy.
Mastalgia	Open	Pye[58] 1985	291	NA	NA	NA	26%	4	Comparison of 4 drugs.
Multiple sclerosis	Open, uncontrolled	Horrobin[62] 1979	14	NA	NA	NA	NA	NA	Full trial not published.

E

Continued

Review of the Evidence: Evening Primrose Oil—*cont'd*

Condition Treated*	Study Design	Author, Year	N[†]	SS[†]	Study Quality[‡]	Magnitude of Benefit	ARR[†]	NNT[†]	Comments
Multiple sclerosis	RCT, double-blind	Bates[63] 1978	116	No	3	Small	NA	NA	Marginal effect on severity and duration of exacerbations, but only at very high doses.
Raynaud's phenomenon	Placebo controlled	Belch[64,65] 1985,1986	21	Yes	3	Small	NA	NA	No improvement noted in objective outcomes.
Postviral fatigue syndrome	RCT	Behan[66] 1990	63	Yes	4	Moderate	51-68%	2	EPO plus fish oil vs. placebo; better results at 3 months vs. 1 month.
Chronic fatigue syndrome	RCT	Warren[67] 1999	50	No	4	None	NA	NA	EPO plus fish oil vs. placebo ineffective at 3 months.
Obesity	RCT	Haslett[70] 1983	100	No	4	None	NA	NA	No evidence of efficacy of EPO in combination with calorie restriction.
Ichthyosis vulgaris	RCT	Chalmers[71] 1983	30	No	3	None	NA	NA	No benefit shown; may not have been adequately powered.
PMS	Systematic review	Budeiri[73] 1996	452	NA	NA	NA	NA	NA	Heterogeneous trials.
PMS	RCT	Collins[82] 1993	49	No	4	NA	NA	NA	Crossover design.
PMS	RCT	Khoo[81] 1990	38	No	3	NA	NA	NA	Crossover design; no carryover effect noted.
PMS	RCT	Puolakka[75] 1985	30	Yes	3	Small	22%	5	Crossover design.
Psoriasis	RCT	Strong 1993	51	No	4	NA	NA	NA	Large drop-out rate; concomitant medication.
Psoriasis	RCT	Oliwiecki[84] 1994	37	No	3	NA	NA	NA	EPO + fish oil given.
Asthma & atopic dermatitis	RCT	Hederos[87] 1996	60	No	4	NA	NA	NA	Crossover design; study in children; concomitant medications.
Asthma	RCT	Ebden[85] 1989	12	No	3	NA	NA	NA	Concomitant medications.
Asthma	RCT	Stenius-Aarniala[86] 1989	36	No	3	NA	28%	4	Subjective evaluation scale; crossover; concomitant medications; blinding likely not adequate.
ADHD	RCT	Arnold[89] 1989	18	No	3	NA	NA	NA	Latin-square, double-crossover; order effect possible.
ADHD	RCT	Aman[88] 1987	31	No	3	NA	NA	NA	Crossover design.
Schizophrenia	Systematic review	Joy[93] 2000	45	NA	NA	NA	NA	NA	Only 2 trials included; small samples.
Schizophrenia	RCT	Peet[94] 1996	29	No	3	None	NA	NA	Subset of 43-patient study no benefit of EPO vs. placebo on PANSS scale; non-significant advantage of fish oil over EPO.
Schizophrenia	RCT	Vaddadi[96] 1989	39	Mixed	3	Small to moderate	NA	NA	Subset of 48-patient study; significant improvement on CPRS subset rating, not on AIMS; Crossover; antidyskinetic effect; concomitant medication.
Schizophrenia	Placebo-controlled	Holman[12] 1983	23	No	3	NA	NA	NA	Crossover design.
Menopausal flushing	RCT	Chenoy[97] 1994	56	No	3	NA	NA	NA	Negative trial; no power calculation performed, but likely sufficiently powered.
Bone metabolism	RCT	Bassey[98] 2000	85	No	4	NA	NA	NA	Pre- and post menopausal women; EPO + fish oil + calcium vs. calcium alone.

*Primary or secondary outcome.
[†]*N*, Number of patients; *SS*, statistically significant; *ARR*, absolute risk reduction; *NNT*, the number of patients who need to undergo a specific intervention in order to observe an outcome in one individual.
[‡]0-2 = poor; 3-4 = good; 5 = excellent.
NA, Not applicable; *ADHD*, attention deficit hyperactivity disorder; *AIMS*, abnormal involuntary movement scale; *CPRS*, comprehensive psychopathological rating scale; *PANSS*, positive and negative syndrome scale; *PMS*, premenstrual syndrome; *RCT*, randomized, controlled trial.
For an explanation of each category in this table, please see Table 3 in the Introduction.

by a placebo-controlled, double-blind trial involving 51 children with a mean age of 4.4 years.[16] All children continued their usual therapy (weak topical steroids and emollients) throughout the study. Low- (0.25 g/kg/day) and high- (0.5 g/kg/day) dose EPO were compared to placebo for 8 weeks. The authors found significant improvement in clinical severity assessment in the high-dose group only at the 8-week end point ($p = 0.046$). Immune status of the children (IgE-mediated) was not correlated with response to EPO. In addition, the authors did not find significant change in red blood cell membrane fluidity and suggested that change in membrane fluidity is thus an unlikely mechanism of action.

- Humphreys et al. conducted a trial with specific emphasis on women with premenstrual worsening of eczema.[33] Fifty-eight subjects entered this double-blind placebo-controlled study of EPO. Significant benefit in erythema and "surface change" were reported after 4 months of treatment, without significant benefit relative to menses.

- Biagi et al. reported the results of an open-label, uncontrolled investigation in 12 children (ages 2 to 4 years).[34] Improvement in eczema symptoms was noted at 4 weeks of therapy, and was maintained throughout a 20-week treatment period. Although these findings were promising, the lack of a control group limits the clinical usefulness of these results.

Negative Trials

- Bamford et al. found that EPO treatment was not associated with any significant response in patients (n = 154) with atopic eczema.[26] The authors completed a double-blind placebo-controlled crossover trial over a 6-month period, evaluating doses higher than those utilized in many other studies (up to 8 g in adults). Patients were allowed to continue to use emollients, topical steroids, and oral antihistamines throughout the trial period. The investigators observed no significant effect of EPO on erythema, scale, excoriation, lichenification, or overall severity. The sample size was likely sufficient (in light of known positive trials with fewer subjects). A re-analysis of data from this study by Morse et al.[29] suggests that assignments to the placebo and EPO treatment may have been confused, thus contaminating the data and perhaps accounting for the negative result. This criticism has not been confirmed.

- Whitaker et al. completed a 24-week double-blind, placebo-controlled trial of the effect of Epogam (dose equivalent to 600 mg/day of GLA) on 39 patients with chronic stable hand dermatitis.[35] No statistical difference in clinical parameters was noted between the placebo group and the EPO group. It is not clear if this sample size was adequate to detect a difference in effect.

- A parallel-group, controlled trial by Berth-Jones et al. reported no significant effect of EPO given in combination with fish oil vs. EPO alone vs. placebo for atopic dermatitis.[36] Patients (n = 123) received the study product for 16 weeks. The interpretation of data and methodology have been challenged elsewhere[37]; however, the authors have provided adequate explanation of their methodology and analysis techniques to support the integrity of these results.[38]

Diabetes and Diabetic Peripheral Neuropathy
Summary

- Animal studies[39-41] and small controlled human trials[42-44] have demonstrated beneficial effects of evening primrose oil (EPO) on serum markers in diabetes mellitus, including prostaglandin levels and serum fatty acids. Changes have not been observed in hemoglobin A1c. It has been hypothesized that EPO may have a role in the prevention of vascular or neurologic complications associated with diabetes mellitus. Notably, gamma-linolenic acid (GLA), one of the components of EPO, has been demonstrated as beneficial for diabetic neuropathy. Additional confirmatory studies are required before a strong therapeutic recommendation can be made.

Evidence

- Arisaka et al. studied 11 diabetic children in a double-blind, placebo-controlled study.[43] Over an 8-month period, treatment arm subjects received EPO (each capsule containing 360 mg of linoleic acid and 45 mg of GLA), 2 capsules/day for 4 months, then 4 capsules/day for 4 months. At the study's end, there were significant decreases in prostaglandin E2/E2-alpha levels and increases in dihomo-gamma-linolenic acid (DGLA) levels (also observed by Takahashi et al.).[44] These favorable effects on lipid metabolism are promising.

- Takahashi et al. conducted a controlled trial in 28 subjects with type 2 diabetes, in which 7 patients received 4 g of EPO, 2.4 g of fish (sardine) oil, and 200 mg of vitamin E.[44] It was noted that EPO subjects experienced significant increases in eicosapentaenoic acid vs. placebo. Although hemoglobin A1c levels fell as well, there was no significant difference from placebo. The benefits of EPO cannot be separated from possible effects of fish oil or vitamin E.

- The Gamma Linolenic Acid Multicenter Trial Group reported on a multicenter, double-blind, controlled trial of 111 patients with mild diabetic neuropathy.[45] Patients were assessed with neurophysiologic and biochemical measurements, and neurologic exams at intervals over 12 months. GLA was administered at a dose of 480 mg/day. Changes in 8/10 neurophysiologic and 5/6 neurologic parameters were significantly better in the treatment group vs. placebo. The authors reported that baseline hemoglobin A1c influenced the degree of response, as subjects with hemoglobin A1c had ≤10% greater improvement. The authors concluded that overall GLA supplementation had a beneficial effect on the course of diabetic neuropathy.

Rheumatoid Arthritis
Summary

- Clinical trials of evening primrose oil (EPO) for arthritis began in the early 1980s, focusing over the following years on patients with rheumatoid arthritis (RA). Studies have been small with high attrition rates and poor descriptions of methodology. Available research has not demonstrated consistent support for this indication, and currently there is not adequate evidence to recommend for or against this use of EPO.

Review

- Joe and Hart[46] reviewed four studies of the effectiveness of EPO in relieving rheumatoid arthritis[47-50] and concluded that all are limited by significant design flaws, including lack of placebo controls, no standardization of concomitant medications, inappropriate statistical analysis, and high number of patient dropouts. Although some subjective benefits were noted in the studies reviewed, changes in conventional, objective measures of disease activity were not identified. Thus, the authors conclude that "EPO cannot be advocated

242 Evening Primrose Oil

for the treatment of RA until its efficacy has been proven by prospective, double-blind, placebo-controlled trials." Additional details regarding the trials reviewed therein are provided here.

Positive Trials

- Belch et al. conducted a double-blind placebo-controlled 15-month trial of 49 patients with RA.[50] EPO (540 mg of gamma-linolenic acid [GLA]), EPO with fish oil (450 mg of GLA, 240 mg of eicosapentaenoic acid [EPA]) and placebo were compared as patients attempted to taper their baseline nonsteroidal anti-inflammatory drug (NSAID) therapy regimens. Significantly more patients taking EPO and EPO/ fish oil reduced their NSAID use vs. placebo and felt subjective improvement, but without significant objective improvement. The authors suggested that EPO might serve as a possible substitute for NSAIDs, based on its beneficial effects on inflammatory prostaglandins. Although this study suggests possible improvement in subjective symptoms, its small size and inadequate description of methodology make results difficult to interpret.
- Jantti et al. reported on changes in serum lipids with EPO treatment in a 12-week randomized, placebo-controlled trial of EPO (20 mL) in 2 patients with rheumatoid arthritis.[48] Neither objective nor subjective symptom changes were assessed in this trial. The authors suggested that the observed increase in the pro-inflammatory precursor arachidonic acid (AA) and the decrease in EPA associated with EPO ingestion might not be beneficial for RA. However, Horrobin[1] has argued that an increase in AA is not harmful in and of itself, because a rise in AA is not tantamount to a rise in its conversion to undesirable metabolites.

Negative Trials

- Brzeski et al. conducted a 6-month double-blind controlled study of EPO (6 g/day = 540 mg of GLA) in patients (n = 40) with RA and NSAID-related upper gastrointestinal symptoms/lesions.[49] The authors did not find a significant reduction in NSAID use compared to placebo (olive oil). Blinding was not adequately described, although this design flaw would likely not account for the result.
- Veale et al. investigated the effects of Efamol Marine (8% EPO l containing 73% linoleic acid [LA] and 9% GLA; 20% fish oil containing 18% EPA and 20% docosahexaenoic acid) in the treatment of 38 patients with psoriatic arthritis.[51] Patients in this double-blind, placebo-controlled trial took either Efamol Marine (12 capsules daily) or placebo for 9 months, followed by 3 months of placebo treatment in both groups. Efamol Marine had no effect on any measure of skin disease activity or arthritis symptoms.

Pre-eclampsia/Pregnancy-induced Hypertension
Summary

- Basic science research has suggested that prostaglandins play a role in the development of pre-eclampsia (characterized by the triad of hypertension, edema, and proteinuria), or pregnancy-induced hypertension. Because of the proposed effect of evening primrose oil (EPO) on prostaglandin metabolism, it has been theorized that EPO therapy may benefit or prevent this condition. Currently, there are limited trials of EPO for this application. Available studies have not been adequately powered or methodologically sound enough to support a recommendation for or against EPO for this indication. There is preliminary evidence that the combination of EPO and fish oil may be equally efficacious as magnesium oxide for pre-eclampsia, but definitive evidence from adequately powered trials is lacking.

Evidence

- Early studies proposed a decreased vascular response to angiotensin II (A2) following dietary supplementation with EPO, suggesting a potential anti-hypertensive effect during pregnancy.[52,53]
- Moodley and Norman conducted a double-blind, placebo-controlled clinical study of 47 primigravid African women with pre-eclampsia.[54] Women were randomly assigned to placebo or EPO (8 capsules containing 500 mg of EPO/day). No significant difference was found for EPO-treated subjects compared to placebo for blood pressure measurements, drug intervention, or outcome.
- In a study of the prevention of pre-eclampsia, D'Almeida et al. reported on 150 pregnant women randomized to placebo (olive oil), EPO plus fish oil, or magnesium oxide.[55] The study was conducted in Angola, South Africa, from 1986 to 1987. A majority (61%) of subjects were assessed as having fair baseline nutritional status. Weight gain during pregnancy was significantly greater for the two experimental groups compared to placebo. Five subjects in the control group developed the triad of pre-eclampsia (hypertension, edema, proteinuria), compared to 2 cases each in the experimental groups. This study suggests that the combination of EPO and fish oil may be equally efficacious to magnesium oxide for pre-eclampsia. However, because of the low event rate and likely underpowering, a larger trial is needed to provide more definitive support.

Breast Pain (Mastalgia)
Summary

- Evening primrose oil (EPO) is officially licensed for the treatment of mastalgia (breast pain) in the United Kingdom and considered first-line therapy in several European countries. However, no high-quality, randomized, placebo-controlled trials investigating the use of EPO for this indication have been published. Therefore, the available evidence does not support a recommendation either for or against EPO in the management of mastalgia.

Evidence

- Blommers et al. evaluated the effect of evening primrose oil and fish oil on breast pain in premenopausal women with severe chronic mastalgia, in a randomized, controlled, double-blind trial, employing a two-by-two factorial design.[56] During a 6-month period, 120 women were assigned to receive one of four treatment regimens: (1) fish oil and control oil, (2) EPO and control oil, (3) fish oil and EPO, or (4) both control oils during 6 months. Corn oil and corn oil with wheat germ oil were used as control oils. The change in percentage of days with breast pain was analyzed on an intention-to-treat basis. The authors reported that the decrease in days with pain was not significantly different between groups: 12.3% for evening primrose oil and 13.8% for the control oil ($p = 0.73$). Similarly, the decrease in days with pain was 15.5% for fish oil and 10.6% for the control oil ($p = 0.28$). All groups demonstrated a decrease in pain, but there were no significant differences between groups.
- In a published abstract, Pashby et al. reported a study of EPO in 73 patients with mastalgia, using a randomized, double-blind crossover design.[57] Patients ingested EPO

or placebo over a 3-month period, and the authors noted that pain and tenderness were significantly reduced in both cyclical and noncyclical mastalgia patients vs. baseline. However, this abstract does not provide adequate information to assess design or statistical analyses.

- Pye et al. reviewed their experience with the treatment of mastalgia.[58] They combined results from randomized trials (details not provided) and open studies that included a total of 291 women. They reported that their data indicate a 45% response rate to EPO in the management of cyclical mastalgia (compared to a 19% response rate to placebo). In addition, they reported a 27% response rate to EPO among patients with noncyclical mastalgia (compared to a placebo response rate of 9%). This publication does not provide sufficient detail to assess the quality of the trials conducted. Thus, the data are of limited clinical utility.

- In a randomized trial, Gateley et al. noted changes in essential fatty acid profiles in patients with mastalgia treated with EPO, but no consistent clinical improvements.[18,19] Thirty-six women with severe cyclic or noncyclic mastalgia were randomly allocated to either EPO (8 capsules of Efamol orally/day, corresponding to 320 mg of gamma-linolenic acid/day) or placebo for 4 months. No blinding protocol was described, but presumably only patients were blinded to the treatment. After 4 months, the most noteworthy change in terms of essential fatty acid profile was seen in those with a "useful" response to EPO treatment, in whom pretreatment low levels of dihomo-gamma-linolenic acid significantly increased. However, a similar, less pronounced increase was seen in the placebo group. The clinical significance of these observations is not clear.

- In an earlier series, Gateley et al. conducted an open-label, uncontrolled study of 126 patients with mastalgia who had failed to respond to first line therapy.[59] They reported that women who have not responded to previous therapies are unlikely to respond to EPO. In contrast, danazol was noted to maintain a high response rate (57% for second line therapy and 25% for third line therapy). Without controls, this study is of limited clinical utility.

Breast Cysts
Summary

- Literature review identifies one randomized, controlled trial that has examined the efficacy of evening primrose oil (EPO) for recurrent breast cysts. This study did not find a statistically significant positive effect. Additional data are required before a conclusion can be drawn.

Evidence

- Mansel et al. reported a slight but statistically insignificant reduction of breast cyst recurrence associated with EPO therapy.[60] Two hundred women with proven aspiratable breast cysts were randomly allocated in a double-blind fashion to either EPO (Efamol, 6 capsules/day) or placebo (paraffin oil). After 1 year, there were slightly fewer cysts observed in the EPO group (92 vs. 113), the difference being statistically insignificant.

Multiple Sclerosis (MS)
Summary

- Investigation of linoleic acid (LA) and gamma-linolenic acid (GLA) (components of evening primrose oil [EPO]) in the management of MS began in the 1970s.[61] Early work suggested that dietary manipulation might increase serum fatty acid levels and alter fatty acid brain composition, which sparked interest in EPO for this indication. However, no randomized controlled studies have been conducted to either confirm or reject this hypothesis. Thus, the use of EPO in the management of MS cannot be either supported or rejected at this time.

Evidence

- Horrobin has reviewed the rationale for this treatment and presented results from preliminary clinical research in a small sample of severely disabled MS patients (n = 14).[62] Although he described improvements in some patients treated with EPO (either alone or in conjunction with colchicine), this open-label, uncontrolled, unpublished study is not described in enough detail to allow the validity of these findings to be adequately assessed.

- In a poorly described randomized trial, Bates et al. reported a marginal effect of very-high-dose LA (20 g/day), well above the amount ingested with "therapeutic doses" of EPO, on severity and duration of MS exacerbations.[63] No effect was observed in subjects (n = 106) in terms of disability.

Raynaud's Phenomenon
Summary

- There is insufficient evidence regarding the use of evening primrose oil (EPO) for Raynaud's phenomenon.

Evidence

- One small (n = 21) randomized controlled trial suggests that some patients may experience symptomatic relief from EPO (12 capsules of Efamol, each containing 4.32 g of linoleic acid and 0.54 g of gamma-linolenic acid, daily for 8 weeks).[64,65] However, no differences in objective measures (hand temperature or cold challenge plethysmography) were noted between the placebo and EPO groups. Larger, randomized, placebo-controlled trials are required to confirm any benefit that EPO may have in the management of Raynaud's phenomenon.

Postviral/Chronic Fatigue Syndrome
Summary

- There is insufficient evidence regarding the use of evening primrose oil (EPO) for postviral or chronic fatigue syndrome.

Evidence

- One small (n = 63) randomized, double-blind, placebo-controlled trial reported that patients ingesting EPO and fish oil (Efamol Marine; 8 500-mg capsules/day for 3 months, each capsule containing 8% EPO l with 73% linoleic acid [LA] and 9% gamma-linolenic acid [GLA], and 20% fish oil with 18% eicosapentaenoic acid [EPA] and 20% docosahexaenoic acid) significantly improved symptomatically compared to those in the placebo control group.[66] The effects of EPO cannot be separated from those of fish oil. Additional studies are needed before a recommendation can be made.

- No evidence of efficacy of EPO and fish oil was found in a randomized, double-blind trial of 50 patients with chronic fatigue syndrome.[67] After 3 months of treatment with Efamol Marine (see preceding discussion), neither physical symptom checklist scores nor Beck Inventory for Depression scores improved more in the EPO group vs. placebo. Docosahexaenoic acid and EPA contents of red cell membranes increased in EPO subjects compared with placebo, but this difference was not statistically significant. No power calculation was presented, although the lack of difference between groups in terms of symptom scores is not likely attributable to the small sample size alone.

Breast Cancer
Summary

- There is insufficient evidence regarding the use of evening primrose oil (EPO) for breast cancer.

Evidence

- Preliminary animal study evidence suggests a beneficial effect of EPO over corn oil in the development of mammary tumorigenesis.[68]
- An open-label, matched control study investigated the EPO component gamma-linolenic acid (GLA) with tamoxifen as primary treatment for endocrine-sensitive breast cancer.[69] Thirty-eight patients took 8 capsules of GLA (3.8 g daily; source/brand not specified) in addition to tamoxifen (20 mg daily), and their progress was compared with 47 matched controls taking tamoxifen alone. Patients on tamoxifen and GLA experienced a faster clinical response than patients on tamoxifen alone, with greater reduction in estrogen receptor expression as well. These data represent early findings from a pilot series and cannot be considered definitive without further study.

Obesity/Weight Loss
Summary

- Literature review reveals no compelling human evidence of the efficacy of evening primrose oil (EPO) in weight-loss regimes/obesity. Results from one trial suggest lack of effect.

Evidence

- Haslett et al. found no anorectic effect of EPO in obese women.[70] One hundred obese women were randomly allocated in a double-blind fashion to either EPO (600 mL per capsule, 2 capsules four times daily) or placebo for 12 weeks, in combination with a 1000-kcal dietary regime. No difference in terms of weight loss was seen between treatment groups. Poorly reported evidence from an earlier trial suggested a positive effect, but cannot be viewed as conclusive.[25]

Ichthyosis Vulgaris
Summary

- Ichthyosis vulgaris, an inherited disorder of skin cornification (ichthyoses), is characterized by hyperkeratosis and scaling. It is relatively common, occurring in one out of 300 people. Current evidence, albeit preliminary, suggests that evening primrose oil (EPO) is not effective for this condition. However, larger, adequately powered studies are required to confirm this conclusion.

Evidence

- A small open trial and subsequent placebo-controlled double-blind trial of 30 patients with ichthyosis vulgaris found that 2 to 3 g/day of EPO did not significantly improve ichthyosis in patients with or without atopy.[71] Although suggesting lack of effect, this trial may not have been adequately powered to assess for small benefits.

Premenstrual Syndrome (PMS)
Summary

- Evening primrose oil (EPO) is widely used internationally by women for symptoms of premenstrual syndrome (PMS).

A survey of 300 Australian women from 13 general practices found EPO regarded as one of the three most effective treatments for PMS.[72] Despite its popularity, studies have suggested a lack of effect. Because trials have generally been underpowered and methodologically flawed, the weight of available evidence does not support the recommendation of EPO for the management of PMS. An adequately powered, well-designed trial is merited to provide a definitive conclusion about efficacy.

Review

- Budeiri et al.[73] completed a literature review of EPO for treatment of PMS. The authors conducted a survey of publications and relevant information on the topic from 1964 to 1993. A meta-analysis was not performed, due to insufficient data and lack of methodological uniformity in controlled trials. They identified 10 studies, including 7 placebo-controlled trials.[74-83] On review of these trials, only 2 were well designed and conducted, albeit small in size, and are discussed here.[81,82] Notably, these were negative trials. The authors of the review concluded that based on the literature available to them, EPO is of unproven value in PMS management.

Randomized Trials

- Khoo et al. completed a randomized, placebo-controlled double-blind trial over 3-cycle treatment periods, with cross-over after the 3rd cycle.[81] Patients (n = 38) were 20- to 40–year-old women, with a combination of PMS symptoms including fluid retention; breast pain, swelling/tenderness; and mood changes. Patients were not allowed to take concomitant systemic steroids or nonsteroidal anti-inflammatory drugs (NSAIDs). Active treatment consisted of 4 capsules of Efamol twice/day, each tablet containing 4.32 g of linoleic acid (LA) and 0.54 g of gamma-linolenic acid (GLA). The authors did not find a significant reduction in patient reporting of PMS symptoms compared to placebo treatment, nor was there an evident carry-over effect. A strong placebo phenomenon was noted.
- Collins et al. (Collins et al., 1993; included in the review above) completed a randomized, double-blind, crossover trial with 49 women (27 diagnosed with PMS and 22 symptom-free controls) to determine whether Efamol (12 capsules daily, each containing 4.32 g of LA and 0.54 g of GLA) was an effective treatment for PMS.[82] The study found that Efamol did not reduce PMS symptoms and concluded that it was an ineffective treatment for PMS.

Psoriasis
Summary

- The current evidence from small, methodologically flawed trials suggests that evening primrose oil (EPO) has no significant benefit for the management of psoriasis. Studies have been done in combination with fish oil and may not have been properly designed to measure benefit. Nonetheless, at this time, the evidence must be considered negative.

Evidence

- In a double-blind, placebo-controlled study of 51 patients with chronic stable psoriasis, Strong and Hamill (Strong and Hamill, 1993) found no significant difference in the remission rates of patients ingesting 6 g of Efamol Marine (8% EPO 1 containing 73% linoleic acid [LA] and 9% gamma-linolenic acid [GLA] and 20% fish oil containing 18%

eicosapentaenoic acid [EPA] and 20% docosahexaenoic acid) compared to placebo. There was significant dropout (only 23 patients [45%] were included in the final data analysis), which casts serious questions about the results.

- Oliwiecki and Burton completed a similar double-blind placebo-controlled trial of combination EPO (430 mg) and fish oil (107 mg) in 37 patients with chronic stable plaque psoriasis.[84] No overall significant benefit was found, although the study may not have been adequately powered to assess for effect. The authors cited unpublished data with similar lack of efficacy of this combination treatment in eczema and suggested that the combination of essential fatty acids may somehow interfere with the efficacy of fish oil. The merits of this unpublished information cannot be assessed.

Asthma
Summary

- Small, randomized, placebo-controlled trials of patients with asthma (with or without atopic dermatitis) have demonstrated lack of efficacy of evening primrose oil (EPO). Larger, adequately powered trials are necessary to confirm this conclusion.

Evidence

- A small 8-week placebo-controlled study of 12 adult patients with mild asthma[85] did not find significant benefit associated with EPO treatment (Efamol, 2 capsules taken four times daily, each containing 4.32 g of linoleic acid and 0.54 g of gamma-linolenic acid [GLA]). Subjective responses and objective measures (bronchodilator use, histamine challenge, peak expiratory flow) were included in the assessment of treatment effect. Efamol ingestion was not associated with a rise in arachidonic acid concentrations.
- Similarly, a 10-week crossover study of supplementary EPO (15 to 20 mL) compared to fish oil or placebo in 36 moderately severe asthmatics did not find a significant difference between the three treatment arms.[86]
- Hederos and Berg conducted a 16-week, double-blind, placebo-controlled trial of 60 children with atopic dermatitis, 22 of whom had concomitant asthma.[87] Epogam tablets (each containing 500 mg of EPO with 40 mg of GLA and 10 mg of Vitamin E) given at a dose of 12 tablets daily did not demonstrate a statistically significant benefit compared to placebo in the primary outcome measure of parental evaluation of itch, or in the parental/clinician assessments for asthmatic symptoms. Fifty patients received concomitant medications, which may have confounded results.

Attention Deficit Hyperactivity Disorder (ADHD)
Summary

- Small clinical trials have found evening primrose oil (EPO) to have no significant benefit greater than placebo for the treatment of ADHD. Although these studies may not have had adequate statistical power, at this time the weight of the evidence must be considered negative. Additional, adequately powered studies are warranted to confirm this conclusion.

Evidence

- Aman et al. conducted a double-blind, placebo-controlled crossover trial of EPO in 31 children (27 boys) with ADHD.[88] EPO was administered as 3 capsules (each containing 360 mg of linoleic acid [LA] and 45 mg of gamma-linolenic acid [GLA]) twice a day. There was no significant difference between the majority of the behavioral measure scores for patients ingesting EPO and those ingesting placebo. In addition, response to EPO did not appear to be associated with baseline fatty acid levels. The authors concluded that EPO supplementation produces minimal or no improvements in hyperactive children selected without regard to baseline essential fatty acid concentrations.

- In a double-blind, double-crossover (placebo vs. EPO vs. d-amphetamine) trial of ADHD children (n = 18), Arnold et al. found no significant effect of EPO supplementation (8 capsules of Efamol, each containing 4.32 g of LA and 0.54 g of GLA) on the majority of outcome measures assessed.[89] The authors concluded that this study "does not establish Efamol as an effective treatment" for ADHD. However, they noted a possible "order-effect," suggesting that ingestion of d-amphetamine immediately prior to EPO might have neutralized any EPO benefit. It is not clear what the appropriate washout period for d-amphetamine should be, and these results merit confirmation.

Schizophrenia
Summarys

- Based on studies demonstrating abnormal membrane phospholipid metabolism in patients with schizophrenia, it has been theorized that essential fatty acids (EFAs), including evening primrose oil (EPO) and fish oil, may play a role in the treatment of schizophrenia.[90-92] Several methodologically weak studies have been conducted in this area with varied results, although the majority of evidence from well-conducted studies is negative. Additional, adequately powered and properly designed clinical trials are warranted before EPO can be recommended for the management of this disease. In contrast, fish oils have shown some promise in this disease, and further study is merited.

Evidence

- Joy et al. conducted a review of randomized controlled trials assessing the efficacy of EFAs in the management of schizophrenia.[93] Two trials met inclusion criteria.[94,95] One of these, published by Peet et al., reported no difference in mental status score (PANSS) between EPO and placebo.[94] A small, non-significant benefit of fish oil over EPO was noted. This trial was conducted in a 29-subject subset of a 43-patient study that was said to be randomized and double-blinded, although neither blinding nor randomization was adequately reported. Two trials of EPO were excluded from the Joy et al. review because of inadequate reporting of data, both of which are discussed here.[12,96]
- Holman and Bell. found no significant therapeutic effect when they administered EPO (8 Efamol capsules daily, each containing 4.32 g of linoleic acid and 0.54 g of gamma-linolic acid) for 2 to 4 months to 13 schizophrenics in a double-blind, crossover study.[12] The size of the study may not have been adequate to detect a large effect.
- Vaddadi et al. conducted a double-blind controlled trial of EPO (Efamol) in patients with tardive dyskinesia (TD) and neuroleptic exposure.[96] Of the sample of 48 patients, 39 had schizophrenia. Schizophrenic patients had significantly lower essential fatty acid (arachidonic acid) levels than healthy controls. No significant treatment effects were observed on the AIMS (abnormal involuntary movement scale). However, the schizophrenia subscale of the comprehensive psychopathological rating scale demonstrated a significant treatment effect in favor of EPO, as did memory scores.

Additional study is warranted before EPO can be considered efficacious for schizophrenia.

Menopause
Summary

- Literature review reveals no evidence that evening primrose oil (EPO) is useful in the management of symptoms associated with menopause. Small trials investigating its effects on flushing and bone mineral density have been negative. Adequately powered studies are necessary to confirm this conclusion.

Evidence

- Chenoy et al. completed a randomized, double-blind, placebo-controlled trial (n = 56) to assess the efficacy of EPO (4 500-mg capsules daily) in the treatment of hot flashes and sweating associated with menopause.[97] The authors found that EPO offered no benefit greater than placebo in treating menopausal flushing. Although this was a small sample size, it likely would have been adequate to detect differences between groups if present.
- Bassey et al. investigated the use of Efacal (total daily dose contained 1000 mg of calcium, 4000 mg of EPO, and 440 mg of marine fish oil) compared to calcium alone (1000 mg daily) on total bone mineral density in both pre- and postmenopausal women.[98] Efacal was not found to have any benefit over calcium supplementation alone.

FORMULARY: BRANDS USED IN CLINICAL TRIALS
Brands Used in Clinical Trials

- Efamol (4.32 g of linoleic acid [LA] and 0.54 g of gamma-linolenic acid [GLA]) (USA, UK, Canada, Italy).
- Efamol Marine (8% evening primrose oil containing 73% LA and 9% GLA; 20% fish oil containing 18% eicosapentaenoic acid and 20% docosahexaenoic acid) (USA, UK, Canada).
- Naudicelle (UK).
- Epogam (UK).
- Efamast (UK).

References

1. Horrobin DF. Nutritional and medical importance of gamma-linolenic acid. Prog Lipid Res 1992;31(2):163-194.
2. Hamburger M, Riese U, Graf H, et al. Constituents in evening primrose oil with radical scavenging, cyclooxygenase, and neutrophil elastase inhibitory activities. J Agric Food Chem 2002;50(20):5533-5538.
3. Chapkin RS, Fan Y, Ramos KS. Dietary GLA retards atherosclerotic progression. Abstracts from the International Symposium on Gamma Linolenic Acid, American Oil Chemists Society, Health and Nutrition Division Annual Conference, San Diego, CA, 2000.
4. Gonzalez CA, Sanz JM, Marcos G, et al. Borage consumption as a possible gastric cancer protective factor. Cancer Epidemiol Biomarkers Prev 1993;2(2):157-158.
5. van der Merwe CF, Booyens J, Joubert HF, et al. The effect of gamma-linolenic acid, and in vitro cytostatic substance contained in evening primrose oil, on primary liver cancer. A double-blind placebo controlled trial. Prostaglandins Leukot Essent Fatty Acids 1990;40(3):199-202.
6. Viikari J, Lehtonen A. Effect of primrose oil on serum lipids and blood pressure in hyperlipidemic subjects. Int J Clin Pharmacol Ther Toxicol 1986;24(12):668-670.
7. Oxholm P, Manthorpe R, Prause JU, et al. Patients with primary Sjogren's syndrome treated for two months with evening primrose oil. Scand J Rheumatol 1986;15(2):103-108.
8. Guivernau M, Meza N, Barja P, et al. Clinical and experimental study on the long-term effect of dietary gamma-linolenic acid on plasma lipids, platelet aggregation, thromboxane formation, and prostacyclin production. Prostaglandins Leukot Essent Fatty Acids 1994;51(5):311-316.
9. Yoshimoto-Furuie K, Yoshimoto K, Tanaka T, et al. Effects of oral supplementation with evening primrose oil for six weeks on plasma essential fatty acids and uremic skin symptoms in hemodialysis patients. Nephron 1999; 81(2):151-159.
10. Buck AC, Jenkins A, Lingham K, et al. The treatment of idiopathic recurrent urolithiasis with fish oil (EPA) and evening primrose oil (GLA)—a double blind study. J Urol 1993;149:253A.
11. Tulloch I, Smellie WS, Buck AC. Evening primrose oil reduces urinary calcium excretion in both normal and hypercalciuric rats. Urol Res 1994; 22(4):227-230.
12. Holman CP, Bell AF. A trial of evening primrose oil in the treatment of chronic schizophrenia. J Orthomolecular Psych 1983;12:302-304.
13. Vaddadi KS. The use of gamma-linolenic acid and linoleic acid to differentiate between temporal lobe epilepsy and schizophrenia. Prostaglandins Med 1981;6(4):375-379.
14. Kleijnen J. Evening primrose oil. BMJ 1994;309(6958):824-825.
15. Barber A. Evening primrose oil: a panacea? Pharmaceutical J 1988;723-725.
16. Biagi PL, Bordoni A, Hrelia S, et al. The effect of gamma-linolenic acid on clinical status, red cell fatty acid composition and membrane microviscosity in infants with atopic dermatitis. Drugs Exp Clin Res 1994;20(2):77-84.
17. Gateley CA, Pye JK, Harrison BJ, et al. Evening primrose oil (Efamol), a safe treatment option for breast disease. Breast Cancer Res Treat 2001;(14):161.
18. Gateley CA, Maddox PR, Pritchard GA, et al. Plasma fatty acid profiles in benign breast disorders. Br J Surg 1992;79(5):407-409.
19. Gateley CA, Miers M, Mansel RE, et al. Drug treatments for mastalgia: 17 years experience in the Cardiff Mastalgia Clinic. J R Soc Med 1992; 85(1):12-15.
20. Engler MM, Engler MB, Erickson SK, et al. Dietary gamma-linolenic acid lowers blood pressure and alters aortic reactivity and cholesterol metabolism in hypertension. J Hypertens 1992;10(10):1197-1204.
21. Engler MM. Comparative study of diets enriched with evening primrose, black currant, borage or fungal oils on blood pressure and pressor responses in spontaneously hypertensive rats. Prostaglandins Leukot Essent Fatty Acids 1993;49(4):809-814.
22. Engler MM. The hypotensive effect of dietary gamma-linolenic acid and associated alterations in tissue fatty acid composition and the Renin-Angiotensin system. Abstracts from the International Symposium on Gamma Linolenic Acid, American Oil Chemists Society, Health and Nutrition Division Annual Conference, San Diego, CA, 2000.
23. Engler MM, Schambelan M, Engler MB, et al. Effects of dietary gamma-linolenic acid on blood pressure and adrenal angiotensin receptors in hypertensive rats. Proc Soc Exp Biol Med 1998;218(3):234-237.
24. Scholkens BA, Gehring D, Schlotte V, et al. Evening Primrose oil, a dietary prostaglandin precursor diminishes vascular reactivity to resin and angiotensin II in rats. Prostaglandins Leukot Med 1982;8:273-285.
25. Garcia C, Carter J, Chou A. Gamma linolenic acid causes weight loss and lower blood pressure in overweight patients with family history of obesity. Swed J Biol Med 1986;4:8-11.
26. Bamford JT, Gibson RW, Renier CM. Atopic eczema unresponsive to evening primrose oil (linoleic and gamma- linolenic acids). J Am Acad Dermatol 1985;13(6):959-965.
27. Poisson J, Germain-Bellenger S, Engler M, et al. Gamma-linolenic acid: A pharmacological nutrient for hypertension? Abstracts from the International Symposium on Gamma Linolenic Acid, American Oil Chemists Society, Health and Nutrition Division Annual Conference, San Diego, CA, 2000.
28. Martens-Lobenhoffer J, Meyer FP. Pharmacokinetic data of gamma-linolenic acid in healthy volunteers after the administration of evening primrose oil (Epogam). Int J Clin Pharmacol Ther 1998;36(7):363-366.
29. Morse PF, Horrobin DF, Manku MS, et al. Meta-analysis of placebo-controlled studies of the efficacy of Epogam in the treatment of atopic eczema. Relationship between plasma essential fatty acid changes and clinical response. Br J Dermatol 1989;121(1):75-90.
30. Wright S, Burton JL. Oral evening-primrose-seed oil improves atopic eczema. Lancet 1982;2(8308):1120-1122.
31. Schalin-Karrila M, Mattila L, Jansen CT, et al. Evening primrose oil in the treatment of atopic eczema: effect on clinical status, plasma phospholipid fatty acids and circulating blood prostaglandins. Br J Dermatol 1987; 117(1):11-19.
32. Bordoni A, Biagi PL, Masi M, et al. Evening primrose oil (Efamol) in the treatment of children with atopic eczema. Drugs Exp Clin Res 1988; 14(4): 291-297.
33. Humphreys F, Symons J, Brown H, et al. The effects of gamolenic acid on adult atopic eczema and premenstrual exacerbation of eczema. Eur J Dermatol 1994;4(598):603.
34. Biagi PL, Bordoni A, Masi M, et al. A long-term study on the use of evening primrose oil (Efamol) in atopic children. Drugs Exp Clin Res 1988;14(4): 285-290.
35. Whitaker DK, Cilliers J, de Beer C. Evening primrose oil (Epogam) in the treatment of chronic hand dermatitis: disappointing therapeutic results. Dermatology 1996;193(2):115-120.
36. Berth-Jones J, Graham-Brown RA. Placebo-controlled trial of essential fatty acid supplementation in atopic dermatitis. Lancet 1993;341(8860): 1557-1560.
37. Horrobin DF, Morse PF. Evening primrose oil and atopic eczema. Lancet 1995;345(8944):260-261.
38. Berth-Jones J, Thompson J, Graham-Brown RA. Evening primrose oil and atopic eczema. Lancet 1995;345(8948):520.
39. Jamal GA. The use of gamma linolenic acid in the prevention and treatment of diabetic neuropathy. Diabet Med 1994;11(2):145-149.

40. Hounsom L, Horrobin DF, Tritschler H, et al. A lipoic acid-gamma linolenic acid conjugate is effective against multiple indices of experimental diabetic neuropathy. Diabetologia 1998;41(7):839-843.
41. Jamal GA, Carmichael H, Weir AI. Gamma-linolenic acid in diabetic neuropathy. Lancet 1986;1(8489):1098.
42. van Doormaal JJ, Idema IG, Muskiet FA, et al. Effects of short-term high dose intake of evening primrose oil on plasma and cellular fatty acid compositions, alpha-tocopherol levels, and erythropoiesis in normal and type 1 (insulin-dependent) diabetic men. Diabetologia 1988;31(8):576-584.
43. Arisaka M, Arisaka O, Yamashiro Y. Fatty acid and prostaglandin metabolism in children with diabetes mellitus. II. The effect of evening primrose oil supplementation on serum fatty acid and plasma prostaglandin levels. Prostaglandins Leukot Essent Fatty Acids 1991;43(3):197-201.
44. Takahashi R, Inoue J, Ito H, et al. Evening primrose oil and fish oil in non-insulin-dependent-diabetes. Prostaglandins Leukot Essent Fatty Acids 1993;49(2):569-571.
45. Keen H, Payan J, Allawi J, et al. Treatment of diabetic neuropathy with gamma-linolenic acid. The Gamma-Linolenic Acid Multicenter Trial Group. Diabetes Care 1993;16(1):8-15.
46. Joe LA, Hart LL. Evening primrose oil in rheumatoid arthritis. Ann Pharmacother 1993;27(12):1475-1477.
47. Hansen TM, Lerche A, Kassis V, et al. Treatment of rheumatoid arthritis with prostaglandin E1 precursors cis-linoleic acid and gamma-linolenic acid. Scand J Rheumatol 1983;12(2):85-88.
48. Jantti J, Nikkari T, Solakivi T, et al. Evening primrose oil in rheumatoid arthritis: changes in serum lipids and fatty acids. Ann Rheum Dis 1989;48(2):124-127.
49. Brzeski M, Madhok R, Capell HA. Evening primrose oil in patients with rheumatoid arthritis and side-effects of non-steroidal anti-inflammatory drugs. Br J Rheumatol 1991;30(5):370-372.
50. Belch JJ, Ansell D, Madhok R, et al. Effects of altering dietary essential fatty acids on requirements for non-steroidal anti-inflammatory drugs in patients with rheumatoid arthritis: a double blind placebo controlled study. Ann Rheum Dis 1988;47(2):96-104.
51. Veale DJ, Torley HI, Richards IM, et al. A double-blind placebo controlled trial of Efamol Marine on skin and joint symptoms of psoriatic arthritis. Br J Rheumatol 1994;33(10):954-958.
52. O'Brien PM, Pipkin FB. The effect of essential fatty acid and specific vitamin supplements on vascular sensitivity in the mid-trimester of human pregnancy. Clin Exp Hypertens B 1983;2(2):247-254.
53. O'Brien PM, Morrison R, Broughton PF. The effect of dietary supplementation with linoleic and gammalinolenic acids on the pressor response to angiotensin II—a possible role in pregnancy-induced hypertension? Br J Clin Pharmacol 1985;19(3):335-342.
54. Moodley J, Norman RJ. Attempts at dietary alteration of prostaglandin pathways in the management of pre-eclampsia. Prostaglandins Leukot Essent Fatty Acids 1989;37(3):145-147.
55. D'Almeida A, Carter JP, Anatol A, et al. Effects of a combination of evening primrose oil (gamma linolenic acid) and fish oil (eicosapentaenoic + docahexaenoic acid) versus magnesium, and versus placebo in preventing pre-eclampsia. Women Health 1992;19(2-3):117-131.
56. Blommers J, de Lange-De Klerk ES, Kuik DJ, et al. Evening primrose oil and fish oil for severe chronic mastalgia: a randomized, double-blind, controlled trial. Am J Obstet Gynecol 2002;187(5):1389-1394.
57. Pashby N, Mansel R, Hughes L, et al. A clinical trial of evening primrose in mastalgia. Br J Surg 1981;68:801.
58. Pye JK, Mansel RE, Hughes LE. Clinical experience of drug treatments for mastalgia. Lancet 1985;2(8451):373-377.
59. Gateley CA, Maddox PR, Mansel RE, et al. Mastalgia refractory to drug treatment. Br J Surg 1990;77(10):1110-1112.
60. Mansel RE, Harrison BJ, Melhuish J, et al. A randomized trial of dietary intervention with essential fatty acids in patients with categorized cysts. Ann N Y Acad Sci 1990;586:288-294.
61. Field EJ, Joyce G. Effect of prolonged ingestion of gamma-linolenate by MS patients. Eur Neurol 1978;17(2):67-76.
62. Horrobin DF. Multiple sclerosis: the rational basis for treatment with colchicine and evening primrose oil. Med Hypotheses 1979;5(3):365-378.
63. Bates D, Fawcett PRW, Shaw DA, et al. Polyunsaturated fatty acids in treatment of acute remitting multiple sclerosis. Br Med J 1978;ii:1390-1391.
64. Belch JJ, Shaw B, O'Dowd A, et al. Evening primrose oil (Efamol) in the treatment of Raynaud's phenomenon: a double blind study. Thromb Haemost 1985;54(2):490-494.
65. Belch JJ, Shaw B, O'Dowd A, et al. Evening primrose oil (Efamol) as a treatment for cold-induced vasospasm (Raynaud's phenomenon). Pre Lipid Res 1986;25:335-340.
66. Behan PO, Behan WM, Horrobin D. Effect of high doses of essential fatty acids on the postviral fatigue syndrome. Acta Neurol Scand 1990;82(3):209-216.
67. Warren G, McKendrick M, Peet M. The role of essential fatty acids in chronic fatigue syndrome. A case-controlled study of red-cell membrane essential fatty acids (EFA) and a placebo-controlled treatment study with high dose of EFA. Acta Neurol Scand 1999;99(2):112-116.
68. el Ela SH, Prasse KW, Carroll R, et al. Effects of dietary primrose oil on mammary tumorigenesis induced by 7,12-dimethylbenz(a)anthracene. Lipids 1987;22(12):1041-1044.
69. Kenny FS, Pinder SE, Ellis IO, et al. Gamma linolenic acid with tamoxifen as primary therapy in breast cancer. Int J Cancer 2000;85(5):643-648.
70. Haslett C, Douglas JG, Chalmers SR, et al. A double-blind evaluation of evening primrose oil as an antiobesity agent. Int J Obes 1983;7(6):549-553.
71. Chalmers RJ, Shuster S. Evening primrose seed oil in ichthyosis vulgaris. Lancet 1983;1(8318):236-237.
72. Campbell EM, Peterkin D, O'Grady K, et al. Premenstrual symptoms in general practice patients. Prevalence and treatment. J Reprod Med 1997;42(10):637-646.
73. Budeiri D, Li Wan PA, Dornan JC. Is evening primrose oil of value in the treatment of premenstrual syndrome? Controlled Clin Trials 1996;17(1):60-68.
74. Brush MG. Efamol (evening primrose oil) in the treatment of the premenstrual syndrome. In Horrobin DF (ed): Clinical Uses of Essential Fatty Acids. Montreal, Eden Press Inc, 1982, pp 155-161.
75. Puolakka J, Makarainen L, Viinikka L, et al. Biochemical and clinical effects of treating the premenstrual syndrome with prostaglandin synthesis precursors. J Reprod Med 1985;30(3):149-153.
76. Ockerman PA, Bachrack I, Glans S, et al. Evening primrose oil as a treatment of premenstrual syndrome. Rec Adv Clin Nutr 1986;2:404-405.
77. Casper RF, Powell AM. Effects of evening primrose oil in the treatment of premenstrual syndrome. Proc 2nd International Symposium on Premenstrual, Postpartum and Menopausal Mood Disorders, 1987; abstract 46.
78. Hunter JO, Wilson AJ. A double-blind controlled trial of gammalinolenic acid (GLA) in the management of pre-menstrual gastrointestinal symptoms. Proc 2nd International Symposium on Premenstrual, Postpartum and Menopausal Mood Disorders, 1987; abstract 44.
79. Massil H, Brush M, Manku M, et al. Polyunsaturated fatty acid levels in premenstrual syndrome and the effect of dietary supplementation on symptoms. Proc 2nd International Symposium on Premenstrual, Postpartum and Menopausal Mood Disorders, 1987; abstract 39.
80. Larsson B, Jonasson A, Fianu S. Evening primrose oil in the treatment of premenstrual syndrome. Curr Ther Res 1989;46(1):58-63.
81. Khoo SK, Munro C, Battistutta D. Evening primrose oil and treatment of premenstrual syndrome. Med J Aust 1990;153(4):189-192.
82. Collins A, Cerin A, Coleman G, et al. Essential fatty acids in the treatment of premenstrual syndrome. Obstet Gynecol 1993;81(1):93-98.
83. Mansel RE, Pye JK, Hughes LE. A controlled trial of evening primrose oil (Efamol) in cyclic premenstrual mastalgia. Proc 2nd International Symposium on Premenstrual, Postpartum and Menopausal Mood Disorders, 1987; abstract 47.
84. Oliwiecki S, Burton JL. Evening primrose oil and marine oil in the treatment of psoriasis. Clin Exp Dermatol 1994;19(2):127-129.
85. Ebden P, Bevan C, Banks J, et al. A study of evening primrose seed oil in atopic asthma. Prostaglandins Leukot Essent Fatty Acids 1989;35(2):69-72.
86. Stenius-Aarniala B, Aro A, Hakulinen A, et al. Evening primrose oil and fish oil are ineffective as supplementary treatment of bronchial asthma. Ann Allergy 1989;62(6):534-537.
87. Hederos CA, Berg A. Epogam evening primrose oil treatment in atopic dermatitis and asthma. Arch Dis Child 1996;75(6):494-497.
88. Aman MG, Mitchell EA, Turbott SH. The effects of essential fatty acid supplementation by Efamol in hyperactive children. J Abnorm Child Psychol 1987;15(1):75-90.
89. Arnold LE, Kleykamp D, Votolato NA, et al. Gamma-linolenic acid for attention-deficit hyperactivity disorder: placebo-controlled comparison to D-amphetamine. Biol Psychiatry 1989;25(2):222-228.
90. Horrobin DF. The membrane phospholipid hypothesis as a biochemical basis for the neurodevelopmental concept of schizophrenia. Schizophr Res 1998;30(3):193-208.
91. Horrobin DF. Lipids and schizophrenia. Br J Psychiatry 1999;175:88.
92. Laugharne JD, Mellor JE, Peet M. Fatty acids and schizophrenia. Lipids 1996;31 Suppl:S163-S165.
93. Joy CB, Mumby-Croft R, Joy LA. Polyunsaturated fatty acid (fish or evening primrose oil) for schizophrenia. Cochrane Database Syst Rev 2000;(2):CD001257.
94. Peet M, Laugharne JD, Mellor J, Ramchand CN. Essential fatty acid deficiency in erythrocyte membranes from chronic schizophrenic patients, and the clinical effects of dietary supplementation. Prostaglandins Leukot Essent Fatty Acids 1996;55(1-2):71-75.
95. Wolkin A, Jordan B, Peselow E, et al. Essential fatty acid supplementation in tardive dyskinesia. Am J Psychiatry 1986;143(7):912-914.
96. Vaddadi KS, Courtney P, Gilleard CJ, et al. A double-blind trial of essential fatty acid supplementation in patients with tardive dyskinesia. Psychiatry Res 1989;27(3):313-323.
97. Chenoy R, Hussain S, Tayob Y, et al. Effect of oral gamolenic acid from evening primrose oil on menopausal flushing. BMJ 1994;308(6927):501-503.
98. Bassey EJ, Littlewood JJ, Rothwell MC, et al. Lack of effect of supplementation with essential fatty acids on bone mineral density in healthy pre- and postmenopausal women: two randomized controlled trials of Efacal v. calcium alone. Br J Nutr 2000;83(6):629-635.

Eyebright
(Euphrasia officinalis)

SYNONYMS/COMMON NAMES/RELATED SUBSTANCES

- Adhib, ambrosia, augentrost, augentrostkraut, augstenzieger, brise-lunettes, casse-lunettes, clary, clary wort, clear eye, eufragia, eufrasia, euphraise, euphraisiae herba (eyebright herb), *Euphrasia*, *Euphrasia mollis*, *Euphrasia rostkoviana*, *Euphrasia sibirica*, euphrasy, ewfras, frasia, herbe d'euphrase, herbe d'euphraise officinale, hirnkraut, laegeojentrost luminella, meadow eyebright, muscatel sage, red eyebright, sage, *Salvia sclarea*, schabab, Scrophulariaceae, see bright, weisses ruhrkraut, wiesenaugetrost, zwang-kraut.

CLINICAL BOTTOM LINE
Background

- In Europe, the herb eyebright (*Euphrasia officinalis*) has been used for centuries as a rinse, compress, or bath against eye infections and other eye-related irritations (a use reflected in many of its vernacular names). When taken orally, eyebright has been used to treat inflammation of nasal mucous membranes and sinusitis.
- Eyebright is high in iridoid glycosides such as aucubin. In several *in vitro* investigations, this constituent has been found to possess hepatoprotective and antimicrobial activity. There is limited clinical research assessing the efficacy of eyebright in the treatment of conjunctivitis, and the use of eyebright for other indications has not been studied in clinical trials.
- Few data exist regarding the safety and toxicity of eyebright. A concern regarding the ophthalmologic use of eyebright is the potential for contamination.

Scientific Evidence for Common/Studied Uses	Grade*
Anti-inflammatory	C
Conjunctivitis	C
Hepatoprotection	C

*Key to grades: A: Strong scientific evidence for this use; B: Good scientific evidence for this use; C: Unclear scientific evidence for this use; D: Fair scientific evidence against this use (it may not work); F: Strong scientific evidence against this use (it likely does not work). For a more detailed explanation of efficacy criteria, see "Natural Standard Evidence-Based Validated Grading Rationale" in the Introduction.

Historical or Theoretical Uses That Lack Sufficient Evidence

- Allergies, antibacterial, antihelmintic, antiviral, appetite stimulant, asthma, astringent, blepharitis, bronchitis (chronic), cancer, cataracts, catarrh of the eyes, common cold, congestion, cough, digestive aid, earaches, epilepsy, expectorant, flavoring agent, gastric acid secretion stimulation, hay fever, headache, hoarseness, jaundice, liver disease, measles, memory loss, middle ear problems, ocular compress, ocular fatigue, ocular inflammation (acute, subacute, blood vessels of eye, eyelids), ocular rinse, ophthalmia, respiratory infections, rhinitis, sinusitis, skin conditions, sneezing (chronic), sore throat, styes, visual disturbances.

Expert Opinion and Folkloric Precedent

- Eyebright's medicinal properties date back to the 14th century, during which it was believed by some to "cure all evils of the eye." Eyebright continues to be used as a topical treatment for eye inflammatory disorders, such as blepharitis, conjunctivitis, and styes (hordeolum), although safety and efficacy information is lacking.
- Herbalists sometimes recommend its use for respiratory tract disorders, including sinus infections, cough, and sore throat. Anthroposophical practitioners use eyebright for "restructuring of the fluid organism of the eye," such as in conjunctivitis.[1]
- The expert German panel, Commission E, suggests that eyebright has not been proven safe and effective and does not recommend the topical application of eyebright for hygienic reasons. The Council of Europe lists eyebright as a natural source for food flavoring. In the United Kingdom, eyebright is included on the General Sale List. The U.S. Food and Drug Administration (FDA) has not evaluated eyebright for a generally recognized as safe (GRAS) status.

Safety Summary

- **Possibly safe:** When used in amounts commonly found in foods or when used as a flavoring agent.
- **Possibly unsafe:** When used in recommended medicinal doses for ophthalmic indications, because of potential microbial contamination.
- **Likely unsafe:** When "home-made" preparations are used for ophthalmic indications, because of the likelihood of microbial contamination; when used in greater than studied doses or duration, because of lack of safety data; when used during pregnancy and lactation, or in pediatric patients.

DOSING/TOXICOLOGY
General

- Recommended doses are based on those most commonly used in available trials, or on historical practice. However, with natural products, the optimal doses needed to balance efficacy and safety often have not been determined. Formulations and preparation methods may vary from manufacturer to manufacturer, and from batch to batch of a specific product made by a single manufacturer. Because often the active components of a product are not known, standardization may not be possible, and the clinical effects of different brands may not be comparable.

Standardization

- There is no widely accepted standardization for eyebright formulations.

Dosing: Adult (18 Years and Older)
Oral

- **General:** 2 to 4 g of dried herb three times daily has been suggested for multiple indications.

Topical

- **Conjunctivitis:** One drop of *Euphrasia* 1 to 5 times daily for 3 to 17 days for inflammatory or catarrhal conjunctivitis was used in a prospective, cohort trial.[1] Traditional use has included application of an eyebright-soaked compress.

Dosing: Pediatric (Younger Than 18 Years)
Topical

- **Conjunctivitis:** Children have tolerated 4 to 5 homeopathic pills of *Euphrasia* 30C daily for 3 days for prevention of viral conjunctivitis in a randomized, controlled trial.[2] However, there are insufficient available safety or efficacy data to recommend for or against eyebright use in children for any indication.

Toxicology

- Anecdotal reports have noted that as little as 10 drops of eyebright tincture may result in a variety of adverse effects, including confusion, constipation, cough, diaphoresis, dyspnea, headache, hoarse voice, insomnia, nausea, ocular changes, ocular itching, redness and inflammation, photophobia, polyuria, toothache, and yawning.

ADVERSE EFFECTS/PRECAUTIONS/CONTRAINDICATIONS
Allergy

- Known allergy/hypersensitivity to eyebright or to any of its constituents.
- Hypersensitivity to members of the Scrophulariaceae family may lead to a cross-sensitivity reaction (theoretical).

Adverse Effects

- **General:** Systematic study of clinical safety and tolerability has been limited. Both children and adults have tolerated short-term ophthalmologic use of eyebright for conjunctivitis.[1,2] However, the potential exists for contamination of ophthalmologic preparations of eyebright, and eyebright tincture has been anecdotally associated with pruritus, redness, and swelling of the eye, vision changes, and photophobia. Other symptoms reported anecdotally include toothache, sneezing, yawning, insomnia, and diaphoresis.
- **Neurologic:** Eyebright has been associated with confusion and headache anecdotally.
- **Ocular:** Anecdotal reports have included raised ocular pressure, lacrimation, pruritus, redness, swelling of eyelid margins, vision changes, and photophobia.
- **Pulmonary:** Eyebright has been associated with cough, dyspnea, nasal congestion, hoarseness, and expectoration in anecdotal reports.
- **Gastrointestinal:** Nausea and constipation have been described with eyebright use anecdotally.
- **Endocrine:** In a rat study, eyebright was found to exert no hypoglycemic effects in normal animals, although in rats with chemically induced diabetes, glucose levels were reduced.[3] The clinical implications in humans are not clear.
- **Genitourinary:** Polyuria has been reported anecdotally.

Precautions/Warnings/Contraindications

- Use cautiously as an ophthalmic treatment, particularly homemade preparations, due to the risk of ophthalmic infection from lack of sterility.
- Use cautiously in patients with diabetes, due to an animal study that demonstrated alterations in blood glucose.
- Use cautiously in patients taking medications metabolized by the cytochrome P450 system, due to an animal study that demonstrated inhibition of CYP P450.

Pregnancy and Lactation

- Not recommended, due to insufficient data.

INTERACTIONS
Eyebright/Drug Interactions

- **Cytochrome P450 (CYP450) metabolized agents:** Theoretically, eyebright may interact with medications that are metabolized by CYP450. An animal study conducted on rat livers demonstrated inhibition of CYP450 by the aglycone of aucubin.[4] However, this effect has not been evaluated in humans.
- **Hypoglycemic agents, insulin:** Theoretically, eyebright may interact with medications that alter blood glucose levels. In a rat study, eyebright was found to exert no hypoglycemic effects in normal animals, although in rats with chemically induced diabetes, glucose levels were reduced.[3]

Eyebright/Herb/Supplement Interactions

- **Cytochrome P450 (CYP450) metabolized herbs and supplements:** Theoretically, eyebright may interact with agents that are metabolized by CYP450. An animal study conducted on rat livers demonstrated inhibition of CYP450 by the aglycone of aucubin.[4] However, this effect has not been evaluated in humans.
- **Hypoglycemic herbs/supplements:** Theoretically, eyebright may interact with medications that alter blood glucose levels. In a rat study, eyebright was found to exert no hypoglycemic effects in normal animals, although in rats with chemically induced diabetes, glucose levels were reduced.[3]

Eyebright/Food Interactions

- Insufficient available data.

Eyebright/Lab Interactions

- Insufficient available data.

MECHANISM OF ACTION
Pharmacology

- **Constituents:** Eyebright contains iridoid glycosides, including aucubin[5,6] and flavonoids, including quercetin, apigenin, and tannins. The most studied constituent of eyebright is aucubin and its aglycone, aucubigenin. However, a mechanism of therapeutic action is not known at this time.
- **Anti-inflammatory effects:** In an animal study of inflammation, an oral dose of aucubin (100 mg/kg) demonstrated an anti-inflammatory effect comparable to that of indomethacin.[7] A more recent *in vitro* study suggested that iridoid glycosides might act through inhibition of thromboxane-synthase enzyme.[8]
- **Antimicrobial effects:** Aucubigenin, the aglycone of aucubin, has been shown *in vitro* to possess antibacterial effects against *Staphylococcus aureus*, *Proteus mirabilis*, and *Bacillus subtilis*, antifungal activity against *Candida albicans* and *Penicillium italicum*,[9,10] as well as anti–hepatitis B virus activity.[11]
- **Hepatoprotective effects:** Aucubigenin, the aglycone of aucubin, inhibited hepatic RNA polymerase and protein synthesis *in vivo* and *in vitro*.[12,13] In a study conducted on rat livers, aucubin inhibited the cytochrome P450 enzyme system through a glutaraldehyde-like protein cross-linking mechanism.[4] Such mechanisms may mediate hepatoprotective properties against liver toxins such as carbon tetrachloride and alpha-amanitin.[14]

Pharmacodynamics/Kinetics

- **Bioavailability:** Aucubin, a constituent of eyebright, has shown linear pharmacokinetic behavior when administered intravenously to rats at doses of 40 to 400 mg/kg.[15] The half-life of aucubin in the post-distributive phase was 42.5 minutes, total body clearance was 7.2 mL/min/kg, and the volume of distribution was 346.9 mL/kg at a given dose of 40 mg/kg.[15] When 100 mg/kg of aucubin was administered orally, intraperitoneally, and hepatoportally to rats, bioavailability was 19.3%, 76.8% and 83.5%, respectively, with a low plasma protein binding of 9%.[15]

- **Metabolism:** Both fecal flora and bacterial strains isolated from human feces transformed aucubin to aucubigenin, aucubinine A, and aucubinine B.[16] Aucubin is thought to be initially hydrolyzed to aucubigenin and glucose by bacterial β-glucosidase. Aucubigenin may then react with an ammonia model to form a base, which may be further subjected to reduction of the double bond and the hydroxymethyl group, oxidation of the hydroxyl group, and aromatization of the nitrogen-containing ring, to give aucubinines A and B. It is not known whether these compounds are pharmacologically active.

HISTORY

- Eyebright (*Euphrasia officinalis*) is a small, downy herb that grows annually to a height of 28 inches in grassy areas, with small white or red flowers that are sometimes streaked with purple.
- Eyebright's genus name, *Euphrasia*, is derived from the Greek "Euphrosyne," the name of one of the three graces, who was distinguished for joy and mirth. Eyebright was used as early as the time of Theophrastus and Dioscorides, who prescribed infusions for topical applications in the treatment of eye infections. During the Middle Ages, eyebright was widely prescribed by medical practitioners as an eye medication and as a cure for "all evils of the eye."
- Eyebright was used by Queen Elizabeth as ale, and as a component of British herbal tobacco, which was smoked in order to alleviate chronic bronchial conditions and colds.

REVIEW OF THE EVIDENCE: DISCUSSION

Conjunctivitis

Summary

- Eyebright has been used in ophthalmic solutions for centuries, in the management of multiple eye conditions. Beyond historical and anecdotal reports, one controlled study in children and one open-label trial in adults have investigated eyebright for conjunctivitis. There are insufficient safety data for this indication, with concerns regarding potential contamination of products and risk of infection. There is currently insufficient scientific evidence to recommend for or against the use of eyebright in the treatment of conjunctivitis.

Evidence

- Mokkapatti conducted a randomized, double-blind, placebo-controlled study evaluating approximately 1300 school-aged children to evaluate the efficacy of *Euphrasia* in preventing viral conjunctivitis.[2] During an epidemic of viral conjunctivitis, children were recruited and randomized to receive placebo or 4 or 5 tablets of a homeopathic preparation of *Euphrasia* 30C daily for 3 days. One week following the third dose, a total of 994 children (available for follow-up) were re-examined for conjunctivitis. The authors reported that in the *Euphrasia* group, 48 children exhibited signs and/or symptoms of conjunctivitis, compared to 43 children in the placebo group. Severe conjunctivitis was seen more frequently in the placebo group, whereas the incidence of mild symptoms was higher in the experimental group. However, none of the results reached statistical significance. Limitations of this study included a poor description of randomization or blinding methods.

- Stoss et al. conducted a prospective, open-label, one-armed, multi-center cohort trial examining the safety and efficacy of single-dose eyebright eye drops in 80 patients with conjunctivitis.[1] Anthroposophical general practitioners and ophthalmologists in Germany and Switzerland participated. Patients were prescribed 1 drop 1 to 5 times daily for 3 to 17 days. The study used *Euphrasia* single-dose eye drops (WALA Heilmittel GmbH, Eck-walden/Bad Boll, Germany). Efficacy measures included assessment of the occurrence of redness, swelling, secretion, burning, and foreign body sensation. Tolerability measures included conjunctival redness or burning, veiled vision and foreign body sensation; data from 65 patients were evaluated. Fifteen patients were excluded; 1 patient did not use the medication and 14 patients reported a time period from baseline to follow-up examination greater than 17 days. Results indicated that 81.5% experienced a "complete recovery." Only 1 patient experienced slight worsening of symptoms. A majority of patients (86%) evaluated the efficacy of eyebright as good to very good. These results were comparable to the physician assessment. A greater majority of patients, by self-report (94%) and physician assessment (97%), described tolerability as "good" to "very good." The limitations of this study included the lack of a placebo group and use of subjective outcome measures.

Anti-inflammatory

Summary

- Limited evidence from animal research suggests that several iridoid glycosides isolated from eyebright, particularly aucubin, possess anti-inflammatory properties comparable to

Review of the Evidence: Eyebright

Condition Treated*	Study Design	Author, Year	N[†]	SS[†]	Study Quality[‡]	Magnitude of Benefit	ARR[†]	NNT[†]	Comments
Conjunctivitis (Prevention)	RCT	Mokkapatti[2] 1992	1300	No	2	NA	NA	NA	Study during viral conjunctivitis epidemic; *Euphrasia* vs. placebo for 3 days.
Conjunctivitis (Inflammatory)	Prospective cohort study	Stoss[1] 2000	80	NA	NA	Small	NA	NA	*Euphrasia* efficacy and tolerability assessed by patients and clinicians.

*Primary or secondary outcome.
[†] *N*, Number of patients; *SS*, statistically significant; *ARR*, absolute risk reduction; *NNT*, the number of patients who need to undergo a specific intervention in order to observe an outcome in one individual.
[‡] 0-2 = poor; 3-4 = good; 5 = excellent.
NA, Not applicable; *RCT*, randomized, controlled trial.
For an explanation of each category in this table, please see Table 3 in the Introduction.

those of indomethacin. The mechanism of action may be the inhibition of thromboxane synthase.[7,8] The clinical relevance in humans is unclear, and there are no known human clinical observations or controlled trials in this area. Therefore, there is currently insufficient evidence to recommend for or against eyebright as an anti-inflammatory agent.

Hepatoprotection
Summary

• Limited evidence from animal studies suggests that aucubin, a constituent of eyebright, may inhibit hepatic RNA and protein syntheses *in vivo*. These properties have been associated with protective effects in carbon tetrachloride and alpha-amanitine–induced hepatotoxicity in mice. Conversion of aucubin to its aglycone appears to be a prerequisite step for these hepatic effects to occur.[11,12,17] The clinical relevance of these findings for humans is unclear, and there is currently insufficient evidence to recommend for or against the use of eyebright as a hepatoprotective agent.

References

1. Stoss M, Michels C, Peter E, et al. Prospective cohort trial of Euphrasia single-dose eye drops in conjunctivitis. J Altern Complement Med 2000;6(6):499-508.
2. Mokkapatti R. An experimental double-blind study to evaluate the use of *Euphrasia* in preventing conjunctivitis. Brit Homeopath J 1992;1(81):22-24.
3. Porchezhian E, Ansari SH, Shreedharan NK. Antihyperglycemic activity of *Euphrasia officinale* leaves. Fitoterapia 2000;71(5):522-526.
4. Bartholomaeus A, Ahokas J. Inhibition of P-450 by aucubin: is the biological activity of aucubin due to its glutaraldehyde-like aglycone? Toxicol Lett 1995;80(1-3):75-83.
5. Salama O, Sticher O. Iridoid glucosides from *Euphrasia rostkoviana*. Part 4. Glycosides from *Euphrasia* species. Planta Med 1983;47:90-94.
6. Ersoz T, Berkman MZ, Tasdemir D, et al. An iridoid glucoside from *Euphrasia pectinata*. J Nat Prod 2000;63(10):1449-1450.
7. Recio MC, Giner RM, Manez S, et al. Structural considerations on the iridoids as anti-inflammatory agents. Planta Med 1994;60(3):232-234.
8. Bermejo BP, Diaz Lanza AM, Silvan Sen AM, et al. Effects of some iridoids from plant origin on arachidonic acid metabolism in cellular systems. Planta Med 2000;66(4):324-328.
9. Rombouts JE, Links J. The chemical nature of the antibacterial substance present in *Aucuba japonica* Thunbg. Experientia 1956;12(2):78-80.
10. Ulubelen A, Topcu G, Eris C, et al. Terpenoids from *Salvia sclarea*. Phytochemistry 1994;36(4):971-974.
11. Chang IM. Liver-protective activities of aucubin derived from traditional oriental medicine. Res Commun Mol Pathol Pharmacol 1998;102(2):189-204.
12. Chang IM, Ryu JC, Park YC, et al. Protective activities of aucubin against carbon tetrachloride-induced liver damage in mice. Drug Chem Toxicol 1983;6(5):443-453.
13. Lee DH, Cho IG, Park MS, et al. Studies on the possible mechanisms of protective activity against alpha- amanitin poisoning by aucubin. Arch Pharm Res 2001;24(1):55-63.
14. Chang I, Yamaura Y. Aucubin: a new antidote for poisonous amanita mushrooms. Phytother Res 1993;7:53-56.
15. Suh NJ, Shim CK, Lee MH, et al. Pharmacokinetic study of an iridoid glucoside: aucubin. Pharm Res 1991;8(8):1059-1063.
16. Hattori M, Kawata Y, Inoue K, et al. Transformation of aucubin to new pyridine monoterpene alkaloids, aucubinines A and B, by human intestinal bacteria. Phytother Res 1990;4(2):66-70.
17. Chang I. Antiviral activity of Aucubin against Hepatitis B virus replication. Phytother Res 1997;11(3):189-192.

E

Fenugreek
(Trigonella foenum-graecum L. Leguminosae)

SYNONYMS/COMMON NAMES/RELATED SUBSTANCES

- Abish, alholva, bird's foot, bockhornsklover, bockshornsamen, bockshornklee, cemen, chilbe, fenegriek, fenogrego, fenugree, fenugreek seed, fenogreco, fenigreko, fenu-thyme, foenugraeci semen, gorogszena, graine de fenugrec, gray hay, Greek hay seed, griechische heusamen, fieno greco, halba, hilbeh, hulba, hu lu ba, kasoori methi, kozieradka pospolita, kreeka lambalaats, mente, mentikura, mentula, methi, methika, methini, methri, methro, mithiguti, pazhitnik grecheskiy, penantazi, sag methi, sambala, sarviapila, shabaliidag, shambelile, trogonella semen, trigonelline, uluhaal, uwatu, vendayam, venthiam.

CLINICAL BOTTOM LINE
Background

- Fenugreek has a long history of medical uses in Indian and Chinese medicine and has been used for numerous indications, including labor induction, aiding digestion, and as a general tonic to improve metabolism and health.
- Preliminary animal and methodologically weak human trials have suggested possible hypoglycemic and antihyperlipidemic properties of oral fenugreek seed powder. However, at this time, the evidence is not sufficient to recommend either for or against fenugreek for diabetes or hyperlipidemia. Nonetheless, caution is warranted in patients taking hypoglycemic agents, in whom blood glucose levels should be monitored. Hypokalemia has also been reported, and potassium levels should be followed in patients taking concomitant hypokalemic agents, or with underlying cardiac disease.

Scientific Evidence for Common/Studied Uses	Grade*
Diabetes mellitus type 1	C
Diabetes mellitus type 2	C
Hyperlipidemia	C

*Key to grades: *A:* Strong scientific evidence for this use; *B:* Good scientific evidence for this use; *C:* Unclear scientific evidence for this use; *D:* Fair scientific evidence against this use (it may not work); *F:* Strong scientific evidence against this use (it likely does not work). For a more detailed explanation of efficacy criteria, see "Natural Standard Evidence-Based Validated Grading Rationale" in the Introduction.

Historical or Theoretical Uses That Lack Sufficient Evidence

- Abortifacient, abscesses, antioxidant,[1] aphthous ulcers, appetite stimulant, asthenia, atherosclerosis, baldness, beriberi, boils, breast enhancement,[2] bronchitis, burns, cancer,[3] cellulitis, chapped lips, colic, colon cancer,[1] constipation, convalescence, cough (chronic), dermatitis, diarrhea, digestion, dropsy, dysentery, dyspepsia, eczema, flatulence, furunculosis, galactagogue (lactation stimulant), gastritis, gastric ulcers,[4] gout, hepatic disease, hepatomegaly, hernia, hypertension, immunomodulator,[5] impotence, indigestion, infections, inflammation, inflammatory bowel disease, labor induction (uterine stimulant), leg edema, leg ulcers, leukemia,[6]

lice, low energy, lymphadenitis, menopausal symptoms, myalgia, postmenopausal vaginal dryness, protection against alcohol toxicity, rickets, splenomegaly, stomach upset, thyroxine-induced hyperglycemia,[7] tuberculosis, vitamin deficiencies, wound healing.

Expert Opinion and Folkloric Precedent

- In India, fenugreek is commonly consumed as a condiment.[8] It is also used medicinally as a lactation stimulant (galactagogue) and during pregnancy.[9] Fenugreek has been recommended for a variety of other ailments, ranging from diabetes to indigestion and baldness. Fenugreek is purported to contain an estrogenic constituent and has been recommended for menstrual disorders and menopausal symptoms. However, there is scant evidence in this area.[10] In the United States, fenugreek has been used since the 19th century for menstrual pain and postmenopausal vaginal dryness. The German expert panel, the Commission E, has approved the use of fenugreek seed to treat loss of appetite and local inflammation.

Safety Summary

- **Likely safe:** When used in the amounts commonly found in food. In a 24-week study of 25 g/day of powdered fenugreek seeds in 60 diabetics, no hepatic, renal, or hematologic abnormalities were detected, although the size of this study is likely too small to generalize results.[11]
- **Possibly safe:** When used in recommended amounts for up to 3 months.[12,13]
- **Possibly unsafe:** When used by individuals taking hypoglycemic agents, due to the risk of precipitating hypoglycemia, and when used in patients taking hypokalemic agents, prone to hypokalemia, taking cardiac glycoside drugs, or with underlying cardiac disease.

DOSING/TOXICOLOGY
General

- Recommended doses are based on available clinical trials or historical practice. However, with natural products, the optimal doses needed to balance efficacy and safety often have not been determined. Formulations and preparation methods may vary from manufacturer to manufacturer, and from batch to batch of a specific product made by a single manufacturer. Because often the active components of a product are not known, standardization may not be possible, and the clinical effects of different brands may not be comparable.

Standardization

- Different clinical trials have used different doses of fenugreek preparations. Because the active ingredient(s) of fenugreek is yet to be identified, it is impossible to relate these preparations to a standard dose. The preparation doses, where known, are listed here.

Dosing: Adult (18 Years and Older)
Oral

- **Type 1 diabetes:** 100 g of debitterized powdered fenugreek seeds divided into 2 equal doses.[14]

- **Type 2 diabetes:** 2.5 g of fenugreek seed powder in capsule form, twice daily for 3 months[15]; 25 g of seed powder, divided into 2 equal doses.[11-13]
- **Hyperlipidemia:** 2.5 g of fenugreek seed powder in capsule form, twice daily for 3 months[15]; or 100 g of debittered powdered seeds divided into 2 equal doses.[14,16]
- *Note:* Products rich in fenugreek fiber may interfere with the absorption of oral medications due to its mucilaginous fiber content and high viscosity in the gut. Medications should be taken separately from such products. However, it should be noted that fenugreek is rarely used for its fiber content.

Dosing: Pediatric (Younger Than 18 Years)

- Insufficient data available.

Toxicology

- Toxicological evaluation in 60 diabetic patients taking 25 grams/day of powdered fenugreek seeds for 24 weeks reported no clinical hepatic or renal toxicity and no hematological abnormalities.[11] However, the size of this study is likely too small to generalize results.
- The acute oral LD_{50} was found to be >5 g/kg in rats, and the acute dermal LD_{50} was >2 g/kg in rabbits.[17] Debittered fenugreek powder failed to induce any signs of toxicity or mortality following acute and subchronic regimens in mice and rats.[18] When given fenugreek seeds for 90 days, weanling rats did not experience significant hematologic, hepatic, or histopathologic changes.[19]

ADVERSE EFFECTS/PRECAUTIONS/CONTRAINDICATIONS
Allergy

- Caution is warranted in patients with known fenugreek allergy or with allergy to chickpeas, because of possible cross-reactivity.[9]
- Fenugreek contained in curry powder was found to be an allergen in a patient who reported severe bronchospasm, wheezing, and diarrhea.[20] Inhaling fenugreek seed powder elicited allergic rhinitis, wheezing and syncope in two patients.[9] A single application of fenugreek to the scalp of a patient with chronic asthma caused numbness of the head, facial angioedema, and wheezing.[9]

Adverse Effects/Postmarket Surveillance

- **General:** Literature review reveals no reports of clinically significant harmful adverse effects. Fenugreek has traditionally been considered safe and well tolerated.
- **Dermatologic:** A single application of fenugreek to the scalp of a patient with chronic asthma was noted to cause numbness of the head, facial angioedema, and wheezing.[9]
- **Neurologic/CNS:** Inhaling fenugreek seed powder caused syncope in two patients who may have had allergies to the powder.[9] However, these reactions occurred in an occupational setting following recurrent exposure to large amounts of powder, and thus may be of limited relevance to general use. Dizziness was rarely reported in a small, methodologically weak clinical study of fenugreek aqueous extract.[21]
- **Pulmonary/Respiratory:** Inhaling fenugreek seed powder has been reported to elicit bronchospasm[20] and wheezing[9] in some individuals. However, these reactions have often occurred in an occupational setting following recurrent exposure to large amounts of powder, and thus may be of limited relevance to general use.

- **Gastrointestinal:** Transient diarrhea and flatulence have been reported.[11,22,23] Fenugreek fibers are not fermented by human colonic bacteria, and therefore may possess a laxative effect.[24]
- **Renal:** A fenugreek aqueous extract was found to reduce potassium levels by 14% in a small, poorly described study of healthy humans.[21] No changes were observed in serum creatinine or blood urea nitrogen (BUN) in a series of 60 diabetic patients given fenugreek powder for 12 weeks.[11] Theoretically, fenugreek may decrease calcium oxalate deposition and stone formation.[9] Increased frequency of micturition was noted in a small, poorly described clinical study of fenugreek aqueous extract.[21]
- **Endocrine (hypoglycemia):** Multiple preclinical studies and small, methodologically weak human investigations have reported both acute and chronic hypoglycemic properties of fenugreek seed powder and aqueous extract.[14-16,21,22,25-27]
- **Endocrine (thyroid):** Decreased serum T_3 and T_3/T_4 ratio, as well as increased T_4 levels, have been observed in mice and rats.[28] Decreased body weight has also been reported and was attributed to decreases in T_3.[28] TFG seed extract has been shown to reduce thyroid hormone concentrations and serum glucose (attributed to thyroxine-induced hyperglycemia) in rats.[7]
- **Hematologic:** Fenugreek preparations may contain coumarin derivatives that can raise prothrombin time (PT) or international normalized ratio (INR) and may increase the risk of bleeding. There is one report of a patient taking warfarin for atrial fibrillation, who was noted to have an increased INR while also using the herbs fenugreek and boldo.[29] Bleeding was not noted.

Precautions/Warnings/Contraindications

- Use cautiously in patients using hypoglycemic agents, and follow blood sugars.[14-16,21,22,25-27]
- Use cautiously in patients taking hypokalemic agents, prone to hypokalemia, using cardiac glycoside drugs, or with underlying cardiac disease (due to risk of hypokalemia).[21]
- Use cautiously in patients who are allergic to chickpeas, due to possible cross-reactivity.[9]
- Use cautiously in patients taking anticoagulants, due to a theoretical increased bleeding risk.[29]
- Use cautiously in children, due to the risk of hypoglycemia.[30]
- Avoid use during pregnancy, due to uterine stimulant properties reported in animals.[31,32]

Pregnancy and Lactation

- Literature review reveals no reliable human data or systematic study of fenugreek during pregnancy or lactation. Caution is warranted during pregnancy because of potential hypoglycemic effects. In addition, both water and alcoholic extracts of fenugreek exert a stimulating effect on the isolated guinea pig uterus, especially during late pregnancy.[31] Therefore, fenugreek may possess abortifacient effects and is usually not recommended for use during pregnancy in doses higher than found in foods.[32]

INTERACTIONS
Fenugreek/Drug Interactions

- **General:** Products rich in fenugreek fiber may interfere with the absorption of oral medications, due to its mucilaginous fiber content and high viscosity in the gut. Medications should be taken separately from such products.
- **Anticoagulants, antiplatelet drugs, nonsteroidal anti-inflammatory drugs (NSAIDs):** Fenugreek preparations

may contain coumarin derivatives which can raise prothrombin time (PT) or international normalized ratio (INR), and may increase the risk of bleeding. There is one report of a patient taking warfarin for atrial fibrillation, who was noted to have an increased INR while also using the herbs fenugreek and boldo.[29] Bleeding was not noted. Concomitant use of fenugreek and anticoagulants/antiplatelet agents is not advised.

- **Hypoglycemic drugs, insulin:** Data from preclinical studies and small, methodologically weak human investigations suggest that fenugreek possesses both acute and chronic hypoglycemic properties. Concomitant use with other hypoglycemic agents may lower serum glucose more than expected, and levels should be monitored closely.[14-16,21,22,25-27]
- **Hypokalemic agents:** A fenugreek aqueous extract was found to reduce potassium levels by 14% in a small, poorly described study of healthy humans, and may precipitate hypokalemia when used with some diuretics, laxatives, mineralocorticoids, or other hypokalemic agents.[21]
- **Hormone replacement therapy (HRT), oral contraceptives (OCPs):** Fenugreek is purported to contain an estrogenic constituent, although there are limited data in this area. Based on such anecdotes, caution is warranted in patients using estrogenic therapies.
- **Laxatives:** Fenugreek fibers are not fermented by human colonic bacteria, and therefore may possess laxative effects.[24] Therefore, concomitant use of high-fiber fenugreek products with other laxatives may precipitate loose stools or diarrhea. However, it should be noted that fenugreek is rarely used for its fiber content.
- **Monoamine oxidase inhibitors (MAOIs):** Fenugreek has been theorized to possibly potentiate the activity of MAOIs, although there are no reliable human data in this area.
- **Thyroid replacement therapy, anti-thyroid therapy:** Decreased serum T_3 and T_3/T_4 ratio, as well as increased T_4 levels, have been observed in mice and rats given fenugreek.[28] In theory, these effects may interfere with thyroid therapies, although there are no reliable human data in this area. TFG seed extract has been shown to reduce thyroid hormone concentrations and serum glucose (thyroxine induced hyperglycemia) in rats.[7]
- **Cardiac glycosides (digoxin, digitoxin):** Fenugreek aqueous extract was found to reduce potassium levels by 14% in a small, poorly described study of healthy humans, and theoretically may precipitate toxicity in patients taking cardiac glycoside agents.[21]
- **Corticosteroids:** Based on its constituents, fenugreek has been theorized to potentially inhibit the activity of corticosteroid drugs, although there are no reliable human data in this area.

Fenugreek/Herb Interactions

- **General:** Products rich in fenugreek fiber may interfere with the absorption of oral agents due to its mucilaginous fiber content and high viscosity in the gut. Medications should be taken separately from such products.
- **Anticoagulant and antiplatelet agents:** Fenugreek preparations may contain coumarin derivatives that can raise prothrombin time (PT) or international normalized ratio (INR), and may increase the risk of bleeding. There is one report of a patient taking warfarin for atrial fibrillation, who was noted to have an increased INR while also using the herbs fenugreek and boldo.[29] Bleeding was not noted to occur. Concomitant use of fenugreek with agents that increase risk of bleeding, such as garlic, ginger, and ginkgo, is not advised.

- **Cardiac glycoside herbs:** Fenugreek aqueous extract was found to reduce potassium levels by 14% in a small, poorly described study of healthy humans and theoretically may precipitate toxicity in patients taking cardiac glycoside agents.[21]
- **Hypoglycemic herbs and supplements:** Data from preclinical studies and small, methodologically weak human investigations suggest that fenugreek possesses hypoglycemic properties. Concomitant use with other hypoglycemic agents may lower serum glucose more than expected, and levels should be monitored closely.
- **Laxatives:** Fenugreek fibers are not fermented by human colonic bacteria and therefore may possess laxative effects.[24] Therefore, concomitant use of high-fiber fenugreek products with other laxatives may precipitate loose stools or diarrhea. However, it should be noted that fenugreek is rarely used for its fiber content.
- **Monoamine oxidase inhibitor (MAOI) herbs and supplements:** Fenugreek has been theorized to possibly potentiate the activity of MAOIs, although there are no available human data in this area.
- **Phytoestrogens:** Fenugreek is purported to contain an estrogenic constituent, although there are limited data in this area. Based on such anecdotes, caution may be warranted in patients using other estrogenic therapies.
- **Thyroid-active herbs and supplements:** TFG seed extract has been shown to reduce thyroid hormone concentrations and serum glucose (attributed to thyroxine-induced hyperglycemia) in rats.[7]

Fenugreek/Food Interactions

- Review of the literature reveals no reported serious reactions in humans, although fenugreek may affect key enzymes of carbohydrate metabolism.[33] The effects of domestic processing and cooking methods on total HCl-extractable iron from fenugreek leaves have been studied *in vitro*.[34]

Fenugreek/Lab Interactions

- **Serum glucose:** Data from preclinical studies and small preliminary human investigations suggest that fenugreek possesses hypoglycemic properties.[14-16,21,22,25-27]
- Glucose levels should be monitored in patients using other hypoglycemic agents.
- **Serum potassium:** A fenugreek aqueous extract was found to reduce potassium levels by 14% in a small, poorly described study of healthy humans.[21]
- **Sotolone (pseudo–maple syrup urine disease):** False diagnoses of maple syrup urine disease have been published in case reports, based on the excretion of sotolone following ingestion of fenugreek herbal tea (sotolone is the compound responsible for the aroma in maple syrup urine disease).[30,35] Fenugreek has also been implicated in the production of a body odor similar to that produced by maple syrup urine disease in an infant.[36]
- **Thyroid panel:** Decreased serum T_3 and T_3/T_4 ratio, as well as increased T_4 levels, have been observed in mice and rats given fenugreek.[28]

MECHANISM OF ACTION
Pharmacology

- **Hypoglycemic effects:** Hypoglycemic effects of fenugreek observed in animal studies have been associated with a fraction that contains the testa and endosperm of the defatted seeds, called the A subfraction. These effects have not been observed with lipid extracts.[37,38] Hypoglycemic effects have been attributed to several mechanisms: Sauvaire et al. demonstrated that the amino acid 4-hyroxyisoleucine in fenugreek seeds increases glucose-induced insulin release *in vitro* in human and rat pancreatic islet cells.[39] This amino acid appeared to act only on pancreatic beta cells, as somatostatin and glucagon were not altered in the study. In human studies, fenugreek reduced the area under the curve (AUC) for plasma glucose and increased the number of insulin receptors via an unclear mechanism.[13] Fenugreek seeds have also been postulated to exert hypoglycemic effects by stimulating glucose-dependent insulin release by beta cells[40] or via inhibition of α-amylase and sucrase activity.[41]

- **Lipid-lowering effects:** In animal studies, fenugreek has been found to lower triglycerides, total cholesterol, and low-density lipoprotein (LDL) levels.[42-46] These effects may be due to saponins, a class of molecules present in fenugreek that are transformed in the gastrointestinal tract to sapogenins. Sapogenins increase biliary cholesterol secretion, potentially leading to lower serum cholesterol levels.[42,47-49]

Pharmacodynamics/Kinetics

- Pharmacokinetic data are not available for all components of fenugreek, or for the compound as a whole. Saponins present in fenugreek are believed to be primarily absorbed in the terminal ileum.[50]

HISTORY

- Fenugreek is one of the oldest medicinal plants, and originated in India and Northern Africa. This annual plant grows to an average height of two feet. Fenugreek leaves and seeds, which mature in long pods, are used to prepare extracts or powders for medicinal use.
- Medicinal applications of fenugreek were documented in ancient Egypt, where it was used in incense and for embalming mummies. In modern Egypt, fenugreek is still used as a supplement to wheat and maize flour for bread-making.[8]
- In ancient Rome, fenugreek was purportedly used to aid labor and delivery. In Chinese traditional medicine, fenugreek

seeds have been used as a tonic, as well as for weakness and edema of the legs.[49]

- In India, fenugreek is commonly consumed as a condiment.[8] It is also used medicinally as a lactation stimulant.[9] There are numerous other folkloric uses of fenugreek, ranging from indigestion to baldness.

REVIEW OF THE EVIDENCE: DISCUSSION

Type 2 Diabetes
Summary

- In animal studies and in several small, methodologically weak human trials, fenugreek has been found to lower serum glucose levels both acutely and chronically. Although promising, these data cannot be considered definitive, and at this time there is insufficient evidence to recommend either for or against fenugreek for type 2 diabetes. Trials have used a diversity of preparations, dosing regimens, and outcomes measures. No long-term investigations have been conducted. Additional study is warranted in this area.

Evidence

- Gupta et al. reported the results of a small, randomized, controlled, double-blind trial to evaluate the effects of fenugreek seeds on glycemic control.[51] Over a 2-month period, 25 patients with newly diagnosed type 2 diabetes were assigned to receive either 1 g/day of a hydroalcoholic extract of fenugreek seeds or "usual care" (dietary discretion and exercise). Outcome measures included mean changes in fasting glucose, oral glucose tolerance, insulin resistance, and lipid levels. Baseline values were similar between groups. After 2 months, mean fasting blood glucose levels were reduced in both groups without significant differences between groups (148.3 to 119.9 in the fenugreek group vs. 137.5 to 113.0 in the "usual care" group). In addition, there were no significant differences between groups in mean glucose tolerance test values at the study's end (210.6 to 181.1 vs. 219.9 to 241.6). The authors did note differences

Review of the Evidence: Fenugreek

Condition Treated*	Study Design	Author, Year	N[†]	SS[†]	Study Quality[‡]	Magnitude of Benefit	ARR[†]	NNT[†]	Comments
Type 2 diabetes, hyperlipidemia	RCT, double-blind	Gupta[51] 2001	25	Yes	3	None	NA	NA	Improved fasting glucose and GTT with fenugreek seeds or diet/exercise, without differences between groups; Altered AUC and insulin resistance with fenugreek.
Type 2 diabetes	RTC, crossover	Raghuram[13] 1994	10	Yes	1	Large	NA	NA	Improved peripheral glucose utilization with fenugreek seed supplementation.
Type 2 diabetes	RCT, crossover	Sharma[16] 1990	15	Yes	1	Small	NA	NA	Improvement in reported diabetic symptoms.
Type 2 diabetes	Case series with matched controls	Neeraja[52] 1996	12	Yes	1	Medium	NA	NA	Improvement of acute glycemic response, most notable with raw fenugreek seed powder.
Type 1 diabetes, hyperlipidemia	RCT, crossover	Sharma[14] 1990	10	Yes	1	Large	NA	NA	Fasting blood glucose levels and GTT improved; serum insulin levels unchanged.

*Primary or secondary outcome.
[†]N, Number of patients; SS, statistically significant; ARR, absolute risk reduction; NNT, the number of patients who need to undergo a specific intervention in order to observe an outcome in one individual.
[‡]0-2 = poor; 3-4 = good; 5 = excellent.
AUC, Area under the curve; GTT, glucose torerance test; NA, not applicable; RCT, randomized, controlled trial.
For an explanation of each category in this table, please see Table 3 in the Introduction.

between groups in the area under the curve (AUC) for blood glucose (2375 vs. 2759) and insulin levels (2492 vs. 2428). Beta-cell secretion and insulin resistance were reported as improved in the fenugreek group, based on HOMA-modeling. Significant decreases in triglyceride levels and increases in high-density lipoproteins ("good cholesterol") were also reported, although total cholesterol and low-density lipoproteins ("bad cholesterol") were not significantly altered. Although these measures of insulin resistance are mechanistically interesting, this study reports a lack of significant differences between groups in fasting sugars or glucose tolerance. It suggests that fenugreek seed extract and diet/exercise may be equally effective strategies for attaining glycemic control in type 2 diabetes. However, the trial may have been too small or brief to detect significant mean differences between groups. In addition, it is not clear if mean glucose values would have normalized without any intervention. Randomization and statistical methods were not well reported, which limits the clinical relevance of the results.

- Raghuram et al. reported a randomized, controlled, crossover trial of fenugreek in 10 patients with type 2 diabetes.[13] For 15 days, patients were given 25 g of powdered fenugreek seeds (into 2 equal doses) with meals, or meals without fenugreek. Subjects were then crossed over for an additional 15 days. In the fenugreek-treated patients, statistically significant mean improvements were reported for glucose tolerance test scores and serum clearance rates of glucose. Although these results are promising, it is not clear that this study was properly randomized or blinded, creating the possibility of bias and confounding. Methodology and statistical analysis were not adequately described. In addition, the correlation between dose and response was not clear, and the specific preparation of fenugreek was not described. Therefore, the clinical applicability of these results is limited.

- Sharma et al. conducted a randomized, controlled, crossover study in 15 patients with type 2 diabetes.[16] For 10 days, subjects were administered meals containing 100 g of defatted fenugreek seed powder (divided into 2 equal doses), or meals without fenugreek. Patients were then crossed over for an additional 10 days. Significant mean improvements in fasting blood glucose levels and glucose tolerance test results were described in the fenugreek-treated patients. A 64% mean reduction was noted in 24-hour urine glucose levels. The fenugreek patient group also reported subjective improvements in polydipsia and polyuria. However, these results can only be considered preliminary because of methodological weaknesses, which include inadequate description of blinding, randomization, baseline patient characteristics, statistical analysis, and standardization data for the therapy used.

- Neeraja and Rajyalakshmi reported a poorly designed, complex case series in six male type 2 diabetics and six non-diabetics.[52] Subjects fasted overnight and were fed a traditional Indian meal (*pongal*) either without fenugreek or with the addition of 12.5 to 20 g of powdered fenugreek seeds (raw, boiled, or germinated). Fasting serum glucose levels were then measured every 30 minutes for 2 hours. Mean increases in fasting blood sugar were seen in the non-diabetic group following the *pongal* meal, without impressive differences with boiled or germinated fenugreek seed powder. However, a mean reduction in fasting glucose was seen with raw fenugreek seeds on the order of 15%. In diabetics, improvements in blood sugars were similarly seen, with even more dramatic decreases when using raw fenugreek seed

powder between 30 and 120 minutes. However, statistical analysis was not performed, and significance of the results was not clear. In addition, blinding was not noted, thus introducing possible bias. Although the method of preparing fenugreek powder was described in detail, the methodology was incompletely reported. Therefore, although these results are suggestive, they cannot be considered conclusive.

- Results from several additional case series have also suggested that fenugreek seeds may improve glycemic control in type 2 diabetes. As with all case series, however, the lack of controls increases the possibility of results being due to chance and the likelihood of introducing bias or confounders. Therefore, the conclusions can only be considered preliminary. Madar et al. reported significantly improved glycemic responses in 21 type 2 diabetics after taking 15 g of powdered fenugreek seeds for 4 to 7 days.[25] Bordia et al. studied the effects of 2.5 g of fenugreek seed powder given twice daily for 3 months to a sub-group of 40 subjects.[15] The authors reported significant decreases in fasting and post-prandial glucose levels in patients with mild type 2 diabetes and coronary artery disease. No changes in serum glucose were observed in non-diabetics, and smaller, non-significant improvements were seen in severe diabetics. Methodology was not clearly documented. In a poorly described study, Sharma et al. reported significant improvements in glucose tolerance, insulin secretion, and 24-hour urinary glucose concentration (from 26 g to 7 g; $p < 0.05$) during 21 days of therapy with 25 g/day of oral fenugreek.[22] In a different study, Sharma et al. investigated 60 type 2 diabetics taking 25 g/day of fenugreek and reported improved mean glycemic responses, decreased HbA1c, decreased 24-hour urinary glucose levels, and subjective improvements in polyuria, polydipsia, peripheral neuropathy, and skin infections after 8 and 24 weeks ($p < 0.001$).[27]

Type 1 Diabetes
Summary

- Review of the literature reveals animal studies and a small, methodologically weak human trial that suggest possible efficacy of fenugreek in type 1 diabetics. Although promising, these data cannot be considered definitive. At this time there is insufficient evidence to recommend either for or against the use of fenugreek for type 2 diabetes.

Evidence

- Sharma et al. conducted a randomized, controlled, crossover trial in 10 patients with type 1 diabetes.[14] Over a 10-day period, meals were served to subjects either with or without defatted fenugreek seed powder added (100 g in 2 divided doses each day). At the study's end, significant improvement in several parameters were noted in the fenugreek group, including a 54% reduction in 24-hour urine glucose levels and mean reductions in fasting glucose levels and glucose tolerance test values. However, the study's inadequate description of blinding and randomization raise questions about the possibility of bias or confounding being introduced. Although promising, these results can only be considered preliminary.

Hyperlipidemia
Summary

- There is insufficient evidence to support the use of fenugreek as a hyperlipidemic agent. Most available studies are case reports without proper controls, randomization, or blinding.

Evidence

- Sharma et al. conducted a randomized, controlled, crossover trial in 10 patients with type 1 diabetes.[14] Over a 10-day period, meals were served to subjects either with or without defatted fenugreek seed powder added (100 g in 2 divided doses each day). At the study's end, small statistically significant reductions were noted in total cholesterol and in low-density lipoprotein (LDL) levels, but high-density lipoprotein (HDL) levels remained unchanged. Although the results are suggestive, this study's inadequate description of blinding and randomization raise questions about the possibility of bias or confounding being introduced. Therefore, the results can only be considered preliminary.

- Several case series have also reported hypocholesterolemic effects associated with oral fenugreek. As with all case series, however, the lack of controls increases the possibility of results being due to chance, as well as the likelihood of introducing bias or confounders. Therefore, the conclusions can only be considered preliminary. Sharma et al. investigated 15 nonobese, nonsymptomatic hyperlipidemic adults.[53] After ingesting 100 g of defatted fenugreek powder per day for 3 weeks, subjects were reported to have lower triglyceride and LDL cholesterol levels vs. baseline. Slight decreases in HDL levels were also noted. In a later study, normalization of lipid profiles was observed in 60 type 2 diabetic patients whose diets were supplemented with 25 g of powdered fenugreek seeds per day for 24 weeks.[11,12] While mean total cholesterol, LDL, and triglyceride levels decreased by 14% to 16% over the study period, mean HDL cholesterol levels increased by 10%. Similarly, Sowmya et al. observed significant reductions in total cholesterol and LDL levels in 20 hypercholesterolemic adults who received 12.5 to 18 g of powder of germinated fenugreek seeds for 1 month, although no change in HDL, very-low-density lipoprotein (VLDL), or triglyceride levels was observed.[54] Sharma also reported a decrease in total cholesterol levels in five diabetic patients treated with fenugreek seed powder (25 g orally per day) for 21 days.[23] Bordia et al. studied the effects of 2.5 g of fenugreek seed powder administered twice daily for 3 months to a subgroup of 40 subjects.[15] In patients with coronary artery disease and type 2 diabetes, the authors reported significant decreases in total cholesterol and triglycerides, but no change in HDL levels. Methodology was not clearly documented.

FORMULARY: BRANDS USED IN CLINICAL TRIALS
Brands Used in Statistically Significant Clinical Trials

- No specific brands of fenugreek have been used in the available human trials. Preparations used have included debitterized seeds and seed powder.

References

1. Devasena T, Menon VP. Enhancement of circulatory antioxidants by fenugreek during 1,2-dimethylhydrazine–induced rat colon carcinogenesis. J Biochem Mol Biol Biophys 2002;6(4):289-292.
2. Fugh-Berman A. "Bust enhancing" herbal products. Obstet Gynecol 2003;101(6):1345-1349.
3. Sur P, Das M, Gomes A, et al. *Trigonella foenum graecum* (fenugreek) seed extract as an antineoplastic agent. Phytother Res 2001;15(3):257-259.
4. Pandian RS, Anuradha CV, Viswanathan P. Gastroprotective effect of fenugreek seeds (*Trigonella foenum graecum*) on experimental gastric ulcer in rats. J Ethnopharmacol 2002;81(3):393-397.
5. Bin-Hafeez B, Haque R, Parvez S, et al. Immunomodulatory effects of fenugreek (*Trigonella foenum graecum* L.) extract in mice. Int Immunopharmacol 2003;3(2):257-265.
6. Hibasami H, Moteki H, Ishikawa K, et al. Protodioscin isolated from fenugreek (*Trigonella foenum graecum* L.) induces cell death and morphological change indicative of apoptosis in leukemic cell line H-60, but not in gastric cancer cell line KATO III. Int J Mol Med 2003;11(1):23-26.
7. Tahiliani P, Kar A. Mitigation of thyroxine-induced hyperglycaemia by two plant extracts. Phytother Res 2003;17(3):294-296.
8. Zia T, Hasnain SN, Hasan SK. Evaluation of the oral hypoglycaemic effect of *Trigonella foenum-graecum* L. (methi) in normal mice. J Ethnopharmacol 2001;75(2-3):191-195.
9. Patil SP, Niphadkar PV, Bapat MM. Allergy to fenugreek (*Trigonella foenum graecum*). Ann Allergy Asthma Immunol 1997;78(3):297-300.
10. Israel D, Youngkin EQ. Herbal therapies for perimenopausal and menopausal complaints. Pharmacotherapy 1997;17(5):970-984.
11. Sharma RD, Sarkar A, Hazra DK, et al. Toxicological evaluation of fenugreek seeds: a long term feeding experiment in diabetic patients. Phytother Res 1996;10(6):519-520.
12. Sharma RD, Sarkar DK, Hazra B, et al. Hypolipidaemic effect of fenugreek seeds: a chronic study in non-insulin dependent diabetic patients. Phytother Res 1996;10:332-334.
13. Raghuram TC, Sharma RD, Sivakumar B, et al. Effect of fenugreek seeds on intravenous glucose disposition in non-insulin dependent diabetic patients. Phytother Res 1994;8(2):83-86.
14. Sharma RD, Raghuram TC, Rao NS. Effect of fenugreek seeds on blood glucose and serum lipids in type I diabetes. Eur J Clin Nutr 1990;44(4):301-306.
15. Bordia A, Verma SK, Srivastava KC. Effect of ginger (*Zingiber officinale* Rosc.) and fenugreek (*Trigonella foenumgraecum* L.) on blood lipids, blood sugar and platelet aggregation in patients with coronary artery disease. Prostaglandins Leukot Essent Fatty Acids 1997;56(5):379-384.
16. Sharma RD, Raghuram TC. Hypoglycaemic effect of fenugreek seeds in non-insulin dependant diabetic subjects. Nutr Res 1990;10:731-739.
17. Opdyke DL. Fenugreek absolute. Food Cosmet Toxicol 1978;16(Suppl 1):755-756.
18. Muralidhara, Narasimhamurthy K, Viswanatha S, et al. Acute and subchronic toxicity assessment of debitterized fenugreek powder in the mouse and rat. Food Chem Toxicol 1999;37(8):831-838.
19. Rao PU, Sesikeran B, Rao PS, et al. Short term nutritional and safety evaluation of fenugreek. Nutr Res 1996;16(9):1495-1505.
20. Ohnuma N, Yamaguchi E, Kawakami Y. Anaphylaxis to curry powder. Allergy 1998;53(4):452-454.
21. Abdel-Barry JA, Abdel-Hassan IA, Jawad AM, et al. Hypoglycaemic effect of aqueous extract of the leaves of *Trigonella foenum-graecum* in healthy volunteers. East Mediterr Health J 2000;6(1):83-88.
22. Sharma RD. Effect of fenugreek seeds and leaves on blood glucose and serum insulin responses in human subjects. Nutr Res 1986;6:1353-1364.
23. Sharma R. An evaluation of hypocholesterolemic factor of fenugreek seeds (*T foenum graecum*) in rats. Nutrit Rep Internat 1986;33:669-677.
24. Al Khaldi SF, Martin SA, Prakash L. Fermentation of fenugreek fiber, psyllium husk, and wheat bran by *Bacteroides ovatus* V975. Curr Microbiol 1999;39(4):231-232.
25. Madar Z, Abel R, Samish S, et al. Glucose-lowering effect of fenugreek in non-insulin dependent diabetics. Eur J Clin Nutr 1988;42(1):51-54.
26. Mishkinsky J, Joseph B, Sulman FG. Hypoglycemic effect of trigonelline. Lancet 1967;2(7529):1311-1312.
27. Sharma RD, Sarkar A, Hazra DK, et al. Use of fenugreek seed powder in the management of non-insulin dependent diabetes mellitus. Nutrit Res 1996;16(8):1331-1339.
28. Panda S, Tahiliani P, Kar A. Inhibition of triiodothyronine production by fenugreek seed extract in mice and rats. Pharmacol Res 1999;40(5):405-409.
29. Lambert JP, Cormier A. Potential interaction between warfarin and boldo-fenugreek. Pharmacotherapy 2001;21(4):509-512.
30. Sewell AC, Mosandl A, Bohles H. False diagnosis of maple syrup urine disease owing to ingestion of herbal tea. N Engl J Med 1999;341(10):769.
31. Abdo MS, al Kafawi AA. Experimental studies on the effect of *Trigonella foenum-graecum*. Planta Med 1969;17(1):14-18.
32. Farnsworth NR, Bingel AS, Cordell GA, et al. Potential value of plants as sources of new antifertility agents I. J Pharm Sci 1975;64(4):535-598.
33. Vats V, Yadav SP, Grover JK. Effect of T. foenumgraecum on glycogen content of tissues and the key enzymes of carbohydrate metabolism. J Ethnopharmacol 2003;85(2-3):237-242.
34. Yadav SK, Sehgal S. Effect of domestic processing and cooking methods on total, HCl extractable iron and *in vitro* availability of iron in bathua and fenugreek leaves. Nutr Health 2003;17(1):61-63.
35. Bartley GB, Hilty MD, Andreson BD, et al. "Maple-syrup" urine odor due to fenugreek ingestion. N Engl J Med 1981;305(8):467.
36. Topaloglu AK, Zeller WP, Andersen BD, et al. Maternal fenugreek ingestion simulating maple syrup urine odor in the infant. Ann Med Sci 1996;5(1):41-42.
37. Ribes G, Sauvaire Y, Baccou JC, et al. Effects of fenugreek seeds on endocrine pancreatic secretions in dogs. Ann Nutr Metab 1984;28(1):37-43.
38. Ribes G, Sauvaire Y, Da Costa C, et al. Antidiabetic effects of subfractions from fenugreek seeds in diabetic dogs. Proc Soc Exp Biol Med 1986;182(2):159-166.
39. Sauvaire Y, Petit P, Broca C, et al. 4-Hydroxyisoleucine: a novel amino acid potentiator of insulin secretion. Diabetes 1998;47(2):206-210.

40. Ajabnoor MA, Tilmisany AK. Effect of *Trigonella foenum graecum* on blood glucose levels in normal and alloxan-diabetic mice. J Ethnopharm 1988; 22:45-49.

41. Amin R, Abdul-Ghani AS, Suleiman MS. Effect of *Trigonella feonum graecum* on intestinal absorption. Proc. of the 47th Annual Meeting of the American Diabetes Association (Indianapolis U.S.A.). Diabetes 1987; 36(Supp 1):211a.

42. Stark A, Madar Z. The effect of an ethanol extract derived from fenugreek (*Trigonella foenum-graecum*) on bile acid absorption and cholesterol levels in rats. Br J Nutr 1993;69(1):277-287.

43. Petit P, Sauvaire Y, Ponsin G, et al. Effects of a fenugreek seed extract on feeding behaviour in the rat: metabolic-endocrine correlates. Pharmacol Biochem Behav. 1993;45(2):369-374.

44. Al-Habori M, Al-Aghbari AM, Al-Mamary M. Effects of fenugreek seeds and its extracts on plasma lipid profile: a study on rabbits. Phytother Res 1998;12(8):572-575.

45. Al-Habori M, Raman A. Antidiabetic and hypocholesterolaemic effects of fenugreek. Phytother Res 1998;12(4):233-242.

46. Valette G, Sauvaire Y, Baccou JC, et al. Hypocholesterolaemic effect of fenugreek seeds in dogs. Atherosclerosis 1984;50(1):105-111.

47. Sauvaire Y, Ribes G, Baccou JC, et al. Implication of steroid saponins and sapogenins in the hypocholesterolemic effect of fenugreek. Lipids 1991;26(3):191-197.

48. Varshney IP, Sharma SC. Saponins and sapogenins: part XXXII. Studies on *Trigonella foenum-graecum* Linn. Seeds. J Indian Chem Soc 1966;43(8): 564-567.

49. Yoshikawa M, Murakami T, Komatsu H, et al. Medicinal foodstuffs. IV. Fenugreek seed. (1): structures of trigoneosides Ia, Ib, IIa, IIb, IIIa, and IIIb, new furostanol saponins from the seeds of Indian *Trigonella foenum-graecum* L. Chem Pharm Bull (Tokyo) 1997;45(1):81-87.

50. Sidhu GS, Oakenfull DG. A mechanism for the hypocholesterolaemic activity of saponins. Br J Nutr 1986;55(3):643-649.

51. Gupta A, Gupta R, Lal B. Effect of *Trigonella foenum-graecum* (fenugreek) seeds on glycaemic control and insulin resistance in type 2 diabetes mellitus: a double blind placebo controlled study. J Assoc Physicians India 2001; 49:1057-1061.

52. Neeraja A, Pajyalakshmi P. Hypoglycemic effect of processed fenugreek seeds in humans. J Food Sci Technol 1996;33(5):427-430.

53. Sharma RD, Raghuram TC, Dayasagar Rao V. Hypolipidaemic effect of fenugreek seeds. A clinical study. Phytother Res 1991;3(5):145-147.

54. Sowmya P, Rajyalakshmi P. Hypocholesterolemic effect of germinated fenugreek seeds in human subjects. Plant Foods Hum Nutr 1999;53(4): 359-365.

Feverfew
(*Tanacetum parthenium* L. Schultz-Bip.)

SYNONYMS/COMMON NAMES/RELATED SUBSTANCES

- Altamisa, bachelor's button, camomille grande, crysanthemum parthenium, featherfew, featherfoil, febrifuge plant, federfoy, flirtwort, *Leucanthemum parthenium*, *Matricaria capensis*, matricaria eximia hort, *Matricaria parthenium* L., midsummer daisy, mother herb, mutterkraut, nosebleed, parthenolide, *Pyrenthrum parthenium* L., santa maria, wild chamomile, wild quinine.

CLINICAL BOTTOM LINE
Background

- Feverfew is an herb that has been used traditionally as an antipyretic, as its name denotes, although this effect has not been well studied.
- Feverfew is most commonly used orally for the prevention of migraine headache. There is a biochemical basis for this use in preclinical studies reporting anti-inflammatory and vascular (inhibition of vasoconstriction) effects. Several controlled human trials have been conducted with mixed results. Overall, these studies suggest that feverfew taken daily as dried leaf capsules may reduce the incidence of headache attacks in patients who experience chronic migraines. However, this research has been poorly designed and reported. Evidence from an adequately powered randomized trial comparing feverfew to placebo and other migraine therapies is warranted before a strong recommendation can be made.
- There is currently inconclusive evidence regarding the use of feverfew for symptoms associated with rheumatoid arthritis.
- Feverfew appears to be well tolerated in clinical trials, with a mild and reversible side effects profile. The most common adverse effect appears to be mouth ulceration and inflammation with direct exposure to leaves. Pre-clinical reports of platelet aggregation inhibition suggest a theoretical increased risk of bleeding.

Scientific Evidence for Common Studied Uses	Grade*
Migraine headache prophylaxis	B
Rheumatoid arthritis	C

*Key to grades: *A:* Strong scientific evidence for this use; *B:* Good scientific evidence for this use; *C:* Unclear scientific evidence for this use; *D:* Fair scientific evidence against this use (it may not work); *F:* Strong scientific evidence against this use (it likely does not work). For a more detailed explanation of efficacy criteria, see "Natural Standard Evidence-Based Validated Grading Rationale" in the Introduction

Historical or Theoretical Uses That Lack Sufficient Evidence

- Abdominal pain, abortifacient, anemia, anti-inflammatory, asthma, cancer, central nervous system diseases, colds, constipation, diarrhea, digestion, fever, gastrointestinal distress, insect bites, insect repellent,[1] labor induction, leukemia,[2] menstrual cramps,[3] myocardial injury, neurological complications of malaria, painful joints,[3] promotion of menstruation, skin rash, tinnitus, toothache, tranquilizer, uterine disorders, vasodilator, vertigo.

Expert Opinion and Historic Precedent:

- Feverfew has been used for centuries as an antipyretic. Other traditional uses include asthma, headache, gynecological disorders, "rheumatism," stomach ache, toothache, and insect bites. The herb was considered to be one of the most effective headache treatments available in 18th-century Europe.
- There is anecdotal evidence supporting the usefulness of feverfew, popularized since the 1970s, in the prevention of migraine headache (largely in Great Britain). People have typically ingested the native fresh or dried leaf.

Safety Summary

- **Possibly safe:** When used in recommended doses for a limited duration by healthy individuals.
- **Possibly unsafe:** With long-term use, due to limited longitudinal data. When used in conjunction with warfarin or other anticoagulant agents, in individuals at risk for bleeding, or prior to some surgical or dental procedures, because of a theoretical risk of bleeding. With abrupt cessation of the herb in chronic users, there may be a withdrawal syndrome, characterized by rebound headache, anxiety, fatigue, muscle stiffness, and joint pain.[4] A risk of immediate hypersensitivity to the feverfew constituent parthenolide has been estimated in 2% to 3% of the population.

DOSING/TOXICOLOGY
General

- Recommended doses are based on those most commonly used in available trials, or on historical practice. However, with natural products, the optimal doses needed to balance efficacy and safety often have not been determined. Formulations and preparation methods may vary from manufacturer to manufacturer, and from batch to batch of a specific product made by a single manufacturer. Because often the active components of a product are not known, standardization may not be possible, and the clinical effects of different brands may not be comparable.

Standardization

- The active agent in feverfew has been thought to be a sesquiterpene lactone, parthenolide, although this has been recently questioned. Parthenolide content may vary accordingly to the origin of the plant or the parts of the plant included in the preparation. For example, Mexican-grown feverfew has been found to be devoid of parthenolide.[5] In general, sesquiterpene lactone concentrations in feverfew ethanol extracts have been found to be ~0.5%, and ~0.3% in aqueous extracts (parthenolide being the principal sesquiterpene lactone in these preparations).[6]
- In Great Britain and Canada, feverfew products are standardized to contain at least 0.2% parthenolide. In France, standardized products must contain at least 0.1% parthenolide.[7]
- Quantitative methods, including IR and TLC/FID, have been used to determine total sesquiterpene lactone and

parthenolide levels, respectively, in feverfew preparations and may be used for chemical standardization of the raw material and its preparations.[6]

Adult Dosing (18 Years and Older)
Oral

- **Migraine headache prophylaxis:** Traditional doses include 2 to 3 dried leaves (approximately 60 mg) or 50 to 250 mg per day of a dried leaf preparation taken daily, standardized to 0.2% parthenolide (a common dose is 125 mg daily). Clinical trials have used 50 to 114 mg of feverfew powdered leaves daily, packed into capsules, standardized to 0.2% parthenolide,[4,8-10] or 0.50 mg of parthenolide daily.[11]
- **Rheumatoid arthritis:** One clinical trial of rheumatoid arthritis used a mean dose of 76 mg of dried feverfew leaf, corresponding to 2 to 3 μmol of parthenolide, in capsules.[12] Traditional doses include 70 to 86 mg of dried chopped feverfew leaves taken once daily.

Pediatric Dosing (Younger Than 18 Years)

- Insufficient available evidence.

Toxicology

- Limited toxicology data are available. No significant mutagenic effects were noted to the chromosomes of patients treated with feverfew for a mean of 2.9 years; no effects have been noted on the Ames mutagenicity test.[13,14]

ADVERSE EFFECTS/PRECAUTIONS/CONTRAINDICATIONS
Allergy

- Feverfew may elicit an allergic response in patients sensitive to chrysanthemums, daisies, and marigolds. There is potential cross-reactivity with other members of the Compositae family, including ragweed.[15]
- There have been multiple reports of allergic reactions to feverfew in Europe, Asia, and the United States.[13,16-27] Allergy to feverfew, determined by skin prick or patch test, has been reported in patients with rhinitis and asthma. Positive allergic responses have been noted in patients with a history of allergic contact dermatitis. Immediate hypersensitivity may occur in up to 2% to 3% of the population.

Adverse Effects

- **General:** Several clinical trials have reported an occurrence of adverse effects similar to or less than placebo,[4,9] typically mild and reversible.[28,29] Authors have noted clinical use of feverfew for more than 10 years in some patients, with adverse effects occurring in up to 18% of self-reporting samples (most common effects include mouth inflammation and ulceration).[4] There is a risk of feverfew withdrawal in chronic users who stop use abruptly, including headache, anxiety, sleep disturbances, muscle stiffness, and pain.[4]
- **Dermatologic:** Occupational irritant contact eczema has been reported in gardeners.[26,27] Feverfew can elicit allergic contact dermatitis.[30-37] Photosensitivity may occur.
- **Neurologic:** In one study, rebound headaches were reported in two patients when feverfew was discontinued after chronic use.[4] In a controlled trial, dizziness was reported with feverfew use, albeit no more frequently than with placebo.[9]
- **Cardiovascular:** One small study in migraine patients reported a significant increase in mean heart rate from baseline.[4] However, these results were skewed by two patients whose heart rates increased by 20 to 26 beats/minute each. Palpitations were also reported by one patient.

- **Gastrointestinal:** In a self-reporting sample, the most common and troublesome adverse event (11%) was mouth inflammation and ulceration, which occurred following direct contact with the leaves. Associated symptoms included swelling of the lips and loss of taste.[4] One patient reported minor ulceration and tongue soreness in a study of arthritis using dried leaf prepared in capsules.[12] Another controlled trial (n = 76) using leaves packed in capsules reported 10 occurrences of mouth ulceration in the feverfew group. However, in this study, mouth ulceration was also reported 16 times with placebo.[9] Gingival bleeding may occur. Indigestion, nausea, flatulence, constipation, diarrhea, abdominal bloating, and heartburn have been reported infrequently in controlled studies (each in 1 to 4 patients).[9,38] One subject withdrew from a trial because of diarrhea, attributed to feverfew.[11]

Precautions/Warnings/Contraindications

- Use cautiously prior to some surgeries or dental procedures, due to a theoretical increased risk of bleeding.
- Use cautiously in patients taking warfarin or other anticoagulants, or anti-platelet agents, due to a theoretical increased risk of bleeding.
- Do not abruptly stop use of the herb in chronic users, due to risk of a withdrawal syndrome characterized by rebound headache, anxiety, fatigue, muscle stiffness, and joint pain.[4]

Pregnancy and Lactation

- There is insufficient available safety information to recommend use. Traditional experience suggests possible emmenagogic (menstrual flow–stimulating) and abortifacient effects.

INTERACTIONS
Feverfew/Drug Interactions

- **Anticoagulant/antiplatelet drugs, nonsteroidal anti-inflammatory drugs (NSAIDs):** Feverfew has been shown to inhibit platelet secretory and aggregation activity and may theoretically increase the risk of bleeding if used concomitantly with anticoagulant or antiplatelet agents.[39-43] Feverfew has been demonstrated to inhibit prostaglandins.[44,45]
- Feverfew may increase the risk of photosensitivity. Caution is advised with concomitant use of other photosensitizing agents.

Feverfew/Herb Interactions

- **Anticoagulant/anti-platelet herbs and supplements:** Feverfew has been shown to inhibit platelet secretory and aggregation activity and may theoretically increase the risk of bleeding if used concomitantly with anticoagulant or antiplatelet agents.[39-43] Feverfew has been demonstrated to inhibit prostaglandins.[44,45]
- Feverfew may increase the risk of photosensitivity. Caution is advised with concomitant use of other photosensitizing agents.

Feverfew/Food Interactions

- Insufficient available data.

Feverfew/Lab Interactions

- Insufficient available data.

MECHANISM OF ACTION
Pharmacology

- **Constituents:** The active agent in feverfew has been thought to be a sesquiterpene lactone, parthenolide, although this has been recently questioned. Parthenolide content may vary according to the origin of the plant or the parts of the plant included in the preparation. For example, Mexican-grown feverfew has been found to be devoid of parthenolide.[5] In general, sesquiterpene lactone concentrations in feverfew ethanol extracts have been found to be ~0.5%, and ~0.3% in aqueous extracts (parthenolide being the principal sesquiterpene lactone in these preparations).[6] The bioactivity of feverfew leaf extract has been analyzed to assess the relative contributions of solvent extraction and parthenolide content. Extracts prepared in acetone-ethanol contained significantly more parthenolide than extracts in chloroform-PBS or PBS alone. The identical and elevated bioactivity-parthenolide ratios for both organic and aqueous-phase leaf extracts suggest that a proportion of the other bioactive compounds have solubilities similar to those of parthenolide.[46]

- Following the reported lack of efficacy of feverfew in a headache trial,[11] it was proposed that parthenolide may not be the active agent, and that whole leaf and extracts of a broad range of feverfew types should be evaluated.[47] Other possible active agents include melatonin, found in feverfew samples,[48] tanetin, a lipophilic flavonoid glycoside characterized in feverfew,[49] sesquiterpenes, monoterpenes, and tannins. In a study of volatiles emitted from the aerial parts of feverfew plants, a total of 41 compounds, primarily monoterpenes, were identified and quantified.[50] Alpha-pinene, camphene, limonene, gamma-terpinene, (E)-beta-ocimene, linalool, p-cymene, (E)-chrysanthenol, camphor and (E)-chrysanthenyl acetate were the predominant monoterpenes, accounting for nearly 88% of the total volatiles emitted. No parthenolide or other sesquiterpene lactones were detected. Other research has reported that lipophilic flavonoids in feverfew leaf and flower include methyl ethers of the flavonols 6-hydroxykaempferol and quercetagetin; vacuolar flavonoids include apigenin and luteolin 7-glucuronides.[51]

- **Platelet secretion/aggregation effects:** Inhibition of platelet aggregation and serotonin (5-hydroxytryptamine [5-HT]) release by extracts of feverfew has been demonstrated. In one study, release of serotonin from platelets induced by various aggregating agents was inhibited. Platelet aggregation was consistently inhibited, but thromboxane synthesis was not.[52] Additional research suggested that inhibition of platelets may involve neutralization of sulfhydryl groups.[40,41] Other work demonstrated similarities between the effects of feverfew extract and of parthenolide on 5-HT secretion and platelet aggregation.[53] Effects on the protein kinase C pathway were suggested. Extracts of feverfew have also been reported to modify the interaction of platelets with collagen substrates.[54] Feverfew extracts appear to inhibit both platelet spreading and formation of thrombus-like platelet aggregates on collagen surfaces, and to inhibit the deposition of [^{51}Cr]-labeled platelets on human collagens CIII and CIV in a dose-dependent manner. Similar concentrations of feverfew were needed to inhibit formation of surface-bound aggregates in CIII and platelet spreading on CIV in both platelet-rich plasma and GFP.[43]

- Studies in isolated rat stomach have been used as a model to study the effects of parthenolide on 5-HT storage and release, and on stimulation of the 5-HT2B receptor.[55] Cumulative-concentration response curves to 5-HT and the indirect-acting serotonergics fenfluramine and dextroamphetamine on fundus suggested that parthenolide does not exhibit agonist effects nor antagonism toward 5-HT. However, parthenolide did appear to inhibit 5-HT release.[55]

- **Anti-inflammatory/antihistamine/cytokine effects:** In the 1980s, feverfew was proposed as an inhibitor of prostaglandin synthesis,[44,56] with observed inhibition of cyclo-oxygenase and lipoxygenase activity.[51,57] *In vitro* inhibition of prostaglandin synthetase–mediated prostaglandin E_2 (PGE_2) production from arachidonic acid by the feverfew constituents parthenolide, michefuscalide, and chrysanthenyl acetate was reported.[58] Extracts of feverfew leaves and commercially available powdered leaves produced dose-dependent inhibition of the generation of thromboxane B_2 (TXB_2) and leukotriene B_4 (LTB_4) by stimulated rat and human leukocytes.[59]

- Feverfew extract has demonstrated dose-dependent inhibition of histamine release from stimulated rat peritoneal mast cells.[60]

- Oral administration of feverfew extract has produced significant dose-dependent antinociceptive and anti-inflammatory effects in rodents.[61] Parthenolide has also produced antinociceptive and anti-inflammatory effects. Naloxone, an opiate antagonist, failed to reverse feverfew and parthenolide-induced antinociception. Feverfew extract in higher doses (40 to 60 mg/kg orally) neither altered the locomotor activity nor potentiated pentobarbitone-induced sleep time in mice.

- A parthenolide affinity reagent was synthesized and shown to bind directly to and inhibit IkappaB kinase beta (IKKbeta), a kinase subunit known to play a vital role in cytokine-mediated signaling. Mutation of cysteine 179 in the activation loop of IKKbeta abolished sensitivity to parthenolide. It was demonstrated that parthenolide's *in vitro* and *in vivo* anti-inflammatory activity are mediated through the alpha-methylene gamma-lactone moiety. The multi-subunit IKK complex has been shown responsible for cytokine-mediated stimulation of genes involved in inflammation. The finding that parthenolide targets this kinase complex provides a possible molecular basis for the anti-inflammatory properties of feverfew.[62] Modulation of adhesion molecule expression may be an alternate mechanism of anti-inflammatory action.[63]

- **Vascular smooth muscle effects:** Investigations of the effects of feverfew on rabbit aortic walls demonstrate protection of the endothelial cell monolayer from perfusion-induced injury, and a reversible increase in the cyclic adenosine monophosphate (cAMP) content of aortic segments.[54] Other investigations have reported *in situ* protection of the aorta monolayer from spontaneous injury,[43] suggesting anti-thrombotic potential. Extracts of feverfew and parthenolide have been reported to inhibit smooth muscle contractility in a time-dependent, nonspecific, and irreversible manner, possibly mediated by parthenolide and cynaropicrin.[64]

- Samples prepared from chloroform extracts of fresh leaves of feverfew have strongly inhibited responses of rabbit aortic rings to phenylephrine, 5-hydroxytryptamine, thromboxane mimetic, and angiotensin II, in a concentration-dependent, time-dependent, noncompetitive, and irreversible manner.[65] These extracts were also associated with progressive loss of tone of precontracted aortic rings and appeared to impair the ability of acetylcholine to induce endothelium-dependent relaxation of tissue. These effects were mimicked by a purified preparation of parthenolide. A chloroform feverfew extract also reduced the inactivating voltage-dependent potassium current in a concentration-related manner in smooth muscle cells, suggesting blockade of open potassium channels.[66,67]

- **Cytotoxic effects:** Parthenolide has been reported to inhibit the growth of mouse fibrosarcoma and human lymphoma cell lines in an irreversible fashion.[68] Extracts of feverfew have been found to inhibit mitogen-induced tritiated thymidine ([3H]-TdR) uptake by human peripheral blood mononuclear cells (PBMCs), interleukin 2-induced [3H]-TdR uptake by lymphoblasts, and PGE_2 release by interleukin 1–stimulated synovial cells.[69] Parthenolide blocked [3H]-TdR uptake by mitogen-induced PBMC. Feverfew extracts and parthenolide were cytotoxic to mitogen-induced PBMCs and interleukin 1–stimulated synovial cells, the cytotoxic effects being functionally indistinguishable from the inhibitory effects. It is unclear to what extent the pharmacologic properties of feverfew may be due to cytotoxicity.

Pharmacodynamics/Kinetics

- Insufficient available evidence.

HISTORY

- Feverfew, an herb of the genus *Tanacetum*, is a short perennial bush reaching a height of 15 to 60 cm. The leaves have a strong smell and bitter taste. Because of feverfew's chrysanthemum-like leaves and yellow daisy-like flowers, it is often mistakenly identified as chamomile.
- Feverfew grows naturally throughout Europe and the Americas. The plant was likely initially introduced into the British Isles from the Balkan peninsula. Feverfew has traditionally been used to treat fevers, colds, constipation, diarrhea, headaches, difficulty in labor, and vertigo. Its botanical name, *Tanacetum parthenium*, is said to be derived from its medicinal use by a Greek workman who had fallen, injuring himself while constructing the Parthenon. The 17th-century English herbalist Culpeper wrote of the effectiveness of the herb for headache and uterine disorders.

REVIEW OF THE EVIDENCE: DISCUSSION
Migraine Headache Prophylaxis
Summary

- Feverfew leaves have long been used orally for the treatment or prevention of headache, and there is a biochemical basis for this use in preclinical studies that have reported anti-inflammatory and vascular (inhibition of vasoconstriction) effects. Several controlled human trials have been conducted in this area, with mixed results. Overall, these studies suggest that feverfew taken daily as dried leaf capsules may reduce the incidence of attacks in patients who experience chronic migraine headaches. However, this research has been poorly designed and reported. Evidence from an adequately powered randomized trial comparing feverfew to placebo and other migraine therapies is warranted before a strong recommendation can be made.

Systematic Reviews

- A well-designed systematic review of placebo-controlled trials of feverfew in the prophylactic treatment of migraine headache was published in 1998 by Vogler et al.[70] The authors included five randomized, double-blind, placebo-controlled trials published through April 1998.[4,8-11] A meta-analysis could not be performed due to the heterogeneity of outcome measures. The authors acknowledged a paucity of data and methodological limitations of the literature, although the data were concluded to be suggestive of feverfew's efficacy compared to placebo. An update of this review was published in 2000 by Ernst and Pittler[28,29] and included one additional multicenter trial by Pfaffenrath et al. (published in abstract form only at the time of the review).[71]

Inclusion of this study did not alter the conclusions of the prior review.

Randomized Controlled Trials (Positive Results)

- Pfaffenrath et al. enrolled 147 patients with migraine headache (diagnosed by International Headache Society criteria) in a 12-week double-blind multi-center trial to assess the efficacy of feverfew as prophylaxis.[71,72] Three dosages of a CO_2 feverfew extract called MIG-99 were compared to placebo: 2.08 mg, 6.25 mg, or 18.75 mg taken three times daily. The primary outcome was the number of migraine headaches that occurred during the last 28 days of the 12-week study period, compared to baseline incidence. Secondary outcomes included mean duration and intensity of attacks and number of days with symptoms, and number of missed work-days. In an intention-to-treat analysis, no differences were found in primary or secondary outcomes between the feverfew and placebo groups. However, a statistically significant benefit was found in a planned sub-group of patients with greater than four headaches during a 4-week run-in period ($p = 0.001$). In addition, the highest absolute change in symptoms was observed with the 6.25-mg (middle) dose. Due to the small number of patients in each subgroup, the results of stratified analysis cannot be considered conclusive. Nonetheless, these results suggest that feverfew may be beneficial in those patients with the most frequent number of migraines. Further study is merited.
- Palevitch et al. evaluated the efficacy of Israeli-grown feverfew as a headache prophylactic treatment.[10] The authors enrolled 57 patients from a hospital-based outpatient pain clinic in this trial. The study was divided into three phases: an initial 60-day open-label trial; a 30-day double-blind, randomized, controlled phase; and crossover to the alternate therapy for an additional 30 days. Outcome measures included pain intensity ratings and evaluation of accompanying symptoms (vomiting, photophobia). Subjects received 100 mg daily of feverfew powdered leaves packed in capsules (standardized to 0.2% parthenolide). Parsley served as the control agent. After 60 days of open-label feverfew treatment, the average pain intensity rating declined significantly with feverfew, by 4.3 points on a 10-point scale, compared to baseline. In the blinded 30-day phases, a 15% mean reduction in pain intensity was associated with feverfew use vs. a 15% mean increase in pain intensity with parsley ($p < 0.01$). Associated symptoms of vomiting and photophobia were significantly reduced with feverfew in both study phases. Although the results are suggestive, limitations of this study include the lack of description of baseline characteristics of the sample and the possible impact of feverfew withdrawal headaches during the second phase of the study in the parsley group.
- Murphy et al. conducted a randomized, double-blind, placebo-controlled crossover study in 72 individuals with chronic migraine headaches.[9] A majority (92%) of subjects had sought treatment in the past. Of 18 patients who had tried feverfew previously, 11 had founsd it to be "effective" and 5 were still taking it prior to study entry. All migraine medications were stopped prior to the trial. After a 1-month single-blind placebo run-in in 76 volunteers, 72 subjects remained who were randomly allocated to receive either 1 capsule of dried feverfew leaves (standardized to 2.19 μmol of parthenolide) or matching placebo (dried cabbage) daily for 4 months, followed by crossover to the alternate therapy for 4 months. Frequency and severity of attacks were determined by diary cards issued every 2 months, and efficacy of

Review of the Evidence: Feverfew

Condition Treated*	Study Design	Author, Year	N[†]	SS[†]	Study Quality[‡]	Magnitude of Benefit	ARR[†]	NNT[†]	Comments
Migraine prevention	Systematic review	Ernst[28] 2000	5 studies	NA	NA	Small	NA	NA	Well-designed systematic review; variable results; no meta-analysis possible due to heterogeneous outcome measures.
Migraine prevention	Systematic review	Vogler[70] 1998	6 studies	NA	NA	Small	NA	NA	Well-designed systematic review; variable results; no meta-analysis possible due to heterogeneous outcome measures.
Migraine prevention	RCT, crossover	De Weerdt[11] 1996	50	No	5	None	NA	NA	Feverfew alcohol extract used, not dry leaves, taken for 16 weeks vs. placebo; concomitant medications allowed for acute attacks; study may have been underpowered.
Migraine prevention	RCT crossover	Murphy[9] 1988	72	Yes	4	Large	NA	NA	Dried feverfew leaves in capsules taken for 16 weeks vs. placebo.
Migraine prevention	RCT (pilot study)	Johnson[4] 1985	17	Yes	4	Small	NA	NA	Dried feverfew leaves in capsules taken for 24 weeks vs. placebo; enrollees had been chronic feverfew users prior to trial; rebound headaches in placebo group may have exaggerated results.
Migraine prevention	RCT, crossover	Palevitch[10] 1997	57	Yes	3	Strong	NA	NA	Powdered feverfew leaves in capsules taken for 4 weeks vs. parsley (placebo); open-label feverfew phase was followed by controlled trial; rebound headaches in placebo group may have exaggerated results.
Migraine prevention	RCT (published abstract)	Pfaffenrath[71,72] 1999, 2002	147	Mixed	2	Medium	NA	NA	CO_2 feverfew extract (MIG-99) taken for 12 weeks vs. placebo; benefit only seen in patients with at least 4 migraines per month; no benefits seen in feverfew recipients overall; mid-range dose (6.25mg TID) most effective.
Migraine prevention	RCT (published abstract)	Kuritzky[8] 1994	20	No	2	None	NA	NA	Feverfew taken for 8 weeks vs. placebo; study may have been underpowered.
Migraine prevention	Case series	Prusinski[74] 1999	24	NA	NA	Medium	NA	NA	Feverfew sap taken for 4-8 weeks by female subjects.
Rheumatoid arthritis	RCT	Pattrick[12] 1989	40	No	3	None	NA	NA	Dried feverfew leaves in capsules taken for 16 weeks vs. placebo; concomitant anti-inflammatory drugs and 1 steroid injection allowed; study may have been underpowered.

*Primary or secondary outcome.
[†]N, Number of patients; SS, statistically significant; ARR, absolute risk reduction; NNT, the number of patients who need to undergo a specific intervention in order to observe an outcome in one individual.
[‡]0-2 = poor; 3-4 = good; 5 = excellent.
NA, Not applicable; RCT, randomized, controlled trial.
For an explanation of each category in this table, please see Table 3 in the Introduction.

treatment was assessed by visual analog scores. Sixty patients completed the study, and full information was available for 59. The authors reported that treatment with feverfew was associated with a 24% reduction in the mean number of headaches, with a significant reduction in nausea and vomiting ($p < 0.02$). There was a nonsignificant trend toward milder headaches with feverfew ($p = 0.06$). Duration of individual attacks was not significantly altered. Visual analog scores indicated a significant global improvement with feverfew compared to placebo ($p < 0.0001$). After study completion, 59% of patients reported feverfew to have been "more effective" compared to 24% who chose placebo. No serious adverse effects were reported.

- In a small pilot trial reported by Johnson et al., 17 patients who had been taking feverfew for migraine prophylaxis were enrolled in a 6-month controlled trial.[4] Subjects had a history of common or classic migraine for at least 2 years and had been taking raw feverfew leaves daily (mean, 60 mg) for at least 3 months. Concomitant medications, started prior to feverfew, were allowed. Outcomes were measured by patient self-reporting. Feverfew was packaged into two 25 mg capsules taken daily. The authors reported fewer headaches in the feverfew group compared to placebo (mean number of attacks, 1.69 and 3.13, respectively). These results represented an increase in headache frequency in the placebo group and no change in the feverfew group. The authors also reported a reduction in associated symptoms of nausea and vomiting with feverfew compared to placebo. Although the benefits of feverfew were statistically significant compared to baseline values, direct comparisons were not made between groups for statistical significance. This point was highlighted by Waller and Ramsay,[73] who suggested that when groups were compared directly, there was no statistically significant benefit of feverfew. Notably, discontinuation of chronic feverfew has been associated with rebound headaches, which may have increased the headache incidence in the placebo group.

Randomized Controlled Trials (Negative/ Nonsignificant Results)

- De Weerdt et al. conducted a randomized, controlled crossover trial of an alcoholic extract of feverfew (not dry leaves) for migraine prevention in 50 outpatients (42 women) in The Netherlands.[11] All subjects had experienced migraines since early youth, described headaches at least once per month with or without aura, and had used various drug treatments and prophylaxis in the past. Following a 1-month washout (placebo) period, subjects entered a crossover trial of alternating 4-month treatments with feverfew extract (standardized to 0.50 mg of parthenolide) or placebo. Enrollees could not use other prophylactic agents, but could take medications to treat acute attacks. The primary outcome measured was self-reported headache. One feverfew subject withdrew due to diarrhea, 3 withdrew due to lack of efficacy (2 taking feverfew), and 2 withdrew for unrelated reasons. The authors reported no significant benefit of feverfew in the primary outcome vs. placebo. All patients used medications to treat acute attacks during the study; 7 feverfew subjects used fewer treatment medications, although the significance vs. placebo was not clear. The lack of a measured difference between groups may have been due to a true lack of efficacy, underpowering (too small sample size), use of a nonstandardized measurement scale that may not have been sufficiently sensitive, heterogeneity of the patient population, or use of an alcoholic feverfew extract rather than dry leaves (reported as efficacious in other studies). Awang suggested that this negative trial provides evidence that parthenolide may not be the active agent in feverfew.[47]
- Kuritzky et al. also reported lack of significant effects in an abstract published in a supplement issue of *Neurology*.[8] In this Israeli study, 20 patients with migraine, diagnosed by International Headache Society criteria, entered a randomized, double-blind, crossover trial. Subjects received 100 mg of feverfew daily or placebo over 2 months. No significant effect was reported in the outcome measurement of headache prevention. In addition, no significant effect was observed on platelet serotonin uptake and activity. Insufficient information was provided in this published abstract to further assess methods, findings, or statistical analysis.

Case Series

- In a Polish case series, Prusinski et al. presented data regarding the efficacy of feverfew in migraine treatment.[74] At a migraine headache center between 1994 and 1996, the authors administered feverfew (5 mL sap) daily for 30 to 60 days to 24 women. Significant reductions in a nonstandardized "Migraine Index" were observed in 8 subjects (33%).

Rheumatoid Arthritis
Summary

- Feverfew has been associated with anti-inflammatory activity in preclinical studies. However, there is only limited study in humans regarding the efficacy of feverfew for the management of joint inflammation. Currently, there is insufficient evidence to recommend for or against the use of feverfew in patients with rheumatoid arthritis.

Evidence

- In 1989, Pattrick et al. conducted a randomized, placebo-controlled trial in 41 women with rheumatoid arthritis.[12] Subjects were outpatients of a hospital rheumatology unit in Nottingham, England, who had been diagnosed with "classical" or "definite" rheumatoid arthritis. Ongoing non-steroidal anti-inflammatory medications and other analgesic medications were maintained during the trial, although subjects with deteriorating symptoms were offered 1 steroid injection halfway through the 6-week trial. Subjects were administered feverfew capsules containing a mean of 76 mg of dried leaf daily (range 70 to 86 mg), corresponding to 2 to 3 μmol of parthenolide. Outcome measures included 21 measures assessed by patients, observers, and serologically, including joint stiffness, pain, grip strength, articular index, erythrocyte sedimentation rate, C-reactive protein, rheumatoid factor, functional capacity, and patient/observer global improvements. The authors reported that the only significant finding was an increase in grip strength in the feverfew group compared to baseline and to placebo at 6 weeks ($p = 0.047$). The sample size may have been too small to detect differences between groups, particularly in the setting of concomitant use of other anti-inflammatory agents. Blinding and randomization procedures were not well described.

FORMULARY: BRANDS USED IN CLINICAL TRIALS
U.S. Equivalents of Most Commonly Recommended European Brands

- Herbal Labs (Tanacet feverfew 125).

Other Brands That May Be Available in the United States

- Nottingham capsules, Green Products, Herbal Labs Powder, Nottingham leaves, Nottingham seeds.

References

1. DePooter H, Vermeesch J, Schamp N. Essential oils of *Tanacetum vulgare* L and *Tanacetum parthenium* L. J Essent Oil Res 1989;1:9-13.
2. Cory AH, Cory JG. Lactacystin, a proteasome inhibitor, potentiates the apoptotic effect of parthenolide, an inhibitor of NFkappaB activation, on drug-resistant mouse leukemia L1210 cells. Anticancer Res 2002;22(6C):3805-3809.
3. Awang DV. Feverfew products. CMAJ 1997;157(5):510-511.
4. Johnson ES, Kadam NP, Hylands DM, et al. Efficacy of feverfew as prophylactic treatment of migraine. Br Med J (Clin Res Ed) 1985;291(6495):569-573.
5. Awang DV, Dawson BA, Kindack DG, et al. Parthenolide content of feverfew (Tanacetum partheniun) assessed by HPLC and H-NMR spectroscopy. J Nat Prod 1991;54:1516-1521.
6. Gromek D, Kisiel W, Stojakowska A, et al. Attempts of chemical standardizing of *Chrysanthemum parthenium* as a prospective antimigraine drug. Pol J Pharmacol Pharm 1991;43(3):213-217.
7. Heptinstall S, Awang DV, Dawson BA, et al. Parthenolide content and bioactivity of feverfew (*Tanacetum parthenium* (L.) Schultz-Bip.). Estimation of commercial and authenticated feverfew products. J Pharm Pharmacol 1992;44(5):391-395.

8. Kuritzky A, Elhacham Y, Yerushalmi Z, et al. Feverfew in the treatment of migraine: its effect on serotonin uptake and platelet activity. Neurology 1994;44(Suppl 2):A201.

9. Murphy JJ, Heptinstall S, Mitchell JR. Randomised double-blind placebo-controlled trial of feverfew in migraine prevention. Lancet 1988;2(8604): 189-192.

10. Palevitch D, Earon G, Carasso R. Feverfew (*Tanacetum parthenium*) as a prophylactic treatment for migraine: a double-blind placebo-controlled study. Phytother Res 1997;11(7):508-511.

11. De Weerdt CJ, Bootsman H, Hendricks H. Herbal medicines in migraine prevention. Randomized double-blind placebo-controlled crossover trial of a feverfew preparation. Phytomed 1996;3(3):225-230.

12. Pattrick M, Heptinstall S, Doherty M. Feverfew in rheumatoid arthritis: a double blind, placebo controlled study. Ann Rheum Dis 1989;48(7): 547-549.

13. Anderson D, Jenkinson PC, Dewdney RS, et al. Chromosomal aberrations and sister chromatid exchanges in lymphocytes and urine mutagenicity of migraine patients: a comparison of chronic feverfew users and matched non-users. Hum Toxicol 1988;7(2):145-152.

14. Johnson ES, Kadam NP, Anderson D, et al. Investigation of possible genotoxic effects of feverfew in migraine patients. Hum Toxicol 1987;6(6):533-534.

15. Sriramarao P, Rao PV. Allergenic cross-reactivity between Parthenium and ragweed pollen allergens. Int Arch Allergy Immunol 1993;100(1):79-85.

16. Rodriguez E, Epstein WL, Mitchell JC. The role of sesquiterpene lactones in contact hypersensitivity to some North and South American species of feverfew (Parthenium-Compositae). Contact Dermatitis 1977;3(3): 155-162.

17. Hausen BM. [Occupational contact allergy to feverfew *Tanacetum parthenium* (L.) Schultz-Bip.; Asteraceae]. Derm Beruf Umwelt 1981; 29(1):18-21.

18. Hausen BM, Osmundsen PE. Contact allergy to parthenolide in *Tanacetum parthenium* (L.) Schulz- Bip. (feverfew, Asteraceae) and cross-reactions to related sesquiterpene lactone containing Compositae species. Acta Derm Venereol 1983;63(4):308-314.

19. Fernandez de Corres L. Contact dermatitis from Frullania, Compositae and other plants. Contact Dermatitis 1984;11(2):74-79.

20. Wedner HJ, Zenger VE, Lewis WH. Allergic reactivity of *Parthenium hysterophorus* (Santa Maria feverfew) pollen: an unrecognized allergen. Int Arch Allergy Appl Immunol 1987;84(2):116-122.

21. Sriramarao P, Selvakumar B, Damodaran C, et al. Immediate hypersensitivity to *Parthenium hysterophorus*. I. Association of HLA antigens and Parthenium rhinitis. Clin Exp Allergy 1990;20(5):555-560.

22. Sriramarao P, Nagpal S, Rao BS, et al. Immediate hypersensitivity to *Parthenium hysterophorus*. II. Clinical studies on the prevalence of Parthenium rhinitis. Clin Exp Allergy 1991;21(1):55-62.

23. Hausen BM. A 6-year experience with composite mix. Am J Contact Dermat 1996;7(2):94-99.

24. Goulden V, Wilkinson SM. Patch testing for Compositae allergy. Br J Dermatol 1998;138(6):1018-1021.

25. Orion E, Paulsen E, Andersen KE, et al. Comparison of simultaneous patch testing with parthenolide and sesquiterpene lactone mix. Contact Dermatitis 1998;38(4):207-208.

26. Paulsen E, Sogaard J, Andersen KE. Occupational dermatitis in Danish gardeners and greenhouse workers (III). Compositae-related symptoms. Contact Dermatitis 1998;38(3):140-146.

27. Paulsen E. Occupational dermatitis in Danish gardeners and greenhouse workers (II). Etiological factors. Contact Dermatitis 1998;38(1):14-19.

28. Ernst E, Pittler MH. The efficacy and safety of feverfew (*Tanacetum parthenium* L.): an update of a systematic review. Public Health Nutr 2000; 3(4A):509-514.

29. Pittler MH, Vogler BK, Ernst E. Feverfew for preventing migraine (Cochrane Review). The Cochrane Library 2000;(4):CD002286.

30. Mitchell JC, Geissman TA, Dupuis G, et al. Allergic contact dermatitis caused by Artemisia and Chrysanthemum species. The role of sesquiterpene lactones. J Invest Dermatol 1971;56(2):98-101.

31. Burry JN. Compositae dermatitis in South Australia: contact dermatitis from *Chrysanthemum parthenium*. Contact Dermatitis 1980;6:445.

32. Arlette J, Mitchell JC. Compositae dermatitis. Current aspects. Contact Dermatitis 1981;7(3):129-136.

33. Senff H, Kuhlwein A, Hausen BM. Aerogene Kontaktdermatitis. Akt Dermatol 1986;12:153-154.

34. Guin JD, Skidmore G. Compositae dermatitis in childhood. Arch Dermatol 1987;123(4):500-502.

35. Mattes H, Hamada K, Benezra C. Stereospecificity in allergic contact dermatitis to simple substituted methylene lactone derivatives. J Med Chem 1987;30(11):1948-1951.

36. Talaga P, Schaeffer M, Mattes H, et al. Synthesis of Boc-Cys-Ala-OMe and its stereoselective addition to alpha-methylene-gamma-butyrolactones. Tetrahedron 1989;45:5029-5038.

37. Lamminpaa A, Estlander T, Jolanki R, et al. Occupational allergic contact dermatitis caused by decorative plants. Contact Dermatitis 1996;34(5): 330-335.

38. Awang DV. Prescribing therapeutic feverfew (*Tanacetum parthenium* (L.)

39. Schultz Bip., Syn. *Chrysanthemum parthenium* (L.) Bernh.). Integrative Med 1998;1:11-13.

39. Makheja AN, Bailey JM. The active principle in feverfew. Lancet 1981; 2(8254):1054.

40. Heptinstall S, Groenewegen WA, Spangenberg P, et al. Extracts of feverfew may inhibit platelet behaviour via neutralization of sulphydryl groups. J Pharm Pharmacol 1987;39(6):459-465.

41. Heptinstall S, Groenewegen WA, Spangenberg P, et al. Inhibition of platelet behaviour by feverfew: a mechanism of action involving sulphydryl groups. Folia Haematol Int Mag Klin Morphol Blutforsch 1988;115(4): 447-449.

42. Loesche W, Mazurov AV, Voyno-Yasenetskaya TA, et al. Feverfew—an antithrombotic drug? Folia Haematol Int Mag Klin Morphol Blutforsch 1988;115(1-2):181-184.

43. Loesche W, Groenewegen WA, Krause S, et al. Effects of an extract of feverfew (*Tanacetum parthenium*) on arachidonic acid metabolism in human blood platelets. Biomed Biochim Acta 1988;47(10-11):S241-S243.

44. Collier HO, Butt NM, McDonald-Gibson WJ, et al. Extract of feverfew inhibits prostaglandin biosynthesis. Lancet 1980;2(8200):922-923.

45. Miller LG. Herbal medicinals: selected clinical considerations focusing on known or potential drug-herb interactions. Arch Intern Med 1998;158(20): 2200-2211.

46. Brown AMC, Edwards CM, Davey MR, et al. Pharmacological activity of feverfew (*Tanacetum parthenium* (L.) Schultz- Bip.): assessment by inhibition of human polymorphonuclear leukocyte chemiluminescence in-vitro. J Pharm Pharmacol 1997;49(5):558-561.

47. Awang DV. Parthenocide: the demise of a facile theory of feverfew activity. J Herbs Spices Med Plants 1998;5(4):95-98.

48. Murch SJ, Simmons CB, Saxena PK. Melatonin in feverfew and other medicinal plants. Lancet 1997;350(9091):1598-1599.

49. Williams CA, Hoult JR, Harborne JB, et al. A biologically active lipophilic flavonol from *Tanacetum parthenium*. Phytochemistry 1995;38(1): 267-270.

50. Christensen LP, Jakobsen HB, Paulsen E, et al. Airborne Compositae dermatitis: monoterpenes and no parthenolide are released from flowering *Tanacetum parthenium* (feverfew) plants. Arch Dermatol Res 1999; 291(7-8):425-431.

51. Williams CA, Harborne JB, Geiger H, et al. The flavonoids of *Tanacetum parthenium* and *T. vulgare* and their anti-inflammatory properties. Phytochemistry 1999;51(3):417-423.

52. Heptinstall S, White A, Williamson L, et al. Extracts of feverfew inhibit granule secretion in blood platelets and polymorphonuclear leucocytes. Lancet 1985;1(8437):1071-1074.

53. Groenewegen WA, Heptinstall S. A comparison of the effects of an extract of feverfew and parthenolide, a component of feverfew, on human platelet activity in-vitro. J Pharm Pharmacol 1990;42(8):553-557.

54. Voyno-Yasenetskaya TA, Loesche W, Groenewegen WA, et al. Effects of an extract of feverfew on endothelial cell integrity and on cAMP in rabbit perfused aorta. J Pharm Pharmacol 1988;40(7):501-502.

55. Bejar E. Parthenolide inhibits the contractile responses of rat stomach fundus to fenfluramine and dextroamphetamine but not serotonin. J Ethnopharmacol 1996;50(1):1-12.

56. Makheja AN, Bailey JM. A platelet phospholipase inhibitor from the medicinal herb feverfew (*Tanacetum parthenium*). Prostaglandins Leukot Med 1982;8(6):653-660.

57. Capasso F. The effect of an aqueous extract of *Tanacetum parthenium* L. on arachidonic acid metabolism by rat peritoneal leucocytes. J Pharm Pharmacol 1986;38(1):71-72.

58. Pugh WJ, Sambo K. Prostaglandin synthetase inhibitors in feverfew. J Pharm Pharmacol 1988;40(10):743-745.

59. Sumner H, Salan U, Knight DW, et al. Inhibition of 5-lipoxygenase and cyclo-oxygenase in leukocytes by feverfew. Involvement of sesquiterpene lactones and other components. Biochem Pharmacol 1992;43(11): 2313-2320.

60. Hayes NA, Foreman JC. The activity of compounds extracted from feverfew on histamine release from rat mast cells. J Pharm Pharmacol 1987;39(6): 466-470.

61. Jain NK, Kulkarni SK. Antinociceptive and anti-inflammatory effects of *Tanacetum parthenium* L. extract in mice and rats. J Ethnopharmacol 1999; 68(1-3):251-259.

62. Kwok BH, Koh B, Ndubuisi MI, et al. The anti-inflammatory natural product parthenolide from the medicinal herb Feverfew directly binds to and inhibits IkappaB kinase. Chem Biol 2001;8(8):759-766.

63. Piela-Smith TH, Liu X. Feverfew extracts and the sesquiterpene lactone parthenolide inhibit intercellular adhesion molecule-1 expression in human synovial fibroblasts. Cell Immunol 2001;209(2):89-96.

64. Hay AJ, Hamburger M, Hostettmann K, et al. Toxic inhibition of smooth muscle contractility by plant-derived sesquiterpenes caused by their chemically reactive alpha-methylenebutyrolactone functions. Br J Pharmacol 1994;112(1):9-12.

65. Barsby RW, Salan U, Knight DW, et al. Feverfew extracts and parthenolide irreversibly inhibit vascular responses of the rabbit aorta. J Pharm Pharmacol 1992;44(9):737-740.

66. Barsby RW, Knight DW, McFadzean I. A chloroform extract of the herb

feverfew blocks voltage-dependent potassium currents recorded from single smooth muscle cells. J Pharm Pharmacol 1993;45(7):641-645.

67. Barsby RW, Salan U, Knight DW, et al. Feverfew and vascular smooth muscle: extracts from fresh and dried plants show opposing pharmacological profiles, dependent upon sesquiterpene lactone content. Planta Med 1993; 59(1):20-25.

68. Ross JJ, Arnason JT, Birnboim HC. Low concentrations of the feverfew component parthenolide inhibit in vitro growth of tumor lines in a cytostatic fashion. Planta Med 1999;65(2):126-129.

69. O'Neill LA, Barrett ML, Lewis GP. Extracts of feverfew inhibit mitogen induced human peripheral blood mononuclear cell proliferation and cytokine mediated responses: a cytotoxic effect. Br J Clin Pharmacol 1987; 23(1):81-83.

70. Vogler BK, Pittler MH, Ernst E. Feverfew as a preventive treatment for migraine: a systematic review. Cephalalgia 1998;18(10):704-708.

71. Pfaffenrath V, Fischer M, Friede M, et al. Clinical dose-response study for the investigation of efficacy and tolerability of *Tanacetum parthenium* in migraine prophylaxis. Deutscher Schmerzkongress; October 20-24, 1999, Munich, Germany.

72. Pfaffenrath V, Diener HC, Fischer M, et al. The efficacy and safety of *Tanacetum parthenium* (feverfew) in migraine prophylaxis—a double-blind, multicentre, randomized placebo-controlled dose-response study. Cephalalgia 2002;22(7):523-532.

73. Waller PC, Ramsay LE. Efficacy of feverfew as prophylactic treatment of migraine. Br Med J (Clin Res Ed) 1985;291(6502):1128.

74. Prusinski A, Durko A, Niczyporuk-Turek A. [Feverfew as a prophylactic treatment of migraine]. Neurol Neurochir Pol 1999;33(Suppl 5):89-95.

Fish Oil/Omega-3 Fatty Acids

SYNONYMS/COMMON NAMES/RELATED SUBSTANCES

- Alpha-linolenic acid (ALA, C18:3n-3), α-linolenic acid, cod liver oil, coldwater fish, docosahexaenoic acid (DHA, C22:6n-3), eicosapentaenoic acid (EPA, C20:5n-3), fish oil fatty acids, fish body oil, fish liver oil, fish extract, halibut oil, long-chain polyunsaturated fatty acids, mackerel oil, marine oil, menhaden oil, n-3 fatty acids, n-3 polyunsaturated fatty acids, omega fatty acids, omega-3 oils, polyunsaturated fatty acids (PUFAs), salmon oil, shark liver oil, w-3 fatty acids.
- *Note:* Should not be confused with omega-6 fatty acids.

CLINICAL BOTTOM LINE
Background

- Dietary sources of omega-3 fatty acids include fish oil and certain plant/nut oils. Fish oil contains both docosahexaenoic acid (DHA) and eicosapentaenoic acid (EPA), and some nuts (English walnuts) and vegetable oils (canola, soybean, flaxseed/linseed, olive) contain alpha-linolenic acid (ALA).
- There is evidence from multiple large-scale population (epidemiologic) studies and randomized, controlled trials that intake of recommended amounts of DHA and EPA in the form of dietary fish or fish oil supplements lowers triglycerides; reduces the risk of death, heart attack, dangerous abnormal heart rhythms, and strokes in people with known cardiovascular disease; slows the buildup of atherosclerotic plaques ("hardening of the arteries"); and lowers blood pressure slightly. However, high doses may have harmful effects, such as an increased risk of bleeding. Although similar benefits are proposed for alpha-linolenic acid, scientific evidence is less compelling, and beneficial effects may be less pronounced.
- Some species of fish carry a high risk of environmental contamination, such as with methylmercury.

Scientific Evidence for Common/Studied Uses	Grade*
Hypertension	A
Hypertriglyceridemia (fish oil / EPA plus DHA)	A
Secondary cardiovascular disease prevention (fish oil / EPA plus DHA)	A
Primary cardiovascular disease prevention (fish intake)	B
Protection from cyclosporine toxicity in organ transplant patients	B
Rheumatoid arthritis (fish oil)	B
Angina pectoris	C
Asthma	C
Atherosclerosis	C
Bipolar disorder	C
Cancer prevention	C
Cardiac arrhythmias (abnormal heart rhythms)	C
Colon cancer	C
Crohn's disease	C
Cystic fibrosis	C
Depression	C
Dysmenorrhea	C
Eczema	C
IgA nephropathy	C
Infant eye/brain development	C
Lupus erythematosus	C
Nephrotic syndrome	C
Preeclampsia	C
Prevention of graft failure after heart bypass surgery	C
Prevention of restenosis after coronary angioplasty (percutaneous transluminal coronary angioplasty [PTCA])	C
Primary cardiovascular disease prevention (alpha-linolenic acid [ALA])	C
Psoriasis	C
Schizophrenia	C
Secondary cardiovascular disease prevention (alpha-linolenic acid [ALA])	C
Stroke prevention	C
Ulcerative colitis	C
Appetite / weight loss in cancer patients	D
Diabetes	D
Hypercholesterolemia	D
Transplant rejection prevention (kidney and heart)	D

*Key to grades: *A:* Strong scientific evidence for this use; *B:* Good scientific evidence for this use; *C:* Unclear scientific evidence for this use; *D:* Fair scientific evidence against this use (it may not work); *F:* Strong scientific evidence against this use (it likely does not work). For a more detailed explanation of efficacy criteria, see "Natural Standard Evidence-Based Validated Grading Rationale" in the Introduction.

Historical or Theoretical Uses That Lack Sufficient Evidence

- Acute myocardial infarction (heart attack), acute respiratory distress syndrome (ARDS), age-related macular degeneration, aggressive behavior, agoraphobia, AIDS, allergies, Alzheimer's disease, anticoagulation, antiphospholipid syndrome, attention deficit hyperactivity disorder (ADHD), anthracycline-induced cardiac toxicity, autoimmune nephritis, bacterial infections, Behçet's syndrome, borderline personality disorder,[1] breast cysts, breast tenderness, cartilage destruction, chronic fatigue syndrome, chronic obstructive pulmonary disease, cirrhosis, common cold, congestive heart failure, critical illness, dementia,[2] dermatomyositis, diabetic nephropathy, diabetic neuropathy, dyslexia, dyspraxia, exercise performance enhancement, fibromyalgia, gallstones, gingivitis, glaucoma, glomerulonephritis, glycogen storage diseases, gout, hay fever, headache, hepatorenal syndrome, hypoxia, ichthyosis, immunosuppression, isotretinoin drug toxicity protection, kidney disease prevention, kidney stones, leprosy, leukemia, malaria, male infertility, mastalgia (breast pain), memory enhancement, menopausal symptoms, menstrual cramps, multiple sclerosis, myopathy, neuropathy, night vision enhancement, obesity, omega-3 fatty acid deficiency, osteoarthritis, osteoporosis, otitis media (ear infection), panic disorder, peripheral vascular disease, post-viral fatigue syndrome, pregnancy nutritional supplement, premature birth prevention, premenstrual syndrome, prostate cancer prevention, Raynaud's phenomenon, Refsum's syndrome, Reye's syndrome, seizure disorder,[3] systemic lupus erythematosus, tardive dyskinesia, tennis elbow, urolithiasis (bladder stones), vision enhancement, wound healing.[4]

Expert Opinion and Folkloric Precedent

- The American Heart Association (AHA) recommends including fish in the diet for all individuals, and fish oil supplements for those with a history of cardiovascular disease. The U.S. Food and Drug Administration allows products containing omega-3 fatty acids to state: "The scientific evidence about whether omega-3 fatty acids may reduce the risk of coronary heart disease is suggestive, but not conclusive."
- In England, the Task Force of the British Nutrition Foundation suggests a daily intake of omega-3 fatty acids ranging from 0.5% to 2.5% of energy requirements, which corresponds to 1 to 6 g daily for men and to 1 to 5 g daily for women.
- Fish oil has been suggested as beneficial in conditions associated with low levels of omega-3 fatty acids (in plasma and/or membrane phospholipids) such as some psychiatric disorders. For mood disorders, Stoll has recommended 3 to 10 g daily of EPA and DHA, in three divided doses with meals. Dean Ornish has recommended 2 g per day of fish oil (MaxEPA) for "cardiovascular improvement."

Safety Summary

- **Likely safe:** When taken as a supplement in recommended doses for limited duration (up to 2 to 3.5 years) or when incorporated into the diet (1 to 2 fish meals per week) chronically. Daily doses of EPA plus DHA of 3 g or less are generally believed to be safe in otherwise healthy individuals. Fish oils have been granted GRAS (generally recognized as safe) status by the U.S. Food and Drug Administration.
- **Possibly safe:** When used orally in amounts found in foods during pregnancy and lactation. There is insufficient reliable information available about the safety of fish oil during pregnancy and breastfeeding when used in amounts greater than that found in foods. Up to 20 g of fish can be well tolerated by most adults, although some experts recommend against this dose due to the theoretical risk of bleeding complications. Slight increases in fasting blood glucose levels have been noted in patients with type 2 diabetes.

- **Possibly unsafe:** When used orally in high doses (greater than 3 g daily of DHA plus EPA or more than 10 g of fish oil). High doses may inhibit blood coagulation and potentially increase the risk of bleeding. In theory, doses greater than 3 g per day may also suppress immune responses. Caution is advised in individuals taking anticoagulant or antiplatelet agents, with bleeding disorders, or during the perioperative period.
- **Likely unsafe:** When taken during active bleeding.

DOSING/TOXICOLOGY

General

- Recommended doses are based on those most commonly used in available trials or on historical practice. However, with natural products, the optimal doses needed to balance efficacy and safety often have not been determined. Formulations and preparation methods may vary from manufacturer to manufacturer, and from batch to batch of a specific product made by a single manufacturer. Because often the active components of a product are not known, standardization may not be possible, and the clinical effects of different brands may not be comparable.

Standardization

- **General:** For fish oil supplements, dosing should be based on the amount of EPA and DHA (omega-3 fatty acids) in a product, not on the total amount of fish oil. Supplements vary in the amounts and ratios of EPA and DHA. A common amount of omega-3 fatty acids in fish oil capsules is 0.18 g (180 mg) of EPA and 0.12 g (120 mg) of DHA. Five g of fish oil contains approximately 0.17 to 0.56 g (170 to 560 mg) of EPA and 0.072 to 0.31 g (72 to 310 mg) of DHA. Different types of fish contain variable amounts of omega-3 fatty acids, and different types of nuts or oil contain variable amounts of alpha-linolenic acid (ALA).
- **Amounts of seafood necessary to provide 1 g of DHA + EPA** (based on USDA Nutrient Data Laboratory information): cod (Pacific), 23 g; haddock, 15 g; catfish, 15 to 20 g; flounder/sole. 7 g; shrimp, 11 g; lobster, 7.5 to 42.5 g; sardines, 2 to 3 g; crab, 8.5 g; cod (Atlantic), 12.5 g; clams, 12.5 g; scallops, 17.5 g; trout, 3 to 3.5 g; salmon, 1.4 to 4.5 g; herring, 1.5 to 2 g; oysters, 2.5 to 8 g; tuna (fresh), 2.5 to 12 g; tuna (canned, light), 12 grams; tuna (canned, white), 4 grams; halibut, 3-7.5 grams; mackerel, 2 to 8.5 g.
- **Amounts of alpha-linolenic acid in nuts and vegetable oils** (based on USDA Nutrient Data Laboratory information): canola oil, 1.3 g/tbsp; flaxseed/linseed oil, 8.5 g/tbsp; flaxseed, 2.2 g/tbsp; olive oil, 0.1 g/tbsp; soybean oil, 0.9 g/tbsp; walnut oil, 1.4 g/tbsp; walnuts (English), 0.7 g/tbsp.
- **Calories:** Fish oils contain approximately 9 calories per g of oil.
- **Vitamin E:** Fish oil taken for many months may cause a deficiency of vitamin E, and therefore vitamin E is added to many commercial fish oil products.

Dosing: Adults (18 Years and Older)

- **Average dietary intake of omega-3/omega-6 fatty acids:** Americans consume approximately 1.6 g of omega-3 fatty acids each day, of which about 1.4 g (~90%) comes from alpha-linolenic acid, and only 0.1 to 0.2 g (~10%) from EPA and DHA. In Western diets, people consume roughly 10 times more omega-6 fatty acids than omega-3 fatty acids. These large amounts of omega-6 fatty acids come from the commonly used vegetable oils containing linoleic acid (e.g., corn oil, evening primrose oil, pumpkin oil, safflower oil, sesame oil, soybean oil, sunflower oil, walnut oil, wheatgerm oil). Because omega-6 and omega-3 fatty acids compete with each other to be converted to active metabolites in the body, benefits can be reached either by decreasing intake of omega-6 fatty acids or by increasing intake of omega-3 fatty acids.

- **Recommended daily intake of omega-3 fatty acids (healthy adults):** For healthy adults with no history of heart disease, the American Heart Association recommends eating fish at least twice a week.[5] In particular, fatty fish are recommended, such as anchovies, bluefish, carp, catfish, halibut, herring, lake trout, mackerel, pompano, salmon, striped sea bass, tuna (albacore), and whitefish. It is also recommended to consume plant-derived sources of alpha-linolenic acid, such as tofu/soybeans, walnuts, flaxseed oil, and canola oil.[5] The World Health Organization and governmental health agencies of several countries recommend consuming 0.3 to 0.5 g daily of EPA + DHA and 0.8 to 1.1 g daily of alpha-linolenic acid.[5]

- **Hypertriglyceridemia:** The effects of omega-3 fatty acid intake on triglyceride-lowering is dose-responsive (higher doses have greater effects). Benefits are seen at doses less than 2 g per day of omega-3 fatty acids from EPA and DHA, although higher doses may be necessary in people with marked hypertriglyceridemia (>750 mg/dL). The American Heart Association, in its 2003 recommendations, reports that supplementation with 2 to 4 grams of EPA + DHA each day can lower triglycerides by 20% to 40%.[5] Effects appear to be additive, with HMG-CoA reductase inhibitor (statin) drugs such as simvastatin (Zocor),[6] pravastatin (Pravachol),[7,8] and atorvastatin (Lipitor).[9] Because of the risk of bleeding from omega-3 fatty acids (particularly at doses greater than 3 g per day), a physician should be consulted prior to starting treatment with supplements.

- **Heart disease (secondary prevention):** In people with a history of heart attack, regular consumption of oily fish (200 to 400 g of fish each week equal to 0.5 to 0.8 g [500 to 800 mg] of daily omega-3 fatty acids) or fish oil/omega-3 supplements (containing 0.85 to1.8 g [850 to 1800 mg] of EPA + DHA) appear to reduce the risk of non-fatal heart attack, fatal heart attack, sudden death, and all-cause mortality (death due to any cause). The American Heart Association, in its 2003 recommendations, suggests that people with known coronary heart disease consume approximately 1 g of EPA + DHA each day.[5] This may be obtained from eating fish or from fish oil capsule supplements. Because of the risk of bleeding from omega-3 fatty acids (particularly at doses greater than 3 g per day), a physician should be consulted prior to starting treatment with supplements.

- **Hypertension:** The effects of omega-3 fatty acids on blood pressure appear to be dose-responsive (higher doses have greater effects).[10] However, intakes of greater than 3 g of omega-3 fatty acids per day may be necessary to obtain clinically relevant effects, and at this dose level, there is an increased risk of bleeding. Therefore, a physician should be consulted prior to starting treatment with supplements.

- **Rheumatoid arthritis:** Clinical trials have used a range of doses, most commonly between 3 and 5 g of EPA + DHA daily (1.7 to 3.8 g of EPA, and 1.1 to 2.0 g of DHA). Effects beyond 3 months of treatment have not been well evaluated.

- **Protection from cyclosporine toxicity in organ transplant patients:** Studies have used 6 g of fish oil per day for up to 1 year. Doses in some research have started at 3 g daily for 6 weeks, followed by 6 g per day.[11] Up to 12 g per day have been used.

- **Other:** Omega-3 fatty acids are used for numerous other indications, although effective doses are not clearly established.

Dosing: Pediatric (Younger Than 18 Years)

- Omega-3 fatty acids are used in some infant formulas, although effective doses are not clearly established. Ingestion of fresh fish should be limited in young children, due to the presence of potentially harmful environmental contaminants. Fish oil capsules should not be used in children except under the direction of a physician.

Toxicology

- In clinical trials, toxicity appears to be minimal both in short- and long-term studies. Fish liver oil (e.g., cod liver oil) contains vitamins A and D, which can be toxic in excess (vitamin A > 50,000 IU and vitamin D > 2000 IU). Some fish oil products are supplemented with vitamin E, which in excess can also accumulate and lead to toxicity.

- In a study of cancer patients, the maximum tolerated dose of omega-3 fatty acid lipid esters was 0.3 g/kg. Dose-limiting toxicity was gastrointestinal, principally diarrhea.[12]

- Potentially harmful contaminants such as dioxins, methylmercury, and polychlorinated biphenyls (PCBs) are found in some species of fish. Methylmercury accumulates in fish meat more than in fish oil, and fish oil supplements appear to contain almost no mercury. Therefore, safety concerns apply to eating fish but likely not to ingesting fish oil supplements. Heavy metals are most harmful in young children and pregnant and nursing women. For sport-caught fish, the U.S. Environmental Protection Agency recommends that intake be limited in pregnant and nursing women to a single 6-ounce meal per week, and in young children to less than 2 ounces per week. For farm-raised, imported, or marine fish, the U.S. Food and Drug Administration recommends that pregnant and nursing women and young children avoid eating types with higher levels of methylmercury (approximately 1 part per million [ppm]), such as mackerel, shark, swordfish, and tilefish, and eat less than 12 ounces per week of other fish types. Women who might become pregnant are advised to eat 7 ounces or less per week of fish with higher levels of methylmercury (up to 1 ppm) and up to 14 ounces per week of fish types with approximately 0.5 ppm, such as marlin, orange roughy, red snapper, and fresh tuna. Unrefined fish oil preparations may contain pesticides.

- There have been concerns regarding rancidity of poorly manufactured products.

ADVERSE EFFECTS/PRECAUTIONS/CONTRAINDICATIONS
Allergy

- People with allergy or hypersensitivity to fish should avoid fish oil and omega-3 fatty acid products derived from fish. Skin rash has been reported rarely.[13,14]

- People with allergy or hypersensitivity to nuts should avoid alpha-linolenic acid or omega-3 fatty acid products that are derived from the types of nuts to which they react.

Adverse Effects/Postmarket Surveillance

- **General:** The U.S. Food and Drug Administration classifies intake of up to 3 g per day of omega-3 fatty acids from fish as GRAS (generally regarded as safe). Caution may be warranted, however, in diabetic patients because of potential (albeit unlikely) increases in blood sugar levels, in patients at risk of bleeding, and in those with high levels of low-density lipoprotein (LDL). Fish meat may contain methylmercury, and caution is warranted in young children and pregnant and breastfeeding women.

- **Neurologic/psychiatric effects:** There are rare reports of mania in patients with bipolar disorder or major depression.[15] Restlessness and formication (the sensation of ants crawling on the skin) have also been reported.[14]
- **Cardiovascular (blood pressure effects):** Multiple human trials report small reductions in blood pressure with intake of omega-3 fatty acids.[10,16-21] Reductions of 2 to 5 mm Hg have been observed, and effects appear to be dose-responsive (higher doses have greater effects).[10] DHA may have greater effects than EPA.[22] Caution is warranted in patients with low blood pressure or in those taking blood-pressure lowering medications.
- **Cardiovascular (cholesterol levels):** Increases (worsening) in low-density lipoprotein levels ("bad cholesterol") by 5% to 10% are observed with intake of omega-3 fatty acids. Effects are dose-dependent, with effects likely to occur at 1 g per day or greater of omega-3 fatty acids.
- **Gastrointestinal (GI upset):** Gastrointestinal upset is common with the use of fish oil supplements, occurring in up to 5% of patients in clinical trials, with nausea in up to 1.5% of patients.[7,13,14,18,23,24] Diarrhea may also occur, with potentially severe diarrhea at very high doses.[25] There are also reports of increased burping,[13] acid reflux/heartburn/ indigestion,[26] abdominal bloating,[21] and abdominal pain.[27] Fishy aftertaste is a common effect.[13,24] Gastrointestinal side effects can be minimized if fish oils are taken with meals and if doses are started low and gradually increased.
- **Gastrointestinal (hepatic effects):** Mild elevations in liver function tests (alanine aminotransferase) have been reported rarely.[28]
- **Gastrointestinal (vitamin A, D, E levels):** Fish oil taken for many months may cause a deficiency of vitamin E,[29-31] and therefore vitamin E is added to many commercial fish oil products. As a result, regular use of vitamin E–enriched products may lead to elevated levels of this fat-soluble vitamin. Fish liver oil contains the fat-soluble vitamins A and D, and therefore fish liver oil products (such as cod liver oil) may increase the risk of vitamin A or D toxicity.
- **Gastrointestinal (calories):** Fish oils contain approximately 9 calories per g of oil.
- **Hematologic (bleeding):** Intake of 3 g per day or greater of omega-3 fatty acids may increase the risk of bleeding, although there is little evidence of significant bleeding risk at lower doses.[32-34] Very large intakes of fish oil/omega-3 fatty acids ("Eskimo" amounts) may increase the risk of hemorrhagic (bleeding) stroke.[35] High doses have also been associated with nosebleed and blood in the urine.[36] Fish oils appear to decrease platelet aggregation and prolong bleeding time and increase fibrinolysis (breaking down of blood clots), and they may reduce von Willebrand factor.
- **Endocrine (blood sugar levels/diabetes):** Although slight increases in fasting blood glucose levels have been noted in patients with type 2 (adult-onset) diabetes, the available scientific evidence suggests that there are no significant long-term effects of fish oil in patients with diabetes, including no changes in hemoglobin A_{1c} levels.[37,38] Limited reports in the 1980s of increased insulin needs in diabetic patients taking long-term fish oils may be related to other dietary changes or weight gain.[36,39]
- **Dermatologic:** Skin rashes have been reported rarely.[13,14]

- **Oncologic:** Based on preliminary evidence, fish oils may further increase the risk of colon cancer in individuals with familial adenomatous polyposis (FAP): three patients with a pre-existing diagnosis of FAP were found to have malignant lesions during a course of long-term fish oil therapy.[40] However, given the high risk for the development of colon cancer in patients with FAP, the specific role of fish oil in mediating risk of malignancy is not clear.
- **Environmental contamination:** Potentially harmful contaminants such as dioxins, methylmercury, and polychlorinated biphenyls (PCBs) are found in some species of fish. Methylmercury accumulates in fish meat more than in fish oil, and fish oil supplements appear to contain almost no mercury. Therefore, safety concerns apply to eating fish but likely not to ingesting fish oil supplements. Heavy metals are most harmful in young children and pregnant/nursing women. For sport-caught fish, the U.S. Environmental Protection Agency recommends that intake be limited in pregnant/nursing women to a single 6-ounce meal per week, and in young children to less than 2 ounces per week. For farm-raised, imported, or marine fish, the U.S. Food and Drug Administration recommends that pregnant/nursing women and young children avoid eating types with higher levels of methylmercury (approximately 1 part per million [ppm]), such as mackerel, shark, swordfish, or tilefish, and limit their intake to less than 12 ounces per week of other fish types. Women who might become pregnant are advised to eat 7 ounces or less per week of fish with higher levels of methylmercury (up to 1 ppm) and up to 14 ounces per week of fish types with approximately 0.5 ppm (such as marlin, orange roughy, red snapper, or fresh tuna). Unrefined fish oil preparations may contain pesticides.

Precautions/Warnings/Contraindications

- Avoid in patients during active bleeding.
- Use cautiously (particularly 3 g per day or greater of omega-3 fatty acids) in patients receiving anticoagulant or antiplatelet therapy due to a potential increase in bleeding risk.
- Use cautiously during the perioperative period (particularly 3 g per day or greater of omega-3 fatty acids), due to the increased risk of bleeding.
- Use cautiously in diabetic patients, as hypoglycemic medication doses may require adjustment. Slight increases in fasting blood glucose levels have been noted in patients with type 2 diabetes; limited reports in the 1980s of increased insulin needs in diabetic patients taking fish oils long-term may be related to other dietary changes or weight gain.
- Use cautiously in patients with low blood pressure, due to small drops in blood pressure observed with intake of omega-3 fatty acids.
- In general, doses greater than 3 g per day of omega-3 fatty acids should be used cautiously.

Pregnancy and Lactation

- **Concerns regarding contaminants:** Potentially harmful contaminants such as dioxins, methylmercury, and polychlorinated biphenyls (PCBs) are found in some species of fish, and may be harmful in pregnant/nursing women. Methylmercury accumulates in fish meat more than in fish oil, and fish oil supplements appear to contain almost no mercury. Therefore, these safety concerns apply to eating fish but likely not to ingesting fish oil supplements. However, unrefined fish oil preparations may contain pesticides. For sport-caught fish, the U.S. Environmental Protection

Agency recommends that intake be limited in pregnant/ nursing women to a single 6-ounce meal per week. For farm-raised, imported, or marine fish, the U.S. Food and Drug Administration recommends that pregnant and nursing women avoid eating types with higher levels of methylmercury (approximately 1 part per million), such as mackerel, shark, swordfish, or tilefish, and no more than 12 ounces per week of other fish types. Women who might become pregnant are advised to eat no more than 7 ounces per week of fish with higher levels of methylmercury (up to 1 part per million), and no more than 14 ounces per week of fish types with approximately 0.5 parts per million (such as marlin, orange roughy, red snapper, or fresh tuna).

- **Fetal transmission:** Long-chain omega-3 fatty acid levels in plasma and erythrocyte phospholipids in mothers and neonates have been significantly correlated.[41] Administration of fish oil during pregnancy appears to promote higher concentrations of DHA in the newborn infant.[42,43] Relatively low maternal intake of dietary DHA seems to significantly elevate DHA content in human milk.[44]
- **Fetal growth:** It is not known conclusively if omega-3 fatty acid supplementation in women during pregnancy or breastfeeding is beneficial to infants. It has been suggested that high intake of omega-3 fatty acids during pregnancy, particularly DHA, may increase birth weight and gestational length.[45] However, higher doses may not be advisable, due to the potential risk of bleeding.
- **Nervous system development:** DHA has been reported as integral in the growth and functional development of the brain in infants and appears to be taken up by the brain in preference to other fatty acids.[46-48] DHA and arachidonic acid are often included in infant formulas. DHA in the diet has also been associated with visual (retinal) development in infants,[49-52] and with retinal pathology during aging.[53] In animal studies, chronic administration of DHA is reported to improve reference memory–related learning ability correlated with the DHA/arachidonic acid ratio in the hippocampus and cerebral cortex.[54] In a case of severe deficiency, supplementation was reported to alleviate severe growth retardation.[55] In contrast, it has been reported that high doses of EPA in addition to DHA may be harmful in pre-term infants,[56] who frequently appear to be DHA-deficient.[50] Daily supplementation with 500 to 1000 mg of omega-3 fatty acids, taken as a milk-based supplement or as fish oil capsules, has been noted to increase fetal omega-3 fatty acid status without affecting omega-6 fatty acid status.[57] The consequences of deficiency in alpha-linolenic acid (ALA), a precursor of DHA, include anomalies in the composition of nervous membranes, perturbation of electrophysiologic parameters, and greater sensitivity to neurotoxins.[58]

INTERACTIONS
Interactions with Drugs

- **Anticoagulants, antiplatelet agents:** In theory, omega-3 fatty acids may increase the risk of bleeding when taken with drugs that increase the risk of bleeding. Some examples include aspirin, anticoagulants ("blood thinners") such as warfarin (Coumadin) and heparin, antiplatelet drugs such as clopidogrel (Plavix), and nonsteroidal anti-inflammatory drugs such as ibuprofen (Motrin, Advil) and naproxen (Naprosyn, Aleve).
- **Antihypertensives:** Based on human studies, omega-3 fatty acids may lower blood pressure and add to the effects of drugs that may also affect blood pressure.[59,60]

- **Hypoglycemic agents:** Fish oil supplements may lower blood sugar levels a small amount. Caution is advised when using medications that may also lower blood sugar. Patients taking drugs for diabetes by mouth or insulin should be monitored closely by a qualified healthcare professional. Medication adjustments may be necessary.
- **Cholesterol lowering agents:** Omega-3 fatty acids lower triglyceride levels, but can actually increase (worsen) low-density lipoprotein (LDL/"bad cholesterol") levels by a small amount. Therefore, omega-3 fatty acids may add to the triglyceride-lowering effects of agents such as niacin/nicotinic acid, fibrates such as gemfibrozil (Lopid), and resins such as cholestyramine (Questran). However, omega-3 fatty acids may work against the LDL-lowering properties of "statin" drugs such as atorvastatin (Lipitor) and lovastatin (Mevacor).

Interactions with Herbs and Dietary Supplements

- **Anticoagulant herbs and supplements:** In theory, omega-3 fatty acids may increase the risk of bleeding when taken with herbs and supplements that are believed to increase the risk of bleeding. Multiple cases of bleeding have been reported with the use of *Ginkgo biloba*, and fewer cases with garlic and saw palmetto. Numerous other agents may theoretically increase the risk of bleeding, although this has not been proven in most cases. Some examples are alfalfa, American ginseng, angelica, anise, *Arnica montana*, asafetida, aspen bark, bilberry, birch, black cohosh, bladderwrack, bogbean, boldo, borage seed oil, bromelain, capsicum, cat's claw, celery, chamomile, chaparral, clove, coleus, cordyceps, danshen, devil's claw, dong quai, evening primrose oil, fenugreek, feverfew, flaxseed/flax powder (not a concern with flaxseed oil), ginger, grapefruit juice, grapeseed, green tea, guggul, gymnestra, horse chestnut, horseradish, licorice root, lovage root, male fern, meadowsweet, nordihydro-guaiaretic acid (NDGA), onion, papain, *Panax ginseng*, parsley, passion flower, poplar, prickly ash, propolis, quassia, red clover, reishi, rue, Siberian ginseng, sweet birch, sweet clover, turmeric, vitamin E, white willow, wild carrot, wild lettuce, willow, wintergreen, and yucca.
- **Blood pressure lowering herbs/supplements:** Based on human studies, omega-3 fatty acids may lower blood pressure and theoretically may add to the effects of agents that may also affect blood pressure. Examples include aconite/monkshood, arnica, baneberry, betel nut, bilberry, black cohosh, bryony, calendula, California poppy, coleus, curcumin; eucalyptol, eucalyptus oil, flaxseed/flaxseed oil, garlic, ginger, ginkgo, goldenseal, green hellebore, hawthorn, Indian tobacco, jaborandi, mistletoe, night-blooming cereus, oleander, pasque flower, periwinkle, pleurisy root, *Polypodium vulgare*, shepherd's purse, Texas milkweed, turmeric, and wild cherry.
- **Hypoglycemic herbs and supplements:** Fish oil supplements may lower blood sugar levels a small amount. Caution is advised when using herbs or supplements that may also lower blood sugar. Blood glucose levels may require monitoring, and doses may need adjustment. Possible examples are *Aloe vera*, American ginseng, bilberry, bitter melon, burdock, fenugreek, gymnema, horse chestnut seed extract (HCSE), maitake mushroom, marshmallow, milk thistle, *Panax ginseng*, rosemary, shark cartilage, Siberian ginseng, stinging nettle, and white horehound. Agents that may raise blood sugar levels include arginine, cocoa, and ephedra (when combined with caffeine).

- **Lipid lowering herbs and supplements:** Omega-3 fatty acids lower triglyceride levels but can actually increase (worsen) low-density lipoprotein (LDL/"bad cholesterol") levels by a small amount. Therefore, omega-3 fatty acids may add to the triglyceride-lowering effects of agents such as niacin/nicotinic acid but may work against the potential LDL-lowering properties of agents such as barley, garlic, guggul, niacin, psyllium, soy, and sweet almond.
- **Vitamin E:** Fish oil taken for many months may cause a deficiency of vitamin E,[29-31] and therefore vitamin E is added to many commercial fish oil products. As a result, regular use of vitamin E–enriched products may lead to elevated levels of this fat-soluble vitamin.
- **Vitamins A and D:** Fish liver oil contains the fat-soluble vitamins A and D, and therefore fish liver oil products (such as cod liver oil) may increase the risk of vitamin A or D toxicity. Because fat-soluble vitamins can build up in the body and cause toxicity, patients taking multiple vitamins regularly or in high doses should discuss this risk with their healthcare practitioners.

MECHANISM OF ACTION
Pharmacology

- **Omega-3 fatty acids:** Sources of oil containing omega-3 fatty acids include anchovy, black cod, bluefish, halibut, kipper, mackerel, menhaden, mullet, herring, pilchard, sable fish, salmon, sardine, seal blubber, sturgeon, trout, tuna, and whale blubber. These types of fish contain oil with long-chain polyunsaturated acids of the omega-3 family: alpha-linolenic acid (ALA; C 18:3, omega-3), eicosapentaenoic acid (EPA; C 20:5, omega-3), and docosahexaenoic acid (DHA; C 22:6, omega-3). This nomenclature is based on the number of carbon atoms in the fatty acid molecule (18, 20, 22), the number of double bonds (3, 5, 6), and the number of carbon atoms counting from the methyl end before the first double bond (omega-3). ALA is the parent compound of all of the omega-3 fatty acids. However, only a small percentage of ALA (<10%) is converted to EPA and DHA, making this an inefficient source of omega-3 fatty acids in the body. Unlike ALA (found mainly in green vegetables, canola oil, and soybeans), EPA and DHA originate almost exclusively from fish oil and other seafoods. Fish oil supplements contain varying amounts of EPA and DHA (18% to 51% and 12% to 32%, respectively).
- **Omega-6 fatty acids:** Omega-6 is the "second" family of polyunsaturated acids. These are derived from linoleic acid, found primarily in vegetable oils: linoleic (C 18:2, omega-6), arachidonic (C 20:4, omega-6), and docosapentaenoic (C 22:5, omega-6). There is no practical interconversion between the two families of fatty acids.[61-64] Some omega-3 and omega-6 fatty acids may be essential components of the diet, as hepatic synthesis may not be sufficient, potentially yielding deficiency syndromes.
- **EPA and DHA:** Although fish oil from herring, cod liver, salmon, mackerel, and sardines is rich in omega-3 fatty acids, these contain varying levels of EPA and DHA. In the United States, the percentage of EPA (20:5) and DHA (22:6) has been found to be lower than in other nations with lower cardiac disease incidence, such as Japan.[65] The source of EPA and DHA found in most marine foodstuffs is phytoplankton. Commercial fish foods contain less DHA and EPA, and pond-reared/cultured fish tend to contain lower levels of EPA/DHA.
- **Arachidonic acid and eicosanoids:** Specific regulatory stimuli can trigger the release of arachidonic acid from cell membranes via the stimulation of phospholipase A_2. Arachidonic acid serves as a substrate for cyclooxygenase and lipoxygenase enzyme systems and thereby is a source of eicosanoids (prostaglandins, leukotrienes, thromboxanes). There is competitive inhibition between omega-3 and omega-6 fatty acids for active enzyme sites, and the quantity and chemical structure of eicosanoids depends on the ratio of these two main families of polyunsaturated fatty acids. Pharmacologic activity of fish oil may be based on the ability to serve both as a source of active eicosanoids and as an inhibitor of the synthesis of eicosanoids from arachidonic acid.[61,62,64,66-71]
- **Neurologic effects:** There is evidence that alterations of omega-3 fatty acid metabolism and the composition of phospholipids in serum and membranes are involved in the pathogenesis of some neurologic conditions. For example, in hepatic encephalopathy, low plasma levels of DHA related to impaired metabolism of omega-3 fatty acids have been observed.[72] A greater frequency of behavior problems assessed by the Conner Rating Scale, temper tantrums, and sleep disturbances have been registered in boys with lower total omega-3 fatty acids in plasma phospholipids.[43] In moderate to severe depression, a significant positive correlation between severity of depression and the ratio of erythrocyte phospholipid arachidonic acid to EPA has been observed.[74] Major depression has been associated with an increased serum C 20:4 omega-6 to C 20:5 omega-3 ratio, attributed to lowered omega-3 polyunsaturated fatty acids.[75] The biochemical bases of these phenomena remain obscure. In autosomal dominant retinitis pigmentosa, it has been demonstrated that there is a metabolic defect in the final stages of DHA biosynthesis from its EPA precursor.[76]
- **Hypotensive effects:** Cod liver oil (approximately 10 g of omega-3 polyunsaturated fatty acid) has been found to decrease blood pressure ($p < 0.05$) and blood pressure response to norepinephrine ($p < 0.01$)[77]; these effects disappear 4 weeks after discontinuing therapy. Linoleic acid and fish oil fatty acids (administered by subcutaneous injection) were equally potent in reducing the rise in systolic arterial pressure induced by the chronic infusion of angiotensin II in rats.[78] Multiple human trials report small reductions in blood pressure with intake of omega-3 fatty acids.[10,16-21] Reductions of 2 to 5 mm Hg have been observed, and effects appear to be dose-responsive.[10] DHA may have greater effects than EPA.[22]
- **Hypolipidemia:** The inclusion of fish oil in the diet of animals produces significant increases in levels of EPA and DHA in plasma lipids; a decrease in plasma triglycerides; reduction in total cholesterol, low-density lipoproteins (LDLs), and very-low-density lipoproteins (VLDLs); and an increase in high-density lipoproteins (HDLs).[63,79] The first studies in healthy humans described a significant lowering effect of fish oil on plasma total cholesterol, triglycerides, LDLs, and VLDLs.[80-88] Even low doses of fish oil–derived omega-3 acids (0.40 g/dL) were demonstrated to be incorporated into blood lipids of elderly subjects,[89] and to decrease fasting and postprandial triglyceride levels in young subjects.[90] It was initially suggested that fish oil fatty acids are utilized in the liver for the synthesis of phospholipids, located on the surface of lipoproteins.[91] However, in the majority of studies reporting reductions in total cholesterol and LDLs, saturated fat intake was lowered when switching from a control diet to a fish oil diet. When fish oil was administered to subjects under constant saturated fat intake, there was no effect on total cholesterol levels.[92] Nevertheless,

there were reports that even under such rigorously controlled conditions (e.g., at low and high fixed concentrations of saturated fatty acids), fish oil was capable of lowering plasma total cholesterol, VLDLs, and LDLs.[93-95] The decrease in triglycerides associated with fish oil dietary consumption or supplementation has been confirmed in numerous human trials.[96-110] Fish oils are thought to lower triglycerides by decreasing secretion of VLDLs, increasing VLDL apolipoprotein B secretion, and possibly by increasing VLDL clearance, decreasing VLDL size, and reducing triglyceride transport. Fish oils appear to decrease synthesis of VLDL by inhibiting 1,2-diacylglycerol-sterol-o-acyltransferase or phosphatidate phosphatase. Fish oils may also decrease chylomicron concentrations; triacylglycerol concentrations significantly decrease after 28 days of supplementation with EPA/DHA in women.[111] Increases in HDL concentrations have been observed less frequently and at higher doses of EPA-DHA mixtures.[63,112-117] In a primate study, a group of African green monkeys fed fish oil developed less atherosclerosis in the coronary arteries and aorta and had lower LDLs and higher HDLs compared with a group fed lard.[118]

- **Oxidative damage:** There is limited evidence that ingestion of high doses of fish oil may increase the susceptibility of cellular membranes and plasma lipids to oxidative damage.[119-121] Human trials conducted with moderate doses of fish oil (2 g of EPA daily vs. 7 to 10 g in previous studies) did not reproduce these findings[122,123] and in some cases reported antioxidant effects.[124] It has been suggested that oxidative damage may be caused by reductions in vitamin E concentrations elicited by large doses of fish oil.[29-31] Fish oils may increase fatty acid oxidation by peroxisomal and mitochondrial routes, reduce fatty acid synthesis, divert fatty acids into phospholipid synthesis, increase hepatic uptake of triglycerides, and downregulate fatty acid esterifying enzymes.

- **Platelet aggregation/adhesion:** In the 1980s it was suggested that the fatty acid composition of platelet phospholipids is significantly altered by fish oil supplementation,[125] and that platelet aggregation in response to adenosine diphosphate (ADP) and collagen is independent of fatty acid composition.[126,127] Decreased aggregation was found to continue for weeks after normalization in phospholipid chemistry.[63] A single dose of omega-3 fatty acids reduced aggregation without any detectable incorporation into platelet membranes.[128] EPA (20:5 omega-3) and DHA (22:6 omega-3) both were noted to inhibit ADP-induced aggregation of platelets.[129] It was not clear why ingestion of both EPA and DHA resulted in reduced aggregation in response to collagen,[130] whereas response to ADP was lowered significantly only by DHA.[131] A more consistent picture emerged in subsequent studies.[132,133] Analysis demonstrated that after ingestion of diets high in linolenic acid (the precursor to omega-6 fatty acid), there was an increase in platelet aggregation. In contrast, intake of alpha-linolenic acid (an omega-3 fatty acid precursor) either had no effect or led to decreased aggregation compared to linoleic acid.[132] Cod liver oil (containing approximately 10 g of omega-3 fatty acids) also decreased platelet aggregation upon ADP and collagen administration,[77] as well as thrombin-induced platelet aggregation.[125] It was further demonstrated that after normalization of plasma fatty acid composition, there was a normalization of platelet aggregation,[134] and the platelet ratio of EPA to arachidonic acid was associated with a decrease in ADP-, collagen-, and adrenalin-induced platelet aggregation.[135] It is now thought that

following incorporation of EPA and DHA into platelet and endothelium phospholipids, a significant change occurs in the operation of key enzyme systems: Instead of pro-aggregatory and vasoconstrictive thromboxane A_2 (often registered as its metabolite thromboxane B_2), activated platelets generate thromboxane A_3 (or its metabolite B_2) with weak aggregatory effects.[136,137] This is augmented by synthesis (in the endothelium) of prostaglandin I_3 from EPA, which also possesses anti-aggregatory properties.[138-140] This mechanism is supported by the finding of a decrease in basic or collagen (thrombin)-stimulated generation of thromboxane B_2 from platelets.[141-144] A similar effect is directly registered by thromboxane A_2 measurements.[145-149] Accumulation of thromboxane A_3 and prostaglandin I_3 has also been noted.[146-149] A fish oil diet has been associated with a significant inhibition of platelet adhesion to collagen I- or fibrinogen-coated surfaces.[68,150] A high consumption of omega-3 polyunsaturated fatty acids (such as cis-5, 8, 11, 14, 17-EPA [C20:5]) has been found to increase the proportion of omega-3 polyunsaturated fatty acids in the platelets of Eskimos.[151]

- **Bleeding time:** Diets containing salmon oil, mackerel, or cod liver oil have been reported to significantly prolong bleeding times in healthy volunteers.[34,77,125,152,153] However, in other studies, no effects of 3-omega fatty acid supplementation have been observed.[140,154] Increased bleeding time is suggested to be due to either less thromboxane (TXA_2) or higher prostacyclin I_3 levels.

- **Fibrinolytic and coagulation effects:** Although no effects on fibrinolysis have been observed in some studies of omega-3 fatty acids,[158-163] other investigations have found increased fibrinolysis and vascular plasminogen activator levels, as well as altered levels of inhibitors of vascular plasminogen activator[158-163] and prothrombin fragment 1-2.[164]

- **Endothelial adhesion:** It has been suggested that EPA may impair induction/expression of endothelial adhesion molecules, based on a pig model[165] and *in vitro* studies.[166,167] There is some evidence that fish oil may suppress intimal smooth muscle cell proliferation by decreasing the production of endothelial paracrine growth factor[168,169]/platelet-derived growth factor.[170,171]

- **Antiarrhythmic properties:** EPA may block fast voltage-dependent sodium channels via specific binding, which results in prolongation of the inactivated states of these channels.[172,173] In dogs, the frequency of ectopic beats after myocardial infarction decreased from 80% to less than 30% with omega-3 fatty acid ingestion.[174] There is promising evidence that omega-3 fatty acids may decrease the risk of cardiac arrhythmias in humans.[175-177]

- **Anti-inflammatory effects:** Inflammation involves synthesis and release of prostaglandins and leukotrienes,[178,179] interleukin-1 and tumor necrosis factor,[180] interferon-gamma,[75] and eicosanoids.[63] Omega-3 fatty acids from fish oil compete with arachidonic acid in the cyclooxygenase and lipoxygenase pathways and inhibit leukotriene synthesis. Fish oils may suppress mediators of immune function by reducing the production of cytokines.[181,182] Synthesis of interleukin-1 (alpha and beta) and tumor necrosis factor can be suppressed in healthy humans by dietary supplementation with omega-3 fatty acids.[180,183-185] However, other research has not confirmed these results.[186] Reduction of inflammation has been observed in various animal models[187-193] and in humans.[194]

- **Immunologic properties:** A fish oil–enriched diet increased survival of mice following *Klebsiella pneumoniae* infection compared to a control diet (olive oil– or corn oil–enriched diet).[195] Fish oil as the exclusive source of lipid-suppressed autoimmune lupus erythematosus (LE) in MKL-lpR mice by decreasing lymphoid hyperplasia and macrophage surface I_a expression and delaying the onset of renal disease.[196] In another mouse model of LE, suppression of autoimmune disease by DHA and EPA was felt to be related to a decrease in interleukin-1 beta gene transcription.[197-199] In animal studies post-transplant, intravenous alimentation with fish oil–derived lipid emulsions prolonged heart transplant survival compared to omega-6 lipids.[200] A fish oil diet was found to inhibit experimental amyloidosis and decrease macrophage arachidonate metabolism in mice.[201]

- **Antiproliferative properties:** In animal and *in vitro* investigations, dietary fish oils have been shown to inhibit the development of mammary,[202-204] pancreatic, intestinal, prostatic,[205,206] and colorectal[207-211] carcinoma and lymphoma.[212]
- **Neuropathy:** In rats with streptozotocin-induced diabetes, dietary supplementation with fish oil increased depressed nerve condition velocity and NaK-ATPase activity in the sciatic nerve compared to olive oil supplementation.[213]
- **Renal function:** In 10 young healthy subjects whose diets were supplemented with 6 g/day of n-3 polyunsaturated fatty acids (3.6 g of EPA and 2.4 g of DHA), a significant increase in renal plasma flow and glomerular filtration rate as well as decreased vascular resistance occurred.[214] However, no such effects were observed in elderly subjects who took 1.7 g/day of EPA over a 4-week period.[215] Mice fed fish oil exhibited higher renal levels of catalase, glutathione peroxidase, and superoxide dismutase mRNAs compared to mice fed corn oil.[216]

Pharmacodynamics/Kinetics

- **Dosing/serum levels:** A 1992 study was conducted that included two different fish oil preparations: Ameu (Omega Pharma GmbH, Berlin, Germany) and MaxEPA (Fresenius AG, Bad Homburg, Germany).[217] Plasma concentrations of eicosapentaenoic acid (EPA) and docosahexaenoic acid (DHA) were evaluated at three dosages (3, 6, and 12 g). During 28 days of ingestion of Ameu and an equally long wash-out period, there was a dose-dependent increase in EPA plasma concentration to maximal levels from 7.2 ± 2.2 mg/dL (3-g subgroup) to 20.6 ± 2.5 mg/dL (12-g subgroup). DHA demonstrated almost identical increases and peak values at all doses (maximal concentrations ranged from 10.3 ± 26 mg/dL (3-g subgroup) to 15.1 ± 2.7 mg/dL (12-g subgroup). During the wash-out period, there was a rapid return of EPA and DHA levels to baseline. EPA and DHA from MaxEPA behaved similarly. The ratio of the area under the curve for both products ranged within 0.8 to 1.2. After 4 weeks, saturation was reached at low doses (3 to 6 g daily). These data suggest that the optimal dose should be 3 to 6 g daily.

- **Absorption:** Emulsified fish oils are often preferred, as they are believed to be better absorbed in humans. A preliminary single-dose absorptive study reported increased plasma omega-3 fatty acid levels 2 to 8 hours after ingestion of 8 1-g capsules of ethyl ester concentrate of fish oil.[218] The capsules contained 3.2 g of EPA and 2.2 g of DHA; 5/6 of patients were observed to experience the increased levels.

- **Distribution:** Dietary omega-3 fatty acids are incorporated into fat tissues.[219]

HISTORY

- Ingestion of cod liver oil became popular in 19th-century England as a source of vitamin D for sun-deprived children.
- Recently, interest in fish oil as a cardiovascular protectant has stemmed from observations that Greenland Eskimos enjoy an unusually low incidence of heart disease despite a diet high in fat. It has been recognized that their diet is rich in omega-3 fatty acids and relatively lower in omega-6 fatty acids and saturated fatty acids compared to Western populations.
- The American Heart Association Nutrition Committee released a report in 1996 stating that the inclusion of marine sources of omega-3 fatty acids in the diet is reasonable and potentially beneficial.
- Food sources of omega-3 fatty acids include tuna (2.3 g of omega-3 per 4 ounces of fish), pink salmon (1 g per 4 ounces of fish), mackerel (1.8-2.6 g per 4 ounces of fish), herring (1 to 2 g per 4 ounces of fish), king crab (0.6 g per 4 ounces of fish), shrimp (0.5 g per 4 ounces of fish), cod (0.3 g per 4 ounces of fish), menhaden oil (6.9 g per ounce), salmon oil (6.6 g per ounce), cod liver oil (6 g per ounce), canola oil (3 g per ounce), soybean oil (2.1 g per ounce), butter fat oil (0.6 g per ounce), and corn oil (0.3 g per ounce).

Review of the Evidence: Fish Oil/Omega-3 Fatty Acids

Condition Treated*	Study Design	Author, Year	N[†]	SS[†]	Study Quality[‡]	Magnitude of Benefit	ARR[†]	NNT[†]	Comments
Primary hyperlipidemia	RCT	Nordoy[9] 2001	422	Yes	4	Medium	NA	NA	Ethyl esters of omega-3 acids, 1.68 g.
Primary hyperlipidemia	RCT	Nordoy[6] 2000	41	Yes	4	Medium	NA	NA	3.36 g omega-3 acids.
Primary hyperlipidemia	RCT	Ezaki 2000	20	No	4	Medium	NA	NA	Perilla oil.
Primary hyperlipidemia	RCT	Bemelmans 2000	266	Yes	4	Medium	NA	NA	Decrease in diastolic pressure observed.
Primary hyperlipidemia	RCT	Goodfellow 2000	30	Yes	4	Medium	NA	NA	4 g omega-3 acids.
Primary hyperlipidemia	RCT	Nakamura[8] 1999	14	Yes	4	Medium	NA	NA	Statins plus EPA (900-1800 mg).

Review of the Evidence: Fish Oil/Omega-3 Fatty Acids—cont'd

Condition Treated*	Study Design	Author, Year	N†	SS†	Study Quality‡	Magnitude of Benefit	ARR†	NNT†	Comments
Primary hyperlipidemia	RCT	Pirich 1999	26	Yes	4	Medium	NA	NA	260 mg EPA, 140 mg DHA.
Primary hyperlipidemia	RCT	Nordoy 1998	41	Yes	4	Medium	NA	NA	Simvastatin plus 4 g omega-3 acids.
Primary hyperlipidemia	RCT	Goode 1997	28	Yes	4	Medium	NA	NA	MaxEPA, 10 capsules.
Primary hyperlipidemia	RCT	Adler 1997	50	Yes	4	Medium	NA	NA	Garlic oil plus fish oil (12 g).
Primary hyperlipidemia	RCT	Mori 1997	120	Yes	4	Medium	NA	NA	1.3 g EPA daily.
Primary hyperlipidemia	RCT	Hau 1996	9	Yes	4	Medium	NA	NA	1 g fish oil daily.
Primary hyperlipidemia	RCT	Grundt 1995	57	Yes	4	Medium	NA	NA	40 g K-85 daily.
Primary hyperlipidemia	RCT	Kasim-Karakas 1995	11	Yes	4	Medium	NA	NA	3 g omega-3 acids.
Primary hyperlipidemia	RCT	Mackness 1994	95	Yes	4	Medium	NA	NA	4 g K-85 daily.
Primary hyperlipidemia	RCT	Mori 1994	138	Yes	4	Medium	NA	NA	6 g fish oil daily.
Primary hyperlipidemia	RCT	Olszewski 1993	15	Yes	4	Medium	NA	NA	12 g fish oil daily.
Primary hyperlipidemia	RCT	Beilin 1993	138	Yes	4	Medium	NA	NA	6 or 12 g fish oil.
Primary hyperlipidemia	RCT	Contacos[7] 1993	32	Yes	4	Medium	NA	NA	3 g omega-3 acids.
Primary hyperlipidemia	RCT	Saynor[400] 1992	365	Yes	4	Medium	NA	NA	1.8 g EPA.
Primary hyperlipidemia	RCT	Naber 1992	17	Yes	4	Medium	NA	NA	1.2 g EPA, 1.2 g DHA.
Primary hyperlipidemia	RCT	Schmidt 1992	11	Yes	4	Medium	NA	NA	2.4 g and 9 g omega-3 acids.
Primary hyperlipidemia	RCT	Deslypere 1992	58	Yes	4	Medium	NA	NA	1.12, 2.24, and 3.37 g omega-3 acids.
Primary hyperlipidemia	RCT	Ernst 1991	44	Yes	4	Medium	NA	NA	3 g fish oil.
Primary hyperlipidemia	RCT	Cobiac 1991	31	Yes	4	Medium	NA	NA	4.5 g EPA and DHA.
Primary hyperlipidemia	RCT	Beil 1991	30	Yes	4	Medium	NA	NA	1.57 or 3.15 g omega-3 acids.
Primary hyperlipidemia	RCT	Terres 1991	30	Yes	4	Medium	NA	NA	10.5 g fish oil.
Primary hyperlipidemia	RCT	Valdini 1990	33	Yes	4	Medium	NA	NA	Fish oil, 6 capsules.
Primary hyperlipidemia	RCT	Molgaard[402] 1990	10	Yes	4	Medium	NA	NA	15 g MaxEPA.
Primary hyperlipidemia	RCT	Radack 1990	25	Yes	4	Medium	NA	NA	1.1-2.2 g Omega-3 acids;. LDL increase observed.
Primary hyperlipidemia	RCT	Haglung 1990	33	Yes	4	Medium	NA	NA	15 or 30 mL fish oil concentrate.
Primary hyperlipidemia	RCT	Harris[417] 1990	10	Yes	4	Medium	NA	NA	4.5, 7.5, and 12 g omega-3 acids.

Continued

Review of the Evidence: Fish Oil/Omega-3 Fatty Acids—*cont'd*

Condition Treated*	Study Design	Author, Year	N[†]	SS[†]	Study Quality[‡]	Magnitude of Benefit	ARR[†]	NNT[†]	Comments
Primary hyperlipidemia	RCT	Green 1990	27	Yes	4	Medium	NA	NA	15 g fish oil.
Primary hyperlipidemia	RCT	Radack 1989	29	Yes	4	Medium	NA	NA	1 or 2.2 g 0mega-3 acids.
Primary hyperlipidemia	RCT	Deck 1989	8	Yes	4	Medium	NA	NA	4.6 g omega-3 acids.
Primary hyperlipidemia	RCT	Wilt[415] 1989	38	Yes	4	Medium	NA	NA	20 g MaxEPA.
Primary hyperlipidemia	RCT	Harris[92] 1989	33	Yes	4	Medium	NA	NA	3-12 g fish oil.
Primary hyperlipidemia	RCT	Schmidt 1989	17	Yes	4	Medium	NA	NA	6 g omega-3 acids daily for 6 weeks.
Primary hyperlipidemia	RCT	Miller[401] 1988	86	Yes	4	Medium	NA	NA	10 g MaxEPA.
Primary hyperlipidemia	Crossover study	Harris 1988 (1)	8	Yes	4	Medium	NA	NA	6.8 g omega-3 acids.
Primary hyperlipidemia	RCT	Harris 1988 (2)	18	Yes	4	Medium	NA	NA	12 g Super EPA.
Primary hyperlipidemia	RCT	Stacpoole[36] 1988	21	Yes	4	Medium	NA	NA	MaxEPA, 15.75% or 3.75% of calories.
Primary hyperlipidemia	RCT	Zucker[416] 1988	25	Yes	4	Medium	NA	NA	3.24 g EPA, 2.16 g DHA.
Primary hyperlipidemia	RCT	Demke 1988	31	Yes	4	Medium	NA	NA	5 g fish oil; adverse effects measured.
Primary hyperlipidemia	RCT	Harris 1987 (1)	8	Yes	4	Medium	NA	NA	18 g MaxEPA.
Primary hyperlipidemia	RCT	Harris 1987 (2)	24	Yes	4	Medium	NA	NA	6-7 g omega-3 acids.
Primary hyperlipidemia	RCT	Simons[413] 1985	25	Yes	4	Medium	NA	NA	6 or 16 g fish oil.
Primary hyperlipidemia	RCT	Boberg[406] 1986	27	Yes	4	Medium	NA	NA	10 g MaxEPA daily, primrose oil.
Primary hyperlipidemia	RCT	Phillipson 1985	20	Yes	4	Medium	NA	NA	Fish oil rich diet vs. vegetable oil diet.
Primary hyperlipidemia	RCT	Sanders 1984	21	Yes	4	Medium	52%	2	15 g MaxEPA; NNT/ARR calculated for triglyceride reduction.
Primary hyperlipidemia	RCT	Chan[225] 2002	58	Yes	3	NA	NA	NA	Fish oil, 4 g daily, or atorvastatin, 40 mg.
Primary hyperlipidemia	RCT	Mori[22] 2000	59	Yes	4	NA	NA	NA	4 g EPA, DHA, or olive oil daily.
Primary hyperlipidemia	RCT	Grimsgaard[224] 1997	234	Yes	4	NA	NA	NA	EPA, 3.8 g, DHA, 3.6 g, or corn oil, 4.0 g daily.
Primary hyperlipidemia	RCT	Stacpoole[36] 1989	27	Yes	3	NA	NA	NA	Diets rich in fish oil (MaxEPA) or vegetable oil.
Primary hyperlipidemia	RCT	Sanders[221] 1997	26	Yes	3	NA	NA	NA	Effect of omega-6 acids vs. omega-3 acids on plasma lipoproteins and hemostatic factors.
Primary hyperlipidemia	RCT	Roche[223] 1996	32	Yes	3	NA	NA	NA	Low-fat dietary treatment with fish oil.
Primary hyperlipidemia	Comparative dose study	Harris[86] 1980	33	Yes	1	Small	NA	NA	3, 6 ,9, or 12 g fish oil.

Review of the Evidence: Fish Oil/Omega-3 Fatty Acids—*cont'd*

Condition Treated*	Study Design	Author, Year	N[†]	SS[†]	Study Quality[‡]	Magnitude of Benefit	ARR[†]	NNT[†]	Comments
Primary hyperlipidemia	Placebo controlled, single-blind	Morcos 1997	40	Yes	3	Medium	NA	NA	1.8 g EPA, 1.2 g DHA.
Primary hyperlipidemia	RCT	Jeyaraj 2000	16	Yes	3	Medium	NA	NA	0.6 g fish oil.
Primary hyperlipidemia	RCT	Warner 1989	34	Yes	3	Medium	NA	NA	50 mL fish oil.
Primary prevention of fatal coronary heart disease	Cohort study	Oomen[280] 2001	667	No	NA	NA	NA	NA	Dietary ALA.
Primary prevention of fatal coronary heart disease	Cohort study	Ascherio[281] 1996	43,757	Yes	NA	NA	NA	NA	ALA dietary intake associated with decreased risk of coronary disease (Health Professionals Follow-Up Study).
Primary prevention of fatal coronary heart disease (women)	Cohort study	Hu[233] 2002	84,688	Yes	NA	Medium	NA	NA	Diet rich in fish and omega-3 acids associated with decreased risk of cardiac disease and cardiac death in women (Nurses' Health Study).
Primary prevention of fatal coronary heart disease	Case control study	Tavani 2001	507	Yes	NA	Medium	NA	NA	Fish oil diet associated with decreased cardiac risk.
Primary prevention of fatal coronary heart disease	Case control study	Guallar[245] 1999	639	Yes	NA	Small	NA	NA	Protective effect of ALA.
Primary prevention of fatal coronary heart disease	Cohort study	Hu[242] 1999	76,283	Yes	NA	Medium	NA	NA	Protective effect for fatal infarction only.
Primary prevention of fatal coronary heart disease	Cohort study	Albert[243] 1998	20,551	Yes	NA	Medium	NA	NA	Fish intake measured (Physicians' Health Study).
Primary prevention of fatal coronary heart disease	Cohort study	Daviglus[239] 1997	1,822	Yes	NA	Medium	NA	NA	Fish consumption measured.
Primary prevention of fatal coronary heart disease	Case control study	Guallar 1995	14,916	No	NA	NA	NA	NA	No effect on incidence of first infarction detected.
Primary prevention of fatal coronary heart disease	Cohort study	Ascherio[281] 1996	44,825	No	NA	NA	NA	NA	No influence on risk of coronary heart disease detected.
Primary prevention of fatal coronary heart disease	Cohort study	Kromhout[235] 1985	852	Yes	NA	Medium	NA	NA	Decrease in mortality observed.
Primary prevention of fatal coronary heart disease	RCT	Dolecek[238] 1992	12,866	No	4	NA	NA	NA	ALA acid yielded no effect on mortality.
Primary prevention of fatal coronary heart disease	Cohort study	Curb 1985	7,615	No	NA	NA	NA	NA	No influence on total and fatal coronary heart disease.
Secondary prevention of fatal coronary heart disease	Meta-analysis	Bucher[226] 2002	15,806	Yes	NA	Medium	NA	NA	11 trials included; reduced overall mortality and cardiovascular death in patients with coronary artery disease taking dietary or supplemental omega-3 acids.
Secondary prevention of fatal coronary heart disease	RCT	Marchioli[230] 2002	11,323	Yes	5	Medium	NA	NA	1 g omega-3 acids.

F

Continued

Review of the Evidence: Fish Oil/Omega-3 Fatty Acids—*cont'd*

Condition Treated*	Study Design	Author, Year	N[†]	SS[†]	Study Quality[‡]	Magnitude of Benefit	ARR[†]	NNT[†]	Comments
Secondary prevention of fatal coronary heart disease	RCT	Anonymous[23] 1999	11,324	Yes	5	Medium	NA	NA	Omega-3 acids daily.
Secondary prevention of fatal coronary heart disease	RCT	Lorgeril[277] 1999	605	Yes	3	Medium	NA	NA	ALA-rich diet; decrease in mortality observed.
Secondary prevention of fatal coronary heart disease	RCT	Burr[227] 1989	2,033	Yes	5	Medium	NA	NA	0.5 g omega-3 acids daily or fish diet; decrease in mortality observed.
Coronary heart disease	RCT	von Schacky[290] 1999	223	Mixed	3	NA	NA	NA	Fish oil concentrate (55% EPA and DHA) significantly decreased progression of coronary artery plaques, although changes in luminal diameter and cardiovascular events were not significantly different between groups.
Coronary heart disease	Cohort study	Yamada[289] 2000	470	Yes	NA	Medium	NA	NA	Comparison of dietary habits.
Coronary heart disease	RCT	Durrington[399] 2001	59	Yes	4	Medium	NA	NA	4 g fish oil concentrate daily.
Coronary heart disease	RCT	Johansen[294] 1999	54	Yes	4	Medium	NA	NA	5.1 g omega-3 acids daily.
Coronary heart disease	RCT	Kothny 1998	18	No	4	NA	NA	NA	18 g fish oil concentrate daily.
Coronary heart disease	RCT	Schindler 1996	20	Yes	4	Medium	NA	NA	0.18-1.1g omega-3 fatty acids.
Coronary heart disease	RCT	Yamamoto 1995	22	Yes	4	Medium	NA	NA	1.8 g EPA daily.
Coronary heart disease	RCT	Eritsland 1995 (1)	511	No	4	NA	NA	NA	4 g fish oil daily.
Coronary heart disease	RCT	Herrmann 1995	35	Yes	4	Medium	NA	NA	12 g fish oil.
Coronary heart disease	RCT	Eritsland 1994 (1)	260	Yes	4	Medium	NA	NA	4 g fish oil concentrate.
Coronary heart disease	RCT	Eritsland 1994 (2)	58	Yes	4	Medium	NA	NA	4 g omega-3 fatty acids.
Coronary heart disease	RCT	Eritsland 1995 (2)	56	Yes	4	Medium	NA	NA	3.4 g EPA and DHA.
Coronary heart disease	RCT	Sacks[291] 1995	59	No	4	NA	NA	NA	6 g omega-3 fatty acids; artery diameter not changed.
Coronary heart disease	RCT	Salachas 1994	39	Yes	4	Medium	NA	NA	10 g fish oil.
Coronary heart disease	RCT	Tomei 1993	39	Yes	4	Medium	NA	NA	Fish oil plus simvastatin vs. simvastatin.
Coronary heart disease	RCT	Fleischhauer 1993	14	Yes	4	Medium	NA	NA	5 g EPA and DHA daily.
Coronary heart disease	RCT	Pyzh 1993	11	Yes	4	Medium	NA	NA	5 g omega-3 fatty acids.
Coronary heart disease	RCT	Aucamp[298] 1993	23	Yes	4	Medium	NA	NA	5 g omega-3 fatty acids.
Coronary heart disease	RCT	Arteaga 1993	21	Yes	3	Medium	NA	NA	2, 4, or 6 g omega-3 fatty acids daily.
Coronary heart disease	RCT	Samsonov 1992	37	Yes	4	Medium	NA	NA	3.4 g omega-3 fatty acids daily.
Coronary heart disease	RCT	Eritsland[296] 1992	370	Yes	4	Medium	NA	NA	3.4 g omega-3 fatty acids daily.

Review of the Evidence: Fish Oil/Omega-3 Fatty Acids—cont'd

Condition Treated*	Study Design	Author, Year	N[†]	SS[†]	Study Quality[‡]	Magnitude of Benefit	ARR[†]	NNT[†]	Comments
Coronary heart disease	RCT	Bairati 1992	125	Yes	4	Medium	NA	NA	4.5 g EPA and DHA.
Coronary heart disease	RCT	Nikkila 1991	32	Yes	4	Medium	NA	NA	2.4 g EPA and DHA.
Coronary heart disease	RCT	Reis 1990	89	Yes	4	Medium	NA	NA	6 g or 7 g fish oil.
Coronary heart disease	RCT	De Caterina 1990	15	Yes	4	Medium	NA	NA	3 g EPA, 1.3 g DHA.
Coronary heart disease	RCT	Reis 1988	67	Yes	4	Medium	NA	NA	6 g omega-3 fatty acids daily.
Coronary heart disease	RCT	Verheught 1986	5	Yes	4	Medium	NA	NA	3 g omega-3 fatty acids daily.
Coronary heart disease	RCT	Vacek 1989	8	No	4	NA	NA	NA	5.4 g EPA, 3.6 g DHA.
Coronary heart disease	RCT	Mehta 1988	8	No	4	NA	NA	NA	3.2 g EPA, 2.2 g DHA.
Coronary heart disease	RCT	Kristensen[299] 1987	36	No	3	Medium	NA	NA	Fish oil supplementation for 12 weeks.
Coronary heart disease	Cohort study	Saynor[405] 1984	107	Yes	NA	Medium	NA	NA	1.8 g or 3.6 g EPA.
Coronary artery bypass graft	RCT	Eritsland[296] 1996	610	Yes	5	Medium	NA	NA	4 g fish oil concentrate daily.
Coronary artery bypass graft	RCT	Roy[297] 1991	120	Yes	4	Medium	NA	NA	Comparison with ASA.
Hypertension	Meta-analysis	Morris 1993	1,356	Yes	NA	Small	NA	NA	31 trials included; dose-response effect found in fish oil dosing.
Hypertension	Meta-analysis	Appel[18] 1993	728	NA	NA	Medium	NA	NA	11 trials included; diets including >3 g daily of omega-3 acids associated with blood pressure reductions.
Hypertension	Meta-analysis	Radack 1989	4 trials	No	NA	Medium	NA	NA	Heterogeneous trials included; inconclusive analysis.
Hypertension	RCT	Mori[19] 1999	59	Yes	5	Medium	NA	NA	4 g DHA or 4 g EPA.
Hypertension	RCT	Howe 1994	56	No	5	NA	NA	NA	No difference between fish and olive oil.
Hypertension	RCT	Margolin 1991	46	No	5	NA	NA	NA	Fish and corn oil associated with decreased blood pressure.
Hypertension	RCT	Prisco 1998	32	Yes	4	Medium	NA	NA	4 g EPA or 4 g DHA.
Hypertension	RCT	Toft 1997	78	No	4	NA	NA	NA	No influence on coagulation.
Hypertension	Cohort study	Pauletto 1996	1308	Yes	NA	Medium	NA	NA	Difference between fish consumers and vegetarians assessed.
Hypertension	RCT	Gray 1996	21	No	4	NA	NA	NA	Drug-treated hypertension observed.
Hypertension	RCT	Toft 1995	78	Yes	4	Medium	NA	NA	4 g EPA and DHA.
Hypertension	Early phase trial; controlled trial	Sacks 1994 (two publications)	350	No	4	NA	NA	NA	Fish and placebo oils decreased blood pressure.
Hypertension	RCT	Lungerhausen 1994	43	Yes	4	Medium	NA	NA	4 g Omacor; not placebo effective in drug-treated patients.
Hypertension	RCT	Sacks 1994	350	No	4	NA	NA	NA	Fish oil 6 g.

F

Continued

Review of the Evidence: Fish Oil/Omega-3 Fatty Acids—cont'd

Condition Treated*	Study Design	Author, Year	N[†]	SS[†]	Study Quality[‡]	Magnitude of Benefit	ARR[†]	NNT[†]	Comments
Hypertension	RCT	Landmark 1993	18	No	4	NA	NA	NA	EPA 4.55 g.
Hypertension	RCT	Grossman 1993	11	No	4	NA	NA	NA	3 g omega-3 acids.
Hypertension	RCT	Morris 1993	16	No	4	NA	NA	NA	6 g or 12 g fish oil.
Hypertension	RCT	Vandongen 1993	120	No	4	NA	NA	NA	3.65 g omega-3 acids.
Hypertension	Cohort study	Cobiac[26] 1992	114	Yes	NA	Medium	NA	NA	Combination of sodium restriction and fish oil.
Hypertension	RCT	Radack 1991	33	Yes	4	Medium	NA	NA	2.4 g omega-3 acids.
Hypertension	RCT	Cobiac 1991	50	Yes	4	Medium	NA	NA	Combination with sodium restriction.
Hypertension	RCT	Wing 1990	20	No	4	NA	NA	NA	15 g fish oil.
Hypertension	RCT	Hughes 1990	26	No	4	NA	NA	NA	5 g omega-3 acids.
Hypertension	RCT	Singer[59] 1990	44	Yes	4	Medium	NA	NA	ALA.
Hypertension	RCT	Levinson 1990	16	Yes	4	Medium	NA	NA	50 g fish oil.
Hypertension	RCT	Singer[59] 1990	47	Yes	4	Medium	NA	NA	9 g fish oil.
Hypertension	RCT	Bonaa[21] 1990	156	Yes	4	Medium	NA	NA	6 g RPA and DHA.
Hypertension	RCT	Knapp[20] 1989	32	Yes	4	Medium	NA	NA	15 g omega-3 acids.
Hypertension	RCT	Steiner 1989	28	Yes	4	Medium	NA	NA	800 mg omega-3 acids.
Hypertension	RCT	Mortensen[403] 1983	20	Yes	4	Medium	NA	NA	4 g omega-3 acids (MaxEPA).
Hypertension	RCT	Norris[404] 1986	16	Yes	4	Medium	NA	NA	16 g MaxEPA.
Rheumatoid arthritis	Meta-analysis	Fortin 1992	317-395	Yes	NA	Medium	NA	NA	9-10 trials included; significant reductions in tender joints and morning stiffness vs. dietary controls.
Rheumatoid arthritis	RCT	Volker[260] 2000	50	Yes	4	Medium	NA	NA	40 mg/kg omega-3 acids.
Rheumatoid arthritis	RCT	Navarro 2000	39	Yes	4	Medium	NA	NA	Increased EPA in joint fluid reported.
Rheumatoid arthritis	Case control study	Shapiro 1996	324	Yes	NA	Medium	NA	NA	Dietary fish observed.
Rheumatoid arthritis	RCT	Lau 1995	45	Yes	4	Medium	NA	NA	1.7 g EPA, 1.1 g DHA.
Rheumatoid arthritis	RCT	Kremer[259] 1995	66	Yes	4	Medium	NA	NA	130 mg/kg omega-3 acids.
Rheumatoid arthritis	RCT	Geusens[258] 1994	90	Yes	4	Medium	NA	NA	2.6 g omega-3 acids daily.
Rheumatoid arthritis	RCT	Faarvang 1994	51	Yes	4	Medium	NA	NA	3.6 g omega-3 fatty acids.

Review of the Evidence: Fish Oil/Omega-3 Fatty Acids—*cont'd*

F

Condition Treated*	Study Design	Author, Year	N[†]	SS[†]	Study Quality[‡]	Magnitude of Benefit	ARR[†]	NNT[†]	Comments
Rheumatoid arthritis	RCT	Lau[257] 1993	64	Yes	4	Medium	NA	NA	10 g MaxEPA.
Rheumatoid arthritis	RCT	Skoldstam[256] 1992	46	Yes	4	Medium	NA	NA	10 g MaxEPA.
Rheumatoid arthritis	RCT	Nielsen[251] 1992	57	Yes	4	Medium	9%	11	3.6 g omega-3 acids.
Rheumatoid arthritis	RCT	Kjeldsenkragh 1992	67	Yes	4	Medium	NA	NA	3.8 g EPA, 2 g DHA.
Rheumatoid arthritis	RCT	van der Tempel 1990	16	Yes	4	Medium	NA	NA	3.36 g omega-3 acids.
Rheumatoid arthritis	RCT	Kremer[248] 1990	49	Yes	4	Medium	NA	NA	27 mg/kg EPA and 18 mg/kg DHA vs. 54 mg/kg EPA and 27 mg/kg DHA
Rheumatoid arthritis	RCT	Kremer 1988	55	Yes	4	Medium	NA	NA	3.2 g EPA, 2 g DHA.
Rheumatoid arthritis	RCT	Cleland[254] 1988	60	Yes	4	Medium	NA	NA	3.2 g EPA, 2 g DHA.
Rheumatoid arthritis	RCT	Belch 1988	16	Yes	4	Medium	54%	2	240 mg EPA, 450 mg DLA.
Rheumatoid arthritis	RCT	Kremer[249] 1987	40	Yes	4	Medium	NA	NA	2.7 g EPA, 1.8 g DHA.
Rheumatoid arthritis	RCT	Kremer 1986	36	Yes	4	Medium	NA	NA	2.7 g MaxEPA.
Rheumatoid arthritis	RCT	Kremer[247] 1985	37	Yes	4	Medium	NA	NA	108 g EPA.
Growth and development of infants	RCT	Carlson[312] 1996	59	Yes	4	Medium	NA	NA	0.2% GHA in infant formula.
Growth and development of infants	RCT	Birch[310] 1992	81	Yes	4	Medium	NA	NA	Fish oil–supplemented formula associated with improved visual development.
Growth and development of infants	RCT	Uauy 1990	42	Yes	4	Medium	NA	NA	Formula containing omega-3 acids ± omega-6 acids.
Growth and development of infants	RCT	Carlson 1987	39	Yes	4	Medium	NA	NA	750 mg/kg EPA.
Growth and development of infants	RCT, comparison	Helland[45] 2001	590	No	3	None	NA	NA	10 mL cod liver oil vs. corn oil during pregnancy associated with no differences in pregnancy outcomes, growth, or development.
Ulcerative colitis	RCT	Dichi[323] 2000	10	Yes	4	Small	NA	NA	5.4 g omega-3 fatty acids.
Ulcerative colitis	RCT	Almallah 2000	18	Yes	4	Medium	NA	NA	3.2 g EPA, 2.4 g DHA.
Ulcerative colitis	RCT	Loeschke[322] 1996	64	No	4	NA	NA	NA	5.1 g omega-3 acids.
Ulcerative colitis	RCT	Aslan[320] 1992	11	Yes	4	Medium	NA	NA	4.2 g omega-3 acids.
Ulcerative colitis	RCT	Hawthorne[319] 1992	87	Yes	4	Medium	NA	NA	4.5 g EPA.
Ulcerative colitis	RCT	Hillier 1991	18	Yes	4	Medium	NA	NA	Changes in colonic lipids.
Ulcerative colitis	RCT	Stenson 1991	18	Yes	4	Medium	NA	NA	18 g MaxEPA.
Ulcerative colitis	RCT	Hawthorne[318] 1990	96	No	4	NA	NA	NA	4.5 g EPA.

Continued

Review of the Evidence: Fish Oil/Omega-3 Fatty Acids—*cont'd*

Condition Treated*	Study Design	Author, Year	N†	SS†	Study Quality‡	Magnitude of Benefit	ARR†	NNT†	Comments
Ulcerative colitis	RCT	Stenson[317] 1990	41	Yes	4	Medium	30%	3	18 g EPA.
Ulcerative colitis	RCT	Lorenz[316] 1989	10	No	4	NA	NA	NA	3.2 g omega-3 acids.
Ulcerative colitis	RCT	McCall 1989	6	Yes	4	Medium	NA	NA	4 g EPA.
Type 2 diabetes	Meta-analysis	Farmer 2001 Montori[38] 2000	823	Yes	NA	Small-medium	NA	NA	18 trials included; 3-18 g fish oil daily for mean of 12 weeks; Significant reduction in triglycerides, but elevated LDL. No effect on HDL or hemoglobin A_{1c}.
Type 2 diabetes	Meta-analysis	Friedberg[37] 1998	423	Yes	NA	Medium	NA	NA	26 trials included; up to 30% reduction in triglycerides with no effects seen on hemoglobin A_{1c} levels; small increase in LDL reported.
Type 2 diabetes	RCT	Frenais[420] 2001	5	Yes	4	Medium	NA	NA	Decrease in HDL-APOA1 production rate.
Type 2 diabetes	RCT	Patti 1999	16	Yes	4	Medium	NA	NA	Decrease in all VLDL subfractions.
Type 2 diabetes	RCT	Sirtori[429] 1997; 1998	935	Yes	4	Medium	NA	NA	2 g omega-3 acids; positive effect on lipid pattern.
Type 2 diabetes	RCT	Dunstan 1997	55	Yes	4	Medium	NA	NA	3.6 g omega-3 acids,.
Type 2 diabetes	RCT	Goh 1997	28	Yes	4	Medium	NA	NA	35 mg/kg EPA and DHA.
Type 2 diabetes	RCT	Sheehan 1997	15	Yes	4	Medium	NA	NA	20 g fish oil.
Type 2 diabetes	RCT	Zak 1996	17	Yes	4	Medium	NA	NA	5.5 g omega-3 acids.
Type 2 diabetes	RCT	Rivellese 1996	16	Yes	4	Medium	NA	NA	2.7 g EPA and DHA.
Type 2 diabetes	RCT	Fasching 1996	10	Yes	4	Medium	NA	NA	4.6 g omega-3 acids.
Type 2 diabetes	RCT	Maffettone 1996	16	Yes	4	Medium	NA	NA	2.7 g EPA and DHA.
Type 2 diabetes	RCT	McManus 1996	11	Yes	4	Medium	NA	NA	35 mg/kg omega-3 acids.
Type 2 diabetes	RCT	McGrath 1996	23	Yes	4	Medium	NA	NA	Increase in lipid peroxidation.
Type 2 diabetes	RCT	Morgan 1995	40	Yes	4	Medium	NA	NA	9 g or 18 g fish oil.
Type 2 diabetes	RCT	McVeigh[409] 1994	16	Yes	4	Medium	NA	NA	1.8 g EPA, 1.2 g DHA.
Type 2 diabetes	RCT	Axelrod 1994	20	Yes	4	Medium	NA	NA	2.5 g omega-3 acids.
Type 2 diabetes	RCT, crossover	McVeigh 1993	23	Yes	4	Medium	NA	NA	Improvement of vascular response to acetylcholine.
Type 2 diabetes	RCT	Takahashi 1993	18	Yes	4	Medium	NA	NA	2.4 g fish oil, 4 g primrose oil.
Type 2 diabetes	RCT	Pelikanova 1993	20	No	4	NA	NA	NA	No effect on glucose homeostasis
Type 2 diabetes	RCT	Connor 1993	16	Yes	4	Medium	NA	NA	4.1 g EPA, 1.9 g DHA.

Review of the Evidence: Fish Oil/Omega-3 Fatty Acids—*cont'd*

Condition Treated*	Study Design	Author, Year	N[†]	SS[†]	Study Quality[‡]	Magnitude of Benefit	ARR[†]	NNT[†]	Comments
Type 2 diabetes	RCT	Donnelly 1994	43	Yes	4	Medium	NA	NA	Increase in lipid peroxidation.
Type 2 diabetes	RCT	Zambon 1992	10	Yes	4	Small	NA	NA	Glyburide and fish oil.
Type 2 diabetes	RCT	Pelikanova 1992	10	No	4	NA	NA	NA	Glucose homeostasis assessed.
Type 2 diabetes	RCT	Boberg 1992	14	Yes	4	Medium	NA	NA	10 g MaxEPA.
Type 2 diabetes	RCT	Hermann 1992	19	Yes	4	Medium	NA	NA	3 g omega-3 acids.
Type 2 diabetes	RCT	Annuzzi 1991	8	Yes	4	Medium	NA	NA	1.8 g EPA, 1.2 g DHA.
Type 2 diabetes	RCT	Fasching 1991	8	Yes	4	Medium	NA	NA	30 ml fish oil; glucose homeostasis assessed.
Type 2 diabetes	RCT	Feskens 1991	175	Yes	4	NA	NA	NA	Glucose intolerance assessed.
Type 2 diabetes	RCT	Vessby 1990	14	Yes	4	Medium	NA	NA	3 g omega-3 acids.
Type 2 diabetes	RCT	Hendra[410] 1990	80	Yes	4	Medium	NA	NA	1.8 g EPA, 1.2 g DHA.
Type 2 diabetes	RCT	Annuzzi 1989	8	Yes	4	Medium	NA	NA	10 g MaxEPA.
Type 2 diabetes	RCT	Borkman 1989	10	Yes	4	Medium	NA	NA	10 g fish oil; adverse effects assessed.
Type 2 diabetes	RCT	Popp-Snijders 1988	11	Yes	4	Medium	NA	NA	Insulin levels assessed.
Type 2 diabetes	RCT	Glauber 1988	6	Yes	4	Medium	NA	NA	Effects on insulin, glucose assessed.
Type 2 diabetes	RCT	Borkman 1988	10	Yes	4	Medium	NA	NA	Increase in fasting glucose observed.
Type 2 diabetes	RCT	Schectman 1988	13	Yes	4	Medium	NA	NA	4 g or 7.5 g omega-3 acids.
Type 2 diabetes	RCT	Popp-Snijders 1987	6	Yes	4	Medium	NA	NA	3 g omega-3 acids.
Type 2 diabetes	RCT	Schectman 1987	8	Yes	4	Medium	NA	NA	4 g omega-3 acids.
Type 1 diabetes	RCT	Stiefel 1999	18	Yes	4	Medium	NA	NA	330 mg DHA, 630 mg EPA.
Type 1 diabetes	RCT	Mori[419] 1991	27	Yes	4	Medium	NA	NA	15 g MaxEPA.
Type 1 diabetes	RCT	Haines[407] 1986	41	Yes	4	Medium	NA	NA	15 g MaxEPA.
Complications of diabetes (diabetic nephropathy)	RCT	Langershausen 1997	32	Yes	4	Medium	NA	NA	3.4 g omega-3 acids.
Complications of diabetes (diabetic nephropathy)	RCT	Rossing 1996	36	Yes	4	Medium	NA	NA	4.6 g omega-3 acids.
Complications of diabetes (diabetic nephropathy)	RCT	Rossing 1995	29	No	4	NA	NA	NA	4.6 g omega-3 acids; renal function.
Complications of diabetes (diabetic nephropathy)	RCT	Jensen 1989	18	Yes	4	Medium	NA	NA	Albumin escape rate assessed.

Continued

Review of the Evidence: Fish Oil/Omega-3 Fatty Acids—*cont'd*

Condition Treated*	Study Design	Author, Year	N[†]	SS[†]	Study Quality[‡]	Magnitude of Benefit	ARR[†]	NNT[†]	Comments
IgA nephropathy	Meta-analysis	Dillon[328] 1997	202	No	NA	No	NA	NA	5 trials included; analysis suggested possible benefits in patients with proteinuria.
IgA nephropathy	Cohort study	Donadio[330] 2001	73	Yes	NA	Medium	NA	NA	3.76 g EPA, 2.94 g DHA.
IgA nephropathy	Cohort from RCT	Donadio 1999	106	Yes	NA	Medium	38%	3	Fish oil supplementation assessed.
IgA nephropathy	RCT	Pettersson 1994	32	Yes	4	Small	NA	NA	6 g fish oil.
IgA nephropathy	RCT	Donadio 1994	106	Yes	4	Medium	30%	3	1.2 g fish oil; NNT/ARR for survival.
IgA nephropathy	Controlled trial	Bennett 1989	37	Yes	3	Medium	NA	NA	10 g EPA vs. no treatment for 2 years.
Crohn's disease	RCT	Belluzzi 1997	50	Yes	4	Medium	28%	3	2.7 g omega-3 acids; Purepa.
Crohn's disease	RCT	Belluzzi[426] 1996	78	Yes	4	Medium	33%	3	2.7 g omega-3 acids.
Crohn's disease	RCT	Lorenz-Meyer 1996	204	No	4	NA	NA	NA	3 g fish oil concentrate.
Crohn's disease	RCT	Belluzzi[327] 1994	50	Yes	4	Medium	NA	NA	Various preparations of EPA and DHA in Purepa capsules, with pH 5.5 and 60-min time release showing best integration into phospholipid membranes.
Crohn's disease	RCT	Ikehata 1992	10	Yes	4	Medium	NA	NA	Lipid emulsion with EPA vs. placebo.
Crohn's disease	RCT	Lorenz[316] 1989	39	Yes	4	Medium	NA	NA	3.2 g omega-3 acids.
Crohn's disease	Case control	Mate 1991	38	Yes	NA	Medium	34%	3	Free diet without drugs vs. fish diet without drugs (100-200 g of fish oil or 250 g of fish oil per week) for 2 years.
Restenosis after coronary angioplasty	Meta-analysis	Gapinski 1993	951	Yes	NA	Medium	13.9%	7	7 trials included; omega-3 fatty acids (fish oil) trials pooled, with dose-response effect observed.
Restenosis after coronary angioplasty	Meta-analysis	O'Connor 1992	951	Yes	NA	Medium	NA	NA	7 trials included; omega-3 fatty acid (fish oil) trials pooled, with 12-month odds-ratio 0.71 (95% CI, 0.54-0.94).
Restenosis after coronary angioplasty	RCT	Johansen[294] 1999	500	No	4	NA	NA	NA	5.1 g Omacor.
Restenosis after coronary angioplasty	RCT	Cairns[293] 1996 (EMPAR Study)	814	No	4	NA	NA	NA	5.4 g omega-3 acids.
Restenosis after coronary angioplasty	RCT	Franzen[113] 1993	212	No	4	NA	NA	NA	3.15 g omega-3 acids.
Restenosis after coronary angioplasty	RCT	Bairati 1992	205	Yes	4	Medium	25%	4	2.7 g EPA, 1.8 g DHA.
Restenosis after coronary angioplasty	RCT	Kaul 1992	107	No	4	NA	NA	NA	1.8 g EPA, 1.2 g DHA.
Restenosis after coronary angioplasty	RCT	Maresta[27] 2002	339	Yes	4	Medium	10%	10	6 capsules omega-3 fatty acids (Esapent: 50% EPA, 35% DHA, 3 mg Vitamin E) daily prior/after PTCA.
Restenosis after coronary angioplasty	RCT	Reis 1989	204	No	4	None	NA	NA	6 g omega-3 acids.

Review of the Evidence: Fish Oil/Omega-3 Fatty Acids—cont'd

Condition Treated*	Study Design	Author, Year	N[†]	SS[†]	Study Quality[‡]	Magnitude of Benefit	ARR[†]	NNT[†]	Comments
Restenosis after coronary angioplasty	RCT	Nye 1990	108	Yes	4	Medium	19%	5	MaxEPA.
Restenosis after coronary angioplasty	RCT	Leaf[295] 1994	551	No	4	None	NA	NA	4.1 g EPA and 2.8 g DHA for 6 months vs. corn oil.
Restenosis after coronary angioplasty	RCT	Milner 1989	194	Yes	4	Medium	16%	6	4.5 g omega-3 acid.
Restenosis after coronary angioplasty	RCT	Grigg 1989	108	No	4	NA	NA	NA	1.8 g EPA, 1.2 g DHA.
Restenosis after coronary angioplasty	RCT	Dehmer 1988	82	Yes	4	Medium	20%	5	3.2 g EPA.
Restenosis after coronary angioplasty	RCT	Reis 1988	300	No	3	NA	NA	NA	6 g omega-3 acids.
Restenosis after coronary angioplasty	Randomized, single-blind	Cheng 1990	50	No	3	NA	NA	NA	10 g MaxEPA.
Cancer	Cohort study	Terry[306] 2001	6,272	Yes	NA	NA	NA	NA	Protective effect of fish oil.
Cancer	RCT	Aronson 2001	9	Yes	4	NA	NA	NA	Expression of COX-2 assessed.
Cancer	RCT	Gee 1999	49	No	4	NA	NA	NA	1.4 g EPA.
Cancer	RCT	Gogos 1998	60	Yes	4	Medium	NA	NA	Increase in survival observed.
Cancer	RCT	Swails 1997	20	Yes	4	Medium	NA	NA	Eicosanoids decreased.
Cancer	Placebo controlled	Anti 1994	60	Yes	3	Medium	NA	NA	Proliferative index assessed.
Cancer	RCT	Anti 1992	20	Yes	4	Medium	NA	NA	4 g EPA; proliferation assessed.
Cancer prevention	Prospective cohort	Augustsson[300] 2003	47, 882	Yes	3	Small	NA	NA	Fish consumption measured; possibly confounded by other environmental factors.
Cancer (anorexia, cachexia)	RCT	Bruera[397] 2003	60	No	3	None	NA	NA	1.8 g EPA, 1.2 g DHA.
Cancer (cachexia)	RCT	Fearon[398] 2003	200	Yes	3	Medium	NA	NA	Supplement drink with vitamin E or C plus 2.2 g EPA.
Cancer (weight loss)	Uncontrolled clinical trial	Wigmore[396] 2000	26	Yes	2	Medium	NA	NA	6 g EPA.
Cancer mortality	Cohort	Caygill[303] 1995	24 countries	Mixed	NA	Medium	NA	NA	Fish oil consumption followed.
Hemodialysis and peritoneal dialysis	RCT	Donnelly 1992	16	No	4	NA	NA	NA	3.6 g omega-3 acids.
Systemic lupus erythematosus	RCT	Clark[333] 1993	26	Yes	4	Medium	NA	NA	Lipid changes assessed; no effect on renal function.
Systemic lupus erythematosus	RCT	Clark[334] 1994	26	No	4	NA	NA	NA	Renal function assessed.
Systemic lupus erythematosus	RCT	Walton[332] 1991	27	Yes	4	Medium	59%	2	20 g MaxEPA.
Heart transplantation	RCT	Holm[276] 2001	45	Yes	4	Medium	NA	NA	Increase in TNF-alpha.
Renal transplantation	RCT	Santos[272] 2000	30	No	4	NA	NA	NA	No effect on renal function.
Renal transplantation	RCT	Castro 1997	43	Yes	4	Medium	NA	NA	Decrease in hyperlipidemia.

Continued

Review of the Evidence: Fish Oil/Omega-3 Fatty Acids—*cont'd*

Condition Treated*	Study Design	Author, Year	N[†]	SS[†]	Study Quality[‡]	Magnitude of Benefit	ARR[†]	NNT[†]	Comments
Renal transplantation	RCT	Kooijmans-Coutinho[273] 1996	50	No	4	NA	NA	NA	6 g fish oil.
Renal transplantation	RCT	Maachi[266] 1995	83	Yes	4	Medium	NA	NA	Improved renal function.
Renal transplantation	RCT	Kooijmans-Coutinho 1994	50	No	4	NA	NA	NA	6 g fish oil.
Renal transplantation	RCT	van der Heide[265] 1993	66	Yes	4	Medium	36%	3	6 g fish oil.
Renal transplantation	RCT	Homan van der Heide[264] 1992	88	Yes	4	Medium	NA	NA	6 g fish oil.
Renal transplantation	RCT	Berthoux[263] 1992	32	Yes	4	Medium	NA	NA	Improved renal function.
Renal transplantation (hemodynamics, rejection)	RCT	van der Heide[264] 1993	31	No	4	NA	NA	NA	6 g fish oil.
Renal transplantation	RCT	Homan van der Heide[262] 1990	21	Yes	4	Medium	NA	NA	6 g fish oil.
Renal transplantation	RCT	Badalamenti[268] 1995	26	Yes	3	Medium	NA	NA	12 g fish oil.
Renal transplantation	RCT	van der Heide[265] 1993	88	Yes	3	Medium	NA	NA	6 g fish oil.
Drug toxicity (cyclosporine)	RCT	Holm[276] 2001	45	Yes	4	Medium	NA	NA	3.4 g omega-3 acids.
Drug toxicity (cyclosporine)	RCT	Andreassen[271] 1997	28	Yes	4	Medium	28%	3	4 g omega-3 acids.
Drug toxicity (cyclosporine)	RCT	Bennett[275] 1995	90	Yes	4	Medium	NA	NA	9 or 18 g EPA.
Drug toxicity (cyclosporine)	RCT	Badalamenti[268] 1995	27	Yes	4	Medium	NA	NA	12 g MaxEPA.
Drug toxicity (cyclosporine)	RCT	Hansen 1995	27	No	4	NA	NA	NA	6 g fish oil.
Drug toxicity (cyclosporine)	RCT	Ventura[270] 1993	20	Yes	4	Medium	NA	NA	3 g omega-3 acids.
Drug toxicity (cyclosporine)	RCT	Brouwer[11] 1991	17	Yes	4	Medium	NA	NA	3 g or 6 g omega-3 acids.
Drug toxicity (cyclosporine)	RCT	Hansen 1995	12	No	3	NA	NA	NA	6 g fish oil.
AIDS	RCT	Luis Roman 2001	38	Yes	4	Medium	NA	NA	9 g omega-3 acids.
AIDS	RCT	Pilchard 1998	64	No	4	NA	NA	NA	No change in immune parameters.
AIDS	RCT	Bell 1996	19	Yes	4	Medium	NA	NA	Change in prostaglandins.
Psoriasis	RCT	Danno[346] 1998	40	Yes	4	Medium	NA	NA	1.8 g EPA.
Psoriasis	RCT	Bittiner[335] 1987	29	Yes	4	Medium	38%	3	ARR/NNT for results at 8 weeks.
Psoriasis	RCT	Mayser[345] 1998	83	Yes	4	Medium	14%	7	4.2 g EPA.
Psoriasis	RCT	Soyland[343] 1993	145	No	4	NA	NA	NA	5 g EPA and DHA.

Review of the Evidence: Fish Oil/Omega-3 Fatty Acids—cont'd

Condition Treated*	Study Design	Author, Year	N[†]	SS[†]	Study Quality[‡]	Magnitude of Benefit	ARR[†]	NNT[†]	Comments
Psoriasis	RCT	Henneicke-von Zepelin[342] 1993	52	Yes	4	Medium	NA	NA	1%-10% omega-3 acids in ointment.
Psoriasis	RCT	Grimminger[341] 1993	20	Yes	4	Medium	NA	NA	Infusions of 2.1 g EPA, 21 g DHA.
Psoriasis	RCT	Escobar[340] 1992	25	Yes	4	Medium	NA	NA	Ointment administered.
Psoriasis	RCT	Gupta[339] 1990	25	No	4	NA	NA	NA	5.4 g EPA, 3.6 g DHA.
Psoriasis	RCT	Gupta[338] 1989	18	Yes	4	Medium	NA	NA	Fish oil or placebo (olive oil) for 15 weeks.
Psoriasis	RCT	Bjorneboe[337] 1988	30	No	4	NA	NA	NA	1.8 g EPA.
Psoriasis	RCT	Bittiner[336] 1988	28	Yes	4	Medium	NA	NA	1.8 g EPA.
Atopic dermatitis (eczema)	RCT	Soyland 1994	45	No	4	NA	NA	NA	6 g omega-3 acids.
Atopic dermatitis (eczema)	RCT	Bjorneboe[348] 1989	23	Yes	4	Medium	NA	NA	1.8 g EPA.
Atopic dermatitis (eczema)	RCT	Bjorneboe[347] 1987	23	Yes	4	Medium	NA	NA	1.8 g EPA.
Bronchial asthma	RCT	Hodge 1998	39	No	4	NA	NA	NA	1.2 g omega-3 acids.
Bronchial asthma	RCT	Okamoto[358] 2000	14	Yes	4	Medium	NA	NA	10-20 mg perilla oil.
Bronchial asthma	RCT	Nagakura[357] 2000	29	Yes	4	Medium	NA	NA	17-26.8 mg/kg EPA, 7.3-11.5 mg/kg DHA; study in children.
Bronchial asthma	Case control	Hodge 1996	574	Yes	NA	NA	NA	NA	Fish diet; reduced risk in children.
Bronchial asthma	Case control	Schwartz 1994	2526	Yes	NA	NA	NA	NA	Association between fish diet and FEV$_1$.
Bronchial asthma	RCT	Thien[355] 1993	37	No	4	NA	NA	NA	MaxEPA, 3.2g daily.
Bronchial asthma	RCT	Dry[356] 1991	12	Yes	4	Medium	NA	NA	1 g omega-3 acids daily.
Bronchial asthma	RCT	McDonald[354] 1990	15	No	4	NA	NA	NA	2.7 g EPA, 1.8 g DHA.
Bronchial asthma	RCT	Stenius-Aarhiala 1989	29	No	4	NA	NA	NA	Primrose and fish oils.
Bronchial asthma	RCT	Arm[352] 1989	25	Yes	4	Medium	NA	NA	Attenuation of allergen response observed.
Bronchial asthma	RCT	Arm[351] 1988	25	No	4	NA	NA	NA	No clinical effect observed.
Acute respiratory distress syndrome	RCT	Gadek 1999	146	Yes	4	Medium	20%	5	EPA and GLA.
Pregnancy-induced hypertension and preeclampsia	Cohort study	Olsen[367] 2002	8729	Yes	NA	NA	NA	NA	Protective effect of fish oil observed.
Pregnancy-induced hypertension and preeclampsia	RCT	Olsen[366] 2000	1619	Yes	4	Medium	NA	NA	Reduced risk of preterm delivery observed.
Pregnancy-induced hypertension and preeclampsia	RCT	Onwude[365] 1995	230	No	4	NA	NA	NA	MaxEPA.

F

Review of the Evidence: Fish Oil/Omega-3 Fatty Acids—*cont'd*

Condition Treated*	Study Design	Author, Year	N[†]	SS[†]	Study Quality[‡]	Magnitude of Benefit	ARR[†]	NNT[†]	Comments
Pregnancy-induced hypertension and preeclampsia	RCT	Williams 1995	62	Yes	4	Medium	NA	NA	Reduced risk of pre-eclampsia observed.
Pregnancy-induced hypertension and preeclampsia	RCT	Salvig[364] 1996	533	No	4	NA	NA	NA	No effect on blood pressure observed.
Pregnancy-induced hypertension and preeclampsia	RCT	Bulstra-Ramarrers[363] 1994	63	No	4	NA	NA	NA	3 g EPA, DHA daily.
Pregnancy-induced hypertension and preeclampsia	RCT	Sorensom 1993	47	Yes	4	Medium	NA	NA	Effects on thromboxanes reported.
Pregnancy-induced hypertension and preeclampsia	RCT	Olsen[361] 1992 1994	533	Yes	4	Medium	NA	NA	2.7 g omega-3 acids.
Pregnancy-induced hypertension and preeclampsia	RCT	D'Almeida[362] 1992	150	Yes	4	Medium	16%	6	Primrose oil plus fish oil.
Pregnancy-induced hypertension and preeclampsia	Case control	Olsen 1990	5644	Yes	NA	Medium	NA	NA	Reduction in preterm delivery observed.
Cystic fibrosis	RCT	Henderson 1994	12	No	4	NA	NA	NA	3.2 g EPA, 2.2 g DHA.
Cystic fibrosis	RCT	De Vizia[383] 2003	50	Yes	3	Small	NA	NA	EPA/DHA = 1.3% of daily dietary intake.
Schizophrenia	RCT	Fenton[370] 2001	87	No	4	NA	NA	NA	3 g EPA.
Bipolar disorder	RCT	Stoll[373] 1999	30	Yes	4	Medium	NA	NA	6.2 g EPA, 3.4 g DHA.
Depression	RCT	Nemets[378] 2002	20	Yes	4	Medium	50%	2	2 g EPA.
Peripheral vascular disease	RCT	Leng 1998	120	No	4	NA	NA	NA	No effect on walking distance observed.
Peripheral vascular disease	RCT	Gazso 1992	19	Yes	4	Medium	NA	NA	Effect on platelet aggregation observed.
Peripheral vascular disease	RCT	Mori 1992	32	Yes	4	Medium	NA	NA	Platelet aggregation measured.
Arrhythmia	RCT	Christensen[176] 1996	55	Yes	4	Medium	NA	NA	4.3 g EPA and DHA.
Arrhythmia	RCT	Christensen[175] 1995	24	No	4		NA	NA	4.3 g EPA and DHA.
Stroke	Cohort study	Iso[285] 2001	79,839	Yes	NA	NA	NA	NA	Lower risk of stroke in fish consumers observed.
Stroke	Case control	Simon[286] 1995	96	Yes	NA	NA	NA	NA	Association of stroke decrease with omega-3 acids in lipids.
Stroke	Cohort study	Keli[283] 1994	550	Yes	NA	NA	NA	NA	Lower risk of stroke observed.
Stroke	RCT	Green 1985	11	Yes	4	Medium	NA	NA	Decrease in triglycerides, no effects on hemostasis observed.
Multiple sclerosis	RCT	Bates[411] 1989	312	No	4	NA	NA	NA	1.7 g EPA, 1.1 g DHA.
Migraine	RCT	Pradalier 2001	96	No	4	NA	NA	NA	6 g omega-3 acids.
Tardive dyskinesia	RCT	Vaddadi 1989	45	Yes	4	Medium	NA	NA	Improvement in psychopathology observed.
Raynaud's phenomenon	RCT	Digiacomo 1989	32	Yes	4	Medium	NA	NA	3.96 g EPA, 2.64 g DHA.
Intensive care unit patients	RCT	Braga 1999	206	Yes	4	Medium	16%	6	Enteral diet with omega-3 acids.

Review of the Evidence: Fish Oil/Omega-3 Fatty Acids—*cont'd*

Condition Treated*	Study Design	Author, Year	N†	SS†	Study Quality‡	Magnitude of Benefit	ARR†	NNT†	Comments
Intensive care unit patients	RCT	Weimann 1998	29	Yes	4	Medium	NA	NA	Enteral diet with omega-3 acids, arginine, and nucleotides.
Intensive care unit patients	RCT	Wachtler 1997	40	Yes	4	Medium	NA	NA	Decrease in leukotriene B_4 observed.
Intensive care unit patients	RCT	Roulet 1997	10	Yes	4	Medium	NA	NA	Decrease in platelet aggregation observed.
Intensive care unit patients	RCT	Schilling 1996	41	Yes	4	Medium	NA	NA	Enteral diet with omega-3 acids, arginine, and nucleotides.
Intensive care unit patients	RCT	Senkal 1995	42	Yes	4	Medium	NA	NA	Decrease in TNF-alpha observed.
Intensive care unit patients	RCT	Bower 1995	296	Yes	4	Medium	NA	NA	Decrease in hospital stay reported.
Serum lipids in postmenopausal women	RCT	Stark 2000	36	Yes	4	Medium	NA	NA	Improvement in risk factors with 2.4 g EPA, 1.6 g DHA.
Serum lipids in postmenopausal women	RCT	Wander 1996	48	Yes	4	Medium	NA	NA	Protection against LDL oxidation reported.
Dysmenorrhea	RCT	Deutch[13] 2000	78	Yes	4	Medium	NA	NA	5 g fish oil.
Dysmenorrhea	RCT	Harel[381] 1996	42	Yes	4	Medium	NA	NA	720 mg DHA, 1080 mg EPA.
Dysmenorrhea	Case control	Deutch 1995	181	Yes	NA	NA	NA	NA	Association of fish oil and menstrual pain observed.
Postviral fatigue syndrome	RCT	Behan 1990	63	Yes	4	Medium	51%	2	Combination of ALA, DHA, and EPA.
Familial hyper-cholesterolemia	RCT	Balestrieri[391] 1996	14	No	4	NA	NA	NA	6 g fish oil.
Familial hyper-cholesterolemia	RCT	Tato[390] 1993	9	Yes	4	Medium	NA	NA	3 g EPA, 4.5 g DHA daily.
Familial hyper-cholesterolemia	RCT	Ullmann[389] 1990	10	Yes	4	Medium	NA	NA	Additive effects of fish oil and statin therapy observed.
Familial hyper-cholesterolemia	RCT	Chan[225] 2002	58	Yes	3	NA	NA	NA	40 mg atorvastatin, 4 g fish oil daily.
Obesity	RCT	Mori[19] 1999	69	Yes	4	Medium	NA	NA	3.65 g omega-3 acids.
Obesity	RCT	Riserus 2001	25	Yes	4	Medium	NA	NA	4.2 g conjugated linoleic acid.
Aggression in young adults	RCT	Hamazaki 1996	41	Yes	4	Medium	NA	NA	25-18 g DHA.
Osteoarthritis	RCT	Stammers 1992	86	No	4	NA	NA	NA	10 mL cod liver oil.
Primary cardiac arrest	Case control	Siscovick 1995	493	Yes	NA	NA	NA	NA	Fish oil associated with reduced risk.
Maximal aerobic performance	RCT	Leaf[424] 1988	19	No	3	NA	NA	NA	6 g or 12 g omega-3 acids.
Acute myocardial infarction	RCT	Singh[229] 1997	122	Yes	4	Medium	10%	10	2.9 g ALA.
Idiopathic recurrent urolithiasis	RCT	Buck 1993	40	Yes	4	Medium	NA	NA	Reduction in urinary calcium observed.

*Primary or secondary outcome.
†*N*, Number of patients; *SS*, statistically significant; *ARR*, absolute risk reduction; *NNT*, the number of patients who need to undergo a specific intervention in order to observe an outcome in one individual.
‡0-2 = poor; 3-4 = good; 5 = excellent.
ASA, Alpha-linolenic acid; *APOA1*, apolipoprotein A1; *COX-2*, cyclooxygenase-2; *DHA*, docosahexaenoic acid; *EPA*, eicosapentaenoic acid; *GLA*, gamma-linolenic acid; *HDL*, high-density lipoprotein; *LDL*, Low-density lipoprotein; *NA*, not applicable; *PTCA*, percutaneous transluminal coronary angioplasty; *RCT*, randomized, controlled trial; *TNF*, tumor necrosis factor; *VLDL*, very-low-density lipoprotein.
For an explanation of each category in this table, please see Table 3 in the Introduction.

REVIEW OF THE EVIDENCE: DISCUSSION
Hypertriglyceridemia (Fish Oil/EPA Plus DHA)

- There is strong scientific evidence from human trials that omega-3 fatty acids from fish or fish oil supplements (EPA + DHA) significantly reduce blood triglyceride levels.[38,220-224] Benefits appear to be dose-dependent, with effects at doses as low as 2 g of omega-3 fatty acids per day. Higher doses have greater effects, and 4 g per day can lower triglyceride levels by 25% to 40%. Effects appear to be additive with HMG-CoA reductase inhibitor ("statin") drugs such as simvastatin,[6] pravastatin,[7,8] and atorvastatin.[9] The effects of fish oil on hypertriglyceridemia are similar in patients with or without diabetes[38] and in those with kidney disease receiving dialysis. It is not clear how fish oil therapy compares to other agents used for hypertriglyceridemia, such as fibrates (e.g., gemfibrozil and fenofibrate) and niacin/nicotinic acid.
- Fish oil supplements appear to cause small improvements in high-density lipoprotein (HDL/"good cholesterol") levels by 1% to 3%. However, increases (worsening) in low-density lipoprotein (LDL/"bad cholesterol") levels by 5% to 10% are also observed. Therefore, for individuals with high blood levels of total cholesterol or LDLs, significant improvements will likely not be seen, and a different treatment should be selected. Fish oil does not appear to affect C-reactive protein (CRP) levels.[225]
- It is not clear if alpha-linolenic acid significantly affects triglyceride levels, and there is conflicting evidence in this area.
- The American Heart Association, in its 2003 recommendations, reports that supplementation with 2 to 4 g of EPA + DHA each day can lower triglycerides by 20% to 40%.[5] Because of the risk of bleeding from omega-3 fatty acids (particularly at doses greater than 3 g per day), a physician should be consulted prior to starting treatment with supplements.

Secondary Cardiovascular Disease Prevention (Fish Oil/ EPA Plus DHA)

- Several well-conducted randomized, controlled trials report that in people with a history of heart attack, regular consumption of oily fish (200 to 400 g of fish each week, equal to 500 to 800 mg of daily omega-3 fatty acids) or fish oil/omega-3 supplements (containing 850 to 1800 mg of EPA + DHA) reduces the risk of non-fatal heart attack, fatal heart attack, sudden death, and all-cause mortality (death due to any cause).[5,23,226-230] Most patients in these studies were also using conventional heart drugs, suggesting that the benefits of fish oils may add to the effects of other therapies. Benefits have been reported after 3 months of use, and after up to 3.5 years of follow-up. Benefits of supplements may not occur in populations that already consume large amounts of dietary fish.[231]
- Multiple mechanisms have been proposed for the beneficial effects of omega-3 fatty acids. These include reduced triglyceride levels, reduced inflammation, slightly lowered blood pressure, reduced blood clotting, reduced tendency of the heart to develop abnormal rhythms, and diminished buildup of atherosclerotic plaques in arteries of the heart. Experiments suggest that omega-3 fatty acids may reduce platelet-derived growth factor (PDGF), decrease platelet aggregation, inhibit the expression of vascular adhesion molecules, and stimulate relaxation of endothelial cells in the walls of blood vessels.[232]
- The American Heart Association, in its 2003 recommendations, suggests that people with known coronary heart disease take approximately 1 g of EPA and DHA (combined) each day.[5] This may be obtained from eating fish or from fish oil capsule supplements. Because of the risk of bleeding from omega-3 fatty acids (particularly at doses greater than 3 g per day), a physician should be consulted prior to starting treatment with supplements.

Hypertension

- Multiple human trials report small reductions in blood pressure with intake of omega-3 fatty acids.[10,15-21] Reductions of 2 to 5 mm Hg have been observed, and benefits may be greater in those with higher blood pressure. Effects appear to be dose-responsive (higher doses have greater effects).[10] DHA may have greater benefits than EPA.[22]
- Intakes of greater than 3 g of omega-3 fatty acids per day may be necessary to obtain clinically relevant effects, and at this dose level there is an increased risk of bleeding. Therefore, a physician should be consulted prior to starting treatment with supplements. Other approaches are known to have greater effects on blood pressure, such as salt reduction, weight loss, exercise, and antihypertensive drug therapy. Therefore, although omega-3 fatty acids do appear to have effects in this area, their role in the management of high blood pressure is limited.

Primary Cardiovascular Disease Prevention (Fish Intake)

- Several large studies of populations (epidemiologic studies) report a significantly lower rate of death from heart disease in men and women who regularly eat fish.[233-242] Other epidemiologic research reports no such benefits.[243-245] It is not clear if reported benefits only occur in certain groups of people, such as those at risk of developing heart disease. Overall, the evidence suggests benefits of regular consumption of fish oil. However, well-designed, randomized, controlled trials that classify people by their risk of developing heart disease are necessary before a firm conclusion can be drawn.
- The American Heart Association, in its 2003 recommendations, suggests that all adults eat fish at least two times per week.[5] In particular, fatty fish are recommended, including mackerel, lake trout, herring, sardines, albacore tuna, and salmon.

Rheumatoid Arthritis (Fish Oil)

- Multiple randomized, controlled trials report improvements in morning stiffness and joint tenderness with the regular intake of fish oil supplements for up to 3 months.[246-260] Benefits have been reported as additive with anti-inflammatory medications such as NSAIDs (e.g., ibuprofen and aspirin). However, because of weaknesses in study designs and reporting, better-quality research is necessary before a strong favorable recommendation can be made. Effects beyond 3 months of treatment have not been well evaluated.

Protection from Cyclosporine Toxicity in Organ Transplant Patients

- There are multiple studies of heart transplant and kidney transplant patients taking cyclosporine (Neoral) who were administered fish oil supplements. The majority of trials report improvements in kidney function (glomerular filtration rate, serum creatinine)[11,261-269] and less hypertension[61,270,271] compared to patients not taking fish oil. Although several recent studies report no benefits on kidney function,[272-276] the weight of scientific evidence favors the beneficial effects of fish oil. No changes have been found in rates of rejection or graft survival.

Secondary Cardiovascular Disease Prevention (Alpha-Linolenic Acid [ALA])

- Several randomized, controlled trials have examined the effects of ALA in people with a history of heart attack. Although some studies suggest benefits,[229,242,277] others do not.[278-280] Weaknesses in some of this research, such as the use of other foods that may also be beneficial, make results difficult to interpret. Additional research is necessary before a conclusion can be drawn in this area.

Primary Cardiovascular Disease Prevention (Alpha-Linolenic Acid [ALA])

- Several large studies of populations (epidemiologic studies) report a significantly reduced risk of fatal or non-fatal heart attack in men and women who regularly consume foods high in ALA.[242,281,282] Other epidemiologic research reports no such benefits.[245,280] Although the existing research is compelling, weaknesses in this research, such as the use of other foods that may also be beneficial and effects of risk factors for heart disease such as smoking, make results difficult to interpret. Additional research is necessary before a conclusion can be drawn in this area.
- The American Heart Association, in its 2003 recommendations, suggests that in addition to eating fish at least twice a week, all adults should consume plant-derived sources of omega-3 fatty acids, such as tofu/soybeans, walnuts, flaxseed oil, and canola oil.[5]

Stroke Prevention

- Several large studies of populations (epidemiologic studies) have examined the effects of omega-3 fatty acid intake on stroke risk. Some studies suggest benefits,[283-285] although others do not.[277,286-288] Effects are likely on ischemic or thrombotic stroke risk, and very large intakes of omega-3 fatty acids ("Eskimo" amounts) may actually increase the risk of hemorrhagic stroke.[35] At this time, it is unclear if there are benefits in people with or without a history of stroke, or if effects of fish oil are comparable to other treatment strategies.
- Multiple mechanisms have been proposed for the beneficial effects of omega-3 fatty acids. These include reduced triglyceride levels, reduced inflammation, slightly lowered blood pressure, reduced blood clotting, and diminished buildup of atherosclerotic plaques in blood vessels. Experiments suggest that omega-3 fatty acids may reduce platelet-derived growth factor (PDGF), decrease platelet aggregation, inhibit the expression of vascular adhesion molecules, and stimulate relaxation of endothelial cells in the walls of blood vessels.[232]

Atherosclerosis

- Some research reports that regular intake of fish or fish oil supplements reduces the risk of developing atherosclerotic plaques in the arteries of the heart,[289,290] although other research reports no effects.[291] Additional evidence is necessary before a firm conclusion can be drawn in this area.

Prevention of Restenosis after Coronary Angioplasty

- Several randomized controlled trials have evaluated whether omega-3 fatty acid intake reduces blockage of arteries in the heart following balloon angioplasty (percutaneous transluminal coronary angioplasty [PTCA]). Some research has reported small significant benefits,[27,292] although other investigations have not found benefits.[293-295] The evidence in this area remains inconclusive.

Prevention of Graft Failure after Heart Bypass Surgery

- There is limited study of the use of fish oils in patients after undergoing coronary artery bypass grafting (CABG). Initial research suggests possible small benefits in reducing blood clot formation in vein grafts.[296,297] Additional evidence is necessary before a firm conclusion can be drawn in this area.

Angina Pectoris

- Preliminary studies report reductions in angina associated with fish oil intake.[298,299] Better research is necessary before a firm conclusion can be drawn.

Cardiac Arrhythmias

- There is promising evidence that omega-3 fatty acids may decrease the risk of cardiac arrhythmias.[175-177] This is one proposed mechanism behind the reduced number of heart attacks in people who regularly ingest fish oil or EPA + DHA. Additional research is needed in this area specifically before a firm conclusion can be reached.

Prevention of Cancer

- Several population (epidemiologic) studies report that dietary omega-3 fatty acids or fish oil may reduce the risk of developing breast, colon, or prostate cancer.[300-306] Randomized, controlled trials are necessary before a clear conclusion can be drawn.

Colon Cancer

- Omega-3 fatty acids are commonly taken by cancer patients.[307] Although preliminary studies report that growth of colon cancer cells may be reduced by taking fish oil, effects on survival or remission have not been measured adequately.

Infant Eye/Brain Development

- It has been suggested that fatty acids, particularly DHA, may be important for normal neurologic development. Fatty acids are added to some infant formulas. Several studies have examined the effects of DHA on development of vision in preterm infants.[308-313] Short-term benefits have been reported, compared to formulas without DHA, although these benefits may not be meaningful in the long term. Well-designed research is necessary before a clear conclusion can be reached.

Ulcerative Colitis

- It has been suggested that effects of omega-3 fatty acids on inflammation may be beneficial in patients with ulcerative colitis when added to standard therapy, and several studies have been conducted in this area.[67,314-324] Although results have been promising, the majority of trials are small and not well designed. Therefore, better research is necessary before a clear conclusion can be drawn.

Crohn's Disease

- It has been suggested that effects of omega-3 fatty acids on inflammation may be beneficial in patients with Crohn's disease when added to standard therapy, and several studies have been conducted in this area.[316,325-327] Results are conflicting, and no clear conclusion can be drawn at this time.

IgA Nephropathy

- There are conflicting results from several poorly designed trials in this area.[328-330]

Nephrotic Syndrome

- There is not enough reliable evidence to form a clear conclusion in this area.[36,331]

Lupus Erythematosus

- There is not enough reliable evidence to form a clear conclusion in this area.[332-334]

Psoriasis

- Several studies in this area do not provide enough reliable evidence to form a clear conclusion.[335-346]

Eczema

- Several studies of EPA for eczema do not provide enough reliable evidence to form a clear conclusion.[347-349]

Asthma

- Several studies in this area do not provide enough reliable evidence to form a clear conclusion, with some studies reporting no effects,[350-355] and others finding benefits.[356-359] Because most studies have been small without clear descriptions of design or results, the results cannot be considered conclusive.[360]

Preeclampsia

- Several studies of fish oil do not provide enough reliable evidence to form a clear conclusion in this area.[361-367]

Schizophrenia

- There is promising preliminary evidence from several randomized, controlled trials in this area.[368-371] Additional research is necessary before a firm conclusion can be reached.[372]

Bipolar Disorder

- Several studies in this area do not provide enough reliable evidence to form a clear conclusion.[373-375]

Depression

- Several studies in this area do not provide enough reliable evidence to form a clear conclusion.[376-378] Promising initial evidence[379] requires confirmation with larger, well-designed trials.

Dysmenorrhea

- It has been suggested that anti-inflammatory or prostaglandin-mediated mechanisms associated with omega-3 fatty acids may play a role in the management of dysmenorrhea. There is preliminary evidence suggesting possible benefits of fish oil/omega-3 fatty acids in patients with dysmenorrhea.[13,380,381] Additional research is necessary before a firm conclusion can be reached.

Cystic Fibrosis

- A small amount of research in this area does not provide enough reliable evidence to form a clear conclusion.[218,382-388]

Diabetes

- Although slight increases in fasting blood glucose levels have been noted in patients with type 2 (adult-onset) diabetes, the available scientific evidence suggests that there are no significant long-term effects of fish oil in patients with diabetes, including no changes in progression of diabetic nephropathy (kidney disease), albuminuria (protein in the urine), or hemoglobin A_{1c} levels.[37,38] Most studies in this area are not well designed.
- The effects of fish oil on hypertriglyceridemia are similar in patients with or without diabetes.[38]

Hypercholesterolemia

- Although fish oil is able to reduce triglycerides, beneficial effects on blood cholesterol levels have not been demonstrated. Fish oil supplements appear to cause small improvements in high-density lipoprotein (HDL/"good cholesterol") levels by 1% to 3%. However, increases (worsening) in low-density lipoprotein (LDL/"bad cholesterol") levels by 5% to 10% are also observed (dose-dependent, with effects likely to occur at 1 g/day or greater of omega-3 fatty acids). Therefore, for individuals with high blood levels of total cholesterol or LDL, significant improvements will likely not be seen, and a different treatment should be selected. Fish oil does not appear to affect C-reactive protein (CRP) levels.[225]
- Several randomized trials in patients with familial hypercholesterolemia yielded conflicting results.[389-393]

Transplant Rejection Prevention (Kidney and Heart)

- There are multiple studies of heart transplant and kidney transplant patients taking cyclosporine (Neoral) who were administered fish oil supplements. The majority of trials report improvements in kidney function (glomerular filtration rate, serum creatinine)[11,261-269] and less hypertension[261,270,271] compared to patients not taking fish oil. However, several recent studies report no benefits on kidney function,[272-276] and no changes have been found in rates of rejection or graft survival.

Appetite/Weight Loss in Cancer Patients

- There is preliminary evidence that fish oil supplementation does not improve appetite or prevent weight loss in cancer patients.[394-398]

FORMULARY: BRANDS USED IN CLINICAL TRIALS/THIRD-PARTY TESTING

Brands Used in Clinical Trials

- Omacor: Pronova, AS, Oslo, Norway.[294,399]
- EICOSAPEN: Hormon-Chemie Munchen GmbH, Germany.[14]
- MaxEPA: Seven Seas Ltd[333,336,347,351-353,371,392,400-407] and Marfleet Refining,[332,411] Hull, UK; Fresenius, Bad Homburg, Germany[408]; Duncan Flockhart[409,410]; RP Scherer Pty, Melbourne, Australia[412,414]; RP Scherer, Clearwater, FL,[24,320] and Troy, MI, USA[339,412,419]; Reckitt and Colman Pharmaceuticals, Sydney, Australia[412,419]; Zyma, Saronno, Italy[268]; Pierre Fabre Sante, Castres, France[420]; RP Scherer Canada Inc., Windsor, Ontario, Canada.[421]
- Pikasol: Pronova Biocare A/S Norway[175]; EPAX 5500, Pronova Biocare A/S Norway[176]; Lube Ltd, Hadsund, Denmark.[422,423]
- Promega: Warner-Lambert Parke Davis, Hanover, NJ, USA.[17,424]
- Purepa: Tillotts Pharma AG.[324,425,426]
- Super-EPA: Pharmacaps Inc., Marlow, Buckinghamshire, UK.[427]
- K-85 (capsules of ethyl-esters of n-3 PUFA, each containing 1000 mg of fish oil): Fresenius, Bad Homburg, Germany.[408]
- Fish oil capsules (180 mg of EPA and 120 mg of DHA per capsule): RP Scherer do Brasil Encapsulacoes Ltda, Sao Paulo, Brazil.[323]

- Trienyl: Lek, International Pharmaceutical group, Republic of Slovenia.[428]
- ESAPENT: Pharmacia and Upjohn.[27,429]
- Efamol Marine(combination of fish oil and evening primrose oil): Scotia Pharmaceuticals Ltd.[344]

Brands Shown to Contain Claimed Ingredients Through Third-Party Testing

- Generally, a high-quality oil will be certified as organic by a reputable third party, will be found in light-resistant containers, may be refrigerated, and will be dated.
- MaxEPA (18% EPA and 12% DHA), and other fish oil supplements (e.g., blue-fin tuna oil, which contains 7% EPA and 25% DHA), are derived from cold-water ocean fish.
- **Consumerlab:** Six of the 20 products failed to pass the review due to inadequate amounts of DHA, which ranged from 50% to 83% of the amounts stated on the labels. Two of these six products were also found to contain only 33% and 82%, respectively, of the labeled amounts of EPA. Two of the products that failed made claims on the labels that their "potency" had been "tested" or "verified."
- Consumerlab.com approved the following omega-3 fatty acids (EPA/DHA) from fish/marine oil products: Health From the Sun The Total EFA Essential Fatty Acid Dietary Supplement (72 mg of EPA, 46 mg of DHA per capsule)—marketed from Health From The Sun, A Division of Arkopharma; Jarrow Formulas MaxDHA Purified by Molecular Distillation, 80% omega-3 Fish Oil, 50% DHA, 20% EPA (500 mg of fish oil, 100 mg of EPA, 250 mg of DHA per softgel)—manufactured by Jarrow Formulas, Inc; Member's Mark Omega 3 Fish Oil, 1000 mg Natural Concentrate (1000 mg of fish oil, 180 mg of EPA, 120 mg of DHA per softgel)—distributed by SWC; Nutrilite Omega 3 Complex Dietary Supplement (300 mg of fish oil, 65 mg of EPA, 45 mg of DHA per softgel)—distributed by Access Business Group International LLC; Pure Encapsulations EPA/DHA essentials (1000 mg of fish oil, 300 mg of EPA, 200 mg of DHA per capsule)—manufactured by Pure Encapsulations, Inc; Puritan's Pride Inspired By Nature Salmon Oil 500 mg (500 mg of fish oil, 40 mg of EPA, 60 mg of DHA per softgel)—manufactured by Puritan's Pride, Inc.; Shaklee EPA Omega-3 Fatty Acid Dietary Supplement (182 mg of EPA, 78 mg of EPA, 240 mg of DHA per softgel)—manufactured by Shaklee Corp; Solgar Omega-3 "700" EPA & DHA from Cold Water Fish (700 mg of fish oil, 360 mg of EPA, 240 mg of DHA per softgel)—manufactured by Solgar Vitamin and Herb; Spectrum Essentials Omega 3 Cold Processed Norwegian Fish Oil (1000 mg of fish oil, 180 mg of EPA, 120 mg of DHA per capsule)—distributed by Spectrum Organic Products, Inc.; The Vitamine Shoppe EPA-DHA Omega-3 Fish Oil 500 (1000 mg of fish oil, 300 mg of EPA, 200 of mg DHA per softgel)—manufactured for the Vitamine Shoppe; Trader Darwin's Molecularly Distilled Omega-34 Fatty Acids Dietary Supplement (1100 mg of fish oil, 300 mg of EPA, 200 mg of DHA per softgel) – manufactured by Trader Joe's; Vitamin World Naturally Inspired EPA Natural Fish Oil 1000 mg (1000 mg of fish oil, 180 mg of EPA, 120 mg of DHA per softgel)—manufactured by Vitamin World, Inc.; ZonePerfect Omega 3 Molecular Distilled Fish Oil and Vitamin E Supplement (1000 mg of fish oil, 160 mg of EPA, 107 mg of DHA per capsule)—distributed by ZonePerfect Nutrition Co.; Dale Alexander Omega-3 Fish Oil Concentrate (234 mg of EPA, 125 mg of DHA per softgel)—manufactured by Twin Laboratories, Inc.; Nutrilite Omega 3 Complex Dietary Supplement (300 mg of fish oil, 65 mg of EPA, 45 mg of DHA per softgel)—distributed by Access Business Group International LLC.
- Analysis of the following samples revealed no detectable total mercury (the analysis could detect as little as 0.1 µg of total mercury per g): Twinlab Emulsified Super Max EPA; Twinlab EPA New & Improved; Twinlab Omege-3 [sic] Concentrate; Nature's Way Max EPA Fish Oil; Amni Omega-3 Marine Fish Oil; Nordic Naturals DHA Junior; Atkins Diet Essential Oils; Health from The Sun Ultra DHA 50; Kyolic-EPA (Aged Garlic & Fish Oil).

References

1. Zanarini MC, Frankenburg FR. Omega-3 fatty acid treatment of women with borderline personality disorder: a double-blind, placebo-controlled pilot study. Am J Psychiatry 2003;160(1):167-169.
2. Barberger-Gateau P, Letenneur L, Deschamps V, et al. Fish, meat, and risk of dementia: cohort study. BMJ 2002;325(7370):932-933.
3. Schlanger S, Shinitzky M, Yam D. Diet enriched with omega-3 fatty acids alleviates convulsion symptoms in epilepsy patients. Epilepsia 2002;43(1):103-104.
4. Terkelsen LH, Eskild-Jensen A, Kjeldsen H, et al. Topical application of cod liver oil ointment accelerates wound healing: an experimental study in wounds in the ears of hairless mice. Scand J Plast Reconstr Surg Hand Surg 2000;34(1):15-20.
5. Kris-Etherton PM, Harris WS, Appel LJ. Fish consumption, fish oil, omega-3 fatty acids, and cardiovascular disease. Arterioscler Thromb Vasc Biol 2003;23(2):e20-e30.
6. Nordoy A, Bonaa KH, Sandset PM, et al. Effect of omega-3 fatty acids and simvastatin on hemostatic risk factors and postprandial hyperlipemia in patients with combined hyperlipemia. Arterioscler Thromb Vasc Biol 2000;20(1):259-265.
7. Contacos C, Barter PJ, Sullivan DR. Effect of pravastatin and omega-3 fatty acids on plasma lipids and lipoproteins in patients with combined hyperlipidemia. Arterioscler Thromb 1993;13(12):1755-1762.
8. Nakamura N, Hamazaki T, Ohta M, et al. Joint effects of HMG-CoA reductase inhibitors and eicosapentaenoic acids on serum lipid profile and plasma fatty acid concentrations in patients with hyperlipidemia. Int J Clin Lab Res 1999;29(1):22-25.
9. Nordoy A, Hansen JB, Brox J, et al. Effects of atorvastatin and omega-3 fatty acids on LDL subfractions and postprandial hyperlipemia in patients with combined hyperlipemia. Nutr Metab Cardiovasc Dis 2001;11(1):7-16.
10. Morris MC, Sacks F, Rosner B. Does fish oil lower blood pressure? A meta-analysis of controlled trials. Circulation 1993;88(2):523-533.
11. Brouwer RM, Wenting GJ, Pos B, et al. Fish oil ameliorates established cyclosporin A nephrotoxicity after heart transplantation [abstract]. Kidney Int 1991;40:347-348.
12. Burns CP, Halabi S, Clamon GH, et al. Phase I clinical study of fish oil fatty acid capsules for patients with cancer cachexia: cancer and leukemia group B study 9473. Clin Cancer Res 1999;5(12):3942-3947.
13. Deutch B, Jorgensen EB, Hansen JC. Menstrual discomfort in Danish women reduced by dietary supplements of omega-3 PUFA and B12 (fish oil or seal oil capsules). Nutr Res 2000;20(5):621-631.
14. Kuenzel U, Bertsch S. Clinical experiences with a standardized commercial fish oil product containing 33.5% omega-3 fatty acids—field trial with 3958 hyperlipemic patients in general practitioner practice. In Chandra RK (ed): Health Effects of Fish and Fish Oils. New Foundland, ARTS Biomedical Publishers and Distributors, 1989, pp 567-579.
15. Kinrys G. Hypomania associated with omega 3 fatty acids. Arch Gen Psychiatry 2000;57(7):715-716.
16. Howe PR. Dietary fats and hypertension. Focus on fish oil. Ann N Y Acad Sci 1997;827:339-352.
17. Morris MC, Taylor JO, Stampfer MJ, et al. The effect of fish oil on blood pressure in mild hypertensive subjects: a randomized crossover trial. Am J Clin Nutr 1993;57(1):59-64.
18. Appel LJ, Miller ER, III, Seidler AJ, et al. Does supplementation of diet with 'fish oil' reduce blood pressure? A meta-analysis of controlled clinical trials. Arch Intern Med 1993;153(12):1429-1438.
19. Mori TA, Bao DQ, Burke V, et al. Docosahexaenoic acid but not eicosapentaenoic acid lowers ambulatory blood pressure and heart rate in humans. Hypertension 1999;34(2):253-260.
20. Knapp HR, FitzGerald GA. The antihypertensive effects of fish oil. A controlled study of polyunsaturated fatty acid supplements in essential hypertension. N Engl J Med 1989;320(16):1037-1043.
21. Bonaa KH, Bjerve KS, Straume B, et al. Effect of eicosapentaenoic and docosahexaenoic acids on blood pressure in hypertension. A population-based intervention trial from the Tromso study. N Engl J Med 1990;322(12):795-801.

22. Mori TA, Watts GF, Burke V, et al. Differential effects of eicosapentaenoic acid and docosahexaenoic acid on vascular reactivity of the forearm microcirculation in hyperlipidemic, overweight men. Circulation 2000;102(11): 1264-1269.

23. Anonymous. Dietary supplementation with n-3 polyunsaturated fatty acids and vitamin E after myocardial infarction: results of the GISSI-Prevenzione trial. Gruppo Italiano per lo Studio della Sopravvivenza nell'Infarto miocardico. Lancet 1999;354(9177):447-455.

24. Salomon P, Kornbluth AA, Janowitz HD. Treatment of ulcerative colitis with fish oil n-3-omega-fatty acid: an open trial. J Clin Gastroenterol 1990; 12(2):157-161.

25. Glaum M, Metzelthin E, Junker S, et al. [Comparative effect of oral fat loads with saturated, omega-6 and omega- 3 fatty acids before and after fish oil capsule therapy in healthy probands]. Klin Wochenschr 1990; 68(Suppl 22):103-105.

26. Cobiac L, Nestel PJ, Wing LM, et al. A low-sodium diet supplemented with fish oil lowers blood pressure in the elderly. J Hypertens 1992;10(1):87-92.

27. Maresta A, Balduccelli M, Varani E, et al. Prevention of postcoronary angioplasty restenosis by omega-3 fatty acids: main results of the Esapent for Prevention of Restenosis Italian Study (ESPRIT). Am Heart J 2002; 143(6):E5.

28. Henderson WR, Jr., Astley SJ, Ramsey BW. Liver function in patients with cystic fibrosis ingesting fish oil. J Pediatr 1994;125(3):504-505.

29. Sanders TA, Hinds A. The influence of a fish oil high in docosahexaenoic acid on plasma lipoprotein and vitamin E concentrations and haemostatic function in healthy male volunteers. Br J Nutr 1992;68(1):163-173.

30. Meydani M, Natiello F, Goldin B, et al. Effect of long-term fish oil supplementation on vitamin E status and lipid peroxidation in women. J Nutr 1991;121(4):484-491.

31. Haglund O, Luostarinen R, Wallin R, et al. The effects of fish oil on triglycerides, cholesterol, fibrinogen and malondialdehyde in humans supplemented with vitamin E. J Nutr 1991;121(2):165-169.

32. Knapp HR. Dietary fatty acids in human thrombosis and hemostasis. Am J Clin Nutr 1997;65(5 Suppl):1687S-1698S.

33. Archer SL, Green D, Chamberlain M, et al. Association of dietary fish and n-3 fatty acid intake with hemostatic factors in the coronary artery risk development in young adults (CARDIA) study. Arterioscler Thromb Vasc Biol 1998;18(7):1119-1123.

34. Weksler BB. Omega 3 fatty acids have multiple antithrombotic effects. World Rev Nutr Diet 1994;76:47-50.

35. Kromann N, Green A. Epidemiological studies in the Upernavik district, Greenland. Incidence of some chronic diseases 1950-1974. Acta Med Scand 1980;208(5):401-406.

36. Stacpoole PW, Alig J, Ammon L, et al. Dose-response effects of dietary marine oil on carbohydrate and lipid metabolism in normal subjects and patients with hypertriglyceridemia. Metabolism 1989;38(10):946-956.

37. Friedberg CE, Janssen MJ, Heine RJ, et al. Fish oil and glycemic control in diabetes. A meta-analysis. Diabetes Care 1998;21(4):494-500.

38. Montori VM, Farmer A, Wollan PC, et al. Fish oil supplementation in type 2 diabetes: a quantitative systematic review. Diabetes Care 2000;23(9): 1407-1415.

39. Stacpoole PW, Alig J, Ammon L, et al. Dose-response effects of dietary fish oil on carbohydrate and lipid metabolism in hypertriglyceridemia [abstract]. Diabetes 1988;37 (Suppl 1):12A.

40. Akedo I, Ishikawa H, Nakamura T, et al. Three cases with familial adenomatous polyposis diagnosed as having malignant lesions in the course of a long-term trial using docosahexaenoic acid (DHA)-concentrated fish oil capsules. Jpn J Clin Oncol 1998;28(12):762-765.

41. Matorras R, Perteagudo L, Sanjurjo P, et al. Intake of long chain w3 polyunsaturated fatty acids during pregnancy and the influence of levels in the mother on newborn levels. Eur J Obstet Gynecol Reprod Biol 1999; 83(2):179-184.

42. van Houwelingen AC, Sorensen JD, Hornstra G, et al. Essential fatty acid status in neonates after fish-oil supplementation during late pregnancy. Br J Nutr 1995;74(5):723-731.

43. Connor WE, Lowensohn R, Hatcher L. Increased docosahexaenoic acid levels in human newborn infants by administration of sardines and fish oil during pregnancy. Lipids 1996;31 Suppl:S183-S187.

44. Harris WS, Connor WE, Lindsey S. Will dietary omega-3 fatty acids change the composition of human milk? Am J Clin Nutr 1984;40(4):780-785.

45. Helland IB, Saugstad OD, Smith L, et al. Similar effects on infants of n-3 and n-6 fatty acids supplementation to pregnant and lactating women. Pediatrics 2001;108(5):E82.

46. Wainwright PE. Alpha-linolenic acid, long-chain n-3 fatty acids, and neonatal brain development. Nutrition 1991;7(6):443-446.

47. Birch EE, Garfield S, Hoffman DR, et al. A randomized controlled trial of early dietary supply of long-chain polyunsaturated fatty acids and mental development in term infants. Dev Med Child Neurol 2000;42(3):174-181.

48. Willatts P, Forsyth JS, DiModugno MK, et al. Effect of long-chain polyunsaturated fatty acids in infant formula on problem solving at 10 months of age. Lancet 1998;352(9129):688-691.

49. Horrocks LA, Yeo YK. Health benefits of docosahexaenoic acid (DHA). Pharmacol Res 1999;40(3):211-225.

50. Lothaller MA, Widhalm K. [Are omega-3-fatty acids essential for newborn infants?]. Infusionstherapie 1991;18(6):280-282.

51. Innis SM, Nelson CM, Rioux MF, et al. Development of visual acuity in relation to plasma and erythrocyte omega-6 and omega-3 fatty acids in healthy term gestation infants. Am J Clin Nutr 1994;60(3):347-352.

52. Birch EE, Hoffman DR, Uauy R, et al. Visual acuity and the essentiality of docosahexaenoic acid and arachidonic acid in the diet of term infants. Pediatr Res 1998;44(2):201-209.

53. Bazan NG. The metabolism of omega-3 polyunsaturated fatty acids in the eye: the possible role of docosahexaenoic acid and docosanoids in retinal physiology and ocular pathology. Prog Clin Biol Res 1989;312:95-112.

54. Gamoh S, Hashimoto M, Sugioka K, et al. Chronic administration of docosahexaenoic acid improves reference memory-related learning ability in young rats. Neuroscience 1999;93(1):237-241.

55. Bjerve KS, Thoresen L, Borsting S. Linseed and cod liver oil induce rapid growth in a 7-year-old girl with N-3- fatty acid deficiency. JPEN J Parenter Enteral Nutr 1988;12(5):521-525.

56. Bjerve KS, Brubakk AM, Fougner KJ, et al. Omega-3 fatty acids: essential fatty acids with important biological effects, and serum phospholipid fatty acids as markers of dietary omega 3-fatty acid intake. Am J Clin Nutr 1993;57(5 Suppl):801S-806S.

57. Velzing-Aarts FV, van der Klis FR, van der Dijs FP, et al. Effect of three low-dose fish oil supplements, administered during pregnancy, on neonatal long-chain polyunsaturated fatty acid status at birth. Prostaglandins Leukot Essent Fatty Acids 2001;65(1):51-57.

58. Bourre J, Dumont OL, Piciotti MJ, et al. Comparison of vegetable and fish oil in the provision of N-3 polyunsaturated fatty acids for nervous tissue and selected organs. J Nutr Biochem 1997;8:472-478.

59. Singer P, Melzer S, Goschel M, et al. Fish oil amplifies the effect of propranolol in mild essential hypertension. Hypertension 1990;16(6): 682-691.

60. Lungershausen YK, Abbey M, Nestel PJ, et al. Reduction of blood pressure and plasma triglycerides by omega-3 fatty acids in treated hypertensives. J Hypertens 1994;12(9):1041-1045.

61. Plotnick AN. The role of omega-3 fatty acids in renal disorders. J Am Vet Med Assoc 1996;209(5):906-910.

62. Sorensen JD, Olsen SF. Effects of fish oil supplementation in late pregnancy on prostaglandin metabolism. World Rev Nutr Diet 1994; 76:122-125.

63. Herold PM, Kinsella JE. Fish oil consumption and decreased risk of cardiovascular disease: a comparison of findings from animal and human feeding trials. Am J Clin Nutr 1986;43(4):566-598.

64. Schwartz J. Role of polyunsaturated fatty acids in lung disease. Am J Clin Nutr 2000;71(1 Suppl):393S-396S.

65. Yamori Y, Nara Y, Iritani N, et al. Comparison of serum phospholipid fatty acids among fishing and farming Japanese populations and American inlanders. J Nutr Sci Vitaminol (Tokyo) 1985;31(4):417-422.

66. d'Ivernois C, Couffinhal T, Le Metayer P, et al. [Potential value of omega-3 polyunsaturated fatty acids in the prevention of atherosclerosis and cardiovascular diseases]. Arch Mal Coeur Vaiss 1992;85(6):899-904.

67. Stenson WF, Cort D, Rodgers J, et al. Dietary supplementation with fish oil in ulcerative colitis. Ann Intern Med 1992;116(8):609-614.

68. Andrioli G, Carletto A, Guarini P, et al. Differential effects of dietary supplementation with fish oil or soy lecithin on human platelet adhesion. Thromb Haemost 1999;82(5):1522-1527.

69. Ritter JM, Taylor GW. Fish oil in asthma. Thorax 1988;43(2):81-83.

70. Gibson RA. The effect of diets containing fish and fish oils on disease risk factors in humans. Aust NZ J Med 1988;18(5):713-722.

71. Secher NJ, Olsen SF. Fish-oil and pre-eclampsia. Br J Obstet Gynaecol 1990;97(12):1077-1079.

72. Watanabe A, Saito S, Tsuchida T, et al. Low plasma levels of docosahexaenoic acid in patients with liver cirrhosis and its correction with a polyunsaturated fatty acid-enriched soft oil capsule. Nutrition 1999; 15(4):284-288.

73. Stevens LJ, Zentall SS, Abate ML, et al. Omega-3 fatty acids in boys with behavior, learning, and health problems. Physiol Behav 1996;59(4-5): 915-920.

74. Adams PB, Lawson S, Sanigorski A, et al. Arachidonic acid to eicosapentaenoic acid ratio in blood correlates positively with clinical symptoms of depression. Lipids 1996;31 Suppl:S157-S161.

75. Maes M, Christophe A, Delanghe J, et al. Lowered omega 3 polyunsaturated fatty acids in serum phospholipids and cholesteryl esters of depressed patients. Psychiatry Res 1999;85(3):275-291.

76. Hoffman DR, Uauy R, Birch DG. Metabolism of omega-3 fatty acids in patients with autosomal dominant retinitis pigmentosa. Exp Eye Res 1995; 60(3):279-289.

77. Lorenz R, Spengler U, Fischer S, et al. Platelet function, thromboxane formation and blood pressure control during supplementation of the Western diet with cod liver oil. Circulation 1983;67(3):504-511.

78. Hui R, St Louis J, Falardeau P. Antihypertensive properties of linoleic acid and fish oil omega-3 fatty acids independent of the prostaglandin system. Am J Hypertens 1989;2(8):610-617.

79. Niyongabo A, Youyou A, Leger CL, et al. Effects of dietary crude palm oil, fish oil and their association on cholesterol and lipoprotein constants in rats

which could be beneficial in humans. Int J Vitam Nutr Res 1999;69(5): 330-336.

80. Chan JK, Bruce VM, McDonald BE. Dietary alpha-linolenic acid is as effective as oleic acid and linoleic acid in lowering blood cholesterol in normolipidemic men. Am J Clin Nutr 1991;53(5):1230-1234.

81. DeLany JP, Vivian VM, Snook JT, et al. Effects of fish oil on serum lipids in men during a controlled feeding trial. Am J Clin Nutr 1990;52(3): 477-485.

82. Harris WS, Connor WE, Inkeles SB, et al. Dietary omega-3 fatty acids prevent carbohydrate-induced hypertriglyceridemia. Metabolism 1984; 33(11):1016-1019.

83. Lox CD. The effects of dietary marine fish oils (omega-3 fatty acids) on coagulation profiles in men. Gen Pharmacol 1990;21(2):241-246.

84. von Lossonczy TO, Ruiter A, Bronsgeest-Schoute HC, et al. The effect of a fish diet on serum lipids in healthy human subjects. Am J Clin Nutr 1978; 31(8):1340-1346.

85. Nestel PJ. Fish oil attenuates the cholesterol induced rise in lipoprotein cholesterol. Am J Clin Nutr 1986;43(5):752-757.

86. Harris WS, Connor WE. The effects of salmon oil upon plasma lipids, lipoproteins, and triglyceride clearance. Trans Assoc Am Physicians 1980; 93:148-155.

87. Harris WS, Connor WE, McMurry MP. The comparative reductions of the plasma lipids and lipoproteins by dietary polyunsaturated fats: salmon oil versus vegetable oils. Metabolism 1983;32(2):179-184.

88. Sanders TA, Vickers M, Haines AP. Effect on blood lipids and haemostasis of a supplement of cod-liver oil, rich in eicosapentaenoic and docosahexaenoic acids, in healthy young men. Clin Sci (Lond) 1981;61(3): 317-324.

89. Rodriguez-Palmero M, Lopez-Sabater MC, Castellote-Bargallo AI, et al. Administration of low doses of fish oil derived N-3 fatty acids to elderly subjects. Eur J Clin Nutr 1997;51(8):554-560.

90. Agren JJ, Hanninen O, Julkunen A, et al. Fish diet, fish oil and docosahexaenoic acid rich oil lower fasting and postprandial plasma lipid levels. Eur J Clin Nutr 1996;50(11):765-771.

91. Sekine K. Hepatic role in the storage and utilization of fish oil fatty acids in humans: studies on liver surgery patients. Intern Med 1995;34(3): 139-143.

92. Harris WS. Fish oils and plasma lipid and lipoprotein metabolism in humans: a critical review. J Lipid Res 1989;30(6):785-807.

93. Nordoy A, Hatcher LF, Ullmann DL, et al. Individual effects of dietary saturated fatty acids and fish oil on plasma lipids and lipoproteins in normal men. Am J Clin Nutr 1993;57(5):634-639.

94. Lehtonen A, Raiha I, Puumalainen R, et al. The effect of the short-term administration of fish oil on serum lipoproteins in old people. Gerontology 1989;35(5-6):311-314.

95. Abbey M, Clifton P, Kestin M, et al. Effect of fish oil on lipoproteins, lecithin:cholesterol acyltransferase, and lipid transfer protein activity in humans. Arteriosclerosis 1990;10(1):85-94.

96. Sanders TA, Roshanai F. The influence of different types of omega 3 polyunsaturated fatty acids on blood lipids and platelet function in healthy volunteers. Clin Sci (Colch) 1983;64(1):91-99.

97. Rogers S, James KS, Butland BK, et al. Effects of a fish oil supplement on serum lipids, blood pressure, bleeding time, haemostatic and rheological variables. A double blind randomised controlled trial in healthy volunteers. Atherosclerosis 1987;63(2-3):137-143.

98. Svaneborg N, Moller JM, Schmidt EB, et al. The acute effects of a single very high dose of n-3 fatty acids on plasma lipids and lipoproteins in healthy subjects. Lipids 1994;29(2):145-147.

99. Bruckner G, Webb P, Greenwell L, et al. Fish oil increases peripheral capillary blood cell velocity in humans. Atherosclerosis 1987;66(3): 237-245.

100. Bronsgeest-Schoute HC, van Gent CM, Luten JB, et al. The effect of various intakes of omega 3 fatty acids on the blood lipid composition in healthy human subjects. Am J Clin Nutr 1981;34(9):1752-1757.

101. Brown AJ, Roberts DC, Pritchard JE, et al. A mixed Australian fish diet and fish-oil supplementation: impact on the plasma lipid profile of healthy men. Am J Clin Nutr 1990;52(5):825-833.

102. Zampelas A, Peel AS, Gould BJ, et al. Polyunsaturated fatty acids of the n-6 and n-3 series: effects on postprandial lipid and apolipoprotein levels in healthy men. Eur J Clin Nutr 1994;48(12):842-848.

103. Bonaa KH, Bjerve KS, Nordoy A. Docosahexaenoic and eicosapentaenoic acids in plasma phospholipids are divergently associated with high density lipoprotein in humans. Arterioscler Thromb 1992;12(6):675-681.

104. Harris WS, Connor WE, Alam N, et al. Reduction of postprandial triglyceridemia in humans by dietary n-3 fatty acids. J Lipid Res 1988; 29(11):1451-1460.

105. Layne KS, Goh YK, Jumpsen JA, et al. Normal subjects consuming physiological levels of 18:3(n-3) and 20:5(n- 3) from flaxseed or fish oils have characteristic differences in plasma lipid and lipoprotein fatty acid levels. J Nutr 1996;126(9):2130-2140.

106. Marckmann P, Bladbjerg EM, Jespersen J. Dietary fish oil (4 g daily) and cardiovascular risk markers in healthy men. Arterioscler Thromb Vasc Biol 1997;17(12):3384-3391.

107. Kestin M, Clifton P, Belling GB, et al. n-3 fatty acids of marine origin lower systolic blood pressure and triglycerides but raise LDL cholesterol compared with n-3 and n-6 fatty acids from plants. Am J Clin Nutr 1990; 51(6):1028-1034.

108. Haglund O, Mehta JL, Saldeen T. Effects of fish oil on some parameters of fibrinolysis and lipoprotein(a) in healthy subjects. Am J Cardiol 1994; 74(2):189-192.

109. Bulliyya G, Reddy KK, Reddy GP, et al. Lipid profiles among fish-consuming coastal and non-fish-consuming inland populations. Eur J Clin Nutr 1990;44(6):481-485.

110. Hirai A, Hamazaki T, Terano T, et al. Eicosapentaenoic acid and platelet function in Japanese. Lancet 1980;2(8204):1132-1133.

111. Laidlaw M, Holub BJ. Effects of supplementation with fish oil-derived n-3 fatty acids and gamma-linolenic acid on circulating plasma lipids and fatty acid profiles in women. Am J Clin Nutr 2003;77(1):37-42.

112. Foulon T, Richard MJ, Payen N, et al. Effects of fish oil fatty acids on plasma lipids and lipoproteins and oxidant-antioxidant imbalance in healthy subjects. Scand J Clin Lab Invest 1999;59(4):239-248.

113. Franzen D, Geisel J, Hopp HW, et al. [Long-term effects of low dosage fish oil on serum lipids and lipoproteins]. Med Klin 1993;88(3):134-138.

114. Blonk MC, Bilo HJ, Nauta JJ, et al. Dose-response effects of fish-oil supplementation in healthy volunteers. Am J Clin Nutr 1990;52(1):120-127.

115. Franceschini G, Calabresi L, Maderna P, et al. Omega-3 fatty acids selectively raise high-density lipoprotein 2 levels in healthy volunteers. Metabolism 1991;40(12):1283-1286.

116. Schmidt EB, Varming K, Ernst E, et al. Dose-response studies on the effect of n-3 polyunsaturated fatty acids on lipids and haemostasis. Thromb Haemost 1990;63(1):1-5.

117. Sanders TA, Hochland MC. A comparison of the influence on plasma lipids and platelet function of supplements of omega 3 and omega 6 polyunsaturated fatty acids. Br J Nutr 1983;50(3):521-529.

118. Parks JS, Rudel LL. Effect of fish oil on atherosclerosis and lipoprotein metabolism. Atherosclerosis 1990;84(2-3):83-94.

119. Tsai PJ, Lu SC. Fish oil lowers plasma lipid concentrations and increases the susceptibility of low density lipoprotein to oxidative modification in healthy men. J Formos Med Assoc 1997;96(9):718-726.

120. Garrido A, Garrido F, Guerra R, et al. Ingestion of high doses of fish oil increases the susceptibility of cellular membranes to the induction of oxidative stress. Lipids 1989;24(9):833-835.

121. Harats D, Dabach Y, Hollander G, et al. Fish oil ingestion in smokers and nonsmokers enhances peroxidation of plasma lipoproteins. Atherosclerosis 1991;90(2-3):127-139.

122. Higdon JV, Du SH, Lee YS, et al. Supplementation of postmenopausal women with fish oil does not increase overall oxidation of LDL ex vivo compared to dietary oils rich in oleate and linoleate. J Lipid Res 2001; 42(3):407-418.

123. Turley E, Wallace JM, Gilmore WS, et al. Fish oil supplementation with and without added vitamin E differentially modulates plasma antioxidant concentrations in healthy women. Lipids 1998;33(12):1163-1167.

124. Fisher M, Upchurch KS, Levine PH, et al. Effects of dietary fish oil supplementation on polymorphonuclear leukocyte inflammatory potential. Inflammation 1986;10(4):387-392.

125. Ahmed AA, Holub BJ. Alteration and recovery of bleeding times, platelet aggregation and fatty acid composition of individual phospholipids in platelets of human subjects receiving a supplement of cod-liver oil. Lipids 1984;19(8):617-624.

126. Thorngren M, Gustafson A. Effects of 11-week increases in dietary eicosapentaenoic acid on bleeding time, lipids, and platelet aggregation. Lancet 1981;2(8257):1190-1193.

127. Salonen R, Nikkari T, Seppanen K, et al. Effect of omega-3 fatty acid supplementation on platelet aggregability and platelet produced thromboxane. Thromb Haemost 1987;57(3):269-272.

128. Silverman DI, Ware JA, Sacks FM, et al. Comparison of the absorption and effect on platelet function of a single dose of n-3 fatty acids given as fish or fish oil. Am J Clin Nutr 1991;53(5):1165-1170.

129. Smith DL, Willis AL, Nguyen N, et al. Eskimo plasma constituents, dihomo-gamma-linolenic acid, eicosapentaenoic acid and docosahexaenoic acid inhibit the release of atherogenic mitogens. Lipids 1989;24(1):70-75.

130. Siess W, Roth P, Scherer B, et al. Platelet-membrane fatty acids, platelet aggregation, and thromboxane formation during a mackerel diet. Lancet 1980;1(8166):441-444.

131. von Schacky C, Weber PC. Metabolism and effects on platelet function of the purified eicosapentaenoic and docosahexaenoic acids in humans. J Clin Invest 1985;76(6):2446-2450.

132. Mutanen M, Freese R. Polyunsaturated fatty acids and platelet aggregation. Curr Opin Lipidol 1996;7(1):14-19.

133. Gorlin R. The biological actions and potential clinical significance of dietary omega-3 fatty acids. Arch Intern Med 1988;148(9):2043-2048.

134. Elmadfa I, Stroh S, Brandt K, et al. Influence of a single parenteral application of a 10% fish oil emulsion on plasma fatty acid pattern and the function of thrombocytes in young adult men. Ann Nutr Metab 1993;37(1):8-13.

135. Nagakawa Y, Orimo H, Harasawa M, et al. Effect of eicosapentaenoic acid on the platelet aggregation and composition of fatty acid in man. A double blind study. Atherosclerosis 1983;47(1):71-75.

136. Galloway JH, Cartwright IJ, Woodcock BE, et al. Effects of dietary fish oil supplementation on the fatty acid composition of the human platelet membrane: demonstration of selectivity in the incorporation of eicosapentaenoic acid into membrane phospholipid pools. Clin Sci (Colch) 1985;68(4):449-454.

137. Goodnight SH, Jr. Effects of dietary fish oil and omega-3 fatty acids on platelets and blood vessels. Semin Thromb Hemost 1988;14(3):285-289.

138. Kinsella JE, Lokesh B, Stone RA. Dietary n-3 polyunsaturated fatty acids and amelioration of cardiovascular disease: possible mechanisms. Am J Clin Nutr 1990;52(1):1-28.

139. Dyerberg J, Bang HO, Stoffersen E, et al. Eicosapentaenoic acid and prevention of thrombosis and atherosclerosis? Lancet 1978;2(8081):117-119.

140. Kristensen SD, Schmidt EB, Dyerberg J. Dietary supplementation with n-3 polyunsaturated fatty acids and human platelet function: a review with particular emphasis on implications for cardiovascular disease. J Intern Med Suppl 1989;225(731):141-150.

141. Malle E, Sattler W, Prenner E, et al. Effects of dietary fish oil supplementation on platelet aggregability and platelet membrane fluidity in normolipemic subjects with and without high plasma Lp(a) concentrations. Atherosclerosis 1991;88(2-3):193-201.

142. Hansen JB, Olsen JO, Wilsgard L, et al. Comparative effects of prolonged intake of highly purified fish oils as ethyl ester or triglyceride on lipids, haemostasis and platelet function in normolipaemic men. Eur J Clin Nutr 1993;47(7):497-507.

143. Prisco D, Filippini M, Francalanci I, et al. Effect of n-3 fatty acid ethyl ester supplementation on fatty acid composition of the single platelet phospholipids and on platelet functions. Metabolism 1995;44(5):562-569.

144. Braden GA, Knapp HR, Fitzgerald DJ, et al. Dietary fish oil accelerates the response to coronary thrombolysis with tissue-type plasminogen activator. Evidence for a modest platelet inhibitory effect in vivo. Circulation 1990;82(1):178-187.

145. Gazso A, Kaliman J, Horrobin D, et al. Effects of omega-3 fatty acids on the prostaglandin system in healthy volunteers. Progress in Clin Biol Res 1989;301:517-521.

146. von Schacky C, Fischer S, Weber PC. Long-term effects of dietary marine omega-3 fatty acids upon plasma and cellular lipids, platelet function, and eicosanoid formation in humans. J Clin Invest 1985;76(4):1626-1631.

147. Fischer S, Weber PC. Thromboxane A3 (TXA3) is formed in human platelets after dietary eicosapentaenoic acid (C20:5 omega 3). Biochem Biophys Res Commun 1983;116(3):1091-1099.

148. Fischer S, Weber PC. Prostaglandin I3 is formed in vivo in man after dietary eicosapentaenoic acid. Nature 1984;307(5947):165-168.

149. Nordoy A, Hatcher L, Goodnight S, et al. Effects of dietary fat content, saturated fatty acids, and fish oil on eicosanoid production and hemostatic parameters in normal men. J Lab Clin Med 1994;123(6):914-920.

150. Li XL, Steiner M. Dose response of dietary fish oil supplementations on platelet adhesion. Arterioscler Thromb 1991;11(1):39-46.

151. Dyerberg J, Bang HO. Haemostatic function and platelet polyunsaturated fatty acids in Eskimos. Lancet 1979;2(8140):433-435.

152. Goodnight SH, Jr., Harris WS, Connor WE. The effects of dietary omega 3 fatty acids on platelet composition and function in man: a prospective, controlled study. Blood 1981;58(5):880-885.

153. Houwelingen R, Nordoy A, van der BE, et al. Effect of a moderate fish intake on blood pressure, bleeding time, hematology, and clinical chemistry in healthy males. Am J Clin Nutr 1987;46(3):424-436.

154. Mueller BA, Talbert RL, Tegeler CH, et al. The bleeding time effects of a single dose of aspirin in subjects receiving omega-3 fatty acid dietary supplementation. J Clin Pharmacol 1991;31(2):185-190.

155. Chamberlain JG. Omega-3 fatty acids and bleeding problems. Am J Clin Nutr 1992;55(3):760-761.

156. Freese R, Mutanen M. Small effects of linseed oil or fish oil supplementation on postprandial changes in hemostatic factors. Thromb Res 1997; 85(2):147-152.

157. Hellsten G, Boman K, Saarem K, et al. Effects on fibrinolytic activity of corn oil and a fish oil preparation enriched with omega-3-polyunsaturated fatty acids in a long-term study. Curr Med Res Opin 1993;13(3):133-139.

158. Barcelli U, Glas-Greenwalt P, Pollak VE. Enhancing effect of dietary supplementation with omega-3 fatty acids on plasma fibrinolysis in normal subjects. Thromb Res 1985;39(3):307-312.

159. Brown AJ, Roberts DC. Fish and fish oil intake: effect on haematological variables related to cardiovascular disease. Thromb Res 1991;64(2): 169-178.

160. Flaten H, Hostmark AT, Kierulf P, et al. Fish-oil concentrate: effects on variables related to cardiovascular disease. Am J Clin Nutr 1990;52(2): 300-306.

161. Emeis JJ, van Houwelingen AC, van den Hoogen CM, et al. A moderate fish intake increases plasminogen activator inhibitor type-1 in human volunteers. Blood 1989;74(1):233-237.

162. Moller JM, Svaneborg N, Lervang HH, et al. The acute effect of a single very high dose of N-3 fatty acids on coagulation and fibrinolysis. Thromb Res 1992;67(5):569-577.

163. Marckmann P, Jespersen J, Leth T, et al. Effect of fish diet versus meat diet on blood lipids, coagulation and fibrinolysis in healthy young men. J Intern Med 1991;229(4):317-323.

164. Seljeflot I, Johansen O, Arnesen H, et al. Procoagulant activity and cytokine expression in whole blood cultures from patients with atherosclerosis supplemented with omega-3 fatty acids. Thromb Haemost 1999;81(4):566-570.

165. Kim DN, Eastman A, Baker JE, et al. Fish oil, atherogenesis, and thrombogenesis. Ann N Y Acad Sci 1995;748:474-480.

166. Lehr HA, Hubner C, Finckh B, et al. Dietary fish oil reduces leukocyte/endothelium interaction following systemic administration of oxidatively modified low density lipoprotein. Circulation 1991;84(4):1725-1731.

167. Kontogiannea M, Gupta A, Ntanios F, et al. Omega-3 fatty acids decrease endothelial adhesion of human colorectal carcinoma cells. J Surg Res 2000;92(2):201-205.

168. Fox PL, DiCorleto PE. Fish oils inhibit endothelial cell production of platelet-derived growth factor-like protein. Science 1988;241(4864): 453-456.

169. Sarris GE, Fann JI, Sokoloff MH, et al. Mechanisms responsible for inhibition of vein-graft arteriosclerosis by fish oil. Circulation 1989; 80(3 Pt 1):I109-I123.

170. Baumann KH, Hessel F, Larass I, et al. Dietary omega-3, omega-6, and omega-9 unsaturated fatty acids and growth factor and cytokine gene expression in unstimulated and stimulated monocytes. A randomized volunteer study. Arterioscler Thromb Vasc Biol 1999;19(1):59-66.

171. Landymore RW, MacAulay M, Sheridan B, et al. Comparison of cod-liver oil and aspirin-dipyridamole for the prevention of intimal hyperplasia in autologous vein grafts. Ann Thorac Surg 1986;41(1):54-57.

172. Kang JX, Leaf A. Antiarrhythmic effects of polyunsaturated fatty acids. Recent studies. Circulation 1996;94(7):1774-1780.

173. Kang JX, Leaf A. The cardiac antiarrhythmic effects of polyunsaturated fatty acid. Lipids 1996;31 Suppl:S41-S44.

174. Culp BR, Lands WE, Lucches BR, et al. The effect of dietary supplementation of fish oil on experimental myocardial infarction. Prostaglandins 1980;20(6):1021-1031.

175. Christensen JH, Gustenhoff P, Ejlersen E, et al. n-3 fatty acids and ventricular extrasystoles in patients with ventricular tachyarrhythmias. Nutr Res 1995;15(1):1-8.

176. Christensen JH, Gustenhoff P, Korup E, et al. Effect of fish oil on heart rate variability in survivors of myocardial infarction: a double blind randomised controlled trial. BMJ 1996;312(7032):677-678.

177. Sellmayer A, Witzgall H, Lorenz RL, et al. Effects of dietary fish oil on ventricular premature complexes. Am J Cardiol 1995;76(12):974-977.

178. Heller A, Koch T. [Immunonutrition with omega-3-fatty acids. Are new anti-inflammatory strategies in sight?]. Zentralbl Chir 2000;125(2): 123-136.

179. Vilaseca J, Salas A, Guarner F, et al. Dietary fish oil reduces progression of chronic inflammatory lesions in a rat model of granulomatous colitis. Gut 1990;31(5):539-544.

180. Endres S, Ghorbani R, Kelley VE, et al. The effect of dietary supplementation with n-3 polyunsaturated fatty acids on the synthesis of interleukin-1 and tumor necrosis factor by mononuclear cells. N Engl J Med 1989;320(5):265-271.

181. Jeng KC, Fernandes G. Effect of fish oil diet on immune response and proteinuria in mice. Proc Natl Sci Counc Repub China B 1991;15(2): 105-110.

182. Venkatraman JT, Chu WC. Effects of dietary omega-3 and omega-6 lipids and vitamin E on serum cytokines, lipid mediators and anti-DNA antibodies in a mouse model for rheumatoid arthritis. J Am Coll Nutr 1999;18(6):602-613.

183. Meydani SN, Lichtenstein AH, Cornwall S, et al. Immunologic effects of national cholesterol education panel step-2 diets with and without fish-derived N-3 fatty acid enrichment. J Clin Invest 1993;92(1):105-113.

184. Gallai V, Sarchielli P, Trequattrini A, et al. Cytokine secretion and eicosanoid production in the peripheral blood mononuclear cells of MS patients undergoing dietary supplementation with n-3 polyunsaturated fatty acids. J Neuroimmunol 1995;56:143-153.

185. Meydani SN, Endres S, Woods MM, et al. Oral (n-3) fatty acid supplementation suppresses cytokine production and lymphocyte proliferation: comparison between young and older women. J Nutr 1991;121(4):547-555.

186. Blok WL, Deslypere JP, Demacker PN, et al. Pro- and anti-inflammatory cytokines in healthy volunteers fed various doses of fish oil for 1 year. Eur J Clin Invest 1997;27(12):1003-1008.

187. Empey LR, Jewell LD, Garg ML, et al. Fish oil-enriched diet is mucosal protective against acetic acid- induced colitis in rats. Can J Physiol Pharmacol 1991;69(4):480-487.

188. Shoda R, Matsueda K, Yamato S, et al. Therapeutic efficacy of N-3 polyunsaturated fatty acid in experimental Crohn's disease. J Gastroenterol 1995;30 Suppl 8:98-101.

189. Cathcart ES, Gonnerman WA. Fish oil fatty acids and experimental arthritis. Rheum Dis Clin North Am 1991;17(2):235-242.

190. Leslie CA, Conte JM, Hayes KC, et al. A fish oil diet reduces the severity of collagen induced arthritis after onset of the disease. Clin Exp Immunol 1988;73(2):328-332.

191. Verbey NL, van Haeringen NJ. The influence of a fish oil dietary supplement on immunogenic keratitis. Invest Ophthalmol Vis Sci 1990; 31(8):1526-1532.

F

192. Campan P, Planchand PO, Duran D. Pilot study on n-3 polyunsaturated fatty acids in the treatment of human experimental gingivitis. J Clin Periodontol 1997;24(12):907-913.

193. Campan P, Planchand PO, Duran D. [Polyunsaturated omega-3 fatty acids in the treatment of experimental human gingivitis]. Bull Group Int Rech Sci Stomatol Odontol 1996;39(1-2):25-31.

194. Kremer JM, Malamood H, Maliakkal B, et al. Fish oil dietary supplementation for prevention of indomethacin induced gastric and small bowel toxicity in healthy volunteers. J Rheumatol 1996;23(10):1770-1773.

195. Bjornsson S, Hardardottir I, Gunnarsson E, et al. Dietary fish oil supplementation increases survival in mice following Klebsiella pneumoniae infection. Scand J Infect Dis 1997;29(5):491-493.

196. Kelley VE, Ferretti A, Izui S, et al. A fish oil diet rich in eicosapentaenoic acid reduces cyclooxygenase metabolites, and suppresses lupus in MRL-lpr mice. J Immunol 1985;134(3):1914-1919.

197. Robinson DR, Xu LL, Tateno S, et al. Suppression of autoimmune disease by dietary n-3 fatty acids. J Lipid Res 1993;34(8):1435-1444.

198. Robinson DR, Knoell CT, Urakaze M, et al. Suppression of autoimmune disease by omega-3 fatty acids. Biochem Soc Trans 1995;23(2):287-291.

199. Robinson DR, Prickett JD, Makoul GT, et al. Dietary fish oil reduces progression of established renal disease in (NZB x NZW)F1 mice and delays renal disease in BXSB and MRL/1 strains. Arthritis Rheum 1986; 29(4):539-546.

200. Grimminger F, Grimm H, Fuhrer D, et al. Omega-3 lipid infusion in a heart allotransplant model. Shift in fatty acid and lipid mediator profiles and prolongation of transplant survival. Circulation 1996;93(2):365-371.

201. Cathcart ES, Leslie CA, Meydani SN, et al. A fish oil diet retards experimental amyloidosis, modulates lymphocyte function, and decreases macrophage arachidonate metabolism in mice. J Immunol 1987;139(6): 1850-1854.

202. Borgeson CE, Pardini L, Pardini RS, et al. Effects of dietary fish oil on human mammary carcinoma and on lipid- metabolizing enzymes. Lipids 1989;24(4):290-295.

203. Gonzalez MJ, Schemmel RA, Dugan L, Jr., et al. Dietary fish oil inhibits human breast carcinoma growth: a function of increased lipid peroxidation. Lipids 1993;28(9):827-832.

204. Moore NG, Wang-Johanning F, Chang PL, et al. Omega-3 fatty acids decrease protein kinase expression in human breast cancer cells. Breast Cancer Res Treat 2001;67(3):279-283.

205. Carroll KK. Biological effects of fish oils in relation to chronic diseases. Lipids 1986;21(12):731-732.

206. Pandalai PK, Pilat MJ, Yamazaki K, et al. The effects of omega-3 and omega-6 fatty acids on in vitro prostate cancer growth. Anticancer Res 1996;16(2):815-820.

207. Minoura T, Takata T, Sakaguchi M, et al. Effect of dietary eicosapentaenoic acid on azoxymethane-induced colon carcinogenesis in rats. Cancer Res 1988;48(17):4790-4794.

208. Deschner EE, Lytle JS, Wong G, et al. The effect of dietary omega-3 fatty acids (fish oil) on azoxymethanol- induced focal areas of dysplasia and colon tumor incidence. Cancer 1990;66(11):2350-2356.

209. Reddy BS, Maruyama H. Effect of dietary fish oil on azoxymethane-induced colon carcinogenesis in male F344 rats. Cancer Res 1986;46(7): 3367-3370.

210. Reddy BS, Burill C, Rigotty J. Effect of diets high in omega-3 and omega-6 fatty acids on initiation and postinitiation stages of colon carcinogenesis. Cancer Res 1991;51(2):487-491.

211. Bartram HP, Gostner A, Scheppach W, et al. Effects of fish oil on rectal cell proliferation, mucosal fatty acids, and prostaglandin E2 release in healthy subjects. Gastroenterology 1993;105(5):1317-1322.

212. Ogilvie GK, Fettman MJ, Mallinckrodt CH, et al. Effect of fish oil, arginine, and doxorubicin chemotherapy on remission and survival time for dogs with lymphoma: a double-blind, randomized placebo-controlled study. Cancer 2000;88(8):1916-1928.

213. Gerbi A, Maixent JM, Ansaldi JL, et al. Fish oil supplementation prevents diabetes-induced nerve conduction velocity and neuroanatomical changes in rats. J Nutr 1999;129(1):207-213.

214. Dusing R, Struck A, Gobel BO, et al. Effects of n-3 fatty acids on renal function and renal prostaglandin E metabolism. Kidney Int 1990;38(2): 315-319.

215. Adam O, Schubert A, Adam A, et al. Effects of omega-3 fatty acids on renal function and electrolyte excretion in aged persons. Eur J Med Res 1998; 3(1-2):111-118.

216. Chandrasekar B, Fernandes G. Decreased pro-inflammatory cytokines and increased antioxidant enzyme gene expression by omega-3 lipids in murine lupus nephritis. Biochem Biophys Res Commun 1994;200(2): 893-898.

217. Marsen TA, Pollok M, Oette K, et al. Pharmacokinetics of omega-3-fatty acids during ingestion of fish oil preparations. Prostaglandins Leukot Essent Fatty Acids 1992;46(3):191-196.

218. Henderson WR. Omega-3 supplementation in CF [abstract]. 6th North American Cystic Fibrosis Conference 1992;s21-s22.

219. Leaf DA, Connor WE, Barstad L, et al. Incorporation of dietary n-3 fatty acids into the fatty acids of human adipose tissue and plasma lipid classes. Am J Clin Nutr 1995;62(1):68-73.

220. Harris WS. n-3 fatty acids and serum lipoproteins: human studies. Am J Clin Nutr 1997;65(5 Suppl):1645S-1654S.

221. Sanders TA, Oakley FR, Miller GJ, et al. Influence of n-6 versus n-3 polyunsaturated fatty acids in diets low in saturated fatty acids on plasma lipoproteins and hemostatic factors. Arterioscler Thromb Vasc Biol 1997; 17(12):3449-3460.

222. Harris WS, Dujovne CA, Zucker M, et al. Effects of a low saturated fat, low cholesterol fish oil supplement in hypertriglyceridemic patients. A placebo-controlled trial. Ann Intern Med 1988;109(6):465-470.

223. Roche HM, Gibney MJ. Postprandial triacylglycerolaemia: the effect of low-fat dietary treatment with and without fish oil supplementation. Eur J Clin Nutr 1996;50(9):617-624.

224. Grimsgaard S, Bonaa KH, Hansen JB, et al. Highly purified eicosapentaenoic acid and docosahexaenoic acid in humans have similar triacylglycerol-lowering effects but divergent effects on serum fatty acids. Am J Clin Nutr 1997;66(3):649-659.

225. Chan DC, Watts GF, Barrett PH, et al. Effect of atorvastatin and fish oil on plasma high-sensitivity C- reactive protein concentrations in individuals with visceral obesity. Clin Chem 2002;48(6 Pt 1):877-883.

226. Bucher HC, Hengstler P, Schindler C, et al. N-3 polyunsaturated fatty acids in coronary heart disease: a meta- analysis of randomized controlled trials. Am J Med 2002;112(4):298-304.

227. Burr ML, Fehily AM, Gilbert JF, et al. Effects of changes in fat, fish, and fibre intakes on death and myocardial reinfarction: diet and reinfarction trial (DART). Lancet 1989;2(8666):757-761.

228. Burr ML, Sweetham PM, Fehily AM. Diet and reinfarction. Eur Heart J 1994;15(8):1152-1153.

229. Singh RB, Niaz MA, Sharma JP, et al. Randomized, double-blind, placebo-controlled trial of fish oil and mustard oil in patients with suspected acute myocardial infarction: the Indian experiment of infarct survival—4. Cardiovasc Drugs Ther 1997;11(3):485-491.

230. Marchioli R, Barzi F, Bomba E, et al. Early protection against sudden death by n-3 polyunsaturated fatty acids after myocardial infarction. Time-course analysis of the results of the gruppo italiano per lo studio della sopravvivenza nell'infarto miocardico (GISSI)-prevenzione. Circulation 2002;105(16):1897-1903.

231. Nilsen DW, Albrektsen G, Landmark K, et al. Effects of a high-dose concentrate of n-3 fatty acids or corn oil introduced early after an acute myocardial infarction on serum triacylglycerol and HDL cholesterol. Am J Clin Nutr 2001;74(1):50-56.

232. Connor WE. Importance of n-3 fatty acids in health and disease. Am J Clin Nutr 2000;71(1 Suppl):171S-175S.

233. Hu FB, Bronner L, Willett WC, et al. Fish and omega-3 fatty acid intake and risk of coronary heart disease in women. JAMA 2002;287(14): 1815-1821.

234. Stone NJ. Fish consumption, fish oil, lipids, and coronary heart disease. Circulation 1996;94(9):2337-2340.

235. Kromhout D, Bosschieter EB, de Lezenne CC. The inverse relation between fish consumption and 20-year mortality from coronary heart disease. N Engl J Med 1985;312(19):1205-1209.

236. Kromhout D, Menotti A, Bloemberg B, et al. Dietary saturated and trans fatty acids and cholesterol and 25-year mortality from coronary heart disease: the Seven Countries Study. Prev Med 1995;308-315.

237. Shekelle RB, Missell L, Paul O, et al. Fish consumption and mortality from coronary heart disease. N Engl J Med 1985;313:820.

238. Dolecek TA. Epidemiological evidence of relationships between dietary polyunsaturated fatty acids and mortality in the multiple risk factor intervention trial. Proc Soc Exp Biol Med 1992;200(2):177-182.

239. Daviglus ML, Stamler J, Orencia AJ, et al. Fish consumption and the 30-year risk of fatal myocardial infarction. N Engl J Med 1997;336(15): 1046-1053.

240. Zhang J, Sasaki S, Amano K, et al. Fish consumption and mortality from all causes, ischemic heart disease, and stroke: an ecological study. Prev Med 1999;28(5):520-529.

241. Mizushima S, Moriguchi EH, Ishikawa P, et al. Fish intake and cardiovascular risk among middle-aged Japanese in Japan and Brazil. J Cardiovasc Risk 1997;4(3):191-199.

242. Hu FB, Stampfer MJ, Manson JE, et al. Dietary intake of alpha-linolenic acid and risk of fatal ischemic heart disease among women. Am J Clin Nutr 1999;69(5):890-897.

243. Albert CM, Hennekens CH, O'Donnell CJ, et al. Fish consumption and risk of sudden cardiac death. JAMA 1998;279(1):23-28.

244. Kromhout D, Bloemberg BP, Feskens EJ, et al. Alcohol, fish, fibre and antioxidant vitamins intake do not explain population differences in coronary heart disease mortality. Int J Epidemiol 1996;25(4):753-759.

245. Guallar E, Aro A, Jimenez FJ, et al. Omega-3 fatty acids in adipose tissue and risk of myocardial infarction: the EURAMIC study. Arterioscler Thromb Vasc Biol 1999;19(4):1111-1118.

246. Fortin PR, Lew RA, Liang MH, et al. Validation of a meta-analysis: the effects of fish oil in rheumatoid arthritis. J Clin Epidemiol 1995;48(11): 1379-1390.

247. Kremer JM, Bigauoette J, Michalek AV, et al. Effects of manipulation of dietary fatty acids on clinical manifestations of rheumatoid arthritis. Lancet 1985;1(8422):184-187.

248. Kremer JM, Lawrence DA, Jubiz W, et al. Dietary fish oil and olive oil supplementation in patients with rheumatoid arthritis. Clinical and immunologic effects. Arthritis Rheum 1990;33(6):810-820.

249. Kremer JM, Jubiz W, Michalek A, et al. Fish-oil fatty acid supplementation in active rheumatoid arthritis. A double-blinded, controlled, crossover study. Ann Intern Med 1987;106(4):497-503.

250. Kjeldsen-Kragh J, Lund JA, Riise T, et al. Dietary omega-3 fatty acid supplementation and naproxen treatment in patients with rheumatoid arthritis. J Rheumatol 1992;19(10):1531-1536.

251. Nielsen GL, Faarvang KL, Thomsen BS, et al. The effects of dietary supplementation with n-3 polyunsaturated fatty acids in patients with rheumatoid arthritis: a randomized, double blind trial. Eur J Clin Invest 1992;22(10):687-691.

252. van der TH, Tulleken JE, Limburg PC, et al. Effects of fish oil supplementation in rheumatoid arthritis. Ann Rheum Dis 1990;49(2):76-80.

253. Tulleken JE, Limburg PC, Muskiet FA, et al. Vitamin E status during dietary fish oil supplementation in rheumatoid arthritis. Arthritis Rheum 1990;33(9):1416-1419.

254. Cleland LG, French JK, Betts WH, et al. Clinical and biochemical effects of dietary fish oil supplements in rheumatoid arthritis. J Rheumatol 1988; 15(10):1471-1475.

255. Sperling RI, Weinblatt M, Robin JL, et al. Effects of dietary supplementation with marine fish oil on leukocyte lipid mediator generation and function in rheumatoid arthritis. Arthritis Rheum 1987;30(9):988-997.

256. Skoldstam L, Borjesson O, Kjallman A, et al. Effect of six months of fish oil supplementation in stable rheumatoid arthritis. A double-blind, controlled study. Scand J Rheumatol 1992;21(4):178-185.

257. Lau CS, Morley KD, Belch JJ. Effects of fish oil supplementation on non-steroidal anti-inflammatory drug requirement in patients with mild rheumatoid arthritis—a double- blind placebo controlled study. Br J Rheumatol 1993;32(11):982-989.

258. Geusens P, Wouters C, Nijs J, et al. Long-term effect of omega-3 fatty acid supplementation in active rheumatoid arthritis. A 12-month, double-blind, controlled study. Arthritis Rheum 1994;37(6):824-829.

259. Kremer JM, Lawrence DA, Petrillo GF, et al. Effects of high-dose fish oil on rheumatoid arthritis after stopping nonsteroidal antiinflammatory drugs. Clinical and immune correlates. Arthritis Rheum 1995;38(8):1107-1114.

260. Volker D, Fitzgerald P, Major G, et al. Efficacy of fish oil concentrate in the treatment of rheumatoid arthritis. J Rheumatol 2000;27(10):2343-2346.

261. Homan van der Heide JJ, Bilo HJ, Tegzess AM, et al. Omega-3 poly-unsaturated fatty acids improve renal function in renal transplant recipients treated with cyclosporin-A [abstract]. Kidney Int 1989;35:516A.

262. Homan van der Heide JJ, Bilo HJ, Donker AJ, et al. Dietary supplementation with fish oil modifies renal reserve filtration capacity in postoperative, cyclosporin A-treated renal transplant recipients. Transpl Int 1990;3(3):171-175.

263. Berthoux FC, Guerin C, Burgard G, et al. One-year randomized controlled trial with omega-3 fatty acid-fish oil in clinical renal transplantation. Transplant Proc 1992;24(6):2578-2582.

264. Homan van der Heide JJ, Bilo HJ, Donker AJ, et al. The effects of dietary supplementation with fish oil on renal function and the course of early postoperative rejection episodes in cyclosporine-treated renal transplant recipients. Transplantation 1992;54(2):257-263.

265. van der Heide JJ, Bilo HJ, Donker JM, et al. Effect of dietary fish oil on renal function and rejection in cyclosporine-treated recipients of renal transplants. N Engl J Med 1993;329(11):769-773.

266. Maachi K, Berthoux P, Burgard G, et al. Results of a 1-year randomized controlled trial with omega-3 fatty acid fish oil in renal transplantation under triple immunosuppressive therapy. Transplant Proc 1995;27(1): 846-849.

267. Sweny P, Wheeler DC, Lui SF, et al. Dietary fish oil supplements preserve renal function in renal transplant recipients with chronic vascular rejection. Nephrol Dial Transplant 1989;4(12):1070-1075.

268. Badalamenti S, Salerno F, Lorenzano E, et al. Renal effects of dietary supplementation with fish oil in cyclosporine- treated liver transplant recipients. Hepatology 1995;22(6):1695-1770.

269. Stoof TJ, Korstanje MJ, Bilo HJ, et al. Does fish oil protect renal function in cyclosporin-treated psoriasis patients? J Intern Med 1989;226(6): 437-441.

270. Ventura HO, Milani RV, Lavie CJ, et al. Cyclosporine-induced hypertension. Efficacy of omega-3 fatty acids in patients after cardiac transplantation. Circulation 1993;88(5 Pt 2):II281-II285.

271. Andreassen AK, Hartmann A, Offstad J, et al. Hypertension prophylaxis with omega-3 fatty acids in heart transplant recipients. J Am Coll Cardiol 1997;29(6):1324-1331.

272. Santos J, Queiros J, Silva F, et al. Effects of fish oil in cyclosporine-treated renal transplant recipients. Transplant Proc 2000;32(8):2605-2608.

273. Kooijmans-Coutinho MF, Rischen-Vos J, Hermans J, et al. Dietary fish oil in renal transplant recipients treated with cyclosporin-A: no beneficial effects shown. J Am Soc Nephrol 1996;7(3):513-518.

274. Hansen JM, Lokkegaard H, Hoy CE, et al. No effect of dietary fish oil on renal hemodynamics, tubular function, and renal functional reserve in long-term renal transplant recipients. J Am Soc Nephrol 1995;5(7): 1434-1440.

275. Bennett WM, Carpenter CB, Shapiro ME, et al. Delayed omega-3 fatty acid supplements in renal transplantation. A double-blind, placebo-controlled study. Transplantation 1995;59(3):352-356.

276. Holm T, Andreassen AK, Aukrust P, et al. Omega-3 fatty acids improve blood pressure control and preserve renal function in hypertensive heart transplant recipients. Eur Heart J 2001;22(5):428-436.

277. de Lorgeril M, Salen P, Martin JL, et al. Mediterranean diet, traditional risk factors, and the rate of cardiovascular complications after myocardial infarction: final report of the Lyon Diet Heart Study. Circulation 1999;99(6):779-785.

278. Natvig H, Borchgrevink CF, Dedichen J, et al. A controlled trial of the effect of linolenic acid on incidence of coronary heart disease. The Norwegian vegetable oil experiment of 1965- 66. Scand J Clin Lab Invest Suppl 1968;105:1-20.

279. Bemelmans WJ, Broer J, Feskens EJ, et al. Effect of an increased intake of alpha-linolenic acid and group nutritional education on cardiovascular risk factors: the Mediterranean Alpha-linolenic Enriched Groningen Dietary Intervention (MARGARIN) study. Am J Clin Nutr 2002;75(2):221-227.

280. Oomen CM, Ocke MC, Feskens EJ, et al. alpha-Linolenic acid intake is not beneficially associated with 10-y risk of coronary artery disease incidence: the Zutphen Elderly Study. Am J Clin Nutr 2001;74(4):457-463.

281. Ascherio A, Rimm EB, Giovannucci EL, et al. Dietary fat and risk of coronary heart disease in men: cohort follow up study in the United States. BMJ 1996;313(7049):84-90.

282. Djousse L, Pankow JS, Eckfeldt JH, et al. Relation between dietary linolenic acid and coronary artery disease in the National Heart, Lung, and Blood Institute Family Heart Study. Am J Clin Nutr 2001;74(5):612-619.

283. Keli SO, Feskens EJ, Kromhout D. Fish consumption and risk of stroke. The Zutphen Study. Stroke 1994;25(2):328-332.

284. Gillum RF, Mussolino ME, Madans JH. The relationship between fish consumption and stroke incidence. The NHANES I Epidemiologic Follow-up Study (National Health and Nutrition Examination Survey). Arch Intern Med 1996;156(5):537-542.

285. Iso H, Rexrode KM, Stampfer MJ, et al. Intake of fish and omega-3 fatty acids and risk of stroke in women. JAMA 2001;285(3):304-312.

286. Simon JA, Fong J, Bernert JT, Jr., et al. Serum fatty acids and the risk of stroke. Stroke 1995;26(5):778-782.

287. Orencia AJ, Daviglus ML, Dyer AR, et al. Fish consumption and stroke in men. 30-year findings of the Chicago Western Electric Study. Stroke 1996;27(2):204-209.

288. Morris MC, Manson JE, Rosner B, et al. Fish consumption and cardiovascular disease in the physicians' health study: a prospective study. Am J Epidemiol 1995;142(2):166-175.

289. Yamada T, Strong JP, Ishii T, et al. Atherosclerosis and omega-3 fatty acids in the populations of a fishing village and a farming village in Japan. Atherosclerosis 2000;153(2):469-481.

290. von Schacky C, Angerer P, Kothny W, et al. The effect of dietary omega-3 fatty acids on coronary atherosclerosis. A randomized, double-blind, placebo-controlled trial. Ann Intern Med 1999;130(7):554-562.

291. Sacks FM, Stone PH, Gibson CM, et al. Controlled trial of fish oil for regression of human coronary atherosclerosis. HARP Research Group. J Am Coll Cardiol 1995;25(7):1492-1498.

292. Gapinski JP, VanRuiswyk JV, Heudebert GR, et al. Preventing restenosis with fish oils following coronary angioplasty. A meta-analysis. Arch Intern Med 1993;153(13):1595-1601.

293. Cairns JA, Gill J, Morton B, et al. Fish oils and low-molecular-weight heparin for the reduction of restenosis after percutaneous transluminal coronary angioplasty. The EMPAR Study. Circulation 1996;94(7): 1553-1560.

294. Johansen O, Brekke M, Seljeflot I, et al. N-3 fatty acids do not prevent restenosis after coronary angioplasty: results from the CART study. Coronary Angioplasty Restenosis Trial. J Am Coll Cardiol 1999;33(6): 1619-1626.

295. Leaf A, Jorgensen MB, Jacobs AK, et al. Do fish oils prevent restenosis after coronary angioplasty? Circulation 1994;90(5):2248-2257.

296. Eritsland J, Arnesen H, Gronseth K, et al. Effect of dietary supplementation with n-3 fatty acids on coronary artery bypass graft patency. Am J Cardiol 1996;77(1):31-36.

297. Roy I, Meyer F, Gingras L, et al. A double blind randomized controlled study comparing the efficacy of fish oil and low dose ASA to prevent coronary saphenous vein graft obstruction after CABG [abstract]. Circulation 1991;84:II-285.

298. Aucamp AK, Schoeman HS, Coetzee JH. Pilot trial to determine the efficacy of a low dose of fish oil in the treatment of angina pectoris in the geriatric patient. Prostaglandins Leukot Essent Fatty Acids 1993;49(3): 687-689.

299. Kristensen SD, Schmidt EB, Andersen HR, et al. Fish oil in angina pectoris. Atherosclerosis 1987;64(1):13-19.

300. Augustsson K, Michaud DS, Rimm EB, et al. A prospective study of intake of fish and marine fatty acids and prostate cancer. Cancer Epidemiol Biomarkers Prev 2003;12(1):64-67.

301. Rose DP, Connolly JM. Omega-3 fatty acids as cancer chemopreventive agents. Pharmacol Ther 1999;83(3):217-244.

302. de Deckere EA. Possible beneficial effect of fish and fish n-3 poly-

unsaturated fatty acids in breast and colorectal cancer. Eur J Cancer Prev 1999;8(3):213-221.

303. Caygill CP, Hill MJ. Fish, n-3 fatty acids and human colorectal and breast cancer mortality. Eur J Cancer Prev 1995;4(4):329-332.

304. Norrish AE, Skeaff CM, Arribas GL, et al. Prostate cancer risk and consumption of fish oils: a dietary biomarker- based case-control study. Br J Cancer 1999;81(7):1238-1242.

305. Klein V, Chajes V, Germain E, et al. Low alpha-linolenic acid content of adipose breast tissue is associated with an increased risk of breast cancer. Eur J Cancer 2000;36(3):335-340.

306. Terry P, Lichtenstein P, Feychting M, et al. Fatty fish consumption and risk of prostate cancer. Lancet 2001;357(9270):1764-1766.

307. Mehrotra B, Ronquillo J. Dietary supplementation in hem/onc out-patients at a tertiary care hospital. American Society of Clinical Oncology 38th Annual Meeting, Orlando, Florida, May 18-21, 2002. 1.

308. Carlson SE, Werkman SH, Rhodes PG, et al. Visual-acuity development in healthy preterm infants: effect of marine- oil supplementation. Am J Clin Nutr 1993;58(1):35-42.

309. Birch DG, Birch EE, Hoffman DR, et al. Retinal development in very-low-birth-weight infants fed diets differing in omega-3 fatty acids. Invest Ophthalmol Vis Sci 1992;33(8):2365-2376.

310. Birch EE, Birch DG, Hoffman DR, et al. Dietary essential fatty acid supply and visual acuity development. Invest Ophthalmol Vis Sci 1992;33(11):3242-3253.

311. Hoffman DR, Birch EE, Birch DG, et al. Effects of supplementation with omega 3 long-chain polyunsaturated fatty acids on retinal and cortical development in premature infants. Am J Clin Nutr 1993;57(5 Suppl):807S-812S.

312. Carlson SE, Werkman SH, Tolley EA. Effect of long-chain n-3 fatty acid supplementation on visual acuity and growth of preterm infants with and without bronchopulmonary dysplasia. Am J Clin Nutr 1996; 63(5):687-697.

313. Carlson SE, Werkman SH. A randomized trial of visual attention of preterm infants fed docosahexaenoic acid until two months. Lipids 1996; 31(1):85-90.

314. Ross E. The role of marine fish oils in the treatment of ulcerative colitis. Nutr Rev 1993;51(2):47-49.

315. Lorenz R, Loeschke K. Placebo-controlled trials of omega 3 fatty acids in chronic inflammatory bowel disease. World Rev Nutr Diet 1994;76:143-145.

316. Lorenz R, Weber PC, Szimnau P, et al. Supplementation with n-3 fatty acids from fish oil in chronic inflammatory bowel disease—a randomized, placebo-controlled, double- blind cross-over study. J Intern Med Suppl 1989;225(731):225-232.

317. Stenson WF, Cort D, Beeken W, et al. A trial of fish oil supplemented diet in ulcerative colitis [abstract]. Gastroenterology 1990;98(Suppl):A475.

318. Hawthorne AB, Daneshmend TK, Hawkey CJ, et al. Fish oil in ulcerative colitis: final results of a controlled clinical trial [abstract]. Gastroenterology 1990;98(5 pt 2):A174.

319. Hawthorne AB, Daneshmend TK, Hawkey CJ, et al. Treatment of ulcerative colitis with fish oil supplementation: a prospective 12 month randomised controlled trial. Gut 1992;33(7):922-928.

320. Aslan A, Triadafilopoulos G. Fish oil fatty acid supplementation in active ulcerative colitis: a double-blind, placebo-controlled, crossover study. Am J Gastroenterol 1992;87(4):432-437.

321. Greenfield SM, Green AT, Teare JP, et al. A randomized controlled study of evening primrose oil and fish oil in ulcerative colitis. Aliment Pharmacol Ther 1993;7(2):159-166.

322. Loeschke K, Ueberschaer B, Pietsch A, et al. n-3 fatty acids only delay early relapse of ulcerative colitis in remission. Dig Dis Sci 1996;41(10):2087-2094.

323. Dichi I, Frenhane P, Dichi JB, et al. Comparison of omega-3 fatty acids and sulfasalazine in ulcerative colitis. Nutrition 2000;16(2):87-94.

324. Belluzzi A, Brignola C, Boschi S, et al. A novel enteric coated preparation of omega-3 fatty acids in a group of steroid-dependent ulcerative colitis: an open study [abstract]. Gastroenterology 1997;112(Suppl):A930.

325. Kim YI. Can fish oil maintain Crohn's disease in remission? Nutr Rev 1996;54(8):248-252.

326. Koretz RL. Maintaining remissions in Crohn's disease: a fat chance to please. Gastroenterology 1997;112(6):2155-2156.

327. Belluzzi A, Brignola C, Campieri M, et al. Effects of new fish oil derivative on fatty acid phospholipid-membrane pattern in a group of Crohn's disease patients. Dig Dis Sci 1994;39(12):2589-2594.

328. Dillon JJ. Fish oil therapy for IgA nephropathy: efficacy and interstudy variability. J Am Soc Nephrol 1997;8(11):1739-1744.

329. Donadio JV, Jr. Use of fish oil to treat patients with immunoglobulin A nephropathy. Am J Clin Nutr 2000;71(1 Suppl):373S-375S.

330. Donadio JV. The emerging role of omega-3 polyunsaturated fatty acids in the management of patients with IgA nephropathy. J Ren Nutr 2001; 11(3):122-128.

331. Bakker DJ, Haberstroh BN, Philbrick DJ, et al. Triglyceride lowering in nephrotic syndrome patients consuming a fish oil concentrate. Nutrit Res 1989;9:27-34.

332. Walton AJ, Snaith ML, Locniskar M, et al. Dietary fish oil and the severity of symptoms in patients with systemic lupus erythematosus. Ann Rheum Dis 1991;50(7):463-466.

333. Clark WF, Parbtani A, Naylor CD, et al. Fish oil in lupus nephritis: clinical findings and methodological implications. Kidney Int 1993;44(1):75-86.

334. Clark WF, Parbtani A. Omega-3 fatty acid supplementation in clinical and experimental lupus nephritis. Am J Kidney Dis 1994;23(5):644-647.

335. Bittiner SB, Tucker WF, Bleehen S. Fish oil in psoriasis - a double-blind randomized placebo-controlled trial. Br J Dermatol 1987;117:25-26.

336. Bittiner SB, Tucker WF, Cartwright I, et al. A double-blind, randomised, placebo-controlled trial of fish oil in psoriasis. Lancet 1988;1(8582):378-380.

337. Bjorneboe A, Smith AK, Bjorneboe GE, et al. Effect of dietary supple-mentation with n-3 fatty acids on clinical manifestations of psoriasis. Br J Dermatol 1988;118(1):77-83.

338. Gupta AK, Ellis CN, Tellner DC, et al. Double-blind, placebo-controlled study to evaluate the efficacy of fish oil and low-dose UVB in the treatment of psoriasis. Br J Dermatol 1989;120(6):801-807.

339. Gupta AK, Ellis CN, Goldfarb MT, et al. The role of fish oil in psoriasis. A randomized, double-blind, placebo- controlled study to evaluate the effect of fish oil and topical corticosteroid therapy in psoriasis. Int J Dermatol 1990;29(8):591-595.

340. Escobar SO, Achenbach R, Iannantuono R, et al. Topical fish oil in psoriasis—a controlled and blind study. Clin Exp Dermatol 1992; 17(3):159-162.

341. Grimminger F, Mayser P, Papavassilis C, et al. A double-blind, randomized, placebo-controlled trial of n-3 fatty acid based lipid infusion in acute, extended guttate psoriasis. Rapid improvement of clinical manifestations and changes in neutrophil leukotriene profile. Clin Invest 1993;71(8):634-643.

342. Henneicke-von Zepelin HH, Mrowietz U, Farber L, et al. Highly purified omega-3-polyunsaturated fatty acids for topical treatment of psoriasis. Results of a double-blind, placebo-controlled multicentre study. Br J Dermatol 1993;129(6):713-717.

343. Soyland E, Funk J, Rajka G, et al. Effect of dietary supplementation with very-long-chain n-3 fatty acids in patients with psoriasis. N Engl J Med 1993;328(25):1812-1816.

344. Strong AM, Hamill E. The effect of combined fish oil and evening primrose oil (Efamol Marine) on the remission phase of psoriasis: a 7 month double-blind randomized placebo-controlled trial. J Derm Treatment 1993;4:33-36.

345. Mayser P, Mrowietz U, Arenberger P, et al. Omega-3 fatty acid-based lipid infusion in patients with chronic plaque psoriasis: results of a double-blind, randomized, placebo-controlled, multicenter trial. J Am Acad Dermatol 1998;38(4):539-547.

346. Danno K, Sugie N. Combination therapy with low-dose etretinate and eicosapentaenoic acid for psoriasis vulgaris. J Dermatol 1998;25(11):703-705.

347. Bjorneboe A, Soyland E, Bjorneboe GE, et al. Effect of dietary supple-mentation with eicosapentaenoic acid in the treatment of atopic dermatitis. Br J Dermatol 1987;117(4):463-469.

348. Bjorneboe A, Soyland E, Bjorneboe GE, et al. Effect of n-3 fatty acid supplement to patients with atopic dermatitis. J Intern Med Suppl 1989; 225(731):233-236.

349. Kunz B, Ring J, Braun-Falco O. Eicosapentaenoic acid (EPA) treatment in atopic eczema (AE): a prospective double-blind trial [abstract]. J Allergy Clin Immunol 1989;83:196.

350. Palat D, Rudolph D, Rothstein M. A trial of fish oil in asthma [abstract]. Am Rev Respir Dis 1988;137(Suppl 4 part 2):329.

351. Arm JP, Horton CE, Mencia-Huerta JM, et al. Effect of dietary supple-mentation with fish oil lipids on mild asthma. Thorax 1988;43(2):84-92.

352. Arm JP, Horton CE, Spur BW, et al. The effects of dietary supple-mentation with fish oil lipids on the airways response to inhaled allergen in bronchial asthma. Am Rev Respir Dis 1989;139(6):1395-1400.

353. Stenius-Aarniala B, Aro A, Hakulinen A, et al. Evening primrose oil and fish oil are ineffective as supplementary treatment of bronchial asthma. Ann Allergy 1989;62(6):534-537.

354. McDonald CF, Vecchie L, Pierce RJ, et al. Effect of fish-oil derived omega-3 fatty acid supplements on asthma control [abstract]. Austral New Zealand J Med 1990;20:526.

355. Thien FC, Mencia-Huerta JM, Lee TH. Dietary fish oil effects on seasonal hay fever and asthma in pollen- sensitive subjects. Am Rev Respir Dis 1993;147(5):1138-1143.

356. Dry J, Vincent D. Effect of a fish oil diet on asthma: results of a 1-year double-blind study. Int Arch Allergy Appl Immunol 1991;95(2-3):156-157.

357. Nagakura T, Matsuda S, Shichijyo K, et al. Dietary supplementation with fish oil rich in omega-3 polyunsaturated fatty acids in children with bronchial asthma. Eur Respir J 2000;16(5):861-865.

358. Okamoto M, Mitsunobu F, Ashida K, et al. Effects of dietary supplementation with n-3 fatty acids compared with n-6 fatty acids on bronchial asthma. Intern Med 2000;39(2):107-111.

359. Masuev KA. [The effect of polyunsaturated fatty acids of the omega-3 class on the late phase of the allergic reaction in bronchial asthma patients]. Terapevticheskii Arkhiv 1997;69(3):31-33.

360. Woods RK, Thien FC, Abramson MJ. Dietary marine fatty acids (fish oil) for asthma in adults and children. Cochrane Database Syst Rev 2002;(3):CD001283.

361. Olsen SF, Sorensen JD, Secher NJ, et al. Randomised controlled trial of effect of fish-oil supplementation on pregnancy duration. Lancet 1992;339(8800):1003-1007.

362. D'Almeida A, Carter JP, Anatol A, et al. Effects of a combination of evening primrose oil (gamma linolenic acid) and fish oil (eicosapentaenoic + docahexaenoic acid) versus magnesium, and versus placebo in preventing pre-eclampsia. Women Health 1992;19(2-3):117-131.

363. Bulstra-Ramakers MT, Huisjes HJ, Visser GH. The effects of 3 g eicosapentaenoic acid daily on recurrence of intrauterine growth retardation and pregnancy induced hypertension. Br J Obstet Gynaecol 1994;102:123-126.

364. Salvig JD, Olsen SF, Secher NJ. Effects of fish oil supplementation in late pregnancy on blood pressure: a randomised controlled trial. Br J Obstet Gynaecol 1996;103(6):529-533.

365. Onwude JL, Lilford RJ, Hjartardottir H, et al. A randomised double blind placebo controlled trial of fish oil in high risk pregnancy. Br J Obstet Gynaecol 1995;102(2):95-100.

366. Olsen SF, Secher NJ, Tabor A, et al. Randomised clinical trials of fish oil supplementation in high risk pregnancies. Fish Oil Trials In Pregnancy (FOTIP) Team. BJOG 2000;107(3):382-395.

367. Olsen SF, Secher NJ. Low consumption of seafood in early pregnancy as a risk factor for preterm delivery: prospective cohort study. BMJ 2002; 324(7335):447.

368. Joy CB, Mumby-Croft R, Joy LA. Polyunsaturated fatty acid (fish or evening primrose oil) for schizophrenia. Cochrane Database Syst Rev 2000;(2):CD001257.

369. Peet M, Mellor J. Double-blind placebo controlled trial of N-3 polyunsaturated fatty acids as an adjunct to neuroleptics [abstract]. Schizophrenia Res 1998;29(1-2):160-161.

370. Fenton WS, Dickerson F, Boronow J, et al. A placebo-controlled trial of omega-3 Fatty Acid (ethyl eicosapentaenoic Acid) supplementation for residual symptoms and cognitive impairment in schizophrenia. Am J Psychiatry 2001;158(12):2071-2074.

371. Mellor J, Laugharne JD, Peet M. Omega-3 fatty acid supplementation in schizophrenic patients. Human Psychopharmacol 1996;11:39-46.

372. Horrobin DF. Omega-3 Fatty acid for schizophrenia. Am J Psychiatry 2003;160(1):188-189.

373. Stoll AL, Severus WE, Freeman MP, et al. Omega 3 fatty acids in bipolar disorder: a preliminary double-blind, placebo-controlled trial. Arch Gen Psychiatry 1999;56(5):407-412.

374. Calabrese JR, Rapport DJ, Shelton MD. Fish oils and bipolar disorder: a promising but untested treatment. Arch Gen Psychiatry 1999;56(5): 413-414.

375. Tanskanen A, Hibbeln JR, Hintikka J, et al. Fish consumption, depression, and suicidality in a general population. Arch Gen Psychiatry 2001; 58(5):512-513.

375. Chiu CC, Huang SY, Shen WW, et al. Omega-3 fatty acids for depression in pregnancy. Am J Psychiatry 2003;160(2):385.

377. Mischoulon D, Fava M. Docosahexaenoic acid and omega-3 fatty acids in depression. Psychiatr Clin North Am 2000;23(4):785-794.

378. Nemets B, Stahl Z, Belmaker RH. Addition of omega-3 fatty acid to maintenance medication treatment for recurrent unipolar depressive disorder. Am J Psychiatry 2002;159(3):477-479.

379. Su KP, Huang SY, Chiu CC, et al. Omega-3 fatty acids in major depressive disorder. A preliminary double-blind, placebo-controlled trial. Eur Neuropsychopharmacol 2003;13(4):267-271.

380. Deutch B. [Painful menstruation and low intake of n-3 fatty acids]. Ugeskr Laeger 1996;158(29):4195-4198.

381. Harel Z, Biro FM, Kottenhahn RK, et al. Supplementation with omega-3 polyunsaturated fatty acids in the management of dysmenorrhea in adolescents. Am J Obstet Gynecol 1996;174(4):1335-1338.

382. Beckles WI, Elliott TM, Everard ML. Omega-3 fatty acids (from fish oils) for cystic fibrosis. Cochrane Database Syst Rev 2002;(3):CD002201.

383. De Vizia B, Raia V, Spano C, et al. Effect of an 8-month treatment with omega-3 fatty acids (eicosapentaenoic and docosahexaenoic) in patients with cystic fibrosis. JPEN J Parenter Enteral Nutr 2003;27(1):52-57.

384. Beckles WN, Elliott TM, Everard ML. Omega-3 fatty acids for cystic fibrosis (Protocol for a Cochrane Review). The Cochrane Library 2001;(3)

385. Kurlandsky LE, Bennink MR, Webb PM, et al. The absorption and effect of dietary supplementation with omega-3 fatty acids on serum leukotriene B4 in patients with cystic fibrosis. Pediatr Pulmonol 1994;18(4):211-217.

386. Henderson WR, Jr., Astley SJ, McCready MM, et al. Oral absorption of omega-3 fatty acids in patients with cystic fibrosis who have pancreatic insufficiency and in healthy control subjects. J Pediatr 1994;124(3): 400-408.

387. Katz DP, Manner T, Furst P, et al. The use of an intravenous fish oil emulsion enriched with omega-3 fatty acids in patients with cystic fibrosis. Nutrition 1996;12(5):334-339.

388. Lawrence R, Sorrell T. Eicosapentaenoic acid in cystic fibrosis: evidence of a pathogenetic role for leukotriene B4. Lancet 1993;342(8869):465-469.

389. Ullmann D, Connor WE, Illingworth DR, et al. Additive effects of lovastatin and fish oil in familial hypercholesterolemia [abstract]. Arteriosclerosis 1990;10(5):846a.

390. Tato F, Keller C, Wolfram G. Effects of fish oil concentrate on lipoproteins and apolipoproteins in familial combined hyperlipidemia. Clin Investig 1993;71(4):314-318.

391. Balestrieri GP, Maffi V, Sleiman I, et al. Fish oil supplementation in patients with heterozygous familial hypercholesterolemia. Recenti Prog Med 1996;87(3):102-105.

392. Clarke JT, Cullen-Dean G, Regelink E, et al. Increased incidence of epistaxis in adolescents with familial hypercholesterolemia treated with fish oil. J Pediatr 1990;116(1):139-141.

393. Salvi A, Di Stefano O, Sleiman I, et al. Effects of fish oil on serum lipids and lipoprotein(a) levels in heterozygous familial hypercholesterolemia. Curr Ther Res Clin Exp 1993;53(6):717-721.

394. Barber MD, Ross JA, Voss AC, et al. The effect of an oral nutritional supplement enriched with fish oil on weight-loss in patients with pancreatic cancer. Br J Cancer 1999;81(1):80-86.

395. Barber MD, Ross JA, Preston T, et al. Fish oil-enriched nutritional supplement attenuates progression of the acute-phase response in weight-losing patients with advanced pancreatic cancer. J Nutr 1999;129(6): 1120-1125.

396. Wigmore SJ, Barber MD, Ross JA, et al. Effect of oral eicosapentaenoic acid on weight loss in patients with pancreatic cancer. Nutr Cancer 2000; 36(2):177-184.

397. Bruera E, Strasser F, Palmer JL, et al. Effect of fish oil on appetite and other symptoms in patients with advanced cancer and anorexia/cachexia: a double-blind, placebo- controlled study. J Clin Oncol 2003;21(1): 129-134.

398. Fearon KC, Von Meyenfeldt MF, Moses AG, et al. Effect of a protein and energy dense n-3 fatty acid enriched oral supplement on loss of weight and lean tissue in cancer cachexia: a randomised double blind trial. Gut 2003; 52(10):1479-1486.

399. Durrington PN, Bhatnagar D, Mackness MI, et al. An omega-3 poly-unsaturated fatty acid concentrate administered for one year decreased triglycerides in simvastatin treated patients with coronary heart disease and persisting hypertriglyceridaemia. Heart 2001;85(5):544-548.

400. Saynor R, Gillott T. Changes in blood lipids and fibrinogen with a note on safety in a long term study on the effects of n-3 fatty acids in subjects receiving fish oil supplements and followed for seven years. Lipids 1992;27(7):533-538.

401. Miller JP, Heath ID, Choraria SK, et al. Triglyceride lowering effect of MaxEPA fish lipid concentrate: a multicentre placebo controlled double blind study. Clin Chim Acta 1988;178(3):251-259.

402. Molgaard J, von Schenck H, Lassvik C, et al. Effect of fish oil treatment on plasma lipoproteins in type III hyperlipoproteinaemia. Atherosclerosis 1990;81(1):1-9.

403. Mortensen JZ, Schmidt EB, Nielsen AH, et al. The effect of N-6 and N-3 polyunsaturated fatty acids on hemostasis, blood lipids and blood pressure. Thromb Haemost 1983;50(2):543-546.

404. Norris PG, Jones CJ, Weston MJ. Effect of dietary supplementation with fish oil on systolic blood pressure in mild essential hypertension. Br Med J (Clin Res Ed) 1986;293(6539):104-105.

405. Saynor R, Verel D, Gillott T. The long-term effect of dietary supplementation with fish lipid concentrate on serum lipids, bleeding time, platelets and angina. Atherosclerosis 1984;50(1):3-10.

406. Boberg M, Vessby B, Selinus I. Effects of dietary supplementation with n-6 and n-3 long-chain polyunsaturated fatty acids on serum lipoproteins and platelet function in hypertriglyceridaemic patients. Acta Med Scand 1986;220(2):153-160.

407. Haines AP, Sanders TA, Imeson JD, et al. Effects of a fish oil supplement on platelet function, haemostatic variables and albuminuria in insulin-dependent diabetics. Thromb Res 1986;43(6):643-655.

408. De Caterina R, Caprioli R, Giannessi D, et al. n-3 fatty acids reduce proteinuria in patients with chronic glomerular disease. Kidney Int 1993; 44(4):843-850.

409. McVeigh GE, Brennan GM, Cohn JN, et al. Fish oil improves arterial compliance in non-insulin-dependent diabetes mellitus. Arterioscler Thromb 1994;14(9):1425-1429.

410. Hendra TJ, Britton ME, Roper DR, et al. Effects of fish oil supplements in NIDDM subjects. Controlled study. Diabetes Care 1990;13(8):821-829.

411. Bates D, Cartlidge NE, French JM, et al. A double-blind controlled trial of long chain n-3 polyunsaturated fatty acids in the treatment of multiple sclerosis. J Neurol Neurosurg Psychiatry 1989;52(1):18-22.

412. Mori TA, Vandongen R, Masarei JR, et al. Dietary fish oils increase serum lipids in insulin-dependent diabetics compared with healthy controls. Metabolism 1989;38(5):404-409.

413. Simons LA, Hickie JB, Balasubramaniam S. On the effects of dietary n-3 fatty acids (Maxepa) on plasma lipids and lipoproteins in patients with hyperlipidaemia. Atherosclerosis 1985;54(1):75-88.

414. Vandongen R, Mori TA, Codde JP, et al. Hypercholesterolaemic effect of fish oil in insulin-dependent diabetic patients. Med J Aust 1988;148(3): 141-143.

415. Wilt TJ, Lofgren RP, Nichol KL, et al. Fish oil supplementation does not lower plasma cholesterol in men with hypercholesterolemia. Results of a randomized, placebo-controlled crossover study. Ann Intern Med 1989;111(11):900-905.

416. Zucker ML, Bilyeu DS, Helmkamp GM, et al. Effects of dietary fish oil on

platelet function and plasma lipids in hyperlipoproteinemic and normal subjects. Atherosclerosis 1988;73(1):13-22.

417. Harris WS, Rothrock DW, Fanning A, et al. Fish oils in hyper-triglyceridemia: a dose-response study. Am J Clin Nutr 1990;51(3): 399-406.

418. Kettler AH, Baughn RE, Orengo IF, et al. The effect of dietary fish oil supplementation on psoriasis. Improvement in a patient with pustular psoriasis. J Am Acad Dermatol 1988;18(6):1267-1273.

419. Mori TA, Vandongen R, Masarei JR, et al. Comparison of diets supplemented with fish oil or olive oil on plasma lipoproteins in insulin-dependent diabetics. Metabolism 1991;40(3):241-246.

420. Frenais R, Ouguerram K, Maugeais C, et al. Effect of dietary omega-3 fatty acids on high-density lipoprotein apolipoprotein AI kinetics in type II diabetes mellitus. Atherosclerosis 2001;157(1):131-135.

421. Hall AV, Parbtani A, Clark WF, et al. Omega-3 fatty acid supplementation in primary nephrotic syndrome: effects on plasma lipids and coagulopathy. J Am Soc Nephrol 1992;3(6):1321-1329.

422. Sorensen JD, Olsen SF, Pedersen AK, et al. Effects of fish oil supplementation in the third trimester of pregnancy on prostacyclin and thromboxane production. Am J Obstet Gynecol 1993;168(3 Pt 1): 915-922.

423. Hansen JM, Hoy CE, Strandgaard S. Fish oil and cyclosporin A-induced renal hypoperfusion in kidney- transplanted patients. Nephrol Dial Transplant 1995;10(9):1745-1750.

424. Leaf DA, Rauch CR. Omega-3 supplementation and estimated VO2max: a double blind randomized controlled trial in athletes. Ann Sports Med 1988;4(1):37-40.

425. Belluzzi A, Campieri M, Belloli C, et al. A new enteric coated preparation of omega-3 fatty acids for prevention of post-surgical recurrence in Crohn's disease [abstract]. Gastroenterology 1997;112(Suppl):A930.

426. Belluzzi A, Brignola C, Campieri M, et al. Effect of an enteric-coated fish-oil preparation on relapses in Crohn's disease. N Engl J Med 1996; 334(24):1557-1560.

427. Rustemeijer C, Bilo HJ, Beukhof JR, et al. The effect of fish oil concentrate on serum lipids and lipoproteins in patients on maintenance hemodialysis. Curr Ther Res 1988;43(4):559-567.

428. Malyszko JS, Malyszko J, Pawlak K, et al. [Effect of treating glomerulonephritis with omega 3 fatty acids for selected parameters of hemostasis, blood platelet function and lipid metabolism]. Przegl Lek 1996;53(8):600-603.

429. Sirtori CR, Crepaldi G, Manzato E, et al. One-year treatment with ethyl esters of n-3 fatty acids in patients with hypertriglyceridemia and glucose intolerance: reduced triglyceridemia, total cholesterol and increased HDL-C without glycemic alterations. Atherosclerosis 1998;137(2):419-427.

F

Flaxseed and Flaxseed Oil

(Linum usitatissimum)

SYNONYMS/COMMON NAMES/RELATED SUBSTANCES

- Alashi, alpha-linolenic acid, Barlean's Flax Oil, Barlean's Vita-Flax, brazen, common flax, eicosapentaenoic acid, flachssamen, flax, gamma-linolenic acid, graine de lin, leinsamen, hu-ma-esze, Linaceae, linen flax, lini semen, lino, lino usuale, linseed, linseed oil, lint bells, linum, linum catharticum, linum humile seeds, keten, omega-3 fatty acid, phytoestrogen, sufulsi, tesi-mosina, type I flaxseed/flaxseed (51%-55% alpha-linolenic acid), type II flaxseed/CDC-flaxseed (2%-3% alpha-linolenic acid), winterlien.

CLINICAL BOTTOM LINE

Background

- Flaxseed and its derivative flaxseed oil/linseed oil are rich sources of the essential fatty acid alpha-linolenic acid, which is a biologic precursor to omega-3 fatty acids such as eicosapentaenoic acid. Although omega-3 fatty acids have been associated with improved cardiovascular outcomes, evidence from human trials is mixed regarding the efficacy of flaxseed products for coronary artery disease or hyperlipidemia.
- The lignan constituents of flaxseed (not flaxseed oil) possesses *in vitro* anti-oxidant and possible estrogen receptor agonist/antagonist properties, prompting theories of efficacy for the treatment of breast cancer. However, there is not sufficient human evidence to make a recommendation. As a source of fiber mucilage, oral flaxseed (not flaxseed oil) may possess laxative properties, although only one human trial has been conducted for this indication. In large doses, or when taken with inadequate water, flaxseed may precipitate bowel obstruction via a mass effect. The effects of flaxseed on blood glucose levels are not clear, although hyperglycemic effects have been reported in one case series.
- Flaxseed oil contains only the alpha-linolenic acid component of flaxseed, and not the fiber or lignan components. Therefore, flaxseed oil may share the purported lipid-lowering properties of flaxseed, but not the proposed laxative or anticancer abilities.
- Preliminary evidence suggests that alpha-linolenic acid may be associated with an *increased* risk of prostate cancer.

Scientific Evidence for Common/Studied Uses	Grade*
Constipation/laxative (flaxseed, not flaxseed oil)	B
Atherosclerosis/coronary artery disease (flaxseed and flaxseed oil)	C
Breast cancer (flaxseed, not flaxseed oil)	C
Cyclic mastalgia (breast pain) (flaxseed, not flaxseed oil)	C
HIV/AIDS	C
Hyperglycemia/diabetes (flaxseed, not flaxseed oil)	C
Hyperlipidemia (flaxseed and flaxseed oil)	C
Hypertension (flaxseed, not flaxseed oil)	C

Lupus nephritis (flaxseed, not flaxseed oil)	C
Menopausal symptoms	C
Prostate cancer (flaxseed, not flaxseed oil)	D

*Key to grades: *A:* Strong scientific evidence for this use; *B:* Good scientific evidence for this use; *C:* Unclear scientific evidence for this use; *D:* Fair scientific evidence against this use (it may not work); *F:* Strong scientific evidence against this use (it likely does not work). For a more detailed explanation of efficacy criteria, see "Natural Standard Evidence-Based Validated Grading Rationale" in the Introduction.

Historical or Theoretical Uses That Lack Sufficient Evidence:

- Abdominal pain, acute respiratory distress syndrome (ARDS),[1] allergic reactions (delayed hypersensitivity reactions), anticoagulant, anti-platelet agent, benign prostatic hypertrophy (BPH), bladder inflammation, bipolar disorder,[2] boils, bronchial irritation, burns (poultice), colon cancer,[3,4] cough suppressant, cystitis, depression, diabetic nephropathy,[5] diarrhea, diverticulitis, dry skin, dysentery, eczema, emollient, enteritis, expectorant, foreign body removal from the eye, gastritis, glomerulonephritis, gonorrhea, hepatoprotection,[6] interstitial nephritis,[7] irritable bowel syndrome, laxative-induced colon damage, melanoma,[8] menstrual luteal phase disorders, mucolytic, ovarian disorders, pimples, pharyngitis, psoriasis, rheumatoid arthritis, skin infections, sore throat, systemic lupus erythematosus, ulcerative colitis,[9] upper respiratory tract infection, skin inflammation, stomach upset, urinary tract infection, vision improvement,[10] vaginitis, weight loss.

Expert Opinion and Historic Precedent

- Flaxseed products are used widely for numerous indications. The expert German panel, the Commission E, has sanctioned the use of flax for chronic constipation, laxative-damaged colons, irritable bowel, diverticulitis, and enteritis.

Safety Summary

- **Likely safe:** The U.S. Food and Drug Administration has not granted a GRAS ("generally regarded as safe") status to flaxseed or cold-pressed flaxseed oil, although it does allow up to 12% flaxseed in food (by weight). Based on the available data, it appears that both flaxseed and flaxseed oil are safe when used orally in recommended doses for under 4 months by healthy individuals. Although long-term studies on the safety of flaxseed or flaxseed oil are scarce in the available literature, a major component of flaxseed, alpha-linolenic acid (ALA), has been well tolerated for up to 5 years as part of the Mediterranean diet (used for secondary prevention of coronary artery disease). Flaxseed should be ingested with adequate fluid intake (1:10, seed:liquid). Topical application of the seed form or poultice is also reported to be generally well tolerated, although antigen sensitization may occur in up to 50% of adult handlers.
- **Possibly safe:** When flaxseed or flaxseed oil is used for >4 months, the safety is not clear, due to lack of data.

- **Possibly unsafe:** Flaxseed (not flaxseed oil) contains lignans that may possess estrogen receptor agonist or antagonist properties, with unclear effects on hormone-sensitive conditions such as breast, uterine, and prostate cancer and endometriosis.[11] Avoid flaxseed in men with prostate cancer or at risk for developing prostate cancer, based on case-control studies associating alpha-linolenic acid intake with the development of prostate cancer.[12-14] In theory, flaxseed and flaxseed oil may increase the risk of bleeding, based on trial evidence showing decreased platelet aggregation.[15-17]
- **Likely unsafe:** Immature flaxseed seed pods may be poisonous and should not be consumed. Anecdotally, intestinal obstruction may occur from mass effect when large amounts of flaxseed are ingested or taken with inadequate amounts of water/liquid (1:10, seed:liquid, is recommended).

DOSING/TOXICOLOGY
General

- Recommended doses are based on those most commonly used in available trials, or on historical practice. However, with natural products, the optimal doses needed to balance efficacy and safety often have not been determined. Formulations and preparation methods may vary from manufacturer to manufacturer, and from batch to batch of a specific product made by a single manufacturer. Because often the active components of a product are not known, standardization may not be possible, and the clinical effects of different brands may not be comparable.

Standardization

- Flaxseed products are not standardized based on specific chemical components, but rather are evaluated with a number of identity and quality tests. Tests may include microscopic/macroscopic inspection and organoleptic evaluation.
- Flaxseed is approximately 35% oil, of which 55% is alpha-linolenic acid[18-22]; 58% to 60% of flaxseed is omega-3 fatty acid, and 18% to 20% is omega-6 fatty acid. Flaxseed and linseed oil contain 30% to 45% unsaturated fatty acids, and approximately 8% of the plant contains soluble fiber mucilage.[23] The plant also contains 20% protein. Flaxseed oil is composed of 73% polyunsaturated fatty acids, 18% monounsaturated fatty acids, and 9% saturated fatty acids.
- As a substitute for fish oil, a dose of 7.2 g of flaxseed is anecdotally equivalent to 1 g of fish oil.

Special Considerations

- **Consumption with other medications:** Consumption of flaxseed (*not* flaxseed oil) may decrease the absorption of co-administered oral medications/vitamins/minerals. Therefore, oral medications should be taken an hour before or 2 hours after a dose of flaxseed to prevent decreased absorption. Anecdotally, the chance of bowel obstruction and adverse reactions with the use of flaxseed is greatly reduced when each dose is mixed with sufficient amounts of liquid.
- **Storage:** Flaxseed oil should be kept refrigerated in an opaque bottle, as it may degrade with exposure to light, oxygen, or heat. Whole flaxseed can be stored for up to 1 year in a dry location. Ground flaxseed can be kept in a refrigerator for up to 3 months and in freezer for 6 months.

Dosing: Adult (18 Years and Older)
Oral

- **Flaxseed oil (liquid form):** Flaxseed oil contains only the alpha-linolenic acid (ALA) component of flax, not the fiber or lignan components found in flaxseed. Flaxseed oil is most often used in a liquid form, which contains approximately 7 g of ALA per tablespoon (15 mL) and contains approximately 130 calories (anecdotal).
- **Flaxseed oil (capsule form):** Flaxseed oil is available in a capsule form, which often contains 500 mg of ALA per 1000-mg capsule (10 calories).
- **Flaxseed powder/flour/soluble fiber:** There are no uniform dosing standards for flaxseed in the treatment of specific disorders in adults. In several studies, adults have consumed up to 50 g/day of ground, raw flaxseeds for periods not exceeding 4 weeks. Study doses for shorter periods of time (<2 weeks) have ranged from 10 to 60 g/day. A dose of 50 g/day of flaxseeds may correlate with 250 g of flaxseed flour. Anecdotally, the dose of flaxseed for gastritis or enteritis is 1 tablespoon of whole or bruised seed mixed with 150 mL of liquid, taken 2 to 3 times/day. As a laxative, the dose of flaxseed used anecdotally is 2 to 3 tablespoons of bulk seed mixed in 10 times the amount of water, although 45 g/day have been noted to have laxative effects in human studies. For lupus nephritis, 30 g/day of flaxseed has been studied.[24] For menopausal symptoms, 40 g of flaxseed daily has been studied.[25]
- **Flaxseed liquid:** The whole or bruised (not ground) flaxseed can be mixed with water or juice and ingested. Generally, 1 tablespoon in this form can be mixed with 6 to 12 ounces of liquid and taken up to three times a day. Some studies have used up to 60 to 80 g/kg of soluble flaxseed mucilage/fiber. These forms of flaxseed should not be confused with preparations of flaxseed oil.
- **Leaf:** There is insufficient evidence available to recommend the use of flaxseed leaves to treat or prevent any medical condition.
- **In foods:** At high temperatures, such as cooking, flaxseed oil and powder/flour will degrade. It has been shown that eating four eggs per day from chickens fed flaxseed results in elevated serum levels of total omega-3 fatty acids and docosahexaenoic acid (DHA).[26] Long-term effects are not clear.

Topical

- **Flaxseed poultice:** Anecdotally, 30 to 100 g of flaxseed flour can be mixed with warm or hot water to form a moist compress and can be used up to three times a day. It is unclear how long a flaxseed poultice should be used.

Ophthalmic

- **Flaxseed:** Flaxseeds have been used for foreign body removal in the eye by placing a single whole flaxseed under the eyelid, allowing the foreign body/mucus to adhere to it, thereby facilitating removal. This process may be unsafe, and it is recommended to consult a healthcare professional for removal of foreign bodies from the eye.

Dosing: Pediatric (Younger Than 18 Years)

- Currently there is insufficient evidence to recommend the use of flaxseed or flaxseed oil in children.

Toxicology

- Based on animal studies, overdoses of flaxseed may cause dyspnea, tachypnea, weakness, or unsteady gait, and may progress to seizure or paralysis. Immature flaxseed pods are reported to be poisonous and should not be consumed. When flaxseed is consumed raw, there may be an increase in blood levels of thiocyanate, which can inhibit oxidative phosphorylation by mitochondria. This effect has not been observed at recommended doses. The flaxseed plant may contain cyanogenic glycosides (linamarin, linustatin, and neolinustatin) which can be converted *in vivo* to cyanide. However, up to 100 g of flaxseed have been consumed without alterations of serum cyanide levels.

- Theoretically, flaxseed (*not* flaxseed oil) may increase lipid peroxidation and thus increase oxidative injury.[23] Diets supplemented with defatted flaxseed have been associated with a decrease in protein thiol groups, suggesting an increase in oxidative stress.[23] Other *in vitro* studies have documented antioxidant effects.

ADVERSE EFFECTS/PRECAUTIONS/CONTRAINDICATIONS
Allergy

- Known allergy or hypersensitivity to flaxseed, flaxseed oil or any other members of the Linaceae plant family or *Linum* genus plant family.
- Hypersensitivity reactions to flaxseed following occupational exposure to the powder have been reported anecdotally. In a case report, a 40-year-old woman experienced palmar pruritus, generalized urticaria, ocular pruritus/weeping, and nausea/vomiting 10 minutes after consuming a spoonful of linseed oil (from flaxseed); a skin prick test confirmed a type I hypersensitivity reaction.[27] In another case report, a skin prick test confirmed that a 40-year-old man had a type I hypersensitivity reaction to linseed oil. He had experienced 5 or 6 episodes of intestinal/abdominal pain, vomiting, diarrhea, generalized urticaria, acute dyspnea without bronchospasm, hydrorrhea, successive sneezing, nasal obstruction, pruritus, and intense general malaise 2 to 3 minutes after eating multigrain bread.[28]

Adverse Effects/Postmarket Surveillance

- **General:** In the few human case reports available, flaxseed and flaxseed oil appear to be well tolerated. Although limited human safety data exist, there is long-standing historical use, with few reports of adverse events.
- **Dermatologic:** One case of palmar pruritus and generalized urticaria was reported in a 40-year-old woman 10 minutes after she ingested a spoonful of linseed oil (from flaxseed).[27] She was treated in an emergency room, where her symptoms resolved. A skin prick test confirmed type I hypersensitivity to linseed. In another case report, a 40-year-old man experienced generalized urticaria and pruritus 2 to 3 minutes after eating multigrain bread.[28] A skin prick test confirmed type I hypersensitivity to linseed oil.
- **Neurologic/CNS:** Anecdotally, an overdose of flaxseed or flaxseed oil may result in weakness, unstable gait, paralysis or seizures. Malaise has been reported in an individual 2 to 3 minutes after eating multigrain bread; type I hypersensitivity to linseed was later confirmed.[28] The physiologic balance between linolenic acid and linoleic acid may be relevant, and linolenic acid deficiency may cause neurological abnormalities. A 6-year-old girl who had 300 cm of bowel removed was maintained on total parenteral nutrition (TPN) rich in linoleic acid but low in linolenic acid. After 5 months she began to experience numbness, paresthesia, weakness, inability to walk, pain in her legs, and blurred vision. The TPN was changed to an emulsion with high linolenic acid, and her symptoms resolved.[29]
- **Ocular/otic:** There is one report of ocular pruritus and weeping following ingestion of linseed oil; type I hypersensitivity to linseed (flaxseed) was later confirmed.[27]

- **Psychiatric:** In theory, consumption of flaxseed or flaxseed oil may precipitate episodes of mania or hypomania in bipolar patients.[2]
- **Pulmonary/respiratory:** Anecdotally, an overdose of flaxseed or flaxseed oil may result in shortness of breath or tachypnea. In a case report, a 40-year-old man experienced acute dyspnea without bronchospasm 2 to 3 minutes after eating multigrain bread; type I hypersensitivity to linseed was later confirmed.[28]
- **Cardiovascular:** Preliminary evidence suggests that higher levels of linolenic acid in human adipose tissues may correlate with lower blood pressure.[30] Because flaxseed contains alpha-linolenic acid, it has been proposed that flaxseed may lower blood pressure. Flaxseed-supplemented diets have had mixed effects on blood pressure in rats.[31,32] Evidence from one poor-quality human study suggests that 2 weeks of flaxseed supplementation lowers blood pressure.[33]
- **Gastrointestinal (nausea/vomiting):** Severe nausea was reported in one patient enrolled in a flaxseed study.[2] Nausea, vomiting, and abdominal pain have been reported in two individuals shortly after ingestion of flaxseed products; these reactions may have been due to an allergic response.[27,28]
- **Gastrointestinal (laxative):** In theory, due to the laxative effects of flaxseed (*not* flaxseed oil), prolonged diarrhea, increased number of bowel movements, and gastrointestinal distress may occur. Laxative effects of flaxseed were observed in one small human trial.[34] A 30% increase in bowel movements was seen in a study of young adults consuming 50 g of flaxseed daily for 4 weeks.[35] Loose stool was the most common side effect in a study evaluating the effects of omega-3 acids in bipolar patients.[2] In a different study, laxative effects were reported by two patients consuming 30 g of flaxseed daily.[36]
- **Gastrointestinal (obstruction):** Anecdotally, intestinal obstruction may occur from mass effect when large amounts of flaxseed are ingested, or when flaxseed (*not* flaxseed oil) is taken with inadequate amounts of water/liquid (1:10, seed:liquid is recommended). Anecdotally, consumption of large quantities of flaxseed may result in ileus.
- **Endocrine:** The omega-3 fatty acids in flaxseed and flaxseed oil may cause hyperglycemia. Six men with type 2 diabetes experienced increases in fasting glucose levels following 1 month of treatment with omega-3 fatty acids (which are present in flaxseed).[37] However, a small case series found no effects of flaxseed (50 g) on postprandial glucose levels.[19] Prolonged luteal phases have been reported in 18 healthy women consuming 10 g of flaxseed powder daily for three menstrual cycles.[38]
- **Hematologic:** Flaxseed and flaxseed oil may increase the risk of bleeding, based on trial evidence showing decreased platelet aggregation.[15-17] Patients taking alpha-linolenic acid, a component of flaxseed, have been noted to have a prolonged bleeding time vs. placebo.[39] No incidents of bleeding have been reported in the available literature. Flaxseed consumption may increase total red blood cell counts, based on animal data.[40]
- **Genitourinary:** Several case-control studies have associated the intake of alpha-linolenic acid (which is present in flaxseed) with an increased risk of developing prostate cancer.[12-14] One brief, small case series in patients with prostate cancer found no effect of flaxseed supplementation on serum prostate specific antigen (PSA) levels.[41] In human prostate cancer cells, the flaxseed constituent linolenic acid promotes cell growth, whereas the constituent eicosapentaenoic acid

(EPA) promotes growth at low concentrations and inhibits growth at high concentrations.[42] Until better evidence is available, flaxseed and alpha-linolenic acid supplements should be avoided in patients with prostate cancer or at risk for prostate cancer.

Precautions/Warnings/Contraindications

- Avoid flaxseed (*not* flaxseed oil) in patients with esophageal stricture, ileus, gastrointestinal stricture, or bowel obstruction. Ingestion of flaxseed without adequate fluids may precipitate bowel obstruction.
- Because of the potential laxative effect of flaxseed, its use should be avoided in patients with acute or chronic diarrhea, irritable bowel disease, diverticulitis, or inflammatory bowel disease.
- Topical flaxseed should be avoided in open wounds or abraded surfaces.
- Flaxseed (*not* flaxseed oil) should be used cautiously in women with hormone-sensitive conditions because of its possible estrogenic properties (breast, uterine, and ovarian cancer, endometriosis, polycystic ovary syndrome, uterine fibroids).[43,44]
- Use flaxseed and flaxseed oil products cautiously in patients with bleeding disorders or taking anticoagulants/antiplatelet agents, due to the theoretical risk of bleeding from platelet aggregation inhibition.[15,16,39]
- Avoid flaxseed *and* flaxseed oil in patients with hypertriglyceridemia, due to unclear effects on triglyceride levels (may raise or lower).[16,40]
- Some natural medicine textbooks advise caution in patients with hypothyroidism, although there are scant data in this area.
- Use flaxseed cautiously in patients with diabetes, based on a case series showing hyperglycemia associated with omega-3 fatty acid consumption (present in flaxseed).
- Avoid flaxseed in men with prostate cancer or at risk for developing prostate cancer, based on studies associating alpha-linolenic acid intake with the development of prostate cancer.[12-14]

Pregnancy and Lactation

- The use of flaxseed or flaxseed oil during pregnancy and lactation is not recommended. Animal studies show possible harmful effects, and there are insufficient human data. Flaxseed may stimulate menstruation or exert other hormonal effects and could be detrimental to pregnancy.
- Male offspring of female rats fed 20% to 40% flaxseed or 13% to 26% flaxmeal during pregnancy and lactation had increased levels of luteinizing hormone and testosterone, increased cauda epididymal weight and cauda epididymal sperm number, and decreased prostatic weight.[45] However, they experienced no effects on testis structure or spermatogenesis.[46] Female rats exposed to 5% flaxseed during gestation and lactation had altered mammary gland structural development, delayed onset of puberty, and a reduced number of estrous cycles; when exposed to a 10% flaxseed diet during gestation and lactation, female rats experienced earlier puberty onset and lengthened estrous cycles.[47]

INTERACTIONS
Flaxseed/Drug Interactions

- **General:** Consumption of flaxseed (*not* flaxseed oil) may decrease the absorption of co-administered oral medications/vitamins/minerals. Oral drugs should be taken an hour before or 2 hours after taking flaxseed to prevent decreased absorption.

- **Laxatives/stool softeners** (flaxseed, *not* flaxseed oil): Laxatives and stool softeners may increase or enhance the laxative effects of flaxseed.[34]
- **Anticoagulants, antiplatelet agents, nonsteroidal anti-inflammatory drugs (NSAIDs)** (flaxseed *and* flaxseed oil): Based on trial evidence of decreased platelet aggregation [15,16] and increased bleeding time,[39] flaxseed may increase the risk of bleeding when taken with anticoagulants or antiplatelet drugs. However, no clinical cases are reported in the available literature.
- **Mood stabilizers, lithium** (flaxseed *and* flaxseed oil): Based on one study, consumption of flaxseed may increase episodes of mania and hypomania in bipolar patients.[2]
- **Oral hypoglycemic agents and insulin:** The omega-3 fatty acids in flaxseed and flaxseed oil may cause hyperglycemia, countering the effects of hypoglycemic agents: six men with type 2 diabetes experienced increases in fasting glucose levels following 1 month of treatment with omega-3 fatty acids (which are present in flaxseed).[37] However, a small case series found no effects of flaxseed (50 g) on postprandial glucose levels.[19]
- **Anti-hyperlipidemic agents:** In theory, flaxseed may act additively with other agents that lower serum lipid levels. Flaxseed and flaxseed oil have been demonstrated to possess lipid-lowering properties *in vitro* and in animals.[22,48,49] Multiple poor-quality human studies have administered flaxseed products and measured effects on lipids, with mixed results.[16,19,21,23,24,26,33,36,41,50-56] It has been reported that defatted flaxseed (equivalent to the fiber component of flaxseed) can significantly reduce levels of total cholesterol and low-density lipoproteins (LDLs).[23]
- **Oral contraceptive pills (OCPs), hormone replacement therapy (HRT):** Flaxseed (*not* flaxseed oil) is a rich source of plant lignans.[22,49] Lignans are often referred to as phytoestrogens and may possess estrogen receptor agonist or antagonist properties,[11] with unclear interactions with oral contraceptive agents and hormone replacement therapies. Enterolactone and enterodiol (metabolized from flaxseed in the bowel) may inhibit aromatase, 5-alpha-reductase, and 17-beta-hydroxysteroid dehydrogenase activity.[57] It has also been shown that lignans increase sex hormone—binding globulin synthesis.[57] In humans, flaxseed has been reported to significantly reduce serum levels of 17-beta-estradiol and estrone sulfate and increase prolactin levels,[57] increase the urinary ratio of the two estrogen metabolites 2-hydroxyestrogen and 16 alpha-hydroxyestrone,[43,44] increase urinary excretion levels of enterodiol and enterolactone,[58] and increase fecal excretion of enterodiol, enterolactone, and matairesinol.[59]
- **Antihypertensive drugs:** In theory, flaxseed may potentiate the blood pressure–lowering effects of antihypertensive agents. Preliminary evidence suggests that higher levels of linolenic acid in human adipose tissues may correlate with lower blood pressure.[30] Since flaxseed contains alpha-linolenic acid, it has been proposed that flaxseed may lower blood pressure. Flaxseed-supplemented diets have had mixed effects on blood pressure in rats.[31,32] Evidence from one poor-quality human study suggests that 2 weeks of flaxseed supplementation lowers blood pressure.[33]

Flaxseed/Herb/Supplement Interactions

- **Psyllium** (flaxseed, *not* flaxseed oil): Both flaxseed and psyllium may reduce the absorption of oral medications and may act additively.

- **Laxative herbs and supplements** (flaxseed, *not* flaxseed oil): Flaxseed may possess laxative properties that could act additively with other laxative agents.[34]
- **Anticoagulant agents** (flaxseed *and* flaxseed oil): Based on trial evidence of decreased platelet aggregation[15,16] and increased bleeding time,[39] flaxseed may have additive effects with herbs considered to predispose patients to bleeding via effects on platelets, bleeding time, or the coagulation cascade.
- **Mood stabilizers** (flaxseed *and* flaxseed oil): Theoretically, consumption of flaxseed may potentially increase episodes of mania and hypomania in bipolar patients, based on evidence from a study done by Stoll et al.[2] Theoretically, there may be an additive effect if flaxseed is used in conjunction with other mood-altering herbs, including St. John's wort (*Hypericum perforatum*), kava (*Piper methysticum*), and valerian (*Valeriana officinalis*).
- **Vitamin E** (flaxseed, *not* flaxseed oil): Consumption of flaxseed may result in increased liver vitamin E levels, as shown in one animal study.[40]
- **Hypoglycemic agents:** The omega-3 fatty acids in flaxseed and flaxseed oil may cause hyperglycemia, countering the effects of hypoglycemic agents: six men with type 2 diabetes experienced increases in fasting glucose levels following 1 month of treatment with omega-3 fatty acids (which are present in flaxseed).[37] However, a small case series found no effects of flaxseed (50 g) on postprandial glucose levels.[19]
- **Antihyperlipidemic agents:** In theory, flaxseed may act additively with other agents that lower serum lipid levels, such as niacin, garlic (*Allium sativum* L.), guggul (*Commifora mukul*), or fish oil. Flaxseed and flaxseed oil have been demonstrated to possess lipid-lowering properties *in vitro* and in animals.[22,48,49] Multiple poor-quality human studies have administered flaxseed products and measured effects on lipids, with mixed results.[16,19,21,23,24,26,33,36,41,50-56] It has been reported that defatted flaxseed (equivalent to the fiber component of flaxseed) can significantly reduce levels of total cholesterol and low-density lipoproteins (LDLs).[23]
- **Phytoestrogens:** Flaxseed (*not* flaxseed oil) is a rich source of plant lignans.[22,60] Lignans are often referred to as phytoestrogens and may possess estrogen receptor agonist or antagonist properties,[11] with unclear interactions with herbs and supplements purported also to possess estrogenic properties. Enterolactone and enterodiol (metabolized from flaxseed in the bowel) may inhibit aromatase, 5-alpha-reductase, and 17-beta-hydroxysteroid dehydrogenase activity.[57] It has also been shown that lignans increase sex hormone–binding globulin synthesis.[57] In humans, flaxseed has been reported to significantly reduce serum levels of 17-beta-estradiol and estrone sulfate and increase prolactin levels,[57] increase the urinary ratio of the two estrogen metabolites 2-hydroxyestrogen and 16 alpha-hydroxyestrone,[43,44] increase urinary excretion levels of enterodiol and enterolactone,[58] and increase fecal excretion of enterodiol, enterolactone, and matairesinol.[59]
- **Hypotensive herbs and supplements:** In theory, flaxseed may potentiate the blood pressure–lowering effects of other agents. Preliminary evidence suggests that higher levels of linolenic acid in human adipose tissues may correlate with lower blood pressure.[30] Because flaxseed contains alpha-linolenic acid, it has been proposed that flaxseed may lower blood pressure. Flaxseed-supplemented diets have had mixed effects on blood pressure in rats.[31,32] Evidence from one poor-quality human study suggests that 2 weeks of flaxseed supplementation lowers blood pressure.[33]

Flaxseed/Food Interactions

- Processing and cooking may alter the lipid content and stability of alpha-linolenic acid in spaghetti containing ground flaxseed.[61]

Flaxseed/Lab Interactions

- **Serum lipids:** Consumption of flaxseed or flaxseed oil may decrease total cholesterol levels.[16,19,23,24,33,41,50,56] Flaxseed may lower low-density lipoprotein (LDL) levels.[16,19,23,33,50,56] Human and animal data suggest triglyceride-lowering properties of flaxseed,[16,33,49] although some animal data report increases in triglycerides.[40]
- **Bleeding time:** Flaxseed or flaxseed oil may increase bleeding time.[39]
- **Serum glucose:** The use of flaxseed may cause hyperglycemia, based on a case series showing hyperglycemia associated with the intake of omega-3 fatty acids (which are present in flaxseed).[37] However, a small case series found no effects of flaxseed (50 g) on postprandial glucose levels.[19]
- **Serum testosterone, luteinizing hormone (LH):** In theory, the use of flaxseed (*not* flaxseed oil) may increase serum levels of LH or testosterone.[45]
- **Hematocrit, hemoglobin:** Based on animal data, flaxseed (*not* flaxseed oil), may increase total red blood cell counts.[40]
- **Alkaline phosphatase:** The use of flaxseed (*not* flaxseed oil) may decrease alkaline phosphatase levels.[40]

MECHANISM OF ACTION
Pharmacology

- **Components of flaxseed:** Alpha-linolenic acid (ALA), cyanogenic glycosides (linamarin, linustatin, neolinustin), unsaturated fatty acids (linolenic acid, linoleic acid, oleic acid), soluble flaxseed fiber mucilage (D-xylose, L-galactose, L-rhamnose, D-galacturonic acid), lignan (secoisolariciresinol diglycoside), monoglycerides, triglycerides, free sterols, sterol esters, hydrocarbons (protein), balast, phenylpropane derivatives.
- **Components of flaxseed oil:** Alpha-linolenic acid (ALA), unsaturated fatty acids (linolenic acid, linoleic acid, oleic acid).
- **Overview:** Flaxseed is composed of multiple chemical constituents, the mechanisms of which are slowly being elucidated. Studies have attributed different properties to the plant, seed, oil, and individual plant components. The plant, seed, and oil contain polyunsaturated fatty acids (PUFAs), including alpha-linolenic acid (ALA) and linoleic acid. They also contain monounsaturated fatty acids (MUFAs), such as oleic acid. ALA and linoleic acid, are essential fatty acids (EFAs), meaning that they cannot be synthesized by the human body and must be derived from the diet.[62-64] ALA is a precursor of eicosapentaenoic acid (EPA),[65,66] and ingestion of flaxseed has been shown to increase cellular EPA levels in a linear manner.[66,67] However, the linoleic component of flaxseed (an omega-6 fatty acid) is reportedly capable of antagonizing the conversion of ALA to EPA.[66] Flaxseed is a concentrated food source of the lignan secoisolariciresinol diglycoside (SDG).[57,68] Flaxseed also contains small quantities of the lignan matairesinol.[57] SDG and matairesinol can be converted into "mammalian lignans" such as enterodiol and enterolactone by colonic bacteria.[57,69]
- **Inflammation/immune function:** Flaxseed and flaxseed oil may possess anti-inflammatory properties, due to the presence of EPA and docosahexaenoic acid (DHA), which

inhibit neutrophil inflammatory responses in humans.[70] These abilities may also result from the inactivation of LTA (leukotriene) epoxide hydrolase which decreases leukotriene B_4 (LTB_4) formation, and from the inhibition of LTB_4 and platelet-activating factor–stimulated chemotaxis via attenuation of the formation of [^{3}H] inositol tris-phosphate by the phosphatidylinositol-selective phospholipase C. It has also been found that ALA decreases the production of arachidonic acid, thereby causing a reduction in inflammation.[71] ALA may suppress cell-mediated immunity/T-cell function without affecting humoral immunity/B-cell function (shown in immunocompromised patients).[72]

- **Antioxidant:** Omega-3 fatty acids have been shown to suppress oxygen free radicals from neutrophils and monocytes, as well as the production of interleukin-1 (IL-1), tumor necrosis factor (TNF), and leukotriene B_4 (LTB_4).[48] Lignans can act as platelet-activating factor–receptor antagonists and inhibit the production of oxygen free radicals by neutrophils.[22,49] Secoisolariciresinol diglycoside (SDG), a plant lignan found in flaxseed, has been found to possess antioxidant properties.[22] Pattanaik and Prasad demonstrated that cardiac cellular damage was attenuated when dogs were given an endotoxin with flaxseed vs. endotoxin alone.[60] Theoretically, flaxseed (*not* flaxseed oil) may increase lipid peroxidation and thus increase oxidative injury.[23] Diets supplemented with defatted flaxseed have been associated with a decrease in protein thiol groups, suggesting an increase in oxidative stress.[23]

- **Lipid-lowering effects:** Proposed lipid-lowering effects of flaxseed (*not* flaxseed oil) have been attributed to the fiber component consisting of D-xylose, L-galactose, L-rhamnose, D-galacturonic acid, and galactose.[23] It has been reported that defatted flaxseed (equivalent to the fiber component of flaxseed) can significantly reduce levels of total cholesterol, low-density lipoproteins (LDLs),[23] and triglycerides.[73] The fiber portion of flaxseed has been proposed to exert lipid-lowering effects by enhancing gastric emptying time, altering transit time, interfering with bulk-phase diffusion of fat, and increasing excretion of bile acids. It is thought that flaxseed may exert a beneficial effect on atherosclerotic plaque formation because of the antioxidant properties of lignans and omega-3 fatty acids.[48]

- **Hormonal effects:** Flaxseed (*not* flaxseed oil) is a rich source of plant lignans.[22,49] Lignans are often referred to as phytoestrogens and may possess estrogen receptor agonist or antagonist properties, with unclear effects on hormone-sensitive cancers such as breast, uterine, and prostate cancer.[11] Flaxseed is a concentrated food source of the lignan secoisolariciresinol diglycoside (SDG).[57] Enterolactone and enterodiol (metabolized from flaxseed in the bowel) may decrease cell proliferation and inhibit aromatase, 5-alpha-reductase, and 17-beta-hydroxysteroid dehydrogenase activity, which may offer a reduction in the risk of breast, prostate, and other hormone-sensitive cancers.[57] It has also been shown that lignans increase sex hormone–binding globulin synthesis.[57] In humans, flaxseed has been reported to significantly reduce serum levels of 17-beta-estradiol and estrone sulfate and increase prolactin levels,[57] increase the urinary ratio of the two estrogen metabolites 2-hydroxyestrogen and 16 alpha-hydroxyestrone,[43,44] increase urinary excretion levels of enterodiol and enterolactone,[58] and increase fecal excretion of enterodiol, enterolactone, and matairesinol.[59] It has been suggested that flaxseed has more potent effects on estrogen metabolism than soy.[74]

- **Platelet aggregation:** In a small study of healthy men, 40 g of daily flaxseed oil was associated with diminished platelet aggregation vs. treatment with sunflower oil.[15] Alpha-linolenic acid, a component of both flaxseed and flaxseed oil, has been associated with increased bleeding time in a small human study.[39]

- **Arterial compliance:** In a case series including 15 obese patients, it was found that a 4-week diet high in alpha linolenic acid (20 g from margarine products based on flax oil) improves arterial compliance.[54]

- **Renoprotection:** Flaxseed fed to rats with polycystic kidneys increases citrate excretion and reduces histologic damage.[75] A diet supplemented with 15% flaxseed for 14 weeks delayed the onset of proteinuria and significantly reduced mortality in a mouse model of lupus nephritis.[76]

- **Laxative:** Flaxseed (*not* flaxseed oil) may produce laxative effects by increasing volume and stimulating peristalsis, due to stretch reflexes. Flaxseed does not appear to be affected by gastric acid or intestinal alkaline conditions. It has also been suggested that flaxseed may coat and protect intestinal mucosa.

Pharmacodynamics/Kinetics

- Limited data are available in this area. Urinary excretion of lignan metabolites has been reported as a dose-dependent biomarker of flaxseed intake.[77] Diets consisting of 5 to 10 g of ground flaxseed per day significantly increase the urinary excretion of enterodiol, enterolactone, and total lignans vs. a diet without flaxseed. Increases in lignan excretion are dose-dependent in a linear fashion.

- Processing and cooking may alter the lipid content and stability of alpha-linolenic acid in spaghetti containing ground flaxseed.[61]

HISTORY

- Flaxseed is an annual plant growing up to three feet in height. It has small, light-green alternate leaves on the stems and branches, and small blue flowers on the ends of the branches that bloom throughout the spring and summer. Originating in Egypt, it was subsequently introduced to North America and now is found extensively throughout Canada and the Northwestern United States.

- Seeds from the plant have historically been used for a variety of maladies, including upper respiratory infections, constipation, abdominal pain, urinary infections, and skin inflammation. Oil (linseed or flaxseed oil) derived from the seeds of the plant has been used in a variety of medicinal ways, including topically as a skin salve/demulcent and orally for constipation, arthritis, cancers, vaginitis, weight loss, heart disease, and benign prostatic hypertrophy.

- Non-medicinal uses of the oil include use in paints and varnishes, as a waterproofing agent, and as a cooking oil. Veterinary uses include flaxseed cakes as cattle feed, as a laxative, and for skin wounds/infections. Fiber strands from the stem of the plant are used to form linen cloth and have been used for over 10,000 years for this purpose.

REVIEW OF THE EVIDENCE: DISCUSSION
Constipation/Laxative
Summary

- It has been proposed that flaxseed (*not* flaxseed oil) produces laxative effects. Loose stools have been observed in patients participating in studies of flaxseed for other indications,[2,6] noted at doses of 45 g/day (more than 30 g/day).[24]

Review of the Evidence: Flaxseed and Flaxseed Oil

Condition Treated*	Study Design	Author, Year	N[†]	SS[†]	Study Quality[‡]	Magnitude of Benefit	ARR[†]	NNT[†]	Comments
Constipation	RCT, equivalence study	Tarpila[34] 1997	55	Yes	3	Medium	NA	NA	Flaxseed more effective laxative than psyllium in irritable bowel; published abstract only.
	RCT, double-blind, crossover	Tarpila[79] 2002	80	Yes	3	Medium	NA	NA	Studied effects of flaxseed supplementation in processed foods on serum fatty acids and enterolactone.
Hyperlipidemia (flaxseed)	RCT, double-blind, equivalence, crossover	Clandinin[52] 1997	26	No	3	None	NA	NA	May have been underpowered; no true placebo group.
Hyperlipidemia (flaxseed)	RCT, crossover	Jenkins[23] 1999	29	Yes	2	Small	NA	NA	Small study; methods poorly described.
Hyperlipidemia (flaxseed)	RCT, double-blind, crossover	Arjmandi[50] 1998	38	Yes	2	Small	NA	NA	Included only post-menopausal women; small study.
Hyperlipidemia	Randomized, controlled	Layne[53] 1996	26	No	2	None	NA	NA	Small study; negative results.
Hyperlipidemia and hyperglycemia (flaxseed)	RCT, crossover	Cunnane[35] 1995	10	Yes	2	Small	NA	NA	Small study; participants were healthy young adults.
Hyperlipidemia (flaxseed)	RCT, prospective,	Ferrier[26] 1995	28	No	2	Small	NA	NA	Small study of consumption of enriched eggs.
Hyperlipidemia	RCT, crossover	Kelley[21] 1993	10	No	2	None	NA	NA	Small study; methods poorly described.
Hyperlipidemia and hypertension	RCT, blinded	Singer[33] 1990	40	Yes	2	Small	NA	NA	Small study; only male patients.
Hyperlipidemia (flaxseed)	Case series	Bierenbaum[16] 1993	15	Yes	NA	None	NA	NA	Small sample size; not randomized.
Hyperlipidemia and hyperglycemia (flaxseed)	Case series	Cunnane[19] 1993	9	Yes	NA	Small	NA	NA	Small study; female volunteers.
Hyperlipidemia (flaxseed)	Case series	Chan[56] 1991	8	Yes	NA	Small	NA	NA	Small study; only men.
Breast cancer (flaxseed)	RCT, crossover	Hutchins[57] 2001	28	Yes	2	Small	NA	NA	Small study; methods poorly described.
Breast cancer	RCT, crossover	Haggans[44] 1999	28	Yes	2	Small	NA	NA	Small study; included only healthy postmenopausal women.
Breast cancer	Prospective, cohort	Bougnoux[94] 1994	121	No	NA	Small	NA	NA	No treatment; fatty acid levels measured in tissue samples.
Cyclic mastalgia (breast pain)	RCT, double-blind	Gross[95] 2000	116	Yes	3	Medium	NA	NA	Published abstract only; unclear if hormonal effects of flaxseed correlated with reduced pain and tenderness.
Menopausal symptoms	RCT, crossover	Lemay[25] 2002	25	Yes	3	Medium	NA	NA	Flaxseed versus hormone replacement therapy in hyper-cholesterolemic menopausal women; 40 g of flaxseed reported equal to HRT for mild menopausal symptoms and to lower glucose/insulin levels (no effects on cholesterol); likely underpowered to detect between-group difference.
Hyperlipidemia	Case series (4 phases)	Nestel[54] 1997	15	No	2	Small	NA	NA	Low-fat diet with flaxseed oil or Sunola oil studied in 4-week test periods; no effect on total cholesterol; rise in HDLs and decrease in LDLs oxidation. Decreased insulin sensitivity.

Review of the Evidence: Flaxseed and Flaxseed Oil—cont'd

Condition Treated*	Study Design	Author, Year	N[†]	SS[†]	Study Quality[‡]	Magnitude of Benefit	ARR[†]	NNT[†]	Comments
Hyperglycemia	Case series	Glauber[37] 1988	9	No	1	Small	NA	NA	Small study; men only, negative effects.
Hypertension	Regression analysis	Berry[30] 1986	399	No	NA	Small	NA	NA	No specific intervention studied.
Lupus nephritis and hyperlipidemia	RCT, crossover	Clark[36] 2001	23	No	2	None	NA	NA	Small study; likely underpowered, poor compliance, large dropout.
Lupus nephritis and hyperlipidemia (flaxseed)	Case series (4 phases)	Clark[24] 1995	9	No	0	NA	NA	NA	30 g/day of flaxseed associated with improved GFR and creatinine.
Lupus nephritis	RCT, double-blind, placebo-controlled, crossover	Clark[67] 1994	26	No	2	NA	NA	NA	Small study; methods poorly described.
HIV/AIDS (weight gain)	RCT, double-blind	Suttmann 1996	10	Yes	2	NA	NA	NA	Pilot study; reported significant increases in weight and TNF receptor proteins.
Prostate cancer	Case-control, prospective	Harvei[13] 1997	141	No	NA	Small	NA	NA	Showed only an association, no cause and effect.
Prostate cancer	Nested, retrospective, case-control	Gann[14] 1994	240	No	NA	Small	NA	NA	Retrospective; showed an association but no cause and effect.
Prostate cancer	Prospective cohort	Giovannucci[12] 1993	300	No	NA	Small	NA	NA	Showed an association, no cause and effect.
Prostate cancer and hyperlipidemia	Case series	Demark-Wahnefried[14] 2001	25	Yes	NA	Small	NA	NA	Small study; lack of comparison group, likely underpowered.

*Primary or secondary outcome.
[†] N, Number of patients; SS, statistically significant; ARR, absolute risk reduction; NNT, the number of patients who need to undergo a specific intervention in order to observe an outcome in one individual.
[‡] 0-2 = poor; 3-4 = good; 5 = excellent.
NA, Not applicable; GFR, glomerulation filtration rate; HIV/AIDS, human immunodeficiency virus/acquired immunodeficiency syndrome; HDLs, high-density lipoproteins; HRT, hormone replacement therapy; LDLs, low-density lipoproteins; RCT, randomized, controlled trial; TNF, tumor necrosis factor.
For an explanation of each category in this table, please see Table 3 in the Introduction.

Additional human evidence is available from a small trial that reported that flaxseed is a more effective treatment for constipation than the popular laxative agent psyllium. The sum of these preliminary human reports, plus a plausible mechanism, suggests that flaxseed does possess laxative properties. However, further evidence is warranted to establish efficacy and dosing. Notably, in large doses, or when taken with inadequate water, flaxseed may precipitate bowel obstruction via a mass effect.

Evidence

- In a published abstract, Tarpila and Kivinen reported a double-blind equivalence trial in 55 individuals with irritable bowel syndrome and constipation.[34] For 3 months, subjects received daily doses of ground flaxseed or psyllium. Significant improvements in constipation, bloating, and abdominal pain were noted in the flaxseed group vs. psyllium. Although the results are promising, the limited description of methods, baseline patient characteristics, compliance, dropout, and statistical analysis limits the ability to apply these results to clinical practice.

Hyperlipidemia
Summary

- Flaxseed and flaxseed oil have been reported to possess lipid-lowering properties *in vitro* and in animals.[22,48,49] Multiple

poor-quality human studies have administered flaxseed products and measured effects on lipids, with mixed results. There are no well-designed human trials in this area, and no evidence-based recommendation can be made at this time.

Positive Trials

- Lucas et al. reported the results of a randomized, double-blind trial, designed to determine the effects of flaxseed consumption on lipids and bone metabolism in postmenopausal women.[78] Women were recruited who were postmenopausal, younger than 65 years, not on hormone replacement therapy, and without major comorbidities (cancer, diabetes, liver disease, thyroid disease, pelvic inflammatory disease, endometrial polyps, or current hospitalization). The site of subject recruitment was not described. The authors randomized 58 such women to receive either 40 g of ground flaxseed or a wheat-based comparative control regimen daily for 3 months. All subjects also received 1000 mg of calcium and 400 IU of vitamin D daily and nutritional counseling. Baseline characteristics of the two groups were comparable for age, weight, body mass index (BMI), nutritional intake, and lipid levels. Primary outcomes measured included fasting cholesterol, low-density lipoproteins (LDLs), high-density lipoproteins (HDLs), triglycerides (TGs), and several serum levels that the authors correlated with bone metabolism (alkaline phosphatase, calcium, IGF-1, tartrate-resistant acid phosphatase). After 3 months, a 6% reduction in mean fasting cholesterol levels was noted in the flaxseed group, whereas no significant mean reduction was noted in controls. Differences between groups were statistically significant. However, no significant differences were noted in LDL, HDL, TG, or bone metabolism markers. Prior to data analysis, 38% of subjects dropped out, with limited analysis of dropouts. Weaknesses in the design and reporting of this trial limit the clinical relevance of its results. The study suggests that a small mean reduction in total cholesterol may occur after 3 months of flaxseed oral therapy, with statistically significant superiority to a wheat-based control. However, the large dropout may limit the validity of results. Statistical significance was not reached for possible changes in other measures, possibly due to the small sample size. No power calculation was conducted to determine the adequacy of sample size for such measures, and as a result this issue remains unclear. Without significant changes in LDL, HDL, or TG values, the clinical relevance of a change in total cholesterol is unclear, as is the potential impact on hard morbidity and mortality outcomes (stroke, myocardial infarction, hospitalization, death). The observed reduction in total cholesterol levels is somewhat less than has been reported with other agents, such as 3-hydroxy 3-methylglutaryl coenzyme A (HMG-CoA) reductase inhibitors ("statins").

- Arjmandi et al. conducted a double-blind, crossover study evaluating the effects of a flaxseed-supplemented diet on the lipid profiles of postmenopausal women.[50] Thirty-eight postmenopausal women with mild to severe hypercholesterolemia were included. Subjects were randomly assigned to receive flaxseed or sunflower seed, and were provided with 38 g of either treatment in the form of breads and muffins. Treatment was administered for 6 weeks followed by a 2-week washout period, then crossover for an additional 6 weeks. After 14 weeks, significant reductions in total cholesterol were noted in both treatment groups; however, only flaxseed showed significant reductions in low-density lipoproteins (LDLs). Both treatments failed to alter the levels of triglycerides or high-density lipoproteins (HDLs).

- In a small double-blind study, 10 patients were asked to consume two 25-g flaxseed muffins daily for 4 weeks, followed by a 2-week washout period, then crossover for 4 more weeks.[35] After 2 weeks, LDL and total cholesterol levels were reduced by 9% and 6%, respectively, compared to baseline or placebo, although after 4 weeks the effects on cholesterol disappeared. The clinical relevance of this study is not clear, particularly in light of the small sample size and unclear baseline patient characteristics.

- Forty mildly hypertensive male inpatients were randomly and blindly assigned to receive diets including olive oil (n = 15), sunflower seed oil (n = 14), or linseed (flaxseed) oil (n = 14).[33] Subjects received 60 mL of their assigned oil daily for 2 weeks. At the study's end it was found that linseed oil treatment significantly lowered total cholesterol, LDL, LDL/HDL ratio, and serum triglycerides. However, methods of this study were poorly described, with incomplete descriptions of randomization or blinding. Thus, bias or confounding may have affected results.

- Jenkins et al. conducted a randomized crossover study of 29 hyperlipidemic men and women in order to determine the effects of partially defatted flaxseed on serum lipids.[23] Subjects completed two 3-week treatment periods consisting of a National Cholesterol Education Program II (NCEP II) diet supplemented with either 20 g of flaxseed or control

(wheat bran). It was found that partially defatted flaxseed was effective in reducing serum total cholesterol, LDL, and apolipoprotein B vs. control.[23] However, this study did not adequately describe methodology and was characterized by incomplete reporting of baseline patient characteristics, randomization, blinding, and dropouts. Therefore, the results can only be considered preliminary.

- Tarpila et al. studied the effects of flaxseed supplementation as a part of daily diet on serum lipids, fatty acids and plasma enterolactone[79] Eighty volunteers participated in this controlled, double-blind, crossover clinical nutrition study. Subjects were randomized to diet sequences "AB" or "BA." Diet A meals contained 1.3 g/100 g of ground flaxseed and 5 g/100 g of flaxseed oil. In addition, 3 to 4 g/100 g of inulin and wheat fiber were added. The AB diet with nonsupplemented foods served as a control. Test subjects were on each diet for 4 weeks, separated by a 4-week washout period. Fifteen test subjects continued an open part of the study for 4 additional months. The dietary intake, basic serum chemistries, serum lipids, fatty acids, and enterolactone were measured at baseline, after both intervention periods, and during the open study at baseline and after 2 and 4 months. Serum thiocyanate and blood cadmium were controlled after both intervention periods. The percentage of flaxseed-supplemented test food out of total dietary intake was 20% of energy. The test food contained significantly higher amounts of fiber, polyunsaturated fatty acids (PUFAs), and alpha-linolenic acid compared with the control food. The authors reported no significant changes in basic laboratory values or blood lipids. However, there was a significant increase in serum alpha-linolenic acid, eicosapentaenoic acid and docosapentaenoic acid. Serum enterolactone concentration was doubled during flaxseed supplementation. Serum thiocyanate and blood cadmium values did not exceed reference values, and there was no mean difference in these levels between the diets.

Negative Trials

- Clandinin et al. conducted a crossover equivalence study of the effects of omega-3 fatty acids (fish oil and flaxseed oil) on plasma lipids.[52] Twenty-six patients were given an olive oil supplement for 3 months, which served as a baseline measurement. Patients were then randomized to receive either fish oil or flaxseed oil for 3 months, then switched to the alternative for 3 additional months. Blood samples were drawn for lipid and lipoprotein analysis at the end of each 3-month period. Neither flaxseed oil nor fish oil treatments significantly lowered total cholesterol or LDL levels. However, this study may have been underpowered to detect differences between groups. Without a true placebo arm, the possible benefits of either therapy are not clear. Therefore, these results are inconclusive.

- Clark et al. conducted a randomized, controlled crossover study in 23 patients with lupus nephritis.[36] Subjects were randomized to receive 30 g of flaxseed or control daily for 1 year, followed by a 12-week washout period, then reversal of therapies for an additional year. Eight subjects dropped out. In the remaining patients, no change in plasma lipids was associated with flaxseed use. However, this trial was small and possibly not adequately powered to detect differences between groups. In addition, the significant dropout without adequate follow-up of dropouts weakens the results.

- Ten healthy men were included in a 126-day controlled crossover trial evaluating the effects of dietary alpha-linolenic acid (from flaxseed oil) on fatty acid composition and lipids.[21] Subjects received either their baseline diet or their diet plus alpha-linolenic acid for 56 days, and then the groups were crossed over for an additional 56 days. Alpha-linolenic acid was found not to alter serum triglycerides, cholesterol, HDLs, LDLs, apoprotein A-I, or apoprotein B when compared to the basal diet. However, it is not clear whether this small study was adequately powered to detect benefits, and no power calculation was performed.

- In an unusual study design, Ferrier et al. examined the effects of human consumption of eggs from hens fed diets containing flaxseed.[26] Endpoints measured were plasma lipid levels and platelet lipids. Diets containing 0%, 10%, or 20% flaxseed were found to increase the fatty acid content of eggs but did not alter the cholesterol content of the yolks. Twenty-eight male volunteers were randomized to receive eggs from one of the three groups. No significant changes in total cholesterol, HDL cholesterol, or plasma triglycerides were observed. The relevance of this study to flaxseed supplementation overall is remote, and ingestion of four eggs per day may not be feasible for many patients.

- Layne et al. conducted a study evaluating the effects of low-dose fatty acids from fish or flaxseed oil on plasma lipid levels in 26 healthy individuals.[53] Participants initially received supplements of olive oil and were then randomized to receive flaxseed oil or fish oil for 3 months. At the end of the study it was found that flaxseed oil did not alter plasma concentrations of total cholesterol, LDLs, HDLs, or triglycerides. However, it is not clear how the comparison was conducted, how the statistics were performed, and how randomization was conducted.

Case Series

- Although case series may provide suggestive information, their results are not directly applicable to clinical practice. Their lack of blinding or randomization allows for the introduction of bias and confounders that may alter results.

- Bierenbaum et al. conducted a 3-month open-label study in 15 subjects evaluating the effects of flaxseed and vitamin E supplementation on lipids and lipid peroxidation.[16] Patients were given 800 IU/day of vitamin E and replaced normal breads and cereals in their diets with 15 g of ground flaxseed (3.4 g of alpha-linolenic acid and 5.5 g of fiber) and three slices of 10% flaxseed-containing bread (1.2 g of alpha-linolenic acid and 10 g of fiber) once daily for 3 months. The study resulted in a significant drop in total serum cholesterol, low-density lipoproteins (LDLs), and triglycerides, whereas high-density lipoprotein (HDL) levels remained constant throughout the study.

- In a case series study of nine healthy female volunteers, it was shown that diets supplemented with 50 g of ground raw flaxseed daily for 4 weeks resulted in a 9% decrease in total serum cholesterol levels and an 18% decrease in LDL cholesterol.[19]

- In a study by Chan et al., eight healthy men were given a diet with 75% of its fat supplied by canola oil, sunflower oil, olive oil, flax oil, and soybean oils.[56] It was found that mean total plasma cholesterol, LDLs, very low-density lipoproteins (VLDLs), apolipoprotein B, and apolipoprotein A-I were all significantly lowered. However, the effects of flaxseed alone are not clear.

- Demark-Wahnefried et al. conducted a case series in 25 men with prostate cancer.[41] Patients were given a low-fat diet (20% kilocalories or less) with 30 g of flaxseed supplementation daily for an average of 34 days. Results showed significant reductions in total serum cholesterol levels from baseline, although it is not clear what the contribution may have been of diet vs. flaxseed. Because this was an uncontrolled open study, bias or confounding may have altered results.

- In a case series by Clark et al., 15 to 45 g of flaxseed was administered to nine patients with lupus nephritis daily for 4 weeks.[24] The authors reported significant decreases in total cholesterol and LDL levels in subjects, most notable with the 30 g/day dose, with effects lasting up to 5 weeks after cessation of therapy. The 45 g/day dose was less well tolerated, due to possible laxative effects.

- In a case series by Nestel et al., 15 obese patients were administered a diet high in alpha-linolenic acid (20 g daily from margarine products based on flax oil).[54] After 4 weeks, subjects were found to have decreased HDL, no change in total cholesterol, and increased LDL peroxidation. However, this was a poorly described study, with four treatment periods using different diets.

- Ezaki et al. conducted a trial in 20 Japanese elderly subjects assessing effects of dietary alpha-linolenic acid. Results did not show any significant changes in LDL or total cholesterol levels in patients treated with alpha-linolenic acid.[55]

- *Note:* A study by Riserus et al. is sometimes cited as part of this body of evidence.[80] However, this research examined conjugated linoleic acid, which is derived from a different source and may not be comparable.

Coronary Artery Disease and Atherosclerosis
Summary

- It has been proposed that flaxseed may exert a beneficial effect on atherosclerotic plaque formation or cardiovascular outcomes, based on purported antioxidant and lipid-lowering properties.[48] There is a paucity of high-quality direct human data in this area. However, there is promising evidence regarding the role of n-3 polyunsaturated fatty acids (n-3 PUFAs) and alpha-linolenic acid (present in flaxseed) for improving outcomes in individuals with coronary artery disease (CAD). In addition, there are animal studies suggesting beneficial effects of flaxseed on atherosclerotic plaque formation. Diets rich in alpha-linolenic acid, such as the Mediterranean diet, have been associated with improved outcomes in patients who have already had a myocardial infarction.[81] Despite this evidence, it remains unclear whether flaxseed supplementation improves human cardiovascular end points, and dosing regimens are not established.

Human Studies

- A prospective cohort study was conducted in 667 men aged 64 to 84 years of age from the Zutphen Elderly Study who were free of coronary artery disease (CAD) at baseline.[82] During a 10-year follow-up period, 98 individuals developed CAD. Dietary alpha-linolenic acid as not significantly associated with the risk of developing CAD. However, it was difficult to separate the intake of alpha-linolenic acid from that of trans fatty acids.

- There is a growing body of evidence that n-3 polyunsaturated fatty acids (n-3 PUFAs) may be beneficial as both primary and secondary prevention for cardiovascular events (myocardial infarction and stroke). For example, a high-quality, large randomized trial assessed the effects of n-3 PUFA or vitamin E on myocardial infarction survivors as secondary prevention.[83] Over a 2-year period, 11,324 patients who had survived a recent (<3 months) myocardial infarction were randomized to receive 1 g of n-3 PUFAs, 300 mg of vitamin E, both agents, or neither each day. The combined primary end point included death, non-fatal myocardial infarction, and stroke. In the n-3 PUFA group, the authors found a statistically significant 10% decrease in the combined end point, attributed to a 14% mortality reduction. Results showed that treatment with n-3 PUFAs, but not vitamin E, had significant effects on decreasing the risk of the primary combined efficacy end point of death, nonfatal myocardial infarction, and stroke. Vitamin E did not improve outcomes. These results suggest a possible role for flaxseed for secondary prevention, but studies of flaxseed specifically are necessary before a firm conclusion can be drawn.

- Alpha-linolenic acid, present in flaxseed, has also been assessed. For example, Hu et al. conducted a prospective, cohort study in women to assess the effects of alpha-linolenic acid on the risk of fatal ischemic heart disease.[84] It was found that intake of alpha-linolenic acid correlates with a decreased relative risk of fatal cardiac events. Additional studies of flaxseed specifically are warranted to establish efficacy and dosing.

Animal Studies

- In an 8-week rabbit study, Prasad et al. found that a high-flaxseed diet (7.5 mg/kg/day) reduced aortic atherosclerosis by 46% without significantly lowering serum cholesterol.[48] A follow-up rabbit study tested 7.5 mg/kg/day of "type II flaxseed" which has the same lignan and oil content of flaxseed but contains much lower levels of alpha-linolenic acid.[49] Reductions in total cholesterol and low-density lipoproteins (LDLs) were observed without an effect on high-density lipoproteins, and there was similarly a reduction in aortic plaque formation. The effects of the lignan secoisolariciresinol diglycoside (SDG), present in flaxseed,[57] were assessed in rabbits.[22] The authors reported that 15 mg/kg/day of SDG reduced levels of total cholesterol and LDLs by 33% and 35%, respectively.

Breast Cancer
Summary

- It has been proposed that the lignan components of flaxseed may offer protection against hormone-sensitive cancers by antagonizing estrogen receptors or inhibiting enzymes involved with the synthesis of sex hormones[11,57] or via effects on epidermal growth factor receptors.[85,86] However, it is unclear if flaxseed possesses estrogen receptor agonist or antagonist properties. Rat studies have reported mixed effects of oral flaxseed on mammary tumors; tumor size was reduced in some studies but increased in others.[4,87-93] Human studies have largely focused on the effects of flaxseed on hormone levels, and there is currently no direct human evidence that supplementation with flaxseed is beneficial in the prevention or treatment of breast cancer.

Evidence

- Hutchins et al. conducted a randomized crossover trial in 28 postmenopausal women (ages 52 to 82 years).[57] During three 7-week feeding periods, subjects consumed their normal diets with or without the addition of ground flaxseed (5 to 10 g). It was found that flaxseed diets significantly reduced 17-beta-estradiol and estrone sulfate levels and increased prolactin levels. Serum levels were unchanged for androstenedione, estrone, sex hormone–binding globulin, progesterone, testosterone, free testosterone, dehydro-epiandrosterone, and dehydroepiandrosterone sulfate.

- In a randomized crossover trial of 16 premenopausal women ingesting flaxseed, the urinary ratio of the two estrogen metabolites 2-hydroxyestrogen and 16 alpha-hydroxyestrone was found to be increased.[44] It has been proposed that women who have an increased ratio may have a reduced risk of breast cancer. In a prior randomized trial of 28 postmenopausal women given 5 to 10 g/day of ground flaxseed for 7 weeks, the ratio of 2-hydroxyestrogen to 16 alpha-hydroxyestrone was also improved, in a dose-dependent fashion.[43]

- In a study of 18 women, Phipps et al. found that subjects who supplemented their diets with 10 g of flaxseed daily (vs. a low-fiber diet) for three menstrual cycles experienced prolongation of their luteal phase and had fewer anovulatory cycles.[38]

- Kurzer et al. conducted a small study in 13 women over the course of three menstrual cycles.[59] Daily diets were supplemented with 10 g of ground flaxseed. Feces were collected on days 7 to 11 of the last menstrual cycle, and it was found that flaxseed consumption significantly increased the excretion of enterodiol, enterolactone, and matairesinol (compared to baseline values).

- Bougnoux et al. reported an association between levels of serum alpha-linolenic acid and metastatic carcinoma (alpha-linoleic acid is present in flaxseed).[94] This study included 121 patients with localized breast cancer. Adipose breast tissue was obtained during surgery, and fatty acid content was analyzed. It was found that there was an association between low levels of alpha-linoleic acid and positive axillary lymph node status/vascular invasion. After an average follow-up of 31 months, 21 patients developed metastases. It was found that large tumor size and low level of alpha-linoleic acid were associated with the development of metastasis.[94] However, it is unclear from this study what is the clinical relevance of low alpha-linolenic acid levels and whether supplementation with sources of alpha-linolenic acid, such as flaxseed, would confer any benefit.

- There is preliminary evidence that flaxseed may improve the symptoms of cyclic mastalgia.[95] Although it has been suggested that cyclic mastalgia is a risk factor for breast cancer,[96] it is not clear that flaxseed reduces this risk.

Cyclic Mastalgia (Breast Pain)
Summary

- Flaxseed (*not* flaxseed oil) contains lignans that may possess estrogen receptor agonist or antagonist properties, and may inhibit enzymes involved with the synthesis of sex hormones.[11,57] Human studies have reported reduced levels of serum estrogens associated with flaxseed use.[57] It has been hypothesized that the hormonal effects of flaxseed may improve the symptoms of cyclic mastalgia, a condition characterized by breast pain and tenderness in women. Preliminary evidence from a human trial published as an abstract only suggests that 25 g of flaxseed daily reduces these symptoms. However, further study is warranted before a recommendation can be made.

Evidence

- In a published abstract, Goss et al. reported the results of a randomized, double-blind study in 116 premenopausal women with severe cyclic mastalgia.[95] Subjects were randomized to receive a muffin containing 25 g of flaxseed or a placebo muffin daily for 6 months. Visual analogue scales

(VASs) were used for assessment of breast pain, swelling, and lumps at each menstrual cycle. Severity of breast pain was recorded daily. Breast pain improved in both groups, but there was a significant reduction in the VAS score in the flaxseed group. Although these results are promising, because this was only a published abstract there was no description of methods or statistical analysis. As a result, the quality of this study cannot be adequately evaluated. Further study is warranted in this area.

Menopausal Symptoms
Summary

- There is preliminary research examining the effects of flaxseed on menopausal symptoms and cholesterol levels in menopausal women. Additional research is necessary before a clear conclusion can be drawn, and this remains an area of controversy.

Evidence

- Lemay et al. conducted a randomized, controlled trial in 25 hypercholesterolemic menopausal women to assess the effects on menopausal symptoms and serum lipids of a phytoestrogen dietary supplement compared with oral estrogen-progesterone replacement.[25] Subjects with total cholesterol greater than 6.2 mmol/L (240 mg/dL), a cholesterol/high-density lipoprotein cholesterol ratio greater than 4.5, and triglycerides less than 3.5 mmol/L (310 mg/dL) after a 4-month controlled diet were randomized to add 40 g/day of crushed flaxseed to their diet or to take daily 0.625 mg of conjugated equine estrogens alone (hysterectomy, n = 10) or combined with 100 mg of micronized progesterone (intact uterus, n = 15). After 2 months of treatment, both groups continued the diet alone for a 2-month washout period before crossing over to the alternate treatment for 2 additional months. The authors reported a significant benefit in terms of high-density lipoprotein levels in the hormone replacement therapy (HRT) group compared to flaxseed (1.6 ± 0.04 mmol/L versus 1.3 ± 0.03 mmol/L; this is the same as 62 ± 1 mg/dL versus 50 ± 1 mg/dL; $p = 0.001$), and similar superiority of HRT for apolipoprotein A-1 levels (1.71 ± 0.07 versus 1.42 ± 0.05 g/L; $p = 0.003$). However, no significant difference was detected between groups in low-density lipoprotein cholesterol levels (3.8 ± 0.2 mmol/L versus 4.4 ± 0.2 mmol/L; this is the same as 148 ± 8 mg/dL versus 170 ± 8 mg/dL; $p = 0.10$). Both treatments produced similar decreases in menopausal symptoms and in glucose and insulin levels. Only HRT induced an elevation of sex hormone–binding globulin ($p = 0.004$), and lowered fibrinogen ($p = 0.08$) as well as plasminogen activator inhibitor type 1 ($p = 0.01$). Because of the small size of this trial, the results cannot be considered conclusive.

Hyperglycemia/Diabetes
Summary

- A small number of poor-quality human studies report mixed effects of oral flaxseed on serum glucose levels. One small case series actually reported hyperglycemia in patients taking omega-3 fatty acids (which are contained in flaxseed). Flaxseed cannot be recommended as a treatment for hyperglycemia or diabetes at this time.

Evidence

- A controlled, double-blind, crossover study in 10 patients assessed the effects of two 25-g flaxseed muffins daily for 4-week periods (separated by a 2-week washout).[35] After 4 weeks of therapy, no significant differences were found between groups in measurements of fasting blood glucose concentrations, peak blood glucose, or total area under the curve (after 4 hours). However, it is not clear that this sample size was adequate to detect differences between therapies, and therefore the results cannot be considered definitive. In addition, it is not known if a 2-week washout period was adequate between treatment periods.

- Cunnane et al. conducted a case series in nine healthy female volunteers.[19] The primary focus of this study was the measurement of serum lipids following 4 weeks of daily flaxseed supplementation (50 g), but it was also reported that following meals with flaxseed, postprandial glucose was reduced by 27%.

- Glauber et al. conducted a case series in six men with type 2 diabetes.[37] Subjects consumed omega-3 fatty acids for 1 month. The results showed increases in fasting glucose levels and a 22% increase in mixed meal glucose levels. Because flaxseed contains omega-3 fatty acids, these results may be extrapolated to flaxseed and flaxseed oil.

- In a case series including 15 obese patients, Nestel et al. reported that a four-week diet high in alpha-linolenic acid (20 g from margarine products based on flaxseed oil) diminished insulin sensitivity.[54] However, this was a poorly described study which focused more on lipid and arterial compliance effects, rather than insulin characteristics.

- **Note:** A study by Riserus et al. is sometimes cited as part of this body of evidence.[80] However, this research examined conjugated linoleic acid which is derived from a different source and may not be comparable.

Hypertension
Summary

- Preliminary evidence suggests that higher levels of linolenic acid in human adipose tissues may correlate with lower blood pressure.[30] Because flaxseed contains alpha-linolenic acid, it has been proposed that flaxseed may lower blood pressure. Flaxseed-supplemented diets have had mixed effects on blood pressure in rats.[31,32] Evidence from one poor-quality human study suggests that 2 weeks of flaxseed supplementation lowers blood pressure. However, at this time there are insufficient data to recommend for or against this use of flaxseed.

Evidence

- Forty mildly hypertensive male inpatients were randomly and blindly assigned to receive diets including olive oil (n = 15), sunflower seed oil (n = 14), or linseed oil (from flaxseed) (n = 14).[33] Subjects received 60 mL of their assigned oil daily for 2 weeks. At the study's end, it was found that linseed oil treatment significantly lowered systolic blood pressure, measured by a "psychophysiological stress test." However, details were limited and methods of the study were poorly described, with incomplete descriptions of randomization or blinding. Thus, bias or confounding may have affected results.

- Sample adipose tissue was analyzed for linolenic acid content in 339 healthy male subjects, average age 47 years (range of 20 to 78), with no history of heart disease, smoking, alcohol, or use of antihypertensive medications.[30] It was reported that the tissue content of linolenic acid (found in flaxseed oil) correlated with blood pressure; for every 1% increase in linolenic acid, there was a drop of 5 mm Hg in mean arterial blood pressure. However, it is not clear whether these measured adipose levels of linolenic acid are causative, benign markers of disease, or adaptive. It is also not apparent whether these levels would be altered by supplementation with flaxseed, or what the long-term effects of supplementation would be.

Lupus Nephritis

Summary

- In animal models of nephritis, mice fed diets supplemented with flaxseed or the flaxseed constituent secoisolariresinol diglucoside have had a delay in the development of proteinuria, and better preservation of glomerular filtration rate (GFR) than controls.[76,97-99] Several low-quality human studies have been conducted by the same lead author (WF Clark), suggesting possible improvements in GFR and serum creatinine levels in patients treated with 30 g/day of flaxseed. However, further evidence is warranted in this area before a recommendation can be made.

Evidence

- Clark et al. conducted a controlled crossover study in 23 patients with lupus nephritis.[36] Subjects were randomized to receive 30 g of flaxseed or control (no flaxseed) daily for 1 year, followed by a 12-week washout period, and then reversal of therapies for an additional year. Eight subjects dropped out. In the remaining patients, flaxseed was associated with a small statistically significant mean reduction in serum creatinine levels (0.03 mg/dL) vs. an increase in creatinine in the placebo group (0.06 mg/dL). Although promising, this study was not adequately described, with incomplete descriptions of methods. The significant dropout without adequate follow-up weakens the results.

- In a case series, 15 to 45 g of flaxseed was administered to nine patients with lupus nephritis daily for 4 weeks.[24] Small improvements in creatinine clearance and serum urea levels were reported with 30 to 45 g of flaxseed/day, although these changes were not statistically significant from baseline values. Small statistically significant improvements in serum creatinine were reported with 30 to 45 g of flaxseed/day, which resolved after 5 weeks off therapy. The 30-g dose was better tolerated than 45 g, due to laxative effects of the latter dose. Although this case series is suggestive, the results are not directly applicable to clinical practice; the lack of blinding or randomization allows for the introduction of bias and confounders that can alter results.

- In a prior study, the same principal author conducted a study of renal function in lupus patients ingesting omega-3 fatty acids from fish oils rather than from flaxseed (also a source of omega-3 fatty acids).[97] This double-blind crossover study lasted for 2 years. Patients were randomized to receive 1 year of fish oil or placebo, followed by a 10-week washout period, and then 1 year of the alternate therapy. Five subjects dropped out. The study reported no improvements in renal function. However, it is not clear that these results are applicable to flaxseed.

HIV/AIDS

Summary

- It has been hypothesized that constituents of flaxseed such as gamma-linolenic and eicosapentaenoic acids may determine an individual's susceptibility to AIDS.[100] In one study, ingestion of alpha-linolenic acid (derived from flax) in combination with arginine and yeast RNA was associated with weight gain in HIV patients. No recommendation can be made without further research.

Evidence

- Weight gain in HIV patients was assessed in a controlled, double-blind study of the effects of a fortified formula consisting of alpha-linolenic acid (derived from flax), arginine, and yeast RNA administered for 4 months.[101] The trial included 10 men with symptomatic HIV on stable medication regimens. Results showed that the fortified formula resulted in significant increases in weight as well as concentrations of soluble tumor necrosis factor receptor proteins. However, the effects of alpha-linolenic acid without the addition of arginine or yeast RNA are not clear. Nonetheless, these results are promising.

Prostate Cancer

Summary

- Several case-control studies have associated the intake of alpha-linolenic acid (which is present in flaxseed) with an *increased* risk of developing prostate cancer. One brief, small case series in patients with prostate cancer found no effect of flaxseed supplementation on serum prostate specific antigen (PSA) levels. In human prostate cancer cells, the flaxseed constituent linolenic acid promotes cell growth, whereas the constituent eicosapentaenoic acid (EPA) promotes growth at low concentrations and inhibits growth at high concentrations.[42] Preclinical studies report effects of flaxseed on epidermal growth factor receptors.[85,86] In a mouse model, a diet supplemented with flaxseed inhibited the growth and development of prostate cancer.[102] Until better human evidence is available, based on the available research, flaxseed and alpha-linolenic acid supplements should be avoided in patients with prostate cancer or at risk for prostate cancer.

Evidence

- Demark-Wahnefried et al. conducted a case series in 25 men with prostate cancer awaiting prostatectomy.[41] Patients were given a low-fat diet (20% kilocalories or less) with 30 g of flaxseed supplementation daily for an average of 34 days. Results showed significant reductions in total testosterone, free androgens, and total serum cholesterol. Prostate cell proliferation was reduced, and rates of apoptosis increased. Overall, there was no change in serum PSA levels. It is not clear what the contribution may have been of diet vs. flaxseed. Because this was an uncontrolled open study, bias or confounding may have affected results. The brief follow-up period and small sample size may not have been sufficient to detect effects, either beneficial or harmful.

- Giovannucci et al. reported data from the Health Professionals Follow-up Study, which included a prospective cohort of 51,529 men ages 40-75.[12] Subjects answered a food frequency questionnaire in 1986 and a follow-up questionnaire in 1990 to document any new cases of diseases. Three hundred new cases of prostate cancer were discovered. It was found that total fat consumption was directly related to the risk of prostate cancer, including intake of saturated fat, monosaturated fat, and alpha-linolenic acid (but not linoleic acid). However, cohort studies are subject to confounding, and it is not clear to what extent supplementation with alpha-linolenic acid sources such as flaxseed impact the incidence of disease.

- Harvei et al. also reported an association between levels of fatty acids and the risk of prostate cancer.[13] This nested case-control study of 141 matched sets (2 controls for every case) reported a positive association between alpha-linolenic acid consumption and the risk of prostate cancer.

• Gann et al. conducted a retrospective nested case-control study to evaluate the association between plasma alpha-linolenic acid levels and the development of prostate cancer.[14] Plasma samples from 14,916 U.S. male physicians were frozen in 1982. Fatty acid compositions in plasma in 120 men who developed prostate cancer were compared to those in 120 men who did not. Men who had higher levels of alpha-linolenic acid had a higher risk of developing prostate cancer than those who had levels that were undetectable. However, these results were not statistically significant and therefore cannot be considered conclusive.

References

1. Gadek JE, DeMichele SJ, Karlstad MD, et al. Effect of enteral feeding with eicosapentaenoic acid, gamma-linolenic acid, and antioxidants in patients with acute respiratory distress syndrome. Enteral Nutrition in ARDS Study Group. Crit Care Med 1999;27(8):1409-1420.

2. Stoll AL, Severus WE, Freeman MP, et al. Omega 3 fatty acids in bipolar disorder: a preliminary double-blind, placebo-controlled trial. Arch Gen Psychiatry 1999;56(5):407-412.

3. Jenab M, Thompson LU. The influence of flaxseed and lignans on colon carcinogenesis and beta-glucuronidase activity. Carcinogenesis 1996;17(6):1343-1348.

4. Serraino M, Thompson LU. Flaxseed supplementation and early markers of colon carcinogenesis. Cancer Lett 1992;63(2):159-165.

5. Velasquez MT, Bhathena SJ, Ranich T, et al. Dietary flaxseed meal reduces proteinuria and ameliorates nephropathy in an animal model of type II diabetes mellitus. Kidney Int 2003;64(6):2100-2107.

6. Endoh D, Okui T, Ozawa S, et al. Protective effect of a lignan-containing flaxseed extract against CCl(4)-induced hepatic injury. J Vet Med Sci 2002;64(9):761-765.

7. Ogborn MR, Nitschmann E, Weiler H, et al. Flaxseed ameliorates interstitial nephritis in rat polycystic kidney disease. Kidney Int 1999;55(2):417-423.

8. Yan L, Yee JA, Li D, et al. Dietary flaxseed supplementation and experimental metastasis of melanoma cells in mice. Cancer Lett 1998;124(2): 181-186.

9. Nieto N, Torres MI, Rios A, et al. Dietary polyunsaturated fatty acids improve histological and biochemical alterations in rats with experimental ulcerative colitis. J Nutr 2002;132(1):11-19.

10. Makrides M, Neumann MA, Jeffrey B, et al. A randomized trial of different ratios of linoleic to alpha-linolenic acid in the diet of term infants: effects on visual function and growth. Am J Clin Nutr 2000;71(1):120-129.

11. Adlercreutz H. Epidemiology of phytoestrogens. Baillieres Clin Endocrinol Metab 1998;12(4):605-623.

12. Giovannucci E, Rimm EB, Colditz GA, et al. A prospective study of dietary fat and risk of prostate cancer. J Natl Cancer Inst 1993;85(19):1571-1579.

13. Harvei S, Bjerve KS, Tretli S, et al. Prediagnostic level of fatty acids in serum phospholipids: omega-3 and omega-6 fatty acids and the risk of prostate cancer. Int J Cancer 1997;71(4):545-551.

14. Gann PH, Hennekens CH, Sacks FM, et al. Prospective study of plasma fatty acids and risk of prostate cancer. J Natl Cancer Inst 1994;86(4):281-286.

15. Allman MA, Pena MM, Pang D. Supplementation with flaxseed oil versus sunflowerseed oil in healthy young men consuming a low fat diet: effects on platelet composition and function. Eur J Clin Nutr 1995;49(3):169-178.

16. Bierenbaum ML, Reichstein R, Watkins TR, et al. Reducing atherogenic risk in hyperlipemic humans with flax seed supplementation: a preliminary report. J Am Coll Nutr 1993;12:501-504.

17. Gruver DI. Does flaxseed interfere with the clotting system? Plast Reconstr Surg 2003;112(3):934.

18. Carter J. Flax seed as a source of alpha linolenic acid. J Am Coll Nutr 1993;12(5):551.

19. Cunnane SC, Ganguli S, Menard C, et al. High alpha-linolenic acid flaxseed (*Linum usitatissimum*): some nutritional properties in humans. Br J Nutr 1993;69(2):443-453.

20. Harris WS. n-3 fatty acids and serum lipoproteins: human studies. Am J Clin Nutr 1997;65(5 Suppl):1645S-1654S.

21. Kelley DS, Nelson GJ, Love JE, et al. Dietary alpha-linolenic acid alters tissue fatty acid composition, but not blood lipids, lipoproteins or coagulation status in humans. Lipids 1993;28(6):533-537.

22. Prasad K. Reduction of serum cholesterol and hypercholesterolemic atherosclerosis in rabbits by secoisolariciresinol diglucoside isolated from flaxseed. Circulation 1999;99(10):1355-1362.

23. Jenkins DJ, Kendall CW, Vidgen E, et al. Health aspects of partially defatted flaxseed, including effects on serum lipids, oxidative measures, and ex vivo androgen and progestin activity: a controlled crossover trial. Am J Clin Nutr 1999;69(3):395-402.

24. Clark WF, Parbtani A, Huff MW, et al. Flaxseed: a potential treatment for lupus nephritis. Kidney Int 1995;48(2):475-480.

25. Lemay A, Dodin S, Kadri N, et al. Flaxseed dietary supplement versus hormone replacement therapy in hypercholesterolemic menopausal women. Obstet Gynecol 2002;100(3):495-504.

26. Ferrier LK, Caston LJ, Leeson S, et al. Alpha-Linolenic acid- and docosahexaenoic acid-enriched eggs from hens fed flaxseed: influence on blood lipids and platelet phospholipid fatty acids in humans. Am J Clin Nutr 1995;62(1):81-86.

27. Alonso L, Marcos ML, Blanco JG, et al. Anaphylaxis caused by linseed (flaxseed) intake. J Allergy Clin Immunol 1996;98(2):469-470.

28. Lezaun A, Fraj J, Colas C, et al. Anaphylaxis from linseed. Allergy 1998;53(1):105-106.

29. Holman RT, Johnson SB, Hatch TF. A case of human linolenic acid deficiency involving neurological abnormalities. Am J Clin Nutr 1982;35(3):617-623.

30. Berry EM, Hirsch J. Does dietary linolenic acid influence blood pressure? Am J Clin Nutr 1986;44(3):336-340.

31. Brandle M, Al Makdessi S, Weber RK, et al. Prolongation of life span in hypertensive rats by dietary interventions. Effects of garlic and linseed oil. Basic Res Cardiol 1997;92:223-232.

32. Talom RT, Judd SA, McIntosh DD, et al. High flaxseed (linseed) diet restores endothelial function in the mesenteric arterial bed of spontaneously hypertensive rats. Life Sci 1999;64(16):1415-1425.

33. Singer P, Jaeger W, Berger I, et al. Effects of dietary oleic, linoleic and alpha-linolenic acids on blood pressure, serum lipids, lipoproteins and the formation of eicosanoid precursors in patients with mild essential hypertension. J Hum Hypertens 1990;4(3):227-233.

34. Tarpila S, Kivinen A. Ground flaxseed is an effective hypolipidemic bulk laxative [published abstract]. Gastroenterology 1997;112:A836.

35. Cunnane SC, Hamadeh MJ, Liede AC, et al. Nutritional attributes of traditional flaxseed in healthy young adults. Am J Clin Nutr 1995;61(1):62-68.

36. Clark WF, Kortas C, Heidenheim AP, et al. Flaxseed in lupus nephritis: a two-year nonplacebo-controlled crossover study. J Am Coll Nutr 2001;20(2 Suppl):143-148.

37. Glauber H, Wallace P, Griver K, et al. Adverse metabolic effect of omega-3 fatty acids in non-insulin- dependent diabetes mellitus. Ann Intern Med 1988;108(5):663-668.

38. Phipps WR, Martini MC, Lampe JW, et al. Effect of flax seed ingestion on the menstrual cycle. J Clin Endocrinol Metab 1993;77(5):1215-1219.

39. Nordstrom DC, Honkanen VE, Nasu Y, et al. Alpha-linolenic acid in the treatment of rheumatoid arthritis. A double- blind, placebo-controlled and randomized study: flaxseed vs. safflower seed. Rheumatol.Int. 1995;14(6):231-234.

40. Babu US, Mitchell GV, Wiesenfeld P, et al. Nutritional and hematological impact of dietary flaxseed and defatted flaxseed meal in rats. Int J Food Sci Nutr. 2000;51(2):109-117.

41. Demark-Wahnefried W, Price DT, Polascik TJ, et al. Pilot study of dietary fat restriction and flaxseed supplementation in men with prostate cancer before surgery: exploring the effects on hormonal levels, prostate-specific antigen, and histopathologic features. Urology 2001;58(1):47-52.

42. Pandalai PK, Pilat MJ, Yamazaki K, et al. The effects of omega-3 and omega-6 fatty acids on *in vitro* prostate cancer growth. Anticancer Res 1996;16(2):815-820.

43. Haggans CJ, Hutchins AM, Olson BA, et al. Effect of flaxseed consumption on urinary estrogen metabolites in postmenopausal women. Nutr Cancer 1999;33(2):188-195.

44. Haggans CJ, Travelli EJ, Thomas W, et al. The effect of flaxseed and wheat bran consumption on urinary estrogen metabolites in premenopausal women. Cancer Epidemiol Biomarkers Prev 2000;9(7):719-725.

45. Sprando RL, Collins TF, Black TN, et al. The effect of maternal exposure to flaxseed on spermatogenesis in F(1) generation rats. Food Chem Toxicol. 2000;38(4):325-334.

46. Sprando RL, Collins TF, Wiesenfeld P, et al. Testing the potential of flaxseed to affect spermatogenesis: morphometry. Food Chem Toxicol. 2000;38(10):887-892.

47. Tou JC, Thompson LU. Exposure to flaxseed or its lignan component during different developmental stages influences rat mammary gland structures. Carcinogenesis 1999;20(9):1831-1835.

48. Prasad K. Dietary flax seed in prevention of hypercholesterolemic atherosclerosis. Atherosclerosis 1997;132(1):69-76.

49. Prasad K, Mantha SV, Muir AD, et al. Reduction of hypercholesterolemic atherosclerosis by CDC-flaxseed with very low alpha-linolenic acid. Atherosclerosis 1998;136(2):367-375.

50. Arjmandi BH, Khan DA, Juma S, et al. Whole flaxseed consumption lowers serum LDL-cholesterol and lipoprotein (a) concentrations in postmenopausal women. Nutrit Res 1998;18(7):1203-1214.

51. Cunnane S. Metabolism and function of alpha-linolenic acid in humans. In: Cunnane S, Thompson L, editors. Flaxseed in Human Nutrition. Champagne: AOCS Press, 1995: 99-127.

52. Clandinin MT, Foxwell A, Goh YK, et al. Omega-3 fatty acid intake results in a relationship between the fatty acid composition of LDL cholesterol ester and LDL cholesterol content in humans. Biochim Biophys Acta 1997;1346(3):247-252.

53. Layne KS, Goh YK, Jumpsen JA, et al. Normal subjects consuming physiological levels of 18:3(n-3) and 20:5(n- 3) from flaxseed or fish oils

F

have characteristic differences in plasma lipid and lipoprotein fatty acid levels. J Nutr 1996;126(9):2130-2140.

54. Nestel PJ, Pomeroy SE, Sasahara T, et al. Arterial compliance in obese subjects is improved with dietary plant n- 3 fatty acid from flaxseed oil despite increased LDL oxidizability. Arterioscler Thromb Vasc Biol 1997; 17(6):1163-1170.

55. Ezaki O, Takahashi M, Shigematsu T, et al. Long-term effects of dietary alpha-linolenic acid from perilla oil on serum fatty acids composition and on the risk factors of coronary heart disease in Japanese elderly subjects. J Nutr Sci Vitaminol (Tokyo) 1999;45(6):759-772.

56. Chan JK, Bruce VM, McDonald BE. Dietary alpha-linolenic acid is as effective as oleic acid and linoleic acid in lowering blood cholesterol in normolipidemic men. Am J Clin Nutr 1991;53(5):1230-1234.

57. Hutchins AM, Martini MC, Olson BA, et al. Flaxseed consumption influences endogenous hormone concentrations in postmenopausal women. Nutr Cancer 2001;39(1):58-65.

58. Shultz T, Bonorden W, Seaman W. Effects of short-term flaxseed consumption on lignan and sex hormone metabolism. Nutr Res 1991;11:1089-1100.

59. Kurzer MS, Lampe JW, Martini MC, et al. Fecal lignan and isoflavonoid excretion in premenopausal women consuming flaxseed powder. Cancer Epidemiol Biomarkers Prev 1995;4(4):353-358.

60. Pattanaik U, Prasad K. Oxygen Free Radicals and Endotoxic Shock: Effect of Flaxseed. J Cardiovasc.Pharmacol Ther 1998;3(4):305-318.

61. Manthey FA, Lee RE, Hall CA, III. Processing and cooking effects on lipid content and stability of alpha-linolenic acid in spaghetti containing ground flaxseed. J Agric Food Chem 2002;50(6):1668-1671.

62. Dyerberg J. Linolenate-derived polyunsaturated fatty acids and prevention of atherosclerosis. Nutr Rev 1986;44(4):125-134.

63. Siguel EN. Essential and trans fatty acid metabolism in health and disease. Compr Ther 1994;20(9):500-510.

64. Stoll AL, Locke CA, Marangell LB, et al. Omega-3 fatty acids and bipolar disorder: a review. Prostaglandins Leukot Essent Fatty Acids 1999;60(5-6): 329-337.

65. Mantzioris E, James MJ, Gibson RA, et al. Nutritional attributes of dietary flaxseed oil. Am J Clin Nutr 1995;62(4):841.

66. Mantzioris E, James MJ, Gibson RA, et al. Differences exist in the relationships between dietary linoleic and alpha-linolenic acids and their respective long-chain metabolites. Am J Clin Nutr 1995;61(2):320-324.

67. Mantzioris E, James MJ, Gibson RA, et al. Dietary substitution with an alpha-linolenic acid-rich vegetable oil increases eicosapentaenoic acid concentrations in tissues. Am J Clin Nutr 1994;59(6):1304-1309.

68. Degenhardt A, Habben S, Winterhalter P. Isolation of the lignan secoisolariciresinol diglucoside from flaxseed (Linum usitatissimum L.) by high-speed counter-current chromatography. J Chromatogr A 2002; 943(2):299-302.

69. Rickard SE, Orcheson LJ, Seidl MM, et al. Dose-dependent production of mammalian lignans in rats and in vitro from the purified precursor secoisolariciresinol diglycoside in flaxseed. J Nutr 1996;126(8):2012-2019.

70. Sperling RI, Benincaso AI, Knoell CT, et al. Dietary omega-3 polyunsaturated fatty acids inhibit phosphoinositide formation and chemotaxis in neutrophils. J Clin Invest 1993;91(2):651-660.

71. Wagner W, Nootbaar-Wagner U. Prophylactic treatment of migraine with gamma-linolenic and alpha- linolenic acids. Cephalalgia 1997;17(2): 127-130.

72. Kelley DS, Branch LB, Love JE, et al. Dietary alpha-linolenic acid and immunocompetence in humans. Am J Clin Nutr 1991;53(1):40-46.

73. Bhathena SJ, Ali AA, Haudenschild C, et al. Dietary flaxseed meal is more protective than soy protein concentrate against hypertriglyceridemia and steatosis of the liver in an animal model of obesity. J Am Coll Nutr 2003; 22(2):157-164.

74. Brooks JD, Ward WE, Lewis JE, et al. Supplementation with flaxseed alters estrogen metabolism in postmenopausal women to a greater extent than does supplementation with an equal amount of soy. Am J Clin Nutr 2004; 79(2):318-325.

75. Ogborn MR, Nitschmann E, Bankovic-Calic N, et al. The effect of dietary flaxseed supplementation on organic anion and osmolyte content and excretion in rat polycystic kidney disease. Biochem Cell Biol 1998;76(2-3): 553-559.

76. Hall AV, Parbtani A, Clark WF, et al. Abrogation of MRL/lpr lupus nephritis by dietary flaxseed. Am J Kidney Dis 1993;22(2):326-332.

77. Hutchins AM, Martini MC, Olson BA, et al. Flaxseed influences urinary lignan excretion in a dose-dependent manner in postmenopausal women. Cancer Epidemiol Biomarkers Prev 2000;9(10):1113-1118.

78. Lucas EA, Wild RD, Hammond LJ, et al. Flaxseed improves lipid profile without altering biomarkers of bone metabolism in postmenopausal women. J Clin Endocrinol Metab 2002;87(4):1527-1532.

79. Tarpila S, Aro A, Salminen I, et al. The effect of flaxseed supplementation in processed foods on serum fatty acids and enterolactone. Eur J Clin Nutr 2002;56(2):157-165.

80. Riserus U, Berglund L, Vessby B. Conjugated linoleic acid (CLA) reduced abdominal adipose tissue in obese middle-aged men with signs of the metabolic syndrome: a randomised controlled trial. Int J Obes Relat Metab Disord 2001;25(8):1129-1135.

81. de Lorgeril M, Renaud S, Mamelle N, et al. Mediterranean alpha-linolenic acid-rich diet in secondary prevention of coronary heart disease. Lancet 1994;343(8911):1454-1459.

82. Oomen CM, Ocke MC, Feskens EJ, et al. Alpha-Linolenic acid intake is not beneficially associated with 10-y risk of coronary artery disease incidence: the Zutphen Elderly Study. Am J Clin Nutr 2001;74(4):457-463.

83. Anonymous. Dietary supplementation with n-3 polyunsaturated fatty acids and vitamin E after myocardial infarction: results of the GISSI-Prevenzione trial. Gruppo Italiano per lo Studio della Sopravvivenza nell'Infarto miocardico. Lancet 1999;354(9177):447-455.

84. Hu FB, Stampfer MJ, Manson JE, et al. Dietary intake of alpha-linolenic acid and risk of fatal ischemic heart disease among women. Am J Clin Nutr 1999;69(5):890-897.

85. Chen J, Stavro PM, Thompson LU. Dietary flaxseed inhibits human breast cancer growth and metastasis and downregulates expression of insulin-like growth factor and epidermal growth factor receptor. Nutr Cancer 2002; 43(2):187-192.

86. Dabrosin C, Chen J, Wang L, et al. Flaxseed inhibits metastasis and decreases extracellular vascular endothelial growth factor in human breast cancer xenografts. Cancer Lett 2002;185(1):31-37.

87. Thompson LU, Rickard SE, Orcheson LJ, et al. Flaxseed and its lignan and oil components reduce mammary tumor growth at a late stage of carcinogenesis. Carcinogenesis 1996;17(6):1373-1376.

88. Serraino M, Thompson LU. The effect of flaxseed supplementation on early risk markers for mammary carcinogenesis. Cancer Lett 1991;60(2): 135-142.

89. Serraino M, Thompson LU. The effect of flaxseed supplementation on the initiation and promotional stages of mammary tumorigenesis. Nutr Cancer 1992;17(2):153-159.

90. Rose DP, Hatala MA, Connolly JM, et al. Effect of diets containing different levels of linoleic acid on human breast cancer growth and lung metastasis in nude mice. Cancer Res 1993;53(19):4686-4690.

91. Rickard SE, Yuan YV, Chen J, et al. Dose effects of flaxseed and its lignan on N-methyl-N-nitrosourea-induced mammary tumorigenesis in rats. Nutr Cancer 1999;35(1):50-57.

92. Rose DP, Connolly JM, Liu XH. Effects of linoleic acid on the growth and metastasis of two human breast cancer cell lines in nude mice and the invasive capacity of these cell lines in vitro. Cancer Res 1994;54(24): 6557-6562.

93. Fritsche KL, Johnston PV. Effect of dietary alpha-linolenic acid on growth, metastasis, fatty acid profile and prostaglandin production of two murine mammary adenocarcinomas. J Nutr 1990;120(12):1601-1609.

94. Bougnoux P, Koscielny S, Chajes V, et al. alpha-Linolenic acid content of adipose breast tissue: a host determinant of the risk of early metastasis in breast cancer. Br J Cancer 1994;70(2):330-334.

95. Goss PE, Li T, Theriault M, et al. Effects of dietary flaxseed in women with cyclical mastalgia. Breast Cancer Res Treat 2000;64:49.

96. Plu-Bureau, Thalabard JC, Sitruk-Ware R, et al. Cyclical mastalgia as a marker of breast cancer susceptibility: results of a case-control study among French women. Br J Cancer 1992;65(6):945-949.

97. Clark WF, Parbtani A. Omega-3 fatty acid supplementation in clinical and experimental lupus nephritis. Am J Kidney Dis 1994;23(5):644-647.

98. Clark WF, Muir RD, Westcott ND, et al. A novel treatment for lupus nephritis: lignan precursor derived from flax. Lupus 2000;9(6):429-436.

99. Ingram AJ, Parbtani A, Clark WF, et al. Effects of flaxseed and flax oil diets in a rat-5/6 renal ablation model. Am J Kidney Dis 1995;25(2):320-329.

100. Begin ME, Das UN. A deficiency in dietary gamma-linolenic and/or eicosapentaenoic acids may determine individual susceptibility to AIDS. Med Hypotheses 1986;20(1):1-8.

101. Suttmann U, Ockenga J, Schneider H, et al. Weight gain and increased concentrations of receptor proteins for tumor necrosis factor after patients with symptomatic HIV infection received fortified nutrition support. J Am Diet Assoc 1996;96(6):565-569.

102. Lin X, Gingrich JR, Bao W, et al. Effect of flaxseed supplementation on prostatic carcinoma in transgenic mice. Urology 2002;60(5):919-924.

Garlic

(*Allium sativum* L.)

SYNONYMS/COMMON NAMES/RELATED SUBSTANCES

- Aged garlic extract, aglio, ail, ail commun, ajo, ajoene, akashneem, alisat, allicin, allii sativi bulbus, alliinase, allium, allyl mercaptan, alubosa elewe, Amaryllidaceae (family), ayo-ishi, ayu, banlasun, camphor of the poor, clove garlic, dai toan, dasuan, da-suan, dawang, diallyl sulfide, diallyl sulphide, dipropyl disulfide, dipropyl sulphide, dra thiam, foom, garlic clove, garlic corns, garlic extract, garlic oil, gartenlauch, hom khaao, hom kia, hom thiam, hua thiam, kesumphin, kitunguu-sumu, knoblauch, kra thiam, krathiam, krathiam cheen, krathiam khaao, Kwai, Kyolic, l'ail, lahsun, lai, la-juan, lasan, lashun, la-suan, lasun, lasuna, lauch, lay, layi, lehsun, lesun, Liliaceae (family), lobha, majo, naharu, nectar of the gods, ninniku, pa-se-waa, poor man's treacle, 2-propenesulfenic acid, rason, rasonam, rasun, rust treacle, rustic treacles, *S*-allylcysteine (SAC), seer, skordo, sluon, stinking rose, sudulunu, tafanuwa, ta-suam, ta-suan, tellagada, tellagaddalu, thiam, thioallyl derivative, thiosulfinates, toi thum, tum, umbi bawang putih, vallaippundu, velluli, vellulli, verum, vinyldithiin.

CLINICAL BOTTOM LINE

Background

- Numerous controlled trials have examined the effects of oral garlic on serum lipids. Most studies have been small (<100 subjects), with poorly described design and results, and most have reported nonsignificant modest benefits. Several overlapping meta-analyses have pooled these studies,[1-5] suggesting that non–enteric-coated tablets containing dehydrated garlic powder (standardized to 1.3% alliin) elicit modest reductions in total cholesterol compared with levels noted with placebo (<20 mg/dL) in the short term (4 to 12 weeks), with unclear effects after 20 weeks. Small reductions in low-density lipoprotein (LDL) (by <10 mg/dL) and triglycerides (by <20 mg/dL) may also occur in the short term, although results have been variable. High-density lipoprotein (HDL) levels are not significantly affected. Long-term effects on lipids or cardiovascular morbidity and mortality remain unknown. Other preparations (such as enteric-coated or raw garlic) have not been well studied.
- Small reductions in blood pressure (<10 mm Hg), inhibition of platelet aggregation, and enhancement of fibrinolytic activity have been reported; such changes may exert effects on cardiovascular outcomes, although evidence is preliminary in these areas.[6]
- Numerous case-control/population-based studies suggest that regular consumption of garlic (particularly unprocessed garlic) may reduce the risk of developing several types of cancer, including gastric and colorectal malignancies. However, prospective controlled trials are lacking.
- Multiple cases of bleeding have been associated with garlic use, and caution is warranted in patients at risk of bleeding or prior to some surgical/dental procedures. Garlic does not appear to significantly affect blood glucose levels.

Scientific Evidence for Common/Studied Uses	Grade*
Hyperlipidemia (modest effects)	B
Antifungal (topical)	C
Antiplatelet effects	C
Atherosclerosis	C
Cancer prevention	C
Cardiac disease/events: secondary prevention	C
Cryptococcal meningitis	C
Familial hyperlipidemia	C
Hypertension	C
Peripheral vascular disease	C
Tick repellent	C
Upper respiratory tract infection	C
Helicobacter pylori infection	D
Type 2 diabetes mellitus	D

*Key to grades: *A*: Strong scientific evidence for this use; *B*: Good scientific evidence for this use; *C*: Unclear scientific evidence for this use; *D*: Fair scientific evidence against this use (it may not work); *F*: Strong scientific evidence against this use (it likely does not work). For a more detailed explanation of efficacy criteria, see "Natural Standard Evidence-Based Validated Grading Rationale" in the Introduction.

Historical or Theoretical Uses That Lack Sufficient Evidence

- Abortifacient, age-related memory disorders,[7] acquired immunodeficiency syndrome (AIDS),[8] allergies, ameba infections, anthrax,[9] antifungal (topical), anthelminthic, antioxidant,[10-15] antisecretory, antispasmodic, antitoxin, antiviral,[16,17] aphrodisiac, antipyretic, arthritis,[18] asbestos lung protection,[19] ascaridiasis,[20] asthma, athlete's foot, bloody urine, bronchitis, cardiac arrhythmia,[21] cholagogue, cholera, claudication,[22] colds, cough,[23] cytomegalovirus infection,[24] dental pain,[25] diabetes,[26] diaphoretic, digestive aid, diphtheria, diuretic, doxorubicin cardiotoxicity,[27] dysentery, dyspepsia,[28] earache,[29] emmenagogue, fatigue, fever, gallstones,[30] gastrointestinal hypermotility,[31] gentamicin-induced nephrotoxicity,[32,33] hair growth, headache, hemorrhoids, hepatoprotection,[34-36] hepatopulmonary syndrome,[37,38] hormonal effects, human immunodeficiency virus (HIV) infection, immunostimulant,[8,39] inflammation, inflammatory bowel disease, influenza, intermittent claudication, larvicidal, leukemia, lymphangitis,[40] malaria,[41] methicillin-resistant *Staphylococcus aureus* infection,[42] mucolytic, mycostatic, nephrotic syndrome,[43] neuroprotection,[44,45] obesity, parasites, peptic ulcer disease, pneumonia, psoriasis, Raynaud's disease, scalp ringworm, sedative, sinus congestion, snake venom protection,[36] spermicide,[46,47] stomachache, stress, stroke, thrush,[48] tinea corporis, tinea cruris, toothache, traveler's diarrhea, tuberculosis, vaginal trichomoniasis, verruca vulgaris,[49] typhus, urinary tract infections, vaginitis, well-being,[50] whooping cough, yeast infection.

Expert Opinion and Folkloric Precedent

- The medicinal use of garlic dates back to Greek physicians, traditional Chinese healers, and American physicians in the 1800s. Garlic was recognized by Louis Pasteur and Albert Schweitzer and was utilized during both World Wars as an antimicrobial agent.
- The expert German panel Commission E supports garlic use for hyperlipidemia in addition to dietary measures, and to prevent age-related vascular changes. The European Scientific Cooperative on Phytotherapy (ESCOP) lists the following indications for garlic: prophylaxis of atherosclerosis, treatment of elevated blood lipids, improvement of circulation in peripheral arterial vascular disease, upper respiratory tract infections, and catarrhal conditions. The World Health Organization (WHO) reports the following garlic uses supported by clinical data: adjuvant to dietary management for hyperlipidemia, prevention of age-dependent atherosclerosis, and possibly mild hypertension.

Safety Summary

- **Likely safe:** When consumed in amounts usually found in foods.
- **Possibly safe:** When used as a dietary supplement in recommended doses in healthy adults.
- **Possibly unsafe:** When used in large amounts orally or when used topically. When taken by patients on anticoagulants, nonsteroidal anti-inflammatory drugs (NSAIDs)/antiplatelet agents, or herbs/supplements that may increase the risk of bleeding such as *Ginkgo biloba*; by patients with known bleeding disorders; or perioperatively, because of an increased risk of bleeding. When used in large doses during pregnancy or lactation. When used by patients taking antihypertensive agents, because of potential mild hypotensive effects of garlic. Garlic does not appear to significantly affect blood glucose levels.

DOSING/TOXICOLOGY
General

- Recommended doses are based on those most commonly used in available trials, or on historical practice. However, with natural products, the optimal doses needed to balance efficacy and safety often have not been determined. Formulations and preparation methods may vary from manufacturer to manufacturer, and from batch to batch of a specific product made by a single manufacturer. Because often the active components of a product are not known, standardization may not be possible, and the clinical effects of different brands may not be comparable.

Preparations and Constituents

- Dried garlic powder is considered approximately equal in activity to fresh garlic homogenates. However, steam-distilled oils and oil macerates have shown substantially decreased antiplatelet activity, and aged garlic in aqueous alcohol has demonstrated no antiplatelet activity.[51]
- It is likely not true, as previously believed, that allicin is the major active constituent. It is thought that some or all of the sulfur-containing moieties, including allicin, exert some

pharmacologic effect. The magnitude of effect attributed to each constituent is not clear.

- There is variation in the main organosulfur compounds that are present in commercially available preparations of fresh garlic (S-alkylcysteine sulfoxides [mainly alliin]; gamma-glutamyl-S-alkylcysteines; alkylalkane thiosulfinates [mainly allicin]), dried extract (S-alkylcysteine sulfoxides [mainly alliin]; gamma-glutamyl-S-alkylcysteines; alkylalkane thiosulfinates [mainly allicin]; thiosulfinate transformation compounds [diallyl, allylmethyl, dimethyl sulfides]), steam-distilled garlic oil (thiosulfinate transformation compounds [diallyl, allylmethyl, dimethyl sulfides]), and aged garlic extract (gamma-glutamyl-S-alkylcysteines).[52]

Standardization

- The Lichtwer Pharma GmbH (Berlin, Germany) standardized garlic powder product Kwai has been often used in studies utilizing fresh garlic and is standardized to 1.3% alliin content. Other trials have used a standardized preparation that contains 220 mg of garlic powder and produces 2.4 mg of allicin *in vitro*.[53] U.S. pharmacopeial-grade garlic must contain 0.3% (powdered) to 0.5% (fresh, dried) allicin, whereas European pharmacopeial-grade garlic must yield not less than 0.45% allicin. Notably, few of the >2000 articles on garlic have utilized a chemically characterized product.[54]

Dosing: Adult (18 Years and Older)
Oral

- **Tablets/capsules:** 600 to 900 mg per day of non–enteric-coated, dehydrated garlic powder in three divided doses, standardized to 1.3% allicin content, has been used in multiple clinical trials of hyperlipidemia, peripheral vascular disease, and hypertension (many studies have used the product Kwai).[1-5] The European Scientific Cooperative on Phytotherapy (ESCOP) 1997 monograph recommends 3 to 5 mg of allicin daily (1 clove or 0.5 to 1.0 g of dried powder) for prophylaxis of atherosclerosis. The World Health Organization (WHO) 1999 monograph recommends 2 to 5 g of fresh garlic, 0.4 to 1.2 g of dried powder, 2 to 5 mg of oil, 300 to 1000 mg of extract, or other formulations corresponding to 2 to 5 mg of allicin.
- **Oil:** Garlic oil preparations have been included in clinical trials, with doses ranging between 4 and 12.3 mg daily,[55-59] but use and pharmacokinetics have been subsequently debated.[60-62] Steam-distilled oils and oil macerates have been shown to substantially decrease antiplatelet activity, and aged garlic in aqueous alcohol has demonstrated no antiplatelet activity.[51]
- **Tincture:** The ESCOP 1997 monograph recommends 2 to 4 g of dried bulb or 2 to 4 mL of tincture (1:5, 45% ethanol) three times a day for upper respiratory tract infections.

Dosing: Pediatric (Younger Than 18 Years)

- Safety or efficacy of garlic supplementation has not been established in children. One study in 31 children (ages 8 to 18 years) with possible familial hyperlipidemia (total cholesterol levels >185 mg/dL) assigned subjects to receive 900 mg of dehydrated garlic powder tablets (Kwai) in three divided daily doses or placebo.[63] No significant effects of garlic were observed on lipid levels, although the trial may have been too small to detect effects.

Toxicology

- Garlic appears to be generally well tolerated when consumed in the diet and at recommended medicinal doses. Toxicity studies have been limited. Toxic effects on gastrointestinal mucosa have been demonstrated in an animal study of three garlic preparations delivered directly onto gastric mucosa via endoscopy; a raw garlic powder preparation caused severe mucosal damage, whereas aged garlic extract caused no effects.[64] In mice, the LD_{50} for allicin has been reported as 120 mg/kg given subcutaneously and 60 mg/kg given intravenously[65]; the LD_{50} for garlic extract has been reported as >30 mL/kg intraperitoneally.[66] Oral doses up to 2000 mg/kg five times per week have been tolerated by rats for up to 6 months.[67]

- Ingestion of a large amount of garlic was associated with an acute myocardial infarction in a 23-year-old man with no known history of cardiac disease or known risk factors.[68]

ADVERSE EFFECTS/PRECAUTIONS/CONTRAINDICATIONS
Allergy

- Patients should avoid garlic if they have a known allergy/hypersensitivity to garlic or any of its constituents, or to other members of the Liliaceae (lily) family, including hyacinth, tulip, onion, leek, and chives.[69]
- Allergic responses have been associated with oral, topical, and inhaled garlic preparations. There are multiple published case reports of garlic allergy characterized by broncho-constriction/asthmatic responses,[70-74] dermatologic reactions such as contact dermatitis,[69,75-87] systemic reactions,[88,89] angioedema, anaphylaxis, and possible coronary artery spasm.[90] A case of immunoglobulin E (IgE)-mediated anaphylaxis occurred in a 23-year-old woman following ingestion of young garlic.[91] Fresh garlic may be more likely than garlic extract to elicit topical reactions; most reactions have resolved following withdrawal of garlic therapy.
- Topical patch testing with diallyl disulfide, a compound implicated in garlic-induced contact dermatitis, elicited a positive skin reaction in 16% of persons tested.[92] An allergen, "alliin lyase," has been identified via mass spectrometry.[93]
- It has been suggested that some cases of asthmatic reactions related to garlic dust inhalation may be due to infestation of garlic by mites.[94]

Adverse Effects

- **General:** A review of 45 randomized trials and 73 studies of garlic use found limited detailed information relating to adverse effects.[2] One review noted that malodorous breath, body odor, and allergic reactions appear to be the most commonly reported effects.[95] Potential reactions of concern associated with oral garlic use include bleeding (multiple case reports and a scientific basis) and hypoglycemia (likely not clinically significant); topical exposure may elicit dermatitis or burns (multiple reports).
- **Dermatologic:** It has been reported since the 1950s that topical application or exposure to garlic can result in contact dermatitis,[75,79,84,86,87,90,96] as well as numerous other dermatologic reactions.[97] Fresh garlic may be more likely than garlic extract to elicit a reaction. Most reactions have resolved following withdrawal of garlic therapy. Cases of occupational eczema or dermatitis have been reported in cooks[98] and caterers.[99] Second- and third-degree burns have been reported in children and infants[100-103] as well as in adults[104-107] exposed to topical garlic.[108] Other reactions have included blisters, ulcers, necrotic lesions, and local irritation. Oral garlic was associated with a case of pemphigus in a 49-year-old man with type 2 diabetes mellitus.[109]
- **Neurologic:** Dizziness and diaphoresis have been noted in anecdotal reports; fever and chills have also been reported.[110]

- **Pulmonary/respiratory:** Cases of garlic-related asthma and rhinitis have been reported since the 1940s.[73]
- **Cardiovascular:** Numerous studies have reported small mean reductions in systolic and diastolic blood pressures associated with the use of oral garlic vs. placebo.[1,2,6,57,59,63,111-139] In general, mean differences have been less than 10 mm Hg (<10%), and a majority of the studies have been small (<100 subjects), with poor descriptions of methodology and results. Ingestion of a large amount of garlic was associated with an acute myocardial infarction in a 23-year-old man with no known history of cardiac disease or known risk factors.[68]
- **Gastrointestinal:** Effects of oral dehydrated garlic preparations or raw garlic ingestion may include malodorous breath (more common with garlic than with placebo in several controlled trials),[134,140-142] abdominal pain or fullness, anorexia, diarrhea, flatulence, belching, and bowel obstruction[2,3,110]; one case of bowel obstruction was reported in a 66-year-old man who ingested an entire garlic bulb.[143] Other reactions have included nausea, vomiting, alteration of gastrointestinal flora, gastrointestinal irritation/burning (affecting mouth, esophagus, and stomach), acute or chronic stomach mucosal inflammation, and gastroenteritis. Diarrhea and constipation have also been noted in human trials.[144]
- **Endocrine (glycemic effects):** Animal studies have reported that garlic or its constituents (such as S-allyl cysteine sulfoxide [SACS]) may decrease glucose concentrations and increase insulin secretion.[145,146] However, multiple human trials have failed to demonstrate significant effects of oral garlic preparations on measures of glycemic control in diabetic or nondiabetic patients, when measured both as primary outcomes[26,130] and as secondary outcomes.[56,112,116,121-123,128,141] One poor-quality study that was designed to measure platelet aggregation noted a small significant reduction in mean blood glucose levels in patients taking 800 mg of daily dehydrated garlic (Kwai), from 89 mg/dL to 79 mg/dL over 4 weeks.[126] Although the available studies have been small (<100 subjects) with methodologic weaknesses, it appears that garlic likely does not exert clinically relevant effects on glucose levels.
- **Endocrine (lipid effects):** Multiple trials have demonstrated modest lipid-lowering properties of oral garlic supplementation, including decreases in total cholesterol and low-density lipoprotein.[1-5]
- **Endocrine (thyroid effects):** Hypothyroidism and reduced iodine uptake by the thyroid have been reported anecdotally. Intake of *Allium* vegetables such as garlic has been linked epidemiologically to a decreased risk of developing nodular disease or thyroid tumors.[147]
- **Hematologic (bleeding risk):** Bleeding has been associated with garlic use in several studies and case reports (including postoperative bleeding), possibly related to impaired platelet aggregation or increased fibrinolysis. There is a case report of a spontaneous spinal epidural hematoma and platelet dysfunction associated with ingestion of fresh garlic in a healthy 87-year-old man who consumed an average of four cloves of garlic per day. This man developed sudden paralysis caused by the spinal bleeding. The patient's platelet count was normal, but bleeding time was prolonged at 11.5 minutes.[148,149] A 72-year-old man hospitalized for acute urinary retention underwent transurethral resection for benign prostatic hypertrophy and developed excessive bleeding requiring four units of blood.[150] His clotting time and prothrombin time were normal. The only known agent the patient was taking was garlic (tablets). The patient continued to take garlic, and 3 months later a study of his

platelet function demonstrated impaired aggregation. There have been additional suggestions of prolonged bleeding associated with garlic,[151,152] postoperative hemorrhage,[153,154] and *in vitro* and clinical reports of impaired platelet aggregation.[22,116,127,155-157] One placebo-controlled trial found that 800 mg of garlic daily led to a decrease in thrombocyte aggregation in patients with peripheral vascular disease.[22] A similar study demonstrated that patients consuming 800 mg of garlic daily for 4 weeks experienced a significant decrease in spontaneous platelet aggregation.[127] Harenberg et al. reported increased fibrinolytic activity in hyperlipidemic patients consuming 600 mg of dried garlic daily.[158] Other trials have reported prolonged clotting time for garlic vs. placebo.[144,159]

- **Hematologic (increased INR):** There is a report of two patients who experienced an increase in a previously stabilized international normalized ratio (INR) with concomitant oral garlic and warfarin use; this report has been subsequently debated because of limited clinical information.[151,160] In a small controlled study, no significant change in INR values was found in a group of patients stabilized on warfarin (Coumadin) therapy (INR target 2 to 3) who received 1200 mg of aged garlic extract (AGE) for 2 months, compared with a placebo group.[161] However, clinical outcomes such as increased bleeding were not assessed, and the study was likely too small and brief to significantly measure such outcomes.
- **Genitourinary:** Chronic garlic ingestion for 70 days has been associated with suppression of spermatogenesis in rats.[162] Effects in humans are not clear.
- **Contamination:** An outbreak of botulism in Vancouver, British Columbia, was associated with ingestion of commercial chopped garlic.[163] Botulism was also reported in a 38-year-old man who ingested canned "garlic in chilli oil."[164] Colchicine overdose and death have occurred following the accidental ingestion of meadow saffron (*Colchicum autumnale*), which was mistaken for wild garlic (*Allium ursinum*).[165]
- **Other (body odor):** Garlic odor has been associated with garlic use in multiple anecdotal and historical accounts and has been noted in several trials, although the incidence has not been clearly greater than that with placebo.[55,135]

Precautions/Warnings/Contraindications

- Avoid in patients with known allergy to garlic or to other members of the Liliaceae (lily) family, including hyacinth, tulip, onion, leek, and chives.
- Avoid topical use in infants/young children, and use cautiously in adults, because of multiple case reports of burns and dermatitis.
- Avoid oral use in patients prior to some surgical or dental procedures[166] because of an increased risk of bleeding.
- Use cautiously in patients with bleeding disorders or taking anticoagulants, NSAIDs/antiplatelet agents, or herbs/supplements that increase risk of bleeding such as *Ginkgo biloba*, because of an increased risk of bleeding.
- Use cautiously in patients with peptic ulcer disease or prone to gastric irritation, because of possibility of gastrointestinal irritation as noted in clinical trials.

Pregnancy and Lactation

- **Pregnancy:** Garlic is likely safe during pregnancy in amounts usually ingested in food, based on historical use. Garlic supplementation should be avoided during pregnancy because of a theoretical increased risk of bleeding. In addition, uterine

stimulant activity was reported in early animal research.[167] In a controlled study of 10 pregnant women, the odor of amniotic fluid samples was reported to smell more like garlic in women who had ingested capsules containing the essential oil of garlic 45 minutes prior to amniocentesis than in women who had not ingested garlic.[168]

- **Lactation:** Garlic is likely safe during lactation in amounts usually ingested in food, based on historical use. However, maternal consumption of garlic supplements has been associated with increases in nursing time, milk odor,[169] and milk consumption.[170] Safety during lactation has not been established.

INTERACTIONS
Garlic/Drug Interactions

- **Anticoagulants, antiplatelet drugs, nonsteroidal anti-inflammatory drugs (NSAIDs):** Bleeding, including intraoperative bleeding, has been associated with oral garlic use in several studies and case reports, possibly related to impaired platelet aggregation or increased fibrinolysis.[22,116,127,144,148,150,151,153-159] By contrast, there is a report of two cases, with limited clinical information provided, of an increase in a previously stabilized international normalized ratio (INR) with concomitant garlic and warfarin use, which has been subsequently debated due to limited clinical information.[151,160] However, in a small controlled study, no significant change in INR values was found in a group of patients stabilized on warfarin (Coumadin) therapy (INR target 2 to 3) who received 1200 mg of aged garlic extract (AGE) for 2 months, compared with a placebo group (clinical outcomes such as increased bleeding were not assessed, and the study was likely too small and brief to significantly measure such outcomes).[161] In theory, the risk of bleeding may be increased by concomitant use of garlic and anticoagulant or antiplatelet agents, although anticoagulant effects of warfarin may be reduced by garlic use.
- **Antihypertensive drugs:** Numerous studies have reported small mean reductions in systolic and diastolic blood pressure associated with the use of oral garlic vs. placebo, and combination use with antihypertensives may result in additive effects.[1,2,6,57,63,111-139] In general, mean differences have been less than 10 mm Hg (<10%), and a majority of the studies have been small (<100 subjects), with poor descriptions of methodology and results.
- **Hypoglycemic drugs:** The available evidence suggests that garlic does not lower blood glucose levels in humans. Although animal studies have reported that garlic or its constituents (such as *S*-allyl cysteine sulfoxide [SACS]) may decrease glucose concentrations and increase insulin secretion,[145,146] multiple human trials have failed to demonstrate significant effects of oral garlic preparations on measures of glycemic control in diabetic or nondiabetic patients.[26,56,112,116,121-123,128,130,141] One poor-quality study noted a small significant reduction in mean blood glucose levels in patients taking 800 mg of daily dehydrated garlic (Kwai), from 89 mg/dL to 79 mg/dL over 4 weeks.[126] Although the available studies have been small (<100 subjects) with methodologic weaknesses, it appears that garlic likely does not exert clinically relevant effects on glucose levels. Possible interactions with hypoglycemic agents have not been systematically evaluated.
- **Saquinavir, ritonavir (protease inhibitors):** Garlic supplementation was shown to cause a significant decrease in plasma concentrations of saquinavir taken at a dose of 1200 mg three times daily by 10 healthy volunteers.[172-174] Combination use may result in diminished effects of saquinavir.

However, a preliminary study in 10 healthy adults found no significant effects on ritonavir levels following eight doses of 10 mg of Natural Source Odourless Garlic.[175]

- **Thyroid drugs, iodine:** Hypothyroidism and reduced iodine uptake by the thyroid have been reported anecdotally with garlic use and may alter the effects of thyroid agents.
- **Lipid-lowering drugs:** Multiple trials have demonstrated modest lipid-lowering properties of oral garlic supplementation, including decreases in total cholesterol and low-density lipoprotein (LDL).[1-5] Effects may be additive with those of other lipid-lowering agents.
- **Cytochrome P450–metabolized drugs:** Although animal studies suggest possible induction or inhibition of various P450 enzymes,[176,177] preliminary human evidence in 14 healthy volunteers administered garlic extract 1800 mg twice daily found no effects on metabolism of alprazolam (P450 3A4) or dextromethorphan (P450 2D6).[178]

Garlic/Herb/Supplement Interactions

- **Fish oil, eicosapentaenoic acid (EPA):** EPA is found in deep-sea fish oils. Garlic may potentiate antithrombotic effects of EPA, and theoretically, concomitant use of these agents may increase the risk of bleeding. Garlic and fish oil may have additive lipid-lowering effects.
- **Anticoagulant herbs and supplements:** Bleeding, including intraoperative bleeding, has been associated with garlic use in several studies and case reports, possibly related to impaired platelet aggregation or increased fibrinolysis.[22,116,127,144,148,151,153,154-159,179] In contrast, there is a report of two cases, with limited clinical information, of an increase in a previously stabilized INR with concomitant garlic and warfarin use, which has been subsequently debated because of limited clinical information.[151,160] However, in a small controlled study, no significant change in INR values was found in a group of patients stabilized on warfarin (Coumadin) therapy (INR target 2 to 3) who received 1200 mg of aged garlic extract (AGE) for 2 months, compared with a placebo group (clinical outcomes such as increased bleeding were not assessed, and the study was likely too small and brief to significantly measure such outcomes).[161] In theory, the risk of bleeding may be increased by concomitant use of garlic and herbs and supplements with anticoagulant or antiplatelet effects.
- **Hypotensive herbs and supplements:** Numerous studies have reported small mean reductions in systolic and diastolic blood pressure associated with the use of oral garlic vs. placebo, and combination use with antihypertensive agents may result in additive effects.[1,2,6,57,63,111-139] In general, mean differences have been less than 10 mm Hg (<10%), and a majority of the studies have been small (<100 subjects), with poor descriptions of methodology and results.
- **Hypoglycemic herbs and supplements:** The available evidence suggests that garlic does not lower blood glucose levels in humans. Although animal studies have reported that garlic or its constituents (such as S-allyl cysteine sulfoxide [SACS]) may decrease glucose concentrations and increase insulin secretion,[145,146] multiple human trials have failed to demonstrate significant effects of oral garlic preparations on measures of glycemic control in diabetic or nondiabetic patients.[26,56,112,116,121-123,128,130,141] One poor-quality study noted a small significant reduction in mean blood glucose levels in patients taking 800 mg of daily dehydrated garlic (Kwai), from 89 mg/dL to 79 mg/dL over 4 weeks.[126] Although the available studies have been small (<100 subjects) with methodologic weaknesses, it appears that garlic likely

does not exert clinically relevant effects on glucose levels. Possible interactions with hypoglycemic agents have not been systematically evaluated.

- **Lipid-lowering herbs and supplements:** Multiple trials have demonstrated modest lipid-lowering properties of oral garlic supplements, including decreases in total cholesterol and LDL.[1-5] Effects may be additive with those of other lipid-lowering agents such as fish oil, guggul, and niacin.
- **Pycnogenol:** Garlic and pycnogenol have been shown to increase human growth hormone secretion in laboratory experiments .

Garlic/Food Interactions

- Insufficient available evidence.

Garlic/Lab Interactions

- **Prothrombin time/INR:** There is a report of two cases, with limited clinical information, of an increase in a previously stabilized INR with concomitant garlic and warfarin use, which has been subsequently debated because of limited clinical information.[151,160] However, in a small controlled study, no significant change in INR values was found in a group of patients stabilized on warfarin (Coumadin) therapy (INR target 2 to 3) who received 1200 mg of aged garlic extract (AGE) for 2 months, compared with a placebo group (clinical outcomes such as increased bleeding were not assessed, and the study was likely too small and brief to significantly measure such outcomes).[161]
- **Serum glucose:** The available evidence suggests that garlic does not significantly lower blood glucose levels in humans. Although animal studies have reported that garlic may decrease glucose concentrations and increase insulin secretion,[145,146] multiple human trials have failed to demonstrate significant effects of oral garlic preparations on measures of glycemic control in diabetic or nondiabetic patients,[26,56,112,116,121-123,128,130,141] with the exception of one poor-quality study that noted a small significant reduction in mean blood glucose levels in patients taking 800 mg of daily dehydrated garlic (Kwai), from 89 mg/dL to 79 mg/dL over 4 weeks.[126]
- **Serum lipid profile:** Multiple trials have demonstrated modest lipid-lowering properties of oral garlic supplementation, including decreases in total cholesterol, LDL, and triglycerides.[1-5] Results have been inconsistent regarding effects of garlic on levels of high-density lipoprotein (HDL), although a meta-analysis of randomized controlled trials did not demonstrate a statistically significant effect when data were pooled.[1]
- **Urine allylmercapturic acid:** Garlic tablets and fresh garlic can result in urinary excretion of allylmercapturic acid (N-acetyl-S-allyl-L-cysteine), which may interfere with urinary monitoring of workers for industrial exposure to allyl halides.[180]

MECHANISM OF ACTION
Pharmacology

- **Constituents:** Chemical analysis in the 1800s attributed garlic's activity to the sulfur-containing garlic oil. In the mid 1900s an American chemist named the strong-smelling liquid "allicin."[181] The sulfur compound alliin (S-allyl-L-cysteine sulfoxide) produces allicin (diallyl thiosulfinate) via the enzyme allinase when the bulb is crushed or ground. Other sulfur compounds—peptides, steroids, terpenoids, flavonoids, and phenols—have increasingly been identified as possible active ingredients[54,182,183] as allicin is metabolized.

G

The exact mechanism of action underlying garlic's effects remains unknown and may vary according to the preparation[184] and the therapeutic effect.

- Garlic appears to exert numerous effects on the cardiovascular system, and atherosclerosis in particular, beyond the reduction of serum lipids. There are possibly multiple protective effects of garlic,[141,185,186] including inhibition of platelet aggregation and enhancement of fibrinolysis. Wild garlic (*Allium ursinum*) has been reported to contain amounts of sulfur-containing compounds (thiosulfinates and ajoenes) similar to those found in garlic (*Allium sativum*), and to exert similar effects on cyclooxygenase, 5-lipoxygenase, angiotensin-converting enzyme, and platelet aggregation.[187]

- **Lipid-lowering effects:** Garlic's lipid-lowering effects may occur via inhibition of hydroxymethyl glutarate–coenzyme A (HMG-CoA) reductase or other enzymes,[188-195] possibly by diallyl di- and trisulfide components of garlic.[196,197] Other suggested mechanisms include increased loss of bile salts in feces and mobilization of tissue lipids into circulation,[198] as garlic has a profound effect on postprandial hyperlipidemia.[199] Wild garlic (*Allium ursinum*) has shown to be similar in efficacy to garlic (*Allium sativum*) in decreasing hepatocyte cholesterol synthesis *in vitro*.[187,200] Aged garlic extract and its constituents have been shown to inhibit Cu^{2+}-induced oxidative modification of LDL.[201] Aged garlic extract and its constituent *S*-allylcysteine have been found to protect vascular endothelial cells from injury caused by oxidized LDL.[202]

- Animal and human cell lines have demonstrated reductions in vascular tissue lipids,[203,204] fatty streak formation, and atherosclerotic plaque size.[141,185,203,205-208] The mechanism of action may include reduction in lipoprotein oxidation, as demonstrated *in vitro*[201,202,209] and *in vivo*,[201] possibly because of organosulfur compounds in garlic.[211] However, this hypothesis has been in dispute, because a 6-month trial in moderately hypercholesterolemic volunteers failed to demonstrate any effects of garlic supplementation on lipoprotein oxidation.[212]

- **Platelet effects:** Garlic and its derived compound ajoene have demonstrated inhibition of platelet aggregation *in vitro* and in animals.[51,157,213-222] and reduction in platelet-dependent thrombus formation.[223,224] Research has demonstrated inhibition of platelet aggregation in hypercholesterolemic men,[225] in healthy subjects, in patients with coronary artery disease,[226-230] and in subjects with cerebrovascular risk factors.[22,115] However, a study using a low dietary dosage found no such effects.[231] Raw garlic has been shown to inhibit platelet cyclooxygenase *in vitro*.[213] Dose-dependent inhibition of cyclooxygenase in human placenta villi was observed with garlic and with allicin-negative (acid-washed) garlic.[232] Antiplatelet activity may be attributable to garlic constituents including adenosine, allicin, and paraffinic polysulfides.[233] Compared with raw garlic, a boiled aqueous garlic extract demonstrated an approximately 50% decrease in platelet aggregation at identical concentrations,[213,222] suggesting that cooking garlic may reduce antiplatelet effects. Raw garlic has been shown to reduce serum thromboxane B_2 in animal and human research,[198,226] at a dose of 1 clove per day.[234] However, boiling garlic prior to administration appears to reduce or abolish this effect,[227] again suggesting a negative impact of cooking on garlic's antiplatelet activity.

- **Fibrinolytic effects:** Increased fibrinolytic activity may account for some degree of garlic's anticlotting effects,[183,235,236] involving fibrinogen and plasminogen.[158] Both raw garlic

and fried garlic have demonstrated significant increases in fibrinolytic activity in humans,[237] as well as essential oil from raw garlic.[199] An increase in fibrinolytic activity in patients with ischemic heart disease was found to be maintained after 7 to 8 weeks of continued therapy.[238,239] However, one study reported that fibrinolytic activity returned to pretreatment levels after 12 weeks of continuous garlic therapy.[239]

- **Vascular effects:** Vasorelaxant properties of garlic have been noted in multiple preclinical studies.[240-242] Cutaneous microperfusion is increased in humans following ingestion of 600 mg of garlic,[243-245] and vasodilation of conjunctival arterioles and venules occurs at 900 mg.[246] Garlic may act on the nitric oxide system[247-249] to exert effects on the elastic properties of vasculature,[250] yielding changes in systemic blood pressure.[249] It has been suggested that allicin is the component of garlic responsible for nitric oxide–mediated effects.[251] Prostaglandins have been identified in garlic extracts that may exert pharmacologic effects,[252] although such effects have not been demonstrated *in vivo*.

- **Chemoprotective/antitumor effects:** Animal studies have reported protective effects of garlic against hepatotoxins,[34-36,253] cyclophosphamide,[254] doxorubicin (Adriamycin),[255] methylcholanthrene,[256] gentamicin,[32] 4-nitroquinoline 1-oxide,[257] and bromobenzene.[258,259] Garlic has demonstrated strong inhibition of cancer development in the presence of known tumor promoters including 12-*O*-tetradecanoylphorbol-13-acetate,[260,261] 7,12-dimethylbenzanthracene,[262] and phorbol-myristate-acetate,[263] as well as tumor inducers such as 7,12-dimethylbenzanthracene[261] and 1,2 dimethylhydrazine.[264,265] There is some evidence that the chemical constituents containing allyl groups may be responsible for chemoprotective properties.[266] Research has provided evidence of antiproliferative effects of garlic on human cancer cell lines,[267] including induction of apoptosis,[268-272] regulation of cell cycle progression,[273] and signal transduction modification. Both cellular proliferation[274,275] and immune function appear to be affected.[276,277]

- **Immunologic effects:** The immunologic activity of garlic may include enhanced phagocytosis, lymphocyte proliferation, enhanced killer cell activity and cytokine production, and prevention of immune suppression.[278-283] There has been suggestion that heating may adversely affect this benefit, related to a loss of alliinase activity,[284] and that different preparations have differing pharmacologic activities.[184]

- **Antimicrobial effects (bacteria, fungi, yeast):** Garlic has been demonstrated *in vitro* to exert activity against multiple pathogens, including bacteria,[54,150,285-290] including resistant strains,[291] mycobacteria,[292-294] *Helicobacter pylori*,[54,295,296] and fungi.[297,298] Garlic extract has been found to be bactericidal to *Histoplasma capsulatum*.[299] Ajoene alone possesses antibacterial activity against both gram-positive and gram-negative bacterial species and inhibits yeast growth *in vitro*, and the disulfide bond in ajoene may be responsible for these effects.[289] The substrate alliin and its enzyme are found in separate but adjacent compartments of the garlic clove and appear to exert antimicrobial activity when they are joined. Allicin may act via inhibition of thiol-containing and other enzyme systems and of DNA, RNA, and protein synthesis.[183,287,300,301] It has been suggested that garlic oil's antimicrobial activity is more potent than that of garlic powder on a unit weight basis.[302] In one study,[301] the minimum inhibitory concentration (MIC) of aqueous garlic extract (AGE) against six clinical yeast isolates ranged between 0.8 and 1.6 mg/mL. Garlic appeared to alter the structure and integrity of the outer surface of yeast cells and to decrease their total lipid content. Garlic was also shown to increase phosphatidylserines while decreasing phosphatidylcholines. Oxygen consumption of yeast cells was also reduced by garlic. The anticandidal activity of AGE was antagonized by thiols including L-cysteine, glutathione and 2-mercaptoethanol. The effect of AGE on the macromolecular synthesis of *Candida albicans* revealed protein and nucleic acid synthesis to be inhibited, and lipid synthesis to be arrested.[303] Antagonism of lipid synthesis may be a component of the anticandidal activity of garlic.

- **Antiviral effects:** *In vitro* studies have demonstrated effects against several viruses,[304] including influenza B virus, herpes simplex virus type 1,[304] herpes simplex virus type 2, parainfluenza virus type 3, vaccinia virus, vesicular stomatitis virus, human rhinovirus type 2,[16,17] and cytomegalovirus.[24] Weber reported that the compound ajoene, found in oil macerates of garlic, possesses a high level of antiviral activity followed by allicin, allyl methyl thiosulfinate, and methyl allyl thiosulfinate.[17]
- **Glycemic effects:** *S*-allyl cysteine sulfoxide (SACS), an antioxidant isolated from garlic, has been found to significantly stimulate insulin secretion from beta cells isolated from normal rats.[145] However, multiple human studies have failed to demonstrate glycemic effects of garlic.
- **Genitourinary effects:** Chronic garlic ingestion for 70 days has been associated with suppression of spermatogenesis in rats.[162]

Pharmacodynamics/Kinetics

- Garlic compounds are rapidly absorbed through mucous membranes and skin. Excretion is primarily via liver, kidney, and intestines.[138]
- Nagae[305] described the pharmacokinetics of *S*-allylcysteine in animal models. The authors demonstrated a first-pass effect following rapid gastrointestinal absorption, with liver and kidney metabolism.
- The pharmacokinetics of the vinyldithiins, transformation products of allicin, have been described; maximal concentrations are reached 15 to 30 minutes after oral absorption.[306]

HISTORY

- Garlic is a member of the lily family, which also includes hyacinth, tulip, onion, leek, and chives. The bulb, which has a white skin encasing multiple individual cloves, is used both medicinally and as a spice. Garlic may be used fresh or in dehydrated form.
- The *Codex Ebers*, an Egyptian medical papyrus dating from 1550 BC, mentions garlic as a remedy for a number of ailments, including hypertension, worms, and tumors. The contents of King Tutankhamen's tomb included cloves of garlic.[307] Garlic was used in ancient Greece (Hippocrates), Rome, India, China, and Japan for multiple indications, including performance enhancement, pulmonary and digestive complaints, abnormal growths, cardiovascular health, emotional health and potency, and as an anti-infective agent.[307] Garlic was used in Native American medicine, and by early European settlers in America.
- The widespread contemporary use and scientific interest in garlic may stem from antibiotic applications by Louis Pasteur and Albert Schweitzer. Garlic was used during both World Wars to prevent gangrene.[181] Research on garlic began with study of its antibacterial activity in the 1930s, with subsequent investigations into cancer inhibition beginning in the late 1940s.[308] Currently, garlic is one of the most widely used herbal compounds in the United States, with ongoing research in several areas related to cardiovascular health, oncology, and infectious disease. Its mechanism of action appears to be related to multiple compounds and not only to allicin, as was previously believed.

Review of the Evidence: Garlic

Condition Treated*	Study Design	Author, Year	N[†]	SS[†]	Study Quality[‡]	Magnitude of Benefit	ARR[†]	NNT[†]	Comments
Cardiovascular outcomes, cancer (prevention), adverse effects	Systematic review, meta-analysis	Mulrow[1] 2000	NA	Variable	NA	Variable	NA	NA	High-quality analysis; pooled results showed small reduction in TC, LDL, triglycerides after 4-12 weeks, no significant difference after 20 weeks; early evidence for cancer prevention suggested by case-control trials. Also noted: small overall hypotensive effects, platelet aggregation inhibition; no significant glycemic effects.
Cardiovascular outcomes	Meta-analysis	Ackermann[2] 2001	1798	Variable	NA	Variable	NA	NA	Reformulation, update of Mulrow[1] data with similar conclusions.
Hyperlipidemia	Meta-analysis	Stevinson[3] 2000	796	Yes	NA	Small	NA	NA	Pooled results showed modest reductions in TC, but analysis of 6 highest-quality trials showed no significant difference between garlic and placebo (low power).
Hyperlipidemia	Meta-analysis	Silagy[5] 1994	952	Yes	NA	Small	NA	NA	Pooled results showed larger effect on lipids than later analyses; heterogeneous studies included.

Continued

Review of the Evidence: Garlic—*cont'd*

Condition Treated*	Study Design	Author, Year	N[†]	SS[†]	Study Quality[‡]	Magnitude of Benefit	ARR[†]	NNT[†]	Comments
Hyperlipidemia	Meta-analysis	Warshafsky[4] 1993	410	Yes	NA	Small	NA	NA	Pooled results showed larger effect on lipids than later analyses; heterogeneous studies included.
Hyperlipidemia	Systematic review	Alder[371] 2003	10 studies	Yes	NA	Small	NA	NA	Positive results in 6 studies with 9.9% mean reduction in TC; 11.4% mean reduction in LDL.
Hyperlipidemia	RCT, double-blind	Gardner[319] 2001	51	No	5	NA	NA	NA	500-1000 mg dehydrated garlic daily for 12 weeks. No significant difference in multiple lipid parameters; study powered to detect effect size of 10%.
Familial hyperlipidemia (children), hypertension	RCT, double-blind	McCrindle[63] 1998	31	No	5	None	NA	NA	900 mg dehydrated garlic daily in 3 divided doses for 8 weeks. Powered to detect effect size of 10%.
Hyperlipidemia	RCT, double-blind	Neil[140] 1996	115	No	5	NA	NA	NA	900 mg dehydrated garlic daily in 3 divided doses for 24 weeks. Intention-to-treat analysis (14% dropout).
Hyperlipidemia, hypertension	Randomized, comparison study	Holzgartner[119] 1992	98	Yes	5	Medium	NA	NA	900 mg dehydrated garlic vs. 600 mg bezafibrate daily for 12 weeks; low-fat diet in both groups. No significant difference between groups, but no placebo group, unclear if adequately powered.
Hyperlipidemia, hypertension	RCT	Kannar[53] 2001	46	Yes	4	Small	NA	NA	880 mg garlic powder (9.6 mg allicin) daily for 12 weeks. Small significant benefit of enteric-coated garlic on TC and LDL but not triglycerides.
Hyperlipidemia, hypertension	RCT, double-blind	Isaacsohn[120] 1998	40	No	4	NA	NA	NA	300 mg dehydrated garlic daily for 12 weeks. May not have been adequately powered.
Hyperlipidemia, hypertension	RCT, double-blind	Steiner[135] 1996	52	Yes	4	Small	NA	NA	2400 mg "aged garlic extract" powder 3 times daily for 16-24 weeks. Significant reductions in TC and LDL. 20% dropout.
Hyperlipidemia, hypertension	RCT, double-blind	Simons[134] 1995	30	No	4	None	NA	NA	900 mg dehydrated garlic daily in 3 divided doses for 12 weeks. Study may have been underpowered.
Hyperlipidemia, hypertension	RCT, double-blind	Saradeth[133] 1994	68	Yes	4	Small	NA	NA	600 mg dehydrated garlic daily for 15 weeks. Significant drop in cholesterol but not triglycerides.
Hyperlipidemia	RCT, double-blind	Rotzsch[316] 1992	24	Yes	4	Medium	NA	NA	900 mg dehydrated garlic daily for 6 weeks. Reduced triglycerides with garlic vs. placebo.
Hyperlipidemia	RCT, placebo-controlled, double-blind	Mader[142] 1990	261	Yes	4	Medium	NA	NA	800 mg garlic powder daily for 16 weeks. Significant reduction in lipids vs. placebo.
Hyperlipidemia	RCT	Zhang[58] 2001	51	No	3	NA	NA	NA	8.2 mg garlic oil daily for 11 weeks. Effects of garlic significantly more effective in female than in male subjects.
Hyperlipidemia, hypertension	Randomized, controlled trial	Zhang[59] 2001	30	No	3	NA	NA	NA	12.3 mg garlic oil daily for 16 weeks. No significant difference in multiple lipid parameters, but possibly underpowered.

Review of the Evidence: Garlic—cont'd

Condition Treated*	Study Design	Author, Year	N[†]	SS[†]	Study Quality[‡]	Magnitude of Benefit	ARR[†]	NNT[†]	Comments
Hyperlipidemia, hypertension	RCT, double-blind	Superko[136] 2000	50	No	3	None	NA	NA	900 mg dehydrated garlic powder daily in 3 divided doses for 12 weeks.
Atherosclerosis	RCT, double-blind	Koscielny[141] 1999	280	Yes	3	Small	NA	NA	900 mg dehydrated garlic daily for 4 years. Plaque size reduction with garlic vs. increase in placebo. Controversial study, has been criticized; 46% dropout.
Hyperlipidemia	RCT, double-blind	Berthold[55] 1998	26	No	3	None	NA	NA	5 mg steam-distilled coated garlic oil tablets twice daily for 12 weeks. Study may not have been adequately powered.
Peripheral vascular disease, atherosclerosis, hypertension, hyperlipidemia, blood glucose	RCT, double-blind	Czerny[116] 1996	100	Yes	3	Small	NA	NA	400 mg garlic oil plus hawthorn and wheat germ for 4 weeks. Improved walking distance, reduced blood pressure, reduced lipids reported. No significant change in blood glucose (secondary outcome). Unclear effects of other agents (hawthorn has cardiac activity).
Hyperlipidemia	RCT, double-blind	Melvin[313] 1996	34	Yes	3	Small	NA	NA	900 mg daily in three divided doses for 4 weeks. Significant reduction in cholesterol, nonsignificant rise in HDL; 15 subjects became unblinded and switched to garlic (not included in study results).
Hyperlipidemia, hypertension, blood glucose	RCT, double-blind	Jain[121] 1993	42	Yes	3	Small	NA	NA	900 mg dehydrated garlic daily in 3 divided doses for 12 weeks. Significant TC and LDL reductions noted; no significant change in blood glucose (secondary outcome). Between-group comparisons not clearly described.
Peripheral vascular disease, hyperlipidemia, hypertension	RCT, double-blind	Kiesewetter[127] 1993	80	Mixed	3	Mixed	NA	NA	800 mg dehydrated garlic daily for 12 weeks; physical therapy in all subjects. Significant increase in walking distance at 6 weeks but not at 12 weeks; reduction in lipids reported. 20% dropout.
Hyperlipidemia, type 2 diabetes mellitus	RCT, double-blind	Sitprija[26] 1987	40	No	3	None	NA	NA	700 mg dehydrated garlic daily in 2 divided doses for 4 weeks. 17.5% dropout.
Hyperlipidemia, coagulation parameters, hypertension, blood glucose	RCT, double-blind (2 trials reported)	Luley[128] 1986	34, 51	No	3	None	NA	NA	198 mg or 450 mg dehydrated garlic three times daily yielded no effects vs. placebo. Studies may have been underpowered.
Hyperlipidemia	RCT, placebo-controlled, double-blind	Gardner[118] 1999	51	No	2	NA	NA	NA	500 mg or 1000 mg dried, powdered garlic daily for 12 weeks. No significant differences in plasma lipids vs. placebo. May have been underpowered.
Hyperlipidemia (renal transplant patients)	RCT, double-blind	Lash[311] 1998	35	Yes	2	Small	NA	NA	1360 mg dehydrated garlic tablets daily in 2 divided doses. Small reduction in LDL vs. placebo.
Hyperlipidemia, hypertension	RCT (unclear blinding)	Adler[111] 1997	50	Yes	2	Small	NA	NA	900 mg dehydrated garlic daily for 12 weeks. Significant reductions in total cholesterol, LDL, triglycerides; better triglyceride effects in combination with fish oil.

G

Continued

Review of the Evidence: Garlic—*cont'd*

Condition Treated*	Study Design	Author, Year	N[†]	SS[†]	Study Quality[‡]	Magnitude of Benefit	ARR[†]	NNT[†]	Comments
Hyperlipidemia, hypertension, blood glucose	RCT, double-blind	Auer[112] 1990	47	Yes	2	Small	NA	NA	600 mg dehydrated garlic powder daily for 12 weeks. Significant reductions in cholesterol and triglycerides. No significant change in blood glucose (secondary outcome). Methodology described poorly.
Hyperlipidemia	RCT, double-blind	Plengvidhya[315] 1988	30	No	2	Small	NA	NA	700 mg spray-dried garlic daily in 2 divided doses for 8 weeks. Nonsignificant trend to reduce TC and triglycerides and increase HDL.
Hyperlipidemia, hypertension	RCT, placebo-controlled, double-blind	Barrie[113] 1987	20	Yes	2	Medium	NA	NA	18 mg garlic oil daily for 4 weeks with crossover. Significant reductions in cholesterol and blood pressure; increase in HDL. No mention of dropouts.
Hyperlipidemia	RCT, placebo-controlled, double-blind	Satitvipawee[321] 2003	136	No	2	None	NA	NA	5.6 mg allicin daily for 12 weeks in hyperlipidemic subjects not associated with changes in TC, LDL, or HDL. Design and methods not well described.
Hyperlipidemia	Randomized, comparison study	Kannar[124] 1998	90	Yes	1	Small	NA	NA	880 mg enteric-coated dehydrated garlic vs. inulin for 12 weeks; low-fat diet in all subjects. No placebo group; unclear if adequately powered.
Hyperlipidemia, hypertension	Randomized, comparison study (different garlic preparations)	de Santos[57] 1995	80	Unclear	1	Small	NA	NA	Dehydrated garlic vs. garlic oil for 16 weeks. Favorable results reported, but unclear methodology and results.
Hyperlipidemia	Before and after study	Gadkari[159] 1991	50	Mixed	1	Small	NA	NA	10 g raw garlic daily for 8 weeks. Significant reduction in TC, but no direct comparison to placebo.
Hyperlipidemia	Nonrandomized, controlled trial	Bimmermann[144] 1988	60	Mixed	1	NA	NA	NA	3.6-5.4 g garlic daily for 12 weeks. Significant rise in HDL but no significant change in LDL or triglycerides. 18% dropout.
Hyperlipidemia	Placebo-controlled trial	Lau[312] 1987	56	Yes	1	Small	NA	NA	4 capsules (1 mL each) of liquid garlic extract for 6 months. Significant reductions in LDL, TC, VLDL, and increase in HDL vs. placebo. No randomization or blinding.
Hyperlipidemia	Placebo-controlled trial	Peleg[320] 2003	33	No	1	None	NA	NA	22.4 mg alliin daily for 16 weeks resulted in no significant change in TC or LDL. Likely underpowered; poorly conceived statistical approach.
Hyperlipidemia	Comparison study	Ghorai[323] 2000	30	Mixed	0	Small	NA	NA	Dosing unclear. Garlic significantly reduced TC more than Bengal gram seeds, less than guggul. Between-group comparisons not clear.
Hyperlipidemia	Controlled, nonrandomized trial	Bordia[198] 1998	40	Unclear	0	Medium	NA	NA	Garlic oil for 12 weeks associated with reduction in TC and triglycerides, increase in HDL.
Hyperlipidemia (type 2 diabetes mellitus), hypertension, glycemic control	Controlled trial	Mansell[322] 1991	60	No	0	Small	NA	NA	900 mg dehydrated garlic daily in 3 divided doses for 12 weeks. No significant effects on LDL, TC, blood glucose, hemoglobin A_{1c}, C-peptide, or insulin levels.

Review of the Evidence: Garlic—*cont'd*

Condition Treated*	Study Design	Author, Year	N[†]	SS[†]	Study Quality[‡]	Magnitude of Benefit	ARR[†]	NNT[†]	Comments
Hyper-triglyceridemia, hypertension, coronary artery disease, blood glucose	Controlled, double-blind trial (unclear randomization)	Bordia[56] 1981	62	Unclear	0	NA	NA	NA	0.25 mg/kg garlic ether extract for 40 weeks. Poorly described methods and results.
Hyper-triglyceridemia	Before and after trial	Bhushan[324] 1979	25	Yes	0	Small	NA	NA	10 g garlic daily for 8 weeks associated with reduced serum cholesterol; no change in placebo group, but between-group comparison not conducted.
Atherosclerosis	Controlled, double-blind trial, nonrandomized	Orekhov[331] 1996	23	Yes	1	Medium	NA	NA	300 mg dehydrated garlic in single dose or 3 times daily for 3-4 weeks associated with "decreased atherogenicity."
Atherosclerosis	Cross-sectional, observational study	Siegel[330] 2001	202	Yes	0	Medium	NA	NA	900 mg dehydrated garlic daily associated with reduced carotid or femoral artery plaque growth on ultrasound study.
Cutaneous microcirculation	RCT, double-blind	Jung[243] 1991	10	Yes	2	Small	NA	NA	900 mg dehydrated garlic associated with increased cutaneous microcirculation.
Coronary artery disease (secondary prevention)	Controlled trial, unclear blinding or randomization	Bordia[114] 1989	432	Unclear	1	Small	NA	NA	6-8 g garlic ether extract daily for 3 years, with concomitant "standard" postinfarction therapy. Favorable results noted, but not clearly reported.
Hypertension	Meta-analysis	Silagy[6] 1994	415	Yes	NA	Small	NA	NA	600-900 mg dehydrated garlic used in 8 trials; heterogeneous measurements and reporting.
Cancer (prevention)	"Meta-analysis"	Fleischauer[334,352] 2001, 2000	22 studies	NA	NA	Mixed	NA	NA	Association suggested between garlic ingestion and reduced risk of gastric, colorectal cancer.
Cryptococcal meningitis	Case series	Anonymous[110] 1980	21	NA	NA	Large	NA	NA	Oral plus parenteral garlic associated with positive outcomes; some patients given other therapies concomitantly. No controls.
Tinea cruris	Equivalence trial	Ledezma[373] 1996	60	Unclear	2	Large	NA	NA	Topical ajoene vs. terbinafine for 7 days. Unclear blinding, unclear if adequately powered to detect between-group differences.
Tinea pedis	Equivalence trial	Ledezma[374] 1999	70	Unclear	1	Large	NA	NA	Topical ajoene vs. terbinafine for 7 days. Unclear blinding, unclear if adequately powered to detect between-group differences. 33% dropout.
Tick repellent	Controlled trial	Stjernberg[378] 2000	100	Yes	2	Medium	NA	NA	1200 mg allium daily for 8 weeks. No comparison to standard repellant. Methodology has been criticized.
URTI	RCT, double-blind	Josling[23] 2001	146	Yes	4	Medium	NA	NA	Garlic for 12 weeks associated with decreased frequency and duration of colds vs. placebo.
URTI (prevention)	RCT, double-blind	Andrianova[382] 2003	41	Yes	2	Medium	NA	NA	Garlic for 5 months associated with reduced URTI symptoms in children vs. placebo.
Type 2 diabetes mellitus	RCT, double-blind	Sitprija[26] 1987	40	No	3	None	NA	NA	700 mg dehydrated garlic daily in 2 divided doses for 4 weeks. 17.5% dropout.

Continued

G

Review of the Evidence: Garlic—*cont'd*

Condition Treated*	Study Design	Author, Year	N[†]	SS[†]	Study Quality[‡]	Magnitude of Benefit	ARR[†]	NNT[†]	Comments
Blood glucose, platelet aggregation, lipid levels	RCT, double-blind	Kiesewetter[126] 1991	60	Unclear	2	Small	NA	NA	800 mg dehydrated garlic daily for 4 weeks. Drop in blood glucose in nondiabetic subjects by 10 mg/dL; inadequate reporting of methods or statistical analysis; large dropout.
H. pylori infection	Case series	McNulty[384] 2001	5	No	NA	None	NA	NA	4-mg garlic oil capsule 4 times daily for 2 weeks. 5 subjects completed study.
H. pylori infection	Case series	Graham[383] 1999	12	No	NA	None	NA	NA	12 garlic cloves and capsaicin with meals, or bismuth, or no therapy. Subjects served as self controls; methodologically weak design.

*Primary or secondary outcome.
[†]*N*, Number of patients; *SS*, statistically significant; *ARR*, absolute risk reduction; *NNT*, the number of patients who need to undergo a specific intervention in order to observe an outcome in one individual.
[‡]0-2 = poor; 3-4 = good; 5 = excellent.
HDL, High-density lipoprotein; *LDL*, low-density lipoprotein; *NA*, not applicable; *RCT*, randomized, controlled trial; *TC*, total cholesterol; *URTI*, upper respiratory tract infection; *VLDL*, very-low-density lipoprotein.
For an explanation of each category in this table, please see Table 3 in the Introduction.

REVIEW OF THE EVIDENCE: DISCUSSION
Hyperlipidemia
Summary

- Oral tablets containing dehydrated garlic powder appear to elicit modest reductions in total cholesterol compared with levels noted with placebo (<20 mg/dL) in the short term (4 to 12 weeks), with unclear effects after 20 weeks. Small reductions in low-density lipoprotein (LDL) (by <10 mg/dL) and triglycerides (by < 20 mg/dL) may also occur in the short term, although results have been variable. High-density lipoprotein (HDL) values have not been found to change significantly. Numerous controlled trials have examined the effects of oral garlic on serum lipids. Most studies have been small (<100 subjects), with poorly described design and results, and most have reported non-significant modest benefits of garlic therapy. Several overlapping meta-analyses have pooled studies and reported significant mean decreases in total cholesterol between 4 and 12 weeks, and variable significance of reductions in LDL and triglycerides.[1-5] The statistical significance of these effects disappears after 20 weeks,[1] which may be due to low statistical power. The optimal dose and preparation for maximal benefit are not clear, and most studies have used non–enteric-coated dehydrated garlic powder tablets standardized to 1.3% alliin content (Kwai), 900 mg daily in three divided doses. Criticisms of existing trials include the frequent use of the non–enteric-coated preparations, which may allow for degradation of alliinase by gastric acid (although there are scant reliable data on the efficacy of enteric-coated preparations).[53,124] There is also preliminary evidence that aged garlic extract may elicit superior resistance to LDL oxidation compared with fresh garlic.[209] The long-term maintenance of effects remains unclear, and ultimate effect on cardiovascular morbidity and mortality is not known. One study of familial hyperlipidemia in children did not demonstrate significant effects on lipids, although this trial was not designed to detect small effect sizes.

Meta-analyses

- In 2000, Mulrow et al. for the Agency for Health Care Research and Quality prepared a high-quality systematic review and meta-analysis of garlic for cardiovascular disease, cancer prevention, and adverse effects.[1] Literature searches were conducted in 11 electronic databases using accepted synonyms and were not restricted to English-language articles; selection criteria included randomized controlled trials of at least 4 weeks' duration. The authors included 44 studies of lipid outcomes in 42 published articles of garlic for hyperlipidemia.[22,26,55-57,63,111-113,115-125,128-130,133-142,198,309-316] There was variability between trials in terms of method and timing of lipid measurements as a primary or secondary outcome. Quality of design and reporting was also variable, with unclear reporting of randomization techniques in 82% of studies, and unclear blinding in 25%. A majority of the trials included fewer than 100 participants. Most trials were conducted in Germany or the United States and were sponsored by industry. Of these trials, 5 were not placebo controlled,[57,119,122,123,309] and 5 evaluated combination products.[116,129,137,314,319] Meta analyses were conducted of placebo-controlled trials that reported total cholesterol outcomes at 4 to 6 weeks, 8 to 12 weeks, and 20 to 24 weeks. Pooled data demonstrated a significant average reduction in total cholesterol levels of 7.2 mg/dL (95% confidence interval [CI] 1.2 to 13.2) after 4 to 6 weeks of any type of garlic therapy vs. placebo, which increased when only studies using standardized dehydrated preparations were analyzed, to 10.2 mg/dL (95% CI 3.1 to 17.3). Combined data from studies with reported outcomes at 8 to 12 weeks showed a significant average reduction in total cholesterol levels for garlic vs. placebo of 17.1 mg/dL (95% CI 13.0 to 25.4). By contrast, combining the results of eight trials with reported outcomes at 20 to 24 weeks did not demonstrate significant cholesterol reductions compared with levels with placebo (1.2 mg/dL; 95% CI –8.2 to 10.7). This lack of significance may be due to true lack of effect or to low statistical power. These results suggest a need for further study of outcomes beyond 12 weeks.

- This publication also included the results of an analysis of 13 trials reporting LDL changes at 8 to 12 weeks. This analysis revealed a significant reduction of 6.2 mg/dL for garlic vs. placebo (95% CI 0.8 to 11.7), with greater benefits when the analysis was limited to 10 trials using dehydrated garlic preparations (6.7 mg/dL; 95% CI 0 to 13.5). Pooled data from 17 studies measuring triglyceride changes after 8 to 12 weeks showed a significant reduction of 19.1 mg/dL (95% CI 7.6 to 30.4), with greater benefits when analysis was limited to the 13 trials of dehydrated garlic preparations (21.1 mg/dL; 95% CI, 8.3 to 34.0). Analysis of 14 trials that measured HDL levels at 8 to 12 weeks found a nonsignificant reduction of 0.9 mg/dL (95% CI, −1.0 to 2.8).

- In 2001, the results of the analysis of lipid effects by Mulrow et al. were slightly reformulated and published in *Archives of Internal Medicine*.[2] This meta-analysis included 34 randomized trials representing 1798 patient records. The authors noted effects of garlic vs. placebo similar to those in the earlier analysis: small reductions in total cholesterol at 1 month (range of average pooled reductions 1.2 to 17.3 mg/dL), small reductions at 3 months (range of average pooled reductions, 12.4 to 25.4 mg/dL), and no significant differences between garlic and control groups at 6 months. Changes in LDL and triglyceride levels paralleled total cholesterol level results, but no statistically significant changes in HDL were observed. The authors noted that their conclusions were limited by the small sample sizes and low overall quality of the included trials.

- Stevinson et al. conducted a 2000 meta-analysis of garlic therapy for hypercholesterolemia,[3] using more stringent inclusion criteria, analyzing 13 trials including 796 subjects.[55,56,111,112,117,120,121,133,138,140,142,171,315] Trials were excluded that were not randomized, double-blinded, or placebo-controlled; all studies administered oral garlic monotherapy, examined patients with mean baseline cholesterol levels ≥200 mg/dL, and used total cholesterol as an end point. Ten of the 13 studies used the same garlic product (Kwai) in daily doses between 600 and 900 mg, administered over 8 to 24 weeks. Pooling of data revealed a significant reduction in total cholesterol levels for garlic vs. placebo of 15.7 mg/dL (95% CI 5.7 to 25.6). Notably, this analysis included one study of children with familial hypercholesterolemia,[171] a genetic defect that may be more refractory to treatment than other underlying causes of hyperlipidemia, which may have reduced the calculated magnitude of effect. A subanalysis was conducted that pooled data from the six included trials of highest methodologic quality and found a nonsignificant difference between garlic and placebo, although this analysis was of low power. Lawson[317] criticized this meta-analysis, citing the use in most included studies of the product Kwai, which does not have a protective coating to prevent degradation of alliinase by gastric acid. Lack of inclusion of other products and uncertain bioavailability were also noted as potential weaknesses.

- Earlier meta-analyses reported more impressive benefits of garlic over placebo. In 1993, Warshafsky et al. analyzed 5 studies with 410 subjects,[4] and in 1994, Silagy and Neil analyzed 16 studies with 952 subjects.[5] Warshafsky et al. reported a significant reduction in total cholesterol of 23 mg/dL for garlic vs. placebo (95% CI 17 to 29), whereas Silagy and Neil noted a reduction of 29.7 mg/dL for garlic vs. placebo, with no significant difference between daily garlic doses of 600 mg and of 900 mg. Dried garlic was also associated with a moderate decrease in triglyceride levels compared with levels noted with placebo. However, the trials included in these meta-analyses were of heterogeneous design and quality, including inappropriate randomization, lack of dietary control, short duration, and inadequate explanation of statistical analysis in most trials. A 1996 follow-up to the Silagy and Neil meta-analysis reported the results

of a 6-month, randomized controlled trial in 115 patients with moderate hyperlipidemia (total cholesterol 6.0 to 8.5 mmol/L and LDL ≥3.5 mmol/L). Subjects received either placebo or 900 mg of daily dried garlic powder (standardized to 1.3% allicin content). The authors reported no significant benefit of garlic vs. placebo in levels of total cholesterol, LDL, or HDL.[140] A meta-analysis including this trial showed a slightly less significant reduction in total cholesterol levels for garlic vs. placebo than was reported in the earlier Silagy and Neil meta-analysis.

Systematic Review

- In 2003, Alder et al. published a systematic review of 10 randomized controlled trials evaluating garlic for hyperlipidemia.[318] Six studies reported positive effects, with a mean 9.9% reduction in total cholesterol, 11.4% reduction in LDL, and 9.9% reduction in triglycerides. The authors noted small sample sizes, lack of power calculations, and lack of control of diet during studies as limitations of the studies described in existing literature.

Trials Published after the Mulrow and Stevinson Meta-analyses (Post-2000)

- Gardner et al. conducted a randomized, double-blind, placebo-controlled trial to assess the effects of garlic on lipid profiles in 51 moderately hypercholesterolemic subjects.[319] Subjects were randomized to receive placebo or a garlic botanical blend providing 500 to 1000 mg of dehydrated garlic powder daily. The study was designed with calculated power to detect a 10% difference in LDL-C values between groups. The primary outcome parameter was plasma lipid concentration. After 12 weeks of therapy, the authors noted a small significant mean reduction in LDL-C from baseline in the 1000-mg garlic group, no significant changes in LDL-C values in the 500-mg and placebo groups from baseline, and no significant changes in total cholesterol, HDL, or triglyceride levels in any group. There were no significant differences between groups for any measures. These results suggest that the effect of this garlic preparation on lipid values may be less than 10%.

- Kannar et al. conducted a randomized, double-blind, controlled trial to assess the effects of an enteric-coated garlic powder tablet in 46 hyperlipidemic patients.[53] The subjects had mild to moderate hyperlipidemia and had failed or were not compliant with drug therapy. Patients were randomized to receive 880 mg of garlic powder (9.6 mg of allicin) or placebo. After 12 weeks of treatment, the garlic supplement group experienced significant mean reductions in total cholesterol of 4.2% and in LDL of 6.6%, vs. nonsignificant increases in total cholesterol and LDL in the placebo group. Differences between groups were significant. In addition, no significant difference in triglycerides or LDL/HDL ratio was observed between groups. A limitation of this study is the lack of a study arm using non–enteric-coated garlic. Randomization was not clearly described.

- In a poorly described trial, Zhang et al. compared the effects of garlic oil, garlic powder, and placebo in 51 subjects (mean age of 27 years).[58] An initial group of subjects were randomly assigned to receive either 8.2 mg daily of garlic oil (allyl sulfides) or placebo for 11 weeks. Subsequently, an additional group of subjects were recruited and administered garlic powder (7.8 mg of allicin daily). In the garlic groups, significant increases in HDL and decreases in triglycerides were measured in female subjects but not in male subjects. Notably, the differences between female and male patients were statistically significant. It is not clear if other factors may have contributed to differences in the gender-based subgroups, and baseline patient characteristics were not well described. Randomization and blinding were not clearly reported.

- A different publication by the same group described a randomized, placebo-controlled, double-blind trial to assess the effects of garlic oil in 30 male runners.[59] Subjects were randomized to receive either placebo or 12.3 mg of garlic oil daily for 16 weeks. Results were reported as mean differences (95% CIs) between the garlic and the placebo groups. Mean differences were not statistically significant for any outcome parameter: plasma total cholesterol 0.01 mmol/L (–0.34 to 0.37; p = 0.95); plasma triglycerides –0.20 mmol/L (–0.43 to 0.03; p = 0.09), LDL density 0.0019 g/mL (–0.0005 to 0.0043; p = 0.12). The major limitation of this trial was its small sample size.

- Peleg et al. reported the results of a 16-week controlled trial in 33 patients, 13 of whom received garlic (alliin 22.4 mg/day) and 20 who received placebo.[320] Both groups received dietary counselling. No changes were observed in total cholesterol or LDL levels at the study's end. However, the small sample size and poorly conceived statistical analysis make these results clinically limited in value.

- Satitvipawee et al. performed a randomized, placebo-controlled, double-blind trial in 136 hyperlipidemic subjects.[321] Participants were assigned either to receive an enteric-coated garlic tablet once daily (standardized to 5.6 mg [1.12%] allicin content per tablet) or placebo for 12 weeks. At the study's end, the authors reported no significant differences between groups in total cholesterol, LDL, or HDL levels. However, the methods and statistical analysis were not well described.

Randomized, Placebo-Controlled Trials (Pre-2001)

- Adler et al. conducted a randomized, double-blind, controlled trial assessing the effects of garlic in 50 moderately hyperlipidemic men.[111] Subjects were randomized to one of four groups: placebo, 900 mg of a dehydrated garlic preparation (Kwai, containing 1.3% alliin), 12 g of fish oil, or the combination of fish oil and garlic. End points included total cholesterol, LDL, and triglyceride levels. Following 12 weeks of therapy, mean total cholesterol decreased by 12.2% in the combination group and 11.5% in the garlic group, with no change in the placebo and fish oil monotherapy groups. Mean LDL levels decreased by 14.2% in the garlic monotherapy group, decreased by 9.5% in the combination group, increased by 8.5% with fish oil, and did not change with placebo. Mean triglycerides decreased by 37.3% with fish oil, 34.3% with combination therapy, and 6.1% with garlic, with no change with placebo. It is not clear that differences between groups were statistically significant, although reported effect sizes are sufficient that these differences would likely be significant. Blinding and randomization procedures were not well described.

- Isaacsohn et al. conducted a randomized, double-blind, placebo-controlled parallel trial examining the effects of garlic in 28 patients with hyperlipidemia.[120] Subjects were randomized to receive placebo or tablets containing 300 mg of dehydrated garlic powder (Kwai) three times per day (equivalent to approximately 2.7 g or 1 clove of fresh garlic daily) given with meals for 12 weeks. Outcome measures included total cholesterol, triglycerides, LDL, and HDL. The authors reported no significant lipid or lipoprotein

changes in either the placebo or the garlic group, and no significant differences between groups. The sample size of this trial may have been too small to adequately detect between-group differences. Blinding and randomization were adequately described.

- Saradeth et al. conducted a randomized, controlled, double-blind study that evaluated effects of garlic in 68 subjects with normal blood cholesterol.[133] Subjects were randomized to receive either placebo or 600 mg of dried garlic (Kwai) daily for 15 weeks. End points included plasma concentrations of lipids. Results indicated that garlic reduced mean total cholesterol from 223 mg/dL to 214 mg/dL after 10 weeks of treatment, with statistical significance for this therapy vs. placebo. A nonsignificant reduction in mean triglycerides was noted for garlic vs. placebo. This study suggests that garlic may affect lipids in individuals with normal cholesterol profiles.

- Plengvidhya et al. conducted a randomized, controlled, double-blind trial assessing the effects of garlic in 30 patients with primary hyperlipidemia.[315] Patients were randomized to receive placebo or 2 garlic capsules of a spray-dried preparation (350 mg/capsule) daily for 2 months. End points included plasma lipid concentrations. Results revealed nonsignificant trends toward lowering mean total cholesterol and triglyceride concentrations while increasing HDL concentrations for garlic vs. placebo. The sample size may have been too small to detect between-group differences.

- Melvin et al. conducted a randomized, double-blind trial evaluating the effects of garlic in 30 hyperlipidemic subjects (mean age range of 41 to 77 years) who were not receiving any drug therapy.[313] Patients were randomized to receive either placebo or Kwai tablets (dehydrated garlic powder tablets) at a dose of 300 mg three times daily for 30 days. At day 30, both groups were switched to receive a different garlic formulation (LI-114 powder tablets, 300 mg three times daily). On day 60, dosing from the blindly labeled bottles of either placebo or garlic powder tablets was resumed. Lipoprotein profiles were obtained at each 30-day visit. A significant decrease in serum cholesterol was noted within 1 month of treatment with 900 mg daily of LI-114 garlic powder tablets. A 12% reduction in cholesterol levels from baseline over 120 days was achieved, and HDL levels rose, although not to a statistically significant degree. There was no significant effect on serum triglycerides. Patients' weights remained reasonably controlled, and no other drugs were used. Notably, 15 patients became unblinded during the study and were not included in the analysis, which could affect the results. Randomization was not adequately described.

- Mansell et al. investigated the effect of dried garlic tablets (Kwai) in a group of patients with type 2 diabetes mellitus.[322] A total of 60 (46 male and 14 female) subjects, whose diabetes was well controlled on diet or oral medications (median age of 63 years), were included. Baseline serum total cholesterol levels were between 6.0 and 8.0 mmol/L. Patients were randomized to receive placebo or 900 mg of garlic with main meals. After 6 weeks, the results revealed a marginal nonsignificant reduction in mean total cholesterol by 0.3 mmol/L in the garlic group vs. the placebo group (p < 0.07); no difference between groups was detected at 12 weeks. A similar trend was noted for LDL cholesterol values. An increase in HDL concentration by 0.07 mmol/L was noted in the garlic group, vs. a reduction in HDL by 0.04 mmol/L in the placebo group. No differences in serum total or subfractional triglycerides or in apolipoprotein A1 or B were noted between the garlic and the placebo groups. Garlic tablets also had no significant effect on fasting blood glucose, hemoglobin A_{1c}, serum insulin, or C peptide. An odor was noted at least once weekly by 9 of 29 patients on garlic, compared with 1 of 31 on placebo, and by relatives and friends of 10 of 29 patients on garlic, compared with none of the 31 placebo group patients. Blinding and randomization were not clearly described.

- Auer et al. evaluated the effects of garlic in 47 outpatients with mild hypertension in a randomized, placebo-controlled, double-blind trial.[112] Included were patients with diastolic blood pressures between 95 and 104 mm Hg after a 2-week acclimatization phase. Subjects were randomized to receive 600 mg of dehydrated garlic powder (Kwai) or placebo for 12 weeks. The authors reported significant reductions in mean total cholesterol and triglyceride levels in the garlic group vs. the placebo group. However, this report did not adequately describe randomization method or results.

- A 1988 study not included in the Stevinson or Mulrow meta-analysis was reported by Bimmermann et al. These authors conducted a nonrandomized, controlled trial in 60 subjects comparing the effects of placebo, 3.6 g of daily garlic (Carisan), and 5.4 g of daily garlic (Carisan) for 12 weeks.[144] Outcome measures included serum concentrations of LDL, HDL, and triglycerides. No statistically significant effects on LDL or triglycerides were noted, although HDL was found to increase significantly by 24%. Of note, there was an 18% dropout rate secondary to gastrointestinal complaints such as diarrhea, flatulence, fetor, and constipation. The lack of randomization allows for the potential introduction of confounding factors.

- In a randomized, placebo-controlled, double-blind study, Rotzsch et al. examined the efficacy of a standardized dehydrated garlic powder preparation (Sapec, Kwai) on alimentary hypertriglyceridemia in 24 healthy volunteers after consumption of a standardized fatty test meal containing 100 g of butter.[316] Subjects with reduced HDL2-cholesterol concentrations (<10 mg/dL for men and <15 mg/dL for women) were randomized to receive placebo or 900 mg of garlic for 6 weeks. Control measurements were made on days 1, 22, and 43 of treatment, at 0, 3, and 5 hours after intake of the meal. The primary outcome measure was plasma triglyceride concentrations. Results showed a reduced mean postprandial increase of triglycerides in the garlic group vs. the placebo group. The area-under-the-curve (AUC) values for the triglycerides were up to 35% lower in the garlic group than in the placebo group. Randomization was not well described, and dropouts were not discussed.

- A 1991 controlled trial not included in the Stevinson or Mulrow meta-analysis was reported by Gadkari and Joshi.[159] In this study, the effects of raw garlic were assessed in 50 medical students aged 17 to 22 years.[159] Subjects received either 10 g of raw garlic taken daily after breakfast or no treatment for 2 months. In the raw garlic group, there was a significant decrease in serum total cholesterol levels. In the control group, there were not any significant changes noted. However, it is not clear that adequate and significant between-group differences occurred.

- A significant decrease in cholesterol levels was associated with aged garlic extract (AGE) powder administered in capsules in a trial reported by Steiner et al.[135] In a double-blind, crossover fashion, 2400 mg (3 capsules) of AGE was taken three times a day by 52 subjects with hypercholesterolemia.

The active treatment phase was 4 to 6 months long. Serum cholesterol levels were assessed at 4-week intervals. At maximal decrease, total cholesterol was reportedly reduced by 7% from baseline, and LDL was reduced 4% from baseline ($p < 0.05$).[135] This is one of few studies with a sample size <100 that demonstrated statistically significant results. Limitations included a 20% dropout rate and lack of description of randomization.

- Simons et al. conducted a double-blind, 12-week trial evaluating the effects of garlic in 30 hyperlipidemic patients.[134] Subjects were randomized to receive placebo or dehydrated garlic powder tablets (Kwai, 300 mg each) three times daily for 12 weeks, followed by a 28-day washout, and then crossover regimen for an additional 12 weeks. All subjects were maintained on a low-cholesterol diet during the trial period. Outcome parameters included plasma cholesterol concentrations, lipoprotein(a) concentrations, and blood pressure. No significant changes in outcome measures were noted at the study's completion (mean LDL with garlic 4.64 + 0.52 mmol/L vs. with placebo 4.60 + 0.59 mmol/L). The sample size may have been too small to detect between-group differences, and the effect size may have been further diminished by the use of a low-cholesterol diet in both groups. Method of randomization was not clearly described.

- A significant decrease in cholesterol levels was associated with the use of a dehydrated garlic tablet, Pure-Gar, in a study by Lash et al.[311] This randomized, controlled trial was conducted in 35 subjects who had undergone renal transplantation >6 months earlier and had elevated lipid levels. Garlic tablets 680 mg twice a day or placebo tablets were administered for 12 weeks in a blinded fashion; however, it is not clear that the investigators were blinded to treatment assignment. Overall, there was a 5.2% decrease in both total and LDL cholesterol from baseline in the subjects who received garlic, compared with no decrease in those assigned to the placebo group ($p < 0.05$).[311]

- Berthold et al. assessed the effects of garlic in 26 patients with moderate hyperlipidemia and no history of coronary disease in a randomized, double-blind, crossover trial.[55] Subjects were not receiving any medications that could potentially affect lipid metabolism and were otherwise healthy. The study design included two crossover sequences, each starting with a 4-week single-blind placebo phase, which was then followed by a double-blind 12-week treatment phase. Patients were randomized to receive placebo or 1 coated garlic tablet (Tegra, a commercially available preparation of steam-distilled garlic oil 5 mg, approximately equivalent to 4 to 5 g of fresh garlic cloves or 4000 units of allicin) twice daily. Outcome measures included plasma concentrations of total cholesterol, LDL, HDL, and triglycerides. Results did not show any significant differences in outcome measures. In addition, fractional cholesterol absorption from the intestine was 39.3 + 10.7% with placebo treatment and 37.5 + 10.5% with garlic treatment, without significant differences between groups. Because of the small size of this trial, lack of adequate power calculation, and the small effect size noted in other trials, the sample size in this trial may not have been sufficient to detect between-group differences.

- Superko et al. conducted a double-blind, randomized, placebo-controlled trial in 50 moderately hypercholesterolemic patients (mean LDL level of 166 mg/dL) to assess effects of garlic on hyperlipidemia.[136] The study included 22 patients characterized as having LDL subclass pattern A (predominantly large LDL) and 28 subjects classified as having subpattern B (predominantly small LDL). After a 2-month stabilization phase, subjects were randomized to receive placebo or 300 mg of a standardized dehydrated garlic tablet (Kwai) three times daily for 3 months. Results revealed that for all subjects (LDL pattern A and pattern B subjects combined), garlic treatment produced no significant changes in total cholesterol, LDL cholesterol, HDL cholesterol, HDL subclass distribution, postprandial triglycerides, apolipoprotein B, lipoprotein(a), LDL peak particle diameter, or LDL subclass distribution.

- Bordia published the results of a poorly designed/reported double-blind, randomized trial in 62 subjects with coronary artery disease and triglyceride levels of 250 to 350 mg/dL.[56] Patients were administered placebo or a garlic ether extract (0.25 mg/kg) for 10 months. Although favorable outcomes were reported (significant decreases in total cholesterol and triglycerides and increases in HDL in the garlic group), the authors did not clearly describe the process of randomization or blinding, baseline patient characteristics, dropouts, or statistical analysis.
- In a larger study, Bordia administered 6 to 10 g of a garlic ether extract or placebo for 3 years to 432 subjects with a history of myocardial infarction.[115] These patients received concomitant "standard" postinfarction therapy according to the study. Primary outcomes included reinfarction and death, although lipids were also evaluated. Although superior outcomes were reported in the garlic group, randomization and blinding were not discussed, baseline patient characteristics were not specified (although stated to be equivalent), dropouts were not noted, and statistical analysis was not clearly conducted.
- Jain et al. reported a controlled, double-blind trial of dehydrated garlic (Kwai) 900 mg vs. placebo daily in three divided doses in 42 outpatients with hypercholesterolemia (total cholesterol >220 mg/dL).[121] After 12 weeks of therapy, a significant mean reduction in total cholesterol, by 6%, was noted in the garlic group, whereas no significant changes were noted in the placebo group. LDL values dropped by 11% in the garlic group, whereas no significant change occurred in the placebo group. However, it is not clear that between-group differences were appropriately measured for statistical significance. Blinding was not clearly described.
- Kiesewetter et al. reported the results of a double-blind, placebo-controlled trial in 60 patients who were believed to have increased levels of platelet aggregation (13% were smokers).[126] Subjects were randomized to receive dehydrated garlic powder tablets (Kwai) 800 mg daily or placebo for 4 weeks. The primary end point was the effect on platelet aggregation, although the authors reported significant decreases in several parameters related to cardiovascular risk, including serum cholesterol. The results, statistical analysis, and randomization for this trial were not clearly reported, and >20% of subjects dropped out without adequate explanation or analysis.
- Kiesewetter et al. conducted a double-blind, controlled trial in 80 patients with (Fontaine stage II) peripheral vascular disease.[22] Subjects were administered 800 mg of dehydrated garlic daily (Kwai) or placebo for 12 weeks, in addition to physical therapy in both groups. The primary end point was effect on walking distance, although the authors also reported significant decreases in several parameters related to cardiovascular risk, including serum cholesterol and blood pressure. It is not clear that results were compared between groups adequately, and randomization was not well described.

- Neil et al. conducted a double-blind, placebo-controlled trial in 115 patients with hyperlipidemia (total cholesterol >230 mg/dL and LDL >130 mg/dL).[140] Following 6 weeks of dietary counseling, subjects were randomized to receive dehydrated garlic powder tablets (Kwai) 900 mg in three divided daily doses or placebo for 6 months. In an intention-to-treat analysis, the authors reported no significant differences between groups in terms of mean concentration of serum lipids, lipoproteins, or apolipoprotein A1 or B. Randomization and blinding were well described.
- Mader et al. reported a randomized, placebo-controlled, double-blind trial assessing the effects of dehydrated garlic powder (Kwai) in 261 patients with hyperlipidemia.[142] Patients were randomized to receive either placebo or 800 mg of garlic powder for 16 weeks. Outcome parameters included mean serum concentrations of cholesterol and of triglycerides. Results indicated that mean serum cholesterol levels decreased in the garlic group from 266 mg/dL to 235 mg/dL, whereas mean triglyceride values decreased from 226 mg/dL to 188 mg/dL. The difference between the garlic and the placebo groups was significant ($p < 0.001$). Randomization and blinding were well described.
- Similar results have been reported by additional small trials comparing various garlic preparations with placebo, often reporting nonsignificant trends toward lipid-lowering properties of garlic, with questionable statistical power to detect between-group differences. Barrie et al. conducted a randomized, placebo-controlled trial in 20 healthy subjects (mean age of 26 years).[113] Subjects were administered either placebo or 18 mg of a garlic oil macerate for 4 weeks. Randomization and blinding were well described. De Santos and Grunwald reported a placebo-controlled, double-blind trial in 60 patients with hypertriglyceridemia.[117] Subjects were assigned to receive placebo or dehydrated garlic (Kwai) 900 mg over 24 weeks. All patients were on a low-fat diet. Results were limited by small sample size and unclear descriptions of randomization or statistical analysis. Gardner et al. compared dehydrated garlic 500 to 1000 mg with placebo in 53 hyperlipidemic patients (LDL 130 to 190 mg/dL) over a 12-week period.[118] Double-blinding was well described, although randomization was unclear; dropout rates were low. Kandziora et al. conducted two trials of similar design, each in 40 patients with hypercholesterolemia (total cholesterol >280 mg/dL), both for 12 weeks. The first study was single-blinded with unclear randomization and compared dehydrated garlic (Kwai) 600 mg daily with placebo.[123] The second trial was double-blinded with unclear randomization and compared Kwai plus an antihypertensive medication with placebo.[122] Lau et al. reported two trials in a single publication, in which 32 subjects with hyperlipidemia and 14 subjects with normal cholesterol levels were assigned to receive either 4 mL of Aged Garlic Extract (a proprietary commercial formulation containing 250 mg/mL of garlic) or placebo for 26 weeks.[312] Primary outcomes included change in serum lipid levels. Plengvidhya et al. administered 700 mg of a dried garlic powder preparation or placebo to 30 patients with mild to moderate hyperlipidemia in a 6-week double-blind trial.[315] Methods and results were not clearly reported. Sitprija et al. assigned 40 outpatients with diabetes to receive 700 mg of dried garlic or placebo for 4 weeks.[26] Dropout rate was >20% without adequate descriptions of dropouts. Randomization was not well described. Vorberg and Schneider[138] administered 900 mg of dehydrated garlic (Kwai) or placebo in three divided daily

doses to 40 nondiabetic patients with hyperlipidemia (total cholesterol >230 mg/dL). Double-blinding was described, although randomization was unclear. Yeh et al. reported the results of a double-blind trial in 34 hyperlipidemic outpatients without other health problems.[139] Subjects received placebo or 7200 mg of Aged Garlic Extract (a proprietary formulation) daily for 20 weeks. Randomization and statistical analysis were not well described.

Randomized Comparison Trials (Pre-2001)

- Luley et al. conducted two 6-week, randomized, controlled, double-blind studies to assess the effects of dried garlic on blood lipids, apolipoproteins, and blood coagulation in hyperlipidemic patients.[128] Study I (n = 34) randomized patients to receive placebo or 198 mg of dried garlic three times daily, whereas Study II (n = 51) randomized patients to receive placebo or 450 mg of dried garlic three times daily. Primary end points for both studies included total cholesterol, HDL, LDL, triglycerides, coagulation end points, and tolerance. Results showed that neither dose of garlic produced any significant effects on any of the primary end points. Lack of effect may have been related to the form of garlic used, as it has been hypothesized that dried garlic may not be as efficacious as other garlic preparations. A small sample size may have led to inadequate power to detect differences between groups.

- A 2000 study not included in the Stevinson or Mulrow meta-analysis was reported by Ghorai et al. This was a comparison trial examining the efficacy of guggulipid, Bengal gram seed, and garlic (allicin) in 30 normal volunteers for 8 weeks.[323] The primary end point was total cholesterol concentration. Results showed that guggulipid therapy significantly reduced mean serum cholesterol levels by 33%, allicin significantly reduced mean total cholesterol levels by 13%, and whole germinated Bengal gram seeds resulted in a reduction of 13%. Outcomes were compared with baseline values, and results were not compared statistically between groups. Another limitation of this trial was the lack of a separate placebo group.

- Holzgartner compared the efficacy of a dehydrated garlic preparation (Sapec, Kwai) with that of bezafibrate in a randomized, double-blind, multicenter trial including 98 patients with primary hyperlipoproteinemia.[119] After a preplacebo phase of 6 weeks, patients were randomized to receive daily doses of 900 mg of garlic powder (standardized as to 1.3% alliin) or 600 mg of bezafibrate for 12 weeks. In addition to drug treatment, patients were advised to follow a low-fat "Step 1" diet. Outcome measures included plasma values of LDL, HDL, total cholesterol, and triglyceride concentrations. The authors reported a highly statistically significant rise in HDL cholesterol with both garlic (from 34.3 mg/dL to 48.6 mg/dL) and bezafibrate, as well as a significant decrease in LDL cholesterol (from 195.3 mg/dL to 130.2 mg/dL) and triglycerides (from 306 mg/dL to 207.5 mg/dL) in both groups. There was no significant difference between the two treatments. There was no correlation between the perception of garlic odor and effects on cholesterol levels. This trial was limited by lack of a separate placebo group.

- A comparison between two different garlic preparations was reported by de Santos et al.[57] This study was a randomized, double-blind trial in 80 patients with mild hypercholesterolemia, conducted over 16 weeks. Subjects were randomized to receive either dehydrated garlic (Kwai) or Hoefels Original

Garlic Oil (1.98 mg). Although favorable lipid outcomes were reported in both groups, the lack of a placebo arm, unclear randomization, 15% dropout rate, and unclear statistical analysis reduce the clinical utility of the results.

- Kannar reported the results of a three-arm randomized, double-blind trial in an unpublished dissertation, in which 90 subjects with total cholesterol >250 mg/dL were randomized to receive an enteric-coated dehydrated garlic tablet 880 mg or inulin, or a combination of both for 12 weeks.[124] A low-fat diet was observed by all participants. Reductions in cholesterol levels were noted with the use of garlic, although the lack of a placebo arm diminishes the clinical applicability of this study.

Controlled, Nonrandomized Trials

- Bordia et al. evaluated the effects of a garlic ether extract on lipid parameters in 40 patients with coronary artery disease, over 3 months.[198] Patients received either placebo or garlic oil. Outcome parameters included plasma lipid concentrations. The authors reported that total cholesterol was reduced by 12.8% and triglycerides by 15.2% from baseline, and HDL increased by 22.3% from baseline, at 3 months in the garlic group. Between-group comparisons were not clearly evaluated, and the design was limited by a lack of apparent randomization and unclear blinding.

- In a controlled, nonblinded trial with unclear randomization, Bhushan et al. studied the effect of raw garlic on cholesterol levels in 25 young males with triglyceride levels 160 to 250 mg/dL (ages 18 to 35 years).[324] Subjects who had never ingested garlic were recruited and either were administered 10 g of garlic daily as a part of their diet for 2 months or received a diet without garlic. Fasting blood samples were drawn before and after 2 months of garlic intake. The authors reported that serum total cholesterol concentration decreased significantly in all subjects taking garlic, whereas no significant changes occurred with placebo. Between-group comparisons were not conducted.

Combination Products

- Although most literature in this area has focused on the effects of garlic used in monotherapy for hypercholesterolemia, several studies have examined combination treatments consisting of garlic and one or more additional agents, such as fish oil,[111,314,325] in which significant and greater effects on multiple lipid parameters were reported in comparison with garlic treatment alone. In one study, a combination tablet containing 120 mg of *Ginkgo biloba* extract and 200 mg of garlic extract was compared with placebo for a 2-month period in 43 subjects with hypercholesterolemia.[310] No significant difference in total cholesterol levels was observed, although this trial may have been too small to detect between-group differences. Notably, there is no evidence elsewhere that ginkgo exerts clinical effects on cholesterol levels. A poorly designed and reported small study administered 50 mg of hawthorn and 150 mg of garlic three times daily vs. placebo and reported a small decrease in total cholesterol levels after 2 months.[137] Czerny and Samochowiec administered a combination of hawthorn, wheat germ, and garlic oil macerate (400 mg) to 100 hyperlipidemic patients for 16 weeks and reported small improvements of unclear statistical significance.[116] Blinding and randomization were not clearly described. In a poorly designed and reported study, Lutomski administered a combination therapy including garlic (Ilja Rogoff) 300 mg daily or placebo to 102 subjects

G

with clinical diagnoses believed to be related to atherosclerosis.[129] After 12 weeks of therapy, significant beneficial effects on cholesterol were reported, although it is not clear that these results were compared between groups. Randomization was not clear, and >15% of subjects dropped out. Morcos conducted a single-blind comparison of placebo with a combination therapy including fish oil (1800 mg of eicosapenteanoic acid plus 1200 mg of docosahexaenoic acid) and garlic powder (1200 mg).[314] In 40 hyperlipidemic subjects (total cholesterol >200 mg/dL), after 4 weeks of therapy, garlic was associated with an 11% decrease in triglycerides, 34% reduction in triglycerides, and 10% decrease in LDL from baseline. No significant changes occurred in the placebo group, although between-group comparisons were not conducted, and it is therefore not clear if changes in the garlic group were significantly superior to results with placebo. Ventura et al. assigned 40 patients with hypercholesterolemia (total cholesterol >200 mg/dL) to receive either Fitoaglio (a combination of dried garlic 450 mg and hawthorn 150 mg) in three divided daily doses or placebo for 8 weeks.[137] The authors reported a 10% decrease in total cholesterol levels, although statistical analysis was not provided, between-group differences were not calculated, and descriptions of randomization or blinding were absent.

Case Series

- Brosche et al. conducted a study evaluating the effect of a dried garlic powder preparation (standardized to 1.3% alliin content) on the composition of plasma lipoproteins.[326] A total of 40 volunteers (aged 70 years and older) received 600 mg of garlic powder daily for 3 months. In 11 participants with initially normal total cholesterol levels (<200 mg/dL) after 3 months of garlic tablet administration, little or no change in values was noted. By contrast, in 29 volunteers with initially elevated total cholesterol (>200 mg/dL), levels were reduced by 7.7% ($p < 0.001$). Triglycerides (−15.9%; $p < 0.05$) and plasma choline phospholipids (−4.6%; $p < 0.01$) were also reduced. No changes in the LDL/HDL ratio were observed. In the absence of a control group, the clinical applicability of these results is limited.

Familial Hyperlipidemia
Summary

- One small study of familial hyperlipidemia in children did not demonstrate significant effects on lipids, although this trial was not designed to detect small effect sizes. Therefore, it is possible that small reductions in total cholesterol and LDL may occur, although such reductions may not be of significant clinical benefit. Further study in this area may be merited.

Evidence

- McCrindle et al. conducted a randomized, double-blind, placebo-controlled trial in 31 children (ages 8 to 18 years) with historical evidence of familial hyperlipidemia and total cholesterol levels >185 mg/dL.[63] Subjects without evidence of smoking or alcohol use were included. Patients were randomized to receive either 900 mg of dehydrated garlic powder tablets (Kwai) in three divided daily doses or placebo. The groups had similar baseline characteristics, and all subjects were on a low-cholesterol diet. Primary outcomes measures included fasting lipid values. After 8 weeks of therapy, the authors reported no statistically significant effect

of garlic therapy compared with placebo in levels of total cholesterol (+0.6%; 95% CI −5.8% to +6.9%) or LDL (−0.5%; 95% CI −8.7% to +7.6%). The study was designed to detect an effect size of >10% in the garlic group vs. the placebo group. In addition, no significant effects were seen on levels of HDL, triglycerides, apolipoprotein B-100, lipoprotein(a), fibrinogen, homocysteine, or blood pressure. A small significant effect on apolipoprotein A-I was seen (+10.0%; 95% CI +1.2% to +16.5%; $p = 0.03$). These results suggest that garlic monotherapy may not have a role in the management of familial hyperlipidemia. However, the short duration of this study and the small sample size may have allowed for delayed or small effect sizes to be missed. Randomization, blinding, and statistical analysis were well described.

Atherosclerosis
Summary

- Meta-analyses of garlic trials suggest modest short-term reductions in total cholesterol and LDL levels with oral garlic supplements.[1-5] Long-term effects on lipids are not clear. There is limited evidence regarding the effects of garlic on the prevention or treatment of atherosclerosis. A small number of studies have explored this issue and reported favorable results, although overall these studies have been poorly designed and reported, with unclear descriptions of randomization, blinding, plaque measurement methods, and statistical analysis.[2,327] There is currently insufficient evidence demonstrating effects of garlic on atherosclerosis, and further study is warranted in this area.

Evidence

- Koscielny et al. reported the results of a double-blind, placebo-controlled trial in 280 subjects with significant but asymptomatic atherosclerotic disease of the carotid or femoral artery without limitations on blood flow.[141] Greater than 60% of subjects had elevated total cholesterol, 30% were smokers, and 40% were hypertensive. Subjects were assigned to receive 900 mg of a standardized dehydrated garlic powder tablet (Kwai) or placebo daily for 4 years. The authors reported a mean reduction in plaque volume of 2.6% with garlic vs. an increase in volume by 15.6% with placebo (measured by B-mode ultrasound examination). Subgroup analysis by gender revealed markedly better results in women than in men, with a large, 53% increase in plaque size among women taking placebo. A subsequent letter conducting a statistical reevaluation showed significant values confirmed in women but not in combined results of men and women.[327] Although these results are compelling, multiple questions have been raised about the results of this study. Baseline characteristics between groups were not equivalent, with a younger average age of women in the placebo group, and 46% of subjects dropped out before study completion. Concerns have also been raised regarding the accuracy and authenticity of ultrasound measurements reported in the trial.[328,329]

- Siegel et al. conducted a cross-sectional observational study assessing effect of garlic on plaque volumes in the carotid and femoral arteries of 202 subjects.[330] A total of 101 healthy adults who had been taking ≥300 mg daily or a greater amount of garlic for ≥2 years were included and compared with 101 age- and sex-matched control subjects. Patients were administered 900 mg of daily dehydrated garlic (Kwai, Sapec). The primary outcome measure of plaque volume was determined by B-mode ultrasound. The authors reported a significantly lower mean growth of plaque volume with garlic than with placebo (7% and 18%, respectively). Regression of plaque was noted in some patients using garlic. However, this study was not comprehensively reported, and the adequacy of design and statistical analysis are not clear.

- Orekhov et al. conducted a nonrandomized, double-blind, placebo-controlled trial to assess the effects of garlic on "atherogenicity" (the effects of treated patients' serum on cultured human aortic smooth muscle cells) in 23 patients with coronary artery disease.[331] Subjects received either placebo or dehydrated garlic powder tablets (Kwai). In an evaluation of acute effects, the authors reported that at 2 to 4 hours following a single 300-mg dose of Kwai, there was reduced atherogenicity in garlic patients' blood, resulting in less cholesterol accumulation in the cultured cells. Following 3 to 4 weeks of a regimen of Kwai 300 mg three times daily, blood serum atherogenicity was reported as significantly lower compared with baseline (as low as half of baseline). Although the placebo group experienced no significant changes throughout the observation period, the significance of differences between groups was not clearly reported. This study was poorly designed and reported, with unclear blinding, and lacked randomization, thus allowing for the possible introduction of bias and confounding variables.

Peripheral Vascular Disease
Summary

- Meta-analyses of garlic trials suggest modest short-term reductions in total cholesterol and LDL levels with oral garlic supplements.[1-5] Long-term effects on lipids and atherosclerosis are not clear. Vasorelaxation is also reported in preclinical studies.[240-242] There is limited evidence regarding the effects of garlic in patients with peripheral vascular disease or claudication. A small number of studies have explored this issue and reported favorable results, including increased walking distances. However, these studies have overall been poorly designed and reported, with unclear descriptions of randomization, blinding, and statistical analysis.[2,327] There is currently insufficient evidence demonstrating effects of garlic on peripheral vascular disease, and further study is warranted in this area.

Claudication

- Kiesewetter et al. conducted a double-blind controlled trial in 80 patients with Fontaine stage II peripheral vascular disease and lower extremity vascular lesions with >60% occlusion of vessels.[22] Subjects were administered 800 mg of dehydrated garlic daily (Kwai) or placebo for 12 weeks, in addition to physical therapy (in both groups). The primary end point was effect on walking distance, although the authors also reported significant decreases in several parameters related to cardiovascular risk, including serum cholesterol and blood pressure. The authors reported a significant increase ($p < 0.05$) in mean walking distance compared with that noted with placebo only during the last 6 weeks of treatment (46 m vs. 31 m); however, the difference at 12 weeks was not significant (range, 161 to 207 m in the garlic group vs. 172 to 203 m in placebo group). A total of 16 patients did not complete the trial (20%), descriptions of dropouts were limited, and an intention-to-treat analysis was not conducted. Review of the results by a different group reported lack of statistical significance.[1]

- Czerny et al. conducted a randomized, double-blind, placebo-controlled study in 100 patients with hyperlipidemia, hypertension, and "atherosclerotic disease," including patients with Fontaine stage II peripheral vascular disease (unclear distribution).[116] Subjects were administered placebo or Preparation R, which includes 400 mg of garlic oil, hawthorn, and wheat germ, for 4 weeks. Primary end points included walking range (determined using a belt ergometer) and blood pressure. Serum lipids were also measured. The authors reported that patients taking Preparation R experienced a statistically significant mean improvement in walking distance of 114%, vs. 17% with placebo ($p < 0.05$). Significant improvements were also reported in lipid status (total cholesterol, triglycerides) and in systolic and diastolic blood pressures. Notably, hawthorn has been associated with improved exercise tolerance in patients with congestive heart failure, although it is unclear if this effect played a role in this study. Randomization, blinding, and statistical analysis were not well described.

- Notably, in 2001, Jepson et al. conducted a systematic review to assess the effects of garlic (both dried and nonpowdered preparations) in the treatment of peripheral arterial occlusive disease.[332] Selection criteria included randomized trials in patients with lower limb atherosclerosis, and outcomes included objective measures of progression of underlying atherosclerosis as well as subjective measures. This review found one trial[22] (discussed earlier) that fit eligibility requirements.

Peripheral Circulation

- Jung et al. conducted a randomized, placebo-controlled, double-blind, crossover trial examining the effects of garlic powder on cutaneous microcirculation.[243,244] Ten healthy volunteers were recruited and received either placebo or dehydrated garlic powder tablets (Kwai, Sapec) 900 mg daily. Results showed that 5 hours after garlic powder consumption, a significant increase in capillary skin perfusion by 55% occurred. Similar changes did not occur in the placebo group, although it is not clear that a direct comparison was made between groups. Limitations of this study include poor descriptions of randomization and blinding methods.

- Siegel et al. conducted a cross-sectional observational study comparing 101 health adults taking a standardized dehydrated garlic powder (Kwai, Sapec), in a daily dose of 300 mg or greater for >2 years, with a group of 101 age/sex-matched control subjects.[330] Outcome parameters included pulse wave velocity and pressure-standardized elastic vascular resistance, which allow assessments of the elastic properties of the aorta. Results showed significantly lower pulse wave velocity and pressure-standardized elastic vascular resistance in the garlic group than in the control group. Garlic appeared to elicit superior results in older patients and those with higher systolic blood pressures. Limitations of this study include lack of prospective randomization and blinding.

Cardiac Secondary Prevention
Summary

- Meta-analyses of garlic trials suggest modest short-term reductions in total cholesterol and LDL levels with oral garlic supplements.[1-5] Long-term effects on lipids and atherosclerosis are not clear. There is limited evidence regarding the effects of garlic on cardiac morbidity and mortality, and it is currently unclear if garlic reduces the incidence of myocardial infarction or cardiac death.

Evidence

- Bordia administered 6 to 10 g of a garlic ether extract or placebo for 3 years to 432 subjects with a history of myocardial infarction.[115] All patients received concomitant "standard" 1989 postinfarction therapy according to the study. Primary outcomes included reinfarction and death, and lipids were also evaluated. Superior outcomes were reported in the garlic group vs. the placebo group, although these results do not appear to be statistically significant between groups (reinfarction rate 7% with garlic vs. 10% with placebo; death rate 5% with garlic vs. 10% with placebo). Randomization and blinding were not discussed, baseline patient characteristics were not specified (although stated to be equivalent), and dropouts were not noted.

Hypertension
Summary

- Numerous studies have reported small mean reductions in systolic and diastolic blood pressures associated with the use of oral garlic vs. placebo. In general, mean differences have been less than 10 mm Hg (<10%). A majority of the studies have been small (<100 subjects), with poor descriptions of methodology and results. Blood pressure measurements have often not been measured as primary outcomes, and in many cases, specific blood pressure numbers have not been provided. Methods and timing of measurement have been variable. A 1994 meta-analysis of 8 trials[6] reported a small mean reduction of 7.7 mm Hg in systolic blood pressure with use of a standardized dehydrated garlic formulation (Kwai) 600 to 900 mg daily, whereas a 2000 systematic review of 27 studies[1,2] was not able to pool studies because of heterogeneity of results (although most studies reported small reductions in systolic blood pressure of variable significance; most trials used Kwai). Preliminary data suggest that dehydrated garlic products such as Kwai may be more efficacious than garlic oil.[57] It has also been proposed that enteric-coated formulations may be more effective than non–enteric-coated products such as Kwai. Overall, it appears that oral garlic may exert a small blood pressure–lowering effect, although the currently available evidence in this area is weak. It is not clear if effects are more pronounced in hypertensive than in normotensive individuals.

Meta-analysis and Systematic Review

- A meta-analysis of the effects of garlic on blood pressure was performed by Silagy and Neil in 1994.[6] Studies were included that were prospective, randomized, and controlled; were >4 weeks in duration (range, 4 to 40 months); and specified both diastolic and systolic blood pressure readings. The authors included eight trials with a total of 415 subjects (both hypertensive and normotensive). One study was single-blinded,[122,123] whereas all others were self-described as double-blinded.[112,117,119,121,123,126,138] All trials used the non–enteric-coated dehydrated garlic powder preparation Kwai in a daily dosage between 600 and 900 mg. Results were reported as the difference between mean changes in blood pressure in garlic and control groups (in mm Hg). Mean systolic blood pressure was found to be 7.7 mm Hg lower in the garlic treatment group than in the placebo group. Mean diastolic blood pressure was found to be 5.0 mm Hg lower with garlic than with placebo. Effects were

greatest when analysis was limited to two trials with samples that only included hypertensive subjects.[112,123] The authors concluded that effects with garlic appeared to be less than with standard antihypertensive medications, although this finding has not been well studied.[123] Overall, the included studies did not include adequate descriptions of blinding methods or compliance, samples were heterogeneous, sample sizes were small (<100), and methods of blood pressure measurement were not consistently well described.

- In 2000, Mulrow et al. for the Agency for Health Care Research and Quality prepared a high-quality systematic review of garlic for cardiovascular disease, cancer prevention, and adverse effects.[1] Literature searches were conducted in 11 electronic databases using accepted synonyms and were not restricted to English-language articles; selection criteria included randomized, controlled trials of at least 4 weeks in duration. The authors included 28 studies (in 27 published articles) that measured blood pressure, although a majority of the trials reported blood pressure as a secondary outcome.[22,57,63,111-125,128-130,133-139] There was variability between trials in terms of method and timing of measurements. Quality of design and reporting was also variable, with unclear reporting of randomization techniques in 79% of studies. A majority of the trials included fewer than 100 participants. Most studies were conducted in Germany or the United States and were sponsored by industry. A majority of the trials used non–enteric-coated dehydrated garlic powder tablets (Kwai). Four studies were not placebo controlled,[57,119,122,123] one of which compared garlic with an antihypertensive medication[123]; the remaining three studies evaluated combination products.[116,129,137] Statistically significant reductions in systolic blood pressure of 2% to 7% were reported by three studies at 10 to 13 weeks of follow-up[111,112,138] and in three studies at 5 to 6 months.[117,135,139] Methods of assessing blood pressures were variable, and more than half of the studies did not report specific blood pressure measurements. Therefore, the results were not pooled by Mulrow et al. In 2001, the results of the analysis by Mulrow et al. were slightly reformulated and published in Archives of Internal Medicine, with similar conclusions.[2]

Additional Studies (Not Included in Analyses by Silagy et al. and Mulrow et al.)

- Additional studies of low methodologic quality have been reported, which do not alter the level of evidence available in this area.
- Zhang et al. described a randomized, placebo-controlled, double-blind trial to assess the effects of garlic oil in 30 male runners.[59] Subjects were randomized to receive either placebo or 12.3 mg of garlic oil daily for 16 weeks. A nonsignificant small mean reduction in systolic blood pressure was observed in the garlic group (–4.5 mm Hg; 95% CI –10.8 to 1.9; $p = 0.16$). The sample size may have been too small to detect between-group differences.
- McMahon[131] conducted an open, uncontrolled trial of the acute effects of high-dose garlic (2400 mg of Kwai, single dose) in a small sample of "severely hypertensive" subjects. Subjects' diastolic blood pressures were reported as significantly reduced over the 24-hour period following the dose with a peak effect at 5 hours.
- A small observational study by Qidwai et al. reported benefits of dietary garlic on blood pressure.[132] The authors administered a dietary questionnaire to 101 healthy adults (who did not have hypertension, obesity, or coronary heart

disease and did not use antihypertensive medications). Average daily garlic use was 134 g. The authors reported that individuals with lower systolic and diastolic blood pressures consumed greater amounts of garlic on average.

Cancer Prevention
Summary

- Numerous case-control/population-based studies have examined the relationship between the consumption of specific food types and cancer incidence. Questionnaires in several of these studies have assessed consumption of garlic, garlic supplements, or *Allium* vegetables (garlic, onions). Results suggest that regular consumption of garlic may be associated with a lower risk of developing several types of cancer, including gastric and colorectal malignancies. However, this type of research is subject to confounding by environmental and lifestyle factors, as well as by recall bias. The effects of garlic on cancer incidence remain unclear, and prospective intervention trials are required before a firm conclusion can be drawn. It has been suggested that raw garlic may be more effective than supplements, although this difference has not been proven.

Reviews

- Fleischauer and Arab reviewed epidemiologic literature through August 1999 and reported on 22 trials that included relative risk estimates.[334] Although most studies reported risk reductions, the results of many were not statistically significant, or confidence intervals were not reported. Four case-control studies of stomach cancer suggested a protective effect,[335-338] whereas one cohort study[339] did not find an association between garlic and stomach cancer. There appeared to be greater benefits from consumption of raw garlic than from use of garlic in supplement form. Colorectal cancer was examined in four case-control trials and in three cohort studies.[340-342] All case-control trials and two of the cohort trials demonstrated an inverse association between garlic consumption and cancer, whereas one study[340] that utilized garlic in supplement form did not find a similar relationship. Because of the heterogeneity of five trials of head and neck cancer and sporadic reporting of actual garlic consumption,[338,343-346] the authors could not draw firm conclusions. Case-control trials and cohort studies were also presented regarding lung cancer,[347] breast cancer,[348-350] and prostate cancer.[351] Associations were not found in two of these studies (both from the large Netherlands Cohort Study)[347,348]; in the prostate cancer study,[351] results were not significant after garlic consumption was adjusted for social class. However, high intake of garlic was associated with a decreased risk in two of the case-control studies assessing breast cancer.[349,350]

- Fleischauer et al. subsequently conducted a "meta-analysis" of 18 epidemiologic studies of the association of dietary garlic consumption with the incidence of colorectal and stomach cancers.[352] All included studies reported relative risk data. The pooled relative risk for colorectal cancer was calculated as 0.69 (95% CI 0.55 to 0.89) and for stomach cancer, as 0.53 (95% CI 0.31 to 0.92). However, analysis of the included studies revealed publication bias, heterogeneity of effect estimates, variations in dosing, and possible confounding by other lifestyle choices.

- A 1997 review by Ernst drew similar conclusions, finding preliminary epidemiologic evidence for benefits of garlic that may merit prospective study.[353]

Gastric Cancer

- A case-control study was conducted in high- and low-risk areas of Italy to evaluate significance of geographic variations in gastric cancer–related incidence and mortality rates.[335] The study included 1016 persons with histologically confirmed gastric cancer and 1159 population controls. Lower risk was associated with consumption of spices, olive oil, and garlic (odds ratio 0.4 to -0.6; CIs not provided). High-risk areas were found to be loci for higher consumption of food associated with elevated risk (traditional soups, cold cuts) and lower consumption of foods associated with reduced risk (raw vegetables, citrus fruits, garlic).

- To evaluate factors contributing to a low incidence of gastric cancer, a comparative study was conducted of ecologic factors in a high-risk area of China (Yangzhong) and a low-risk area of China (Pizhou).[354] Subjects included 414 residents of Yangzhong and 425 residents of Pizhou. Ecologic factors were compared for the two areas using a questionnaire and analysis by the Cochran-Mantel-Haenszel method, age-adjusted. Results showed that *Allium* vegetables were consumed in Pizhou more frequently (as well as raw vegetables, fruit, tomatoes, kidney beans, and soybean products). People who consumed large quantities of garlic three times or more per week comprised 82% of men and 75% of women in the Pizhou area and 1% of men and women in Yangzhong.

- You et al., in a dietary survey conducted in garlic-producing Cangshan county, China, found consumption of garlic to correlate with a protective effect against chronic gastritis (odds ratio 0.5 to 0.7) and intestinal metaplasia/dysplasia (odds ratio 0.5 to –0.6).[355] However, there was not a significant linear trend. Garlic consumption was associated with a lower incidence of *H. pylori* infection (a known risk factor for gastrointestinal malignancy).

- Gail et al. presented a study design and initial data for a study of progression of precancerous gastric lesions in Shandong, China.[356] In 1995, 3411 persons in 13 rural villages in China entered a blinded, randomized trial to assess the effects of three treatments: antibiotics, dietary supplementation with vitamins C and E plus selenium, and garlic supplementation (Kyolic, aged extract and oil). Endoscopic examinations began in 1999.

Esophageal and Stomach Cancer

- Cook-Mozaffari compared 324 subjects in Iran with esophageal cancer with 648 controls to determine history of raw garlic consumption.[357] A questionnaire was used, and no significant difference in history of garlic intake was found.

- In contrast, Gao et al. matched 81 cases of esophageal cancer and 153 cases of stomach cancer with 234 controls in Shanghai, China.[338] A questionnaire was used to collect data, including frequency of intake of *Allium* vegetables, tea, smoking, and alcohol. Weekly garlic consumption was associated with an odds ratio of 0.3 (95% CI 0.19 to 0.47) for esophageal cancer and 0.31 (95% CI 0.22 to 0.44) for stomach cancer vs. consumption of garlic less than once per week. It is not clear if there are differences in cancer etiology or specific environmental factors between China and Iran that may account for these differences.

Colon Cancer

- Steinmetz et al. reported a set of results from the Iowa Women's Health Study, which included 41,837 women aged 55 to 69 years who completed a 127-item food frequency questionnaire in 1986 and were followed for the development of cancer over 5 years.[342] The authors matched 212 women who developed colorectal cancer with the available study population as controls and determined an inverse relationship of garlic consumption with risk of developing cancer, with an age-adjusted relative risk of 0.68 (95% CI 0.46 to 1.02) when the uppermost and lowermost consumption levels were compared.

- Witte et al. used case-control data from 488 matched pairs to evaluate associations of vegetables, fruits, and grains with colorectal polyps.[358] After adjustment for potentially anti-carcinogenic constituents of foods, inverse associations were identified for high-carotenoid vegetables, cruciferous vegetables, garlic, and soy.
- Dorant et al. matched 443 cases of colorectal cancer with 3123 controls as part of the large (n = 120,852) prospective Netherlands Cohort Study of dietary factors and cancer.[340] Dietary intake was measured with a 150-item food frequency questionnaire. After 3.3 years of follow-up, an analysis was conducted and demonstrated that the use of garlic supplements was not significantly associated with colon or rectal carcinoma in men and women combined.

Thyroid Cancer

- Thyroid nodularity following continuous low-dose environmental radiation exposure (330 mR/year) in China was identified in 1001 women aged 50 to 65 years, and in 1005 comparison subjects exposed to normal levels of radiation (114 mR/year).[147] Cumulative doses to the thyroid were estimated to be on the order of 14cGy and 5cGy, respectively. Personal interviews were conducted, and measurements were made of serum thyroid hormone levels, urinary iodine concentrations, and chromosome aberrations in circulating lymphocytes. Increased intake of *Allium* vegetables (garlic, onions) was associated with a decreased risk of nodular disease.
- Swanson et al. found that among male residents of a mining community in Yunnan Province, China, the relative risk of lung cancer across increasing quartiles of consumption of dark-green, leafy vegetables was 1.00, 0.62, 0.52, and 0.41 ($p < 0.01$ for this trend).[359] However, specific dietary constituent(s) responsible for the protective effect of vegetable consumption could not be identified.

Breast Cancer

- Dorant et al. reported results from a large prospective cohort study in the Netherlands (n = 120,852), designed to assess the effects of diet on the development of cancer.[348] After 3.3 years of follow-up, breast cancer was identified in 469 women. These subjects were matched with 1713 controls and asked via a questionnaire for their history of garlic supplement use. Use of a garlic supplement daily was associated with a risk reduction of 0.75 in women who had used no other supplements; however, the 95% CI was 0.41 to 1.38.

Endometrial Cancer

- Shu et al. examined the relationship between diet and endometrial cancer in a population-based case-control study conducted in Shanghai, China, between 1988 and 1990, involving interviews with 268 women with the cancer and 268 controls, aged 18 to 74 years.[360] After adjustment for total calories, no significant association of risk was found with intake of vegetables or dark green/yellow vegetables, although consumption of fruit and of *Allium* vegetables was associated with a small reduction in risk.

- Levi et al. conducted a study in Italy and Switzerland in which 274 women with endometrial cancer were matched with 572 controls.[361] Intake of various foods was assessed in a structured questionnaire. Weekly intake of garlic was associated with a risk reduction of 0.71, although confidence intervals were not provided.

Prostate Cancer

- Key et al. matched 328 men with prostate cancer with 328 controls and administered a questionnaire regarding garlic consumption. The authors noted an odds ratio of 0.64 for those who ingested garlic or garlic supplements more than twice weekly, although 95% CIs were 0.38 to 1.09.

Preclinical Data

- Animal research[278,362] and *in vitro* studies[363] have suggested efficacy of garlic as a treatment for cancer, and for the reduction of adverse effects associated with chemotherapeutic agents such as doxorubicin[364] and methotrexate.[365] It has been suggested that garlic possesses antiproliferative effects on human cancers,[267] including induction of apoptosis,[268] regulation of cell cycle progression, and signal transduction modification.

Cryptococcal Meningitis
Summary

- One observational study documented potential benefits of oral plus intravenous garlic in the management of cryptococcal meningitis. Further research is needed before a recommendation can be made for or against the use of garlic in the treatment of this potentially serious condition, for which other therapies are available.

Evidence

- A 1980 case series described 21 subjects with cryptococcal meningitis who were encountered during a 5-year period.[110] A total of 16 patients received treatment with garlic alone and 5 with garlic in addition to other drugs. All but 2 patients were given garlic orally and intramuscularly/intravenously (>40 intravenous garlic infusions in each case). The author reported that among the 16 patients, 6 were cured and 5 improved, with greater reported efficacy with garlic monotherapy (11 of 16 cases). Four patients were lost to follow-up, and 11 stayed on treatment from 7 months to 19.5 years. Of the six deaths that occurred, five resulted from brain herniation. Although these results are compelling, other treatments are available for this potentially serious condition, and garlic remains an unproven agent for this indication.

Antifungal (Topical)
Summary

- Garlic has been used topically to treat fungal infections[183,366] and antifungal effects have been demonstrated *in vitro* against *Candida*,[289,367] *Aspergillus*,[368] *Cryptococcus neoformans*,[369] and dermatophytes.[370] Diminished adherence of *Candida* to buccal epithelial cells has been demonstrated,[371] and antagonism of lipid synthesis has also been suggested as a possible mechanism of action.[303] A small number of human studies have suggested possible efficacy of topical garlic or ajoene (an organosulfur constituent of garlic) for the treatment of fungal infections. However, there is currently insufficient scientific evidence in this area to make a recommendation.

Evidence

- A randomized controlled trial of topical ajoene (an organosulfur constituent of garlic) for the short-term management of tinea cruris and tinea corporis was conducted by Ledezma et al., who reported a healing rate equivalent to that achieved with terbinafine.[372] Subjects included 60 soldiers with diagnosed dermatophytosis, treated topically with 0.6% ajoene or 1% terbinafine for a period of 7 days. However, there was no placebo arm, and it is not clear that this trial was sufficiently large to detect between-group differences. This trial followed an initial positive observational study of ajoene in the treatment of tinea pedis, in which 27 of 34 patients experienced a "complete cure" after 7 days of treatment.[373]

- In a different publication, Ledezma et al. reported on the safety and effectiveness of twice-daily topical application of ajoene or terbinafine, administered to 70 soldiers with tinea pedis over a 1-week period.[374] Subjects were randomly distributed into three treatment groups: 0.6% ajoene, 1% ajoene, or 1% terbinafine. Outcome measures included mycologic cure and clinical improvement as demonstrated by decrease in symptoms. Although 70 patients were enrolled, only 47 were available for final evaluation. The authors reported a rapid decrease in signs and symptoms in all groups. Mycologic cure rates 60 days after therapy completion were reported as 72% in the ajoene 0.6% group, 100% for ajoene 1%, and 94% for terbinafine.

- A case report involved culture-confirmed lesions of *Microsporum canis* infection on the arms of a young woman.[375] Freshly cut garlic was applied to the lesions on one arm and tolnaftate to the lesions on the other arm. The arm treated with garlic took 10 days to heal; the other took 4 weeks. A different case report cited the successful treatment of culture-confirmed sporotrichosis.[376] Following garlic treatment, a patient was cured (without recurrence after 6 months).

- In five healthy volunteers, 10 to 25 mL of garlic extract exerted antifungal activity against *Candida*, *Cryptococcus*, *Aspergillus*, and other organisms in serum samples at 30 and 60 minutes after ingestion; this effect disappeared after 2 hours.[298]

- Campos et al. evaluated the usefulness of garlic in the treatment of ascariasis.[28] Children known to be infected with *Ascaris lumbricoides* were given an 8-g infusion daily for 5 days. Results failed to show efficacy.

- The effect of serial dilutions of crude garlic extract on adult *Hymenolepis nana* was studied *in vitro* to detect the minimal lethal concentration, which was determined to be 1:20.[377] Garlic was then evaluated in the treatment of fungal infection in 10 children infected with *H. nana* and 26 infected with *Giardia lamblia* (as a 5-mL crude garlic extract in 100 mL of water in two doses per day, or a commercial preparation consisting of 1.2 mg of garlic twice daily for 3 days). Garlic was reported to shorten the duration of garlic of treatment. No control group was used.

Antiplatelet Effects
Summary

- The effects of garlic on platelet aggregation have been assessed in several human trials. Although these studies have overall been methodologically weak, garlic does appear to possess some platelet-inhibiting properties. Dosing, safety, comparison with other agents, duration of effects, and clinical outcomes are not known, and the potential benefits of using garlic for this purpose are not clear. Because garlic has been associated with several cases of bleeding, therapy should be applied with caution (particularly in patients using other agents that may precipitate bleeding).

Evidence

- Several preclinical studies and controlled human trials have reported impaired platelet aggregation associated with oral garlic use.[22,116,127,154-157,207] Two trials by Kiesewetter et al. reported that 800 mg of garlic daily led to a decrease in platelet aggregation in patients with peripheral vascular disease who were studied for 4 or 12 weeks.[22,127] In most cases, platelet aggregation has been measured by assessing the effects of adenosine diphosphate (ADP) on patients' serum. A majority of these studies have been methodologically flawed, with vague descriptions of design and methods. Comparisons with established antiplatelet agents have not been assessed, doses are not established, duration of effect is not clear, and clinical outcomes are not known. It should be kept in mind that garlic has been associated with several case reports of bleeding and may increase fibrinolytic activity[158] and prolong clotting time.[144,159] Garlic has also been associated with one case of an *increase* in a previously stabilized INR when used concomitantly with warfarin.[151,160]

Tick Repellent
Summary

- There is a lack of sufficient data to recommend for or against the use of garlic as an insect repellent.

Evidence

- Garlic has been studied as a tick repellent in a controlled trial in 100 Swedish marines.[378] Subjects were assigned to receive 1200 mg of daily *Allium* capsules or placebo for 8 weeks. Self-reports of tick bites were significantly fewer in individuals receiving garlic vs. placebo. The methodology of this trial has been challenged because of the lack of comparison with a standard repellent,[379] flawed statistical analysis,[380] and limited information regarding the form of garlic used.[381]

Upper Respiratory Tract Infection
Summary

- Garlic has a long history of use in the treatment of infections due to various microorganisms, including bacteria, fungi, and viruses. Garlic has been effective *in vitro* against numerous gram-negative and gram-positive bacteria, including resistant strains,[54,150,286-289] mycobacteria,[292-294] and *Helicobacter* species.[54,295,296] *In vitro* studies have also demonstrated effects against several viruses,[304] including influenza B virus, herpes simplex virus type 1,[304] herpes simplex virus type 2, parainfluenza virus type 3, vaccinia virus, vesicular stomatitis virus, human rhinovirus type 2,[16,17] and cytomegalovirus.[24] However, there is limited available evidence in humans. One trial has reported reduced frequency and duration of cold symptoms with daily garlic vs. placebo.[23] Further study may be warranted in this area.

Evidence

- Josling randomly assigned 146 volunteers to receive placebo or an allicin-containing garlic supplement, 1 capsule daily, over a 12-week winter-time period.[23] A 5-point subjective questionnaire was administered to all subjects in the form of a daily diary, in order to assess health status and identify common cold symptoms. The garlic group experienced significantly fewer colds than were reported by the placebo group (24 vs. 65, $p < 0.001$). In the placebo group, when colds occurred, they lasted significantly longer than in the garlic group (5.01 vs. 1.52 days, $p < 0.001$).

- Andrianova et al. conducted a two-phase study in which the tolerance of extended-release garlic tablets (Allicor 600 mg) was assessed in 172 children over a 5-month period, followed by a 5-month randomized, double-blind, placebo-controlled trial in 41 children.[382] In the first phase, therapy was reported as well tolerated, without significant gastrointestinal distress, compared with 468 matched controls. In the second phase, measured symptoms thought to be associated with viral upper respiratory tract infection were reported as reduced by 1.7-fold compared with placebo. Lack of use of established scales and unclear reporting of statistical analysis limit the value of these results.

Type 2 Diabetes Mellitus
Summary

- Animal studies have reported that garlic or its constituents (such as S-allyl cysteine sulfoxide [SACS]) may decrease glucose concentrations and increase insulin secretion.[145,146] However, multiple human trials have failed to demonstrate significant effects of oral garlic preparations on measures of glycemic control in diabetic or nondiabetic patients. Two trials have studied the effects of oral garlic in patients with type 2 diabetes mellitus as primary outcomes and found no significant effects.[26,130] Several other trials have measured glucose levels as a secondary outcome (largely in nondiabetic individuals) and found no significant effects, with the exception of a small significant reduction noted in one poor-quality trial (from a mean blood glucose of 89 mg/dL to 79 mg/dL over 4 weeks).[126] Overall, the available studies have been small (<100 subjects), with unclear descriptions of methods and statistical analysis. Nonetheless, it appears that garlic does not exert clinically relevant effects on glucose levels and is likely not a viable therapy for the management of type 2 diabetes mellitus.

Evidence

- A total of 40 patients with type 2 (non–insulin dependent) diabetes from an outpatient clinic were divided into two groups by Sitprija et al. to participate in a double-blind trial.[26] Patients were randomly administered 350 mg of a dehydrated garlic preparation or placebo twice daily for a period of 1 month. Outcomes were measured via a glucose tolerance test, fasting blood glucose, serum insulin, liver function tests, blood total cholesterol, and triglycerides. Seven patients (17.5%) failed to complete the study. All subjects were reported to have tolerated the drug, and no adverse effects were reported. Results did not show any statistically significant responses in blood glucose, insulin, total cholesterol, HDL lipoprotein, or triglyceride levels. Limitations include high dropout rate, small sample size, and unclear reporting of results and statistical analysis.
- Masell et al. conducted a controlled, double-blind trial in 60 subjects (median age of 63 years) with type 2 diabetes mellitus that was well controlled on diet or oral medications.[130] Subjects were randomized to receive a dehydrated garlic preparation (Kwai) 900 mg daily or placebo for 12 weeks. The authors reported no significant effects at 6 or 12 weeks on measures of serum glucose control including fasting glucose, hemoglobin A_{1c} (glycosylated hemoglobin), insulin levels, or C peptide. Notably, an odor was noted at least once weekly by 31% of patients taking garlic vs. 3% of placebo, which may have led to bias. The effects of garlic, if

any, may have been blunted by the concomitant use of drugs or dietary discretion to control blood sugars. Blinding and randomization were not clearly described.

- Kiesewetter et al. reported glucose levels as a secondary outcome in a double-blind, placebo-controlled trial that was designed to measure platelet aggregation in 60 nondiabetic patients believed to have increased levels of platelet aggregation (13% were smokers).[126] Subjects were randomized to receive dehydrated garlic powder tablets (Kwai) 800 mg daily or placebo for 4 weeks. Patients in the garlic group demonstrated a mean reduction in serum glucose levels from a mean of 89 mg/dL to 79 mg/dL. However, the results, statistical analysis, and randomization of this trial were not clearly reported, and >20% of subjects dropped out without adequate explanation or analysis.
- Numerous other human trials of garlic have measured serum glucose levels or indices of glycemic control as secondary outcomes (primarily in nondiabetic subjects).[56,112,116,121-123,128,141] None of these studies has found significant changes in blood glucose levels, although overall they have not been designed to measure this outcome and were small in size (<100 subjects).

Helicobacter pylori Infection
Summary

- Garlic has a long history of use in the treatment of infections due to various microorganisms, including bacteria, fungi, and viruses. Garlic has been effective *in vitro* against numerous gram-negative and gram-positive bacteria, including resistant strains,[54,150,286-289] mycobacteria,[292-294] and *Helicobacter* species.[54,295,296] Several human case studies have examined the effects of garlic on *H. pylori* infection and found a lack of benefit. This preliminary negative evidence may merit follow-up with more rigorous trials.

Evidence

- In a poorly designed study, Graham et al. investigated the effects of garlic and capsaicin (jalapeno peppers) on 12 subjects who served as their own controls (ages 27 to 51 years), all with *H. pylori* infections.[383] Patients were excluded if they had undergone a recent treatment with antibiotics, bismuth, or antacids. Subjects ate a test meal containing 10 cloves of garlic and 6 jalapeno peppers, or 2 tablets of bismuth, or no treatment (control). Subsequently, some subjects underwent a 2-day washout period before receiving the alternate therapies. The test meal was administered three times on each testing day. Outcome measures included results from a urea breath test (UBT). Ten patients took the garlic cloves and six took jalapeno peppers. The authors reported that garlic and jalapeno ingestion tended to increase *H. pylori* activity, whereas bismuth decreased it. Limitations of this study included lack of a separate control group, use of self-controls for a condition that may be significantly affected by the tested interventions, small sample size, and inconsistent application of the interventions.
- McNulty et al. conducted a pilot study examining effects of garlic oil on dyspeptic patients who were seropositive for *H. pylori*.[384] Treatment consisted of one 4-mg garlic oil capsule four times per day for 14 days (taken with food). The primary outcome measure was *H. pylori* eradication, defined as a negative ^{13}C UBT at two follow-up appointments. Suppression was defined as a 50% fall in ^{13}C excess between baseline and follow-up. Among the five patients who completed the study, no evidence of either eradication or

suppression of *H. pylori* or symptom improvement was noted. Limitations of this study include lack of a control group and small sample size.

- Similar negative results have been reported in two additional case series. Aydin et al. did not find significant reductions in symptoms, gastritis grade, and *H. pylori* density in a trial of 20 infected dyspeptic patients who received garlic for 2 weeks.[385] Ernst did not report efficacy in an 8-week open trial.[386] The methodologic limitations of these studies have been noted elsewhere.[387]

- Salih et al. evaluated the potential preventive effects of garlic dietary consumption against *H. pylori* infection by retrospectively correlating garlic consumption levels with incidence of infection and antibody titer levels.[388] In a cohort of 81 garlic-eating and 80 non–garlic-eating individuals in Turkey, the authors found a high prevalence of infection in both groups (79% and 81%, respectively) but lower antibody titers in persons with higher and longer-duration garlic intake. The clinical implications of these results are not clear.

FORMULARY: BRANDS USED IN CLINICAL TRIALS
Brands Used in Statistically Significant Clinical Trials

- Kwai (Lichtwer Pharma) is a non–enteric-coated dehydrated garlic powder formulation standardized for 1.3% alliin content and is the product most often used in clinical trials. Another standardized dehydrated garlic powder preparation is Sapec (produced by the same manufacturer).
- Kyolic (Wakunaga of America) is the product most often used in studies with aged garlic extract (AGE).

References

1. Mulrow C, Lawrence V, Ackerman R, et al. Garlic: effects on cardiovascular risks and disease, protective effects against cancer, and clinical adverse effects. Evidence Report/Technology Assessment No. 20 (Contract 290-97-0012 to the San Antonio Evidence-based Practice Center based at The University of Texas Health Science Center at San Antonio and the Veterans Evidence-based Research, Dissemination, and Implementation Center, a Veterans Affairs Health Services Research and Development Center of Excellence). AHRQ Publication No. 01-E023. Rockville, Md, Agency for Healthcare Research and Quality, October 2000.
2. Ackermann RT, Mulrow CD, Ramirez G, et al. Garlic shows promise for improving some cardiovascular risk factors. Arch Intern Med 2001;161(6):813-824.
3. Stevinson C, Pittler MH, Ernst E. Garlic for treating hypercholesterolemia. A meta-analysis of randomized clinical trials. Ann Intern Med 2000;133(6):420-429.
4. Warshafsky S, Kamer RS, Sivak SL. Effect of garlic on total serum cholesterol. A meta-analysis. Ann Intern Med 1993;119(7 Pt 1):599-605.
5. Silagy C, Neil A. Garlic as a lipid lowering agent—a meta-analysis. J R Coll Physicians Lond 1994;28(1):39-45.
6. Silagy CA, Neil HA. A meta-analysis of the effect of garlic on blood pressure. J Hypertension 1994;12(4):463-468.
7. Moriguchi T, Saito H, Nishiyama N. Aged garlic extract prolongs longevity and improves spatial memory deficit in senescence-accelerated mouse. Biol Pharm Bull 1996;19(2):305-307.
8. Abdullah T, Kirkpatrick DV, Carter J. Enhancement of natural killer cell activity in AIDS with garlic. Dtsch Zeit Onkol 1989;21:52-53.
9. Sasaki J, Kita J. Bacteriocidal activity of garlic powder against *Bacillus anthracis*. J Nutr Sci Vitaminol (Tokyo) 2003;49(4):297-299.
10. Imai J, Ide N, Nagae S, et al. Antioxidant and radical scavenging effects of aged garlic extract and its constituents. Planta Med 1994;60(5):417-420.
11. Banerjee SK, Mukherjee PK, Maulik SK. Garlic as an antioxidant: the good, the bad and the ugly. Phytother Res 2003;17(2):97-106.
12. Betancor-Fernandez A, Perez-Galvez A, Sies H, et al. Screening pharmaceutical preparations containing extracts of turmeric rhizome, artichoke leaf, devil's claw root and garlic or salmon oil for antioxidant capacity. J Pharm Pharmacol 2003;55(7):981-986.
13. Dillon SA, Burmi RS, Lowe GM, et al. Antioxidant properties of aged garlic extract: an in vitro study incorporating human low density lipoprotein. Life Sci 2003;72(14):1583-1594.
14. Ichikawa M, Ryu K, Yoshida J, et al. Identification of six phenylpropanoids from garlic skin as major antioxidants. J Agric Food Chem 2003;51(25):7313-7317.
15. Sener G, Satyroglu H, Ozer SA, et al. Protective effect of aqueous garlic extract against oxidative organ damage in a rat model of thermal injury. Life Sci 2003;73(1):81-91.
16. Hughes BG, Murray BK, North JA, et al. Antiviral constituents from *Allium sativum*. Planta Med 1989;55:114.
17. Weber ND, Andersen DO, North JA, et al. *In vitro* virucidal effects of *Allium sativum* (garlic) extract and compounds. Planta Med 1992;58(5):417-423.
18. Denisov LN, Andrianova IV, Timofeeva SS. [Garlic effectiveness in rheumatoid arthritis]. Ter Arkh 1999;71(8):55-58.
19. Ameen M, Musthapa MS, Abidi P, et al. Garlic attenuates chrysotile-mediated pulmonary toxicity in rats by altering the phase I and phase II drug metabolizing enzyme system. J Biochem Mol Toxicol 2003;17(6):366-371.
20. Campos R, Amato N, V, Castanho RE, et al. [Treatment of ascaridiasis with garlic (*Allium sativum*)]. Rev Hosp Clin Fac Med Sao Paulo 1990;45(5):213-215.
21. Martin N, Bardisa L, Pantoja C, et al. Anti-arrhythmic profile of a garlic dialysate assayed in dogs and isolated atrial preparations. J Ethnopharmacol 1994;43(1):1-8.
22. Kiesewetter H, Jung F, Jung EM, et al. Effects of garlic coated tablets in peripheral arterial occlusive disease. Clin Investig 1993;71(5):383-386.
23. Josling P. Preventing the common cold with a garlic supplement: a double-blind, placebo-controlled survey. Adv Ther 2001;18(4):189-193.
24. Guo NL, Lu DP, Woods GL, et al. Demonstration of the anti-viral activity of garlic extract against human cytomegalovirus *in vitro*. Chin Med J (Engl) 1993;106(2):93-96.
25. Diaz MR, Sembrano JM. A comparative study of the efficacy of garlic and eugenol as palliative agents against dental pain of pulpal origin. J Philipp Dent Assoc 1985;35(1):3-10.
26. Sitprija S, Plengvidhya C, Kangkaya V, et al. Garlic and diabetes mellitus phase II clinical trial. J Med Assoc Thai 1987;70(Suppl 2):223-227.
27. Mukhrejee S, Banerjee SK, Maulik M, et al. Protection against acute Adriamycin-induced cardiotoxicity by garlic: role of endogenous antioxidants and inhibition of TNF-alpha expression. BMC Pharmacol 2003;3(1):16.
28. Damrau F, Ferguson EA. The modus operandi of carminatives. The therapeutic value of garlic in functional gastrointestinal disorder. Rev Gastroentrol 1949;16:411-419.
29. Sarrell EM, Mandelberg A, Cohen HA. Efficacy of naturopathic extracts in the management of ear pain associated with acute otitis media. Arch Pediatr Adolesc Med 2001;155:796-799.
30. Nijhawan S, Agarwal V, Sharma D, et al. Evaluation of garlic oil as a contact dissolution agent for gallstones: comparison with monooctanoin. Trop Gastroenterol 2000;21(4):177-179.
31. Joshi DJ, Dikshit RK, Mansuri SM. Gastrointestinal actions of garlic oil. Phytother Res 1987;1(3):140-141.
32. Pedraza-Chaverri J, Maldonado PD, Medina-Campos ON, et al. Garlic ameliorates gentamicin nephrotoxicity: relation to antioxidant enzymes. Free Radic Biol Med 2000;29(7):602-611.
33. Maldonado PD, Barrera D, Medina-Campos ON, et al. Aged garlic extract attenuates gentamicin induced renal damage and oxidative stress in rats. Life Sci 2003;73(20):2543-2556.
34. Hikino H, Tohkin M, Kiso Y, et al. Antihepatotoxic actions of *Allium sativum* bulbs. Planta Med 1986;(3):163-168.
35. Wang EJ, Li Y, Lin M, et al. Protective effects of garlic and related organosulfur compounds on acetaminophen-induced hepatotoxicity in mice. Toxicol Appl Pharmacol 1996;136(1):146-154.
36. Rahmy TR, Hemmaid KZ. Prophylactic action of garlic on the histological and histochemical patterns of hepatic and gastric tissues in rats injected with a snake venom. J Nat Toxins 2001;10(2):137-165.
37. Abrams GA, Fallon MB. Treatment of hepatopulmonary syndrome with *Allium sativum* L. (garlic): a pilot trial. J Clin Gastroenterol 1998;27(3):232-235.
38. Caldwell SH, Jeffers LJ, Narula OS, et al. Ancient remedies revisited: does *Allium sativum* (garlic) palliate the hepatopulmonary syndrome? J Clin Gastroenterol 1992;15(3):248-250.
39. Brosche T, Platt D. Garlic therapy and the immune defense of the elderly. Phytotherapy 1994;15:23-24.
40. Zhou W. Acute lymphangitis treated by moxibustion with garlic in 118 cases. J Tradit Chin Med 2003;23(3):198.
41. Perez HA, De la RM, Apitz R. *In vivo* activity of ajoene against rodent malaria. Antimicrob Agents Chemother 1994;38(2):337-339.
42. Tsao SM, Hsu CC, Yin MC. Garlic extract and two diallyl sulphides inhibit methicillin-resistant *Staphylococcus aureus* infection in BALB/cA mice. J Antimicrob Chemother 2003;52(6):974-980.
43. Pedraza-Chaverri J, Medina-Campos ON, Granados-Silvestre MA, et al. Garlic ameliorates hyperlipidemia in chronic aminonucleoside nephrosis. Mol Cell Biochem 2000;211(2):69-77.
44. Ito Y, Ito M, Takagi N, et al. Neurotoxicity induced by amyloid beta-peptide and ibotenic acid in organotypic hippocampal cultures: protection by *S*-allyl-L-cysteine, a garlic compound. Brain Res 2003;985(1):98-107.
45. Ito Y, Kosuge Y, Sakikubo T, et al. Protective effect of *S*-allyl-L-cysteine, a garlic compound, on amyloid beta-protein–induced cell death in nerve growth factor-differentiated PC12 cells. Neurosci Res 2003;46(1):119-125.

46. Qian YX, Shen PJ, Xu RY, et al. Spermicidal effect in vitro by the active principle of garlic. Contraception 1986;34(3):295-302.

47. Chakrabarti K, Pal S, Bhattacharyya AK. Sperm immobilization activity of *Allium sativum* L. and other plant extracts. Asian J Androl 2003;5(2): 131-135.

48. Zhang RS. [A clinical study on allicin in the prevention of thrush in newborn infants]. Zhongguo Zhong Xi Yi Jie He Za Zhi (Chin J Integr Tradit West Med) 1992;12(1):28-9, 6.

49. Anon. Garlic cloves for verruca vulgaris. Pediatr Dermatol 2002; 19(2): 183.

50. Kade F, Miller W. Standardised garlic-ginkgo combination product improves well-being—a placebo controlled double blind study. Eur J Clin Res 1993;4:49-55.

51. Lawson LD, Ransom DK, Hughes BG, et al. Inhibition of whole blood platelet-aggregation by compounds in garlic clove extracts and commercial garlic products. Thrombosis Res 1992;65(2):141-156.

52. Spigelski D, Jones PJ. Efficacy of garlic supplementation in lowering serum cholesterol levels. Nutr Rev 2001;59(7):236-241.

53. Kannar D, Wattanapenpaiboon N, Savige GS, et al. Hypocholesterolemic effect of an enteric-coated garlic supplement. J Am Coll Nutr 2001;20(3): 225-231.

54. Sivam GP. Protection against *Helicobacter pylori* and other bacterial infections by garlic. J Nutr 2001;131(3s):1106S-1108S.

55. Berthold HK, Sudhop T, von Bergmann K. Effect of a garlic oil preparation on serum lipoproteins and cholesterol metabolism: a randomized controlled trial. JAMA 1998;279(23):1900-1902.

56. Bordia A. Effect of garlic on blood lipids in patients with coronary heart disease. Am J Clin Nutr 1981;34(10):2100-2103.

57. de Santos AO, Jones RA. Effects of garlic powder and garlic oil preparations on blood lipids, blood pressure and well-being. Br J Clin Res 1995; 6:91-100.

58. Zhang XH, Lowe D, Giles P, et al. Gender may affect the action of garlic oil on plasma cholesterol and glucose levels of normal subjects. J Nutr 2001;131(5):1471-1476.

59. Zhang XH, Lowe D, Giles P, et al. A randomized trial of the effects of garlic oil upon coronary heart disease risk factors in trained male runners. Blood Coagul Fibrinolysis 2001;12(1):67-74.

60. Lawson LD. Effect of garlic on serum lipids. JAMA 1998;280(18):1568.

61. Lawson LD. Garlic powder for hyperlipidemia: analysis of recent negative results. Q Rev Nat Med 1998;187-189.

62. Berthold HK, Sudhop T, von Bergmann K. Effect of garlic on serum lipids. JAMA 1998;280(18):1568.

63. McCrindle BW, Helden E, Conner WT. Garlic extract therapy in children with hypercholesterolemia. Arch Pediatr Adolesc Med 1998;152(11): 1089-1094.

64. Hoshino T, Kashimoto N, Kasuga S. Effects of garlic preparations on the gastrointestinal mucosa. J Nutr 2001;131(3s):1109S-1113S.

65. Cavallito CJ, Bailey JH. Allicin, the antibacterail principle of *Allium sativum*. 1. Isolation, physical properties and antibacterial action. J Am Chem Soc 1944;66:1950-1954.

66. Nakagawa S, Masamoto K, Sumiyoshi H, et al. [Acute toxicity test of garlic extract]. J Toxicol Sci 1984;9(1):57-60.

67. Sumiyoshi H, Kanezawa A, Masamoto K, et al. [Chronic toxicity test of garlic extract in rats]. J Toxicol Sci 1984;9(1):61-75.

68. Gupta MK, Mittal SR, Mathur AK, et al. Garlic—the other side of the coin. Int J Cardiol 1993;38(3):333.

69. Bleumink E, Nater JP. Contact dermatitis to garlic; crossreactivity between garlic, onion and tulip. Arch Dermatol Forsch 1973;247(2):117-124.

70. Anibarro B, Fontela JL, De La HF. Occupational asthma induced by garlic dust. J Allergy Clin Immunol 1997;100(6 Pt 1):734-738.

71. Couturier P, Bousquet J. Occupational allergy secondary inhalation of garlic dust. J Allergy Clin Immunol 1982;70(2):145.

72. Lybarger JA, Gallagher JS, Pulver DW, et al. Occupational asthma induced by inhalation and ingestion of garlic. J Allergy Clin Immunol 1982;69(5): 448-454.

73. Seuri M, Taivanen A, Ruoppi P, et al. Three cases of occupational asthma and rhinitis caused by garlic. Clin Exp Allergy 1993;23(12):1011-1014.

74. Falleroni AE, Zeiss CR, Levitz D. Occupational asthma secondary to inhalation of garlic dust. J Allergy Clin Immunol 1981;68(2):156-160.

75. Bleumink E, Doeglas HM, Klokke AH, et al. Allergic contact dermatitis to garlic. Br J Dermatol 1972;87(1):6-9.

76. Bojs G, Svensson A. Contact allergy to garlic used for wound healing. Contact Dermatitis 1988;18(3):179-181.

77. Delaney TA, Donnelly AM. Garlic dermatitis. Austr J Dermatol 1996; 37(2):109-110.

78. Lembo G, Balato N, Patruno C, et al. Allergic contact dermatitis due to garlic (*Allium sativum*). Contact Dermatitis 1991;25(5):330-331.

79. Mitchell JC. Contact sensitivity to garlic (*Allium*). Contact Dermatitis 1980;6(5):356-357.

80. Papageorgiou C, Corbet JP, Menezes-Brandao F, et al. Allergic contact dermatitis to garlic (*Allium sativum* L.). Identification of the allergens: the role of mono-, di-, and trisulfides present in garlic. A comparative study in man and animal (guinea-pig). Arch Dermatol Res 1983;275(4): 229-234.

81. Sanchez-Hernandez MC, Hernandez M, Delgado J, et al. Allergenic cross-reactivity in the Liliaceae family. Allergy 2000;55(3):297-299.

82. Eming SA, Piontek JO, Hunzelmann N, et al. Severe toxic contact dermatitis caused by garlic. Br J Dermatol 1999;141(2):391-392.

83. Kaplan B, Schewach-Millet M, Yorav S. Factitial dermatitis induced by application of garlic. Int J Dermatol 1990;29(1):75-76.

84. Lee TY, Lam TH. Contact dermatitis due to topical treatment with garlic in Hong Kong. Contact Dermatitis 1991;24(3):193-196.

85. Kurzen M, Bayerl C. [Immediate-type hypersensitivity to garlic]. Aktuelle Dermatol 1997;23:145-147.

86. Fleischer S, Bayerl C, Jung EG. [Occupational allergic hand dermatitis to garlic in a pizza baker]. Aktuelle Dermatol 1996;22:278-279.

87. Gaddoni G, Selvi M, Resta F, et al. Allergic contact dermatitis to garlic in a cook. Ann Ital Dermatol Clin Sperimentale 1994;48:120-121.

88. Asero R, Mistrello G, Roncarolo D, et al. A case of garlic allergy. J Allergy Clin Immunol 1998;101(3):427-428.

89. Burden AD, Wilkinson SM, Beck MH, et al. Garlic-induced systemic contact dermatitis. Contact Dermatitis 1994;30(5):299-300.

90. Edelstein AJ, Johnstown PA. Dermatitis caused by garlic. Arch Dermatol 1950;61:111.

91. Perez-Pimiento AJ, Moneo I, Santaolalla M, et al. Anaphylactic reaction to young garlic. Allergy 1999;54(6):626-629.

92. Fernandez-Vozmediano JM, Armario-Hita JC, Manrique-Plaza A. Allergic contact dermatitis from diallyl disulfide. Contact Dermatitis 2000;42(2): 108-109.

93. Kao SH, Hsu CH, Su SN, et al. Identification and immunologic characterization of an allergen, alliin lyase, from garlic (*Allium sativum*). J Allergy Clin Immunol 2004;113(1):161-168.

94. Armentia A, Vega JM. Can inhalation of garlic dust cause asthma? Allergy 1996;51(2):137-138.

95. Morbidoni L, Arterburn J, Young V et al. Garlic: its history and adverse effects. J Herbal Pharmacother 2001;1(1):63-83.

96. Bruynzeel DP. Bulb dermatitis. Dermatological problems in the flower bulb industries. Contact Dermatitis 1997;37(2):70-77.

97. Jappe U, Bonnekoh B, Hausen BM, et al. Garlic-related dermatoses: case report and review of the literature. Am J Contact Dermatit 1999;10(1): 37-39.

98. van Ketel WG, de Haan P. Occupational eczema from garlic and onion. Contact Dermatitis 1978;4(1):53-54.

99. McFadden JP, White IR, Rycroft RJ. Allergic contact dermatitis from garlic. Contact Dermatitis 1992;27(5):333-334.

100. Canduela V, Mongil I, Carrascosa M, et al. Garlic: always good for the health? Br J Dermatol 1995;132(1):161-162.

101. Garty BZ. Garlic burns. Pediatrics 1993;91(3):658-659.

102. Parish RA, McIntire S, Heimbach DM. Garlic burns: a naturopathic remedy gone awry. Pediatr Emerg Care 1987;3(4):258-260.

103. Rafaat M, Leung AK. Garlic burns. Pediatr Dermatol 2000;17(6):475-476.

104. Farrell AM, Staughton RC. Garlic burns mimicking herpes zoster. Lancet 1996;347(9009):1195.

105. Lachter J, Babich JP, Brookman JC, et al. Garlic: a way out of work. Mil Med 2003;168(6):499-500.

106. Roberge RJ, Leckey R, Spence R, et al. Garlic burns of the breast. Am J Emerg Med 1997;15(5):548.

107. Hviid K, Alsbjorn B. ["Burns" caused by local application of garlic]. Ugeskr Laeger 2000;162(50):6853-6854.

108. Cronin E. Dermatitis of the hands in caterers. Contact Dermatitis 1987; 17(5):265-269.

109. Ruocco V, Brenner S, Lombardi ML. A case of diet-related pemphigus. Dermatology 1996;192(4):373-374.

110. Anonymous. Garlic in cryptococcal meningitis: a preliminary report of 21 cases. Chin Med J (Engl) 1980;93(2):123-126.

111. Adler AJ, Holub BJ. Effect of garlic and fish-oil supplementation on serum lipid and lipoprotein concentrations in hypercholesterolemic men. Am J Clin Nutr 1997;65(2):445-450.

112. Auer W, Eiber A, Hertkorn E, et al. Hypertension and hyperlipidaemia: garlic helps in mild cases. Br J Clin Pract Suppl 1990;69:3-6.

113. Barrie SA, Wright JV, Pizzorno JE. Effects of garlic oil on platelet aggregation, serum lipids and blood pressure in humans. J Orthomolec Med 1987;2(1):15-21.

114. Bordia A. Knoblauch und koronare Herzkrankheit: Wirkungen einer dreijahrigen Behandlung min Knoblauchextrakt auf die Reinfarkt und Mortalitatsrate. Dtsch Apoth Ztg 1989;129(suppl 15):1-25.

115. Bordia A. [Garlic and coronary heart disease. Results of a 3-year treatment with garlic extract on the reinfarction and mortality rate]. Dtsch Apoth Zeit 1989;129(28 suppl 15):16-17.

116. Czerny B, Samochowiec J. Klinische Untersuchungen mit einem Knoblauch-Lezithin-Präparat. Arztezeitschr Naturheilverf 1996;37: 126-129.

117. De Santos O, Grunwald J. Effect of garlic powder tablets on blood lipids and blood pressure: a six month placebo controlled double blind study. Br J Clin Res 1993;4:37-44.

118. Gardner CD, Chatterjee L, Carlson J. Effect of garlic supplementation on plasma lipids in hypercholesterolemic men and women. Circulation 1999; 99(8):1123.

119. Holzgartner H, Schmidt U, Kuhn U. Comparison of the efficacy and tolerance of a garlic preparation vs. bezafibrate. Arzneimittelforschung 1992;42(12):1473-1477.

120. Isaacsohn JL, Moser M, Stein EA, et al. Garlic powder and plasma lipids and lipoproteins: a multicenter, randomized, placebo-controlled trial. Arch Intern Med 1998;158(11):1189-1194.

121. Jain AK, Vargas R, Gotzkowsky S, et al. Can garlic reduce levels of serum lipids? A controlled clinical study. Am J Med 1993;94(6):632-635.

122. Kandziora J. Blutdruck und lipidsenkende Wirkung eines Knoblauch-praparates in kombination mit einem Diuretikum. Arztliche Forschung 1988;3:3-8.

123. Kandziora J. Antihypertensive Wirksamkeit und Vertraglichkeit eines Knoblauch-preparates. Arztliche Forschung 1988;1:1-8.

124. Kannar D. Clinical evaluation of Australian based garlic and its combination with inulin in mild and moderate hyperlipidaemia [dissertation]. Clayton, Australia, Monash University, 1998, i-vi(6), pp. 67-114.

125. Kiesewetter H, Jung F, Mrowietz C, et al. Effects of garlic on blood fluidity and fibrinolytic activity: a randomised, placebo-controlled, double-blind study. Br J of Clin Prac 1990;69:24-29.

126. Kiesewetter H, Jung F, Pindur G, et al. Effect of garlic on thrombocyte aggregation, microcirculation, and other risk factors. Int J Clin Pharmacol Ther Toxicol 1991;29(4):151-155.

127. Kiesewetter H, Jung F, Jung EM, et al. Effect of garlic on platelet aggregation in patients with increased risk of juvenile ischaemic attack. Eur J Clin Pharmacol 1993;45(4):333-336.

128. Luley C, Lehmann-Leo W, Moller B, et al. Lack of efficacy of dried garlic in patients with hyperlipoproteinemia. Arzneimittelforschung 1986;36(4):766-768.

129. Lutomski J. Klinische Untersuchungen zur therapeutischen Wirksamkeit von Ilha Rogoff Knobauchpillen mit Rutin. Z Phytother 1984;5:938-942.

130. Mansell P, Reckless PD, Lloyd L. The effect of dried garlic powder tablets on serum lipids in non-insulin dependent diabetic patients. Eur J Clin Res 1996;8:25-26.

131. McMahon FG, Vargas R. Can garlic lower blood pressure? A pilot study. Pharmacotherapy 1993;13(4):406-407.

132. Qidwai W, Qureshi R, Hasan SN, et al. Effect of dietary garlic (*Allium sativum*) on the blood pressure in humans—a pilot study. J Pak Med Assoc 2000;50(6):204-207.

133. Saradeth T, Seidl S, Resch KL, et al. Does garlic alter the lipid pattern in normal volunteers? Phytomedicine 1994;1:183-185.

134. Simons LA, Balasubramaniam S, von Konigsmark M, et al. On the effect of garlic on plasma lipids and lipoproteins in mild hypercholesterolaemia. Atherosclerosis 1995;113(2):219-225.

135. Steiner M, Khan AH, Holbert D, et al. A double-blind crossover study in moderately hypercholesterolemic men that compared the effect of aged garlic extract and placebo administration on blood lipids. Am J Clin Nutr 1996;64(6):866-870.

136. Superko HR, Krauss RM. Garlic powder, effect on plasma lipids, post-prandial lipemia, low-density lipoprotein particle size, high-density lipoprotein subclass distribution and lipoprotein(a). J Am Coll Cardiol 2000;35(2):321-326.

137. Ventura P, Girola M, Lattuada V. [Clinical evaluation and tolerability of a drug with garlic and hawthorn]. Acta Toxicol Ther 1990;11(4):365-372.

138. Vorberg G, Schneider B. Therapy with garlic: results of a placebo-controlled, double-blind study. Br J Clin Pract Suppl 1990;69:7-11.

139. Yeh YY, Lin RI, Yeh SM, et al. Garlic reduces plasma cholesterol in hypercholesterolemic men maintaining habitual diets. In Ohigashi H, Osawa T, Terao J, et al (eds): Food Factors for Cancer Prevention. Tokyo, Springer-Verlag, 1997, pp. 226-230.

140. Neil HA, Silagy CA, Lancaster T, et al. Garlic powder in the treatment of moderate hyperlipidaemia: a controlled trial and meta-analysis. J R Coll Physicians Lond 1996;30(4):329-334.

141. Koscielny J, Klussendorf D, Latza R, et al. The antiatherosclerotic effect of *Allium sativum*. Atherosclerosis 1999;144:237-249.

142. Mader FH. Treatment of hyperlipidaemia with garlic-powder tablets. Arzneim Forsch/Drug Res 1990;40(II):1111-1116.

143. Szybejko J, Zukowski A, Herbec R. [Unusual cause of obturation of the small intestine]. Wiad Lek 1982;35(2):163-164.

144. Bimmermann A, Weingart K, Schwartzkopff W. *Allium sativum*: Studie zur Wirksamkeit bei Hyperlipoproteinamie. Therapiewoche 1988;38:3885-3890.

145. Augusti KT, Sheela CG. Antiperoxide effect of S-allyl cysteine sulfoxide, an insulin secretagogue, in diabetic rats. Experientia 1996;52(2):115-120.

146. Sheela CG, Augusti KT. Antidiabetic effects of S-allyl cysteine sulphoxide isolated from garlic Allium sativum Linn. Indian J Exp Biol 1992;30(6):523-526.

147. Wang ZY, Boice JD, Jr., Wei LX, et al. Thyroid nodularity and chromosome aberrations among women in areas of high background radiation in China. J Natl Cancer Inst 1990;82(6):478-485.

148. Rose KD, Croissant PD, Parliament CF, et al. Spontaneous spinal epidural hematoma with associated platelet dysfunction from excessive garlic ingestion: a case report. Neurosurgery 1990;26(5):880-882.

149. Fedder SL. Spinal epidural hematoma and garlic ingestion. Neurosurgery 1990;27(4):659.

150. Kumar M, Berwal JS. Sensitivity of food pathogens to garlic (*Allium sativum*). J Appl Microbiol 1998;84(2):213-215.

151. Vaes LP, Chyka PA. Interactions of warfarin with garlic, ginger, ginkgo, or ginseng: nature of the evidence. Ann Pharmacother 2000;34(12):1478-1482.

152. Jain RC. Effect of garlic on serum lipids, coagulability and fibrinolytic activity of blood. Am J Clin Nutr 1977;30(9):1380-1381.

153. Burnham BE. Garlic as a possible risk for postoperative bleeding. Plast Reconstr Surg 1995;95(1):213.

154. German K, Kumar U, Blackford HN. Garlic and the risk of TURP bleeding. Br J Urol 1995;76(4):518.

155. Petry JJ. Garlic and postoperative bleeding. Plast Reconstr Surg 1995;96(2):483-484.

156. el Sabban F, Radwan GM. Influence of garlic compared to aspirin on induced photothrombosis in mouse pial microvessels, in vivo. Thromb Res 1997;88(2):193-203.

157. Apitz-Castro R, Escalante J, Vargas R, et al. Ajoene, the antiplatelet principle of garlic, synergistically potentiates the antiaggregatory action of prostacyclin, forskolin, indomethacin and dypiridamole on human platelets. Thromb Res 1986;42(3):303-311.

158. Harenberg J, Giese C, Zimmermann R. Effect of dried garlic on blood coagulation, fibrinolysis, platelet aggregation and serum cholesterol levels in patients with hyperlipoproteinemia. Atherosclerosis 1988;74(3):247-249.

159. Gadkari JV, Joshi VD. Effect of ingestion of raw garlic on serum cholesterol level, clotting time and fibrinolytic activity in normal subjects. J Postgrad Med 1991;37(3):128-131.

160. Sunter WH. Warfarin and garlic. Pharm J 1991;246:722.

161. Rozenfeld V, Sisca TS, Callahan AK, et al. Double blind, randomized, placebo controlled trial of aged garlic extract in patients stabilized on warfarin therapy [abstract]. ASHP Midyear Clinical Meeting 2000;35:P-26E.

162. Dixit VP, Joshi S. Effects of chronic administration of garlic (*Allium sativum* Linn.) on testicular function. Indian J Exp Biol 1982;20(7):534-536.

163. St Louis ME, Peck SH, Bowering D, et al. Botulism from chopped garlic: delayed recognition of a major outbreak. Ann Intern Med 1988;108(3):363-368.

164. Lohse N, Kraghede PG, Molbak K. [Botulism in a 38-year-old man after ingestion of garlic in chilli oil]. Ugeskr Laeger 2003;165(30):2962-2963.

165. Klintschar M, Beham-Schmidt C, Radner H, et al. Colchicine poisoning by accidental ingestion of meadow saffron (*Colchicum autumnale*): pathological and medicolegal aspects. Forensic Sci Int 1999;106(3):191-200.

166. Murphy JM. Preoperative considerations with herbal medicines. AORN J 1999;69(1):173-8, 180.

167. Velasquez BL, Garcia PS, Minjan CD, et al. Vascular effect of garlic extract: its mechanism of action. Arch Inst Farmacol Exp (Madrid) 1958;10:15-22.

168. Mennella JA, Johnson A, Beauchamp GK. Garlic ingestion by pregnant women alters the odor of amniotic fluid. Chem Senses 1995;20(2):207-209.

169. Mennella JA, Beauchamp GK. Maternal diet alters the sensory qualities of human milk and the nursling's behavior. Pediatrics 1991;88(4):737-744.

170. Mennella JA, Beauchamp GK. The effects of repeated exposure to garlic-flavored milk on the nursling's behavior. Pediatr Res 1993;34(6):805-808.

171. McCrindle BW, Helden E, Conner WT. Alternative medicine—randomized double blind placebo-controlled clinical trial of garlic in hypercholesterolemic children [white diamond suit] 661. Pediatric Res 1998;43(4 suppl 2):115.

172. Piscitelli SC, Burstein AH, Welden N, et al. The effect of garlic supplements on the pharmacokinetics of saquinavir. Clin Infect Dis 2002;34(2):234-238.

173. Anonymous. Garlic supplements can impede HIV medication. J Am Coll Surg 2002;194(2):251.

174. Anonymous. NIH studies link between saquinavir and garlic pills. Aids Alert 2002;17(2):26.

175. Gallicano K, Foster B, Choudhri S. Effect of short-term administration of garlic supplements on single-dose ritonavir pharmacokinetics in healthy volunteers. Br J Clin Pharmacol 2003;55(2):199-202.

176. Chen HW, Tsai CW, Yang JJ, et al. The combined effects of garlic oil and fish oil on the hepatic antioxidant and drug-metabolizing enzymes of rats. Br J Nutr 2003;89(2):189-200.

177. Le Bon AM, Vernevaut MF, Guenot L, et al. Effects of garlic powders with varying alliin contents on hepatic drug metabolizing enzymes in rats. J Agric Food Chem 2003;51(26):7617-7623.

178. Markowitz JS, Devane CL, Chavin KD, et al. Effects of garlic (*Allium sativum* L.) supplementation on cytochrome P450 2D6 and 3A4 activity in healthy volunteers. Clin Pharmacol Ther 2003;74(2):170-177.

179. Pathak A, Leger P, Bagheri H, et al. Garlic interaction with fluindione: a case report. Therapie 2003;58(4):380-381.

180. de Rooij BM, Boogaard PJ, Rijksen DA, et al. Urinary excretion of N-acetyl-S-allyl-L-cysteine upon garlic consumption by human volunteers. Arch Toxicol 1996;70(10):635-639.

181. Block E. The chemistry of garlic and onions. Sci Am 1985;252(3):114-119.

182. Agarwal K. Therapeutic actions of garlic constituents. Med Res Rev 1996; 16(1):111-124.
183. Reuter HD, Sendl A. *Allium sativum* and *Allium ursinum*: chemistry, pharmacology and medicinal applications. In: Wagner H, Farnsworth NR, editors. Economic and Medicinal Research. London, Academic Press Ltd, 1994, pp. 55-103.
184. Kasuga S, Uda N, Kyo E, et al. Pharmacologic activities of aged garlic extract in comparison with other garlic preparations. J Nutr 2001;131(3s): 1080S-1084S.
185. Campbell JH, Efendy JL, Smith NJ, et al. Molecular basis by which garlic suppresses atherosclerosis. J Nutr 2001;131(3s):1006S-1009S.
186. Patumraj S, Tewit S, Amatyakul S, et al. Comparative effects of garlic and aspirin on diabetic cardiovascular complications. Drug Deliv 2000;7(2): 91-96.
187. Sendl A, Elbl G, Steinke B, et al. Comparative pharmacological investigations of *Allium ursinum* and *Allium sativum*. Planta Med 1992;58(1):1-7.
188. Chi MS. Effects of garlic products on lipid metabolism in cholesterol-fed rats (41494). Proc Soc Exper Biol Med 1982;171:174-178.
189. Chi M, Koh ET, Stewart TJ. Effects of garlic on lipid metabolism in rats fed cholesterol or lard. J Nutrit 1982;112(2):241-248.
190. Qureshi A, Abuirmeileh N, Din Z, et al. Inhibition of cholesterol and fatty acid biosynthesis in liver enzymes and chicken hepatocytes by polar fractions of garlic. Lipids 1983;18:343-348.
191. Qureshi AA, Crenshaw TD, Abuirmeileh N. Influence of minor plant constituents on porcine hepatic lipid metabolism. Atherosclerosis 1987;64:109-115.
192. Gebhardt R, Beck H, Wagner K. Inhibition of cholesterol biosynthesis by allicin and ajoene in rat hepatocytes and HepG2 cells. Biochim Biophys Acta 1994;1213(1):57-62.
193. Yeh YY, Yeh SM. Garlic reduces plasma lipids by inhibiting hepatic cholesterol and triacylglycerol synthesis. Lipids 1994;29(3):189-193.
194. Gupta N, Porter TD. Garlic and garlic-derived compounds inhibit human squalene monooxygenase. J Nutr 2001;131(6):1662-1667.
195. Yeh YY, Liu L. Cholesterol-lowering effect of garlic extracts and organosulfur compounds: human and animal studies. J Nutr 2001;131(3s): 989S-993S.
196. Gebhardt R, Beck H. Differential inhibitory effects of garlic-derived organosulfur compounds on cholesterol biosynthesis in primary rat hepatocyte cultures. Lipids 1996;31(12):1269-1276.
197. Liu L, Yeh YY. Inhibition of cholesterol biosynthesis by organosulfur compounds derived from garlic. Lipids 2000;35(2):197-203.
198. Bordia A, Verma SK, Srivastava KC. Effect of garlic (*Allium sativum*) on blood lipids, blood sugar, fibrinogen and fibrinolytic activity in patients with coronary artery disease. Prostaglandins Leukot Essent Fatty Acids 1998;58(4):257-263.
199. Bordia A, Bansal HC. Letter: Essential oil of garlic in prevention of atherosclerosis. Lancet 1973;2(7844):1491-1492.
200. Sendl A, Schliack M, Loser R, et al. Inhibition of cholesterol synthesis in vitro by extracts and isolated compounds prepared from garlic and wild garlic. Atherosclerosis 1992;94(1):79-85.
201. Ide N, Nelson AB, Lau BHS. Aged garlic extract and its constituents inhibit Cu^{2+}-induced oxidative modification of low density lipoprotein. Planta Med 1997;63:263-264.
202. Ide N, Lau BH. Garlic compounds protect vascular endothelial cells from oxidized low density lipoprotein-induced injury. J Pharm Pharmacol 1997; 49(9):908-911.
203. Orekhov A, Tertov V. *In vitro* effect of garlic powder extract on lipid content in normal and atherosclerotic human aortic cells. Lipids 1997;32: 1055-1060.
204. Orekhov AN, Tertov VV, Sobenin IA, et al. Direct anti-atherosclerosis-related effects of garlic. Ann Med 1995;27(1):63-65.
205. Efendy JL, Simmons DL, Campbell GR, et al. The effect of the aged garlic extract, 'Kyolic', on the development of experimental atherosclerosis. Atherosclerosis 1997;132(1):37-42.
206. Jain RC, Konar DB. Effect of garlic oil in experimental cholesterol atherosclerosis. Atherosclerosis 1978;29(2):125-129.
207. Kiesewetter H. Long-term effect of garlic powder tablets on the development of plaque formation in the carotid branches of both femoral arteries—a preliminary report. Eur J Clin Res 1996;8:34-35.
208. Durak İ, Öztürk HS, Olcay E, et al. Effects of garlic extract supplementation on blood lipid and antioxidant parameters and atherosclerotic plaque formation process in cholesterol-fed rabbits. J Herbal Pharmacother 2002;2(2):19-32.
209. Munday JS, James KA, Fray LM, et al. Daily supplementation with aged garlic extract, but not raw garlic, protects low density lipoprotein against in vitro oxidation. Atherosclerosis 1999;143(2):399-404.
210. Phelps S, Harris WS. Garlic supplementation and lipoprotein oxidation susceptibility. Lipids 1993;28(5):475-477.
211. Dwivedi C, John LM, Schmidt DS, et al. Effects of oil-soluble organosulfur compounds from garlic on doxorubicin-induced lipid peroxidation. Anticancer Drugs 1998;9(3):291-294.
212. Byrne DJ, Neil HA, Vallance DT, et al. A pilot study of garlic consumption shows no significant effect on markers of oxidation or sub-fraction composition of low-density lipoprotein including lipoprotein(a) after allowance for non-compliance and the placebo effect. Clin Chim Acta 1999; 285(1-2):21-33.
213. Ali M. Mechanism by which garlic (*Allium sativum*) inhibits cyclo-oxygenase activity. Effect of raw versus boiled garlic extract on the synthesis of prostanoids. Prostaglandins Leukot Essent Fatty Acids 1995;53(6): 397-400.
214. Teranishi K, Apitz-Castro R, Robson SC, et al. Inhibition of baboon platelet aggregation *in vitro* and *in vivo* by the garlic derivative, ajoene. Xenotransplantation 2003;10(4):374-379.
215. Apitz-Castro R, Cabrera S, Cruz MR, et al. Effects of garlic extract and of three pure components isolated from it on human platelet aggregation, arachidonate metabolism, release reaction and platelet ultrastructure. Thromb Res 1983;32(2):155-169.
216. Makheja AN, Vanderhoek JY, Bailey JM. Inhibition of platelet aggregation and thromboxane synthesis by onion and garlic. Lancet 1979;1(8119):781.
217. Srivastava KC, Tyagi OD. Effects of a garlic-derived principle (ajoene) on aggregation and arachidonic acid metabolism in human blood platelets. Prostaglandins Leukot Essent Fatty Acids 1993;49(2):587-595.
218. Boullin DJ. Garlic as a platelet inhibitor. Lancet 1981;1(8223):776-777.
219. Jamaluddin MP, Krishnan LK, Thomas A. Ajoene inhibition of platelet aggregation: possible mediation by a hemoprotein. Biochem Biophys Res Communicat 1988;153(1):479-486.
220. Rendu F, Daveloose D, Debouzy JC, et al. Ajoene, the antiplatelet compound derived from garlic, specifically inhibits platelet release reaction by affecting the plasma membrane internal microviscosity. Biochem Pharmacol 1989;38(8):1321-1328.
221. Oshiba S, Sawai H, Tamada T, et al. [Inhibitory effect of orally administered inclusion complex of garlic oil on platelet aggregation in man]. Igaku no Ayuma 1990;155(3):199-200.
222. Ali M, Bordia T, Mustafa T. Effect of raw versus boiled aqueous extract of garlic and onion on platelet aggregation. Prostaglandins Leukot Essent Fatty Acids 1999;60(1):43-47.
223. Apitz-Castro R, Badimon JJ, Badimon L. Effect of ajoene, the major antiplatelet compound from garlic, on platelet thrombus formation. Thromb Res 1992;68(2):145-155.
224. Apitz-Castro R, Badimon JJ, Badimon L. A garlic derivative, ajoene, inhibits platelet deposition on severely damaged vessel wall in an in vivo porcine experimental model. Thromb Res 1994;75(3):243-249.
225. Steiner M, Lin RS. Changes in platelet function and susceptibility of lipoproteins to oxidation associated with administration of aged garlic extract. J Cardiovasc Pharmacol 1998;31(6):904-908.
226. Bordia A, Verma SK, Srivastava KC. Effect of garlic on platelet aggregation in humans: a study in healthy subjects and patients with coronary artery disease. Prostaglandins Leukot Essent Fatty Acids 1996;55(3):201-205.
227. Bordia T, Mohammed N, Thomson M, et al. An evaluation of garlic and onion as antithrombotic agents. Prostaglandins Leukot Essent Fatty Acids 1996;54(3):183-186.
228. Legnani C, Frascaro M, Guazzaloca G, et al. Effects of a dried garlic preparation on fibrinolysis and platelet aggregation in healthy subjects. Arzneimittelforschung 1993;43(2):119-122.
229. Rahman K, Billington D. Dietary supplementation with aged garlic extract inhibits ADP-induced platelet aggregation in humans. J Nutr 2000; 130(11):2662-2665.
230. Steiner M, Li W. Aged garlic extract, a modulator of cardiovascular risk factors: a dose-finding study on the effects of AGE on platelet functions. J Nutr 2001;131(3s):980S-984S.
231. Morris J, Burke V, Mori TA, et al. Effects of garlic extract on platelet aggregation: a randomized placebo-controlled double-blind study. Clin Exp Pharmacol Physiol 1995;22(6-7):414-417.
232. Das I, Patel S, Sooranna SR. Effects of aspirin and garlic on cyclooxygenase-induced chemiluminescence in human term placenta. Biochem Soc Trans 1997;25(1):99S.
233. Makheja AN, Bailey JM. Antiplatelet constituents of garlic and onion. Agents Actions 1990;29(3-4):360-363.
234. Ali M, Thomson M. Consumption of a garlic clove a day could be beneficial in preventing thrombosis. Prostaglandins Leukot Essent Fatty Acids 1995;53(3):211-212.
235. Kendler BS. Garlic (*Allium sativum*) and onion (*Allium cepa*): a review of their relationship to cardiovascular disease. Prev Med 1987;16(5):670-685.
236. Srivastava KC, Bordia A, Verma SK. Garlic (*Allium sativum*) for disease prevention. S Afr J Sci 1995;91:68-77.
237. Chutani SK, Bordia A. The effect of fried versus raw garlic on fibrinolytic activity in man. Atherosclerosis 1981;38(3-4):417-421.
238. Bordia AK, Joshi HK, Sanadhya YK, et al. Effect of essential oil of garlic on serum fibrinolytic activity in patients with coronary artery disease. Atherosclerosis 1977;28(2):155-159.
239. Arora RC, Arora S, Gupta RK. The long-term use of garlic in ischemic heart disease—an appraisal. Atherosclerosis 1981;40(2):175-179.
240. Ashraf MZ, Hussain ME, Fahim M. Endothelium-mediated vasorelaxant response of garlic in isolated rat aorta: role of nitric oxide. J Ethnopharmacol 2004;90(1):5-9.
241. Baluchnejadmojarad T, Roghani M, Homayounfar H, et al. Beneficial effect of aqueous garlic extract on the vascular reactivity of streptozotocin-diabetic rats. J Ethnopharmacol 2003;85(1):139-144.

242. Baluchnejadmojarad T, Roghani M. Endothelium-dependent and -independent effect of aqueous extract of garlic on vascular reactivity on diabetic rats. Fitoterapia 2003;74(7-8):630-637.

243. Jung EM, Jung F, Mrowietz C, et al. Influence of garlic powder on cutaneous microcirculation. A randomized placebo-controlled double-blind cross-over study in apparently healthy subjects. Arzneimittelforschung 1991;41(6):626-630.

244. Jung F, Jung EM, Mrowietz C, et al. [The effects of garlic powder on cutaneous microcirculation. A cross-over test with healthy test persons]. Med Welt 1991;42:28-30.

245. Wohlrab J, Wohlrab D, Marsch WC. Acute effect of a dried ethanol-water extract of garlic on the microhaemovascular system of the skin. Arzneimittelforschung 2000;50(7):606-612.

246. Wolf S, Reim M, Jung F. Effect of garlic on conjunctival vessels: a randomised, placebo- controlled, double-blind trial. Br J Clin Pract Suppl 1990;69:36-39.

247. Das I, Khan NS, Sooranna SR. Potent activation of nitric oxide synthase by garlic: a basis for its therapeutic applications. Curr Med Res Opin 1995; 13(5):257-263.

248. Dirsch VM, Kiemer AK, Wagner H, et al. Effect of allicin and ajoene, two compounds of garlic, on inducible nitric oxide synthase. Atherosclerosis 1998;139:333-339.

249. Pedraza-Chaverri J, Tapia E, Medina-Campos O. Garlic prevents hypertension induced by chronic inhibition of nitric oxide synthesis. Life Sciences 1998;62(6):71-77.

250. Breithaupt-Grogler K, Ling M, Boudoulas H, et al. Protective effect of chronic garlic intake on elastic properties of aorta in the elderly. Circulation 1997;96(8):2649-2655.

251. Ku DD, Abdel-Razek TT, Dai J, et al. Mechanisms of garlic induced pulmonary vasorelaxation: role of allicin. Circulation 1997;96(8S):6-I.

252. Al-Naghdy SA, Abdel-Rahman MO, Heiba HI. Evidence for some prostag-landins in Allium sativum extracts. Phytother Res 1988;2(4):196-197.

253. Kweon S, Park KA, Choi H. Chemopreventive effect of garlic powder diet in diethylnitrosamine-induced rat hepatocarcinogenesis. Life Sci 2003; 73(19):2515-2526.

254. Unnikrishnan MC, Soudamini KK, Kuttan R. Chemoprotection of garlic extract toward cyclophosphamide toxicity in mice. Nutr Cancer 1990; 13(3):201-207.

255. Thabrew MI, Samarawickrema NA, Chandrasena LG, et al. Protection by garlic against adriamycin induced alterations in the oxido-reductive status of mouse red blood cells. Phytother Res 2000;14(3):215-217.

256. Hussain SP, Jannu LN, Rao AR. Chemopreventive action of garlic on methylcholanthrene-induced carcinogenesis in the uterine cervix of mice. Cancer Lett 1990;49(2):175-180.

257. Balasenthil S, Ramachandran CR, Nagini S. Prevention of 4-nitroquinoline 1-oxide–induced rat tongue carcinogenesis by garlic. Fitoterapia 2001; 72(5):524-531.

258. Wang BH, Zuzel KA, Rahman K, et al. Protective effects of aged garlic extract against bromobenzene toxicity to precision cut rat liver slices. Toxicology 1998;126(3):213-222.

259. Wang BH, Zuzel KA, Rahman K, et al. Treatment with aged garlic extract protects against bromobenzene toxicity to precision cut rat liver slices. Toxicology 1999;132(2-3):215-225.

260. Nishino H, Iwashima A, Itakura Y, et al. Antitumor-promoting activity of garlic extracts. Oncology 1989;46(4):277-280.

261. Dwivedi C, Rohlfs S, Jarvis D, et al. Chemoprevention of chemically induced skin tumor development by diallyl sulfide and diallyl disulfide. Pharm Res 1992;9(12):1668-1670.

262. Balasenthil S, Rao KS, Nagini S. Retinoic acid receptor-beta mRNA expression during chemoprevention of hamster cheek pouch carcinogenesis by garlic. Asia Pac J Clin Nutr 2003;12(2):215-218.

263. Belman S. Onion and garlic oils inhibit tumor promotion. Carcinogenesis 1983;4(8):1063-1065.

264. Wargovich MJ. Diallyl sulfide, a flavor component of garlic (Allium sativum), inhibits dimethylhydrazine-induced colon cancer. Carcinogenesis 1987;8(3):487-489.

265. Wargovich MJ, Uda N, Woods C, et al. Allium vegetables: their role in the prevention of cancer. Biochem Soc Trans 1996;24(3):811-814.

266. Sparnins VL, Barany G, Wattenberg LW. Effects of organosulfur compounds from garlic and onions on benzo[a]pyrene-induced neoplasia and glutathione S-transferase activity in the mouse. Carcinogenesis 1988; 9(1):131-134.

267. Pinto JT, Rivlin RS. Antiproliferative effects of allium derivatives from garlic. J Nutr 2001;131(3s):1058S-1060S.

268. Dirsch VM, Gerbes AL, Vollmar AM. Ajoene, a compound of garlic, induces apoptosis in human promyeloleukemic cells, accompanied by generation of reactive oxygen species and activation of nuclear factor kappaB. Mol Pharmacol 1998;53(3):402-407.

269. Xiao D, Pinto JT, Soh JW, et al. Induction of apoptosis by the garlic-derived compound S-allylmercaptocysteine (SAMC) is associated with microtubule depolymerization and c-Jun NH(2)-terminal kinase 1 activation. Cancer Res 2003;63(20):6825-6837.

270. Bradley R, Endres J, Hockenberry D, et al. Investigation of garlic-induced apoptosis in breast cancer cell lines [poster presentation]. International Scientific Conference on Complementary, Alternative and Integrative Medicine Research, Boston, MA, 2002.

271. Hu X, Cao BN, Hu G, et al. Attenuation of cell migration and induction of cell death by aged garlic extract in rat sarcoma cells. Int J Mol Med 2002;9(6):641-643.

272. Tilli CM, Stavast-Kooy AJ, Vuerstaek JD, et al. The garlic-derived organosulfur component ajoene decreases basal cell carcinoma tumor size by inducing apoptosis. Arch Dermatol Res 2003;295(3):117-123.

273. Li M, Ciu JR, Ye Y, et al. Antitumor activity of Z-ajoene, a natural compound purified from garlic: antimitotic and microtubule-interaction properties. Carcinogenesis 2002;23(4):573-579.

274. Morioka N, Sze LL, Morton DL, et al. A protein fraction from aged garlic extract enhances cytotoxicity and proliferation of human lymphocytes mediated by interleukin-2 and concanavalin A. Cancer Immunol Immunother 1993;37(5):316-322.

275. Siegers CP, Steffen B, Robke A, et al. The effects of garlic preparation against human tumour cell proliferation. Phytomedicine 1999;6(1):7-11.

276. Milner JA. A historical perspective on garlic and cancer. J Nutr 2001;131(3s):1027S-1031S.

277. Lau BH, Tadi PP, Tosk JM. Allium sativum (garlic) and cancer prevention. Nutrit Res 1990;10:937-948.

278. Lamm DL, Riggs DR. The potential application of Allium sativum (garlic) for the treatment of bladder cancer. Urol Clin North Am 2000;27(1):157-162, xi.

279. Hassan ZM, Yaraee R, Zare N, et al. Immunomodulatory affect of R10 fraction of garlic extract on natural killer activity. Int Immunopharmacol 2003;3(10-11):1483-1489.

280. Keiss HP, Dirsch VM, Hartung T, et al. Garlic (Allium sativum L.) modulates cytokine expression in lipopolysaccharide-activated human blood thereby inhibiting NF-kappaB activity. J Nutr 2003;133(7):2171-2175.

281. Lamm DL, Riggs DR. Enhanced immunocompetence by garlic: role in bladder cancer and other malignancies. J Nutr 2001;131(3s):1067S-1070S.

282. Salman H, Bergman M, Bessler H, et al. Effect of a garlic derivative (alliin) on peripheral blood cell immune responses. Int J Immunopharmacol 1999;21(9):589-597.

283. Mel'chinskaia EN, Popovtseva ON, Gromnatskii NI. [Immunologic aspects of alisate in diabetes mellitus patients]. Biull Eksp Biol Med 1997;124(11):595-597.

284. Song K, Milner JA. The influence of heating on the anticancer properties of garlic. J Nutr 2001;131(3s):1054S-1057S.

285. Yoshida H, Iwata N, Katsuzaki H, et al. Antimicrobial activity of a compound isolated from an oil-macerated garlic extract. Biosci Biotechnol Biochem 1998;62(5):1014-1017.

286. Hughes BG, Lawson LD. Antimicrobial effects of Allium sativum L. (garlic), Allium ampeloprasum L. (elephant garlic), and Allium cepa L. (onion), garlic compounds and commercial garlic supplement products. Phytother Res 1991;5:154-158.

287. Ankri S, Mirelman D. Antimicrobial properties of allicin from garlic. Microbes Infect 1999;1(2):125-129.

288. Sasaki J, Kita T, Ishita K, et al. Antibacterial activity of garlic powder against Escherichia coli O-157. J Nutr Sci Vitaminol (Tokyo) 1999; 45(6):785-790.

289. Naganawa R, Iwata N, Ishikawa K, et al. Inhibition of microbial growth by ajoene, a sulfur-containing compound derived from garlic. Appl Environ Microbiol 1996;62(11):4238-4242.

290. Rao R, Rao S, Natarajan S, et al. Inhibition of Mycobacterium tuberculosis by garlic extract. Nature 1946; (3988):441.

291. Sharma VD, Sethi MS, Kumar A, et al. Antibacterial property of Allium sativum Linn.: in vivo & in vitro studies. Indian J Exper Biol 1977;15:466-468.

292. Abbruzzese MR, Delaha EC, Garagusi VF. Absence of antimycobacterial synergism between garlic extract and antituberculosis drugs. Diagn Microbiol Infect Dis 1987;8(2):79-85.

293. Delaha EC, Garagusi VF. Inhibition of mycobacteria by garlic extract (Allium sativum). Antimicrob Agents Chemother 1985;27(4):485-486.

294. Deshpande RG, Khan MB, Bhat DA, et al. Inhibition of Mycobacterium avium complex isolates from AIDS patients by garlic (Allium sativum). J Antimicrob Chemother 1993;32(4):623-626.

295. Jonkers D, van den BE, van D, I, et al. Antibacterial effect of garlic and omeprazole on Helicobacter pylori. J Antimicrob Chemother 1999;43(6):837-839.

296. O'Gara EA, Hill DJ, Maslin DJ. Activities of garlic oil, garlic powder, and their diallyl constituents against Helicobacter pylori. Appl Environ Microbiol 2000;66(5):2269-2273.

297. Moore GS, Atkins RD. The fungicidal and fungistatic effects of an aqueous garlic extract on medically important yeast-like fungi. Mycologia 1977;69(2):341-348.

298. Caporaso N, Smith SM, Eng RH. Antifungal activity in human urine and serum after ingestion of garlic (Allium sativum). Antimicrob Agents Chemother 1983;23(5):700-702.

299. Fliermans CB. Inhibition of Histoplasma capsulatum by garlic. Mycopathol Mycol Appl 1973;50(3):227-231.

G

300. Feldberg RS, Chang SC, Kotik AN, et al. *In vitro* mechanism of inhibition of bacterial cell growth by allicin. Antimicrob Agents Chemother 1988; 32(12):1763-1768.

301. Ghannoum MA. Studies on the anticandidal mode of action of *Allium sativum* (garlic). J Gen Microbiol 1988;134 (Pt 11):2917-2924.

302. Ross ZM, O'Gara EA, Hill DJ, et al. Antimicrobial properties of garlic oil against human enteric bacteria: evaluation of methodologies and comparisons with garlic oil sulfides and garlic powder. Appl Environ Microbiol 2001;67(1):475-480.

303. Adetumbi M, Javor GT, Lau BH. *Allium sativum* (garlic) inhibits lipid synthesis by *Candida albicans*. Antimicrob Agents Chemother 1986; 30(3):499-501.

304. Tsai Y, Cole LL, Davis LE, et al. Antiviral properties of garlic: in vitro effects on influenza B, herpes simplex and coxsackie viruses. Planta Med 1985;(5):460-461.

305. Nagae S, Ushijima M, Hatono S, et al. Pharmacokinetics of the garlic compound S-allylcysteine. Planta Med 1994;60(3):214-217.

306. Egen-Schwind C, Eckard R, Jekat FW, et al. Pharmacokinetics of vinyldithiins, transformation products of allicin. Planta Med 1992;58:8-13.

307. Rivlin RS. Historical perspective on the use of garlic. J Nutr 2001;131(3s): 951S-954S.

308. Dausch JG, Nixon DW. Garlic: a review of its relationship to malignant disease. Prev Med 1990;19(3):346-361.

309. Buhsan S, Sharma SP, Singh SP, et al. Effect of garlic on normal blood cholesterol level. Indian J Physiol Pharmacol 1979;23:211-214.

310. Kenzelmann R, Kade F. Limitation of the deterioration of lipid parameters by a standardized garlic-ginkgo combination product. A multicenter placebo-controlled double-blind study. Arzneimittelforschung 1993;43(9): 978-981.

311. Lash JP, Cardoso LR, Mesler PM, et al. The effect of garlic on hypercholesterolemia in renal transplant patients. Transplant Proc 1998;30(1): 189-191.

312. Lau BH, Lam F, Wang-Cheng R, et al. Effect of odor-modified garlic preparation on blood lipids. Nutrition Research 1987;7:139-149.

313. Melvin KR. Effects of garlic powder tablets on patients with hyperlipidaemia in Canadian clinical practice. Eur J Clin Res 1996;8:30-32.

314. Morcos NC. Modulation of lipid profile by fish oil and garlic combination. J Natl Med Assoc 1997;89(10):673-678.

315. Plengvidhya C, Sitprija S, Chinayon S, et al. Effects of spray dried garlic preparation on primary hyperlipoproteinemia. J Med Assoc Thai 1988; 71(5):248-252.

316. Rotzsch W, Richter V, Rassoul F, et al. [Postprandial lipemia under treatment with *Allium sativum*. Controlled double-blind study of subjects with reduced HDL2-cholesterol]. Arzneimittelforschung 1992;42(10): 1223-1227.

317. Lawson LD. Garlic for total cholesterol reduction. Ann Intern Med 2001; 135(1):65-66.

318. Alder R, Lookinland S, Berry JA, et al. A systematic review of the effectiveness of garlic as an anti-hyperlipidemic agent. J Am Acad Nurse Pract 2003;15(3):120-129.

319. Gardner CD, Chatterjee LM, Carlson JJ. The effect of a garlic preparation on plasma lipid levels in moderately hypercholesterolemic adults. Atherosclerosis 2001;154(1):213-220.

320. Peleg A, Hershcovici T, Lipa R, et al. Effect of garlic on lipid profile and psychopathologic parameters in people with mild to moderate hypercholesterolemia. Isr Med Assoc J 2003;5(9):637-640.

321. Satitvipawee P, Rawdaree P, Indrabhakti S, et al. No effect of garlic extract supplement on serum lipid levels in hypercholesterolemic subjects. J Med Assoc Thai 2003;86(8):750-757.

322. Mansell P, Reckless JP. Garlic. BMJ 1991;303(6799):379-380.

323. Ghorai M, Mandal SC, Pal M, et al. A comparative study on hypocholesterolaemic effect of allicin, whole germinated seeds of Bengal gram and guggulipid of gum gugglu. Phytother Res 2000;14(3):200-202.

324. Bhushan S, Sharma SP, Singh SP, et al. Effect of garlic on normal blood cholesterol level. Indian J Physiol Pharmacol 1979;23(3):211-214.

325. Jeyaraj S, Shivaji G, Jeyaraj SD. Effect of a combined supplementation of fish oil (MEGA-3) with garlic pearls on the serum lipid profile, blood pressure and body mass index of hypercholesterolemic subjects. Heart 2000;83(suppl 2):A4.

326. Brosche T, Platt D. [Garlic as phytogenic antilipemic agent. Recent studies with a standardized dry garlic powder substance]. Fortschr Med 1990; 108(36):703-706.

327. Siegel G, Klussendorf D. The anti-atheroslerotic effect of *Allium sativum*: statistics re-evaluated. Atherosclerosis 2000;150(2):437-438.

328. Schiermeier Q. German garlic study under scrutiny. Nature 1999; 401(6754):629.

329. Koscielny J, Schmitt R, Radtke H, et al. Garlic study vindicated by official investigation. Nature 2000;404(6773):542.

330. Siegel G. Long-term effect of garlic in preventing arteriosclerosis—results of two controlled clinical trials. Eur Phytojournal 2001;Symposium posters(1):1.

331. Orekhov AN, Pivovarova EM, Tertov VV. Garlic powder tablets reduce atherogenicity of low density lipoprotein. A placebo-controlled double-blind study. Nutr Metab Cardiovascular Dis 1996;6:21-31.

332. Jepson RG, Kleijnen J, Leng GC. Garlic for peripheral arterial occlusive disease. Cochrane Database Syst Rev 2000;(2):CD000095. Review.

333. Kandziora J. The blood pressure lowering and lipid lowering effect of a garlic preparation in combination with a diuretic. Arzliche Forschung 1988;3:1-8.

334. Fleischauer AT, Arab L. Garlic and cancer: a critical review of the epidemiologic literature. J Nutr 2001;131(3s):1032S-1040S.

335. Buiatti E, Palli D, Decarli A, et al. A case-control study of gastric cancer and diet in Italy. Int J Cancer 1989;44(4):611-616.

336. Hansson LE, Nyren O, Bergstrom R. Diet and risk of gastric cancer: a population-based case-control study in Sweden. Int J Cancer 1993;55: 181-189.

337. You WC, Blot WJ, Chang YS, et al. *Allium* vegetables and reduced risk of stomach cancer. J Natl Cancer Inst 1989;81(2):162-164.

338. Gao CM, Takezaki T, Ding JH, et al. Protective effect of allium vegetables against both esophageal and stomach cancer: a simultaneous case-referent study of a high-epidemic area in Jiangsu Province, China. Jpn J Cancer Res 1999;90(6):614-621.

339. Dorant E, van den Brandt PA, Goldbohm RA, et al. Consumption of onions and a reduced risk of stomach carcinoma. Gastroenterology 1996; 110(1):12-20.

340. Dorant E, van den Brandt PA, Goldbohm RA. A prospective cohort study on the relationship between onion and leek consumption, garlic supplement use and the risk of colorectal carcinoma in The Netherlands. Carcinogenesis 1996;17(3):477-484.

341. Giovannucci E, Rimm EB, Stampfer MJ, et al. Intake of fat, meat, and fiber in relation to risk of colon cancer in men. Cancer Res 1994;54:2390-2397.

342. Steinmetz KA, Kushi LH, Bostick RM, et al. Vegetables, fruit, and colon cancer in the Iowa women's health study. Am J Epidemiol 1994;139(1):1-15.

343. Hu J, Nyren O, Wolk A, et al. Risk factors for oesophageal cancer in northeast China. Int J Cancer 1994;57(1):38-46.

344. Zheng W, Blot WJ, Shu XO, et al. A population-based case-control study of cancers of the nasal cavity and paranasal sinuses in Shanghai. Int J Cancer 1992;52(4):557-561.

345. Gao YT, McLaughlin JK, Gridley G. Risk factors for esophageal cancer in Shanghai, China. Role of diet and nutrients. Int J Cancer 1994;58:197-202.

346. Zheng W, Blot WJ, Shu XO, et al. Diet and other risk factors for laryngeal cancer in Shanghai, China. Am J Epidemiol 1992;136(2):178-191.

347. Dorant E, van den Brandt PA, Goldbohm RA. A prospective cohort study on *Allium* vegetable consumption, garlic supplement use, and the risk of lung carcinoma in The Netherlands. Cancer Res 1994;54(23):6148-6153.

348. Dorant E, van den Brandt PA, Goldbohm RA. *Allium* vegetable consumption, garlic supplement intake, and female breast carcinoma incidence. Breast Cancer Res Treat 1995;33(2):163-170.

349. Levi F, La Vecchia C, Gulie C, et al. Dietary factors and breast cancer risk in Vaud, Switzerland. Nutr Cancer 1993;19(3):327-335.

350. Challier B, Perarnau JM, Viel JF. Garlic, onion and cereal fibre as protective factors for breast cancer: a French case-control study. Eur J Epidemiol 1998;14(8):737-747.

351. Key TJ, Silcocks PB, Davey GK, et al. A case-control study of diet and prostate cancer. Br J Cancer 1997;76(5):678-687.

352. Fleischauer AT, Poole C, Arab L. Garlic consumption and cancer prevention: meta-analyses of colorectal and stomach cancers. Am J Clin Nutr 2000;72(4):1047-1052.

353. Ernst E. Can allium vegetables prevent cancer? Phytomedicine 1997; 4(1):79-83.

354. Takezaki T, Gao CM, Ding JH, et al. Comparative study of lifestyles of residents in high and low risk areas for gastric cancer in Jiangsu Province, China; with special reference to allium vegetables. J Epidemiol 1999;9(5): 297-305.

355. You WC, Zhang L, Gail MH, et al. *Helicobacter pylori* infection, garlic intake and precancerous lesions in a Chinese population at low risk of gastric cancer. Int J Epidemiol 1998;27(6):941-944.

356. Gail M, You WC, Chang YS, et al. Factorial trial of three interventions to reduce the progression of precancerous gastric lesions in Shandong, China: Design issues and initial data. Controlled Clin Trials 1998;19:352-369.

357. Cook-Mozaffari PJ, Azordegan F, Day NE, et al. Oesophageal cancer studies in the Caspian Littoral of Iran: results of a case-control study. Br J Cancer 1979;39(3):293-309.

358. Witte JS, Longnecker MP, Bird CL, et al. Relation of vegetable, fruit, and grain consumption to colorectal adenomatous polyps. Am J Epidemiol 1996;144(11):1015-1025.

359. Swanson CA, Mao BL, Li JY, et al. Dietary determinants of lung-cancer risk: results from a case-control study in Yunnan Province, China. Int J Cancer 1992;50(6):876-880.

360. Shu XO, Zheng W, Potischman N, et al. A population-based case-control study of dietary factors and endometrial cancer in Shanghai, People's Republic of China. Am J Epidemiol 1993;137(2):155-165.

361. Levi F, Franceschi S, Negri E, et al. Dietary factors and the risk of endometrial cancer. Cancer 1993;71(11):3575-3581.

362. Marsh CL, Torrey RR, Woolley JL, et al. Superiority of intravesical immunotherapy with *Corynebacterium parvum* and *Allium sativum* in control of murine bladder cancer. J Urol 1987;137(2):359-362.

363. Sigounas G, Hooker J, Anagnostou A, et al. *S*-allylmercaptocysteine inhibits cell proliferation and reduces the viability of erythroleukemia, breast, and prostate cancer cell lines. Nutr Cancer 1997;27(2):186-191.

364. Mostafa MG, Mima T, Ohnishi ST, et al. *S*-allylcysteine ameliorates doxorubicin toxicity in the heart and liver in mice. Planta Med 2000; 66(2):148-151.

365. Horie T, Matsumoto H, Kasagi M, et al. Protective effect of aged garlic extract on the small intestinal damage of rats induced by methotrexate administration. Planta Med 1999;65(6):545-548.

366. Sovova M, Sova P. [Pharmaceutical significance of *Allium sativum* L. 4. Antifungal effects]. Ceska Slov Farm 2003;52(2):82-87.

367. Sandhu DK, Warraich MK, Singh S. Sensitivity of yeasts isolated from cases of vaginitis to aqueous extracts of garlic. Mykosen 1980;23(12):691-698.

368. Pai ST, Platt MW. Antifungal effects of *Allium sativum* (garlic) extract against the Aspergillus species involved in otomycosis. Lett Appl Microbiol 1995;20(1):14-18.

369. Davis LE, Shen J, Royer RE. In vitro synergism of concentrated *Allium sativum* extract and amphotericin B against *Cryptococcus neoformans*. Planta Med 1994;60:546-549.

370. Venugopal PV, Venugopal TV. Antidermatophytic activity of garlic (*Allium sativum*) *in vitro*. Int J Dermatol 1995;34(4):278-279.

371. Ghannoum MA. Inhibition of *Candida* adhesion to buccal epithelial cells by an aqueous extract of *Allium sativum* (garlic). J Appl Bacteriol 1990; 68(2):163-169.

372. Ledezma E, Marcano K, Jorquera A, et al. Efficacy of ajoene in the treatment of tinea pedis: a double-blind and comparative study with terbinafine. J Am Acad Dermatol 2000;43(5 Pt 1):829-832.

373. Ledezma E, DeSousa L, Jorquera A, et al. Efficacy of ajoene, an organosulphur derived from garlic, in the short-term therapy of tinea pedis. Mycoses 1996;39(9-10):393-395.

374. Ledezma E, Lopez JC, Marin P, et al. Ajoene in the topical short-term treatment of tinea cruris and tinea corporis in humans. Randomized comparative study with terbinafine. Arzneimittelforschung 1999;49(6): 544-547.

375. Rich GE. Garlic an antibiotic? Med J Aust 1982;1(2):60.

376. Tutakne MA, Satyanarayanan G, Bhardwaj JR, et al. Sporotrichosis treated with garlic juice. A case report. Indian J Dermatol 1983;28(1):41-45.

377. Soffar SA, Mokhtar GM. Evaluation of the antiparasitic effect of aqueous garlic (*Allium sativum*) extract in hymenolepiasis nana and giardiasis. J Egypt Soc Parasitol 1991;21(2):497-502.

378. Stjernberg L, Berglund J. Garlic as an insect repellent. JAMA 2000; 284(7):831.

379. McHugh CP. Garlic as a tick repellent. JAMA 2001;285(1):41-42.

380. Ranstam J. Garlic as a tick repellent. JAMA 2001;285(1):41-42.

381. Tunon H. Garlic as a tick repellent. JAMA 2001;285(1):41-42.

382. Andrianova IV, Sobenin IA, Sereda EV, et al. [Effect of long-acting garlic tablets "Allicor" on the incidence of acute respiratory viral infections in children]. Ter Arkh 2003;75(3):53-56.

383. Graham DY, Anderson SY, Lang T. Garlic or jalapeno peppers for treatment of *Helicobacter pylori* infection. Am J Gastroenterol 1999;94(5): 1200-1202.

384. McNulty CA, Wilson MP, Havinga W, et al. A pilot study to determine the effectiveness of garlic oil capsules in the treatment of dyspeptic patients with *Helicobacter pylori*. Helicobacter 2001;6(3):249-253.

385. Aydin A, Ersoz G, Tekesin O, et al. Garlic oil and *Helicobacter pylori* infection. Am J Gastroenterol 2000;95(2):563-564.

386. Ernst E. Is garlic an effective treatment for *Helicobacter pylori* infection? Arch Intern Med 1999;159(20):2484-2485.

387. Mahady GB, Pendland S. Garlic and *Helicobacter pylori*. Am J Gastroenterol 2000;95(1):309.

388. Salih BA, Abasiyanik FM. Does regular garlic intake affect the prevalence of *Helicobacter pylori* in asymptomatic subjects? Saudi Med J 2003;24(8): 842-845.

G

Ginger
(Zingiber officinale Roscoe)

SYNONYMS/COMMON NAMES/RELATED SUBSTANCES

- 4-gingesulfonic acid, 8-ginerol, african ginger, *Amomum zingiber* L., black ginger, chayenne ginger, cochin ginger, EV.EXT35, gan jiang, gegibre, gingembre, gingerall, Ginger BP, Ginger Power BP, ginger root, ginger trips, gingerly, ingwer, Jamaica ginger, kankyo, Myanmar ginseng, *Panax zingiberensis*, race ginger, rhizoma zingeberis, sheng jiang, shogasulfonic acid, shokyo, zerzero, *Zingiber capitatum, Zingiber officinale* Roscoe, *Zingiber zerumbet* Smith, *Zingiber blancoi* Massk, *Zingiber majus* Rumph, zingiberis rhizome, Zintona EC.

CLINICAL BOTTOM LINE
Background

- The rhizomes (underground stem) and stems of ginger have assumed significant roles in Chinese, Japanese and Indian medicine since the 1500s. The oleoresin of ginger is often contained in digestive, antitussive, antiflatulent, laxative, and antacid compounds.
- There is supportive evidence from one randomized controlled trial and an open-label study that ginger reduces the severity and duration of chemotherapy-induced nausea/emesis. Effects appear to be additive to prochlorperazine (Compazine). The optimal dose remains unclear. Ginger's effects on other types of nausea/emesis, such as postoperative nausea or motion sickness, remain indeterminate.
- Ginger is used orally, topically, and intramuscularly for a wide array of other conditions, without scientific evidence of benefit.
- Ginger may inhibit platelet aggregation/decrease platelet thromboxane production, thus theoretically increasing bleeding risk.

Scientific Evidence for Common/Studied Uses	Grade*
Hyperemesis gravidarum, nausea/vomiting of pregnancy	B
Motion sickness/seasickness	C
Nausea (chemotherapy-induced)	C
Nausea and vomiting (postoperative)	C
Rheumatic diseases (rheumatoid arthritis, osteoarthritis, arthralgias, muscle pain)	C

*Key to grades: *A:* Strong scientific evidence for this use; *B:* Good scientific evidence for this use; *C:* Unclear scientific evidence for this use; *D:* Fair scientific evidence against this use (it may not work); *F:* Strong scientific evidence against this use (it likely does not work). For a more detailed explanation of efficacy criteria, see "Natural Standard Evidence-Based Validated Grading Rationale" in the Introduction.

Historical or Theoretical Uses That Lack Sufficient Evidence

- Acute bacterial dysentery, alcohol withdrawal, analgesic, antacid, antibacterial,[1,2] antioxidant,[3] antiseptic, anti-spasmodic, antitussive, antiviral, aphrodisiac, asthma, atherosclerosis, athlete's foot, baldness, bile secretion, body warming, bronchitis, burns (topical), cancer,[4] carminative (antiflatus), cholera, colds, colic, coronary artery disease, cough suppressant, depression, diaphoresis, diarrhea, digestive aid,[5,6] diminished appetite (anorexia), diuresis, dysmenorrhea, dyspepsia, expectorant, fungicide, flatulence, flu, general stimulant, gonarthritis,[7] headache, heart disease, *Helicobacter pylori* infection,[8] hepatitis,[9] high blood pressure, hypercholesterolemia,[5,6,10] hyperglycemia-evoked dysrhythmias,[11] immune system stimulation,[12] impotence, increased drug absorption, increased metabolism, insecticide, intestinal parasites,[13] Kawasaki's disease, kidney disease, laxative, leukemia,[3] liver disease, liver toxicity, low blood pressure, migraines, malaria, nephrotoxicity, neuroblastoma,[14] orchitis, pain relief, perspiration, poisonous snake bites, promotion of menstruation, psoriasis (topical), rubefacient, selective serotonin reuptake inhibitor (SSRI) discontinuation or tapering,[15] serotonin-induced hypothermia, small intestinal transport,[16] stimulant, stomachache, stomach ulcers,[8] testicular inflammation, tonic, toothache, ulcers, upper respiratory infections,[1] "warming."

Expert Opinion and Folkloric Precedent

- Reports on the beneficial effects of ginger date back to the 9th and 10th centuries. In Asia, ginger has been recommended in the treatment of stomachaches, diarrhea, and nausea for thousands of years.
- In modern times, ginger is often recommended to alleviate nausea, vomiting, and gastrointestinal discomfort. It is believed by some to increase gastric motility and cause absorption of toxins/gastric acid, thereby modifying gastrointestinal reactions and feedback responsible for nausea.
- Ginger has been listed in the United States Pharmacopoeia (USP) and the National Formulary as a carminative (antiflatus agent), aromatic, and stimulant.
- Ginger is widely used as a seasoning or fragrance in foods, beverages, soaps, candles and cosmetics. There is generally <0.5% ginger in average baked goods.

Safety Summary

- **Likely safe:** When the fresh or dried root/stem is used in culinary quantities (0.023%), including during pregnancy. Ginger has a long history of human consumption and topical use in both the East and West, with minimal evidence of harm. Ginger gained U.S. Food and Drug Administration (FDA) status as "generally recognized as safe" (GRAS) in the United States. However, mechanism of action and dosing standards are not known definitively.
- **Possibly safe:** When the fresh or dried root is used orally (encapsulated) in recommended doses.
- **Possibly unsafe:** When used in pregnancy at doses exceeding 1 g daily and in patients perioperatively, due to theoretical increased risk of bleeding. There are multiple theoretical herb/drug and herb/herb interactions when ingested in high doses.
- **Maximum recommended daily dose:** 4.0 g (accepted by many experts, but clinical data are limited).

DOSING/TOXICOLOGY
General

- Recommended doses are based on those most commonly used in available trials, or on historical practice. However, with natural products, the optimal doses needed to balance efficacy and safety often have not been determined. Formulations and preparation methods may vary from manufacturer to manufacturer, and from batch to batch of a specific product made by a single manufacturer. Because often the active components of a product are not known, standardization may not be possible, and the clinical effects of different brands may not be comparable.
- Common forms of ginger include fresh root, dried root, powdered root, tablets, capsules, liquid extract, tincture, tea, and use in foods.
- Maximum daily recommended dose of ginger is 4.0 g, based on expert opinion.

Standardization

- Although consensus is limited for formal standardization, ginger products are increasingly being standardized to gingerol content.

Dosing: Adult (18 Years and Older)
Oral

- *Note:* The mild gastrointestinal distress sometimes associated with ginger may be reduced by ingesting encapsulated (rather than powdered) ginger.[17]
- **General use:** Powder/tablets/capsules or fresh-cut ginger, 1 to 4 g/day in divided doses (dose recommended by most experts, including the European Scientific Cooperative on Phytotherapy, and the German expert panel, the Commission E).
- **Post-operative nausea:** 1 g given 1 hour prior to surgery.[18,19] *Note:* Use in the peri-operative period should be approached with caution: ginger may inhibit platelet aggregation/decrease platelet thromboxane production, thus theoretically increasing perioperative bleeding risk. Increased prothrombin time (PT) and international normalized ratio (INR) have been reported in a woman taking both warfarin and ginger, although the contribution of ginger is not clear.[20]
- **Hyperemesis gravidarum:** 1 to 2 g/day in divided doses.[21,22] *Note:* Consumption of ginger during pregnancy in amounts greater than those commonly found in food [<1 g dry weight/day] is not advised by some authors, due to concerns about mutagenicity or abortifacient properties.[23] However, others report no scientific or medical evidence for a pregnancy contraindication.[24] This matter is sometimes confusing because ginger is cautioned against during pregnancy in traditional Chinese medicine. However, in Chinese medicine, much higher doses are generally used. Nonetheless, supervision by a qualified healthcare provider is recommended for pregnant women considering use of ginger.
- **Motion sickness/seasickness:** 1 to 2 g daily in divided doses.[17]
- **Anticoagulation:** 5 g/day in 2 divided doses.[25] Insufficient safety or efficacy data.
- **Rheumatic diseases:** 1 to 2 g/day of powdered ginger.[26] *Note*: In one study,[26] patients who mistakenly took 2 to 4 g/day of ginger (number of patients not specified) reported faster and superior pain relief.

Dosing: Pediatric (Younger Than 18 Years)

- Insufficient evidence to recommend.

Toxicology

- It has been suggested by expert panels that a maximum dose of 4.0 g/day of ginger is associated with few adverse effects, although this has not been tested in reliable human trials. When used topically, the oil of ginger is usually well tolerated, with the possible exception of atopic individuals.
- The acute oral LD_{50} in rats was found to exceed 5 g of ginger oil/day, as reported by the European Scientific Cooperative on Phytotherapy.
- Mice have tolerated doses of 2.5 g/kg of a concentrated ethanolic extract (85%) of ginger over a 7-day period.[27]

ADVERSE EFFECTS/PRECAUTIONS/CONTRAINDICATIONS
Allergy

- Known allergy/hypersensitivity to ginger and possibly other members of the Zingiberaceae family, including alpinia formosana, alpinia purpurata (red ginger), alpinia zerumbet (shell ginger), costus barbatus, costus malortieanus, costus pictus, costus productus, dimerocostus strobilaceus, elettaria cardamomum (green cardamom). Contact dermatitis has been reported,[28] with a prevalence of 6% among patients with known allergy to balsam of Peru (used as a screening substance for spice allergy).

Adverse Effects

- **General:** Ginger has a long history of oral and topical use with minimal reports of toxicity or serious reactions. Adverse effects have usually been reported for dosage amounts exceeding (usually far exceeding) recommended doses.[29] Some of the mild gastrointestinal symptoms may be reduced by ingesting encapsulated (rather than powdered) ginger.[17]
- **Dermatologic:** Dermatitis may occur in individuals with sensitive skin when ginger is applied topically. In a study of 55 patients with suspected localized/generalized contact dermatitis, seven subjects responded positively to patch tests with ginger (10% to 25%). One of these patients worked with ginger plants and presented with hand eczema.[30] Allergic contact dermatitis to ginger has been reported,[27] with a prevalence of 6% among patients allergic to balsam of Peru (used as a screening substance for spice allergy).
- **Neurologic/CNS:** Central nervous system depression has been reported as a potential result of large overdoses, although human data are scant.
- **Ocular/Otic:** Conjunctivitis developed in one of 75 patients in a crossover trial of ginger,[31] although this appears to be an isolated report.
- **Cardiovascular:** Arrhythmias are theoretically possible at high doses, based on *in vitro* and *in vivo* studies showing components of ginger to activate Ca^{2+}-ATPase, and to have dose-dependent positive inotropic effects.[32] Anecdotally, some experts report hemodynamic effects of large doses, including hypertension or hypotension, although scientific data are lacking in this area.
- **Gastrointestinal:** Oral/esophageal irritation described as "pepper-like," heartburn, belching, bloating, flatulence, nausea, and "bad taste" have been reported occasionally, primarily with powdered forms of ginger.[31,33-35] When encapsulated ginger is ingested, reports of adverse effects are minimized.[17] Four cases of small bowel obstruction due to ginger bolus have been reported following ingestion of raw ginger without sufficient mastication (chewing). In each case, the bolus was removed by enterotomy. Ginger is composed of cellulose, and therefore is resistant to digestion

and absorbs water, which may cause it to swell and become lodged in narrow areas of the digestive tract.[36]

- **Genitourinary:** An "intense" urge to urinate after 30 minutes was reported in two of eight patients given 0.5 to 1.0 g of ginger in a placebo-controlled trial,[34] although this effect has not been corroborated elsewhere.
- **Endocrine:** Ginger is purported to possess hypoglycemic properties, particularly at high doses, although scientific data are lacking in this area.[37]
- **Hematologic:** Ginger has been shown to decrease platelet aggregation in randomized controlled studies, and concern has been raised that ginger may prolong bleeding time due to its inhibition of thromboxane synthetase.[38,39] There is one case report of inhibition of platelet aggregation following chronic consumption of a large quantity of marmalade containing 15% raw ginger; platelet function spontaneously returned to normal one week after discontinuation of ginger. There is also a European case report of a 75-year-old woman taking chronic warfarin whose international normalized ratio(INR) rose after initiating therapy with ginger, and was complicated by epistaxis.[20] Her INR normalized after discontinuation of ginger and treatment with vitamin K. It is not clear to what extent ginger was responsible for this rise in INR.

Precautions/Warnings/Contraindications

- Avoid in patients using anticoagulation therapy due to theoretical increased bleeding risk.[38,39]
- Avoid large quantities of fresh-cut ginger in patients with inflammatory bowel disease or history of intestinal obstruction, due to potential mechanical bowel obstruction.[36]
- Use cautiously in patients prior to surgery due to theoretical risk of increased bleeding (inhibition of thromboxane synthetase and induction of prostacyclin).[38,39]
- Use cautiously in patients with gastric or duodenal ulcers, due to reports of gastric/esophageal irritation (encapsulated ginger is better tolerated).
- Use cautiously in patients with gallstones, due to the cholagogic effects of ginger.[40]
- Long-term use is cautioned against, although reliable human research is not available.[41]

Pregnancy and Lactation

- **General:** Consumption during pregnancy of ginger in amounts greater than those commonly found in food (<1 g dry weight/day) is not advised by some authors, due to purported emmenagogic effects (menstrual discharge-promoting), as well as abortifacient, mutagenic, and antiplatelet effects.[23] However, others have reported no scientific or medical evidence for a pregnancy contraindication.[23,24] Literature review reveals scant reliable data in this area. This matter is sometimes confusing because ginger is cautioned against in pregnancy in traditional Chinese medicine. However, in Chinese medicine, much higher doses are generally used.
- **Human evidence:** In a double-blind randomized crossover trial of 25 pregnant women given 250 mg of powdered ginger root four times daily for 4 days to treat hyperemesis gravidarum, no teratogenicity was observed. One woman in the study experienced a spontaneous abortion in her 12th week of pregnancy, although the role of ginger is not clear.[21] A randomized placebo-controlled study of 70 women (32 in the ginger group) did not detect ginger to have an adverse

effect on pregnancy with oral administration of 1 g/day for 4 days.[22] A different placebo-controlled study in 120 women (half receiving ginger) noted normal ranges of birth weights, gestational ages, Apgar scores, and frequencies of congenital abnormalities when ginger group infants were compared to the general population of infants born at the Royal Hospital for Women during 1999 to 2000.[42] In a prospective cohort study with matched controls, 187 pregnancies and births to women ingesting ginger during the first trimester of pregnancy were observed.[43] There were 181 live births, 2 stillbirths, 3 spontaneous abortions, and 1 therapeutic abortion. The mean birth weight was 3542 ± 543 g, mean gestational age was 39 ± 2 weeks, and there were three major malformations. There were no statistically significant differences in birth outcomes when this group was compared to a comparison group (exposed to nonteratogenic drugs that were not antiemetics), except that there were more infants weighing less than 2500 g in the comparison group (12 vs. 3; $p = 0.001$).
- **Preclinical evidence:** The mutagenicity of ginger has not been systematically examined in mammalian cell cultures.[44] Both mutagenic ([6]-gingerol and shogaol) and antimutagenic (zingerone) components have been identified in ginger as a result of *in vitro* studies in bacteria.[45-48] Presently, the net effect of ginger on mutagenicity in humans is unknown. It has been proposed that, through inhibition of thromboxane synthetase, ginger may affect testosterone receptor binding in the fetus, possibly affecting sex steroid differentiation of the fetal brain.[38]

INTERACTIONS
Ginger/Drug Interactions

- **Gastric acid-inhibiting drugs/antacids:** There is evidence that ginger rhizome (underground stem) increases stomach acid production. Therefore, it may interfere with antacids, sucralfate (Carafate), H-2 antagonists or proton pump inhibitors. In contrast, other *in vitro* and animal studies have revealed gastroprotective properties.[49,50]
- **Anticoagulants, antiplatelet drugs, NSAIDs:** In theory, since ginger has been observed to inhibit thromboxane synthetase, and because decreased platelet aggregation has been reported in clinical trials, concurrent use of ginger with agents that predispose to bleeding could enhance their effect and increase the risk of bleeding.[38,39,51,52] In addition, there is also a European case report of a 75-year-old woman taking chronic warfarin whose international normalized ratio/ INR rose after initiating therapy with ginger, complicated by epistaxis.[20] Her INR normalized after discontinuation of ginger and treatment with vitamin K. It is not clear to what extent ginger was responsible for this rise in INR.
- **Barbiturates, benzodiazepines, CNS depressants:** In theory, since large doses of ginger have been reported to depress the central nervous system (CNS), it may enhance the CNS depressant effects of other drugs.
- **Digoxin, beta-blockers, positive inotropic agents:** Due to its inotropic properties, ginger may interfere with cardiac drug therapy/negative inotropes, or act in a synergistic manner with other inotropes.[32]
- **Insulin, oral hypoglycemic agents:** Theoretically, due to its purported hypoglycemic effects, ginger may interfere with diabetes therapy, potentially requiring dosing adjustments.[37]
- **Cytochrome P450, xanthine oxidase:** The Chinese herbal medicine sho-saiko-to contains ginger and six other herbs

(bupleurum, pinellia tuber, scutellaria root, jujube fruit, ginseng, licorice root), and has been associated in healthy humans with reduced activity of cytochrome P450 1A2, P450 3A, and xanthine oxidase (in 26 healthy subjects).[53] The contribution of ginger to this effect is not clear.

Ginger/Herb/Supplement Interactions:

- **Anticoagulant herbs and supplements:** In theory, since ginger has been observed to inhibit thromboxane synthetase, concurrent use of ginger with agents that predispose to bleeding could enhance their effect and increase the risk of bleeding.[38,39,51,52] In addition, there is also a European case report of a 75-year-old woman taking chronic warfarin whose international normalized ratio/INR rose after initiating therapy with ginger, complicated by epistaxis.[20] Her INR normalized after discontinuation of ginger and treatment with vitamin K. It is not clear to what extent ginger was responsible for this rise in INR.
- **Calcium:** Ginger or ginger extracts may stimulate calcium uptake in both skeletal and cardiac muscle. *In vitro* studies of gingerol involving canine cardiac tissue and rabbit skeletal muscle demonstrated gingerol to activate the Ca^{2+}-ATPase pump in a dose-dependent manner.[54] In theory, ginger coupled with high serum levels of calcium could cause hyperexcitability of cardiac muscle.
- **Hypoglycemic agents:** Theoretically, due to its purported hypoglycemic effects, ginger may lower blood glucose levels when taken concomitantly with hypoglycemic/anti-hyperglycemic herbs or supplements.[37]
- **Cytochrome P450, xanthine oxidase:** The Chinese herbal medicine sho-saiko-to contains ginger and six other herbs (bupleurum, pinellia tuber, scutellaria root, jujube fruit, ginseng, licorice root), and has been associated in healthy humans with reduced activity of cytochrome P450 1A2, P450 3A, and xanthine oxidase (in 26 healthy subjects).[53] The contribution of ginger to this effect is not clear.

Ginger/Lab Interactions

- **International normalized ratio/INR:** There is a European case report of a 75-year-old woman taking chronic warfarin whose international normalized ratio/INR rose after initiating therapy with ginger, and was complicated by epistaxis.[20] Her INR normalized after discontinuation of ginger and treatment with vitamin K. It is not clear to what extent ginger was responsible for this rise in INR.

MECHANISM OF ACTION
Pharmacology

- The "pungent principles" or nonvolatile constituents of ginger are considered responsible for its flavor, aromatic properties, and pharmacological activity. These include: gingerols (usually <1% of the root's weight), (6)-shogaol (a dehyroxylated analog of (6)-gingerol), (6)- and (10)-dehydro-gingerdione, (6)- and (10)-gingerdione, and zingerone. Other compounds present include carbohydrates, fats, minerals, oleoresins, vitamins, waxes and zingibain (a proteolytic enzyme).
- *In vitro* research indicates that gingerols and the related shogaols exhibit cardiodepressant activity at low doses and cardiotonic properties at higher doses.[55] Both (6)-shogaol and (6)-gingerol, and the gingerdiones, are reportedly potent enzymatic inhibitors of prostaglandin, thromboxane and leukotriene biosynthesis.

- Ginger has been shown to inhibit platelet aggregation[51,52] and to decrease platelet thromboxane production *in vitro*.[56-58] However, its effects *in vivo* have not been well studied. Although Verma found ginger to decrease platelet aggregation,[25] Lumb found no effect of ginger on platelet count, bleeding time, or platelet aggregation.[59] Similarly, Bordia found ginger to have no effect on platelet aggregation, fibrinolytic activity or fibrinogen levels.[60] Janssen showed no effect of oral ginger on platelet thromboxane B2 production,[61] while Srivastava found thromboxane levels to be decreased by ginger ingestion in a small study.[62]
- Oral ingestion of ginger extract has been shown to have hypocholesterolemic, hypolipidemic and antiatherosclerotic effects in cholesterol-fed rabbits[63] and in rats.[64] Inhibition of LDL oxidation and attenuated development of atherosclerosis has also been observed in apolipoprotein E-deficient mice.[65]
- (6)-Shogaol, generally more potent than (6)-gingerol, has exhibited antitussive effects, inhibited intestinal motility in intravenous preparations, and facilitated gastrointestinal motility in oral preparations.
- The mechanism of action of ginger's effect on nausea and vomiting remains uncertain. Using gastroduodenal manometry, Micklefield demonstrated that oral ginger increases antral motility during phase III of the migrating motor complex (MMC), and increases motor response to a test meal in the corpus.[66] However, ginger had no significant effect in the antrum or corpus during other phases, except for a significant decrease in the amplitude of antral contractions during phase II of the MMC. Additionally, there was no effect of ginger on duodenal contractions, or on the "motility index."
- In a randomized, placebo-controlled, crossover trial of 16 healthy volunteers, ginger (1g orally) had no effect on gastric emptying.[67] It appears unlikely that ginger's anti-emetic or anti-nausea effects are mediated through increased gastroduodenal motility or through increased gastric emptying.
- Lumb proposed that ginger's antiemetic effect could be mediated through central 5-hydroxytryptamine-3 ($5-HT_3$) antagonism.[68] *In vitro* studies have shown that both ginger extract and galanolactone, a diterpenoid of ginger, antagonize the $5-HT_3$ receptor.[69,70]
- Ginger extract, zingiberene, and (6)-gingerol have been observed to afford cytoprotection against chemically-induced ulceration in rats,[49,50] and ginger extract has been reported to inhibit the growth of *Helicobacter pylori in vitro*.[8] However, Desai observed a significant increase in the exfoliation of gastric surface epithelial cells following consumption of 6 g or more of ginger (after examining gastric aspirates in 10 healthy volunteers).[71]
- (6)-shogaol has produced anti-nociception and inhibited the release of substance P in rats, seemingly via the same receptor to which capsaicin binds. However, it was observed to be 100 times less potent and to elicit half the maximal effect of capsaicin.[72]
- Inhibition of prostaglandin and thromboxane formation by human platelets, and the subsequent production of lipid peroxides, have been proposed as possible mechanisms by which ginger might provide relief of rheumatoid arthritis symptoms.[73]
- There is evidence that ginger rhizome (root) increases stomach acid production. If so, it may interfere with antacids, sucralfate (Carafate), H-2 antagonists or proton pump

inhibitors. In contrast, other *in vitro* and animal studies have revealed gastroprotective properties.[49,50]

Pharmacodynamics/Kinetics

- Insufficient reliable data available.

HISTORY

- Ginger is a perennial commonly found in warmer climates, including China, India, and Jamaica. Its green-purple flowers are similar in appearance to orchids. The rhizome (root) is aromatic and is usually the most valued portion of the plant. Herbal preparations are obtained by cutting the fresh plant, by powdering the dried root (or stem), or via extraction with acetone, ethanol, or methanol.
- Ginger is popular as a seasoning and has played a prominent role in Chinese, Indian, and Japanese medicine since the 1500s, due to its purported carminative, stimulant, diuretic, and antiemetic properties.

Review of the Evidence: Ginger

Condition Treated*	Study Design	Author, Year	N[†]	SS[†]	Study Quality[‡]	Magnitude of Benefit	ARR[†]	NNT[†]	Comments
Nausea and vomiting	Systematic review	Ernst[44] 2000	6 studies	NA	NA	NA	NA	NA	Well designed, although studies analyzed nausea/vomiting of multiple etiologies; pooled analysis with positive trend.
Hyperemesis gravidarum	RCT, double-blind comparison study	Sripramote[35] 2003	138	NA	3	Medium	NA	NA	Comparison of 500 mg of ginger vs. 10 mg of Vitamin B_6; improvements seen with both therapies, but lack of placebo arm makes results difficult to interpret.
Hyperemesis gravidarum	RCT, double-blind, placebo-controlled	Willetts[42] 2003	120	Yes	4	Medium	NA	NA	Significant improvements in nausea and retching but not vomiting with ginger (1.5 g) daily for 4 days compared to placebo.
Hyperemesis gravidarum	Prospective cohort study with matched controls	Portnoi[43] 2003	187	Unclear	2	Small	NA	NA	Pregnancy outcomes of women ingesting ginger found no significant differences vs. control women taking nonteratogenic drugs, except that infants weighed less in the control group.
Hyperemesis gravidarum	RCT	Vutyavanich[22] 2001	70	Yes	4	High	28%	4	Ginger found superior to placebo for reduction of nausea of pregnancy.
Hyperemesis gravidarum	RCT, crossover	Fischer-Rasmussen[21] 1990	30	Yes	2	Medium	NA	NA	250 mg of powdered ginger root superior to placebo in subjective improvement of symptoms.
Nausea and vomiting (chemotherapy-induced)	RCT, unclear blinding	Pace[74] 1987	41	Yes	2	Small	NA	NA	Reduction in self-reported nausea, but not vomiting; unclear dose.
Nausea and vomiting (chemotherapy-induced)	Case series	Meyer[75] 1995	11	NA	NA	NA	NA	NA	Open-label, uncontrolled.
Nausea and vomiting (postoperative)	RCT, double-blind	Eberhart[76] 2003	184	No	4	None	NA	NA	No decrease seen in nausea and vomiting with ginger (100 mg or 200 mg) pre-medication for laparoscopic surgery.
Nausea and vomiting (postoperative)	RCT, double-blind, placebo-controlled, comparison study	Visalyaputra[77] 1998	111	No	4	None	NA	NA	No benefit of ginger (2 g) for perioperative nausea compared to placebo or droperidol; however, no effects of droperidol either, raising question about study design and outcomes measurements.
Nausea and vomiting (postoperative)	RCT	Arfeen[33] 1995	108	No	4	None	NA	NA	Ginger powder (500 mg or 1 g) vs. placebo; increased nausea trend with 1 g of ginger.
Nausea and vomiting (postoperative)	Equivalence trial	Phillips[18] 1993	120	Yes	3	Medium	12%	8	Equal efficacy to metoclopramide; inadequate power calculation.

Review of the Evidence: Ginger—cont'd

Condition Treated*	Study Design	Author, Year	N[†]	SS[†]	Study Quality[‡]	Magnitude of Benefit	ARR[†]	NNT[†]	Comments
Nausea (postoperative)	Equivalence trial	Bone[19] 1990	60	Yes	3	Medium	NA	NA	Ginger (1 g) vs. metoclopramide (10 mg) vs. placebo.
Motion sickness	Equivalence trial	Schmid[78] 1994	1741	No	5	NA	NA	NA	No difference between ginger (1000 mg; 2 doses 4 hours apart) and 6 common medications.
Motion sickness, gastric function	RCT, crossover	Stewart[34] 1991	28	No	1	None	NA	NA	No protection against motion sickness.
Motion sickness	RCT	Holtmann[79] 1989	38	No	2	None	NA	NA	No effect on induced nystagmus.
Motion sickness	RCT	Wood[80] 1988	56	No	2	NA	NA	NA	Ginger not more effective than placebo.
Motion sickness	RCT	Mowrey[81] 1982	36	Yes	3	Medium	NA	NA	Likely improper blinding.
Seasickness	RCT	Grontved[17] 1988	80	Yes	4	Medium	NA	NA	Decreased vomiting and cold sweating, but no decrease in nausea or vertigo.
Osteoarthritis (knee)	RCT, double-blind, intention-to-treat	Altman[82] 2001	261	Mixed	5	Small	13%	8	Significant small mean improvement in pain on standing, but no significant difference in WOMAC scores (well-established scale).
Osteoarthritis (hip and knee)	RCT, crossover	Bliddal[31] 2000	75	No	4	None	NA	NA	No effect of ginger extract (170 mg, 4 times daily for 3 weeks).
Arthritis, muscular discomfort	Case series	Srivastava[26] 1992	56	NA	NA	Small	NA	NA	Limited quality, due to no placebo.
Rheumatoid arthritis	Case series	Srivastava[73] 1989	7	NA	NA	Medium	NA	NA	Limited quality, due to no placebo.

*Primary or secondary outcome.

[†]N, Number of patients; SS, statistically significant; ARR, absolute risk reduction; NNT, the number of patients who need to undergo a specific intervention in order to observe an outcome in one individual.

[‡]0-2 = poor; 3-4 = good; 5 = excellent.

NA, Not applicable; RCT, randomized, controlled trial; WOMAC, Western Ontario and McMaster Universities Osteoarthritis Composite Index.

For an explanation of each category in this table, please see Table 3 in the Introduction.

REVIEW OF THE EVIDENCE: DISCUSSION

Hyperemesis Gravidarum, Nausea/Vomiting of Pregnancy

Summary

- A limited number of randomized controlled trials suggests that 1 g/day of ginger may be safe and effective for pregnancy-associated nausea and vomiting when used for short periods (≤4 days). Doses between 500 mg and 1500 mg (1.5 g) have been evaluated. However, consumption of ginger during pregnancy in amounts greater than commonly found in food (>1 g dry weight/day) is not advised by some authors, due to purported emmenagogic effects (menstrual discharge–promoting), as well as abortifacient, mutagenic, and antiplatelet effects.[23] However, others have reported no scientific or medical evidence for a pregnancy contraindication.[23,24] Additional research is warranted regarding the safety and efficacy of ginger during pregnancy before it can be routinely recommended to patients for extended courses.

Evidence

- Sripramote and Lekhyananda conducted a randomized, double-blind controlled trial to compare the efficacy of ginger to vitamin B_6 in the treatment of nausea and vomiting of pregnancy.[35] Women were included who presented to an antenatal clinic complaining of nausea and vomiting of pregnancy at or before 16 weeks of gestation, were otherwise healthy, and did not require hospitalization for their symptoms. The study included 138 subjects, who were randomly allocated to receive either 500 mg of ginger or 10 mg of vitamin B_6, taken orally for three days. No placebo arm was included. Outcomes included subjective grading of nausea severity, using a visual analog scale, and frequency of vomiting episodes. Baseline characteristics were equivalent between groups. The authors reported that both ginger and vitamin B_6 significantly reduced mean nausea scores from 5.0 to 3.6 and 5.3 to 3.3, respectively ($p < 0.001$). There was no statistically significant difference between groups ($p = 0.136$). The frequency of daily vomiting episodes also decreased from baseline in both groups without significant differences between groups (1.9 to 1.2 and 1.7 to 1.2, respectively; $p < 0.01$). Because no placebo arm was included, it is not clear to what extent the improvements in both groups were due to a "placebo effect" or to the natural tendency of this condition to improve. Therefore, these results cannot be considered conclusive.

- Willetts et al. conducted a randomized, double-blind, placebo-controlled trial to investigate the effects of ginger extract "EV.EXT35" on symptoms of morning sickness in 120 women who were fewer than 20 weeks pregnant.[42] Subjects were recruited from a tertiary metropolitan teaching hospital, and experienced morning sickness daily for at least 1 week without relief through dietary modification. Patients were assigned to receive either 125 mg of EV.EXT35 (equivalent to 1.5 g of dried ginger) or placebo, administered four times daily for 4 days. Nausea, vomiting, and retching were measured by the "Rhodes Index of Nausea, Vomiting, and Retching." The authors reported that after 4 days, significant improvements in nausea and retching occurred in the ginger group compared to placebo, although no significant differences in vomiting were observed. Follow-up of pregnancies and deliveries revealed normal ranges of birth weights, gestational ages, Apgar scores, and frequencies of congenital abnormalities when ginger group infants were compared to the general population of infants born at the Royal Hospital for Women during 1999 to 2000.

- Vutyavanich conducted a randomized, double-blind, placebo-controlled trial in 70 women at or before 17 weeks of gestation, with nausea and vomiting of pregnancy.[22] Subjects were administered either 1g of ginger or placebo orally for 4 days. After baseline nausea scores were subtracted, post-therapy visual analog scores of nausea were significantly decreased in the ginger group compared to placebo ($p = 0.014$). The number of vomiting episodes also significantly decreased among women in the ginger group ($p < 0.001$). No adverse effects on pregnancy outcomes were detected.

- Fischer-Rasmussen conducted a double-blind, randomized, crossover trial comparing powdered ginger root with placebo in the treatment of hyperemesis gravidarum.[21] Thirty women were given either 250 mg of ginger or lactose four times daily for 4 days with a 2-day washout between treatment periods. A significant subjective improvement was reported among the women when they were taking ginger ($p = 0.003$). Relief scores also revealed significantly greater relief from symptoms after treatment with ginger than placebo ($p = 0.035$). Three women were excluded due to noncompliance and a diagnosis of gallstone. No side effects were observed. One woman had a spontaneous abortion in her 12th week of gestation which was not considered "suspicious," although details are limited. Blinding and randomization were not adequately reported.

- Portnoi et al. conducted a prospective cohort study with matched controls to assess the use of ginger in women with nausea and vomiting of pregnancy.[43] Subjects included pregnant women who called the "Motherisk Program," who were already taking ginger during the first trimester of pregnancy. A control group included women who were exposed to nonteratogenic drugs that were not antiemetics. Both groups were followed to ascertain subjective impressions of the outcome of the pregnancy and the health of infants. A total of 187 pregnancies in the ginger group were monitored. Among these subjects, there were 181 live births, 2 stillbirths, 3 spontaneous abortions, and 1 therapeutic abortion. The mean birth weight was 3542 ± 543 g, mean gestational age was 39 ± 2 weeks, and there were three major malformations. However, there were no statistically significant differences in birth outcomes when this group was compared to the comparison group, except that there were more infants weighing less than 2500 g in the comparison group (12 vs. 3; p = 0.001). When subjects were asked, on a scale of 0 to 10, how effective the ginger was for their symptoms, mild improvements were reported, although the statistical significance of these responses is not clear.

Nausea (Chemotherapy Induced)
Summary

- There is supportive evidence from one randomized controlled trial and an open-label study that ginger reduces the severity and duration of self-reported nausea (but not vomiting) during chemotherapy. Effects appear to be additive to those of prochlorperazine (Compazine). The optimal dose remains unclear. Long-term randomized controlled trials are warranted to confirm these results and to establish safety.

Evidence

- Pace and Conlin conducted a double-blind, randomized pair, placebo-controlled study to examine the effect of encapsulated ginger on relief of chemotherapy-associated nausea and vomiting in 41 patients with leukemia.[74] A control group of 21 patients was given scheduled doses of placebo in conjunction with a prochlorperazine (Compazine) injection over 2 days. Another 20 patients were given scheduled doses of encapsulated ginger (dose not specified) in conjunction with a prochlorperazine (Compazine) injection over 2 days. A significant decline in self-reported symptoms (severity and duration of nausea) was noted among the experimental group. However, a significant difference was not observed with respect to severity and duration of vomiting.

- In a case series, 530-mg ginger capsules were administered to 11 patients with cutaneous T-cell lymphoma and frequent nausea 30 minutes prior to 8-MOP dosing.[75] Nausea was measured using a linear analog scale, and was found to be reduced by two thirds overall.

Nausea and Vomiting (Postoperative)
Summary

- A limited number of randomized controlled studies have found a significant decrease in postoperative nausea and/or vomiting following administration of preoperative ginger prophylaxis, whereas other research reports perioperative ginger to be no more efficacious than placebo. Additional studies are warranted before a definitive recommendation can be made. *Note:* Use of ginger in the perioperative period should be approached with caution: ginger may inhibit platelet aggregation/decrease platelet thromboxane production, thus theoretically increasing perioperative bleeding risk; increased prothrombin time (PT) and international normalized ratio (INR) have been reported in a woman taking both warfarin and ginger, although the contribution of ginger is not clear.[20]

Systematic Review

- Ernst and Pittler[44] conducted a systematic review of the efficacy of ginger for nausea and vomiting. They restricted their review to randomized, double-blind, placebo-controlled trials and excluded studies that induced nausea or vomiting through experimental methods. Only six studies met inclusion criteria, of which three assessed ginger's ability to prevent postoperative nausea and vomiting.[18,19,33] In a pooled analysis of ginger's effect on the incidence of postoperative nausea, there was a nonsignificant difference between the 1 g of powdered ginger group versus placebo. The absolute risk reduction was 0.052, with a 95% confidence interval which included zero (−0.082 to +0.186).

Positive Trials

- Phillips conducted a randomized, controlled double-blind trial of 120 women having elective laparoscopic gynecologic day surgery.[18] Group A (n = 40) received 10 mg of oral metoclopramide, group B (n = 40) received 1 g of powdered ginger root, and group C (n = 40) received 1 g of lactulose as placebo. All medications were taken 1 hour prior to induction of anesthesia. The incidence of postoperative nausea and vomiting was 27% in group A, 21% in group B, and 41% in the placebo group. Antiemetics were required by only 15% of patients treated with ginger, compared to 32% of patients treated with metoclopramide and 38% of patients treated with placebo ($p < 0.05$ for ginger vs. placebo). This study suggests that preoperative ginger is as effective in decreasing the incidence of postoperative nausea and vomiting as metoclopramide and superior to placebo. There were no side effects attributed to ginger.

- Bone conducted a double-blind, randomized, placebo-controlled study of ginger vs. metoclopramide in women undergoing major gynecologic surgery.[19] Patients received either 1 g of ginger root and a placebo injection (group 1; n = 20), 1 g of lactulose (as placebo) and 10 mg of intravenous metoclopramide (group 2; n = 20), or 1 g of lactulose and placebo injection (group 3; n = 20) prior to induction of anesthesia. Patients in group 1 had 23 total incidences of nausea in the first 24 hours postoperatively, patients in group 2 had 24, and patients in the placebo group (group 3) had a total of 41 ($p < 0.05$). No patients in group 1 required postoperative metoclopramide for treatment of nausea, and 6 patients in group 3 required metoclopramide postoperatively ($p < 0.05$). This study suggests that prophylactic preoperative ginger is as effective as prophylactic metoclopramide, and superior to placebo, in the treatment of postoperative nausea. Although the authors stated that vomiting was assessed, they did not report the incidence of vomiting.

Negative Trials

- Eberhart et al. conducted a randomized, placebo-controlled trial to compare two different doses of ginger root extract (100 mg, 200 mg) vs. placebo for the prevention of postoperative nausea in 184 patients undergoing gynecologic laparoscopy.[76] Subjects were randomly allocated to receive ginger or placebo tablets both before and after the procedure. The authors reported no differences between groups in terms of nausea and vomiting following the procedures.

- Arfeen et al. conducted a double-blind randomized controlled trial of patients undergoing laparoscopic gynecologic surgery.[33] Patients received either placebo (n = 36), 500 mg of ginger powder BP (n = 36), or 1 g of ginger powder BP (n = 36) 1 hour prior to surgery. Ginger was ineffective in reducing the incidence of postoperative nausea and vomiting (assessed 3 hours postoperatively). There was a trend (not statistically significant) toward increased nausea in patients receiving 1g of ginger.

- Visalyaputra et al. conducted a randomized, double-blind placebo-controlled study in 111 women undergoing diagnostic laparoscopic gynecologic surgery.[77] Patients received either an oral placebo plus 0.5 mL of intravenous normal saline prior to anesthesia, an oral placebo plus 1.25 mg of intravenous droperidol, 2 g of oral ginger plus intravenous normal saline, or 2 g of oral ginger plus 1.25 mg of intravenous droperidol. The authors reported that ginger did not significantly decrease the incidence of postoperative nausea or vomiting compared to placebo or droperidol. However, droperidol also had no significant effect, raising questions about the measurement instrument and study design. The sample size may have been too small to adequately stratify into four treatment groups.

Motion Sickness/Seasickness
Summary

- Several studies have found ginger to have no effect on motion sickness, whereas a study of naval cadets found ginger to reduce vomiting (but not nausea or vertigo). Additional studies are warranted before a definitive recommendation can be made.

Evidence

- Schmid et al. conducted a randomized, double-blind, controlled study to compare the effects of ginger (100 mg total given as 2 divided doses 4 hours apart) with six other medications: a combination of cinnarizine (20 mg) and domperidone (15 mg) given twice, 4 hours apart; cyclizine (50 mg); a combination of dimenhydrinate (50 mg) and caffeine (50 mg); a combination of meclizine (12.3 mg) and caffeine (10 mg); cinnarizine (25 mg); and scopolamine (0.5 mg).[78] In total, 1741 tourists on a whaling expedition agreed to participate in the trial, and 1489 completed questionnaires. None of the study medications offered complete protection from nausea and vomiting associated with motion. However, there was no significant difference in the incidence of nausea and vomiting between the medications tested. The questionnaire was not validated. There was no assessment of baseline characteristics of subjects, dropouts, or compliance.

- Stewart et al. conducted a randomized, placebo-controlled crossover study of the effect of ginger (500 mg or 1000 mg of ginger powder or 1000 mg of fresh ginger root) or scopolamine (0.6 mg orally) on motion sickness induced by a rotating chair and gastric motility.[34] In this study of 28 subjects, ginger had no effect on motion sickness or on gastric function during motion sickness. However, blinding and randomization were inadequately described, and no power calculation was conducted.

- Holtmann et al. conducted a randomized, placebo-controlled double-blind study of ginger root (1 g) or dimenhydrinate (100 mg) vs. placebo in 38 subjects who were subjected to optokinetic testing, caloric testing, and rotary testing.[79] Although dimenhydrinate was able to decrease nystagmus in response to the various stimuli, ginger had no effect on nystagmus. The authors suggested that ginger likely does not reduce symptoms of motion sickness through a central nervous system mechanism.

- Grontved et al. conducted a double-blind, placebo-controlled study of 80 naval cadets who were randomized to either placebo or 1 g of ginger while on the high seas.[17] Ginger significantly reduced vomiting and cold sweating, but did not reduce symptoms of nausea or vertigo.

- Wood et al. examined the effect of three different doses of ginger (1000 mg of fresh ginger, 500 mg of dried ginger, 1000 mg of dried ginger) in comparison with several other antimotion sickness medications, including scopolamine (0.6 mg), D-amphetamine (10 mg), amitriptyline (25 mg), dimenhydrate (50 mg), and promethazine (25 mg), on prevention of motion sickness in a double-blind crossover study (Latin square design) of 56 subjects (7 groups of

8 subjects).[80] Standardized National Aeronautics and Space Administration (NASA) techniques were used to evaluate motion sickness by measuring tolerance to head movements in a revolving chair. None of the doses of ginger root increased tolerance to motion above that of placebo in this study.

• In a randomized, placebo-controlled study designed to simulate sea/motion sickness (kinetosis) by using a revolving chair, doses of dimenhydrinate (100 mg), ginger root (940 mg) or placebo (chickweed herb) were given to 36 blindfolded, kinetosis-prone subjects just prior to the chair trials.[81] Although the participants appear to have been blinded with respect to which product they ingested, it is not clear if the investigators were blinded. Subjects in the dimenhydrinate and placebo groups tolerated the trial for an average of 3.5 and 1.5 minutes, respectively. Subjects receiving ginger root tolerated the trial for an average of 5.5 minutes, and 50% managed the full 6 minutes ($p < 0.001$). Vomiting occurred in 3 subjects in the chickweed group. Notably, subjects were told that they were taking either dimenhydrinate or capsules of "a mixture of harmless garden herbs," and it is unclear how subjects' views on herbal medications may have biased the results (although subjects were blinded). It is not clear if the susceptibility to motion sickness at baseline was comparable between the three groups.

Osteoarthritis (Hip and Knee)
Summary

• The use of ginger in rheumatic diseases is still under preliminary investigation. One randomized, controlled trial observed ginger to have no effect on the relief of osteoarthritic symptoms.[82] However, a retrospective analysis of the data obtained in this study (using a different method of analysis) found ginger to be of statistically greater benefit than placebo. A controlled crossover trial found no benefits of ginger, although post hoc analysis of the data reported effects prior to crossover, suggesting possible carry-over confounding results.[31] The results of two case series support the role of ginger as an analgesic in patients with rheumatic disease. However, additional randomized controlled trials are required to confirm if ginger possesses analgesic properties in rheumatic patients.

Evidence

• In a well-designed trial, Altman and Marcussen studied a highly concentrated Danish ginger preparation in 261 patients (mean age, 64) with knee osteoarthritis.[82] One capsule was given twice/day (each capsule containing 255 mg of EV.EXT 77 extract, manufactured from 2500 to 4000 mg of dried ginger roots and 500 to 1500 mg of galanga roots) for 6 weeks. Randomization and blinding were well described and properly conducted; baseline characteristics of patients were adequately described; and analysis was by intention-to-treat. Results were mixed. Statistically significant positive results were noted for the study's primary outcome, reduction in knee pain on standing: Reduced pain on standing was noted in 63% of ginger subjects vs. 50% of controls ($p = 0.048$). This yields an absolute risk reduction of 13% and a number of patients needed to treat of 8. However, when the data are analyzed in terms of mean difference in pain, the gap between ginger and placebo is relatively small. In addition, as an editorial in the same journal issue points out, this is not the gold standard measurement of osteoarthritis therapy benefit.[83] Rather, the Western Ontario and McMaster

Universities Osteoarthritis Composite Index (WOMAC) is more commonly used, and for this measure no statistically significant difference between ginger and placebo was observed ($p = 0.087$). Therefore, even if there is some benefit of this preparation of ginger for symptoms of knee osteoarthritis, it is likely small and may not occur in all patients.

• Bliddal et al. conducted a controlled, double-blind, double-dummy crossover trial in 75 patients with hip/knee osteoarthritis.[31] Subjects were administered either 400 mg of ibuprofen, 170 mg of ginger extract, or placebo three times daily for 3 weeks, with 1 week washout between crossovers. The authors reported no significant difference between groups in multiple measures of function. Twenty-five percent of subjects dropped out prior to assessment. Despite these negative results, the authors note that analysis of the first treatment period before crossover revealed both ibuprofen and ginger extract to be more effective than placebo ($p < 0.05$), thus suggesting possible carry-over effects (inadequate washout) leading to a null result.

Rheumatoid Arthritis
Summary

• There is insufficient evidence to recommend for or against the use of ginger for rheumatoid arthritis.

Evidence

• In a case series, Srivastava and Mustafa studied powdered ginger in 56 patients with rheumatoid arthritis (n = 28), osteoarthritis (n = 18), or muscular discomfort (n = 10).[26] The majority of patients took 0.5 to 1 teaspoon of powdered ginger per day (approximately 1 to 2 g). Seventy-five percent of patients with arthritis experienced relief from pain and swelling to varying degrees after taking ginger (varying doses). All patients with muscular discomfort reported pain relief after taking ginger. Although the results are promising, the lack of placebo makes interpretation difficult. In a prior case series, the same authors reported benefit of ginger when added to the existing regimen of seven patients with rheumatoid arthritis.[73] Given the small size of this case series and the lack of placebo, it is difficult to interpret these results.

FORMULARY: BRANDS USED IN CLINICAL TRIALS
Brands Used in Statistically Significant Clinical Trials

• Most available clinical trials have not identified the brands of ginger used. Some studies have tested fresh ginger purchased from local grocery stores.

References

1. Akoachere JF, Ndip RN, Chenwi EB, et al. Antibacterial effect of *Zingiber officinale* and Garcinia kola on respiratory tract pathogens. East Afr Med J 2002;79(11):588-592.
2. Jagetia GC, Baliga MS, Venkatesh P, et al. Influence of ginger rhizome (*Zingiber officinale* Rosc) on survival, glutathione and lipid peroxidation in mice after whole-body exposure to gamma radiation. Radiat Res 2003; 160(5):584-592.
3. Wang CC, Chen LG, Lee LT, et al. Effects of 6-gingerol, an antioxidant from ginger, on inducing apoptosis in human leukemic HL-60 cells. In Vivo 2003;17(6):641-645.
4. Vimala S, Norhanom AW, Yadav M. Anti-tumour promoter activity in Malaysian ginger rhizobia used in traditional medicine. Br J Cancer 1999; 80(1-2):110-116.
5. Tanabe M, Chen YD, Saito K, et al. Cholesterol biosynthesis inhibitory component from *Zingiber officinale* Roscoe. Chem Pharm Bull (Tokyo) 1993;41(4):710-713.
6. Giri J, Devi TK, Meerarani S. Effect of ginger on serum cholesterol levels. Indian J Nutrition Diet 1984;21:433-436.
7. Wigler I, Grotto I, Caspi D, et al. The effects of Zintona EC (a ginger extract) on symptomatic gonarthritis. Osteoarthritis Cartilage 2003;11(11): 783-789.

8. Mahady GB, Pendland SL, Yun GS, et al. Ginger (*Zingiber officinale* Roscoe) and the gingerols inhibit the growth of Cag A+ strains of *Helicobacter pylori*. Anticancer Res 2003;23(5A):3699-3702.

9. Bean P. The use of alternative medicine in the treatment of hepatitis C. Am Clin Lab 2002;21(4):19-21.

10. Gujral S, Bhumra H, Swaroop M. Effect of ginger (*Zingebar officinale* Roscoe) oleoresin on serum and hepatic cholesterol levels in cholesterol fed rats. Nut Report Internat 1978;17(2):183-189.

11. Gonlachanvit S, Chen YH, Hasler WL, et al. Ginger reduces hyperglycemia-evoked gastric dysrhythmias in healthy humans: possible role of endogenous prostaglandins. J Pharmacol Exp Ther 2003;307(3):1098-1103.

12. Dugenci SK, Arda N, Candan A. Some medicinal plants as immunostimulant for fish. J Ethnopharmacol 2003;88(1):99-106.

13. Taroeno BJ, Noerhajati S, Sutarjadi. Anthelmintic activities of some hydrocarbons and oxygenated compounds in the essential oil of Zingiber purpureum. Planta Medica 1989;55:105.

14. Kim DS, Kim DS, Oppel MN. Shogaols from *Zingiber officinale* protect IMR32 human neuroblastoma and normal human umbilical vein endothelial cells from beta-amyloid(25-35) insult. Planta Med 2002;68(4):375-376.

15. Schechter JO. Treatment of disequilibrium and nausea in the SRI discontinuation syndrome. J Clin Psychiatry 1998;59(8):431-432.

16. Hashimoto K, Satoh K, Murata P, et al. Component of *Zingiber officinale* that improves the enhancement of small intestinal transport. Planta Med 2002;68(10):936-939.

17. Grontved A, Brask T, Kambskard J, et al. Ginger root against seasickness. A controlled trial on the open sea. Acta Otolaryngol 1988;105(1-2):45-49.

18. Phillips S, Ruggier R, Hutchinson SE. Zingiber officinale (ginger)—an antiemetic for day case surgery. Anaesthesia 1993;48(8):715-717.

19. Bone ME, Wilkinson DJ, Young JR, et al. Ginger root—a new antiemetic. The effect of ginger root on postoperative nausea and vomiting after major gynaecological surgery. Anaesthesia 1990;45(8):669-671.

20. Kruth P, Brosi E, Fux R, et al. Ginger-associated overanticoagulation by phenprocoumon. Ann Pharmacother 2004;38(2):257-260.

21. Fischer-Rasmussen W, Kjaer SK, Dahl C, et al. Ginger treatment of hyperemesis gravidarum. Eur J Obstet Gynecol Reprod Biol 1990;38(1):19-24.

22. Vutyavanich T, Kraisarin T, Ruangsri R. Ginger for nausea and vomiting in pregnancy: randomized, double-masked, placebo-controlled trial. Obstet Gynecol 2001;97(4):577-582.

23. McGuffin M, Hobbs C, Upton R, et al. American Herbal Products Associations Botanical Safety Handbook. Boca Raton: CRC Press, 1997.

24. Fulder S, Tenne M. Ginger as an anti-nausea remedy in pregnancy: the issue of safety. Herbalgram 1996;38:47-50.

25. Verma SK, Singh J, Khamesra R, et al. Effect of ginger on platelet aggregation in man. Indian J Med Res 1993;98:240-242.

26. Srivastava KC, Mustafa T. Ginger (*Zingiber officinale*) in rheumatism and musculoskeletal disorders. Med Hypotheses 1992;39(4):342-348.

27. Mascolo N, Jain R, Jain SC, et al. Ethnopharmacologic investigation of ginger (*Zingiber officinale*). J Ethnopharmacol 1989;27(1-2):129-140.

28. Kanerva L, Estlander T, Jolanki R. Occupational allergic contact dermatitis from spices. Contact Dermatitis 1996;35(3):157-162.

29. Vaes LP, Chyka PA. Interactions of warfarin with garlic, ginger, ginkgo, or ginseng: nature of the evidence. Ann Pharmacother 2000;34(12):1478-1482.

30. Futrell JM, Rietschel RL. Spice allergy evaluated by results of patch tests. Cutis 1993;52(5):288-290.

31. Bliddal H, Rosetzsky A, Schlichting P, et al. A randomized, placebo-controlled, cross-over study of ginger extracts and ibuprofen in osteoarthritis. Osteoarthritis Cartilage 2000;8(1):9-12.

32. Cupp MJ. Toxicology and Clinical Pharmacology of Herbal Products. New Jersey: Humana Press, 2000:

33. Arfeen Z, Owen H, Plummer JL, et al. A double-blind randomized controlled trial of ginger for the prevention of postoperative nausea and vomiting. Anaesth Intensive Care 1995;23(4):449-452.

34. Stewart JJ, Wood MJ, Wood CD, et al. Effects of ginger on motion sickness susceptibility and gastric function. Pharmacology 1991;42(2):111-120.

35. Sripramote M, Lekhyananda N. A randomized comparison of ginger and vitamin B$_6$ in the treatment of nausea and vomiting of pregnancy. J Med Assoc Thai 2003;86(9):846-853.

36. Liu PH, Ho HL. Ginger and drug bezoar induced small bowel obstruction. J R Coll Surg Edinb 1983;28(6):397-398.

37. Miller LG. Herbal medicinals: selected clinical considerations focusing on known or potential drug-herb interactions. Arch Intern Med 1998;158(20):2200-2211.

38. Backon J. Ginger in preventing nausea and vomiting of pregnancy; a caveat due to its thromboxane synthetase activity and effect on testosterone binding. Eur J Obstet Gynecol Reprod Biol 1991;42(2):163-164.

39. Backon J. Ginger as an antiemetic: possible side effects due to its thromboxane synthetase activity. Anaesthesia 1991;46(8):705-706.

40. Yamahara J, Miki K, Chisaka T, et al. Cholagogic effect of ginger and its active constituents. J Ethnopharmacol 1985;13(2):217-225.

41. Muller JL, Clauson KA. Pharmaceutical considerations of common herbal medicine. Amer J Managed Care 1997;3(11):1753-1770.

42. Willetts KE, Ekangaki A, Eden JA. Effect of a ginger extract on pregnancy-induced nausea: a randomised controlled trial. Aust N Z J Obstet Gynaecol 2003;43(2):139-144.

43. Portnoi G, Chng LA, Karimi-Tabesh L, et al. Prospective comparative study of the safety and effectiveness of ginger for the treatment of nausea and vomiting in pregnancy. Am J Obstet Gynecol 2003;189(5):1374-1377.

44. Ernst E, Pittler MH. Efficacy of ginger for nausea and vomiting: a systematic review of randomized clinical trials. Br J Anaesth 2000;84(3):367-371.

45. Nakamura H, Yamamoto T. Mutagen and anti-mutagen in ginger, *Zingiber officinale*. Mutat Res 1982;103(2):119-126.

46. Nakamura H, Yamamoto T. The active part of the [6]-gingerol molecule in mutagenesis. Mutat Res 1983;122(2):87-94.

47. Nagabhushan M, Amonkar AJ, Bhide SV. Mutagenicity of gingerol and shogaol and antimutagenicity of zingerone in Salmonella/microsome assay. Cancer Lett 1987;36(2):221-233.

48. Sivaswamy SN, Balachandran B, Balanehru S, et al. Mutagenic activity of south Indian food items. Indian J Exp Biol 1991;29(4):730-737.

49. al Yahya MA, Rafatullah S, Mossa JS, et al. Gastroprotective activity of ginger, *Zingiber officinale* rosc., in albino rats. Am J Chin Med 1989;17(1-2):51-56.

50. Yamahara J, Mochizuki M, Rong HQ, et al. The anti-ulcer effect in rats of ginger constituents. J Ethnopharmacol 1988;23(2-3):299-304.

51. Srivastava KC. Effects of aqueous extracts of onion, garlic and ginger on platelet aggregation and metabolism of arachidonic acid in the blood vascular system: in vitro study. Prostagland Leukotrienes Med 1984;13:227-235.

52. Srivastava KC. Aqueous extracts of onion, garlic and ginger inhibit platelet aggregation and alter arachidonic acid metabolism. Biomed Biochim Acta 1984;43:S 335-S 346.

53. Saruwatari J, Nakagawa K, Shindo J, et al. The in-vivo effects of sho-saiko-to, a traditional Chinese herbal medicine, on two cytochrome P450 enzymes (1A2 and 3A) and xanthine oxidase in man. J Pharm Pharmacol 2003;55(11):1553-1559.

54. Kobayashi M, Shoji N, Ohizumi Y. Gingerol, a novel cardiotonic agent, activates the Ca2+-pumping ATPase in skeletal and cardiac sarcoplasmic reticulum. Biochim Biophys Acta 1987;903(1):96-102.

55. Shoji N, Iwasa A, Takemoto T, et al. Cardiotonic principles of ginger (*Zingiber officinale* Roscoe). J Pharm Sci 1982;71(10):1174-1175.

56. Guh JH, Ko FN, Jong TT, et al. Antiplatelet effect of gingerol isolated from *Zingiber officinale*. J Pharm Pharmacol 1995;47(4):329-332.

57. Srivastava KC. Isolation and effects of some ginger components on platelet aggregation and eicosanoid biosynthesis. Prostaglandins Leukot Med 1986;25(2-3):187-198.

58. Nurtjahja-Tjendraputra E, Ammit AJ, Roufogalis BD, et al. Effective anti-platelet and COX-1 enzyme inhibitors from pungent constituents of ginger. Thromb Res 2003;111(4-5):259-265.

59. Lumb AB. Effect of dried ginger on human platelet function. Thromb Haemost 1994;71(1):110-111.

60. Bordia A, Verma SK, Srivastava KC. Effect of ginger (*Zingiber officinale* Rosc.) and fenugreek (Trigonella foenumgraecum L.) on blood lipids, blood sugar and platelet aggregation in patients with coronary artery disease. Prostaglandins Leukot Essent Fatty Acids 1997;56(5):379-384.

61. Janssen PL, Meyboom S, van Staveren WA, et al. Consumption of ginger (*Zingiber officinale* Roscoe) does not affect *ex vivo* platelet thromboxane production in humans. Eur J Clin Nutr 1996;50(11):772-774.

62. Srivastava KC. Effect of onion and ginger consumption on platelet thromboxane production in humans. Prostaglandins Leukot Essent Fatty Acids 1989;35(3):183-185.

63. Bhandari U, Sharma JN, Zafar R. The protective action of ethanolic ginger (Zingiber officinale) extract in cholesterol fed rabbits. J Ethnopharmacol 1998;61(2):167-171.

64. Thomson M, Al Qattan KK, Al Sawan SM, et al. The use of ginger (*Zingiber officinale* Rosc.) as a potential anti-inflammatory and antithrombotic agent. Prostaglandins Leukot Essent Fatty Acids 2002;67(6):475-478.

65. Fuhrman B, Rosenblat M, Hayek T, et al. Ginger extract consumption reduces plasma cholesterol, inhibits LDL oxidation and attenuates development of atherosclerosis in atherosclerotic, apolipoprotein E–deficient mice. J Nutr 2000;130(5):1124-1131.

66. Micklefield GH, Redeker Y, Meister V, et al. Effects of ginger on gastroduodenal motility. Int J Clin Pharmacol Ther 1999;37(7):341-346.

67. Phillips S, Hutchinson S, Ruggier R. *Zingiber officinale* does not affect gastric emptying rate. A randomised, placebo-controlled, crossover trial. Anaesthesia 1993;48(5):393-395.

68. Lumb AB. Mechanism of antiemetic effect of ginger. Anaesthesia 1993;48(12):1118.

69. Yamahara J, Rong HQ, Iwamoto M, et al. Active components of ginger exhibiting anti-serotonergic action. Phytotherapy Res 1989;3(2):70-71.

70. Huang Q, Iwamoto M, Aoki S, et al. Anti-5-hydroxytryptamine3, effect of galanolactone, diterpenoid isolated from ginger. Chem Pharm Bull 1991;39(2):397-399.

71. Desai HG, Kalro RH, Choksi AP. Effect of ginger & garlic on DNA content of gastric aspirate. Indian J Med Res 1990;92:139-141.

72. Onogi T, Minami M, Kuraishi Y, et al. Capsaicin-like effect of (6)-shogaol on substance P–containing primary afferents of rats: a possible mechanism of its analgesic action. Neuropharmacology 1992;31(11):1165-1169.

G

73. Srivastava KC, Mustafa T. Ginger (*Zingiber officinale*) and rheumatic disorders. Med Hypotheses 1989;29(1):25-28.

74. Pace J, Conlin DS. Oral ingestion of encapsulated ginger and reported self-care actions for the relief of chemotherapy-associated nausea and vomiting. Dissertation Abstracts International 1987;47(8):3297-B.

75. Meyer K, Schwartz J, Crater D, et al. *Zingiber officinale* (ginger) used to prevent 8-Mop associated nausea. Dermatol Nurs 1995;7(4):242-244.

76. Eberhart LH, Mayer R, Betz O, et al. Ginger does not prevent postoperative nausea and vomiting after laparoscopic surgery. Anesth Analg 2003;96(4): 995-8, table.

77. Visalyaputra S, Petchpaisit N, Somcharoen K, et al. The efficacy of ginger root in the prevention of postoperative nausea and vomiting after outpatient gynaecological laparoscopy. Anaesthesia 1998;53(5):506-510.

78. Schmid R, Schick T, Steffen R, et al. Comparison of seven commonly used agents for prophylaxis of seasickness. J Travel Med 1994;1:102-106.

79. Holtmann S, Clarke AH, Scherer H, et al. The anti-motion sickness mechanism of ginger. A comparative study with placebo and dimenhydrinate. Acta Otolaryngol 1989;108(3-4):168-174.

80. Wood CD, Manno JE, Wood MJ, et al. Comparison of efficacy of ginger with various antimotion sickness drugs. Clin Res Pr Drug Regul Aff 1988;6(2):129-136.

81. Mowrey DB, Clayson DE. Motion sickness, ginger, and psychophysics. Lancet 1982;1(8273):655-657.

82. Altman RD, Marcussen KC. Effects of a ginger extract on knee pain in patients with osteoarthritis. Arthritis Rheum 2001;44(11):2531-2538.

83. Marcus DM, Suarez-Almazor ME. Is there a role for ginger in the treatment of osteoarthritis? Arthritis Rheum 2001;44(11):2461-2462.

Ginkgo
(*Ginkgo biloba* L.)

SYNONYMS/COMMON NAMES/RELATED SUBSTANCES

- Adiantifolia, arbre aux quarante écus, baiguo, bai guo ye, BN-52063, duck foot tree, elefantenohr, EGb, EGb 761, eun-haeng, facherblattbaum, fossil tree, GBE, GBE 24, GBX, ginan, gin-nan, Ginkgoaceae, ginkgo balm, ginkgoblätter, ginkgo folium, *Ginkgo biloba* blätter, ginkgogink, ginkgold, ginkgopower, ginkyo, icho, ityo, japanbaum, Japanese silver apricot, kew tree, kung sun shu, LI 1370, maidenhair tree, noyer du Japon, Oriental plum tree, pei kuo, pei-wen, Pterophyllus, *Pterophyllus salisburiensis*, rokan, salisburia, *Salisburia adiantifolia*, *Salisburia macrophylla*, sophium, silver apricot, tempeltrae, tanakan, tanakene, tebofortan, tebonin, temple balm, tramisal, valverde, vasan, vital, ya chio, yin-guo, yin-hsing.

CLINICAL BOTTOM LINE
Background

- *Ginkgo biloba* has been used medicinally for thousands of years. Today, it is one of the top-selling herbs in the United States, accounting for $140 million of sales in 1998.[1]
- Ginkgo is used for the treatment of numerous conditions, many which are under scientific investigation. Available evidence demonstrates ginkgo's efficacy in the management of intermittent claudication, Alzheimer's/multi-infarct dementia, and "cerebral insufficiency" (a syndrome thought to be secondary to atherosclerotic disease, characterized by impaired concentration, confusion, decreased physical performance, fatigue, headache, dizziness, depression, and anxiety).
- Although not definitive, there is promising early evidence favoring use of ginkgo for memory enhancement in healthy subjects, altitude (mountain) sickness, symptoms of premenstrual syndrome (PMS), and reduction of chemotherapy-induced end-organ vascular damage.
- Although still controversial, a recent large trial has shifted the evidence against the use of ginkgo for tinnitus.
- The herb is generally well tolerated, but due to multiple case reports of bleeding, should be used cautiously in patients on anticoagulant therapy and those with known coagulopathy. Ginkgo should be discontinued before some surgical or dental procedures.

Scientific Evidence for Common/Studied Uses	Grade*
Claudication (peripheral vascular disease)	A
Dementia treatment (multi-infarct and Alzheimer's type)	A
Cerebral insufficiency	B
Age-associated memory impairment (AAMI)	C
Altitude (mountain) sickness	C
Chemotherapeutic adjunct (reduce adverse vascular effects)	C
Decreased libido and erectile dysfunction (impotence)	C

Depression and seasonal affective disorder (SAD)	C
Glaucoma	C
Macular degeneration	C
Memory enhancement (in healthy patients)	C
Multiple sclerosis	C
Premenstrual syndrome (PMS)	C
Tinnitus	C
Vertigo	C
Acute ischemic stroke	D

*Key to grades: A: Strong scientific evidence for this use; B: Good scientific evidence for this use; C: Unclear scientific evidence for this use; D: Fair scientific evidence against this use (it may not work); F: Strong scientific evidence against this use (it likely does not work). For a more detailed explanation of efficacy criteria, see "Natural Standard Evidence-Based Validated Grading Rationale" in the Introduction.

Historical or Theoretical Uses That Lack Sufficient Evidence

- Acidosis, acrocyanosis (circulatory insufficiency of the extremities), aging, alcoholism, allergies,[2] angina, antibacterial,[3] antifungal, antioxidant,[4-10] anti-parasitic, antitussive, anxiety, atherosclerosis, asthma,[11-14] attention deficit hyperactivity disorder (HDAD),[15] benign breast diseases, breast tenderness, bronchitis, cancer,[16,17] cardiac arrhythmias,[18] chilblains (inflammation of the toes, fingers, ears, or face upon exposure to cold), chronic rhinitis, cocaine dependence,[20] cochlear deafness,[19] congestive heart failure, cyanosis, dementia prevention,[21,22] dermatitis,[23] diabetes, diabetic neuropathy, diabetic retinopathy,[24] digestive aid, dizziness, dysentery, dysmenorrhea, eczema,[25] edema,[26,27] expectorant, fatigue, filariasis, freckle removal, genitourinary disorders, headache,[31,32] hearing loss,[28-30] heart disease, hepatitis B,[33] hyperlipidemia, hypertension,[34,35] hypoxia, insomnia, labor induction, menopausal symptoms,[36] migraine, mood disturbances, myocardial ischemia,[37] neuropathy,[38,39] postphlebitis syndrome, Raynaud's phenomenon, respiratory tract illnesses, scabies (topical), schizophrenia,[40-42] sepsis,[43] skin sores (topical), thrombosis, traumatic brain injury,[44] ulcerative colitis,[45] varicose veins, vascular congestion, vitiligo.[46]

Expert Opinion and Folkloric Precedent

- Ginkgo has been used in traditional Chinese medicine (TCM) to treat pulmonary diseases, circulatory disorders, and memory loss and topically for skin lesions. Currently, ginkgo is most commonly used in Europe and the United States for dementia, memory enhancement, and claudication. The German expert panel, the Commission E, has approved ginkgo for the symptomatic treatment of "disturbed performance in organic brain syndrome" (memory deficits, disturbances in concentration), claudication, vertigo, and tinnitus.

Safety Summary

- **Likely safe:** Ginkgo appears to be generally safe when taken orally in recommended doses by otherwise healthy adults for up to six months.
- **Possibly unsafe:** Ginkgo may increase risk of bleeding. It therefore should be used with caution in patients taking anticoagulants or with known clotting disorders and should be discontinued 2 weeks prior to some surgical and dental procedures. Ginkgo may be unsafe in large doses, based on case reports of seizures after ingestion of ≥50 unprocessed seeds (believed to be an effect of ginkgotoxin [4-O-methylpyridoxine]), or when used during pregnancy or lactation.
- **Likely unsafe:** When ginkgo is consumed as fresh seeds, as they are toxic and potentially deadly (possibly due to 4-metoxypyridoxine).[47] Ginkgo is likely unsafe when administered intravenously. The intravenous ginkgo product Tebonin, which was available in Germany, was removed from the German market because of significant adverse effects.

DOSING/TOXICOLOGY
General

- Recommended doses are based on those most commonly used in available trials, or on historical practice. However, with natural products, the optimal doses needed to balance efficacy and safety often have not been determined. Formulations and preparation methods may vary from manufacturer to manufacturer, and from batch to batch of a specific product made by a single manufacturer. Because often the active components of a product are not known, standardization may not be possible, and the clinical effects of different brands may not be comparable.

Standardization

- Ginkgo is available as ginkgo leaf, ginkgo leaf extract, and ginkgo seed. Ginkgo leaf extract is the most commonly used form.
- Products that utilize standardized extracts referred to as EGb 761 should contain 24% ginkgo flavone glycosides and 6% terpenoids.
- Products that utilize standardized extracts referred to as LI 1370 should contain 25% ginkgo flavone glycosides and 6% terpenoids.

Dosing: Adult (18 Years and Older)
Oral

- **Tablets/capsules:** In general, 80 to 240 mg of a 50:1 standardized leaf extract taken daily by mouth in 2 to 3 divided doses has been used traditionally and in studies (standardized to 24% to 25% ginkgo flavone glycosides and 6% terpine lactones). For intermittent claudication, there is evidence that 240 mg daily is more beneficial than 120 mg daily.[48] For dementia, doses of 120 to 240 mg daily in three divided doses have been studied.[49-53] For memory enhancement in healthy individuals, doses of 240 to 360 mg daily in three divided doses have been studied.[54-59]
- **Liquid/fluid:** A dose of 3 to 6 mL of 40 mg/mL of extract taken daily by mouth in three divided doses has been used. There is evidence that 6 mL/day is more efficacious than 3 mL/day for intermittent claudication.[48]
- **Tea:** Tea bags usually contain approximately 30 mg of *Ginkgo biloba* extract. There are no reliable safety or efficacy data specific to teas.

- **Functional foods:** There is no evidence that the small concentrations of ginkgo found in "fortified" foods yields any clinical benefit.
- **Seeds:** Ginkgo seeds are potentially toxic and should be avoided.
- *Note:* Beneficial effects may take 4 to 6 weeks to appear.

Intravenous

- *Note:* The intravenous ginkgo product Tebonin, which was available in Germany, was removed from the German market because of significant adverse effects. The ginkgo product Tanakan has been studied at a dose of 100 mg in 500 cc of normal saline, administered parenterally twice daily for peripheral vascular disease.[60] Safety has not been established.

Dosing: Pediatric (Younger Than 18 Years)

- Insufficient evidence to recommend.

Toxicology

- Ingestion of ginkgo seeds is potentially fatal, secondary to tonic-clonic seizure activity and loss of consciousness.[47] This adverse effect (sometimes referred to as "gin-nan food poisoning") has been documented in as many as 70 case reports between 1930 and 1970, with the worst outcomes seen in infants. Seizure activity has been attributed to 4-metoxypyridoxine (4-O-methylpyridoxine), also known as "ginkgotoxin," which is present in much higher doses in seeds than in commercial products.[61] In several reviews of ginkgo taken at recommended doses, no seizure activity was noted,[49,62-64] although there is a published case report of two patients with well-controlled seizure disorder who presented with recurrent seizures following commencement of ginkgo therapy, which subsided with cessation of ginkgo.[65]
- Severe allergic skin reactions and gastrointestinal (anal) sphincter spasms have occurred after direct contact with the fleshy fruit pulp. An allergic cross-reaction in a person allergic to poison ivy has been reported.[66]
- Colchicine has been isolated in commercial preparations of *Ginkgo biloba*.[67]

ADVERSE EFFECTS/PRECAUTIONS/CONTRAINDICATIONS
Allergy

- The use of ginkgo should be avoided with persons with known allergy/hypersensitivity to *Ginkgo biloba* or the Ginkgoaceae family. Cross-sensitivity is possible in people allergic to urusiols (mango rind, sumac, poison ivy, poison oak, cashews). There is a case report of Stevens-Johnson syndrome, characterized by blistering and exfoliative rash, occurring with use of the ginkgo product One-A-Day Memory and Concentration, which contains 60 mg of ginkgo leaf extract as well as vitamins B_6, B_{12}, and choline bitartrate.[68] Ginkgo fruit or pulp is considered to be a potent contact allergen. Intravenous products may induce a skin allergy, phlebitis and circulatory disturbances.

Adverse Effects

- **General:** Ginkgo appears to be well tolerated in most healthy adults when taken at recommended doses for up to 6 months. In several reviews, ginkgo use was associated with similar rates of adverse effects as placebo.[49,62-64,69] Postmarket surveillance of more than 10,000 subjects found a 1.69% incidence of minor symptoms, including headache, nausea, and gastrointestinal complaints.[70] The most concerning

G

potential complication is bleeding, which has been life-threatening in a small number of case reports. Ginkgo in the form of fresh seeds has been associated with toxicity in anecdotal reports, and regulations in some countries do not allow ginkgo seeds in foods.

- **Dermatologic:** Allergic hypersensitivity has been reported in few case reports and rarely in clinical trials; dermatitis, stomatitis, and cheilitis have been noted in case reports.[66,71] There is one case report of Stevens-Johnson syndrome, characterized by blistering and exfoliative rash, which occurred with use of the combination product One-A-Day Memory and Concentration (60 mg of ginkgo leaf extract as well as vitamins B_6, B_{12}, and choline bitartrate).[68]
- **Neurologic:** Headache, dizziness, and restlessness have been reported infrequently in clinical trials.[49,62,63] Ginkgo should be used cautiously in patients with known seizure disorder.[72] A case report has described two patients with well-controlled seizure disorder who presented with recurrent seizures following commencement of ginkgo therapy, which subsided with cessation of ginkgo.[65] Ingestion of large quantities of raw seeds (>50) may result in seizure activity and loss of consciousness, particularly in infants.[47,61] Seizure activity has been attributed to 4-metoxypyridoxine (4-O-methyl-pyridoxine), also known as "ginkgotoxin," which is present in much higher doses in seeds than in commercial products. Deaths associated with ginkgo seed ingestion have been reported in infants. There is a case report of "coma" in an elderly Alzheimer's patient taking trazodone and ginkgo; however, the patient responded to flumazenil, which raises questions about whether this effect is related to ginkgo.[73] Monoamine oxidase (MAO) inhibition by ginkgo was reported in one animal study[74] but was not confirmed by subsequent study in animals[75] or in humans.[76]
- **Ocular:** Spontaneous hyphema was reported in a 70-year-old-man taking 80 mg/day of ginkgo for 1 week; however, the patient was also taking 325 mg of daily aspirin.[77]
- **Cardiovascular:** Ginkgo has been found to decrease systolic and diastolic blood pressure in healthy volunteers[34,35] and to possess vasodilatory effects, possibly due to inhibition of nitric oxide.[78] However, paradoxical hypertension has been documented in a male patient taking a thiazide diuretic and ginkgo. Palpitations have been associated with ginkgo ingestion in anecdotal reports and clinical reviews.
- **Hematologic:** Several case reports have documented bleeding associated with ginkgo use, both as a monotherapy, and in combination with other agents that may predispose to bleeding. Spontaneous bilateral subdural hematoma occurred in a 33-year-old woman taking 120 mg/day of ginkgo for 2 years with no other medications.[79] Subarachnoid hemorrhage was documented in a 61-year-old man taking 120 to 160 mg/day of ginkgo for >6 months.[80,81] Spontaneous intracerebral hemorrhage occurred in a 56-year-old man who regularly self-medicated with an herbal preparation including ginkgo.[82] Spontaneous hyphema (bleeding into the eye) occurred in a 70-year-old man taking 80 mg/day of ginkgo for 1 week concomitantly with 325 mg of daily aspirin.[77] Intracerebral hemorrhage occurred in a 78-year-old woman taking ginkgo for 2 months in addition to chronic warfarin administration. Subdural hematoma was reported in a 72-year-old woman using ginkgo.[84] Postoperative bleeding has been reported following laparoscopic cholecystectomy in a patient using ginkgo.[85] Bleeding of an intracerebral mass in a patient taking ginkgo and ibuprofen has been

reported.[86] In addition, bleeding reactions have been reported anecdotally by practitioners, including epistaxis and ocular bleeding complications. Preclinical data support anticoagulant properties as well.[87] Caution is warranted in patients predisposed to bleeding, and prior to some surgical or dental procedures. Notably, an investigation in 32 healthy volunteers administered ginkgo extract EGb 761 (120, 240, and 480 mg/day for 14 days) did not reveal any alteration of platelet function or coagulation parameters.[88]

- **Gastrointestinal:** Infrequent mild gastrointestinal discomfort has been reported in clinical studies, particularly when ginkgo is taken with selective serotonin reuptake inhibitors.[89] Occasional nausea, diarrhea, vomiting, stomatitis, and proctitis have been reported in trials.[70] Ingestion of ginkgo pulp has been associated with perioral erythema, rectal burning, and anal sphincter spasms.
- **Genitourinary:** In theory, high concentrations of ginkgo may reduce male and female fertility.
- **Endocrine:** Ginkgo has been reported to increase plasma insulin concentrations in healthy volunteers[34] and to decrease these concentrations in subjects with type 2 diabetes.[90] Effects on serum glucose concentrations have not been evaluated.
- **Musculoskeletal:** Muscle weakness and loss of tone have been reported anecdotally in association with ginkgo use.

Precautions/Warnings/Contraindications

- Avoid in patients at risk of bleeding, taking anticoagulants, or with clotting disorders, based on case reports of bleeding.
- Discontinue use 2 to 3 weeks prior to some surgical and dental procedures because of increased risk of bleeding.
- Use cautiously in patients with history of seizure, based on reports of seizure due to ginkgo seed ingestion.
- Use cautiously in children.
- Avoid use in couples who are trying to conceive, based on theoretical reduction of fertility.
- Avoid handling ginkgo fruit pulp, due to possible adverse reactions.
- Avoid ingesting ginkgo seeds, due to toxicity.

Pregnancy and Lactation

- Not recommended due to lack of sufficient data. Use with caution in pregnancy because of increased bleeding risk. In one report, colchicine identified in placental blood at concentrations of 49 to 763 µg/L was traced to colchicine present in a commercial preparation of ginkgo.[67]
- In theory, high concentrations of ginkgo may reduce male and female fertility.

INTERACTIONS
Ginkgo/Drug Interactions

- **Acetylcholinesterase inhibitor drugs:** In theory, drugs such as donepezil (Aricept) and tacrine (Cognex) may have an additive effect when used concurrently with ginkgo, potentially precipitating cholinergic effects.
- **Anticonvulsant drugs:** Ingestion of ginkgo seeds has been associated with seizure and may lower seizure threshold and antagonize the effect of antiseizure therapies.[61] The protective effects of sodium valproate and carbamazepine on seizures in mice was diminished with the administration of *Ginkgo biloba*.[91]
- **Anticoagulants, antiplatelet drugs, NSAIDs, pentoxifylline (Trental):** Concurrent use of ginkgo with drugs that increase clotting time or inhibit platelet function may increase

the risk of bleeding, based on several case reports of spontaneous bleeding in patients using ginkgo as a monotherapy or concomitantly with warfarin or aspirin.[77,79,80,83] One case report documents a possible increase in the antiplatelet effect of ticlopidine (Ticlid) during ginkgo use.[92]

- **Antihypertensive medications:** Ginkgo has been found to decrease systolic and diastolic blood pressure in healthy volunteers.[34] Theoretically, ginkgo may have additive effects when used with antihypertensive medications. However, paradoxical hypertension has been documented in a male patient taking a thiazide diuretic and ginkgo. No pharmacokinetic interaction has been found between ginkgo and digoxin.[93]
- **Antipsychotic drugs (positive interaction):** Based on anecdotal reports, ginkgo may reduce some side effects of antipsychotic drugs, although scientific data in this area are not available.
- **Colchicine:** Colchicine has been isolated in commercial preparations of *Ginkgo biloba*, and may increase serum concentrations in patients using colchicine.[67]
- **Hypoglycemic oral agents, insulin:** Ginkgo has been found to increase plasma insulin concentrations in healthy volunteers[34] and to decrease these concentrations in subjects with type 2 diabetes.[90] Effects on serum glucose concentrations have not been evaluated, and possible interactions with hypoglycemic agents are not clear.
- **Monoamine oxidase inhibitors (MAOIs):** MAO inhibition by ginkgo was reported in one animal study[74] but was not confirmed by subsequent study in animals[75] or in humans.[76] Based on preclinical research, ginkgo may act additively with MAOIs, with a risk of causing serotonin syndrome, a condition characterized by rigidity, tachycardia, hyperthermia, restlessness, and diaphoresis.[94]
- **Papaverine, yohimbine, sildenafil (Viagra) (positive interaction):** *Ginkgo biloba* may potentiate the actions of other drugs used in the management of vascular erectile dysfunction.[95]
- **Selective serotonin reuptake inhibitors (SSRIs):** Based on preclinical research, ginkgo may act additively with SSRIs, with a risk of causing serotonin syndrome, a condition characterized by rigidity, tachycardia, hyperthermia, restlessness, and diaphoresis. Human data are not available in this area. Ginkgo has also been reported to relieve genital anesthesia associated with the SSRI fluoxetine.[96]
- **Thiazide diuretics:** Although paradoxical hypertension was documented in a male patient taking a thiazide diuretic and ginkgo, ginkgo has been found to decrease systolic and diastolic blood pressure in healthy volunteers.[34,35]
- **Trazodone:** There is a case report of "coma" in an elderly Alzheimer's patient taking trazodone and ginkgo; however, the patient responded to flumazenil, which raises questions about whether this effect is related to ginkgo.[73]
- **5-fluorouracil, cyclosporine:** 5-Fluorouracil–induced adverse effects and cyclosporine nephrotoxicity may be alleviated by ginkgo, although evidence is preliminary in this area.[97]

Ginkgo/Herb/Supplement Interactions

- **Anticoagulant herbs and supplements:** Ginkgo may act additively with other agents that increase the risk of bleeding, based on several case reports of spontaneous bleeding in patients using ginkgo as a monotherapy or concomitantly with warfarin or aspirin.[77,79,80,83] Isolated case reports have associated bleeding with the use of garlic (*Allium sativum*) or saw palmetto (*Serenoa repens*). There are numerous herbs that may theoretically increase bleeding risk, based on

laboratory and animal research. High-dose vitamin E may increase the risk of bleeding if used concomitantly with ginkgo.

- **Hypoglycemic herbs and supplements:** Ginkgo has been found to increase plasma insulin concentrations in healthy volunteers[34] and to decrease these concentrations in subjects with type 2 diabetes.[90] Effects on serum glucose concentrations have not been evaluated, and possible interactions with hypoglycemic agents are not clear.
- **Hypotensive herbs and supplements:** Ginkgo has been found to decrease systolic and diastolic blood pressure in healthy volunteers.[34] Theoretically, ginkgo may have additive effects when used with agents that lower blood pressure.
- **Monoamine oxidase inhibitor (MAOI) herbs and supplements:** MAO inhibition by ginkgo was reported in one animal study,[74] but was not confirmed by subsequent study in animals[75] or in humans.[76] Based on preclinical research, ginkgo may act additively with agents that inhibit monoamine oxidase, with a risk of causing serotonin syndrome, a condition characterized by rigidity, tachycardia, hyperthermia, restlessness, and diaphoresis.[94] Human data are not available in this area.
- **Selective serotonin reuptake inhibitor (SSRI) herbs and supplements:** Based on preclinical research, ginkgo may act additively with SSRI agents, with a risk of causing serotonin syndrome, a condition characterized by rigidity, tachycardia, hyperthermia, restlessness, and diaphoresis.[94] Human data are not available in this area.
- **Yohimbe bark extract, yohimbine (positive interaction):** Ginkgo may potentiate the actions of other agents used in the management of erectile dysfunction.[95]

Ginkgo/Food Interactions

- **Tyramine-containing foods:** Based on the possible monoamine oxidase inhibitor (MAOI) properties of ginkgo (suggested in some animal research but refuted in other animal and human studies), high doses of ginkgo may lead to hypertensive crisis when ingested with tyramine-containing foods such as wine or cheeses.

Ginkgo/Lab Interactions

- **Blood C-peptide levels:** Ginkgo has been found to increase C-peptide concentrations in a preliminary study of healthy volunteers.[34]
- **Blood insulin levels:** Ginkgo has been found to increase plasma insulin concentrations in a preliminary study of healthy volunteers.[34]

MECHANISM OF ACTION
Pharmacology

- **Constituents:** Flavonoids (glycosides) and terpenoids (ginkgolide, bilobalide) are considered to be ginkgo's primary active components.[98-101] Most studies have been conducted with the standardized ginkgo preparation EGb 761 (24% ginkgo flavone glycosides, 6% terpenoids) or LI 1370 (25% ginkgo flavone glycosides, 6% terpenoids).
- **Antioxidant/anti-inflammatory effects:** Flavonoids serve as free radical scavengers, and have been shown to reduce oxidative stress in human models.[6,8,102-108] This mechanism is hypothesized to reduce oxidative cellular damage in Alzheimer's disease and has prompted theories that ginkgo may have favorable effects on reperfusion injury.[109-115] Ginkgolides inhibit receptor binding of platelet-activating factor (PAF), which may mediate beneficial clinical effects.[116-128] PAF is pro-inflammatory, induces platelet aggregation, and

contracts bronchial smooth muscle.[129] Ginkgo has been found to increase corticosteroid secretion in rats.[130]

- **Neurotransmitter effects:** Neuroprotective properties have been attributed to inhibition of age-related decline of adrenergic and cholinergic receptors.[131-134] Ginkgo has also been found to increase serotonin levels, increase muscarinic binding sites, and increase serum levels of acetylcholine and norepinephrine.[135]
- **Vascular effects:** Ginkgo has been found to have vasodilatory effects, which have been attributed to stimulation of endothelium-derived relaxing factor (EDRF) and prostacyclin release. Studies have suggested that ginkgo inhibits nitric oxide, causing vascular relaxation.[78,136,137] In a controlled single-blind study of 10 healthy human subjects[138] and a controlled crossover study of patients with known claudication,[139] ginkgo was shown to significantly increase blood capillary flow and decrease erythrocyte aggregation.
- **Monoamine oxidase inhibitor (MAOI) effects:** MAO inhibition by ginkgo has been reported in animals[74] but has not been confirmed by subsequent animal research.[75] One study of a small human sample did not demonstrate significant changes in human brain MAO A or B, measured by positron emission tomography after subjects had taken 120 mg of ginkgo daily for 1 month.[76]
- **Other effects:** *In vitro* study has demonstrated that ginkgo promotes proliferation of human skin fibroblasts.[92]

Pharmacodynamics/Kinetics

- Oral bioavailability of the terpene lactones ginkgolide A, ginkgolide B, and bilobalide are 98% to 100%, 79% to 93%, and 70%, respectively. Absorption has been found to occur principally via the small intestine. The half-lives of ginkgolides A and B and bilobalide have been found to be 4.5, 10.6, and 3.2 hours, respectively, with peak plasma levels at 2 to 3 hours. Approximately 70% of ginkgolide A, 50% of ginkolide B, and 30% of bilobalide are excreted unchanged in urine, with seven other metabolites detectable in the urine but undetectable in serum. Toxicity is low, with an oral LD_{50} in mice of 7725 mg.[140,141] Duration of action has been reported as 7 hours.

HISTORY

- *Ginkgo biloba* extract is obtained from the ginkgo tree, which is believed to be the oldest living tree, dating back more than 200 million years. Ginkgo has been used for thousands of years in Asia, with traditional use for respiratory complaints, memory loss, and circulatory problems, as well as culinary usage of the seed. Ginkgo was introduced by Chen Noung in the first pharmacopoeia, *Chen Noung Pen T'sao.*
- The ginkgo tree, although native to China, is now cultivated in Europe, Japan, Southeast Asia, and the United States. Known for its hearty nature and resilience against infection and pollution, it has been planted along city streets in the United States since the 1700s.
- Many of ginkgo's current uses originate from research and clinical observations during the 1950s in Europe. In 1994, a standardized extract of *Ginkgo biloba* was approved by the health authorities in Germany for treatment of dementia. Today, use of ginkgo is widespread in the Americas, Europe, and Asia.

Review of the Evidence: Ginkgo

Condition Treated*	Study Design	Author, Year	N[†]	SS[†]	Study Quality[‡]	Magnitude of Benefit	ARR[†]	NNT[†]	Comments
Claudication	Meta-analysis	Pittler[62] 2000	415	Yes	NA	Medium	NA	NA	Eight trials included in analysis; pooled data showed an increase in pain-free walking vs. placebo (34 meters, 95% CI, 26-43 meters); analysis limited by methodologic flaws in included studies.
Claudication	Meta-analysis	Moher[155] 2000	213 (5 trials)	Mixed	NA	Small	NA	NA	Out of 52 studies of therapies for claudication, 5 using ginkgo were included; pooled data for ginkgo studies found no short-term benefits of ginkgo, but significant longer-term (24-week) effect size of 0.7, with improved mean walking distance of 32 meters (95% CI, 0.2-1.1).
Claudication	Meta-analysis	Schneider[157] 1992	5 studies	Yes	NA	Medium	NA	NA	Trials between 1975-1988; mean increase in pain-free walking distance of 0.75 standard deviations greater than placebo; analysis limited by methodologic quality.
Claudication (PVD)	RCT, double-blind	Blume[146] 1996	60	Yes	4	Medium	NA	NA	Improvement in pain-free and maximum walking distances with 6 months of ginkgo vs. placebo.
Claudication	RCT, double-blind	Bauer[147,159,160] 1984, 1986	79	Yes	4	Large	NA	NA	Improvement in pain-free and maximum walking distances with 6 months of ginkgo vs. placebo; similar promising results after 2-3 years of follow-up.

Continued

Review of the Evidence: Ginkgo—cont'd

Condition Treated*	Study Design	Author, Year	N[†]	SS[†]	Study Quality[‡]	Magnitude of Benefit	ARR[†]	NNT[†]	Comments
Claudication	RCT, double-blind, crossover	Salz[149] 1980	29	Yes	3	Large	NA	NA	Improvement in pain-free and maximum walking distances with 6 weeks of ginkgo vs. placebo.
Claudication	RCT, double-blind	Draboek[150] 1996	20	No	3	NA	NA	NA	No improvement in walking distance after 12 weeks of ginkgo vs. placebo; sample size may have been too small to detect between-group differences.
Claudication	RCT, double-blind	Blume[151] 1998	41	Yes	3	Large	NA	NA	Improvement in pain-free walking distance with 24 weeks of ginkgo vs. placebo.
Claudication	RCT, double-blind	Peters[152] 1998	111	Yes	2	Small	NA	NA	Improvement in pain-free walking distance after 8, 12, and 24 weeks of ginkgo vs. placebo.
Claudication	RCT, double-blind	Thomson[148] 1990	37	Yes	2	Small	NA	NA	Improvement in pain-free walking distance with 6 months of ginkgo vs. placebo; groups were dissimilar at baseline.
Claudication	RCT, double-blind	Mouren[154] 1994	20	Yes	2	Large	NA	NA	Decreased mean lower leg ischemia (38% reduction measured by transcutaneous Po_2) during exercise with 4 weeks of ginkgo vs. placebo.
Claudication	RCT, double-blind	Saudreau[60] 1989	64	No	2	None	NA	NA	No change in pain at rest after 8 days of IV ginkgo in patients with severe peripheral vascular disease.
Claudication	RCT	Rudofsky[139] 1987	10	Yes	2	Small	NA	NA	Serum measurements recorded after 1 IV dose of 35 mg of ginkgo; improved serum pH and "plasma viscosity," with unclear clinical implications.
Claudication	Dosing trial	Schweizer[48] 1999	74	Yes	2	Medium	NA	NA	Higher-dose ginkgo (240 mg daily) yielded better walking distance results than standard dose (120 mg daily).
Claudication	Randomized, double-blind comparison trial	Böhmer[166] 1988	27	Unclear	2	None	NA	NA	Ginkgo compared to pentoxifylline over 24 weeks; improvements in walking distance occurred in both groups, but unclear if sample size was adequate to measure between-group differences.
Dementia, cognitive impairment	Meta-analysis	Birks[69] 2003	33 trials	Yes	NA	Mixed	NA	NA	33 trials analyzed, including patients with dementia and cognitive impairment; significant benefits of ginkgo vs. placebo reported for CGI, cognition, and ADL with doses of less than 200 mg/day at 12, 24, and 52 weeks; heterogeneity and poor methodologic quality of many included trials limit results.
Dementia	Meta-analysis	Oken[49] 1998	430	Yes	NA	Small	NA	NA	4 trials analyzed, including patients with Alzheimer's and multi-infarct dementia; small mean effect size reported (0.413); studies used 120-240 mg ginkgo daily for 3-6 months.
Dementia, age-related memory impairment	RCT	Van Dongen[187] 2003	214	No	4	None	NA	NA	No benefits seen after 24 weeks in psychometric functioning, CGI, or ADL; study included a heterogeneous population of which 36 were diagnosed with dementia; possibly underpowered to detect planned end points.

Review of the Evidence: Ginkgo—cont'd

Condition Treated*	Study Design	Author, Year	N[†]	SS[†]	Study Quality[‡]	Magnitude of Benefit	ARR[†]	NNT[†]	Comments
Dementia	RCT, double-blind	Le Bars[53] 1997	309	Mixed	4	Medium	NA	NA	Improvement in cognitive performance on standardized scales after 1 year of ginkgo vs. placebo; intention-to-treat analysis; high attrition rate (50%).
Dementia	RCT, double-blind	van Dongen[186] 2000	214	No	4	None	NA	NA	No cognitive benefits found with ginkgo vs. placebo after 24 weeks; non-dementia patients included in sample, and older mean age may have skewed outcomes toward negative results.
Dementia	RCT, double-blind	Kanowski[52,189] 1996, 1997	216	Yes	4	Medium	13%	8	Improvement in cognitive performance on standardized scales after 24 weeks of ginkgo vs. placebo; intention-to-treat analysis; high attrition rate (30%).
Dementia	RCT, double-blind	Rai[190] 1991	31	Yes	4	Small	NA	NA	Improved cognitive functioning on standardized scales after 24 weeks of daily ginkgo vs. placebo.
Dementia	RCT, double-blind	Hofferberth[51] 1994	40	Yes	3	Medium	NA	NA	Improvement in cognitive performance on standardized scales after 12 weeks of ginkgo vs. placebo.
Dementia	RCT, double-blind	Wesnes[50] 1987	54	Yes	3	NA	NA	NA	Improved cognitive functioning on non-validated scales after 12 weeks of daily ginkgo vs. placebo.
Cerebral insufficiency	Systematic review	Kleijnen[140] 1992	885 (8 trials)	NA	NA	NA	NA	NA	Of 40 trials identified, 8 met methodological criteria; overall positive results were associated with ginkgo vs. placebo, although cerebral insufficiency is a clinical diagnosis that may capture patients with heterogeneous disease processes.
Cerebral insufficiency	Meta-analysis	Hopfenmüller[199] 1994	6 trials	Yes	NA	Small	NA	NA	Of 11 initial studies, 5 excluded for methodological weaknesses; overall positive results reported, although pooled data calculation was unclear.
AAMI	RCT, double-blind	Brautigam[170] 1998	241	Mixed	3	Mixed	NA	NA	Improvement in short-term visual memory, but not in attention, concentration, or global short-term memory in patients with self-reported AAMI after 24 weeks of ginkgo vs. placebo; inclusion criteria for patients were poorly defined.
AAMI	RCT, double-blind	Winther[35] 1998	60	Mixed	3	Small	NA	NA	Improved cognitive function after 12 weeks of ginkgo (120 mg daily) vs. placebo, but no significant benefits with 240 mg of ginkgo; subgroups may have been too small to detect between-group differences.
AAMI	RCT, double-blind, crossover	Allain[217] 1993	18	Yes	3	Medium	NA	NA	Improvement on a "dual coding" test with 320-600 mg of ginkgo vs. placebo; inclusion criteria for patients were poorly defined.
Memory enhancement (older individuals)	RCT, double-blind	Solomon[219] 2002	230	Yes	5	None	None	None	No significant benefits in multiple standardized tests of memory and attention after 6 weeks of ginkgo (120 mg daily) vs. placebo; well-designed study with adequate power calculation.

Continued

G

Review of the Evidence: Ginkgo—cont'd

Condition Treated*	Study Design	Author, Year	N[†]	SS[†]	Study Quality[‡]	Magnitude of Benefit	ARR[†]	NNT[†]	Comments
Memory enhancement	RCT, double-blind	Moulton[226] 2001	60	Mixed	3	Small	NA	NA	Significant benefits on only 1 of multiple standardized tests of memory after 5 days of ginkgo (60 mg daily) vs. placebo.
Memory enhancement	RCT, double-blind	Mix[225] 2000	48	Mixed	3	Small	NA	NA	Significant improvement in subjective memory and processing but not in objective measures of memory after 6 weeks of ginkgo vs. placebo.
Memory enhancement	RCT, double-blind	Rigney[54] 1999	31	Mixed	3	Small	NA	NA	Significant improvement in short-term memory with 2 300-mg doses of ginkgo vs. placebo and lower doses of ginkgo.
Memory enhancement	RCT, double-blind	Kennedy[55] 2000	20	Yes	2	Small	NA	NA	Significant improvement in short-term memory with a single dose (240-360 mg) of ginkgo vs. placebo and 120 mg of ginkgo.
Tinnitus	Systematic review	Holstein[235] 2001	19 trials	NA	NA	Small	NA	NA	Of 19 trials identified, 5 were randomized, placebo-controlled, and double-blind; positive results reported.
Tinnitus	Systematic review	Ernst[64] 1999	541 (5 trials)	NA	NA	Mixed	NA	NA	4 trials reported positive results; 1 trial was negative but possibly underpowered[233]; 1 trial was unpublished (Juretzck, 1998).
Tinnitus	RCT	Drew[231] 2001	1121	Yes	4	None	NA	NA	In contrast to prior small positive studies, this trial found no benefits from ginkgo (LI 1370, 150 mg/day) for 12 weeks; outcomes were measured by telephone/mail questionnaires, and compliance was not clear.
Tinnitus	RCT	Meyer[197] 1986	103	Yes	3	Medium	10	10	Improvement after 12 weeks of ginkgo (150 mg daily) vs. placebo.
Tinnitus	RCT	Meyer[232] 1986	259	Yes	0	Small	NA	NA	Improvement observed by a clinician after at least 1 year of ginkgo (Tanakan).
Tinnitus	RCT	Morgenstern[234] 1997	99	Yes	3	Small	NA	NA	Improvement measured by audiometry after 12 weeks of ginkgo (150 mg daily) vs. placebo.
Tinnitus	Randomized, controlled trial	Holgers[233] 1994	20	No	3	NA	NA	NA	No benefit from ginkgo, but results may have been affected by the low daily dose (29.2 mg) and small sample size.
Altitude (mountain) sickness	RCT	Roncin[245] 1996	44	Yes	3	Large	41%	3	Improvement in subjective cerebral and respiratory symptoms with ginkgo (160 mg daily) vs. placebo.
Vertigo	Controlled, non-randomized trial	Haguenauer[196] 1986	70	Yes	1	Small	29%	3	Improvement in symptoms measured by clinical assessment with ginkgo (160 mg daily) vs. placebo.
Macular degeneration	RCT	Lebuisson[253] 1986	20	Yes	3	Small	NA	NA	Small improvement in long-distance vision identified; inadequately blinded study.
PMS	RCT	Tamborini[257] 1993	165	Yes	2	Medium	NA	NA	Subjective improvement in symptoms with ginkgo (160 mg daily) for 20 days vs. placebo.

Review of the Evidence: Ginkgo—cont'd

Condition Treated*	Study Design	Author, Year	N[†]	SS[†]	Study Quality[‡]	Magnitude of Benefit	ARR[†]	NNT[†]	Comments
SAD	RCT, double-blind	Lingaerde 1999	27	No	2	None	NA	NA	Not effective in preventing symptoms vs. placebo; sample size may have been too small to detect between-group differences.
Depression	RCT, double-blind	Schubert[266] 1993	40	Yes	2	Small	NA	NA	Small improvement in symptoms on validated scales after 8 weeks of ginkgo (240 mg daily) vs. placebo.
Acute ischemic stroke	RCT, double-blind	Garg[274] 1995	55	No	3	None	NA	NA	No improvement on standardized neurologic assessment scale after 4 weeks of ginkgo (160 mg daily) vs. placebo.

*Primary or secondary outcome.
[†] N, Number of patients; SS, statistically significant; ARR, absolute risk reduction; NNT, the number of patients who need to undergo a specific intervention in order to observe an outcome in one individual.
[‡] 0-2 = poor; 3-4 = good; 5 = excellent.
AAMI, Age-associated memory impairment; ADL, activities of daily living; CGI, clinical global improvement; IV, intravenous; NA, not applicable; PMS, premenstrual syndrome; PVD, peripheral vascular disease; RCT, randomized, controlled trial; SAD, seasonal affective disorder.
For an explanation of each category in this table, please see Table 3 in the Introduction.

REVIEW OF THE EVIDENCE: DISCUSSION

Claudication (Peripheral Vascular Disease)

Summary

- Data from multiple small, randomized, controlled trials and two meta-analyses suggest that oral *Ginkgo biloba* modestly improves symptoms of intermittent claudication. Most statistically significant studies have administered 120 mg/day (in 2 to 3 divided doses), although one dosing trial found better results with 240 mg/day.[48] Treatment has been evaluated for up to 6 months. Most of the available studies have had methodological weaknesses, including unclear blinding and randomization. It should be noted that exercise therapy likely yields a greater improvement in symptoms than either ginkgo or available prescription drug therapies,[142-144] and therefore ginkgo should be recommended as an adjunct to an exercise regimen when possible. Initial comparisons of ginkgo to drug therapy with pentoxifylline have not yielded conclusive results. Additional evidence from a high-quality trial using standardized outcomes measures and comparing/combining ginkgo with drug and exercise therapies is warranted in this area.

Systematic Reviews/Meta-analyses

- In 2000, Pittler and Ernst performed a literature review and meta-analysis of controlled trials of ginkgo for intermittent claudication.[62,145] Seven published studies[146-152] and one internal report by the manufacturer Schwabe[153] were included that were placebo-controlled, double-blind, used ginkgo monotherapy, included walking distance as an outcome measure, and employed a standardized outcome measurement instrument. Three studies were excluded for which walking distance was not an outcome.[60,139,154] Seven studies demonstrated weighted mean differences compared to placebo. Four trials reported mean differences in pain-free walking distance from baseline, with 95% confidence intervals (CI) that did not overlap zero. Pooled data from all trials showed an increase in pain-free walking greater than placebo (34 meters, 95% CI, 26-43 meters). On review of included studies, limitations included poorly defined randomization, lack of washout between crossover periods,

lack of detailed descriptions of study subjects, and inconsistent specification of extracts used.

- In a 2000 meta-analysis of 52 randomized, double-blind, placebo-controlled trials of multiple therapies for claudication, Moher et al.[155] included five studies of ginkgo (n = 213).[146,148,150,152,156] Pooled data found no significant short-term benefits of ginkgo, and a longer-term (24-week) improvement in effect size of 0.7 (95% CI, 0.2-1.1). At 24 weeks, ginkgo therapy was associated with an improvement in walking distance of 32 meters vs. placebo (95% CI, 14.0-50.5). This improvement was relatively small compared to other therapies such as pentoxifylline (208.0 meters; 95% CI, 66.6-482.5). The small number of subjects in the included ginkgo trials may not have been sufficient (as evidenced by the conflicting short- and longer-term effect size data).

- An earlier meta-analysis by Schneider evaluated five placebo controlled trials of ginkgo for PVD and reported a mean increase in pain-free walking distance of 0.75 standard deviations greater than placebo.[157] This 1992 review included trials from 1975 through 1988.

Placebo-Controlled Trials Included in Pittler Meta-analysis

- Blume et al. conducted a randomized, placebo-controlled, double-blind study comparing *Ginkgo biloba* extract EGb 761 to placebo, using objective and subjective parameters of walking performance in PVD.[146] Sixty patients diagnosed with mild-to-moderate intermittent claudication (Fontaine stage IIb) of at least 6 months' duration were given 120 mg/day of ginkgo extract EGb 761 or placebo over 24 weeks. EGb 761–treated patients demonstrated significant improvement compared to placebo, with a clinically relevant difference between groups of 20% (p = 0.008). Although well designed with clear descriptions of outcomes, this study was limited by poor documentation of blinding procedures.

- Bauer et al. conducted a randomized, double-blind trial examining the effects of ginkgo in 79 patients diagnosed with PVD (Fontaine stage IIb).[147] Patients were randomized to receive 40 mg of ginkgo three times daily or placebo over a 24-week period. Outcome parameters included measurements of mean pain-free walking distance and mean maximum walking distance. Results showed ginkgo to significantly increase pain-free walking distance by 64 meters and maximum walking distance by 112 meters, vs. placebo (28 meters and 29 meters, respectively). This study was limited by an incomplete description of blinding procedures. Similar favorable results were documented by the authors after 2 to 3 years of follow-up.[158-160]

- In a randomized, double-blind, crossover study, Salz administered 160 mg of ginkgo daily to 29 individuals with moderate claudication according to the Fontaine scale.[149] After 6 weeks of therapy, mean pain-free walking distance increased by 113 meters with ginkgo vs. 4 meters with placebo. These impressive results are limited by incomplete descriptions of baseline patient characteristics, statistical analysis, and randomization technique.

- Draboek et al. conducted a controlled, double-blind trial in 20 patients with intermittent claudication of moderate severity (baseline pain-free walking distance, 96 meters).[150] Subjects were randomized to receive 120 mg of ginkgo daily or placebo over a 12-week period. At the study's end, no significant difference was found between groups in pain-free walking capacity (equal slight improvement from baseline in each group) or maximum distance walking (no significant improvement in either group). This small study may not have been adequately powered to detect between-group differences, despite the medium to large effect sizes reported in other studies.

- Blume et al. conducted a follow-up randomized, placebo-controlled trial of their prior study in 41 patients with mild to moderate (Fontaine stage IIb) claudication.[151] After 24 weeks of administration of ginkgo (EGb 761) dosed at 80 mg/day, pain-free walking distance was reported as significantly improved in the ginkgo group vs. placebo (46 meters and 5 meters, respectively). Blinding and randomization were not well described.

- Peters performed a trial of 111 patients with angiographically demonstrated PVD and mild to moderate symptomatic claudication (Fontaine stage IIb).[152] Subjects were enrolled in a 24-week, multicenter, randomized, placebo-controlled, double-blind study, using ginkgo extract EGb 761. Mean pain-free walking distances increased from 108.5 meters to 153.2 meters in the EGb 761 group, and from 105.2 meters to 126.6 meters in the placebo group at the end of the treatment period. Significant differences were found at 8-, 16-, and 24-week visits. Maximum walking distance and increases in pain-free walking distance were also significantly higher in the EGb 761 group.

- Thomson et al. examined the effects of ginkgo in 37 patients with intermittent claudication due to PVD (Fontaine stage II).[148] Subjects were randomized to receive 120 mg of ginkgo daily or placebo over a 6-month period. The groups were dissimilar at baseline, including better mean walking distance capacity in the ginkgo group vs. the placebo group. At the study's completion, small significant improvements were seen in mean pain-free walking distance scores in the ginkgo group vs. placebo, as measured by an analogue scale (38 meters vs. 33 meters). Statistical analysis, blinding, and randomization were not well described.

Placebo Controlled Trials Not Included in Pittler Meta-analysis

- Trials using outcomes measures other than walking distance have been published, providing additional supportive evidence.

- Mouren et al. conducted a randomized, double-blind, placebo-controlled trial assessing the effects of EGb 761 in patients with peripheral vascular disease.[154] Twenty patients with claudication (Fontaine stage II) who had been diagnosed for ≥1 year and were symptomatically stable for 3 months were selected. During a pre-randomization period, subjects received placebo for 15 days, followed by assignment to receive placebo or ginkgo extract EGb 761 at a dose of 320 mg daily for 4 weeks. Degree of lower limb ischemia was assessed via measures of transcutaneous partial pressure of oxygen ($TcPO_2$) during treadmill exercise. The authors report that areas of ischemia were reduced by 38% in the ginkgo group, although degree of ischemia was unchanged in the placebo group. Between-group differences were statistically significant. Although this study did not report a clinical outcome, the results provide support to the assertion that ginkgo improves circulation in peripheral vascular disease. Notably, the daily dose of ginkgo used (320 mg) was higher than the dose used in most clinical studies (120 mg).

- Saudreau et al. conducted a multicenter, randomized, controlled trial examining the effects of parenteral ginkgo (Tanakan, 100 mg in 500 cc of normal saline, twice daily) in patients with PVD and pain at rest (Fontaine stage III).[60] Sixty-four patients received either ginkgo or placebo for 8 days. The primary outcome measure was scored on the validated McGill Pain Questionnaire. No statistically significant difference in pain scores was found between groups. However, it is not clear if an 8-day duration is sufficient for potential effects of ginkgo to occur. This study suggests that ginkgo may not be an effective therapy for relieving pain in patients with arterial occlusive disease of the lower extremities and pain at rest.

- In a randomized, controlled trial, Rudofsky administered a single 35-mg dose of intravenous Tenorbin forte or placebo to 10 patients with intermittent claudication.[139] Several outcomes were measured, with the aim to quantify levels of limb ischemia. The author reported statistically significant benefits with ginkgo therapy vs. baseline or placebo, including improvements in blood pH and "plasma viscosity." However, this trial was poorly described, with incomplete descriptions of blinding and randomization, and it is unclear if the measurements employed can be clinically correlated.

- Additional studies have yielded data that do not affect the level of available evidence in this area.[161-165]

Dosing Trial

- Schweizer and Hautmann conducted a multicenter, randomized, double-blind trial of a higher dose of ginkgo EGb 761 in patients with peripheral vascular disease and symptomatic claudication (Fontaine stage IIb).[48] Thirty-eight patients received the dosage of ginkgo used in most other trials (120 mg daily), and 36 patients received a higher dose (240 mg daily). A mean increase in pain-free walking distance of 60.6 meters was found in the group of patients who received 120 mg, compared to a statistically significantly higher mean increase of 107.0 meters in the group that received 240 mg ($p = 0.025$). No adverse drug reactions were noted in the higher-dose group.

Comparison Trials

- Böhmer et al. conducted a poor-quality randomized, double-blind comparison trial of the ginkgo product Rökan (Interstan GmbH, Ettlingen, Germany) and pentoxifylline.[166] Over a 24-week period, 27 subjects with PVD were dosed with either

160 mg of daily ginkgo or 1200 mg of daily pentoxifylline. Significant improvements in walking distance were noted in both groups. Although the results are suggestive, no power calculation was conducted prior to initiating this trial, and it is thus not clear that this study had an adequate sample size to discern differences between groups. No placebo arm was included, which might have clarified this issue. Blinding and randomization were not adequately described. Due to weaknesses in the design and reporting of this trial, its results cannot be extrapolated to clinical practice.

- Letzel and Schoop conducted a 1992 review of placebo-controlled trials of ginkgo extract Egb 761 for claudication, as well as placebo-controlled trials of pentoxifylline for claudication.[167] The authors assert that comparable effect sizes were reported in the respective studies of these two therapies. However, no formal meta-analysis or pooled analysis of effect sizes was conducted, and these results can only be considered a review of available 1992 research, with the opinion of the authors offered as analysis.

Dementia (Multi-Infarct and Alzheimer Type)
Summary

- Research has produced an abundance of *in vitro*, *in vivo*, and clinical trial data examining ginkgo as a therapy for dementia and cognitive impairment. Although more than 50 human trials have been published to date (particularly early studies), almost all have methodological deficiencies, including vague classification, pseudo-randomization, improper blinding, limited sample size, and inadequate description of dropouts and treatment effects. Pooled analyses of research in this area report significant benefits over placebo with small effect sizes using ginkgo at a dose of less than 200 mg/day over 12 to 54 weeks,[46,69] although due to the heterogeneity of included studies and broad inclusion criteria of many trials, firm conclusions about which specific patient groups or diagnoses may benefit from ginkgo are difficult to formulate. It remains unclear if there is any difference in effect between the 120-mg and 240-mg daily dosing regimens of ginkgo for these indications. Some authors allude to the preferable side-effect profile of ginkgo compared to drugs such as cholinesterase inhibitors,[168] although the availability of direct comparisons is limited.[52,53,169] Preliminary evidence from a retrospective case-control study suggests possible protective effects of ginkgo against the development of Alzheimer's disease, although these results are preliminary.[22]

Systematic Review/Meta-analysis

- In a Cochrane systematic review and meta-analysis, Birks et al. analyzed data from 33 controlled trials of ginkgo for acquired cognitive impairment, including dementia.[69] Studies were included with doses between 80 and 600 mg/day (most were 200 mg/day or less), standardized to 24 mg of total flavone glycosides and 6 mg ginkgolides per day in all cases but one, which used very low concentrations,[170] with separate analyses for treatment durations of <12, 12, 24, and 52 weeks. Numerous studies included patients based on non-specific symptoms such as headache, dizziness, depression, fatigue, memory deficits, and tinnitus, in some cases measuring symptoms using subjective assessments rather than validated instruments, although CGI (clinical global improvement) was able to be used for pooled analysis.[35,42,171-180] Other studies used various standardized scales, resulting in heterogeneity among included studies particularly in the

12-week analysis.[42,50,53,180-186] Because most included trials did not utilize intention-to-treat analyses, pooled results were based on subjects who completed the various studies. The authors reported that based on the CGI scale (dichotomized between those who improved versus those who remained unchanged or got worse), ginkgo showed improvement over placebo in a dose less than 200 mg/day in less than 12 weeks (OR, 15.32; 95% CI, 5.90 to 39.80; $p < 0.0001$) and at 24 weeks (OR, 2.16; 95% CI, 1.11 to 4.20; $p = 0.02$). Significant improvements were also seen in cognitive measures and activities of daily living (ADL) for doses of less than 200 mg/day at 12, 24, and 52 weeks, and for mood/emotional status at 12 weeks. No significant differences in dropouts between ginkgo and placebo subjects were detected, and incidence of adverse events was similar between pooled groups. There were not sufficient data to assess quality of life, depression, or dependency. Although these results are suggestive, they are limited by the heterogeneity of included trials, particularly regarding the broad range of criteria for inclusion of patients. As a result, generalization is somewhat limited. Nonetheless, the analysis points to a need for research that investigates the impact of ginkgo in patients with more rigorously defined diagnoses. The inclusion of studies of patients diagnosed with age-related memory impairment, for which the available evidence of efficacy is less compelling than for dementia, may have pulled the pooled results closer to the null.

- A well-designed meta-analysis by Oken et al.[49] and a review by Ernst[63] have examined randomized, double-blind, placebo-controlled trials of ginkgo for Alzheimer's dementia. In the meta-analysis by Oken, only 4 of 57 trials identified met methodologic criteria for inclusion (n = 430).[50-53] The majority of studies were excluded because of heterogeneous inclusion criteria and/or unclear definitions of dementia (or study of conditions other than dementia). For included studies, heterogeneous outcome measures had been employed, and thus individual effect sizes were initially calculated. The authors reported a weighted mean effect size equivalent to less than half a standard deviation improvement (0.413) in measures of cognitive function. This was considered to be demonstrative of a small improvement, in this well-done meta-analysis. Included studies used either 120 mg/day or 240 mg/day of ginkgo for 3 to 6 months of therapy; both doses yielded significant results, although no comparison was made between the two doses.

Placebo-Controlled Trials

- Van Dongen et al. report the results of a randomized, placebo-controlled trial in patients with dementia or age-associated memory impairment (a syndrome that may be a distinct entity from dementia, although there is likely diagnostic crossover).[187] Subjects were administered either placebo or ginkgo extract EGb 761 (160 mg or 240 mg daily) over a 24-week period. Only 36 of the 214 total participants were diagnosed with dementia. The authors reported no significant benefits in terms of psychometric functioning, CGI, or ADL via validated scales. However, the study was likely underpowered for its two subgroups, particularly in light of small effect sizes previously reported for the use of ginkgo in dementia, and lack of clearly demonstrated benefits in patients with age-associated memory impairment. Therefore, the results cannot be considered conclusive. The same lead author previously reported negative results of ginkgo use in a similar heterogeneous group of patients.[186]

- Le Bars conducted a randomized, double-blind, placebo controlled, parallel-group, multicenter study in 309 patients with mild to severe dementia.[53] This well-designed trial included patients with Alzheimer's disease or multi-infarct dementia, without other significant medical conditions. Subjects received ginkgo EGb 761 (120 mg daily) or placebo during a 52-week trial period. By the end point of this intention-to-treat study, 202 subjects remained in the analysis. Overall, the ginkgo group scored better than placebo ($p = 0.04$) on the Alzheimer's Disease Assessment Scale-Cognitive subscale (ADAS-Cog), and better than placebo ($p = 0.004$) on the Geriatric Evaluation by Relative's Rating Instrument (GERRI). Effects were seen at up to 1 year. However, the actual clinical significance of these findings is questionable because of the lack of statistical significance in measured CGI. In addition, the study was limited by exclusion of patients with significant medical or psychiatric illnesses, and a significant attrition rate (almost 50%). A follow-up to this study[188] reported statistically significant improvement in 244 completers in the ADAS-Cog and GERRI.
- Kanowski et al. examined the efficacy of ginkgo EGb 761 in outpatients with pre-senile and senile primary degenerative dementia of the Alzheimer type, and multi-infarct dementia.[52,189] There were 216 patients included in this 24-week randomized, double-blind, placebo controlled, multi-center trial. Subjects received a daily dose of 240 mg of ginkgo or placebo. The frequency of therapy responders was significant in favor of ginkgo, yielding an absolute risk reduction of 13% and a number needed to treat of 8 patients. Intention-to-treat analysis of 205 patients yielded similar results. Therapy responders demonstrated improvement in two of three primary variables: the Clinical Global Impression scale; an attention and memory scale (Syndrom-Kurztest [SKT]); and a behavioral assessment of ADL (Nurnberger Alters-Beobachtungsskala).
- Hofferberth studied the efficacy of ginkgo in a randomized, double-blind trial in 40 hospitalized patients with Alzheimer's dementia diagnosed by the "Blessed Dementia Scale."[51] Subjects were randomized to receive either ginkgo (Tebonin forte) (240 mg daily) or placebo over a 3-month period. Outcomes were measured by the Skt Brief Cognitive Evaluation Instrument (memory and attention) and the Sandoz Clinical Assessment Geriatric Scale. The authors report that memory, attention, and psychomotor performance improved moderately in the ginkgo group vs. placebo, with statistical significance. Weaknesses of this study include unclear descriptions of blinding and randomization.
- Wesnes et al. conducted a double-blind, placebo-controlled trial in 54 elderly outpatients with mild cognitive impairment as measured by the Crichton Geriatric Behavioural Scale for Dementia.[50] Subjects were randomized to receive ginkgo (Tanakan), 40 mg three times daily, or placebo for a 12-week period. Outcomes were measured via several "psychometric" tests of cognitive ability, including digit span, number matching, rapid visual information processing, choice reaction, and word recognition. The authors reported significant small to moderate improvements in all measures of cognitive functioning in the ginkgo group vs. placebo. However, standardized measures of global improvement were not employed, making it difficult to compare these results to other clinical studies.
- In 2000, a double-blind, placebo-controlled, multicenter trial reported no significant neurocognitive benefits in 214 elderly patients with mild to moderate dementia treated with ginkgo for 24 weeks.[186] Subjects (mean age, 83) were randomized to receive either placebo or ginkgo extract EGb 761 (160 mg or 240 mg) in two divided daily doses. Multiple types of dementia classifications were included in this study; patients with Alzheimer's dementia, multi-infarct/vascular dementia, and age-related memory impairment (AAMI) were studied together, without adequate statistical power to conduct subgroup analyses. Outcomes were assessed after 12 and 24 weeks, utilizing neuropsychological testing (trail-making speed, digit memory span, verbal learning), clinical assessment (presence and severity of geriatric symptoms [SCAG], depressive mood [GDS], self-perceived health and memory status), and self-reported behavioral assessment. No differences were reported between ginkgo and placebo in any of the measures. This negative result may be due to the inclusion of patients with AAMI. Although other studies have revealed statistically significant improvements in neuro-cognitive tests for patients with Alzheimer's and vascular dementia, benefits have not been found for AAMI. The inclusion of the latter group in this study may have skewed results toward statistical insignificance. This factor, and the relatively older patient population in this study (14 years older than the mean in the study by Le Bars[53]), may account for the discrepant result. This issue would be clarified by a study adequately powered for subgroup analysis of dementia patients.
- Rai et al. conducted a double-blind placebo-controlled trial in 31 patients older than 50 years with mild to moderate memory impairment of unclear etiology, as measured by a standardized instrument (NINCDS-ADRDA) and lasting for greater than 3 months.[190] Subjects were randomized to receive ginkgo (Tanakan), 40 mg three times daily, or placebo over a 6-month period. Measures of cognitive outcomes included the Kendrick digit copying task, object learning task, classification task, and digit recall. At the study's completion, significant small improvements were noted on the Kendrick digit copying task and classification task, although other "psychometric" tests did not demonstrate benefits of ginkgo. Weaknesses of this study are heterogeneous patients with unclear baseline characteristics, and unclear descriptions of statistical analysis.
- A number of additional studies have examined the effects of oral ginkgo on cognitive function in patients with dementia of various etiologies.[35,172,181,182,185,191-195] However, these trials have been small, poorly designed, and inadequately reported. Although overall their results have been positive, thus lending further support for better-quality positive trials, methodological weaknesses limit the application of their results to clinical practice.

Comparison Study

- Wettstein reported a comparison of study results between trials of ginkgo and acetylcholinesterase inhibitors.[169] Historical results from ginkgo trials by Le Bars[53] and Kanowski[52] were compared to four trials of acetylcholinesterase inhibitors (donepezil, tacrine, rivastigmine, and metrifonate). Studies included were of a randomized, placebo-controlled design. Wettstein reported that acetylcholinesterase inhibitors and ginkgo yielded similar improvements in dementia symptoms on the same validated scale (ADAS-Cog) compared to placebo. He suggested that ginkgo may be equally as effective as acetylcholinesterase inhibitors. However, baseline characteristics of patients across trials were dissimilar, and adequacy of blinding and randomization varied between studies. Although this report is suggestive, a head-to-head comparison of agents is necessary in order to conclude equivalence.

Cerebral Insufficiency
Summary

- Multiple clinical trials have been conducted to evaluate *Ginkgo biloba* for a syndrome called "cerebral insufficiency." This condition, which is more commonly diagnosed in Europe than in the United States, is characterized by a complex of symptoms, including impaired concentration, confusion, absent-mindedness, decreased physical performance, fatigue, headaches, dizziness, depression, and anxiety. The diagnosis is often made clinically. It is believed that the etiology of cerebral insufficiency is decreased cerebral circulation due to fixed atherosclerotic disease. In Europe, ginkgo is often used to treat these symptoms when they are suspected manifestations of cerebral insufficiency. Meta-analyses and clinical reviews have demonstrated efficacy, but suffer from significant methodological limitations, including inconsistent inclusion criteria, inadequate blinding in included studies, and inaccurate translation of foreign-language articles. Few trials document imaging or other studies that confirm vascular compromise. Therefore, it is difficult to discern if subjects' symptoms are truly due to poor cerebral circulation or to other etiologies such as early Alzheimer's or multi-infarct dementia (for which there is evidence of efficacy). Nonetheless, there is good support in the literature for this syndrome, as defined symptomatically.

Systematic Review and Meta-analysis

- Kleijnen reviewed 40 trials of ginkgo for symptoms and signs consistent with a diagnosis of cerebral insufficiency, beginning in the mid-1970s.[140] Studies originated in Germany, France, Italy and the United Kingdom. Patients were of a heterogeneous sampling, with a variety of the diverse symptoms of cerebral insufficiency. While most trials reported positive findings, only eight trials met methodologic criteria.[50,173,174,179,180,196-198] These studies were not pooled because of their heterogeneity. On review of these articles, there is unclear blinding in each. The authors concluded that ginkgo is applicable for patients with mild to moderate symptoms of cerebral insufficiency, found in several studies to be comparable to Hydergine (ergoloid mesylates), an FDA-approved medication for Alzheimer's disease and cerebral vascular insufficiency.

- Hopfenmüller conducted a meta-analysis of placebo-controlled, randomized, double-blind studies.[199] Eleven studies were initially included via less rigorous inclusion criteria (based on study design only),[70,173,177-180,200-204] and 5 trials were excluded because of "methodological weakness." Daily dosages of the ginkgo extract LI 1370 (Kaveri forte) ranged from 112 to 160 mg, using 150 mg of extract in the majority of trials. The 7 included studies demonstrated greater efficacy of *Ginkgo biloba* compared to placebo in treating a range of clinical symptoms associated with cerebral insufficiency, although pooled data were not sufficiently reported.

Controlled Trials

- A number of randomized, controlled trials were conducted during the 1980s and 1990s to examine the efficacy of ginkgo in cerebral insufficiency.[50,70,172-174,177,179,180,183,191,196-198,201-216] In the majority of these studies, this diagnosis was made clinically, based on a symptom complex. The majority of trials reported benefits associated with ginkgo administration at doses between 112 and 160 mg daily in three divided doses for up to 12 weeks, including improved concentration and functional status, and reduced headaches, dizziness, depression, and anxiety. However, classification of patients was uneven, sample sizes were small (<150), and randomization, blinding, and statistical analysis were not clearly described. Further evidence is warranted in this area in patients with diagnoses correlated with specific pathophysiologic processes.

Age-Associated Memory Impairment (AAMI)
Summary

- AAMI is a nonspecific syndrome, likely resulting from any one of several pathophysiologic etiologies. Some patients may suffer from early manifestations of Alzheimer's disease or multi-infarct dementia, conditions for which ginkgo has been shown to yield some benefit. There is promising early evidence showing small improvements in short-term visual memory and response to stimuli for patients with AAMI. However, it is not clear if these improvements are due to effects on patient subsets with early Alzheimer's disease or multi-infarct dementia. Despite these preliminary results, there is currently not sufficient evidence to recommend for or against ginkgo for this indication.

Evidence

- Brautigam conducted a multicenter, randomized, placebo-controlled trial in 241 subjects, ages 55 to 86 years, with age-related memory and/or concentration complaints (self-reported).[170] After 24 weeks of therapy, no improvement was found in attention, concentration, global short-term memory, or learning curve. An 11% improvement in short-term visual memory was seen in the placebo group, compared with 18% in the low-dose ginkgo group (0.9 mL three times daily), and 26% in the high-dose group (1.9 mL three times daily). The improvements with ginkgo were statistically significant and may suggest a dose-response. However, the isolated small improvement in one measure makes it difficult to draw broad conclusions from this study. The inclusion criterion of self-reported memory/concentration complaints makes the results difficult to generalize. In addition, there were notable differences in baseline characteristics between the three study groups: The high-dose ginkgo group had fewer baseline memory complaints and lower levels of alcohol consumption (57% vs. 65% in the placebo group). These factors raise questions about randomization and serve as potential confounders.

- Van Dongen et al. report the results of a randomized, controlled trial in patients with AAMI or dementia who were administered placebo versus ginkgo extract EGb 761 (160 mg or 240 mg daily) over a 24-week period.[187] In this group of 214 total subjects, 87 were diagnosed with AAMI. The authors reported no significant benefits in terms of psychometric functioning, clinical global improvement (CGI), or activities of daily living (ADL) via validated scales. However, the study may have been underpowered for its subgroup analyses. Therefore, the results cannot be considered conclusive. The same lead author previously reported negative results of ginkgo use in a similar heterogeneous group of patients.[186]

- Winther et al. examined the effects of ginkgo on 60 patients aged 61-88 years with mild-to-moderate "mental impairment"

(Mini Mental Status Exam score >22) in a randomized, placebo controlled, double-blinded trial.[35] Patients received one of three treatment options: placebo, 120 mg or 240 mg of ginkgo daily for the duration of 3 months. Ginkgo dosed at 120 mg daily was associated with significantly improved cognitive function as measured by validated scales compared to placebo. However, the higher dose of ginkgo (240 mg) did not produce any significant changes over placebo. In a 2002 follow-up double-blind study by Winther et al., 60 patients with Mini Mental Status Exam scores between 0 and 22 were randomized to receive ginkgo therapy (GB-8, undocumented dose) or placebo for 12 months.[192] No significant improvements were noted in long-term memory. Effects on motor and intellectual functions were variable depending on what measurement scale was used for assessment. This was a published abstract only, with limited description of results or analysis.

- Allain et al. conducted a double-blind, crossover trial assessing the impact of ginkgo in 18 patients with mild AAMI.[217] Patients received placebo or ginkgo extract EGb 761 at a dose of 320 mg or 600 mg prior to performing a "dual-coding test." The ginkgo groups required significantly shorter times in "break point" and dual coding, both of which were interpreted as an improvement in speed of information processing. However, baseline subject characteristics were not well described in this small study.
- Semlitsch studied the effects on electroencephalography (EEG) of ginkgo in patients with AAMI. Forty-eight subjects, ages 51 to 79 years, were randomized to treatment for 57 days of 120 mg of Ginkobene in three divided daily doses or placebo.[218] A finding of shortened latency of event-related potentials measured on EEG led the authors to conclude that ginkgo may accelerate stimulus evaluation time.

Memory Enhancement (in Healthy Patients)
Summary
- A well-designed 2002 trial demonstrated no benefits of ginkgo (120 mg daily) on multiple measures of memory and concentration after 6 weeks of therapy in older individuals. However, prior evidence from smaller, less rigorous studies suggests that ginkgo in doses greater than or equal to 240 mg daily for up to 6 weeks may play a role in general enhancement of memory and other cognitive functions in healthy individuals. Therefore, although it remains unclear if higher doses of ginkgo are effective, it seems unlikely that 120 mg has significant benefits.

Evidence
- In 2002, Solomon et al. conducted a well-designed and reported study of ginkgo for memory and concentration in a population of healthy individuals older than 60 years.[219] A power calculation determined that a sample size of 172 participants would be necessary to detect differences of 0.5 SD with a power of 90%. Therefore, a sample of 230 community-dwelling participants was randomized to receive either ginkgo (Ginkoba, Boehringer Ingelheim Pharmaceuticals) (40 mg three times daily) or placebo for 6 weeks. Participants were included if their baseline Mini-Mental State Examination score was >26 and were excluded for a history of psychiatric or neurologic disorder in the last 5 years. Outcome measures included standardized tests of learning and memory (California Verbal Learning Test, Logical Memory subtest of the Wechsler Memory Scale–Revised,

Visual Reproduction subscale, Memory Questionnaire, and a global evaluation completed by a spouse or companion); attention and concentration (Digit Symbol subscale of the Wechsler Adult Intelligence Scale–Revised, Stroop Test, Digit Span, Mental Control test); expressive language (Controlled Category Fluency Test; Boston Naming Test); and mental status (Mini-Mental State Examination). After 6 weeks, a total of 203 participants (88%) completed the protocol, and a modified intention-to-treat analysis was performed. The authors reported that no statistically significant differences were detected between groups on any measure. This trial suggests that ginkgo at a dose of 120 mg daily for 6 weeks does not enhance memory and attention in healthy older individuals. However, extensive baseline characteristics of the population were not provided, and the results may not be widely generalizable. Most notably, the dose used is lower than the dose suggested in prior trials to be efficacious in healthy individuals (240 mg daily or greater), although notably these other studies have been methodologically flawed with small sample sizes.

- Rigney conducted a randomized, double-blind, placebo-controlled five-way crossover study of 31 asymptomatic volunteers ages 30 to 59 years.[54] Subjects were treated with ginkgo (LI 1370, 120, 240, or 300 mg in three divided doses) or placebo for 2 days and then underwent a battery of established memory and cognitive tests. No statistically significant improvements were seen in word recall, choice reaction, digit substitution, or sleep quality. A small statistically significant improvement was seen in the Sternberg Short-Term Memory Scanning Test with the 300-mg dose only; lower doses yielded no differences from placebo. In younger subjects (ages 30 to 39 years), scores on the Stroop color task worsened, while Stroop scores improved in those 50 to 59 years of age. This small study, which tested healthy subjects after only 2 days of therapy, suggests that there may be a small benefit of ginkgo when taken in doses >300 mg/day (in three divided doses). Weaknesses include small sample size and a relatively short washout period (5 days).
- A study by Mix examined the efficacy of ginkgo extract for enhancement of cognitive abilities in 48 healthy adults, ages 55 years or older.[225] Subjects received ginkgo (EGb 761, 60 mg three times daily) or placebo in double-blind fashion during a 6-week trial. Compared with placebo, the ginkgo group demonstrated a statistically significant improvement in processing (Stroop color task), as well as a subjective memory benefit. However, no significant differences were found in objective memory assessments. The study was limited by small sample size, which may have precluded finding subtle differences in this healthy population.
- Kennedy et al. conducted a randomized, placebo-controlled, double-blind, crossover trial to assess the effects of ginkgo on enhancing cognition in healthy adults.[55] Twenty subjects received ginkgo (120 mg, 240 mg, or 360 mg) or placebo. Primary outcome parameters included standardized measures of attention and memory. When compared to placebo, a significant dose-dependent improvement in these parameters was found 2.5 hours (still present at 6 hours) following administration of 240 mg and 360 mg of ginkgo. Methods and statistical analysis were inadequately described in this publication, which limits the clinical application of the results.
- Moulton et al. conducted a double-blind, placebo-controlled trial in 60 healthy adults.[226] Subjects were randomized to

receive BioGinkgo (LI 1370, 60 mg daily) or placebo. Outcomes were measured via the Sternberg Memory Scanning Test, a reaction time control test, the vocabulary and digit span subtests of the revised Wechsler Adult Intelligence Scale, a reading span test, and a prose recall test. After 5 days of therapy, a small significant mean improvement was observed in the ginkgo group on the Sternberg Memory Scanning Test vs. placebo, but no other significant benefits on any scale were measured. Notably, this study used a lower dose of ginkgo than most other studies.

- Other studies of limited methodological quality report benefits but are limited in their clinical relevance because of poor design and reporting of results.[36,227,228]

Combination Products

- Wesnes et al. reported a significant benefit of an herbal combination containing ginkgo and ginseng on memory in 256 healthy middle-aged subjects.[229] Subjects were recruited into this randomized, placebo-controlled, double-blind trial and assigned to receive either 160 or 320 mg of ginkgo (GK 501) plus ginseng (G 115), or placebo in 1 daily dose for 12 weeks. Cognitive performance was assessed by a computer-based test system (CDR computerized performance tests), subjective "psycho-physical state" (alertness, calmness, contentment) via the Bond-Lader Visual Analog Scale, and stimulus processing capacity was measured by the Hannover form of the Vienna Determination Unit (Emotional Overload Test). Assessments were conducted at weeks 0, 4, 8, 12, and 14, each time 1 hour before and 1, 3, and 6 hours after taking the study medication(s). The main outcome variable was the quality of memory index, and no differences were found between the two dosing groups. The authors report that memory performance was significantly better in the ginkgo-ginseng group vs. placebo, and that this effect was most pronounced 6 hours after medication dosing at week 14. These results were similar to those found in a prior study by the same principal author in 64 patients with "neurasthenic" complaints.[230] These results are limited by the use of a combination product and by incomplete description of blinding procedures.

- Kennedy et al. reported a study of the effects of ginkgo, ginseng, and their combination in healthy individuals in a placebo-controlled, double-blind, crossover trial.[56,57,59] Twenty subjects received 360 mg of ginkgo, 400 mg of ginseng, a combination of the two agents, or placebo. Ginkgo was found to significantly improve "episodic secondary memory" at 1 and 6 hours post-dosing. The combination formula was associated with improved quality of "episodic memory" at 1 and 2.5 hours and of "working memory" at 1 and 6 hours. Paradoxically, the combination was found to decrease the speed of attention at 4 hours. Ginseng alone was shown to improve the quality of secondary memory at 4 and 6 hours, accuracy of attention at 2.5 hours, and the speed of retrieval of information at 4 hours.

Tinnitus
Summary

- There is conflicting evidence regarding the efficacy of ginkgo for tinnitus. Traditional use and multiple small, methodologically weak trials conducted during the 1980s and 1990s have reported efficacy of ginkgo for this indication. However, a large 2001 trial found no evidence of efficacy. This area remains controversial, and the data remain equivocal. A

well-designed controlled trial utilizing standardized outcomes measurement instruments and assuring compliance is warranted.

Evidence

- In the 1980s, publicity surrounding the use of ginkgo for tinnitus and hearing loss was based on the results of a low-quality 9-week open trial that reported reduction or resolution of tinnitus in 17 of 33 patients and hearing improvements in 22 of 66 patients.[231] This prompted the initiation of a number of randomized trials.

- In 1999, Ernst and Stevinson conducted a systematic review of ginkgo for tinnitus.[64] Five randomized, controlled trials met inclusion criteria (four published and one unpublished).[197,232-234] These studies collectively treated 541 patients. In three trials, patients treated with ginkgo were reported to experience statistically significant improvements in loudness or severity of tinnitus compared to placebo. In one study,[232] there was improvement in symptoms compared to treatment with almitrine-raubasine or nicergoline. Another study[233] found no improvement over placebo. Regarding this negative study, possible explanations advanced by the reviewers included small daily dose (29.2 mg daily in two doses) and underpowering to detect between-group differences (n = 20). Two of the studies included in the systematic review did not provide clear explanations of methods or blinding.[197,232] One trial by Juretzck (1998) was a *Schwabe* internal report, which was submitted to the reviewers but never formally published and therefore cannot be externally critiqued. One included trial appeared to be well designed with clear reporting of methods and results, but the provided citation information was not correct for this study.[234] This trial reportedly utilized 120 mg daily of EGb 761 in three divided doses. After 12 weeks, audiometry detected a small (3dB) average reduction in loudness of tinnitus compared to placebo.

- A 2001 systematic review by Holstein identified 19 studies of ginkgo (Egb 761) for tinnitus, including studies of multiple designs and symptom etiologies.[235] The review's search strategy was described, but inclusion and exclusion criteria were not well defined. Overall, the identified studies reported small to moderate benefits of ginkgo in the reduction of tinnitus. Five placebo-controlled, double-blind, randomized trials were described that overall reported similar positive results.[174,175,197,232-234] However, in two cases, tinnitus was associated with "cerebrovascular insufficiency"[174,175] and tinnitus was not a primary outcome measure of those trials.

- In 2001, Drew conducted a larger randomized, controlled trial (n = 1121) and found no significant differences between treatment and placebo on a subjective five-point tinnitus scale after 12 weeks of 150 mg/day of ginkgo (LI 1370) in three divided doses.[236] This study was conducted by telephone and mail, and measures of tinnitus were based on results of a subjective questionnaire. This questionnaire was based on a previously validated instrument. The primary methodological weakness of this otherwise well-designed study was the inability to assure compliance with the dosage regimen. Although there was a compliance question on the questionnaire, the level of compliance was not reported in the results. Despite this negative study, many experts believe, based on clinical experience and prior studies, that there may be efficacy for this indication. A well-designed trial with objective measurements might resolve this controversy.

- Additional data have been published in methodologically weak trials that do not affect the equivocal nature of the scientific evidence in this area.[237-244]

Altitude (Mountain) Sickness
Summary
- There is inconclusive evidence regarding the efficacy of ginkgo for the treatment of altitude (mountain) sickness. Benefits of ginkgo have been reported by a methodologically weak trial.

Evidence
- Altitude sickness, which can include vertigo, headache, nausea, insomnia, microcirculatory disturbance, and pulmonary edema, was studied in 44 mountain climbers.[245] Subjects were randomized to 160 mg daily of ginkgo (EGb 761) or placebo. No subjects in the treatment group developed cerebral symptoms of altitude sickness, and 40.9% of the placebo group did. Respiratory symptoms were notable in 13.6% of the ginkgo group, and 81.8% of the placebo group. These differences were statistically significant. However, results were based on subjective reporting of symptoms rather than on serum or physiologic measurements.

Vertigo
Summary
- There is inconclusive evidence regarding the efficacy of ginkgo for the treatment of vertigo. Benefits of ginkgo have been reported by a methodologically weak trial.

Evidence
- Haguenauer et al. conducted a placebo-controlled, double-blind, non-randomized study in 70 patients with vertigo.[196] Subjects were assigned to receive either ginkgo (Egb 761, 160 mg daily) or placebo. After three months of treatment, the authors reported significant mean improvements in the ginkgo group in terms of intensity and frequency and duration of symptoms, as measured by a clinical assessment. A standardized protocol was not used to measure outcomes. At the end of the trial, 47% of the patients treated with ginkgo were reported as rid of their symptoms, vs. 18% in the placebo group. The lack of randomization of this trial allows for the possible introduction of confounders. The method of blinding was not described, and inadequate blinding could allow for bias.
- Additional poor-quality research has been presented that does not affect the level of available evidence.[246-250]

Macular Degeneration
Summary
- The available evidence is not sufficient to recommend for or against the use of ginkgo for macular degeneration.

Evidence
- Investigators have reported on ginkgo-associated improvements in ocular blood flow in healthy volunteers[251] and on the antioxidant effect of ginkgo on the retina in animal models.[5,252] Lebuisson conducted a randomized, controlled trial in 20 subjects with age-related macular degeneration.[253] Patients were randomized to receive either ginkgo (EGb 761, 160 mg daily in 2 divided doses) or placebo over a 6-month period. Outcomes were assessed via fundoscopic examination and measurements of visual acuity and visual fields. A small statistically significant improvement in long-distance visual acuity was reported in the ginkgo group. However, limitations of this trial include its small sample size and lack of adequate blinding of acuity measurers. In 2000, a Cochrane systematic review identified only the Lebuisson trial in this area and concluded that insufficient evidence exists to recommend for or against the use of ginkgo for macular degeneration.[254]
- Merte et al. conducted a case series to assess the effects of ginkgo in 46 patients with visual field disturbances and/or retinal vascular degeneration.[255] Subjects received 160 mg of ginkgo daily for 4 weeks, after which time the dose was decreased to 120 mg daily. Outcome parameters included measurements of visual acuity, visual fields, fundoscopic examination, intraocular pressure, blood pressure, and heart rate. The authors reported mild, non-significant improvements in these measures.
- A low-quality double-blind trial in 20 patients reported an increase in ophthalmic artery blood flow and diameter of ocular arterial capillaries after 6 weeks of treatment with ginkgo extract LI 1370 (100 mg three times daily) vs. placebo.[265] However, these types of external measurements are generally inaccurate, and the measurement techniques, statistical analysis, and blinding were not described by the authors.

Premenstrual Syndrome (PMS)
Summary
- The available evidence is not sufficient to recommend for or against the use of ginkgo for symptoms associated with PMS.

Evidence
- A double-blind, placebo-controlled trial reported efficacy of ginkgo in the treatment of women who had experienced symptoms associated with PMS or breast pain/tenderness for more than 3 months.[257] Women between the ages of 18 and 45 years were followed for two menstrual cycles. Each of the 143 subjects received either 80 mg twice daily of ginkgo extract (EGb 761) or placebo, starting on day 16 of the first cycle, until day 5 of the following cycle. The authors reported that ginkgo significantly relieved major PMS symptoms, including breast pain and emotional disturbance. However, outcomes were assessed subjectively by patients and clinicians, without the use of standardized scales. In addition, randomization was not described. Additional studies are warranted before a recommendation can be made in this area.

Decreased Libido and Erectile Dysfunction (Impotence)
Summary
- Ginkgo has been used and evaluated for the treatment of sexual dysfunction in men and women. It has been postulated that ginkgo may be efficacious in the treatment of erectile dysfunction, based on reports of vasodilatory effects (possibly related to inhibition of nitric oxide).[78] However, there is inconclusive evidence regarding the efficacy of ginkgo for decreased libido or erectile dysfunction.

Erectile Dysfunction
- Ginkgo has been reported in animal and human models as possessing vascular smooth muscle relaxant properties, which may act on corpus cavernosum tissue [258] and improve penile blood flow in patients with erectile dysfunction.[95] Ginkgo has also been reported to be effective in antidepressant-induced sexual dysfunction, including reduction of fluoxetine-induced "genital anesthesia."[96]

- In a published abstract, Sikora et al. documented the results of a case report in 60 men with erectile dysfunction.[95] Subjects had not responded to intracavernous papaverine injections of up to 50 mg. Ginkgo extract (60 mg daily) was administered for 12 to 18 months, during which time penile blood flow was assessed via ultrasonography. The authors reported that perfusion improved in most patients after 6 to 8 weeks, and that after 6 months, 50% of patients were able to achieve an erection. In an additional 20% of patients, papaverine injections became successful. Without a control group, it is not clear if these results may have been due to the natural history of erectile dysfunction to resolve in some subjects. Baseline patient characteristics and etiology of erectile dysfunction were not described in this brief publication.
- Similar results were noted in a subsequent published case series by the same lead authors.[259] Fifty patients with vascular erectile dysfunction were assigned to receive ginkgo (Egb 761, 240 mg daily). After 6 months of therapy, 40% of subjects were capable of achieving an erection. Notably, these subjects had responded to intracavernous injections of papaverine prior to the study. Improved blood flow was noted in all subjects via ultrasonography compared to baseline, although statistical analysis was not documented.
- In a published abstract, Sikora et al. described a randomized, placebo-controlled, double-blind study in 32 men with vascular erectile dysfunction.[260] Following 24 weeks of therapy with either ginkgo (Egb 761, 240 mg daily) or placebo, 39% of subjects dropped out of the trial. Analysis of the remaining patients revealed a decline in erectile functioning in the placebo group, as measured by a "Rigiscan" device, and no significant improvements over baseline in the ginkgo group. This poorly described study with a high dropout rate cannot be considered conclusive.

Decreased Libido

- Cohen et al. conducted an open trial of ginkgo for antidepressant-induced sexual dysfunction.[89] This study involved a small mixed sample of patients (n = 63) receiving antidepressants, with symptoms including decreased libido (76%), delayed or inhibited orgasm (54%), erectile dysfunction (19%), and ejaculatory failure, based on clinical assessment and subjective reporting. Patients received a mean dose of 207 mg of ginkgo daily for 4 weeks. Efficacy was reported in 91% of the female sample and in 76% of male subjects, with a reported statistically significant positive effect in all phases of the sexual response cycle. As critiqued in an editorial,[261] this study has multiple limitations, including limited description of patient population and unclear outcome measures.
- A published letter documented a case series of 22 patients with antidepressant-induced sexual dysfunction who were treated in a psychiatric clinic with ginkgo.[263] Three of the 13 female patients experienced partial improvement in sexual function, and none of the men in the study improved.
- Ito et al. administered the herbal combination therapy ArginMax or placebo to 77 adult women with self-reported sexual dysfunction.[264] ArginMax contains extracts of ginkgo, ginseng, damiana, L-arginine, multivitamins, and minerals. After 4 weeks, subjective improvement in overall sexual satisfaction was reported by 73.5% of ArginMax subjects vs. 37.2% of placebo patients ($p < 0.01$). These results cannot be extrapolated to ginkgo monotherapy, due to the use of a combination formula. In addition, because of inadequate description of blinding, randomization, and statistical analysis and lack of use of a standardized evaluation instrument, the clinical utility of these results is limited.
- In a case series, Waynberg and Brewer administered the combination product Herbal vX, which contains muira puama and ginkgo, to 202 healthy women with decreased libido.[264] Following 1 month of therapy, 65% of subjects demonstrated significant improvement over baseline, based on a self-assessment questionnaire designed to assess frequency and degree of sexual desire, sexual intercourse, sexual fantasies, satisfaction with sex life, and ability to reach orgasm. Because of the lack of a control group and use of validated measurement criteria, these results can only be considered preliminary.

Depression and Seasonal Affective Disorder (SAD)
Summary

- The available evidence is not sufficient to recommend for or against the use of ginkgo for depression and SAD.

Evidence

- Ginkgo has been studied as a preventive therapy in patients with a history of SAD. In a double-blind trial, 27 subjects were randomized to receive either ginkgo or placebo for a 10-week period.[265] Outcome measures included the Montgomery-Asberg Depression Rating Scale and subject self-ratings. Ginkgo was not found to be significantly effective in preventing the development of symptoms of winter depression. However, the sample size in this trial may not have been adequate to detect between-group difference.
- Schubert and Halama conducted a randomized, double-blind trial in 40 elderly patients with depression who had failed therapy with tricyclic antidepressants.[266] Notably, these patients had also been clinically diagnosed with "mild to moderate cerebral dysfunction." Subjects were randomized to receive either ginkgo (240 mg daily) or placebo while continuing their prior antidepressant regimen. Outcomes were measured via the Hamilton Rating Scale for Depression (HAM-D) and a clinical assessment of cognitive function. After 8 weeks of therapy, small significant changes were reported in HAM-D scores as well as in measures of cognitive function. These results cannot be extrapolated to clinical practice because of methodological weaknesses, including unclear baseline patient characteristics, blinding, randomization, and statistical analysis.
- Improvements in sleep architecture have been reported following the addition of ginkgo to trimipramine therapy in patients with major depression.[267]

Chemotherapeutic Adjunct (Reduction of Vascular Adverse Effects)
Summary

- There is inconclusive evidence regarding the efficacy of ginkgo to reduce the vascular adverse effects associated with some chemotherapeutic agents, such as 5-fluorouracil (5-FU).

Evidence

- Based on reports of vasodilatory effects, ginkgo was examined as an adjunct to 5-fluorouracil (5-FU) in the treatment of pancreatic cancer.[97] In 32 evaluable patients, cancer response rates with the addition of ginkgo were comparable to those with chemotherapy alone, and treatment was well tolerated. A follow-up study of similar design in patients with advanced colorectal cancer yielded similar results.[268] These results may merit further investigation in a controlled trial.

Multiple Sclerosis (MS)
Summary
- It has been postulated that ginkgo's anti-inflammatory and platelet-activating factor (PAF)–inhibiting properties may exert beneficial effects in MS. However, the available evidence is not sufficient to recommend for or against the use of ginkgo in MS.

Evidence
- In a case series by Brochet et al., 10 patients with relapsing-remitting MS were treated for 5 days with intravenous ginkgolide B, a ginkgo constituent.[269] Eight subjects demonstrated neurocognitive improvement after 2 to 6 days, as assessed clinically, with sustained effects in 5 patients. No serious adverse effects were noted.
- In a follow-up double-blind study, Brochet et al. randomized 104 patients with exacerbations of MS to receive either placebo, 240 mg of daily ginkgolide B, or 360 mg of ginkgolide B.[270] No statistically significant difference was observed between the three groups on the Rankin, Kurtzke Expanded Disability Status Scale (EDSS), or Hauser Ambulation Index (AI) scores, although there was a trend toward improvement in the ginkgolide groups on the Rankin and AI scales.
- Preliminary results of a randomized, controlled trial have been presented.[271]

Glaucoma
Summary
- The available evidence is not sufficient to recommend for or against the use of ginkgo for glaucoma.

Evidence
- Chung et al. conducted a phase I, placebo-controlled, crossover trial assessing the effects of ginkgo in the treatment of glaucoma.[251] Eleven healthy volunteers were administered either placebo or ginkgo (40 mg three times daily). Following a 2-week washout period, subjects crossed over to the other treatment regimen. The authors reported that ginkgo therapy was associated with significant increases in mean end-diastolic ophthalmic artery blood velocity vs. placebo. However, no significant mean effects were noted in intraocular pressure.
- Raabe et al. conducted a randomized, double-blind trial in 24 elderly patients to assess the effects of ginkgo (EGb 761) on retinal perfusion.[272] Subjects were randomized to receive placebo, or EGB 761 at a dose of 80 mg or 160 mg. Patients receiving 160 mg, but not 80 mg, were reported to experience a significant mean increase in "retinal sensitivity" after 4 weeks, as measured by the "octopus 2000 P," an electronic device designed to measure retinal perfusion noninvasively. The authors noted that increased "retinal sensitivity" may correlate with improved retinal circulation. This measurement technique has not been widely validated and has unclear clinical implications. It should be noted that indirect measurements of mean end diastolic ophthalmic artery blood velocity are often inaccurate.
- Merte et al. conducted a case series to assess the effects of ginkgo in 46 patients with visual field disturbances and/or retinal vascular degeneration.[255] Subjects received ginkgo (160 mg daily) for 4 weeks, after which time the dose was decreased to 120 mg daily. Outcome parameters included measurements of visual acuity, visual fields, fundoscopic examination, intraocular pressure, blood pressure, and heart rate. The authors reported mild, non-significant improvements in these measures.
- A low-quality double-blind trial in 20 patients reported an increase in ophthalmic artery blood flow and diameter of ocular arterial capillaries after 6 weeks of treatment with ginkgo extract LI 1370 (100 mg three times daily) vs. placebo.[256] However, these types of external measurements are generally inaccurate, and the measurement techniques, statistical analysis, and blinding were not described by the authors.

Acute Ischemic Stroke
Summary
- It has been postulated that ginkgo therapy may be beneficial following acute ischemic stroke, because of vascular and/or antioxidant properties.[273] However, the limited available evidence suggests that ginkgo does not elicit clinical improvement in patients following ischemic cerebral vascular accidents.

Evidence
- A double-blind, placebo-controlled trial was conducted on 55 patients with computerized tomographic evidence of acute ischemic infarction.[274] Twenty-one patients were initiated on ginkgo (40 mg four times daily) for 4 weeks. At 2- and 4-week intervals, no difference was noted between the ginkgo and placebo groups in scores on the validated Matthew's Neurologic Assessment Scale.

FORMULARY: BRANDS USED IN CLINICAL TRIALS/ THIRD-PARTY TESTING
Brands Used in Statistically Significant Clinical Trials
- **Standardized extracts referred to as EGb 761:** 24% ginkgo flavone glycosides, 6% terpenoids) Tebonin, Tanakan, Rokan.
- **Standardized extracts referred to as LI 1370:** (25% ginkgo flavone glycosides, 6% terpenoids) Kaveri, Kaver, Ginkgold (Nature's Way), Ginkoba (Pharmaton), Quanterra Mental Sharpness.

Brands Shown to Contain Claimed Ingredients Through Third-Party Testing
- **Consumer Reports (May 2000):** American Fare Vita-Smart, Health's Finest, Lichtwer Pharma Ginkai, Natural Brand, Nature Made, Nature's Resource, Nature's Way Ginkgold, Pharmanex BioGinkgo, Pharmaton Ginkoba, Rite Aid, Sundown Ginkgo Alert, Your Life.

U.S. Equivalents to Most Commonly Recommended European Brands
- Ginkgold (Nature's Way), Ginkoba (Pharmaton), Quanterra, Ginkai (Lichtwer).

Additional Trade Names
- BioGinkgo, Gincosan Ginexin Remind, Ginkai Ginkgo Go, Ginkgold, Ginkgo Phytosome, Ginkgo Powder, Ginkopur, Gingopret, Rö Kan.

References
1. Brevoort P. The booming US botanical market–a new overview. Herbalgram 1998;44:33-47.
2. Guinot P, Braquet P, Duchier J, et al. Inhibition of PAF-acether induced

heal and flare reaction in man by a specific PAF antagonist. Prostaglandins 1986;32(1):160-163.

3. Atzori C, Bruno A, Chichino G, et al. Activity of bilobalide, a sesquiterpene from *Ginkgo biloba*, on *Pneumocystis carinii*. Antimicrob Agents Chemother 1993;37(7):1492-1496.

4. Bridi R, Crossetti FP, Steffen VM, et al. The antioxidant activity of standardized extract of *Ginkgo biloba* (EGb 761) in rats. Phytother Res 2001;15(5):449-451.

5. Droy-Lefaix MT, Cluzel J, Menerath JM, et al. Antioxidant effect of a *Ginkgo biloba* extract (EGb 761) on the retina. Int J Tissue React 1995;17(3):93-100.

6. Droy-Lefaix MT. Effect of the antioxidant action of *Ginkgo biloba* extract (EGb 761) on aging and oxidative stress. Age 1997;20:141-149.

7. Maitra I, Marcocci L, Droy-Lefaix MT, et al. Peroxyl radical scavenging activity of *Ginkgo* biloba extract EGb 761. Biochem Pharmacol 1995; 49(11):1649-1655.

8. Marcocci L, Packer L, Droy-Lefaix MT, et al. Antioxidant action of *Ginkgo biloba* extract EGb 761. Methods Enzymol 1994;234:462-475.

9. Wei T, Ni Y, Hou J, et al. Hydrogen peroxide-induced oxidative damage and apoptosis in cerebellar granule cells: protection by *Ginkgo biloba* extract. Pharmacol Res 2000;41(4):427-433.

10. Yoshikawa T, Naito Y, Kondo M. *Ginkgo biloba* leaf extract: review of biological actions and clinical applications. Antioxid Redox Signal 1999; 1(4):469-480.

11. Guinot P, Brambilla C, Duchier J, et al. Effect of BN 52063, a specific PAF-acether antagonist, on bronchial provocation test to allergens in asthmatic patients. A preliminary study. Prostaglandins 1987;34(5):723-731.

12. Li MH, Zhang HL, Yang BY. [Effects of ginkgo leaf concentrated oral liquor in treating asthma]. Zhongguo Zhong Xi Yi Jie He Za Zhi 1997;17(4):216-218.

13. Wilkens H, Wilkens JH, Uffmann J, et al. [Effect of the platelet-activating factor antagonist BN 52063 on exertional asthma]. Pneumologie 1990;44 Suppl 1:347-348.

14. Wilkens JH, Wilkens H, Uffmann J, et al. Effects of a PAF-antagonist (BN 52063) on bronchoconstriction and platelet activation during exercise induced asthma. Br J Clin Pharmacol 1990;29(1):85-91.

15. Lyon MR, Cline JC, Totosy dZ, et al. Effect of the herbal extract combination *Panax quinquefolium* and *Ginkgo biloba* on attention-deficit hyperactivity disorder: a pilot study. J Psychiatry Neurosci 2001;26(3): 221-228.

16. Emerit I, Oganesian N, Sarkisian T, et al. Clastogenic factors in the plasma of Chernobyl accident recovery workers: anticlastogenic effect of *Ginkgo biloba* extract. Radiat Res 1995;144(2):198-205.

17. Emerit I, Arutyunyan R, Oganesian N, et al. Radiation-induced clastogenic factors: anticlastogenic effect of *Ginkgo biloba* extract. Free Radic Biol Med 1995;18(6):985-991.

18. Koltai M, Tosaki A, Hosford D, et al. Ginkgolide B isolated hearts against arrhythmias induced by ischemia but not reperfusion. Eur J Pharmacol 1989;164(2):293-302.

19. Dubreuil C. [Therapeutic trial in acute cochlear deafness. A comparative study of *Ginkgo biloba* extract and nicergoline]. Presse Med 1986;15(31): 1559-1561.

20. Kampman K, Majewska MD, Tourian K, et al. A pilot trial of piracetam and *Ginkgo biloba* for the treatment of cocaine dependence. Addict Behav 2003;28(3):437-448.

21. Ahlemeyer B, Krieglstein J. Neuroprotective effects of *Ginkgo biloba* extract. Cell Mol Life Sci 2003;60(9):1779-1792.

22. Andrieu S, Gillette S, Amouyal K, et al. Association of Alzheimer's disease onset with *Ginkgo biloba* and other symptomatic cognitive treatments in a population of women aged 75 years and older from the EPIDOS study. J Gerontol A Biol Sci Med Sci 2003;58(4):372-377.

23. Castelli D, Colin L, Camel E, et al. Pretreatment of skin with a *Ginkgo biloba* extract/sodium carboxymethyl- beta-1,3-glucan formulation appears to inhibit the elicitation of allergic contact dermatitis in man. Contact Dermatitis 1998;38(3):123-126.

24. Lanthony P, Cosson JP. [The course of color vision in early diabetic retinopathy treated with *Ginkgo biloba* extract. A preliminary double-blind versus placebo study]. J Fr Ophtalmol 1988;11(10):671-674.

25. Chung KF, Dent G, McCusker M, et al. Effect of a ginkgolide mixture (BN 52063) in antagonising skin and platelet responses to platelet activating factor in man. Lancet 1987;1(8527):248-251.

26. Lagrue G, Behar A, Kazandjian M, et al. [Idiopathic cyclic edema. The role of capillary hyperpermeability and its correction by *Ginkgo biloba* extract]. Presse Med 1986;15(31):1550-1553.

27. Lagrue G, Behar A, Laurent J, et al. [*Ginkgo biloba* extract in the treatment of idiopathic orthostatic edema]. Gaz Medicale 1992;99(8):40-43.

28. Burschka MA, Hassan HA, Reineke T, et al. Effect of treatment with *Ginkgo biloba* leaf extract EGb 761 (oral) on unilateral idiopathic sudden hearing loss in a prospective randomized double-blind study of 106 outpatients. Eur Arch Otorhinolaryngol 2001;258(5):213-219.

29. Reisser CH, Weidauer H. *Ginkgo biloba* extract EGb 761 or pentoxifylline for the treatment of sudden deafness: a randomized, reference-controlled, double-blind study. Acta Otolaryngol 2001;121(5):579-584.

30. Hoffmann F, Beck C, Schutz A, et al. [Ginkgo extract EGb 761 (tenobin)/

HAES versus naftidrofuryl (Dusodril)/HAES. A randomized study of therapy of sudden deafness]. Laryngorhinootologie 1994;73(3):149-152.

31. Dalet R. Essai du Tanakan dans les cephalees et les migraines. Vie Med 1974;2:2971-2972.

32. De Mattos GR. [The *Ginkgo biloba* extract (EGb 761) in the treatment of chronic headache]. Rev Brasil Neurol 1991;27(6):203-206.

33. Li W, Dai QT, Liu ZE. [Preliminary study on early fibrosis of chronic hepatitis B treated with *Ginkgo biloba* Composita]. Zhongguo Zhong Xi Yi Jie He Za Zhi 1995;15(10):593-595.

34. Kudolo GB. The effect of 3-month ingestion of *Ginkgo biloba* extract on pancreatic beta-cell function in response to glucose loading in normal glucose tolerant individuals. J Clin Pharmacol 2000;40(6):647-654.

35. Winther KA, Randlov C, Rein E, et al. Effects of *Ginkgo biloba* extract on cognitive function and blood pressure in elderly subjects. Curr Ther Res 1998;59(12):881-888.

36. Hartley DE, Heinze L, Elsabagh S, et al. Effects on cognition and mood in postmenopausal women of 1-week treatment with *Ginkgo biloba*. Pharmacol Biochem Behav 2003;75(3):711-720.

37. Guillon JM, Rochette L, Baranes J. [Effects of *Ginkgo biloba* extract on 2 models of experimental myocardial ischemia]. Presse Med 1986;15(31): 1516-1519.

38. Koltringer P, Langsteger W, Lind P, et al. [*Ginkgo biloba* extract and folic acid in the therapy of changes caused by autonomic neuropathy]. Acta Med Austriaca 1989;16(2):35-37.

39. Husstedt IW, Thumler R, Roder R, et al. Treatment of polyneuropathies. Investigations on efficacy of *Ginkgo biloba* extract EGb 761 in patients with polyneuropathy. Zeitschr Allgemeinmed 1993;69(26):714-717.

40. Zhang XY, Zhou DF, Zhang PY. A double-blind, placebo-controlled trial of extract of *Ginkgo biloba* added to haloperidol in treatment-resistant patients with schizophrenia. J Clin Psychiatry 2001;62(11):878-883.

41. Zhang XY, Zhou DF, Su JM, et al. The effect of extract of *Ginkgo biloba* added to haloperidol on superoxide dismutase in inpatients with chronic schizophrenia. J Clin Psychopharmacol 2001;21(1):85-88.

42. Hofferberth B. [The effect of *Ginkgo biloba* extract on neurophysiological and psychometric measurement results in patients with psychotic organic brain syndrome. A double-blind study against placebo]. Arzneimittelforschung 1989;39(8):918-922.

43. Canturk NZ, Utkan NZ, Canturk Z, et al. The effects of prostaglandin E2 indomethacin & *Ginkgo biloba* extract on resistance to experimental sepsis. Indian J Med Res 1998;108:88-92.

44. Stein DG, Hoffman SW. Chronic administration of *Ginkgo biloba* extract (EGb 761) can enhance recovery from traumatic brain injury. *In* Christen Y, Costentin J, Lacour M (eds): Effects of *Ginkgo biloba* Extract (EGb 76) on the Central Nervous System. Paris, Elsevier, 1992, pp 95-104.

45. Sandberg-Gertzen H. An open trial of Cedemin, a *Ginkgo biloba* extract with PAF-antagonistic effects for ulcerative colitis. Am J Gastroenterol 1993;88(4):615-616.

46. Parsad D, Pandhi R, Juneja A. Effectiveness of oral *Ginkgo biloba* in treating limited, slowly spreading vitiligo. Clin Exp Dermatol 2003;28(3): 285-287.

47. Kajiyama Y, Fujii K, Takeuchi H, et al. Ginkgo seed poisoning. Pediatrics 2002;109(2):325-327.

48. Schweizer J, Hautmann C. Comparison of two dosages of *Ginkgo biloba* extract EGb 761 in patients with peripheral arterial occlusive disease Fontaine's stage IIb. A randomised, double-blind, multicentric clinical trial. Arzneimittelforschung 1999;49(11):900-904.

49. Oken BS, Storzbach DM, Kaye JA. The efficacy of *Ginkgo biloba* on cognitive function in Alzheimer disease. Arch Neurol 1998;55(11):1409-1415.

50. Wesnes K, Simmons D, Rook M, et al. A double-blind placebo-controlled trial of Tanakan in the treatment of idiopathic cognitive impairment in the elderly. Hum Psychopharm 1987;2:159-169.

51. Hofferberth B. The efficacy of EGb 761 in patients with senile dementia of the Alzheimer type, a double-blind, placebo-controlled study on different levels of investigation. Hum Psychopharm 1994;9(3):215-222.

52. Kanowski S, Herrmann WM, Stephan K, et al. Proof of efficacy of the *Ginkgo biloba* special extract EGb 761 in outpatients suffering from mild to moderate primary degenerative dementia of the Alzheimer type or multi-infarct dementia. Pharmacopsychiatry 1996;29(2):47-56.

53. Le Bars PL, Katz MM, Berman N, et al. A placebo-controlled, double-blind, randomized trial of an extract of *Ginkgo biloba* for dementia. North American EGb Study Group. JAMA 1997;278(16):1327-1332.

54. Rigney U, Kimber S, Hindmarch I. The effects of acute doses of standardized *Ginkgo biloba* extract on memory and psychomotor performance in volunteers. Phytother Res 1999;13(5):408-415.

55. Kennedy DO, Scholey AB, Wesnes KA. The dose-dependent cognitive effects of acute administration of *Ginkgo biloba* to healthy young volunteers. Psychopharmacology (Berl) 2000;151(4):416-423.

56. Kennedy DO, Scholey AB, Wesnes KA. Differential, dose dependent changes in cognitive performance following acute administration of a *Ginkgo biloba/Panax ginseng* combination to healthy young volunteers. Nutrit Neurosci 2001;4:399-412.

57. Kennedy DO, Scholey AB, Wesnes K. A direct comparison of the cognitive effects of acute doses of ginseng, *Ginkgo biloboa* and their combination in healthy volunteers. J Psychopharm 2001;15(Suppl):A56.

58. Scholey AB, Kennedy DO. Acute, dose-dependent cognitive effects of *Ginkgo biloba*, *Panax ginseng* and their combination in healthy young volunteers: differential interactions with cognitive demand. Human Psychopharmacology 2002;17(1):35-44.

59. Kennedy DO, Scholey AB, Wesnes K. A direct comparison of the cognitive effects of acute doses of ginseng, *Ginkgo biloba* and their combination in healthy volunteers. 8th Annual Symposium on Complementary Health Care, 6th-8th December 2001.

60. Saudreau F, Serise JM, Pillet J, et al. [Efficacy of an extract of *Ginkgo biloba* in the treatment of chronic obliterating arteriopathies of the lower limbs in stage III of Fontaine's classification]. J Mal Vasc 1989;14(3):177-182.

61. Arenz A, Klein M, Fiehe K, et al. Occurrence of neurotoxic 4'-*O*-methylpyridoxine in *Ginkgo biloba* leaves, ginkgo medications, and Japanese ginkgo food. Planta Med 1996;62:548-551.

62. Pittler MH, Ernst E. *Ginkgo biloba* extract for the treatment of intermittent claudication: a meta-analysis of randomized trials. Am J Med 2000; 108(4):276-281.

63. Ernst E, Pittler MH. *Ginkgo biloba* for dementia. A systematic review of double-blind, placebo-controlled trials. Clin Drug Invest 1999;17(4): 301-308.

64. Ernst E, Stevinson C. *Ginkgo biloba* for tinnitus: a review. Clin Otolaryngol 1999;24(3):164-167.

65. Granger AS. *Ginkgo biloba* precipitating epileptic seizures. Age Ageing 2001;30(6):523-525.

66. Tomb RR, Foussereau J, Sell Y. Mini-epidemic of contact dermatitis from ginkgo tree fruit (*Ginkgo biloba* L.). Contact Dermatitis 1988;19(4): 281-283.

67. Petty HR, Fernando M, Kindzelskii AL, et al. Identification of colchicine in placental blood from patients using herbal medicines. Chem Res Toxicol 2001;14(9):1254-1258.

68. Davydov L, Stirling AL. Stevens-Johnson syndrome with *Ginkgo biloba*. J Herbal Pharmacother 2001;1(3):65-69.

69. Birks J, Grimley EV, Van Dongen M. *Ginkgo biloba* for cognitive impairment and dementia. Cochrane Database Syst Rev 2003;(4): CD003120.

70. Burkard G. [The efficacy and safety of *Ginkgo biloba* extract in dementia]. Fortschr Med [Supp] 1991;109(107):6-8.

71. Becker LE, Skipworth GB. Ginkgo-tree dermatitis, stomatitis, and proctitis. JAMA 1975;231(11):1162-1163.

72. Gregory PJ. Seizure associated with *Ginkgo biloba*? Ann Intern Med 2001; 134(4):344.

73. Galluzzi S, Zanetti O, Binetti G, et al. Coma in a patient with Alzheimer's disease taking low dose trazodone and *Gingko biloba*. J Neurol Neurosurg Psychiatry 2000;68(5):679-680.

74. White HL, Scates PW, Cooper BR. Extracts of *Ginkgo biloba* leaves inhibit monoamine oxidase. Life Sci 1996;58(16):1315-1321.

75. Porsolt RD, Roux S, Drieu K. Evaluation of a *Ginkgo biloba* extract (EGb 761) in functional tests for monoamine oxidase inhibition. Arzneimittelforschung 2000;50(3):232-235.

76. Fowler JS, et al. Evidence that *Gingko biloba* extract does not inhibit MAO A and B in living human brain. Life Sci 2000;66:141-146.

77. Rosenblatt M, Mindel J. Spontaneous hyphema associated with ingestion of *Ginkgo biloba* extract. N Engl J Med 1997;336(15):1108.

78. Chen X, Salwinski S, Lee TJ. Extracts of *Ginkgo biloba* and ginsenosides exert cerebral vasorelaxation via a nitric oxide pathway. Clin Exp Pharmacol Physiol 1997;24(12):958-959.

79. Rowin J, Lewis SL. Spontaneous bilateral subdural hematomas associated with chronic *Ginkgo biloba* ingestion. Neurology 1996;46(6):1775-1776.

80. Vale S. Subarachnoid haemorrhage associated with *Ginkgo biloba*. Lancet 1998;352(9121):36.

81. Skogh M. Extracts of *Ginkgo biloba* and bleeding or haemorrhage. Lancet 1998;352(9134):1145-1146.

82. Benjamin J, Muir T, Briggs K, et al. A case of cerebral haemorrhage—can *Ginkgo biloba* be implicated? Postgrad Med J 2001;77(904):112-113.

83. Matthews MK, Jr. Association of *Ginkgo biloba* with intracerebral hemorrhage. Neurology 1998;50(6):1933-1934.

84. Gilbert GJ. *Ginkgo biloba*. Neurology 1997;48(4):1137.

85. Fessenden JM, Wittenborn W, Clarke L. *Ginkgo biloba*: a case report of herbal medicine and bleeding postoperatively from a laparoscopic cholecystectomy. Am Surg 2001;67(1):33-35.

86. Meisel C, Johne A, Roots I. Fatal intracerebral mass bleeding associated with *Ginkgo biloba* and ibuprofen. Atherosclerosis 2003;167(2):367.

87. Bourgain RH, Maes L, Andries R, et al. Thrombus induction by endogenic paf-acether and its inhibition by *Ginkgo biloba* extracts in the guinea pig. Prostaglandins 1986;32(1):142-144.

88. Bal Dit SC, Caplain H, Drouet L. No alteration in platelet function or coagulation induced by EGb761 in a controlled study. Clin Lab Haematol 2003;25(4):251-253.

89. Cohen AJ, Bartlik B. *Ginkgo biloba* for antidepressant-induced sexual dysfunction. J Sex Marital Ther 1998;24(2):139-143.

90. Kudolo GB. The effect of 3-month ingestion of *Ginkgo biloba* extract (EGb 761) on pancreatic beta-cell function in response to glucose loading in individuals with non-insulin-dependent diabetes mellitus. J Clin Pharmacol 2001;41(6):600-611.

91. Manocha A, Pillai KK, Husain SZ. Influence of *Ginkgo biloba* on the effect of anticonvulsants. Indian J Pharmacol 1996;28:84-87.

92. Kim YS, Pyo MK, Park KM, et al. Antiplatelet and antithrombotic effects of a combination of ticlopidine and *Ginkgo biloba* ext (EGb 761). Thromb Res 1998;91(1):33-38.

93. Mauro VF, Mauro LS, Kleshinski JF, et al. Impact of *Ginkgo biloba* on the pharmacokinetics of digoxin. Am J Ther 2003;10(4):247-251.

94. Ramassamy C, Christen Y, Clostre F, et al. The *Ginkgo biloba* extract, EGb761, increases synaptosomal uptake of 5-hydroxytryptamine: in-vitro and *ex-vivo* studies. J Pharm Pharmacol 1992;44(11):943-945.

95. Sikora R, Sohn M, Deutz FJ, et al. *Ginkgo biloba* extract in the therapy of erectile dysfunction. J Urol 1989;141:188A.

96. Ellison JM, DeLuca P. Fluoxetine-induced genital anesthesia relieved by *Ginkgo biloba* extract. J Clin Psychiatry 1998;59(4):199-200.

97. Hauns B, Haring B, Kohler S, et al. Phase II study with 5-fluorouracil and *Ginkgo biloba* extract (GBE 761 ONC) in patients with pancreatic cancer. Arzneimittelforschung 1999;49(12):1030-1034.

98. Biber A. Pharmacokinetics of *Ginkgo biloba* extracts. Pharmacopsychiatry 2003;36 Suppl 1:S32-S37.

99. Deng F, Zito SW. Development and validation of a gas chromatographic-mass spectrometric method for simultaneous identification and quantification of marker compounds including bilobalide, ginkgolides and flavonoids in *Ginkgo biloba* L. extract and pharmaceutical preparations. J Chromatogr A 2003;986(1):121-127.

100. Diamond BJ, Shiflett SC, Feiwel N, et al. *Ginkgo biloba* extract: mechanisms and clinical indications. Arch Phys Med Rehabil 2000;81(5):668-678.

101. Sticher O. Quality of ginkgo preparations. Planta Med 1993;59(1):2-11.

102. Pietri S, Seguin JR, D'Arbigny P, et al. *Ginkgo biloba* extract (EGb 761) pretreatment limits free radical-induced oxidative stress in patients undergoing coronary bypass surgery. Cardiovasc Drugs Ther 1997;11(2): 121-131.

103. Pietri S, Maurelli E, Drieu K, et al. Cardioprotective and anti-oxidant effects of the terpenoid constituents of *Ginkgo biloba* extract (EGb 761). J Mol Cell Cardiol 1997;29(2):733-742.

104. Artmann GM, Schikarski C. *Ginkgo biloba* extract (EGb 761) protects red blood cells from oxidative damage. Clin Hemorheol 1993;13(4):529-539.

105. Akiba S, Kawauchi T, Oka T, et al. Inhibitory effect of the leaf extract of *Ginkgo biloba* L. on oxidative stress-induced platelet aggregation. Biochem Mol Biol Int 1998;46(6):1243-1248.

106. Dumont E, Petit E, Tarrade T, et al. UV-C irradiation-induced peroxidative degradation of microsomal fatty acids and proteins: protection by an extract of *Ginkgo biloba* (EGb 761). Free Radic Biol Med 1992; 13(3):197-203.

107. Marcocci L, Maguire JJ, Droy-Lefaix MT, et al. The nitric oxide-scavenging properties of *Ginkgo biloba* extract EGb 761. Biochem Biophys Res Commun 1994;201(2):748-755.

108. Pincemail J, Dupuis M, Nasr C, et al. Superoxide anion scavenging effect and superoxide dismutase activity of *Ginkgo biloba* extract. Experientia 1989;45(8):708-712.

109. Szabo ME, Droy-Lefaix MT, Doly M. Direct measurement of free radicals in ischemic/reperfused diabetic rat retina. Clin Neurosci 1997;4(5): 240-245.

110. Janssens D, Michiels C, Delaive E, et al. Protection of hypoxia-induced ATP decrease in endothelial cells by *Ginkgo biloba* extract and bilobalide. Biochem Pharmacol 1995;50(7):991-999.

111. Koltringer P, Langsteger W, Eber O. Dose-dependent hemorheological effects and microcirculatory modifications following intravenous administration of *Ginkgo biloba* special extract EGb 761. Clin Hemorheol 1995;15(4):649-656.

112. Kose K, Dogan P. Lipoperoxidation induced by hydrogen peroxide in human erythrocyte membranes. 1. Protective effect of *Ginkgo biloba* extract (EGb 761). J Int Med Res 1995;23(1):1-8.

113. Oberpichler H, Beck T, Abdel-Rahman MM, et al. Effects of *Ginkgo biloba* constituents related to protection against brain damage caused by hypoxia. Pharmacol Res Commun 1988;20(5):349-368.

114. Szabo ME, Droy-Lefaix MT, Doly M, et al. Free radical-mediated effects in reperfusion injury: a histologic study with superoxide dismutase and EGB 761 in rat retina. Ophthalmic Res 1991;23(4):225-234.

115. Szabo ME, Droy-Lefaix MT, Doly M. EGb 761 and the recovery of ion imbalance in ischemic reperfused diabetic rat retina. Ophthalmic Res 1995;27(2):102-109.

116. Braquet P, Bourgain RH. Anti-anaphylactic properties of BN 52021: a potent platelet activating factor antagonist. Adv Exp Med Biol 1987; 215:215-235.

117. Braquet P. The ginkgolides: Potent platelet-activating factor antagonists isolated from *Ginkgo biloba* L.: Chemistry, pharmacology and clinical applications. Drugs Future 1987;12:643-688.

118. Braquet P. Proofs of involvement of PAF-acether in various immune disorders using BN 52021 (ginkgolide B): a powerful PAF-acether antagonist isolated from *Ginkgo biloba* L. Adv Prostaglandin Thromboxane Leukot Res 1986;16:179-198.

119. Desquand S, Touvay C, Randon J, et al. Interference of BN 52021 (Ginkgolide B) with the bronchopulmonary effects of PAF-acether in the guinea-pig. Eur J Pharm 1986;127:83-95.

120. Guinot P, Summerhayes C, Berdah L, et al. Treatment of adult systemic mastocytosis with a PAF-acether antagonist BN52063. Lancet 1988; 2(8602):114.

121. Guinot P, Caffrey E, Lambe R, et al. Tanakan inhibits platelet-activating-factor-induced platelet aggregation in healthy male volunteers. Haemostasis 1989;19(4):219-223.

122. Lamant V, Mauco G, Braquet P, et al. Inhibition of the metabolism of platelet activating factor (PAF- acether) by three specific antagonists from *Ginkgo biloba*. Biochem Pharmacol 1987;36(17):2749-2752.

123. Markey AC, Barker JN, Archer CB, et al. Platelet activating factor-induced clinical and histopathologic responses in atopic skin and their modification by the platelet activating factor antagonist BN52063. J Am Acad Dermatol 1990;23(2 Pt 1):263-268.

124. Oberpichler H, Sauer D, Rossberg C, et al. PAF antagonist ginkgolide B reduces postischemic neuronal damage in rat brain hippocampus. J Cereb Blood Flow Metab 1990;10(1):133-135.

125. Prehn JH, Krieglstein J. Platelet-activating factor antagonists reduce excitotoxic damage in cultured neurons from embryonic chick telencephalon and protect the rat hippocampus and neocortex from ischemic injury *in vivo*. J Neurosci Res 1993;34(2):179-188.

126. Roberts NM, McCusker M, Chung KF, et al. Effect of a PAF antagonist, BN52063, on PAF-induced bronchoconstriction in normal subjects. Br J Clin Pharmacol 1988;26(1):65-72.

127. Roberts NM, Page CP, Chung KF, et al. Effect of a PAF antagonist, BN52063, on antigen-induced, acute, and late-onset cutaneous responses in atopic subjects. J Allergy Clin Immunol 1988;82(2):236-241.

128. Smith PF, Maclennan K, Darlington CL. The neuroprotective properties of the *Ginkgo biloba* leaf: a review of the possible relationship to platelet-activating factor (PAF). J Ethnopharmacol 1996;50(3):131-139.

129. Dutta-Roy AK, Gordon MJ, Kelly C, et al. Inhibitory effect of *Ginkgo biloba* extract on human platelet aggregation. Platelets 1999;10:298-305.

130. Marcilhac A, Dakine N, Bourhim N, et al. Effect of chronic administration of *Ginkgo biloba* extract or ginkgolide on the hypothalamic-pituitary-adrenal axis in the rat. Life Sci 1998;62(25):2329-2340.

131. DeFeudis FV. *Ginkgo biloba* extract (EGb 761): pharmacological activities and clinical applications. Paris: Elsevier, 1991: 133-134.

132. Huguet F, Tarrade T. Alpha 2-adrenoceptor changes during cerebral ageing. The effect of *Ginkgo biloba* extract. J Pharm Pharmacol 1992; 44(1):24-27.

133. Huguet F, Drieu K, Piriou A. Decreased cerebral 5-HT1A receptors during ageing: reversal by *Ginkgo biloba* extract (EGb 761). J Pharm Pharmacol 1994;46(4):316-318.

134. Zhu L, Gao J, Wang Y, et al. Neuron degeneration induced by verapamil and attenuated by EGb761. J Basic Clin Physiol Pharmacol 1997;8(4): 301-314.

135. Amri H, Drieu K, Papadopoulos V. *Ex vivo* regulation of adrenal cortical cell steroid and protein synthesis, in response to adrenocorticotropic hormone stimulation, by the *Ginkgo biloba* extract EGb 761 and isolated ginkgolide B. Endocrinology 1997;138(12):5415-5426.

136. Cheung F, Siow YL, Chen WZ, et al. Inhibitory effect of *Ginkgo biloba* extract on the expression of inducible nitric oxide synthase in endothelial cells. Biochem Pharmacol 1999;58(10):1665-1673.

137. Kudolo GB, Blodgett J. Effect of *Ginkgo biloba* ingestion on arachidonic acid metabolism in the platelets of type 2 diabetic subjects [abstract]. International Scientific Conference on Complementary, Alternative and Integrative Medicine Research, April 12-14 2002.

138. Jung F, Mrowietz C, Kiesewetter H, et al. Effect of *Ginkgo biloba* on fluidity of blood and peripheral microcirculation in volunteers. Arzneimittelforschung 1990;40(5):589-593.

139. Rudofsky G. [Effect of *Ginkgo biloba* extract in arterial occlusive disease. Randomized placebo controlled crossover study]. Fortschr Med 1987;105(20):397-400.

140. Kleijnen J, Knipschild P. *Ginkgo biloba* for cerebral insufficiency. Br J Clin Pharmacol 1992;34(4):352-358.

141. Pietta PG, Gardana C, Mauri PL. Identification of *Gingko biloba* flavonol metabolites after oral administration to humans. J Chromatogr B Biomed Sci Appl 1997;693(1):249-255.

142. Girolami B, Bernardi E, Prins MH, et al. Treatment of intermittent claudication with physical training, smoking cessation, pentoxifylline, or nafronyl: a meta-analysis. Arch Intern Med 1999;159(4):337-345.

143. Gardner AW, Poehlman ET. Exercise rehabilitation programs for the treatment of claudication pain. A meta-analysis. JAMA 1995;274(12): 975-980.

144. Ernst E, Fialka V. A review of the clinical effectiveness of exercise therapy for intermittent claudication. Arch Intern Med 1993;153(20):2357-2360.

145. Ernst E. [*Ginkgo biloba* in treatment of intermittent claudication. A systematic research based on controlled studies in the literature]. Fortschr Med 1996;114(8):85-87.

146. Blume J, Kieser M, Holscher U. [Placebo-controlled double-blind study of the effectiveness of *Ginkgo biloba* special extract EGb 761 in trained patients with intermittent claudication]. Vasa 1996;25(3):265-274.

147. Bauer U. Six-month double-blind randomised clinical trial of *Ginkgo biloba* extract versus placebo in two parallel groups in patients suffering from peripheral arterial insufficiency. Arzneimittelforschung 1984;34(6):716-720.

148. Thomson GJ, Vohra RK, Carr MH, et al. A clinical trial of *Ginkgo biloba* extract in patients with intermittent claudication. Int Angiol 1990;9(2): 75-78.

149. Salz H. [The effectiveness of a *Ginkgo biloba* preparation in arterial ischemic diseases of the leg. Controlled double-blind cross-over study]. Therapie der Gegenwart 1980;119(II):1345-1356.

150. Drabæk H, Petersen JR, Wiinberg N, et al. Effekten af *Ginkgo biloba*-ekstrakt hos patienter med claudicatio intermittens. Ugeskr Læger 1996; 158(27):3928-3931.

151. Blume VJ, Kieser M, Hölscher U. Ginkgo-spezialextrakt EGb 761 bei peripherer arterieller Verschlußkrankheit. Fortschr Med 1998;116:137-143.

152. Peters H, Kieser M, Holscher U. Demonstration of the efficacy of *Ginkgo biloba* special extract EGb 761 on intermittent claudication—a placebo-controlled, double-blind multicenter trial. Vasa 1998;27(2):106-110.

153. Natali J, Boissier P. Internal report (*Ginkgo biloba*); Schwabe, 1985.

154. Mouren X, Caillard P, Schwartz F. Study of the antiischemic action of EGb 761 in the treatment of peripheral arterial occlusive disease by TcPo2 determination. Angiology 1994;45(6):413-417.

155. Moher D, Pham B, Ausejo M, et al. Pharmacological management of intermittent claudication: a meta-analysis of randomised trials. Drugs 2000;59(5):1057-1070.

156. Bulling B, von Bary S. The treatment of chronic peripheral arterial occlusion disease with physical training and *Ginkgo biloba* extract 761, results of a placebo-controlled, double-blind study. Die Medizin Welt 1991;42:702-708.

157. Schneider B. [*Ginkgo biloba* extract in peripheral arterial diseases. Meta-analysis of controlled clinical studies]. Arzneimittelforschung 1992;42(4): 428-436.

158. Bauer U. [*Ginkgo biloba* extract in the treatment of arteriopathy of the lower extremities. A 65-week trial]. Presse Med 1986;15(31):1546-1549.

159. Bauer U. Long-term treatment of peripheral occlusive arterial disease with *Ginkgo biloba* extract (GBE). A three year study. Vasa 1986; (Suppl)15:26.

160. Bauer U. A two-year study of *Ginkgo-biloba* extract in the treatment of peripheral arterial disease (Fontaigne stage IIb). Proc 14th World Congr Int Union Angiol, 1986.

161. Frileux C, Cope R. [The concentrated extract of *Ginkgo biloba* in peripheral vascular disease]. Cahiers d'Arteriol Royat 1975;3:117-122.

162. Courbier R, Jausseran JM, Reggi M. [Double-blind crossover study of Tanakan in arteriopathies of the lower extremities]. Mediter Medicale 1977;126:61-64.

163. Garzya G, Picari M. Trattamento delle vasculopatie periferiche con una nuova sostanza estrattiva: il Tanakan. Clin Europea 1981;20(5):936-944.

164. Lauliac M, Bernasconi P. [Clinical study of Tanakan in peripheral vascular disorders]. Lille Med 1976;21(7 Suppl 3):620-622.

165 Palade R, Vasile D, Grigoriu M, et al. [Treatment with Ginkor Fort in varicose veins]. Chirurgia (Bucur) 1997;92(4):249-255.

166. Böhmer D, Kalinski S, Michaelis P et al. Behandlung der PAVK mit *Ginkgo-biloba*-extrakt (GBE) oder Pentoxifyllin. Herz Kreislauf 1988; 20(1):5-8.

167. Letzel H, Schoop W. [*Gingko biloba* extract EGb 761 and pentoxifylline in intermittent claudication. Secondary analysis of the clinical effectiveness]. Vasa 1992;21(4):403-410.

168. Schulz V. Ginkgo extract or cholinesterase inhibitors in patients with dementia: what clinical trials and guidelines fail to consider. Phytomedicine 2003;10 Suppl 4:74-79.

169. Wettstein A. Cholinesterase inhibitors and Gingko extracts—are they comparable in the treatment of dementia? Comparison of published placebo-controlled efficacy studies of at least six months' duration. Phytomedicine 2000;6(6):393-401.

170. Brautigam MR, Blommaert FA, Verleye G, et al. Treatment of age-related memory complaints with *Ginkgo biloba* extract: a randomized double blind placebo-controlled study. Phytomed 1998;5(6):425-434.

171. Arrigo A, Cattaneo S. Clinical and psychometric evaluation of *Ginkgo biloba* extract in chronic cerebro-vascular diseases. *In* Agnoli A, Rapin JF, Scapagnini V, et al. (eds): Effects of *Ginkgo biloba* Extracts on Organic Cerebral Impairment. London, John Libbey Eurotext Ltd, 1985, pp 71-76.

172. Arrigo A. Treatment of chronic cerebrovascular insufficiency with *Ginkgo biloba* extract. Therapiewoche 1986;36:5208-5218.

173. Brüchert E, Heinrich SE, Ruf-Kohler P. Wirksamkeit von LI 1370 bei älteren Patienten mit Hirnleistungsschwäche. Multizentrische Doppelblindstudie des Fachverbandes Deutscher Allgemeinärzte. Munch Med Wochenschr 1991;133(Suppl 1):S9-S14.

174. Eckmann VF, Schlag H. Kontrollierte doppelblind-studie zum wirksamkeitsnachweis von tebonin forte bei patienten mit zerebrovaskulärer insuffizienz. Fortschr Med 1982;100(31):1474-1478.

175. Halama VP, Bartsch G, Meng G. Hirnleistungsstörungen vaskulärer genese. Fortschr Med 1988;106(19):408-412.

176. Halama P, Bartsch G, Meng G. [Disturbances of cerebral performance of vascular origin. Randomized, double-blind study on the efficacy of *Ginkgo biloba* extract]. Revista Brasileira de Neurologia 1991;27(2):73-78.

177. Hartmann A, Frick M. Wirkung eines ginkgo-spezial-extraktes auf psychometrische parameter bei patienten mit vaskular bedingter demenz. Munch Med Wochenschr 1991;133(Suppl):S23-S25.

178. Hofferberth B. *Ginkgo-biloba*-spezialekstrakt bei patienten mit hirnorganischem psychosyndrom. Prufung der wirksamkeit mit neurophysiologischen und psychometrischen methoden. Munch Med Wochenschr 1991;133(Suppl 1):30-33.
179. Schmidt U, Rabinovici K, Lande S. Einfluss eines Ginkgo-spezial-extraktes auf die befindlichkeit bei zerebraler insuffizienz. Munch Med Wochenschr 1991;133(Suppl 1):S15-S18.
180. Vorberg G, Schenk N, Schmidt U. Efficacy of a new *Ginkgo biloba* extract in 100 patients affected by cerebral insufficiency. Herz Gefasse, Periodical Prac Cardioangiol 1989;7:1-10 (936-941).
181. Weitbrecht WV, Jansen W. Double-blind and comparative (*Gingko biloba* versus placebo) therapeutic study in geriatric patients with primary degenerative dementia —a preliminary evaluation. *In* Agnoli A, Rapin JF, Scapagnini V, et al. (eds):. Effects of Gingko Biloba Extract On Organic Cerebral Impairment. London, John Libbey Eurotext Ltd., 1985.
182. Mancini M, Agozzino B, Bompani R. [Clinical and therapeutic effects of *Ginkgo biloba* extract (GBE) versus placebo in the treatment of psychoorganic senile dementia of arteriosclerotic origin]. Gazz Med Italiana 1993;152:69-80.
183. Grassel E. [Effect of *Ginkgo-biloba* extract on mental performance. Double-blind study using computerized measurement conditions in patients with cerebral insufficiency]. Fortschr Med 1992;110(5):73-76.
184. Maurer K, Ihl R, Dierks T, et al. Clinical efficacy of *Ginkgo biloba* special extract EGb 761 in dementia of the Alzheimer type. J Psychiatr Res 1997;31(6):645-655.
185. Maurer K, Ihl R, Dierks T, et al. Clinical efficacy of *Ginkgo biloba* special extract EGb 761 in dementia of the Alzheimer type. Phytomed 1998;5(6):417-424.
186. van Dongen MC, van Rossum E, Kessels AG, et al. The efficacy of ginkgo for elderly people with dementia and age- associated memory impairment: new results of a randomized clinical trial. J Am Geriatr Soc 2000;48(10):1183-1194.
187. Van Dongen M, van Rossum E, Kessels A, et al. Ginkgo for elderly people with dementia and age-associated memory impairment: a randomized clinical trial. J Clin Epidemiol 2003;56(4):367-376.
188. Le Bars PL, Kieser M, Itil KZ. A 26-week analysis of a double-blind, placebo-controlled trial of the *Ginkgo biloba* extract EGb 761 in dementia. Dement Geriatr Cogn Disord 2000;11(4):230-237.
189. Kanowski S, Herrmann WM, Stephan K, et al. Proof of efficacy of the *Ginkgo biloba* special extract EGb 761 in outpatients suffering from mild to moderate primary degenerative dementia of the Alzheimer type or multi-infarct dementia. Phytomed 1997;4(1):3-13.
190. Rai GS, Shovlin C, Wesnes KA. A double-blind, placebo controlled study of *Ginkgo biloba* extract ('tanakan') in elderly outpatients with mild to moderate memory impairment. Curr Med Res Opin 1991;12(6):350-355.
191. Augustin P. [*Ginkgo biloba* extract in geriatrics. Clinical and psychometric study of 189 patients]. Psychologie Med 1976;8(1):123-130.
192. Winther K, Randlov C, Rein E, et al. *Ginkgo biloba* (GB-8) enhances motor and intellectual function in patients with dementia when evaluated by local nurses [abstract]. Inter Scientific Conf Complement Altern Integr Med Res, April 12-14, 2002.
193. Chartres JP, Bonnan P, Martin G. Réduction de posologie de médicaments psychotropes chez des personnes âgées vivant en institution. Étude à double-insu chez des patients prenant soit de l'extrait de *Ginkgo biloba* 761 soit du placebo. Psychologie Med 1987;19(8):1365-1375.
194. Natali J, Critol R. Experimentation clinique d'un extrait de *Ginkgo biloba* dans les insuffisances arterielles peripheriques. Vie Med 1976;17:1023.
195. Weitbrecht WU, Jansen W. [Primary degenerative dementia: therapy with *Ginkgo biloba* extract. Placebo-controlled double-blind and comparative study]. Fortschr Med 1986;104(9):199-202.
196. Haguenauer JP, Cantenot F, Koskas H, et al. [Treatment of equilibrium disorders with *Ginkgo biloba* extract. A multicenter double-blind drug vs. placebo study]. Presse Med 1986;15(31):1569-1572.
197. Meyer B. [Multicenter randomized double-blind drug vs. placebo study of the treatment of tinnitus with *Ginkgo biloba* extract]. Presse Med 1986;15(31):1562-1564.
198. Taillandier J, Ammar A, Rabourdin JP, et al. Treatment of cerebral aging disorders with *Ginkgo biloba* extract. A longitudinal multicenter double-blind drug vs. placebo study. Presse Med 1986;15(31):1583-1587.
199. Hopfenmüller W. [Evidence for a therapeutic effect of *Ginkgo biloba* special extract. Meta-analysis of 11 clinical studies in patients with cerebrovascular insufficiency in old age]. Arzneimittelforschung 1994;44(9):1005-1013.
200. Halama P. *Ginkgo biloba*. Wirksamkeit eines spezialextrakts bei patienten mit zerebraler insuffizienz. Munch Med Wochenschr 1991;133(12):190-194.
201. Eckmann F. [Cerebral insufficiency—treatment with *Ginkgo-biloba* extract. Time of onset of effect in a double-blind study with 60 inpatients]. Fortschr Med 1990;108(29):557-560.
202. Maier-Hauff K. LI 1370 nach cerebraler aneurysma-operation. Wirksamkeit bei ambulanten patienten mit storungen der hirnleistungsfahigkeit. Munch Med Wochenschr 1991;133(Suppl 1):34-37.
203. Schulz V. Placebo-controlled double-blind study on the efficacy of *Ginkgo biloba* extract in general practice. Fortschr Med [Supp] 1991;109(107):8-11.
204. Vesper J, Hansgen KD. Efficacy of *Ginkgo biloba* in 90 outpatients with cerebral insufficiency caused by old age. Results of a placebo-controlled double-blind trial. Phytomed 1994;1:9-16.
205. Gessner B, Voelp A, Klasser M. Study of the long-term action of a *Ginkgo biloba* extract on vigilance and mental performance as determined by means of quantitative pharmaco-EEG and psychometric measurements. Arzneimittelforschung 1985;35(9):1459-1465.
206. Vorberg G. *Ginkgo biloba* extract (GBE): a long-term study of chronic cerebral insufficiency in geriatric patients. Clin Trials J 1985;22(2):149-157.
207. Gerhardt G, Rogalla K, Jaeger J. [Drug therapy of disorders of cerebral performance. Randomized comparative study of dihydroergotoxine and *Ginkgo biloba* extract]. Fortschr Med 1990;108(19):384-388.
208. Schaffler K, Reeh PW. [Double blind study of the hypoxia protective effect of a standardized *Ginkgo biloba* preparation after repeated administration in healthy subjects]. Arzneimittelforschung 1985;35(8):1283-1286.
209. D'Avila JL. [A multicenter study on the efficacy of *Ginkgo biloba* extract (EGb 761) in patients with cerebral and peripheral vascular insufficiency]. Arquivos Brasileiros de Medicina 1992;66(1):87-91.
210. Dieli G, LaMantia V, Saetta E, et al. Studio clinico in doppio cieco del tanakan nell' insufficienza cerebrale cronica. Lavoro Neuropsich 1981;68:3-15.
211. Eckmann F. Ergebnis einer placebokontrollierten crossover doppelblindstudie mit Tebonin-Dragees bei patienten mit zerebrovaskularer Insuffizienz infolge prasklerotischer Gefaßveranderungen. Klinischer Bericht 1984.
212. Halama P. [*Ginkgo biloba* extract (EGb 761) in the treatment of patients with cerebrovascular insufficiency and therapy-resistant depressive symptoms]. Therapiewoche 1990;40(51-52):3760-3765.
213. Kade F, Miller W. Dose-dependent effects of *Ginkgo biloba* extraction on cerebral, mental and physical efficiency: a placebo controlled double blind study. Brit J Clin Res 1993;4:97-103.
214. Knipschild P, van Dongen M, van Rossum E, et al. Clinical experience with ginkgo in patients with cerebral insufficiency. Rev Bras Neurol 1994;30 (suppl 1):18S-25S.
215. Rudenko AE, Lushchik UB, Dzhumik VA. The clinical efficacy of Tanakan in patients with stage-I atherosclerotic circulatory encephalopathy. Lik Sprava 1997;2:99-101.
216. Tea S, Celsis P, Clanet M, et al. Effets clinique, hemodynamique et metaboliques de l'extrait de *Ginkgo biloba* en pathologie vasculaire cerebrale. Gaz Med Fr 1979;86(35):4149-4152.
217. Allain H, Raoul P, Lieury A, et al. Effect of two doses of *Ginkgo biloba* extract (EGb 761) on the dual-coding test in elderly subjects. Clin Ther 1993;15(3):549-558.
218. Semlitsch HV, Anderer P, Saletu B, et al. Cognitive psychophysiology in nootropic drug research: effects of *Ginkgo biloba* on event-related potentials (P300) in age-associated memory impairment. Pharmacopsychiatry 1995;28(4):134-142.
219. Solomon PR, Adams F, Silver A, et al. Ginkgo for memory enhancement: a randomized controlled trial. JAMA 2002;288(7):835-840.
220. Cheuvront SN, Carter R, III. Ginkgo and memory. JAMA 2003;289(5):547-548.
221. Wheatley D. Ginkgo and memory. JAMA 2003;289(5):546-547.
222. Arnold KR. Ginkgo and memory. JAMA 2003;289(5):546-548.
223. Nathan PJ, Harrison BJ, Bartholomeusz C. Ginkgo and memory. JAMA 2003;289(5):546-548.
224. PM, Pomara N. Ginkgo and memory. JAMA 2003;289(5):547-548.
225. Mix JA, Crews WD, Jr. An examination of the efficacy of *Ginkgo biloba* extract EGb761 on the neuropsychologic functioning of cognitively intact older adults. J Altern Complement Med 2000;6(3):219-229.
226. Moulton PL, Boyko LN, Fitzpatrick JL, et al. The effect of *Ginkgo biloba* on memory in healthy male volunteers. Physiol Behav 2001;73(4):659-665.
227. Cieza A, Maier P, Poppel E. Effects of *Ginkgo biloba* on mental functioning in healthy volunteers. Arch Med Res 2003;34(5):373-381.
228. Cieza A, Maier P, Poppel E. [*Ginkgo biloba* works in healthy persons, too. Older people feel more mentally fit]. Fortschr Med 2003; 145(10):51.
229. Wesnes KA, Ward T, McGinty A, et al. The memory enhancing effects of a *Ginkgo biloba/Panax ginseng* combination in healthy middle-aged volunteers. Psychopharmacology (Berl) 2000;152(4):353-361.
230. Wesnes KA, Faleni RA, Hefting NR, et al. The cognitive, subjective, and physical effects of a *Ginkgo biloba/Panax ginseng* combination in healthy volunteers with neurasthenic complaints. Psychopharmacol Bull 1997;33(4):677-683.
231. Sprenger FH. Gute therapie ergebnisse mit *Ginkgo biloba*. Arztlich Praxis 1986;38:938-940.
232. Meyer B. [A multicenter study of tinnitus. Epidemiology and therapy]. Ann Otolaryngol Chir Cervicofac 1986;103(3):185-188.
233. Holgers KM, Axelsson A, Pringle I. *Ginkgo biloba* extract for the treatment of tinnitus. Audiology 1994;33(2):85-92.
234. Morgenstern C, Biermann E. Ginkgo Spezialextrakt EGb 761 in der Behandlung des Tinnitus aureum. Fortschr Med 1997;115:7-11.
235. Holstein N. [Ginkgo special extract EGb 761 in tinnitus therapy. An overview of results of completed clinical trials]. Fortschr Med 2001;118(4):157-164.
236. Drew S, Davies E. Effectiveness of *Ginkgo biloba* in treating tinnitus: double blind, placebo controlled trial. BMJ 2001;322(7278):73-75.

237. Coles R. Trial of an extract of *Ginkgo biloba* (EGB) for tinnitus and hearing loss. Clin Otolaryngol 1988;13(6):501-502.

238. Fucci JM. Effects of *Ginkgo biloba* extract on tinnitus: A double blind study. St Petersberg Assoc Res Otolaryngol 1992;57:336.

239. Enrique Gomez A. [Multicenter study with standardized extract of *Ginkgobiloba* EGB 761 in the treatment of memory alteration, vertigo and tinnitus]. Invest Med Internacional 1997;24(2):31-39.

240. Jastreboff PJ, Zhou S, Jastreboff MM, et al. Attenuation of salicylate-induced tinnitus by *Ginkgo biloba* extract in rats. Audiol Neurootol 1997; 2(4):197-212.

241. Olivier J, Plath P. Combined low power laser therapy and extracts of *Ginkgo biloba* in a blind trial of treatment for tinnitus. Laser Ther 1993; 5(3):137-139.

242. Partheniadis-Stumpf M, Maurer J, Mann W. [Soft laser therapy in combination with tebonin i.v. in tinnitus]. Laryngorhinootologie 1993; 72(1):28-31.

243. Plath P, Olivier J. Results of combined low-power laser therapy and extracts of *Ginkgo biloba* in cases of sensorineural hearing loss and tinnitus. Adv Otorhinolaryngol 1995;49:101-104.

244. von Wedel H, Calero L, Walger M, et al. Soft-laser/Ginkgo therapy in chronic tinnitus. A placebo-controlled study. Adv Otorhinolaryngol 1995; 49:105-108.

245. Roncin JP, Schwartz F, D'Arbigny P. EGb 761 in control of acute mountain sickness and vascular reactivity to cold exposure. Aviat Space Environ Med 1996;67(5):445-452.

246. Claussen CF. Etude randomisee, conduite en double insu, des effets de l'extrait de *Ginkgo biloba* et du placebo. La craniocorpographie montre une reduction statistiquement significative de la symptomatologie vertigineuse et ataxique. Arztl Praxis 1984;36:1.

247. Claussen CF, Kirtane MV. Randomized double-blind study of the effect of *Ginkgo biloba* extract on dizziness and unsteady gait in the elderly. *In* Claussen CF (ed): Dizziness, Ataxia and Tinnitus of Old Age: Disorders of Balance and Sensory Impairment in the Elderly. Berlin, Springer-Verlag, 1985, pp 103-115.

248. Claussen CF. [Diagnostic and practical value of craniocorpography in vertiginous syndromes]. Presse Med 1986;15(31):1565-1568.

249. Hamann KF. Physical treatment of vestibular vertigo in relation with *Ginkgo biloba* extract. Therapiewoche 1985;35(40):4586-4590.

250. Lacour M, Ez-Zaher L, Raymond J. Plasticity mechanisms in vestibular compensation in the cat are improved by an extract of *Ginkgo biloba* (EGb 761). Pharmacol Biochem Behav 1991;40(2):367-379.

251. Chung HS, Harris A, Kristinsson JK, et al. *Ginkgo biloba* extract increases ocular blood flow velocity. J Ocul Pharmacol Ther 1999;15(3):233-240.

252. Droy-Lefaix MT, Menerath JM, Szabo-Tosaki E, et al. Protective effect of EGb 761 on ischemia-reperfusion damage in the rat retina. Transplant Proc 1995;27(5):2861-2862.

253. Lebuisson DA, Leroy L, Rigal G. [Treatment of senile macular degeneration with *Ginkgo biloba* extract. A preliminary double-blind drug vs. placebo study]. Presse Med 1986;15(31):1556-1558.

254. Evans JR. *Ginkgo biloba* extract for age-related macular degeneration. Cochrane Database Syst Rev 2000;(2):CD001775. Review.

255. Merte HJ, Merkle W. Long-term treatment of circulatory disturbances of the retina and optic nerve with Rökan. Klin Monatsbl Augenheilkd 1980;177(5):577-583.

256. Blaeser-Kiel G. [Therapeutic trial with *Ginkgo biloba* in ocular hypertension]. Fortschr Med 1991;109(26):102.

257. Tamborini A, Taurelle R. [Value of standardized *Ginkgo biloba* extract (EGb 761) in the management of congestive symptoms of premenstrual syndrome]. Rev Fr Gynecol Obstet 1993;88(7-9):447-457.

258. Paick JS, Lee JH. An experimental study of the effect of *Ginkgo biloba* extract on the human and rabbit corpus cavernosum tissue. J Urol 1996; 156(5):1876-1880.

259. Sohn M, Sikora R. *Ginkgo biloba* extract in the therapy of erectile dysfunction. J Sex Ed Ther 1991;17(1):53-61.

260. Sikora R, Sohn MH, Engelke B, et al. Randomized placebo-controlled study on the effects of oral treatment with *Gingko biloba* extract in patients with erectile dysfunction. J Urology 1998;159(Suppl 5):240.

261. Balon R. *Gingko biloba* for antidepressant-induced sexual dysfunction? J Sex Marital Ther 1999;25(1):1-2.

262. Ashton AK, Ahrens K, Gupta S, et al. Antidepressant-induced sexual dysfunction and *Ginkgo biloba*. Am J Psychiatry 2000;157(5):836-837.

263. Ito TY, Trant AS, Polan ML. A double-blind placebo-controlled study of ArginMax, a nutritional supplement for enhancement of female sexual function. J Sex Marital Ther 2001;27(5):541-549.

264. Waynberg J, Brewer S. Effects of Herbal vX on libido and sexual activity in premenopausal and postmenopausal women. Adv Ther 2000;17(5): 255-262.

265. Lingaerde O, Foreland AR, Magnusson A. Can winter depression be prevented by *Ginkgo biloba* extract? A placebo- controlled trial. Acta Psychiatr Scand 1999;100(1):62-66.

266. Schubert H, Halama P. Depressive episode primarily unresponsive to therapy in elderly patients. Efficacy of *Ginkgo biloba* (Egb 761) in combination with antidepressants. Geriatre Forschung 1993;3(1):45-53.

267. Hemmeter U, Annen B, Bischof R, et al. Polysomnographic effects of adjuvant *Ginkgo biloba* therapy in patients with major depression medicated with trimipramine. Pharmacopsychiatry 2001;34(2):50-59.

268. Hauns B, Haring B, Kohler S, et al. Phase II study of combined 5-fluorouracil/*Ginkgo biloba* extract (GBE 761 ONC) therapy in 5-fluorouracil pretreated patients with advanced colorectal cancer. Phytother Res 2001;15(1):34-38.

269. Brochet B, Orgogozo JM, Guinot P, et al. [Pilot study of ginkgolide B, a PAF-acether specific inhibitor in the treatment of acute outbreaks of multiple sclerosis]. Rev Neurol (Paris) 1992;148(4):299-301.

270. Brochet B, Guinot P, Orgogozo JM, et al. Double blind placebo controlled multicentre study of ginkgolide B in treatment of acute exacerbations of multiple sclerosis. The Ginkgolide Study Group in multiple sclerosis. J Neurol Neurosurg Psychiatry 1995;58(3):360-362.

271. Kenney C, Norman M, Jacobson M, et al. A double-blind, placebo-controlled, modified crossover pilot study of the effects of *Ginkgo biloba* on cognitive and functional abilities in multiple sclerosis. Am Acad Neurology 54th Ann Meeting, April 13-20 2002; P06.081.

272. Raabe A, Raabe M, Ihm P. [Therapeutic follow-up using automatic perimetry in chronic cerebroretinal ischemia in elderly patients. Prospective double-blind study with graduated dose *Ginkgo biloba* treatment (EGb 761)]. Klin Monatsbl Augenheilkd 1991;199(6):432-438.

273. Clostre F. [Protective effects of a *Ginkgo biloba* extract (EGb 761) on ischemia- reperfusion injury]. Therapie 2001;56(5):595-600.

274. Garg RK, Nag D, Agrawal A. A double blind placebo controlled trial of *Ginkgo biloba* extract in acute cerebral ischaemia. J Assoc Physicians India 1995;43(11):760-763.

G

Ginseng

(*Panax species* including *Panax ginseng* (Asian ginseng), *Panax quinquefolius* (American ginseng); excluding *Eleutherococcus senticosus* (Siberian ginseng))

SYNONYMS/COMMON NAMES/RELATED SUBSTANCES

- **General:** Allheilkraut, Araliaceae (family), chikusetsu ginseng, chosen ninjin, dwarf ginseng, five-fingers, five-leaf ginseng, G115, ginseng radix, ginsengwurzel, ginsenosides (Rb1, Rb2, Rc, Rd, Re, Rf, and Rg1), hakusan, hakushan, higeninjin, hongshen, hua qi shen, hungseng, hungsheng, hunseng, insam, jenseng, jenshen, jinpi, kao-li-seng, Korean ginseng, kraftwurzel, man root, minjin, nhan sam, ninjin, ninzin, niuhan, Oriental ginseng, otane ninjin, panax de chine, panax ginseng, panax notoginseng, panax vietnamensis (Vietnamese ginseng), *Panax pseudoginseng*, *Panax pseudoginseng* Wall. var. *notoginseng*, *Panax pseudoginseng* var. *major*, *Panax trifolius* L., pannag, racine de ginseng, renshen, sanchi ginseng, sang, san-pi, schinsent, sei yang sam, seng, shanshen, shen-sai-seng, shenshaishanshen, shenghaishen, siyojin, t'ang-sne, tartar root, true ginseng, tyosenninzin, Western ginseng, Western sea ginseng, xi shen, xi yang shen, yakuyo ninjin, yakuyo ninzin, yang shen, yeh-shan-seng, yuanseng, yuansheng, zhuzishen.
- **Asian/panax ginseng (*Panax ginseng*) synonyms:** Asiatic ginseng, Chinese ginseng, ginseng asiatique, ginseng radix, ginseng root, Japanese ginseng, jintsam, Korean red, Korean red ginseng, ninjin, Oriental ginseng, *Panax schinseng*, red ginseng, ren shen, sang, shen.
- **American ginseng (*Panax quinquefolius*) synonyms:** Anchi ginseng, Canadian ginseng, North American ginseng, Ontario ginseng, red berry, ren shen, sang, tienchi ginseng, Wisconsin ginseng.
- **Siberian ginseng (*Eleutherococcus senticosus*) synonyms:** *Acanthopanax senticosus*, ci wu jia (ciwujia), devil's bush, devil's shrub, eleuthera, eleuthero, eleuthero ginseng, eleutherococ, eleutherococcus, eleutherococci radix, shigoka, touch-me-not, wild pepper, wu-jia, wu-jia-pi, ussuri, ussurian thorny pepperbrush.

CLINICAL BOTTOM LINE

Background

- The term *ginseng* refers to several species of the genus *Panax*. For more than 2000 years, the roots of this slow-growing plant have been valued in Chinese medicine. The two most commonly used species are Asian ginseng (*Panax ginseng* C.A. Meyer), which is mostly extinct in its natural range but is still cultivated, and American ginseng (*Panax quinquefolius* L.), which is both harvested from the wild and cultivated. *Panax ginseng* should not be confused with Siberian ginseng (*Eleutherococcus senticosus*). In Russia, Siberian ginseng was promoted as a cheaper alternative to ginseng and was believed to have identical benefits. However, Siberian ginseng does not contain the ginsenosides that are present in the *Panax* species, which are believed to be active ingredients and have been studied scientifically.

Uses Based on Scientific Evidence	Grade*
Mental performance Several studies report that ginseng can modestly improve thinking or learning at doses of 200 to 400 mg	B

of standardized extract G115, taken by mouth daily for up to 12 weeks. Mental performance has been assessed using standardized measurements of reaction time, concentration, learning, math, and logic. Benefits have been seen both in healthy young people and in older, ill patients. Effects also have been reported for the combined use of ginseng with *Ginkgo biloba*. Although this evidence is promising, most studies have been small and not well designed or reported. There is also a small amount of negative evidence, reporting that ginseng actually may not significantly affect thinking processes. It is not clear if people with certain conditions may benefit more than others. Therefore, although the available scientific evidence does suggest some effectiveness of short-term use of ginseng for enhancing thinking or learning, better research is necessary before a strong recommendation can be made.

Type 2 diabetes mellitus Several studies in humans report that ginseng may lower blood sugar levels in patients with type 2 diabetes mellitus (adult-onset diabetes), both in the fasting state and after eating. Long-term effects are not clear, and it is not known what doses are safe or effective. Preliminary research suggests that ginseng may not carry a significant risk of causing dangerously low blood sugar levels (hypoglycemia). Additional studies are needed that measure long-term effects of ginseng in patients with diabetes and that also examine interactions with standard prescription drugs for diabetes. People with diabetes should seek the care of a qualified healthcare practitioner and should not use ginseng instead of more proven therapies. Effects of ginseng in type 1 diabetes mellitus (insulin-dependent diabetes) are not well studied.	B
Cancer prevention A small number of studies report that ginseng taken by mouth may lower the risk for various cancers, especially if ginger powder or extract is used. However, most of these studies have been published by the same research group and have used a type of research design (the case-control study) that limits usefulness of results, and the findings can only be considered preliminary. Results may have been affected by other lifestyle choices in people who use ginseng, such as exercise and dietary habits. Additional trials are necessary before a clear conclusion can be reached.	C
Chronic obstructive pulmonary disease (COPD) Ginseng was reported to improve pulmonary function and exercise capacity in patients with COPD in one study. Further research is needed to confirm these results.	C

Continued

Uses Based on Scientific Evidence	Grade*
Congestive heart failure Evidence from a small amount of research is unclear regarding use of ginseng in patients with congestive heart failure	C
Coronary artery (heart) disease Several studies from China report that ginseng in combination with various other herbs may reduce symptoms of coronary artery disease such as anginal chest pain and may correct abnormalities seen on the electrocardiogram. Most studies have not been well described or reported. Without further evidence of the effects of ginseng specifically, a firm conclusion cannot be reached.	C
Erectile dysfunction Preliminary study reports that a cream containing ginseng may be helpful for men who have difficulty with erections or decreased libido. Additional research is necessary before a clear conclusion can be reached.	C
Exercise performance Ginseng is commonly used by athletes with the intention of improving stamina. However, it remains unclear if ginseng taken by mouth significantly affects exercise performance. Numerous studies of this use have been published, with mixed results. Most research has not been well designed or reported, and results cannot be considered reliable. Trials in the 1980s reported benefits, whereas more recent research found no effects. Better studies are necessary before a clear conclusion can be reached.	C
Fatigue Limited research using ginseng extract G115 (with or without multivitamins) reports improvement in patients with fatigue of various causes. However, these results are preliminary, and studies have not been of high quality. Additional research is necessary before a clear conclusion can be reached.	C
High blood pressure Preliminary research suggests that ginseng may lower blood pressure (systolic and diastolic). It is not clear what doses are safe or effective. Well-conducted studies are needed to confirm these early results.	C
Immune system enhancement A small number of studies report that ginseng may stimulate activity of immune cells in the body (T-lymphocytes and neutrophils), improve the effectiveness of antibiotics in people with acute bronchitis, and enhance the body's response to influenza vaccines. Most research in this area has been published by the same lead author. Additional studies that examine the effects of ginseng on specific types of infections are necessary before a clear conclusion can be reached.	C
Low white blood cell counts Poorly described preliminary research reports improved blood counts in patients with aplastic anemia using ginseng in combination with other herbs, and improved	C

white blood cell counts in patients with neutropenia using high doses of ginsenosides. Reliable studies are needed before a conclusion can be reached. Of note, decreased blood cell counts after ginseng use have been reported.

Menopausal symptoms Evidence from a small amount of research on use of ginseng for relief of menopausal symptoms is unclear. Some studies report less depression and improved sense of well-being, without changes in hormone levels.	C
Methicillin-resistant *Staphylococcus aureus* (MRSA) In patients taking the herbal preparation hochu-ekki-to, which contains ginseng and several other herbs, urinary MRSA decreased after a 10-week treatment period. Further study of ginseng alone is necessary before firm conclusions can be drawn.	C
Multi-infarct dementia A small study conducted in patients with multi-infarct dementia reports that a herbal combination known as Fuyuan mixture, which contains ginseng, may have therapeutic benefits. The effects of ginseng alone are not clear, and no firm conclusion can be drawn.	C
Sense of well-being Several studies have examined the effects of ginseng (with or without multivitamins) on overall sense of well-being in healthy and ill patients, when taken for up to 12 weeks. Most trials are not of high quality, and results are mixed. Preliminary research suggests that benefits may occur in people with the worst baseline quality of life. However, it remains unclear if ginseng is beneficial for this purpose in any patient group.	C

*Key to grades: *A:* Strong scientific evidence for this use; *B:* Good scientific evidence for this use; *C:* Unclear scientific evidence for this use; *D:* Fair scientific evidence against this use (it may not work); *F:* Strong scientific evidence against this use (it likely does not work). For a more detailed explanation of efficacy criteria, see "Natural Standard Evidence-Based Validated Grading Rationale" in the Introduction.

Historical or Theoretical Indications That Lack Sufficient Evidence

Adrenal tonic, aerobic fitness, aging, aggression, Alzheimer's disease, allergy, anemia, antidepressant, anti-inflammatory, antioxidant, antiplatelet, antitumor, anxiety, aphrodisiac, aplastic anemia, appetite stimulant, asthma, atherosclerosis, athletic stamina, attention-deficit hyperactivity disorder (ADHD), bleeding disorders, breast cancer, breast enlargement, breathing difficulty, bronchodilation, burns, cancer prevention, chemotherapy support, cold limbs, colitis, convulsions, dementia, diabetic nephropathy (kidney disease), digestive complaints, diuretic (water pill) effect, dizziness, dysentery, estrogen-like activity, fatigue, fever, gynecologic disorders, fibromyalgia, hangover relief, headaches, heart damage, hepatitis/hepatitis B infection, herpes, high blood pressure, HIV, inflammation, influenza, insomnia, kidney disease, learning enhancement, liver diseases, liver health, long-term debility, low sperm count, male infertility, malignant tumors, memory and thinking enhancement after menopause, menopausal

Continued

Uses Based on Tradition, Theory, or Limited Scientific Evidence (cont'd)

symptoms, migraine, morphine tolerance, neuralgia (pain due to nerve damage or inflammation), neurosis, organ prolapse, oxygen absorption, pain relief, palpitations, physical work capacity increase, premature ejaculation, prostate cancer, *Pseudomonas* infection in cystic fibrosis, psychoasthenia, prostate cancer, qi deficiency and blood stasis syndrome in heart disease (Eastern medicine), quality of life enhancement, recovery from irradiation, rehabilitation, sedative, senile dementia, sexual arousal, sexual symptoms, spontaneous sweating, stomach cancer, stomach upset, stress, strokes, surgical recovery, upper respiratory tract infection, vomiting.

DOSING/TOXICOLOGY

The following doses are based on scientific research, publications, traditional use, or expert opinion. Many herbs and supplements have not been thoroughly tested, and their safety and effectiveness may not be proven. Brands may be made differently, with variable ingredients even within the same brand. The doses shown may not apply to all products. It is important to always read product labels and discuss doses with a qualified healthcare provider before therapy is started.

Standardization

- Standardization involves measuring the amount of certain chemicals in products to try to make different preparations similar to each other. It is not always known if the chemicals being measured are the "active" ingredients.
- Ginseng extracts may be standardized to 4% ginsenosides content (for example, in G115) or 7% total ginsenosides content. Standardized products have been used in studies, although tests of commercially available ginseng products have found that many brands do not contain the claimed ingredients, and some include detectable pesticides.

Adults (18 Years and Older)

- **Tablets/Capsules:** 100 to 200 mg of a standardized ginseng extract (4% ginsenosides) taken by mouth once or twice daily has been used in studies for up to 12 weeks. Doses of 0.5 to 2 g of dry ginseng root, taken daily by mouth in divided doses, also have been used. Higher doses are sometimes given in studies or under the supervision of a qualified healthcare provider. Many different doses are used traditionally. Some practitioners recommend that after taking ginseng continuously for 2 to 3 weeks, the patient should stop use of this herb for 1 or 2 weeks, and that long-term dosing should not exceed 1 g of dry root daily.
- **Decoction/Fluid Extract/Tincture:** The following dosages have been used: decoction of 1 to 2 g added to 150 ml of water, taken by mouth daily; a 1:1 (grams per milliliter) fluid extract taken as 1 to 2 ml by mouth daily; 5 to 10 ml (approximately 1 to 2 teaspoons) of a 1:5 (grams per milliliter) tincture taken by mouth daily. Some practitioners recommend that after taking ginseng continuously for 2 to 3 weeks, the patient should stop use of this herb for 1 or 2 weeks.

Children (Younger Than 18 Years)

- There is not enough scientific information available to recommend the safe use of ginseng in children.

SAFETY

The U.S. Food and Drug Administration does not strictly regulate herbs and supplements. There is no guarantee of strength, purity, or safety of products, and effects may vary. It is important to always read product labels. People who have a medical condition, or are taking other drugs, herbs, or supplements, should consult a qualified healthcare provider before starting a new therapy. A healthcare provider should be consulted immediately about any side effects.

Allergies

- People with known allergy to plants in the Araliaceae family should avoid ginseng.

Side Effects and Warnings

- Ginseng has been well tolerated by most people in scientific studies when used at recommended doses, and serious side effects appear to be rare.
- Based on limited evidence, long-term use may be associated with skin rash or spots, itching, diarrhea, sore throat, loss of appetite, excitability, anxiety, depression, or insomnia. Less common reported side effects include headache, fever, dizziness/vertigo, blood pressure abnormalities (increases or decreases), chest pain, heart palpitations, rapid heart rate, leg swelling, nausea/vomiting, and manic episodes in people with bipolar disorder.
- Research in humans indicates that ginseng may lower blood sugar levels. This effect may be greater in patients with diabetes than in nondiabetic persons. Caution is advised in patients with diabetes or hypoglycemia and in those taking drugs, herbs, or supplements that affect blood sugar. Serum glucose levels may need to be monitored by a healthcare provider, and medication adjustments may be necessary.
- There are anecdotal reports of nosebleeds and vaginal bleeding with ginseng use, although scientific study of this potential risk is limited. In one report, ginseng reduced the effectiveness of the blood-thinning medication warfarin (Coumadin). Caution is advised regarding use of ginseng in patients with bleeding disorders or taking drugs that may affect the risk of bleeding or blood clotting. Dosing adjustments may be necessary. Severe drops in white blood cell counts were reported in several people using a combination product containing ginseng in the 1970s; this effect may have been due to contamination.
- Ginseng may have estrogen-like effects. Use of ginseng has been associated with reports of breast tenderness, loss of menstrual periods, vaginal bleeding after menopause, breast enlargement (reported in men), difficulty developing or maintaining an erection, and increased sexual responsiveness. Ginseng should be avoided by patients with hormone-sensitive conditions such as breast cancer, uterine cancer, and endometriosis.
- Ginseng may produce manic symptoms: In a single case report involving a 56-year-old woman with a previously diagnosed affective disorder, a manic episode occurred during ginseng intake. Symptoms disappeared rapidly with low doses of neuroleptics and benzodiazepines.
- A severe life-threatening rash known as Stevens-Johnson syndrome occurred in one patient and may have been due to contaminants in a ginseng product. A case report describes liver damage (cholestatic hepatitis) in a patient who took a combination product containing ginseng. High doses of ginseng have been associated with rare cases of temporary inflammation of blood vessels in the brain (cerebral arteritis),

abnormal dilation of the pupils of the eye, confusion, or depression.

- There is preliminary evidence that ginseng, at doses of 200 mg of extract daily, may increase the QTc interval as seen on the electrocardiogram (thus increasing the risk of abnormal heart rhythms) and decrease diastolic blood pressure 2 hours after ingestion in healthy adults.

Pregnancy and Breastfeeding

- Ginseng traditionally has been used in pregnant and breast-feeding women. Studies in animals and preliminary research in humans suggest possible safety, although safety has not been clearly established in humans. Therefore, ginseng use cannot be recommended during pregnancy or the period of breastfeeding. There is a report of neonatal death and the development of male sex characteristics in a baby girl whose mother had taken ginseng during pregnancy.
- Many tinctures contain high levels of alcohol and should be avoided during pregnancy.

INTERACTIONS

Most herbs and supplements have not been thoroughly tested for interactions with other herbs, supplements, drugs, or foods. The interactions listed here are based on reports in scientific publications, laboratory experiments, or traditional use. It is important to always read product labels. People who have a medical condition, or are taking other drugs, herbs, or supplements, should consult a qualified healthcare provider before starting a new therapy.

Interactions with Drugs

- As suggested by research in humans, ginseng may lower blood sugar levels. This effect may be greater in patients with diabetes than in nondiabetic persons. Caution is advised with use of medications that also may lower blood sugar. Patients taking drugs for diabetes by mouth or insulin should be monitored closely by a qualified healthcare provider. Medication adjustments may be necessary.
- Headache, tremors, mania, or insomnia may occur if ginseng is combined with prescription antidepressant drugs called monoamine oxidase inhibitors (MAOIs), such as isocarboxazid (Marplan), phenelzine (Nardil), and tranylcypromine (Parnate).
- As described in case reports, ginseng may alter the effects of blood pressure or heart medications, including calcium channel blockers such as nifedipine (Procardia). There is preliminary evidence that ginseng, at doses of 200 mg of extract daily, may increase the QTc interval as seen on the electrocardiogram (thus increasing the risk of abnormal heart rhythms) and decrease diastolic blood pressure 2 hours after ingestion in healthy adults. Therefore, caution is advised with use of other medications that may alter the QTc interval. In one case report, effects of the diuretic drug furosemide (Lasix) were decreased when the drug was used with ginseng. A Chinese study reports that the effects of the cardiac glycoside drug digoxin (Lanoxin) may be increased when it is used with ginseng in patients with heart failure. Ginseng must not be combined with heart or blood pressure medications without the advice of a qualified healthcare provider.
- As suggested by limited animal research and anecdotal reports of nosebleeds and vaginal bleeding in humans, ginseng may increase the risk of bleeding when taken with drugs that also increase the risk of bleeding. Some examples are aspirin, anticoagulants (blood thinners) such as warfarin (Coumadin) and heparin, antiplatelet drugs such as clopidogrel (Plavix),

and nonsteroidal anti-inflammatory drugs such as ibuprofen (Motrin, Advil) and naproxen (Naprosyn, Aleve). By contrast, in one reported case, the effectiveness of the blood thinner warfarin (Coumadin) was reduced when ginseng was taken at the same time, with a decrease in the international normalized ratio (INR), a blood test used to measure warfarin effects.

- Limited laboratory evidence indicates that ginseng may contain estrogen-like chemicals and may affect medications with estrogen-like or estrogen-blocking properties. This effect has not been demonstrated in humans.
- In theory, ginseng may interfere with how the body uses the liver's cytochrome P450 enzyme system to process components of some drugs. As a result, blood levels of these components may be elevated, causing increased effects or potentially serious adverse reactions. People who are taking any medications should always read the package insert and consult with their healthcare provider and pharmacist about possible interactions.
- The analgesic effect of opioids may be inhibited by ginseng.
- Many tinctures contain high levels of alcohol and may cause nausea or vomiting when taken with metronidazole (Flagyl) or disulfiram (Antabuse). In a preliminary study, ginseng was reported to increase the removal of alcohol from the blood, although this effect has not been substantiated.

Interactions with Herbs and Dietary Supplements

- According to research in humans, ginseng may lower blood sugar levels. This effect may be greater in patients with diabetes than in nondiabetic persons. Caution is advised with use of herbs or supplements that also may lower blood sugar. Blood glucose levels may require monitoring, and doses may need adjustment. Possible examples include *Aloe vera*, bilberry, bitter melon, burdock, fenugreek, fish oil, gymnema, horse chestnut seed extract (HCSE), marshmallow, maitake mushroom, milk thistle, rosemary, stinging nettle, and white horehound.
- Headache, tremors, mania, and insomnia may occur if ginseng is combined with supplements that have MAOI activity or that interact with MAOI drugs. Some examples are 5-hydroxytryptophan (5-HTP), California poppy, chromium, dehydroepiandrosterone (DHEA), DL-phenylalanine (DLPA), ephedra, evening primrose oil, fenugreek, *Ginkgo biloba*, hops, mace, St. John's wort, S-adenosylmethionine (SAMe), sepia, tyrosine, valerian, vitamin B_6, and yohimbe bark extract. In theory, ginseng can increase the stimulatory effects of caffeine, coffee, tea, cocoa, chocolate, guarana, cola nut, and yerba mate.
- As described in case reports, ginseng may raise or lower blood pressure. Caution is advised with use of ginseng in combination with other products that can affect blood pressure. Some herbs that may lower blood pressure are aconite/monkshood, arnica, baneberry, betel nut, bilberry, black cohosh, bryony, calendula, California poppy, coleus, curcumin, eucalyptol, eucalyptus oil, evening primrose oil, flaxseed, garlic, ginger, ginkgo, goldenseal, green hellebore, hawthorn, Indian tobacco, jaborandi, mistletoe, night-blooming cereus, oleander, pasque flower, periwinkle, pleurisy root, shepherd's purse, Texas milkweed, turmeric, and wild cherry. Herbs that may increase blood pressure include arnica, bayberry, betel nut, blue cohosh, broom, cayenne, cola, coltsfoot, ephedra/ma huang, ginger, licorice, *Polypodium vulgare*, and yerba mate.

- Preliminary evidence indicates that ginseng, at doses of 200 mg of extract daily, may increase the QTc interval as seen on the electrocardiogram (thus increasing the risk of abnormal heart rhythms) and decrease diastolic blood pressure 2 hours after ingestion in healthy adults. Therefore, caution is advised with use of other agents that may cause abnormal heart rhythms.
- As suggested by limited animal research and anecdotal reports of nosebleeds and vaginal bleeding in humans, ginseng may increase the risk of bleeding when taken with herbs and supplements that are believed to increase the risk of bleeding. Multiple cases of bleeding have been reported with the use of *Ginkgo biloba*, some cases with garlic, and fewer cases with saw palmetto. Numerous other agents may theoretically increase the risk of bleeding, although this effect has not been proven in most cases. Some examples are alfalfa, angelica, anise, *Arnica montana*, asafetida, aspen bark, bilberry, birch, black cohosh, bladderwrack, bogbean, boldo, borage seed oil, bromelain, capsicum, cat's claw, celery, chamomile, chaparral, clove, coleus, cordyceps, danshen, devil's claw, dong quai, eicosapentaenoic acid (EPA), evening primrose oil, fenugreek, feverfew, fish oil, flaxseed/flaxseed powder (not a concern with flaxseed oil), ginger, grapefruit juice, grapeseed, green tea, guggul, gymnestra, horse chestnut, horseradish, licorice root, lovage root, male fern, meadowsweet, nordihydroguaiaretic acid (NDGA), onion, papain, parsley, passion flower, poplar, prickly ash, propolis, quassia, red clover, reishi, rue, sweet birch, sweet clover, turmeric, vitamin E, white willow, wild carrot, wild lettuce, willow, wintergreen, and yucca.
- In theory, ginseng may decrease the effects of diuretic herbs such as horsetail and licorice.
- In theory, ginseng may interfere with how the body uses the liver's cytochrome P450 enzyme system to process certain components of other herbs or supplements. As a result, blood levels of these components may be elevated. It also may alter the effects of other herbs or supplements on the cytochrome P450 system. Examples of such herbs are bloodroot, cat's claw, chamomile, chaparral, chasteberry, damiana, *Echinacea angustifolia*, goldenseal, grapefruit juice, licorice, oregano, red clover, St. John's wort, wild cherry, and yucca. People who are taking any herbal medications or dietary supplements should check the package insert and consult their healthcare provider or pharmacist about possible interactions.
- Limited laboratory evidence suggests that ginseng may contain estrogen-like chemicals and may affect agents with estrogen-like or estrogen-blocking properties. This effect has not been demonstrated in humans. Examples of herbs with possible estrogen-like effects are alfalfa, black cohosh, bloodroot, burdock, hops, kudzu, licorice, pomegranate, red clover, soy, thyme, white horehound, and yucca.

Selected References

Natural Standard developed the preceding evidence-based information based on a systematic review of more than 600 scientific articles. For comprehensive information about alternative and complementary therapies on the professional level, go to www.naturalstandard.com. Selected references are listed here.

Abebe W. Herbal medication: potential for adverse interactions with analgesic drugs. J Clin Pharm Ther 2002;27(6):391-401.

Allen JD, McLung J, Nelson AG, et al. Ginseng supplementation does not enhance healthy young adults' peak aerobic exercise performance. J Am Coll Nutr 1998;17(5):462-466.

Anderson GD, Rosito G, Mohustsy MA, et al. Drug interaction potential of soy extract and *Panax ginseng*. J Clin Pharmacol 2003;43(6):643-648.

Attele AS, Wu JA, Yuan CS. Ginseng pharmacology: multiple constituents and multiple actions. Biochem Pharmacol 1999;58(11):1685-1693.

Awang DV. Maternal use of ginseng and neonatal androgenization. JAMA 1991;266(3):363.

Bahrke MS, Morgan WR. Evaluation of the ergogenic properties of ginseng: an update. Sports Med 2000;29(2):113-133.

Banskota AH, Tezuka Y, Le Tran Q, et al. Chemical constituents and biological activities of Vietnamese medicinal plants. Curr Top Med Chem 2003;3(2): 227-248.

Belogortseva NI, Yoon JY, Kim KH. Inhibition of *Helicobacter pylori* hemagglutination by polysaccharide fractions from roots of *Panax ginseng*. Planta Med 2000;66(3):217-220.

Cardinal BJ, Engels HJ. Ginseng does not enhance psychological well-being in healthy, young adults: results of a double-blind, placebo-controlled, randomized clinical trial. J Am Diet Assoc 2001;101(6):655-660.

Caron MF, Hotsko AL, Robertson S, et al. Electrocardiographic and hemodynamic effects of *Panax ginseng*. Ann Pharmacother 2002;36(5): 758-763.

Chang TK, Chen J, Benetton SA. *In vitro* effect of standardized ginseng extracts and individual ginsenosides on the catalytic activity of human CYP1A1, CYP1A2, and CYP1B1. Drug Metab Dipos 2002;30(4):378-384.

Chan RY, Chen WF, Dong A, et al. Estrogen-like activity of ginsenoside Rg1 derived from *Panax notoginseng*. J Clin Endocrinol Metab 2002;87(8): 3691-3695.

Chavez M. Treatment of diabetes mellitus with ginseng. J Herb Pharm 2001;1(2):99-113.

Cherdrungsi P, Rungroeng K. Effects of standardized ginseng extract and exercise training on aerobic and anaerobic exercise capacities in humans. Korean J Ginseng Sci 1995;19(2):93-100.

Choi CH, Kang G, Min YD. Reversal of P-glycoprotein–mediated multidrug resistance by protopanaxatriol ginsenosides from Korean red ginseng. Planta Med 2003;69(3):235-240.

Choi HK, Seong DH, Rha KH. Clinical efficacy of Korean red ginseng for erectile dysfunction. Int J Impot Res 1995;7(3):181-186.

Choi HK, Jung GW, Moon KH, et al. Clinical study of SS-cream in patients with lifelong premature ejaculation. Urology 2000;55(2):257-261.

Choi SE, Choi S, Lee JH, et al. Effects of ginsenosides on GABA(A) receptor channels expressed in *Xenopus* oocytes. Arch Pharm Res 2003;26(1):28-33.

Choi S, Lee JH, Oh S, et al. Effects of ginsenoside Rg2 on the 5-HT3a receptor–mediated ion current in *Xenopus* oocytes. Mol Cells 2003;15(1):108-113.

Choo MK, Park EK, Han MJ, et al. Antiallergic activity of ginseng and its ginsenosides. Planta Med 2003;69(6):518-522.

Chow L, Johnson M, Wells A, et al. Effect of the traditional Chinese medicines chan su, lu-shen-wan, dan shen, and Asian ginseng on serum digoxin measurement by Tina-quant (Roche) and Synchron LX system (Beckman) digoxin immunoassays. J Clin Lab Anal 2003;17(1):22-27.

Chung WY, Yow CM, Benzie IF. Assessment of membrane protection by traditional Chinese medicines using a flow cytometric technique: preliminary findings. Redox Rep 2003;8(1):31-33.

Cicero AF, Vitale G, Savino G, et al. *Panax notoginseng* (Burk.) effects on fibrinogen and lipid plasma level in rats fed on a high-fat diet. Phytother Res 2003;17(2):174-178.

Coleman CI, Hebert JH, Reddy P. The effects of *Panax ginseng* on quality of life. J Clin Pharm Ther 2003;28(1):5-15.

Cui XM, Lo CK, Yip KL, et al. Authentication of *Panax notoginseng* by 5S-rRNA spacer domain and random amplified polymorphic DNA (RAPD) analysis. Planta Med 2003;69(6):584-586.

Dasgupta A, Wu S, Actor J, et al. Effect of Asian and Siberian ginseng on serum digoxin measurement by five digoxin immunoassays. Significant variation in digoxin-like immunoreactivity among commercial ginsengs. Am J Clin Pathol 2003;119(2):298-303.

Donovan JL, DeVane CL, Chavin KD, et al. Siberian ginseng (*Eleutheroccus senticosus*) effects on CYP2D6 and CYP3A4 activity in normal volunteers. Drug Metab Dispos 2003;31(5):519-522.

Dragun Z, Puntaric D, Prpic-Majic D, et al. Toxic metals and metalloids in dietetic products. Croat Med J 2003;44(2):214-218.

Ellis JM, Reddy P. Effects of *Panax ginseng* on quality of life. Ann Pharmacother 2002;36:375-379.

Engels HJ, Wirth JC. No ergogenic effects of ginseng (*Panax ginseng* C.A. Meyer) during graded maximal aerobic exercise. J Am Diet Assoc 1997; 97(10):1110-1115.

Engels HJ, Kolokouri I, Cieslak TJ, et al. Effects of ginseng supplementation on supramaximal exercise performance and short-term recovery. J Strength Cond Res 2001;15(3):290-295.

Faleni R, Soldati F. Ginseng as cause of Stevens-Johnson syndrome? Lancet 1996;348(9022):267.

Gingrich PM, Fogel CI. Herbal therapy use by perimenopausal women. J Obstet Gynecol Neonatal Nurs 2003;32(2):181-189.

Glenn MB, Lexell J. Ginseng. J Head Trauma Rehabil 2003;18(2):196-200.

Gonzalez-Seijo JC, Ramos YM, Lastra I. Manic episode and ginseng: report of a possible case. J Clin Psychopharmacol 1995;15(6):447-448.

Gross D, Shenkman Z, Bleiberg B, et al. Ginseng improves pulmonary functions and exercise capacity in patients with COPD. Monaldi Arch Chest Dis 2002; 57(5-6):242-246. Comment in: Monaldi Arch Chest Dis 2002;57(5-6): 225-226.

Han KH, Choe SC, Kim HS, et al. Effect of red ginseng on blood pressure in patients with essential hypertension and white coat hypertension. Am J Chin Med 1998;26(2):199-209.

Hong B, Ji YH, Hong JH, et al. A double-blind crossover study evaluating the efficacy of Korean red ginseng in patients with erectile dysfunction: a preliminary report. J Urol 2002;168(5):2070-2073.

Hopkins MP, Androff L, Benninghoff AS. Ginseng face cream and unexplained vaginal bleeding. Am J Obstet Gynecol 1988;159(5):1121-1122.

Janetzky K, Morreale AP. Probable interaction between warfarin and ginseng. Am J Health Syst Pharm 1997;54(6):692-693.

Jin YH, Yim H, Park JH, et al. Cdk2 activity is associated with depolarization of mitochondrial membrane potential during apoptosis. Biochem Biophys Res Commun 2003;305(4)974-980.

Kennedy D, Scholey AB, Wesnes K. A direct cognitive comparison of the acute effects of ginseng, ginkgo and their combination in healthy volunteers. J Psychopharm 2001;15(Suppl):A56.

Kennedy D, Scholey A. A direct cognitive comparison of the acute effects of ginseng, ginkgo and their combination in healthy volunteers. Presented at Scientific Conference on Complementary, Alternative & Integrative Medicine Research, Boston, 2002.

Keum YS, Han SS, Chun KS, et al. Inhibitory effects of the ginsenoside Rg3 on phorbol ester–induced cyclooxygenase-2 expression, NF-kappaB activation and tumor promotion. Mutat Res 2003;523-524:75-85.

Kim SW, Kwon HY, Chi DW, et al. Reversal of P-glycoprotein–mediated multidrug resistance by ginsenoside Rg(3). Biochem Pharmacol 2003;65(1):75-82.

Kolokouri I, Engels H, Cieslak T, et al. Effect of chronic ginseng supplementation on short duration, supramaximal exercise test performance [abstract]. Med Sci Sports Exerc 1999;31(5 Suppl):S117.

Ko SR, Choi KJ, Uchida K, et al. Enzymatic preparation of ginsenosides Rg2, Rh1, and F1 from protopanaxatriol-type ginseng saponin mixture. Planta Med 2003;69(3):285-286.

Kuo SC, Teng CM, Lee JC, et al. Antiplatelet components in Panax ginseng. Planta Med 1990;56(2):164-167.

Kwan CY. Vascular effects of selected antihypertensive drugs derived from traditional medicinal herbs. Clin Exp Pharmacol Physiol 1995;22(Suppl 1): S297-S299.

Lee EH, Cho SY, Kim SJ, et al. Ginsenoside F1 protects human HaCaT keratinocytes from ultraviolet-B–induced apoptosis by maintaining constant levels of Bcl-2. J Invest Dermatol 2003;121(3):607-613.

Lee Y, Jin Y, Lim W, et al. A ginsenoside-Rh1, a component of ginseng saponin, activates estrogen receptor in human breast carcinoma MCF-7 cells. J Steroid Biochem Mol Biol 2003;84(4):463-468.

Lee YJ, Jin YR, Lim WC, et al. Ginsenoside-Rb1 acts as a weak phytoestrogen in MCF-7 human breast cancer cells. Arch Pharm Res 2003;26(1):58-63.

Lifton B, Otto RM, Wygand J. The effect of ginseng on acute maximal aerobic exercise. Med Sci Sports Exerc 1997;29(Suppl 5):249.

Lun X, Rong L, Yang WH. Observation on efficacy of CT positioning scalp circum-needling combined with Chinese herbal medicine in treating poly-infarctional vascular dementia. Zhongguo Zhong Xi Yi Jei He Za Zhi 2003; 23(6):423-425.

Mahady GB, Parrot J, Lee C, et al. Botanical dietary supplement use in peri- and postmenopausal women. Menopause 2003;10(1):65-72.

Morris CA, Avorn J. Internet marketing of herbal products. JAMA 2003; 290(11):1505-1509.

Nishida S. Effect of hochu-ekki-to on asymptomatic MRSA bacteriuria. J Infect Chemother 2003;9(1):58-61.

Noh JH, Choi S, Lee JH, et al. Effects of ginsenosides on glycine receptor alpha1 channels expressed in Xenopus oocytes. Mol Cells 2003;15(1):34-39.

Palazon J, Mallol A, Eibl R, et al. Growth and ginsenoside production in hairy root cultures of Panax ginseng: a novel bioreactor. Planta Med 2003;69(4): 344-349.

Pharand C, Ackman ML, Jackevicius CA, et al. Use of OTC and herbal products in patients with cardiovascular disease. Ann Pharmacother 2003;37(6):899-904.

Rosado MF. Thrombosis of a prosthetic aortic valve disclosing a hazardous interaction between warfarin and a commercial ginseng product. Cardiology 2003;99(2):111.

Rowland DL, Tai W. A review of plant-derived and herbal approaches to the treatment of sexual dysfunctions. J Sex Marital Ther 2003;29(3):185-205.

Ryu SJ, Chien YY. Ginseng-associated cerebral arteritis. Neurology 1995;45(4): 829-830.

Scaglione F, Weiser K, Alessandria M. Effects of the standardised ginseng extract G115(R) in patients with chronic bronchitis: a nonblinded, randomised, comparative pilot study. Clin Drug Invest 2001;21(1):41-45.

Scholey AB, Kennedy DO. Acute, dose-dependent cognitive effects of Ginkgo biloba, Panax ginseng and their combination in healthy young volunteers: differential interactions with cognitive demand. Hum Psychopharmacol 2002;17(1):35-44.

Sievenpiper JL, Arnason JT, Leiter LA, et al. Variable effects of American ginseng: a batch of American ginseng (Panax quinquefolius L.) with a depressed ginsenoside profile does not affect postprandial glycemia. Eur J Clin Nutr 2003;57(2):243-248.

Sievenpiper JL, Stavro MP, Leiter LA, et al. Variable effects of ginseng: American ginseng (Panax quinquefolius L.) with a low ginsenoside content does not affect postprandial glycemia in normal subjects. Diabetes 2001;50:A425.

Sorensen H, Sonne J. A double-masked study of the effects of ginseng on cognitive function. Curr Ther Res 1996;57(12):959-968.

Sotaniemi EA, Haapakoski E, Rautio A. Ginseng therapy in non–insulin-dependent diabetic patients. Diabetes Care 1995;18(10):1373-1375.

Sundgot-Brogen J, Berglund B, Torstveit MK. Nutritional supplements in Norwegian elite athletes—impact of international rank and advisors. Scand J Med Sci Sports 2003;13(2):138-144.

Taik-koo Y, Soo-Yong C. Preventive effect of ginseng intake against various human cancers: a case-control study on 1987 pairs. Cancer Epidemiol Biomarkers Prev 1995;4:401-408.

Tesch BJ. Herbs commonly used by women: an evidence-based review. Am J Obstet Gynecol 2003;188(5 Suppl):S44-S55.

Thommessen B, Laake K. No identifiable effect of ginseng (Gericomplex) as an adjuvant in the treatment of geriatric patients. Aging (Milano) 1996;8(6): 417-420.

Thompson Coon J, Ernst E. Panax ginseng: a systematic review of adverse effects and drug interactions. Presented at the 8th Annual Symposium on Complementary Health Care, Exeter, England, December 6-8, 2001.

Vazquez I, Aguera-Ortiz LF. Herbal products and serious side effects: a case of ginseng-induced manic episode. Acta Psychiatr Scand 2002;105(1): 76-77;discussion 77-78.

Vogler BK, Pittler MH, Ernst E. The efficacy of ginseng. A systematic review of randomised clinical trials. Eur J Clin Pharmacol 1999;55(8):567-575.

Vuksan V, Xu Z, Jenkins AL, et al. American ginseng (Panax quinquefolius L.) improves long term glycemic control in type 2 diabetes. Diabetes 2000; 49:A95.

Vuksan V, Stavro MP, Sievenpiper JL, et al. Similar postprandial glycemic reductions with escalation of dose and administration time of American ginseng in type 2 diabetes. Diabetes Care 2000;23(9):1221-1226.

Vuksan V, Sievenpiper JL, Koo VY, et al. American ginseng (Panax quinquefolius L.) reduces postprandial glycemia in nondiabetic subjects and subjects with type 2 diabetes mellitus. Arch Intern Med 2000;160(7):1009-1013.

Vuksan V, Sievenpiper JL, Wong J, et al. American ginseng (Panax quinquefolius L.) attenuates postprandial glycemia in a time-dependent but not dose-dependent manner in healthy individuals. Am J Clin Nutr 2001;73(4): 753-758.

Wiklund IK, Mattsson LA, Lindgren R, et al. Effects of a standardized ginseng extract on quality of life and physiological parameters in symptomatic postmenopausal women: a double-blind, placebo-controlled trial. Swedish Alternative Medicine Group. Int J Clin Pharmacol Res 1999;19(3):89-99.

Wong HC. Probable false authentication of herbal plants: ginseng. Arch Intern Med 1999;159(10):1142-1143.

Yeh GY, Eisenberg DM, Kaptchuk TJ, et al. Systematic review of herbs and dietary supplements for glycemic control in diabetes. Diabetes Care 2003; 26(4):1277-1294.

Youl Kang H, Hwan Kim S, Jun Lee W, Byrne HK. Effects of ginseng ingestion on growth hormone, testosterone, cortisol, and insulin-like growth factor 1 responses to acute resistance exercise. J Strength Cond Res 2002;16(2): 179-183.

Yun TK. Experimental and epidemiological evidence of the cancer-preventive effects of Panax ginseng C.A. Meyer. Nutr Rev 1996;54(11 Pt 2):S71-S81.

Yun TK. Experimental and epidemiological evidence on non-organ specific cancer preventative effect of Korean ginseng and identification of active compounds. Mutat Res 2003;523-524:63-74.

Zeilmann CA, Dole EJ, Skipper BJ, et al. Use of herbal medicine by elderly Hispanic and non-Hispanic white patients. Pharmacotherapy 2003;23(4): 526-532.

Zhu M, Chan KW, Ng LS, et al. Possible influences of ginseng on the pharmaco-kinetics and pharmacodynamics of warfarin in rats. J Pharm Pharmacol 1999;51(2):175-180.

Ziemba AW, Chmura J, Kaciuba-Uscilko H, et al. Ginseng treatment improves psychomotor performance at rest and during graded exercise in young athletes. Int J Sport Nutr 1999;9(4):371-377.

Glucosamine
(*N*-acetyl D-glucosamine)

SYNONYMS/COMMON NAMES/RELATED SUBSTANCES

- 2-acetamido-2-deoxyglucose, acetylglucosamine, Arth-X Plus, chitosamine, D-glucosamine, enhanced glucosamine sulfate, Flexi-Factors, glucosamine chlorohydrate, Glucosamine Complex, glucosamine hydrochloride, glucosamine hydroiodide, Glucosamine Mega, glucosamine *N*-acetyl, glucosamine sulfate, glucosamine sulphate, Joint Factors, *N*-acetyl D-glucosamine (NAG, N-A-G), Nutri-Joint, Poly-NAG, Ultra Maximum Strength Glucosamine Sulfate.

CLINICAL BOTTOM LINE

Background

- Glucosamine is an amino-monosaccharide that is naturally produced in humans. It is one of the principal substrates used in the biosynthesis of macromolecules that comprise articular cartilage, such as glycosaminoglycans, proteoglycans, and hyaluronic acid.
- Available evidence from randomized, controlled trials supports the use of glucosamine (sulfate) in the treatment of osteoarthritis, particularly of the knee. It is believed that sulfate moiety provides clinical benefit in the synovial fluid by strengthening cartilage and aiding glycosaminoglycan synthesis. If this hypothesis is confirmed, it would mean that only the glucosamine sulfate form is effective and nonsulfated glucosamine forms are not effective.[1]
- Glucosamine is commonly taken in combination with chondroitin, a glycosaminoglycan derived from articular cartilage. Use of complementary therapies, including glucosamine, is frequently observed in patients with osteoarthritis[2] and may allow for reduced doses of nonsteroidal anti-inflammatory agents.[3]
- Hypotheses of beneficial effects of glucosamine or chemically related compounds on wound healing,[4,5] psoriasis,[6] inflammatory bowel disease,[5,7,8] and migraine prophylaxis[9] have been proposed, but little rigorous research has been done in these areas.
- Numerous studies demonstrate that glucosamine is well tolerated for up to 3 years, although it should be avoided by patients with shellfish allergy. Initial concerns about effects on insulin levels or glycemic control have been tempered by more recent human evidence suggesting no significant effects, although this remains an area of controversy.

Scientific Evidence for Common/Studied Uses	Grade*
Knee osteoarthritis (mild to moderate)	A
Osteoarthritis (general)	B
Chronic venous insufficiency	C
Diabetes	C
Inflammatory bowel disease (Crohn's disease, ulcerative colitis)	C
Rheumatoid arthritis	C
Temporomandibular joint (TMJ) disorders	C

*Key to grades: *A:* Strong scientific evidence for this use; *B:* Good scientific evidence for this use; *C:* Unclear scientific evidence for this use; *D:* Fair scientific evidence against this use (it may not work); *F:* Strong scientific evidence against this use (it likely does not work). For a more detailed explanation of efficacy criteria, see "Natural Standard Evidence-Based Validated Grading Rationale" in the Introduction.

Historical or Theoretical Uses That Lack Sufficient Evidence

- AIDS, athletic injuries, back pain, bleeding esophageal varices (injection),[10] cancer, congestive heart failure, depression, immunosuppression,[11] inflammatory bowel disease, fibromyalgia, joint pain, kidney stones, knee pain, migraine headache, migraine prophylaxis, osteoporosis, pain, psoriasis, skin rejuvenation, spondylosis deformans, hypopigmenting agent, ulcerative colitis, wound healing.

Expert Opinion and Historic/Folkloric Precedent

- Glucosamine has been used extensively for the treatment of osteoarthritis for more than a decade in Europe.
- In response to the growing popularity of glucosamine in the United States, the National Institutes of Health (NIH) has sponsored a large Phase III clinical trial to rigorously test the efficacy of glucosamine (alone and in combination with chondroitin) in treating symptoms of osteoarthritis. The NIH, in collaboration with the National Center for Complementary and Alternative Medicine (NCCAM) and the National Institute of Arthritis and Musculoskeletal and Skin Diseases (NIAMSD), awarded the University of Utah School of Medicine a 4-year research contract to coordinate a nine-center study of the effectiveness of glucosamine (and chondroitin) in over 1000 patients with osteoarthritis of the knee. Subjects will be randomized to receive either glucosamine, chondroitin, glucosamine and chondroitin together, celecoxib, or placebo for 16 weeks. The primary outcome measure will be pain improvement.

Safety Summary

- **Likely safe:** When used orally in studied doses of standardized products (500 mg taken three times daily or 1500 mg once daily) for short durations by otherwise healthy adults. When given as intra-articular injections of glucosamine sulfate at recommended doses for up to 6 weeks (not available in the United States).[12]
- **Possibly safe:** When used orally at recommended doses for up to 3 years[13,14] or when used short-term intramuscularly[15] or intravenously.[16] A physician has reported using doses of up to 3 g daily and higher in patients with osteoarthritis.[17] Despite initial concerns about use in diabetic patients, based largely on *in vitro* and rat studies noting insulin resistance and possible glycemic effects[18-24] and on preliminary human

work,[25] more recent human research reports no significant effects (including on hemoglobin A1c levels in patients with type 2 diabetes after 90 days of therapy).[26,27]

- **Possibly unsafe:** Due to lack of sufficient data, may be unsafe when used in patients during pregnancy and lactation. Glucosamine is not recommended for children under the age of 2 years. Patients with shellfish allergies should avoid glucosamine; poor processing during the manufacturing process can lead to traces of intact proteins that can contribute to allergic reactions. The injectable forms of glucosamine are not available in the United States.

DOSING/TOXICOLOGY
General

- Recommended doses are based on those most commonly used in available trials, or on historical practice. However, with natural products, the optimal doses needed to balance efficacy and safety often are not clear.
- Glucosamine is not considered a drug in the United States and is therefore not required to be tested for quality by any agency (governmental or otherwise) prior to sale. Therefore, glucosamine preparations in the United States may vary in quality among different manufacturers and from batch to batch of a specific product made by a single manufacturer. In parts of Europe, glucosamine sulfate is available as a prescription drug of defined chemical nature.

Standardization

- Most studies of orally administered glucosamine have used glucosamine sulfate. Multiple salts of glucosamine are available, including glucosamine sulfate, glucosamine hydrochloride, and glucosamine hydroiodide. It is not clear if formulations other than glucosamine sulfate confer differences in efficacy or safety.
- In December 1999 and January 2000, ConsumerLabs conducted quality tests on 23 glucosamine and glucosamine-chondroitin products. All 10 of the glucosamine-only products passed testing. However, 6 out of 13 glucosamine-chondroitin products did not pass, primarily due to low chondroitin levels.

Dosing: Adult (18 Years and Older)
Oral

- **Osteoarthritis:** In most clinical trials, 500 mg of glucosamine sulfate three times daily (tablets or capsules) has been used for up to 90 days,[28-34] with limited long-term study for up to 3 years.[13] In one clinical trial, 1500 mg daily (crystalline powder for oral solution) was used.[35] In another trial, glucosamine hydrochloride (HCl) was given to patients at doses of 500 mg three times daily.[36] There are anecdotal reports that dosing adjustments may be necessary in obese patients, (20 mg/kg of body weight daily has been recommended); however, clinical studies to support this recommendation are lacking. A dose of 2000 mg per day for 12 weeks has also been administered in a study. Note: Full therapeutic benefit may take several weeks or up to 1 month in some patients. Glucosamine HCl provides more glucosamine than the glucosamine sulfate salt form on a molar level, although this difference becomes irrelevant when glucosamine is formulated to provide 500 mg of glucosamine per tablet. A higher dose of the sulfate salt of glucosamine than of the hydrochloride salt is required to provide a dose of 1500 mg of glucosamine.[37]

Intramuscular

- **Osteoarthritis:** Doses of 400 mg twice weekly have been used in clinical trials.[15]

Intra-articular

- **Osteoarthritis:** Doses of 400 mg of glucosamine sulfate daily for 7 days have been used.[16]

Intravenous

- **Osteoarthritis:** One 400-mg ampule of glucosamine sulfate has been administered intravenously daily for 7 days.[16]

Dosing: Pediatric (Younger Than 18 Years)

- Often not recommended, due to lack of sufficient evidence.
- In one study, 12 children with inflammatory bowel disease were treated with 3 to 6 g of N-acetyl-glucosamine.[7]

Toxicology

- According to anecdotal reports, no LD_{50} has been established for glucosamine; doses as high as 5000 mg/kg orally, 3000 mg/kg intramuscularly, and 1500 mg/kg intravenously have not been lethal in mice or rats.
- Glucosamine was found to inhibit beta-cell glucokinase activity *in vitro* and impair glucose-induced insulin secretion.[19]

ADVERSE EFFECTS/PRECAUTIONS/CONTRAINDICATIONS
Allergy/Hypersensitivity

- A case report describes an immediate hypersensitivity reaction (angioedema) to glucosamine sulfate.[38] Glucosamine should be avoided by individuals with known or suspected allergy/hypersensitivity to glucosamine sulfate or any of its constituents. Because glucosamine is derived from shells of shrimp, crab, and other shellfish, individuals with shellfish allergy or iodine hypersensitivity should avoid glucosamine.
- There are reported cases suggesting a link between glucosamine/chondroitin products and asthma exacerbations.[39] Until more reliable data exist, patients with a history of asthma should use glucosamine supplements cautiously.

Adverse Effects

- **General:** In most clinical trials, glucosamine sulfate at a dose of 500 mg three times daily (tablets or capsules) has been tolerated for 30 to 90 days.[28-34] In a 3-year double-blind study of 212 patients, incidence of adverse events in patients taking glucosamine was not significantly different from that of patients taking placebo.[13] Short-term studies including more than 150 patients in each trial report similar findings.[15,29,30,34]
- **Central nervous system:** Glucosamine has been reported to cause drowsiness, somnolence, insomnia, and headache.[40,41]
- **Ophthalmic:** An increased risk for cataract formation associated with glucosamine has been suggested in a bovine model,[42] but evidence in humans is lacking.
- **Dermatologic:** Photosensitization that was reproducible with rechallenge was reported in one case report.[43] Fingernail and toenail toughening, with increased rate of growth, has also been reported.[44] Several studies have reported skin reactions with the use of glucosamine.[40,41] Rash has been reported anecdotally.
- **Cardiovascular:** In a published letter, Danao-Camara noted three case reports of reversible elevations in systolic blood pressure by 20 to 30 mm Hg associated with glucosamine/

chondroitin products.[43] Specific brands were not mentioned in the letter; however, it was noted that effects may have been due to other concurrent medications or to impurities in glucosamine/chondroitin products. One patient developed tachycardia, and another became edematous.[41] Palpitations have also been reported with glucosamine use.[40]

- **Respiratory:** There are reported cases suggesting a link between glucosamine/chondroitin products and asthma exacerbations.[39] Until more reliable data exist, patients with a history of asthma should use glucosamine supplements cautiously.
- **Gastrointestinal:** Abdominal pain and diarrhea have been reported in clinical trials, but the incidence was no higher than with placebo.[13,30] A study conducted in 80 patients with osteoarthritis receiving 1500 mg of glucosamine sulfate daily reported two cases of constipation and one patient with mild heartburn.[28] There have been other instances of digestive problems associated with glucosamine, including epigastric pain/tenderness, heartburn, diarrhea, nausea, dyspepsia, vomiting, constipation, gastric heaviness, anorexia, abdominal pain, and flatulence.[27,41]
- **Hematologic:** Earlier forms of glucosamine formulations for injection (glucosaminoglycans) may cross-react with antibodies of patients with heparin-induced thrombocytopenia. This reaction has not been observed with the use of glucosamine sulfate.[45]
- **Endocrine:** The effects of glucosamine on glucose levels and insulin resistance have been controversial. Despite initial concerns about use in diabetic patients, based largely on *in vitro* and rat studies noting insulin resistance and possible glycemic effects[18-24] and on preliminary human work,[25] more recent human research reports no significant effects (including on hemoglobin A1c levels in patients with type 2 diabetes after 90 days of therapy).[26,27] Clinically relevant effects on blood sugar levels have not been noted in several clinical trials.[13,17,26,46]
- **Renal:** In a published letter, Danao-Camara noted four cases of 1+ to 2+ proteinuria in patients receiving glucosamine/chondroitin products.[43] Specific brands were not mentioned in the letter; however, it was noted that effects may have been due to other concurrent medications or to impurities in glucosamine/chondroitin products. Glucosamine is excreted mainly in urine,[47] with only small amounts excreted in feces,[48] and notable amounts are also metabolized to carbon dioxide and are excreted in expired air.[48] Elimination is delayed in renal insufficiency.[49]
- **Skeletal/Muscle:** In a published letter, Danao-Camara noted three instances of modestly elevated creatine phosphokinase (1 to 2 times above upper limit) in patients receiving glucosamine/chondroitin products.[43] Specific brands were not mentioned in the letter; however, it was noted that effects may have been due to other concurrent medications or to impurities in glucosamine/chondroitin products.

Precautions/Warnings/Contraindications

- Avoid in women who are or wish to become pregnant.
- Use cautiously in patients with diabetes mellitus.
- Use cautiously in patients with shellfish allergies.
- Use cautiously in renally impaired patients, due to renal excretion of glucosamine hydrochloride.[49]
- Use cautiously in patients with active peptic ulcer disease, as glucosamine may contribute to gastrointestinal upset.[41]

Pregnancy and Lactation

- Not recommended, due to lack of sufficient evidence.

INTERACTIONS

Glucosamine/Drug Interactions

- **Hypoglycemic agents:** The effect of glucosamine on glucose levels or insulin resistance has been controversial, and it remains unclear if interactions with agents possessing glycemic properties may occur. Despite initial concerns about use in diabetic patients, based largely on *in vitro* and rat studies noting insulin resistance and possible glycemic effects[18-24] and on preliminary human work,[25] more recent human research reports no significant effects (including on hemoglobin A1c levels in patients with type 2 diabetes after 90 days of therapy).[26,27] Clinically relevant effects on blood sugar levels have not been noted in several clinical trials.[13,17,26,46]
- **Diuretics:** Patients receiving concomitant therapy of glucosamine and a diuretic may have an increased risk of side effects associated with glucosamine use, although the evidence for this interaction is minimal.[41]

Glucosamine/Herb/Supplement Interactions

- **Hypoglycemic herbs and supplements:** The effect of glucosamine on glucose levels or insulin resistance has been controversial, and it remains unclear if interactions with agents possessing glycemic properties may occur. Despite initial concerns about use in diabetic patients based largely on *in vitro* and rat studies noting insulin resistance and possible glycemic effects[18-24] and on preliminary human work,[25] more recent human research reports no significant effects (including on hemoglobin A1c levels in patients with type 2 diabetes after 90 days of therapy).[26,27] Clinically relevant effects on blood sugar levels have not been noted in several clinical trials.[13,17,26,46]
- **Diuretic herbs and supplements:** Patients receiving concomitant therapy of glucosamine and a diuretic may have an increased risk of side effects associated with glucosamine use, although the evidence for this interaction is minimal.[41]
- **Bromelain (positive influence):** There are anecdotal reports that the concomitant use of bromelain and glucosamine may result in synergistic effects (anecdotal). It is unclear if a specific form of glucosamine has been implicated in this interaction.
- **Chondroitin sulfate (positive influence):** There are numerous studies evaluating the concomitant use of glucosamine and chondroitin sulfate,[50-53] suggesting that they may work synergistically.
- **Fish oil (positive influence):** One study evaluated the effects of glucosamine as a treatment for psoriasis and found that glucosamine with concomitant use of fish oil may have additive effects.[6]
- **Vitamin C:** There are anecdotal reports that concomitant use of glucosamine with vitamin C may lead to increased glucosamine effects. Vitamin C strengthens collagen and is an essential co-factor for collagen fibers; collagen is an essential component in the extracellular matrix of cartilage.
- **Manganese (positive influence):** There are anecdotal reports of concomitant use of glucosamine with manganese, due to the role of manganese as an essential co-factor for bone and joint formation. Manganese is thought to improve glucosamine utilization within chondrocytes and potentially lead to increased glucosamine effects.

Glucosamine/Food Interactions

- Insufficient available evidence.

Glucosamine/Lab Interactions

- **Serum glucose:** Animal models suggest that glucosamine may decrease the effectiveness of insulin and other oral hypoglycemics by increasing insulin resistance.[22] Limited human studies suggest that glucosamine has no clinically important effects on glucose metabolism.[46] Theoretically, glucosamine may increase blood glucose levels and alter test results.

MECHANISM OF ACTION
Pharmacology

- **General:** Glucosamine is an amino-monosaccharide naturally produced in humans. It is one of the principal substrates used in the biosynthesis of macromolecules that constitute articular cartilage, such as glycosaminoglycans, proteoglycans, and hyaluronic acid. It is believed to play a role in cartilage formation and repair.
- **Anti-inflammatory effects:** Unlike prostaglandin inhibitors, which have been associated with deterioration of joints in osteoarthritis, glucosamine sulfate increases synthesis of proteoglycans in *in vitro* cultures of normal human chondrocytes,[54,55] and of chondrocytes isolated from human osteoarthritic articular cartilage[55,56] and may be associated with disease-modifying effects clinically.[13] Clinical trials suggest that the disease-modifying effect is limited to patients with mild to moderate disease.[50,57]
- Although glucosamine is neither an analgesic nor an anti-inflammatory agent, it may exert mild anti-inflammatory effects. Glucosamine has a beneficial effect in animal models of experimental arthritis [58,59] and also appears to display mild anti-inflammatory activity.[60-62]
- **Hematologic effects:** A study conducted in eight heparinized dogs with bleeding esophageal varices greater than 2 mm in diameter were given glucosamine gel.[10] The dogs were given 2.5% to 3.5% of poly-*N*-acetyl glucosamine gel intravariceally and paravariceally. Results showed that in all cases the variceal hemorrhage was stopped with three to four injections that had a mean total gel volume of 1.9 mL. The authors concluded that the endoscopic injection of bleeding esophageal varices in the dogs with the use of poly-*N*-acetyl glucosamine gel was an effective and safe method for stopping the hemorrhage and inducing permanent varix obliteration.
- **Endocrine effects:** The effects of glucosamine on insulin resistance and serum glucose levels have been controversial. Initial research *in vitro* and in rats reported insulin resistance,[18-24] with some suggestion that there may be a small effect on glucose levels in humans,[25] although more recent studies in humans report no significant effects.[26,27] Scroggie et al. conducted a placebo-controlled, double-blind, randomized trial to evaluate possible effects of glucosamine supplementation on glycemic control in a population of patients with type 2 diabetes mellitus.[27] Included subjects were typically elderly and being treated with one or two drugs to maintain glycemic control. Over a 90-day period, patients received either placebo or a combination of 1500 mg of glucosamine hydrochloride with 1200 mg chondroitin sulfate (Cosamin DS; Nutramax Laboratories Inc, Edgewood, Md). The primary outcome measure was the hemoglobin A1c level. The authors reported that mean hemoglobin A1c concentrations did not significantly differ between groups or within groups.

Pharmacodynamics/Kinetics

- **Bioavailability:** The bioavailability of intramuscular administration of glucosamine sulfate in healthy adults was found to be approximately 96%.[63] The bioavailability of oral glucosamine sulfate is 26%, indicating a significant first-pass metabolism of glucosamine by the liver.[63]
- **Absorption:** A small, brief evaluation of *N*-acetylglucosamine (NAG) and the polymeric form (sustained action) of NAG suggests that NAG is readily absorbed, with the polymeric form producing sustained levels.[64] No detailed studies on the absorption of other forms of glucosamine (for example, glucosamine hydrochloride) by humans are available. The maximum concentration (C_{max}) of plasma proteins after glucosamine sulfate administered orally to healthy adults is 31 µmol/L, administered intravenously is 130 µmol/L, and administered intramuscularly is 128 µmol/L.[63]
- **Distribution:** The volume of distribution after intravenous administration of glucosamine in humans has been reported as 71 mL/kg.[48] Glucosamine is incorporated into plasma glycoproteins and distributed into liver, kidney, and skeletal tissues.[65] Due to the substantial mass of the skeleton (bones and cartilage), it has been estimated that approximately 30% of administered glucosamine is taken up by the skeletal tissues in the rat.[65]
- **Elimination:** The plasma levels of glucosamine sulfate (800 mg) administered intravenously falls rapidly, with an initial half-life of 6.1 minutes and a terminal half-life of 2.1 hours.[48] In a study conducted in 6 healthy men, the terminal half-life in plasma proteins for intravenous administration of glucosamine was 70 hours, for intramuscular 57 hours, and for oral 68 hours.[63] Larger doses of 12 to 30 g exhibit a beta elimination half-life of 120 to 150 minutes, suggesting a linear pharmacokinetic profile.[47,49]
- **Excretion:** Glucosamine is excreted mainly in urine,[47] with only small amounts excreted in feces.[48] Notable amounts are also metabolized to carbon dioxide and are excreted in expired air.[48] Elimination is delayed in renal insufficiency.[49]

HISTORY

- German physicians first reported the use of glucosamine as a therapeutic agent for osteoarthritis in 1969. In several uncontrolled trials, the administration of glucosamine sulfate given intravenously, intra-articularly, and intramuscularly was reported to diminish pain and increase mobility. More controlled trials became feasible after the introduction of glucosamine sulfate tablets by Rotta Research Laboratorium, an Italian pharmaceutical company. Notably, the majority of the clinical and pharmacokinetic studies, conducted in Europe during the 1980s and 1990s, have been conducted with glucosamine sulfate supplied by researchers affiliated with Rotta. Public enthusiasm for glucosamine as a treatment for osteoarthritis increased substantially in 1997 largely because of the best-selling book, *The Arthritis Cure*, by Jason Theodosakis, MD. In 1998, over one billion capsules of glucosamine were sold in the United States.[36]

REVIEW OF THE EVIDENCE: DISCUSSION
Knee Osteoarthritis
Summary

- There is compelling evidence from available randomized, controlled trials to support the use of oral glucosamine sulfate in the treatment of mild to moderate knee osteoarthritis. Notably, nearly all statistically significant studies

Review of the Evidence: Glucosamine

Condition Treated*	Study Design	Author, Year	N[†]	SS[†]	Study Quality[‡]	Magnitude of Benefit	ARR[†]	NNT[†]	Comments
Knee osteoarthritis	Systematic review	Richy[66] 2003	NA	Yes	NA	Medium	NA	NA	High level of efficacy reported across included trials in terms of Lequesne index, WOMAC osteoarthritis index, visual analog scale for pain, mobility, safety, and response to treatment; limited study found of effects on joint space narrowing.
Knee/hip osteoarthritis	Meta-analysis	McAlindon[66] 2000	1710	Yes	NA	Medium	44%	3	Possible overestimation of benefits; 30% effect size in knee osteoarthritis of mild to moderate severity; 2 abstracts included in analysis.
Knee osteoarthritis	RCT	Reginster[13] 2001	212	Yes	5	Medium	22%	5	Glucosamine oral solution (1500 mg) daily vs. placebo for 3 years; no significant radiologic joint-space loss with glucosamine vs. loss with placebo; significant improvement in WOMAC pain score vs. placebo.
Knee osteoarthritis	RCT	Reginster[13,68] 1999, 2001	212	Yes	4	Medium	NA	NA	Glucosamine (1500 mg) daily vs. placebo for 3 years; significant improvements in WOMAC osteoarthritis index and joint space narrowing.
Knee osteoarthritis	Sub-analysis of RCT by Reginster[13]	Bruyere[91] 2003	212	Yes	NA	Small	NA	NA	In sub-study of RCT, patients with the least severe joint space narrowing at baseline experienced the greatest deterioration over 3 years and appeared to be the most responsive to glucosamine sulfate therapy.
Knee osteoarthritis	RCT	Pavelka[14,69] 2000, 2002	202	Yes	4	Small	9%	11	Glucosamine (1500 mg) daily vs. placebo for 3 years; significant improvements in Lequesne index and absence of joint-space narrowing vs. placebo.
Knee osteoarthritis	RCT	Rindone[57] 2000	114	No	4	None	NA	NA	Glucosamine (1500 mg) vs. placebo for 2 months; no significant difference between groups; study in patients with advanced disease; salt form of glucosamine used not specified.
Knee osteoarthritis	RCT, combination therapy	Das[50] 2000	93	Yes	4	Medium	24%	4	Glucosamine (1000 mg), chondroitin (800 mg), manganese ascorbate (152 mg) twice daily for 6 months; benefit limited to individuals with mild to moderate osteoarthritis; study sponsored by manufacturer.
Knee osteoarthritis	RCT	Cohen[93] 2003	63	Unclear	2	Medium	NA	NA	Topical glucosamine/chondroitin combination vs. placebo for 8 weeks associated with improved symptoms.
Knee osteoarthritis	RCT	Hughes[70,71] 2000, 2002	80	No	3	None	NA	NA	Glucosamine (1500 mg) daily vs. placebo for 3 years; large placebo effect noted (33%); possibly underpowered to detect between-group differences.
Knee osteoarthritis	RCT	Houpt[36] 1999	118	No	5	NA	9%	11	Glucosamine HCl (1500 mg) vs. placebo for 8 weeks; improved mobility but no significant difference between groups in pain and stiffness; unique trial of glucosamine HCl, with trend toward improvement late in trial.

Review of the Evidence: Glucosamine—*cont'd*

Condition Treated*	Study Design	Author, Year	N[†]	SS[†]	Study Quality[‡]	Magnitude of Benefit	ARR[†]	NNT[†]	Comments
Knee osteoarthritis	RCT	Noack[30] 1994	252	Yes	5	Small	17%	6	1500 mg of glucosamine vs. placebo daily for 4 weeks; responder rate significantly higher with glucosamine than with placebo.
Knee osteoarthritis	RCT (published abstract)	Förster[72] 1996	329	Yes	3	Medium	34%	3	Glucosamine (1500 mg) vs. piroxicam (20 mg) vs. glucosamine + piroxicam vs. placebo daily for 90 days; limited description of methodology or statistical analysis.
Knee osteoarthritis	Equivalence trial	Muller-Fassbender[29] 1994	200	Yes	5	Medium	NA	NA	Glucosamine sulfate (1500 mg) vs. ibuprofen (1200 mg) daily for 4 weeks; improvement in both groups vs. baseline; no significant difference between groups; no placebo arm.
Knee osteoarthritis	RCT	Rovati[32] 1994	329	Yes	4	Medium	NA	NA	Glucosamine (1500 mg) vs. piroxicam (20 mg) vs. glucosamine + piroxicam vs. placebo daily.
Knee osteoarthritis	RCT	Reichelt[15] 1994	155	Yes	4	Small	22%	5	Glucosamine (400 mg) IM injections twice weekly for 6 weeks vs. placebo; intention-to-treat analysis.
Knee osteoarthritis	Combined data of three RCTs	Rovati[73] 1992	606	Yes	3	Small	Oral, 15%; IM, 19%	Oral, 7; IM, 5	Combined data of three 4- to 6-week trials of glucosamine (oral or IM) vs. ibuprofen vs. placebo; methodologically limited analysis.
Knee osteoarthritis	RCT	Raatikainen[74] 1990	31	Yes	3	Small	38%	3	12 IM glycosaminoglycan (Arteparon) injections given over 6 weeks; patients followed for 1 year.
Knee osteoarthritis	RCT	Ishikowa[75] 1982	120	Yes	2	Small	0%	33	Intra-articular glycosaminoglycan polysulfate studied; randomization not specified; outcomes assessment tool not clearly standardized.
Knee osteoarthritis		Vajaradul[12] 1981	54	Yes	1	Medium	39%	3	Intra-articular glucosamine injections vs. placebo for 4 weeks; incomplete dosing information.
Knee osteoarthritis	Equivalence trial	Qiu[34] 1998	178	Yes	4	Medium	NA	NA	1500 mg glucosamine vs. 1200 mg ibuprofen daily for 4 weeks. Broad range of patient ages (28-78 years).
Knee osteoarthritis	Equivalence trial	Lopes[33] 1982	40	Yes	2	Small	29%	4	Glucosamine(1500 mg) vs. ibuprofen (1200 mg) daily for 8 weeks; significantly lower pain scores with glucosamine; subjective measures of efficacy used; blinding not described.
Knee osteoarthritis	RCT	Pujalte[31] 1980	20	Yes	4	Large	60%	2	Glucosamine (1500 mg) vs. placebo daily for 6-8 weeks; significant reductions in articular pain, joint tenderness, swelling in glucosamine group vs. placebo.
Knee pain (suspected osteoarthritis)	RCT	Braham[92] 2003	46	Mixed	4	Mixed	NA	NA	Glucosamine (2000 mg) daily improved subjective accounts of knee pain but not objective measures of function vs. placebo after 12 weeks.
Osteoarthritis	Meta-analysis	Towheed[76] 2001	3021	No	NA	Medium	NA	NA	Pooled data from 16 trials showed mean difference for pain reduction vs. placebo to be 1.40; mean difference in Lequesne index was 0.63.
Osteoarthritis	Meta-analysis	Towheed[77] 1999	9 trials	NA	NA	Small	NA	NA	Pooled data from 5 placebo-controlled trials found effect size for pain relief vs. placebo to be 1.23.

Continued

Review of the Evidence: Glucosamine—cont'd

Condition Treated*	Study Design	Author, Year	N[†]	SS[†]	Study Quality[‡]	Magnitude of Benefit	ARR[†]	NNT[†]	Comments
Osteoarthritis	Meta-analysis	Denham[51] 2000	15 trials	NA	NA	Medium	NA	NA	Pooled data from 15 trials found effect size for pain to be 0.44.
Osteoarthritis	Meta-analysis	Kreder[48] 2000	911	NA	NA	Medium	NA	NA	Pooled data from 16 trials found effect size for pain to be 0.44.
Osteoarthritis	Systematic review	Barclay[40] 1998	275	NA	NA	Medium	NA	NA	Benefits reported in pain and mobility. Analysis excluded studies with >30 subjects or with poor design.
Osteoarthritis	Systematic review	Gottleib[79] 1997	6 trials	NA	NA	Small	NA	NA	Positive trends in osteoarthritis symptoms reported; vaguely described study.
Osteoarthritis	Systematic review	Da Camara[80] 1998	2537	NA	NA	Small	NA	NA	Positive trends in osteoarthritis symptoms reported from 11 trials; vaguely described study.
Osteoarthritis	Systematic review	Brief[81] 2001	984	NA	NA	Medium	NA	NA	Positive trends in osteoarthritis symptoms reported from 9 trials; vaguely described study.
Osteoarthritis (temporo-mandibular joint)	Equivalence trial	Thie[82] 2001	45	Yes	5	Medium	10%	10	Glucosamine sulfate (1500 mg) vs. ibuprofen (1200 mg) daily for 3 months.
Osteoarthritis (knee and spinal degenerative joint disease)	RCT	Leffler[52] 1999	34	Mixed	3	Small	48%	2	Glucosamine HCl (1500 mg), chondroitin sulfate (1200 mg), and manganese (228 mg) daily for 16 weeks; significant results for knee, but not for back; study was sponsored by manufacturer.
Osteoarthritis	Equivalence trial	D'Ambrosio[16] 1981	30	Yes	2	Medium	NA	NA	Glucosamine (400 mg) injection for 1 week, followed by glucosamine (500 mg) 3 times daily for 2 weeks OR piperazine/ chlorbutanol injection for 1 week followed by 2 weeks of placebo; inconsistent routes of administration; comparisons made with unproven therapies.
Osteoarthritis	RCT	Drovanti[28] 1980	80	Yes	2	Medium	32%	3	Glucosamine (1500 mg) or placebo daily for 30 days; significantly better scores for articular pain, joint tenderness, swelling, and restriction of active movements in glucosamine group.
Osteoarthritis	RCT	Mund-Hoym[83] 1980	80	Yes	1	Small	NA	NA	IM glucosamine (400 mg) 3 times weekly, then 250 mg orally 4 times weekly OR IM phenylbutazone (600 mg) daily, then 200 mg orally 4 times weekly or 250 mg orally twice daily; both groups showed improvements.
Osteoarthritis	Equivalence trial	Crolle[84] 1980	30	Yes	1	Medium	27%	4	IM glucosamine (400 mg) for 1 week, followed by glucosamine (500 mg) 3 times daily for 2 weeks OR piperazine/ chlorbutanol injection for 1 week followed by 2 weeks of placebo; inconsistent routes of administration; comparisons made with unproven therapies.
Osteoarthritis	Equivalence trial	Hehne[85] 1984	68	No	1	Small	NA	NA	Intra-articular glucosamine sulfate associated with superior effect vs. glycosaminoglycan polysulfate in mild osteoarthritis.

Review of the Evidence: Glucosamine—cont'd

Condition Treated*	Study Design	Author, Year	N[†]	SS[†]	Study Quality[‡]	Magnitude of Benefit	ARR[†]	NNT[†]	Comments
Osteoarthritis	Dosing study	Dettmer[86] 1979	100	No	0	Small	NA	NA	Intra-articular injection vs. intramuscular injection, with similar clinical response.
Osteoarthritis	Open cohort study	Tapadinhas[41] 1982	1208	Yes	2	Medium	NA	NA	Glucosamine (1500 mg) daily for 6-8 weeks; no placebo arm.
Rheumatoid arthritis	RCT	Giordano[87] 1975	15	No	2	Small	NA	NA	Glucosamine (420 mg) OR 100 mg indomethacin (100 mg) daily for 14 days; both groups with significantly improved pain on pressure; no difference between groups, but possibly underpowered.
Venous insufficiency	Before and after	Gosetti[88] 1986	60	No	3	Small	NA	NA	Perclar (glycosaminoglycan) administered at various daily doses: (48 mg, 72 mg, 96 mg); treatment associated with improvements in 70%-96% of subjects.
Inflammatory bowel disease (Crohn's, ulcerative colitis)	Pilot study	Salvatore[7] 2000	12	No	0	Small	NA	NA	3-6 g daily of N-acetyl glucosamine in children; mixed results.
TMJ disorders	Case series	Shankland[53] 1998	50	No	0	Small	NA	NA	Glucosamine (1600 mg), chondroitin (200 mg), and calcium (1000 mg) twice daily; mixed results.

*Primary or secondary outcome.
[†]N, Number of patients; SS, statistically significant; ARR, absolute risk reduction; NNT, the number of patients who need to undergo a specific intervention in order to observe an outcome in one individual.
[‡]0-2 = poor; 3-4 = good; 5 = excellent.
IM, Intramuscular; NA, not applicable; RCT, randomized, controlled trial; TMJ, temporomandibular joint; WOMAC, Western Ontario and MacMaster Universities Osteoarthritis Composite Index.
For an explanation of each category in this table, please see Table 3 in the Introduction.

have used glucosamine sulfate supplied by one European manufacturer (Rotta Research Laboratorium). Therefore, it is unknown whether glucosamine preparations sold by different manufacturers are equally effective. Studies not demonstrating statistically significant efficacy have often either included patients with severe osteoarthritis or utilized formulations other than glucosamine sulfate. Additional high-quality studies, conducted independently of glucosamine manufacturers, are warranted to confirm the efficacy of glucosamine. Full therapeutic benefit may take several weeks or up to 1 month to occur.

Systematic Review and Meta-analysis

- Richy et al. conducted a systematic review of controlled trials of glucosamine sulfate and chondroitin sulfate in patients with knee osteoarthritis.[66] A literature search was conducted to include placebo-controlled trials published or performed between January 1980 and March 2002 via MEDLINE, PREMEDLINE, EMBASE, the Cochrane Database of Systematic Reviews, Current Contents, BIOSIS Previews, HealthSTAR, and EBM Reviews, as well as a manual review of the literature and congressional abstracts, and direct contact with authors and manufacturers of glucosamine and chondroitin products. Outcomes of interest included joint space narrowing, Lequesne Index, Western Ontario and MacMaster Universities Arthritis Index (WOMAC) osteoarthritis index, visual analog scale for pain, mobility, safety, and response to treatment. Data abstraction was performed systematically by two independent reviewers who were

blinded to sources and authors. The authors reported highly significant efficacy of glucosamine overall in terms of all assessed outcomes, although limited results were available in included studies for joint space narrowing.

- McAlindon et al. conducted a meta-analysis and systematic quality assessment of clinical trials of glucosamine in knee and/or hip osteoarthritis.[67] Human clinical trials were identified via a search of MEDLINE (1966 to June 1999), and were included if they were published or unpublished double-blind, randomized, placebo-controlled trials of 4 or more weeks' duration that studied glucosamine for knee or hip osteoarthritis,, and that reported extractable data on the effects of treatment on symptoms. Inclusion criteria also required reporting of at least one of the following outcomes: global pain score for index joint, pain on walking for index joint, WOMAC osteoarthritis index pain subscale, Lequesne index, or pain in index joint during activities other than walking. Six studies met inclusion criteria.[12,15,30,31,36,89] Each trial was evaluated with a quality assessment instrument measuring 14 aspects of clinical trial conduct. Pooled analysis revealed a moderate treatment effect for glucosamine of 0.44 (95% CI, 0.24-0.64). Although these results are suggestive, methodological flaws and publication bias of the individual trials may have exaggerated estimates of clinical benefit. Notably, two abstracts[36,39] were included in the meta-analysis that were not subjected to peer review prior to publication and did not include detailed accounts of statistical analyses, and one[36] used glucosamine hydrochloride, which may not be clinically comparable to glucosamine sulfate. Other limitations include a lack of detailed descriptions of patients enrolled in the individual trials. The safety profiles of glucosamine sulfate and chondroitin sulfate were not reviewed in the meta-analysis.[90]

Controlled Trials of Oral Glucosamine (Long-Term Results)

• Reginster et al. assessed the effects of glucosamine on the long-term progression of osteoarthritis joint structure changes and symptoms.[13,68] A total of 212 patients with knee osteoarthritis were studied in this well-designed and reported randomized, double-blind, placebo-controlled trial. Subjects were administered a daily oral solution containing glucosamine sulfate (1500 mg) or placebo for 3 years. The primary measure of biologic effect was change in width of medial tibiofemoral joint space, a radiographic measurement of outcome recommended by expert consensus. Clinical symptoms were scored by the validated WOMAC osteoarthritis index. An intent-to-treat analysis demonstrated a progressive joint-space loss in the placebo group (by an average of 20 mm), whereas no significant joint-space loss was observed in the glucosamine group. Patients treated with glucosamine also experienced significant improvements in WOMAC pain and physical function subscales when compared to placebo. No significant differences from placebo were found in terms of adverse effects, suggesting fairly long-term safety of oral glucosamine sulfate. The glucosamine used in this study was a prescription formulation (Dona, Viartril-S, or Xicil; Rotta Research Group, Monza, Italy) of defined chemical composition. Glucosamine sulfate cannot be generalized to other glucosamine products (or compound mixtures) that are available as dietary supplements in some countries. Limitations of this trial include a large dropout rate of approximately one third of the subjects (38 in treatment group and 35 in placebo group). The authors note that the reasons for dropout did not differ significantly between groups and were not directly attributable to symptoms, although detailed follow-up of dropouts was not clearly described.

• Pavelka et al. published results of a three-year randomized, placebo controlled trial of glucosamine sulfate 1500 mg once daily for osteoarthritis of the knee.[14,69] This study was conducted in 202 patients with mild to moderate knee osteoarthritis confirmed by physical and radiographic diagnosis, using American College of Rheumatology criteria, with baseline average joint space widths of slightly less than 4 mm and a Lequesne index score of less than 9 points. The primary outcome was progression of osteoarthritis, measured via the Lequesne index and joint space measurements. Changes in radiographic minimum joint space width were measured in the medial compartment of the tibiofemoral joint, and symptoms were assessed using the algo-functional indexes of Lequesne and WOMAC. The authors reported that after 3 years of treatment, the placebo group experienced progression of mean joint space narrowing of −0.19 mm (95% confidence interval, −0.29 to −0.09 mm), whereas there was no average change with glucosamine sulfate use (0.04 mm; 95% confidence interval, −0.06 to 0.14 mm). Differences between the groups were statistically significant ($p = 0.001$). In addition, fewer patients treated with glucosamine sulfate experienced predefined severe narrowings (>0.5 mm): 5% versus 14% (p = 0.05). Symptoms improved modestly with placebo use but by as much as 20% to 25% with glucosamine sulfate, with significant final differences on the Lequesne index and the WOMAC total

index and pain, function, and stiffness subscales. There was no significant difference in adverse events between groups.

• Bruyere et al. investigated the relationship between baseline radiographic severity of knee osteoarthritis and long-term joint space narrowing, reporting that those with the least severe joint space narrowing at baseline experience the greatest deterioration over three years and appeared to be the most responsive to glucosamine sulfate.[91] This study was a sub-analysis of the previously published 3-year randomized, placebo-controlled, prospective study in 212 patients with knee osteoarthritis, recruited from outpatient clinics by Reginster et al.[13,68] Mean joint space width (JSW) was assessed by a computer-assisted method using weight-bearing anteroposterior knee radiographs. The authors reported that in the placebo group, baseline JSW was significantly negatively correlated with joint space narrowing measured after 3 years ($p = 0.003$). Also, in the placebo group, among patients in the lowest quartile of baseline mean JSW values (<4.5 mm), JSW increased by a mean of 3.8%, compared to 6.2% in the glucosamine sulfate group, although this difference was not statistically significant ($p = 0.70$). In the highest quartile of baseline mean JSW values (>6.2 mm), joint space narrowing of 14.9% occurred in the placebo group, compared to 6.0% in the glucosamine sulfate group. Patients with the most severe osteoarthritis at baseline had a risk ratio (relative risk) of 0.42 to experience 0.5 mm of joint space narrowing over 3 years, compared to those with less severely affected joints. In patients with mild osteoarthritis (highest quartile of baseline mean JSW), glucosamine sulfate use was associated with a nonsignificant trend toward reduction in joint space narrowing ($p = 0.10$).

Controlled Trials of Oral Glucosamine (Short-Term Results)

• Rindone et al. conducted a randomized, controlled trial comparing the effects of glucosamine and placebo in the treatment of 98 patients with knee osteoarthritis.[57] Patients were randomized by a computer generated code to receive placebo or glucosamine 500 mg three times daily for 2 months. The primary outcome was pain intensity at rest and while walking, as assessed by a visual analog scale, measured at baseline and after 30 and 60 days of treatment. The authors reported no statistical difference between glucosamine and placebo at either 30 or 60 days. It is unclear if the negative results are related to inclusion of patients with more advanced disease or if the study was not sufficiently powered. Of note, the salt form of glucosamine was not specified, and the American manufacturer is no longer in business at the address indicated in the study.

• A randomized, double-blind, placebo-controlled trial was conducted in 80 patients with radiographic diagnosis of osteoarthritis who were recruited from a rheumatology outpatient clinic, to evaluate the effects of glucosamine sulfate (1500 mg daily) or a placebo for 6 months.[70,71] Patients were excluded if they had prosthetic material in both knees, had previously taken glucosamine, had received arthroscopic surgery of the knee in the past 3 months, or had any intra-articular injection in the last month. The study assessed safety and efficacy at 0, 6, 12, and 24 weeks. The assessment included 100-mm visual analog scale (VAS) pain scores for global pain, pain on movement, and pain at rest; the McGill pain questionnaire; WOMAC, range of movement, use of rescue analgesics, and adherence to trial medication. The primary outcome was patients' global assessment of pain in the knee. The results of the primary outcome global assessment of pain in the knee demonstrated no statistically significant difference between glucosamine and placebo, based on area under the curve analysis (mean difference, 0.15 mm; 95% CI, –8.78 to 9.07). However, there was a 33% response in the placebo group, and therefore the sample size may not have been adequate to detect true between-group differences. No significant differences were found between groups with regard to pain, range of movement, or use of rescue analgesia. A small significant difference was found between groups in knee flexion (mean difference, 13 degrees; 95% CI, –23.13 to –1.97). A subgroup of patients with mild to moderate pain experienced a trend toward analgesia with glucosamine sulfate.

- Houpt et al. conducted a double-blind, randomized, placebo-controlled trial of glucosamine in which 118 patients with knee osteoarthritis were given glucosamine hydrochloride (500 mg three times daily) or placebo for 8 weeks.[36] The primary outcome was a difference in total scores of the Western Ontario and McMaster Universities osteoarthritis index (WOMAC) at week 0 and week 8. The secondary outcomes assessed were pain reductions measured by daily diary and knee examination. Although positive trends were seen in subjects treated with glucosamine, no significant differences were observed in WOMAC scores between the glucosamine hydrochloride and placebo groups. However, positive trends were seen in the glucosamine group in 23 of 24 WOMAC questions. The secondary outcomes did reach statistical significance from weeks 5 to 8, suggesting improvements in knee examinations ($p = 0.026$) and in the responses to a daily diary pain question ($p = 0.018$). Although mobility did improve, pain and stiffness did not reach a statistically significant difference between the two groups. The wide confidence intervals suggest very low precision, possibly suggesting too much heterogeneity. This trial is unique because it used glucosamine hydrochloride instead of the more common glucosamine sulfate. The study was well designed and reported, reporting no significant difference in WOMAC scores compared to placebo. However, the results of the secondary outcomes should be viewed cautiously; due to the subjective nature of the questions, variations in patient understanding may lead to bias.

- Noack et al. performed a double-blind, randomized, placebo controlled trial of glucosamine in 252 patients with knee osteoarthritis.[30] Patients received glucosamine sulfate (500 mg three times daily) or placebo for 4 weeks. Responders were defined as patients with a reduction of at least 3 points in the Lequesne index with a positive overall assessment by the investigator. The responder rate was significantly higher in the glucosamine group (55%) than in placebo (38%). The overall result did not change after analysis of the data by intention-to-treat.

- Förster et al. presented an abstract of a randomized controlled trial comparing glucosamine, piroxicam, and placebo.[72] In this 90-day analysis, patients were assigned to receive daily placebo, 1500 mg of glucosamine, 20 mg of piroxicam, or the combination of 1500 mg of glucosamine and 20 mg of piroxicam. The primary outcome measure was the Lequesne index of severity. Improvements in this index were noted in 48% of glucosamine patients, 39% of piroxicam patients, 46% of patients receiving the combination, and 14% of patients receiving placebo. Because only an abstract was published, data regarding methodology and statistical analysis are limited.

- Muller-Fassbender et al. compared the efficacy of glucosamine to ibuprofen in treating symptoms of knee osteoarthritis in a randomized, controlled, double-blind trial.[29] In this study, 200 patients were randomized to receive either 500 mg of glucosamine sulfate or 400 mg of ibuprofen three times daily for 4 weeks. Inclusion criteria were based on medical and medication history, physical examination, and radiographic evaluation. The exclusion criteria included significant hematologic disorders, history of renal or hepatic impairment, peptic ulcer disease, hypersensitivity to nonsteroidal anti-inflammatory drugs (NSAIDs), recent injury to the involved knee, and intra-articular corticosteroid use in the past 2 months. Patients were not permitted to take NSAIDs, corticosteroids, analgesics or any other medication for the treatment of osteoarthritis but were allowed to receive physical therapy if it was recorded in their profiles. The primary outcome of the study was clinical improvement in symptoms and a decrease in the Lequesne index. After 4 weeks, significant reductions in symptoms (defined as a reduction of at least 2 points in the Lequesne index) were observed in both groups; however, significantly more adverse events were noted in the ibuprofen group (35%) than in the glucosamine group (6%) ($p < 0.05$). Limitations of this trial include poorly described randomization methods.

- An abstract by Rovati et al. describes a double-blind, randomized, placebo-controlled trial of 329 patients with knee osteoarthritis.[32] Subjects were randomized to receive either 1500 mg of glucosamine sulfate, 20 mg of piroxicam, 1500 mg of glucosamine plus 20 mg of piroxicam, or placebo, all administered once daily. The primary outcome measure was the Lequesne index. The study results were based on an intention-to-treat approach in 310 evaluable patients, including dropouts for worsening, inefficiency, or concomitant use of other symptomatic drugs. The glucosamine and glucosamine-piroxicam group showed significant decreases in the Lequesne index. The results are promising, although descriptions of methods and statistical analysis were limited in this abstract.

- Qiu et al. conducted a randomized, double-blind trial comparing glucosamine to ibuprofen in 178 patients with knee osteoarthritis.[34] Both glucosamine sulfate (500 mg, three times daily) and ibuprofen (400 mg, three times daily) significantly reduced pain and swelling of the knee after 2 and 4 weeks of treatment. Patients taking ibuprofen reported significantly more adverse effects than those taking glucosamine ($p = 0.01$). This study is promising, although there is possible bias due to association with the glucosamine manufacturer Rotta Research Laboratorium.

- Lopes et al. conducted a trial comparing tolerance and efficacy of glucosamine to ibuprofen in 40 patients with osteoarthritis of the knee.[33] Patients were randomized to receive 500 mg of glucosamine sulfate or 400 mg of ibuprofen three times daily with meals for 8 weeks. The primary outcomes assessed were articular pain and presence of swelling. Results showed that pain scores initially decreased more slowly in the glucosamine group than in the ibuprofen group (during the first 2 weeks). However, pain scores in the glucosamine group continued to decrease until becoming significantly lower than in the ibuprofen group by week 8 ($p < 0.05$). Four patients with inflammation in the ibuprofen group showed no reduction in inflammation, while two of seven patients in the glucosamine group returned to normal. This study is limited by the use of highly subjective efficacy measures.

- Pujalte et al. performed a double-blind, randomized, placebo-controlled trial of glucosamine in 20 patients with knee osteoarthritis.[31] Patients were randomized to receive placebo or 500 mg of glucosamine three times daily for 6 to 8 weeks. Results revealed significant reductions in the primary outcomes measured (articular pain, joint tenderness, swelling) in the glucosamine group compared to placebo ($p < 0.01$). The clinical relevance of these results is limited by the lack of accounting for dropouts and by the small sample size.

- Braham et al. conducted a randomized, placebo-controlled trial to assess the effects of oral glucosamine supplementation on functional ability and degree of pain in 46 individuals with regular knee pain felt to be due to previous articular cartilage damage and osteoarthritis.[92] Subjects were assigned to receive either glucosamine (2000 mg) or placebo daily for 12 weeks. During this period, four testing sessions were conducted, with changes in knee pain and function assessed by clinical and functional tests (joint line palpation, a 3-meter "duck walk," repeated walking stair climb), two questionnaires (knee injury and osteoarthritis outcome score [KOOS] and knee pain scale [KPS]), and participant subjective evaluation. At the completion of the study period, the authors reported significant improvements in clinical and functional test scores in the glucosamine group compared to baseline, but there were no significant differences between groups. Significant improvements were observed in the glucosamine group compared to placebo in questionnaire results ($p < 0.05$), KOOS quality of life scores ($p < 0.05$), and KPS scores ($p < 0.05$). On self-report evaluations of knee pain, improvements were reported by 88% of glucosamine patients versus 17% of placebo patients. Most improvements were observed at 8 weeks.

Controlled Trials of Parenteral (Injection) Glucosamine

- Rovati reported on combined data of three trials of 4 to 6 weeks' duration comparing glucosamine sulfate against placebo or ibuprofen in the treatment of osteoarthritis of the knee.[73] In the first trial, glucosamine sulfate (500 mg three times daily for 4 weeks) was compared to placebo in 241 patients, with improvement in 52% of subjects receiving glucosamine and 37% of those receiving placebo (based on intention-to-treat). In the second trial, glucosamine sulfate (400 mg) or placebo was administered intramuscularly twice weekly for 6 weeks to 155 individuals, with 51% of glucosamine subjects responding and 32% of placebo subjects responding (again based on intention-to-treat). A third trial of glucosamine sulfate (500 mg three times daily) vs. ibuprofen (400 mg three times daily) was evaluated in 199 hospitalized patients for 4 weeks, with 48% responding to glucosamine and 51% responding to ibuprofen. The studies were limited in that randomization procedures and accountability for dropouts were not clearly specified.
- Reichelt et al. studied the efficacy of intramuscular injections of glucosamine in 155 patients with knee osteoarthritis in a multi-center, double-blind, randomized, placebo-controlled trial.[15] Patients were randomized to twice-weekly injections of either glucosamine sulfate (400 mg) or placebo for 6 weeks. Efficacy was assessed at weekly intervals using the Lequesne index. Therapy responders were considered those patients with a decrease in the Lequesne index of at least 3 points from basal value, together with an investigator overall judgment of efficacy rated "good" or "moderate." The authors reported that the frequency of therapy responders was significantly greater in the glucosamine sulfate group ($p = 0.012$). An intention-to-treat analysis of the data yielded

similar results. However, one cannot necessarily extrapolate the relative efficacy between intramuscular and oral formulations of glucosamine sulfate.

- A small study by Raatikainen et al. evaluated the effects of 12 intramuscular injections of glycosaminoglycan polysulfonate (Arteparon) given over 6 weeks to relatively young patients with damaged patellar cartilage and arthroscopically verified chondromalacia.[74] The patients were followed for 1 year. Improvement was seen in macroscopic evaluation of patellar cartilage at 1 year in 8 of 13 patients treated with glycosaminoglycan and in 3 of 13 patients receiving placebo. Limitations of the study include the small study size, questions as to randomization (randomization method not specified, trend toward heavier patients in placebo group), and no accountability for dropouts.
- Vajaradul studied the effect of intra-articular injections of glucosamine on symptoms of knee osteoarthritis.[12] In this double-blind, randomized, placebo-controlled trial, 54 patients received a weekly injection of glucosamine (Viartril, dosage unspecified) or placebo in the affected knee for 5 consecutive weeks. Although both treatments significantly reduced pain, the action of glucosamine was greater than that of placebo. Four weeks after the last injection, 13 of 26 glucosamine-treated patients were completely pain-free, compared to only 2 of 26 placebo-treated patients ($p < 0.001$). The clinical utility of these results is limited due to the lack of reported dosing information and limited description of methods.

Controlled Trials of Combination Therapy (Glucosamine/Chondroitin)

- Das et al. performed a 6-month manufacturer-sponsored evaluation of a combination of 1000 mg of glucosamine hydrochloride (FCHG49), 800 mg of low-molecular-weight sodium chondroitin sulfate (TRH122), and 152 mg of manganese ascorbate (Cosamin DS).[50] Each agent was administered twice daily to patients with radiographically defined osteoarthritis of the knee. Exclusion criteria for the study included pregnancy, severe activity-limiting diseases, type 2 diabetes, alcoholism, history of significant hematologic disorder, history of hepatic or renal impairment, active peptic ulcer, metabolic diseases, musculoskeletal disease other than osteoarthritis, injury or surgery to the involved knee in the past 6 months, intra-articular corticosteroids within the last 2 months, and regular use of nonsteroidal anti-inflammatory drugs (NSAIDs) in the past 2 months. Patients included had at least a Lequesne index of severity of osteoarthritis of 7, and a radiograph grade of 2 or more, based on the Keligren and Lawrence grading system. Further inclusion criteria were ability to walk, willingness to comply with study protocol, arthritic symptoms for greater than 6 months, and age between 45 and 75 years. The primary outcome of this study was the Lequesne index of severity of osteoarthritis of the knee (ISK). The secondary outcome was the Western Ontario and McMaster Universities osteoarthritis index (WOMAC). Response to treatment was defined as a 25% improvement in the parameters studied (ISK, WOMAC score, or patients' global assessment, with ISK as the primary outcome). Patients with mild to moderate osteoarthritis displayed significant improvement in the ISK for osteoarthritis of the knee compared to placebo at 4 months ($p = 0.003$). The patients' global assessments were used to evaluate the results in 70% of the intervention group vs. 46% of the placebo group ($p = 0.04$). The WOMAC results were used in 58% of the treated group vs. 41% of the placebo group ($p = 0.2$). Patients with severe osteoarthritis did not show significant improvement in any of the index methods used. A methodological limitation of this study was the use of data from prior visits to fill in for missing data elements (accounting for 16% of data points). In addition, this trial used doses greater than those commonly used in other clinical trials (2000 mg of glucosamine/1600 mg of chondroitin sulfate daily rather than 1500 mg of glucosamine/1200 mg of chondroitin sulfate daily.

Topical Glucosamine/Chondroitin

- Cohen et al. assessed the ability of a topical preparation of glucosamine sulfate and chondroitin sulfate to reduce pain related to osteoarthritis of the knee.[93] In this randomized controlled trial, 63 patients were assigned to receive either topical glucosamine/chondroitin or placebo over an 8-week period. At the end of the study period, the authors reported a greater mean reduction in visual analog scale (VAS) pain scores in the glucosamine/chondroitin group (mean change, –3.4 cm) compared to the placebo group (mean change, –1.6 cm), with effects also seen after 4 weeks. However, statistical analysis was not well described.

Open Trials

- An open trial was conducted by Wein et al. to evaluate the use of glucosamine hydrochloride in the treatment of pain associated with osteoarthritis of the knee.[94] The study was conducted in 110 individuals who received either an unknown amount of glucosamine hydrochloride or placebo tablets for 2 months. Outcomes were evaluated using a patient questionnaire (2 pain questions and 3 function questions). The authors reported that the only statistically significant difference between the treated group and placebo was a decrease in pain when using stairs in the glucosamine group ($p = 0.043$). This was an open (unblinded) trial, which may have allowed for the introduction of bias.
- A case series was reported in 190 patients from 1978 through December 1982 to evaluate the efficacy of glucosamine in the treatment of knee osteoarthritis.[95] Patients received a total of five intra-articular injections containing 200 mg of glucosamine sulfate, 200 mg of glucosamine hydrochloride, and 50 mg of lidocaine. Following the injections, patients received 500 mg of glucosamine sulfate twice daily for 12 consecutive weeks. The authors reported that after the second intra-articular injection, and following use of oral glucosamine, improvements occurred in overall pain and function of joints.

Osteoarthritis (General)
Summary

- Several controlled trials have reported benefits of glucosamine in the management of osteoarthritis at sites other than the knee. However, the evidence is less plentiful than that for knee osteoarthritis. Overall, trials have not been well designed or reported, and many have compared the efficacy of glucosamine to that of other agents (without proven efficacy), without placebo comparison. A number of meta-analyses and systematic reviews have reported beneficial effects, although most have included trials of knee osteoarthritis. Notably, knee osteoarthritis tends to respond better than other osteoarthritic joints to any treatment (it is possible that the make-up and structure of the knee joint plays a role). Future studies are warranted to assess the efficacy of glucosamine in treating osteoarthritis of different specific joints at different stages of severity.

Meta-analyses and Systematic Reviews

- In 2000, McAlindon et al. conducted a meta-analysis and systematic quality assessment of clinical trials of glucosamine in knee and/or hip osteoarthritis.[67] Human clinical trials were identified via a search of MEDLINE (1966 to June 1999), and were included if they were published or unpublished double-blind, randomized, placebo controlled trials of 4 or more weeks' duration that studied glucosamine for knee or hip osteoarthritis, and reported extractable data on the effects of treatment on symptoms. Inclusion criteria also required reporting of at least one of the following outcomes: global pain score for index joint, pain on walking for index joint, Western Ontario and McMaster Universities (WOMAC) osteoarthritis index pain subscale, Lequesne index, or pain in index joint during activities other than walking. Six studies met inclusion criteria.[12,15,31,36,89] Each trial was evaluated with a quality assessment instrument measuring 14 aspects of clinical trial conduct. Pooled analysis revealed a moderate treatment effect for glucosamine of 0.44 (95% CI, 0.24 to 0.64). Although these results are suggestive, methodological flaws and publication bias of the individual trials may have exaggerated estimates of clinical benefit. Notably, two abstracts[36,89] were included in the meta-analysis that were not subjected to peer review prior to publication and did not include detailed accounts of statistical analyses, and one[36] used glucosamine hydrochloride, which may not be clinically comparable. Other limitations include a lack of detailed descriptions of patients enrolled in the individual trials. The safety profiles of glucosamine sulfate and chondroitin sulfate were not reviewed in the meta-analysis.[90]
- In 2000, Denham and Newton conducted a meta-analysis of 15 randomized double-blind placebo controlled trials of glucosamine and chondroitin either given as separate agents or together for patients with osteoarthritis of the knee or hip.[51] Trials were included if they lasted longer than 4 weeks and used standardized osteoarthritis outcome measures. Two independent reviewers examined outcomes, quality, and financial sponsorship of the studies, and disagreements were resolved by discussion. Pooled effect size was calculated by dividing the difference in mean outcomes between treatment group and control group by the standard deviation of the outcome value in the control group. The resulting effect measure combined disability outcomes with pain outcomes; the primary outcome was improvement of symptoms at 4 weeks, measured by either a pain scale or a disability index. None of the studies had affiliation with government agencies or companies that might bias the results toward positive trials. Glucosamine therapy was reported to be associated with an effect size of 0.44 (95% CI, 0.24 to 0.64). Limitations of this meta-analysis include the poor design and reporting of the included trials and pooling of heterogeneous outcomes.
- In 2000, Kreder conducted a meta-analysis of controlled trials published between 1966 and June 1999.[78] Studies were included in any language that compared oral/parenteral glucosamine sulfate or glucosamine hydrochloride with placebo, lasted for ≥4 weeks, were conducted in patients with knee or hip osteoarthritis, and measured outcomes using a standardized tool. Two reviewers used a 14-point scale to evaluate studies and to resolve any scoring discrepancies. Six studies were included in the pooled analysis, involving

911 patients. The combined results of this meta-analysis showed a moderate benefit of glucosamine, with an effect size of 0.44 (95% CI, 0.24 to 0.64). However, due to inconsistencies in the designs of included studies, the result cannot be considered definitive.

- In 2001, Towheed et al. conducted a systematic review and meta-analysis of randomized controlled trials evaluating the effectiveness and toxicity of glucosamine in the treatment of osteoarthritis, for the Cochrane Collaboration.[76] Literature searches were conducted in MEDLINE, Embase, and Current Contents through November 1999, as well as the Cochrane Library Controlled Trials Register. The authors also contacted experts and searched reference lists of randomized control trials and pertinent review articles. Trials were included if they evaluated effectiveness and safety of glucosamine in osteoarthritis, included a placebo or equivalent agent, and were single- or double-blinded. Sixteen trials met inclusion criteria, representing 11 published articles.[12,15,16,28-31,33,34,36,84] Outcomes data were pooled using standardized mean differences. The standardized mean difference for pain reduction comparing glucosamine to placebo was found to be 1.40, representing a clinically significant treatment benefit. The pooled standardized mean difference for pain reduction comparing glucosamine to placebo for Lequesne index was 0.63, and for pain reduction comparing glucosamine to nonsteroidal anti-inflammatory drugs (NSAIDs) was 0.86. The authors suggested that there is evidence that glucosamine is both effective and safe in the short-term management of osteoarthritis, but long-term safety and efficacy are not known. It is also unknown whether different glucosamine preparations/brands are equally effective: 81% of the included trials had some affiliation with Rotta, an Italian manufacturer of glucosamine sulfate.

- In 1999, Towheed and Anastassiades reported a systematic review and meta-analysis of randomized controlled trials evaluating the efficacy of glucosamine sulfate in the management of osteoarthritis.[77] The review consisted of a MEDLINE search from 1966 to 1997, in order to identify controlled trials published in English. A meta-analysis was conducted and effect sizes were used to synthesize data measured with various scales, and odds ratio was used to pool dichotomous data. The search strategy identified nine clinical trials with a mean duration of 5.4 weeks. In seven trials that compared glucosamine to placebo, glucosamine was reported as superior in all. In two trials that compared glucosamine to ibuprofen, glucosamine was superior in one and equivalent in one. The combined effect for pain relief comparing glucosamine to placebo in five studies was 1.23 (95% CI, 0.93 to 1.53). The odds ratio for overall favorable response comparing glucosamine to placebo, which was comparable in two trials, was 2.04 (95% CI, 1.38 to 3.02). A limitation of this analysis was the heterogeneity of included studies, in terms of osteoarthritis definitions and outcome measures used.

- Several additional reviews have been conducted, in most cases without quantitative analyses, and concluded with promising results of glucosamine in the treatment of osteoarthritis.[40,79-81] In general, the trials included have used heterogeneous measurement techniques, and the reviews have not utilized comprehensive, systematic search strategies or inclusion criteria.

Placebo-Controlled Trial

- Drovanti et al. performed a double-blind, randomized, placebo-controlled trial of glucosamine in 80 patients with osteoarthritis.[28] Patients received either oral glucosamine sulfate (500 mg three times daily) or placebo (lactose) for 30 days. The primary outcomes were evaluation of clinical signs of osteoarthritis after glucosamine use. Scores for articular pain, joint tenderness, swelling, and restriction of active movements were reported as significantly lower in glucosamine-treated patients at 14, 21, and 30 days ($p < 0.01$). At the study's end, physicians rated improvements in 29 of 40 glucosamine-treated patients as excellent or good overall, compared with 17 of 40 for placebo ($p = 0.005$).

Comparison Trials (Various Routes of Administration)

- Thie et al. compared glucosamine sulfate to ibuprofen in the management of osteoarthritis of the temporomandibular joint.[82] A total of 45 patients were randomized to receive glucosamine sulfate (500 mg) or ibuprofen (400 mg) three times daily for 3 months. The authors reported that both groups experienced improved pain scores and voluntary maximal mouth opening over baseline. At 3 months, 71% of those receiving glucosamine sulfate and 61% of those receiving ibuprofen displayed at least a 20% improvement in clinical response. Limitations include the lack of a placebo group.

- Leffler et al. reviewed the daily use of glucosamine hydrochloride (1500 mg), chondroitin sulfate (1200 mg), or manganese ascorbate (228 mg) in a 16-week crossover trial, to evaluate treatment of degenerative joint disease of the knee and low back.[52] Thirty-four males from the U.S. Navy diving and special warfare community, with a mean age of 44 years, were assessed. The primary outcomes included results of pain and functional questionnaires, physical examination scores, and running times. The authors reported that knee osteoarthritis symptoms were relieved as measured by summary disease score ($p = 0.05$), patient assessment of treatment ($p = 0.02$), visual analog scale for pain recorded at clinic visits ($p = 0.05$) and in a diary ($p = 0.02$), and physical examination score ($p = 0.01$). There was no difference noted in running times. The study did not report a benefit or exclude a benefit for spinal degenerative joint disease. Generalizability to clinical practice is limited by the small study size.

- Using virtually identical study designs, Crolle et al. and D'Ambrosio et al. published trials comparing the efficacy of glucosamine sulfate to piperazine/chlorbutanol, a combination registered in Italy as an anti-arthritic drug (without anti-inflammatory properties).[16,84] In each study, 30 patients with chronic osteoarthritis received either 400 mg of glucosamine sulfate daily (by intramuscular, intravenous, or intra-articular routes) for 1 week, followed by 2 weeks of oral glucosamine sulfate (500 mg three times daily), or an intramuscular daily injection of piperazine/chlorbutanol for 1 week, followed by 2 weeks of placebo. In both studies, semiquantitative scores of pain improved in both treatments during the first week; however, in the following 2 weeks, further significant reductions in pain scores were noted only in the glucosamine group. Crolle et al. reported results that were significantly different from placebo at 21 days in pain at rest, pain on active movement, and restricted function ($p < 0.01$).[84] D'Ambrosio et al. reported significant results in a decrease in mean symptoms scores with injectable glucosamine treatment by 58% ($p < 0.05$) and by a further 13% with oral maintenance therapy ($p < 0.01$) compared to piperazine/chlorbutanol.[16] Interpretation of the results from these studies is limited because of inconsistent routes of administration of glucosamine, inadequate descriptions of the severity of osteoarthritis, heterogeneous durations of disease, and the use of subjective measures of efficacy.

- Mund-Hoym conducted a randomized comparison trial comparing the efficacy of Dona 200-S (glucosamine sulfate) or phenylbutazone for arthritis-induced changes in spinal column flexibility and pain in 80 arthritic patients.[83] Subjects received either 400 mg of intramuscular Dona 200-S three times weekly followed by 250 mg orally 4 times weekly, or 600 mg of intramuscular phenylbutazone daily followed by 200 mg orally 4 times weekly or 250 mg twice daily. The authors reported improvements with both treatment therapies, although Dona 200-S demonstrated greater improvements in paravertebral tension and pain intensity over a shorter period of time than phenylbutazone. Limitations of this study included lack of a placebo arm, unclear randomization methods, and lack of blinding.

- Hehne et al. reported a comparative study in 68 patients with mild-to-moderate osteoarthritis.[85] Subjects were administered intra-articular injections of glucosamine sulfate or glycosaminoglycan polysulfate for 6 weeks to evaluate differences between the two forms of drug. The authors reported that therapy was successful in two-thirds of patients treated: Initial pain was eliminated or improved in 80% of subjects, "getting going" pain was reduced in approximately 64%, signs of synovitis decreased in 66%, and gait function and motility improved. In subjects with "mild" osteoarthritis, reduction of pain occurred in 90% of subjects using glucosamine, whereas glycosaminoglycan polysulfate was more beneficial in advanced cases. Limitations of this study include lack of a placebo arm and incomplete description of statistical analysis.

Case Series

- Tapadinhas et al. reported a study in 1208 patients with osteoarthritis to evaluate the clinical effectiveness of glucosamine sulfate.[41] Patients received 500 mg of glucosamine sulfate three times daily for 6 to 8 weeks. Outcomes were assessed by physician ratings. Physicians rated patient progress as being "good" in 694 patients (58.7%), "sufficient" in 426 (36%), and "insufficient" in 63 (5.3%). A significant proportion of patients (9.3%) who had not responded to previous treatments reportedly benefited from oral glucosamine sulfate treatment. However, lack of a control group and use of subjective assessment measures limit the clinical applicability of these results.

Dosing/Route of Administration

- Dettmer evaluated the effects of Arteparon (Glycosaminoglycan polysulfuric acid [GAGPS]) at different doses and routes of administration in 100 patients with osteoarthritis of the hip joint.[86] Subjects were divided evenly to receive either 6 intra-articular injections of 125 mg/0.5 mL of Arteparon or 10 intramuscular injections of 125 mg/0.5 mL of Arteparon. The results showed that there are no significant differences between dosing administration. and both groups reported positive results. The study has some flaws that limit the interpretation of the data, such as no explanation of blinding or randomization and the lack of statistical analysis.

Rheumatoid Arthritis
Summary

- There is not sufficient evidence from human trials to recommend for or against the use of glucosamine in the management of rheumatoid arthritis. Only limited, preliminary study has been conducted in this area.

Evidence

- Giordano et al. reported a double-blind crossover study in 15 rheumatoid arthritis patients to compare the actions of Teoremac (glucosamine) and indomethacin.[87] Total daily doses of 420 mg of Teoremac and 100 mg of indomethacin were administered for 14 days. Primary outcomes measured included number of painful joints on pressure and intensity of pain, number of painful joints on passive movement and intensity of pain, number of swollen joints and amount of swelling, and number of joints with functional limitation and the degree of functional limitation. The authors reported that both Teoremac and indomethacin significantly improved pain on pressure, with no difference between the two drugs ($p < 0.01$). Teoremac elicited a slightly better effect in pain on passive movement, whereas the action of both drugs on limitations of function and swelling were not significant ($p > 0.05$). Notably, the sample size in this trial may have been too small to detect significant differences in outcomes between groups. There was no placebo arm as a reference for comparisons of efficacy. Therefore, these results can only be considered preliminary.

Chronic Venous Insufficiency
Summary

- Chronic venous insufficiency is a syndrome characterized by failure of venous valves of the legs. Clinically this may include lower extremity edema, varicosities, pain, pruritus, atrophic skin changes, and ulcerations. The term is more commonly used in Europe than in the United States. Currently, there is a lack of sufficient evidence to recommend for or against the use of glucosamine in the treatment of this syndrome.

Evidence

- Gosetti et al. reported a case series evaluating daily doses of 48 mg, 72 mg, or 96 mg of Perclar (glycosaminoglycan) in the treatment of 60 patients diagnosed with venous insufficiency of the lower limbs.[88] After 30 days of treatment, the authors reported an improvement in edema and pain in all evaluable patients, reduction in venous pressure values in 97% of cases, and activation of the fibrinolytic system in 90% of patients. Although the results are promising, the lack of a placebo group limits the clinical applicability of these findings.

Inflammatory Bowel Disease
Summary

- There is a lack of sufficient evidence to recommend for or against the use of glucosamine in the treatment of inflammatory bowel disease (Crohn's disease or ulcerative colitis).

Evidence

- A pilot study was conducted in 12 children to evaluate the effects of N-acetyl glucosamine as an adjunct therapy in treating inflammatory bowel disease.[7] Subjects had all been diagnosed with refractory inflammatory bowel disease, 10 with Crohn's disease and 2 with ulcerative colitis. All patients were administered oral N-acetyl glucosamine, 3-6 g daily. The authors reported that 8 children demonstrated "clear improvements," while 4 required bowel resection. In 7 children diagnosed with symptomatic Crohn's strictures prior to the trial, 3 required surgery over a mean follow-up of >2.5 years, and endoscopic exam detected "improvements" in the other 4 children. Rectal administration of N-acetyl glucosamine was associated with remission in 2 cases, "clear improvement" in 3 cases, and no effect in 2 cases. Although the results are suggestive, the lack of a control group makes it difficult to distinguish these results from the possible natural history of these diseases. The small sample size, heterogeneous baseline diagnoses, subjective measures used, and lack of statistical analysis limit the clinical utility of these results.

Temporomandibular Joint (TMJ) Disorders

Summary

- There is a lack of sufficient evidence to recommend for or against the use of glucosamine (or the combination of glucosamine and chondroitin) in the treatment of temporomandibular joint disorders.

Evidence

- Shankland conducted a study in 50 patients diagnosed with TMJ disorders to evaluate the clinical effects of treatment with chondroitin and glucosamine.[53] Subjects all received a mixture of 1200 mg of chondroitin sulfate-4 and chondroitin sulfate-6 twice daily, 1600 mg of glucosamine hydrochloride twice daily, and 1000 mg of calcium ascorbate. Patients were instructed to take all three supplements together and were also permitted to take over-the-counter ibuprofen or aspirin if needed. The authors found that 40 patients (80%) reported decreased joint inflammation and pain, 1 patient (2%) reported worsened symptoms, 4 patients (8%) reported no change, and 5 patients (10%) did not comply with the study protocol. These preliminary results are limited by the lack of a control group, use of a combination therapy, and subjective outcomes measurements.

FORMULARY: BRANDS USED IN CLINICAL TRIALS/ THIRD-PARTY TESTING

Brands Used in Statistically Significant Clinical Trials

- Glucosamine sulfate preparations manufactured by Rotta Research Group, Monza, Italy: Dona,[13,15,30] Viartril,[12] Viartril-S,[13,34] Xicil.[13]
- Glucosamine/chondroitin preparations manufactured by Nutramax: Cosamin,[52] CosaminDS.[50]

Third-Party Testing

- **Consumer Reports (January 2002):** Out of 19 products that were tested, most were well standardized and were reported to deliver at least 90% of the amount of glucosamine or chondroitin as labeled.

References

1. Hoffer LJ, Kaplan LN, Hamadeh MJ, et al. Sulfate could mediate the therapeutic effect of glucosamine sulfate. Metabolism 2001;50(7):767-770.
2. Rao JK, Mihaliak K, Kroenke K, et al. Use of complementary therapies for arthritis among patients of rheumatologists. Ann Intern Med 1999;131(6):409-416.
3. Zupanets IA, Drogovoz SM, Bezdetko NV, et al. [The influence of glucosamine on the antiexudative effect of nonsteroidal anti-inflammatory agents]. Farmakol Toksikol 1991;54(2):61-63.
4. McCarty MF. Glucosamine may retard atherogenesis by promoting endothelial production of heparan sulfate proteoglycans. Med Hypotheses 1997;48(3):245-251.
5. Russell AL. Glucosamine in osteoarthritis and gastrointestinal disorders: an exemplar of the need for a paradigm shift. Med Hypotheses 1998;51(4):347-349.
6. McCarty MF. Glucosamine for psoriasis? Med Hypotheses 1997;48(5):437-441.
7. Salvatore S, Heuschkel R, Tomlin S, et al. A pilot study of N-acetyl glucosamine, a nutritional substrate for glycosaminoglycan synthesis, in paediatric chronic inflammatory bowel disease. Aliment Pharmacol Ther 2000;14(12):1567-1579.
8. Anderson PM, Schroeder G, Skubitz KM. Oral glutamine reduces the duration and severity of stomatitis after cytotoxic cancer chemotherapy. Cancer 1998;83(7):1433-1439.
9. Russell AL, McCarty MF. Glucosamine for migraine prophylaxis? Med Hypotheses 2000;55(3):195-198.
10. Kulling D, Vournakis JN, Woo S, et al. Endoscopic injection of bleeding esophageal varices with a poly-N-acetyl glucosamine gel formulation in the canine portal hypertension model. Gastrointest Endosc 1999;49(6):764-771.
11. Ma L, Rudert WA, Harnaha J, et al. Immunosuppressive effects of glucosamine. J Biol Chem 2002;277(42):39343-39349.
12. Vajaradul Y. Double-blind clinical evaluation of intra-articular glucosamine in outpatients with gonarthrosis. Clin Ther 1981;3(5):336-343.
13. Reginster JY, Deroisy R, Rovati LC, et al. Long-term effects of glucosamine sulphate on osteoarthritis progression: a randomised, placebo-controlled clinical trial. Lancet 2001;357(9252):251-256.
14. Pavelka K, Gatterova J, Olejarova M, et al. Glucosamine sulfate use and delay of progression of knee osteoarthritis: a 3-year, randomized, placebo-controlled, double-blind study. Arch Intern Med 2002;162(18):2113-2123.
15. Reichelt A, Forster KK, Fischer M, et al. Efficacy and safety of intramuscular glucosamine sulfate in osteoarthritis of the knee. A randomised, placebo-controlled, double-blind study. Arzneimittelforschung 1994;44(1):75-80.
16. D'Ambrosio E, Casa B, Bompani R, et al. Glucosamine sulphate: a controlled clinical investigation in arthrosis. Pharmatherapeutica 1981;2(8):504-508.
17. Russell AI, McCarty MF. Glucosamine in osteoarthritis. Lancet 1999;354(9190):1641-1642.
18. Holmang A, Nilsson C, Niklasson M, et al. Induction of insulin resistance by glucosamine reduces blood flow but not interstitial levels of either glucose or insulin. Diabetes 1999;48(1):106-111.
19. Balkan B, Dunning BE. Glucosamine inhibits glucokinase in vitro and produces a glucose-specific impairment of in vivo insulin secretion in rats. Diabetes 1994;43(10):1173-1179.
20. Virkamaki A, Yki-Jarvinen H. Allosteric regulation of glycogen synthase and hexokinase by glucosamine-6-phosphate during glucosamine-induced insulin resistance in skeletal muscle and heart. Diabetes 1999;48(5):1101-1107.
21. Baron AD, Zhu JS, Zhu JH, et al. Glucosamine induces insulin resistance in vivo by affecting GLUT 4 translocation in skeletal muscle. Implications for glucose toxicity. J Clin Invest 1995;96(6):2792-2801.
22. Giaccari A, Morviducci L, Zorretta D, et al. In vivo effects of glucosamine on insulin secretion and insulin sensitivity in the rat: possible relevance to the maladaptive responses to chronic hyperglycaemia. Diabetologia 1995;38(5):518-524.
23. Nelson BA, Robinson KA, Buse MG. High glucose and glucosamine induce insulin resistance via different mechanisms in 3T3-L1 adipocytes. Diabetes 2000;49(6):981-991.
24. Shankar RR, Zhu JS, Baron AD. Glucosamine infusion in rats mimics the beta-cell dysfunction of non-insulin-dependent diabetes mellitus. Metabolism 1998;47(5):573-577.
25. Monauni T, Zenti MG, Cretti A, et al. Effects of glucosamine infusion on insulin secretion and insulin action in humans. Diabetes 2000;49(6):926-935.
26. Pouwels MJ, Jacobs JR, Span PN, et al. Short-term glucosamine infusion does not affect insulin sensitivity in humans. J Clin Endocrinol Metab 2001;86(5):2099-2103.
27. Scroggie DA, Albright A, Harris MD. The effect of glucosamine-chondroitin supplementation on glycosylated hemoglobin levels in patients with type 2 diabetes mellitus: a placebo-controlled, double-blinded, randomized clinical trial. Arch Intern Med 2003;163(13):1587-1590.
28. Drovanti A, Bignamini AA, Rovati AL. Therapeutic activity of oral glucosamine sulfate in osteoarthrosis: a placebo-controlled double-blind investigation. Clin Ther 1980;3(4):260-272.
29. Muller-Fassbender H, Bach GL, Haase W, et al. Glucosamine sulfate compared to ibuprofen in osteoarthritis of the knee. Osteoarthritis Cartilage 1994;2(1):61-69.
30. Noack W, Fischer M, Förster KK, et al. Glucosamine sulfate in osteoarthritis of the knee. Osteoarthritis Cartilage 1994;2(1):51-59.
31. Pujalte JM, Llavore EP, Ylescupidez FR. Double-blind clinical evaluation of oral glucosamine sulphate in the basic treatment of osteoarthrosis. Curr Med Res Opin 1980;7(2):110-114.
32. Rovati LC, Giacovelli G, Annefeld M, et al. A large, randomised, placebo controlled, double-blind study of glucosamine sulfate vs. piroxicam and vs. their association, on the kinetics of the symptomatic effect in knee osteoarthritis [abstract]. Osteoarthritis Cartilage 1994;2(Suppl 1):56.
33. Lopes VA. Double-blind clinical evaluation of the relative efficacy of ibuprofen and glucosamine sulphate in the management of osteoarthrosis of the knee in out-patients. Curr Med Res Opin 1982;8(3):145-149.
34. Qiu GX, Gao SN, Giacovelli G, et al. Efficacy and safety of glucosamine sulfate versus ibuprofen in patients with knee osteoarthritis. Arzneimittelforschung 1998;48(5):469-474.
35. Reginster JY. Review: glucosamine and chondroitin improve outcomes in osteoarthritis, but the magnitude of effect is unclear. ACP Journal Club 2000;(133):58.
36. Houpt JB, McMillan R, Wein C, et al. Effect of glucosamine hydrochloride in the treatment of pain of osteoarthritis of the knee. J Rheumatol 1999;26(11):2423-2430.
37. Deal CL, Moskowitz RW. Nutraceuticals as therapeutic agents in

osteoarthritis. The role of glucosamine, chondroitin sulfate, and collagen hydrolysate. Rheum Dis Clin North Am 1999;25(2):379-395.

38. Matheu V, Gracia Bara MT, Pelta R, et al. Immediate-hypersensitivity reaction to glucosamine sulfate. Allergy 1999;54(6):643.

39. Tallia AF, Cardone DA. Asthma exacerbation associated with glucosamine-chondroitin supplement. J Am Board Fam Pract 2002;15(6):481-484.

40. Barclay TS, Tsourounis C, McCart GM. Glucosamine. Ann Pharmacother 1998;32(5):574-579.

41. Tapadinhas MJ, Rivera IC, Bignamini AA. Oral glucosamine sulphate in the management of arthrosis: report on a multi-centre open investigation in Portugal. Pharmatherapeutica 1982;3(3):157-168.

42. Ajiboye R, Harding JJ. The non-enzymic glycosylation of bovine lens proteins by glucosamine and its inhibition by aspirin, ibuprofen and glutathione. Exp Eye Res 1989;49(1):31-41.

43. Danao-Camara T. Potential side effects of treatment with glucosamine and chondroitin. Arthritis Rheum 2000;43(12):2853.

44. Swinburne LM. Glucosamine sulphate and osteoarthritis. Lancet 2001; 357(9268):1617.

45. Weimann G, Lubenow N, Selleng K, et al. Glucosamine sulfate does not crossreact with the antibodies of patients with heparin-induced thrombocytopenia. Eur J Haematol 2001;66(3):195-199.

46. Rovati LC, Annefeld M, Giacovelli G, et al. Glucosamine in osteoarthritis. Lancet 1999;354(9190):1640-1642.

47. Levin RM, Krieger NN, Winzler RJ. Glucosamine and acetylglucosamine tolerance in man. J Lab Clin Med 1961;58(6):927-932.

48. Setnikar I, Giacchetti C, Zanolo G. Pharmacokinetics of glucosamine in the dog and in man. Arzneimittelforschung 1986;36(4):729-735.

49. Weiden S, Wood IJ. The fate of glucosamine hydrochloride injected intravenously in man. J Clin Pathol 1958;11:343-349.

50. Das A Jr, Hammad TA. Efficacy of a combination of FCHG49 glucosamine hydrochloride, TRH122 low molecular weight sodium chondroitin sulfate and manganese ascorbate in the management of knee osteoarthritis. Osteoarthritis Cartilage 2000;8(5):343-350.

51. Denham AC, Newton WP. Are glucosamine and chondroitin effective in treating osteoarthritis? J Fam Pract 2000;49(6):571-572.

52. Leffler CT, Philippi AF, Leffler SG, et al. Glucosamine, chondroitin, and manganese ascorbate for degenerative joint disease of the knee or low back: a randomized, double-blind, placebo-controlled pilot study. Mil Med 1999;164(2):85-91.

53. Shankland WE. The effects of glucosamine and chondroitin sulfate on osteoarthritis of the TMJ: a preliminary report of 50 patients. Journal of Craniomandibular Practice 1998;16(4):230-235.

54. Vacha J, Pesakova V, Krajickova J, et al. Effect of glycosaminoglycan polysulphate on the metabolism of cartilage ribonucleic acid. Arzneimittelforschung 1984;34(5):607-609.

55. Bassleer C, Henrotin Y, Franchimont P. In-vitro evaluation of drugs proposed as chondroprotective agents. Int J Tissue React 1992;14(5):231-241.

56. Jimenez SA, Dodge GR. The effects of glucosamine sulfate (GSO$_4$) on human chondrocyte gene expression [abstract]. Osteoarthritis Cartilage 1997;5:72.

57. Rindone JP, Hiller D, Collacott E, et al. Randomized, controlled trial of glucosamine for treating osteoarthritis of the knee. West J Med 2000; 172(2):91-94.

58. Vanharanta H. Glycosaminoglycan polysulphate treatment in experimental osteoarthritis in rabbits. Scand J Rheumatol 1983;12(3):225-230.

59. Setnikar I, Pacini MA, Revel L. Antiarthritic effects of glucosamine sulfate studied in animal models. Arzneimittelforschung 1991;41(5):542-545.

60. Setnikar I, Cereda R, Pacini MA, et al. Antireactive properties of glucosamine sulfate. Arzneimittelforschung 1991;41(2):157-161.

61. Johnson KA, Hulse DA, Hart RC, et al. Effects of an orally administered mixture of chondroitin sulfate, glucosamine hydrochloride and manganese ascorbate on synovial fluid chondroitin sulfate 3B3 and 7D4 epitope in a canine cruciate ligament transection model of osteoarthritis. Osteoarthritis Cartilage 2001;9(1):14-21.

62. Kalbhen DA. [Experimental confirmation of the antiarthritic activity of glycosaminoglycan polysulfate]. Z Rheumatol 1983;42(4):178-184.

63. Setnikar I, Palumbo R, Canali S, et al. Pharmacokinetics of glucosamine in man. Arzneimittelforschung 1993;43(10):1109-1113.

64. Talent JM, Gracy RW. Pilot study of oral polymeric N-acetyl-D-glucosamine as a potential treatment for patients with osteoarthritis. Clin Ther 1996; 18(6):1184-1190.

65. Setnikar I, Giachetti C, Zanolo G. Absorption, distribution and excretion of radioactivity after a single intravenous or oral administration of [14C] glucosamine to the rat. Pharmatherapeutica 1984;3(8):538-550.

66. Richy F, Bruyere O, Ethgen O, et al. Structural and symptomatic efficacy of glucosamine and chondroitin in knee osteoarthritis: a comprehensive meta-analysis. Arch Intern Med 2003;163(13):1514-1522.

67. McAlindon TE, LaValley MP, Gulin JP, et al. Glucosamine and chondroitin for treatment of osteoarthritis: a systematic quality assessment and meta-analysis. JAMA 2000;283(11):1469-1475.

68. Reginster JY, Deroisy R, Paul l, et al. Glucosamine sulfate significantly reduces progression of the knee osteoarthritis over 3 years: a large random-ised, placebo-controlled, double-blind, prospective trial. Arthritis Rheum 1999;42(9):S400.

69. Pavelka K, Gatterova J, Olejarova M, et al. Glucosamine sulfate decreases progression of knee osteoarthritis in a long-term randomized placebo-controlled, independent, confirmatory trial. Arthritis Rheum 2000;43(9 (suppl)):S384.

70. Hughes RA, Chertsey AJ. A randomised, double-blind, placebo-controlled trial of glucosamine to control pain in osteoarthritis of the knee [abstract]. Arthritis Rheum 2000;43(9 (suppl)):S384.

71. Hughes R, Carr A. A randomized, double-blind, placebo-controlled trial of glucosamine sulphate as an analgesic in osteoarthritis of the knee. Rheumatology (Oxford) 2002;41(3):279-284.

72. Förster KK, Schmid K, Rovati LC, et al. Longer-term treatment of mild-to-moderate osteoarthritis of the knee with glucosamine sulfate: a randomized, controlled, double-blind clinical study [abstract]. Eur J Clin Pharmacol 1996;50(6):542.

73. Rovati LC. Clinical research in osteoarthritis: design and results of short-term and long-term trials with disease-modifying drugs. Int J Tissue React 1992;14(5):243-251.

74. Raatikainen T, Vaananen K, Tamelander G. Effect of glycosaminoglycan polysulfate on chondromalacia patellae. A placebo-controlled 1-year study. Acta Orthop Scand 1990;61(5):443-448.

75. Ishikawa K, Kitagawa T, Tanaka T, et al. [Clinical testing of intra-articularly injected glycosaminoglycan polysulfate in gonarthrosis (a controlled multicenter double-blind study)]. Z Orthop Ihre Grenzgeb 1982;120(5): 708-716.

76. Towheed TE, Anastassiades TP, Shea B, et al. Glucosamine therapy for treating osteoarthritis (Cochrane Review). Cochrane Database Syst Rev. 2001;(1):CD002946.

77. Towheed TE, Anastassiades TP. Glucosamine therapy for osteoarthritis. J Rheumatol 1999;26(11):2294-2297.

78. Kreder HJ. Glucosamine and chondroitin were found to improve outcomes in patients with osteoarthritis. J Bone Joint Surg Am 2000;82(9):1323.

79. Gottlieb MS. Conservative management of spinal osteoarthritis with glucosamine sulfate and chiropractic treatment. J Manipulative Physiol Ther 1997;20(6):400-414.

80. da Camara CC, Dowless GV. Glucosamine sulfate for osteoarthritis. Ann Pharmacother 1998;32(5):580-587.

81. Brief AA, Maurer SG, Di Cesare PE. Use of glucosamine and chondroitin sulfate in the management of osteoarthritis. J Am Acad Orthop Surg 2001;9(2):71-78.

82. Thie NM, Prasad NG, Major PW. Evaluation of glucosamine sulfate compared to ibuprofen for the treatment of temporomandibular joint osteoarthritis: a randomized double blind controlled 3 month clinical trial. J Rheumatol 2001;28(6):1347-1355.

83. Mund-Hoym WD. Konservative Behandlung von Wirbelsäulenarthrosen mit Glukosaminsulfat und Phenylbutazon. Eine kontrollierte Studie. Therapiewoche 1980;30:5922-5928.

84. Crolle G, D'Este E. Glucosamine sulphate for the management of arthrosis: a controlled clinical investigation. Curr Med Res Opin 1980;7(2): 104-109.

85. Hehne HJ, Blasius K, Ernst HU. [Therapy of gonarthrosis using chondro-protective substances. Prospective comparative study of glucosamine sulphate and glycosaminoglycan polysulphate]. Fortschr Med 1984; 102(24):676-682.

86. Dettmer N. [The therapeutic effect of glycosaminoglycan polysulfate (Arteparon) in arthroses depending on the mode of administration (intraarticular or intramuscular)]. Z Rheumatol 1979;38(5-6):163-181.

87. Giordano M, Capelli L, Chianese U. The therapeutic activity of 1-(p-chlorobenzoyl)-5-methoxy-2-methylindole-3-acetic acid monohydrate glucosamide in rheumatoid arthritis (double blind trial). Arzneimittelforschung 1975;25(3):435-437.

88. Gossetti B, Gattuso R, Irace L, et al. [Venous insufficiency of the legs. Pharmacologic treatment with glycosamine-glycan (Perclar)]. Minerva Med 1986;77(41):1915-1918.

89. Rovati LC. The clinical profile of glucosamine sulfate as a selective symptom modifying drug in osteoarthritis: current data and perspectives. Osteoarthritis Cartilage 1997;5:72.

90. osteoarthritis: evidence is widely touted but incomplete. JAMA 2000; 283(11):1483-1484.

91. Bruyere O, Honore A, Ethgen O, et al. Correlation between radiographic severity of knee osteoarthritis and future disease progression. Results from a 3-year prospective, placebo-controlled study evaluating the effect of glucosamine sulfate. Osteoarthritis Cartilage 2003;11(1):1-5.

92. Braham R, Dawson B, Goodman C. The effect of glucosamine supplemen-tation on people experiencing regular knee pain. Br J Sports Med 2003; 37(1):45-49.

93. Cohen M, Wolfe R, Mai T, et al. A randomized, double blind, placebo con-trolled trial of a topical cream containing glucosamine sulfate, chondroitin sulfate, and camphor for osteoarthritis of the knee. J Rheumatol 2003; 30(3):523-528.

94. Wein CR, Houpt JB, McMillan R, et al. Open trial of glucosamine hydrochloride (GHCl) in the treatment of pain of osteoarthritis of the knee. J Rheumatol 1998;25(Supplement 52):8.

95. Vajranetra P. Clinical study of glucosamine compounds for osteoarthrosis of knee joints. J Med Assoc Thai 1984;67(7):409-418.

Goldenseal

(Hydrastis canadensis L.)*

SYNONYMS/COMMON NAMES/RELATED SUBSTANCES

- Berberine, berberine bisulfate, curcuma, eye balm, eye root, golden root, goldensiegel, goldsiegel, ground raspberry, guldsegl, hydrastidis rhizoma, hydrophyllum, Indian dye, Indian paint, Indian plant, Indian turmeric, jaundice root, kanadische gelbwurzel, kurkuma, Ohio curcuma, orange root, tumeric root, warnera, wild curcuma, wild turmeric, yellow eye, yellow Indian plant, yellow paint, yellow paint root, yellow puccoon, yellow root, yellow seal, yellow wort.
- **Note:** Goldenseal is sometimes referred to as "Indian turmeric" or "curcuma" but should not be confused with turmeric (*Curcuma longa* L.).

CLINICAL BOTTOM LINE
Background

- Goldenseal is currently one of the five top-selling herbal products in the United States. However, little scientific evidence regarding its efficacy or toxicity is available. It can be found in dietary supplements, eardrops, feminine cleansing products, cold/flu remedies, allergy remedies, laxatives, and digestive aids. Goldenseal is often found in combination with echinacea in treatments for upper respiratory infections, and is suggested to enhance the effects of echinacea; however, the effects when these agents are combined are scientifically unproven. Goldenseal preparations have also been used popularly because it is believed that detection of illicit drugs in urine may be masked by use of the herb, although data are scant in this area.
- The popularity of goldenseal has led to a higher demand for the herb than cultivation can supply. This high demand has led to the substitution of other isoquinoline alkaloid-containing herbs, including Chinese goldthread (*Coptis chinensis* Fransch.) and Oregon grape (*Mahonia aquifolium* [Pursh] Nutt.), that do not contain exactly the same isoquinoline alkaloids, and consequently may not share the same activity, as goldenseal.[1]
- Efficacy studies regarding goldenseal are limited to one of its main constituents, berberine salts, and there are few published clinical studies evaluating the use of goldenseal itself in humans. Due to the small amount of berberine actually available from goldenseal preparations (0.5% to 6%), it is difficult to extrapolate the available evidence regarding berberine salts to the use of goldenseal. Thus, there is insufficient scientific evidence to support the use of goldenseal in humans for any indication. Recent promising evidence suggests possible benefits in patients with chronic heart failure.

Scientific Evidence for Common/Studied Uses	Grade*
Chloroquine-resistant malaria	C
Heart failure	C
Immunostimulant	C
Infectious diarrhea	C
Narcotic concealment (urinalysis)	C
Trachoma (*Chlamydia trachomatis* eye infection)	C
Upper respiratory tract infection	C

*Key to grades: *A:* Strong scientific evidence for this use; *B:* Good scientific evidence for this use; *C:* Unclear scientific evidence for this use; *D:* Fair scientific evidence against this use (it may not work); *F:* Strong scientific evidence against this use (it likely does not work). For a more detailed explanation of efficacy criteria, see "Natural Standard Evidence-Based Validated Grading Rationale" in the Introduction.

Historical or Theoretical Indications That Lack Sufficient Evidence

- Abortifacient, acne, AIDS, alcoholic liver disease, amoebiasis,[2-4] anal fissures, anesthetic, anorexia, antiarrhythmic,[5-10] antibacterial,[11,12] anticoagulant, antifungal,[13,14] antiheparin, antihistamine, antihyperglycemic, antihypertensive, anti-inflammatory,[15] antineoplastic,[16-18] antipyretic,[19] antiseptic, anxiety, appetite stimulant, arthritis,[15] asthma, astringent, atherosclerosis, athlete's foot, bile flow stimulant, boils, bronchitis, cancer,[20,21] candidiasis, canker sores, cardiac arrhythmias, cervicitis, chickenpox,[22-24] cholecystitis, chronic fatigue syndrome, circulatory stimulant, cirrhosis, cleansing vital organs, cold sores, colitis, common cold, congestion, conjunctivitis, constipation, cough, Crohn's disease, croup, cystic fibrosis, cystitis, dandruff, deafness, diabetes mellitus (type 2),[25-28] diarrhea,[29,30] digestive disorders, diphtheria, diuretic, dysmenorrhea, dyspepsia, eczema, expectorant, eyewash, fistula, flatulence, gallstones, gangrene, gastritis, gastroenteritis,[31] genitourinary disorders, giardiasis,[32,33] gingivitis, headache, *Helicobacter pylori* infection,[34] hepatic congestion, hemorrhage, hemorrhoids, hepatitis, herpes labialis, herpetic uveitis, hiatal hernia, hypercholesterolemia, hypertyraminemia,[35] hypoglycemia, immunostimulant,[36,37] impetigo, influenza, insulin potentiation, jaundice, keratitis, leishmaniasis,[38-42] leukopenia,[37] leukorrhea, lupus erythematosus, menorrhagia, morning sickness, mouthwash, muscle pain, night sweats, obesity, osteoporosis,[43] otorrhea, oxytocic agent, peptic ulcer disease, periodontal disease, pneumonia, postpartum hemorrhage, premenstrual syndrome, prostatitis, pruritus, rhinitis, psoriasis,[44] ringworm, sciatica, scratchy throat, seborrhea, sedative, sinusitis, skin infections, stimulantt, stomachache, strep throat, syphilis, tetanus,[45] thrombocytopenia,[46] thrush, tinnitus, tonsillitis, trichomoniasis, tuberculosis,[47] tumors, urinary disorders, uterine inflammation, uterine stimulant,[48,49] whooping cough, vaginal irritation, vaginitis, varicose veins,[50] ventricular tachyarrhythmias.[51,52]

Expert Opinion and Folkloric Precedent

- Goldenseal was first used in the United States by Native Americans as a diuretic and stimulant, to treat stomach ulcers, and as a wash for irritated eyes and mouth sores. Cherokee, Iroquois, Crow, Seminole and Blackfoot tribes used goldenseal as a dye, paint, and wash. It was noted in

1804 by settlers who used it to increase appetite, to facilitate digestion, and as a mouth and eye wash.

- Common traditional medicinal uses of goldenseal include bronchitis, cystitis, and as a digestive aid. The use of goldenseal to treat the common cold is a recent development, and this was not a traditional use of this herb. It has been referred to as "king of the mucous membranes" because of its use for inflammation of mucosal tissue.

Safety Summary

- **Possibly safe:** When used short-term in recommended doses. There is little available safety and efficacy information regarding goldenseal use in humans.
- **Possibly unsafe:** When used long-term or in higher than recommended doses.
- **Possibly unsafe:** When taken by patients with cardiovascular disease or at risk of developing arrhythmias, because berberine, one of the active constituents of goldenseal, has been associated with ventricular tachycardia/torsades de pointes in patients with heart failure.[53]
- **Likely unsafe:** When administered to infants with increased bilirubin levels or individuals with glucose-6-phosphate deficiency, because berberine, an active constituent found in goldenseal, has been shown to displace bilirubin from albumin in both *in vitro* and animal studies, resulting in an increase in serum total and direct bilirubin concentrations.[54]

DOSING/TOXICOLOGY
General

- Recommended doses are based on historical practice or clinical trials, although there is a paucity of scientific research evaluating the safety or efficacy of goldenseal. With natural products, the optimal doses needed to balance efficacy and safety often have not been determined. Formulation and preparation methods may vary from manufacturer to manufacturer, and from batch to batch of a specific product made by a single manufacturer. Because often the active components of a product are not known, standardization may not be possible, and the clinical effects of different brands may not be comparable.

Standardization

- Published analyses of various commercially available goldenseal-containing products by high-performance liquid chromatography have found no consistency in the content of hydrastine and berberine, the proposed active constituents of goldenseal, with hydrastine concentrations ranging from 0% to 2.93% and berberine concentrations ranging from 0.82% to 5.86%.[55,56] Utilizing spectrophotometric analysis, a different study reported the mean alkaloid concentrations of a goldenseal tincture to include hydrastine 0.223 g %, canadine 0.056 g %, and berberine 0.263 g %.[57]
- Some sources have noted standardization to isoquinoline alkaloids (5% to 10% total alkaloids, including hydrastine, berberine, and canadine).
- Contaminants have been found in commercial goldenseal preparations.[58]

Dosing: Adult (18 Years and Older)
Goldenseal Dosing

- **Tablets/capsules:** 0.5 to 1 g of goldenseal three times daily has been used historically, although safety and efficacy have not been demonstrated in clinical trials. One trial administered 4 goldenseal capsules (535 mg each) (Nature's Herbs, Utah) plus 1 gallon of water in the evaluation of urinalysis narcotic concealment.[59]
- **Liquid/fluid extract (1:1 in 60% ethanol):** 0.3 to 1 mL taken three times daily has been used historically, although safety and efficacy have not been demonstrated in clinical trials.
- **Dried root:** 0.5 to 1 g taken three times daily as a decoction has been used historically, although safety and efficacy have not been demonstrated in clinical trials.
- **Tea:** One trial administered 1 gallon of Naturally Klean Herbal Tea (Klean Tea, Arizona) in the evaluation of urinalysis narcotic concealment.[59] Safety and efficacy have not been demonstrated.
- **Tincture (1:10 in 60% ethanol):** 2 to 4 mL taken three times daily has been used historically, although safety and efficacy have not been demonstrated in clinical trials.

Berberine Salts (Including Hydrochloride) Dosing

- **Tablets:** 100 to 200 mg of berberine hydrochloride four times daily [60,61] or a single 400-mg dose[62] has been used in clinical trials for the treatment of infectious diarrhea, although efficacy and safety have not been demonstrated definitively. Berberine sulfate is often used as well, and the hydrochloride and sulfate forms are generally considered interchangeably.

Dosing: Pediatric (Younger Than 18 Years)
Goldenseal Dosing

- Insufficient available evidence to recommend.

Berberine Dosing

- 25 to 50 mg of berberine four times daily has been studied in the management of diarrhea, although safety and efficacy have not been established.[63,64]

Toxicology

- Limited toxicology information is available for goldenseal itself. However, LD_{50} values have been determined for its active constituents, berberine and hydrastine. The LD_{50} of berberine sulfate has been found to be 205 mg/kg when administered intraperitoneally in rats[3] and 24.3 mg/kg in mice.[65] In mice, the oral LD_{50} dose is 329 mg/kg of berberine and the subcutaneous LD_{50} dose is 18 mg/kg.[66] In rats, the intramuscular and oral LD_{50} doses of berberine sulfate have been found to be 14.5 mg/kg and >1000 mg/kg, respectively.[67] The LD_{50} dose of intraperitoneal hydrastine in rats is 104 mg/kg.[66]
- Although not from goldenseal, berberine has been shown to displace bilirubin from albumin both *in vitro* and in animal studies, resulting in an increase in serum total and direct bilirubin concentrations.[54] This effect may also occur with the use of goldenseal and theoretically may lead to brain damage in infants with increased bilirubin levels or glucose-6-phosphate deficiency.
- Toxic doses of berberine, an active constituent of goldenseal, may cause convulsions and irritation of the upper gastrointestinal tract when taken orally; however, the dose range for this toxicity is not clear.[68]
- **Adulteration:** The popularity of goldenseal has led to a higher demand for the herb than cultivation can supply. This high demand has led to the substitution of other alkaloid-containing herbs, including Chinese goldthread (*Coptis chinensis* Fransch.) and Oregon grape (*Mahonia aquifolium* [Pursh] Nutt.), that do not contain the exact same isoquinoline alkaloids as goldenseal and may not share

G

the same activity as goldenseal.[1] Cases of jaundice have been associated with the use of a traditional Chinese patent formula that included Chinese goldthread. Adulteration of goldenseal products and the substitution of other berberine-containing herbs may increase the risk of serious toxicity or adverse events.

ADVERSE EFFECTS/PRECAUTIONS/CONTRAINDICATIONS
Allergy

- Known allergy/hypersensitivity to goldenseal (*Hydrastis canadensis*) or any of its constituents, including berberine and hydrastine.

Adverse Effects/Postmarket Surveillance

- **General:** Goldenseal has been reported to cause drying of mucous membranes, nausea, vomiting, hypertension, respiratory failure, and paresthesias; however, clinical evidence of such adverse effects is not prominent in the literature.[69] Adverse effects including headache, hypotension, bradycardia, nausea, vomiting, and leukopenia have been reported with the use of berberine (an active constituent of goldenseal) in both animals and humans.[32,53,63,70-72]
- **Dermatologic:** Photosensitivity has been reported in a 32-year-old woman taking a combination herbal preparation containing goldenseal as well as ginseng and bee pollen.[73] The contribution of goldenseal or any of its constituents to this reaction is not clear, and this is not a commonly reported adverse effect of goldenseal. Traditionally, goldenseal is said to commonly cause drying of mucous membranes at therapeutic doses and to elicit skin and mucous membrane ulcers with topical or internal use of large doses. Literature review reveals no published cases.
- **Neurologic/CNS:** Headache was experienced by three of 25 subjects taking berberine (5 mg/kg daily) for the treatment of giardiasis.[32] Paresthesias have been reported anecdotally in association with large doses of goldenseal. Literature review reveals no available published cases.
- **Cardiovascular:** Numerous animal studies have shown berberine, a constituent of goldenseal, to elicit transient hypotension and bradycardia, although these effects may or may not occur in humans.[70] In contrast, the constituent hydrastine may theoretically induce vasoconstriction, resulting in hypertension. Marin-Neto et al. administered intravenous berberine at a rate of 0.2 mg/kg/min to twelve patients with congestive heart failure, and four subjects developed ventricular tachycardia (torsades de pointes).[53]
- **Respiratory/pulmonary:** Respiratory failure has been reported anecdotally in association with large doses of goldenseal. Traditionally, goldenseal is said to commonly cause drying of mucous membranes at therapeutic doses. Literature review reveals no available published cases.
- **Gastrointestinal:** Nausea and vomiting have been reported with the use of goldenseal. Three of 25 subjects taking 5 mg/kg of the goldenseal constituent berberine daily for the treatment of giardia infection experienced abdominal distention.[32] Three out of 50 children taking berberine for the treatment of diarrhea developed vomiting after berberine ingestion.[63] One subject of 82 receiving pyrimethamine and berberine for the treatment of chloroquine-resistant malaria experienced nausea and abdominal discomfort during the 3-day study period.[72] Anecdotally, large doses of goldenseal have been associated with mucous membrane irritation and possible exacerbation of peptic ulcer disease (via increased acid production), although literature review reveals no published cases in this area.

- **Hematologic:** In theory, the use of goldenseal or berberine could increase the risk of bleeding, based on *in vitro* and animal research reporting inhibition of platelet aggregation.[74,75] However, the literature review reveals no reports of bleeding in humans. Berberine has been reported to stimulate platelet formation in human subjects with thrombocytopenia.[46] One practitioner observed leukopenia in patients using goldenseal for periods of 2 to 3 weeks.[71]

Precautions/Warnings/Contraindications

- Use cautiously in patients with cardiovascular disease. Goldenseal has been shown to elicit hypotension and bradycardia in animals.[65] Berberine, a constituent of goldenseal, has been associated with ventricular arrhythmias in subjects with congestive heart failure.[53]

Pregnancy and Lactation

- The oral administration of goldenseal or its active constituent hydrastine may induce labor and should not be use by pregnant women.[49] Berberine-containing herbs such as goldenseal have been suggested historically as abortifacients, although literature review reveals no available published cases in this area. Adulteration of goldenseal preparations with Chinese goldthread (*Coptis chinensis*) was associated with multiple cases of kernicterus in Asia in the 1970s and 1980s.
- Use is not recommended during breastfeeding, due to lack of sufficient data.

INTERACTIONS
Goldenseal/Drug Interactions

- **Antiplatelet agents, nonsteroidal anti-inflammatory drugs (NSAIDs), anticoagulants:** In theory, the use of goldenseal or its constituent berberine could increase the risk of bleeding, based on *in vitro* and animal research reporting inhibition of platelet aggregation.[74,75] However, literature review reveals no reports of bleeding in humans and no systematic evaluation of patients using berberine with other anticlotting agents.
- **Beta-blockers:** Timolol has been shown to partially inhibit the smooth muscle relaxant activity of a goldenseal alcoholic extract in animals, and this inhibition may also apply to other beta-blocking agents and their actions in humans.[76] Propranolol inhibits the increase in slow-response action potentials seen with berberine *in vitro*.[77]
- **Cytochrome P450-3A4 (CYP3A4)–metabolized drugs:** *In vitro*, goldenseal extract has been shown to weakly inhibit CYP3A4, and theoretically may increase serum levels of drugs metabolized by this enzyme.[78,79] This interaction has not been sufficiently evaluated in humans, although one study found no significant interaction between goldenseal root and the pharmacokinetics of the antiretroviral drug indinavir, which is metabolized by CYP3A4.[80] Nonetheless, goldenseal should be used cautiously in patients taking agents metabolized by CYP3A4.
- **L-Phenylephrine:** The goldenseal constituent berberine and L-phenylephrine have demonstrated additive effects in animals when administered concurrently.[81]
- **Neostigmine (Prostigmin):** Administration of the goldenseal constituent berberine has been shown to reverse the secretory effects of neostigmine in animals.[81] It is not clear if any interaction occurs in humans.
- **Tetracycline antibiotics:** One double-blind study found 100 mg of berberine (a constituent of goldenseal) to "decrease the efficacy" of tetracycline in the treatment of cholera.[60]

- **Yohimbine:** Berberine, an alkaloid present in goldenseal, has been shown to competitively inhibit the binding of yohimbine, which may or may not affect its pharmacologic actions when the two agents are administered concurrently.[82]
- **1,3-bis (2-chloroethyl)-1-nitosourea (BCNU):** Berberine and BCNU have been shown to have additive effects against human brain tumor cell lines *in vitro.*[18]

Goldenseal/Herb/Supplement Interactions

- **Anticoagulant herbs and supplements:** In theory, the use of goldenseal or its constituent berberine may increase the risk of bleeding, based on *in vitro* and animal research reporting inhibition of platelet aggregation.[74,75] However, the literature review reveals no reports of bleeding in humans and no systematic evaluation of patients using berberine with other anticlotting agents.
- **Cytochrome P450-3A4 (CYP3A4)–metabolized agents:** *In vitro,* goldenseal extract has been shown to weakly inhibit CYP3A4 and theoretically may increase serum levels of herbs and supplements metabolized by this enzyme.[78-80] This interaction has not been sufficiently evaluated in humans. Nonetheless, goldenseal should be used cautiously in patients taking agents metabolized by CYP3A4.

Goldenseal/Food Interactions

- Insufficient available evidence.

Goldenseal/Lab Interactions

- **Bilirubin:** Berberine, a constituent of goldenseal, has been shown to displace bilirubin from albumin both *in vitro* and in animal studies, resulting in an increase in serum total and direct bilirubin concentrations.[54]

MECHANISM OF ACTION
Pharmacology

- **Constituents:** The active ingredients of goldenseal include lisoquinoline alkaloids such as berberine, canadine, and hydrastine. Goldenseal has been reported to contain these alkaloids in the ranges of 1.5% to 4% hydrastine, 0.5% to 6% berberine, and 2% to 3% berberastine.[68] Most of the actions of goldenseal have been attributed to hydrastine and berberine. Because of the lack of clinical evidence regarding the use of goldenseal itself, it is unclear whether the actions of its constituents are also attributable to goldenseal preparations.
- **Antibacterial effects:** *In vitro* research assessing the antibacterial activity of berberine has found an aqueous extract containing berberine to have a minimum inhibitory concentration (MIC) of 50 µg/mL for *Clostridium tetani*,[45] and an MIC of <4 µg/mL for *Candida krusei*.[83] The MIC for *Streptococcus pyogenes* was found to be 30 µg/mL; berberine inhibits the adherence of *S. pyogenes* to epithelial cells, possibly by immobilizing fibronectin and hexadecane at concentrations below the MIC.[84] Berberine is bactericidal against *Vibrio cholera* at an MIC of 35 µg/mL, and against *Staphylococcus aureus* at an MIC of 50 µg/mL.[85] Berberine sulfate has been shown to possess antimicrobial activity against gram-positive, gram-negative, fungal and protozoal organisms *in vitro* through inhibition of RNA and protein synthesis.[85] *In vitro,* a methanol extract of berberine has demonstrated "cidal activity" against *Trichomonas vaginalis, Giardia lamblia,* and *Entamoeba histolytica.*[86] Subsequent *in vitro* study has found that berberine sulfate (1 mg/mL) causes nuclear chromatin clumping in *E. histolytica* after 24 hours of exposure, irregular shaped vacuoles in *G. lamblia* after 3 hours of incubation, and an increased number of autophagic vacuoles in *T. vaginalis.*[87] Berberine (0.5 mg) injected into chick embryos reduced the mortality rate of the embryos due to the introduction of trachoma organisms into the yolk sac.[24]

- **Anti-leishmaniasis effects:** *In vitro* study has demonstrated the ability of berberine to completely inhibit the growth of promastigotes at a concentration of 5 mcg/mL, possibly by inhibiting endogenous respiration of the organism and inhibiting nucleic acid and protein synthesis.[88] Subsequent study has shown berberine chloride to interact with *Leishmania donovani* nuclear DNA, inhibiting the multiplication of amastigotes in macrophage culture *in vitro* and decreasing parasitic load in animals.[39]
- **Anti-fungal effects:** Berberine, at concentrations of 10 mg/mL, has exhibited antifungal activity versus *Alternaria, Candida albicans, Curvularia, Drechslera, Fusarium, Mucor,* and *Rhizopus oryzae*; concentrations of 25 mg/mL have inhibited growth of *Aspergillus flavus* and *Asp. fumigates in vitro.*[14]
- **Gastrointestinal effects:** Oral berberine sulfate (40 to 80 mg/kg) has significantly decreased the occurrence of diarrhea induced by ingestion of castor oil and *Cassia angustifolia* in mice.[89] In 20 healthy subjects, the oral administration of 1.2 g of berberine significantly delayed small intestinal transit time of a meglucamine diatrizoate and sorbitol test mixture (71.10 ± 22.04 minutes in control vs. 98.25 ± 29.03 minutes with berberine; $p < 0.01$).[90] Berberine has significantly potentiated apomorphine-induced emesis in dogs.[91]
- **Anti-inflammatory effects:** Berberine sulfate administered subcutaneously in the ears of mice in doses of 4 to 8 mg/kg has significantly inhibited xylene-induced swelling.[89] Berberine has inhibited edema and inflammation induced in guinea pig paw by carrageenan or zymosan solution.[15] Rats treated with 6.6 g of goldenseal extract in drinking water were repeatedly exposed to a known antigen (keyhole limpet hemocyanin); goldenseal was associated with increased production of IgM following antigen exposure.[36] COX-2 regulation has been implicated as a possible mechanism.[92,93]
- **Antiproliferative effects:** Berberine was shown *in vitro* to inhibit DNA fragmentation and apoptosis of thymocytes induced by etoposide and camptothecin,[94] to affect the cell cycle and apoptosis in HeLa/L1210 cells,[21] and to inhibit synthesis of DNA, RNA, protein, and lipids in ascitic tumor cell lines; however, this inhibition did not carry over to experiments performed in mice.[95] Berberine significantly inhibited the transformation of lymphocytes despite the presence of known mitogens *in vitro*, as measured by [³H]thymidine uptake by lymphocytes.[96] After 3 days of continuous exposure *in vitro*, berberine significantly inhibited hepatoma cell growth in a dose-dependent manner and inhibited the release of alpha-fetoprotein after 18 hours of exposure.[97] In concentrations of 25 µg/mL, berberine induced apoptosis during the S-phase of the cell cycle in promyelocytic leukemia HL-60 cells.[98] An *in vitro* study found that 9-ethoxycarbonyl berberine significantly inhibits topoisomerase II.[99] Protoberberines are organic cations that are able to intercalate DNA and inhibit topoisomerase I.[100] Berberine has also been found to activate macrophages to act against the growth of tumor cells at concentrations above 0.15 µg/mL.[102] Additionally, at concentrations above 1.5 µg/mL, berberine successfully inhibited DNA synthesis in tumor cells. Berberine was shown to induce differentiation of human teratocarcinoma cells into cells with neuronal

cell morphology, beginning 1 day after the addition of 0.1 mg/mL of berberine to the culture medium.[102] In an experiment on mouse skin, berberine inhibited activity of the tumor promoters teleocidin and 12-O-tetradecanoylphorbol-13-acetate.[20] In a murine model of Lewis lung carcinoma, oral administration of berberine for 2 weeks significantly inhibited mediastinal lymph node metastases; however, there was no inhibition of tumor growth in lung parenchyma.[103] The addition of berberine to a culture of human brain tumor cell lines resulted in a mean 91% rate of cell death.[18] In a rat model of gliosarcoma, berberine administration resulted in a mean 80.9% rate of cell death.[18]

- **Antiplatelet effects:** *In vitro* study has found that berberine inhibits platelet-activating factor and aggregation of platelets, with a reported 50% inhibition at a concentration of 38 µg/mL, and inhibits the binding of platelet-activating factor to rabbit platelets with 50% inhibition seen at a concentration of 480 µg/mL.[74] Other animal research has reported that berberine inhibits platelet aggregation caused by adenosine diphosphate, arachidonic acid, and collagen and decreases thromboxane-B_2 in rats with ischemic cerebral artery occlusion, at doses of 20 mg/kg for 1 to 5 days.[75]

- **Antisecretory effects:** Berberine sulfate administered orally in doses of 60 mg/kg significantly decreases vascular permeability caused by 0.7% acetic acid in mice.[89] Subcutaneous administration of berberine sulfate in doses of 20 to 50 mg/kg decreases vascular permeability induced by histamine.[89] Berberine significantly reduces the secretory response of pig jejunal segments to *E. coli* heat-stable enterotoxin or neostigmine.[81,104,105]

- **Cardiovascular effects:** A 30-minute infusion of berberine in 12 patients with congestive heart failure at a rate of 0.2 mg/kg has been shown to significantly improve systemic and pulmonary vascular resistance, right atrial and left ventricular end-diastolic pressures, cardiac index, and left ventricular ejection fraction.[53] Intravenous berberine at a concentration of 0.2 mg/kg/minute significantly raised left ventricular end-diastolic pressure in anesthetized dogs with embolized left main coronary arteries.[106] Berberine has exhibited positive inotropic effects in dogs and prevents/reverses ouabain-induced ventricular arrhythmias.[5,6] Berberine plasma concentrations greater than 0.11 mg/L have been associated with a significant decrease in the occurrence of ventricular premature beats and a significant increase in left ventricular ejection fraction in patients with congestive heart failure vs. plasma concentrations less than 0.11 mg/L.[107] Animal experiments have reported that berberine restores ventricular arrhythmias and atrial fibrillation to normal sinus rhythm.[7] Berberine (0.2 to 0.7 mg/kg/minute) increases cardiac output and decreases total peripheral resistance and heart rate in animals; doses of 0.02 mg/kg/minute only increase cardiac output.[108] Berberine sulfate bolus injection (1 mg/kg), administered to rats 1 minute after undergoing coronary artery occlusion significantly reduced early mortality from ventricular fibrillation or complete atrioventricular block (36% mortality vs. 66% mortality in a control group).[9] Berberine sulfate solution (5 mg/mL) produced a dose-dependent decrease in blood pressure in anesthetized dogs, cats, frogs, and rats that was not inhibited by intravenous atropine, mepyramine maleate, pentolinium tartrate, propranolol, or phenoxybenzamine.[65] Intravenous berberine caused a significant decrease in systolic and diastolic blood pressure in rats at doses of 2 to 8 mg/kg.[70] Berberine has caused bradycardia in isolated right and left atria excised

from guinea pigs, which was not reversible by atropine.[109] An alcoholic extract of goldenseal has been shown *in vitro* to cause dose-dependent inhibition of epinephrine, serotonin, and histamine-induced aortic contraction.[110] Dose dependent vasoconstriction was observed beginning at a concentration of 50 µg/mL of goldenseal, although neither berberine nor hydrastine alone demonstrated this effect. Extract of berberine alone showed inhibitory activity on adrenaline-induced aortic contraction (hydrastine alone was ineffective).

- Berberine has been found to competitively inhibit the binding of yohimbine in a fashion similar to that of clonidine, suggesting that berberine may possess partial agonist activity at platelet alpha-2 receptors.[82]

- **Glycemic effects:** Berberine was reported to improve insulin resistance and liver glycogen levels similarly to metformin in rats fed a high-fat diet.[25] Rats with alloxan-induced diabetes mellitus treated with berberine had significantly lower blood sugar concentrations than control rats.[26] Goldenseal has also reduced hyperphagia and polydipsia associated with streptozotocin-induced diabetes mellitus in animals.[27] *In vitro* study reports decreased glucose absorption by Caco-2 cells.[28]

- **Muscle relaxant effects:** Goldenseal extract, at a cumulative dose of 5 µg/mL, caused complete relaxation of carbachol-precontracted guinea pig trachea *in vitro* and a significant increase in cAMP levels.[111] Berberine sulfate (20 µg/mL) pretreatment blocked the response of ileum, trachea, and rectal muscles to acetylcholine in animals.[3] Similarly, an ethanol extract of goldenseal induced relaxation in rabbit bladder muscle *in vitro*.[112] This relaxation was partly blocked by the addition of propranolol to the medium, suggesting a mechanism partially mediated through β-adrenoreceptors. An alcoholic extract of goldenseal inhibited acetylcholine, oxytocin, and serotonin-induced contractions of rat uterus cells in a dose-dependent fashion *in vitro*.[76] Berberine inhibited muscle contractions of guinea pig ileum and rat uterus induced by acetylcholine, carbachol, histamine, potassium chloride, and bradykinin.[65] Berberine increased the amplitude of slow-response action potentials induced by histamine by 6.2%, increased the maximum rate of depolarization by 21.1%, increased the action potential duration (APD) by 50.1% (APD 50) and 47.2% (APD 100) and effective refractory period by 92.2%.[77]

- **Osteoporotic effects:** Berberine, an active component of goldenseal, has been shown to inhibit parathyroid hormone–stimulated bone resorption in animal study.[113] Berberine, in doses of 30 to 50 mg/kg daily, has demonstrated an ability to prevent a decrease in bone mineral density of lumbar vertebrae in ovariectomized rats and induce apoptosis of osteoclastic cells.[113]

- **Sedative effects:** In animals, berberine produced sedation and potentiated the sedative effects of pentobarbitone when administered via intraperitoneal or intraventricular routes.[114] Berberine has been shown to reduce spontaneous motor activity and prolong hexobarbitone-induced sleeping time when administered to mice.[65] The administration of berberine (0.1 to 0.5 g/kg) for 14 days was effective in improving scopolamine-induced amnesia in rats, an effect that was augmented by physostigmine and neostigmine[115]

- **Bilirubin effects:** Berberine was shown to increase acutely the secretion of bilirubin in rats with hyperbilirubinemia, although this effect diminished with continued berberine exposure.[116] A subsequent study reported that berberine displaced bilirubin from albumin both *in vitro* and in animals, resulting in an increase in serum total and direct bilirubin concentrations.[54]

Pharmacodynamics/Kinetics

- Goldenseal is traditionally believed to be poorly absorbed from the gastrointestinal tract.
- Berberine plasma concentrations greater than 0.11 mg/L have been associated with a significant decrease in the occurrence of ventricular premature beats and a significant increase in left ventricular ejection fraction in patients with congestive heart failure vs. plasma concentrations less than 0.11 mg/L.[107]
- **Cytochrome P450 (CYP) Effects:** *In vitro*, goldenseal extract has been shown to weakly inhibit CYP3A4 and theoretically may increase serum levels of herbs and supplements metabolized by this enzyme.[78] This interaction has not been sufficiently evaluated in humans. Nonetheless, goldenseal should be used cautiously in patients taking agents metabolized by CYP3A4.

HISTORY

- Goldenseal is a low-growing herbaceous perennial in the buttercup family, notable for a bright yellow rhizome and red fruit. Goldenseal grows naturally in woodland areas across the eastern and midwestern United States. Goldenseal is difficult to cultivate, and over-harvesting has led to a decline in the number of plants available for processing.
- Goldenseal was officially approved as a medicinal herb in the U.S. Pharmacopeia from 1803 to 1840 and 1860 to 1926. It was part of the National Formulary in 1888 and from 1936 to 1955. Eclectic medical doctors promoted the use of goldenseal but were critical of some of its claims, such as the theory that goldenseal could cure cancer. The decline of the eclectic medicine in the 1930s led also to a decline in the use of goldenseal, until interest increased again in the 1970s when it was reported that ingesting the root could mask morphine, cocaine, and marijuana from detection by drug urinalysis.

Review of the Evidence: Goldenseal

Condition Treated*	Study Design	Author, Year	N[†]	SS[†]	Study Quality[‡]	Magnitude of Benefit	ARR[†]	NNT[†]	Comments
Chloroquine-resistant malaria	Equivalence trial	Sheng[72] 1997	215	No	2	Small	7.2%	14	Berberine cleared more parasitemia after 4 days than tetracycline or cotrimoxazole; no statistical analysis done.
Infectious diarrhea	RCT	Khin[60] 1985	400	No	3	None	NA	NA	Berberine vs. tetracycline vs. placebo vs. berberine + tetracycline in watery choleric diarrhea; berberine reduced stool volume, but results were not significant.
Infectious diarrhea	Equivalence trial	Khin[61] 1987	74	No	2	None	NA	NA	Berberine + tetracycline vs. tetracycline alone in the treatment of choleric diarrhea; no significant differences between groups.
Infectious diarrhea	RCT	Rabbani[62] 1987	165	Yes	2	Small	22%	5	Berberine vs. placebo in the treatment of ETEC diarrhea; berberine is effective in resolving diarrhea and reducing fecal volume; berberine added to tetracycline treatment for choleric diarrhea showed no added benefit.
Infectious diarrhea	Equivalence trial	Lahiri[117] 1967	620	No	1	None	NA	NA	Berberine vs. chloramphenicol for the treatment of choleric diarrhea; no significant differences between groups.
Narcotic concealment (urine analysis)	Equivalence trial	Cone[59] 1998	7	No	1	None	NA	NA	Crossover design of 5 treatment groups: Klean Tea, goldenseal capsules, hydrochlorothiazide, water (1 gal or 12 oz); false-negative drug tests for marijuana and cocaine, due solely to dilution of urine.
Heart failure	Placebo-controlled trial	Zeng[118] 2003	156	Yes	4	Medium	NA	NA	Berberine (2 g/day) for 8 weeks associated with improved LVEF, exercise capacity, dyspnea-fatigue index, VPC incidence, and mortality, compared to placebo.

*Primary or secondary outcome.
[†]*N*, Number of patients; *SS*, statistically significant; *ARR*, absolute risk reduction; *NNT*, the number of patients who need to undergo a specific intervention in order to observe an outcome in one individual.
[‡]0-2 = poor; 3-4 = good; 5 = excellent.
LVEF, Left ventricular ejection fraction; *NA*, not applicable; *RCT*, randomized, controlled trial; *VPC*, ventricular premature complex;
For an explanation of each category in this table, please see Table 3 in the Introduction.

REVIEW OF THE EVIDENCE: DISCUSSION
Chloroquine-resistant Malaria
Summary

- A single low-quality, randomized trial has assessed the use of berberine (an alkaloid constituent of goldenseal) in combination with pyrimethamine in the treatment of chloroquine-resistant malaria.[72] A clearance of asexual parasitemia was seen after 4 days of treatment, which was greater than that seen with pyrimethamine plus tetracycline or pyrimethamine plus cotrimoxazole. However, no statistical analysis was performed to impart significance to these results. Due to the small amount of berberine actually available from goldenseal preparations (0.5% to 6%), it is unclear whether goldenseal contains enough berberine to be effective in the treatment of chloroquine-resistant malaria.

Evidence

- Sheng et al. randomized 215 subjects with chloroquine-resistant malaria to treatment with pyrimethamine plus one of three additional agents: berberine (5 g three times daily), tetracycline (500 mg every 6 hours), or cotrimoxazole (200 mg of sulfamethoxazole and 80 mg of trimethoprim per tablet, 2 tablets twice daily) for a period of 3 days.[72] Effectiveness was defined as complete disappearance of symptomatic disease and complete clearance of all asexual forms of the parasite at the end of treatment. After 4 days of treatment, the clearance of asexual parasitemia and symptom resolution was 74.4% in the berberine group, 67.2% in the tetracycline group, and 47.8% in the cotrimoxazole group. However, no statistical analysis was performed to determine the significance of these results. Also limiting the quality of this study was the lack of blinding, which may have allowed for the introduction of bias.

Infectious Diarrhea
Summary

- Berberine, an alkaloid constituent of goldenseal, has been evaluated as a treatment for infectious diarrhea, including choleric diarrhea, in several animal and small preliminary human studies.[29,119] In animals, berberine appears to exert antisecretory effects in the setting of diarrhea induced by *Escherichia coli* enterotoxin or *Vibrio cholera*.[81,89,104,105,120] A review by Rabbani et al. suggests the use of berberine sulfate to treat diarrhea with a number of etiologies.[121] However, human studies have been poorly designed and reported and have provided conflicting data. In addition, because of the small amount of berberine actually available from goldenseal preparations (0.5% to 6%), it is not clear whether the concentrations of berberine in goldenseal are sufficient to elicit clinically significant effects. Therefore, there is currently insufficient evidence regarding the efficacy of berberine or goldenseal in the management of infectious diarrhea.

Evidence

- Khin et al. randomized, in a double-blind fashion, 400 subjects presenting with watery diarrhea to assess the efficacy of berberine hydrochloride (100-mg tablet four times daily), tetracycline (500-mg tablet four times daily), or both tetracycline and berberine hydrochloride.[60] Subjects were assigned to one of five groups: 1 placebo tablet four times daily; 1 placebo capsule four times daily; 1 berberine tablet and 1 placebo capsule four times daily; 1 tetracycline capsule and 1 placebo tablet four times daily; or 1 berberine tablet and 1 tetracycline capsule four times daily. Hourly intravenous and oral fluid intake as well as stool, urine, and vomit output were recorded; stool samples were tested for the presence of cholera. Cholera-induced diarrhea was diagnosed in 185 patients (there were no significant baseline differences between these and the 215 non-cholera subjects). In subjects with cholera, after 24 hours those receiving tetracycline or tetracycline plus berberine excreted significantly less cholera in their stool compared to the placebo or berberine-only groups. No significant differences were seen between groups in subjects with noncholera diarrhea. Berberine did not result in a significant mean improvement in fluid status. The results of this study suggest no benefit of berberine in the management of watery diarrhea (due to cholera or "noncholera" causes). However, results, blinding, and statistical analysis were not clearly reported.

- Subsequently, Khin et al. investigated the use of tetracycline (500 mg four times daily) and high-dose berberine (200 mg four times daily) vs. tetracycline alone for 48 hours in the treatment of 74 subjects with cholera-induced diarrhea in a randomized, controlled trial.[61] No statistically significant difference was seen between groups in the number of bowel movements, stool volume, or duration of diarrhea during the 48-hour period. The lack of difference may have resulted from equivalent effectiveness or equivalent lack of effectiveness of these therapies; too-brief duration to adequately measure effects; or statistical underpowering. The lack of a berberine monotherapy arm or placebo arm reduces the ability to assess efficacy. Nonetheless, this study suggests lack of efficacy of berberine as an adjunct to antibiotics in the management of cholera. Notably, tetracycline resistance by *Vibrio cholera* has been documented in some areas, and other therapies such as ciprofloxacin are sometimes recommended. The primary treatment of cholera is fluid repletion.

- Rabbani et al. conducted a randomized controlled trial in 175 adult subjects with diarrhea caused by enterotoxigenic *Escherichia coli* (ETEC) or *Vibrio cholera* to assess the efficacy of berberine sulfate for diarrhea.[62] Subjects were administered either a single oral dose of berberine sulfate (400 mg) or placebo. Mean stool volume was assessed in each subject every 8 hours and served as a marker of effectiveness. In subjects with ETEC, berberine sulfate was associated with a significant mean decrease in the volume of stools compared to control. The percentage of patients treated with berberine sulfate in which diarrhea stopped within 24 hours was 42% vs. 20% in the control group ($p < 0.05$). In subjects with diarrhea due to *V. cholera*, after 8 hours the mean stool volume declined significantly compared to controls (2.22 L vs. 2.79 L; $p < 0.05$); however, in a subset of patients treated with 1200 mg of berberine sulfate and tetracycline, the combination treatment was not significantly different from treatment with tetracycline alone. The results of this trial indicate that berberine sulfate may be an effective treatment in ETEC diarrhea, but that berberine may impart no additional benefit to tetracycline in the treatment of diarrhea due to *V. cholera*. However, these results are limited by lack of blinding and confusing methodology.

- Lahri et al. conducted a randomized trial in 620 patients over 2 years, comparing the use of berberine and chloramphenicol in the treatment of cholera and its associated diarrhea.[117] Subjects were randomly assigned to receive either berberine hydrochloride (50 mg every 8 hours for 2 days, followed by 50 mg twice daily until the fifth day) or chloramphenicol (250 mg every 4 hours for the first day, then 250 mg every 6 hours for the second day, then three times daily for 3 days). Every 12 hours, patients were evaluated for fluid intake, diarrhea volume, and number of bowel movements. Also recorded was the presence of *Vibrio cholera* in stool. The authors reported that both chloramphenicol and berberine reduced the volume of bowel movements with no significant differences between groups. There was no significant difference between groups in the detection of *V. cholera* in stool. Methodological weaknesses of this study include lack of blinding, lack of a placebo group, confusing methodology, and unclear statistical analysis.

Studies of Lesser Design Strength

- Sharda et al. alternately assigned 100 children with diarrhea due to various causes to receive either berberine (25 mg four times daily for ages ≤6 months; 50-mg first dose followed by 25 mg every 6 hours for ages >6 months) sulfonamide, sulfonamide plus streptomycin, Chloromycetin plus streptomycin, or furazolidine.[63] Symptoms were monitored every 6 hours, and the frequency and number of bowel movements and number of vomiting episodes were recorded. Overall recovery after 5 days of treatment did not differ significantly between groups, suggesting that berberine may be as effective as sulfonamides, streptomycin, furazolidone and Chloromycetin in the treatment of childhood diarrhea. However, there was no placebo group, and therefore it is not clear that any of these therapies significantly altered the natural course of disease.

- Sharma et al. alternately assigned children with acute diarrhea to treatment with berberine tannate (25 mg every 6 hours), phthalylsulfathiazole plus streptomycin, streptomycin plus chloramphenicol, or sulfaguanidine.[64] Recovery was defined as two or less stools and relief of associated symptoms for 24 hours. Stool samples were also cultured to determine any bacterial causes of diarrhea and to assess the effectiveness of therapies in eradicating any bacteria present. The authors reported that berberine was associated with improved symptoms in 30.76% of subjects within 24 hours vs. 11.71% to 24% in the control groups; berberine appeared to be effective against diarrhea caused by *Escherichia coli*, *Shigella*, *Paratyphoid B*, and *Faecalis aerogenes*. Overall, 94% of subjects in the berberine group responded to treatment, and the control group responses ranged from 88% to 96%, suggesting that berberine may be as effective as these agents. However, there was no placebo group, and therefore it is not clear that any of these therapies significantly altered the natural course of disease. Statistical analysis was not well reported.

Preclinical Studies

- Swabb et al. reported that berberine reduced the secretion of water, sodium, chloride, and bicarbonate induced by cholera toxin in rat ilea and prevented edema, compared to non–berberine-treated controls.[122] Sack et al. studied rabbit ligated intestinal loops and reported that berberine sulfate significantly inhibited the actions of *Vibrio cholera* crude enterotoxin and *Escherichia coli* heat-labile enterotoxin when administered before or up to 4 hours after toxin injection.[123] At concentrations of 0.05 to 0.1 mg, berberine significantly inhibited the secretory response of infant mice to *E. coli* heat-stable enterotoxin.

Narcotic Concealment (Urinalysis)
Summary

- Goldenseal is purported to be effective in masking the detection of illicit drugs by urinalysis and is used popularly for this purpose. However, there is a paucity of data to support this assertion. A methodologically weak human trial

assessing the effectiveness of goldenseal in masking marijuana and cocaine use suggests that it may be dilution of urine that causes false negative results on urinalysis and not goldenseal itself, although conclusions of this study are not definitive.[59] Additional *in vitro* research investigating substances that may interfere with urine-testing methods have had mixed results.[124-126] Based on the available evidence, it is not clear that ingestion of goldenseal conceals narcotics from urinalysis detection. Notably, the ethics of conducting trials to assess the efficacy of concealing illicit substances has not been adequately addressed by authors of studies in this area.

Evidence

- Cone et al. conducted a randomized, crossover equivalence trial to assess the efficacy of goldenseal capsules, goldenseal tea, hydrochlorothiazide, and water in producing false-negative urinalysis results in seven subjects exposed to marijuana and cocaine.[59] Over a period of 7 weeks, subjects smoked one marijuana cigarette (containing 3.58% tetra-hydrocannabinol [THC]) on Tuesdays and inhaled 40 mg of cocaine hydrochloride on Thursdays. On Wednesday and Friday of each week, all subjects received an intervention and were instructed to collect urine for 24 hours, which was then tested for creatinine concentration, specific gravity, and fluorescence polarization immunoassay (a validated test designed to detect cocaine, marijuana, or their metabolites in the urine). Interventions included 1 gallon of goldenseal Naturally Klean Herbal Tea (Klean Tea, Arizona); 4 goldenseal capsules (Nature's Herbs, Utah) plus 1 gallon of water; 50 mg of hydrochlorothiazide (Geneva Pharmaceuticals, CO) plus 1 gallon of water; 1 gallon of water; or 12 ounces of water. Analysis of urine creatinine concentrations and specific gravity demonstrated that all treatments, including the ingestion of 1 gallon of water, produced the same results, with specific gravity decreasing to <1.003 and creatinine concentrations falling to <20 mg/dL, both indicative of dilute urine. Drug and metabolite levels became undetectable after the ingestion of 2 quarts of water and returned to detectable within 2.5 to 10 hours after the cessation of water intake. The results of this study are weakened by a number of methodological flaws, including lack of blinding, small sample size, and a design that is difficult to ethically reproduce, given the need for narcotic ingestion. There was no study arm using goldenseal without water, and therefore it is not clear if goldenseal alone would affect outcomes.

Studies of Lesser Design Strength

- An analysis of various adulterants added *in vitro* to urine samples found that goldenseal tea, at a concentration of 15 g/L, was able to produce a false-negative reading for the presence of marijuana, but the brownish color that the goldenseal tea imparted to the urine sample made the adulteration obvious.[124] These results suggest that goldenseal tea may effectively conceal the presence of marijuana in urine samples; however, the *in vitro* nature of the experiment gives no indication of the effects of goldenseal tea ingestion on human urinalysis.

- Winek et al. conducted an *in vitro* study to examine the effects of 50 common herbal preparations, including goldenseal, on both fluorescence polarization immunoassay (FPIA) and thin-layer chromatography (TLC), two techniques commonly used to perform urinalysis for illicit drug use.[125] Infusions were made of each herbal product and tested for interaction with the testing methods. None of the herbals tested showed any interference with either the FPIA or TLC testing methods.

- Wu et al. screened 13,535 urine samples, using the CEDIA and EMIT II assays, for the presence of amphetamines, cocaine, opiates, phencyclidine hydrochloride (PCP), tetrahydrocannabinol (THC), barbiturates, and benzodiazepines.[126] The urine was also studied for the presence of adulterants aimed at creating false-negative results, namely sodium bicarbonate, bleach, dishwashing detergent, Drano, glutaraldehyde, goldenseal tea, salt, vinegar, Visine, and lemon juice concentrate. Goldenseal tea was found to interfere strongly with the detection of amphetamines and THC by both the CEDIA and EMIT II assays, suggesting that false negatives might occur.

Trachoma (*Chlamydia Trachomatis* Eye Infection)
Summary

- The goldenseal constituent berberine has been found *in vitro* and in animals to possess antimicrobial properties,[24,45,83-87] and there is limited evidence of anti-inflammatory properties in animals.[15,89] Two methodologically weak human studies have reported favorable effects of berberine ophthalmic preparations on trachoma. However, the safety and efficacy of goldenseal or berberine for this indication remains unclear.

Evidence

- Babbar et al. reported an open trial in 51 patients with trachoma lesions.[127] Subjects were assigned to receive 2 drops in each eye three times daily for 3 weeks of either 0.2% berberine chloride solution, 20% sulfacetamide, or a combination of both therapies. The results of this study were not clearly reported, and statistical analysis was not conducted. The authors noted superior short-term resolution of lesions with sulfacetamide with persistent positive *Chlamydia trachomatis* cultures vs. berberine, which yielded a slower recovery and negative *C. trachomatis* cultures. Because of the lack of a placebo group or statistical analysis, it is not clear whether these results were different from the natural course of disease.
- Khosla et al. reported a study in 32 subjects with trachoma.[22] The authors reported that a 0.2% berberine chloride solution was significantly superior to 20% sulfacetamide in reducing number of lesions and positive *C. trachomatis* cultures, although statistical analysis was not clearly documented. This study was neither randomized nor blinded, allowing for the possible introduction of bias and confounding.
- Mohan et al. reported a study in 96 children (ages 9 to 11 years) with trachoma infections.[23] Subjects were assigned to receive topical eye treatments three times daily for 3 months, consisting of either 0.2% berberine drops, 0.2% berberine drops plus 0.5% neomycin ointment, 20% sodium sulfacetamide drops plus 6% sodium sulfacetamide ointment, or saline (placebo). After 3 months of treatment, the authors reported complete resolution of lesions in 83.3% of subjects in the berberine group, 87.5% in the berberine plus neomycin group, and 72.73% in the sulfacetamide group. No cases improved in the placebo group. Although no statistical analysis was conducted, it appears that berberine was substantially superior to placebo; it is unclear if significant differences occurred between the treatment groups. Although these results are compelling, the lack of adequate blinding (single-blinding appears to have been used), randomization,

and statistical analysis weaken the clinical applicability of these results.

- Sabir et al. reported an experiment in chick embryos in which berberine (0.5 mg) was found to be protective against inoculation with *C. trachomatis*, while lesser concentrations were not effective.[24] Berberine was found to be equally effective as sulfadiazine (1 mg).

Upper Respiratory Tract Infection
Summary

- Goldenseal has become a popular treatment for the common cold and upper respiratory tract infections, and is often added to echinacea in commercially sold herbal cold remedies. The goldenseal constituent berberine has been found *in vitro* and in animals to possess antimicrobial properties,[24,45,83-87] and there is limited evidence of anti-inflammatory properties in animals.[15,89] However, there is no human evidence regarding the use of goldenseal or berberine for respiratory tract infections. Goldenseal contains 2% to 4% berberine, which may not be clinically significant, and goldenseal may be poorly absorbed. Therefore, there is insufficient evidence to make a recommendation regarding the efficacy of goldenseal or berberine for this indication.

Immunostimulant
Summary

- Goldenseal is sometimes promoted as a stimulator of the immune system. However, there is scant human or preclinical evidence in this area. It remains unclear whether goldenseal possesses clinically significant activity as an immunostimulant.

Evidence

- Liu et al. reported a case series in 405 patients with leukopenia (white blood cell count <4000).[37] The goldenseal constituent berberine was administered to subjects orally three times daily in a dose of 50 mg for 1 to 4 weeks. The authors reported that leukocyte counts increased to >4000 after 1 week in 40.2% of patients, after 2 weeks in 38.8%, and was "ineffective" in 29%. In subjects with a leukocyte count <1000, 54.8% of patients experienced increases to >4000 after 2 weeks. Although these results are compelling, the lack of a control group and unclear reporting of results weaken their clinical applicability. Further research may be warranted in this area.
- Rats treated with 6.6 g of goldenseal extract in drinking water were repeatedly exposed to a known antigen (keyhole limpet hemocyanin); goldenseal was associated with increased production of IgM following antigen exposure.[36]

Heart Failure
Summary

- Preliminary animal and laboratory research,[8,106,107,109,128] and human studies[53,118] suggest that berberine in addition to a standard prescription drug regimen for chronic congestive heart failure (CHF) may improve quality of life and cardiac function, decrease vascular resistance and incidence of ventricular premature complexes (VPCs), and improve mortality. Further research is necessary before a firm conclusion can be drawn in this area regarding safety, efficacy, and comparative effects with other established drugs for this indication that are often added to standard therapy (such as beta-blockers and spironolactone).

Evidence

- In 2003, Zeng et al. published a placebo-controlled trial in the *American Journal of Cardiology*.[118] In this trial, 156 patients with idiopathic or dilated cardiomyopathy were assigned to receive either placebo or berberine (1.2 to 2.0 g/day) over an 8-week period. Notably, all subjects also received "conventional therapy" (consisting of angiotensin-converting enzyme inhibitors, digoxin, diuretics, and nitrates), and all had been found to have >90 ventricular premature complexes (VPCs) and/or nonsustained ventricular tachycardia (NSVT) during a 24-hour Holter monitor evaluation. The authors reported that the berberine group experienced significant increases in left ventricular ejection fraction, exercise capacity, and dyspnea-fatigue index, as well as decreased VPCs, compared to the placebo group. In addition, significantly fewer deaths occurred in the berberine group (7 vs. 12, respectively; $p < 0.02$). No serious adverse effects were observed. Notably, these patients were not receiving beta-blockers, and it is not clear if all were taking spironolactone. These results are promising and merit further evaluation.

- In 1988, Marin-Neto et al. published a case series in 12 patients with refractory congestive heart failure, in which an intravenous infusion of berberine (either 0.02 or 0.2 mg/kg/minute) was administered for 30 minutes to subjects.[53] Cardiac indices and vascular resistance were measured via cardiac catheterization and contrast angiography. The authors reported that no significant circulatory changes occurred with the lower dose, but at the higher dose, several statistically significant changes were observed: a 48% decrease in systemic vascular resistance, 41% decrease in pulmonary vascular resistance, 28% decrease in right atrial pressures, 32% decrease in left ventricular end-systolic pressures, 45% increase in cardiac index, 45% increase in stroke volume, and 56% increase in left ventricular ejection fraction.

References

1. Betz JM, Miller LJ, Musser SM, et al. Differentiation between goldenseal (*Hydrastis canadensis* L.) and possible adulterants by LC/MCS of the alkaloids. FDA 1997 Science Forum:Abstract A1.
2. Dutta NK, Iyer SN. Anti-amoebic value of berberine and kurchi alkaloids. J Indian Med Assoc 1968;50(8):349-354.
3. Kulkarni SK, Dandiya PC, Varandani NL. Pharmacological investigations of berberine sulphate. Jpn J Pharmacol 1972;22(1):11-16.
4. Subbaiah TV, Amin AH. Effect of berberine sulphate on *Entamoeba histolytica*. Nature 1967;215(100):527-528.
5. Krol R, Zalewski A, Cheung W, et al. additive effects of berberine and ouabain on myocardial contractility. Clin Res 1982;30(3):673A.
6. Krol R, Zalewski A, Maroko PR. Beneficial effects of berberine, a new positive inotropic agent, on digitalis-induced ventricular arrhythmias. Circulation 1982;66(suppl 2):56.
7. Ksiezycka E, Cheung W, Maroko PR. Antiarrhythmic effects of berberine on aconitine-induced ventricular and supraventricular arrhythmias. Clinl Res 1983;31(2):197A.
8. Lau CW, Yao XQ, Chen ZY, et al. Cardiovascular actions of berberine. Cardiovasc Drug Rev 2001;19(3):234-244.
9. Ribeiro LG, Bowker BL, Maroko PR, et al. Beneficial effects of berberine on early mortality after experimental coronary artery occlusion in rats. Circulation 1982;66(II):56.
10. Wang YX, Yao XJ, Tan YH. Effects of berberine on delayed after-depolarizations in ventricular muscles *in vitro* and *in vivo*. J Cardiovasc Pharmacol 1994;23(5):716-722.
11. Freile ML, Giannini F, Pucci G, et al. Antimicrobial activity of aqueous extracts and of berberine isolated from *Berberis heterophylla*. Fitoterapia 2003;74(7-8):702-705.
12. Hwang BY, Roberts SK, Chadwick LR, et al. Antimicrobial constituents from goldenseal (the Rhizomes of *Hydrastis canadensis*) against selected oral pathogens. Planta Med 2003;69(7):623-627.
13. Albal MV, Jadhav S, Chandorkar AG. Clinical evaluation of berberine in mycotic infections. Indian J Ophthalmol 1986;34:91-92.
14. Mahajan VM, Sharma A, Rattan A. Antimycotic activity of berberine sulphate: an alkaloid from an Indian medicinal herb. Sabouraudia 1982;20:79-81.
15. Ivanovska N, Philipov S. Study on the anti-inflammatory action of *Berberis vulgaris* root extract, alkaloid fractions and pure alkaloids. Int J Immunopharmacol 1996;18(10):553-561.
16. Hartwell JL. Plants used against cancer. A survey. Lloydia 1971;34(1):103-160.
17. Hoshi A, Ikekawa T, Ikeda Y, et al. Antitumor activity of berberrubine derivatives. Gann 1976;67(2):321-325.
18. Zhang RX, Dougherty DV, Rosenblum ML. Laboratory studies of berberine used alone and in combination with 1,3-bis(2-chloroethyl)-1-nitrosourea to treat malignant brain tumors. Chin Med J (Engl) 1990;103(8):658-665.
19. Khattak SG, Gilani SN, Ikram M. Antipyretic studies on some indigenous Pakistani medicinal plants. J Ethnopharmacol 1985;14(1):45-51.
20. Nishino H, Kitagawa K, Fujiki H, et al. Berberine sulfate inhibits tumor-promoting activity of teleocidin in two-stage carcinogenesis on mouse skin. Oncology 1986;43:131-134.
21. Jantova S, Cipak L, Cernakova M, et al. Effect of berberine on proliferation, cell cycle and apoptosis in HeLa and L1210 cells. J Pharm Pharmacol 2003;55(8):1143-1149.
22. Khosla PK, Neeraj VI, Gupta SK, et al. Berberine, a potential drug for trachoma. Rev Int Trach Pathol Ocul Trop Subtrop Sante Publique 1992;69:147-165.
23. Mohan M, Pant CR, Angra SK, et al. Berberine in trachoma. (A clinical trial). Indian J Ophthalmol 1982;30(2):69-75.
24. Sabir M, Mahajan VM, Mohapatra LN, et al. Experimental study of the antitrachoma action of berberine. Indian J Med Res 1976;64(8):1160-1167.
25. Gao CR, Zhang JQ, Huang QL. [Experimental study on berberin raised insulin sensitivity in insulin resistance rat models]. Zhongguo Zhong Xi Yi Jie He Za Zhi 1997;17(3):162-164.
26. Ni YX. [Therapeutic effect of berberine on 60 patients with type II diabetes mellitus and experimental research]. Zhong Xi Yi Jie He Za Zhi—Chinese Journal of Modern Developments in Traditional Medicine 1988;8(12):711-3, 707.
27. Swanston-Flatt SK, Day C, Bailey CJ, et al. Evaluation of traditional plant treatments for diabetes: studies in streptozotocin diabetic mice. Acta Diabetol Lat 1989;26:51-55.
28. Pan GY, Huang ZJ, Wang GJ, et al. The antihyperglycaemic activity of berberine arises from a decrease of glucose absorption. Planta Med 2003;69(7):632-636.
29. Desai AB, Shah KM, Shah DM. Berberine in treatment of diarrhoea. Indian Pediatr 1971;8(9):462-465.
30. Li Xie Bin. [Controlled clinical trial in infants and children comparing Lacteol Fort sachets with two antidiarrhoeal reference drugs]. Ann Pediatr 1995;42(2):396-401.
31. Kamat SA. Clinical trials with berberine hydrochloride for the control of diarrhea in acute gastroenteritis. J Assoc Physicians India 1967;15:525-529.
32. Choudhry VP, Sabir M, Bhide VN. Berberine in giardiasis. Indian Pediatr 1972;9(3):143-146.
33. Gupte S. Use of berberine in treatment of giardiasis. Am J Dis child 1975;129(7):866.
34. Mahady GB, Pendland SL, Stoia A, et al. *In vitro* susceptibility of *Helicobacter pylori* to isoquinoline alkaloids from *Sanguinaria canadensis* and *Hydrastis canadensis*. Phytother Res 2003;17(3):217-221.
35. Watanabe A, Obata T, Nagashima H. Berberine therapy of hyper-tyraminemia in patients with liver cirrhosis. Acta Med Okayama 1982;36(4):277-281.
36. Rehman J, Dillow JM, Carter SM, et al. Increased production of antigen-specific immunoglobulins G and M following *in vivo* treatment with the medicinal plants *Echinacea angustifolia* and *Hydrastis canadensis*. Immunol Lett 1999;68:391-395.
37. Liu CX, Xiao PG, Liu GS. Studies on plant resources, pharmacology and clinical treatment with berbamine. Phytother Res 1991;5:228-230.
38. Ahuja A, Purohit SK, Yadav JS, et al. Cutaneous leishmaniasis in domestic dogs. Indian J Public Health 1993;37(1):29-31.
39. Ghosh AK, Bhattacharyya FK, Ghosh DK. *Leishmania donovani*: amastigote inhibition and mode of action of berberine. Exp Parasitol 1985;60:404-413.
40. Purohit SK, Kochar DK, Lal BB, et al. Cultivation of *Leishmania tropica* from untreated and treated cases of oriental sore. Indian J Public Health 1982;26(1):34-37.
41. Saksena HC, Tomar VN, Soangra MR. Efficacy of a new salt of Berberine (Uni-Berberine) in oriental sore. Curr Medl Pract 1970;14:247-252.
42. Vennerstrom JL, Lovelace JK, Waits VB, et al. Berberine derivatives as antileishmanial drugs. Antimicrob Agents Chemother 1990;34(5):918-921.
43. Li H, Miyahara T, Tezuka Y, et al. Effect of berberine on bone mineral density in SAMP6 as a senile osteoporosis model. Biol Pharm Bull 2003;26(1):110-111.
44. Muller K, Ziereis K, Gawlik I. The antipsoriatic *Mahonia aquifolium* and its active constituents; II. Antiproliferative activity against cell growth of human keratinocytes. Planta Med 1995;61:74-75.

45. Palasuntheram C, Iyer KS, de Silva LB, et al. Antibacterial activity of *Coscinium fenestratum* Colebr against *Clostridium tetani.* Ind J Med Res 1982;76(Suppl):71-76.

46. Chekalina SI, Umurzakova RZ, Saliev KK, et al. [Effect of berberine bisulfate on platelet hemostasis in thrombocytopenia patients]. Gematol Transfuziol 1994;39(5):33-35.

47. Gentry EJ, Jampani HB, Keshavarz-Shokri A, et al. Antitubercular natural products: berberine from the roots of commercial *Hydrastis canadensis* powder. Isolation of inactive 8-oxotetrahydrothalifendine, Canadine, beta-Hydrastine, and two new quinic acid esters, hycandinic acid esters-1 and -2. J Nat Prod 1998;61(10):1187-1193.

48. Farnsworth NR, Bingel AS, Cordell GA, et al. Potential value of plants as sources of new antifertility agents I. J Pharm Sci 1975;64(4):535-598.

49. Grismondi GL, Scivoli L, Cetera C. [Induction of labor. I. Review]. Minerva Ginecol 1979;31(1-2):19-32.

50. Royer RJ, Schmidt CL. [Evaluation of venotropic drugs by venous gas plethysmography. A study of procyanidolic oligomers (author's transl)]. Sem Hop 1981;57(47-48):2009-2013.

51. Huang WM, Wu ZD, Gan YQ. [Effects of berberine on ischemic ventricular arrhythmia]. Zhonghua Xin Xue Guan Bing Za Zhi 1989;17(5): 300-301, 319.

52. Huang W. [Ventricular tachyarrhythmias treated with berberine]. Zhonghua Xin Xue Guan Bing Za Zhi 1990;18(3):155-6, 190.

53. Marin-Neto JA, Maciel BC, Secches AL, et al. Cardiovascular effects of berberine in patients with severe congestive heart failure. Clin Cardiol 1988;11(4):253-260.

54. Chan E. Displacement of bilirubin from albumin by berberine. Biol Neonate 1993;63(4):201-208.

55. Abourashed EA, Khan IA. High-performance liquid chromatography determination of hydrastine and berberine in dietary supplements containing goldenseal. J Pharm Sci 2001;90(7):817-822.

56. Edwards DJ, Draper EJ. Variations in alkaloid content of herbal products containing goldenseal. J Am Pharm Assoc (Wash DC) 2003;43(3): 419-423.

57. El-Masry S, Korany MA, Abou-Donia AH. Colorimetric and spectrophotometric determinations of hydrastis alkaloids in pharmaceutical preparations. J Pharm Sci 1980;69(5):597-598.

58. Weber HA, Zart MK, Hodges AE, et al. Chemical comparison of goldenseal (*Hydrastis canadensis* L.) root powder from three commercial suppliers. J Agric Food Chem 2003;51(25):7352-7358.

59. Cone EJ, Lange R, Darwin WD. *In vivo* adulteration: excess fluid ingestion causes false-negative marijuana and cocaine urine test results. J Anal Toxicol 1998;22(6):460-473.

60. Khin MU, Myo K, Nyunt NW, et al. Clinical trial of berberine in acute watery diarrhoea. Br Med J (Clin Res Ed) 1985;291(6509):1601-1605.

61. Khin-Maung U, Myo-Khin, Nyunt-Nyunt-Wai, et al. Clinical trial of high-dose berberine and tetracycline in cholera. J Diarrhoeal Dis Res 1987;5(3):184-187.

62. Rabbani GH, Butler T, Knight J, et al. Randomized controlled trial of berberine sulfate therapy for diarrhea due to enterotoxigenic *Escherichia coli* and *Vibrio cholerae.* J Infect Dis 1987;155(5):979-984.

63. Sharda DC. Berberine in the treatment of diarrhoea of infancy and childhood. J Indian Med Assoc 1970;54(1):22-24.

64. Sharma R, Joshi CK, Goyal RK. Berberine tannate in acute diarrhoea. Indian Pediatr 1970;7(9):496-501.

65. Sabir M, Bhide NK. Study of some pharmacological actions of berberine. Ind J Physiol Pharmacol 1971;15(3):111-132.

66. Tice R. Goldenseal (*Hydrastis canadensis* L.) and two of its constituent alkaloids: berberine [2086-83-1] and Hydrastine [118-08-1]. Review of Toxicological Literature. 1997;i-vi, pp 1-52.

67. Kowalewski Z, Mrozikiewicz A, Bobkiewicz T, et al. [Toxicity of berberine sulfate]. Acta Pol Pharm 1975;32(1):113-120.

68. Hamon N. Goldenseal. CPJ-RPC 1990;508-510.

69. Lewin NA, Howland MA, Goldfrank LR. Herbal Preparations. *In* Goldfrank's Toxicological Emergencies. Norwalk, CT: Appleton & Lange, 1996, pp 963-979.

70. Chun YT, Yip TT, Lau KL, et al. A biochemical study on the hypotensive effect of berberine in rats. Gen Pharmac 1979;10:177-182.

71. Saxe TG. Toxicity of medicinal herbal preparations. Am Fam Physician 1987;35(5):135-142.

72. Sheng WD, Jiddawi MS, Hong XQ, et al. Treatment of chloroquine-resistant malaria using pyrimethamine in combination with berberine, tetracycline or cotrimoxazole. East Afr Medl J 1997;74(5):283-284.

73. Palanisamy A, Haller C, Olson KR. Photosensitivity reaction in a woman using an herbal supplement containing ginseng, goldenseal, and bee pollen. J Toxicol Clin Toxicol 2003;41(6):865-867.

74. Tripathi YB, Shukla SD. *Berberis artistata* inhibits PAF induced aggregation of rabbit platelets. Phytother Res 1996;10:628-630.

75. Wu JF, Liu TP. [Effects of berberine on platelet aggregation and plasma levels of TXB2 and 6-keto-PGF1 alpha in rats with reversible middle cerebral artery occlusion]. Yao Xue Xue Bao 1995;30(2):98-102.

76. Cometa MF, Abdel-Haq H, Palmery M. Spasmolytic activities of *Hydrastis canadensis* L. on rat uterus and guinea-pig trachea. Phytother Res 1998;12(suppl 1):S83-S85.

77. Huang W, Zhang Z, Xu Y. Study of the effects and mechanisms of berberine on slow-response action potentials. J Electrocardiol 1990;23(3): 231-234.

78. Budzinski JW, Foster BC, Vandenhoek S, et al. An *in vitro* evaluation of human cytochrome P450 3A4 inhibition by selected commercial herbal extracts and tinctures. Phytomedicine 2000;7(4):273-282.

79. Chatterjee P, Franklin MR. Human cytochrome p450 inhibition and metabolic-intermediate complex formation by goldenseal extract and its methylenedioxyphenyl components. Drug Metab Dispos 2003;31(11): 1391-1397.

80. Sandhu RS, Prescilla RP, Simonelli TM, et al. Influence of goldenseal root on the pharmacokinetics of indinavir. J Clin Pharmacol 2003;43(11): 1283-1288.

81. Zhu B, Ahrens F. Antisecretory effects of berberine with morphine, clonidine, L- phenylephrine, yohimbine or neostigmine in pig jejunum. Eur J Pharmacol 1983;96(1-2):11-19.

82. Hui KK, Yu JL, Chan WF, et al. Interaction of berberine with human platelet alpha 2 adrenoceptors. Life Sci 1991;49(4):315-324.

83. Park KS, Kang KC, Kim JH, et al. Differential inhibitory effects of protoberberines on sterol and chitin biosyntheses in Candida albicans. J Antimicrob Chemother 1999;43(5):667-674.

84. Sun D, Courtney HS, Beachey EH. Berberine sulfate blocks adherence of *Streptococcus pyogenes* to epithelial cells, fibronectin, and hexadecane. Antimicrob Agents Chemother 1988;32(9):1370-1374.

85. Amin AH, Subbaiah TV, Abbasi KM. Berberine sulfate: antimicrobial activity, bioassay, and mode of action. Can J Microbiol 1969;15(9): 1067-1076.

86. Kaneda Y, Tanaka T, Saw T. Effects of berberine, a plant alkaloid, on the growth of anaerobic protozoa in axenic culture. Tokai J Exp Clin Med 1990;15(6):417-423.

87. Kaneda Y, Torii M, Tanaka T, et al. *In vitro* effects of berberine sulphate on the growth and structure of *Entamoeba histolytica, Giardia lamblia* and *Trichomonas vaginalis.* Ann Trop Med Parasitol 1991;85(4):417-425.

88. Ghosh AK, Rakshit MM, Ghosh DK. Effect of berberine chloride on *Leishmania donovani.* Indian J Med Res 1983;78:407-416.

89. Zhang MF, Shen YQ. [Antidiarrheal and anti-inflammatory effects of berberine]. Zhongguo Yao Li Xue Bao 1989;10(2):174-176.

90. Yuan J, Shen XZ, Zhu XS. [Effect of berberine on transit time of human small intestine]. Zhongguo Zhong Xi Yi Jie He Za Zhi 1994;14(12): 718-720.

91. Sabir M, Akhter MH, Bhide NK. Further studies on pharmacology of berberine. Ind J Physiol Pharmacol 1978;22(1):9-23.

92. Kuo CL, Chi CW, Liu TY. The anti-inflammatory potential of berberine in vitro and in vivo. Cancer Lett 2004;203(2):127-137.

93. Lee DU, Kang YJ, Park MK, et al. Effects of 13-alkyl-substituted berberine alkaloids on the expression of COX-II, TNF-alpha, iNOS, and IL-12 production in LPS-stimulated macrophages. Life Sci 2003;73(11): 1401-1412.

94. Miura N, Yamamoto M, Ueki T, et al. Inhibition of thymocyte apoptosis by berberine. Biochem Pharmacol 1997;53:1315-1322.

95. Creasey WA. Biochemical effects of berberine. Biochem Pharmacol 1979;28(7):1081-1084.

96. Ckless K, Schlottfeldt JL, Pasqual M, et al. Inhibition of *in-vitro* lymphocyte transformation by the isoquinoline alkaloid berberine. J Pharm Pharmacol 1995;47(12A):1029-1031.

97. Chi CW, Chang YF, Chao TW, et al. Flowcytometric analysis of the effect of berberine on the expression of glucocorticoid receptors in human hepatoma HepG2 cells. Life Sci 1994;54(26):2099-2107.

98. Kuo CL, Chou CC, Yung BY. Berberine complexes with DNA in the berberine-induced apoptosis in human leukemic HL-60 cells. Cancer Lett 1995;93:193-200.

99. Krishnan P, Bastow KF. The 9-position in berberine analogs is an important determinant of DNA topoisomerase II inhibition. Anticancer Drug Des 2000;15(4):255-264.

100. Li TK, Bathory E, LaVoie EJ, et al. Human topoisomerase I poisoning by protoberberines: potential roles for both drug-DNA and drug-enzyme interactions. Biochemistry 2000;39(24):7107-7116.

101. Kumazawa Y, Itagaki A, Fukumoto M, et al. Activation of peritoneal macrophages by berberine-type alkaloids in terms of induction of cytostatic activity. Int J Immunopharmacol 1984;6(6):587-592.

102. Chang KS, Gao C, Wang LC. Berberine-induced morphologic differentiation and down-regulation of c- Ki-ras2 protooncogene expression in human teratocarcinoma cells. Cancer Lett 1990;55(2):103-108.

103. Mitani N, Murakami K, Yamaura T, et al. Inhibitory effect of berberine on the mediastinal lymph node metastasis produced by orthotopic implantation of Lewis lung carcinoma. Cancer Lett 2001;165(1):35-42.

104. Zhu B, Ahrens FA. Effect of berberine on intestinal secretion mediated by *Escherichia coli* heat-stable enterotoxin in jejunum of pigs. Am J Vet Res 1982;43(9):1594-1598.

105. Khin MU, Nwe NW. Effect of berberine on enterotoxin-induced intestinal fluid accumulation in rats. J Diarrhoeal Dis Res 1992;10(4):201-204.

106. Vik-Mo H, Faria DB, Cheung W, et al. Beneficial effects of berberine on left ventricular function in dogs with heart failure. Clinical Research 1983;31(2):224a.

107. Zeng X, Zeng X. Relationship between the clinical effects of berberine on severe congestive heart failure and its concentration in plasma studied by HPLC. Biomed Chromatogr 1999;13(7):442-444.

108. Zalewski A, Krol R, Maroko PR. Berberine, a new inotropic agent—distinction between its cardiac and peripheral responses. Clin Res 1983; 31(2):227A.

109. Shaffer JE. Inotropic and chronotropic activity of berberine on isolated guinea pig atria. J Cardiovasc Pharmacol 1985;7(2):307-315.

110. Palmery M, Leone M, Pimpinella G, et al. Effects of *Hydrastis canadensis* L. and the two major alkaloids berberine and hydrastine on rabbit aorta. Pharmacoll Res 1993;27(suppl 1):73-74.

111. Abdel-Haq H, Cometa MF, Palmery M, et al. Relaxant effects of *Hydrastis canadensis* L. and its major alkaloids on guinea pig isolated trachea. Pharmacol Toxicol 2000;87(5):218-222.

112. Bolle P, Cometa MF, Palmery M, et al. Response of rabbit detrusor muscle to total extract and major alkaloids of *Hydrastis canadensis*. Phytother Res 1998;12:S86-S88.

113. Li H, Miyahara T, Tezuka Y, et al. The effect of kampo formulae on bone resorption *in vitro* and *in vivo*. II. Detailed study of berberine. Biol Pharm Bull 1999;22(4):391-396.

114. Shanbhag SM, Kulkarni HJ, Gaitonde BB. Pharmacological actions of berberine on the central nervous system. Jpn J Pharmacol 1970;20(4): 482-487.

115. Peng WH, Hsieh MT, Wu CR. Effect of long-term administration of berberine on scopolamine-induced amnesia in rats. Jpn J Pharmacol 1997; 74(3):261-266.

116. Chan MY. The effect of berberine on bilirubin excretion in the rat. Comp Med East West 1977;5(2):161-168.

117. Lahiri S, Dutta NK. Berberine and chloramphenicol in the treatment of cholera and severe diarrhoea. J Indian Med Assoc 1967;48(1):1-11.

118. Zeng XH, Zeng XJ, Li YY. Efficacy and safety of berberine for congestive heart failure secondary to ischemic or idiopathic dilated cardiomyopathy. Am J Cardiol 2003;92(2):173-176.

119. Dutta NK, Panse MV. Usefulness of berberine (an alkaloid from *Berberis aristata*) in the treatment of cholera (experimental). Indian J Med Res 1962;50(5):732-736.

120. Tai YH, Feser JF, Marnane WG, et al. Antisecretory effects of berberine in rat ileum. Am J Physiol 1981;241:G253-G258.

121. Rabbani G. Mechanism and treatment of diarrhoea due to *Vibrio cholerae* and *Escherichia coli*: roles of drugs and prostaglandins. Dan Med Bull 1996;43:173-185.

122. Swabb EA, Tai YH, Jordan L. Reversal of cholera toxin-induced secretion in rat ileum by luminal berberine. Am J Physiol 1981;241(3):G248-G252.

123. Sack RB, Froehlich JL. Berberine inhibits intestinal secretory response of *Vibrio cholerae* and *Escherichia coli* enterotoxins. Infect Immun 1982; 35(2):471-475.

124. Mikkelsen SL, Ash KO. Adulterants causing false negatives in illicit drug testing. Clin Chem 1988;34(11):2333-2336.

125. Winek CL, Elzein EO, Wahba WW, et al. Interference of herbal drinks with urinalysis for drugs of abuse. J of Anal Toxicol 1993;17:246-247.

126. Wu AH, Forte E, Casella G, et al. CEDIA for screening drugs of abuse in urine and the effect of adulterants. J Forensic Sci 1995;40(4):614-618.

127. Babbar OP, Chhatwal VK, Ray IB, et al. Effect of berberine chloride eye drops on clinically positive trachoma patients. Indian J Med Res 1982; 76(Suppl):83-88.

128. Hong Y, Hui SS, Chan BT, et al. Effect of berberine on catecholamine levels in rats with experimental cardiac hypertrophy. Life Sci 2003;72(22): 2499-2507.

G

Gotu Kola
(*Centella asiatica* Linn.)

SYNONYMS/COMMON NAMES/RELATED SUBSTANCES

- Antanan gede, asiaticoside, Asiatic pennywort, asiatischer wassernabel, bavilacqua, Blasteostimulina, brahmi, brahmi-buti, brahmi manduc(a) parni, calingan rambat, Centasium, Centalase, Centellase, *Centella coriacea, Centella asiatica* triterpenic fraction (CATTF), coda-gam, Emdecassol, Fo-Ti-Teng, gagan-gagan, gang-gagan, HU300, hydrocotyle, *Hydrocotyle asiatica*, hydrocolyte asiatique, idrocotyle, Indian pennywort, Indian water navelwort, indischer wassernabel, kaki kuda, kaki kuta, kerok batok, kos tekosan, lui gong gen, Madecassol, marsh penny, pagaga, panegowan, papaiduh, pegagan, pepiduh, piduh, puhe beta, rending, sheep rot, talepetrako, tete kadho, tete karo, thankuni, thick-leaved pennywort, titrated extract of *Centella asiatica* (TECA), total triterpenic fraction of *Centella asiatica* (TTFCA), Trofolastin, tsubo-kusa, tungchian, tungke-tunfke, water pennyrot, white rot.

CLINICAL BOTTOM LINE
Background

- The most popular use of gotu kola in the United States is the treatment for varicose veins or cellulitis. Preliminary evidence suggests short-term efficacy (6 to 12 months) of the total triterpenic fraction of *Centella asiatica* (TTFCA) in the treatment of "chronic venous insufficiency" (a syndrome characterized by lower extremity edema, varicosities, pain, pruritus, atrophic skin changes, and ulcerations, possibly due to venous valvular incompetence or a post-thrombotic syndrome). Small to moderate benefits on subjective and objective endpoints have been reported. However, the available human trials have been small and methodologically flawed and employed varying dosages. Many have been published by the same group of investigators. Although this evidence is sufficient to suggest efficacy, further research is necessary before a strong recommendation can be made. No other uses of gotu kola are supported by scientific evidence.
- *Note:* Gotu kola is not related to the kola nut (*Cola nitida, Cola acuminata*). Gotu kola is not a stimulant and does not contain caffeine.

Scientific Evidence for Common/Studied Uses	Grade*
Chronic venous insufficiency/varicose veins	B
Anxiety	C
Diabetic microangiopathy	C
Wound healing	C

*Key to grades: *A:* Strong scientific evidence for this use; *B:* Good scientific evidence for this use; *C:* Unclear scientific evidence for this use; *D:* Fair scientific evidence against this use (it may not work); *F:* Strong scientific evidence against this use (it likely does not work). For a more detailed explanation of efficacy criteria, see "Natural Standard Evidence-Based Validated Grading Rationale" in the Introduction.

Historical or Theoretical Indications That Lack Sufficient Evidence

- Abscesses, alcoholic liver disease,[1] Alzheimer's disease,[2,3] amenorrhea, anemia, antidepressant, antifertility agent,[4] anti-infective, antioxidant,[3,5,6] antivenom, anxiety, aphrodisiac, asthma, bladder lesions,[7] blood purifier, bronchitis, bruises, burns,[8,9] cancer,[10] cellulitis,[11] cholera, colds, corneal abrasion,[12] dehydration, diarrhea, diuretic, dysentery, eczema, elephantiasis, energy, epilepsy, eye diseases, fatigue, fever, airline flight–induced lower extremity edema,[13] fungal infections, gastric ulcers,[14] gastric ulcer prophylaxis,[15-17] gastritis, hair growth promoter, hemorrhoids,[18,19] hepatic disorders,[1] hepatitis, herpes simplex virus 2, hot flashes, hypertension, immunomodulator, inflammation, influenza, jaundice, keloid formation prevention,[9] leprosy, leukoderma, libido, longevity, malaria, memory enhancement, menstrual disorders, mental disorders, mood disorders, pain, periodontal disease,[20] peripheral vasodilator, physical exhaustion, psoriasis,[21] radiation-induced behavioral changes,[22] restless leg syndrome, rheumatism, scabies, scar healing,[23] scleroderma,[24,25] shigellosis,[26] shingles (postherpetic neuralgia), skin diseases, skin graft donor wounds,[27] snakebites, striae gravidarum (stretch marks),[28] sunstroke, syphilis, systemic lupus erythematosus, tonsillitis, tuberculosis, urinary retention, urinary tract infection, vaginal discharge, vascular fragility, venous disorders.[29]

Expert Opinion and Folkloric Precedent

- In Ayurveda (the medicinal tradition of India), gotu kola is called *brahmi*, meaning "of divine origin," or "from the god Brahma," and is considered to be a highly spiritual herb. It is said to develop the crown *chakra*, the energy center at the top of the head, and to balance the right and left hemispheres of the brain. Ayurveda regards gotu kola as an important rejuvenating herb for nerve and brain cells, capable of increasing intelligence, longevity, and memory. Traditionally, gotu kola is described as bitter, sweet, and cool. It purportedly affects the heart and liver, rejuvenates *Pitta*, inhibits *Vata*, and helps reduce excessive *Kapha*. It has been traditionally used by yogis as a food for meditation. In Chinese folk medicine, a tea made from gotu kola leaves is used for respiratory and urinary tract infections, and topical gotu kola is applied to treat snakebites, injuries, and postherpetic neuralgia (shingles).

Safety Summary

- **Likely safe:** When used orally for the short-term treatment (6 to 12 months) of venous insufficiency or varicosities of the lower extremities. In patients with lower extremity edema, potentially serious etiologies such as heart failure, liver disease, and nephrotic syndrome should be ruled out.
- **Possibly safe:** When used topically for the short-term treatment of wound healing.
- **Possibly unsafe:** When used orally for the treatment of diabetic microangiopathy, due to the theoretical risk that large doses may increase blood glucose levels.

DOSING/TOXICOLOGY
General
- Recommended doses are based on those most commonly used in available trials, or on historical practice. However, with natural products, the optimal doses needed to balance efficacy and safety often have not been determined. Formulations and preparation methods may vary from manufacturer to manufacturer, and from batch to batch of a specific product made by a single manufacturer. Because often the active components of a product are not known, standardization may not be possible, and the clinical effects of different brands may not be comparable.

Standardization
- Insufficient available evidence.

Dosing: Adult (18 Years and Older)
Oral
- **Chronic venous insufficiency, varicose veins, venous hypertension:** Various dosing regimens of Centellase (TTFCA [total triterpenic fraction of *Centella asiatica*]) have been studied, including 60 to 120 mg daily,[30,31] 30 mg twice daily,[32] 30 mg three times daily,[33] 60 mg twice daily,[32,34,35] and 60 mg three times daily.[32,37] Preliminary studies suggest a dose-dependent response, with better results using 60 mg three times daily.[33] TECA (titrated extract of *Centella asiatica*) has also been studied, at a dose of 60 to 120 mg daily.[38]
- **Diabetic microangiopathy:** 60 mg twice daily of TTFCA has been used.[39,40]

Topical
- Insufficient available evidence.

Intravenous/Intramuscular
- Insufficient available evidence.

Dosing: Pediatric (Younger Than 18 Years)
- Insufficient evidence to recommend.

Toxicology
- There are reports of contamination with aspergillus in a Sri Lankan medicinal factory storing *Centella asiatica* for medicinal use.[41]
- Asiaticoside, a constituent of gotu kola, has been found to be a weak carcinogen when applied twice weekly to mice in a concentration of 0.10% in benzene.[42]
- There are numerous reports of allergic contact dermatitis after topical gotu kola use.[43-49]

ADVERSE EFFECTS/PRECAUTIONS/CONTRAINDICATIONS
Allergy
- Known allergy/hypersensitivity to gotu kola or any of its constituents, including asiaticoside, asiatic acid, and madecassic acid.
- There are numerous reports of allergic contact dermatitis after topical gotu kola use.[43-49] Allergic contact dermatitis has been reported after the use of topical Blasteostimulina cream, containing titrated extract of *Centella asiatica* (TECA) in a 38-year-old male, a 42-year-old woman, and a 59-year-old woman.[43,46,47] Topical Centelase cream also reportedly caused allergic contact dermatitis in nine subjects.[44,48,49] Eun et al. reported four cases of allergic contact

dermatitis after the application of topical Madecassol ointment.[45] After patch testing in 63 normal adults with Madecassol and its components (TECA and asiaticoside), 8% developed an allergic reaction within 4 days.[45] An animal study found that the raw extract of *C. asiatica* and several of its constituents (asiaticoside, asiatic acid, madecassic acid) are weak sensitizers.[50]

Adverse Effects
- **General:** Gotu kola appears to be well tolerated when taken orally for up to 6 to 12 months. Gastric irritation and nausea have been reported after oral administration in controlled trials.[38-51] There are several case reports of allergic contact dermatitis after topical application.[43,45-49] An animal study reported sedating effects, cholesterol elevation, and hyperglycemia after gotu kola administration, but these effects have not been reported in human subjects.[52]
- **Dermatologic:** There have been numerous reports of allergic responses after topical gotu kola use.[43-49] Allergic contact dermatitis has been noted after the use of topical Blasteostimulina cream, containing *Centella asiatica* extract in a 38-year-old male, 42-year-old woman, and a 59-year-old woman.[43,46,47] Topical Centelase cream has been associated with allergic contact dermatitis in nine subjects.[44,48,49] Eun et al. reported four cases of allergic contact dermatitis after the application of topical Madecassol ointment.[45] After patch testing in 63 normal adults with Madecassol and its components (titrated extract of *Centella asiatica* [TECA] and asiaticoside), 8% developed an allergic reaction within 4 days.[45]
- **Neurologic/central nervous system:** An animal study reports gotu kola to be sedating in large doses,[52] although there are limited human data in this area.
- **Gastrointestinal:** In a trial assessing the gotu kola product Centellase in 17 patients with chronic venous insufficiency, three subjects withdrew from the study because of mild gastrointestinal discomfort.[51] In a trial of 94 subjects taking TECA (titrated extract of *Centella asiatica*) daily for chronic venous insufficiency, two patients withdrew because of the development of gastric irritation and nausea.[53]
- **Endocrine:** An animal study has found that large doses of gotu kola can cause hyperglycemia.[52] However, studies in diabetic humans have reported no adverse effects.[39,40,54]
- **Genitourinary:** A 1968 animal study reported a reduction in the fertility of female mice after the ingestion of isothankuniside and its derivative BK compound (isolated from *Centella asiatica*).[4]
- **Oncologic:** Asiaticoside, a constituent of gotu kola, was found to be a weak carcinogen when applied topically twice weekly to mice in a concentration of 0.10% in benzene.[42]

Precautions/Warnings/Contraindications
- Use cautiously in patients with hyperlipidemia, based on animal evidence that gotu kola may elevate cholesterol.[52]
- Use cautiously in patients with diabetes or glucose intolerance, based on animal evidence that gotu kola may cause hyperglycemia.[52]
- Avoid in patients who have developed allergic contact dermatitis after topical use of gotu kola or its constituents (including asiaticoside, asiatic acid, and madecassic acid).
- *Note:* Gotu kola is not related to the kola nut (*Cola nitida, Cola acuminata*). Gotu kola is not a stimulant and does not contain caffeine.

Pregnancy and Lactation

- Not recommended due to lack of sufficient data.

INTERACTIONS
Gotu Kola/Drug Interactions

- **Sedative drugs, CNS depressants:** Based on findings of an animal study,[52] gotu kola may possess sedative qualities that potentiate the effects of other sedative agents.
- **Oral hypoglycemic drugs, insulin:** Gotu kola has been found in large doses to elevate blood glucose levels in an animal study[52] and may counteract the effects of drugs that reduce serum glucose levels. Careful monitoring and dose adjustments may be necessary.
- **Lipid-lowering agents:** Based on findings of an animal study,[52] gotu kola in large doses may possess lipid-lowering properties that potentiate the effects of other antihyperlipidemic agents.
- **Corticosteroids:** In a 1976 animal study of wound healing, observed benefits of intramuscular asiaticoside (from gotu kola) were antagonized by subcutaneous administration of dexamethasone.[55] However, steroids are known to interfere with healing because of immunosuppressant properties, and the observed effects in this study may not be specific to asiaticoside. In addition, asiaticoside has not been demonstrated to improve wound healing in humans, and the safety of intramuscular asiaticoside is not clear.
- **Phenylbutazone:** In a 1976 animal study of wound healing, observed benefits of intramuscular asiaticoside (from gotu kola) were antagonized by subcutaneous administration of phenylbutazone.[55] The application to humans is not clear, and intramuscular asiaticoside has not been demonstrated to be safe or efficacious for wound healing in humans.

Gotu Kola/Herb/Supplement Interactions

- **Sedating herbs and supplements:** Based on findings of an animal study,[52] gotu kola may possess sedative qualities that potentiate the effects of other sedative agents.
- **Lipid-lowering agents:** Based on findings of an animal study,[52] gotu kola in large doses may possess lipid-lowering properties that potentiate the effects of other antihyperlipidemic agents such as garlic (*Allium sativum* L.).
- **Hypoglycemic or hyperglycemic herbs and supplements:** Gotu kola has been found in large doses to elevate blood glucose levels in an animal study,[52] and may counteract the effects of agents that reduce serum glucose levels or add to the effects of hyperglycemic agents. Careful monitoring and dose adjustments may be necessary.

Gotu Kola/Food Interactions

- Insufficient available data.

Gotu Kola/Lab Interactions

- **Serum glucose:** In an animal study, large doses of gotu kola have been found to elevate blood glucose levels.[52]
- **Serum cholesterol:** In an animal study, large doses of gotu kola have been found to increase blood cholesterol levels.[52]

MECHANISM OF ACTION
Pharmacology

- **Constituents:** The purported active components of gotu kola, accounting for 1% to 8% of the constituents, include asiatic acid, madecassic acid, asiaticoside, asiaticoside A, and asiaticoside B.[56] The leaves of *Centella asiatica* have been reported to contain 170 mg of calcium, 30 mg of phosphorus, 3.1 mg of iron, 414 mg of potassium, 6.58 mg

of beta-carotene, 0.15 mg of thiamine, 0.14 mg of riboflavin, 1.2 mg of niacin, and 4 mg of ascorbic acid.[56]

- **Antineoplastic:** *In vitro*, partially purified fractions of *Centella asiatica* crude extract significantly inhibit proliferation of cancerous cells in a dose-dependent fashion, with no toxic effects on human lymphocytes.[10] In mice, oral administration of both crude extract of *C. asiatica* and partially purified fractions of the crude extract slow the development of solid and ascites tumors, and increase the lifespan of mice, with possible action directly on DNA synthesis.[10]
- **Wound/burn healing:** Asiatic acid, madecassic acid, and asiaticoside have been shown to stimulate the *in vitro* synthesis of collagen, both alone and in combination.[57] Titrated extract of *Centella asiatica* (TECA), asiatic acid, and asiaticoside were shown to increase remodeling of a wound collagen matrix after injection into an animal model, through the stimulation of both collagen and glycosaminoglycan synthesis.[58] Asiaticoside isolated from *C. asiatica* increased hydroxyproline content, tensile strength, and collagen content of wounds after topical administration in an animal model.[59,60] Asiaticoside was found to promote angiogenesis in chick chorioallantoic membranes *in vitro*.[59,60] The application of topical 0.2% asiaticoside twice daily for 7 days to cutaneous wounds in rats led to increased levels of antioxidants (superoxide dismutase, catalase, glutathione peroxidase, vitamin E, and ascorbic acid), and decreased lipid peroxide levels.[59,60] Increased cellular proliferation and collagen synthesis were observed at wound sites after treatment with topical or oral extract of *C. asiatica* in rats.[19] An animal study found that application of topical *C. asiatica* extract three times daily for 24 days to open wounds resulted in increased collagen content and tensile strength.[61] An *in vitro* study of the effects of total triterpenoid fraction of *C. asiatica* (TTFCA) on human skin fibroblasts found the extract to have no significant effect on cell proliferation, total protein synthesis, or proteoglycan synthesis; however, a significant increase in the percentage of collagen and cell layer fibronectin was observed.[62] Asiaticoside was found to cause a dose-related increase in tensile strength after intramuscular administration of asiaticoside.[55]
- **Venous disorders:** A controlled study in 21 subjects with postphlebitic limbs or lymphedema reports that daily Centellase (TTFCA) causes a significant decrease in both the lymphatic/plasma protein concentration ratio and distal edema.[63] TTFCA has been noted to reduce ankle edema, foot swelling, and capillary filtration rate, as well as to improve microcirculatory parameters (including resting flux, venoarteriolar response, PO_2, PCO_2) in subjects with reported venous insufficiency of the lower extremities.[64] HU300 (containing 17.5 mg of total triterpenoids derived from *Centella asiatica*), 2 tablets twice daily, is reported to decrease venous distensibility index, reduce venous congestion, and reduce supine venous pressure after 8 months in subjects with venous insufficiency, deep vein thrombosis, or perimalleolar leg ulcers.[65]
- **Carotid plaque stabilization:** In an investigation of oral Centellase (TTFCA) (60 mg three times daily) to stabilize carotid plaques, it was reported that TTFCA regulated and modulated collagen production over the 12-month study period.[66]
- **Antigastric ulcer activity:** In rats, extract of *Centella asiatica* significantly inhibits gastric ulceration induced by cold and resistant stress, similar to the inhibition caused by famotidine and sodium valproate.[15] Titrated extract of *C. asiatica* (TECA) has been shown to have protective and

therapeutic effects on gastric mucosal damage in rats.[16] Fresh juice of *C. asiatica* given in doses of 200 or 600 mg/kg twice daily for 5 days was shown to have protective activity against gastric ulcers induced by ethanol, aspirin, cold-restraint stress, and pyloric ligation.[17] The higher dose resulted in significantly increased mucin secretion and mucus formation, while significantly decreasing cell shedding.

- **Anti-inflammatory:** In rats, Madecassol was shown to decrease the severity of radiation-induced dermatitis vs. control.[67]
- **Antifertility** Animal study shows a consistent reduction of fertility in female mice after the ingestion of isothankuniside and its derivative BK compound, both of which are isolated from *Centella asiatica*.[4]
- **Antimicrobial:** An *in vitro* study of *Centella asiatica* powder found no activity against the acid-fastness or viability of *Mycobacterium tuberculosis*, despite its use in the treatment of leprosy (*M. leprae*).[68] A subsequent *in vitro* study found asiaticoside to have little microbicidal activity against *M. tuberculosis* or *M. leprae*; however, when incorporated into liposomal form, the microbicidal activity of asiaticoside was greatly increased.[69] *C. asiatica* extract and asiaticoside are active against herpes simplex virus *in vitro*.[70,71]
- **Scleroderma:** Madecassol, an asiaticoside-containing compound, inhibited the biosynthesis of acid mucopolysaccharides and collagens in an animal granuloma model.[25] Madecassol also inhibited the proliferation of human embryo fibroblasts *in vitro*.[25]
- **Antioxidant/Alzheimer's disease:** Asiaticoside derivatives, including asiatic acid and asiaticoside 6, were shown to reduce hydrogen peroxide–induced cell death, decrease free radical concentrations, and inhibit beta amyloid cell death *in vitro*, suggesting a possible role for gotu kola in the treatment and prevention of Alzheimer's disease and beta amyloid toxicity.[2]

Pharmacodynamics/Kinetics

- **Absorption:** An animal study found that madecassoside, asiaticoside, asiatic acid, and madecassic acid have a bioavailability between 30% and 50%.[72]
- **Distribution:** Bosse et al. reported that peak plasma levels are reached 2 to 4 hours after oral ingestion, intramuscular injection, or topical application of Madecassol, a gotu kola preparation.[9] Grimaldi et al. found no difference in time to peak plasma concentration with different dosages or single versus chronic dosing in a crossover study of the total triterpenic fraction of *Centella asiatica* (TTFCA).[73] The area under the curve (AUC) significantly increased in a dose-dependent fashion after single doses of either 30 mg or 60 mg of TTFCA in humans.[73]
- After chronic treatment for 7 days with either 30 mg or 60 mg of TTFCA twice daily, it was observed that peak plasma concentrations, AUC_{0-24}, and half-life were significantly higher than after single dose administration, possibly explained by the fact that asiaticoside is transformed into asiatic acid *in vivo*.[73]
- **Metabolism:** A study in 12 healthy volunteers found that asiaticoside is converted to asiatic acid *in vivo* by hydrolytic cleavage of the sugar moiety.[74]
- **Elimination:** Madecassol is predominantly eliminated in the feces within 24 to 76 hours after ingestion, injection, or application, with a small unspecified amount metabolized by the kidneys.[9]

HISTORY

- Gotu kola has a long history of use, dating back to ancient Chinese and Ayurvedic medicine. Gotu kola is mentioned in the *Shennong Herbal*, compiled in China roughly 2000 years ago, and has been widely used medicinally since 1700 AD.[56] It has been used to treat leprosy in Mauritius since 1852; to treat wounds and gonorrhea in the Philippines; and to treat fever and respiratory infections in China. In Sri Lanka, the Singhalese noted that elephants often consumed the gotu kola plant, and given the longevity of elephants, proposed that the plant may hold health benefits for humans. Thus, the Sinhalese proverb: "two leaves a day keeps old age away." Gotu kola was incorporated into the Indian Pharmacopoeia in the 19th century, and has been viewed as a rejuvenating herb. The French accepted it as a drug in the 1880s. Its purported active ingredient, asiaticoside, was first isolated and purified in 1940, and systemic clinical studies with gotu kola began in 1945. After World War II, gotu kola was included in an herb tea blend called fo-ti-teng, which was claimed to boost longevity because the ancient Chinese herbalist Li Ching Yun had used it regularly (and lived for a reported 256 years).
- Gotu kola is from the perennial creeping plant *Centella asiatica* (formerly known as *Hydrocotyle asiatica*), which is a member of the parsley family. It is indigenous to India, Madagascar, Sri Lanka, Africa, Australia, China, and Indonesia. In the Singhalese language of Sri Lanka, "gotu" means cup-shaped and "kola" means leaf.
- Although good-quality human evidence on the efficacy of gotu kola is still lacking, the herb can now be found worldwide as a component of skin creams, lotions, hair conditioners, shampoos, tablets, drops, ointments, powders, and injections.

Review of the Evidence: Gotu Kola

Condition Treated*	Study Design	Author, Year	N[†]	SS[†]	Study Quality[‡]	Magnitude of Benefit	ARR[†]	NNT[†]	Comments
CVI, varicose veins	RCT	Cesarone[35] 2001	40	Yes	3	Medium	NA	NA	Evaluation of TTFCA (60 mg) bid vs. placebo on microcirculation parameters; significant improvement in treatment group.
CVI, varicose veins	RCT	Incandela, Belcaro 2001	99	Yes	3	Medium	NA	NA	60 mg/day. vs. 120 mg/day of Centellase (TTFCA) vs. placebo for 2 months; significant improvement in objective and subjective parameters with TTFCA; greater improvement with higher dose.

Continued

Review of the Evidence: Gotu Kola—cont'd

Condition Treated*	Study Design	Author, Year	N[†]	SS[†]	Study Quality[‡]	Magnitude of Benefit	ARR[†]	NNT[†]	Comments
CVI, varicose veins	RCT	Belcaro[30] 1989	99	Yes	2	Medium	NA	NA	120 mg/day vs. 60 mg/day of Centellase (TTFCA) vs. placebo; significant decrease in symptoms with TTFCA.
CVI, varicose veins	RCT	Belcaro[37] 1990	62	Yes	2	Medium	NA	NA	60 mg t.i.d. vs. 30 mg tid of Centellase vs. placebo; higher dose most effective at improving objective and subjective findings.
CVI, varicose veins	RCT	Cesarone[32] 1994	90	Yes	2	Small	NA	NA	Effect of 60 mg b.i.d vs. 30 mg bid of Centellase vs. placebo for 60 days on peripheral venous microcirculation; significant improvement with Centellase.
CVI, varicose veins	RCT	Cesarone[34] 2001	40	Yes	2	Medium	NA	NA	TTFCA 60 mg bid of TTFCA vs. placebo for 8 weeks; significant improvement in signs and symptoms of venous hypertension.
CVI, varicose veins	RCT; dose comparison	De Sanctis[33] 2001	52	Yes	2	Small	NA	NA	60 mg tid vs. 30 mg tid of TTFCA for 4 months vs. placebo; significant improvement in objective and subjective parameters with TTFCA; greater changes with higher dose.
CVI, varicose veins	RCT	Pointel[38] 1987	94	Yes	2	Small	NA	NA	120 mg/day vs. 60 mg/day of TECA vs. placebo for 2 months; significant improvement in symptoms with TECA.
CVI, varicose veins	Comparative trial	De Sanctis[76] 1994	25	Yes	1	Small	NA	NA	Single dose of Centellase (60 mg or 120 mg) to assess any variation in CFR; dose-related effect on CFR demonstrated.
CVI, varicose veins	Before and after comparison	Marastoni[51] 1982	34	Yes	1	Small	NA	NA	Centellase (2 tablets tid) vs. tribenoside (1 capsule bid) for 30 days; significant decreases in symptoms in both groups from baseline, but interventions not compared to each other.
C, varicose veins	Controlled study	Belcaro, Grimaldi 1990	44	Yes	0	Small	NA	NA	Improvements seen in microcirculatory parameters with TTFCA 60 mg tid vs. no treatment.
Diabetic microangiopathy	RCT	Cesarone, Incandela 2001	50	Yes	3	Medium	NA	NA	TTFCA 60 mg bid vs. placebo vs. no treatment for 6 months. Significant improvement in TTFCA group only.
Diabetic microangiopathy	RCT	Belcaro[37] 1990	50	Yes	2	Medium	NA	NA	TTFCA (60 mg bid) vs. no treatment vs. placebo; significant improvement with TTFCA, but no change in other groups.
Diabetic microangiopathy	RCT	Incandela[54] 2001	140	Yes	2	Medium	NA	NA	TTFCA (60 mg bid) for 12 months vs. placebo; TTFCA significantly improved microcirculation.
Anxiety	RCT	Bradwejn[81] 2000	40	Yes	3	Small	NA	NA	Single oral dose of 12 g of gotu kola vs. placebo; significant decrease in acoustic startle response with gotu kola.

*Primary or secondary outcome.
[†]N, Number of patients; SS, statistically significant; ARR, absolute risk reduction; NNT, the number of patients who need to undergo a specific intervention in order to observe an outcome in one individual.
[‡]0-2 = poor; 3-4 = good; 5 = excellent.
b.i.d., Twice daily; CVI, chronic venous insufficiency; NA, not applicable; RCT, randomized, controlled trial; t.i.d., three times daily; TECA, titrated extract of Centella asiatica; TTFCA, total triterpenic fraction of Centella asiatica.
For an explanation of each category in this table, please see Table 3 in the Introduction.

REVIEW OF THE EVIDENCE: DISCUSSION
Chronic Venous Insufficiency/Varicose Veins
Summary

- Chronic venous insufficiency (CVI) is a term more commonly used in Europe than the United States. It describes a syndrome characterized by lower-extremity edema, varicosities, pain, pruritis, atrophic skin changes, and ulcerations. It may be due to venous valvular incompetence or to a post-thrombotic syndrome. Measurable venous hypertension of the lower extremities may accompany this syndrome. Severity may be measured by rate of blood flow, capillary permeability, venous pressure, leg volume, or the ratio of oxygen to carbon dioxide. Multiple small European trials suggest that the total triterpenoid fraction of *Centella asiatica* (TTFCA) (from gotu kola) may have small to moderate benefits on objective and subjective parameters associated with CVI. However, these trials have been methodologically flawed and inconsistent with dosing, have often used nonclinical end points, and have been brief (1 to 12 months). The same group of investigators has produced much of the available research. Although this evidence is sufficient to suggest efficacy, further research is necessary before a strong recommendation can be made.

Evidence

- Cesarone et al. randomized 40 subjects with diagnosed venous insufficiency to receive either 60 mg of TTFCA twice daily or placebo for a 6-week period, to assess the effect of TTFCA on microcirculation and edema.[35] Parameters measured at baseline and at 6 weeks included resting flux, venoarteriolar response, Po_2, Pco_2, leg volume, ambulatory venous pressure, and refilling time. At the end of the study, the treatment group experienced a significant decrease in resting flux, improvement in venoarteriolar response, increase in Po_2, decrease in Pco_2, and decrease in leg volume. No significant changes were observed in ambulatory venous pressure or refilling time. Although these results are suggestive, they are weakened by the inadequate description of randomization, blinding, and baseline patient characteristics and by the brief period of the trial.

- In a 2-month study of 99 subjects with venous hypertension randomized to receive placebo or 60 mg (30 mg twice daily) or 120 mg (60 mg twice daily) of Centellase (TTFCA) in a single-blind fashion, a significant decrease in the signs, symptoms, and microcirculatory parameters was seen in those taking Centellase vs. placebo.[75] Significantly greater improvement was seen in those taking 120 mg of Centellase daily vs. those taking 60 mg. A significant improvement was also seen in the signs and symptoms of venous insufficiency (venous pain, tired/heavy legs, edema, muscle cramps) as rated by the subjects on an analog scale. The single-blind design of this trial allows for the possibility of bias, and the unclear method of randomization suggests the possible influence of confounders on the results.

- In a similar, earlier single-blind trial, Belcaro et al. compared the efficacy of oral TTFCA to placebo in patients with venous insufficiency.[30] Ninety-nine patients were randomized to receive placebo, 120 mg, or 60 mg daily of oral Centellase for a 2-month period. Patients were blinded as to the study medication. Patients receiving active TTFCA experienced a significant decrease in their symptoms after 2 months. Transcutaneous Po_2 and Pco_2 measurements were significantly improved by TTFCA treatment, as was resting flow, venoarteriolar response, and skin temperature. The 120-mg

dose was reported as more efficacious and better tolerated. This trial is suggestive but did not sufficiently report methods of patient blinding or statistical analysis. The single-blind design allows for the introduction of bias.

- Belcaro et al. randomized 62 subjects with lower extremity venous insufficiency (ambulatory venous pressure >42 mm Hg) to receive 30 mg or 60 mg of Centellase (TTFCA) three times daily or placebo for 4 weeks in order to assess the effects of TTFCA on capillary filtration rate, ankle circumference, and ankle edema.[37] Subjects taking TTFCA experienced significant improvement in the parameters measured and in subjective symptoms vs. placebo. Those taking the higher dose experienced significantly greater improvement than those taking the lower dose. This study lends additional support to the notion that the effects of TTFCA are dose dependent, although the results can only be considered preliminary, due to poor description of methods and statistical analysis.

- In a randomized, controlled trial, Cesarone et al. examined the effects of 30 mg or 60 mg of Centellase (TTFCA) twice daily or placebo on the peripheral venous microcirculation in 90 patients with venous insufficiency.[32] The effects of therapy were measured via laser Doppler analysis of skin flux at rest. After the 60-day study period, a significant improvement in resting flux was observed for both treatment groups vs. placebo. However, it is not clear that Doppler measurements correlate with long-term clinical outcomes such as edema or pain. In addition, the methods of randomization, blinding, and statistical analysis were not adequately described, and the results were not reported clearly. Therefore, this study cannot be applied to clinical practice.

- Cesarone et al. conducted a placebo-controlled trial in which 40 subjects with venous insufficiency were randomized to ingest either TTFCA (60 mg twice daily) or placebo for 8 weeks.[34] Subjects in the TTFCA group experienced significant improvements vs. placebo in reported signs and symptoms of venous hypertension, including decreased resting flux and rate of ankle swelling. However, this study was described only briefly, with inadequate description of patient baseline characteristics, methods, and statistical analysis.

- Fifty-two subjects with venous insufficiency were randomized to receive 30 mg or 60 mg of TTFCA three times daily or placebo in a study assessing the effect of TTFCA on edema, increased capillary filtration rate, and subjective symptoms associated with venous insufficiency (edema, restless legs, pain, cramps, fatigue).[33] Ten healthy subjects were assigned to ingest TTFCA (60 mg three times daily) to gauge its effects on capillary filtration rate in normal individuals. After 4 months, all subjects using TTFCA were found to have significantly decreased capillary filtration rates, ankle edema, and subjective symptoms vs. placebo. The higher-dose group (180 mg daily) experienced greater improvement than the lower–dose group (90 mg daily). The healthy subjects experienced no significant changes after ingesting TTFCA. Although suggestive, this study suffers from a lack of description of blinding and statistical analysis.

- In a randomized, double-blind, placebo-controlled trial in 94 patients with venous insufficiency, Pointel et al. studied the effectiveness of 60 mg or 120 mg of TECA (titrated extract of *Centella asiatica*) orally administered daily in two divided doses.[38] After 2 months, statistically significant decreases in venous "distensibility" (measured by plethysmography) and increases in venous wall tonicity were measured. Subjects reported reduced lower limb heaviness and edema. No statistically significant difference was detected between doses, and doses were similarly well tolerated. Although suggestive, this was a poorly designed and described study, with incomplete descriptions of baseline patient characteristics, randomization, blinding, and statistical analysis.

- In a dosing study without placebo, De Sanctis et al. randomized 20 subjects with venous insufficiency and five normal subjects to receive a single dose of Centellase (TTFCA) (either 60 mg or 120 mg).[76] The investigators studied the acute effects of TTFCA on capillary filtration, as assessed by venous occlusion strain gauge plethysmography. Results showed a significant decrease in capillary filtration rate in both groups 5 hours after ingestion. However, the 120-mg group experienced a significantly lower capillary filtration rate at 10 hours after ingestion, suggesting dose-dependent activity of TTFCA. These results may only be considered preliminary, as the small sample size, lack of blinding, and lack of placebo control limit their application.

- In a comparison study, Marastoni et al. assigned 34 patients with chronic venous insufficiency to take either Centellase (TTFCA) (2 capsules three times daily) or tribenoside (Glyvenol, Alven; used in Europe for the treatment of varicose veins) (1 capsule twice daily).[51] After 1 month of treatment, symptoms improved significantly in both groups, and treatment was well tolerated. However, because of the lack of a placebo group, it is not clear that improvements were due to therapeutic interventions vs. the natural course of disease. In addition, no power calculation was conducted, and it is therefore not clear whether the sample size was adequate to distinguish between-group differences. Blinding and randomization were not well described.

- Belcaro et al. studied the effects of oral TTFCA on capillary permeability and microcirculation in 10 normal subjects, 12 subjects with moderate superficial venous insufficiency, and 12 subjects with severe venous insufficiency/postphlebitic limbs.[36] After two weeks of treatment with either 60 mg of TTFCA three times daily or observation alone, the patients with venous insufficiency receiving TTFCA experienced a significant decrease in the disappearance time of a wheal caused by a vacuum suction chamber (VSC). The patients receiving no treatment did not experience any significant change in capillary permeability or disappearance time of the wheal caused by the VSC device. Patients taking TTFCA reported significant improvement in their symptoms of venous insufficiency. This study was not placebo controlled, thus allowing for the possible introduction of bias. In addition, reproducible clinical end points were not measured.

Diabetic Microangiopathy
Summary

- Studies have suggested beneficial effects of the total triterpenoid fraction of *Centella asiatica* (TTFCA) on subjective and objective parameters of venous insufficiency of the lower extremities. Based on these observations, it has been postulated that there could be a role for gotu kola in the treatment of vascular disease associated with diabetes. However, diabetic patients experience vascular disease that is often different in etiology from venous insufficiency. Nonetheless, initial controlled trials have found oral gotu kola (TTFCA, 60 mg twice daily) to have statistically significant beneficial effects on microcirculatory parameters in patients with diabetic microangiopathy. These studies have been brief and methodologically weak, with limited assessment of clinical

outcomes. Therefore, no recommendation can be made at this time.

Evidence

- Cesarone et al. completed a prospective trial in 50 patients with diabetic microangiopathy, randomizing them to receive 60 mg of TTFCA twice daily, placebo, or no treatment for a period of 6 months.[40] Baseline measurements of laser Doppler parameters, transcutaneous PO_2, PCO_2, and rate of ankle swelling were measured. These measurements were repeated at 3 and 6 months after the start of treatment, with the exception of the rate of ankle swelling, which was measured at 6 months only. In subjects treated with TTFCA, there was a significant increase in PO_2, decrease in PCO_2, decrease in rate of ankle swelling, increase in venoarteriolar reflex, and decrease in resting flow vs. control. It is not clear whether this study's measurements assessed effects on diabetic vascular disease explicitly, rather than lower extremity edema possibly due to other etiologies (such as venous incompetence or low serum albumin). In addition, there was poor description of blinding, randomization, and statistical analysis. Due to these methodological problems, additional study is warranted before a recommendation can be made.

- The effect of TTFCA on patients with diabetic microangiopathy was studied in a randomized, placebo-controlled study.[39] Fifty subjects were given 60 mg of TTFCA twice daily, placebo, or no treatment, and were monitored for 6 months. TTFCA was found to significantly increase microcirculatory parameters and decrease capillary permeability. These findings were similar to that of previous studies by the same research group in patients with venous insufficiency of the lower extremities.[30] It is not clear from this study that the benefits of TTFCA are of particular benefit to diabetic patients, and diabetics may experience vascular disease different in etiology from venous insufficiency. Poor description of blinding and randomization further weakens these results.

- Incandela et al. randomized 100 subjects diagnosed with diabetic microangiopathy (50 with neuropathy and 50 without neuropathy) to receive 60 mg of TTFCA twice daily or placebo for 12 months.[54] All subjects completed the study. Those receiving TTFCA experienced significant decreases in resting flux and rate of ankle swelling vs. placebo. TTFCA appeared to decrease edema and improve symptoms in patients both with neuropathy and without, although a power calculation was not conducted prior to the study to detect differences between these subgroups. This study was described only briefly, with inadequate description of methods, blinding, randomization, and statistical analysis.

Anxiety
Summary

- In Ayurvedic (traditional Indian) medicine, gotu kola is said to develop the crown *chakra*, the energy center at the top of the head, and to balance the right and left hemispheres of the brain. It has traditionally been used by yogis as a food for meditation. Recent animal research has demonstrated anxiolytic properties of gotu kola.[77,78] This anxiolytic activity may or may not apply to humans. A single randomized trial assessing the effects of gotu kola on startle responses in healthy (non-anxious) individuals has reported some benefits. These preliminary findings are promising, although further research using established end points in patients with anxiety is necessary before an evidence-based therapeutic recommendation can be made.

Evidence

- In 40 healthy (non-anxious) subjects, Bradwejn et al. studied the effects of gotu kola on acoustic startle response (ASR), a validated instrument used to measure level of anxiety.[79-81] In this double-blind, placebo-controlled trial, subjects were randomized to receive a single 12-g dose of gotu kola (from crude herb capsules, Nature's Way, Canada, Ltd.) mixed in 300 mL of grape juice, or grape juice alone. At 30 and 60 minutes after intervention, the gotu kola group experienced a significant decrease in their ASR, suggesting the possible ability of gotu kola to decrease anxiety. The small sample size and use of healthy (non-anxious) subjects limit the application of these data but do suggest that gotu kola may possess anxiolytic properties. Further study is warranted to determine the efficacy of gotu kola in the management of anxiety disorders.

Wound Healing
Summary

- Numerous animal and *in vitro* studies have demonstrated the ability of *Centella asiatica* extracts to promote wound healing, possibly through the stimulation of collagen synthesis.[19,25,55,57-62] However, there is a paucity of human evidence regarding the use of gotu kola or *C. asiatica* extract in the treatment of wounds,[20] and no recommendation can be made at this time.

FORMULARY: BRANDS USED IN CLINICAL TRIALS
Brands Used in Statistically Significant Clinical Trials

- Centellase[30,32,37,75,76] Nature's Way Canada, Ltd. Gotu Kola.[81]

References

1. Darnis F, Orcel L, Saint-Maur PP, et al. [Use of a titrated extract of *Centella asiatica* in chronic hepatic disorders (author's transl)]. Sem Hop 1979;55(37-38):1749-1750.
2. Mook-Jung I, Shin JE, Yun SH, et al. Protective effects of asiaticoside derivatives against beta-amyloid neurotoxicity. J Neurosci Res 1999;58(3):417-425.
3. Veerendra Kumar MH, Gupta YK. Effect of *Centella asiatica* on cognition and oxidative stress in an intracerebroventricular streptozotocin model of Alzheimer's disease in rats. Clin Exp Pharmacol Physiol 2003;30(5-6):336-342.
4. Dutta T, Basu UP. Crude extract of *Centella asiatica* and products derived from its glycosides as oral antifertility agents. Indian J Exp Biol 1968;6(3):181-182.
5. Gupta YK, Veerendra Kumar MH, Srivastava AK. Effect of *Centella asiatica* on pentylenetetrazole-induced kindling, cognition and oxidative stress in rats. Pharmacol Biochem Behav 2003;74(3):579-585.
6. Jayashree G, Kurup MG, Sudarslal S, et al. Anti-oxidant activity of *Centella asiatica* on lymphoma-bearing mice. Fitoterapia 2003;74(5):431-434.
7. Fam A. Use of titrated extract of *Centella asiatica* (TECA) in bilharzial bladder lesions. Int Surg 1973;58(7):451-455.
8. Boiteau P, Batsimamanga AR. Asiaticoside extracted from *Centella asiatica*, and its therapeutic uses in the healing of experimental refractory wounds, leprosy, skin tuberculosis and lupus. Therapie 1950;11:125-149.
9. Bosse JP, Papillon J, Frenette G, et al. Clinical study of a new antikeloid agent. Ann Plast Surg 1979;3(1):13-21.
10. Babu TD, Kuttan G, Padikkala J. Cytotoxic and anti-tumour properties of certain taxa of Umbelliferae with special reference to *Centella asiatica* (L.) Urban. J Ethnopharmacol 1995;48(1):53-57.
11. Morganti P, Randazzo SD, Fabrizi G, et al. A new cosmeceutical for the 'orange peel' skin. J Applied Cosmetol 1997;15(4):139-145.
12. Mekkawi MF. Local asiaticoside in the treatment of ulcers & wounds of the cornea. Bull Ophthalmol Soc Egypt 1975;68:77-79.
13. Cesarone MR, Incandela L, De Sanctis MT, et al. Flight microangiopathy in medium- to long-distance flights: prevention of edema and microcirculation alterations with total triterpenic fraction of *Centella asiatica*. Angiology 2001;52(10 suppl 2):S33-S37.
14. Mayall RC, et al. Ulceras troficas—acao cicatrical do extrato titulado da *Centella asiatica*. Rev Brasil Med 1975;32(1):26-29.
15. Chatterjee TK, Chakraborty A, Pathak M, et al. Effects of plant extract *Centella asiatica* (Linn.) on cold restraint stress ulcer in rats. Indian J Exp Biol 1992;30(10):889-891.
16. Ji B, Chen B, Jia B, et al. Effect of titrated extract of Centella asiatica on

17. experimental gastric injury—the mechanism of initial investigation [published abstract]. J Gastroenterol Hepatol 1997;12(Supplement A214): A214.
17. Sairam K, Rao CV, Goel RK. Effect of *Centella asiatica* Linn on physical and chemical factors induced gastric ulceration and secretion in rats. Indian J Exp Biol 2001;39(2):137-142.
18. MacKay D. Hemorrhoids and varicose veins: a review of treatment options. Altern Med Rev 2001;6(2):126-140.
19. Suguna L, Sivakumar P, Chandrakasan G. Effects of *Centella asiatica* extract on dermal wound healing in rats. Indian J Exp Biol 1996;34(12):1208-1211.
20. Sastravaha G, Yotnuengnit P, Booncong P, et al. Adjunctive periodontal treatment with *Centella asiatica* and *Punica granatum* extracts. A preliminary study. J Int Acad Periodontol 2003;5(4):106-115.
21. Natarajan S, Paily PP. Effect of topical *Hydrocotyle Asiatica* in psoriasis. Indian J Dermatol 1973;18(4):82-85.
22. Shobi V, Goel HC. Protection against radiation-induced conditioned taste aversion by *Centella asiatica*. Physiol Behav 2001;73(1-2):19-23.
23. Widgerow AD, Chait LA, Stals R, et al. New innovations in scar management. Aesthetic Plast Surg 2000;24(3):227-234.
24. Guseva NG, Starovoitova MN, Mach ES. [Madecassol treatment of systemic and localized scleroderma]. Ter Arkh 1998;70(5):58-61.
25. Sasaki S, Shinkai H, Akashi Y, et al. Studies on the mechanism of action of asiaticoside (Madecassol) on experimental granulation tissue and cultured fibroblasts and its clinical application in systemic scleroderma. Acta Derm Venereol 1972;52(2):141-150.
26. Haider R, Khan AK, Aziz KM, et al. Evaluation of indigenous plants in the treatment of acute shigellosis. Trop Geogr Med 1991;43(3):266-270.
27. O'Keeffe P. A trial of asiaticoside on skin graft donor areas. Br J Plast Surg 1974;27(2):194-195.
28. Mallol J, Belda MA, Costa D, et al. Prophylaxis of Striae gravidarum with a topical formulation. A double blind trial. Int J Cosmetic Sci 1991;13:51-57.
29. Allegra C, Pollari G, Criscuolo A, et al. [*Centella asiatica* extract in venous disorders of the lower limbs. Comparative clinico-instrumental studies with a placebo]. Clin Ther 1981;99(5):507-513.
30. Belcaro G, Laurora G, Cesarone MR, et al. Efficacy of Centellase in the treatment of venous hypertension evaluated by a combined microcirculatory model. Curr Ther Res 1989;46(6):1015-1026.
31. Incandela L, Cesarone MR, Cacchio M, et al. Total triterpenic fraction of *Centella asiatica* in chronic venous insufficiency and in high-perfusion microangiopathy. Angiology 2001;52(10 suppl 2):S9-S13.
32. Cesarone MR, Laurora G, De Sanctis MT, et al. [The microcirculatory activity of *Centella asiatica* in venous insufficiency. A double-blind study]. Minerva Cardioangiol 1994;42(6):299-304.
33. De Sanctis MT, Belcaro G, Incandela L, et al. Treatment of edema and increased capillary filtration in venous hypertension with total triterpenic fraction of *Centella asiatica*: A clinical, prospective, placebo-controlled, randomized, dose-ranging trial. Angiology 2001;52(10 suppl 2):S55-S59.
34. Cesarone MR, Belcaro G, De Sanctis MT, et al. Effects of the total triterpenic fraction of *Centella asiatica* in venous hypertensive microangiopathy: a prospective, placebo-controlled, randomized trial. Angiology 2001;52(10 suppl 2):S15-S18.
35. Cesarone MR, Belcaro G, Rulo A, et al. Microcirculatory effects of total triterpenic fraction of *Centella asiatica* in chronic venous hypertension: measurement by laser Doppler, TcPO2-CO2, and leg volumetry. Angiology 2001;52(10 suppl 2):S45-S48.
36. Belcaro GV, Grimaldi R, Guidi G. Improvement of capillary permeability in patients with venous hypertension after treatment with TTFCA. Angiology 1990;41(7):533-540.
37. Belcaro GV, Rulo A, Grimaldi R. Capillary filtration and ankle edema in patients with venous hypertension treated with TTFCA. Angiology 1990;41(1):12-18.
38. Pointel JP, Boccalon H, Cloarec M, et al. Titrated extract of *Centella asiatica* (TECA) in the treatment of venous insufficiency of the lower limbs. Angiology 1987;38(1 Pt 1):46-50.
39. Belcaro GV, Grimaldi R, Guidi G, et al. Treatment of diabetic microangiopathy with TTFCA. A microcirculatory study with laser-Doppler flowmetry, PO2/PCO2, and capillary permeability measurements. Curr Ther Res 1990;37(3):421-428.
40. Cesarone MR, Incandela L, De Sanctis MT, et al. Evaluation of treatment of diabetic microangiopathy with total triterpenic fraction of *Centella asiatica*: a clinical prospective randomized trial with a microcirculatory model. Angiology 2001;52(10 suppl 2):S49-S54.
41. Abeywickrama K, Bean GA. Toxigenic *Aspergillus flavus* and aflatoxins in Sri Lankan medicinal plant material. Mycopathologia 1991;113(3):187-190.
42. Laerum OD, Iversen OH. Reticuloses and epidermal tumors in hairless mice after topical skin applications of cantharidin and asiaticoside. Cancer Res 1972;32(7):1463-1469.
43. Bilbao I, Aguirre A, Zabala R, et al. Allergic contact dermatitis from butoxyethyl nicotinic acid and *Centella asiatica* extract. Contact Dermatitis 1995;33(6):435-436.
44. Danese P, Carnevali C, Bertazzoni MG. Allergic contact dermatitis due to *Centella asiatica* extract. Contact Dermatitis 1994;31(3):201.
45. Eun HC, Lee AY. Contact dermatitis due to Madecassol. Contact Dermatitis 1985;13(5):310-313.
46. Izu R, Aguirre A, Gil N, et al. Allergic contact dermatitis from a cream

containing *Centella asiatica* extract. Contact Dermatitis 1992;26(3): 192-193.

47. Morante J, Bujan J, Guemes M, et al. [Allergic contact dermatitis from *Centella asiatica* extract: Report of a new case]. Actas Dermo-Sifiliograficas 1998;89(6):341-343.

48. Santucci B, Picardo M, Cristaudo A. Contact dermatitis due to Centelase. Contact Dermatitis 1985;13(1):39.

49. Vena GA, Angelini G. Contact allergy to Centelase. Contact Dermatitis 1986;15(2):108-109.

50. Hausen BM. *Centella asiatica* (Indian pennywort), an effective therapeutic but a weak sensitizer. Contact Dermatitis 1993;29(4):175-179.

51. Marastoni F, Baldo A, Redaelli G, et al. [*Centella asiatica* extract in venous pathology of the lower limbs and its evaluation as compared with tribenoside]. Minerva Cardioangiol 1982;30(4):201-207.

52. Ramaswamy AS, et al. Pharmacological studies on *Centella asiatica* Linn. (*Brahma manduki*) (N. O. Umbelliferae). J Res Indian Med 1970;4:160-175.

53. Pointel JP, Boccalon H, Cloarec M, et al. Titrated extract of *Centella asiatica* (T.E.C.A.) in the treatment of venous insufficiency of the lower limbs. Phlebology 1986;840-842.

54. Incandela L, Belacaro G, Cesarone MR, et al. Treatment of diabetic microangiopathy and edema with total triterpenic fraction of *Centella asiatica*: a prospective, placebo-controlled randomized study. Angiology 2001; 52(10 suppl 2):S27-S31.

55. Velasco M, Romero E. Drug interaction between asiaticoside and some anti-inflammatory drugs in wound healing of the rat. Curr Ther Res Clin Exp 1976;19(1):121-125.

56. Brinkhaus B, Lindner M, Schuppan D, et al. Chemical, pharmacological and clinical profile of the East Asian medical plant *Centella asiatica*. Phytomedicine 2000;7(5):427-448.

57. Bonte F, Dumas M, Chaudagne C, et al. Influence of asiatic acid, madecassic acid, and asiaticoside on human collagen I synthesis. Planta Med 1994; 60(2):133-135.

58. Maquart FX, Chastang F, Simeon A, et al. Triterpenes from *Centella asiatica* stimulate extracellular matrix accumulation in rat experimental wounds. Eur J Dermatol 1999;9(4):289-296.

59. Shukla A, Rasik AM, Jain GK, et al. *In vitro* and *in vivo* wound healing activity of asiaticoside isolated from *Centella asiatica*. J Ethnopharmacol 1999;65(1):1-11.

60. Shukla A, Rasik AM, Dhawan BN. Asiaticoside-induced elevation of antioxidant levels in healing wounds. Phytother Res 1999;13(1):50-54.

61. Sunilkumar, Parameshwaraiah S, Shivakumar HG. Evaluation of topical formulations of aqueous extract of *Centella asiatica* on open wounds in rats. Indian J Exp Biol 1998;36(6):569-572.

62. Tenni R, Zanaboni G, De Agostini MP, et al. Effect of the triterpenoid fraction of *Centella asiatica* on macromolecules of the connective matrix in human skin fibroblast cultures. Ital J Biochem 1988;37(2):69-77.

63. Cesarone MR, Laurora G, Pomante P, et al. [Efficacy of TTFCA in reducing the ratio between lymphatic and plasma protein concentration in lymphatic and postphlebetic edema]. Minerva Cardioangiol 1991;39(12):475-478.

64. Cesarone MR, Laurora G, De Sanctis MT, et al. [Activity of *Centella asiatica* in venous insufficiency]. Minerva Cardioangiol 1992;40(4):137-143.

65. Mahajani SS, Oberai C, Jerajani H, et al. Study of the venodynamic effect of an Ayurvedic formulation of *Centella asiatica* using venous occlusion plethysmography (VOP) and laser-Doppler velocimetry (LVD). Can J Physiol Pharmacol 1994;72(supplement 1):180.

66. Cesarone MR, Belcaro G, Nicolaides AN, et al. Increase in echogenicity of echolucent carotid plaques after treatment with total triterpenic fraction of *Centella asiatica*: a prospective, placebo-controlled, randomized trial. Angiology 2001;52(10 suppl 2):S19-S25.

67. Chen YJ, Dai YS, Chen BF, et al. The effect of tetrandrine and extracts of *Centella asiatica* on acute radiation dermatitis in rats. Biol Pharm Bull 1999; 22(7):703-706.

68. Herbert D, Paramasivan CN, Prabhakar R, et al. In vitro experiments with *Centella asiatica*: investigation to elucidate the effect of an indigenously prepared powder of this plant on the acid- fastness and viability of *M. tuberculosis*. Indian J Lepr 1994;66(1):65-68.

69. Medda S, Das N, Mahato SB, et al. Glycoside-bearing liposomal delivery systems against macrophage- associated disorders involving *Mycobacterium leprae* and *Mycobacterium tuberculosis*. Indian J Biochem Biophys 1995; 32(3):147-151.

70. Yoosook C, Bunyapraphatsara N, Boonyakiat Y, et al. Anti-herpes simplex virus activities of crude water extracts of Thai medicinal plants. Phytomedicine 1999;6(6):411-419.

71. Zheng MS. An experimental study of the anti-HSV-II action of 500 herbal drugs. J Tradit Chin Med 1989;9(2):113-116.

72. Vogel HG, DeSouza N, D'Sa A. Effects of terpenoids isolated from *Centella* asiatica on granuloma tissue. Acta Therapeutica 1990;16:285-298.

73. Grimaldi R, De Ponti F, D'Angelo L, et al. Pharmacokinetics of the total triterpenic fraction of *Centella asiatica* after single and multiple administrations to healthy volunteers. A new assay for asiatic acid. J Ethnopharmacol 1990;28(2):235-241.

74. Rush WR, Murray GR, Graham DJ. The comparative steady-state bioavailability of the active ingredients of Madecassol. Eur J Drug Metab Pharmacokinet 1993;18(4):323-326.

75. Incandela L, Belcaro G, De Sanctis MT, et al. Total triterpenic fraction of *Centella asiatica* in the treatment of venous hypertension: a clinical, prospective, randomized trial using a combined microcirculatory model. Angiology 2001;52(10 suppl 2):S61-S67.

76. De Sanctis MT, Incandela L, Cesarone MR, et al. Acute effects of TTFCA on capillary filtration in severe venous hypertension. Panminerva Medica 1994;36(2):87-90.

77. DeLucia R, Sertie JAA, Camargo EA, et al. Pharmacologic and toxicological studies on *Centella asiatica* extract. Fitoterapia 1997;68:413-416.

78. Sarma DNK, Khosa RL, Chansauria JPN, et al. Antistress activity of Tinospora cordifolia and *Centella asiatica* extracts. Phytother Res 1996; 10(2):181-189.

79. Bradwejn J, Zhou Y, Koszycki, et al. Effect of acute administration of Gotu-kola (*Centella asiatica*) on acoustic startle response in healthy volunteers. XXIst Collegium Internationale Neuro-psychopharmacologicum, Glascow, Scotland (July 12-16) 1998;(Abstract Ref: NRW001).

80. Bradwejn J, Koszycki D, Shlik J, et al. *Centella asiatica* decreases the acoustic startle response. 152nd Annual Meeting of the American Psychiatric Association, Washington DC, USA (May 15-20) 1999.81. Bradwejn J, Zhou Y, Koszycki D, et al. A double-blind, placebo-controlled study on the effects of Gotu Kola (*Centella asiatica*) on acoustic startle response in healthy subjects. J Clin Psychopharmacol 2000;20(6):680-684.

Green Tea

(Camellia sinensis)

SYNONYMS/COMMON NAMES/RELATED SUBSTANCES

- AR25, camellia, *Camellia assamica*, *Camellia sinensis* L. Kuntze, camellia tea, catechins, Chinese tea, epigallocatechin-3-gallate (ECGC), Exolise, green tea extract (GTE), matsucha tea, *Thea sinensis*, *Thea bohea*, *Thea viridis*, theanine, theifers.

CLINICAL BOTTOM LINE

Background

- Green tea is made from the dried leaves of *Camellia sinensis*, a perennial evergreen shrub. Green tea has a long history of use, dating back to China approximately 5000 years ago. Green tea, black tea, and oolong tea all are derived from the same plant.

- Green tea is a source of caffeine, a methylxanthine that stimulates the central nervous system, relaxes smooth muscle in the airways to the lungs (bronchioles), stimulates the heart, and acts on the kidney as a diuretic (increasing urine). One cup of tea contains approximately 50 mg of caffeine, depending on the strength of the infusion and the size of the cup; by comparison, coffee contains 65 to 175 mg of caffeine per cup. Tea also contains polyphenols (catechins, anthocyanins, phenolic acids), tannin, trace elements, and vitamins.

- The tea plant is native to Southeast Asia; it can grow up to a height of 40 feet but usually is maintained at a height of 2 to 3 feet by regular pruning. The first spring leaf buds, called the *first flush*, are considered the highest-quality leaves. When the first flush leaf bud is picked, another one grows, and this set of leaves is called the *second flush*; the harvesting continues until an *autumn flush*. The older leaves picked farther down the stems are considered to be of poorer quality.

- Tea varieties reflect the growing region (for example, Ceylon or Assam), the district (for example, Darjeeling), the form (for example, pekoe is cut, whereas gunpowder is rolled), and the processing method (for example, black, green, or oolong). India and Sri Lanka are the major producers of green tea.

- Green tea is produced by lightly steaming the freshly cut leaf, so that oxidation of the enzymes within the leaf does not take place. Green tea is produced and consumed primarily in China, Japan, and countries in North Africa and the Middle East. By contrast, allowing the leaves of *Camellia sinensis* to oxidize produces black tea (a fermentation process that alters flavor as well as enzymes present in the tea). Oolong tea is a partially oxidized tea and accounts for less than 5% of all tea produced.

- Historically, tea has been served as a part of various ceremonies and has been used to maintain alertness during long meditations. A legend in India tells the story of Prince Siddhartha Gautama, the founder of Buddhism, who tore off his eyelids in frustration at his inability to stay awake during meditation while journeying through China. A tea plant is said to have sprouted from the spot where his eyelids fell, providing him with the means to stay awake, meditate, and reach enlightenment. Turkish traders reportedly introduced tea to Western cultures in the 6th century.

Uses Based on Scientific Evidence	Grade*
Arthritis Research indicates that green tea may benefit arthritis by reducing inflammation and slowing cartilage breakdown. Further studies are required before a recommendation can be made.	C
Asthma Research has shown caffeine to cause improvement in air flow to the lungs (bronchodilation). However, it is not clear if caffeine or tea consumption has significant clinical benefits in people with asthma. Better research regarding this effect is needed before a conclusion can be drawn.	C
Cancer prevention Several large population-based studies have been undertaken to examine the possible association between green tea consumption and cancer incidence. Cancers of the digestive system (stomach, colon, rectum, pancreas, and esophagus) have primarily been tracked. The risk of prostate cancer, cervical cancer, and breast cancer in women also has been studied. Although much of this research suggests a cancer-protective effect of habitual green tea consumption, some studies have not observed significant benefits. In studies that have shown benefits, it is not clear if other lifestyle choices of people who drink tea may actually be the beneficial factors. If there is a benefit, it may be small and require large amounts of daily consumption (several cups per day). At this time, the scientific evidence remains indeterminate in this area. Laboratory research and studies in animals report that components of tea, such as polyphenols, have antioxidant or free radical scavenging properties and may possess various effects against tumor cells (such as angiogenesis inhibition, hydrogen peroxide generation, or induction of apoptosis). Limited evidence from studies in humans includes reports of lower estrogen levels in women drinking green tea, proposed as possibly beneficial in estrogen receptor–positive breast cancers. However, other animal and laboratory research suggests that components of green tea may actually be carcinogenic, although effects in humans are not clear. Overall, the relationship of green tea consumption and human cancer remains unclear. Evidence from a controlled trial of sufficient size and duration is needed before a recommendation regarding this possible association can be made.	C
Dental caries prevention There is limited study of tea as a gargle (mouthwash) for the prevention of dental caries (tooth decay). It is not clear if this is a beneficial therapy.	C

Continued

Heart attack prevention	C
Early suggestive evidence indicates that regular intake of green tea may reduce the risk of heart attack or atherosclerosis (clogged arteries). Tea may cause a decrease in platelet aggregation or endothelial dysfunction, proposed to be beneficial against blockage of arteries in the heart. Evidence from controlled trials of sufficient size and duration is needed before a recommendation regarding this effect can be made.	
High cholesterol	C
Laboratory evidence, studies in animals, and limited research in humans suggest possible effects of green tea on cholesterol levels. Recent research using a theaflavin-enriched GTE is promising. Better evidence from studies in humans is necessary to confirm a lipid-lowering effect.	
Memory enhancement	C
Several preliminary studies have examined the effects of caffeine, tea, or coffee use on short-term and long-term memory. It remains unclear if tea is beneficial for this use.	
Menopausal symptoms	C
A study conducted in healthy postmenopausal women showed that a morning and evening menopausal formula containing green tea was effective in relieving menopausal symptoms including hot flashes and sleep disturbance. Further studies are needed to confirm these results.	
Mental performance/alertness	C
Limited, low-quality research reports that the use of green tea may improve cognition and sense of alertness. Green tea contains caffeine, which is a stimulant.	
Sun protection	C
There is limited evidence from studies in animals and humans for a protective effect of green tea against ultraviolet light injury of the skin. Well-designed research is needed before a recommendation regarding this effect can be made. Comparisons have not been made with well-established forms of sun protection such as use of ultraviolet light–protective sunscreen.	
Weight loss	C
Several small studies in humans have addressed the use of green tea extract (GTE) capsules for weight loss in overweight people or in persons of average weight. Better research is needed before a recommendation regarding this effect can be made.	

*Key to grades: *A:* Strong scientific evidence for this use; *B:* Good scientific evidence for this use; *C:* Unclear scientific evidence for this use; *D:* Fair scientific evidence against this use (it may not work); *F:* Strong scientific evidence against this use (it likely does not work). For a more detailed explanation of efficacy criteria, see "Natural Standard Evidence-Based Validated Grading Rationale" in the Introduction.

Historical or Theoretical Indications That Lack Sufficient Evidence

Asbestos lung injury protection, alcohol intoxication reversal, antioxidant, astringent, bleeding from gums or tooth sockets, blood flow improvement, body temperature regulation, bone density improvement, cataracts, cognitive performance enhancement, Crohn's disease, detoxification from alcohol or other toxins, diabetes, diarrhea, digestion promotion, disease resistance enhancement, diuretic (increasing urine), fibrosarcoma, flatulence, fungal infections, gastritis, gum swelling, headache, heart disease, *Helicobacter pylori* infection, HIV infection/AIDS, ischemia-reperfusion injury protection, joint pain, kidney stone prevention, liver cancer, longevity promotion, lung cancer, neuroprotection, oral leukoplakia, ovarian cancer, Parkinson's disease prevention, platelet aggregation inhibition, stimulant, stomach disorders, stroke prevention, sunburn, tired eyes, urine flow improvement, vomiting.

DOSING/TOXICOLOGY

The following doses are based on scientific research, publications, traditional use, or expert opinion. Many herbs and supplements have not been thoroughly tested, and their safety and effectiveness may not be proven. Brands may be made differently, with variable ingredients even within the same brand. The doses shown may not apply to all products. It is important to always read product labels and discuss doses with a qualified healthcare provider before therapy is started.

Adults (18 Years and Older)

- Benefits of specific doses of green tea are not established. Most studies have examined green tea taken as a brewed beverage, rather than in capsule form. One cup of tea contains approximately 50 mg of caffeine and 80 to 100 mg of polyphenols, depending on the strength of the infusion and the size of the cup. For cancer prevention, studies have examined the effects of habitually drinking anywhere from 1 to 10 cups daily (or greater). For heart disease prevention, one study reports benefits of drinking greater than 375 ml of tea daily, although evidence in this area remains unclear.
- In capsule form, there is considerable variation in the amount of green tea extract (GTE) per capsule, which may range from 100 to 750 mg per capsule. Extracts of green tea may be standardized to contain anywhere from 60% to 97% polyphenols. A recent phase I study reported that the maximum tolerated dose of oral GTE is 4.2 g/m^2 of body surface area daily, taken once or in three divided doses (equivalent to 7 or 8 Japanese cups), or 120 ml of green tea three times daily. Currently, there is no established recommended dose for GTE capsules.

SAFETY

The U.S. Food and Drug Administration does not strictly regulate herbs and supplements. There is no guarantee of strength, purity, or safety of products, and effects may vary. It is important to always read product labels. People who have a medical condition, or are taking other drugs, herbs, or supplements, should consult a qualified healthcare provider before starting a new therapy. A healthcare provider should be consulted immediately about any side effects.

Allergies

- People with known allergy/hypersensitivity to caffeine or tannin should avoid green tea. Skin rash and hives have been reported with caffeine ingestion.

Side Effects and Warnings

- Studies of the side effects of green tea specifically are limited. However, green tea is a source of caffeine, for which multiple reactions are reported.

- Caffeine is a stimulant of the central nervous system and may cause insomnia in adults, children, and infants (including nursing infants of mothers taking caffeine). Caffeine acts on the kidneys as a diuretic (increasing urine and urine sodium and potassium levels and potentially decreasing blood sodium and potassium levels) and may worsen urge incontinence. Caffeine-containing beverages may increase the production of stomach acid and may worsen ulcer symptoms. Tannin in tea can cause constipation. Caffeine in doses of 250 to 350 mg can increase heart rate and blood pressure, although people who consume caffeine regularly do not seem to experience these effects in the long term.
- An increase in blood sugar levels may occur after consumption of green tea containing the equivalent of 200 mg of caffeine (4 to 5 cups, depending on tea strength and cup size). Caffeine-containing beverages such as green tea should be used cautiously in patients with diabetes. By contrast, lowering of blood sugar levels from drinking green tea also has been reported in preliminary research. Additional study of the effect of green tea on blood sugar is needed.
- People with severe liver disease should use caffeine cautiously, as levels of caffeine in the blood may build up and last longer with impaired liver function. Skin rashes have been associated with caffeine ingestion. In laboratory research and studies in animals, caffeine has been found to affect blood clotting, although effects in humans are not known.
- **Caffeine toxicity/high doses:** When the equivalent of greater than 500 mg of caffeine is consumed (usually more than 8 to 10 cups per day, depending on the strength of the infusion and the size of the cup), symptoms of anxiety, delirium, agitation, psychosis, or detrusor muscle instability (unstable bladder) may occur. Conception may be delayed in women who consume large amounts of caffeine. Seizure, muscle spasm, life-threatening muscle breakdown (rhabdomyolysis), and life-threatening abnormal heart rhythms have been reported with caffeine overdose. Doses greater than 1000 mg may be fatal.
- **Caffeine withdrawal:** Chronic use can result in tolerance and psychological dependence and may be habit forming. Abrupt discontinuation may result in withdrawal symptoms such as headache, irritation, nervousness, anxiety, tremor, and dizziness. In people with psychiatric disorders such as affective disorder or schizoaffective disorder, caffeine withdrawal may worsen symptoms or cause confusion, disorientation, excitement, restlessness, violent behavior, or mania.
- **Chronic effects:** Several population studies initially suggested a possible association between caffeine use and fibrocystic breast disease, although more recent research has not found this connection. Limited research reports a possible relationship between caffeine use and multiple sclerosis, although the evidence for this association is not definitive. Studies in animals report that tannin fractions from tea plants may increase the risk of cancer, although it is not clear that the tannin present in green tea has significant carcinogenic effects in humans.
- Drinking tannin-containing beverages such as tea may contribute to iron deficiency. In infants, tea consumption has been associated with impaired iron metabolism and microcytic anemia.
- In preliminary research, green tea has been associated with decreased levels of estrogens in the body. It is not clear if significant side effects such as hot flashes may occur.

Pregnancy and Breastfeeding

- Large amounts of green tea should be used cautiously in pregnant women, because caffeine crosses the placenta and has been associated with spontaneous abortion, intrauterine growth restriction/retardation, and low birth weight. Heavy caffeine intake (400 mg or greater daily) during pregnancy may increase the risk of sudden infant death syndrome (SIDS). Very high doses of caffeine (1100 mg or greater daily) have been associated with birth defects, including limb and palate malformations.
- Caffeine is readily transferred into breast milk. Caffeine ingestion by infants can lead to sleep disturbances/insomnia. Nursing infants of mothers consuming greater than 500 mg of caffeine daily have been reported to experience tremors and heart rhythm abnormalities. Components present in breast milk may reduce infants' ability to metabolize caffeine, resulting in higher-than-expected blood levels. Tea consumption by infants has been associated with anemia, reductions in iron metabolism, and irritability.

INTERACTIONS

Most herbs and supplements have not been thoroughly tested for interactions with other herbs, supplements, drugs, or foods. The interactions listed here are based on reports in scientific publications, laboratory experiments, or traditional use. It is important to always read product labels. People who have a medical condition, or are taking other drugs, herbs, or supplements, should consult a qualified healthcare provider before starting a new therapy.

Interactions with Drugs

- Studies of the interactions of green tea with drugs are limited. However, green tea is a source of caffeine, for which multiple interactions have been documented.
- The combination of caffeine with ephedrine, an ephedra alkaloid, has been implicated in numerous severe or life-threatening cardiovascular events such as very high blood pressure, stroke, or heart attack. This combination is commonly used in over-the-counter weight loss products and also may be associated with other adverse effects, including abnormal heart rhythms, insomnia, anxiety, headache, irritability, poor concentration, blurred vision, and dizziness. Stroke also has been reported after the nasal ingestion of caffeine with amphetamine.
- Caffeine may add to the effects and side effects of other stimulants including nicotine, beta-adrenergic agonists such as albuterol (Ventolin), and other methylxanthines such as theophylline. Conversely, caffeine can counteract drowsy effects and mental slowness caused by benzodiazepines such as lorazepam (Ativan) and diazepam (Valium). Phenylpropanolamine and caffeine should not be used together, because of reports of numerous potentially serious adverse effects, although forms of phenylpropanolamine taken by mouth have been removed from the U.S. market following reports of bleeding into the head.
- When taken with caffeine, a number of drugs may increase caffeine blood levels or the length of time caffeine acts on the body, including disulfiram (Antabuse), oral contraceptives (OCPs) or agents for hormone replacement therapy (HRT), ciprofloxacin (Cipro), norfloxacin, fluvoxamine (Luvox), cimetidine (Tagamet), verapamil, and mexiletine. Caffeine levels may be lowered with simultaneous use of dexamethasone (Decadron). The metabolism of caffeine by the liver (using the cytochrome P450 isoenzyme 1A2) may be affected by numerous drugs, although the effects in humans are not clear.

- Caffeine may lengthen the effects of carbamazepine or increase the effects of clozapine (Clozaril) and dipyridamole. Caffeine may affect serum lithium levels, and abrupt cessation of caffeine use by regular caffeine users taking lithium may result in high levels of lithium or lithium toxicity. Levels of aspirin or phenobarbital may be lowered in the body, although clinical effects in humans are not clear.
- Although caffeine by itself does not appear to have pain-relieving properties, it is used in combination with ergotamine tartrate in the treatment of migraine or cluster headaches (for example, Cafergot). It has been shown to increase the headache-relieving effects of other pain relievers such as acetaminophen and aspirin (for example, Excedrin). Caffeine also may increase the pain-relieving effects of codeine and ibuprofen (Advil, Motrin).
- As a diuretic, caffeine increases urine and sodium losses through the kidney and may add to the effects of other diuretics such as furosemide (Lasix).
- Green tea may contain vitamin K, which when used in large quantities can reduce the blood-thinning effects of warfarin (Coumadin), a phenomenon that has been reported in a human case.

Interactions with Herbs and Dietary Supplements

- Studies of green tea interactions with herbs and supplements are limited. However, green tea is a source of caffeine, for which multiple interactions have been documented.
- Caffeine may add to the effects and side effects of other stimulants. The combination of caffeine with ephedrine, which is present in ephedra (ma huang), has been implicated in numerous severe or life-threatening cardiovascular events such as sudden onset of very high blood pressure, stroke, or heart attack. This combination is commonly used in over-the-counter weight loss products and also may be associated with other adverse effects, including abnormal heart rhythms, insomnia, anxiety, headache, irritability, poor concentration, blurred vision, and dizziness.
- Cola nut, guarana (*Paullina cupana*), and yerba mate (*Ilex paraguariensis*) also are sources of caffeine and may add to the effects and side effects of caffeine in green tea. A combination product containing caffeine, yerba mate, and damania (*Turnera diffusa*) has been reported to cause weight loss, slowing of the gastrointestinal transit, and a feeling of stomach fullness.
- As a diuretic, caffeine increases urine and sodium losses through the kidney and may add to the effects of other diuretic agents. Herbs with diuretic effects may include artichoke, celery, corn silk, couchgrass, dandelion, elder flower, horsetail, juniper berry, kava, shepherd's purse, uva ursi, and yarrow.

Selected References

Natural Standard developed the preceding evidence-based information based on a systematic review of more than 900 articles. For comprehensive information about alternative and complementary therapies on the professional level, go to www.naturalstandard.com. Selected references are listed here.

Adcocks C, Collin P, Buttle DJ. Catechins from green tea (*Camellia sinensis*) inhibit bovine and human cartilage proteoglycan and type II collagen degradation in vitro. J Nutr 2003;132(3):341-346.

Adhami VM, Ahmad N, Mukhtar H. Molecular targets for green tea in prostate cancer prevention. J Nutr 2003;133(7 Suppl):2417S-2424S.

Afaq F, Adhami VM, Ahmad N, et al. Inhibition of ultraviolet B–mediated activation of nuclear factor kappa B in normal human epidermal karatinocytes by green tea constituent (–)-epigallocatechin-3-gallate. Oncogene 2003;22(7):1035-1044.

Ahmad N, Mukhtar H. Cutaneous photochemoprotection by green tea: a brief review. Skin Pharmacol Appl Skin Physiol 2001;14(2):69-76.

Ahn WS, Huh SW, Bae SM, et al. A major constituent of green tea, EGCG, inhibits the growth of a human cervical cell line, CaSki cells, through apoptosis, G(1) arrest, and regulation of gene expression. DNA Cell Biol 2003;22(3):217-224.

Alic M. Green tea for remission maintenance in Crohn's disease? Am J Gastroenterol 1999;94(6):1710-1711.

Anonymous. Green tea and leukoplakia. The Indian-US Head and Neck Cancer Cooperative Group. Am J Surg 1997;174(5):552-555.

Arimoto-Kobayashi S, Inada N, Sato Y, et al. Inhibitory effects of (–)-epigallocatechin gallate on the mutation, DNA strand cleavage, and DNA adduct formation by heterocyclic amines. J Agric Food Chem 203;51(17):5150-5153.

Arts IC, Hollman PC, Feskens EJ, et al. Catechin intake might explain the inverse relation between tea consumption and ischemic heart disease: the Zutphen Elderly Study. Am J Clin Nutr 2001;74(2):227-232.

Birkett NJ, Logan AG. Caffeine-containing beverages and the prevalence of hypertension. J Hypertens Suppl 1988;6(4):S620-S622.

Brown SL, Salive ME, Pahor M, et al. Occult caffeine as a source of sleep problems in an older population. J Am Geriatr Soc 1995;43(8):860-864.

Cao Y, Cao R. Angiogenesis inhibited by drinking tea. Nature 1999;398(6726):381.

Cerhan JR, Putnam SD, Bianchi GD, et al. Tea consumption and risk of cancer of the colon and rectum. Nutr Cancer 2001;41(1-2):33-40.

Chai PC, Long LH, Halliwell B. Contribution of hydrogen peroxide to the cytotoxicity of green tea and red wines. Biochem Biophys Res Commun 2003;304(4):650-654.

Chang LK, Wei TT, Chiu YF, et al. Inhibition of Epstein-Barr virus lytic cycle by (–)-epigallocatechin gallate. Biochem Biophys Res Commun 2003;301(4):1062-1068.

Chantre P, Lairon D. Recent findings of green tea extract AR25 (Exolise) and its activity for the treatment of obesity. Phytomedicine 2002;9(1):3-8.

Chen C, Shen G, Hebbar V, et al. Epigallocatechin-3-gallate–induced stress signals in HT-29 human colon adenocarcinoma cells. Carcinogenesis 2003;24(8):1369-1378.

Chow HH, Cai Y, Alberts DS, et al. Phase I pharmacokinetic study of tea polyphenols following single-dose administration of epigallocatechin gallate and polyphenon E. Cancer Epidemiol Biomarkers Prev 2001;10(1):53-58.

Chow WH, Blot WJ, McLaughlin JK. Tea drinking and cancer risk: epidemiologic evidence. Proc Soc Exp Biol Med 1999;220(4):197.

Chow WH, Swanson CA, Lissowska J, et al. Risk of stomach cancer in relation to consumption of cigarettes, alcohol, tea and coffee in Warsaw, Poland. Int J Cancer 1999;81(6):871-876.

Chung WY, Yow CM, Benzie IF. Assessment of membrane protection by traditional Chinese medicines using a flow cytometric technique: preliminary findings. Redox Rep 2003;8(1):31-33.

Clausson B, Granath F, Ekbom A, et al. Effect of caffeine exposure during pregnancy on birth weight and gestational age. Am J Epidemiol 2002;155(5):429-436.

Cnattingius S, Signorello LB, Anneren G, et al. Caffeine intake and the risk of first-trimester spontaneous abortion. N Engl J Med 2000;343(25):1839-1845.

Disler PB, Lynch SR, Charlton RW, et al. The effect of tea on iron absorption. Gut 1975;16(3):193-200.

Dlugosz L, Belanger K, Hellenbrand K, et al. Maternal caffeine consumption and spontaneous abortion: a prospective cohort study. Epidemiology 1996;7(3):250-255.

Dona M, Dell'Aica I, Calabrese F, et al. Neutrophil restraint by green tea: inhibition of inflammation, associated angiogenesis, and pulmonary fibrosis. J Immunol 2003;170(8):4335-4341.

Duffy SJ, Vita JA, Holbrook M, et al. Effect of acute and chronic tea consumption on platelet aggregation in patients with coronary artery disease. Arterioscler Thromb Vasc Biol 2001;21(6):1084-1089.

Durlach PJ. The effects of a low dose of caffeine on cognitive performance. Psychopharmacology (Berl) 1998;140(1):116-119.

Esimone CO, Adikwu MU, Nwafor SV, et al. Potential use of tea extract as a complementary mouthwash: comparative evaluation of two commercial samples. J Altern Complement Med 2001;7(5):523-527.

Ewertz M, Gill C. Dietary factors and breast-cancer risk in Denmark. Int J Cancer 1990;46(5):779-784.

Fernandes O, Sabharwal M, Smiley T, et al. Moderate to heavy caffeine consumption during pregnancy and relationship to spontaneous abortion and abnormal fetal growth: a meta-analysis. Reprod Toxicol 1998;12(4):435-444.

Ford RP, Schluter PJ, Mitchell EA, et al. Heavy caffeine intake in pregnancy and sudden infant death syndrome. New Zealand Cot Death Study Group. Arch Dis Child 1998;78(1):9-13.

Fujiki H, Suganuma M, Okabe S, et al. Cancer inhibition by green tea. Mutat Res 1998;402(1-2):307-310.

Fung KF, Zhang ZQ, Wong JW, et al. Aluminum and fluoride concentrations of three tea varieties growing at Lantau Island, Hong Kong. Environ Geochem Health 2003;25(2):219-232.

Gao YT, McLaughlin JK, Blot WJ, et al. Reduced risk of esophageal cancer associated with green tea consumption. J Natl Cancer Inst 1994;86(11):855-858.

Geleijnse JM, Launer LJ, Hofman A, et al. Tea flavonoids may protect against atherosclerosis: the Rotterdam Study. Arch Intern Med 1999;159(18):2170-2174.

Geleijnse JM, Witteman JC, Launer LJ, et al. Tea and coronary heart disease: protection through estrogen-like activity? Arch Intern Med 2000;160(21): 3328-3329.

Grosso LM, Rosenberg KD, Belanger K, et al. Maternal caffeine intake and intrauterine growth retardation. Epidemiology 2001;12(4):447-455.

Gupta S, Ahmad N, Mohan RR, et al. Prostate cancer chemoprevention by green tea: in vitro and *in vivo* inhibition of testosterone-mediated induction of ornithine decarboxylase. Cancer Res 1999;59(9):2115-2120.

Gupta S, Hussain T, Mukhtar H. Molecular pathway for (–)-epigallocatechin-3-gallate–induced cell cycle arrest and apoptosis of human prostate carcinoma cells. Arch Biochem Biophys 2003;410(1):177-185.

Gupta SK, Halder N, Srivastava S, et al. Green tea (*Camellia sinensis*) protects against selenite-induced oxidative stress in experimental cataractogenesis. Opthalmic Res 2003;34(4):258-263.

Hadeed A, Siegel S. Newborn cardiac arrhythmias associated with maternal caffeine use during pregnancy. Clin Pediatr (Phila) 1993;32(1):45-47.

Hartman TJ, Tangrea JA, Pietinen P, et al. Tea and coffee consumption and risk of colon and rectal cancer in middle-aged Finnish men. Nutr Cancer 1998; 31(1):41-48.

Hastak K, Gupta S, Ahmad N, et al. Role of p53 and NF-kappa B in epigallocatechin-3-gallate–induced apoptosis of LNCaP cells. Oncogene 2003; 22(31):4851-4859.

Hegarty VM, May HM, Khaw KT. Tea drinking and bone mineral density in older women. Am J Clin Nutr 2000;71(4):1003-1007.

Hiatt RA, Klatsky AL, Armstrong MA. Pancreatic cancer, blood glucose and beverage consumption. Int J Cancer 1988;41(6):794-797.

Hodgson JM, Puddey IB, Burke V, et al. Effects on blood pressure of drinking green and black tea. J Hypertens 1999;17(4):457-463.

Hodgson JM, Puddey IB, Croft KD, et al. Acute effects of ingestion of black and green tea on lipoprotein oxidation. Am J Clin Nutr 2000;71(5):1103-1107.

Hoshiyama Y, Kawaguchi T, Miura Y, et al. A prospective study of stomach cancer death in relation to green tea consumption in Japan. Br J Cancer 2002; 87(3):309-313.

Hsu S, Bollag WB, Lewis J, et al. Green tea polyphenols induce differentiation and proliferation in epidermal keratinocytes. J Pharmacol Exp Ther 2003; 306(1):29-34.

Hsu S, Lewis J, Singh B, et al. Green tea polyphenol targets the mitochondria in tumor cells inducing caspase 3-dependant apoptosis. Anticancer Res 2003; 23(2B):1533-1539.

Hu J, Nyren O, Wolk A, et al. Risk factors for oesophageal cancer in northeast China. Int J Cancer 1994;57(1):38-46.

Imai K, Suga K, Nakachi K. Cancer-preventive effects of drinking green tea among a Japanese population. Prev Med 1997;26(6):769-775.

Infante-Rivard C, Fernandez A, Gauthier R, et al. Fetal loss associated with caffeine intake before and during pregnancy. JAMA 1993;270(24):2940-2943.

Iwai N, Ohshiro H, Kurozawa Y, et al. Relationship between coffee and green tea consumption and all-cause mortality in a cohort of a rural Japanese population. J Epidemiol 2002;12(3):191-198.

James JE. Chronic effects of habitual caffeine consumption on laboratory and ambulatory blood pressure levels. J Cardiovasc Risk 1994;1(2):159-164.

Jatoi A, Ellison N, Burch PA, et al. A phase II trial of green tea in the treatment of patients with androgen independent metastatic prostate carcinoma. Cancer 2003;97(6):1442-1446.

Jensen OM, Wahrendorf J, Knudsen JB, et al. The Copenhagen case-control study of bladder cancer. II. Effect of coffee and other beverages. Int J Cancer 1986;37(5):651-657.

Ji BT, Chow WH, Hsing AW, et al. Green tea consumption and the risk of pancreatic and colorectal cancers. Int J Cancer 1997;70(3):255-258.

Joseph SL, Joseph SL, Arab L. Tea consumption and the reduced risk of colon cancer—results from a national prospective cohort study. Public Health Nutr 2002;5(3):419-426.

Kakuda T. Neuroprotective effects of the green tea components theanine and catechins. Biol Pharm Bull 2002;25(12):1513-1518.

Katiyar SK, Ahmad N, Mukhtar H. Green tea and skin. Arch Dermatol 2000;136(8):989-994.

Kaundun SS, Matsumoto S. Development of CAPS markers based on three key genes of the phenylpropanoid pathway in tea, *Camellia sinensis* (L.) O. Kuntze, and differentiation between assamica and sinensis varieties. Theor Appl Genet 2003;106(3):375-383.

Kaundun SS, Matsumoto S. Identification of processed Japanese green tea based on polymorphisms generated by STS-RFLP analysis. J Agric Food Chem 2003;51(7):1765-1770.

Kinlen LJ, McPherson K. Pancreas cancer and coffee and tea consumption: a case-control study. Br J Cancer 1984;49(1):93-96.

Kinlen LJ, Willows AN, Goldblatt P, et al. Tea consumption and cancer. Br J Cancer 1988;58(3):397-401.

Klatsky AL, Armstrong MA, Friedman GD. Coffee, tea, and mortality. Ann Epidemiol 1993;3(4):375-381.

Kohlmeier L, Weterings KG, Steck S, et al. Tea and cancer prevention: an evaluation of the epidemiologic literature. Nutr Cancer 1997;27(1):1-13.

Koizumi Y, Tsubono Y, Nakaya N, et al. No association between green tea and the risk of gastric cancer: pooled analysis of two prospective studies in Japan. Cancer Epidemiol Biomarkers Prev 2003;12(5):472-473.

Kono S, Shinchi K, Ikeda N, et al. Green tea consumption and serum lipid

profiles: a cross-sectional study in northern Kyushu, Japan. Prev Med 1992; 21(4):526-531.

Kono S. Green tea and colon cancer. Jpn J Cancer Res 1992;83(6):669.

Kono S. Green tea and gastric cancer in Japan. N Engl J Med 2001;344(24): 1867-1868.

Lambert JD, Yang CS. Cancer chemopreventive activity and bioavailability of tea and tea polyphenols. Mutat Res 2003:523-524:201-208.

Lambert JD, Yang CS. Mechanisms of cancer prevention by tea constituents. J Nutr 2003;133(10):3262S-3267S.

La Vecchia C, Negri E, Decarli A, et al. A case-control study of diet and colo-rectal cancer in northern Italy. Int J Cancer 1988;41(4):492-498.

La Vecchia C, Negri E, Franceschi S, et al. Tea consumption and cancer risk. Nutr Cancer 1992;17(1):27-31.

Lawson DH, Jick H, Rothman KJ. Coffee and tea consumption and breast disease. Surgery 1981;90(5):801-803.

Levites Y, Amit T, Mandel S, et al. Neuroprotection and neurorescue against Abeta toxicity and PKC-dependent release of nonamyloidogenic soluble precursor protein by green tea polyphenol (–)-epifallocatechin-3-gallate. FASEB J 2003;17(8):952-954.

Lee IP, Kim YH, Kang MH, et al. Chemopreventive effect of green tea (*Camellia sinensis*) against cigarette smoke–induced mutations (SCE) in humans. J Cell Biochem Suppl 1997;27:68-75.

Levi M, Guchelaar HJ, Woerdenbag HJ, et al. Acute hepatitis in a patient using a Chinese herbal tea—a case report. Pharm World Sci 1998;20(1):43-44.

Lill G, Voit S, Schror K, et al. Complex effects of different green tea catechins on human platelets. FEBS Lett 2003;546(2-3):265-270.

Lin YS, Tsai YJ, Tsay JS, et al. Factors affecting the levels of tea polyphenols and caffeine in tea leaves. J Agric Food Chem 2003;51(7):1864-1873.

Locher R, Emmanuele L, Suter PM, et al. Green tea polyphenols inhibit human vascular smooth muscle cell proliferation stimulated by native low-density lipoprotein. Eur J Pharmacol 2002;434(1-2):1-7.

Lu H, Meng X, Li C, et al. Glucuronides of tea catechins: enzymology of biosynthesis and biological activities. Drug Metab Dispos 2003;31(4): 452-461.

Maeda K, Kusuya M, Cheng XW, et al. Green tea catechins inhibit the cultured smooth muscle cell invasion through the basement barrier. Atherosclerosis 2003;166(1):23-20.

Maeda-Yamamoto M, Suzuki N, Sawai, et al. Association of suppression of extracellular signal–regulated kinase phosphorylation by epigallocatechin gallate with the reduction of matrix metalloproteinase activities in human fibrosarcoma HT1080 cells. J Agric Food Chem 2003;51(7):1858-1863.

Mameleers PA, Van Boxtel MP, Hogervorst E. Habitual caffeine consumption and its relation to memory, attention, planning capacity and psychomotor performance across multiple age groups. Hum Psychopharmacol 2000;15(8): 573-581.

Maron DJ, Lu GP, Cai NS, et al. Cholesterol-lowering effect of a theaflavin-enriched green tea extract: a randomized controlled trial. Arch Intern Med 2003;163(12):1448-1453.

Martinez-Richa A, Joseph-Nathan P. Carbon-13 CP-MAS nuclear magnetic resonance studies of teas. Solid State Nucl Magn Reson 2003;23(3):119-135.

Mei Y, Wei D, Liu J. Reversal of cancer multidrug resistance by tea polyphenol in KB cells. J Chemother 2003;15(3):260-265.

Morre DJ, Morre DM, Sun H, et al. Tea catechin synergies in inhibition of cancer cell proliferation and of a cancer specific cell surface oxidase (ECTO-NOX). Pharmacol Toxicol 2003;92(5):234-241.

Mukamal KJ, Maclure M, Muller JE, et al. Tea consumption and mortality after acute myocardial infarction. Circulation 2002;105:2476-2481.

Nagano J, Kono S, Preston DL, et al. A prospective study of green tea consumption and cancer incidence, Hiroshima and Nagasaki (Japan). Cancer Causes Control 2001;12(6):501-508.

Nakachi K, Eguchi H, Imai K. Can teatime increase one's lifetime? Ageing Res Rev 2003;2(1):1-10.

Nakachi K, Suemasu K, Suga K, et al. Influence of drinking green tea on breast cancer malignancy among Japanese patients. Jpn J Cancer Res 1998;89(3): 254-261.

Nakagawa K, Ninomiya M, Okubo T, et al. Tea catechin supplementation increases antioxidant capacity and prevents phospholipid hydroperoxidation in plasma of humans. J Agric Food Chem 1999;47(10):3967-3973.

Nyska A, Suttie A, Bakshi S, et al. Slowing tumorigenic progression in TRAMP mice and prostatic carcinoma cell lines using natural anti-oxidant from spinach, NAO—a comparative study of three anti-oxidants. Toxicol Pathol. 2003 Jan-Feb;31(1):39-51.

Ohno Y, Wakai K, Genka K, et al. Tea consumption and lung cancer risk: a case-control study in Okinawa, Japan. Jpn J Cancer Res 1995;86(11):1027-1034.

Park AM, Dong Z. Signal transduction pathways: targets for green and black tea polyphenols. J Biochem Mol Biol 2003;36(1):66-77.

Paschka AG, Butler R, Young CY. Induction of apoptosis in prostate cancer cell lines by the green tea component, (–)-epigallocatechin-3-gallate. Cancer Lett 1998;130(1-2):1-7.

Peters U, Poole C, Arab L. Does tea affect cardiovascular disease? a meta-analysis. Am J Epidemiol 2001;154(6):495-503.

Pezzato E, Dona M, Sartor L, et al. Proteinase-3 directly activates MMP-2 and degrades gelatin and Matrigel; differential inhibition by (–)epigallocatechin-3-gallate. J Leukoc Biol 2003;74(1):88-94.

Pisters KM, Newman RA, Coldman B, et al. Phase I trial of oral green tea extract in adult patients with solid tumors. J Clin Oncol 2001;19(6):1830-1838.

Robinson R. Green tea extract may have neuroprotective effects in Parkinson's disease. Lancet 2001;358:391.

Rosenberg L. Coffee and tea consumption in relation to the risk of large bowel cancer: a review of epidemiologic studies. Cancer Lett 1990;52(3):163-171.

Roy M, Chakrabarty S, Sinha D, et al. Anticlastogenic, antigenotoxic and apoptotic activity of epigallocatechin gallate: a green tea polyphenol. Mutat Res 2003:33-41.

Sadzuka Y, Sugiyama T, Hirota S. Modulation of cancer chemotherapy by green tea. Clin Cancer Res 1998;4(1):153-156.

Saha P, Das S. Regulation of hazardous exposure by protective exposure: modulation of phase II detoxification and lipid peroxidation by *Camellia sinensis* and *Swertia chirata*. Teratog Carcinog Mutagen 2003;Suppl 1:313-322.

Sakanaka S. A novel convenient process to obtain a raw decaffeinated tea polyphenol fraction using a lignocellulose column. J Agric Food Chem 2003; 51(10):3140-3143.

Sano M, Yoshida R, Degawa M, et al. Determination of peroxyl radical scavenging activity of flavonoids and plant extracts using an automatic potentiometric titrator. J Agric Food Chem 2003;51(10):2912-2918.

Sano T, Sasako M. Green tea and gastric cancer. N Engl J Med 2001;344(9): 675-676.

Santos IS, Victora CG, Huttly S, et al. Caffeine intake and pregnancy outcomes: a meta-analytic review. Cad Saude Publica 1998;14(3):523-530.

Sasazuki S, Kodama H, Yoshimasu K, et al. Relation between green tea consumption and the severity of coronary atherosclerosis among Japanese men and women. Ann Epidemiol 2000;10(6):401-408.

Sato D, Matsushima M. Preventive effects of urinary bladder tumors induced by *N*-butyl-*N*-(4-hydroxybutyl)-notrosamine in rat by green tea leaves. Int J Urol 2003;10(3):160-166.

Sato Y, Nakatsuka H, Watanabe T, et al. Possible contribution of green tea drinking habits to the prevention of stroke. Tohoku J Exp Med 1989;157(4): 337-343.

Sesso HD, Gaziano JM, Buring JE, et al. Coffee and tea intake and the risk of myocardial infarction. Am J Epidemiol 1999;149(2):162-167.

Setiawan VW, Zhang ZF, Yu GP, et al. Protective effect of green tea on the risks of chronic gastritis and stomach cancer. Int J Cancer 2001;92(4):600-604.

Shibata K, Moriyama M, Fukushima T, et al. Green tea consumption and chronic atrophic gastritis: a cross-sectional study in a green tea production village. J Epidemiol 2000;10(5):310-316.

Shirlow MJ, Mathers CD. A study of caffeine consumption and symptoms; indigestion, palpitations, tremor, headache and insomnia. Int J Epidemiol 1985;14(2):239-248.

Singh R, Ahmed S, Malemud CJ, et al. Epigallocatechin-3-gallate selectivity inhibits interleukin-1beta–induced activation of mitogen activated protein kinase subgroup c-Jun N-terminal kinase in human osteoarthritis chondrocytes. J Orthop Res;21(1):102-109.

Skrzydlewska E, Ostrowska J, Stankiewicz A, et al. Green tea as a potent antioxidant in alcohol intoxication. Addict Biol 2002;7(3):307-314.

Stavchansky S, Combs A, Sagraves R, et al. Pharmacokinetics of caffeine in breast milk and plasma after single oral administration of caffeine to lactating mothers. Biopharm Drug Dispos 1988;9(3):285-299.

Stoner GD, Mukhtar H. Polyphenols as cancer chemopreventive agents. J Cell Biochem Suppl 1995;22:169-180.

Sun J. Morning/evening menopausal formula relieves menopausal symptoms: a pilot study. J. Altern Complement Med 2003;9(3):403-409.

Sung H, Nah J, Chun S, et al. *In vivo* antioxidant effect of green tea. Eur J Clin Nutr 2000;54(7):527-529.

Suzuki Y, Shioi Y. Identification of chlorophylls and carotenoids in major teas by high-performance liquid chromatography with photodiode array detection. J Agric Food Chem 2003;51(18):5307-5314.

Tavani A, Pregnolato A, La Vecchia C, et al. Coffee and tea intake and risk of cancers of the colon and rectum: a study of 3,530 cases and 7,057 controls. Int J Cancer 1997;73(2):193-197.

Taylor JR, Wilt VM. Probable antagonism of warfarin by green tea. Ann Pharmacother 1999;33(4):426-428.

Tedeschi E, Suzuki H, Menegazzi M. Antiinflammatory action of EGCG, the main component of green tea, through Stat-1 inhibition. Ann N Y Acad Sci 2003:435-437.

Tokunaga S, White IR, Frost C, et al. Green tea consumption and serum lipids and lipoproteins in a population of healthy workers in Japan. Ann Epidemiol 2002;12(3):157-165.

Tombola F, Campello S, De Luca L, et al. Plant polyphenols inhibit VacA, a toxin secreted by the gastric pathogen *Helicobacter pylori*. FEBS Lett 2003; 543(1-3):184-189.

Tsubono Y, Nishino Y, Komatsu S, et al. Green tea and the risk of gastric cancer in Japan. N Engl J Med 2001;344(9):632-636.

Valentao P, Fernandes E, Carvalho F, et al. Hydroxyl radical and hypochlorous acid scavenging activity of small centaury (*Centaurium erythraea*) infusion. A comparative study with green tea (*Camellia sinensis*). Phytomedicine 2003; 10(6-7):517-522.

Vankemmelbeke MN, Jones GC, Fowles C, et al. Selective inhibition of ADAMTS-1, -4, and -5 by catechin gallate esters. Eur J Biochem 2003; 270(11):2394-2403.

Vinson J, Zhang J. Green and black tea inhibit diabetic cataracts by three mechanisms: sorbitol, lipid peroxidation and protein glycation. Diabetes 2001; 50(Suppl 2):A476.

Weber JM, Ruzindana-Umunyana A, Imbeault L, et al. Inhibition of adenovirus infection and adenain by green tea catechins. Antiviral Res 2003;58(2): 167-173.

Wrenn KD, Oschner I. Rhabdomyolysis induced by a caffeine overdose. Ann Emerg Med 1989;18(1):94-97.

Wu AH, Yu MC, Tseng CC, et al. Green tea and risk of breast cancer in Asian Americans. Int J Cancer 2003;106(4):574-579.

Wu CH, Yang YC, Yao WJ, et al. Epidemiological evidence of increased bone mineral density in habitual tea drinkers. Arch Intern Med 2002;162(9): 1001-1006.

Xu J, Yang F, Chen L, et al. Effect of selenium on increasing the antioxidant activity of tea leaves harvested during the early spring tea producing season. J Agric Food Chem 2003;51(4):1081-1084.

Yamamoto T, Hsu S, Lewis J, et al. Green tea polyphenol causes differential oxidative environments in tumor versus normal epithelial cells.. J Pharmacol Exp Ther 2003;301(1):230-236.

Yang TT, Koo MW. Hypocholesterolemic effects of Chinese tea. Pharmacol Res 1997;35(6):505-512.

Yee Y-K KW, Szeto ML. Effect of Chinese tea consumption on *Helicobacter pylori* infection (abstract). J Gastroenterol Hepatol 2000;15:B33-A90.

Yee YK, Koo MW, Szeto ML. Chinese tea consumption and lower risk of *Helicobacter* infection. J Gastroenterol Hepatol 2002;17(5):552-555.

Yu GP, Hsieh CC, Wang LY, et al. Green-tea consumption and risk of stomach cancer: a population-based case-control study in Shanghai, China. Cancer Causes Control 1995;6(6):532-538.

Zhang M, Binns CW, Lee AH. Tea consumption and ovarian cancer risk: a case control study in China. Cancer Epidemiol Biomarkers Prev 2002;11(8): 713-718.

Zheng W, Doyle TJ, Kushi LH, et al. Tea consumption and cancer incidence in a prospective cohort study of postmenopausal women. Am J Epidemiol 1996;144(2):175-182.

Zhong L, Goldberg MS, Gao YT, et al. A population-based case-control study of lung cancer and green tea consumption among women living in Shanghai, China. Epidemiology 2001;12(6):695-700.

Zhou JR, Yu L, Zhong Y, et al. Soy phytochemicals and tea bioactive components synergistically inhibit androgen-sensitive human prostate tumors in mice. J Nutr 2003;133(2):516-521.

Guggul
(Commifora mukul)

SYNONYMS/COMMON NAMES/RELATED SUBSTANCES

- African myrrh, Arabian myrrh, *Commiphora myrrha*, guggal, guggulu, guggulsterone (4,17(20)-pregnadiene-3,16-dione), gum guggul, gum guggulu, guggulsterone, gugulimax, guggulipid C+, guglip, gum myrrh, fraction A, myrrha, Somali myrrh, yemen myrrh.

CLINICAL BOTTOM LINE
Background

- Guggul (gum guggul) is a resin produced by the mukul mirth tree. Guggulipid is extracted from guggul and contains plant sterols (guggulsterones E and Z), which are believed to be its bioactive compounds.
- Prior to 2003, the majority of scientific evidence suggested that guggulipid elicits significant reductions in serum total cholesterol, low-density lipoproteins (LDLs), and triglycerides, as well as elevations in high-density lipoprotein (HDLs).[1-11] However, most published studies were small and not well designed or reported. In August 2003, a well-designed trial reported small significant *increases* in serum LDL levels associated with the use of guggul compared to placebo.[12] No significant changes in total cholesterol, HDLs, or triglycerides were noted. These results are consistent with two prior published case reports.[13,14] Although this evidence provides preliminary evidence against the efficacy of guggul for hypercholesterolemia, because of the precedent of prior research and historical use, further study is necessary before a definitive conclusion can be reached.
- Initial research reports that guggulsterones are antagonists of the farsenoid X receptor (FXR) and the bile acid receptor (BAR), which are nuclear hormones involved in cholesterol metabolism and bile acid regulation.[1,15,16]

Scientific Evidence for Common/Studied Uses	Grade*
Acne	C
Hyperlipidemia	C
Obesity	C
Osteoarthritis	C
Rheumatoid arthritis	C

*Key to grades: A: Strong scientific evidence for this use; B: Good scientific evidence for this use; C: Unclear scientific evidence for this use; D: Fair scientific evidence against this use (it may not work); F: Strong scientific evidence against this use (it likely does not work). For a more detailed explanation of efficacy criteria, see "Natural Standard Evidence-Based Validated Grading Rationale" in the Introduction.

Historical or Theoretical Uses
That Lack Sufficient Evidence

- Asthma, bleeding, colitis, diabetes, gingivitis, hemorrhoids, leprosy, leukorrhoea, menstrual disorders, mouth infections, neuralgia, obesity, pain, psoriasis, rhinitis, sore throat, sores, tumors, weight loss, wound healing.

Expert Opinion and Folkloric Precedent

- Guggul has been used medicinally since at least 600 B.C. for weight loss, heart conditions, and numerous other ailments. Although widely used in India, guggul and its preparations are less well known in the United States. Guggul is believed to have medicinal benefits and minimum toxicity when taken as a soluble extract rather than as a gum resin.[17,18]

Safety Summary

- **Likely safe:** When taken at recommended doses for up to 6 months.[9]
- **Possibly unsafe:** When taken at doses of 2000 mg three times daily standardized to 2.5% guggulsterones (50 mg of guggulsterones three times daily), because of the risk of hypersensitivity skin reactions (which appear to resolve spontaneously within 1 week in most cases).[12] Guggul also is possibly unsafe when used by patients with thyroid disorders, based on guggulipid-induced thyroid stimulation in animal studies,[19] although a recent human trial reports no effects of guggulipid in thyroid-stimulating hormone (TSH) levels after 8 weeks of therapy.[12]
- **Likely unsafe:** When taken during pregnancy, based on studies suggesting the possibility of abortive effects.[20,21]

DOSING/TOXICOLOGY
General

- Recommended doses are based on those most commonly used in available trials, or on historical practice. However, with natural products, the optimal doses needed to balance efficacy and safety often have not been determined. Formulations and preparation methods may vary from manufacturer to manufacturer, and from batch to batch of a specific product made by a single manufacturer. Because often the active components of a product are not known, standardization may not be possible, and the clinical effects of different brands may not be comparable.

Standardization

- Guggulipid preparations are often standardized to contain 2.5% to 5% of guggulsterones.
- In July 2003, ConsumerLab.com evaluated five guggulsterone supplements. They report that Vitamin World Select Herbals Standardized Extract Guggul Plex, 340 mg, Standardized to contain 2.5% Guggulsterones (8.5 mg per capsule, 3 per day) was "approved," based on its claimed constituents. The remaining four brands contained as little as 4% to 74% of the expected ingredient. None of the products was contaminated with lead or arsenic.
- A recent human trial used guggulipid provided by Sabinsa Corp. (Piscataway, NJ), standardized to contain at least 2.5% of guggulsterones E and Z and found the tablets to contain 2.1% guggulsterones (85% of the claimed ingredients). This was considered satisfactory for research and clinical use.[12]

Dosing: Adult 18 Years and Older)
Oral

- **Hyperlipidemia:** 500-1000 mg of guggulipid (standardized to 2.5% guggulsterones) taken twice or three times daily has been used clinically and in research. An equivalent dose of commercially prepared guggulsterone is 25 mg three times daily or 50 mg twice daily by mouth.[2,9,10] A higher dose has been studied (2000 mg three times daily, standardized to 2.5% guggulsterones), although this dose may be associated with a greater risk of hypersensitivity skin reactions.[12]

- **Nodulocystic acne:** A dose of guggulipid equivalent to 25 mg guggulsterone per day has been used.[22]

Dosing: Pediatric (Younger Than 18 Years)

- Insufficient evidence to recommend.

Toxicology

- Insufficient available evidence.

ADVERSE EFFECTS/PRECAUTIONS/CONTRAINDICATIONS
Allergy

- Known allergy/hypersensitivity to guggul or any of its constituents.
- Hypersensitivity skin reactions were noted in a clinical trial, occurring in 5 of 34 patients (15%) receiving 50 mg of guggulsterones three times daily and in 1 of 33 patients (3%) receiving 25 mg of guggulsterones three times daily.[12] In most cases, reactions occurred within 48 hours of starting therapy and resolved spontaneously within 1 week of therapy discontinuation, although one patient required oral steroids. The guggulipid formulation used was prepared by the Sabinsa Corp. (Piscataway, NJ).

Adverse Effects/Postmarket Surveillance

- **General:** Standardized guggulipid is generally regarded as being safe in healthy adults when taken at recommended doses for up to 6 months. Gastrointestinal upset, most commonly loose stools or diarrhea, is the predominant adverse effect that has been described in humans.
- **Neurologic/CNS:** Headache was reported in 22 of 31 patients (71%) in one study.[9] Restlessness and apprehension were noted in 1 of 44 patients in a different study.[23]
- **Gastrointestinal:** In clinical studies and historically, guggul and guggulipid have been associated with diarrhea, loose stools, nausea, vomiting, eructation (belching), and hiccough. Frequency has varied between 10% and 30%; these symptoms have been observed both with guggul[23-25] and with guggulipid.[2,9,12] Most symptoms have been well controlled with supportive care or treatment such as antacids, although discontinuation is occasionally necessary.
- **Endocrine:** Stimulation of thyroid function has been noted in animal studies,[19,26,27] although a recent human trial reports no effects of guggulipid in thyroid-stimulating hormone (TSH) levels after 8 weeks of therapy.[12] Multiple small trials in India and traditional accounts reported lower serum lipid levels with regular use of guggulipid (decreases in cholesterol, triglycerides, and low-density lipoproteins [LDLs] and increases in high-density lipoproteins [HDLs]),[1-11] although subsequent evidence from a well-designed trial in the United States reports small increases in LDLs and no significant changes in total cholesterol, HDLs, or triglycerides.[12] Initial research reports that guggulsterones are antagonists of the farsenoid X receptor (FXR) and the bile acid receptor (BAR), which are nuclear hormones involved in cholesterol metabolism and bile acid regulation.[1,15,16]
- **Hematologic:** Guggulipid administration has been associated with inhibition of platelet aggregation and increased fibrinolysis.[10,28-30] In theory, the risk of bleeding may increase, although there are no reports of bleeding in the available literature.
- **Genitourinary:** Weight reduction and chemical changes in reproductive organs have been observed in female rats.[21]
- **Dermatologic:** Hypersensitivity skin reactions were noted in a clinical trial, occurring in 5 of 34 patients (15%) receiving 50 mg of guggulsterones three times daily, and in 1 of 33 (3%) patients receiving 25 mg of guggulsterones three times daily. In most cases, reactions occurred within 48 hours of starting therapy and resolved spontaneously within 1 week of therapy discontinuation, although one patient required oral steroids.[12] The guggulipid formulation used was prepared by the Sabinsa Corp. (Piscataway, NJ).

Precautions/Warnings/Contraindications

- Use cautiously in patients with thyroid disorders because of potential thyroid stimulating properties.
- Use cautiously in patients at risk for bleeding.

Pregnancy and Lactation

- Not recommended, due to lack of sufficient data.

INTERACTIONS
Guggul/Drug Interaction:

- **Beta-blockers:** Co-administration of guggulipid to humans has been reported to decrease the bioavailability of the beta-blocker propranolol.[31] Effects on other beta-blockers have not been evaluated.
- **Diltiazem (Cardizem, Dilacor, Tiazac):** Co-administration of guggulipid to humans has been found to decrease the bioavailability of the calcium channel blocker diltiazem.[31] The chemical structures of other calcium channel blockers are sufficiently distinct that guggul may not affect other members of this class. Patients taking diltiazem should be monitored for changes in blood pressure and heart rate if guggulipid therapy is initiated.
- **Thyroid drugs:** Data from animal models suggest that the guggul constituent guggulsterone Z may stimulate thyroid function.[19] However, results from a recent randomized, controlled trial in 103 patients reports no difference in thyroid-stimulating hormone (TSH) with the use of guggul.[12] Nonetheless, guggulipid should be used with caution in patients taking thyroid drugs.
- **Lipid-lowering agents:** Initial research reports that guggulsterones are antagonists of the farsenoid X receptor (FXR) and the bile acid receptor (BAR), which are nuclear hormones involved in cholesterol metabolism and bile acid regulation.[1,15,16] Multiple small trials in India and traditional accounts reported lower serum lipid levels with regular use of guggulipid (decreases in cholesterol, triglycerides, and low-density lipoproteins [LDLs] and increases in high-density lipoproteins [HDLs]),[1-11] although subsequent evidence from a well-designed trial in the United States reports small increases in LDLs and no significant changes in total cholesterol, HDLs, or triglycerides.[12] It is not clear if guggulipid affects the action of other agents used for cholesterol reduction.
- **Anticoagulants, antiplatelet drugs:** Guggulipid administration has been associated with inhibition of platelet aggregation and increased fibrinolysis.[10,28-30] In theory, the risk of bleeding may increase, although there are no reports of bleeding in humans in the available literature, including multiple controlled trials.

Guggul/Herb/Supplement Interactions

- **Lipid-lowering agents:** Initial research reports that guggulsterones are antagonists of the farsenoid X receptor (FXR) and the bile acid receptor (BAR), which are nuclear hormones involved in cholesterol metabolism and bile acid regulation.[1,15,16] Multiple small trials in India and traditional accounts reported lower serum lipid levels with regular use of guggulipid (decreases in cholesterol, triglycerides, and low-density lipoproteins [LDLs] and increases in high-density lipoproteins [HDLs]),[1-11] although subsequent evidence from a well-designed trial in the United States reports small increases in LDLs and no significant changes in total cholesterol, HDLs, or triglycerides.[12] It is not clear if guggulipid affects the action of other agents used for cholesterol reduction.

- **Anticoagulant herbs and supplements:** Guggulipid administration has been associated with inhibition of platelet aggregation and increased fibrinolysis.[10,28-30] In theory, the risk of bleeding may increase, although there are no reports of bleeding in humans in the available literature, including multiple controlled trials.

Guggul/Food Interactions

- Insufficient available evidence.

Guggul/Lab Interactions

- **Thyroid panel:** Data from animal models suggest that the guggul constituent guggulsterone Z may stimulate thyroid function.[19] However, results from a recent randomized, controlled trial in 103 patients reports no difference in thyroid-stimulating hormone (TSH) with the use of guggul.[12]

MECHANISM OF ACTION

Pharmacology

- **Lipid-lowering effects:** Guggul (gum guggul) is a resin produced by the mukul mirth tree. Guggulipid is extracted from guggul using ethyl acetate. The preparation produced by extraction with petroleum ether is called fraction A. Typical guggulipid preparations contain 2.5% to 5% of the plant sterols guggulsterones E and Z. These two components

have been reported to exert effects on lipids.[32,33] Several hypotheses have been advanced to explain these effects on lipids. Guggulsterones, particularly guggulsterone 4,17(20)-pregnadiene-3,16-dione, have been reported to function as antagonists of the farsenoid X receptor (FXR) and the bile acid receptor (BAR), which are nuclear hormones involved in cholesterol metabolism and bile acid regulation.[1,15,16] It has been reported that guggulsterone does not exert its lipid effects on mice lacking FXR. Other publications have proposed that guggul may inhibit lipogenic enzymes and HMG-Co A reductase in the liver,[34,35] increase uptake of cholesterol by the liver via stimulation of LDL-receptor binding,[33] directly activate the thyroid gland,[16,26,27,36] and/or increase biliary and fecal excretion of cholesterol.[35]

- **Antioxidant effects:** Guggul extracts have been reported to possess antioxidant properties[37] possibly mediating protection against myocardial necrosis.[38,39]

- **Platelet effects:** Guggulipid has been found to inhibit platelet aggregation and increase fibrinolysis.[10,28-30]

- **Anti-inflammatory effects:** The results of several studies suggest possible anti-inflammatory and antiarthritic activities of guggul.[40-48] On a per-microgram basis, guggulipid appears to be significantly less potent than indomethacin or hydrocortisone.[43] Possible effects on high-sensitivity C-reactive protein (hs-CRP) have recently been observed in a clinical trial.[12]

Pharmacodynamics/Kinetics

- Insufficient available evidence.

HISTORY

- Resin from the guggul (*Commifora mukul*) tree has been used in Ayurvedic medicine since at least 600 BC. This thorny tree has little foliage and is indigenous to Western India. In 1966, the hypolipidemic properties of soluble extracts from the resin were evaluated scientifically. In 1986, guggul oleoresin was approved in India for marketing as a lipid-lowering agent.[49,50] Guggul was introduced more recently to the Western medical literature in 1994.[9]

Review of the Evidence: Guggul

Condition Treated*	Study Design	Author, Year	N[†]	SS[†]	Study Quality[‡]	Magnitude of Benefit	ARR[†]	NNT[†]	Comments
Hyperlipidemia	RCT, placebo-controlled, double-blind	Szapary[12] 2003	103	Yes	5	Negative	NA	NA	Guggulipid (1000 or 2000 mg) (standardized to 2.1%-2.5% guggulsterones) three times daily for 8 weeks elicited small elevation in LDLs vs. placebo and no other significant effects on lipids; skin hypersensitivity in 33% of higher-dose patients.
Hyperlipidemia	RCT double-blind, crossover	Nityanand[2] 1989	125	Mixed	5	Medium	NA	NA	Guggulipid (500 mg) twice daily for 12 weeks vs. clofibrate; both reduced total cholesterol and triglycerides.
Hyperlipidemia	RCT, double-blind	Gaur[10] 1997	68	Mixed	4	Medium	NA	NA	Guggulipid (500 mg) three times daily associated with significant reduction in LDLs and increase in HDLs vs. aspirin.

Continued

Review of the Evidence: Guggul—*cont'd*

Condition Treated*	Study Design	Author, Year	N[†]	SS[†]	Study Quality[‡]	Magnitude of Benefit	ARR[†]	NNT[†]	Comments
Hyperlipidemia	Before-and-after study	Verma[8] 1988	40	Yes	4	Large	NA	NA	Purified gum guggulu (4.5 g daily) for 16 weeks associated with reduced total cholesterol and triglycerides vs. baseline; lesser reductions seen with placebo, but between-group differences were not compared statistically.
Hyperlipidemia	Before-and-after study	Kotiyal[5] 1985	85	Yes	4	Medium	NA	NA	Fraction A (500 mg) three times daily for 12 weeks associated with reduced total cholesterol vs. baseline; lesser reductions seen with placebo, but between-group differences were not compared statistically.
Hyperlipidemia	RCT, double-blind	Kuppurajan[3] 1978	120	Yes	4	Medium	NA	NA	Gum guggulu (2 g) three times daily vs. fraction A (500 mg) twice daily vs. clofibrate (500 mg) three times daily vs. placebo; reduced cholesterol in all guggul groups vs. placebo.
Hyperlipidemia	RCT, double-blind	Ghorai[11] 2000	30	Unclear	3	Large	NA	NA	Guggulipid (25 mg of guggulsterone) twice daily for 8 weeks reduced cholesterol vs. allicin (from garlic); unclear statistical analysis.
Hyperlipidemia	RCT, single-blind	Singh[9] 1994	64	Yes	3	Medium	NA	NA	Guggulipid (50 mg) twice daily associated with significant reduction in total cholesterol vs. baseline, but no significant difference vs. placebo; all subjects were placed on low-fat diets.
Hyperlipidemia	Before-and after-study	Kotiyal[4] 1979	48	Yes	3	Medium	NA	NA	Gum guggulu fraction A (500 mg) three times daily for 4 weeks associated with reduced cholesterol and triglycerides.
Hyperlipidemia	RCT, double-blind	Tripathi[51] 1978	75	Yes	3	Medium	NA	NA	Gum guggulu (10-15 g) daily for 3 months associated with reduced cholesterol vs. placebo.
Hyperlipidemia	Randomized, controlled, double-blind comparison study	Malhotra[24] 1977	51	Unclear	3	Large	NA	NA	Fraction A (1.5 g daily) or clofibrate (2 g daily) for 75 weeks associated with reduced cholesterol levels; no placebo group.
Hyperlipidemia	RCT, double-blind	Malhotra[23] 1971	44	No	3	Medium	NA	NA	Guggul fraction A (500 mg) three times daily no different from ethyl-*p*-chloro- phenoxy-isobutyrate or Ciba-13437 Su; no power calculation performed.
Hyperlipidemia	RCT, double-blind, crossover	Sharma[53] 1976	60	Unclear	2	Medium	NA	NA	Guggul (4 g daily) for 4 weeks associated with reduced cholesterol and triglycerides vs. placebo; large dropout.
Hyperlipidemia	Unclear study design	Upadhyaya[54] 1976	25	Unclear	2	Small	NA	NA	(12-16 g daily) for 3 months associated with reduced cholesterol and triglyceride levels.
Hyperlipidemia	Before-and-after study	Kuppurajan[25] 1973	120	No	2	Medium	NA	NA	Guggul (2 g daily) or fraction A (300 mg three times daily) for 21 days not associated with changes in cholesterol vs. baseline.
Hyperlipidemia	Unclear study design	Beg[55] 1996	50	Unclear	1	NA	NA	NA	Guggulsterone (25 mg three times daily) for 8 weeks associated with reduced LDLs and total cholesterol.

Review of the Evidence: Guggul—cont'd

Condition Treated*	Study Design	Author, Year	N[†]	SS[†]	Study Quality[‡]	Magnitude of Benefit	ARR[†]	NNT[†]	Comments
Hyperlipidemia	Unclear study design	Singh[56] 1993	200	Yes	1	Medium	NA	NA	6-8 g of combination guggul plus pushkarmool daily for 6 months associated with significantly reduced cholesterol and triglycerides.
Hyperlipidemia, obesity	Case series (published abstract)	Jain[57] 1980	93	Yes	NA	NA	NA	NA	Guggul (2 g three times daily) for 1 month associated with significantly reduced cholesterol (not quantified); large dropout.
Hyperlipidemia	Unclear study design	Gopal[6] 1986	22	Yes	NA	Large	NA	NA	Guggulipid (500 mg three times daily) for 6 weeks associated with reduced cholesterol.
Hyperlipidemia	Phase I/II trial (safety, efficacy)	Agarwal[7] 1986	21	Yes	NA	Large	NA	NA	Guggulipid (400-500 mg three times daily) for 4-12 weeks associated with no adverse effects and reduced cholesterol and triglycerides.
Acne vulgaris	Equivalence trial, non-blinded	Thappa[22] 1994	20	No	2	NA	NA	NA	Oral guggulipid no different from tetracycline; no placebo group or power calculation.
Acne vulgaris	Case series	Dogra[58] 1990	30	Unclear	2	NA	NA	NA	Guggulsterone (25 mg twice daily) for 6 weeks associated with "improvement" in most patients.
Obesity	RCT, double-blind	Bhatt[59] 1995	58	No	3	NA	NA	NA	Guggulipid (1.5 g) three times daily plus dietary control for 30 days associated with non-significant weight loss trend vs. diet alone.
Obesity	RCT, double-blind	Kotiyal[5] 1985	85	Mixed	3	Small	NA	NA	Fraction A (500 mg) three times daily associated with small decrease in triceps skin folds.
Obesity	RCT, double-blind, crossover	Sidhu[60] 1976	60	No	3	NA	NA	NA	Gum guggul (4 g) three times daily for 4 weeks associated with non-significant weight loss trend vs. placebo.
Obesity	RCT, unclear blinding	Antonio[61] 1999	20	Mixed	2	Small	NA	NA	Combination therapy with guggulsterone (750 mg daily) plus phosphate for 6 weeks associated with non-significant weight loss trend vs. placebo.
Rheumatoid arthritis	Case series	Mahesh[62] 1981	30	Yes	NA	Medium	NA	NA	Guggul (3 g daily) for 4 months associated with improved arthritis symptoms.
Rheumatoid arthritis	Case series	Kishore[63] 1982	63	Unclear	NA	NA	NA	NA	Combination product including guggulu (1 g) three times daily for 6 weeks associated with "relief" in most subjects; poorly described methods and results.
Arthritis (mixed types, including osteoarthritis)	Case series	Majumdar[64,65] 1984	61	Unclear	NA	Medium	NA	NA	Gum guggul (1-2 g) plus gold therapy for 2-12 weeks associated with "improvement" in half of subjects.
Osteoarthritis (knee)	Case report	Singh[66] 2001	1	NA	NA	NA	NA	NA	Guggul (500 mg) three times daily for 3 months associated with "marked pain relief."

*Primary or secondary outcome.
[†]N, Number of patients; SS, statistically significant; ARR, absolute risk reduction; NNT, the number of patients who need to undergo a specific intervention in order to observe an outcome in one individual.
[‡]0-2 = poor; 3-4 = good; 5 = excellent.
HDLs, High-density lipoproteins; LDLs, low-density lipoproteins; NA, not applicable; RCT, randomized, controlled trial.
For an explanation of each category in this table, please see Table 3 in the Introduction.

REVIEW OF THE EVIDENCE: DISCUSSION
Hyperlipidemia
Summary

- Prior to 2003, the majority of scientific evidence suggested that guggulipid elicits significant reductions in serum total cholesterol, low-density lipoproteins (LDLs), and triglycerides, as well as elevations in high-density lipoprotein (HDL).[1-11] However, most published studies were small and methodologically flawed. In August 2003, a well-designed trial reported small significant *increases* in serum LDL levels associated with the use of guggul compared to placebo.[12] No significant changes in total cholesterol, HDLs, or triglycerides were noted. These results are consistent with two prior published case reports.[13,14] Although this evidence provides preliminary evidence against the efficacy of guggul for hypercholesterolemia, because of the precedent of prior research and historical use, further study is necessary before a definitive conclusion can be reached. There is no reliable research comparing guggul preparations with HMG-CoA reductase inhibitors (statins), or evaluating long-term effects of guggul on cardiac morbidity or mortality outcomes.

Preclinical Research

- Initial research reports that guggulsterones are antagonists of the farsenoid X receptor (FXR) and the bile acid receptor (BAR), which are nuclear hormones involved in cholesterol metabolism and bile acid regulation.[1,15,16]

Controlled Trials

- Szapary et al. report the results of a randomized, double-blind, placebo-controlled trial in which 103 adults with hypercholesterolemia were assigned to receive either 1000 or 2000 mg of a standardized guggul extract (2.5% guggulsterones E and Z), taken three times daily, or placebo.[12] Tablets were tested for constituents using high-pressure liquid chromatography. The study lasted for 8t weeks. The authors report that after 8 weeks, directly measured mean levels of LDL significantly decreased by 5% in the placebo group ($p = 0.01$), but increased in the 1000-mg guggul group by 4%, and in the 2000-mg guggul group by 5% ($p = 0.006$). No significant changes in total cholesterol, HDLs, or triglycerides were noted. A borderline trend toward reduced HDLs was seen in the guggul groups. Notably, in patients with baseline LDL levels greater than 160 mg/dL (4.14 mmol/L), a significant reduction in triglyceride levels by 14% was seen, compared to a 10% increase in the placebo group. A favorable response in LDL levels to guggul was seen in 18% of patients, compared to greater than 80% in prior reports. The discrepancy from prior trials may be due to differences between American and Indian dietary habits, or to other regional environmental or genetic factors. Although this trial provides preliminary evidence against the efficacy of guggul for hypercholesterolemia, because of the precedent of multiple prior trials (of inferior design), further research is necessary before a definitive conclusion can be reached. Also of note, possible effects on high-sensitivity C-reactive protein (hs-CRP) were observed, which merit further evaluation.

- Nityanand described the findings of two multicenter research studies of patients diagnosed with hyperlipidemia (elevated total cholesterol and/or triglycerides) at seven sites in India.[2] The first study, a 12-week case series in 205 individuals, found that guggulipid (500 mg three times daily) yielded a significant reduction in total cholesterol (mean, 22%) and triglycerides (mean, 25%). The second study, a 12-week

double-blind, crossover trial of 125 subjects, compared guggulipid to clofibrate. Significant decreases in total cholesterol (13% to 15%) and triglycerides (16% to 23%) occurred in both groups compared to baseline, without significant differences between groups. Mean HDL levels increased by 16% for guggulipid patients, compared to 8% in clofibrate patients. Effects on cholesterol and triglyceride levels persisted for 6 to 8 weeks after drug withdrawal. Although these results are promising, neither randomization nor blinding procedures were adequately described, no placebo group was utilized, and no power calculation was conducted prior to conducting the latter study (and the sample size may not have been adequate to detect differences between the guggulipid and clofibrate groups).

- Gaur et al. conducted a randomized, controlled trial to assess the effects of guggulipid on cholesterol levels in 68 patients following acute ischemic stroke.[10] Subjects were assigned to receive aspirin monotherapy (320 mg daily) or daily aspirin plus guggulipid (500 mg three times daily). Following 4 weeks of treatment, a significant reduction in LDLs and an increase in HDLs occurred in the aspirin/guggulipid group vs. the aspirin monotherapy group. A non-significant decrease in total cholesterol and triglycerides occurred in the aspirin/guggulipid group vs. the aspirin monotherapy group. Blinding and randomization were not clearly described. Notably, lipid levels can be affected by acute illnesses such as stroke, which potentially could confound results.

- A randomized, controlled, double-blind study was conducted on the cholesterol effects of purified gum guggul in 40 patients with hyperlipidemia.[8] Subjects were randomized to receive placebo or 4.5 g of gum guggul in two divided daily doses. After 16 weeks, total cholesterol levels significantly decreased by 21.75% and triglyceride levels significantly decreased by 27% compared to baseline. Significant decreases were also noted in LDLs and very-low-density lipoproteins (VLDL), whereas HDL levels rose by 35.8%. Significant changes were not noted in the placebo group, although there was a trend toward improved cholesterol levels. Although these results are compelling, direct comparisons were not made between the guggul and placebo groups.

- Kotiyal et al. conducted a randomized, double-blind trial in 85 obese patients.[5] Subjects were given 500 mg of guggul fraction A three times daily, or placebo. After 12 weeks, a significant reduction was noted in the guggul group in levels of cholesterol vs. baseline (15% reduction) and triglycerides vs. baseline (37% reduction). No significant changes were registered in the control group. However, no between-group comparisons were reported. Information on the method of statistical analysis and dropouts was not presented.

- Kuppurajan et al. reported the results of a randomized, placebo-controlled, double-blind trial in 120 patients with hyperlipidemia.[3] Subjects were randomized to receive one of four treatments: gum guggulu (2 g three times daily), guggul fraction A (500 mg twice daily), clofibrate (500 mg three times daily), or placebo. Over a 21-day period, all three treatment groups experienced significant decreases in serum cholesterol levels compared to placebo. However, results were not adequately quantified.

- Ghorai et al. reported a three-arm, double-blind comparison study in 30 healthy individuals.[11] Subjects were assigned to receive either guggulipid (guggulsterone, 25 mg twice daily), allicin (a thioaminoacid from garlic), or germinated Bengal gram seeds. Following 8 weeks of therapy, guggulipid patients experienced a significant mean reduction in cholesterol levels of 32%, vs. 13% with allicin and 17% with Bengal seeds.

Although these results suggest superiority of guggul to this form of garlic therapy, there was no placebo arm, and statistical analysis and dropouts were not well described.

- Singh et al. conducted a randomized, single-blind, placebo-controlled trial in 64 patients with hypercholesterolemia (average baseline total cholesterol, 245 mg/dL; LDL, 150 mg/dL).[9] All subjects were initially placed on a 12-week stringent diet, which excluded meat, eggs, certain oils, and butter. At the end of this run-in period, total cholesterol decreased by 10% to 12% in both groups. Subjects were then randomized to receive either guggulipid (50 mg twice daily) or placebo for 24 weeks. The authors report that an additional 12% to 13% drop occurred in total cholesterol and LDL levels in the guggulipid group, compared with a slight increase in these parameters in the placebo group. Although the changes in the guggulipid group were statistically significant compared to baseline values, they were not statistically significant compared to placebo. This may have been because of the decrease in cholesterol levels that occurred in both groups due to pretreatment with dietary restriction (suggesting that guggul therapy may not provide significant added benefit to dietary discretion). However, the lack of statistical significance between groups may also reflect a sample size too small to detect differences. This trial was not adequately investigator-blinded, and no information was given regarding compliance.
- In a published abstract, Tripathi et al. described the results of a controlled trial in 75 patients.[51] Subjects were assigned to receive either gum guggulu (10 to 15 g daily) (n = 50) or placebo (n = 25) for 3 months. The authors reported a 25% reduction in serum cholesterol and a 30% decrease in triglycerides in the guggul group vs. placebo. However, study methods, baseline patient characteristics, and statistical analysis were not adequately reported.
- Malhotra et al. conducted a comparison trial in 51 patients with hyperlipoproteinemia.[24] Subjects received either guggul (1.5 g daily) (n = 41) or clofibrate (2 g daily) (n = 10). After 75 weeks of treatment, reductions in cholesterol of 37% and triglycerides of 50% were noted in the guggul group compared to baseline values. In the clofibrate group, reductions in cholesterol were 43% and in triglycerides were 50% compared to baseline. However, the results for each group were not compared statistically. There was no placebo arm, and therefore it is not clear that these reported changes in cholesterol levels were not due to confounding factors.
- Malhotra and Ahuja reported a study in 44 patients with hyperlipoproteinemia.[23] Subjects were randomized to receive one of three treatment regimens: fraction A of guggul (500 mg twice daily), ethyl-p-chlorophenoxyisobutyrate (500 mg three times daily), or the formulation Ciba-13437 Su (100 mg three times daily) for 6 to 34 weeks. The fraction A group experienced reductions in serum lipids, cholesterol, and triglycerides of 34%, 27%, and 29%, respectively, compared to baseline, although there were no significant differences in these values compared to the other two treatment groups. It is not clear if this trial was too small to detect between-group differences or if there was true equivalence between these therapies. Without a placebo arm, it is not clear if changes in cholesterol levels might have been due to confounding factors.

Studies of Lesser Design Strength

- A number of additional studies of lesser methodological quality have been conducted. Many of these have included unclear or poor design, reporting of results, and statistical analysis. Using a validated quality measurement scale developed by Jadad et al.,[52] these studies have scored less than "3," which correlates with lower methodological quality. The majority of these trials have reported positive results, although because of methodological weaknesses, their conclusions are of limited clinical value.
- Sharma et al. described the results of a randomized, controlled, crossover trial in 60 obese subjects.[53] Patients received either placebo or guggul (4 g daily) for 4 weeks, followed by crossover to the alternate treatment for 4 weeks. The authors reported decreases in cholesterol and triglyceride levels associated with guggul vs. placebo, although clear quantification and statistical significance were not reported. Descriptions of blinding and randomization were not presented, and there was a 40% dropout in the placebo group.
- Upadhyaya et al. administered guggul (12 to 16 g daily) to 25 subjects for 3 months.[54] The authors reported a decrease in serum cholesterol and triglyceride levels of 28% and 33%, respectively, compared to baseline. However, statistical analysis was not adequately reported.
- Kuppurajan et al. conducted a 21-day study in 120 patients with hypercholesterolemia.[25] Subjects received crude guggul (2 g daily), fraction A (500 mg three times daily), or placebo. After 10 days, a significant decrease in serum cholesterol was observed compared to baseline values for crude guggul but not for fraction A. After 21 days, no significant changes in lipid levels were observed in either guggul group (vs. baseline). However, all values were compared to baseline, not to the placebo arm.
- Beg et al. reported a study in 50 patients with hyperlipidemia associated with nephrotic syndrome.[55] Subjects were administered 25 mg of guggulsterone three times daily. After 8t weeks of therapy, the authors reported mean reductions in total cholesterol of 24% and LDLs of 20%, compared to baseline. Confidence intervals were large for these results, and statistical analysis was not clearly described.
- In a poorly described study, Singh et al. administered a combination therapy to 200 patients with ischemic heart disease.[56] Subjects received a mixture of powders from guggul and puhkarmool root (6 to 8 g daily) for 6 months. The authors noted a significant decrease in cholesterol (39%) and triglycerides (51%). However, limited information regarding study design and statistical analysis was provided.
- In a published abstract, Jain reported the results of a case series of 93 patients with obesity and hyperlipidemia.[57] Patients were given placebo for 1 month, followed by 2 g of guggul three times daily. After 3 months of guggul therapy, a significant fall was observed in cholesterol levels, which persisted for 3 months after guggul cessation. Notably, 50% of subjects dropped out before study completion. This study was not well described, and results were not adequately quantified.
- In a case series, 22 patients with primary hyperlipidemia were administered 500 mg of guggulipid three times daily for 6 weeks.[6] Patients demonstrating a fall in cholesterol levels by ≥2 standard deviations were considered to be therapy "responders," which represented 59% of the sample. Cholesterol-lowering effects reached a plateau at 4 weeks, with a mean reduction of 24.5% compared to baseline. Six weeks after discontinuation of guggul, cholesterol levels returned to pretreatment values. No significant triglyceride lowering was noted. Although a placebo group was noted in the study's description, no details of number of placebo subjects or outcomes were included in the results.

- Agarwal et al. reported the results of a two-part (phase I/II) case series in patients with hyperlipidemia.[7] In the first phase, 400 mg of guggulipid was administered three times daily to 21 patients for 4 weeks, during which time no significant adverse effects were noted. In phase II, 19 subjects ingested 500 mg of guggulipid three times daily for 12 weeks, followed by placebo for 8 weeks. The authors stratified subjects according to whether they "responded" to therapy during the treatment period vs. the placebo period, as defined by a 17.5% reduction in total cholesterol and a 30% reduction in triglycerides. By these criteria, 78.9% of subjects were reported as "responders." It is not clear if there were baseline differences between subjects that were or were not responders.
- Kotiyal et al. conducted a randomized, controlled, crossover trial in 48 subjects with hypercholesterolemia.[4] Patients received either placebo or guggul fraction A (500 mg three times daily) for 4 weeks, followed by crossover for an additional 4 weeks. The authors reported significant reductions in total cholesterol (12%), triglycerides (21%), and non-esterified fatty acids (23%). However, results were reported in comparison to baseline values rather than between-groups. Blinding procedures were not described.

Acne
Summary
- Guggulipid has been found to possess anti-inflammatory properties[40-48] and has been suggested as an oral therapy for nodulocystic acne vulgaris. Preliminary data from small methodologically weak human studies suggest possible short-term improvements in the number of acne lesions. However, further evidence is warranted before a therapeutic recommendation can be made.

Evidence
- Thappa and Dogra conducted a controlled, non-blinded comparison trial between oral guggulipid and tetracycline in 20 patients with nodulocystic acne vulgaris.[22] The authors reported that the agents were equivalent in reducing the number of lesions. However, a validated scale was not used to measure outcomes, and the lack of blinding may have allowed for the introduction of bias. No power calculation was documented, and the sample size may not have been adequate to detect between-group differences. No placebo arm was included, and it is not clear that the improvements observed do not reflect the natural history of this condition to wax and wane periodically.
- Dogra et al. reported a case series in 30 patients with nodulocystic acne vulgaris.[58] Tablets of guggulipid equivalent to 25 mg of guggulsterone were administered twice daily for 6 weeks. The authors reported "excellent" improvement in 30% of cases, "good" results in 47%, and "moderate" results in 23%. However, a validated scale was not used to measure outcomes, and statistical analysis was not adequately reported. Because of the lack of a control group, there is a possibility of the introduction of bias or confounders.

Obesity
Summary
- There is insufficient evidence to support the use of guggul or guggul derivatives for the management of obesity.

Evidence
- Bhatt et al. evaluated guggulipid in 58 patients.[59] Subjects were assigned to receive either dietary control alone or dietary control plus guggulipid (1.5 g) three times daily. After

30 days, the authors noted a modest non-significant trend toward weight loss in a guggulipid sub-group weighing >90 kg. Additional details of design and results were scant, and these results cannot be considered conclusive.
- Sidhu et al. conducted a randomized, controlled, crossover trial in 60 obese subjects.[60] Patients were administered either gum guggul (4 g daily) or placebo for 4 weeks, followed by crossover to the opposite therapy for an additional 4 weeks. Outcome measures included measurements of weight and subcutaneous tissue folds. The authors reported a non-significant trend toward weight loss in the guggul group, but no significant differences between groups.
- A similar study reported by Kotiyal et al. in 85 patients also found negative results, although a small decrease in triceps skin folds was associated with guggul therapy.[5]
- Antonio et al. conducted a randomized, controlled, three-arm trial in 20 overweight subjects.[61] Patients were assigned to receive capsules containing guggulsterone (750 mg), phosphate, and "other possible promoters of weight loss" or a placebo containing maltodextrin or no treatment. All subjects were maintained on a standardized diet and physical exercise program. After 6 weeks, the authors noted a significant 3.2% decrease in body weight and a 20.6% decrease in fat mass in the guggulsterone group compared to baseline values. Fat mass decreased significantly by 8.6% in the control group. Notably, there were no significant differences in any results between groups, suggesting either lack of efficacy or underpowering (sample size too small). Because of the composite nature of the trial therapy, results of this study cannot be directly extrapolated to guggul monotherapy.

Rheumatoid Arthritis
Summary
- There is insufficient evidence to support the use of guggul or guggul derivatives for the management of rheumatoid arthritis.

Evidence
- Mahesh et al. reported a case series in 30 patients with rheumatoid arthritis diagnosed by "American Rheumatism Association" criteria.[62] Guggul pills (3 g daily in divided doses) were administered to all subjects for 4 months. The authors reported "highly significant" improvements in morning stiffness, fatigue, grip-strength, writing, dressing, and walking times. However, a standardized assessment technique was not used. Because this is a case series without a control group, there is the possibility of introduction of bias or confounding variables.
- Kishore et al. reported a case series in 63 patients with rheumatoid arthritis.[63] Guggulu (1 g three times daily) in combination with "other Ayurvedic preparations" was administered for 6 weeks as a combination formula called "sunthi-guggulu." The authors reported complete or partial relief in 66% of cases with this therapy. The clinical applicability of these results is limited by the lack of control group, large dropout, and use of a combination product.

Osteoarthritis
Summary
- There is insufficient evidence to support the use of guggul or guggul derivatives for the management of osteoarthritis.

Evidence
- Majumdar reported a poorly designed study in 61 patients, of which 24 were diagnosed with osteoarthritis, 10 with

"periarthritis," and the others with nonspecific conditions characterized by joint and muscle pains.[64,65] All subjects received either 2 g of gum guggulu plus 75 mg of "incinerated gold" three times daily or 1 g of gum guggulu plus 125 mg of gold twice daily. Duration of treatment varied from 2 to 12 weeks. "Improvements" in symptoms of 50% were reported in 32 patients (18 with osteoarthritis). However, a validated measurement scale was not used, statistical analysis was not conducted, and results were not clearly described. Because this is a case series without a control group, there is a possibility of the introduction of bias or confounding variables.

• A case report published by Singh et al. described a patient with knee osteoarthritis who received 500 mg of guggul three times daily for 3 months.[66] "Marked pain relief" was observed, as well as improvement in function.

FORMULARY: BRANDS USED IN CLINICAL TRIALS/THIRD-PARTY TESTING

Brands Used in Statistically Significant Clinical Trials

• Guglip (Cipla, Bombay, India).[9]

Brands Shown to Contain Claimed Ingredients Through Third-Party Testing

• Vitamin World Select Herbals Standardized Extract Guggul Plex 340 mg, standardized to contain 2.5% guggulsterones (8.5 mg per capsule, 3 per day), manufactured by Vitamin World, Inc. (July 2003, ConsumerLab.com).

• Guggulipid tablets produced by Sabinsa Corp. (Piscataway, NJ), standardized to contain 2.5% of the guggulsterones E and Z, were found to contain at least 2.1% guggulsterones (85% of the claimed ingredients), which was considered satisfactory for research and clinical use.[12]

References

1. Urizar NL, Liverman AB, Dodds DT et al. A natural product that lowers cholesterol as an antagonist ligand for the FXR. Science (Science Express Reports) 2002 (May 3).
2. Nityanand S, Srivastava JS, Asthana OP. Clinical trials with gugulipid. A new hypolipidaemic agent. J Assoc Physicians India 1989;37(5):323-328.
3. Kuppurajan K, Rajagopalan SS, Rao TK, et al. Effect of guggulu (Commiphora mukul—Engl.) on serum lipids in obese, hypercholesterolemic and hyperlipemic cases. J Assoc Physicians India 1978;26(5):367-373.
4. Kotiyal JP, Bisht DB, Singh DS. Double blind cross-over trial of gum guggulu (Commiphora mukul) Fraction A in hypercholesterolemia. J Res Indian Med Yoga Hom 1979;14(2):11-16.
5. Kotiyal JP, Singh DS, Bisht DB. Gum guggulu (Commiphora mukul) fraction 'A' in obesity —a double-blind clinical trial. J Res Ayur and Siddha 1985;6(1,3,4):20-35.
6. Gopal K, Saran RK, Nityanand S, et al. Clinical trial of ethyl acetate extract of gum gugulu (gugulipid) in primary hyperlipidemia. J Assoc Physicians India 1986;34(4):249-251.
7. Agarwal RC, Singh SP, Saran RK, et al. Clinical trial of gugulipid—a new hypolipidemic agent of plant origin in primary hyperlipidemia. Indian J Med Res 1986;84:626-634.
8. Verma SK, Bordia A. Effect of Commiphora mukul (gum guggulu) in patients of hyperlipidemia with special reference to HDL-cholesterol. Indian J Med Res 1988;87:356-360.
9. Singh RB, Niaz MA, Ghosh S. Hypolipidemic and antioxidant effects of Commiphora mukul as an adjunct to dietary therapy in patients with hypercholesterolemia. Cardiovasc Drugs Ther 1994;8(4):659-664.
10. Gaur SP, Garg RK, Kar AM, et al. Gugulipid, a new hypolipidaemic agent, in patients of acute ischaemic stroke: effect on clinical outcome, platelet function and serum lipids. Asia Pacif J Pharm 1997;12:65-69.
11. Ghorai M, Mandal SC, Pal M, et al. A comparative study on hypocholesterolaemic effect of allicin, whole germinated seeds of bengal gram and guggulipid of gum gugglu. Phytother Res 2000;14(3):200-202.
12. Szapary PO, Wolfe ML, Bloedon LT, et al. Guggulipid for the treatment of hypercholesterolemia: a randomized controlled trial. JAMA 2003;290(6):765-772.
13. Das Gupta R. Gugulipid: pro-lipaemic effect. J Assoc Physicians India 1990;38(12):346.
14. Das Gupta RD. Gugulipid: pro-lipaemic effect. J Assoc Physicians India 1990;38(8):598.
15. Cui J, Huang L, Zhao A, et al. Guggulsterone is a farnesoid X receptor antagonist in coactivator association assays but acts to enhance transcription of bile salt export pump. J Biol Chem 2003;278(12):10214-10220.
16. Wu J, Xia C, Meier J, et al. The hypolipidemic natural product guggulsterone acts as an antagonist of the bile acid receptor. Mol Endocrinol 2002;16(7):1590-1597.
17. Morelli V, Zoorob RJ. Alternative therapies: Part II. Congestive heart failure and hypercholesterolemia. Am Fam Physician 2000;62(6):1325-1330.
18. Mashour NH, Lin GI, Frishman WH. Herbal medicine for the treatment of cardiovascular disease: clinical considerations. Arch Intern Med 1998;158(20):2225-2234.
19. Tripathi YB, Malhotra OP, Tripathi SN. Thyroid stimulating action of Z-guggulsterone obtained from Commiphora mukul. Planta Med 1984;(1):78-80.
20. Farnsworth NR, Bingel AS, Cordell GA, et al. Potential value of plants as sources of new antifertility agents I. J Pharm Sci 1975;64(4):535-598.
21. Amma MK, Malhotra N, Suri RK, et al. Effect of oleoresin of gum guggul (Commiphora mukul) on the reproductive organs of female rat. Indian J Exp Biol 1978;16(9):1021-1023.
22. Thappa DM, Dogra J. Nodulocystic acne: oral gugulipid versus tetracycline. J Dermatol 1994;21(10):729-731.
23. Malhotra SC, Ahuja MM. Comparative hypolipidaemic effectiveness of gum guggulu (Commiphora mukul) fraction 'A', ethyl-p-chlorophenoxyisobutyrate and Ciba-13437-Su. Indian J Med Res 1971;59(10):1621-1632.
24. Malhotra SC, Ahuja MM, Sundaram KR. Long term clinical studies on the hypolipidaemic effect of Commiphora mukul (Guggulu) and clofibrate. Indian J Med Res 1977;65(3):390-395.
25. Kuppurajan K, Rajagopalan SS, Koteswara Rao T, et al. Effect of guggulu (Commiphora mukul-Engl) on serum lipids in obese subjects. J Res Indian Med 1973;8(4):1-8.
26. Tripathi SN, Gupta M, Sen SP, et al. Effect of a keto-steroid of Commifora mukul L. on hypercholesterolemia & hyperlipidemia induced by neomercazole & cholesterol mixture in chicks. Indian J Exp Biol 1975;13(1):15-18.
27. Tripathi YB, Tripathi P, Malhotra OP, et al. Thyroid stimulatory action of (Z)-guggulsterone: mechanism of action. Planta Med 1988;54(4):271-277.
28. Mester L, Mester M, Nityanand S. Inhibition of platelet aggregation by "guggulu" steroids. Planta Med 1979;37(4):367-369.
29. Baldwa VS, Sharma RC, Ranka PC, et al. Effect of Commiphora mukul (guggul) on fibrinolytic activity and platelet aggregation in coronary artery disease. Rajas Med J 1980;19(2):84-86.
30. Bordia A, Chuttani SK. Effect of gum guggulu on fibrinolysis and platelet adhesiveness in coronary heart disease. Indian J Med Res 1979;70:992-996.
31. Dalvi SS, Nayak VK, Pohujani SM, et al. Effect of gugulipid on bio-availability of diltiazem and propranolol. J Assoc Physicians India 1994;42(6):454-455.
32. Nityanand S, Kapoor NK. Hypocholesterolemic effect of Commiphora mukul resin (guggal). Indian J Exp Biol 1971;9(3):376-377.
33. Singh V, Kaul S, Chander R, et al. Stimulation of low density lipoprotein receptor activity in liver membrane of guggulsterone treated rats. Pharmacol Res 1990;22(1):37-44.
34. Nityanand S, Kapoor NK. Cholesterol lowering activity of the various fractions of the guggal. Indian J Exp Biol 1973;11(5):395-396.
35. Sheela CG, Augusti KT. Effects of S-allyl cysteine sulfoxide isolated from Allium sativum Linn and gugulipid on some enzymes and fecal excretions of bile acids and sterols in cholesterol fed rats. Indian J Exp Biol 1995;33(10):749-751.
36. Panda S, Kar A. Gugulu (Commiphora mukul) induces triiodothyronine production: possible involvement of lipid peroxidation. Life Sci 1999;65(12):L137-L141.
37. Singh K, Chander R, Kapoor NK. Guggulsterone, a potent hypolipidaemic, prevents oxidation of low density lipoprotein. Phytother Res 1997;11:291-294.
38. Kaul S, Kapoor NK. Reversal of changes of lipid peroxide, xanthine oxidase and superoxide dismutase by cardio-protective drugs in isoproterenol induced myocardial necrosis in rats. Indian J Exp Biol 1989;27(7):625-627.
39. Kaul S, Kapoor NK. Cardiac sarcolemma enzymes & liver microsomal cytochrome P450 in isoproterenol treated rats. Indian J Med Res 1989;90:62-68.
40. Arora RB, Kapoor V, Gupta SK, et al. Isolation of a crystalline steroidal compound from Commiphora mukul & its anti-inflammatory activity. Indian J Exp Biol 1971;9(3):403-404.
41. Arora RB, Taneja V, Sharma RC, et al. Anti-inflammatory studies on a crystalline steroid isolated from Commiphora mukul. Indian J Med Res 1972;60(6):929-931.
42. Singh GB, Atal CK. Pharmacology of an extract of salai guggal ex-Boswellia serrata, a new non-steroidal anti-inflammatory agent. Agents Actions 1986;18(3-4):407-412.
43. Sosa S, Tubaro R, Della Loggia R, et al. Anti-inflammatory activity of Commiphora mukul extracts. Pharmacol Res 1993;27(suppl 1):89-90.
44. Duwiejua M, Zeitlin IJ, Waterman PG, et al. Anti-inflammatory activity of resins from some species of the plant family Burseraceae. Planta Med 1993;59(1):12-16.
45. Gujral ML, Sareen K, Reddy GS, et al. Endocrinological studies on the oleo resin of gum guggul. Indian J Med Sci 1962;16:847-851.

46. Kesava RG, Dhar SC. Effect of a new non-steroidal anti-inflammatory agent on lysosomal stability in adjuvant induced arthritis. Ital J Biochem 1987; 36(4):205-217.

47. Kesava RG, Dhar SC, Singh GB. Urinary excretion of connective tissue metabolites under the influence of a new non-steroidal anti-inflammatory agent in adjuvant induced arthritis. Agents Actions 1987;22(1-2):99-105.

48. Sharma JN, Sharma JN. Comparison of the anti-inflammatory activity of *Commiphora mukul* (an indigenous drug) with those of phenylbutazone and ibuprofen in experimental arthritis induced by mycobacterial adjuvant. Arzneimittelforschung 1977;27(7):1455-1457.

49. Arya VP. Gugulipid. Drugs Fut 1988;13:618-619.

50. Satyavati GV. Gum guggul (*Commiphora mukul*)—the success story of an ancient insight leading to a modern discovery. Indian J Med Res 1988; 87:327-335.

51. Tripathi SN, Upadhyay BN. A clinical trial of *Commiphora mukul* in the patients of ischaemic heart disease. J Mol and Cell Cardiol 1978; 10(suppl 1):124.

52. Jadad AR, Moore RA, Carroll D, et al. Assessing the quality of reports of randomized clinical trials: is blinding necessary? Control Clin Trials 1996; 17(1):1-12.

53. Sharma K, Puri AS, Sharma R, et al. Effect of gum guggul on serum lipids in obese subjects. J Res Indian Med Yoga Hom 1976;11(2):132.

54. Upadhyaya BN, Tripathi SN, Dwivedi LD. Hypocholesterolemic and hypolipidemic action of gum guggulu in patients of coronary heart disease. J Res Indian Med Yoga Hom 1976;11(2):1-8.

55. Beg M, Singhal KC, Afzaal S. A study of effect of guggulsterone on hyperlipidemia of secondary glomerulopathy. Indian J Physiol Pharmacol 1996;40(3):237-240.

56. Singh RP, Singh R, Ram P, et al. Use of Pushkar-Guggul, an indigenous antiischemic combination, in the management of ischemic heart disease. Int J Pharmacog 1993;31(2):147-160.

57. Jain JP. Clinical assessment of the value of oleo-resin of *Commiphora mukul* (Guggul) in obesity and hyperlipidemia. ICMR Bull 1980;10:83-84.

58. Dogra J, Aneja N, Saxena VN. Oral gugulipid in acne vulgaris management. Ind J Dermatol Venereol Leprol 1990;56(1):381-383.

59. Bhatt AD, Dalal DG, Shah SJ, et al. Conceptual and methodologic challenges of assessing the short-term efficacy of Guggulu in obesity: data emergent from a naturalistic clinical trial. J Postgrad Med 1995;41(1):5-7.

60. Sidhu LS, Sharma K, Puri AS, et al. Effect of gum guggul on body weight and subcutaneous tissue folds. J Res Indian Med Yoga Hom 1976;11(2): 16-22.

61. Antonio J, Colker CM, Torina GC, et al. Effects of a standardized guggulsterone phosphate supplement on body composition in overweight adults: A pilot study. Curr Ther Res 1999;60:220-227.

62. Mahesh S, Pandit M, Hakala C. A study of Shuddha Guggulu on rheumatoid arthritis. Rheumatism 1981;16(2):54-67.

63. Kishore P, Devi Das KV, Banarjee S. Clinical studies on the treatment of amavata-rheumatoid arthritis with sunthi-guggulu. J Res Ayur Siddha 1982; 3(3-4):133-146.

64. Majumdar KA. Role of gum guggulu with gold in rheumatic and other allied disorders. Rheumatism 1984;20(1):9-15.

65. Majumdar KA. A clinical study of R-Arthritis with A-Compound—a herbal formulation. Rheumatism 1984;19(3):66-74.

66. Singh BB, Mishra L, Aquilina N, et al. Usefulness of guggul (*Commiphora mukul*) for osteoarthritis of the knee: an experimental case study. Altern Ther Health Med 2001;7(2):120, 112-114.

Gymnema
(*Gymnema sylvestre* R. Br.)

SYNONYMS/COMMON NAMES/RELATED SUBSTANCES

- *Asclepias geminata* roxb., Asclepiadaceae, *Gemnema melicida*, GS4 (water soluble extract of the leaves), gur-mar, gurmar, gurmarbooti, *Gymnema inodum*, kogilam, mangala gymnema, merasingi, meshashingi, meshavalli, periploca of the woods, periploca sylvestris, podapatri, Probeta, ram's horn, small Indian ipecac, sarkaraikolli, sirukurinja.

CLINICAL BOTTOM LINE
Background

- Preliminary human evidence suggests that gymnema may be efficacious for the management of serum glucose levels in type 1 and type 2 diabetes, as an adjunct to conventional drug therapy, for up to 20 months. Gymnema appears to lower serum glucose and glycosylated hemoglobin (HbA1c) levels following chronic use but may not have significant acute effects.[1] High-quality human trials are lacking in this area. There is early evidence suggesting possible efficacy of gymnema as a lipid-lowering agent.
- Some of the available research has been conducted by authors affiliated with manufacturers of gymnema products.

Scientific Evidence for Common/Studied Uses	Grade*
Type 1 diabetes mellitus	B
Type 2 diabetes mellitus	B
Hyperlipidemia	C

*Key to grades: A: Strong scientific evidence for this use; B: Good scientific evidence for this use; C: Unclear scientific evidence for this use; D: Fair scientific evidence against this use (it may not work); F: Strong scientific evidence against this use (it likely does not work). For a more detailed explanation of efficacy criteria, see "Natural Standard Evidence-Based Validated Grading Rationale" in the Introduction.

Historical or Theoretical Indications That Lack Sufficient Evidence

- Aphrodisiac, cardiovascular disease, constipation, cough, digestive stimulant, diuresis, gout,[2] hepatoprotection, hyperlipidemia, hypertension,[3,4] laxative, liver disease, malaria, obesity, rheumatoid arthritis,[2] snake venom antidote,[5] stomach ailments, uterine stimulant.

Expert Opinion and Folkloric Precedent

- Gymnema leaves have been used for over 2000 years in India to treat *madhu meha*, or "honey urine." It has been used alone and as a component of the Ayurvedic medicinal compound "tribang shila," a mixture of tin, lead, zinc, gymnema sylvestre leaves, neem leaves (*Melia azadirachta*), enicostemma littorale, and jambul seeds (*Eugenia jambolana*). Traditional healers observed that chewing the leaves of gymnema resulted in a reversible loss of sweet-taste perception.
- The plant has also been used in African healing traditions, for example by Tanzanian healers as an aphrodisiac. Other traditional applications include use as an antimalarial agent, digestive stimulant, laxative, diuretic, and snake venom antidote.

Safety Summary

- **Possibly unsafe:** When used in patients taking other hypoglycemic agents, because of possible potentiation of effects. Hypoglycemic effects associated with gymnema have been noted in both diabetic and non-diabetic individuals.[6]

DOSING/TOXICOLOGY
General

- Listed doses are based on those most commonly used in available trials, on historical practice, or on manufacturer recommendations. However, with natural products, the optimal doses needed to balance efficacy and safety often have not been determined. Formulations and preparation methods may vary from manufacturer to manufacturer, and from batch to batch of a specific product made by a single manufacturer. Because often the active components of a product are not known, standardization may not be possible, and the clinical effects of different brands may not be comparable.

Standardization

- At least one manufacturer offers an extract of gymnema standardized to 25% gymnemic acid, but this extract has not yet been clinically evaluated.
- An ethanolic acid–precipitated extract from gymnema, labeled GS4, has been used in human trials.[1,7] GS4 has since been patented as the product Proβeta by a research team that includes the Drs. Shanmugasundaram, who have conducted some of the research in this area. According to the makers of Proβeta, the preparation is standardized to possess a specific biological result, as measured by a test developed by the company that evaluates "pancreotropic" effects.

Dosing: Adult (18 Years and Older)
Oral

- **Type 1 diabetes:** 200 mg of extract GS4 orally, twice daily,[7] under careful continuation of insulin. Doses of insulin or other concomitant hypoglycemic drugs may have to be adjusted or discontinued under the supervision of a healthcare professional.
- **Type 2 diabetes:** 200 mg of extract GS4 orally, twice daily,[1] or 2 mL of an aqueous decoction (10 g of shade-dried powdered leaves per 100 mL), three times daily.[6] Doses of insulin or other concomitant hypoglycemic drugs may have to be adjusted or discontinued under the supervision of a healthcare professional.
- *Note:* The manufacturer PharmaTerra recommends the dose for their product Proβeta (GS4) to be two 250-mg capsules taken twice daily at mealtimes for adults weighing >100 pounds, or one 250-mg capsule taken twice daily at mealtimes for adults weighing <100 pounds.

Dosing: Pediatric (Younger Than 18 Years)

- Insufficient available evidence.

Toxicology

- Insufficient available evidence.

ADVERSE EFFECTS/PRECAUTIONS/CONTRAINDICATIONS
Allergy

- No allergy/hypersensitivity to gymnema has been reported in the available literature. In theory, allergic cross-reactivity may occur with members of the Asclepiadaceae (milkweed) family.

Adverse Effects

- **General:** Aside from hypoglycemia and potentiation of the effects of hypoglycemic drugs following chronic use of gymnema, no clinically significant adverse effects have been associated with oral gymnema in the available literature, in studies up to 20 months in duration.
- **Endocrine:** Multiple animal studies have reported hypoglycemic effects associated with ingestion of gymnema leaves. Gymnema reduced hyperglycemia in experimentally and spontaneously diabetic rats and rabbits,[8-14] as well as in non-diabetic and diabetic humans.[1,5-7,11] One subject with brittle diabetes had to discontinue gymnema in a clinical trial because of repeated hypoglycemic episodes.[7] Hypoglycemic effects have been noted in both diabetic and non-diabetic individuals.[6]
- **Oral (taste effects):** Gymnema has been reported to possess a sweet taste–suppressing effect, attributed to the peptide gurmarin.[15-19] This phenomenon has been observed historically, prompting the Hindi name *gurmar* or "sugar destroyer."

Precautions/Warnings/Contraindications

- Use cautiously in diabetic patients taking hypoglycemic medications, because of possible potentiation of effects. Serum glucose levels should be monitored, and doses of concomitant hypoglycemic drugs may require adjustment under the supervision of a healthcare professional. Hypoglycemia may also occur in non-diabetic patients.[6]

Pregnancy and Lactation

- Not recommended, due to insufficient available safety information.

INTERACTIONS
Gymnema/Drug Interactions

- **Hypoglycemic agents, insulin:** Gymnema may potentiate the effects of hypoglycemic drugs in diabetic patients.[1,7] Doses of such medications may therefore need adjustment. Serum glucose levels should be monitored, and doses of concomitant hypoglycemic drugs may require adjustment under the supervision of a healthcare professional. Multiple animal studies have reported hypoglycemic effects associated with ingestion of gymnema leaves. Gymnema reduced hyperglycemia in experimentally and spontaneously diabetic rats and rabbits,[8-14] as well as in non-diabetic and diabetic humans.[1,5-7,11]
- **Lipid-lowering agents:** Reductions in levels of serum triglycerides, total cholesterol, very- low-density lipoprotein (VLDL), and low-density lipoprotein (LDL) have been observed in animals following administration of gymnema.[20,21] A study of gymnema in type 2 diabetes patients reported decreased cholesterol and triglyceride levels as a secondary outcome.[1] Concomitant use of gymnema with other lipid-lowering agents may potentiate these effects.

Gymnema/herb/supplement interactions

- **Hypoglycemic herbs and supplements:** Gymnema may potentiate the effects of hypoglycemic herbs or supplements in diabetic patients.[1,7] Doses of these agents may therefore need adjustment. Serum glucose levels should be monitored, and doses of concomitant hypoglycemic agents may require adjustment under the supervision of a healthcare professional. Multiple animal studies have reported hypoglycemic effects associated with ingestion of gymnema leaves. Gymnema reduced hyperglycemia in experimentally and spontaneously diabetic rats and rabbits,[8-14] as well as in non-diabetic and diabetic humans.[1,5-7,11]
- **Lipid-lowering herbs and supplements:** Reductions in levels of serum triglycerides, total cholesterol, very-low-density lipoprotein (VLDL), and low-density lipoprotein (LDL) have been observed in animals following administration of gymnema.[20,21] A study of gymnema in type 2 diabetes patients reported decreased cholesterol and triglyceride levels as a secondary outcome.[1] Concomitant use of gymnema with other lipid-lowering agents may potentiate these effects.

Gymnema/Food Interactions

- **Fat absorption:** In an animal study, absorption of oleic acid (a fatty acid) was decreased by gymnema.[22] It is unknown whether gymnema exerts these effects in humans or affects the absorption of other nutritionally important lipids or fat-soluble vitamins (A, D, E, and K).

Gymnema/Lab Interactions

- **Serum glucose, glycosylated hemoglobin (HbA1c):** Based on animal research and preliminary human data, ingestion of gymnema may cause hypoglycemia in diabetic patients and reductions over time in HbA1c levels.[1,5-14] Hypoglycemic effects have been noted in patients without diabetes as well as in patients with diabetes.[6]
- **Serum lipids:** In a small human study, patients with type 2 diabetes taking gymnema in addition to oral hypoglycemic drugs experienced reductions in cholesterol, triglycerides, and free fatty acids, whereas subjects taking oral hypoglycemic agents alone did not.[1] Serum triglycerides, total cholesterol, very-low-density lipoprotein (VLDL), and low-density lipoprotein (LDL) cholesterol-lowering effects have been observed in animals.[20,21] The mechanism may be via a decrease in the synthesis or increase in the metabolism of cholesterol, or through decreased fat absorption.[22]

MECHANISM OF ACTION
Pharmacology

- **Constituents:** Few studies have closely evaluated the constituents of *Gymnema sylvestre* leaf. Proposed active components include gurmarin, conduritol A, and triterpene glycosides.[23-25] Gymnemoside b[25] and gymnema acids V and VII appear to be the key saponin constituents.[26]
- **Hypoglycemic effects:** Multiple animal studies have reported hypoglycemic effects associated with the ingestion of gymnema leaves. Gymnema reduced hyperglycemia in experimentally and spontaneously diabetic rats and rabbits[8-14] as well as in normal and diabetic humans.[1,5-7,11,27-33] Gymnema may act by enhancing insulin secretion through increased pancreatic β-cell number and through improved cell function[4,11]. However, insulin resistance was not improved by gymnema in one animal model of diabetes.[14] Other proposed mechanisms include stimulation of the release of endogenous insulin[1,23] via interactions with insulinotropic enteric

hormones or increases in glucose utilization.[9] Such activities may explain the observed hypoglycemic effects in individuals with type 2 diabetes. Gymnema has also been reported to restore levels of glycoproteins in diabetic rats to normal, thereby potentially preventing diabetic microangiopathy and other pathologic organ changes.[34]

- **Lipid effects:** Serum triglycerides, total cholesterol, very-low-density lipoprotein (VLDL), and low-density lipoprotein (LDL) cholesterol-lowering effects have been observed in animals.[20,21] The mechanism may be via a decrease in the synthesis or increase in the metabolism of cholesterol, or through decreased intestinal fat absorption.[22]
- **Taste effects:** Gymnema has been reported to possess a sweet taste–suppressing effect, attributed to the peptide gurmarin.[15-17] This effect may result from interference with Na^+/K^+ ATPase activity of taste receptors[18] or from neural inhibition.[19] This phenomenon has been observed historically, prompting the Hindi name *gurmar* or "sugar destroyer."

Pharmacodynamics/Kinetics

- Limited available data.
- In one small human study, it was reported that oral administration of gymnema did not have acute effects on fasting serum glucose levels (after 45 minutes).[1]

HISTORY

- *Gymnema sylvestre* is a woody, climbing plant native to India. The leaves are most commonly used medicinally, although the stem is believed also to possess some pharmacologic action. The leaves have been used for over 2000 years in India to treat *madhu meha*, or "honey urine." Chewing the leaves was noted to diminish the ability to discriminate sweet tastes, which along with hypoglycemic properties may have prompted the Hindi name *gurmar*, or "sugar destroyer." Gymnema has a long history of use in individuals with diabetes.

- Gymnema has become a popular natural product used in the management of blood sugar levels in individuals with diabetes and is believed by some to play a role in reducing serum lipids.

REVIEW OF THE EVIDENCE: DISCUSSION
Type 1 Diabetes
Summary

- Multiple animal studies have noted that gymnema lowers serum glucose levels.[8-14,27-33] Preliminary evidence from small, methodologically flawed human trials suggest hypoglycemic effects of chronic oral gymnema when used in patients with type 1 or type 2 diabetes, as an adjunct to insulin or oral hypoglycemic drugs. The onset of effect has not been clearly described, although one study noted that oral administration of gymnema did not have acute effects on fasting serum glucose levels (after 45 minutes).[1] The available studies have assessed effects of gymnema after 10 days, up to 20 months. Although it appears that gymnema may act to lower serum glucose levels, further studies of dosing, safety, and efficacy are merited before a strong recommendation can be made. Multiple drugs are available that have been demonstrated to establish good long-term control of blood glucose levels, and gymnema has not been thoroughly evaluated as a safe or effective alternative or adjunct to these agents.

Evidence

- Shanmugasundaram et al. conduced a study in 64 individuals with type 1 diabetes.[7] All subjects were continued on insulin therapy during the trial, and 27 patients were concurrently started on 200 mg twice daily of GS4 (an ethanolic acid–precipitated extract of gymnema). Outcomes measures included fasting glucose levels, glycosylated hemoglobin (HbA1c) levels, and insulin requirements. The gymnema subjects were followed for a period that varied from 6 to 30 months, whereas the 37 insulin-only controls were tracked

Review of the Evidence: Gymnema

Condition Treated*	Study Design	Author, Year	N[†]	SS[†]	Study Quality[‡]	Magnitude of Benefit	ARR[†]	NNT[†]	Comments
Type 1 diabetes	Controlled trial, non-randomized, non-blinded	Shanmugasundaram[7] 1990	64	Yes	0	Large	59	2	GS4 (gymnema) plus insulin vs. insulin alone; 11 dropouts; 40 non-diabetics also studied; author affiliated with manufacturer.
Type 2 diabetes	Case series	Kothe[5] 1997	21	NA	0	NA	NA	NA	Gymnema administered over 6-month period; uncontrolled; limited reporting of numerical results.
Type 2 diabetes (glucose and lipid levels)	Before and after study, non-randomized, non-blinded	Baskaran[1] 1990	47	Yes	1	Large	23	4	GS4 (gymnema) added to oral hypoglycemic drugs improved fasting glucose and HbA1c levels.
Type 2 diabetes	Case series	Khare[6] 1983	16	Yes	0	Large	NA	NA	Gymnema for 10 days reduced serum glucose levels in both diabetic and non-diabetic patients.

*Primary or secondary outcome.
[†]N, Number of patients; SS, statistically significant; ARR, absolute risk reduction; NNT, the number of patients who need to undergo a specific intervention in order to observe an outcome in one individual.
[‡]0-2 = poor; 3-4 = good; 5 = excellent.
NA, Not applicable.
For an explanation of each category in this table, please see Table 3 in the Introduction.

for 10 to 12 months. Eleven subjects dropped out during the initial 6 months (10 for non-medical reasons, 1 because of brittle diabetes). In the gymnema group, mean insulin requirements were reduced by 50%, accompanied by significant reductions in mean fasting blood glucose levels, from 232 mg/dL to 152 mg/dL. HbA1c levels were also reportedly reduced. The insulin-only group exhibited no significant mean decreases in insulin requirements or blood sugar levels. Subjective measures of well-being (alertness, work and school performance) were also reported to improve with gymnema therapy. A secondary outcome of C-peptide level was measured in the two groups, and compared to values for 40 non-diabetic individuals. A statistically significant lower mean C-peptide value was found in the gymnema plus insulin group (0.185) vs. insulin alone (0.272), but was higher than the mean value in non-diabetic group (0.105). During the study, no adverse effects other than hypoglycemia were observed. Although these results are promising, the lack of blinding allows the possible introduction of bias, and lack of randomization may allow the influence of confounding factors. Baseline patient characteristics and statistical analysis were not well described. The principal author is involved with a company that produces a GS4 product.

Type 2 Diabetes
Summary
- Multiple animal studies have noted that gymnema lowers serum glucose levels.[8-14,27-33] Preliminary evidence from small, methodologically flawed human trials suggests hypoglycemic effects of chronic oral gymnema when used in patients with type 1 or type 2 diabetes, as an adjunct to insulin or oral hypoglycemic drugs. The onset of effect has not been clearly described, although one study noted that oral administration of gymnema did not have acute effects on fasting serum glucose levels (after 45 minutes).[1] The available studies have assessed effects of gymnema after 10 days, up to 20 months. Although it appears that gymnema may act to lower serum glucose levels, further studies of dosing, safety, and efficacy are merited before a strong recommendation can be made. Multiple drugs are available that have been demonstrated to establish good long-term control of blood glucose levels, and gymnema has not been thoroughly evaluated as a safe or effective alternative or adjunct to these agents.

Evidence
- Baskaran et al. performed a controlled, non-randomized, non-blinded study in 47 patients with type 2 diabetes.[1] GS4 extract (400 mg daily) was administered for 18 to 20 months to 22 patients, in addition to baseline conventional oral hypoglycemic agents. The control group remained on conventional drug therapy alone without GS4 and was followed for 12 months. After 18 to 20 months, fasting glucose levels in the gymnema group were reported to be 29% lower than baseline ($p < 0.001$), and mean glycosylated hemoglobin (HbA1c) levels decreased from a baseline value of 11.91% to 8.48% ($p < 0.001$). Insulin responses ware reported as being superior in the gymnema-supplemented group ($p < 0.01$). Five subjects in the gymnema group were able to discontinue hypoglycemic medications. After 8-10 months, no significant changes in glucose levels or HbA1c were observed in patients continued on oral hypoglycemic medications alone. As a secondary outcome, blood lipid levels were evaluated. In

the GS4 group, there were significant reductions in plasma lipid levels, including cholesterol, triglycerides, and free fatty acids, whereas lipid levels in patients on conventional drug therapy alone remained elevated. Methodological limitations of this study include the lack of randomization and blinding. Glucose and HbA1c levels were compared to baseline values in each group, rather than compared between groups, making this a "before-and-after" study design (a methodologically weaker design than a between-group comparison).

- A briefly described case series by Kothe and Uppal examined the use of gymnema in 21 subjects with type 2 diabetes over a 6-month period.[5] This paper was presented at the Scientific Session of the 9th Annual International Homeopathic Conference of the Asian Homeopathic Medical League, Jaipur, India. All subjects received 6 to 15 drops of *Gymnema sylvestre* "Q" with 0.25-cup of water, taken 2 to 4 times daily, on a sliding scale based on blood sugar measurements. Additional homeopathic remedies were allowed in "complicated" cases. The authors reported that 16 of 21 patients demonstrated "moderate" to "excellent" blood glucose control. Although suggestive, the lack of a control group and vague description of baseline patient characteristics raises questions about whether these results were due to the natural course of disease, rather than a result of gymnema therapy. Details were not provided regarding methodology or data analysis, and glucose levels during the study period were provided for only 2 patients. Results may have been confounded by the use of additional homeopathic remedies in some patients, which were not described.

- In a 10-day study described in a letter to the editor, Khare et al. investigated the effects of gymnema on glucose levels in 10 healthy young adults (ages 19 to 25) and 6 diabetic adults (ages 35 to 50) with mild to moderate baseline hyperglycemia but without diagnosed diabetic complications.[6] Subjects were not receiving diabetes treatment prior to the trial. Glucose tolerance tests were performed before and after administration of gymnema (2 g, three times daily. of a 10 g/100 mL aqueous decoction of shade-dried powdered leaves). Administration of gymnema for 10 days significantly reduced fasting blood sugar levels compared to baseline in both normal and diabetic subjects and significantly reduced mean glucose levels in diabetics after oral glucose load at both 30 minutes (110.7 mg/dL vs. 135.7 mg/dL) and 120 minutes (180.7 mg/dL vs. 220.0 mg/dL). As a case series, this study lacked comparison to controls receiving placebo or a comparison agent. Methodology and statistical analysis were not well described in this brief publication.

Hyperlipidemia
Summary
- Reductions in levels of serum triglycerides, total cholesterol, very low-density lipoprotein (VLDL), and low-density lipoprotein (LDL) have been observed in animals following administration of gymnema.[20,21] The mechanism may be via a decrease in the synthesis or increase in the metabolism of cholesterol, or through decreased intestinal fat absorption.[22] One study of gymnema in type 2 diabetes patients reported decreased cholesterol and triglyceride levels as a secondary outcome.[1] Further study is warranted in this area before an evidence-based recommendation can be made.

Evidence
- Baskaran et al. performed a controlled, non-randomized, unblinded study in 47 patients with type 2 diabetes.[1]

Gymnema extract GS4 (400 mg daily) was administered for 18 to 20 months to 22 patients, in addition to baseline conventional oral hypoglycemic agents. The control group remained on conventional drug therapy alone without GS4 and was followed for 12 months. Although this study was designed to evaluate the effects of gymnema on serum glucose levels, the measurement of plasma lipids was a secondary outcome assessed. In the GS4 group, statistically significant reductions in plasma lipid levels were observed vs. baseline, including cholesterol (18% reduction), triglycerides (16% reduction), and free fatty acids (22% reduction), whereas lipid levels in patients on conventional drug therapy alone remained unchanged. Methodological limitations of this study include the lack of randomization or blinding. Lipid levels appear to have been compared to baseline values in each group, rather than compared between groups, making this a "before-and-after" study design (a methodologically weaker design than a between-group comparison).

FORMULARY: BRANDS USED IN CLINICAL TRIALS/THIRD-PARTY TESTING

Brands Used in Statistically Significant Clinical Trials

- Proβeta (PharmaTerra, Inc, Bellevue, WA): A patented ethanolic acid–precipitated extract from gymnema, also called GS4. According to the makers of Proβeta, the preparation is standardized to possess a specific biological result, as measured by a test developed by the company that evaluates "pancreotropic" effects.

Brands Shown to Contain Claimed Ingredients Through Third-Party Testing

- Beta Fast GXR (Informulab): 400 mg standardized to 25% gymnemic acids.
- Gymnesyl (Nature's Herbs): Extract standardized for 150 mg of crude gymnemic acids.
- Gymnema (Nature's Way): 260 mg standardized to 75% gymnemic acids.

References

1. Baskaran K, Ahamath B, Shanmugasundaram K, et al. Antidiabetic effect of a leaf extract from *Gymnema sylvestre* in non-insulin-dependent diabetes mellitus patients. J Ethnopharm 1990;30:295-305.
2. Shimizu K, et al. Suppression of glucose absorption by extracts from the leaves of *Gymnema inodorum*. J Vet Med Sci 1997;59:753-757.
3. Preuss HG, Gondal JA, Bustos E, et al. Effect of chromium and guar on sugar-induced hypertension in rats. Clin Neph 1995;44:170-177.
4. Preuss HG, Jarrell ST, Scheckenbach R, et al. Comparative effects of chromium, vanadium and *Gymnema sylvestre* on sugar-induced blood pressure elevations in SHR. J Amer Coll Nutrit 1998;17(2):116-123.
5. Kothe A, Uppal R. Antidiabetic effects of *Gymnema sylvestre* in NIDDM—a short study. Indian J Homeopath Med 1997;32(1-2):61-62, 66.
6. Khare AK, Tondon RN, Tewari JP. Hypoglycaemic activity of an indigenous drug (*Gymnema sylvestre*, "Gurmar") in normal and diabetic persons. Indian J Physiol Pharm 1983;27:257-258.
7. Shanmugasundaram ERB, Rajeswari G, Baskaran K, et al. Use of *Gymnema sylvestre* leaf extract in the control of blood glucose in insulin-dependent diabetes mellitus. J Ethnopharm 1990;30(3):281-294.
8. Srivastava Y, Bhatt HV, Prem AS, et al. Hypoglycemic and life-prolonging properties of *Gymnema sylvestre* leaf extract in diabetic rats. Israel J Med Sci 1985;21:540-542.
9. Shanmugasundaram KR, Panneerselvam C, Samudram P, et al. Enzyme changes and glucose utilisation in diabetic rabbits: the effect of *Gymnema sylvestre*, R.Br. J Ethnopharm 1983;7:205-234.
10. Okabayashi Y, Tani S, Fujisawa T, et al. Effect of *Gymnema sylvestre*, R.Br. on glucose homeostasis in rats. Diabetes Res Clin Pract 1990;9(2):143-148.
11. Shanmugasundaram ERB, Gopinath KL, Shanmugasundaram KR, et al. Possible regeneration of the islets of Langerhans in streptozotocin-diabetic rats given *Gymnema sylvestre* leaf extracts. J Ethnopharm 1990;30:265-279.
12. Chattopadhyay RR. Possible mechanism of antihyperglycemic effect of *Gymnema sylvestre* leaf extract, Part I. Gen Pharm 1998;31(3):495-496.
13. Gupta SS, Variyar MC. Experimental studies on pituitary diabetes IV. Effect of *Gymnema sylvestre* and *Coccinia indica* against the hyperglycemia response of somatotrophin and corticotrophin hormones. Indian J Med Res 1964;52:200-207.
14. Tominaga M, Kimura M, Sugiyama K, et al. Effects of seishin-renshi-in and *Gymnema sylvestre* on insulin resistance in streptozotocin-induced diabetic rats. Diabet Res Clin Pract 1995;29:11-17.
15. Kamei K, Takano R, Miyasaka A, et al. Amino acid sequence of sweet-taste-suppressing peptide (gurmarin) from the leaves of *Gymnema sylvestre*. J Biochem 1992;111:109-112.
16. Imoto T, Miyasaka A, Ishima R, et al. A novel peptide isolated from the leaves of *Gymnema sylvestre*— I. Characterization and its suppressive effect on the neural responses to sweet taste stimuli in the rat. Comp Biochem Physiol A 1991;100(2):309-314.
17. Brala P, Hagen R. Effects of sweetness perception and caloric value of a preload on short term intake. Physiol Behav 1983;30:1-9.
18. Koch RB, Desaiah D, Cutkomp LK. Inhibition of ATPases by gymnemic acid. Chem Biol Interact 1973;7:121-125.
19. Lawless HT. Evidence for neural inhibition in bittersweet taste mixtures. J Comp Physiol Psychol 1979;93(3):538-547.
20. Bishayee A, Chatterjee M. Hypolipidaemic and antiatherosclerotic effects of oral gymnema sylvestre R. Br. leaf extract in albino rats fed a high fat diet. Phytother Res 1994;8:118-120.
21. Terasawa H, Miyoshi M, Imoto T. Effects of long-term administration of *Gymnema sylvestre* watery-extract on variations of body weight, plasma glucose, serum triglyceride, total cholesterol and insulin in Wistar fatty rats. Yonago Acta Med 1994;37:117-127.
22. Wang LF, Luo H, Miyoshi M, et al. Inhibitory effect of gymnemic acid on intestinal absorption of oleic acid in rats. Can J Physiol Pharmacol 1998;76: 1017-1023.
23. Persaud SJ, Al Majed H, Raman A, et al. *Gymnema sylvestre* stimulates insulin release *in vitro* by increased membrane permeability. J Endocrinol 1999;163(2):207-212.
24. Sinsheimer JE, Rao GS, McIlhenny HM. Constituents from *Gymnema sylvestre* leaves. V. Isolation and preliminary characterization of the gymnemic acids. J Pharm Sci 1970;59(5):622-628.
25. Yoshikawa M, Murakami T, Kadoya M, et al. Medicinal foodstuffs. IX. The inhibitors of glucose absorption from the leaves of *Gymnema sylvestre* R. BR. (Asclepiadaceae): structures of gymnemosides a and b. Chem Pharm Bull (Tokyo) 1997;45(10):1671-1676.
26. Murakami N, Murakami T, Kadoya M, et al. New hypoglycemic constituents in "gymnemic acid" from *Gymnema sylvestre*. Chem Pharm Bull 1996; 44(2):469-471.
27. Ananthan R, Baskar C, NarmathaBai V, et al. Antidiabetic effect of *Gymnema montanum* leaves: effect on lipid peroxidation induced oxidative stress in experimental diabetes. Pharmacol Res 2003;48(6):551-556.
28. Ananthan R, Latha M, Pari L, et al. Effect of *Gymnema montanum* on blood glucose, plasma insulin, and carbohydrate metabolic enzymes in alloxan-induced diabetic rats. J Med Food 2003;6(1):43-49.
29. Gholap S, Kar A. Effects of Inula racemosa root and *Gymnema sylvestre* leaf extracts in the regulation of corticosteroid induced diabetes mellitus: involvement of thyroid hormones. Pharmazie 2003;58(6):413-415.
30. Jiang H. [Advances in the study on hypoglycemic constituents of *Gymnema sylvestre* (Retz.) Schult]. Zhong Yao Cai 2003;26(4):305-307.
31. Porchezhian E, Dobriyal RM. An overview on the advances of Gymnema sylvestre: chemistry, pharmacology and patents. Pharmazie 2003;58(1):5-12.
32. Satdive RK, Abhilash P, Fulzele DP. Antimicrobial activity of *Gymnema sylvestre* leaf extract. Fitoterapia 2003;74(7-8):699-701.
33. Xie JT, Wang A, Mehendale S, et al. Anti-diabetic effects of *Gymnema yunnanense* extract. Pharmacol Res 2003;47(4):323-329.
34. Rathi AN, Visvanathan A, Shanmugasundaram KR. Studies on protein-bound polysaccharide components & glycosaminoglycans in experimental diabetes—effect of *Gymnema sylvestre*, R.Br. Indian J Exper Biol 1981;19: 715-721.

Hawthorn
(Crataegus laevigata, Crataegus monogyna, Crataegus oxyacantha, Crataegus pentagyna)

SYNONYMS/COMMON NAMES/RELATED SUBSTANCES

- Aubepine, bei shanzha, bianco spino, bread and cheese tree, Cardiplant, Chinese hawthorn, cockspur, cockspur thorn, crataegi flos, crataegi folium, crataegi folium cum flore, crataegi fructus, crataegi herba, Crataegisan, *Crataegus azaerolus, Crataegus cuneata, Crataegus fructi, Crataegus monogyna, Crataegus nigra, Crataegus oxyacanthoides, Crataegus pentagyna, Crataegus pinnatifida, Crataegus sinaica* Boiss, Crataegutt, English hawthorn, epine blanche, epine de mai, Euphytose (EUP) (combination product), fructus oxyacanthae, fructus spinae albae, gazels, haagdorn, hagedorn, hagthorn, halves, harthorne, haw, Hawthorne Berry, Hawthorne Formula, Hawthorne Heart, Hawthorne Phytosome, Hawthorne Power, hawthorn tops, hazels, hedgethorn, huath, ladies' meat, LI 132, may, mayblossoms, maybush, mayhaw, maythorn, mehlbeerbaum, meidorn, nan shanzha, northern Chinese hawthorn, oneseed, oneseed hawthorn, quickset, red haw, RN 30/9, sanza, sanzashi, shanza, shan zha rou, southern Chinese hawthorn, thornapple tree, thorn plum, tree of chastity, Washington thorn, weissdorn, weissdornblaetter mit blueten, whitethorn, whitethorn herb, WS 1442.

CLINICAL BOTTOM LINE

Background

- Hawthorn, a flowering shrub of the rose family, has an extensive history of use in cardiovascular disease, dating back to the 1st century. Modern-day animal and *in vitro* studies suggest that flavonoids and other pharmacologically active compounds found in hawthorn may synergistically improve performance of the damaged myocardium and, further, may prevent or reduce symptoms of coronary artery disease.
- Numerous well-conducted human clinical trials have demonstrated safety and efficacy of hawthorn leaf and flower in New York Heart Association (NYHA) Class I or II heart failure (characterized by slight or no limitation of physical activity). An international, multicenter randomized controlled trial is currently under way to investigate long-term benefits.
- Hawthorn is widely used in Europe for treating NYHA Class I or II heart failure, with standardization of preparations of its leaves and flowers. Overall, hawthorn appears to be safe and well tolerated and, in accordance with its indication, best used under the supervision of a medical professional.
- The therapeutic equivalence of hawthorn extracts to drugs considered standard-of-care for heart failure (such as angiotensin-converting enzyme [ACE] inhibitors, diuretics, or beta-adrenergic receptor blockers) remains to be established, as does the effect of concomitant use of hawthorn with these drugs. Nonetheless, hawthorn is a potentially beneficial therapeutic agent for patients who cannot or will not take prescription drugs and may offer additive benefits to prescription drug therapy.

Scientific Evidence for Common/Studied Uses	Grade*
Congestive heart failure	A
Coronary artery disease (angina)	C
Functional cardiovascular disorders	C

*Key to grades: *A:* Strong scientific evidence for this use; *B:* Good scientific evidence for this use; *C:* Unclear scientific evidence for this use; *D:* Fair scientific evidence against this use (it may not work); *F:* Strong scientific evidence against this use (it likely does not work). For a more detailed explanation of efficacy criteria, see "Natural Standard Evidence-Based Validated Grading Rationale" in the Introduction.

Historical or Theoretical Indications That Lack Sufficient Evidence

- Abdominal colic, abdominal distention, abdominal pain, acne, amenorrhea, angina, antibacterial, antioxidant,[1] anxiety,[2,3] appetite stimulant, asthma, astringent, bladder disorders, Buerger's disease, cancer, cardiac arrhythmia,[4] circulation,[5] diabetes insipidus, diabetes mellitus, diarrhea, diuresis, dysentery, dyspepsia, dyspnea, edema, frostbite, cardiac murmurs, hemorrhoids, human immunodeficiency virus (HIV) infection,[6] hyperlipidemia,[7] hypertension,[8] insomnia, orthostatic hypotension,[9] nephrosis, peripheral artery disease,[10] skin sores, sore throat, spasmolytic, stomachaches, varicose veins.

Expert Opinion and Folkloric Precedent

- Experimental and clinical studies of this century support the efficacy of hawthorn leaf with flower, whereas the edible fruits have a rich history in early medicine, dating back to the 1st century. Modern-day herbalists consider hawthorn leaf to be one of the most specific cardioactive agents.
- Hawthorn is widely used in Europe for treating NYHA Class I or II heart failure, having undergone extensive study in Germany. Numerous preparations are found in Germany and Switzerland. Expert groups such as the German Commission E, an expert committee established by the German Ministry of Health, and the European Scientific Cooperative on Phytotherapy list the indication for hawthorn leaf and flower to be for individuals with declining cardiac performance corresponding to functional capacity Class II of the NYHA heart failure classification system.

Safety Summary

- **Likely safe:** When used in recommended dosages under the supervision of a medical professional for the treatment of mild (NYHA Class I or II) congestive heart failure (CHF).
- **Possibly unsafe:** When used concomitantly with other cardiovascular medications, herbs, or supplements, including antihypertensives, vasodilators, and cardiac glycosides.

DOSING/TOXICOLOGY
General

- Recommended doses are based on those most commonly used in available trials, or on historical practice. However, with natural products, the optimal doses needed to balance efficacy and safety often have not been determined. Formulations and preparation methods may vary from manufacturer to manufacturer, and from batch to batch of a specific product made by a single manufacturer. Because often the active components of a product are not known, standardization may not be possible, and the clinical effects of different brands may not be comparable.

Standardization

- International standardization recommendations range from 0.6% to 1.5% flavonoids, typically calculated as hyperoside.
- Hawthorn extract WS 1442 is standardized to 18.75% oligomeric procyanidines.
- Hawthorn extract LI 132 is standardized to 2.2% flavonoids.

Dosing: Adults (18 Years and Older)
Oral (Congestive Heart Failure)

- **Products containing standardized extract WS 1442** (18.75% oligomeric procyanidines): Statistically significant trials have used doses of 60 mg three times daily[11-13] or 80 mg twice daily.[14] The U.S. brand HeartCare (Nature's Way) is standardized in this fashion.
- **Products containing standardized extract LI 132** (2.2% flavonoids): Statistically significant trials have used doses of 100 mg three times daily,[15,16] 200 mg twice daily,[17] and up to 300 mg three times daily.[18]
- **Dosage range:** The dosage range recommended in review literature is 160 to 900 mg hawthorn extract per day in 2 or 3 divided doses (corresponding to 3.5 to 19.8 mg flavonoids or 30 to 168.8 mg oligomeric procyanidines). Some sources recommend a range of 240 to 480 mg/day for extracts standardized to 18.75% oligomeric procyanidines.

Dosing: Children (Younger Than 18 Years)

- There is insufficient available evidence to recommend hawthorn for children.

Toxicology

- Literature review reveals no evidence of toxicity of hawthorn extracts when given in recommended doses.
- After administration for 6 months of up to 300 mg/kg daily (100 × standard human dose), no target organ toxicity was found in cats or dogs. Standard mutagenic and clastogenic (chromosome-damaging) tests gave negative results as well.[19]
- For the hawthorn preparations Esbericard and Crataegutt, LD_{50} has been estimated to lie in the range between 18 and 24 mL/kg with intravenous administration and 18.5 and 33.8 mL/kg with oral administration.[20-22]

ADVERSE EFFECTS/PRECAUTIONS/CONTRAINDICATIONS
Allergy

- Known allergy/hypersensitivity to hawthorn is a contraindication.
- A case report has described an immediate-type hypersensitivity reaction to hawthorn plants. It is not known if this applies to oral formulations.[23]

Adverse Effects

- **General:** Although systematic analysis of hawthorn's safety profile in humans is lacking, limited adverse effects clearly associated with this agent have been reported. A recent clinical trial reported no side effects.[24] A 24-week multicenter observational trial of 1011 cardiac patients reported 14 total adverse events.[25] A large surveillance study of 3664 patients with Class I or II cardiac insufficiency confirmed a causal relationship for side effects in only 22 patients.[26]
- **Gastrointestinal:** Rare abdominal discomfort has been reported in a large clinical trial and surveillance study, which was of uncertain relationship to hawthorn.[25,26] Mild and rare nausea has been reported.[27]
- **Cardiac:** Tachycardia (with facial pains) of uncertain relationship to hawthorn was reported in a multicenter clinical trial.[25] Palpitations were reported in 3 patients in a large surveillance trial comprising 3664 patients with cardiac failure.[26]
- **Pulmonary:** Dyspnea was reported in one patient in a double-blind trial of cardiac failure. The patient received a hawthorn/passion flower extract.[28]
- **Neurologic:** Headache and dizziness were reported in 2 patients in a large surveillance trial comprising 3664 patients with cardiac failure.[26]
- **Dermatologic:** Fatigue, sweating, and a mild macular skin eruption on the hands were reported in a double-blind trial of hawthorn/passion flower extract for cardiac failure.[28]
- **Other:** Sleeplessness and agitation were reported once each in a large surveillance trial comprising 3664 patients with cardiac failure.[26]

Precautions/Warnings/Contraindications

- Avoid use with known allergy/hypersensitivity to hawthorn or *Crataegus* species, or to any of the herb's components.
- Use cautiously in the elderly, or in individuals at risk for hypotension.
- Use cautiously in combination with other cardiovascular medications, herbs, or supplements, because of the possibility of additive effects.

Pregnancy and Lactation

- There is insufficient available evidence to recommend hawthorn in pregnancy or during lactation.

INTERACTIONS
Hawthorn/Drug Interactions

- **Cardiac glycosides (digoxin, digitoxin):** Hawthorn has been noted to potentiate inotropic effects of cardiac glycoside drugs without toxicity in a study of isolated guinea pig hearts.[29] Hawthorn has been suggested and used concomitantly with cardiac glycosides, to decrease glycoside dosage and potential toxicity.[20-22] A 10-day randomized crossover pharmacokinetic trial in eight healthy volunteers did not detect statistically significant effects of hawthorn on digoxin, suggesting possible safe coadministration, although close monitoring during dose titration is warranted.[30] Data on safe and efficacious dosing in this setting are still limited.
- **Antihypertensives:** Based on animal and clinical data, hawthorn may have additive activity with medications that possess hypotensive action.
- **Coronary vasodilators:** Based on animal data, hawthorn may have additive activity with medications that possess coronary vasodilatory action.[31]

H

- **Alpha receptor agonists:** Based on animal data, which have demonstrated *in vitro* inhibition of phenylephrine-induced vasoconstriction,[32] hawthorn may reduce the vasoconstrictive effects of phenylephrine (Neo-Synephrine) or other alpha receptor agonists such as ephedrine and norepinephrine.
- **Cholesterol-lowering agents:** Based on limited laboratory, animal, and clinical data, hawthorn may have additive activity with medications that reduce cholesterol.[28,33]

Hawthorn/Herb/Supplement Interactions

- **Cardiac glycoside herbs/supplements:** Hawthorn has been noted to potentiate inotropic effects of cardiac glycoside drugs without toxicity in a study of isolated guinea pig hearts.[29] Hawthorn has been used concomitantly with cardiac glycoside drugs, to decrease glycoside dosage and toxicity.[20-22] These data suggest potential synergistic/additive and/or potential toxic effects when hawthorn is taken concomitantly with cardiac glycoside herbs/supplements.
- **Hypotensive herbs/supplements:** Based on animal and clinical data, hawthorn may have additive activity with herbs/supplements that possess hypotensive or coronary vasodilatory action.[31]
- **Hypertensive herbs/supplements:** Based on animal and clinical data, hawthorn may interfere with the activity of herbs/supplements that increase blood pressure.[31,32]
- **Cholesterol-lowering herbs/supplements:** Based on limited laboratory, animal and clinical data, hawthorn may have additive activity with herbs/supplements that reduce cholesterol.[28,33] Examples are niacin, guggul, garlic, and fish oil.

Hawthorn/Food Interactions

- Insufficient data available.

Hawthorn/Lab Interactions

- Insufficient data available.

MECHANISM OF ACTION
Pharmacology

- Hawthorn is a flowering shrub of the rose family, common in Europe. Because of widespread hybridization, the species of *Crataegus* are difficult to distinguish from one another. Multiple species are commonly found in hawthorn preparations, including *C. laevigata*, *C. oxyacantha*, and *C. monogyna*. Major pharmacologically active components are believed to be flavonoids, such as hyperoside and vitexin, and procyanidins.
- Direct effects on the cardiovascular system have been demonstrated. Administration of hawthorn extract has been shown to decrease blood pressure and total peripheral resistance, economize myocardial function, and decrease cardiac preload in healthy subjects.[34,35] More specifically, hawthorn extract (WS 1442) has shown an inotropic effect on myocardial tissue isolated from patients with terminal left ventricular heart failure (CHF).[36] The inotropic effects of hawthorn may be caused by inhibition of 3′,5′-cyclic adenosine monophosphate diesterase,[37] rather than beta-sympathomimetic activity.[38]
- In the isolated perfused guinea pig heart, the inotropic effect of hawthorn extract LI 132 was weaker than that of digoxin and epinephrine. However, the refractory period was prolonged, perhaps as a result of blockage of repolarizing potassium currents. Thus, hawthorn may be potentially less arrhythmogenic than conventional inotropic agents.[39] At a dose of 20 mg/kg, crataemon (flavonoid fraction of hawthorn) stopped barium chloride–induced arrhythmia in animals; at doses greater than 30 mg/kg, hypotensive effects were seen.[31] A hawthorn extract (LI 132) prevented reperfusion arrhythmias and drastically reduced lactate dehydrogenase (LDH) release in isolated rat hearts.[4,40,41] However, in a more recent study, no antiarrhythmic effect on the reperfused rat heart was found.[42] The authors suggested an intracellular increase in calcium as the mechanism for inotropy as well as for the occasional aggravation of arrhythmia.
- Earlier areas of animal study included effects of hawthorn on myocardial perfusion.[43,44] In one experiment, crataemon increased rabbit coronary blood flow by 37% at a dose of 10 mg/kg and decreased myocardial oxygen consumption.[31]
- A preventive effect of hawthorn on coronary artery disease[4,45,46] and cancer[47] has been proposed as being due to hawthorn's antioxidant activities. Free radical properties have been demonstrated *in vivo*[45,48] and may depend on the phenol[49] or flavonoid content of the extract.
- Other pharmacologic properties of hawthorn may include thromboxane A_2 biosynthesis inhibition, observed *in vitro*,[50] reductions in lipids, diuretic activity (inhibition of ACE), antineoplastic activity, and collagen-stabilizing action. In rats, hawthorn tincture has been shown to enhance hepatic LDH receptor activity, to stimulate intrahepatic cholesterol degradation, and to suppress cholesterol biosynthesis.[33] Triterpene-enriched fractions of hawthorn extract have demonstrated almost complete inhibition of cultured larynx cancer cell growth.[51]

Pharmacodynamics/Kinetics

- Overall, there are insufficient available data.
- The pharmacokinetics of another botanical (the common grape) whose constituents, like hawthorn, include procyanidins, have been reviewed elsewhere. In the common grape, large quantities of procyanidins have been found unmetabolized in renal and intestinal elimination pathways, suggesting limited metabolic degradation. The procyanidins of the hawthorn berry are reported to have a higher degree of polymerization, yet a lower concentration of flavonoids and procyanidins.

HISTORY

- The name *Crataegus* is said to be a Greek derivation from the word for "strong" or "always having been there." In the history of Christianity, it has been suggested that hawthorn formed the crown of thorns.
- Medicinal use of hawthorn can be traced back to the 1st century AD. Dioscorides, Pliny, and Galen all referred to hawthorn in their writings but gave little explanation of its use. Quercetanus, physician of Henry IV of France, used syrup made from hawthorn fruit to treat heart ailments.
- Historically, traditional healers have used the fruit of hawthorn, whereas extracts derived from leaves and flowers are more common today. In traditional Chinese medicine, hawthorn berries (shanzha) were used for bloating, indigestion, flatulence, and diarrhea. Native Americans have traditionally used hawthorn as a diuretic for kidney and bladder disorders, as a heart tonic, for stomach aches, as an appetite suppressant, and to improve circulation.
- Hawthorn became popular as a heart medicine in Europe in the late 19th century and remains one of the most popular herbal medicines for cardiovascular use, especially in Germany and Switzerland.

Review of the Evidence: Hawthorne

Condition Treated*	Study Design	Author, Year	N[†]	SS[†]	Study Quality[‡]	Magnitude of Benefit	ARR[†]	NNT[†]	Comments
CHF	Meta-analysis	Pittler[27] 2003	8 trials, 632 patients	Yes	NA	Medium	NA	NA	Pooled data reflect significant benefits of hawthorn over placebo in terms of maximal workload capacity, pressure–heart rate product, and symptoms including dyspnea and fatigue.
CHF	Systematic review	Weihmayr[55] 1996	8	NA	NA	NA	NA	NA	Efficacy of hawthorn in the treatment of NYHA Class II CHF.
CHF	RCT	Forster[16] 1994	72	Yes	5	Medium	NA	NA	Well-conducted trial.
CHF	RCT	Schmidt[17] 1994	78	Yes	5	Large	NA	NA	Improved cardiac and psychological indicators.
CHF	RCT	Iwamoto[57] 1981	80	Yes	4	Small	NA	NA	Improved cardiac function and symptoms.
CHF	RCT	Hanak[11] 1983	60	Yes	4	Large	NA	NA	Statistical methodology insufficient.
CHF	RCT	O'Conolly[12] 1986	36	Yes	4	Medium	NA	NA	Improved cardiac and psychological indicators.
CHF	RCT	O'Conolly[13] 1987	36	Yes	4	Medium	NA	NA	Improved cardiac and psychological indicators.
CHF	RCT	Bodigheimer[15] 1994	85	Yes	4	Large	NA	NA	"Global" improvement observed.
CHF	RCT	Weikl[53] 1993	136	Yes	3	Medium	NA	NA	Nonrandomized, relatively low dosing.
CHF	RCT	Von Eiff[28] 1994	40	Yes	3	Small	NA	NA	Hawthorn/passionflower extract.
CHF	RCT	Beier[56] 1974	63	Yes	2	Medium	NA	NA	Unusual presentation of results.
CHF	RCT	Degenring[58] 2003	143	Yes	3	Small	NA	NA	Standardized extract of fresh berries of *C. oxycantha* and *C. monogyna* Jacq. (Crataegisan) yielded improvements in exercise tolerance but no decrease in subjective symptoms vs. placebo.
CHF	Equivalence trial	Tauchert[18] 1994	132	Yes	5	Large	NA	NA	Hawthorn compared with captopril.
CHF	Non-randomized, cohort, non-inferiority study	Schroder[60] 2003	212	No	1	NA	NA	NA	Homeopathic preparation of hawthorn, Cralonin, found equivalent to standard therapy (ACE/diuretics) for exercise double-product changes, but not for blood pressure reductions.
Coronary artery disease	RCT	Weng[61] 1984	46	Yes	3	Large	54%	2	*C. pinnatifada* in prevention of angina.
Functional cardiovascular disorders	RCT	Schmidt[62] 2000	190	Yes	4	Medium	NA	NA	Hawthorn/camphor combination.
Functional cardiovascular disorders	RCT	Ventura[63] 1990	40	Yes	2	Large	70%	2	Hawthorn/garlic combination.

*Primary or secondary outcome.
[†]*N*, number of patients; *SS*, statistically significant; *ARR*, absolute risk reduction; *NNT*, the number of patients who need to undergo a specific intervention in order to observe an outcome in one individual.
[‡]0-2 = poor; 3-4 = good; 5 = excellent.
CHF, Congestive heart failure; *NA*, not applicable; *RCT*, randomized, controlled trial.
For an explanation of each category in this table, please see Table 3 in the Introduction.

REVIEW OF THE EVIDENCE: DISCUSSION
Congestive Heart Failure
Summary

- Extracts of the leaves and flowers of hawthorn at doses of 160 to 900 mg daily have been reported as efficacious in the treatment of mild to moderate CHF, both improving exercise capacity and alleviating symptoms of cardiac insufficiency. This assessment is based on numerous randomized placebo-controlled clinical trials. However, the therapeutic equivalence of hawthorn extracts to drugs considered standard-of-care for heart failure (such as ACE inhibitors, diuretics, and beta-adrenergic receptor blockers) remains to be established, as does the effect of concomitant use of hawthorn with these drugs. One equivalence trial found hawthorn comparable to captopril but may not have been adequately powered to detect small differences between therapies.[18] Nonetheless, hawthorn is a potentially beneficial therapeutic agent for patients who cannot or will not take prescription drugs and may offer additive benefits to established therapies. Further study of these issues is warranted.

Meta-analysis

- Pittler et al. conducted a systematic review and meta-analysis of controlled trials assessing the use of hawthorn in patients with chronic heart failure.[27] Included studies were randomized, double-blinded, and placebo-controlled and used hawthorn monopreparations. Thirteen trials met all inclusion criteria; most used hawthorn as an adjunct to conventional drug therapy. Eight trials including 632 patients with chronic heart failure (NYHA Classes I to III) provided data suitable for meta-analysis. Hawthorn extract was found to be significantly more beneficial than placebo for the physiologic outcome of maximal workload (weighted mean difference, 7 watts; 95% CI, 3 to 11 watts; $p < 0.01$; n = 310 patients). The pressure-heart rate product results also demonstrated a significant beneficial decrease with hawthorn vs. placebo (weighted mean difference, –20; 95% CI, –32 to –8; n = 264 patients). In addition, symptoms including dyspnea and fatigue decreased significantly with hawthorn treatment compared with placebo. Reported adverse events were infrequent, mild, and transient; they included nausea, dizziness, and cardiac and gastrointestinal complaints.

Systematic Review

- A systematic review of controlled trials in NYHA Class I or II heart failure examined seven studies[11,12,15-17,52-54] and concluded that hawthorn is an effective and safe alternative to conventional approaches in the treatment of NYHA Class I or II CHF. The studies reported clinical improvement with decrease in symptoms due to treatment with hawthorn extract, and most found clear objective evidence of efficacy, usually by exercise ergometry.[55] The seven studies are reviewed separately in the following sections.

Randomized Trials (Included in Systematic Review)

- In an early trial, Hanak assessed the effect of hawthorn extract in 60 patients with mild to moderate untreated NYHA Class I or II CHF.[11] Patients were randomized into two groups for 21 days: Group 1 received hawthorn extract WS 1442 (Crataegutt novo 1 tablet three times daily, corresponding to 180 mg hawthorn extract per day); group 2 received placebo. Exercise tolerance improved in the extract group by 100 watts/min, but remained unchanged (–2.6 watts/min) in the placebo group ($p = 0.08$; statistical method not described). Of 23 patients with abnormal findings on exercise electrocardiogram (ECG) who received hawthorn, 78% improved, including 35% in whom the ECG normalized. In the placebo group, the corresponding proportions were 29% and 10% ($p < 0.001$).

- Similarly, O'Conolly et al. enrolled 36 patients with multisystem problems and mild CHF (NYHA Class I or II) in a 6-week randomized double-blind crossover trial of hawthorn extract WS 1442 (Crattaegutt novo, 1 tablet three times a day) and placebo.[12,13] Patients were evaluated by the heart rate–blood pressure product based on measurements obtained during exercise and by two standardized rating scales (the Nurses Observation Scale for Inpatient Evaluation and the Brief Psychiatric Rating Scale). Improvement in cardiac performance, subjective well-being, and evaluated behavior was more pronounced with hawthorn than with placebo treatment.

- Leuchtgens evaluated the efficacy of a slightly lower dose of the same extract (160 mg WS 1442) in 30 patients with NYHA Class II CHF.[52] Subjects in this double-blind trial were randomly assigned to either hawthorn or placebo and were evaluated before and after 8 weeks of treatment via measurement of blood pressure–heart rate product and a subjective symptom scale (*Beschwerdeliste*, or "well-being"). The heart rate–blood pressure product during 50-watt exercise, and the symptom score significantly improved in the hawthorn group compared with the placebo group.

- In a larger, multicenter study on the efficacy of hawthorn extract WS 1442 in the treatment of CHF, Weikl et al. assigned 136 patients with NYHA Class II disease to either hawthorn (Crataegutt, 160 mg in two equal doses) or placebo.[14] After a 2-week run-in phase, treatment was initiated. The main outcome, heart rate–blood pressure product under exercise, improved in the treatment group significantly but deteriorated in the placebo group ($p = 0.018$). Symptoms improved in 59% of the hawthorn group, but only in 44% of the placebo group (p = 0.05). The findings of this study support results from prior smaller trials. However, baseline differences in the groups' heart rate–blood pressure (higher in treatment group) may have affected the results.

- In a poorly described, randomized, placebo-controlled, double-blind trial, Bodigheimer and Chase investigated the efficacy of a different hawthorn extract (300 mg LI 132 in three equal daily doses) in 85 patients with stable NYHA Class II CHF.[15] Cardiac function was assessed by exercise tolerance during bicycle ergometry at days –7, 0, 14, and 28. Symptoms of CHF were assessed by a 4-point scale (not present, mild, moderate, severe). Patients and physicians rated global therapeutic effect of the treatment. At 4 weeks, more than two thirds of patients and physicians in the hawthorn group reported "very good" or "good" efficacy of hawthorn, compared with only slightly more than a third in the placebo group. Authors of the study did not note the statistical significance. Exercise tolerance increased by 13 watts in the hawthorn group and 3 watts in the placebo group; the baseline value was higher in the placebo group.

- Forster also examined the efficacy of hawthorn extract LI 132. Patients (n = 72) with NYHA II heart failure were randomized to placebo or to 300 mg standardized hawthorn extract LI 132 tablets (Faros) three times daily over 8 weeks.[16] Besides diuretics, no cardioactive drugs were allowed. Assessments included a subjective symptom score and determination of cardiac performance by bicycle ergometry. After 8 weeks, 86% of patients in the treatment group and 47% of the placebo group reported improved subjective state ($p < 0.01$). In the treatment group, anaerobic threshold was reached 30 seconds later, compared with 2 seconds later in the placebo group ($p < 0.05$), and oxygen capacity increased as well ($p < 0.05$). Cardiac performance in the steady-state protocol and oxygen capacity increased in the hawthorn group more than in the placebo group.

- Schmidt performed a similarly designed study.[17,54] Seventy-eight patients with NYHA Class II heart failure were randomly assigned to either hawthorn extract LI 132 (Faros, 600 mg in three equal doses for 8 weeks) or placebo. Patients were evaluated at 0, 28, and 56 days by exercise tolerance (bicycle ergometry) and symptom index. After 8 weeks, patients in the hawthorn group tolerated on average 28 watts more than baseline, whereas in the placebo group, the increase was 5 W ($p < 0.001$). The heart rate–blood pressure product, heart rate, and symptom scores were significantly lower with hawthorn than with placebo.

Randomized Trials (Not Included in Systematic Review)

- In an early (1974) study, Beier evaluated the benefit for patients with CHF by adding hawthorn to a nitrate (penta-erythrityltetranitrate [PETN]).[56] Patients (n = 63) with "relatively severe" coronary sclerosis and unspecified degree of CHF were enrolled in a crossover trial. Patients were first treated for 5 weeks with the combination of PETN 30 mg, hawthorn leaf ("e. fol") 10 mg, hawthorn berry ("e. fructu") 40 mg twice daily, or with PETN 30 mg alone twice daily. After 5 weeks, subjects were crossed over to an alternate treatment. Treatment effect was measured qualitatively. Only 54 patients on long-term glycoside therapy were further analyzed. In 25% of these patients, the combination PETN plus hawthorn was "clearly superior" to PETN alone ($p < 0.001$). This methodologically limited study must be viewed in historical context.

- In a 1984 trial including more impaired patients, Iwamoto et al. randomized 102 subjects with NYHA Class II or III CHF in a double-blind fashion to hawthorn or placebo treatment.[57] During the two initial weeks, hawthorn extract tablets (180 mg/day in three equal doses of 2 tablets) or placebo tablets were administered. The treating physicians were then allowed to vary the active or placebo dose between 6 and 9 tablets per day. Several markers of cardiac performance improved in the group given hawthorn, as compared with the placebo group. Overall cardiac performance was improved in the hawthorn (77%) vs. placebo (49%) group ($p < 0.01$). A more detailed analysis of the data showed that a significant improvement was seen only in patients with NYHA Class II CHF, not in those with NYHA Class III CHF. Clinical improvement was significant only for subjective symptoms of dyspnea, palpitations, and edema. This may have been due to a lack of statistical power. No clear ECG differences were found between the groups. However, radiographic signs of heart failure lessened in 82% of the hawthorn group, compared with 45% of the placebo group ($p < 0.05$).

- Degenning et al. conducted a randomized, placebo-controlled, multicenter trial in 143 adults diagnosed with NYHA Class II heart failure.[58] Over an 8-week period, subjects were randomized to receive either placebo or a standardized extract of fresh berries of C. oxyacantha L. and C. monogyna Jacq. (Crataegisan) taken as 30 drops three times daily. The primary outcome measured was a change in exercise tolerance determined with bicycle exercise testing. A secondary outcome was the blood pressure–heart rate product. Subjective cardiac symptoms at rest and at higher levels of exertion were assessed by patients using a categorical rating scale. The analysis was conducted based on intention-to-treat. The authors reported that after 8 weeks, a significant increase was observed in the hawthorn group compared with placebo in terms of exercise tolerance (8.3-watt difference; $p = 0.045$). Nonsignificant improvements in the blood pressure–heart rate product were observed with hawthorn versus placebo. There were no significant differences between groups in subjective assessments of cardiac symptoms.

- An international multicenter randomized placebo-controlled trial investigating the long-term effect of hawthorn therapy on mortality and prognosis of patients with CHF is currently under way.[59]

Equivalence Trials

- Direct comparison with conventional medications has been limited. Tauchert et al. compared the efficacy of hawthorn and of captopril in the treatment of CHF.[18] One hundred and thirty-two patients with NYHA Class II CHF were randomized to receive hawthorn LI 132 (Faros, 900 mg/day in three doses) or captopril (37.5 mg/day). Patients were evaluated at days −7, 0, 7, 14, 28, and 56 by clinical examination, ergometry, ECG, and symptom index. In both groups, cardiac performance significantly increased, and symptoms decreased. However, differences between the two treatments were not statistically significant. It is not clear if this study had insufficient statistical power to detect minor differences between the two groups. Further study is warranted, since use of angiotensin receptor inhibitors such as captopril is standard-of-care for heart failure, and hawthorn may offer an alternative to patients unable to take ACE inhibitors (e.g., those with significant renal insufficiency).

- Schroder et al. conducted a nonrandomized cohort study in 212 adult patients with NYHA Class II heart failure.[60] This trial was designed as a non-inferiority evaluation between standard therapy (ACE inhibitor plus diuretics) and use of a homeopathic preparation of hawthorn, Cralonin. Patients were divided into two groups at baseline, taking into account underlying disease characteristics. After 8 weeks, no statistically significant differences were detected between groups in 15 variables including exercise double-product, although blood pressure reductions were greater in the standard therapy group.

Combination Product

- Von Eiff et al. conducted a randomized, double-blind study in 53 patients assigned to hawthorn/passion flower extracts (520 mg crataegi herba cum flore, 80 mg crataegi fructus, 280 mg passiflorae herba daily) or placebo.[28] After 6 weeks of treatment, walking distance increased, and both diastolic pressure under exercise and cholesterol plasma levels fell significantly in the treatment compared with the placebo group. Other indicators were not significantly different. Notably, there was no difference in exercise capacity between the two groups. This study, which evaluated a hawthorn/passion flower extract, found beneficial effects on cardiac performance in CHF similar to those reported from studies of hawthorn alone. Based on what is known of the mechanism of action of both herbs, hawthorn is likely to be the active component.

Uncontrolled Trial

- A more recent, uncontrolled trial was conducted by Tauchert et al.[25] The efficacy of hawthorn extract WS 1442 (Crataegutt novo 450, 1 tablet daily for 24 weeks) was assessed in 1011 patients with NYHA Class II CHF. Symptoms markedly decreased over the study period. Ankle edema disappeared in 83% and nocturia in 50% of patients who had suffered from these symptoms at baseline. Mean ejection fraction improved. Percentile "shortening fraction," as determined by M-mode echocardiography, increased. Two thirds of the patients felt subjectively better after treatment. In three fourths, the physician deemed treatment efficacious. This trial had been designed in part as a safety trial; thus, its value is limited because of its methodology (lack of treatment controls or blinding).

Coronary Artery Disease (Angina)
Summary

- Increased myocardial perfusion and performance due to hawthorn have been observed in animals, and one randomized clinical trial indicates that hawthorn may be effective in decreasing frequency or severity of anginal symptoms. However, hawthorn has not been tested in the setting of concomitant use of drugs such as beta-blockers or ACE inhibitors, which are often considered to be standard-of-care. At this time, there is insufficient evidence to recommend for or against hawthorn for coronary artery disease or angina.

Evidence

- In a 1984 study, Weng et al. treated 46 patients suffering from angina pectoris with *Crataegus pinnatifada* extract (100 mg orally three times daily) or placebo for 4 weeks.[61] Treatment assignment was random and in a double-blind fashion. Besides nitroglycerine (NTG) during angina episodes, no beta-blockers, calcium antagonists, or antianginal drugs were used, but digoxin, diuretics, or antihypertensive drugs were continued. After 4 weeks of treatment, angina was decreased in 91% of patients in the hawthorn group, whereas this figure was only 37% ($p < 0.01$) in the placebo group. Accordingly, 45% of the hawthorn group completely stopped NTG, compared with 25% of placebo group. An additional 35% of the hawthorn group reduced intake of NTG, compared with 11% in the placebo group ($p < 0.01$). ECG findings improved in 46% of hawthorn-treated subjects, vs. 3% of the placebo group ($p < 0.01$). These results suggest that hawthorn may be effective in preventing angina in coronary artery disease. However, since most patients did not receive beta-adrenergic receptor blockers or ACE inhibitors regularly, often considered standard-of-care, the results may not be additive or generalizable to patients taking these drugs.

Functional Cardiovascular Disorders
Summary

- Two randomized trials have found efficacy of herbal combinations containing hawthorn in the treatment of functional cardiovascular symptoms. However, because of a lack of controlled information on hawthorn monotherapy, there is insufficient evidence to recommend for or against hawthorn for functional cardiovascular disorders.

Evidence

- Schmidt et al. found an herbal combination of hawthorn and camphor to be effective in the treatment of functional cardiovascular disorders (ICD 10, F 45.3).[62] One hundred and ninety patients were randomized to receive hawthorn plus camphor (Korodin Herz-Kreislauf-Tropfen) or placebo for 4 weeks. The "heart-related symptom complex" score fell from an average baseline value of 10.0 in both groups

to 4.5 and 5.5 points, respectively ($p = 0.017$). Efficacy was rated "good" or "very good" by (blinded) investigators in 70.5% of the treatment group, compared to 49.5% of placebo group. Although these results are promising, the use of an herbal combination makes the isolated effect of hawthorn difficult to evaluate.

- Another combination trial examined garlic with hawthorn on a poorly defined set of functional symptoms attributed to the cardiovascular system.[63] Forty patients with symptoms such as memory loss, vertigo, and "cold hands/feet" were randomized to receive 3 capsules per day containing 150 mg garlic extract plus 50 mg hawthorn extract, or placebo. All patients in the garlic/hawthorn group reported at least some improvement (50% reported "excellent" efficacy), whereas in the placebo group, 70% did not report any improvement. None reported "excellent" improvement. Systolic blood pressure, total cholesterol, triglycerides, and low-density lipoprotein (LDL) cholesterol significantly decreased in the treatment group, whereas no statistically significant changes were seen in the placebo group. However, no intergroup comparison was presented. Because of poor methodologic quality, and the use of a combination product, the effects of hawthorn cannot clearly be evaluated.

FORMULARY: BRANDS USED IN CLINICAL TRIALS
Brands Used in Statistically Significant Clinical Trials

- Adenylocrat f (Gödecke Aktiengesellschaft, Germany)[64]; Crataegutt novo (Schwabe GmbH & Co, Germany)[11-13]; Crataegutt forte (Schwabe GmbH & Co)[52]; Faros 300 (Lichtwer Pharma GmbH, Berlin, Germany).[15-18,54,65]
- **U.S. brand equivalent:** HeartCare (Nature's Way): standardized to 18.75% oligomeric procyanidines.

References

1. Bahorun T, Aumjaud E, Ramphul H, et al. Phenolic constituents and antioxidant capacities of *Crataegus monogyna* (Hawthorn) callus extracts. Nahrung 2003;47(3):191-198.
2. Hanus M, Lafon J, Mathieu M. Double-blind, randomised, placebo-controlled study to evaluate the efficacy and safety of a fixed combination containing two plant extracts (*Crataegus oxyacantha* and *Eschscholtzia californica*) and magnesium in mild-to-moderate anxiety disorders. Curr Med Res Opin 2004;20(1):63-71.
3. Bourin M, Bougerol T, Guitton B, et al. A combination of plant extracts in the treatment of outpatients with adjustment disorder with anxious mood: controlled study versus placebo. Fundam Clin Pharmacol 1997;11(2):127-132.
4. Al Makdessi S, Sweidan H, Dietz K, et al. Protective effect of *Crataegus oxyacantha* against reperfusion arrhythmias after global no-flow ischemia in the rat heart. Basic Res Cardiol 1999;94(2):71-77.
5. Bernatoniene J, Bernatoniene R, Jakstas V, et al. [Production technology and analysis of blood circulation improving tincture]. Medicina (Kaunas) 2003;39(Suppl 2):76-79.
6. Hammouda FM, Ismail SI, Azzam A, et al. Evaluation of the active constituents of *Crataegus sinaica* Boiss as inhibitors of human immunodeficiency virus type 1 (HIV-1). Pharm World Sci 1994;16(6)(suppl 1):18.
7. Chen JD, Wu YZ, Tao ZL, et al. Hawthorn (shan zha) drink and its lowering effect on blood lipid levels in humans and rats. World Rev Nutr Diet 1995;77:147-154.
8. Walker AF, Marakis G, Morris AP, et al. Promising hypotensive effect of hawthorn extract: a randomized double-blind pilot study of mild, essential hypertension. Phytother Res 2002;16(1):48-54.
9. Belz GG, Loew D. Dose-response related efficacy in orthostatic hypotension of a fixed combination of D-camphor and an extract from fresh crataegus berries and the contribution of the single components. Phytomedicine 2003;10(Suppl 4):61-67.
10. Di Renzi L, Cassone R, Lucisano V, et al. [On the use of injectable crataegus extracts in therapy of disorders of peripheral arterial circulation in subjects with obliterating arteriopathy of the lower extremities]. Boll Soc Ital Cardiol 1969;14(4):577-585.
11. Hanack T, Bruckel MH. [The treatment of mild stable forms of angina pectoris using Crategutt novo]. Therapiewoche 1983;33:4331-4333.
12. O'Conolly M, Jansen W, Bernhoft G, et al. [Treatment of decreasing cardiac

performance. Therapy using standardized crataegus extract in advanced age]. Fortschr Med 1986;104(42):805-808.

13. O'Conolly M, Bernhoft G, Bartsch G. [Treatment of stenocardia (angina pectoris) pain in advanced age patients with multi-morbidity]. Therapiewoche 1987;37:3587-3600.

14. Weikl A, Assmus KD, Neukum-Schmidt A, et al. [Crataegus Special Extract WS 1442. Assessment of objective effectiveness in patients with heart failure (NYHA II)]. Fortschr Med 1996;114(24):291-296.

15. Bodigheimer K, Chase D. [Effectiveness of hawthorn extract at a dosage of 3 × 100 mg per day]. Munch Med Wochenschr 1994;136(suppl 1):s7-s11.

16. Forster A, Forster K, Buhring M, et al. [Crataegus for moderately reduced left ventricular ejection fraction. Ergospirometric monitoring study with 72 patients in a double-blind comparison with placebo]. Munch Med Wochenschr 1994;136(suppl 1):s21-s26.

17. Schmidt U, Kuhn U, Ploch M, et al. Efficacy of hawthorn (crataegus) preparation LI 132 in 78 patients with chronic congestive heart failure defined as NYHA functional class II. Phytomedicine 1994;1:17-24.

18. Tauchert M, Ploch M, Hubner WD. Effectiveness of hawthorn extract LI 132 compared with the ACE inhibitor captopril: multicenter double-blind study with 132 NYHA Stage II. Munch Med Wochenschr 1994; 136(suppl 1):S27-S33.

19. Schlegelmilch R, Heywood R. Toxicity of Crataegus (hawthorn) extract (WS 1442). J Am Coll Toxicol 1994;13(2):103-111.

20. Ammon HP, Handel M. [Crataegus, toxicology and pharmacology. Part III: Pharmacodynamics and pharmacokinetics] (author's transl)]. Planta Med 1981;43(4):313-322.

21. Ammon HP, Handel M. [Crataegus, toxicology and pharmacology. Part II: Pharmacodynamics (author's transl)]. Planta Med 1981;43(3):209-239.

22. Ammon HP, Handel M. [Crataegus, toxicology and pharmacology. Part I: Toxicity (author's transl)]. Planta Med 1981;43(2):105-120.

23. Steinman HK, Lovell CR, Cronin E. Immediate-type hypersensitivity to Crataegus monogyna (hawthorn). Contact Dermatitis 1984;11(5):321.

24. Zapfe jG. Clinical efficacy of crataegus extract WS 1442 in congestive heart failure NYHA class II. Phytomedicine 2001;8(4):262-266.

25. Tauchert M, Gildor A, Lipinski J. [High-dose Crataegus extract WS 1442 in the treatment of NYHA stage II heart failure]. Herz 1999;24(6):465-474.

26. Loew D, Albrecht M, Podzuweit H. Efficacy and tolerability of a hawthorn preparation in patients with heart failure Stage I and II according to NYHA—a surveillance study. Phytomedicine 1996;3(Suppl 1):92.

27. Pittler MH, Schmidt K, Ernst E. Hawthorn extract for treating chronic heart failure: meta-analysis of randomized trials. Am J Med 2003;114(8): 665-674.

28. Von Eiff M, Brunner H, Haegeli A, et al. Hawthorn/passion flower extract and improvement in physical exercise capacity of patients with dyspnoea class II of the NYHA functional classification. Acta Therapeutica 1994;20:47-66.

29. Trunzler G, Schuler E. Comparative studies on the effects of a Crataegus extract, digitoxin, digoxin, and G-strophanthin in the isolated heart of homoiothermals. Arzneimittelforschung 1962;12:198-202.

30. Tankanow R, Tamer HR, Streetman DS, et al. Interaction study between digoxin and a preparation of hawthorn (Crataegus oxyacantha). J Clin Pharmacol 2003;43(6):637-642.

31. Petkov V. Plants with hypotensive, antiatheromatous and coronarodilatating action. Am J Chin Med 1979;7(3):197-236.

32. Chen ZY, Zhang ZS, Kwan KY, et al. Endothelium-dependent relaxation induced by hawthorn extract in rat mesenteric artery. Life Sci 1998;63(22): 1983-1991.

33. Rajendran S, Deepalakshmi PD, Parasakthy K, et al. Effect of tincture of Crataegus on the LDL-receptor activity of hepatic plasma membrane of rats fed an atherogenic diet. Atherosclerosis 1996;123(1-2):235-241.

34. Mang C, Herrmann V, Butzer R, et al. Crataegus fructi extract: a placebo-controlled study on haemodynamic effects of single and repetitive doses in normal volunteers. Eur J Clin Pharmacol 1997;52(suppl[abstract 116]):A59.

35. Popping S, Rose H, Ionescu I, et al. Effect of a hawthorn extract on contraction and energy turnover of isolated rat cardiomyocytes. Arzneimittelforschung 1995;45(11):1157-1161.

36. Brixius K, Frank K, Muench G, et al. WG 1442 (Crataegus spezialextrakt) works at the insufficient human myocardium contractible force-increasing. Verh Dtsch Ges Herz Kreisl 1998;30:28-33.

37. Schussler M, Holzl J, Fricke U. Myocardial effects of flavonoids from Crataegus monogyna species. Arzneimittelforschung 1995;45(8):842-845.

38. Muller A, Linke W, Klaus W. Crataegus extract blocks potassium currents in guinea pig ventricular cardiac myocytes. Planta Med 1999;65(4):335-339.

39. Joseph G, Zhao Y, Klaus W. [Pharmacologic action profile of crataegus extract in comparison to epinephrine, amrinone, milrinone and digoxin in the isolated perfused guinea pig heart]. Arzneimittelforschung 1995;45(12): 1261-1265.

40. Al Makdessi S, Sweidan H, Mullner S, et al. Myocardial protection by pretreatment with Crataegus oxyacantha: an assessment by means of the release of lactate dehydrogenase by the ischemic and reperfused Langendorff heart. Arzneimittelforschung 1996;46(1):25-27.

41. Nasa Y, Hashizume H, Hoque AN, et al. Protective effect of crataegus extract on the cardiac mechanical dysfunction in isolated perfused working rat heart. Arzneimittelforschung 1993;43(9):945-949.

42. Rothfuss MA, Pascht U, Kissling G. Effect of long-term application of Crataegus oxyacantha on ischemia and reperfusion induced arrhythmias in rats. Arzneimittelforschung 2001;51(1):24-28.

43. Mavers WH, Hensel H. [Changes in local myocardial blood circulation following oral administration of a Crataegus extract in non-narcotized dogs]. Arzneimittelforschung 1974;24(5):783-785.

44. Roddewig C, Hensel H. [Reaction of local myocardial blood flow in non-anesthetized dogs and anesthetized cats to the oral and parenteral administration of a Crataegus fraction (oligomere procyanidins)]. Arzneimittelforschung 1977;27(7):1407-1410.

45. Chatterjee SS, Koch E, Jaggy H, et al. [In vitro and in vivo studies on the cardioprotective action of oligomeric procyanidins in a Crataegus extract of leaves and blooms]. Arzneimittelforschung 1997;79:821-825.

46. Hertog MG, Feskens EJ, Hollman PC, et al. Dietary antioxidant flavonoids and risk of coronary heart disease: the Zutphen Elderly Study. Lancet 1993; 342:1007-1011.

47. Hertog MG, Kromhout D, Aravanis C, et al. Flavonoid intake and long-term risk of coronary heart disease and cancer in the seven countries study. Arch Intern Med 1995;155(4):381-386.

48. Bahorun T, Gressier B, Trotin F, et al. Oxygen species scavenging activity of phenolic extracts from hawthorn fresh plant organs and pharmaceutical preparations. Arzneimittelforschung 1996;46(2):1086-1089.

49. Rakotoarison DA, Gressier B, Trotin F, et al. Antioxidant activities of polyphenolic extracts from flowers, in vitro callus and cell suspension cultures of Crataegus monogyna. Pharmazie 1997;52(1):60-64.

50. Vibes J, Lasserre B, Gleye J, et al. Inhibition of thromboxane A$_2$ biosynthesis in vitro by the main components of Crataegus oxyacantha (hawthorn) flower heads. Prostaglandins Leukot Essent Fatty Acids 1994;50(4):173-175.

51. Saenz MT, Ahumada MC, Garcia MD. Extracts from Viscum and Crataegus are cytotoxic against larynx cancer cells. Z Naturforsch 1997;52c:42-44.

52. Leuchtgens H. [Crataegus Special Extract WS 1442 in NYHA II heart failure. A placebo controlled randomized double-blind study]. Fortschr Med 1993;111(20-21):352-354.

53. Weikl A, Noh HS. The influence of Crataegus on global cardiac insufficiency. Herz Gefabe 1993;11:516-524.

54. Schmidt U, Kuhn U, Ploch M, et al. Efficacy of the hawthorn extract LI 132 (600 mg/d) during eight weeks' treatment. Placebo-controlled double-blind trial with 78 NYHA stage II heart failure patients. Munch Med Wochenschr 1994;136(suppl 1):s13-s19.

55. Weihmayr T, Ernst E. [Therapeutic effectiveness of Crataegus]. Fortschr Med 1996;114(1-2):27-29.

56. Beier A, Konigstein RP, Samec V. [Clinical experiences with a crataegus–pentaerythrityl-tetranitrate combination drug in heart diseases due to coronary sclerosis in old age]. Wien Med Wochenschr 1974;124(24): 378-381.

57. Iwamoto M, Sato T, Ishizaki T. The clinical effect of Crataegus in heart disease of ischemic or hypertensive origin. A multicenter double-blind study. Planta Med 1981;42(1):1-16.

58. Degenring FH, Suter A, Weber M, et al. A randomised double blind placebo controlled clinical trial of a standardised extract of fresh Crataegus berries (Crataegisan) in the treatment of patients with congestive heart failure NYHA II. Phytomedicine 2003;10(5):363-369.

59. Holubarsch CJ, Colucci WS, Meinertz T, et al. Survival and prognosis: investigation of Crataegus extract WS 1442 in congestive heart failure (SPICE)—rationale, study design and study protocol. Eur J Heart Fail 2000;2(4):431-437.

60. Schroder D, Weiser M, Klein P. Efficacy of a homeopathic Crataegus preparation compared with usual therapy for mild (NYHA II) cardiac insufficiency: results of an observational cohort study. Eur J Heart Fail 2003; 5(3):319-326.

61. Weng WL, Zhang WQ, Liu FZ, et al. Therapeutic effect of Crataegus pinnatifida on 46 cases of angina pectoris—a double blind study. J Tradit Chin Med 1984;4(4):293-294.

62. Schmidt U, Albrecht M, Schmidt S. [Effects of an herbal crataegus-camphor combination on the symptoms of cardiovascular diseases]. Arzneimittelforschung 2000;50(7):613-619.

63. Ventura P, Girola M, Lattuada V. [Clinical evaluation and tolerability of a drug with garlic and hawthorn]. Acta Toxicol Ther 1990;11(4):365-372.

64. Blesken R. [Crataegus in cardiology]. Fortschr Med 1992;110(15): 290-292.

65. Fischer K, Jung F, Koscielny J, et al. [Crataegus extract vs. medigoxin. Effects on rheology and microcirculation in 12 healthy volunteers]. Munch Med Wochenschr 1994;136(suppl 1):s35-s38.

H

Hops

(*Humulus lupulus* L.)

SYNONYMS/COMMON NAMES/RELATED SUBSTANCES

- Common hops, European hops, hop, hop strobile, hopfen, houblon, humulus, lupulin, lupulus, lupuli strobulus, Ze 91019.
- **Selected combination products:** Avena Sativa Compound in Species Sedative Tea, HR 129 Serene, Hova-Filmtabletten, HR 133 Stress, Melatonin with Vitamin B$_6$, Seda-Kneipp, Snuz Plus, Stress Aid, Valverde, Zemaphyte.

CLINICAL BOTTOM LINE
Background

- The hop vine (*Humulus lupulus*) is a member of the Cannabaceae family. Dried hop flowers, called *hops*, are traditionally used for relaxation and sedation and to treat insomnia. A number of methodologically weak human trials have investigated hops in combination with valerian (*Valeriana officinalis*) for the treatment of sleep disturbances, and several animal studies have examined the sedative properties of hops given as monotherapy. However, the results of these studies are equivocal, and there is currently insufficient evidence to recommend hops alone or in combination for any medical condition.
- Hops are also sometimes found in combination products with passionflower (*Passiflora incanata*) or skullcap (potentially hepatotoxic), or with a high percentage of alcohol (up to 70% grain alcohol), confounding the association between the herb and possible sedative or hypnotic effects.
- Hops contain phytoestrogens, which may possess estrogen receptor agonist or antagonist properties, with unclear effects on hormone-sensitive conditions such as breast, uterine, cervical, and prostate cancer and endometriosis.

Scientific Evidence for Studied/Common Uses	Grade*
Insomnia/sleep quality	C
Sedation	C

*Key to grades: *A:* Strong scientific evidence for this use; *B:* Good scientific evidence for this use; *C:* Unclear scientific evidence for this use; *D:* Fair scientific evidence against this use (it may not work); *F:* Strong scientific evidence against this use (it likely does not work). For a more detailed explanation of efficacy criteria, see "Natural Standard Evidence-Based Validated Grading Rationale" in the Introduction.

Historical or Theoretical Uses That Lack Sufficient Evidence

- Analgesic, antidepressant, antibacterial, anti-inflammatory, antispasmodic, anthelmintic, anxiety, aphrodisiac, appetite stimulant, asbestosis,[1] atopic dermatitis,[2] breast cancer,[3] Crohn's disease, diabetes, digestion, dysentery, dyspepsia, estrogenic effects,[3] irritable bowel syndrome, kidney disorders, leprosy, menopausal/perimenopausal-related anxiety, mood disturbances, muscle spasm,[4] restlessness, rheumatic disorders, silicosis, skin ulcers (topical), tuberculosis.

Expert Opinion and Folkloric Precedent

- Expert European panels including the German Commission E, the British Herbal Compendium, and the European Scientific Cooperative on Phytotherapy (ESCOP) have approved hops for mood disturbances (restlessness, anxiety, excitability, tenseness) and for sleep disturbances (insomnia, difficulty falling asleep).

Safety Summary

- **Likely safe:** Hops have been used traditionally for thousands of years, with few anecdotal reports of adverse effects. Most natural medicine experts and textbooks assert that hops are likely safe when consumed in recommended doses; several clinical trials suggest that hops are likely safe when used in combination with valerian for sleep.[5-7]
- **Possibly unsafe:** Some experts believe that hops are possibly unsafe in combination with central nervous system (CNS)-depressant drugs or antipsychotics, because of theoretical potentiation of effects.[8,9] Hops contact dermatitis has been reported, particularly in hops pickers.

DOSING/TOXICOLOGY
General

- Recommended doses are based on those most commonly used in available trials, or on historical practice. However, with natural products, the optimal doses needed to balance efficacy and safety often have not been determined. Formulations and preparation methods may vary from manufacturer to manufacturer, and from batch to batch of a specific product made by a single manufacturer. Because often the active components of a product are not known, standardization may not be possible, and the clinical effects of different brands may not be comparable.

Standardization

- Some hops extracts are standardized to 5.2% bitter acids and/or 4% flavonoids per dose.

Dosing: Adults (18 Years and Older)
Oral

- **Insomnia/sleep disturbances:** 300 to 400 mg of hops extract combined with 240 to 300 mg of valerian (*Valeriana officinalis*) extract taken before bed.[5-7] Hops monopreparations have not been extensively studied, although traditional doses have included 0.5 to 1 g of dried extract and 0.5 to 1 mL of liquid extract (1:1 in 45% alcohol) taken three times daily.

Parenteral (Intravenous/Intramuscular)

- Not recommended. In animals, large parenteral doses have resulted in a soporific effect, followed by death; chronic administration has resulted in weight loss and death.[10]

Topical

- Insufficient available data.

Dosing: Children (Younger Than 18 Years)

- Traditionally, hops are considered as one of the milder sedative herbs, and to be safe for children. However, there is limited research in this area, and safety has not been established in this population. Some natural medicine experts suggest adjusting the dosage according to body weight (e.g., multiply the usual adult dose by the child's weight in pounds; then divide by 150).

Toxicology

- There is one case report of death in a dog 6 hours after ingesting 28 g of a hops plug that had been used for brewing beer; a malignant hyperthermia–like episode also occurred.[11]
- In animals, large parenteral doses have resulted in a soporific effect followed by death; chronic administration has resulted in weight loss and death.[10]

ADVERSE EFFECTS/PRECAUTIONS/CONTRAINDICATIONS
Allergy

- Contact dermatitis from hops is a recognized phenomenon, particularly in hops harvesters. Allergy to the pollen has been reported. In one small clinical study, bronchial hyper-responsiveness was observed among hops packagers, although the incidence was believed to be similar to that in the general population.[12]

Adverse Effects/Postmarket Surveillance

- **General:** Based on traditional use and available clinical trials, there have been no reported serious adverse effects associated with hops.[5-7]
- **Neurologic/CNS:** Hops may possess mild CNS-depressant activities, particularly when used concomitantly with other CNS depressants.[7-9] Scientific data are limited in this area. Large doses of "spent" hops (used for beer-making) ingested by dogs resulted in seizures, hyperthermia, restlessness, panting, vomiting, and signs of abdominal pain, possibly caused by uncoupling oxidative phosphorylation.[11]
- **Dermatologic:** Contact dermatitis from hops is a recognized phenomenon, particularly in hops harvesters. Allergy to hops pollen has been reported.
- **Gastrointestinal:** A stimulant effect on gastric secretion by hops has been demonstrated in laboratory animals.[13] There is no available human research in this area. Large doses of "spent" hops (used for beer-making) ingested by dogs resulted in vomiting, signs of abdominal pain, hyperthermia, restlessness, panting, and seizures, possibly caused by uncoupling oxidative phosphorylation.[11]
- **Pulmonary/respiratory:** An increased prevalence of chronic respiratory symptoms has been reported in brewery workers exposed to dust from hops, barley, and brewery yeast, reported in a study of 97 men.[14]
- **Endocrine (estrogenic effects):** Phytoestrogens in hops may exert estrogenic agonist or antagonist properties, with unknown effects on hormone-sensitive conditions such as breast, uterine, cervical, and prostate cancer and endometriosis.[3,15-18] Phytoestrogens found in hops have been shown to exert direct estrogenic activity *in vitro*,[3] whereas other studies have shown significant competitive binding to the estrogen receptor alpha (ER alpha) and beta (ER beta) *in vitro*[18] and to intracellular receptors for estradiol (ER) in human breast cancer cells.[3] A poorly described paper reported that women started menstruating 2 days after beginning hops collection; however, hormonal activity was not observed in a variety of hops extracts tested in animal models under controlled conditions.[19]
- **Endocrine (glucose effects):** Based on animal studies, hops may increase blood glucose levels in diabetic patients (but

may lower blood sugar in nondiabetic patients). Colupulone from hops has been found to elevate serum glucose levels in diabetic mice, but to have either no effect or to lower serum glucose levels in nondiabetic mice.[20,21] In other mouse studies, hops have not significantly altered the parameters of glucose homeostasis (basal glucose and insulin, insulin-induced hypoglycemia, glycosylated hemoglobin, and pancreatic insulin concentration).[22]

Precautions/Warnings/Contraindications

- Use cautiously in patients receiving CNS depressants or anti-psychotic medications, because of theoretical potentiation of sedative effects.[7-9]
- Use cautiously in patients who will be driving or operating heavy machinery, because of possible slowing of thought process.[7]
- Caution is warranted in patients with hormone-sensitive conditions, such as breast, uterine, cervical, or prostate cancer, or endometriosis because of the presence of phytoestrogens in hops, which may exert estrogen receptor agonist or antagonist properties.[3,15-18]
- Caution is warranted in diabetic patients because of potential increases in blood sugar levels (although hops may lower blood sugars in non-diabetic patients).

Pregnancy and Lactation

- Caution is warranted during pregnancy and lactation because of possible hormonal (estrogenic) and sedative effects of hops or other ingredients found in combination products. There is insufficient evidence regarding safety in these areas.

INTERACTIONS
Hops/Drug Interactions

- **Sedatives and CNS depressants:** Hops may possess mild CNS-depressant activities when used alone or concomitantly with other CNS depressants.[8,9] A study of a hop/valerian combination reported no potentiation of sedation associated with ethanol; a single dose of a combination product (300 mg of hops, 300 mg of valerian) did not yield sedative effects that were different from placebo effects after 12 hours.[7]
- **Oral contraceptives (oral contraceptive pills [OCPs]), hormone replacement therapy (HRT), tamoxifen, raloxifene:** Phytoestrogens in hops may possess estrogen receptor agonist or antagonist properties, with unknown effects on other hormonal therapies.[3,15-18] Phytoestrogens found in hops have been shown to exert direct estrogenic activity *in vitro*.[3]
- **Agents metabolized by P450 (CYP 450):** Hops may cause decreased plasma levels of these agents. *In vitro* and *in vivo* studies have demonstrated induction of cytochrome P450 3A and P450 2B by hops.[23-25]
- **Oral hypoglycemic drugs, insulin:** Based on animal studies, hops may elevate blood glucose levels in diabetic patients and may interfere with the effects of hypoglycemic agents (but may lower blood sugar in nondiabetic patients). Colupulone from hops has been found to elevate serum glucose levels in diabetic mice, but to have either no effect or to lower serum glucose levels in nondiabetic mice.[20,21] In other mouse studies, hops have not significantly altered the parameters of glucose homeostasis (basal glucose and insulin, insulin-induced hypoglycemia, glycated hemoglobin, and pancreatic insulin concentration).[22]
- **Antipsychotic drugs:** Ingestion of hops with phenothiazines has been suggested as possibly increasing the risk of hyperthermia, although there are no supporting human data.

- **Disulfiram (Antabuse):** Some hops preparations may contain high alcohol content and theoretically may elicit a disulfiram reaction.
- **Metronidazole (Flagyl):** A disulfiram-type reaction can occur when metronidazole and alcohol are used concomitantly. Because of the high alcohol content in some hops preparations, this combination theoretically may cause such a reaction.

Hops/Herb/Supplement Interactions

- **Sedative herbs and supplements:** Hops may possess mild CNS-depressant activities when used alone and may potentiate the effects of other CNS depressants.[8,9] Hops are often found in combination products with other herbs such as valerian (*Valeriana officinalis* L.) or passionflower (*Passiflora incarnata* L.), formulated with the intention of eliciting hypnotic or sedative effects. However, preliminary evidence from one study found that a hops/valerian combination product (300 mg of hops, 300 mg of valerian) did not yield sedative effects that were different from placebo effects after 12 hours (although 1 to 2 hours after ingestion there was a mild slowing in the processing of complex thoughts).[7]
- **Phytoestrogenic herbs:** As with many other herbs that contain phytoestrogenic compounds, the phytoestrogens in hops may possess estrogen receptor agonist or antagonist properties, with unknown effects on other hormonal therapies.[3,15-18] Phytoestrogens found in hops have been shown to exert direct estrogenic activity *in vitro*.[3]
- **P450 (CYP 450)-metabolized herbs and supplements:** Hops may cause decreased plasma levels of these agents. *In vitro* and *in vivo* studies have demonstrated induction of cytochrome P450 3A and P450 2B by hops.[23-25]
- **Hypoglycemic herbs and supplements:** Based on animal studies, hops may elevate blood glucose levels in diabetic patients and may oppose the effects of hypoglycemic agents (but may lower blood sugar in nondiabetic patients). Colupulone from hops has been found to elevate serum glucose levels in diabetic mice, but either to have no effect or to lower serum glucose levels in nondiabetic mice.[20,21] In other mouse studies, hops have not significantly altered the parameters of glucose homeostasis (basal glucose and insulin, insulin-induced hypoglycemia, glycated hemoglobin, and pancreatic insulin concentration).[22]

Hops/Food Interactions

- Insufficient available data.

Hops/Lab Interactions

- **Serum glucose:** Based on animal studies, hops may increase blood sugar in diabetic patients (but may lower blood sugar in nondiabetic patients). Colupulone from hops has been found to elevate serum glucose levels in diabetic mice, but either to have no effect or to lower serum glucose levels in nondiabetic mice.[20,21] In other mouse studies, hops have not significantly altered the parameters of glucose homeostasis (basal glucose and insulin, insulin-induced hypoglycemia, glycated hemoglobin, and pancreatic insulin concentration).[22]

MECHANISM OF ACTION
Pharmacology

- **Constituents:** The volatile oils of hops have been associated with the promotion of sleep and with antimicrobial properties *in vitro*. The bitter acids may possess anti-inflammatory and antiproliferative activity, and the flavonoids may also have antiproliferative properties.

- **Sedative/hypnotic effects:** Mouse models have found hops to have sedative, hypnotic, hypothermic, antinociceptive, and anticonvulsant properties.[26] *In vivo*, the 2-methyl-3-butene-2-ol in the volatile fraction has been identified as a principal sedative-hypnotic constituent of hops.[27] In fresh hops, there are only traces of this constituent, but the concentration of 2-methyl-3-butene-2-ol has been shown by other studies to continuously increase after drying, reaching maximum levels (approximately 0.15%) within 2 years with storage at room temperature. Pharmacologically relevant concentrations of this compound may be attained in both tea and bath preparations.[28] In a clinical trial, quantitative topographical electroencephalography (EEG) detected mild effects on the CNS from a high dosage of a valerian/hops combination product.[29] This effect was observed as an increase in delta, decrease in alpha, and a weak decrease in beta power.
- **Hormonal effects:** Zenisek et al. reported a high level of estrogenic activity in the beta bitter acid fraction of hops.[17] The hops component 8-prenylnaringenin has also exhibited estrogenic activity.[16] A poorly described paper reported that women started menstruating 2 days after beginning hops collection; however, hormonal activity was not observed in a variety of hops extracts tested in animal models under controlled conditions.[19] Furthermore, hops have shown significant competitive binding to the estrogen receptor alpha (ER alpha) and beta (ER beta) *in vitro*,[18] and to intracellular receptors for estradiol (ER) in human breast cancer cell.[3]
- **Cytochrome P450 effects:** Hop flavonoids have been shown to be effective and selective inhibitors of the human cytochrome P450, enzymes implicated in the activation of carcinogens.[23,24] These results are corroborated by an *in vivo* study demonstrating hops-mediated induction of P450 3A and P450 2B.[25] The induction of hepatic cytochrome P450 3A is attributed to the lupulone constituent of hops. The hops component 8-prenylnaringenin has been shown to be a potent inhibitor of the 2-amino-3-methylimidazo[4.5-f]quinoline (IQ), a potential carcinogen found in cooked foods that requires initial metabolic activation by P450.[30]
- **Glucose metabolism effects:** Colupulone from hops has been found to elevate serum glucose levels in diabetic mice, but either to have no effect or to lower serum glucose levels in nondiabetic mice.[20,21] In other mouse studies, hops have not significantly altered the parameters of glucose homeostasis (basal glucose and insulin, insulin-induced hypoglycemia, glycated hemoglobin, and pancreatic insulin concentration).[22]
- **Antimicrobial effects:** *In vitro*, the essential oil and chloroform extracts of hops have demonstrated activity against gram-positive bacteria (*Bacillus subtilis* and *Staphylococcus aureus*) and fungi (*Trichophyton mentagrophytes* var. *interdigitale*).[31] Another study found that antibacterial effects associated with weak acids derived from hops increase with decreasing pH.[32]
- **Anti-inflammatory effects:** Humulon, one of the bitter constituents in the hop, has shown anti-inflammatory activity in mouse models, inhibiting activity against 12-*O*-tetradecanopyphorbo-13-acetate (TPA)–induced inflammation and arachidonic acid–induced inflammation.[33]

Pharmacodynamics/Kinetics

- Studies using animal models have found that a sedative-hypnotic constituent of hops, 2-methyl-3-buten-2-ol, diminishes animal motility by 50% when given intraperitoneally at a dose of 206.5 mg/kg.[8,9] The onset of activity occurs within 2 minutes and reaches a maximum response within 2 hours. The effects of this hop constituent were found to be similar to those of the sedative drug methylpentynol.

HISTORY

- As a perennial marsh plant, the hop vine is native to Europe, Asia, and North America. The plant materials used in products come exclusively from the female plants. The hop vine is cultivated primarily in the United States, Germany, Great Britain, the Czech Republic, and China. The common name *hop* is derived from the Anglo-Saxon *hoppan* (to climb). The species name *lupulus* is derived from the Latin *lupus* (wolf), perhaps based on accounts of growth of the plant among willows, which it strangles, as a wolf attacks sheep.
- Hops were perhaps first used as a preservative in brewing beer, where the herb also is responsible for elements of the taste. Subsequently, it was noticed that hop-pickers tire easily, which may have inspired its medicinal use as a sedative. The Cherokee used hops as a sedative and analgesic and for treating rheumatic disorders, breast and uterine conditions, and kidney/urinary problems. In traditional Chinese medicine, hops are used to treat insomnia, restlessness, dyspepsia, intestinal cramps, and lack of appetite. In Germany, hops are licensed as a standard medicinal tea.
- Hop strobile and hops extract were listed in the U.S. National Formulary and unofficially in the United States Pharmacopoeia (USP) from 1831 until 1910.
- Hops essential oils are used in perfumes, cereal, beverages, and tobacco.

REVIEW OF THE EVIDENCE: DISCUSSION
Insomnia/Sleep Quality
Summary

- Hops has been found to possess sedative and hypnotic effects in animal studies. In humans, the effects of hops on sleep quality have been assessed in combination products with valerian (*Valeriana officinalis*). Although these trials have suggested possible hypnotic effects, they have been of low methodologic quality. In addition, in these studies the activity

of hops cannot be separated from the possible benefits of valerian. The evidence is thus equivocal, and it remains unclear if hops are efficacious as a hypnotic. Further study is warranted in this area.

Evidence

- In a double-blind, controlled trial, Müller-Limroth et al. studied the effects of a valerian/hops combination product on sleep disturbances.[5] Patients (n = 12) were given either placebo or 4 capsules of Seda-Kneipp (60 mg of valerian plus 100 mg of hops) each night at bedtime. The study showed a trend for the valerian/hops combination to facilitate sleep vs. placebo, but results were not statistically significant. Limitations of this trial include inadequate descriptions of baseline patient characteristics, lack of randomization, and a sample size that may not have been adequate to detect beneficial effects.
- Schmitz and Jackel conducted a randomized, double-blind trial comparing a hops/valerian combination product (Hova-Filmtabletten) and treatment with benzodiazepines in 46 patients diagnosed with sleep disorders by *Diagnostic and Statistical Manual of Mental Disorders*, 4th edition (DSM-IV), criteria.[6] In the herb treatment group, 2 daily capsules were given, each containing 200 mg of hops extract and 45.5 mg of valerian. After 2 weeks of therapy, the authors report that the "state of health" was observed to improve equally during therapy in both groups, with statistical significance; these benefits deteriorated 1 week after cessation of therapy. No withdrawal symptoms were reported with hops/valerian but were observed with benzodiazepine treatment. The clinical relevance of this study is limited by the inadequate reporting of randomization, blinding procedures, or outcomes measures, and by the small sample size. The effects of hops and of valerian cannot be separated.
- Leathwood et al. conducted a double-blind, randomized, crossover trial using self-rated measures to assess sleep latency and sleep quality in 128 healthy participants.[34] Subjects received either 2 placebo capsules, 2 specially prepared Hova capsules (prepared by grinding Hova tablets and preparing

Review of the Evidence: Hops

Condition Treated*	Study Design	Author, Year	N[†]	SS[†]	Study Quality[‡]	Magnitude of Benefit	ARR[†]	NNT[†]	Comments
Sleep quality	Controlled, double-blind	Muller-Limroth[5] 1977	12	No	3	NA	NA	NA	In healthy patients, a hops/valerian combination caused a nonsignificant trend to facilitate sleep.
Sleep quality	Equivalence study	Schmitz[6] 1998	46	Yes	3	Medium	NA	NA	A hops/valerian combination was found equivalent to a benzodiazepine after 2 weeks of therapy.
Sleep latency and quality	Double-blind, crossover	Leathwood[34] 1982	128	Mixed	3	Small	NA	NA	A single-dose hops/valerian combination was similar to placebo and less effective than valerian monotherapy for several measures of sleep quality.
Sedation, "hangover effect"	Double-blind, controlled, drug-monitoring study	Gerhard[7] 1996	80	Yes	2	Medium	NA	NA	A hops/valerian combination yielded a mild slowing of complex thought processing after 1-2 hours, but no "hangover" after 12 hours.

*Primary or secondary outcome.
[†]N, number of patients; SS, statistically significant; ARR, absolute risk reduction; NNT, the number of patients who need to undergo a specific intervention in order to observe an outcome in one individual.
[‡]0-2 = poor; 3-4 = good; 5 = excellent.
NA, Not applicable.
For an explanation of each category in this table, please see Table 3 in the Introduction.

capsules containing hops 100 mg plus valerian 200 mg in each capsule), or 2 valerian capsules (200 mg of dried powder per capsule) for one night each before bedtime. The alternate therapies were administered on the subsequent two evenings. A questionnaire was filled out by the subjects reflecting back on their sleep quality after each treatment. The study showed a significant improvement in subjective assessments of sleep latency (decreased time until falling asleep) with valerian monotherapy (37% of patients) and Hova (31%) vs. placebo (23%) ($p < 0.05$ for valerian, but results were nonsignificant for Hova). Subgroup analysis revealed the greatest benefit in poor sleepers and older (>40 years) subjects. In the data presented for sleep quality, 43% of respondents reported improved sleep after taking valerian monotherapy vs. 25% for placebo ($p < 0.05$) (there was no significant improvement in the Hova group). The only significant difference between the Hova data and the placebo data was an increased feeling of "sleepiness" the following morning. It is not clear why results were not significant in most categories for the Hova data, since the amounts of valerian were equivalent in each preparation. Possible explanations are that the commercial product Hova actually did not contain the claimed ingredients; that the hops somehow diminished the effects of valerian on sleep; that the study questionnaire was not a valid measure; and that there was random variation in the results. The study was methodologically flawed, with poor description of randomization or blinding, a nonvalidated questionnaire, and a 23% dropout rate (which may have explained the lack of reported benefits in some patients). Study of the effects of hops monotherapy on sleep is warranted.

- A controlled trial was conducted in 80 individuals to assess the effects on vigilance/reaction time in healthy patients taking Valverde (2 capsules, each containing 150 mg of valerian extract and 150 mg of hop extract), or 800 mg of valerian only (Valverde sleeping syrup, 10 mL), or 1 mg of the benzodiazepine flunitrazepam (Rohypnol), or placebo.[7] Doses were taken before bedtime, and effects were measured the following morning. A "hangover" phenomenon was observed in 50% of benzodiazepine subjects and in 10% of the Valverde and placebo groups. The authors concluded that the hops/valerian combination did not cause clinically relevant effects on cognitive function after 12 hours. A substudy of 36 individuals assessed the effects of Valverde or placebo 1 to 2 hours after ingestion, and the authors concluded that valerian monotherapy syrup caused a "very mild" statistically significant impairment of vigilance, whereas the valerian/hops combination caused mild slowing in the processing of complex thoughts. This study was designed to assess adverse effects rather than efficacy. The trial is limited by poor reporting of baseline patient characteristics and lack of proper randomization or blinding.

Sedation
Summary

- Hops have been used traditionally as a sedative. Preliminary evidence from animal studies suggests possible sedative properties, although human data are lacking. At this time, there is insufficient information to adequately evaluate the efficacy of hops for sedation.

Evidence

- Mouse models have found hops to have sedative, hypnotic, hypothermic, antinociceptive, and anticonvulsant properties.[26]

In vivo, the 2-methyl-3-butene-2-ol in the volatile fraction has been identified as a principal sedative-hypnotic constituent of hops.[27] In fresh hops, there are only traces of this constituent, but the concentration of 2-methyl-3-butene-2-ol has been shown by other studies to continuously increase after drying, reaching maximum levels (approximately 0.15%) within 2 years with storage at room temperature. Pharmacologically relevant concentrations of this compound may be attained in both tea and bath preparations.[28] In a clinical trial, quantitative topographical electro-encephalography (EEG) detected mild effects on the CNS from a high dosage of a valerian/hops combination product.[29] This effect was observed as an increase in delta, decrease in alpha, and a weak decrease in beta power.

FORMULARY: BRANDS USED IN CLINICAL TRIALS
Brands Used in Clinical Trials (Combination Hops/Valerian Products)

- Hova-Filmtabletten, Seda-Kneipp, Valverde.

References

1. Chang HM, But PPH. Pharmacology and Applications of Chinese Materia Medica. Philadelphia, World Scientific, 1986, pp 1077-1083.
2. Fung AY, Look PC, Chong LY, et al. A controlled trial of traditional Chinese herbal medicine in Chinese patients with recalcitrant atopic dermatitis. Int J Dermatol 1999;38(5):387-392.
3. Zava DT, Dollbaum CM, Blen M. Estrogen and progestin bioactivity of foods, herbs, and spices. Proc.Soc Exp Biol Med 1998;217(3):369-378.
4. Caujolle F, Pham HC, Duch-Kan P, et al. [Spasmolytic action of hop (*Humulus lupulus*, Cannabinaceae)]. Agressologie 1969;10(5):405-410.
5. Muller-Limmroth W, Ehrenstein W. [Experimental studies of the effects of Seda-Kneipp on the sleep of sleep disturbed subjects; implications for the treatment of different sleep disturbances (author's transl)]. Med Klin 1977;72(25):1119-1125.
6. Schmitz M, Jackel M. [Comparative study for assessing quality of life of patients with exogenous sleep disorders (temporary sleep onset and sleep interruption disorders) treated with a hops-valerian preparation and a benzodiazepine drug]. Wien Med Wochenschr 1998;148(13):291-298.
7. Gerhard U, Linnenbrink N, Georghiadou C, et al. [Vigilance-decreasing effects of 2 plant-derived sedatives]. Schweiz Rundsch Med Prax 1996; 85(15):473-481.
8. Wohlfart R, Wurm G, Hansel R, et al. [Detection of sedative-hypnotic active ingredients in hops. 5. Degradation of bitter acids to 2-methyl-3-buten-2-ol, a hop constituent with sedative-hypnotic activity]. Arch Pharm (Weinheim) 1983;316(2):132-137.
9. Wohlfart R, Hansel R, Schmidt H. [The sedative-hypnotic action of hops. 4. Communication: pharmacology of the hop substance 2-methyl-3-buten-2-ol]. Planta Med 1983;48(2):120-123.
10. Anon. In Bradley PR (ed): British Herbal Compendium. Bournemouth, UK, British Herbal Medicine Association, 1992.
11. Duncan KL, Hare WR, Buck WB. Malignant hyperthermia-like reaction secondary to ingestion of hops in five dogs. J Am Vet Med Assoc 1997; 210(1):51-54.
12. Meznar B, Kajba S. [Bronchial responsiveness in hops processing workers]. Plucne Bolesti 1990;42(1-2):27-29.
13. Tamasdan S, Cristea E, Mihele D. Action upon gastric secretion of Robiniae flores, Chamomilae flores and Strobuli lupuli extracts. Farmacia 1981; 29:71-75.
14. Godnic-Cvar J, Zuskin E, Mustajbegovic J, et al. Respiratory and immunological findings in brewery workers. Am J Ind Med 1999;35(1): 68-75.
15. Milligan SR, Kalita JC, Pocock V, et al. The endocrine activities of 8-prenylnaringenin and related hop (*Humulus lupulus* L.) flavonoids. J Clin Endocrinol Metab 2000;85(12):4912-4915.
16. Milligan SR, Kalita JC, Heyerick A, et al. Identification of a potent phytoestrogen in hops (*Humulus lupulus* L.) and beer. J Clin Endocrinol Metab 1999;84(6):2249-2252.
17. Zenisek A, Bednar IJ. Contribution of the identification of the estrogen activity of hops. Am Perfumer Arom 1960;75:61.
18. Liu J, Burdette JE, Xu H, et al. Evaluation of estrogenic activity of plant extracts for the potential treatment of menopausal symptoms. J Agric Food Chem 2001;49(5):2472-2479.
19. Fenselau C, Talalay P. Is oestrogenic activity present in hops? Food Cosmet Toxicol 1973;11(4):597-602.
20. Mannering GJ, Shoeman JA, Shoeman DW. Effects of colupulone, a component of hops and brewers yeast, and chromium on glucose tolerance

and hepatic cytochrome P450 in nondiabetic and spontaneously diabetic mice. Biochem Biophys Res Commun 1994;200(3):1455-1462.

21. Mannering GJ, Shoeman JA. Murine cytochrome P4503A is induced by 2-methyl-3-buten-2-ol, 3-methyl- 1-pentyn-3-ol(meparfynol), and tert-amyl alcohol. Xenobiotica 1996;26(5):487-493.

22. Swanston-Flatt SK, Day C, Flatt PR, et al. Glycaemic effects of traditional European plant treatments for diabetes. Studies in normal and streptozotocin diabetic mice. Diabetes Res 1989;10(2):69-73.

23. Dixon-Shanies D, Shaikh N. Growth inhibition of human breast cancer cells by herbs and phytoestrogens. Oncol Rep 1999;6(6):1383-1387.

24. Henderson MC, Miranda CL, Stevens JF, et al. *In vitro* inhibition of human P450 enzymes by prenylated flavonoids from hops, *Humulus lupulus.* Xenobiotica 2000;30(3):235-251.

25. Mannering GJ, Shoeman JA, Deloria LB. Identification of the antibiotic hops component, colupulone, as an inducer of hepatic cytochrome P-4503A in the mouse. Drug Metab Dispos 1992;20(2):142-147.

26. Lee KM, Jung JS, Song DK, et al. Effects of *Humulus lupulus* extract on the central nervous system in mice. Planta Med 1993;59(Suppl):A691.

27. Hansel R, Wohlfart R, Coper H. [Sedative-hypnotic compounds in the exhalation of hops, II]. Z.Naturforsch.[C] 1980;35(11-12):1096-1097.

28. Hänsel R, Wohlfart R, Schmidt H. The sedative-hypnotic principle of hops.

3. Communication: contents of 2-methyl-3-butene-2-ol in hops and hop preparations. Planta Med 1982;45:224-228.

29. Vonderheid-Guth B, Todorova A, Brattstrom A, et al. Pharmacodynamic effects of valerian and hops extract combination (Ze 91019) on the quantitative-topographical EEG in healthy volunteers. Eur J Med Res 2000; 5(4):139-144.

30. Miranda CL, Yang YH, Henderson MC, et al. Prenylflavonoids from hops inhibit the metabolic activation of the carcinogenic heterocyclic amine 2-amino-3-methylimidazo[4,5- f] quinoline, mediated by cDNA-expressed human CYP1A2. Drug Metab Dispos 2000;28(11):1297-1302.

31. Langezaal CR, Chandra A, Scheffer JJ. Antimicrobial screening of essential oils and extracts of some *Humulus lupulus* L. cultivars. Pharm Weekbl Sci 1992;14(6):353-356.

32. Simpson WJ, Smith AR. Factors affecting antibacterial activity of hop compounds and their derivatives. J Appl Bacteriol 1992;72(4):327-334.

33. Yasukawa K, Takeuchi M, Takido M. Humulon, a bitter in the hop, inhibits tumor promotion by 12-O-tetradecanoylphorbol-13-acetate in two-stage carcinogenesis in mouse skin. Oncology 1995;52(2):156-158.

34. Leathwood PD, Chauffard F, Heck E, et al. Aqueous extract of valerian root (*Valeriana officinalis* L.) improves sleep quality in man. Pharmacol Biochem Behav 1982;17(1):65-71.

Horse Chestnut
(Aesculus hippocastanum L.)

SYNONYMS/COMMON NAMES/RELATED SUBSTANCES

- Aescin, aescine, aescule, bongay, buckeye, chestnut, conkers, conquerors, eschilo, escin, escine, esculin, fish poison, graine de marronier d'Inde, hestekastanje, hippocastani folium, hippocastani semen, *Hippocastanum vulgare* Gaertn., horse chestnut seed extract (HCSE), horsechestnut, marron europeen, marronier, NV-101, rokastaniensamen, rosskastanie, Spanish chestnut, Venastat, Venoplant, Venostasin.

CLINICAL BOTTOM LINE
Background

- Horse chestnut seed extract (HCSE) is widely used in Europe for chronic venous insufficiency (CVI), a syndrome characterized by lower extremity edema, varicosities, pain, pruritus, atrophic skin changes, and ulceration. Although HSCE is traditionally recommended for a variety of medical conditions, CVI is the only indication for which there is strong supportive scientific evidence.
- Review of the literature reveals 14 randomized controlled trials, of which 7 are well designed (albeit limited by small size and short duration). These studies support the superiority of HCSE over placebo and suggest equivalence to compression stockings.
- Side effects from HCSE have been similar to effects reported with placebo in clinical trials. However, because of increased risk of hypoglycemia, caution is advised in children and diabetics.
- Horse chestnut flower, branch bark, and leaf have not been shown effective for any indication, and it is strongly advised that they be avoided because of known toxicity.

Scientific Evidence for Common/Studied Use(s)	Grade*
Chronic venous insufficiency	A

*Key to grades: *A:* Strong scientific evidence for this use; *B:* Good scientific evidence for this use; *C:* Unclear scientific evidence for this use; *D:* Fair scientific evidence against this use (it may not work); *F:* Strong scientific evidence against this use (it likely does not work). For a more detailed explanation of efficacy criteria, see "Natural Standard Evidence-Based Validated Grading Rationale" in the Introduction.

Historical or Theoretical Indications That Lack Sufficient Evidence

- Benign prostatic hypertrophy (BPH), biliary/gallbladder disease (cholecystitis, cholelithiasis, colic), bladder disorders (incontinence, cystitis), bruising (hematoma), cough (antitussive), deep venous thrombosis, diarrhea, dizziness (vertigo), fever, hemorrhoids, kidney diseases, liver (hepatic) congestion, menstrual spastic pain, neuralgia, nocturnal leg cramps, osteoarthritis, pancreatitis, pulmonary edema, pulmonary embolism, rectal complaints, "rheumatism," rheumatoid arthritis, skin conditions (topical use), postoperative or post-traumatic soft tissue swelling (topical use), tinnitus, ulcers, whooping cough (pertussis).

Expert Opinion and Folkloric Precedent

- Although popular in Europe for CVI, horse chestnut seed extract (HSCE) is less widely used in the Americas. Based on German sales alone, HSCE products were the third best-selling herbal extracts in 1996 (behind *Ginkgo biloba* and St. John's wort), accounting for a $51 million U.S. dollar expenditure. Most experts agree that because of known toxicity and unproven efficacy, oral forms of horse chestnut other than HCSE should be avoided. Topical gel is occasionally recommended for hematomas. Intravenous horse chestnut has been used to treat deep venous thrombosis, but results have varied and this use is generally discouraged.

Safety Summary

- **Likely safe:** When horse chestnut seed extract (HCSE) products standardized to escin (aescin) content are taken under supervision of a health care professional for up to 12 weeks (at recommended doses).
- **Possibly unsafe:** When used by patients with diabetes or glucose intolerance, based on hypoglycemia in animal studies.[1]
- **Likely unsafe:** When any amount of raw horse chestnut seed, flower, branch bark, or leaf is consumed, or when HSCE is taken in amounts greater than recommended, based on known toxicity.

DOSING/TOXICOLOGY
General

- Recommended doses are based on those most commonly used in available trials and on clinical practice patterns. However, with natural products, the optimal doses needed to balance efficacy and safety often have not been determined. Formulations and preparation methods may vary from manufacturer to manufacturer, and from batch to batch of a specific product made by a single manufacturer. Because often the active components of a product are not known, standardization may not be possible, and the clinical effects of different brands may not be comparable.

Standardization

- Horse chestnut seed extract (HCSE) products are normally standardized to contain 16% to 20% triterpene glycosides calculated as escin content.

Dosing: Adults (18 Years and Older)
Oral

- A range of doses for horse chestnut seed extract (HCSE) have been noted in the literature. Clinical trials suggest it is necessary to ingest a standardized product containing 50 to 75 mg escin every 12 hours to obtain benefit. This often results in an HCSE product total dose of 300 mg twice daily.

Topical

- A trial of topical 2% escin gel (three to four times daily) vs. placebo for hematoma failed to demonstrate reduction in tenderness.[2] Therefore, no specific topical concentration or dose can be recommended.

Intravenous

- No reliable data support the use of HCSE intravenously for any indication, and anaphylactic shock has been reported.[3]

Dosing: Children (Younger Than 18 Years)

- No data support the use of horse chestnut seed extract (HCSE) in children, and CVI is generally seen only in adults.
- It is recommended that children not take HCSE, because of potential hypoglycemic effects.
- Children who drank tea from leaves and twigs, or who ate raw horse chestnut seeds, have been poisoned, and death has been reported.[4]

Toxicology

- Unprocessed horse chestnut seeds, leaves, bark, and flowers contain esculin, which has been associated with significant toxicity and death. Horse chestnut seed extract (HCSE) standardized to escin content should not contain clinically relevant levels of esculin, and thus most possible toxic effects will not be a concern.
- Horse chestnut poisoning may cause vomiting, diarrhea, headache, stupor, coma, weakness, muscle fasciculation, malcoordination, or paralysis.[5]
- Aflatoxins, considered potent carcinogens, have been identified in commercial skin products containing horse chestnut, but not in HCSE.[6]
- Intravenous administration of horse chestnut has caused anaphylactic shock.[3]
- The LD_{50} for the water-soluble portion of a nonstandardized alcoholic extract of horse chestnut seeds has been calculated as 10 to 11 mg per gram of body weight in chicks and hamsters. Dried, powdered seeds have been found nontoxic in animals at 80 mg/g.[5]

ADVERSE EFFECTS/PRECAUTIONS/CONTRAINDICATIONS
Allergy

- Horse chestnut seed extract (HCSE) should be avoided in patients with known allergy to horse chestnuts, esculin, or any of the ingredients of HSCE (flavonoids, biosides, trisides of quertins, and oligosaccharides including 1-ketose and 2-ketose).
- Intravenous administration of horse chestnut has caused anaphylactic shock.[3]

Adverse Effects

- **General:** Standardized HCSE is generally regarded as safe. The incidence of adverse effects was 0.6% in an observational study of >5000 subjects,[7] and up to 3.0% in 14 available randomized trials. Gastrointestinal tract upset and calf spasm are the most common symptoms, whereas headache, nausea, and pruritus are less common.
- **Dermatologic:** Pruritus has been rarely documented in the available HCSE randomized trials and is similar in incidence after placebo is given. Contact dermatitis has been reported following topical application of HCSE.[8]
- **Neurologic/CNS:** Occasional headache and dizziness have been reported with HCSE, although the exact frequency is not clear in published clinical trials. One trial (n = 62) reported a composite adverse event rate of 3.2%, in which headache and transient dizziness were listed.[9]
- **Gastrointestinal/hepatic:** Mild nausea and dyspepsia have been documented in few subjects in HCSE trials.[9] Horse chestnut leaf has been associated with hepatitis after intra-

muscular injection.[10] A 69-year-old woman taking Venocapsan containing horse chestnut leaf experienced hepatotoxicity, which resolved after discontinuing the product.[11]

- **Renal:** There have been case reports of nephrotoxicity associated with high parenteral doses of escin (HCSE).[12,13]
- **Endocrine:** Theoretically, HCSE may cause hypoglycemia: HCSE has been noted to inhibit normal increases in serum glucose levels in glucose-loaded rats.[1]
- **Hematologic:** Horse chestnut theoretically may increase bleeding risk because of the hydroxycoumarin content of esculin. Properly prepared HCSE should not contain esculin and therefore should not carry this risk.
- **Musculoskeletal:** Calf spasm has been reported by a small number of subjects in an observational study involving >5000 patients taking HCSE for CVI.[7]

Precautions/Warnings/Contraindications

- Use HCSE with caution in patients with diabetes, because of observed hypoglycemia in rats.
- Use parenteral horse chestnut seed preparations with caution in patients with renal insufficiency, because of rare case reports of renal injury.
- Avoid horse chestnut products other than HCSE because of known toxicity.

Pregnancy and Lactation

- HCSE is generally not recommended during pregnancy or nursing because of limited data. Steiner et al. conducted a brief placebo-controlled, double-blind study of use of HCSE in 52 women with leg edema attributed to pregnancy-induced venous insufficiency and failed to observe any serious adverse effects after 2 weeks.[14] Subjects received 300 mg twice daily of Venostasin retard (240 to 290 mg of HCSE, standardized to 50 mg of escin).

INTERACTIONS
Horse Chestnut/Drug Interactions

- **Anticoagulants, antiplatelet agents, nonsteroidal anti-inflammatory drugs (NSAIDs):** Because of its esculin constituents, horse chestnut (but not horse chestnut seed extract [HCSE], which when properly prepared does not contain esculin) may theoretically increase the risk of bleeding when taken with anticoagulants (warfarin, heparin) or antiplatelet drugs (aspirin, clopidogrel, ticlopidine, NSAIDs). However, no clinical cases are reported in the available literature.
- **Hypoglycemic/antihyperglycemic drugs:** HCSE has been noted to inhibit the normal increase of serum glucose levels in glucose-loaded rats.[1] Thus, HCSE may theoretically have an additive effect with drugs that cause hypoglycemia, including sulfonylureas, insulin, and metformin.
- **Protein-binding drugs:** Escin may theoretically interfere with protein-bound drugs such as phenytoin, warfarin, and amiodarone, although no cases are reported in the available literature.

Horse Chestnut/Herb/Supplement Interactions

- **Anticoagulant herbs/supplements:** Because of its esculin constituents, horse chestnut (but not horse chestnut seed extract [HCSE], which when properly prepared does not contain esculin) may have additive effects with herbs considered to predispose to bleeding via effects on platelets, bleeding time, or the coagulation cascade. These include angelica, anise, arnica, asafetida, bogbean, boldo, capsicum,

H

celery, clove, chamomile, danshen, devil's claw, fenugreek, feverfew, garlic, ginger, ginkgo, gymnestra, horseradish, licorice, meadowsweet, onion, papain, passionflower, poplar, prickly ash, quassia, red clover, turmeric, vitamin E, wild carrot, wild lettuce, and willow.

- **Hypoglycemic herbs/supplements:** Herbs that may lower blood sugar, such as bitter melon, *Panax ginseng*, and American ginseng (*Panax quinquefolius*), should be used cautiously with HCSE, because of a theoretical additive effect. Literature review reveals no cases in humans.

MECHANISM OF ACTION
Pharmacology

- Horse chestnut seed contains 3% to 6% of a triterpene saponin mixture called escin (or aescin), flavonoids, condensed tannins, quinines, sterols and fatty acids (including linolenic, palmitic, and steric acids), and coumarins (including aesculetin, fraxin [fraxetin glucoside], and scopolin [scopoletin glucoside]). The main active ingredient is considered to be escin, which acts on capillary membranes to normalize vascular permeability. Purified escin has been shown to decrease histamine- and serotonin-induced capillary hyperpermeability and to decrease chemically induced inflammation in rats.[15-17]
- Horse chestnut seed extract (HCSE) inhibits enzymes that are implicated in the pathogenesis of CVI.[18] It has been found to contract canine[17] and human[19] isolated saphenous veins *in vitro* in dose-dependent fashion, possibly as a result of preferential formation of the vasoconstrictive eicosanoid prostaglandin F2-alpha (PGF$_{2\alpha}$).[20] HCSE has also been shown to increase femoral venous pressure and flow; to decrease the formation of edema induced in rat paw models;

and to suppress plasma extravasation and leukocyte emigration into the pleural cavity in an experimental rat model of pleurisy.[17] Additionally, the extract has been reported to have antioxidant effects.[17,21] In aggregate, these findings suggest that HCSE increases venous tone, improves venous return, and reduces vascular permeability, all of which lead to the clinical benefit of dependent edema reduction.

- Horse chestnut contains the hydroxycoumarin component esculin, which may have antithrombin activity. Esculin is found in the bark, buds, and other parts of the fruits but should not be present in properly prepared HCSE.

Pharmacodynamics/Kinetics

- Oral escin is not well absorbed and undergoes substantial first-pass metabolism. Half-life is 10 to 20 hours. Peak plasma levels occur 2 to 3 hours after ingestion.[22]

HISTORY

- Horse chestnuts have been used medicinally for centuries. Native Americans roasted, peeled, and mashed chestnut seeds and then leached them in lime in order to render them less toxic. Extracts of the bark have been used as a yellow dye. In European folk medicine, carrying the fruit in the pockets was believed to prevent or cure arthritis.
- Horse chestnut is a member of the genus *Aesculus* and family Hippocastanaceae. The fruit has a thick husk and contains from one to six seeds. The plant has pink and white flowers. Indigenous to the mountains of Greece, Bulgaria, the Caucasus, northern Iran, and the Himalayas, horse chestnut is now cultured internationally, particularly in Europe and Russia.

Review of the Evidence: Horse Chestnut

Condition Treated*	Study Design	Author, Year	N†	SS†	Study Quality‡	Magnitude of Benefit	ARR†	NNT†	Comments
CVI	Systematic review[26]	Pittler[25,26] 1998, 2003	14 trials	Yes	NA	Small-medium	NA	NA	Well designed. Found overall reductions in ankle circumference, leg volume; decreased leg pain, pruritus, fatigue, "tenseness."
CVI	Meta-analysis	Siebert[24] 2002	13 trials	Yes	NA	Medium	NA	NA	Heterogeneous studies analyzed together; incomplete description of methods. Meta-analysis included 1051 patients. Reported overall 1.5-fold decrease in edema; 1.7-fold in itching; 4.1-fold in leg pain.
CVI	RCT, double-blind	Bisler[29] 1986	24	Yes	5	Medium	NA	NA	100 mg escin once daily. Small trial. Examined acute effect on "capillary coefficient."
CVI	RCT	Rudofsky[39] 1986	40	Yes	5	Medium	NA	NA	50 mg escin twice daily. Small trial. Outcome: leg volume.
CVI	Equivalence trial	Rehn[9] 1996	137	Yes	4	NA	NA	NA	50 mg escin twice daily. Equivalent to oxerutins at 4 weeks in reducing leg edema. No power calculation.
CVI	RCT	Diehm[30] 1992	40	Yes	4	Medium	NA	NA	75 mg escin twice daily. Small trial. Outcome: leg volume.
CVI	RCT	Pilz[38] 1990	30	Yes	4	Small	NA	NA	50 mg escin twice daily. Small trial. Outcome: leg circumference.
CVI	Equivalence trial	Kalbfleisch[35] 1989	33	No	4	NA	NA	NA	50 mg escin once daily. Equivalent to oxerutins at 4 weeks in reducing leg edema. No power calculation. Small trial.

Review of the Evidence: Horse Chestnut—*cont'd*

Condition Treated*	Study Design	Author, Year	N†	SS†	Study Quality‡	Magnitude of Benefit	ARR†	NNT†	Comments
CVI	RCT	Friederich[34] 1978	118	Yes	4	Small	NA	NA	50 mg escin twice daily. Large number of dropouts (19%). Outcome: leg pain/spasm.
CVI	Equivalence trial	Diehm[31] 1996	240	Yes	3	Small	NA	NA	HCSE equivalent to compression stockings. Outcome: leg volume.
CVI	RCT	Erler[33] 1991	40	Yes	2	Small	NA	NA	150 mg escin/day. Methodologically weak trial. Outcome: edema.
CVI	RCT	Steiner[14] 1990	20	Yes	2	Small	NA	NA	Methodologically weak trial. Outcome: leg volume.
CVI	Equivalence trial	Erdlen[32] 1989	30	Yes	2	Small	NA	NA	Venostasin retard vs. oxerutins. Methodologically weak trial. Outcome: leg volume.
CVI	RCT	Lohr[36] 1986	80	NA	1	Small	NA	NA	Methodologically weak trial, no *p* values given. Outcome: leg volume.
CVI	RCT	Neiss[37] 1976	233	Yes	1	Medium	NA	NA	Methodologically weak trial. Outcome: leg pain/edema.
CVI	RCT	Alter[28] 1973	96	Yes	1	Small	NA	NA	Methodologically weak trial. Outcome: edema/pruritus.

*Primary or secondary outcome.
†N, Number of patients; SS, statistically significant; ARR, absolute risk reduction; NNT, the number of patients who need to undergo a specific intervention in order to observe an outcome in one individual.
‡0-2 = poor; 3-4 = good; 5 = excellent.
CVI, Chronic venous insufficiency; NA, not applicable; RCT, randomized, controlled trial.
For an explanation of each category in this table, please see Table 3 in the Introduction.

REVIEW OF THE EVIDENCE: DISCUSSION
Chronic Venous Insufficiency
Summary

- There is strong evidence that horse chestnut seed extract (HCSE) reduces symptoms associated with CVI.[23-27] Of 14 identified randomized trials,[9,14,28-39] 6 found statistically significant decreases in lower leg circumference, leg volume, and symptoms of leg pain, pruritus, fatigue, and "tenseness" vs. placebo. The remaining 8 studies compared HCSE with reference medications, most commonly a derivative of the flavonoid rutin (used in Germany for CVI). Although most of these trials found equivalence, their results are tainted by methodologic weaknesses, including lack of power calculations or placebo arms. Results of one trial suggest equivalence of HCSE to compression stockings.[31] A preliminary investigation reported superior efficacy of Pycnogenol (pine bark extract) in the management of CVI compared with horse chestnut, although these results cannot be considered conclusive because of methodologic weaknesses.[40]

Evidence

- Preliminary evidence stemmed from studies by Friederich et al.[34] and Bisler et al.[29] Friederich's group examined symptoms of CVI in a crossover trial of 118 subjects, in which patients received 50 mg of escin twice daily for 3 weeks. Statistically significant reductions in pain, lower leg spasm, and fatigue were found vs. placebo. However, this study was limited by a 19% dropout rate, without ample follow-up or examination of dropouts. In the Bisler trial, 22 patients with documented CVI were randomized to receive 1200 mg of Venostasin (a German preparation containing 100 mg of escin) or placebo and then to proceed to crossover. This double-blind study found a statistically significant 22% decrease in the capillary filtration coefficient 3 hours after taking HCSE. The authors concluded that Venostasin might have an inhibitory effect on edema formation via a decrease in transcapillary filtration.

- Rudofsky conducted a well-designed (albeit small) randomized, double-blind, placebo-controlled study using a parallel design.[39] This trial evaluated HCSE (Venostasin retard, containing 50 mg of escin, 1 tablet twice daily) vs. placebo over 4 weeks in 40 subjects. The results demonstrated a statistically significant reduction in leg volume of 44 mL from baseline as measured by liquid plethysmography in the HSCE treatment group (vs. an increase in volume from baseline in the placebo group). Although this study failed to show a significant effect on venous capacity, it did demonstrate a statistically significant change in both calf and foot circumference ($p < 0.01$). At 28 days, HCSE-treated patients noted a mean decrease in ankle circumference of 6.5 mm, as compared with a 1-mm increase in placebo-treated patients. In addition, there was significant clinical improvement as demonstrated by decrease in pain, pruritus, fatigability, and fullness in the HCSE-treated group on a 5-point Likert scale.

- Pilz conducted a randomized trial in which subjects ingested 50 mg of escin twice daily for 3 weeks and were found to have a statistically significant reduction in ankle circumference of 0.7 cm vs. placebo.[38] This study was limited by small size (n = 30) and unclear level of compliance. Diehm et al. followed this trial with a well-designed placebo-controlled study of 40 patients with CVI.[30] Subjects received either placebo or HCSE (75 mg of escin twice daily) for 6 weeks. Patients who received HCSE had significantly decreased leg volume both at rest and after edema provocation (allowing legs to hang down during sitting for 15 minutes). Patients in the treatment group also had significantly fewer symptoms of venous stasis (feeling of heaviness, leg fatigue, numbness).

- Pilz et al. conducted a second, larger, randomized, "partially double-blinded" study comparing leg compression stockings with oral HCSE (50 mg of escin twice daily) and placebo in 240 patients with CVI.[31] The trial was partially blinded by necessity, since those subjects randomized to compression stockings were aware of their treatment assignment, whereas subjects receiving HCSE or placebo were not (blinded component of the trial). As a result, this trial is considered to be of lesser methodologic quality, revealing the difficulty of blinding in patients using compression stockings. After 12 weeks of therapy, mean lower leg volume decreased by 53.6 mL with HCSE and by 56.6 mL with compression stocking treatment, when compared with the placebo group. HCSE and compression stocking treatments had comparable effects and were well tolerated. Compliance with compression stockings in this trial was 90%, compared with 98% compliance with HCSE. Notably, the compliance with compression stockings outside of a clinical trial has been reported to be 47%.[31] Although some authors have challenged the leg volume measurements used in this study,[41,42] the results lend support to the claim that HCSE can be beneficial in the treatment of venous insufficiency.

- Rehn et al. conducted the longest-duration randomized double-blind study of patients with CVI.[9] Subjects (n = 137) were randomized to three treatment arms: two with oxerutins and one with HCSE (100 mg of escin per day). Outcomes were assessed at 12 weeks and at 6 weeks after cessation of treatment. Patients receiving HCSE experienced a 28-mL mean decrease in leg volume at 12 weeks (compared with mean reductions of 57.9 mL and 40.2 mL in the two control groups). Although results were stated as statistically significant, p values were not reported. Oxerutins were also compared with HCSE in a small (n = 33) trial conducted by Kalbfleisch and Pfalzgraf.[35] Over an 8-week period, 50 mg of escin daily was compared with 500 mg/day of oxerutins. No statistically significant difference was found between the groups, both experiencing reductions in lower leg circumference of 0.18 to 0.20 cm. On review of these two trials,[9,35] it is not clear that either was adequately powered to assess the equivalence of the treatments. A follow-up study utilizing a power calculation in its methodology and a placebo arm might provide further support of these results.

- The remaining seven trials provide additional support, universally reporting superiority of HCSE over placebo or equivalence of HSCE to rutins. However, their results are tainted by inadequate blinding, randomization, or follow-up of dropouts. On a 5-point quality scale validated by Jadad,[43] each of the seven studies scored <4,[14,28,31-33,36,37] generally thought to correlate with lower methodologic quality (see Review of the Evidence table). These conclusions are supported by a well-designed 1998 systematic review by Pittler and Ernst,[25] which followed established standards for locating studies, rating quality, and abstracting data.

- In the future, an adequately powered equivalence trial designed to assesses long-term outcomes and safety would lend further support to this treatment for CVI.

FORMULARY: BRANDS USED IN CLINICAL TRIALS
Brands Used in Statistically Significant Trials

- Venostatin (Klinge-Pharma), Venastat Supro Caps (Pharmaton).

References

1. Yoshikawa M, Murakami T, Yamahara J, et al. Bioactive saponins and glycosides. XII. Horse chestnut. (2): Structures of escins IIIb, IV, V, and VI and isoescins Ia, Ib, and V, acylated polyhydroxyoleanene triterpene oligoglycosides, from the seeds of horse chestnut tree (*Aesculus hippocastanum* L., Hippocastanaceae). Chem Pharm Bull (Tokyo) 1998; 46(11):1764-1769.
2. Calabrese C, Preston P. Report of the results of a double-blind, randomized, single-dose trial of a topical 2% escin gel versus placebo in the acute treatment of experimentally-induced hematoma in volunteers. Planta Med 1993;59(5):394-397.
3. Jaspersen-Schib R, Theus L, Guirguis-Oeschger M, et al. [Serious plant poisonings in Switzerland 1966-1994. Case analysis from the Swiss Toxicology Information Center]. Schweiz Med Wochenschr 1996;126(25): 1085-1098.
4. Hardin J. Human Poisoning from Native and Cultivated Plants. Durham, NC, Duke University Press, 1974.
5. Williams MC, Olsen JD. Toxicity of seeds of three *Aesculus* spp to chicks and hamsters. Am J Vet Res 1984;45(3):539-542.
6. el Dessouki S. Aflatoxins in cosmetics containing substrates for aflatoxin-producing fungi. Food Chem Toxicol 1992;30(11):993-994.
7. Greeske K, Pohlmann BK. [Horse chestnut seed extract—an effective therapy principle in general practice. Drug therapy of chronic venous insufficiency]. Fortschr Med 1996;114(15):196-200.
8. Comaish JS, Kersey PJ. Contact dermatitis to extract of horse chestnut (esculin). Contact Dermatitis 1980;6(2):150-151.
9. Rehn D, Unkauf M, Klein P, et al. Comparative clinical efficacy and tolerability of oxerutins and horse chestnut extract in patients with chronic venous insufficiency. Arzneimittelforschung 1996;46(5):483-487.
10. Takegoshi K, Tohyama T, Okuda K, et al. A case of Venoplant-induced hepatic injury. Gastroenterol Jpn 1986;21(1):62-65.
11. De Smet PA, Van den Eertwegh AJ, Lesterhuis W, et al. Hepatotoxicity associated with herbal tablets. BMJ 1996;313(7049):92.
12. Klose P, Pistor K. Posttraumatisches nierenversagen bei 2 Kindern nach beta-aescin-therapie. Munch Med Wschr 1976;719-720.
13. Grasso A, Covaglia E. Two cases of suspected toxic tubulonephrosis due to escine. Gass Med Ital 1976;135:581-584.
14. Steiner M. Untersuchungen zur odemvermindernden und odemportektiven wirking vonrokastaniensamenextrakt. Phlebol Prokto 1990;19:239-242.
15. Matsuda H, Li Y, Murakami T, et al. Effects of escins Ia, Ib, IIa, and IIb from horse chestnut, the seeds of *Aesculus hippocastanum* L., on acute inflammation in animals. Biol Pharm Bull 1997;20(10):1092-1095.
16. Matsuda H, Yuhao L, Murakami T, et al. Antiinflammatory effects of escins Ia, Ib, IIa, and IIb from horse chestnut, the seeds of *Aesculus hippocastanum* L. Bioorganic Med Chem Lett 1997;7(13):1611-1616.
17. Guillaume M, Padioleau F. Veinotonic effect, vascular protection, antiinflammatory and free radical scavenging properties of horse chestnut extract. Arzneimittelforschung 1994;44(1):25-35.
18. Kreysel HW, Nissen HP, Enghofer E. A possible role of lysosomal enzymes in the pathogenesis of varicosis and the reduction in their serum activity by Venostasin. Vasa 1983;12(4):377-382.
19. Brunner F, Hoffmann C, Schuller-Petrovic S. Responsiveness of human varicose saphenous veins to vasoactive agents. Br J Clin Pharmacol. 2001; 51(3):219-224.
20. Longiave D, Omini C, Nicosia S, et al. The mode of action of aescin on isolated veins: relationship with PGF2 alpha. Pharmacol Res Commun 1978;10(2):145-152.
21. Masaki H, Sakaki S, Atsumi T, et al. Active-oxygen scavenging activity of plant extracts. Biol Pharm Bull 1995;18(1):162-166.
22. Schrader E, Schwankl W, Sieder C, et al. [Comparison of the bioavailability of beta-aescin after single oral administration of two different drug formulations containing an extract of horse-chestnut seeds]. Pharmazie 1995;50(9): 623-627.
23. Tiffany N, Ulbricht C, Bent S, et al. Horse chestnut: a multidisciplinary clinical review. J Herbal Pharmacother 2002;2(1):71-85.
24. Siebert U, Brach M, Sroczynski G, et al. Efficacy, routine effectiveness, and safety of horsechestnut seed extract in the treatment of chronic venous insufficiency. A meta-analysis of randomized controlled trials and large observational studies. Int Angiol 2002;21(4):305-315.
25. Pittler MH, Ernst E. Horse-chestnut seed extract for chronic venous insufficiency. A criteria-based systematic review. Arch Dermatol 1998; 134(11):1356-1360.
26. Pittler MH, Ernst E. Horse-chestnut seed extract for chronic venous insufficiency. Cochrane Database Syst Rev 2003;(1):CD003230.
27. Pittler MH, Ernst E. Efficacy of horse chestnut seed extract for chronic venous insufficiency: a systematic review of randomized trials [abstract]. Altern Ther Health Med 2001;7(3):108.
28. Alter H. Zur medikamentosen therapie der varikosis. Z Allg Med 1973; 49(17):1301-1304.
29. Bisler H, Pfeifer R, Kluken N, et al. [Effects of horse-chestnut seed extract on transcapillary filtration in chronic venous insufficiency]. Dtsch Med Wochenschr 1986;111(35):1321-1329.
30. Diehm C, Vollbrecht D, Amendt K, et al. Medical edema protection—

clinical benefit in patients with chronic deep vein incompetence. A placebo controlled double blind study. Vasa 1992;21(2):188-192.

31. Diehm C, Trampisch HJ, Lange S, et al. Comparison of leg compression stocking and oral horse-chestnut seed extract therapy in patients with chronic venous insufficiency. Lancet 1996;347(8997):292-294.

32. Erdlen F. Klinische wirksamkeit von Venostasin retard im Doppelblindversuch. Med Welt 1989;40:994-996.

33. Erler M. Rokastaniensamenextrakt bei der therapie peripherer venoser odeme: ein klinischer therapievergleich. Med Welt 1991;43:593-596.

34. Friederich HC, Vogelsberg H, Neiss A. [Evaluation of internally effective venous drugs]. Z Hautkr 1978;53(11):369-374.

35. Kalbfleisch W, Pfalzgraf H. Odemprotektiva: aquipotente dosierung: rokastaniensamenextrakt und O-beta- hydroxyethylrutoside im vergleich. Therapiewoche 1989;39:3703-3707.

36. Lohr E, Garanin P, Jesau P, et al. [Anti-edemic therapy in chronic venous insufficiency with tendency to formation of edema]. Munch Med Wochenschr 1986;128:579-581.

37. Neiss A, Bohm C. [Demonstration of the effectiveness of the horse-chestnut-seed extract in the varicose syndrome complex]. MMW Munch Med Wochenschr 1976;118(7):213-216.

38. Pilz E. Odeme bei venenerkrankungen. Med Welt 1990;40:1143-1144.

39. Rudofsky G, et al. Odemprotektive wirkung und klinische wirksamkeit von rokastaniensamenextrakt im doppeltblindversuch. Phleb Prokto 1986;15: 47-54.

40. Koch R. Comparative study of Venostasin(R) and Pycnogenol(R) in chronic venous insufficiency. Phytother Res 2002;16(Suppl 1):1-5.

41. Vayssairat M, Debure C, Maurel A, et al. Horse-chestnut seed extract for chronic venous insufficiency. Lancet 1996;347(9009):1182.

42. Simini B. Horse-chestnut seed extract for chronic venous insufficiency. Lancet 1996;337(9009):1182-1183.

43. Jadad AR, Moore RA, Carroll D, et al. Assessing the quality of reports of randomized clinical trials: is blinding necessary? Control Clin Trials 1996; 17(1):1-12.

H

Horsetail
(*Equisetum arvense* L.)

SYNONYMS/COMMON NAMES/RELATED SUBSTANCES

- Bottle brush, cola de caballo, common horsetail, common scouring rush, corncob plant, corn horsetail, Dutch rush, *Equisetum arvense*, field horsetail, horse willow, horsetail grass, horsetail rush, mokchok, mokuzoku, muzei (*Equisetum hymale*), paddock pipes, pewterwort, prele, pribes des champs, running clubmoss, schachtelhalm, scouring rush, shenjincao, shave grass, toadpipe, wenjing, zinnkraut.
- **Crude drugs:** Crude drugs derived from *E. arvense* include wenjing, jiejiecao, and bitoucai.
- *Note: E. arvense* should not be confused with members of the genus *Laminaria*, kelp, or brown alga, for which "horsetail" has been used as a synonym.

CLINICAL BOTTOM LINE
Background

- Horsetail (*Equisetum arvense*) has traditionally been used in Europe as an oral diuretic for the treatment of edema. The German Commission E expert panel has approved horsetail for this indication. Horsetail is also occasionally used for osteoporosis, nephrolithiasis, urinary tract inflammation, and wound healing (topical). These uses have been based largely on anecdote and clinical tradition, rather than on scientific evidence.
- There is preliminary human evidence supporting the use of horsetail as a diuretic. One poorly designed human trial found horsetail to be as effective as calcium supplements for raising bone density.
- In theory (based on mechanism of action), horsetail ingestion in large amounts may cause thiamine deficiency, hypokalemia, or nicotine toxicity. Reported adverse effects include dermatitis.

Scientific Evidence for Common/Studied Uses	Grade*
Diuresis	B
Osteoporosis	C

*Key to grades: *A*: Strong scientific evidence for this use; *B*: Good scientific evidence for this use; *C*: Unclear scientific evidence for this use; *D*: Fair scientific evidence against this use (it may not work); *F*: Strong scientific evidence against this use (it likely does not work). For a more detailed explanation of efficacy criteria, see "Natural Standard Evidence-Based Validated Grading Rationale" in the Introduction.

Historical or Theoretical Indications That Lack Sufficient Evidence

- Astringent, bladder disturbances, bleeding, brittle fingernails, cancer, cosmetic, cystic ulcers, dyspepsia, edema, enuresis, fever, frostbite, gonorrhea, gout, hair loss, hemorrhage, hematuria, hypothyroidism, kidney disease, kidney stones, leukorrhea, lower extremity edema, malaria, menorrhagia, nephrolithiasis,[1] neurodermatitis, nosebleeds, pulmonary edema, prostatitis, styptic, Reiter's syndrome, rheumatoid arthritis, thyroiditis, tuberculosis, urethritis, urinary incontinence, urinary tract infection (UTI), urinary tract inflammation, urolithiasis (urinary tract stones), vulnerary (wound healing).

Expert Opinion and Folkloric Precedent

- Horsetail has been approved for use in Germany for "post-traumatic and static edema," for "irrigation therapy" in bacterial and inflammatory diseases of the lower urinary tract, and for "renal gravel" (urolithiasis). Topical use of horsetail has also been approved as an aid to wound healing.

Safety Summary

- **Possibly safe:** The German Commission E expert panel considers horsetail to be generally safe when taken in recommended doses for short-term use by otherwise healthy individuals. There are limited safety studies in humans.
- **Possibly unsafe:** Because of theoretical risks of thiamine deficiency, hypokalemia, and nicotine toxicity, horsetail should be used cautiously by patients with preexisting thiamine deficiency, chronic alcoholism, malnutrition, renal insufficiency, or cardiac arrhythmias, and by persons who take digoxin, who smoke, or who are receiving nicotine replacement therapy, and in pregnancy and lactation (especially when taken in large doses).
- **Likely unsafe:** Poisonings in children have been reported anecdotally. Horsetail contains inorganic silica, and the powdered herb may cause toxicity similar to that from nicotine poisonings. However, no documentation of such reactions is found in the available literature.

DOSING/TOXICOLOGY
General

- Recommended doses for horsetail are based on historical practice or expert opinion; there are no available reliable human trials demonstrating safety or efficacy for any specific doses.
- In general, with natural products, the optimal doses needed to balance efficacy and safety often have not been determined. Formulations and preparation methods may vary from manufacturer to manufacturer, and from batch to batch of a specific product made by a single manufacturer. Because often the active components of a product are not known, standardization may not be possible, and the clinical effects of different brands may not be comparable.

Standardization

- Standardized products are not widely available. Standardization can be problematic, as approximately 25 species of *Equisetum* exist, and it is often difficult to differentiate between species. Adulteration of *E. arvense* L. has occurred anecdotally.
- In Europe, the silicon content in horsetail is often required to be less than 15%. Some experts assert that horsetail should be standardized to 10% silicon per dose.

Dosing: Adult (18 Years and Older)
Oral

- **Tablets/capsules:** Variable doses have been recommended by experts, beginning at 300 mg capsules three times a day as needed, up to a maximum of 6 g daily.
- **Tea:** A maximum of 6 cups of tea, containing 1.5 g of dried stem in 1 cup of hot water.
- **Tincture** (1:1 in 25% alcohol): 1 to 4 mL three times daily.

Topical

- **External wash:** Soak 10 teaspoons in cold water for 10 to 12 hours for use as a wash.

Dosing: Children (Younger Than 18 Years)

- There is insufficient evidence to recommend horsetail in children. Avoid use, as anecdotal reports have indicated poisonings in children who used horsetail stems as whistles.

Toxicology

- *Equisetum palustre* (marsh horsetail) contains a toxic alkaloid and should be avoided. Adulteration of *E. arvense* with *E. palustre* has been reported anecdotally.
- Large doses of horsetail may lead to nicotine toxicity. Symptoms may include fever, cold extremities, abnormal heart rate, ataxia, muscle weakness, and weight loss.[2]
- Horsetail possesses thiaminase-like activity, which inactivates thiamine, possibly leading to thiamine deficiency. This may progress to irreversible central nervous system (CNS) toxicity.[3]

ADVERSE EFFECTS/PRECAUTIONS/CONTRAINDICATIONS
Allergy

- Known allergy/hypersensitivity to *E. arvense* or related substances is a contraindication. Avoid horsetail in persons with known hypersensitivity to nicotine. Dermatitis has been reported in a patient taking horsetail who was known to be sensitive to nicotine.[2]

Adverse Effects

- **General:** Horsetail has been associated with few reports of adverse effects. It is more often used in Germany and Canada, where it is regarded as generally safe when taken in therapeutic doses. Currently there are limited clinical trials that assess the dosing and safety of horsetail.
- **Neurologic/CNS:** The thiaminase activity of horsetail may theoretically deplete human thiamine stores, resulting in neurologic changes, including Wernicke-Korsakoff syndrome; the neurologic damage may be irreversible.[3] Wernicke's encephalopathy is characterized by confusion, ataxia, nystagmus; and ophthalmoplegia (weakness of the lateral rectus muscle and conjugate gaze palsies), whereas Korsakoff's psychosis involves confusion, anterograde amnesia, and retrograde amnesia.
- **Dermatologic:** Dermatitis has been linked to horsetail ingestion in a rat study[4] as well as in one human case report.[2] After exposure to horsetail, a patient rapidly developed seborrheic dermatitis, which required local application of epinephrine and oral antihistamines. This patient had previously developed dermatitis after exposure to tobacco smoke. Therefore, it was believed that the cause of the seborrheic dermatitis was the nicotine found in horsetail.[2]
- **Gastrointestinal:** Abdominal distention, increased frequency of bowel movements, and nausea were noted in a trial of horsetail for nephrolithiasis. The frequency and severity among the 34 patients taking horsetail were not reported, nor were the specific doses reported.[1]
- **Renal/endocrine:** Horsetail is believed to have a weak diuretic effect via action of its constituents equisetonin and flavone glycosides and has preliminarily been demonstrated to act as a diuretic in humans.[1] Anecdotal reports from clinical practice and expert opinion suggest that potassium depletion may occur following prolonged use of horsetail. A different horsetail species (*Equisetum myriochaetum*) has reportedly caused low blood sugar levels in patients with type 2 diabetes.[5]
- **Musculoskeletal:** Muscle weakness has been shown to occur in horses and believed to be a result of horsetail-induced thiamine deficiency. Field observations discovered thiamine deficiency in three horses whose feeding had been changed to hay mixed with horsetail. These animals developed "nervousness," malcoordination, and decreased movements. When two of the horses were given thiamine 100 mg subcutaneously for 4 days, their symptoms resolved. Following these observations, a study examined a colt fed *Equisetum*-containing hay for 35 days. The colt developed malcoordination and "nervousness" and had difficulty rising. Despite administration of thiamine starting on the 35th day, the colt became progressively weaker and died on the 40th day.[3] Theoretically, potential hypokalemia caused by horsetail use could cause muscle weakness as well.

Precautions/Warnings/Contraindications

- Use cautiously in patients with cardiac arrhythmias. Because of potassium-depleting effects of horsetail, it may theoretically cause toxicity among patients with underlying cardiac arrhythmias or those taking digoxin. Studies have demonstrated that horsetail likely does not affect blood pressure when taken orally.[6]
- Avoid in patients with thiamine deficiency, malnutrition, or chronic alcohol abuse. Because of its thiaminase-like activity, horsetail may theoretically cause thiamine depletion and thereby elicit CNS toxicity. Alcoholic or malnourished patients are often thiamine deficient. Although no human case reports have been documented, animal studies have noted horsetail-induced CNS toxicity.[3]
- Avoid in patients with kidney disorders, because of the possibility of increased excretion of potassium and diuretic effect of Mexican equisetum found when given orally to mice.[7]
- Avoid use in children, because of anecdotal reports of poisonings in children who used horsetail stems as whistles.

Pregnancy and Lactation

- Not recommended, because of the lack of sufficient data. Caution should be taken during pregnancy and breast-feeding, because of theoretical effects of thiamine depletion, hypokalemia, and nicotine toxicity.

INTERACTIONS
Horsetail/Drug Interactions

- **Nicotine:** Because of the small amounts of nicotine found in horsetail, additive effects are possible when this herb is used with cigarettes or nicotine replacement therapy preparations. Theoretically this may cause nicotine toxicity, characterized by fever, cold extremities, tachycardia, ataxia, muscle weakness, and weight loss. However, there are no available case reports documenting this reaction.

- **CNS stimulants:** Nicotine, contained in horsetail, is a CNS stimulant. Concomitant use of horsetail with other CNS stimulants may produce synergistic effects.
- **Diuretics:** Horsetail is believed to have a weak diuretic effect via action of its constituents equisetonin and flavone glycosides[7] and has preliminarily been demonstrated to act as a diuretic in humans.[1] Theoretically, horsetail may thus reduce potassium levels. Use of horsetail with other diuretics may lead to hypokalemia or dehydration. However, there are no reports of horsetail-associated hypokalemia in the available literature.
- **Corticosteroids:** Use of horsetail with corticosteroids that decrease potassium may theoretically cause hypokalemia. However, there are no reports of this interaction in the available literature.
- **Digoxin, digitoxin:** Horsetail's potassium-depleting properties have been reported anecdotally. Hypokalemia is potentially dangerous in patients using cardiac glycosides, and potassium levels should be monitored in such individuals. There are no documented cases of this interaction in the available literature.
- **Alcohol (chronic use/abuse):** Chronic alcohol abusers may have thiamine deficiency. Because horsetail lowers thiamine levels, there may be an additive effect in alcoholics, leading to neurologic damage.
- **Stimulant laxatives:** Stimulant laxatives used with horsetail may increase risk of potassium depletion, although literature searches have revealed no clinical cases.
- **Hypoglycemic agents:** A different horsetail species (*E. myriochaetum*) has reportedly caused low blood sugar levels in patients with type 2 diabetes.[5] Effects of *E. arvense* are not clear.

Horsetail/Herb/Supplement Interactions

- **Herbs containing cardiac glycosides:** Horsetail theoretically may compound cardiac glycoside toxicity, as a result of the potassium-lowering properties of the herb. No reports of this interaction are found in the available literature.
- **Diuretic herbs/supplements:** Horsetail is believed to have a weak diuretic effect via action of its constituents equisetonin and flavone glycosides and has preliminarily been demonstrated to act as a diuretic in humans.[1] Theoretically, horsetail may thus reduce potassium levels. Use of horsetail with other diuretics may lead to hypokalemia or dehydration. However, there are no reports of horsetail-associated hypokalemia in the available literature.
- **CNS stimulants:** Nicotine contained in horsetail may act as a CNS stimulant. Concomitant use of horsetail with other CNS stimulants, such as ephedra, may produce additive or synergistic effects.
- **Stimulant laxative herbs:** Stimulant laxative herbs used with horsetail may increase risk of potassium depletion, although literature searches have revealed no clinical cases.
- **Hypoglycemic herbs:** A different horsetail species (*E. myriochaetum*) has reportedly caused low blood sugar levels in patients with type 2 diabetes.[5] Effects of *E. arvense* are not clear.
- **Licorice:** Licorice and horsetail both have potassium-depleting properties and theoretically may additively result in hypokalemia. There are no reports of this interaction in the available literature.

Horsetail/Food Interactions

- **Thiamine:** The silicon component of horsetail can break down thiamine, resulting in thiamine deficiency. This has been demonstrated only in animal observations.[3] Currently there are no human clinical cases documenting this interaction.

Horsetail/Lab Interactions

- **Serum potassium level:** Horsetail may possess potassium-depleting properties, resulting in hypokalemia and subsequent electrolyte abnormalities.
- **Serum creatinine, urine pH, urine uric acid:** In one human trial examining patients with a history of nephrolithiasis, an 18% to 24% statistically significant increase in diuresis was noted vs. baseline after 8 to 12 weeks, with an increase in glomerular filtration rate (GFR) of 22%.[1] Horsetail was also noted to lower urine pH. Renal excretion of uric acid increased, although urine uric acid crystal formation also increased.

MECHANISM OF ACTION
Pharmacology

- **Diuretic properties:** There is limited research regarding the mechanism of action of horsetail. Horsetail possesses weak diuretic properties, which are believed to be due to equisetonin and flavone glycosides. In one human trial examining patients with a history of nephrolithiasis, an 18% to 24% statistically significant increase in diuresis was noted vs. baseline after 8 to 12 weeks, with an increase in glomerular filtration rate (GFR) of 22%.[1] Horsetail was also noted to lower urine pH. Renal excretion of uric acid increased, although urine uric acid crystal formation also increased.
- **Steroidal properties:** Sterols contained in *E. arvense* include beta-sitosterol, campesterol, isofucosterol, and trace amounts of cholesterol.[8]
- The benzoic acid derivative hippuric acid and the quercetin derivative homovanillic acid are metabolites of *E. arvense*.[9]
- Crude drugs derived from *E. arvense* include wenjing, jiejiecao, and bitoucai.[10]

Pharmacodynamics/Kinetics

- There are insufficient available data.

HISTORY

- Use of horsetail dates to ancient Roman and Greek medicine. The name *Equisetum* is derived from *equus*, "horse," and *seta*, "bristle." Horsetail was traditionally used in Europe to treat bleeding, ulcers, wounds, inflammation, and kidney stones, and in Ayurvedic medicine for inflammation, benign prostatic hypertrophy, urinary incontinence, and enuresis in children. In traditional Chinese medicine, members of the genus *Equisetum* were used to treat bloody stools and urine, malaria, and sore throat, and the herb was applied externally to treat skin sores. During the 19th century, American physicians tried using horsetail for gonorrhea, prostatitis, and enuresis. Native Americans traditionally prepared horsetail as a urinary aid to treat dysuria, bladder incontinence, and kidney diseases.

REVIEW OF THE EVIDENCE: DISCUSSION
Diuresis
Summary

- Horsetail has traditionally been used as a diuretic. There are limited suggestive human data, supported by *in vitro* studies and theory, regarding the diuretic properties of the constituent equisetonin and flavone glycosides. It appears

Review of the Evidence: Horsetail

Condition Treated*	Study Design	Author, Year	N[†]	SS[†]	Study Quality[‡]	Magnitude of Benefit	ARR[†]	NNT[†]	Comments
Diuresis	Data extracted from equivalence trial	Tiktinskii[1] 1983	34	Yes	1	Small	NA	NA	Not randomized or blinded.
Bone density	RCT	Corletto[11] 1999	122	Yes	1	Medium	NA	NA	Randomization and blinding procedures not described.

*Primary or secondary outcome.
[†] N, Number of patients; SS, statistically significant; ARR, absolute risk reduction; NNT, the number of patients who need to undergo a specific intervention in order to observe an outcome in one individual.
[‡] 0-2 = poor; 3-4 = good; 5 = excellent.
NA, Not applicable; RCT, randomized, controlled trial.
For an explanation of each category in this table, please see Table 3 in the Introduction.

likely that horsetail does possess some diuretic properties, although further human studies comparing horsetail with known diuretics are warranted to determine magnitude of effect and safety.

Evidence

- A 1983 Russian study examined urine parameters in 34 patients taking horsetail (a subset of a larger equivalence trial of horsetail vs. Java tea in 67 patients).[1] All patients had a history of forming uric acid kidney stones. After 8 to 12 weeks, an 18% to 24% statistically significant increase in diuresis was noted vs. baseline, with an increase in GFR of 22%. Horsetail was also noted to lower urine pH. Renal excretion of uric acid increased with horsetail, although uric acid crystal formation also increased. The means of measurement of diuresis/fluid intake were not reported clearly, making results difficult to interpret. Additional studies in this area are needed.

Osteoporosis
Summary

- Animal and *in vitro* studies suggest that silicon plays a role in bone development, may increase the rate of bone mineralization, and may enhance calcium deposition in bone. It has therefore been hypothesized that horsetail, which contains silicon, may be an effective natural treatment for osteoporosis. One poorly designed human trial found horsetail to be as effective as calcium supplements for raising bone density.

Evidence

- In a 1999 Italian randomized trial, 122 women were randomized to receive placebo, no treatment, horsetail dry extract (dose not specified), or Osteosil calcium 270 mg twice daily (a horsetail/calcium combination used in Italy for osteoporosis and fractures).[11] After 40, 80, and 365 days, a statistically significant improvement in bone density was reported in both the horsetail and the Osteosil calcium groups, with an average increase of 2.3% in vertebral bone density in the latter group. This study failed to adequately describe blinding, randomization, or dropouts and cannot be considered methodologically strong. Toxicity and adverse effects were not reported. Without further demonstrations of efficacy or safety, a firm recommendation cannot be made on the use of horsetail for osteoporosis.

FORMULARY: BRANDS USED IN CLINICAL TRIALS/THIRD-PARTY TESTING
Brand(s) Used in Statistically Significant Clinical Trials

- Osteosil calcium (combination of horsetail and calcium, available in Italy).

Brand(s) Shown to Contain Claimed Ingredients through Third-Party Testing

- Goldenrod-Horsetail (Herb Pharm Compounds).

Combination Products

- Goldenrod-Horsetail (Herb Pharm Compounds) (liquid extract including 22.5% goldenrod flowering tips, 22.5% corn silk, 22.5% horsetail, 22.5% pipsissewa leaf, and 10% juniper berry).
- Horsetail has been combined with hydrangea in the treatment of prostate diseases.
- Horsetail is used in cosmetics and shampoos.

References

1. Tiktinskii OL, Bablumian IA. [Therapeutic action of Java tea and field horsetail in uric acid diathesis]. Urol Nefrol (Mosk) 1983;3(1):47-50.
2. Sudan BJ. Seborrhoeic dermatitis induced by nicotine of horsetails (*Equisetum arvense* L.). Contact Dermatitis 1985;13(3):201-202.
3. Henderson JA, Evans EV, McIntosh RA. The antithiamine action of *Equisetum*. J Am Vet Med Assoc 1952;120:375-378.
4. Maeda H, Miyamoto K, Sano T. Occurrence of dermatitis in rats fed a cholesterol diet containing field horsetail (*Equisetum arvense* L.). J Nutr Sci Vitaminol (Tokyo) 1997;43(5):553-563.
5. Revilla MC, Andrade-Cetto A, Islas S, et al. Hypoglycemic effect of *Equisetum myriochaetum* aerial parts on type 2 diabetic patients. J Ethnopharmacol 2002;81(1):117-120.
6. Gibelli C. The hemostatic action of *Equisetum*. Arch Intern Pharmacodyn 1931;41:419-429.
7. Perez Gutierrez RM, Laguna GY, Walkowski A. Diuretic activity of Mexican equisetum. J Ethnopharmacol 1985;14(2-3):269-272.
8. D'Agostino M, Dini A, Pizza C, et al. Sterols from *Equisetum arvense*. Boll Soc Ital Biol Sper 1984;60(12):2241-2245.
9. Graefe EU, Veit M. Urinary metabolites of flavonoids and hydroxycinnamic acids in humans after application of a crude extract from *Equisetum arvense*. Phytomedicine 1999;6(4):239-246.
10. Nitta A, Yoshida S, Tagaeto T. A comparative study of crude drugs in Southeast Asia. X. Crude drugs derived from *Equisetum* species. Chem Pharm Bull (Tokyo) 1977;25(5):1135-1139.
11. Corletto F. [Female climacteric osteoporosis therapy with titrated horsetail (*Equisetum arvense*) extract plus calcium (osteosil calcium): randomized double blind study]. Miner Ortoped Traumatol 1999;50:201-206.

H

Hoxsey Formula

CLINICAL BOTTOM LINE
Background

- "Hoxsey formula" is a misleading name because it is not a single formula, but rather is a therapeutic regimen consisting of an oral tonic, topical (on the skin) preparations, and supportive therapy. The tonic is individualized for cancer patients based on general condition, location of cancer, and previous history of treatment. An ingredient that usually remains constant for every patient is potassium iodide. Other ingredients are then added and may include licorice, red clover, burdock, stillingia root, berberis root, pokeroot, cascara, Aromatic USP 14, prickly ash bark, and buckthorn bark. A red paste may be used, which tends to be caustic (irritating) and contains antimony trisulfide, zinc chloride, and bloodroot. A topical yellow powder may be used, and contains arsenic sulfide, talc, sulfur, and a "yellow precipitate." A clear solution may also be administered, and contains trichloroacetic acid.

Uses Based on Scientific Evidence	Grade*
Cancer The original "Hoxsey formula" was developed in the mid-1800s, when a horse belonging to John Hoxsey was observed to recover from cancer after feeding in a field of wild plants. These plants were collected and used to create a remedy that was initially given to ill animals. Different historical accounts state various herbs included in the original formula. The formula was passed down in the Hoxsey family, and John Hoxsey's great-grandson Harry Hoxsey, an Illinois coal miner, marketed an herbal mixture for cancer and promoted himself as an herbal healer. The first Hoxsey clinic opened in the 1920s in Illinois, and Hoxsey therapy became popular for cancer in the U.S. during the 1940s and 1950s, with clinics operating in multiple states. The Hoxsey clinic in Dallas was one of the largest privately owned cancer hospitals in the world. However, after legal conflicts with the American Medical Association and U.S. Food and Drug Administration, the last U.S. clinic closed in the 1950s. The formula was passed to Mildred Nelson, a nurse in the clinic, who used the formula to open and operate a Hoxsey clinic in Tijuana, Mexico. The modern Hoxsey formula consists of a tonic taken by mouth, preparations placed on the skin, and other supportive therapies. The tonic is individualized for each patient according to cancer type and medical history. An ingredient often present is potassium iodide. Other ingredients are then added and may include licorice, red clover, burdock, stillingia root, berberis root, pokeroot, cascara, Aromatic USP 14, prickly ash bark, and buckthorn bark. A red paste may be used, which tends to be caustic (irritating), and contains antimony trisulfide, zinc chloride, and bloodroot. A topical yellow powder may be used, and contains arsenic sulfide, talc,	C

sulfur, and a "yellow precipitate." A clear solution may also be administered, and contains trichloroacetic acid. There are no well-designed human studies evaluating the safety or effectiveness of Hoxsey formula. A small number of individual human cases and case series have reported miraculous cancer cures with the treatment. However, many of the included patients did not have biopsy proven cancer, were treated with other therapies at the same time as Hoxsey formula, still had cancer after treatment, or died. Because the formula is individualized for each patient, it is not clear which ingredient(s) may be beneficial. Without further well-designed research, a firm conclusion cannot be reached.

*Key to grades: *A:* Strong scientific evidence for this use; *B:* Good scientific evidence for this use; *C:* Unclear scientific evidence for this use; *D:* Fair scientific evidence against this use (it may not work); *F:* Strong scientific evidence against this use (it likely does not work). For a more detailed explanation of efficacy criteria, see "Natural Standard Evidence-Based Validated Grading Rationale" in the Introduction.

Historical or Theoretical Indications That Lack Sufficient Evidence

Breast cancer, cervical cancer, colon cancer, elimination of toxins, improving/normalizing cell metabolism, lung cancer, lymphoma, melanoma, mouth cancer, prostate cancer, sarcomas, tumor regression.

DOSING/TOXICOLOGY

Many herbal components of the Hoxsey formula have not been thoroughly tested, and their safety and effectiveness may not be proven. Formulas are tailored for individual patients and may be made differently, with variable ingredients even within the same formula. It is important to always read product labels and discuss doses with a qualified healthcare provider before therapy is started.

Adults (18 Years and Older)

- **Cancer:** No specific doses can be recommended, based on human use or scientific study.

Children (Younger Than 18 Years)

- There is no reliable scientific evidence to support the safe or effective use of the Hoxsey formula in children.

SAFETY

The U.S. Food and Drug Administration does not strictly regulate herbs and supplements. There is no guarantee of the strength, purity, or safety of products, and effects may vary. It is important to always read product labels. People who have a medical condition, or are taking other drugs, herbs, or supplements, should consult a qualified healthcare provider before starting a new therapy. A healthcare provider should be contacted immediately about any side effects.

Allergies

- People with known allergy/hypersensitivity to burdock root, potassium iodide, licorice, red clover, stillingia root, berberis root, pokeroot, cascara, prickly ash bark, or buckthorn bark (any of which may be contained in the oral Hoxsey tonic) should avoid the use of the Hoxsey formula.

Side Effects and Warnings

- Although no serious side effects have been reported, thorough safety studies of the Hoxsey formula have not been conducted. It is not known if concentrations of the various ingredients are great enough to cause side effects that may be associated with those ingredients when used alone in therapeutic amounts.

Pregnancy and Breastfeeding

- There is no reliable scientific study of the safety of the Hoxsey formula in women who are pregnant or breastfeeding. Therefore, use cannot be recommended.

INTERACTIONS

Most herbs and supplements have not been thoroughly tested for interactions with other herbs, supplements, drugs, or foods. It is important to always read product labels. People who have a medical condition, or are taking other drugs, herbs, or supplements, should consult a qualified healthcare provider before starting a new therapy.

Interactions with Drugs

- There is no published scientific evidence of drug interactions with the Hoxsey formula. It is not known if concentrations of the various ingredients are great enough to cause interactions that may be associated with those ingredients when used alone in therapeutic amounts. The formula may include antimony trisulfide, aromatic USP 14, arsenic sulfide, berberis root, bloodroot, buckthorn bark, burdock, licorice, pokeroot, cascara, potassium iodide, prickly ash bark, red clover, stillingia root, sulfur, talc, trichloroacetic acid, and/or zinc chloride.

Interactions with Herbs and Dietary Supplements

- There is no published scientific evidence of interactions of herbs or supplements with the Hoxsey formula. It is not known if concentrations of the various ingredients are great enough to cause interactions that may be associated with those ingredients when used alone in therapeutic amounts. The formula may include administration of antimony trisulfide, Aromatic USP 14, arsenic sulfide, berberis root, bloodroot, buckthorn bark, burdock, licorice, pokeroot, cascara, potassium iodide, prickly ash bark, red clover, stillingia root, sulfur, talc, trichloroacetic acid, and/or zinc chloride.

Interactions with Foods

- According to Mildred Nelson, who founded a Hoxsey clinic in Mexico, patients on Hoxsey therapy should not consume tomatoes, alcohol, artificial sweeteners, carbonated beverages, pork, bleached flour, salt, sugar, or vinegar to avoid negating the formula's effects. There is no available scientific evidence supporting such interactions.

Selected References

Natural Standard developed the preceding evidence-based information based on a systematic review of the published literature. For comprehensive information about alternative and complementary therapies on the professional level, go to www.naturalstandard.com. Selected references are listed here.

Austin S, Baumgartner E, DeKadt S. Long term follow-up of cancer patients using Contreras, Hoxsey and Gerson therapies. J Naturopathic Med 1995; 5(1):74-76.
Gebland H. The Hoxsey treatment. Unconventional Cancer Treatments. Washington, DC: U.S. Government Printing Office, 1990:75-81.
Hartwell JL. Plants used against cancer. A survey. Lloydia 1971;34(1):103-160.
Morton JF. Medicinal plants—old and new. Bull Med Libr Assoc 1968;56(2): 161-167.

H

Kava
(*Piper methysticum* G. Forst)

SYNONYMS/COMMON NAMES/RELATED SUBSTANCES

- Ava, ava pepper, ava pepper shrub, ava root, awa, cavain, gea, gi, intoxicating long pepper, intoxicating pepper, kao, kava kava rhizome, kava root, kavain, kava kava, kavapiper, kavarod, kave-kave, kawa, kawa kawa, kawa pepper, kawapfeffer, kew, LI 150, long pepper, malohu, maluk, maori kava, meruk, milik, pepe kava, piperis methystici rhizoma, rauschpfeffer, rhizoma piperis methystici, rhizome di kava-kava, sakaua, tonga, wurzelstock, WS 1490, yagona, yangona, yaqona, yongona.

CLINICAL BOTTOM LINE
Background

- Kava beverages, made from the dried root of the shrub *Piper methysticum*, have been used ceremonially and socially in the South Pacific and Europe for hundreds of years. Currently, pharmaceutical preparations of the herb are widely used in Europe and the United States as anxiolytics but have recently been withdrawn in several European markets and Canada because of safety concerns.[1-6]
- Several well-conducted human trials and a meta-analysis[7-10] have demonstrated kava's efficacy in the treatment of anxiety, with effects observed after as few as 1 or 2 doses, and progressive improvement over 1 to 4 weeks. Preliminary evidence suggests possible equivalence to benzodiazepines. Many experts believe that kava is neither sedating nor tolerance forming in recommended doses. Some trials report occasional mild sedation, although preliminary data from small studies suggest lack of neurologic-psychological impairment.
- However, there is widespread concern regarding the potential hepatotoxicity of kava.[11-22] More than 30 cases of liver damage have been reported in Europe, including hepatitis,[23-25] cirrhosis, and fulminant liver failure,[26,27] potentially fatal,[28,29] although some authors have challenged these reports and maintain that kava is safe in most individuals at recommended doses.[30,31] This remains an area of controversy, and it is unclear if the safety profile of kava is comparable to that for other agents used in the management of anxiety.
- Kava is still available in the United States, although the U.S. Food and Drug Administration has issued warnings to consumers and physicians.[15,16,32] It is not clear what dose or duration of use is correlated with the risk of liver damage. The quality of these case reports has been variable; several are vague, describe use of products that do not actually list kava as an ingredient, or include patients who also ingest large quantities of alcohol. Nonetheless, caution is warranted.
- Chronic or heavy use of kava has also been associated with cases of neurotoxicity, pulmonary hypertension, and dermatologic changes. Most human trials have been shorter than 2 months, with the longest study being 6 months in duration.[33]

Historical or Theoretical Indications That Lack Sufficient Evidence

- Analgesia, anesthesia,[34] anorexia, anticonvulsant,[35,36] antifungal, antipsychotic,[34,37] antispasmodic, aphrodisiac, arthritis, asthma, brain damage, cancer,[38] cerebral ischemia, contraception, colds, cystitis, depression, diuretic, dizziness, dyspepsia, filariasis, gonorrhea, hemorrhoids, infections, jet lag, joint pain, kidney disorders, leprosy, menopausal symptoms (hot flashes, sleep disturbances), menstrual disorders, migraine, muscle relaxant,[39] otitis, pain, premenstrual dysphoric disorder (PMDD), premenstrual syndrome (PMS),[40] renal colic, respiratory tract infections, rheumatism, seizures, spasm, stomach upset, syphilis, toothache, tuberculosis, urinary incontinence, urinary tract disorders, uterine inflammation, vaginal prolapse, vaginitis, weight reduction, wound healing.

Expert Opinion and Folkloric Precedent

- Kava has been approved in several European countries as a prescription or over-the-counter agent for the treatment of anxiety. Oral preparations are widely recommended by European physicians and natural medicine practitioners. In the United States, before the publication of adverse hepatic effects, kava had gained popularity among clinicians, although U.S. physicians and pharmacists are more apt to recommend benzodiazepines to patients with anxiety, because of lack of government-enforced safety or manufacturing standards for kava. Self-medication with kava by patients in the United States is widespread.

Safety Summary

- **Possibly unsafe:** In recommended doses over short periods of time (<1 to 2 months), kava has historically been regarded as safe and well tolerated. However, there is widespread concern regarding the potential hepatotoxicity of kava.[11-22] More than 30 cases of liver damage have been reported, including hepatitis,[23-25] cirrhosis, and fulminant liver failure,[26,27] potentially fatal.[28,29] The U.S. Food and Drug Administration has issued warnings to consumers and physicians.[15,16,32] It is not clear what dose or duration of use is correlated with the risk of liver damage. In case reports, chronic and/or heavy use has also been associated with significant neurotoxicity, pulmonary hypertension, seizures, psychotic syndromes, and dermatologic changes.[11,26] As a result of monoamine oxidase inhibitor (MAOI)-like activity, kava may theoretically prolong the effects of anesthesia, and discontinuation should be considered prior to some surgery. Sedation has been reported anecdotally and in some trial subjects, although preliminary studies have found that kava does not impair neurologic-psychological functioning at recommended doses.
- **Likely unsafe:** Kava should be avoided in patients with liver disease.

Scientific Evidence for Common/Studied Use(s)	Grade*
Anxiety	A

*Key to grades: *A:* Strong scientific evidence for this use; *B:* Good scientific evidence for this use; *C:* Unclear scientific evidence for this use; *D:* Fair scientific evidence against this use (it may not work); *F:* Strong scientific evidence against this use (it likely does not work). For a more detailed explanation of efficacy criteria, see "Natural Standard Evidence-Based Validated Grading Rationale" in the Introduction.

DOSING/TOXICOLOGY
General

- Recommended doses are based on those most commonly used in available trials, and/or on historical practice. However, with natural products, the optimal doses needed to balance efficacy and safety often have not been determined. Formulations and preparation methods may vary from manufacturer to manufacturer, and from batch to batch of a specific product made by a single manufacturer. Because often the active components of a product are not known, standardization may not be possible, and the clinical effects of different brands may not be comparable.

Standardization

- Multiple formulations are available, including dried rhizome, cold macerate, fluid extract, dry extract, and soft native extract. Kava extract is typically standardized to 30% kava lactones. The actual lactone content of the root varies between 3% and 20%. Many brands use the standardized preparation WS 1490.
- A review of standardized kava brands in the United States found actual (measured) and labeled amounts of kava lactones to be approximately equivalent in 13 products that listed amounts of constituents (*Consumer Reports*, December 2000). Kava lactones per tablet/capsule ranged from 50 to 110 mg. Two brands that did not label amounts of constituents contained 10 to 15 mg lactones per tablet/capsule. Some tested products are listed later on in the Formulary section.

Dosing: Adults (18 Years and Older)
Oral

- Safety concerns should be carefully reviewed prior to considering therapy with this agent.
- 300 mg/day of kava extract (standardized to WS 1490) in three divided doses is a regimen reported as efficacious and well tolerated in multiple clinical trials.[9,41-43] Typical usage ranges from 70 to 280 mg of kava lactones daily as a single bedtime dose or in divided doses (60 to 120 mg of kava pyrones daily has also been recommended). Many practitioners start the patient at a lower dose and titrate up as needed. Daily doses as high as 800 mg of kava extract have been tolerated for short periods but have not been extensively studied.

Dosing: Children (Younger Than 18 Years)

- Insufficient available safety or efficacy data.

Toxicology

- There is widespread concern regarding the potential hepatotoxicity of kava.[11-22] More than 30 cases of liver damage have been reported, including hepatitis,[23-25] cirrhosis, and fulminant liver failure,[26,27] potentially fatal.[28,29] Two cases in Switzerland involved one specific brand (Leitan, Schwabe, Germany).
- Chronic heavy use of kava has been associated with case reports of renal dysfunction, hematologic abnormalities, pulmonary hypertension, dermopathy, and choreoathetosis (abnormal body movements).[44-46] These effects have been observed primarily in the context of heavy traditional/ceremonial use, and the causal relationship with kava is unclear because of multiple confounders.
- The LD_{50} for kava lactones is approximately 300 to 400 mg/kg in test animals.[47]

ADVERSE EFFECTS/PRECAUTIONS/CONTRAINDICATIONS
Allergy

- Avoid in patients with known allergy/hypersensitivity to kava or kava pyrones.
- Allergic skin reactions have been reported, including systemic/contact-type dermatitis, sebotropic reactions, and generalized erythema with papules following 2 to 3 weeks of use.[48-50]

Adverse Effects

- **General:** In recommended doses over short periods of time (<1 to 2 months), kava has traditionally been regarded as safe and well tolerated. A poorly designed drug-monitoring study of 4049 patients taking 105 mg/day of a 75% kava lactone extract for 7 weeks found side effects in 1.5% of cases, primarily gastrointestinal (GI) complaints or allergic rashes (no serologic measurements were done).[51] A 4-week study of 3029 patients given 800 mg/day of 30% kava lactone extract reported side effects in 2.3% of subjects, including GI distress, allergic rashes, and mild headache. It remains unclear to what extent clinically relevant sedation occurs at recommended doses. Severe adverse effects have been observed with chronic and/or heavy use. More than 30 cases of liver damage have been reported, including hepatitis,[23-25] cirrhosis, and fulminant liver failure,[26,27] potentially fatal.[28,29] The U.S. Food and Drug Administration has issued warnings to consumers and physicians.[15,16,32] The safety of kava use remains unclear; clinicians and patients should understand the risks involved prior to considering use of this agent.
- **Dermatologic:** Chronic use of kava in large quantities may cause dry, scaly skin or yellow skin discoloration, commonly referred to as "kava dermopathy" (called *kani* in Fiji).[45,52] This type of dermopathy appears to be reversible on discontinuation of kava. Since kava dermopathy may mimic the signs and symptoms of liver disease (also a concern with kava use), a thorough clinical assessment is warranted. Although the condition is thought to be related to impaired B vitamin uptake or assimilation, improvement has not been found after niacin supplementation.[53] Cases have been reported of systemic/contact-type dermatitis, sebotropic reactions, and generalized erythema with papules following short-term use (for 2 to 3 weeks).[48-50] Kava dermopathy is believed to result from large doses.[54]
- **Neurologic/CNS (sedation):** It remains unclear to what extent clinically relevant sedation occurs at recommended doses, and it has been theorized that kava selectively acts on limbic structures, promoting anxiolysis without clinically relevant sedation.[55] Sedation has been occasionally reported anecdotally, in case reports, and in trials, although preliminary evidence from three small human studies suggests lack of neurologic-psychological impairment.[56-58] No effect of kava on motor vehicle driving performance was found in two double-blind, placebo-controlled trials.[59,60] There have been two cases in the state of California of drivers arrested for "driving under the influence" after ingesting kava tea; neither case resulted in successful prosecution. In a case report, a 54-year-old man experienced lethargy and disorientation for several hours after taking recommended doses of kava for 3 days, in addition to alprazolam, cimetidine, and terazosin (the independent contribution of kava is unclear).[61] In one study, tracking tasks (maintaining a pointer between parallel lines) and reaction time tasks (with response by pressing correct key) were measured as indicators of cognitive

performance and physiologic function.[62] Results showed no statistically significant differences between kava and placebo. In a small double-blind, placebo-controlled comparison trial of kava and the European benzodiazepine clobazam, synthetic kavain was found to improve intellectual performance, attention, concentration, reaction time, and motor speed reaction time, whereas clobazam produced the opposite effect.[63] Similar results were seen in a small trial evaluating kava extract standardized to 30% kava lactones vs. diazepam and placebo.[57]

- **Neurologic/CNS (extrapyramidal):** Several cases of extrapyramidal side effects (central dopamine antagonism)[37] have been reported after short-term use (for 1 to 4 days), including torticollis, oculogyric crisis, and oral dyskinesias in young to middle-aged people; serious exacerbations of Parkinsonian symptoms[64,65]; and three episodes of generalized choreoathetosis (abnormal body movements) following ingestion of high-dose kava in a 27-year-old Aboriginal man.[46] Tremor and malcoordination, as well as headache, drowsiness, and fatigue, have been reported as infrequent adverse effects in clinical trials and surveys, particularly in association with large oral doses of kava.[9,44]
- **Psychiatric:** Apathy has been associated with traditional heavy kava use.[34]
- **Ocular:** Anecdotally, accommodative (ocular) disturbances have rarely been associated with continuous kava use. There is one case report of impaired accommodation and convergence, increased pupil diameter, and oculomotor disturbance following one-time use.[66] Eye irritation has been reported with heavy consumption.[53]
- **Cardiovascular:** Tachycardia and electrocardiogram (ECG) abnormalities (tall P waves) have been reported in heavy kava users.[44] It has been theorized that these P wave abnormalities reflect pulmonary hypertension, although study is lacking in this area.
- **Pulmonary/respiratory:** In one study, shortness of breath was reported in 72% of heavy Aboriginal kava users vs. 39% of nonusers. Pulmonary hypertension has been proposed as a possible etiology, based on tall P waves on the kava users' ECG tracings.[44]
- **Gastrointestinal (hepatotoxicity):** There is growing concern regarding the potential hepatotoxicity of kava.[11] More than 30 cases of liver damage have been reported, including hepatitis,[23-25] cirrhosis, and fulminant liver failure,[26,27] potentially fatal.[28,29] The U.S. Food and Drug Administration has issued warnings to consumers and physicians,[15,16,32] and has requested that U.S. physicians report cases of hepatotoxicity that may be related to kava use (telephone number: 1-800-332-1088). It is not clear what dose or duration of use is correlated with the risk of liver damage. The quality of these case reports has been variable; several are vague, describe use of products that do not actually list kava as an ingredient, or include patients who also ingest large quantities of alcohol. Nonetheless, caution is warranted. Published case reports include that of a 39-year-old woman taking kava who developed acute hepatitis with confluent necrosis.[67] The product was not analyzed for contaminants, and other causes of hepatitis were not ruled out. A 60-year-old woman required a liver transplant because of fulminant hepatic failure, attributed to kava use (via process of elimination).[27] In heavy Aboriginal kava users (mean 440 g per week), gamma-glutamyl transferase (GGT) levels have been found to be significantly increased,[44] although causality is not clear.[68] Two cases reported from

Switzerland involved one specific brand (Leitan). In November 2001, the German Federal Institute for Drugs and Medical Devices (BfArM) announced that based on 24 cases of kava-associated hepatotoxicity (resulting in 1 death and 3 transplants), it is considering regulation of available kava dosing, to allow only low, "proven-safe" doses.[1]

- **Gastrointestinal (GI discomfort):** Gastrointestinal upset has been reported as an infrequent adverse event in trials.[9,43,69]
- **Musculoskeletal:** A case of rhabdomyolysis has been reported in a 29-year-old man after self-administration of a herbal combination of ginkgo, guarana, and kava.[70] The causal role of kava in this case is unclear.
- **Renal:** There has been a single case report of rhabdomyolysis in a 29-year-old man after self-administration of a herbal combination of ginkgo, guarana, and kava.[70] It is not clear if renal failure occurred. The causal role of kava in this case is unclear.
- **Hematologic:** Chronic and heavy use has been associated with increased red blood cell volume, reduced platelet volume, reduced lymphocyte counts, and reduced serum albumin.[44,71] Hematuria has also been reported anecdotally, with unclear association to hematologic parameters.[44] Racemic kavain, present in kava preparations, has been shown to have antiplatelet effects due to cyclooxygenase inhibition and inhibition of thromboxane synthesis in animals.[72]

Precautions/Warnings/Contraindications

- Avoid long-term use (for >1 to 2 months) or doses greater than recommended (>300 mg/day), based on reports of significant hepatotoxicity, skin changes, neurotoxicity, and possible pulmonary hypertension.
- Avoid in patients with known liver disease, based on more than 30 reports of hepatotoxicity.
- Avoid driving or using heavy machinery while taking kava. Drowsiness has been reported in clinical trials, although no effect on driving motor vehicles has been found in two double-blind, placebo-controlled trials.
- Avoid concomitant use with other CNS depressants, such as alcohol or benzodiazepines, based on theoretical additive sedative effects, although it remains unclear if kava is sedating.
- Avoid concomitant use with hepatotoxic drugs, such as acetaminophen, HMG-CoA reductase inhibitors, isoniazid, and methotrexate.
- Avoid in patients with Parkinson's disease, or in patients with a history of medication-induced extrapyramidal effects, based on reports of extrapyramidal effects in people taking kava.
- Avoid in patients with chronic lung disease, based on reports of dyspnea and pulmonary hypertension after chronic heavy use.
- Use cautiously in patients with endogenous depression, because of purported sedative activity of kava resin and the pyrones dihydrokawain and dihydromethysticin.[45,73]

Pregnancy and Lactation

- Kava has not been systematically studied during pregnancy or lactation. Use is discouraged during pregnancy because of possible decreases in uterine tone, and during lactation because of the possibility of pyrone transport into milk (with unknown effects).[45]

INTERACTIONS
Kava/Drug Interactions

- **Alcohol:** Animal studies have demonstrated marked increases in alcohol's sedative-hypnotic effect when it is taken with kava.[74] However, this effect has not been confirmed in healthy human volunteers.[60]

- **Sedative drugs/CNS depressants:** Kava may potentiate CNS depressants, including barbiturates and benzodiazepines. Lethargy and disorientation were reported in a 54-year-old man taking kava in combination with alprazolam.[61] In the rat, kava does not appear to interact with benzodiazepine/gamma-aminobutyric acid (GABA) receptors.[75,76]
- **Dopamine, dopamine antagonists, dopamine agonists:** Kava has been reported to antagonize the effect of dopamine and elicit extrapyramidal effects.[37,46,64] Therefore, it may interfere with the effects of dopamine or dopamine agonists and may exacerbate the extrapyramidal effects of dopaminergic antagonists such as droperidol, haloperidol, risperidol, and metoclopramide.
- **Monoamine oxidase inhibitors (MAOIs):** The pyrone constituents of kava have been found to have weak monoamine oxidase inhibitory properties *in vitro*.[77] Therefore, there may be an additive effect when kava is used concomitantly with MAOIs, including phenelzine (Nardil) and tranylcypromine (Parnate). This effect has not been confirmed in humans.
- **Anesthetics:** Kava may prolong the sedative action of anesthetic agents via presumed MAOI-like activity. Although numerous anecdotal reports have circulated, no clinical research has confirmed this interaction.[78] Anesthesiologists may recommend that patients stop taking kava 2 to 3 weeks prior to surgery.
- **Antiplatelet agents:** Racemic kavain, present in kava preparations, has been shown to have antiplatelet effects due to cyclooxygenase inhibition and inhibition of thromboxane synthesis.[72] Effects on platelets have not been reported in humans, and clinical relevance is not clear.
- **Hepatotoxic drugs:** More than 30 cases of liver damage have been reported, including hepatitis,[23-25] cirrhosis, and fulminant liver failure,[26,27] potentially fatal.[28,29] Concomitant use with other potentially hepatotoxic drugs, including anabolic steroids, amiodarone, methotrexate, acetaminophen (Tylenol), and antifungal medications such as ketoconazole, is generally not advised.
- **Cytochrome P450 (1A2, 2C9, 2C19, 2D69, 3A4) substrates:** Preliminary evidence suggests that kava may significantly inhibit multiple cytochrome P450 enzymes.[79,80]

Kava/Herb/Supplement Interactions

- **Sedative-hypnotic herbs/supplements:** Kava has been reported occasionally to cause sedation or lethargy[9,44] and may act synergistically with benzodiazepines,[61] although animal studies have revealed no interactions with benzodiazepine/GABA receptor binding.[75,76] It is unclear to what extent kava might act additively or synergistically with other purported sedative herbs, such as calamus, calendula, California poppy, catnip, capsicum, celery, couchgrass, elecampane, ginseng (Siberian), gotu kola, German chamomile, goldenseal, hops, dogwood, kava, lemon balm, sage, sassafras, scullcap, shepherd's purse, St. John's wort, stinging nettle, valerian, wild carrot, wild lettuce, withania root, and yerba mansa.
- **Melatonin:** Theoretically, kava and melatonin taken concomitantly may have additive sedative effects.
- **Monoamine oxidase inhibitory herbs/supplements:** The pyrone constituents of kava have been found to have weak monoamine oxidase inhibitory properties *in vitro*.[77] Therefore, there is a theoretical additive or synergistic effect when kava is used concomitantly with purported monoamine oxidase inhibitory agents, including chromium, ephedra, evening primrose oil, fenugreek, *Ginkgo biloba*, hops, St. John's wort, tyrosine, valerian, yohimbe, 5-hydroxytryptophan (5-HTP), dehydroepiandrosterone (DHEA), DL-phenylalanine (DLPA), S-adenosylmethionine (SAMe), vitamin B_6, and homeopathic remedies including aurum metallicum, kali bromatum, and sepia.
- **Antiplatelet agents:** Racemic kavain, present in kava preparations, has been shown to have antiplatelet effects due to cyclooxygenase inhibition and inhibition of thromboxane synthesis.[72] Effects on platelets have not been reported in humans, and clinical relevance is not clear.
- **Valerian:** In a telephone survey, one woman reported nausea, diaphoresis, muscle cramping, weakness and elevated pulse and blood pressure after a single dose of combination St. John's wort, kava, and valerian (*Valeriana officinalis*).[81]
- **St. John's wort:** In a telephone survey, one woman reported nausea, diaphoresis, muscle cramping, weakness, and elevated pulse and blood pressure after a single dose of combination St. John's wort (*Hypericum perforatum*), kava, and valerian.[81]
- **Cytochrome P450 (1A2, 2C9, 2C19, 2D69, 3A4) substrates:** Preliminary evidence suggests that kava may significantly inhibit multiple cytochrome P450 enzymes.[79,80]

Kava/Food Interactions

- **Tyramine/tryptophan-containing foods/beverages:** Tyramine- or tryptophan-containing foods may pose a risk of hypertensive crisis if eaten by a person who is taking kava, due to the monoamine oxidase inhibitory activity of kava found *in vitro*,[77] although this interaction has not been reported in humans.

Kava/Lab Interactions

- **Serum transaminases:** Kava use has been associated with elevations of liver function test values in animals and humans.[19,20,44,71]
- **Serum bilirubin:** Chronic heavy use of kava has been paradoxically associated with decreased bilirubin.[44]
- **Serum albumin, total protein:** Chronic heavy use of kava has been associated with decreased albumin and total protein.[44] Causality is unclear, and the changes may be due to poor nutrition in chronic kava users or hepatic damage.
- **Lymphocyte count:** Chronic heavy use of kava has been associated with decreased lymphocyte counts.[44,71]
- **Red blood cell volume, platelet size:** Chronic heavy use of kava has been associated with increased red blood corpuscle volume and reduced platelet size.[44] It is not clear if poor nutrition or iron deficiency coincides with chronic kava use, thus confounding these findings.
- **Urine red blood cells:** Hematuria of unclear etiology has been reported anecdotally with kava use, although scientific data are scant.[44]

MECHANISM OF ACTION
Pharmacology

- Kava contains pyrones, lactones (methysticin, dihydromethysticin [DMH], yangonin, dihydrokawain [DHK], kawain), flavonoids, and alkaloids.[82-88]
- Pyrones have been noted for their anticonvulsive, spasmolytic, and antimycotic effects, as well as synergistic hypnotic (barbiturate), analgesic, and local anesthetic effects.[89-96] Pyrones exhibit neuroprotective[97] and "recovery-supporting" effects on neurologic deficits after cerebral infarction in animals.[98] These effects have been attributed to calcium channel agonism,[99,100] sodium channel blocking,[35,101,102] inhibition

of monoamine oxidase,[77] and inhibition of norepinephrine (noradrenaline) uptake.[103] In the rat, kava does not appear to interact with benzodiazepine/GABA receptors.[75,76]

- Kava may selectively act on limbic structures, promoting anxiolysis without sedation.[55] Neurophysiologic studies with EEG have demonstrated activity of kava similar to that of GABA agonists.[58,104]
- Interactions with glutamate,[105] dopamine,[37] norepinephrine (noradrenaline),[103] and serotonin[37,99,100] and their respective receptors may mediate the anxiolytic effect of kava. Neither high single doses nor chronic administration of kavain, from the lipophilic fraction of kava, alter dopaminergic or serotonergic tissue levels in rats.[106] Therefore, dopaminergic or serotonergic effects may reside in the water-soluble fraction of kava.[107,108]
- Kava's analgesic effect is not antagonized by naloxone,[73,109] suggesting a mechanism unrelated to opiate receptors. In an animal model, development of tolerance and dependence has not been demonstrated.[110]

Pharmacodynamics/Kinetics

- A psychophysiologic study of kavain (Klinge Pharma, Munich, Germany) found pharmacodynamic peaks at 1 to 2 hours and 8 hours, suggesting active metabolites. Peak levels occurred at 1.8 hours, with an elimination half-life of approximately 9 hours and a distribution half-life of 50 minutes.[63]
- Absorption of kava root extracts may be faster than absorption of isolated lactones.
- Metabolites and unchanged lactones of kava are excreted in human urine.[111]

HISTORY

- Kava (*Piper methysticum*) is a shrub indigenous to South Sea Pacific islands. A beverage made from the roots of *P. methysticum* has been used as a social, medicinal, and ceremonial drink since the beginning of recorded history in that region. The drink is reported to have pleasant mild psychoactive effects,[45] similar to that of alcoholic beverages in Western societies. The first descriptions of its use were brought to Europe by Captain Cook following his expeditions in the late 1700s.[96] Welcome ceremonies using kava (for local and international political and religious dignitaries) continue in Fiji to the present day.
- Recreational use of kava has spread to Aboriginal communities in Australia,[34] where it is often heavily used in combination with alcohol.[68] Local annual sales in Fiji have been reported in the range of $30 million, with exports amounting to $17 million (Associated Press, June 11, 2000). Reportedly, 350,000 prescriptions for kava are written in Germany every year. Kava has become a popular herbal supplement in the United States, with multimillion dollar sales and several books supporting its use. Pharmacologic and chemical properties of the plant have been studied since the 1960s.[90]

REVIEW OF THE EVIDENCE: DISCUSSION
Anxiety
Summary

- A majority of relevant clinical trials identified by a systematic literature review report at least moderate efficacy of kava in the treatment of anxiety. A recent meta-analysis of randomized controlled trials found a statistically significant overall reduction in anxiety symptoms due to kava (standardized

extract WS 1490, 300 mg orally daily in three equal doses). Preliminary evidence suggests that kava may be equivalent to benzodiazepines in the treatment of nonpsychotic anxiety. Kava's effects were reported to be similar to those of the prescription drug buspirone (Buspar) used for generalized anxiety disorder (GAD) in one study.[112] In the past, the German expert panel Commission E has approved kava for nervous anxiety, stress, and restlessness. Efficacy is discussed below without consideration of potential adverse effects, which should also be considered by clinicians and patients.

Systematic Review and Meta-analysis

- A systematic review and meta-analysis of controlled trials conducted by Pittler and Ernst examined the use of kava monotherapy for anxiety, initially published in 2000[9] and subsequently updated.[7,8] In the initial publication, of 14 identified studies, 7 were excluded because of duplicate reporting, concomitant benzodiazepine use, and use of kavain (an isolated lactone). Seven double-blind, placebo-controlled trials were identified and reviewed, with attention to research methodology. Three German trials with common outcome measures were selected for meta-analysis: those reported by Kinzler et al. (1991), Warnecke (1991), and Volz and Kieser (1997).[41-43] The meta-analysis included 198 patients enrolled from general outpatient practices and a gynecology practice. Only half of the subjects (from one study with 100 patients) were diagnosed by standard criteria from the American Psychiatric Association's *Diagnostic and Statistical Manual of Mental Disorders*, 3rd edition, revised (DSM-III-R). Subjects received 100 mg three times a day of kava extract WS 1490 for the duration of each trial (range, 4 to 25 weeks of treatment). When pooling data from the three studies that used a common outcome measure, the authors of the systematic review found a significant greater reduction in the mean anxiety score (Hamilton Anxiety Rating Scale [HAM-A]) in the kava group compared with the placebo group (weighted mean difference, 9.69 points; 95% confidence interval [CI], 3.54 to 15.83). Four trials, including one American trial, reported significant reduction in anxiety; however, anxiety was not consistently or clearly defined, the dose of kava varied, and the study periods ranged from two doses to 4 weeks of treatment.[96,113,114] In the update of this analysis in 2003,[7] 11 trials with a total of 645 participants met inclusion criteria. A meta-analysis of six studies using the total score on the HAM-A as a common outcome measure suggested a significant reduction in anxiety in patients receiving kava extract compared with patients receiving placebo (weighted mean difference: 5.0, 95% CI, 1.1 to 8.8; $p = 0.01$; n = 345). Adverse effects as reported in the reviewed trials were mild, transient, and infrequent.

Randomized Controlled Trials

- Kinzler et al. conducted a randomized, placebo-controlled, double-blind trial comprising 58 adult patients who received kava for 4 weeks.[41] Inclusion was based on a patient history questionnaire and a baseline HAM-A score ≥19, with exclusions including psychotropic medications that would interfere with efficacy, psychosis, major depression, medical illness, and dementia. Placebo was compared with 300 mg/day WS 1490 (Laitan) kava extract. Outcome measures were HAM-A score, Clinical Global Impression scale (CGI) score, and self-assessment. HAM-A score in the kava group was significantly decreased compared with that in the placebo group at week 1 (mean score 16.2 vs. 21.8, respectively) and week

Review of the Evidence: Kava

Condition Treated*	Study Design	Author, Year	N[†]	SS[†]	Study Quality[‡]	Magnitude of Benefit	ARR[†]	NNT[†]	Comments
Anxiety	Systematic review, meta-analysis	Pittler[7-9] 2000, 2002, 2003	11 trials	Yes	NA	Large	NA	NA	Pooled results reflect a significant reduction in mean anxiety scores (HAM-A).
Anxiety	RCT, double-blind	Malsch[115] 2001	40	Yes	5	Large	NA	NA	Well-conducted trial using WS 1490, up to 300 mg/day while tapering benzodiazepines.
Anxiety	RCT	Lehmann[114] 1996	58	Yes	5	Large	NA	NA	Well-conducted trial using WS 1490, 90 mg three times daily; validated scales used.
Anxiety	RCT	Kinzler[41] 1991	58	Yes	5	Large	NA	NA	Well-conducted trial using WS 1490, 300 mg/day; validated scales used.
Anxiety	RCT	Warnecke[42] 1991	40	Yes	5	Large	NA	NA	Well-conducted trial using WS 1490, 300 mg/day; validated scales used.
Anxiety	RCT	Singh[96] 1997	60	Yes	4	Large	NA	NA	Efficacy demonstrated for nonclinical anxiety.
Anxiety	Equivalence trial	Woelk[120] 1993	172	No	4	NA	NA	NA	WS 1490 300 mg/day found equivalent to two benzodiazepines. No placebo. No power calculation; sample size may be inadequate.
Anxiety	RCT	Volz[43] 1997	108	Yes	3	Medium	NA	NA	WS 1490 300 mg/day; validated scales used; poor description of methodology.
Anxiety (preoperative)	RCT	Bhate[113] 1989	60	Yes	3	Large	NA	NA	60 mg kava extract given prior to surgery. Unequal gender ratio in treatment arms. Unclear measurement scales.
Anxiety: postmenopausal	RCT	De Leo[33,125] 2000, 2001	40	Yes	3	Medium	NA	NA	Benefit for postmenopausal anxiety when kava 100 mg/day was combined with HRT.
Anxiety: perimenopausal	RCT, open study	Cagnacci[116] 2003	68	Yes	2	Medium	NA	NA	Calcium vs. calcium plus kava 100 mg vs. calcium plus kava 200 mg.
Anxiety	RCT	Lehmann[117] 1989	52	Yes	3	Medium	NA	NA	Kavain 400 mg/day in 2 divided doses; poorly described methodology.
Anxiety	Equivalence trial	Lindenberg[119] 1990	38	No	2	None	NA	NA	Comparison with oxazepam, no placebo. No power calculation; sample size may be inadequate.
Anxiety	Case series	Scherer[69] 1998	42	NA	NA	NA	NA	NA	100 mg kava extract/day over ~50 days decreased anxiety (observational study).
Generalized anxiety disorder	RCT, double-blind, multi-center comparison trial	Boerner[112] 2003	129	NA	5	NA	NA	NA	No difference observed between kava, buspirone, and opipramol after 8 weeks, although sample size may not be adequate to discern true differences. No placebo arm.
Generalized anxiety disorder	Randomized, placebo-controlled, double-blind trial	Connor[121] 2002	37	No	4	None	NA	NA	No differences in HAM-A score after 4 weeks, although sample size may not be adequate to discern true differences.
Generalized anxiety disorder	Randomized, placebo-controlled, double-blind trial	Gastpar[122] 2002	141	No	4	None	NA	NA	No differences in primary outcomes observed, although post hoc analysis revealed trends toward benefits of kava.
Anxiety disorder (associated sleep disturbances)	Randomized, placebo-controlled, double-blind trial	Lehrl[123] 2004	61	Yes	4	Small	NA	NA	Kava extract WS 1490 superior to placebo for improvement of sleep measures and HAM-A score.

*Primary or secondary outcome.
[†]N, Number of patients; SS, statistically significant; ARR, absolute risk reduction; NNT, the number of patients who need to undergo a specific intervention in order to observe an outcome in one individual.
[‡]0-2 = poor; 3-4 = good; 5 = excellent.
HAM-A, Hamilton Anxiety Rating Scale; HRT, hormone replacement therapy; NA, not applicable; RCT, randomized, controlled trial.
For an explanation of each category in this table, please see Table 3 in the Introduction.

K

4 (mean score 12.6 vs. 21.0); this difference was significant throughout the study ($p < 0.01$). Although small, this trial was well designed.

- A high-quality trial by Warnecke included 40 female adult patients from a gynecology practice with menopausal-related anxiety syndrome and baseline HAM-A score ≥19.[42] Patients were randomly assigned to placebo or 300 mg/day WS 1490 kava extract for 8 weeks. The HAM-A score decreased an average of 25 points from baseline (mean score 31) in the kava group, compared with a 7.7 point reduction in the placebo group, with statistical significance. The author also reported overall improvements in mood and decrease in menopausal symptoms as secondary outcomes.

- In the largest and longest trial included in the Pittler meta-analysis, 108 patients were randomized to receive WS 1490 kava extract (300 mg in three equal daily doses, corresponding to 210 mg of kava lactones per day) or placebo.[43] Patients were recruited from general outpatient clinics across 10 centers. The heterogeneous sample included patients with DSM-III-R agoraphobia, specific phobia, social phobia, generalized anxiety, and adjustment disorder, with a baseline HAM-A score ≥19. Approximate mean baseline Hamilton anxiety score was 31. By intention-to-treat analysis, Hamilton anxiety rating total scores in the kava group were significantly lower than in the placebo group from week 8 ($p = 0.02$) through week 24, at which time mean HAM-A score was 9.7 in the kava group, compared with 15.2 in the placebo group ($p < 0.001$). This well-designed trial provides strong evidence for the efficacy of kava.

- Bhate et al. evaluated the efficacy of kava as an oral pre-operative medication in 60 patients undergoing hernioplasty, varicose vein stripping, or vaginal hysterectomy.[113] Patients were randomly allocated to receive either kava (60 mg of kava extract the night before and 1 hour preoperatively) or placebo. Anxiety levels were determined by "psychostatus" and a subjective anxiety scale (no descriptions given for these instruments). Following kava administration, anxiety levels were found to be significantly lower, and preoperative sleep quality significantly better, in patients who received kava than in those given placebo. Subjects given kava required less frequent additional anxiolytic medication than those given placebo (7 vs. 14). In the kava group, heart rates remained unchanged postoperatively, whereas in the placebo group, the average heart rate rose to 100 beats/minute postoperatively from 70 beats/minute preoperatively. These findings support the anxiolytic potential of kava in acute settings. Baseline characteristics revealed a significantly greater percentage of women in the placebo (44%) compared with the kava (38%) group, a difference the authors did not adjust for in their analysis. In addition, blinding and randomization procedures were not clearly described.

- Lehmann et al. examined the efficacy of kava in the treatment of anxiety.[114] Fifty-eight outpatients with anxiety, defined by a HAM-A score >19, were randomized in a double-blind fashion to receive kava (WS 1490, 90 mg orally in three equal doses) or placebo. The study duration was 4 weeks. The HAM-A score was the primary outcome measure. Secondary outcome measures included HAM-A subscales, Adjectives Check List (EWL), and Clinical Global Impression scale (CGI). After 1 week of treatment, the mean HAM-A scores were significantly lower in the kava group than in the placebo group (16.2 vs. 21.8; $p = 0.004$). The difference became more pronounced at 4 weeks (study end), with a difference in mean score between groups of 8.4 ($p = 0.004$).

Consistent changes were observed in all secondary outcomes. Singh et al. found similar results in a 60-patient cohort using a comparable design.[96]

- Malsch and Kieser conducted a randomized, placebo-controlled trial comprising 40 patients with anxiety disorder.[115] Subjects received increasing amounts of kava (WS 1490, up to 300 mg/day) as benzodiazepine medications were tapered and discontinued within 2 weeks. In the kava group, anxiety scores (HAM-A) and subjective well-being progressively improved from the first to the fifth week of treatment, whereas no changes were seen in the placebo group. This well-conducted (albeit small) trial supports the efficacy of kava for the treatment of nonpsychotic anxiety, as a potential substitute for benzodiazepines.

- As an expansion of earlier examinations of anxiety in female gynecologic patients, De Leo et al. completed a placebo-controlled trial of kava and hormone replacement therapy (HRT) for "postmenopausal anxiety."[33] Forty women were randomly assigned to HRT plus 100 mg kava or HRT plus placebo for 6 months. HAM-A scores were significantly reduced in all groups, with significantly greater reduction in those patients who received kava plus HRT compared with HRT plus placebo.

- Cagnacci et al. conducted a 3-month randomized, controlled open study in perimenopausal women who received either calcium supplements plus kava 100 mg/day, calcium plus kava 200 mg/day, or calcium alone.[116] Outcomes included anxiety as evaluated by the State Trait Anxiety Inventory (STAI), depression by the Zung scale (SDS), and climacteric symptoms by the Greene scale. Evaluations were performed at baseline and after 1 and 3 months. The authors reported a nonsignificant decline in the control group for anxiety, depression, and climacteric symptoms. Significant improvements over baseline were observed in the kava group for anxiety at 1 and 3 months, depression at 3 months ($p < 0.002$), and climacteric symptoms at 1 and 3 months ($p < 0.0006$). However, when groups were compared, only anxiety levels were significantly superior in the kava group compared with control ($p < 0.009$).

- Lehmann et al. conducted a trial using the kava preparation kavain (400 mg orally in two equal doses daily) instead of WS 1490.[117] Fifty-two patients with symptoms of anxiety disorder significantly improved, compared with those receiving placebo, after 4 weeks. However, description of randomization and blinding were limited, thus reducing the usefulness of this study.

- In a lesser-quality study, Scherer examined the effects of a lower dose of kava in anxiety disorder.[69] Forty-two patients with anxiety disorder were enrolled and treated for an average of 50 days with kava extract (100 mg daily in one oral dose). According to the Global Improvement Scale, 80% of patients improved following treatment. Physician-rated anxiety symptoms (tension, restlessness) markedly decreased after treatment as well. Although the results are consistent with more rigorous clinical trials, because of multiple methodologic limitations, including inadequate blinding and randomization, the results are of limited scientific value.

- In a case series, Wheatley administered kava 120 mg/day (unknown preparation/brand) to 24 patients with "stress-induced anxiety" for 6 weeks, followed by 2 weeks without therapy, and then 600 mg valerian (unknown preparation/brand) for 6 weeks.[118] Five patients (26%) dropped out during the no-therapy period. Measurements of anxiety were assessed via an instrument developed by the author

("Wheatley Stress Profile"), stated to be validated. Although statistically significant reductions in anxiety scale scores were recorded following kava administration, the lack of controls and design flaws make results difficult to interpret.

Comparative Trials

- Lindenberg and Pitule-Schodel compared kavain (Neuronika, a German product) with oxazepam in 38 patients with anxiety over 4 weeks. No statistically significant difference was found between treatments on anxiety outcome measures.[119] The value of this study is limited by its lack of randomization and placebo control. It is not clear that this study was adequately powered to detect differences between groups (lack of power calculation and small sample size), and results can only be considered suggestive.

- Woelk et al. conducted a larger, more methodologically rigorous trial comparing kava with oxazepam and bromazepam.[120] In this randomized, controlled trial, 172 patients with anxiety defined by the International Classification of Diseases (ICD) criteria were randomized to treatment with WS 1490 kava extract (300 mg in three equal daily doses), oxazepam 15 mg/day, or bromazepam 9 mg/day for 6 weeks. All three treatments were similarly effective in lowering anxiety (measured by HAM-A score). However, there was no placebo group, and it is not clear if the sample size was adequate to measure equivalence.

- Boerner et al. conducted an 8-week randomized, controlled, double-blind, multicenter clinical trial that investigated kava formulation LI 150 in generalized anxiety disorder (GAD), as diagnosed by ICD code (ICD-10: F41.1).[112] In this investigation, 129 outpatients were administered either 400 mg of LI 150, 10 mg of buspirone, or 100 mg of opipramol daily for 8 weeks. At week 9, subjects were evaluated for symptoms of withdrawal or relapse. Primary outcome measures included HAM-A score, and secondary measures were the Boerner Anxiety Scale (BOEAS), SAS, CGI, a self-rating scale for well-being (Bf-S), a sleep questionnaire (SF-B), a quality-of-life questionnaire (AL), and global judgments by investigator and patient. In an intention-to-treat analysis, no significant differences were observed regarding all efficacy and safety measures between groups. Approximately 75% of patients were classified as responders (50% reduction in HAM-A score) in each treatment group, and approximately 60% achieved full remission. These results cannot be considered definitive owing to the lack of a placebo arm.

- Connor et al. assessed the efficacy and safety of kava in 37 adults with generalized anxiety disorder diagnosed by DSM-IV (fourth edition of the DSM) criteria in a randomized double-blind trial.[121] Subjects were assigned to receive 4 weeks of kava or a matching placebo. Measured outcomes included HAM-A, Hospital Anxiety and Depression Scale (HADS), Self Assessment of Resilience and Anxiety scale (SARA), and clinician safety evaluations. No differences were found between groups in the principal analysis, although the size of this study was likely too small to detect between-group differences.

- Gastper et al. published a randomized, placebo-controlled, double-blind multicenter trial in 141 adult outpatients with neurotic anxiety (DSM-III-R: 300.02, 300.22, 300.23, 300.29, 309.24).[122] Subjects were assigned to receive either kava extract WS 1490 150 mg or placebo daily for 4 weeks, followed by 2 weeks of observation. Measured outcomes included total score on the Anxiety Status Inventory (ASI),

observer rating scale. The authors reported a nonsignificant improvement in the kava group compared with baseline ($p > 0.05$). An exploratory analysis of variance suggested superiority of kava over placebo ($p < 0.01$; two-sided), although these results can only be considered suggestive. Significant advantages were observed for kava in secondary outcomes, including improved scores on a structured well-being self-rating scale (Bf-S) and the Clinical Global Impression scale (CGI). However, the Erlangen Anxiety, Tension and Aggression Scale (EAAS) and the Brief Test of Personality Structure (KEPS) demonstrated only minimal differences.

- Lehrl published a randomized, double-blind trial of kava extract WS 1490 in 61 patients with sleep disturbances associated with anxiety, tension, and restlessness states of nonpsychotic origin.[123] Subjects received daily doses of either WS 1490 200 mg or placebo over 4 weeks. Efficacy was measured by sleep questionnaire SF-B, Hamilton Anxiety Rating Scale (HAM-A), Bf-S self-rating scale of well-being, and Clinical Global Impression (CGI) scale. The authors reported significant improvements in Sf-B subscores for "Quality of sleep" and "Recuperative effect after sleep" compared with baseline and with placebo. Kava was also significantly superior in the HAM-A psychic anxiety subscore.

- **Absence of sedation/neurologic-psychological performance:** It has been suggested that kava does not possess sedative effects at recommended therapeutic doses, which may be an advantage over benzodiazepines or other sedating anxiolytics. There is preliminary evidence from small, methodologically flawed human studies in support of this assertion, with a suggestion of possible improved psychological-neurologic performance from kava.[56-58,124] However, larger, well-designed trials specifically examining this question are warranted. Munte et al. compared the effects of kava extract and oxazepam on behavior and brain event–related potentials during a memory task.[56] Twelve healthy subjects were given either WS 1490 (600 mg/day for 5 days) or oxazepam (15 mg on the day before testing, then 75 mg on the morning of testing) in this double-blind crossover study. The authors found a significant decrease in the speed and quality of responses under oxazepam as compared with placebo, but no negative effect from kava. There was a suggestion of "enhanced memory performance" in the kava group, although this was not the primary outcome. Notably, the dose of oxazepam given was somewhat higher than the recommended starting dose (10 to 30 mg three times a day), which may have accounted for the degree of sedation in that group. Gessner and Cnota[57] performed a double-blind randomized crossover trial in 12 healthy volunteers given single doses of kava extract (Antares 120), benzodiazepine (10 mg of diazepam) or placebo. Electroencephalographic (EEG) testing demonstrated improvements in reaction time in those subjects given kava compared with reaction times with placebo and diazepam. These results suggest possible improvement of neurologic-psychological function by kava. In a single-blind study of six healthy volunteers given 300 to 600 mg of kava extract for 1 week, improvement in attentiveness and concentration performance was found, as well as lack of restriction on short-term memory.[58]

BRANDS USED IN CLINICAL TRIALS/THIRD-PARTY TESTING
Brands Used in Clinical Trials

- Kavatrol, Laitan, Neuronica, WS 1490 (standardized preparation, available in multiple brands).

Brands Shown to Contain Claimed Ingredients through Third-Party Testing

- **Consumer Reports (December 2000):** Botanic Choice Kava Kava; CVS Herbal Supplement Kava Kava Standardized Herbal Extract; Enzymatic Therapy Kava-30; GNC Herbal Plus Standardized Kava Kava Root; Natrol Kavatrol Standardized Potency Kava Extract; Nature's Bounty Herbal Harvest Kava Kava; Nature's Herbs Power-Herbs Kava Kava-Power Standardized Extract; Nature's Resource Premium Herb Kava Kava Standardized Extract; Nature's Way Standardized Kava Extract Max 55% Potency; Puritan's Pride Kava Kava 250 mg Standardized Herbal Extract; Solaray Kava Kava Two Daily; Spring Valley Kava Kava Root; Sundown Herbals Kava Kava Xtra Advanced Formula; Vitamin Shoppe Kava Kava Extract; Your Life Kava Kava Standardized Herbal Extract.

References

1. Stafford N. Germany may ban kava kava herbal supplement. Reuter's News Service Germany (November 19, 2001).
2. Mills E, Singh R, Ross C, et al. Sale of kava extract in some health food stores. CMAJ 2003;169(11):1158-1159.
3. Schulze J, Raasch W, Siegers CP. Toxicity of kava pyrones, drug safety and precautions—a case study. Phytomedicine 2003;10(Suppl 4):68-73.
4. Anonymous. Kava: first suspended, now prohibited. Prescrire Int 2003;12(66):142.
5. Ernst E. [Recall of the herbal anxiolytic kava. Underestimation of its value or overestimation of its risks?]. MMW Fortschr Med 2002;144(41):40.
6. Boon HS, Wong AH. Kava: a test case for Canada's new approach to natural health products. CMAJ 2003;169(11):1163-1164.
7. Pittler MH, Ernst E. Kava extract for treating anxiety. Cochrane Database Syst Rev 2003;(1):CD003383.
8. Pittler MH, Ernst E. Kava extract for treating anxiety. Cochrane Database Syst Rev 2002;(2):CD003383.
9. Pittler MH, Ernst E. Efficacy of kava extract for treating anxiety: systematic review and meta-analysis. J Clin Psychopharmacol 2000;20(1):84-89.
10. Basch E, Ulbricht C, Hammerness P, et al. Kava monograph. J Herbal Pharmacother 2002;2(4):65-91.
11. Russmann S, Lauterburg BH, Helbling A. Kava hepatotoxicity. Ann Intern Med 2001;135(1):68-69.
12. Anonymous. Kava kava may cause irreversible liver damage. S Afr Med J 2002;92(12):961.
13. Anonymous. Concerns over kava have the FDA's attention. Mayo Clin Health Lett 2002;20(7):4.
14. Anonymous. Kava concerns. FDA, Botanical Council raises safety concerns. AWHONN Lifelines 2002;6(1):13-15.
15. Parkman CA. Another FDA warning: Kava supplements. Case Manager 2002;13(4):26-28.
16. Center for Food Safety and Applied Nutrition (US Food and Drug Administration). Letter to health care professionals: FDA issues consumer advisory that kava products may be associated with severe liver injury (document issued March 25, 2002), contact information for FDA Medwatch program: 1-800-332-1088.
17. De Smet PA. Safety concerns about kava not unique. Lancet 2002;360(9342):1336.
18. Anonymous. From the Centers for Disease Control and Prevention. Hepatic toxicity possibly associated with kava-containing products—United States, Germany, and Switzerland, 1999-2002. JAMA 2003; 289(1):36-37.
19. Clough AR, Bailie RS, Currie B. Liver function test abnormalities in users of aqueous kava extracts. J Toxicol Clin Toxicol 2003;41(6):821-829.
20. Russmann S, Barguil Y, Cabalion P, et al. Hepatic injury due to traditional aqueous extracts of kava root in New Caledonia. Eur J Gastroenterol Hepatol 2003;15(9):1033-1036.
21. Anonymous. Hepatic toxicity possibly associated with kava-containing products—United States, Germany, and Switzerland, 1999-2002. MMWR Morb Mortal Wkly Rep 2002;51(47):1065-1067.
22. Ernst E. Safety concerns about kava. Lancet 2002;359(9320):1865.
23. Bujanda L, Palacios A, Silvarino R, et al. [Kava-induced acute icteric hepatitis]. Gastroenterol Hepatol 2002;25(6):434-435.
24. Humberston CL, Akhtar J, Krenzelok EP. Acute hepatitis induced by kava kava. J Toxicol Clin Toxicol 2003;41(2):109-113.
25. Stickel F, Baumuller HM, Seitz K, et al. Hepatitis induced by kava (Piper methysticum rhizoma). J Hepatol 2003;39(1):62-67.
26. Escher M, Desmeules J, Giostra E, et al. Hepatitis associated with kava, a herbal remedy for anxiety. BMJ 2001;322(7279):139.
27. Kraft M, Spahn TW, Menzel J, et al. [Fulminant liver failure after administration of the herbal antidepressant kava-kava]. Dtsch Med Wochenschr 2001;126(36):970-972.
28. Thomsen M, Vitetta L, Schmidt M, et al. Fatal fulminant hepatic failure induced by a natural therapy containing kava. Med J Aust 2004;180(4):198-199.
29. Gow PJ, Connelly NJ, Hill RL, et al. Fatal fulminant hepatic failure induced by a natural therapy containing kava. Med J Aust 2003;178(9):442-443.
30. Anonymous. Relevant hepatotoxic effects of kava still need to be proven. A statement of the Society for Medicinal Plant Research. Planta Med 2003;69(11):971-972.
31. Denham A, McIntyre M, Whitehouse J. Kava—the unfolding story: report on a work-in-progress. J Altern Complement Med 2002;8(3):237-263.
32. Center for Food Safety and Applied Nutrition (US Food and Drug Administration). Kava-containing dietary supplements may be associated with severe liver injury (document issued March 25, 2002).
33. De Leo V, La Marca A, Lanzetta D, et al. [Assessment of the association of kava-kava extract and hormone replacement therapy in the treatment of postmenopause anxiety]. Minerva Ginecol 2000;52(6):263-267.
34. Cawte J. Parameters of kava used as a challenge to alcohol. Aust N Z J Psychiatry 1986;20(1):70-76.
35. Gleitz J, Friese J, Beile A, et al. Anticonvulsive action of (+/−)-kavain estimated from its properties on stimulated synaptosomes and Na+ channel receptor sites. Eur J Pharmacol 1996;315(1):89-97.
36. Schmitz D, Zhang CL, Chatterjee SS, et al. Effects of methysticin on three different models of seizure like events studied in rat hippocampal and entorhinal cortex slices. Naunyn Schmiedebergs Arch Pharmacol 1995;351(4):348-355.
37. Baum SS, Hill R, Rommelspacher H. Effect of kava extract and individual kavapyrones on neurotransmitter levels in the nucleus accumbens of rats. Prog Neuropsychopharmacol Biol Psychiatry 1998;22(7):1105-1120.
38. Steiner GG. The correlation between cancer incidence and kava consumption. Hawaii Med J 2000;59(11):420-422.
39. Singh YN. Effects of kava on neuromuscular transmission and muscle contractility. J Ethnopharmacol 1983;7(3):267-276.
40. Girman A, Lee R, Kligler B. An integrative medicine approach to premenstrual syndrome. Am J Obstet Gynecol 2003;188(5 Suppl):S56-S65.
41. Kinzler E, Kromer J, Lehmann E. [Effect of a special kava extract in patients with anxiety-, tension-, and excitation states of non-psychotic genesis. Double blind study with placebos over 4 weeks]. Arzneimittelforschung 1991;41(6):584-588.
42. Warnecke G. [Psychosomatic dysfunctions in the female climacteric. Clinical effectiveness and tolerance of kava extract WS 1490]. Fortschr Med 1991;109(4):119-122.
43. Volz HP, Kieser M. Kava-kava extract WS 1490 versus placebo in anxiety disorders—a randomized placebo-controlled 25-week outpatient trial. Pharmacopsychiatry 1997;30(1):1-5.
44. Mathews JD, Riley MD, Fejo L, et al. Effects of the heavy usage of kava on physical health: summary of a pilot survey in an aboriginal community. Med J Aust 1988;148(11):548-555.
45. Singh YN. Kava: an overview. J Ethnopharmacol 1992;37(1):13-45.
46. Spillane PK, Fisher DA, Currie BJ. Neurological manifestations of kava intoxication. Med J Aust 1997;167(3):172-173.
47. Meyer HG. Pharmakologie der wirksamen prinzipien de kawarhizoms (Piper methysticum Forst.). Arch Int Pharmacodyn Ther 1962;138:505-536.
48. Jappe U, Franke I, Reinhold D, et al. Sebotropic drug reaction resulting from kava-kava extract therapy: a new entity? J Am Acad Dermatol 1998;38(1):104-106.
49. Schmidt P, Boehncke WH. Delayed-type hypersensitivity reaction to kava-kava extract. Contact Dermatitis 2000;42(6):363-364.
50. Suss R, Lehmann P. [Hematogenous contact eczema caused by phytogenic drugs exemplified by kava root extract]. Hautarzt 1996;47(6):459-461.
51. Siegers CP, Honold E, Krall B, et al. Results of the drug monitoring L 1090 with Laitan capsules. Arztl Forsch 1992;39:7-11.
52. Norton SA, Ruze P. Kava dermopathy. J Am Acad Dermatol 1994;31(1):89-97.
53. Ruze P. Kava-induced dermopathy: a niacin deficiency? Lancet 1990;335(8703):1442-1445.
54. Keller F, Klohs M. A review of the chemistry and pharmacology of the constituents of Piper methysticum. Lloydia 1963;26:1-15.
55. Holm E, Staedt U, Heep J, et al. [The action profile of D,L-kavain. Cerebral sites and sleep-wakefulness- rhythm in animals]. Arzneimittelforschung 1991;41(7):673-683.
56. Munte TF, Heinze HJ, Matzke M, et al. Effects of oxazepam and an extract of kava roots (Piper methysticum) on event-related potentials in a word recognition task. Neuropsychobiology 1993;27(1):46-53.
57. Gessner B, Cnota P. Extract of the kava-kava rhizome in comparison with diazepam and placebo. Z Phytother 1994;15(1):30-37.
58. Johnson D, Frauendorf A, Stecker K, et al. Neurophysiological active profile and tolerance of kava extract WS 1490. A pilot study with randomized evaluation. TW Neurologie Psychiatrie 1991;5(6):349-354.
59. Herberg KW. Driving ability after intake of kava special extract WS 1490, a double-blind, placebo-controlled study with volunteers. Zeitschrift für Allgemeinmedizin 1991;13:842-846.

60. Herberg KW. [Effect of Kava-Special Extract WS 1490 combined with ethyl alcohol on safety-relevant performance parameters]. Blutalkohol 1993;30(2):96-105.

61. Almeida JC, Grimsley EW. Coma from the health food store: interaction between kava and alprazolam. Ann Intern Med 1996;125(11):940-941.

62. Prescott J, Jamieson D, Emdur N, et al. Acute effects of kava on measures of cognitive performance, physiological function and mood. Drug Alc Rev 1993;12:49-58.

63. Saletu B, Grünberger J, Linzmayer L, et al. EEG-brain mapping, psychometric and psychophysiological studies on central effects of kavain-a kava plant derivative. Hum Psychopharm 1989;4:169-190.

64. Schelosky L, Raffauf C, Jendroska K, et al. Kava and dopamine antagonism. J Neurol Neurosurg Psychiatry 1995;58(5):639-640.

65. Meseguer E, Taboada R, Sanchez V, et al. Life-threatening parkinsonism induced by kava-kava. Mov Disord 2002;17(1):195-196.

66. Garner LF, Klinger JD. Some visual effects caused by the beverage kava. J Ethnopharmacol 1985;13(3):307-311.

67. Strahl S, Ehret V, Dahm HH, et al. [Necrotizing hepatitis after taking herbal remedies]. Dtsch Med Wochenschr 1998;123(47):1410-1414.

68. Douglas W. The effects of heavy usage of kava on physical health. Med J Aust 1988;149:341-342.

69. Scherer J. Kava-kava extract in anxiety disorders: an outpatient observational study. Adv Ther 1998;15(4):261-269.

70. Donadio V, Bonsi P, Zele I, et al. Myoglobinuria after ingestion of extracts of guarana, Ginkgo biloba and kava. Neurol Sci 2000;21(2):124.

71. Clough AR, Jacups SP, Wang Z, et al. Health effects of kava use in an eastern Arnhem Land Aboriginal community. Intern Med J 2003;33(8):336-340.

72. Gleitz J, Beile A, Wilkens P, et al. Antithrombotic action of the kava pyrone (+)-kavain prepared from Piper methysticum on human platelets. Planta Med 1997;63(1):27-30.

73. Jamieson DD, Duffield PH, Cheng D, et al. Comparison of the central nervous system activity of the aqueous and lipid extract of kava (Piper methysticum). Arch Int Pharmacodyn Ther 1989;301:66-80.

74. Jamieson DD, Duffield PH. Positive interaction of ethanol and kava resin in mice. Clin Exp Pharmacol Physiol 1990;17(7):509-514.

75. Davies LP, Drew CA, Duffield P, et al. Kava pyrones and resin: studies on GABAA, GABAB and benzodiazepine binding sites in rodent brain. Pharmacol Toxicol 1992;71(2):120-126.

76. Jussofie A, Schmiz A, Hiemke C. Kavapyrone enriched extract from Piper methysticum as modulator of the GABA binding site in different regions of rat brain. Psychopharmacology (Berl) 1994;116(4):469-474.

77. Uebelhack R, Franke L, Schewe HJ. Inhibition of platelet MAO-B by kava pyrone-enriched extract from Piper methysticum Forster (kava-kava). Pharmacopsychiatry 1998;31(5):187-192.

78. Murphy JM. Preoperative considerations with herbal medicines. AORN J 1999;69(1):173-8, 180.

79. Mathews JM, Etheridge AS, Black SR. Inhibition of human cytochrome P450 activities by kava extract and kavalactones. Drug Metab Dispos 2002;30(11):1153-1157.

80. Unger M, Holzgrabe U, Jacobsen W, et al. Inhibition of cytochrome P450 3A4 by extracts and kavalactones of Piper methysticum (kava-kava). Planta Med 2002;68(12):1055-1058.

81. Beckman SE, Sommi RW, Switzer J. Consumer use of St. John's wort: a survey on effectiveness, safety, and tolerability. Pharmacotherapy 2000;20(5):568-574.

82. Duffield AM, Lidgard RO, Low GK. Analysis of the constituents of Piper methysticum by gas chromatography methane chemical ionization mass spectrometry. New constituents of kava resin. Biomed Environ Mass Spectr 1986;13:305-313.

83. Duffield AM, Lidgard RO. Analysis of kava resin by gas chromatography and electron impact and methane negative ion chemical ionization mass spectrometry. New trace constituents of kava resin. Biomed Environ Mass Spectr 1986;13:621-626.

84. Duve RN. Gas-liquid chromatographic determination of major constituents of Piper methysticum. Analyst 1981;106:160-165.

85. Klohs MW, Keller F, Williams RE, et al. A chemical and pharmacological investigation of Piper methysticum Forst. J Med Pharm Chem 1959;1(1):95-103.

86. Smith RM. Kava lactones in Piper methysticum from Fiji. Phytochemistry 1983;22:1055-1056.

87. Smith RM, Thakrar H, Arowolo A, et al. High-performance liquid chromatography of kava lactones from Piper methysticum. J Chromatography 1984;283:303-308.

88. Young RL, Hylin JW, Plucknett DL, et al. Analysis for kawa pyrones in extracts of piper methysticum. Phytochemistry 1966;5:795-798.

89. Brüggemann F, Meyer HJ. Die analgetische wirkung der Kawa-inhaltsstoffe dihydrokawain und dihydromethystin. Arzneimittelforschung 1963;13:407-409.

90. Hänsel R. Characterization and physiological activity of some Kawa constituents. Pacific Science 1968;22:293-313.

91. Kretzschmar R, Meyer HJ. [Comparative studies on the anticonvulsant activity of the pyrone compounds of Piper methysticum Forst]. Arch Int Pharmacodyn Ther 1969;177(2):261-277.

92. Kretzschmar R, Meyer HJ, Teschendorf HJ. Strychnine antagonistic potency of pyrone compounds of the kavaroot (Piper methysticum Forst). Experientia 1970;26(3):283-284.

93. Kretzschmar R, Teschendorf HJ, Ladous A, et al. On the sedative action of the kava rhizome (piper methyst.). Acta Pharmacol Toxicol 1971;29(4):26.

94. Meyer HJ. [Spasmolytic effect of dihydromethysticin, a constituent of Piper methysticum Forst]. Arch Int Pharmacodyn Ther 1965;154(2):449-467.

95. Meyer HJ, Meyer-Burg J. Hemmung des elektrokrampfes durch die kawa-pyrone dihydromethysticin und dihydrokawain. Arch Int Pharmacodyn 1964;148(1-2):97-110.

96. Singh Y, Blumenthal M. Kava: an overview. Distribution, mythology, botany, culture, chemistry and pharmacology of the South Pacific's most revered herb. HerbalGram 1997;39(Suppl 1):34-56.

97. Backhauss C, Krieglstein J. Extract of kava (Piper methysticum) and its methysticin constituents protect brain tissue against ischemic damage in rodents. Eur J Pharmacol 1992;215(2-3):265-269.

98. Kleiser B, Diepers M, Wagner N, et al. Treatment of intracerebral hematomas with kava in rats. Neurology 1998;50(4):a398.

99. Walden J, von Wegerer J, Winter U, et al. Effects of kawain and dihydromethysticin on field potential changes in the hippocampus. Prog Neuropsychopharmacol Biol Psychiatry 1997;21(4):697-706.

100. Walden J, von Wegerer J, Winter U, et al. Actions of kavain and dihydromethysticin on ipsapirone-induced field potential changes in the hippocampus. Human Psychopharm 1997;12:265-270.

101. Gleitz J, Gottner N, Ameri A, et al. Kavain inhibits non-stereospecifically veratridine-activated Na+ channels. Planta Med 1996;62:580-581.

102. Magura EI, Kopanitsa MV, Gleitz J, et al. Kava extract ingredients, (+)-methysticin and (+/-)-kavain inhibit voltage-operated Na(+)-channels in rat CA1 hippocampal neurons. Neuroscience 1997;81(2):345-351.

103. Seitz U, Schule A, Gleitz J. [3H]-monoamine uptake inhibition properties of kava pyrones. Planta Med 1997;63(6):548-549.

104. Emser W, Bartylla K. Improvement of sleep quality. Effect of kava extract WS 1490 on the sleep pattern in healthy subjects. Neurologie/Psychiatrie 1991;5(11):636-642.

105. Gleitz J, Beile A, Peters T. (+/-)-kavain inhibits the veratridine- and KCl-induced increase in intracellular Ca2+ and glutamate-release of rat cerebrocortical synaptosomes. Neuropharmacology 1996;35(2):179-186.

106. Boonen G, Ferger B, Kuschinsky K, et al. In vivo effects of the kavapyrones (+)-dihydromethysticin and (+/-)-kavain on dopamine, 3,4-dihydroxy-phenylacetic acid, serotonin and 5-hydroxyindoleacetic acid levels in striatal and cortical brain regions. Planta Med 1998;64(6):507-510.

107. Buckley JP, Furgiuele AR, O'Hara MJ. Pharmacology of kava. Ethnopharm Search Psych Drugs 1967;1:141-151.

108. Furgiuele AR, Kinnard WJ, Aceto MD, et al. Central activity of aqueous extracts of Piper methysticum (kava). J Pharm Sci 1965;54:247-252.

109. Jamieson DD, Duffield PH. The antinociceptive actions of kava components in mice. Clin Exp Pharmacol Physiol 1990;17(7):495-507.

110. Duffield PH, Jamieson D. Development of tolerance to kava in mice. Clin Exp Pharmacol Physiol 1991;18(8):571-578.

111. Duffield AM, Jamieson DD, Lidgard RO, et al. Identification of some human urinary metabolites of the intoxicating beverage kava. J Chromatogr 1989;475:273-281.

112. Boerner RJ, Sommer H, Berger W, et al. Kava-kava extract LI 150 is as effective as opipramol and buspirone in generalised anxiety disorder—an 8-week randomized, double-blind multi-centre clinical trial in 129 outpatients. Phytomedicine 2003;10(Suppl 4):38-49.

113. Bhate H, Gerster G, Gracza E. Orale Prämedikation mit Zubereitungen aus Piper methysticum bei operativen Eingriffen in Epiduralanästhesie. Erfahrungsheilkunde 1989;6:339-345.

114. Lehmann E, Kinzler E, Friedemann J. Efficacy of a special Kava extract (Piper methysticum) in patients with states of anxiety, tension and excitedness of non-mental origin—a double-blind placebo-controlled study of four weeks treatment. Phytomedicine 1996;3(2):113-119.

115. Malsch U, Kieser M. Efficacy of kava-kava in the treatment of non-psychotic anxiety, following pretreatment with benzodiazepines. Psychopharm 2001;157(3):277-283.

116. Cagnacci A, Arangino S, Renzi A, et al. Kava-kava administration reduces anxiety in perimenopausal women. Maturitas 2003;44(2):103-109.

117. Lehmann E, Klieser E, Klimke A, et al. The efficacy of Cavain in patients suffering from anxiety. Pharmacopsychiatry 1989;22(6):258-262.

118. Wheatley D. Kava and valerian in the treatment of stress-induced insomnia. Phytother Res 2001;15:549-551.

119. Lindenberg D, Pitule-Schodel H. [D,L-Kavain in comparison with oxazepam in anxiety disorders. A double-blind study of clinical effectiveness]. Fortschr Med 1990;108(2):49-53.

120. Woelk H, Kapoula O, Lehrl S, et al. [Treatment of patients suffering from anxiety—double-blind study: kava special extract versus benzodiazepines]. Z Allg Med 1993;69:271-277.

121. Connor KM, Davidson JR. A placebo-controlled study of kava kava in generalized anxiety disorder. Int Clin Psychopharmacol 2002;17(4):185-188.

122. Gastpar M, Klimm HD. Treatment of anxiety, tension and restlessness states with kava special extract WS 1490 in general practice: a randomized

placebo-controlled double-blind multicenter trial. Phytomedicine 2003; 10(8):631-639.

123. Lehrl S. Clinical efficacy of kava extract WS 1490 in sleep disturbances associated with anxiety disorders. Results of a multicenter, randomized, placebo-controlled, double-blind clinical trial. J Affect Disord 2004; 78(2):101-110.

124. Pfeiffer CC, Murphree HB, Goldstein L. Effect of kava in normal subjects and patients. Psychopharmacol Bull 1967;4(3):12.

125. De Leo V, la Marca A, Morgante G, et al. Evaluation of combining kava extract with hormone replacement therapy in the treatment of postmenopausal anxiety. Maturitas 2001 Aug 25;39(2):185-188.

Lavender
(Lavandula angustifolia Miller)

SYNONYMS/COMMON NAMES/RELATED SUBSTANCES

- Common lavender, English lavender, garden lavender, *Lavandula burnatii*, *Lavandula dentata*, *Lavandula dhofarensis*, *Lavandula latifolia*, *Lavandula officinalis* L., *Lavandula stoechas*, limonene, perillyl alcohol (POH), pink lavender, true lavender, white lavender.

CLINICAL BOTTOM LINE
Background

- Lavender is native to the Mediterranean, the Arabian peninsula, Russia, and Africa. It has been used cosmetically and medicinally throughout history. In modern times, lavender is cultivated around the world, and the fragrant oils of its flowers are used in aromatherapy, baked goods, candles, cosmetics, detergents, jellies, massage oils, perfumes, powders, shampoo, soaps, and tea. English lavender (*Lavandula angustifolia*) is the most common species of lavender used, although other species are in use, including *Lavandula burnatii*, *Lavandula dentata*, *Lavandula dhofarensis*, *Lavandula latifolia*, and *Lavandula stoechas*.
- Many people find lavender aromatherapy to be relaxing, and it has been reported to have anxiolytic effects in several small, methodologically flawed trials. Overall, the weight of the evidence suggests a small positive effect, although additional data from well-designed studies are required before the evidence can be considered strong.
- Lavender as an aromatherapy constituent is also used as a hypnotic, although there is insufficient evidence in support of this use.
- Small phase I human trials of the lavender constituent perillyl alcohol (POH) for cancer have suggested safety and tolerability (up to $1200 \, mg/m^2$ four times a day), although efficacy has not been demonstrated.

Scientific Evidence for Common/Studied Uses	Grade*
Antibiotic (topical)	C
Anxiety (aromatherapy)	C
Cancer (oral perillyl alcohol)	C
Dementia	C
Depression (mild to moderate)	C
Hypnotic/sleep (aromatherapy)	C
Perineal discomfort following childbirth (bathing)	C
Spasmolytic (oral)	C

*Key to grades: *A:* Strong scientific evidence for this use; *B:* Good scientific evidence for this use; *C:* Unclear scientific evidence for this use; *D:* Fair scientific evidence against this use (it may not work); *F:* Strong scientific evidence against this use (it likely does not work). For a more detailed explanation of efficacy criteria, see "Natural Standard Evidence-Based Validated Grading Rationale" in the Introduction.

Historical or Theoretical Uses That Lack Sufficient Evidence

- Acne, alopecia, analgesia, angioprotectant, anticolic, anticonvulsant, antidepressant, antiflatulent, antifungal, anti-inflammatory,[1] antimicrobial,[2] antioxidant,[3] antipyretic, antiseptic, anxiety, aphrodisiac, appetite stimulant, asthma, balneotherapy (for functional circulatory disorders), bronchitis, carpal tunnel syndrome, cholagogue, choleretic, chronic bronchitis, ciatrizant, circulation problems, colic, common cold, cordial, diabetes,[4] diuretic, dizziness, douche, emmenagogue, exercise recovery, fatigue, fever, gas, hair loss, hangovers, heartburn, human immunodeficiency virus (HIV) infection, hypotension, indigestion, infertility, insect repellent, insomnia,[5] lice, low blood pressure, menopause, menstrual problems, migraine, minor burns, motion sickness, muscle spasm, nausea, neuroprotection,[6] nontubercular mycobacteria (NTM),[7] pain, parasitic infection, psychosis, rheumatism, Roemheld's syndrome, rubefacient, seizures/epilepsy, snake repellent,[8] sores, sprains, tension headache, toothache, varicose veins, vomiting, wound healing.

Expert Opinion and Folkloric Precedent

- Lavender is rich in volatile oils and has been used for centuries both as a fragrance and a medicinal herb. Linen bags containing lavender flowers were commonly placed under pillows for their alleged soporific properties.
- Lavender is thought by some experts to possess antibacterial properties. Currently, lavender oil is often used as an aromatherapeutic anxiolytic and hypnotic, including in the hospital setting.[9] Infusions of lavender flowers have been used for similar indications.

Safety Summary

- **Likely safe:** When consumed in amounts commonly found in foods and beverages (lavender received GRAS (generally regarded as safe) status for food use in the United States), or when used in recommended oral/topical doses.
- **Possibly unsafe:** When used concomitantly with central nervous system (CNS) depressants, owing to potential additive effects.[10-12]

DOSING/TOXICOLOGY
General

- Recommended doses are based on those most commonly used in available trials, or on historical practice. These doses have not necessarily been shown to be effective. Anecdotal dosing regimens are based on traditional health practice patterns and/or expert opinion. With natural products, the optimal doses needed to balance efficacy and safety often have not been determined. Formulations and preparation methods may vary from manufacturer to manufacturer, and from batch to batch of a specific product made by a single manufacturer. Because often the active components of a product are not known, standardization may not be possible, and the clinical effects of different brands may not be comparable.

Standardization

- Lavender products are not standardized in the United States.
- Each species of lavender has unique chemical constituents and activity.
- The flowers are the part of the lavender plant most often used medicinally.

Dosing: Adults (18 Years and Older)
Oral

- **Tea:** 1 to 2 teaspoons of the herb taken as a tea (based on anecdote and expert opinion). The tea can be made by steeping 2 teaspoons (10 g) of leaves in 250 mL (1 cup) of boiling water for 15 minutes.
- **Oral perillyl alcohol (POH):** In preliminary (phase I) cancer trials, doses between 800 and 1200 mg/m^2 of body surface area four times a day in a 50:50 POH–soybean oil preparation were tolerated with minimal adverse effects (efficacy has not been demonstrated).[13,14]

Inhalation (Aromatherapy)

- **Aromatherapy:** 2 to 4 drops in 2 to 3 cups of boiling water; the vapors are inhaled. Aromatherapy can be administered intermittently or daily as needed (based on anecdote and expert opinion).

Topical/Infusion

- **Bath additive:** For perianal discomfort after childbirth, 6 drops of lavender oil has been studied as a bath additive (no specific brand).[15] Persons wishing to use the whole flower may add $1/4$ to $1/2$ cup of dried lavender flowers to hot bath water (based on anecdote and expert opinion).
- **Massage therapy:** 1 to 4 drops of lavender oil per tablespoon of base oil (based on anecdote and expert opinion).

Dosing: Children (Younger Than 18 Years)
- Insufficient data available.

Toxicology

- There have been rare reports of sensitization after topical use of lavender.[16,17]
- Lavender has been reported to exert "narcotic-like" effects in both animals[10,11] and humans.[5]

ADVERSE EFFECTS/PRECAUTIONS/CONTRAINDICATIONS
Allergy

- Caution should be exercised in patients with known allergy/hypersensitivity to lavender. Persons with allergy to lavender may experience mild local skin reactions after topical use of lavender oil.[16,18]

Adverse Effects

- **General:** In recommended doses, lavender is generally considered to be well tolerated, with minimal adverse effects.[9,15,19]
- **Dermatologic:** There have been case reports of mild derma-titis following the use of topical lavender oil.[20] One individual developed an itchy dermatitis on his face after using lavender oil on his pillow.[18] Patch testing subsequently confirmed a positive allergy to lavender. There have been reports of photosensitization and changes in skin pigmentation after the use of topical products containing lavender oil.[16,21]
- **Neurologic/CNS:** CNS depression has been noted with lavender aromatherapy,[5,13] including reports of significant decrements in performance of working memory and impaired reaction times.[22] Additive narcotic effects have been noted in rats when lavender is taken orally concomitantly with barbiturates or chloral hydrate.[11,23] Headache has been observed in patients taking lavender tincture, which could be due to alcohol in the formulation (lavender 1:5 in 50% alcohol, 60 drops a day for 4 weeks).[24]
- **Hematologic:** Reversible neutropenia has been noted after large oral doses of perillyl alcohol (POH), a monoterpene constituent of lavender, in patients with untreatable malignancies (on multiple chemotherapy regimens).[13]
- **Gastrointestinal:** Nausea, vomiting, and anorexia have been reported after large oral doses of lavender (>5.0 g daily),[25,26] and after large doses of the lavender constituent POH.[14]

Precautions/Warnings/Contraindications

- Avoid in patients with known allergy/hypersensitivity to lavender, based on several case reports of dermatitis in patients with lavender allergy.[18,21]
- Use cautiously in patients who are currently taking drugs that depress the CNS, because concomitant use of lavender may exacerbate sedation.[5,11,12]

Pregnancy and Lactation

- Use of lavender is not recommended during pregnancy or breastfeeding because of lack of sufficient data.
- Because of its purported properties as an emmenagogue, excessive internal use of lavender should be avoided during pregnancy. However, there is no definitive evidence in this area.

INTERACTIONS
Lavender/Drug Interactions

- **Sedating drugs:** In rats, concomitant use of lavender and pentobarbital or chloral hydrate has significantly increased sleeping time and narcotic effects.[11,23] Concurrent use with other sedative or hypnotic agents theoretically may result in additive or synergistic effects.
- **Anticoagulants, nonsteroidal anti-inflammatory drugs (NSAIDs), antiplatelet agents:** Lavender contains varying amounts of coumarins and may therefore theoretically increase the effect of anticoagulant medications.
- **Antiseizure medications:** Lavender enhances gamma-aminobutyric acid (GABA) effects and may therefore intensify the sedative effects of GABA-dependent anti-epileptics.
- **HMG-CoA reductase inhibitors, niacin, cholesterol-lowering agents** (*theoretical positive interaction*): Lavender may act in an additive fashion with cholesterol-lowering agents: Cineole, a cyclic monoterpene found in lavender, lowers cholesterol in rats via inhibition of the HMG-CoA enzyme; the lavender constituent POH has been shown to inhibit the conversion of lathesterol to cholesterol.[27,28]
- **Antidepressants:** Based on limited evidence, lavender may have additive effects when used with prescription antidepressant medications, including tricyclics such as imipramine (Tofranil).[24]

Lavender/Herb/Supplement Interactions

- **Sedating agents:** Lavender has been found to have sedative effects in animal models and acts additively with sedatives, including pentobarbital and chloral hydrate.[11,23] In theory, it may intensify the effects of other sedative agents such as kava and valerian root.

- **Anticoagulant herbs/supplements:** Lavender contains varying amounts of coumarins and may therefore theoretically increase the effect of anticoagulant medications.

Lavender/Food Interactions

- Insufficient available evidence.

Lavender/Lab Interactions

- **Low-density lipoprotein (LDL), total cholesterol, high-density lipoprotein (HDL):** Based on animal studies, oral lavender may act similarly to HMG-CoA reductase inhibitors, lowering total cholesterol/LDL while raising HDL.[27,28]

MECHANISM OF ACTION
Pharmacology

- Lavender is composed of more than 100 constituents, including linalool, perillyl alcohol (POH), linalyl acetate, camphor, limonene, tannins, triterpenes, coumarins, cineole, and flavonoids.
- Linalool has been shown to reduce motor activity in mice through a dose-related binding to glutamate, a primary excitatory neurotransmitter of the CNS, and it has been suggested that hypnotic and anticonvulsant effects of lavender may be due to the potentiation of the neurotransmitter GABA.[29]
- The mechanism of lavender's spasmolytic activity has not been fully elucidated. Gamez et al. studied the antispasmodic effect of *L. dentata* (a lavender species) *in vitro*.[30] An observed antagonism of acetylcholine-induced muscle contractions was attributed largely to cineole. Lis-Balchin et al. observed that the linalool and linalyl acetate in *L. angustifolia* oil can induce cyclic adenosine monophosphate (cAMP)-mediated relaxation of guinea pig ileum smooth muscle.[31] The authors postulated a cAMP-based mechanism for lavender's purported physiologic effects on sympathetic nervous system activity.
- Components of lavender appear to have cytotoxic properties. Fulton et al. demonstrated cell-proliferating effects of POH on smooth muscle cell cultures.[32] Both limonene and POH have been shown to inhibit tumor growth in rats by blocking initiation and by promoting apoptosis.[33-35] One *in vitro* study evaluated the effects of POH in lung carcinogenesis and described an inhibitory effect on farnesylation, a step toward activation of the oncogene K-*ras*.[36]

- The lipid-lowering effect of lavender has been attributed to the constituent cineole, a cyclic monoterpene that lowers cholesterol in rats via inhibition of the HMG-CoA enzyme.[27] The lavender constituent POH has been shown to inhibit the conversion of lathesterol to cholesterol.[28]
- Caffeic acid, a constituent of lavender, has been demonstrated to possess antioxidant effects *in vitro*.[37]

Pharmacodynamics/Kinetics

- **Topical:** Lavender oil is quickly absorbed by the skin. The constituents linalool and linalyl acetate are detectable in the blood 5 minutes after topical application, peak at 19 minutes, and largely disappear from the blood within 90 minutes.[38]
- **Oral:** The constituents limonene and POH are metabolized into perillic acid (PA) and dihydroperillic acid (DHPA). In rats fed a diet containing POH or limonene, peak levels of PA can be seen at 1 to 2.5 hours, peak levels of DHPA are noted at 2 to 3.5 hours, and half-lives for each metabolite are 1 to 2 hours.[34] POH, PA, and DHPA are detectable in subjects' urine following high oral doses of POH. Approximately 9% of the total dose can be recovered in the first 24 hours. PA is the major metabolite found, with <1% of recovered POH.
- The absorption of POH does not appear to be affected by concomitant ingestion of foods.[13,14]

HISTORY

- The name lavender is derived from the Latin *lavare,* meaning "to wash." In ancient Greece, Persia, and Rome, it was used as a perfume in baths and laundry, and as an antiseptic. Ancient Egyptians created mummification casts by soaking linen in oil of lavender containing asphalt and then wrapping the bodies with these and drying them in the sun until the casts were hard. Lavender has been renowned as a "healing agent" in India and Tibet. In Tibetan Buddhist medicine, lavender is still used to treat insanity and psychoses. Today, in Europe and the Americas, lavender is often used as an anxiolytic and sleep aid.

Review of the Evidence: Lavender

Condition Treated*	Study Design	Author, Year	N[†]	SS[†]	Study Quality[‡]	Magnitude of Benefit	ARR[†]	NNT[†]	Comments
Anxiety (during radiotherapy)	Randomized, double-blind, placebo-controlled	Graham[39] 2003	313	NA	3	None	NA	NA	Inhalation aromatherapy during radiotherapy not found beneficial for reducing anxiety.
Anxiety	Nonrandomized, controlled	Saeki[19] 2000	10	Yes	1	Small	NA	NA	Poor description of methodology; unclear blinding or randomization.
Anxiety	RCT	Dunn[9] 1995	122	Yes	1	Small	NA	NA	Initial benefit dissipated after first session.
Anxiety	Non-randomized, controlled	Motomura[40] 1999	42	Yes	0	Large	NA	NA	Small study; results unclear owing to lack of randomization.
Anxiety	Case series	Itai[41] 2000	14	Yes	NA	Large	NA	NA	No significant difference compared with odorless conditions.
Depression (mild to moderate)	RCT, double-blind	Akhondzadeh[24] 2003	45	Yes	4	Medium	NA	NA	Tincture of lavender vs. imipramine alone vs. combination. Alcohol in tincture may be confounder; 4 weeks may be too brief to assess adequately.

Continued

Review of the Evidence: Lavender—cont'd

Condition Treated*	Study Design	Author, Year	N[†]	SS[†]	Study Quality[‡]	Magnitude of Benefit	ARR[†]	NNT[†]	Comments
Hypnotic	Case series	Hardy[5] 1995	4	NA	NA	None	NA	NA	Small series using aromatherapy.
Dementia	Single-blind, placebo-controlled	Holmes[44] 2002	15	NA	3	Medium	NA	NA	Lavender oil aroma stream with modest efficacy in the treatment of agitated behavior in patients with severe dementia.
Dementia	RCT	Gray[45] 2002	13	NA	1	None	NA	NA	Aromatherapy with *Lavendula officinalis* vs. sweet orange (*Citrus aurantium*) vs. tea tree oil (*Malaleuca alternifolia*) vs. no aroma (control). No observed benefits of lavender on combative behavior, although sample size and study design likely not adequate.
Cognitive performance and mood	RCT	Moss[22] 2003	144	Yes	3	Small	NA	NA	Small improvement observed with lavender.
Perianal relief following childbirth	Double-blind, RCT	Dale[15] 1994	635	No	3	None	NA	NA	Subjective outcome measure; incomplete data; no difference found.
Tumor regression	Case series (phase I clinical trial)	Ripple[13] 1998	18	NA	1	NA	NA	NA	Uncontrolled trial using perillyl alcohol (POH).
Tumor regression	Case series (phase I clinical trial)	Ripple[14] 2000	19	NA	1	NA	NA	NA	Uncontrolled trial using POH.

*Primary or secondary outcome.
[†]*N*, Number of patients; *SS*, statistically significant; *ARR*, absolute risk reduction; *NNT*, the number of patients who need to undergo a specific intervention in order to observe an outcome in one individual.
[‡]0-2 = poor; 3-4 = good; 5 = excellent.
NA, Not applicable; *RCT*, randomized, controlled trial.
For an explanation of each category in this table, please see Table 3 in the Introduction.

REVIEW OF THE EVIDENCE: DISCUSSION
Anxiety (Aromatherapy)
Summary

• In general, the evidence supporting lavender aromatherapy as an anxiolytic is weak. There are conflicting results from methodologically flawed studies, with some showing lack of effect. However, overall, the weight of the evidence suggests a small positive effect in relieving anxiety. Further study through well-designed randomized trials would strengthen this case. However, there are inherent difficulties involved with designing blinding or placebo control for study of an olfactory therapy. These difficulties must be overcome before compelling results can be generated.

Evidence

• Graham et al. conducted a randomized, controlled trial to evaluate the effects of aromatherapy inhalation on anxiety levels during radiotherapy for cancer.[39] In this trial, 313 patients undergoing radiotherapy were randomly assigned to receive either carrier oil with fractionated oils, carrier oil only, or pure essential oils of lavender, bergamot, and cedarwood, administered by inhalation concurrently with radiation. Subjects were assessed via the Hospital Anxiety and Depression Scale (HADS) and the Somatic and Psychological Health Report (SPHERE), both at baseline and at treatment completion. The authors reported no significant differences in HADS depression or SPHERE scores between groups. HADS anxiety scores were marginally significantly lower at treatment completion in the carrier oil–only group than in either of the fragrance arms ($p = 0.04$). The authors concluded that aromatherapy—as administered in this study—is not beneficial for anxiety reduction.

• Saeki et al. attempted to demonstrate that lavender aromatherapy via footbath produced anxiolytic effects comparable to those noted with placebo.[19] This "before and after" study, which consisted of 10 subjects, concluded that a hot footbath with lavender oil is associated with small but significant changes in autonomic activity. However, the incomplete description of methodology and analysis makes results difficult to interpret.

• Dunn et al. conducted a randomized, single-blind study in 122 intensive care unit patients, allocated to receive one of three treatments: body massage with grapeseed oil, body massage with lavender oil, or undisturbed rest.[9] Psychological end points were assessed using an arbitrary 4-point scale, and physiologic end points included blood pressure, heart rate, and breaths per minute. Number of treatments ranged from one to three 30-minute sessions, 24 hours apart. All patients received at least one session; 66 patients completed three sessions. After the first session, patients who had received a massage with lavender oil had significantly less anxiety than the group who rested. This difference was not maintained in the following sessions. It is not clear to what extent the lack of double-blinding, or the high dropout rate, affected results.

- Motomura et al. conducted an experiment in which 42 students were divided into three groups: Group 1 experienced a "stressful condition"; group 2 experienced a "stressful condition" with the addition of lavender odor; group 3 experienced a "nonstressful condition." Stress was evaluated using a Japanese version of Cox and Mackay's stress/arousal adjective checklist. The experiment found that scores in the lavender group were significantly lower than in the group in which subjects were stressed and did not receive lavender therapy.[40] However, blinding and randomization were not clearly described.

- In a case series consisting of 14 female patients with chronic renal failure undergoing hemodialysis, Itai et al. evaluated the effect of lavender oil on mood using the Hamilton rating scale for depression (HAMD) and the Hamilton rating scale for Anxiety (HAMA).[41] Compared with natural smell (baseline), lavender was observed to decrease anxiety as evidenced by the HAMA scale ($p = 0.05$). Lavender did not significantly alter patients' HAMD scores from baseline. When lavender was compared with odorless conditions, the difference in HAMA and HAMD scores was minimal.

- Buckle compared therapeutic benefits of oils from two different species of lavender (L. angustifolia and L. burnatii) applied by massage to 28 hospitalized patients.[42] A semi-structured interview to collect qualitative, subjective data was conducted several days after treatment. The study reported that L. burnatii had significantly more relaxing effects than its counterpart. However, further details of statistical analysis or methodology were incomplete, thus raising questions about the results.

Depression (Mild to Moderate)
Summary

- Preliminary research suggests that lavender tincture may be helpful as an adjunct to prescription antidepressant medications. Alcohol in tinctures may confound these results and may be inadvisable in depressed patients, except in low concentrations. Additional research is necessary before a firm conclusion can be drawn.

Evidence

- Akhondzadeh et al. conducted a 4-week double-blind, randomized, controlled trial comparing tincture of lavender (Lavandula angustifolia Miller) with the tricyclic antidepressant imipramine in the treatment of mild to moderate depression.[24] Participants included 45 adult outpatients who met criteria for major depression based on the structured clinical interview for the Diagnostic and Statistical Manual of Mental Disorders, 4th edition (DSM-IV). Patients had a baseline Hamilton Rating Scale for Depression (HAMD) score of at least 18. In this single-center trial, subjects were randomly assigned to receive lavender tincture (1:5 in 50% alcohol) 60 drops/day plus a placebo tablet (Group A), imipramine 100 mg/day plus placebo drops (Group B), or imipramine 100 mg/day plus lavender tincture 60 drops/day (Group C). The authors reported that lavender tincture at this concentration was significantly less effective than imipramine in the treatment of mild to moderate depression ($p = 0.001$). In the imipramine group, an excess of anticholinergic effects such as dry mouth and urinary retention was observed, whereas headache was observed more often in the lavender tincture group. Notably, the combination

of imipramine and lavender tincture was more effective than imipramine alone ($p < 0.0001$). The authors concluded that lavender tincture may be of therapeutic benefit in the management of mild to moderate depression as an adjunct to prescription medications. However, the study was not conducted with selective serotonin reuptake inhibitors (SSRIs), which are the standard of care, and therefore it is not clear if lavender would be beneficial in conjunction with SSRIs. Furthermore, the presence of alcohol in tinctures may confound results. Therefore, additional research is necessary before a firm conclusion regarding clinical utility can be made.

- Moss et al. conducted a randomized, controlled trial to assess the effects of the essential oils of lavender (L. angustifolia) and rosemary (Rosmarinus officinalis) on cognitive performance and mood in 144 healthy volunteers.[22] Subjects were randomly assigned to receive aromatherapy with lavender, rosemary, or placebo (no odor) and were evaluated using the Cognitive Drug Research (CDR) computerized assessment battery (in a cubicle containing the aromatherapy vapor). Visual analog mood questionnaires were completed at baseline and subsequently after completion of the test battery. Participants were not informed of the genuine aims of the study until completion of testing. Analysis of performance revealed that lavender produced a significant decrement in performance of working memory, and impaired reaction times for both memory- and attention-based tasks compared with controls. By contrast, rosemary produced a significant enhancement of performance for overall quality of memory and secondary memory factors but produced an impairment of speed of memory compared with controls. With regard to mood, comparisons of the change in ratings from baseline to post-test revealed that following the completion of the cognitive assessment battery, both the control and the lavender groups were significantly less alert than the rosemary group. However, the control group was significantly less content on average than either the rosemary or the lavender group. The authors concluded that these essential oils may produce objective effects on cognitive performance, as well as subjective effects on mood. Further investigation is warranted.

Hypnotic/Sleep (Aromatherapy)
Summary

- Many experts and patients believe that lavender as an aromatherapy constituent is an effective hypnotic. Although preliminary evidence suggests some hypnotic effects of lavender, there are no randomized trials in the available literature. Without further study, the current evidence can only be considered equivocal. However, there are inherent difficulties involved with designing blinding or placebo control for study of an olfactory therapy. These difficulties must be overcome before compelling results can be generated.

Evidence

- Hardy et al. evaluated aromatherapeutic lavender as an alternative to conventional hypnotics in four geriatric patients.[5] Sleep hours were monitored during three 2-week phases. During phase I, subjects continued their current hypnotic (temazepam, promazine, clomethiazole [chlormethiazole]). Phase II involved a withdrawal and washout period. During phase III, lavender oil was introduced into the patients' sleeping quarters via an odor diffuser. The results demonstrated that hours asleep were comparable to the number of hours asleep during phase I of the trial for all four participants. However, without controls or blinding, results can only be considered preliminary.

- Diego et al. demonstrated the effects of 3-minute aromatherapy sessions using a 10% lavender oil concentration on participants' brain waves via electroencephalogram (EEG).[43] The EEG reading was recorded before, during, and after sessions. Alpha and beta activity were found to increase after the inhalation of lavender. Notably, increased frontal alpha and beta activity have been associated with increased drowsiness, which provides mechanistic supportive evidence for this purported indication.

Dementia
Summary

- Small randomized, controlled trials investigating the effects of lavender aromatherapy on agitation and behavior in patients with Alzheimer's dementia report conflicting results. Better-quality studies are necessary before a firm conclusion can be drawn.

Evidence

- To investigate the effects of aromatherapy with lavender oil in severely demented patients with agitated behavior, Homes et al. conducted a placebo self-controlled trial with blinded observer rating in a long-stay psychogeriatric ward.[44] This small study included 15 patients meeting International Classification of Diseases (ICD)-10 diagnostic criteria for severe dementia and suffering from agitated behavior defined as a minimum score of 3 points on the Pittsburgh Agitation Scale (PAS). A 2% lavender oil aromatherapy stream was administered on the ward for a 2-hour period, alternating with placebo (water) every other day for a total of 10 treatment sessions. For each subject, 10 total PAS scores were obtained (five during treatment and five during placebo). Nine patients (60%) demonstrated an improvement, five (33%) exhibited no change, and one (7%) showed a worsening of agitated behavior during aromatherapy compared with placebo. A comparison of the group median PAS scores during aromatherapy reflected an improvement in agitated behavior during aromatherapy compared with placebo, which was reported as being significant, although a one-tailed rather than two-tailed p value was calculated, leaving uncertain whether these results are truly statistically significant (median PAS scores 3; one-tailed $p = 0.016$). These results cannot be considered conclusive.
- Gray et al. conducted a randomized self-controlled trial in 13 elderly individuals living in a residential care facility.[45] All participants had histories of confusion due to dementia and were identified by staff as being consistently resistant to medication administration as indicated by vocal outbursts, physical resistance, or combativeness. Subjects were assigned to be exposed to aroma interventions during medication administration, with either (1) lavender vera (*Lavandula officinalis*); (2) sweet orange (*Citrus aurantium*); (3) tea tree oil (*Malaleuca alternifolia*); or (4) no aroma (control). All medication administrations were videotaped for later analysis. Observers were trained to record frequency and duration of resistive behaviors during medication administration in all four interventions for each subject. The authors reported that the measured reliability between observers was very high. The results suggested no statistically significant differences between aromatherapies for either resistive behavior or duration of medication administration. Because

of the small study size, lack of use of validated measurement instruments, and incomplete blinding, these results cannot be considered conclusive.

Perineal Discomfort Following Childbirth (Baths)
Summary

- There is insufficient scientific evidence regarding the use of lavender oil baths for the relief of postpartum perineal discomfort.

Evidence

- Dale and Cornwell examined the effect of lavender oil baths on perineal discomfort in 635 postpartum women in a randomized trial.[15] Subjects were divided into three groups: Group 1 added a natural lavender oil extract to baths, group 2 added a synthetic lavender oil to baths, and the third group used an unspecified control substance that had U.S. Food and Drug Administration GRAS (generally regarded as safe) status. The control was reported to be distinguishable from the other two oils by smell, and in efforts to compensate for this, patients were informed that the trial was testing "different bath additives." To evaluate discomfort, women were asked to complete visual analog scales (VAS) in a subjective questionnaire used to evaluate the degree of discomfort over the 10 days of the experiment. Data were obtained from ~60% (n = 386) of participants. Although this trial found no significant differences in perineal relief between the groups, the large dropout rate and lack of information about the control substance (which could have been active) raise doubts about the validity of results.

Spasmolytic (Oral)
Summary

- Preliminary data from animal and *in vitro* studies indicate a potential spasmolytic effect of lavender oil inhalation. However, human evidence is lacking.

Animal Data

- A variety of lavender species have demonstrated an ability to inhibit stimulated muscle contractions in the ileum and conjunctiva in animal models.[30,31,46-48]

Antibiotic (Topical)
Summary

- Preliminary data from *in vitro* studies suggest that lavender oils possess antibiotic activity. However, this has not been tested in animal or human studies, and results cannot be considered clinically relevant.

In Vitro Data

- Gabbrielli et al. demonstrated *in vitro* activity of lavender oil (*L. angustifolia* and *L. latifolia*) against various strains of nontubercular mycobacteria (NTM).[7] Nelson et al. found documented activity of 2% to 0.12% (vol/vol) lavender oils against both methicillin-resistant *Staphylococcus aureus* (MRSA) and vancomycin-resistant enterococci (VRE).[2]

Cancer (Oral)
Summary

- Preliminary data from animal studies suggest an antineoplastic effect of oral perillyl alcohol (POH) and other monoterpenes found in lavender. Studies have focused on cancers of the pancreas, breast, and intestine. Small phase I studies have been conducted in humans, with results suggesting safety and tolerability of POH (up to 1200 mg/m^2 four times/day), but efficacy has not been established.

Animal Data

- Elegbede et al. and Haag et al. demonstrated regression of primary mammary tumors in rats after supplementing diets with limonene and POH (lavender constituents).[33,34] Burke et al. documented inhibition of pancreatic adenocarcinoma growth in hamsters using a similar diet.[49] Reddy et al. found a significant chemoprotective effect of oral POH against carcinogenesis in the large and small intestines in rats.[50]

Human Evidence

- In a phase I clinical trial, Ripple et al. examined the potential of POH to suppress tumor growth in humans.[13] This study consisted of 18 patients with advanced malignancies of various origins, refractory to standard therapies. POH was formulated in gelatin capsules containing 250 mg of POH and 250 mg of soybean oil. Prior to receiving POH, as a washout, patients did not receive hormonal or immunologic therapy for 2 weeks, or chemotherapy/radiotherapy for 4 weeks. Patients were divided into three groups according to dosage: 800 mg/m^2/dose, 1600 mg/m^2/dose, or 2400 mg/m^2/dose, three times a day. Although no objective tumor responses were noted, disease stabilization was noted in several patients for up to 6 months. POH was generally well tolerated, although dose-dependent gastrointestinal side effects (nausea, early satiety) and fatigue led to withdrawal of one patient from the study.
- In a second case series, the same authors examined the effects of more frequent administration of POH at slightly lower doses.[14] Nineteen patients with various malignancies, refractory to standard treatment, received one of the following doses: 800 mg/m^2/dose, 1200 mg/m^2/dose, or 1600 mg/m^2/dose, four times a day. The maximum tolerated dose of POH given continuously four times a day was 1200 mg/m^2. Patterns of disease progression similar to those observed in the initial trial were observed at all doses. Although promising, these results must be further evaluated through controlled studies before a recommendation can be made. Nonetheless, these small studies suggest safety and tolerability of POH at doses up to 1200 mg/m^2 four times a day.

References

1. Kim HM, Cho SH. Lavender oil inhibits immediate-type allergic reaction in mice and rats. J Pharm Pharmacol 1999;51(2):221-226.
2. Nelson RR. In-vitro activities of five plant essential oils against methicillin-resistant *Staphylococcus aureus* and vancomycin-resistant *Enterococcus faecium*. J Antimicrob Chemother 1997;40(2):305-307.
3. Siurin SA. [Effects of essential oil on lipid peroxidation and lipid metabolism in patients with chronic bronchitis]. Klin Med (Mosk) 1997;75(10):43-45.
4. Gamez MJ, Zarzuelo A, Risco S, et al. Hypoglycemic activity in various species of the genus *Lavandula*. Part 2: *Lavandula dentata* and *Lavandula latifolia*. Pharmazie 1988;43(6):441-442.
5. Hardy M, Kirk-Smith MD, Stretch DD. Replacement of drug treatment for insomnia by ambient odour. Lancet 1995;346(8976):701.
6. Buyukokuroglu ME, Gepdiremen A, Hacimuftuoglu A, et al. The effects of aqueous extract of *Lavandula angustifolia* flowers in glutamate-induced neurotoxicity of cerebellar granular cell culture of rat pups. J Ethnopharmacol 2003;84(1):91-94.
7. Gabbrielli G, Loggini F, Cioni PL, et al. Activity of lavandino essential oil against non-tubercular opportunistic rapid grown mycobacteria. Pharmacol Res Commun 1988;20 Suppl 5:37-40.
8. Clark L, Shivik J. Aerosolized essential oils and individual natural product compounds as brown treesnake repellents. Pest Manag Sci 2002;58(8):775-783.
9. Dunn C, Sleep J, Collett D. Sensing an improvement: an experimental study to evaluate the use of aromatherapy, massage and periods of rest in an intensive care unit. J Adv Nurs 1995;21(1):34-40.
10. Buchbauer G, Jirovetz L, Jager W, et al. Aromatherapy: evidence for sedative
11. Guillemain J, Rousseau A, Delaveau P. [Neurodepressive effects of the essential oil of Lavandula angustifolia Mill]. Ann Pharm Fr 1989;47(6):337-343.
12. Wolfe N. Can aromatherapy oils promote sleep in severely demented patients? Int J Geriatr Psychiatry 1996;11:926-927.
13. Ripple GH, Gould MN, Stewart JA, et al. Phase I clinical trial of perillyl alcohol administered daily. Clin Cancer Res 1998;4(5):1159-1164.
14. Ripple GH, Gould MN, Arzoomanian RZ, et al. Phase I clinical and pharmacokinetic study of perillyl alcohol administered four times a day. Clin Cancer Res 2000;6(2):390-396.
15. Dale A, Cornwell S. The role of lavender oil in relieving perineal discomfort following childbirth: a blind randomized clinical trial. J Adv Nurs 1994;19(1):89-96.
16. Brandao FM. Occupational allergy to lavender oil. Contact Dermatitis 1986;15(4):249-250.
17. Schaller M, Korting HC. Allergic airborne contact dermatitis from essential oils used in aromatherapy. Clin Exp Dermatol 1995;20(2):143-145.
18. Coulson IH, Khan AS. Facial 'pillow' dermatitis due to lavender oil allergy. Contact Dermatitis 1999;41(2):111.
19. Saeki Y. The effect of foot-bath with or without the essential oil of lavender on the autonomic nervous system: a randomized trial. Complement Ther Med 2000;8(1):2-7.
20. Rademaker M. Allergic contact dermatitis from lavender fragrance in Difflam gel. Contact Dermatitis 1994;31(1):58-59.
21. Varma S, Blackford S, Statham BN, et al. Combined contact allergy to tea tree oil and lavender oil complicating chronic vulvovaginitis. Contact Dermatitis 2000;42(5):309-310.
22. Moss M, Cook J, Wesnes K, et al. Aromas of rosemary and lavender essential oils differentially affect cognition and mood in healthy adults. Int J Neurosci 2003;113(1):15-38.
23. Atanassova-Shopova S, Roussinov KS. On certain central neurotropic effects of lavender essential oil. Izv Inst Fiziol (Sofiia) 1970;13:69-77.
24. Akhondzadeh S, Kashani L, Fotouhi A, et al. Comparison of *Lavandula angustifolia* Mill. tincture and imipramine in the treatment of mild to moderate depression: a double-blind, randomized trial. Prog Neuropsychopharmacol Biol Psychiatry 2003;27(1):123-127.
25. Ziegler J. Raloxifene, retinoids, and lavender: "me too" tamoxifen alternatives under study. J Natl Cancer Inst 1996;88(16):1100-1102.
26. Zweibel J, Ho P, Sepelak SB, et al. Clinical trials referral resource. Clinical trials with perillyl alcohol. Oncology (Huntingt) 1997;11(12):1817, 1820.
27. Clegg RJ, Middleton B, Bell GD, et al. The mechanism of cyclic monoterpene inhibition of hepatic 3-hydroxy-3- methylglutaryl coenzyme A reductase in vivo in the rat. J Biol Chem 1982;257(5):2294-2299.
28. Ren Z, Gould MN. Inhibition of ubiquinone and cholesterol synthesis by the monoterpene perillyl alcohol. Cancer Lett 1994;76(2-3):185-190.
29. Elisabetsky E, Marschner J, Souza DO. Effects of linalool on glutamatergic system in the rat cerebral cortex. Neurochem Res 1995;20(4):461-465.
30. Gamez MJ, Jimenez J, Navarro C, et al. Study of the essential oil of *Lavandula dentata* L. Pharmazie 1990;45(1):69-70.
31. Lis-Balchin M, Hart S. Studies on the mode of action of the essential oil of lavender (*Lavandula angustifolia* P. Miller). Phytother Res 1999;13(6):540-542.
32. Fulton GJ, Barber L, Svendsen E, et al. Oral monoterpene therapy (perillyl alcohol) reduces vein graft intimal hyperplasia. J Surg Res 1997;69(1):128-134.
33. Elegbede JA, Elson CE, Qureshi A, et al. Inhibition of DMBA-induced mammary cancer by the monoterpene d-limonene. Carcinogenesis 1984;5(5):661-664.
34. Haag JD, Gould MN. Mammary carcinoma regression induced by perillyl alcohol, a hydroxylated analog of limonene. Cancer Chemother Pharmacol 1994;34(6):477-483.
35. Mills JJ, Chari RS, Boyer IJ, et al. Induction of apoptosis in liver tumors by the monoterpene perillyl alcohol. Cancer Res 1995;55(5):979-983.
36. Lantry LE, Zhang Z, Gao F, et al. Chemopreventive effect of perillyl alcohol on 4-(methylnitrosamino)-1-(3-pyridyl)-1-butanone induced tumorigenesis in (C3H/HeJ X A/J)F1 mouse lung. J Cell Biochem Suppl 1997;27:20-25.
37. Hohmann J, Zupko I, Redei D, et al. Protective effects of the aerial parts of *Salvia officinalis*, *Melissa officinalis* and *Lavandula angustifolia* and their constituents against enzyme-dependent and enzyme-independent lipid peroxidation. Planta Med 1999;65(6):576-578.
38. Jager W, Buchbauer G, Jirovetz L, et al. Percutaneous absorption of lavender oil from massage oil. J Soc Cosmet Chem 1992;43:49-54.
39. Graham PH, Browne L, Cox H, et al. Inhalation aromatherapy during radiotherapy: results of a placebo-controlled double-blind randomized trial. J Clin Oncol 2003;21(12):2372-2376.
40. Motomura N, Sakurai A, Yotsuya Y. A psychophysiological study of lavender odorant. Memoirs of Osaka Kyoiku University Series III 1999;47(2):281-297.
41. Itai T, Amayasu H, Kuribayashi M, et al. Psychological effects of aromatherapy on chronic hemodialysis patients. Psychiatry Clin Neurosci 2000;54(4):393-397.
42. Buckle J. Aromatherapy. Nurs Times 1993;89(20):32-35.

43. Diego MA, Jones NA, Field T, et al. Aromatherapy positively affects mood, EEG patterns of alertness and math computations. Int J Neurosci 1998; 96(3-4):217-224.

44. Holmes C, Hopkins V, Hensford C, et al. Lavender oil as a treatment for agitated behaviour in severe dementia: a placebo controlled study. Int J Geriatr Psychiatry 2002;17(4):305-308.

45. Gray SG, Clair AA. Influence of aromatherapy on medication administration to residential-care residents with dementia and behavioral challenges. Am J Alzheimers Dis Other Demen 2002;17(3):169-174.

46. Ghelardini C, Galeotti N, Salvatore G, et al. Local anaesthetic activity of the essential oil of *Lavandula angustifolia*. Planta Med 1999;65(8):700-703.

47. Lis-Balchin M, Hart S. A preliminary study of the effect of essential oils on skeletal and smooth muscle *in vitro*. J Ethnopharmacol 1997;58(3): 183-187.

48. Yamada K, Kimaki Y, Ashida Y. Anticonvulsive effects of inhaling lavender oil vapour. Biol Pharm Bull 1994;17(2):359-360.

49. Burke YD, Stark MJ, Roach SL, et al. Inhibition of pancreatic cancer growth by the dietary isoprenoids farnesol and geraniol. Lipids 1997;32(2):151-156.

50. Reddy BS, Wang CX, Samaha H, et al. Chemoprevention of colon carcinogenesis by dietary perillyl alcohol. Cancer Res 1997;57(3):420-425.

Licorice
(Glycyrrhiza glabra L.)

SYNONYMS/COMMON NAMES/RELATED SUBSTANCES

- Bois doux, fabaceae, gan cao, glucoliquiritin, glycyrrhetenic acid, glycyrrhiza, *Glycyrrhiza uralensis*, glycyrrhizin, kanzo, lakrids, lakritzenwurzel, leguminose, licorice root, liquiritiae radix, *Liquiritia officinalis,* liquirizia, liquorice, prenyllicoflavone, radix glycyrrhizae, réglisse, sussholzwurzel, sweet root, sweet wood.

CLINICAL BOTTOM LINE
Background

- Licorice is harvested from the root and dried rhizomes of the low-growing shrub *Glycyrrhiza glabra.* Currently, most licorice is produced in Greece, Turkey, and Asia.
- Licorice was used in ancient Greece, China, and Egypt, primarily for gastritis and ailments of the upper respiratory tract. Ancient Egyptians prepared a licorice drink for ritual use to honor spirits of the pharaohs.
- During World War II, the Dutch physician F. E. Revers observed improvement in patients with peptic ulcer disease who were taking a licorice preparation. He also noted facial and peripheral edema, sparking scientific investigation into licorice's properties and adverse effects. In the 1950s, there were reports that patients with Addison's disease had a "craving" for licorice candy, viewed by some as early evidence of steroid-modulating properties of licorice.
- In addition to its medicinal uses, licorice has been used as a flavoring agent, valued for sweetness (glycyrrhizin, a compo-

nent of licorice, is 50 times sweeter than table sugar). The generic name *glycyrrhiza* stems from ancient Greek, meaning "sweet root." It was originally used as flavoring for licorice candies, although most licorice candy is now flavored with anise oil. Licorice is still used in subtherapeutic doses as a sweetening agent in herbal medicines, lozenges, and tobacco products (doses low enough that significant adverse effects are unlikely).

- Licorice has a long history of medicinal use in Europe and Asia. At high doses, potentially severe side effects have been reported, including high blood pressure, hypokalemia (low blood potassium levels) and fluid retention. Most adverse effects have been attributed to the chemical component glycyrrhiza (or glycyrrhizic acid). Licorice can be processed to remove the glycyrrhiza, resulting in deglycyrrhizinated licorice (DGL), which does not appear to have the metabolic disadvantages of unprocessed licorice.
- In Europe, licorice has most often been used to treat cough, bronchitis, gastritis, and peptic ulcer disease. In Chinese medicine, it is felt to benefit *qi,* reduce "fire poison" (sore throat, skin eruptions), and diminish "heat." Specific conditions treated by Chinese herbalists include abdominal pain, abscesses and sores, gastric and duodenal ulcers, pharyngitis, malaria, and tuberculosis. In Ayurveda (traditional medicine practice in India), licorice is believed to be effective in the treatment of constipation, inflamed joints, peptic ulcer disease, and diseases of the eye.

Uses Based on Scientific Evidence	Grade
Aphthous ulcers/canker sores Some research studies suggested that the licorice extracts deglycyrrhizinated licorice (DGL) and carbenoxolone may be beneficial in the treatment of canker sores. However, the studies were small, with design flaws. The safety of DGL makes it an attractive therapy, but it is not clear at this time whether there is truly any benefit.	C
Bleeding stomach ulcers caused by aspirin Although there has been some study of DGL in this area, it is not clear what effects DGL has on gastrointestinal bleeding.	C
Familial Mediterranean fever (FMF) A small clinical pilot study and laboratory study of a multi-ingredient preparation containing licorice, called Immunoguard, suggests possible effects in the management of FMF. Well-designed studies of licorice alone are necessary before a recommendation can be made.	C
Herpes simplex virus infection Laboratory studies have found that DGL may hinder the spread and infection of herpes simplex virus. Studies in humans have been small, but they suggest that topical application of carbenoxolone cream may improve healing and prevent recurrence.	C

	Grade
High potassium levels resulting from hypoaldosteronism In theory, because of the known effects of licorice, there may be some benefits of licorice in the treatment of high potassium levels caused by hypoaldosteronism (abnormally low aldosterone levels). There is early evidence in humans in support of this use. However, research is preliminary and a qualified healthcare provider should supervise treatment.	C
Peptic ulcer disease The licorice extracts DGL and carbenoxolone have been studied for treatment of peptic ulcers. DGL (but not carbenoxolone) may offer some benefits. However, these studies have been small, with design flaws, and results of different studies have disagreed. Therefore, it is unclear whether there is any benefit from licorice for this condition.	C
Viral hepatitis The licorice extracts DGL and carbenoxolone have been proposed as possible therapies for viral hepatitis. Studies in animals have investigated the mechanism of licorice in hepatitis, and studies in humans have shown some benefits with a patented intravenous licorice preparation that is not available in the United States. Studies using oral licorice have been small, with design flaws. Therefore, it is not clear whether there is any benefit from oral licorice for hepatitis treatment.	C

Continued

Genital herpes	D
Available studies have not found any benefit from carbenoxolone cream when applied topically (to the skin) to treat genital herpes infections.	

Historical or Theoretical Indications That Lack Sufficient Evidence

Adrenal insufficiency (Addison's disease), antimicrobial, antioxidant, antispasmodic, aplastic anemia, asthma, bacterial infections, bad breath, body fat reducer, bronchitis, cancer, chronic fatigue syndrome, colitis, colorectal cancer, constipation, coronavirus, cough, dental hygiene, depression, detoxification, diabetes, diuretic, diverticulitis, dropped head syndrome, eczema, Epstein-Barr virus infection, fever, gastroesophageal reflux disease, gentamicin-induced kidney damage, graft healing, high cholesterol, HIV infection, hormone regulation, inflammation, inflammatory skin disorders, laryngitis, liver protection, lung cancer, menopausal symptoms, metabolic abnormalities, methicillin-resistant *Staphylococcus aureus*, muscle cramps, obesity, osteoarthritis, plaque, polycystic ovarian syndrome, rheumatoid arthritis, severe acute respiratory syndrome (SARS), skin disorders, sore throat, stomach upset, urinary tract inflammation.

DOSING/TOXICOLOGY

The following doses are based on scientific research, publications, traditional use, or expert opinion. Many herbs and supplements have not been thoroughly tested, and their safety and effectiveness may not be proven. Brands may be made differently, with variable ingredients even within the same brand. The doses shown may not apply to all products. It is important to always read product labels and discuss doses with a qualified healthcare provider before therapy is started.

Standardization

- Standardization involves measuring the amounts of certain chemicals in products to try to make different products similar to each other. It is not always known if the chemicals being measured are the "active" ingredients.
- The expert panel German Commission E recommends that licorice be used for only 4 to 6 weeks unless it is administered under direct medical supervision. However, this is based on the use of relatively large daily doses (5 to 15 g daily). Many experts believe that extended treatments may be safe if lower doses are used. In a 4-week study in healthy individuals, recommended doses were well tolerated, with few adverse effects. There are no standard or well-studied doses of licorice, and many different doses are used traditionally.

Adults (18 Years and Older)

- **Licorice powdered root (4% to 9% glycyrrhizin):** Doses of 1 to 4 g taken by mouth daily, divided into three or four doses, have been used.
- **Licorice fluid extract (10% to 20% glycyrrhizin):** Doses of 2 to 4 ml daily have been taken by mouth.
- **DGL extract tablets:** Doses of 380 to 1140 mg three times daily taken by mouth 20 minutes before meals have been used.
- **Carbenoxolone gel or cream:** A 2% cream or gel has been applied five times a day for 7 to 14 days for herpes simplex virus skin lesions.

Children (Younger Than 18 Years)

- Licorice is not recommended for use in children because of potential side effects.

SAFETY

The U.S. Food and Drug Administration does not strictly regulate herbs and supplements. There is no guarantee of the strength, purity, or safety of products, and effects may vary. It is important to always read product labels. People who have a medical condition, or are taking other drugs, herbs, or supplements, should consult a qualified healthcare provider before starting a new therapy. A healthcare provider should be contacted immediately about any side effects.

Allergies

- People should avoid the use of licorice if they have a known allergy to licorice, any component of licorice, or any member of the Fabaceae (Leguminosae) plant family (pea family). In one case report, a rash occurred after application of a cosmetic product containing licorice to the skin.

Side Effects and Warnings

- Licorice contains a chemical called glycyrrhizic acid, which is responsible for many of its reported side effects. Deglycyrrhizinated licorice (DGL) has had the glycyrrhizic acid removed and therefore is considered safer for use.
- Many of the adverse effects of licorice result from actions on hormone levels in the body. By altering the activities of certain hormones, licorice may cause electrolyte disturbances. Possible effects include sodium and fluid retention, low potassium levels, and metabolic alkalosis.
- Licorice has been reported to cause dangerously high blood pressure with symptoms such as headache, nausea, vomiting, and hypertensive encephalopathy with stroke-like effects (for example, one-sided weakness).
- Electrolyte abnormalities may also lead to irregular heartbeats, heart attack, kidney damage, muscle weakness, and muscle breakdown. Licorice should be used cautiously by people with congestive heart failure, coronary heart disease, kidney or liver disease, fluid retention (edema), high blood pressure, underlying electrolyte disturbances, or hormonal abnormalities, and by people taking diuretics.
- Hormonal imbalances have been reported with the use of licorice, such as abnormally low testosterone levels in men and high prolactin and estrogen levels in women. These adverse effects may reduce fertility or cause menstrual abnormalities.
- Reduced body fat mass has been observed with the use of licorice.
- High doses of licorice may cause temporary vision problems or loss.

Pregnancy and Breastfeeding

- Licorice cannot be recommended for use in women who are pregnant or breastfeeding because of possible alterations of hormone levels and the possibility of premature labor.
- Hormonal imbalances reported with the use of licorice include abnormally low testosterone levels in men and high prolactin levels/estrogen levels in women.

INTERACTIONS

Most herbs and supplements have not been thoroughly tested for interactions with other herbs, supplements, drugs, or foods. The interactions listed here are based on reports in scientific publications, laboratory experiments, or traditional use. It is important to always read product labels. People who have a medical condition, or are taking other drugs, herbs, or supplements, should consult a qualified healthcare provider before starting a new therapy.

Interactions with Drugs

- In general, prescription drugs should be taken 1 hour before taking licorice or 2 hours after taking licorice because licorice may increase the absorption of many drugs. Increased absorption may increase the activities and side effects of some drugs (for example, nitrofurantoin). Phosphate salts have been shown to increase licorice absorption.

- Because the toxicity of digoxin (Lanoxin) is increased when potassium levels are low, people who take digoxin and are interested in using licorice should discuss this with their healthcare provider. Increased monitoring may be necessary. Other drugs that may increase the tendency for irregular heart rhythms are also best avoided when using licorice.

- Licorice may reduce the effects of blood-pressure or diuretic (urine-producing) drugs, including hydrochlorothiazide and spironolactone. Use of licorice with the diuretics hydrochlorothiazide or furosemide (Lasix) may cause potassium levels to fall very low and lead to dangerous complications. Other drugs that can also cause potassium levels to fall and are best avoided when using licorice include insulin, sodium polystyrene (Kayexalate), and laxatives. Chewing tobacco may increase the toxicity of licorice gums by causing electrolyte disturbances.

- Licorice may increase the adverse effects associated with corticosteroids such as prednisolone, and monoamine oxidase inhibitors such as Isocarboxazid (Marplan), phenelzine (Nardil), and tranylcypromine (Parnate).

- Licorice may reduce the effects of birth control pills, hormone replacement therapies, and testosterone therapy.

- In theory, licorice may increase the risk of bleeding when used with anticoagulants (blood thinners) or antiplatelet drugs. Examples of such drugs are warfarin (Coumadin), heparin, clopidogrel (Plavix), and aspirin.

Interactions with Herbs and Dietary Supplements

- Herbs with potential laxative properties may add to the potassium-lowering effects of licorice. Examples include alder buckthorn, aloe dried leaf sap, black root, blue flag rhizome, butternut bark, dong quai, European buckthorn, eyebright, cascara bark, castor oil, chasteberry, colocynth fruit pulp, dandelion, gamboges bark, horsetail, jalap root, manna bark, plantain leaf, podophyllum root, psyllium, rhubarb, senna, wild cucumber fruit, and yellow dock root.

- Herbs with potential diuretic properties may increase adverse effects associated with licorice. Examples are artichoke, celery, corn silk, couchgrass, dandelion, elder flower, horsetail, juniper berry, kava, shepherd's purse, uva ursi, and yarrow.

- Herbs and supplements that lower blood pressure may add to the blood pressure–lowering effects of licorice. Examples of such agents are aconite/monkshood, arnica, baneberry, betel nut, bilberry, black cohosh, bryony, calendula, California poppy, coleus, curcumin, eucalyptol, eucalyptus oil, flaxseed/flaxseed oil, garlic, ginger, ginkgo, goldenseal, green hellebore, hawthorn, Indian tobacco, jaborandi, mistletoe, night-blooming cereus, oleander, pasque flower, periwinkle, pleurisy root, *Polypodium vulgare*, shepherd's purse, Texas milkweed, turmeric, and wild cherry.

- Herbs with monoamine oxidase inhibitor (MAOI) activity may worsen side effects when used at the same time as licorice. Examples of such herbs are California poppy, chromium, dehydroepiandrosterone (DHEA), (DL-phenylalanine (DLPA), ephedra, evening primrose oil, fenugreek, *Ginkgo biloba*, hops, 5-hydroxytryptophan (5-HTP), mace, S-adenosylmethionine (SAMe), sepia, St. John's wort, tyrosine, valerian, vitamin B_6, and yohimbe bark extract.

- In theory, herbs and supplements that increase the risk of bleeding may further increase the risk of bleeding when taken with licorice. Multiple cases of bleeding have been reported with the use of *Ginkgo biloba*, and fewer cases with garlic and saw palmetto. Numerous other agents may theoretically increase the risk of bleeding, although this has not been proven in most cases. Examples of such agents are alfalfa, American ginseng, angelica, anise, *Arnica montana*, asafetida, aspen bark, bilberry, birch, black cohosh, bladderwrack, bogbean, boldo, borage seed oil, bromelain, capsicum, cat's claw, celery, chamomile, chaparral, clove, coleus, cordyceps, danshen, devil's claw, dong quai, eicosapentaenoic acid (EPA), evening primrose oil, fenugreek, feverfew, fish oil, flaxseed/flax powder (not a concern with flaxseed oil), ginger, grapefruit juice, grape seed, green tea, guggul, gymnestra, horse chestnut, horseradish, lovage root, male fern, meadowsweet, nordihydroguaiaretic acid (NDGA), omega-3 fatty acids, onion, *Panax ginseng*, papain, parsley, passionflower, poplar, prickly ash, propolis, quassia, red clover, reishi, rue, Siberian ginseng, sweet birch, sweet clover, turmeric, vitamin E, white willow, wild carrot, wild lettuce, willow, wintergreen, and yucca.

Interactions with Laboratory Values

- Licorice may decrease cortisol, ACTH, aldosterone, and potassium levels in the blood. Increases in renin and sodium levels also have been observed.

Selected References

Natural Standard developed the preceding evidence-based information based on a systematic review of more than 350 articles. For comprehensive information about alternative and complementary therapies on the professional level, go to www.naturalstandard.com. Selected references are listed here.

Amaryan G, Astvatsatryan V, Gabrielyan E, et al. Double-blind, placebo-controlled, randomized, pilot clinical trial of ImmunoGuard—a standardized fixed combination of *Andrographis paniculata* Nees, with *Eleutherococcus senticosus* Maxim, *Schizandra chinensis* Bail. and *Glycyrrhiza glabra* L. extracts in patients with Familial Mediterranean Fever. Phytomed 2003;10(4):271-285.

Arase Y, Ikeda K, Murashima N, et al. The long term efficacy of glycyrrhizin in chronic hepatitis C patients. Cancer 1997;79(8):1494-1500.

Carbonell-Barrachina AA, Aracil P, Garcia E, Burlo F, et al. Source of arsenic in licorice confectionery products. J Agric Food Chem 2003;51(6):1749-1752.

Cinatl J, Morgenstern B, Bauer G, et al. Glycyrrhizin, an active component of liquorice roots, and replication of SARS-associated coronavirus. Lancet 2003;361(9374):2045-2046.

Elinav E, Chajek-Shaul T. Licorice consumption causing severe hypokalemic paralysis. Mayo Clin Proc 2003;78(6):767-768.

Eriksson JW, Carlberg B, Hillorn V. Life-threatening ventricular tachycardia due to liquorice-induced hypokalaemia. J Intern Med 1999;245(3):307-310.

Fujioka T, Kondou T, Fukuhara A, et al. Efficacy of a glycyrrhizin suppository for the treatment of chronic hepatitis C: a pilot study. Hepatol Res 2003;26(1):10-14.

Harada T, Ohtaki E, Misu K, et al. Congestive heart failure caused by digitalis toxicity in an elderly man taking a licorice-containing Chinese herbal laxative. Cardiology 2002;98(4):218.

Hinoshita F, Ogura Y, Suzuki Y, et al. Effect of orally administered shao-yao-gan-cao-tang (Shakuyaku-kanzo-to) on muscle cramps in maintenance hemodialysis patients: a preliminary study. Am J Chin Med. 2003;31(3):445-453.

Hughes J, Sellick S, King R, et al. Re: "preterm birth and licorice consumption during pregnancy". Am J Epidemiol. 2003;158(2):190-191; author reply, 191.

Kamei J, Nakamura R, Ichiki H, et al. Antitussive principles of Glycyrrhizae radix, a main component of the Kampo preparations Bakumondo-to (Mai-men-dong-tang). Eur J Pharmacol. 2003;469(1-3):159-163.

Kang DG, Sohn EJ, Mun YJ, et al. Glycyrrhizin ameliorates renal function defects in the early-phase of ischemia-induced acute renal failure. Phytother Res 2003;17(8):947-951.

Kang DG, Sohn EJ, Lee HS. Effects of glycyrrhizin on renal functions in association with the regulation of water channels. Am J Chin Med 2003;31(3):403-413.

Lin JC. Mechanism of action of glycyrrhizic acid in inhibition of Epstein-Barr virus replication in vitro. Antiviral Res 2003;59(1):41-47.

Liu J, Manheimer E, Tsutani K, et al. Medicinal herbs for hepatitis C virus infection: a Cochrane hepatobiliary systematic review of randomized trials. Am J Gastroenterol 2003;98(3):538-544.

Nokhodchi A, Nazemiyeh H, Ghafourian T, et al. The effect of glycyrrhizin on the release rate and skin penetration of diclofenac sodium from topical formulations. Farmaco 2002;57(11):883-888.

Ofir R, Tamir S, Khatib S, Vaya J. Inhibition of serotonin re-uptake by licorice constituents. J Mol Neurosci 2003;20(2):135-140.

Oganesyan KR. Antioxidant effect of licorice root on blood catalase activity in vibration stress. Bull Exp Biol Med 2002;134(2):135-136.

Russo S, Mastropasqua M, Mosetti MA, et al. Low doses of liquorice can induce hypertension encephalopathy. Am J Nephrol 2000;20(2):145-148.

Sasaki H, Takei M, Kobayashi M, et al. Effect of glycyrrhizin, an active component of licorice roots, on HIV replication in cultures of peripheral blood mononuclear cells from HIV-seropositive patients. Pathobiol 2002-2003; 70(4):229-236.

Serra A, Uehlinger DE, Ferrari P, et al. Glycyrrhetinic Acid decreases plasma potassium concentrations in patients with anuria. J Am Soc Nephrol 2002; 13(1):191-196.

Sigurjonsdottir HA, Manhem K, Axelson M, et al. Subjects with essential hypertension are more sensitive to the inhibition of 11 beta-HSD by liquorice. J Hum Hypertens 2003;17(2):125-131.

Sohn EJ, Kang DG, Lee HS. Protective effects of glycyrrhizin on gentamicin-induced acute renal failure in rats. Pharmacol Toxicol 2003;93(3):116-122.

Strandberg TE, Andersson S, Jarvenpaa AL. Risk factors for preterm delivery. Lancet 2003;361(9355):436; author reply, 436-437.

van Rossum TG, Vulto AG, Hop WC, et al. Glycyrrhizin-induced reduction of ALT in European patients with chronic hepatitis C. Am J Gastroenterol 2001; 96(8):2432-2437.

Lycopene

(Tomato [*Lycopersicon esculentum*])

SYNONYMS/COMMON NAMES/RELATED SUBSTANCES

- ψ, ψ-carotene, all-trans lycopene, lycopersicon, solanorubin, tomato.

CLINICAL BOTTOM LINE
Background

- Lycopene is a carotenoid and is present in human serum, liver, adrenal glands, lungs, prostate, colon, and skin at higher levels than other carotenoids. Lycopene has been found to possess antioxidant and antiproliferative properties in animal and *in vitro* studies, although activity in humans remains controversial.
- Numerous epidemiologic investigations have correlated high intake of lycopene-containing foods or high lycopene serum levels with reduced incidence of cancer, cardiovascular disease, and macular degeneration. However, estimates of lycopene consumption have been based on reported tomato intake, not on the use of lycopene supplements. Because tomatoes are sources of other nutrients, including vitamin C, folate, and potassium, it is not clear that lycopene itself is beneficial.
- There is no established definition of "lycopene deficiency," and no direct evidence that repletion of low lycopene levels has any benefit.

Scientific Evidence for Common/Studied Uses	Grade*
Age-related macular degeneration prevention	C
Antioxidant	C
Asthma (exercise-induced)	C
Atherosclerosis/hyperlipidemia (lipid peroxidation)	C
Breast cancer prevention	C
Cancer prevention (general)	C
Cervical cancer prevention	C
Lung cancer prevention	C
Prostate cancer prevention	C
Upper gastrointestinal tract and colorectal cancer prevention	C
Immunostimulation (cell-mediated)	D

*Key to grades: *A:* Strong scientific evidence for this use; *B:* Good scientific evidence for this use; *C:* Unclear scientific evidence for this use; *D:* Fair scientific evidence against this use (it may not work); *F:* Strong scientific evidence against this use (it likely does not work). For a more detailed explanation of efficacy criteria, see "Natural Standard Evidence-Based Validated Grading Rationale" in the Introduction.

Historical or Theoretical Uses
That Lack Sufficient Evidence

- AIDS, bladder cancer prevention,[1-6] breast cancer recurrence/secondary prevention,[7,8] cataracts,[9-11] cognitive function,[12]

coronary death prevention,[13,14] coronary event prevention,[15,16] diabetes mellitus, esophageal cancer prevention,[17,18] inflammatory conditions, laryngeal cancer prevention,[19] malignant mesothelioma prevention,[20] melanoma prevention, myocardial infarction prevention,[21-23] ovarian cancer prevention,[24,25] pancreatic cancer prevention,[26-29] pancreatitis,[30] Parkinson's disease,[31] periodontal disease, pharyngeal cancer prevention,[32] skin cancer prevention,[33] stroke prevention,[34,35] stomach cancer,[36] urinary tract cancer.[37]

Expert Opinion and Historic Precedent

- Diets rich in fruits and vegetables have been associated with health benefits in a number of epidemiologic studies and are often recommended by clinicians. Tomatoes and tomato-based products have been specifically investigated, with benefits and observed antioxidant properties often attributed to lycopene. Despite the lack of available evidence for lycopene supplements, their use remains popular.

Safety Summary

- **Likely safe:** There is insufficient available evidence regarding the use of lycopene supplements to specify any safety information concerning their use. Safety has not been systematically assessed. However, tomatoes and tomato-based products have historically been used in human diets with no reported adverse effects.

DOSING/TOXICOLOGY
General

- Recommended doses are based on those most commonly reported in human studies, although prospective trial data are scant. Efficacy and safety have not necessarily been demonstrated. Preparation of products may vary from manufacturer to manufacturer, and from batch to batch of a specific product made by a single manufacturer. The clinical effects of different brands may not be comparable.

Standardization

- Insufficient evidence is available for lycopene supplements.
- The approximate amounts of lycopene found in commonly ingested foods include 3 mg/100 g of canned tomatoes, 17.2 mg/100 g of tomato ketchup, and 18 mg/100 g of tomato sauce.[38]

Dosing: Adult (18 Years and Older)
Oral

- **Cancer prevention:** No specific amounts of lycopene or lycopene-rich vegetables have been clearly established in cancer prevention studies. The efficacy of lycopene for cancer prevention has not been proven. Therefore, no recommendation can be made.
- **Age-related macular degeneration prevention:** No specific doses of lycopene or lycopene-rich vegetables have been clearly established. Therefore, no recommendation can be made.
- **Exercise-induced asthma:** 30 mg lycopene daily, supplied as Lyc-O-Mato (LycoRed Natural Products Industries Ltd., Israel).[39]

- **Atherosclerosis/lipid peroxidation prevention:** 1.243 g of 6% lycopene oleoresin capsules daily (LycoRed Natural Product Industries Ltd., Israel).[40]
- **Immune enhancement (cell-mediated):** 13.3 mg lycopene daily, supplied as Lyco-O-Pen, LycoRed Natural Products Industries Ltd., Israel.[41]

Dosing: Pediatric (Younger Than 18 Years)

- Insufficient evidence to recommend.

Toxicology

- Literature review reveals no reported toxicities associated with the intake of tomatoes or tomato-based products and no toxicities in the few studies utilizing lycopene supplements.[39-41]

ADVERSE EFFECTS/PRECAUTIONS/CONTRAINDICATIONS
Allergy

- Known allergy/hypersensitivity to lycopene or tomatoes.

Adverse Effects/Postmarket Surveillance

- **General:** Literature review reveals no reported adverse effects from the consumption of tomatoes, tomato-based products, or lycopene supplements.[39-41] However, the safety of lycopene supplements has not been systematically studied.

Precautions/Warnings/Contraindications

- Lycopene supplements should be avoided in individuals with known allergy/hypersensitivity to lycopene or tomatoes.
- Tomatoes and tomato-based products may be acidic.

Pregnancy and Lactation

- Not recommended due to lack of sufficient data.
- Lycopene metabolites have been isolated from samples of human breast milk[42] at approximately 10% of serum concentrations.[43] The clinical ramifications are not known.

INTERACTIONS
Lycopene/Drug Interactions

- **HMG CoA reductase inhibitors (statins):** Lycopene may act similarly to statin drugs and potentiate their effects, based on *in vitro* observations that lycopene reduces cellular cholesterol synthesis with a mechanism similar to that of fluvastatin.[44] In addition, the use of statins may reduce serum lycopene levels: Lycopene and other carotenoids are transported in human plasma primarily by lipoproteins.[45] Studies have found plasma lycopene levels to be significantly correlated with plasma low-density lipoprotein (LDL) levels.[46-49] To a lesser extent, lycopene is transported via high-density lipoproteins (HDLs).[50,51] Lowering of LDL levels by statins or other drugs may result in lowering of serum lycopene levels.
- **Bile acid sequestrants (cholestyramine, cholestipol):** Bile acid sequestrants such as cholestyramine (Questran, Prevalite, LoCHOLEST) and cholestipol (Cholestid) may reduce serum levels of lycopene. In a 3-year, randomized, double-blind study, cholestyramine administration was associated with a statistically significant reduction in serum carotenoid levels in 303 hypercholesterolemic patients.[52] It has been theorized that cholestyramine caused a 30% decrease in serum lycopene levels, attributed to impaired gastrointestinal absorption and decreased serum cholesterol levels. It is not clear if these changes in carotenoid levels were harmful, beneficial, or neither, and supplementation was not

given to patients. Therefore, although lycopene supplementation may offset these observed reductions, the potential outcome of such supplementation is not clear.

- **Probucol (available in Canada, not commercially available in U.S.):** In a three-year, randomized, double-blind study, probucol administration was associated with a statistically significant decrease in serum carotenoid levels in 303 hypercholesterolemic patients.[52] It is not clear if these changes in carotenoid levels were harmful, beneficial, or neither. Although supplementation with carotenoids such as lycopene may offset these observed reductions, the potential benefits of supplementation are not clear.
- **Nicotine:** Conflicting evidence exists regarding the influence of cigarette smoking on lycopene levels.[53-56] Although not consistent, it appears that lycopene serum concentrations, unlike other carotenoids, are not influenced by cigarette smoking.[47,55,57-60] However, the inconsistency of study results leaves the concern that cigarette smoking may lead to decreased serum levels of lycopene.[61] In a case-control study examining the relationship between serum carotenoid levels and the risk of myocardial infarction in nearly 500 subjects, it was noted that subjects who smoked ≥25 cigarettes per day had significantly lower serum lycopene levels.[23] In an *in vitro* study of the effect of cigarette smoke on serum carotenoid levels, lycopene was the most susceptible to degradation by the exposure.[62]
- **Alcohol (ethanol):** The serum concentrations of some carotenoids are influenced by alcohol consumption, and it has been theorized that lycopene may also be subject to this interaction. However, a study in 12 healthy, nonsmoking men found that the intake of red wine, beer, or spirits had no significant effect on serum lycopene levels.[60,63]

Lycopene/Herb/Supplement Interactions

- **β-carotene:** There is conflicting evidence regarding the interaction of β-carotene and lycopene. Concomitant ingestion of lycopene and β-carotene has been reported to increase lycopene absorption in human studies.[64,65] Other investigations have found β-carotene to have no effect on lycopene serum levels.[66-71] One study found that subjects receiving β-carotene supplements reduced the concentration of lycopene in an assay of low-density lipoproteins (LDLs).[72] Because of the unclear nature of this potential interaction, these agents should be administered concurrently with caution.
- **Canthaxanthin:** Canthaxanthin, a carotenoid, has been shown to inhibit lycopene uptake from dietary sources and may result in decreased serum levels, with unclear clinical consequences.[73]
- **Vitamin D (calciferol):** Lycopene has been shown *in vitro* to have synergistic effects on the inhibition of cellular proliferation of HL-60 promyelocytes when administered with 1,25-dihydroxy vitamin D_3.[74] These antiproliferative effects may have implications for concurrent administration of these agents in humans.
- **Lutein (*positive interaction*):** The combination of lutein and lycopene demonstrated more efficient antioxidant activity than either compound alone *in vitro*, suggesting synergy when lutein and lycopene are ingested together.[75] Beneficial effects have not been demonstrated in humans.
- **Vitamin E (α-tocopherol)(*positive interaction*):** Lycopene has been shown *in vitro* to act synergistically with α-tocopherol to inhibit the proliferation of prostate carcinoma cells.[76] Beneficial effects have not been demonstrated in humans.

Lycopene/Food Interactions

- **Olestra (Olean):** The fat substitute, Olestra, may decrease serum levels of lycopene by up to 30%.[40,77] Olestra is available commercially in many reduced-fat foods (indicated on product labels).
- **High-fat diet:** Theoretically, because lycopene is a fat-soluble carotenoid, it may be absorbed better with the consumption of fatty foods; however, studies comparing the consumption of a full-fat to a reduced-fat diet showed no effect on plasma lycopene levels.[78,79]

Lycopene/Lab Interactions

- Insufficient available data.

MECHANISM OF ACTION
Pharmacology

- **General:** Lycopene belongs to a group of physiologic compounds known as carotenoids. Carotenoids are fat-soluble hydrocarbon pigments that impart yellow, red and orange colors to birds, fish, crustaceans, vegetables, flowers, and fruits. Most of the known carotenoids are precursors of vitamin A, with the exception of lutein, lycopene, and canthaxanthin. The most predominant carotenoids in human serum include β-carotene, α-carotene, β-cryptoxanthin, lycopene, and lutein. Lycopene makes up half of the carotenoids in human serum, and it is found in the liver, adrenal glands, lungs, prostate, colon, and skin at concentrations higher than all other carotenoids. Average human plasma levels have been reported to be 0.5 mmol/L.
- Lycopene is a red pigment found most abundantly in tomatoes, but it is also present in watermelon,[80,82] apricots, green peppers, carrots, rose hips, guava, pink grapefruit, and autumn olive (*Elaeagnus umbellate*). The most important sources of lycopene in the human diet are tomatoes (3 mg/100 g of fresh tomatoes, 10 mg/100 g of canned tomatoes), ketchup, pizza, tomato sauce, tomato paste (30 mg/100 g), and salsa.
- **Antioxidant:** Like other carotenoids, lycopene is purported to possess antioxidant, antiradical, singlet oxygen quenching, and gap-junction communication enhancement activities. Multiple *in vitro* and *in vivo* studies have demonstrated antioxidant properties,[61] whereas other studies suggest a lack of effects.[15,82] It remains unclear if antioxidant activities depend on other factors that may account for these conflicting results. *In vitro*, lycopene has been demonstrated to possess greater singlet oxygen quenching abilities[83,84] and greater antioxidant activity than other carotenoids.[75] Lycopene has been shown capable of scavenging the ABTS·+ radical cation with the most activity of all the carotenoids[85] and is twice as effective as β-carotene in protecting lymphocytes from nitrogen dioxide radical membrane damage.[86] Studies in humans have yielded conflicting results.[15,59,87-93]
- **Antineoplastic:** Multiple *in vitro* and *in vivo* studies have assessed the ability of lycopene to prevent tumor growth and to reduce serum markers associated with cancer risk. Following supplementation with 15 mg of lycopene twice daily for 3 to 4 weeks, investigators found that insulin-like growth factor I (IGF-I) serum concentrations decreased in 53% of subjects vs. placebo; notably, serum levels of IGF-I have been associated with the development of breast and prostate cancers.[94] The investigators also found lycopene to decrease the IGF-I mediated growth stimulation of mammary cancer cell lines. Lycopene has been shown *in vitro* to inhibit the proliferation of endometrial, mammary, and lung cancer

cells after incubation for 24 hours, effects that persisted for >3 days.[95] *In vitro*, lycopene has also been shown to inhibit cell proliferation of HL-60 promyelocytes in a concentration-dependent fashion, reportedly by arresting cell development at the G_0/G_1 phase.[74] When added to low concentrations of 1,25-dihydroxy vitamin D_3, lycopene synergistically inhibited the cellular proliferation of HL-60 promyelocytes after two days.[74] An animal study found that lycopene, when given to rats in daily doses of 0.001 to 0.1 g/kg for 2 weeks, resulted in modification of antioxidant and drug metabolizing enzymes that are involved in the protection of cells from oxidative stress and malignant growth.[96] A diet supplemented with 5×10^{-5}% lycopene was shown to significantly decrease the development of mammary tumors in rats through a reduction in mammary gland thymidylate synthetase activity and decreased serum free fatty acid and prolactin levels.[97] In an animal study examining tumor induction with 7,12-dimethyl-benz[a]anthracene, Sharoni et al. observed that 16 weeks of twice-weekly lycopene-enriched tomato oleoresin (10 mg/kg) resulted in significantly diminished mammary tumor development in rats.[98] Lycopene has also been shown *in vitro* to inhibit prostate carcinoma cell proliferation in a dose-dependent fashion.[76,99,100] Anticarcinogenic effects of lycopene have been suggested to be due to the regulation of gap-junction communication in mouse embryo fibroblast cells.[101]

- **Hypocholesterolemic:** When added to human macrophage cell lines, lycopene has been found to decrease cholesterol synthesis and augment the activity of macrophage low-density lipoprotein (LDL) receptors with a mechanism similar to that of the HMG-CoA reductase inhibitor fluvastatin.[44] At a dose of 15 mg daily for 26 days, lycopene was found to lower significantly the ratio of polyunsaturated to saturated fatty acid *in vivo*, reportedly through the reduction of plasma linoleic acid.[102]
- **Effects on erythema:** In a 10-week study, consumption of tomato paste (16 mg/day of lycopene) with pasta and olive oil was associated with increased serum lycopene levels and a 40% reduction in skin erythema caused by ultraviolet (UV) light, when compared to controls (pasta and olive oil without tomato paste).[103] In a different study, skin levels of lycopene were significantly decreased after exposure to UV light.[69]
- **Immunomodulation:** Two studies assessing the effects of daily lycopene supplementation (15 mg) found no significant increases in the expression of monocyte cell surface molecules.[104,105]

Pharmacodynamics/Kinetics

- **Absorption:** It appears, from the results of numerous pharmacokinetic studies, that lycopene is better absorbed when ingested in the form of processed tomato-based products than from raw tomatoes.[59,106-109] It is postulated that this increased bioavailability may be due to the isomeric form of lycopene found in processed foods. Lycopene accounts for 80% to 90% of the carotenoids in tomatoes and is found in the all-*trans* conformation.[109] Through the processing of tomatoes into tomato products such as tomato paste and ketchup, the proportion of *cis* isomers greatly increases, while not affecting the stability of lycopene.[110] The increased bioavailability associated with processed tomato products, compared to fresh tomatoes, suggests that the *cis* isomer of lycopene has greater bioavailability.[106,109] The release of carotenoids from their food matrix appears to be the limiting factor in the absorption of these nutrients, and heating or processing these food sources may increase the release of carotenoids like lycopene through protein breakdown.[45,50]

- The evidence is mixed regarding the extent to which supplementation with lycopene-rich foods or supplements affects plasma lycopene levels. Plasma lycopene levels were reported to correlate with dietary intake of lycopene in 19 cancer patients.[111] Paetau et al. reported a significant increase in lycopene concentrations in the buccal mucosa cells of subjects after 4 weeks of ingestion of tomato oleoresin capsules (Lyc-O-Mato) and lycopene beadlets (Lycobeads), but not after the ingestion of tomato juice.[112] Other studies have found no significant changes in serum levels after supplementation with lycopene-rich foods or supplements. A randomized crossover trial in 15 healthy adults found no significant difference in plasma lycopene levels after daily consumption of tomato juice, oleoresin capsules (Lyc-O-Mato), or lycopene beadlets (Lycobeads) (4-week duration separated by 6-week washout).[113] A crossover study randomized 19 healthy human subjects to consume four different diets, each for 9 days, and found that whereas other plasma carotenoid concentrations increased significantly after the consumption of carotenoid-rich diets, lycopene levels remained unchanged.[114] A controlled study randomized 201 patients with recent adenomas to eat their usual diet or ≥8 servings of fruits/vegetables per day for 1 year.[115] The increased fruit/vegetable intake had no significant effect on plasma lycopene levels vs. controls. Similar findings were reported after daily ingestion of 20 to 50 mg of lycopene.[116]

- **Distribution:** Average human plasma lycopene levels have been identified as 0.22 to 1.06 μmol/L.[117] In a study of antioxidant concentrations in 3480 human subjects, average lycopene concentration was determined to be 0.4 μmol/L (95% CI, 0.11 to 0.80).[118]

- One study found lycopene to reach steady state in lymphocytes within 6 hours following a continuous infusion into the duodenum of rats.[119] The concentration of lycopene increased in a dose-dependent fashion. In a human study, peak serum concentrations were reached between 4 and 6 hours after ingestion of 49.5-mg lycopene capsules (supplied by Makhleshim of Israel) with a meal by three healthy volunteers.[120] In another investigation, 10 women were fed single portions of either raw tomatoes or tomato puree, each containing approximately 16.5 mg of lycopene, and their serum levels peaked at 6 to 12 hours.[108] In a study of lycopene uptake in six adults, serum concentrations were found to increase in a dose-dependent fashion after the ingestion of processed tomato juice, with a peak reached in 24 to 48 hours.[121]

- Carotenoids are transported in human plasma by lipoproteins.[45] A study in 59 healthy human subjects demonstrated plasma levels of lycopene to be significantly correlated with plasma low-density lipoprotein (LDL) levels.[46] The percentage of lycopene found on LDLs was 87.4 ± 10.5, indicating that lycopene is predominantly transported by LDLs. Lower non-HDL cholesterol levels have been associated with decreased lycopene levels in samples of healthy individuals.[47-49] It has also been shown that high-density lipoproteins provide lycopene transport to a lesser degree.[50,51]

- No consistent relationship exists between lycopene concentrations found in various human organs.[122] Primary storage areas for lycopene appear to be the adrenal glands and the testes, but high amounts are also found in the liver, fat tissue, prostate gland, kidneys, and ovaries.[50,123] Autopsies of 20 subjects, ages 4 months to 86 years, showed higher concentrations of lycopene in the liver, kidneys, and lungs.[124] Analysis of serum and prostate tissue samples from 10 subjects enrolled in the Health Professionals Follow-up Study showed that lycopene achieved comparable levels in both the serum and malignant prostate tissue.[99] Concentrations of lycopene were found to be greater in the liver, adrenal glands and testes than in the kidneys, ovaries, or fat.[125] In an analysis of cataractous lenses extracted from seven subjects, concentrations of lycopene were found to be undetectable, despite substantial plasma levels of the carotenoid.[126] The investigators concluded that a 50-fold concentration gradient exists between human plasma and eye lenses, indicating an effective barrier to the distribution of lycopene in the eyes. In a study of the relationship between serum and tissue levels of carotenoids in 93 patients with actinic keratoses, lycopene was found in similar concentrations in the skin and plasma.[127]

- Lycopene metabolites have been isolated from samples of human breast milk,[42] at 10% of serum concentrations.[43] Giulianoet al. reported lycopene and β-carotene to be the most predominant carotenoids in an analysis of breast milk, although there was a high degree of within-person variability.[128] In a study of carotenoid levels in mother and umbilical cord blood immediately post partum, lycopene was shown to have the lowest correlation of any of the carotenoids measured.[129] However, when adjusted for triglycerides, the concentration was actually found to be the highest ($p = 0.0047$).

- **Metabolism:** No reliable *in vivo* data exist regarding lycopene and its metabolites. However, the metabolite 5,6-dihydroxy-5,6-dihydrolycopene has been identified *in vitro* and most likely results from the oxidation of lycopene.[130]

- **Elimination:** The half-life of lycopene in women fed controlled diets for 10 weeks was determined to be 26 days, and lycopene was eliminated by first-order kinetics.[13] In another study, the half-life of elimination in six adults ingesting processed tomato juice was determined as 2 to 3 days.[121] The large discrepancy between these results warrants additional research.

- **Patient variables:** An analysis of serum lycopene levels in 638 subjects from the Framingham Heart Study demonstrated serum lycopene concentrations to be inversely correlated with age, with the lowest levels in patients over 80 years.[132] Subsequent studies have confirmed this association.[47,52]

- In a study to determine serum reference ranges for various carotenoids and antioxidants, Olmedilla et al. found 60 men with diabetes mellitus (type 1) to have significantly higher serum lycopene levels than healthy male controls.[133] However, a different study found no difference in the lycopene levels of 54 subjects with diabetes mellitus (type 2) and 450 nondiabetic controls.[134] In a case-control study of 72 patients with diabetes mellitus (type 2) and 72 matched controls, subjects with diabetes had significantly lower serum levels of lycopene and other carotenoids.[135] In a study of serum carotenoid levels in patients with normal glucose tolerance, impaired glucose tolerance, newly diagnosed diabetes, and long-standing diabetes, it was found that diabetics had significantly lower lycopene serum levels than individuals with normal glucose tolerance.[136]

- In a study to assess any differences between the serum carotenoid concentrations of women and men, no significant differences were found for lycopene.[137]

HISTORY

- Humans obtain dietary lycopene primarily from tomatoes and tomato-based products. The tomato originated in South America as a vine berry and was named by 16th-century Spanish explorers after the Aztec word for tomato, *tomatl*. Average annual consumption of tomatoes in the United States is 23 pounds per capita. Lycopene is also found in apricots, pink grapefruit, guava, guava juice, rose hip puree, palm oil, and watermelon.[138,139]

- Lycopene as a dietary supplement has become popular recently because of its purported antioxidant properties and based on initial epidemiologic evidence suggesting benefit against cancer, coronary artery disease, and macular degeneration.

Review Of the Evidence: Lycopene

Condition Treated*	Study Design	Author, Year	N[†]	SS[†]	Study Quality[‡]	Magnitude of Benefit	ARR[†]	NNT[†]	Comments
Cancer prevention (general)	Review of observational studies	Giovannucci[140] 1999	72 studies	Mixed	NA	Small	NA	NA	57 of 72 studies with positive results, but only 35 statistically significant; all based on dietary intake of tomatoes, lycopene, or serum lycopene levels.
Cancer prevention (prostate)	Review of observational studies	Giovannucci[199] 1998	6 studies	Mixed	NA	Small	NA	NA	2 of 6 studies statistically significant; both dietary tomato intake and lycopene serum levels assessed; lycopene supplementation not used.
Cancer prevention (gastrointestinal tract)	Review of observational studies	Franceschi[165] 1994	3 studies	Yes	NA	Small	NA	NA	Calculated odds ratio 0.4-0.7; studies correlated tomato intake with cancer incidence.
Exercise-induced asthma	RCT, double-blindl	Neuman 2000	20	Yes	2	Small	NA	NA	30 mg of Lyc-O-Mato lycopene supplements given daily for 1 week vs. placebo.
Lipid peroxidation	RCT, crossover	Agarwal[40] 1998	19	Yes	1	Small	NA	NA	Study compared lycopene levels from tomato juice vs. spaghetti sauce vs. lycopene oleoresin capsules vs. placebo; lycopene found to significantly decrease LDL oxidation vs. placebo (odds ratio 1.9-2.2).
Lipid peroxidation	RCT, crossover	Sutherland[92] 1999	15	No	1	None	NA	NA	Renal transplant patients given tomato juice or synthetic orange drink (control) daily for 4 weeks each; no significant difference between groups.
Lipid peroxidation	RCT	Steinberg[6] 1998	39	Yes	3	None	NA	NA	Tomato juice supplemented with "antioxidants" superior to unsupplemented tomato juice for LDL peroxidation in smokers; suggests other antioxidants may be preferable to lycopene.
Immunostimulation	RCT, double-blind	Corridan[41] 2001	58	No	2	None	NA	NA	β-Carotene vs. lycopene (Lyc-O-Pen) vs. placebo (α- and γ-tocopherols); no immune enhancement seen in either group.
Immunostimulation	RCT	Watzl[217] 2000	53	No	1	None	NA	NA	Tomato juice vs. mineral water daily for 8 weeks; no significant effect on immunity.
Immunostimulation	RCT, crossover	Hughes[104,105] 1997, 2000	20	No	2	None	NA	NA	Lycopene (15 mg) vs. placebo; no significant increase in monocyte cell-surface molecule expression.

*Primary or secondary outcome.
[†]*N*, Number of patients; *SS*, statistically significant; *ARR*, absolute risk reduction; *NNT*, the number of patients who need to undergo a specific intervention in order to observe an outcome in one individual.
[‡]0-2 = poor; 3-4 = good; 5 = excellent.
NA, Not applicable; *LDL*, low-density lipoprotein; *RCT*, randomized, controlled trial.
For an explanation of each category in this table, please see Table 3 in the Introduction.

L

REVIEW OF THE EVIDENCE: DISCUSSION
Cancer Prevention (General)
Summary

- Numerous epidemiologic studies have suggested an association between diets high in fruits and vegetables and a decreased risk of developing cancer. However, it remains unclear what the causative agent(s) might be, or if fruit/vegetable intake is actually a marker of a "healthy lifestyle" rather than a beneficial factor itself. The role of tomatoes, tomato-based products, and serum lycopene levels (but not lycopene supplements) has also been evaluated in observational studies, with mixed results. Although some of these investigations have correlated lycopene with a lower incidence of cancer, these results can only be considered preliminary until properly controlled, prospective trials are conducted. Animal and *in vitro* studies have similarly produced conflicting results in this area.[19,74,94-99,101] At this time, there is insufficient evidence either for or against the efficacy of lycopene for cancer prevention.

Evidence

- Giovannucci et al. published a review of 72 cohort and case-control studies that evaluated the association between tomatoes, tomato-based products, or serum lycopene levels with cancer incidence.[140] They found that 57 of these investigations showed an inverse relationship between lycopene and the incidence of cancer, but only 35 were statistically significant. The authors noted that most trials reported a similar relative risk reduction (RR) of approximately 40% (RR = 0.6), whether measuring lycopene intake or lycopene blood levels. The data appear to be strongest for prostate, lung, and stomach cancers, although a decreased risk of breast, cervical, pancreatic, colorectal, esophageal, and oral cancers was also demonstrated. Many of these studies drew conclusions based on tomato intake, and therefore any benefits cannot be attributed to lycopene specifically. Although compelling, these results can only be considered preliminary.
- Additional reviews of epidemiologic studies evaluating the association of vegetable, fruit, and carotenoid intake with cancer incidence have also been published (not studying lycopene specifically).[43,123,141-147] Overall, these reviews have found that the consumption of high amounts of fruits/vegetables is associated with a decreased incidence of cancer. Because these studies have not examined specific nutrients and have not been controlled, it remains unclear what the causative agent(s) might be or if fruit/vegetable intake is actually a marker of a "healthy lifestyle" rather than a beneficial factor itself.
- A large case-controlled series analyzing the consumption of vegetables in 8077 cases with various cancers and 6147 controls found that the intake of high amounts of vegetables decreased the risk of developing epithelial cancers.[148] These results may or may not have implications for the recommendation of increased lycopene intake or lycopene supplementation to prevent cancer.

Breast Cancer Prevention
Summary

- Evaluations of lycopene's role in the prevention of breast cancer are limited to observational studies assessing the association between disease incidence and fruit/vegetable intake, tomato consumption, or lycopene serum/tissue levels. Some results have demonstrated significant benefits,[149-153]

whereas other evidence suggests no significant association.[151,154-158] There have been no studies conducted to date that reliably assess the influence of lycopene supplementation on the prevention of breast cancer. Animal and *in vitro* studies also provide conflicting results.[94,95,97,98,159] Until further preclinical and prospective controlled studies are completed assessing the influence of lycopene supplementation on the development of breast cancer, no recommendations can be made regarding the use of lycopene for this indication.

Cervical Cancer Prevention
Summary

- The role of lycopene in the prevention of cervical cancer has been evaluated in observational studies of the association between tomato intake/lycopene serum levels and disease incidence.[54,160-164] Only two of these investigations have found statistically significant benefits of lycopene intake (based on reported tomato consumption).[161,164] The others have found no significant association between lycopene levels and subsequent cervical cancer development.[54,160,162,163] The inconsistency of the available evidence and the lack of prospective controlled studies (or studies of lycopene supplements) point to the need for further research before a firm conclusion can be drawn.

Upper Gastrointestinal Tract and Colorectal Cancer Prevention
Summary

- The role of lycopene in the prevention of digestive tract cancers, including oral, pharyngeal, esophageal, gastric, colon and rectal cancer, is not conclusive. One review of three case-control studies has found that there is a significant decrease in risk associated with high tomato intake.[165] Several additional observational studies also exist for gastric and colorectal cancers specifically, with conflicting results. The lack of prospective randomized data on the use of lycopene supplements for this indication, along with the inconsistency of available data, serves only to emphasize the need for more research before recommendations regarding lycopene for the prevention of digestive tract cancers can be made.

Evidence

- Franceschi et al. analyzed the data from a series of case-control studies concerning the association of tomato consumption on the risk of digestive tract cancers.[165] The studied population included subjects with oral or pharyngeal cancer, esophageal cancer, stomach cancer, colon cancer, and rectal cancer. Comparison was made with 2879 control subjects from three case-controlled studies.[32,166,167] The odds ratios for the upper quartiles of tomato intake ranged from 0.4 to 0.7, and all were significant. While these data appear promising, they do not specifically address the direct effect of lycopene on cancer risk. It remains unclear if lycopene is the agent responsible for a decreased risk of cancer development, as lycopene intake was estimated from dietary intake of tomatoes.
- **Upper gastrointestinal tract cancer:** A case-control study of upper aerodigestive tract cancers (esophagus, oral cavity, pharynx, larynx) assessing the association between dietary tomato intake and cancer risk found a significantly decreased risk of developing digestive tract cancer with an increased intake of tomatoes and tomato-based foods (relative risk reduction [RR] = 0.30; 95% CI, 0.18 to 0.51 for overall

tomato intake).[168] Two additional case-control studies found a significant protective effect against the development of gastric cancer with high dietary tomato consumption.[36,169] Other studies have reported that a diet high in vegetables confers a significant protective effect, but these results were not specific to tomatoes.[166,170-173] In contrast, other studies have found no significant association between vegetable intake and the development of gastric cancer.[174] From the available evidence, it is not possible to recommend either for or against the use of lycopene-rich foods or lycopene supplements in the prevention of upper gastrointestinal tract cancers. Properly randomized trials assessing the influence of lycopene on the development of these cancers are warranted before a firm conclusion can be drawn.

- **Colorectal cancer:** Numerous case-control studies have assessed the association between dietary vegetable intake and the incidence of colorectal cancer, largely finding a statistically significant decreased risk associated with increased vegetable intake.[167,175-179] Of the available studies, two have addressed the intake of lycopene specifically, as estimated from dietary tomato consumption: One found that subjects with tomato consumption in the highest tertile were half as likely to develop colon or rectal cancer as those with low tomato consumption (OR = 0.5 for colon cancer, $p = 0.04$; OR = 0.4 for rectal cancer, $p = 0.03$).[167] However, the second study found no association between dietary lycopene and disease (although intake of lutein, a different carotenoid, was associated with decreased colon cancer risk).[180] From the available evidence, it is not possible to recommend either for or against the use of lycopene-rich foods or lycopene supplements in the prevention of colon cancer. Properly randomized trials assessing the influence of lycopene on colon cancer are warranted before a firm conclusion can be drawn.

Lung Cancer Prevention
Summary
- The role of lycopene in the prevention of lung cancer is not clear. Numerous observational population/cohort studies have yielded inconsistent results. Prospective randomized trials are lacking.

Evidence
- Several population studies have found that increased dietary intake of lycopene, as estimated from reports of tomato consumption, significantly decreases the incidence of lung cancer.[181-186] Others have reported a significant association between the consumption of yellow-orange vegetables and the incidence of lung cancer.[187-189] One case-control study identified a significant inverse association between plasma lycopene levels and lung cancer.[190] However, a number of other studies found no significant association between lycopene intake or lycopene serum levels and the development of lung cancer.[51,191-196] Given the paucity of experimental data specifically examining the use of lycopene supplements, the lack of consistency among the available published studies, and the absence of prospective controlled investigations, no recommendation can be made either for or against this use of lycopene.

Prostate Cancer Prevention
Summary
- The majority of studies evaluating the effects of lycopene on the risk of prostate cancer are observational population investigations. Most have focused on tomato consumption and have yielded mixed results. One uncontrolled study reported reductions in serum prostate-specific antigen (PSA) levels following ingestion of tomato sauce for 3 weeks. At this time, the evidence is not sufficient to recommend for or against the use of lycopene-containing foods or supplements for the prevention of prostate cancer.

Evidence
- Chen et al. reported a case series in 32 subjects with localized prostate adenocarcinoma.[197] All patients consumed tomato sauce–based pasta dishes daily, containing 30 mg of lycopene, for 3 weeks. After 3 weeks, all subjects underwent previously scheduled radical prostatectomy. Primary outcome measures included serum lycopene levels, prostate-specific antigen (PSA) levels, and chemical measures of oxidative damage. When compared to pre-intervention values, the authors reported significant increases in serum lycopene, decreases in PSA (pre-intervention, 10.9 ng/mL [95% CI, 8.7 to 13.2] vs. post-intervention, 8.7 ng/mL [95% CI, 6.8 to 10.6]), and decreases in leukocyte and prostate cell oxidative damage. The results of this prospective intervention are compelling, and warrant follow-up with a controlled trial using a lycopene supplement arm. A duplicate publication of these results has been reported by Bowen et al.[198]

- In 1998, Giovannucci et al. reviewed the existing literature regarding tomatoes, lycopene, and the risk of prostate cancer.[199] They identified only two prospective cohort studies, the Physician's Health Study and the Seventh Day Adventist Study, which found a significantly decreased risk of prostate cancer associated with increased dietary tomato intake.[200,201] However, in four other studies, no significant association was found between tomato intake/serum lycopene levels and prostate cancer incidence.[202-205]

- Additional observational studies have also yielded conflicting results. A significant association between lycopene intake (estimated from tomato consumption) and decreased prostate cancer risk has been found in three studies,[99,100,206] as well as in a prospective study conducted historically using banked serum from the Health Professionals Follow-Up Study.[207] Serum lycopene levels were also correlated with decreased prostate cancer incidence in some series,[99,100,208] but not in several case-control studies evaluating lycopene serum levels [209] or lycopene intake.[210,211] Because of the conflicting nature of these results and the lack of a well-conducted prospective, randomized, controlled trial, the evidence cannot be considered conclusive.

Antioxidant
Summary
- Like other carotenoids, lycopene is purported to possess antioxidant, antiradical, singlet oxygen quenching, and gap-junction communication enhancement activities. Multiple *in vitro* studies have demonstrated antioxidant properties, whereas a limited number of others have suggested a lack of these effects. Overall, lycopene does appear to exert antioxidant properties *in vitro*. In human studies, however, there have been mixed results in this area. Most trials have focused on serum lycopene levels or consumption of tomatoes and tomato-based products rather than intake of lycopene supplements. Therefore, it remains unclear to what extent lycopene supplements exert clinically relevant antioxidant effects in humans, or whether these potential effects alter the progression of any disease.

Antioxidant (Supportive Evidence)

- An investigation in 57 patients with diabetes mellitus (type 2) assessing the intake of 500 mL of tomato juice daily vs. vitamin E and vitamin C over a 4-week period found tomato juice intake to be associated with a significant reduction in the susceptibility of low-density lipoproteins (LDLs) to oxidation.[87] Lymphocytes of 10 women consuming either a tomato-free diet or daily tomato puree in a crossover design experienced a significant decrease of 33% to 42% in oxidative damage after *ex vivo* exposure to hydrogen peroxide.[88] After consuming 25 g of tomato puree daily for 14 days, nine women showed significant increases in plasma and lymphocyte concentrations of lycopene and a significant 50% decrease in oxidative damage to lymphocytes.[89] A crossover study of 19 healthy individuals randomized to consume tomato juice, tomato oleoresin capsules, or spaghetti sauce for 1 week each showed a trend toward decreased protein and DNA oxidation; however, these results were not statistically significant.[59] An analysis of dietary lycopene intake in 20 healthy volunteers showed that after oxidative stresses (namely eating a meal and/or smoking three cigarettes), serum lycopene levels decreased.[90] *In vitro*, lycopene has been demonstrated to possess greater singlet oxygen quenching abilities [83,84] and greater antioxidant activity than other carotenoids.[75] Lycopene has been shown capable of scavenging the $ABTS^+$ radical cation with the most activity of all the carotenoids [85] and is twice as effective as β-carotene in protecting lymphocytes from nitrogen dioxide radical membrane damage.[85] An animal study demonstrated that lycopene, when given to rats in daily doses of 0.001 to 0.1 g/kg for 2 weeks, resulted in modification of antioxidant and drug metabolizing enzymes that are involved in the protection of cells from oxidative stress and malignant growth.[96]

Antioxidant (Negative Evidence)

- Conflicting results regarding lycopene as an antioxidant include a placebo-controlled study in which 175 males ingested 15 mg of lycopene daily for 3 months and experienced no enhancement in the resistance of their low-density lipoproteins (LDLs) to oxidation.[15] Biopsies of gastric mucosa in 44 subjects, 23 with *Helicobacter pylori* gastritis, showed increased concentrations of lycopene in the gastritis patients compared to normal subjects, suggesting that lycopene may have no role in protecting gastric mucosal cells from reactive oxygen species damage.[91] Increased serum lycopene levels were found to have no significant effect on the resistance of LDLs to oxidation in 15 renal transplant patients ingesting 330 mL of tomato juice daily for 4 weeks.[92] Pellegrini et al. instructed 11 women to eat a low-carotenoid diet for 1 week and then ingest 25 g of tomato puree daily.[93] At the end of 14 days, plasma lycopene levels had significantly increased in the women, but the total plasma "antioxidant capacity" had not significantly changed, suggesting that increased serum lycopene concentrations may not correspond with antioxidant activity. In one *in vitro* study evaluating the effect of carotenoids on LDL oxidation, lycopene was found to have no effect.[82]

Age-Related Macular Degeneration Prevention
Summary

- Based on its demonstrated antioxidant properties *in vitro*, lycopene has been suggested as a preventive therapy for age-related macular degeneration (ARMD).[59,61,75,83-89,96,212]

The current evidence is based on a small number of human observational and case-control studies. These investigations have been largely negative but, in the absence of reliable prospective randomized trials, can only be considered preliminary. Therefore, at this time the evidence cannot be considered adequate either for or against this use of lycopene.

Evidence

- A case-control trial found that subjects with serum lycopene levels in the lowest quintile were almost twice as likely to develop ARMD as subjects with lycopene levels in the highest quintile.[11] Of four additional studies, two found no significant association between dietary lycopene intake and the risk of ARMD,[9,213] and two found that increased serum lycopene levels did not result in any significant reduction in the development of ARMD.[10,214] Although this evidence for lycopene as a protectant against ARMD is largely negative, because it is not based on prospective randomized trials, it can only be considered preliminary. Further research may be warranted in this area.

Asthma (Exercise-Induced)
Summary

- A number of *in vitro* studies have demonstrated lycopene to possess antioxidant properties.[61,75,83-90,96] It has been theorized that these antioxidant properties may be beneficial in the prevention of exercise-induced asthma, although the biochemical basis for these theories has not been fully elucidated. A methodologically weak, small, randomized trial has reported beneficial effects of prophylactic lycopene supplementation on exercise-induced asthma. However, further evidence is warranted before a firm conclusion can be drawn.

Evidence

- In a randomized, double-blind trial assessing the effects of daily lycopene supplementation on exercise-induced asthma, 20 patients were randomly assigned to receive either 30 mg of lycopene (Lyc-O-Mato) daily or placebo.[39] Baseline pulmonary function tests (PFTs) were performed for all subjects before and after a period of exercise. Subjects then took their assigned study medication daily for 1 week, at which time PFTs were repeated. All subjects in the placebo group experienced a decreased forced expiratory volume in one second (FEV_1) following exercise, whereas 55% of those in the lycopene group were reported to be significantly protected from exercise-induced asthma. Although this study is suggestive, because of methodological weaknesses (including incomplete descriptions of randomization and blinding) and small sample size, the results can only be considered preliminary (and may not be generalizable). Further study is warranted before a recommendation can be made.

Atherosclerosis/Hyperlipidemia (Lipid Peroxidation)
Summary

- A number of retrospective epidemiologic studies have found lycopene levels in serum and adipose tissue to be inversely associated with the risk of coronary artery disease.[14,22,90] It has been hypothesized that these benefits may be due to the antioxidant properties of lycopene, reported *in vitro*.[61,75,83-90,96,215] Specifically, it has been suggested that antioxidants such as lycopene may reduce the risk of atherosclerosis progression via reduction of lipid peroxidation, although this remains an area of scientific controversy. Several studies have examined the association between lycopene and lycopene-containing foods with lipid peroxidation. Results have been mixed, although the majority of investigations have not found a positive correlation. Established clinical outcomes have not been measured. Therefore, there is currently insufficient evidence to recommend either for or against the use of lycopene for the management of atherosclerosis or hyperlipidemia.

Evidence

- Agarwal et al. randomized 19 healthy adults to receive daily lycopene in the form of 540 mL of tomato juice (H.J. Heinz Co., Canada), 126 g of spaghetti sauce (Hunt-Wesson, Inc., USA), and 1.243 g of 6% lycopene oleoresin capsules (LycoRed Natural Product Industries Ltd., Israel) for 1 week each in a crossover design.[40] The total study duration was 8 weeks and included a 1-week placebo phase and a 1-week washout period between each treatment. Subjects were instructed to avoid tomatoes and tomato-based foods for the duration of the study, and blood samples were analyzed for serum lycopene and serum low-density lipoprotein (LDL) levels at the end of each treatment period. Results showed serum lycopene levels to increase significantly with the daily intake of tomato juice, spaghetti sauce, and tomato oleoresin capsules vs. placebo, with no significant difference between the active treatment groups. No significant effect was seen on the total cholesterol or triglyceride levels between active groups and placebo. However, serum LDL oxidation was significantly decreased in the groups receiving lycopene products vs. placebo (odds ratio 1.9 to 2.2). These early preclinical results appear promising, although correlation with clinical outcomes is necessary before lycopene can be considered in the management of lipids or atherosclerosis.
- There is conflicting evidence from other human studies. Sutherland et al. randomized 15 renal transplant patients to receive either 200 mL of tomato juice or 200 mL of synthetic orange drink twice daily for 4 weeks each, in a crossover study, to assess the effect of plasma lycopene levels on reducing LDL susceptibility to oxidation.[92] The orange drink was used as a comparison to control for the vitamin C content in tomato juice. Serum samples were drawn at baseline, at 4 weeks, and at the end of the study to measure serum thiobarbituric acid–reacting substances (TBARS) and serum protein fluorescence as a measure of circulating lipid oxidation products (FLOP). Results showed that whereas serum lycopene levels increased significantly with tomato juice ingestion vs. control, there was no significant increase in the resistance of LDLs to oxidation.
- A randomized, double-blind, placebo-controlled trial examined the effects of an "antioxidant" tomato juice (supplemented with 600 mg of ascorbic acid, 30 mg of β-carotene, and 400 mg of *all-rac-α* tocopherol) vs. unsupplemented tomato juice (placebo) on LDL peroxidation in 39 smokers.[6] All subjects consumed placebo juice daily for 4 weeks, then ingested their assigned study juice daily for an additional 4 weeks. Measurements of LDL peroxidation were performed at baseline and after 4 and 8 weeks. No significant difference in plasma lycopene levels was found between the groups. The vitamin-supplemented tomato juice group experienced a significant increase in the resistance of LDLs to oxidation vs. placebo. Notably, the subjects consuming tomato juice ("controls") had significantly higher levels of lipid peroxidation, suggesting that lycopene may

not be the agent responsible for lipid peroxidation decreases observed in other trials or may not be as potent as other agents. However, these results can only be considered preliminary, particularly in light of conflicting evidence from other studies. More convincing evidence might be derived from longer-term studies using established clinical outcomes, which study specific lycopene supplement doses rather than tomato juice (which may contain other active agents.)

- Results from a randomized, controlled trial of antioxidant supplementation and its effect on indices of oxidative status in 175 health adult males found that 15 mg of lycopene ingested daily for 3 months caused no enhancement in the resistance of LDL to oxidation *in vitro*.[15]
- In a case-control study assessing the dietary antioxidant intake of two separate populations with significantly different indices of plasma lipid peroxidation, it was found that subjects from Naples, Italy, consumed significantly more tomatoes and tomato products than did the subjects from Bristol, UK.[216] It was hypothesized that this may be a reason for significantly lower indices of plasma lipid peroxidation in the Naples group. As with all studies of similar design, these results can only be considered preliminary and hypothesis-generating, since many potential confounders that cannot be measured (environmental and genetic) may play a role in the differences between two disparate populations.

Immunostimulation (Cell-Mediated)
Summary

- The effect of carotenoids on immune status has been investigated for β-carotene, but studies involving other carotenoids are less common. A small number of randomized, controlled trials have examined the effects of lycopene consumption on human immune function and found a lack of effect, particularly regarding cell-mediated immunity. Although these studies are limited in number and have investigated only a subset of immune functions, the available evidence is sufficient to conclude a lack of efficacy.

Evidence

- Watzl et al. studied the effect of tomato juice consumption (330 mL daily for 8 weeks) vs. water in 53 healthy elderly subjects.[217] Assessment of immune status was based on the number of natural killer cells found in the serum, the secretion of cytokines, lymphocyte proliferation, and delayed-type hypersensitivity. The investigators found that the daily intake of tomato juice by the subjects resulted in no change in cell-mediated immunity compared to the intake of mineral water.
- A randomized, placebo-controlled, crossover study was conducted by Hughes et al. to assess the effect of lycopene on the expression of monocyte cell surface molecules in 20 healthy volunteers.[104] Results showed that supplementation with 15 mg of lycopene daily for 28 days had no effect on the expression of these molecules, making the role of lycopene in immune enhancement questionable. A second study, similar to the first but assessing the effect of 15 mg of lycopene, 15 mg of lutein, or placebo, taken daily for 26 days in a crossover design found the same results.[105]
- Corridan et al. conducted a double-blind, randomized trial comparing daily supplementation with 13.3 mg of lycopene (Lyco-O-Pen; LycoRed Natural Products Industries Ltd., Israel), 8.2 mg of β-carotene (Biocon Caroteen; Quest International, Netherlands), or placebo (containing 0.5 mg of corn oil, 0.06 mg of α-tocopherol, 0.23 mg of γ-tocopherol;

RP Scherer, USA) in 58 healthy, elderly subjects.[41] Both active capsules also contained unspecified amounts of α- and γ-tocopherols. Before and after the 12-week treatment, T-cell subsets and the expression of functionally associated cell surface molecules were measured and compared in blood samples from each subject. The authors reported that neither the β-carotene nor the lycopene groups experienced significant effects on the enhancement of cell-mediated immunity.

Sun Protection
Summary

- Lycopene in combination with other carotenoids, such as beta-carotene, vitamins C and E, selenium, and proanthocyanidins, has been proposed to protect skin from ultraviolet (UV) skin damage—for example, due to sun exposure. Selected protective effects from UV rays have been observed in small, short-term studies.[218-221] Additional research is necessary before a firm conclusion can be drawn.

FORMULARY: BRANDS USED IN CLINICAL TRIALS
Brands Used in Clinical Trials

- Lyc-O-Mato, LycoRed Natural Product Industries Ltd., Israel.[39]
- Lyco-O-Pen, LycoRed Natural Products Industries Ltd., Israel.[41]
- Lycobeads.[113]

References

1. Bruemmer B, White E, Vaughan TL, et al. Nutrient intake in relation to bladder cancer among middle-aged men and women. Am J Epidemiol 1996;144(5):485-495.
2. Helzlsouer KJ, Comstock GW, Morris JS. Selenium, lycopene, alpha-tocopherol, beta-carotene, retinol, and subsequent bladder cancer. Cancer Res 1989;49(21):6144-6148.
3. Okajima E, Ozono S, Endo T, et al. Chemopreventive efficacy of piroxicam administered alone or in combination with lycopene and beta-carotene on the development of rat urinary bladder carcinoma after N-butyl-N-(4-hydroxybutyl)nitrosamine treatment. Jpn J Cancer Res 1997;88(6):543-552.
4. Okajima E, Tsutsumi M, Ozono S, et al. Inhibitory effect of tomato juice on rat urinary bladder carcinogenesis after N-butyl-N-(4-hydroxybutyl)nitrosamine initiation. Jpn J Cancer Res 1998;89(1):22-26.
5. Riboli E, Gonzalez CA, Lopez-Abente G, et al. Diet and bladder cancer in Spain: a multi-centre case-control study. Int J Cancer 1991;49(2):214-219.
6. Steinberg FM, Chait A. Antioxidant vitamin supplementation and lipid peroxidation in smokers. Am J Clin Nutr 1998;68(2):319-327.
7. Pierce JP, Faerber S, Wright FA, et al. Feasibility of a randomized trial of a high-vegetable diet to prevent breast cancer recurrence. Nutr Cancer 1997;28(3):282-288.
8. Rock CL, Flatt SW, Wright FA, et al. Responsiveness of carotenoids to a high vegetable diet intervention designed to prevent breast cancer recurrence. Cancer Epidemiol Biomarkers Prev 1997;6(8):617-623.
9. Brown L, Rimm EB, Seddon JM, et al. A prospective study of carotenoid intake and risk of cataract extraction in US men. Am J Clin Nutr 1999;70(4):517-524.
10. Lyle BJ, Mares-Perlman JA, Klein BE, et al. Serum carotenoids and tocopherols and incidence of age-related nuclear cataract. Am J Clin Nutr 1999;69(2):272-277.
11. Mares-Perlman JA, Brady WE, Klein R, et al. Serum antioxidants and age-related macular degeneration in a population-based case-control study. Arch Ophthalmol 1995;113(12):1518-1523.
12. Schmidt R, Hayn M, Reinhart B, et al. Plasma antioxidants and cognitive performance in middle-aged and older adults: results of the Austrian Stroke Prevention Study. J Am Geriatr Soc 1998;46(11):1407-1410.
13. Knekt P, Reunanen A, Jarvinen R, et al. Antioxidant vitamin intake and coronary mortality in a longitudinal population study. Am J Epidemiol 1994;139(12):1180-1189.
14. Kristenson M, Zieden B, Kucinskiene Z, et al. Antioxidant state and mortality from coronary heart disease in Lithuanian and Swedish men: concomitant cross sectional study of men aged 50. BMJ 1997;314(7081):629-633.
15. Hininger IA, Meyer-Wenger A, Moser U, et al. No significant effects of lutein, lycopene or beta-carotene supplementation on biological markers of oxidative stress and LDL oxidizability in healthy adult subjects. J Am Coll Nutr 2001;20(3):232-238.
16. Morris DL, Kritchevsky SB, Davis CE. Serum carotenoids and coronary heart disease. The Lipid Research Clinics Coronary Primary Prevention Trial and Follow-up Study. JAMA 1994;272(18):1439-1441.
17. Brown LM, Blot WJ, Schuman SH, et al. Environmental factors and high risk of esophageal cancer among men in coastal South Carolina. J Natl Cancer Inst 1988;80(20):1620-1625.
18. Cook-Mozaffari PJ, Azordegan F, Day NE, et al. Oesophageal cancer studies in the Caspian Littoral of Iran: results of a case-control study. Br J Cancer 1979;39(3):293-309.
19. Zheng W, Blot WJ, Shu XO, et al. Diet and other risk factors for laryngeal cancer in Shanghai, China. Am J Epidemiol 1992;136(2):178-191.
20. Muscat JE, Huncharek M. Dietary intake and the risk of malignant mesothelioma. Br J Cancer 1996;73(9):1122-1125.
21. Hak AE, Stampfer MJ, Campos H, et al. Plasma carotenoids and tocopherols and risk of myocardial infarction in a low-risk population of US male physicians. Circulation 2003;108(7):802-807.
22. Kohlmeier L, Kark JD, Gomez-Gracia E, et al. Lycopene and myocardial infarction risk in the EURAMIC Study. Am J Epidemiol 1997;146(8):618-626.
23. Street DA, Comstock GW, Salkeld RM, et al. Serum antioxidants and myocardial infarction. Are low levels of carotenoids and alpha-tocopherol risk factors for myocardial infarction? Circulation 1994;90(3):1154-1161.
24. Cramer DW, Kuper H, Harlow BL, et al. Carotenoids, antioxidants and ovarian cancer risk in pre- and postmenopausal women. Int J Cancer 2001;94(1):128-134.
25. Helzlsouer KJ, Alberg AJ, Norkus EP, et al. Prospective study of serum micronutrients and ovarian cancer. J Natl Cancer Inst 1996;88(1):32-37.
26. Baghurst PA, McMichael AJ, Slavotinek AH, et al. A case-control study of diet and cancer of the pancreas. Am J Epidemiol 1991;134(2):167-179.
27. Bueno de Mesquita HB, Maisonneuve P, Runia S, et al. Intake of foods and nutrients and cancer of the exocrine pancreas: a population-based case-control study in The Netherlands. Int J Cancer 1991;48(4):540-549.
28. Burney PG, Comstock GW, Morris JS. Serologic precursors of cancer: serum micronutrients and the subsequent risk of pancreatic cancer. Am J Clin Nutr 1989;49(5):895-900.
29. Mills PK, Beeson WL, Abbey DE, et al. Dietary habits and past medical history as related to fatal pancreas cancer risk among Adventists. Cancer 1988;61(12):2578-2585.
30. Morris-Stiff GJ, Bowrey DJ, Oleesky D, et al. The antioxidant profiles of patients with recurrent acute and chronic pancreatitis. Am J Gastroenterol 1999;94(8):2135-2140.
31. Jimenez-Jimenez FJ, Molina JA, Fernandez-Calle P, et al. Serum levels of beta-carotene and other carotenoids in Parkinson's disease. Neurosci Lett 1993;157(1):103-106.
32. Franceschi S, Bidoli E, Baron AE, et al. Nutrition and cancer of the oral cavity and pharynx in north-east Italy. Int J Cancer 1991;47(1):20-25.
33. Breslow RA, Alberg AJ, Helzlsouer KJ, et al. Serological precursors of cancer: malignant melanoma, basal and squamous cell skin cancer, and prediagnostic levels of retinol, beta-carotene, lycopene, alpha-tocopherol, and selenium. Cancer Epidemiol Biomarkers Prev 1995;4(8):837-842.
34. Ascherio A, Rimm EB, Hernan MA, et al. Relation of consumption of vitamin E, vitamin C, and carotenoids to risk for stroke among men in the United States. Ann Intern Med 1999;130(12):963-970.
35. Gillman MW, Cupples LA, Gagnon D, et al. Protective effect of fruits and vegetables on development of stroke in men. JAMA 1995;273(14):1113-1117.
36. Boeing H, Jedrychowski W, Wahrendorf J, et al. Dietary risk factors in intestinal and diffuse types of stomach cancer: a multicenter case-control study in Poland. Cancer Causes Control 1991;2(4):227-233.
37. Nomura AM, Kolonel LN, Hankin JH, et al. Dietary factors in cancer of the lower urinary tract. Int J Cancer 1991;48(2):199-205.
38. Beecher GR. Nutrient content of tomatoes and tomato products. Proc Soc Exp Biol Med 1998;218(2):98-100.
39. Neuman I, Nahum H, Ben Amotz A. Reduction of exercise-induced asthma oxidative stress by lycopene, a natural antioxidant. Allergy 2000;55(12):1184-1189.
40. Agarwal S, Rao AV. Tomato lycopene and low density lipoprotein oxidation: a human dietary intervention study. Lipids 1998;33(10):981-984.
41. Corridan BM, O'Donoghue M, Hughes DA, et al. Low-dose supplementation with lycopene or beta-carotene does not enhance cell-mediated immunity in healthy free-living elderly humans. Eur J Clin Nutr 2001;55(8):627-635.
42. Khachik F, Spangler CJ, Smith JC, Jr., et al. Identification, quantification, and relative concentrations of carotenoids and their metabolites in human milk and serum. Anal Chem 1997;69(10):1873-1881.
43. Clinton SK. Lycopene: chemistry, biology, and implications for human health and disease. Nutr Rev 1998;56(2 Pt 1):35-51.
44. Fuhrman B, Elis A, Aviram M. Hypocholesterolemic effect of lycopene and beta-carotene is related to suppression of cholesterol synthesis and augmentation of LDL receptor activity in macrophages. Biochem Biophys Res Commun 1997;233(3):658-662.
45. Parker RS. Absorption, metabolism, and transport of carotenoids. FASEB J 1996;10(5):542-551.
46. Ziouzenkova O, Winklhofer-Roob BM, Puhl H, et al. Lack of correlation

between the alpha-tocopherol content of plasma and LDL, but high correlations for gamma-tocopherol and carotenoids. J Lipid Res 1996; 37(9):1936-1946.

47. Brady WE, Mares-Perlman JA, Bowen P, et al. Human serum carotenoid concentrations are related to physiologic and lifestyle factors. J Nutr 1996; 126(1):129-137.

48. Campbell DR, Gross MD, Martini MC, et al. Plasma carotenoids as biomarkers of vegetable and fruit intake. Cancer Epidemiol Biomarkers Prev 1994;3(6):493-500.

49. Casso D, White E, Patterson RE, et al. Correlates of serum lycopene in older women. Nutr Cancer 2000;36(2):163-169.

50. Johnson EJ. Human studies on bioavailability and plasma response of lycopene. Proc Soc Exp Biol Med 1998;218(2):115-120.

51. Steinmetz KA, Potter JD, Folsom AR. Vegetables, fruit, and lung cancer in the Iowa Women's Health Study. Cancer Res 1993;53(3):536-543.

52. Elinder LS, Hadell K, Johansson J, et al. Probucol treatment decreases serum concentrations of diet-derived antioxidants. Arterioscler Thromb Vasc Biol 1995;15(8):1057-1063.

53. Palan PR, Mikhail MS, Goldberg GL, et al. Plasma levels of beta-carotene, lycopene, canthaxanthin, retinol, and alpha- and tau-tocopherol in cervical intraepithelial neoplasia and cancer. Clin Cancer Res 1996;2(1):181-185.

54. Potischman N, Hoover RN, Brinton LA, et al. The relations between cervical cancer and serological markers of nutritional status. Nutr Cancer 1994;21(3):193-201.

55. Mayne ST, Cartmel B, Silva F, et al. Plasma lycopene concentrations in humans are determined by lycopene intake, plasma cholesterol concentrations and selected demographic factors. J Nutr 1999;129(4):849-854.

56. Marangon K, Herbeth B, Lecomte E, et al. Diet, antioxidant status, and smoking habits in French men. Am J Clin Nutr 1998;67(2):231-239.

57. Pamuk ER, Byers T, Coates RJ, et al. Effect of smoking on serum nutrient concentrations in African-American women. Am J Clin Nutr 1994;59(4):891-895.

58. Peng YM, Peng YS, Lin Y, et al. Concentrations and plasma-tissue-diet relationships of carotenoids, retinoids, and tocopherols in humans. Nutr Cancer 1995;23(3):233-246.

59. Rao AV, Agarwal S. Bioavailability and in vivo antioxidant properties of lycopene from tomato products and their possible role in the prevention of cancer. Nutr Cancer 1998;31(3):199-203.

60. Tsubono Y, Tsugane S, Gey KF. Differential effects of cigarette smoking and alcohol consumption on the plasma levels of carotenoids in middle-aged Japanese men. Jpn J Cancer Res 1996;87(6):563-569.

61. Arab L, Steck S. Lycopene and cardiovascular disease. Am J Clin Nutr 2000;71(6 Suppl):1691S-1695S.

62. Handelman GJ, Packer L, Cross CE. Destruction of tocopherols, carotenoids, and retinol in human plasma by cigarette smoke. Am J Clin Nutr 1996;63(4):559-565.

63. van der Gaag MS, van den BR, van den BH, et al. Moderate consumption of beer, red wine and spirits has counteracting effects on plasma antioxidants in middle-aged men. Eur J Clin Nutr 2000;54(7):586-591.

64. Johnson EJ, Qin J, Krinsky NI, et al. Ingestion by men of a combined dose of beta-carotene and lycopene does not affect the absorption of beta-carotene but improves that of lycopene. J Nutr 1997;127(9):1833-1837.

65. Wahlqvist ML, Wattanapenpaiboon N, Macrae FA, et al. Changes in serum carotenoids in subjects with colorectal adenomas after 24 mo of beta-carotene supplementation. Australian Polyp Prevention Project Investigators. Am J Clin Nutr 1994;60(6):936-943.

66. Micozzi MS, Brown ED, Edwards BK, et al. Plasma carotenoid response to chronic intake of selected foods and beta- carotene supplements in men. Am J Clin Nutr 1992;55(6):1120-1125.

67. Nierenberg DW, Dain BJ, Mott LA, et al. Effects of 4 y of oral supplementation with beta-carotene on serum concentrations of retinol, tocopherol, and five carotenoids. Am J Clin Nutr 1997;66(2):315-319.

68. Palan PR, Chang CJ, Mikhail MS, et al. Plasma concentrations of micronutrients during a nine-month clinical trial of beta-carotene in women with precursor cervical cancer lesions. Nutr Cancer 1998;30(1):46-52.

69. Ribaya-Mercado JD, Garmyn M, Gilchrest BA, et al. Skin lycopene is destroyed preferentially over beta-carotene during ultraviolet irradiation in humans. J Nutr 1995;125(7):1854-1859.

70. Ribaya-Mercado JD, Ordovas JM, Russell RM. Effect of beta-carotene supplementation on the concentrations and distribution of carotenoids, vitamin E, vitamin A, and cholesterol in plasma lipoprotein and non-lipoprotein fractions in healthy older women. J Am Coll Nutr 1995;14(6):614-620.

71. van den Berg H, van Vliet T. Effect of simultaneous, single oral doses of beta-carotene with lutein or lycopene on the beta-carotene and retinyl ester responses in the triacylglycerol-rich lipoprotein fraction of men. Am J Clin Nutr 1998;68(1):82-89.

72. Gaziano JM, Johnson EJ, Russell RM, et al. Discrimination in absorption or transport of beta-carotene isomers after oral supplementation with either all-trans- or 9-cis-beta- carotene. Am J Clin Nutr 1995;61(6):1248-1252.

73. Blakely SR, Brown ED, Babu U, et al. Bioavailability of carotenoids in tomato paste and dried spinach and their interactions with canthaxanthin. FASEB J 1994;8:192.

74. Amir H, Karas M, Giat J, et al. Lycopene and 1,25-dihydroxyvitamin D3

cooperate in the inhibition of cell cycle progression and induction of differentiation in HL-60 leukemic cells. Nutr Cancer 1999;33(1):105-112.

75. Stahl W, Junghans A, de Boer B, et al. Carotenoid mixtures protect multilamellar liposomes against oxidative damage: synergistic effects of lycopene and lutein. FEBS Lett 1998;427(2):305-308.

76. Pastori M, Pfander H, Boscoboinik D, et al. Lycopene in association with alpha-tocopherol inhibits at physiological concentrations proliferation of prostate carcinoma cells. Biochem Biophys Res Commun 1998;250(3):582-585.

77. Koonsvitsky BP, Berry DA, Jones MB, et al. Olestra affects serum concentrations of alpha-tocopherol and carotenoids but not vitamin D or vitamin K status in free-living subjects. J Nutr 1997;127(8 Suppl):1636S-1645S.

78. Velthuis-te Wierik EJ, van den BH, Weststrate JA, et al. Consumption of reduced-fat products: effects on parameters of anti- oxidative capacity. Eur J Clin Nutr 1996;50(4):214-219.

79. Weststrate JA, het Hof KH, van den BH, et al. A comparison of the effect of free access to reduced fat products or their full fat equivalents on food intake, body weight, blood lipids and fat-soluble antioxidants levels and haemostasis variables. Eur J Clin Nutr 1998;52(6):389-395.

80. Edwards AJ, Vinyard BT, Wiley ER, et al. Consumption of watermelon juice increases plasma concentrations of lycopene and beta-carotene in humans. J Nutr 2003;133(4):1043-1050.

81. Fish WW, Davis AR. The effects of frozen storage conditions on lycopene stability in watermelon tissue. J Agric Food Chem 2003;51(12):3582-3585.

82. Dugas TR, Morel DW, Harrison EH. Dietary supplementation with beta-carotene, but not with lycopene, inhibits endothelial cell-mediated oxidation of low-density lipoprotein. Free Radic Biol Med 1999;26(9-10):1238-1244.

83. Tinkler JH, Bohm F, Schalch W, et al. Dietary carotenoids protect human cells from damage. J Photochem Photobiol B 1994;26(3):283-285.

84. Di Mascio P, Kaiser S, Sies H. Lycopene as the most efficient biological carotenoid singlet oxygen quencher. Arch Biochem Biophys 1989;274(2):532-538.

85. Miller NJ, Sampson J, Candeias LP, et al. Antioxidant activities of carotenes and xanthophylls. FEBS Lett 1996;384(3):240-242.

86. Bohm F, Tinkler JH, Truscott TG. Carotenoids protect against cell membrane damage by the nitrogen dioxide radical. Nat Med 1995;1(2):98-99.

87. Upritchard JE, Sutherland WH, Mann JI. Effect of supplementation with tomato juice, vitamin E, and vitamin C on LDL oxidation and products of inflammatory activity in type 2 diabetes. Diabetes Care 2000;23(6):733-738.

88. Riso P, Pinder A, Santangelo A, et al. Does tomato consumption effectively increase the resistance of lymphocyte DNA to oxidative damage? Am J Clin Nutr 1999;69(4):712-718.

89. Porrini M, Riso P. Lymphocyte lycopene concentration and DNA protection from oxidative damage is increased in women after a short period of tomato consumption. J Nutr 2000;130(2):189-192.

90. Rao AV, Agarwal S. Effect of diet and smoking on serum lycopene and lipid peroxidation. Nutrit Research 1998;18(4):713-721.

91. Sanderson MJ, White KL, Drake IM, et al. Vitamin E and carotenoids in gastric biopsies: the relation to plasma concentrations in patients with and without Helicobacter pylori gastritis. Am J Clin Nutr 1997;65(1):101-106.

92. Sutherland WH, Walker RJ, De Jong SA, et al. Supplementation with tomato juice increases plasma lycopene but does not alter susceptibility to oxidation of low-density lipoproteins from renal transplant recipients. Clin Nephrol 1999;52(1):30-36.

93. Pellegrini N, Riso P, Porrini M. Tomato consumption does not affect the total antioxidant capacity of plasma. Nutrition 2000;16(4):268-271.

94. Levy J, Sharoni Y. Lycopene interferes in vivo and in vitro with the IGF system. Brit Med J 2001;54(1):46.

95. Levy J, Bosin E, Feldman B, et al. Lycopene is a more potent inhibitor of human cancer cell proliferation than either alpha-carotene or beta-carotene. Nutr Cancer 1995;24(3):257-266.

96. Breinholt V, Lauridsen ST, Daneshvar B, et al. Dose-response effects of lycopene on selected drug-metabolizing and antioxidant enzymes in the rat. Cancer Lett 2000;154(2):201-210.

97. Nagasawa H, Mitamura T, Sakamoto S, et al. Effects of lycopene on spontaneous mammary tumour development in SHN virgin mice. Anticancer Res 1995;15(4):1173-1178.

98. Sharoni Y, Giron E, Rise M, et al. Effects of lycopene-enriched tomato oleoresin on 7,12-dimethyl- benz[a]anthracene-induced rat mammary tumors. Cancer Detect Prev 1997;21(2):118-123.

99. Clinton SK, Emenhiser C, Giovannucci EL, et al. Cis-trans isomers of lycopene in the human prostate: a role in cancer prevention? FASEB J 1995;9:A442.

100. Clinton SK, Emenhiser C, Schwartz SJ, et al. cis-trans lycopene isomers, carotenoids, and retinol in the human prostate. Cancer Epidemiol Biomarkers Prev 1996;5(10):823-833.

101. Zhang LX, Cooney RV, Bertram JS. Carotenoids enhance gap junctional communication and inhibit lipid peroxidation in C3H/10T1/2 cells: relationship to their cancer chemopreventive action. Carcinogenesis 1991;12(11):2109-2114.

102. Wright AJ, Hughes DA, Bailey AL, et al. Beta-carotene and lycopene, but

not lutein, supplementation changes the plasma fatty acid profile of healthy male non-smokers. J Lab Clin Med 1999;134(6):592-598.

103. Stahl W, Heinrich U, Wiseman S, et al. Dietary tomato paste protects against ultraviolet light-induced erythema in humans. J Nutr 2001;131(5): 1449-1451.

104. Hughes DA, Wright AJ, Finglas PM, et al. Comparison of effects of beta-carotene and lycopene supplementation on the expression of functionally associated molecules on human monocytes. Biocheml Soc Trans 1997; 25(2):206S.

105. Hughes DA, Wright AJ, Finglas PM, et al. Effects of lycopene and lutein supplementation on the expression of functionally associated surface molecules on blood monocytes from healthy male nonsmokers. J Infect Dis 2000;182(Suppl 1):S11-S15.

106. Gartner C, Stahl W, Sies H. Lycopene is more bioavailable from tomato paste than from fresh tomatoes. Am J Clin Nutr 1997;66(1):116-122.

107. Holloway DE, Yang M, Paganga G, et al. Isomerization of dietary lycopene during assimilation and transport in plasma. Free Radic Res 2000; 32(1):93-102.

108. Porrini M, Riso P, Testolin G. Absorption of lycopene from single or daily portions of raw and processed tomato. Br J Nutr 1998;80(4):353-361.

109. Shi J, Le Maguer M. Lycopene in tomatoes: chemical and physical properties affected by food processing. Crit Rev Food Sci Nutr 2000; 40(1):1-42.

110. Nguyen ML, Schwartz SJ. Lycopene stability during food processing. Proc Soc Exp Biol Med 1998;218(2):101-105.

111. Le Marchand L, Hankin JH, Carter FS, et al. A pilot study on the use of plasma carotenoids and ascorbic acid as markers of compliance to a high fruit and vegetable dietary intervention. Cancer Epidemiol Biomarkers Prev 1994;3(3):245-251.

112. Paetau I, Rao D, Wiley ER, et al. Carotenoids in human buccal mucosa cells after 4 wk of supplementation with tomato juice or lycopene supplements. Am J Clin Nutr 1999;70(4):490-494.

113. Paetau I, Khachik F, Brown ED, et al. Chronic ingestion of lycopene-rich tomato juice or lycopene supplements significantly increases plasma concentrations of lycopene and related tomato carotenoids in humans. Am J Clin Nutr 1998;68(6):1187-1195.

114. Martini MC, Campbell DR, Gross MD, et al. Plasma carotenoids as biomarkers of vegetable intake: the University of Minnesota Cancer Prevention Research Unit Feeding Studies. Cancer Epidemiol Biomarkers Prev 1995;4(5):491-496.

115. Smith-Warner SA, Elmer PJ, Tharp TM, et al. Increasing vegetable and fruit intake: randomized intervention and monitoring in an at-risk population. Cancer Epidemiol Biomarkers Prev 2000;9(3):307-317.

116. Garg V, Stacewicz-Sapuntzakis M. Lycopene absorption kinetics after a single dose of tomato oleoresin. FASEB J 1994;8:A192.

117. Stahl W, Sies H. Lycopene: a biologically important carotenoid for humans? Arch Biochem Biophys 1996;336(1):1-9.

118. Sowell AL, Huff DL, Yeager PR, et al. Retinol, alpha-tocopherol, lutein/zeaxanthin, beta-cryptoxanthin, lycopene, alpha-carotene, trans-beta-carotene, and four retinyl esters in serum determined simultaneously by reversed-phase HPLC with multiwavelength detection. Clin Chem 1994; 40(3):411-416.

119. Clark RM, Yao L, She L, et al. A comparison of lycopene and canthaxanthin absorption: using the rat to study the absorption of non-provitamin A carotenoids. Lipids 1998;33(2):159-163.

120. O'Neill ME, Thurnham DI. Intestinal absorption of beta-carotene, lycopene and lutein in men and women following a standard meal: response curves in the triacylglycerol- rich lipoprotein fraction. Br J Nutr 1998;79(2):149-159.

121. Stahl W, Sies H. Uptake of lycopene and its geometrical isomers is greater from heat- processed than from unprocessed tomato juice in humans. J Nutr 1992;122(11):2161-2166.

122. Kaplan LA, Lau JM, Stein EA. Carotenoid composition, concentrations, and relationships in various human organs. Clin Physiol Biochem 1990;8(1):1-10.

123. Gerster H. The potential role of lycopene for human health. J Am Coll Nutr 1997;16(2):109-126.

124. Schmitz HH, Poor CL, Wellman RB, et al. Concentrations of selected carotenoids and vitamin A in human liver, kidney and lung tissue. J Nutr 1991;121(10):1613-1621.

125. Stahl W, Schwarz W, Sundquist AR, et al. cis-trans isomers of lycopene and beta-carotene in human serum and tissues. Arch Biochem Biophys 1992; 294(1):173-177.

126. Bates CJ, Chen SJ, Macdonald A, et al. Quantitation of vitamin E and a carotenoid pigment in cataractous human lenses, and the effect of a dietary supplement. Int J Vitam Nutr Res 1996;66(4):316-321.

127. Peng YM, Peng YS, Lin Y, et al. Micronutrient concentrations in paired skin and plasma of patients with actinic keratoses: effect of prolonged retinol supplementation. Cancer Epidemiol Biomarkers Prev 1993;2(2): 145-150.

128. Giuliano AR, Neilson EM, Yap H, et al. Quantitation of and inter/intra-individual variability in major carotenoids of mature human milk. J Nutr Biochem 1994;5:551-556.

129. Yeum KJ, Ferland G, Patry J, et al. Relationship of plasma carotenoids, retinol and tocopherols in mothers and newborn infants. J Am Coll Nutr 1998;17(5):442-447.

130. Khachik F, Beecher GR, Smith JC, Jr. Lutein, lycopene, and their oxidative metabolites in chemoprevention of cancer. J Cell Biochem Suppl 1995; 22:236-246.

131. Burri BJ, Neidlinger TR, Clifford AJ. Serum carotenoid depletion follows first-order kinetics in healthy adult women fed naturally low carotenoid diets. J Nutr 2001;131(8):2096-2100.

132. Vogel S, Contois JH, Tucker KL, et al. Plasma retinol and plasma and lipoprotein tocopherol and carotenoid concentrations in healthy elderly participants of the Framingham Heart Study. Am J Clin Nutr 1997;66(4): 950-958.

133. Olmedilla B, Granado F, Gil-Martinez E, et al. Reference values for retinol, tocopherol, and main carotenoids in serum of control and insulin-dependent diabetic Spanish subjects. Clin Chem 1997;43(6 Pt 1):1066-1071.

134. Granado F, Olmedilla B, Gil-Martinez E, et al. Carotenoids, retinol and tocopherols in patients with insulin-dependent diabetes mellitus and their immediate relatives. Clin Sci (Colch) 1998;94(2):189-195.

135. Polidori MC, Mecocci P, Stahl W, et al. Plasma levels of lipophilic antioxidants in very old patients with type 2 diabetes. Diabetes Metab Res Rev 2000;16(1):15-19.

136. Ford ES, Will JC, Bowman BA, et al. Diabetes mellitus and serum carotenoids: findings from the Third National Health and Nutrition Examination Survey. Am J Epidemiol 1999;149(2):168-176.

137. Olmedilla B, Granado F, Blanco I, et al. Seasonal and sex-related variations in six serum carotenoids, retinol, and alpha-tocopherol. Am J Clin Nutr 1994;60(1):106-110.

138. Mangels AR, Holden JM, Beecher GR, et al. Carotenoid content of fruits and vegetables: an evaluation of analytic data. J Am Diet Assoc 1993; 93(3):284-296.

139. Micozzi MS, Beecher GR, Taylor PR, et al. Carotenoid analyses of selected raw and cooked foods associated with a lower risk for cancer. J Natl Cancer Inst 1990;82(4):282-285.

140. Giovannucci E. Tomatoes, tomato-based products, lycopene, and cancer: review of the epidemiologic literature. J Natl Cancer Inst 1999;91(4): 317-331.

141. Block G, Patterson B, Subar A. Fruit, vegetables, and cancer prevention: a review of the epidemiological evidence. Nutr Cancer 1992;18(1):1-29.

142. Rao AV, Agarwal S. Role of lycopene as antioxidant carotenoid in the prevention of chronic diseases: a review. Nutrit Research 1999;19(2): 305-323.

143. Sengupta A, Das S. The anti-carcinogenic role of lycopene, abundantly present in tomato. Eur J Cancer Prev 1999;8(4):325-330.

144. Sies H, Stahl W. Vitamins E and C, beta-carotene, and other carotenoids as antioxidants. Am J Clin Nutr 1995;62(6 Suppl):1315S-1321S.

145. Sies H, Stahl W. Lycopene: antioxidant and biological effects and its bio-availability in the human. Proc Soc Exp Biol Med 1998;218(2):121-124.

146. Steinmetz KA, Potter JD. Vegetables, fruit, and cancer. II. Mechanisms. Cancer Causes Control 1991;2(6):427-442.

147. Ziegler RG. Vegetables, fruits, and carotenoids and the risk of cancer. Am J Clin Nutr 1991;53(1 Suppl):251S-259S.

148. Negri E, La Vecchia C, Franceschi S, et al. Vegetable and fruit consumption and cancer risk. Int J Cancer 1991;48(3):350-354.

149. Colditz GA, Branch LG, Lipnick RJ, et al. Increased green and yellow vegetable intake and lowered cancer deaths in an elderly population. Am J Clin Nutr 1985;41(1):32-36.

150. Dorgan JF, Sowell A, Swanson CA, et al. Relationships of serum carotenoids, retinol, alpha-tocopherol, and selenium with breast cancer risk: results from a prospective study in Columbia, Missouri (United States). Cancer Causes Control 1998;9(1):89-97.

151. Potischman N, McCulloch CE, Byers T, et al. Breast cancer and dietary and plasma concentrations of carotenoids and vitamin A. Am J Clin Nutr 1990;52(5):909-915.

152. Zhang S, Tang G, Russell RM, et al. Measurement of retinoids and carotenoids in breast adipose tissue and a comparison of concentrations in breast cancer cases and control subjects. Am J Clin Nutr 1997;66(3): 626-632.

153. Zhang S, Hunter DJ, Forman MR, et al. Dietary carotenoids and vitamins A, C, and E and risk of breast cancer. J Natl Cancer Inst 1999;91(6): 547-556.

154. Freudenheim JL, Marshall JR, Vena JE, et al. Premenopausal breast cancer risk and intake of vegetables, fruits, and related nutrients. J Natl Cancer Inst 1996;88(6):340-348.

155. Jarvinen R, Knekt P, Seppanen R, et al. Diet and breast cancer risk in a cohort of Finnish women. Cancer Lett 1997;114(1-2):251-253.

156. Levi F, La Vecchia C, Gulie C, et al. Dietary factors and breast cancer risk in Vaud, Switzerland. Nutr Cancer 1993;19(3):327-335.

157. London SJ, Stein EA, Henderson IC, et al. Carotenoids, retinol, and vitamin E and risk of proliferative benign breast disease and breast cancer. Cancer Causes Control 1992;3(6):503-512.

158. Simon MS, Djuric Z, Dunn B, et al. An evaluation of plasma antioxidant levels and the risk of breast cancer: a pilot case control study. Breast J 2000;6(6):388-395.

159. Cohen LA, Zhao Z, Pittman B, et al. Effect of dietary lycopene on

N-methylnitrosourea–induced mammary tumorigenesis. Nutr Cancer 1999;34(2):153-159.

160. Batieha AM, Armenian HK, Norkus EP, et al. Serum micronutrients and the subsequent risk of cervical cancer in a population-based nested case-control study. Cancer Epidemiol Biomarkers Prev 1993;2(4):335-339.

161. de Vet HC, Knipschild PG, Grol ME, et al. The role of beta-carotene and other dietary factors in the aetiology of cervical dysplasia: results of a case-control study. Int J Epidemiol 1991;20(3):603-610.

162. Kantesky PA, Gammon MD, Mandelblatt J, et al. Dietary intake and blood levels of lycopene: association with cervical dysplasia among non-Hispanic, black women. Nutr Cancer 1998;31(1):31-40.

163. Potischman N, Herrero R, Brinton LA, et al. A case-control study of nutrient status and invasive cervical cancer. II. Serologic indicators. Am J Epidemiol 1991;134(11):1347-1355.

164. VanEenwyk J, Davis FG, Bowen PE. Dietary and serum carotenoids and cervical intraepithelial neoplasia. Int J Cancer 1991;48(1):34-38.

165. Franceschi S, Bidoli E, La Vecchia C, et al. Tomatoes and risk of digestive-tract cancers. Int J Cancer 1994;59(2):181-184.

166. La Vecchia C, Negri E, Decarli A, et al. A case-control study of diet and gastric cancer in northern Italy. Int J Cancer 1987;40(4):484-489.

167. Bidoli E, Franceschi S, Talamini R, et al. Food consumption and cancer of the colon and rectum in north-eastern Italy. Int J Cancer 1992;50(2):223-229.

168. De Stefani E, Oreggia F, Boffetta P, et al. Tomatoes, tomato-rich foods, lycopene and cancer of the upper aerodigestive tract: a case-control in Uruguay. Oral Oncol 2000;36(1):47-53.

169. Correa P, Fontham E, Pickle LW, et al. Dietary determinants of gastric cancer in south Louisiana inhabitants. J Natl Cancer Inst 1985;75(4):645-654.

170. Buiatti E, Palli D, Decarli A, et al. A case-control study of gastric cancer and diet in Italy. Int J Cancer 1989;44(4):611-616.

171. Graham S, Haughey B, Marshall J, et al. Diet in the epidemiology of gastric cancer. Nutr Cancer 1990;13(1-2):19-34.

172. Gonzalez CA, Sanz JM, Marcos G, et al. Dietary factors and stomach cancer in Spain: a multi-centre case-control study. Int J Cancer 1991;49(4):513-519.

173. Tuyns AJ, Kaaks R, Haelterman M, et al. Diet and gastric cancer. A case-control study in Belgium. Int J Cancer 1992;51(1):1-6.

174. Ramon JM, Serra L, Cerdo C, et al. Dietary factors and gastric cancer risk. A case-control study in Spain. Cancer 1993;71(5):1731-1735.

175. Cronin KA, Krebs-Smith SM, Feuer EJ, et al. Evaluating the impact of population changes in diet, physical activity, and weight status on population risk for colon cancer (United States). Cancer Causes Control 2001;12(4):305-316.

176. Centonze S, Boeing H, Leoci C, et al. Dietary habits and colorectal cancer in a low-risk area. Results from a population-based case-control study in southern Italy. Nutr Cancer 1994;21(3):233-246.

177. Franceschi S, Favero A, La Vecchia C, et al. Food groups and risk of colorectal cancer in Italy. Int J Cancer 1997;72(1):56-61.

178. Freudenheim JL, Graham S, Marshall JR, et al. A case-control study of diet and rectal cancer in western New York. Am J Epidemiol 1990;131(4):612-624.

179. Hu JF, Liu YY, Yu YK, et al. Diet and cancer of the colon and rectum: a case-control study in China. Int J Epidemiol 1991;20(2):362-367.

180. Slattery ML, Benson J, Curtin K, et al. Carotenoids and colon cancer. Am J Clin Nutr 2000;71(2):575-582.

181. Holick CN, Michaud DS, Stolzenberg-Solomon R, et al. Dietary carotenoids, serum beta-carotene, and retinol and risk of lung cancer in the alpha-tocopherol, beta-carotene cohort study. Am J Epidemiol 2002;156(6):536-547.

182. Bond GG, Thompson FE, Cook RR. Dietary vitamin A and lung cancer: results of a case-control study among chemical workers. Nutr Cancer 1987;9(2-3):109-121.

183. Forman MR, Yao SX, Graubard BI, et al. The effect of dietary intake of fruits and vegetables on the odds ratio of lung cancer among Yunnan tin miners. Int J Epidemiol 1992;21(3):437-441.

184. Kvale G, Bjelke E, Gart JJ. Dietary habits and lung cancer risk. Int J Cancer 1983;31(4):397-405.

185. Le Marchand L, Yoshizawa CN, Kolonel LN, et al. Vegetable consumption and lung cancer risk: a population-based case-control study in Hawaii. J Natl Cancer Inst 1989;81(15):1158-1164.

186. Voorrips LE, Goldbohm RA, Brants HA, et al. A prospective cohort study on antioxidant and folate intake and male lung cancer risk. Cancer Epidemiol Biomarkers Prev 2000;9(4):357-365.

187. Agudo A, Esteve MG, Pallares C, et al. Vegetable and fruit intake and the risk of lung cancer in women in Barcelona, Spain. Eur J Cancer 1997;33(8):1256-1261.

188. Knekt P, Jarvinen R, Seppanen R, et al. Dietary antioxidants and the risk of lung cancer. Am J Epidemiol 1991;134(5):471-479.

189. Ziegler RG, Mason TJ, Stemhagen A, et al. Carotenoid intake, vegetables, and the risk of lung cancer among white men in New Jersey. Am J Epidemiol 1986;123(6):1080-1093.

189. Li Y, Elie M, Blaner WS, et al. Lycopene, smoking and lung cancer. Proc Am Assoc Cancer Res 1997;38:113.

190. Candelora EC, Stockwell HG, Armstrong AW, et al. Dietary intake and risk of lung cancer in women who never smoked. Nutr Cancer 1992;17(3):263-270.

192. Comstock GW, Alberg AJ, Huang HY, et al. The risk of developing lung cancer associated with antioxidants in the blood: ascorbic acid, carotenoids, alpha-tocopherol, selenium, and total peroxyl radical absorbing capacity. Cancer Epidemiol Biomarkers Prev 1997;6(11):907-916.

193. Harris RW, Key TJ, Silcocks PB, et al. A case-control study of dietary carotene in men with lung cancer and in men with other epithelial cancers. Nutr Cancer 1991;15(1):63-68.

194. Key TJ, Silcocks PB, Davey GK, et al. A case-control study of diet and prostate cancer. Br J Cancer 1997;76(5):678-687.

195. Le Marchand L, Hankin JH, Kolonel LN, et al. Intake of specific carotenoids and lung cancer risk. Cancer Epidemiol Biomarkers Prev 1993;2(3):183-187.

196. Mayne ST, Janerich DT, Greenwald P, et al. Dietary beta carotene and lung cancer risk in U.S. nonsmokers. J Natl Cancer Inst 1994;86(1):33-38.

197. Chen L, Stacewicz-Sapuntzakis M, Duncan C, et al. Oxidative DNA damage in prostate cancer patients consuming tomato sauce-based entrees as a whole-food intervention. J Natl Cancer Inst 2001;93(24):1872-1879.

198. Bowen P, Chen L, Stacewicz-Sapuntzakis M, et al. Tomato sauce supplementation and prostate cancer: lycopene accumulation and modulation of biomarkers of carcinogenesis. Exp Biol Med (Maywood) 2002;227(10):886-893.

199. Giovannucci E, Clinton SK. Tomatoes, lycopene, and prostate cancer. Proc Soc Exp Biol Med 1998;218(2):129-139.

200. Giovannucci E, Ascherio A, Rimm EB, et al. Intake of carotenoids and retinol in relation to risk of prostate cancer. J Natl Cancer Inst 1995;87(23):1767-1776.

210. Mills PK, Beeson WL, Phillips RL, et al. Cohort study of diet, lifestyle, and prostate cancer in Adventist men. Cancer 1989;64(3):598-604.

202. Hsing AW, Comstock GW, Abbey H, et al. Serologic precursors of cancer. Retinol, carotenoids, and tocopherol and risk of prostate cancer. J Natl Cancer Inst 1990;82(11):941-946.

203. Le Marchand L, Hankin JH, Kolonel LN, et al. Vegetable and fruit consumption in relation to prostate cancer risk in Hawaii: a reevaluation of the effect of dietary beta-carotene. Am J Epidemiol 1991;133(3):215-219.

204. Nomura AM, Stemmermann GN, Lee J, et al. Serum micronutrients and prostate cancer in Japanese Americans in Hawaii. Cancer Epidemiol Biomarkers Prev 1997;6(7):487-491.

205. Schuman LM, Bastyr NA, Radke A, et al. Some selected features of the epidemiology of prostatic cancer: Minneapolis-St. Paul, Minnesota case-control study, 1976-1979. *In* Knut M (ed): Trends in Cancer Incidence: Causes and Practical Implications. Washington, Hemisphere Publishing Corp, 1982, pp 345-354.

206. Cerhan J, Chiu B, Putnam S, et al. A cohort study of diet and prostate cancer risk. Cancer Epidem Biomark Preven 1998;7:175.

207. Giovannucci E, Rimm EB, Liu Y, et al. A prospective study of tomato products, lycopene, and prostate cancer risk. J Natl Cancer Inst 2002;94(5):391-398.

208. Rao AV, Fleshner N, Agarwal S. Serum and tissue lycopene and biomarkers of oxidation in prostate cancer patients: a case-control study. Nutr Cancer 1999;33(2):159-164.

209. Huang HY, Alberg AJ, Norkus EP, et al. Prospective study of antioxidant micronutrients in the blood and the risk of developing prostate cancer. Am J Epidemiol 2003;157(4):335-344.

210. Gann PH, Ma J, Giovannucci E, et al. Lower prostate cancer risk in men with elevated plasma lycopene levels: results of a prospective analysis. Cancer Res 1999;59(6):1225-1230.

211. Norrish AE, Jackson RT, Sharpe SJ, et al. Prostate cancer and dietary carotenoids. Am J Epidemiol 2000;151(2):119-123.

212. Flood V, Smith W, Wang JJ, et al. Dietary antioxidant intake and incidence of early age-related maculopathy. Ophthalmology 2002;109(12):2272-2278.

213. Seddon JM, Ajani UA, Sperduto RD, et al. Dietary carotenoids, vitamins A, C, and E, and advanced age-related macular degeneration. JAMA 1994;272(18):1413-1420.

214. Anonymous. Antioxidant status and neovascular age-related macular degeneration. Eye Disease Case-Control Study Group. Arch Ophthalmol 1993;111(1):104-109.

215. Gianetti J, Pedrinelli R, Petrucci R, et al. Inverse association between carotid intima-media thickness and the antioxidant lycopene in atherosclerosis. Am Heart J 2002;143(3):467-474.

216. Parfitt VJ, Rubba P, Bolton C, et al. A comparison of antioxidant status and free radical peroxidation of plasma lipoproteins in healthy young persons from Naples and Bristol. Eur Heart J 1994;15(7):871-876.

217. Watzl B, Bub A, Blockhaus M, et al. Prolonged tomato juice consumption has No effect on cell-mediated immunity of well-nourished elderly men and women. J Nutr 2000;130(7):1719-1723.

218. Heinrich U, Gartner C, Wiebusch M, et al. Supplementation with beta-carotene or a similar amount of mixed carotenoids protects humans from UV-induced erythema. J Nutr 2003;133(1):98-101.

219. Greul AK, Grundmann JU, Heinrich F, et al. Photoprotection of UV-irradiated human skin: an antioxidative combination of vitamins E and

L

C, carotenoids, selenium and proanthocyanidins. Skin Pharmacol Appl Skin Physiol 2002;15(5):307-315.

220. Eichler O, Sies H, Stahl W. Divergent optimum levels of lycopene, beta-carotene and lutein protecting against UVB irradiation in human fibroblastst. Photochem Photobiol 2002;75(5):503-506.

221. Offord EA, Gautier JC, Avanti O, et al. Photoprotective potential of lycopene, beta-carotene, vitamin E, vitamin C and carnosic acid in UVA-irradiated human skin fibroblasts. Free Radic Biol Med 2002;32(12): 1293-1303.

Maitake Mushroom
(Grifola frondosa)

SYNONYMS/COMMON NAMES/RELATED SUBSTANCES

- Beta-glucan, cloud mushroom, dancing mushroom, grifolan, Grifon Pro Maitake D Fraction Extract, king of mushroom, Maitake Gold 404, MD-fraction, MDF, my-take.

CLINICAL BOTTOM LINE
Background

- Maitake is the Japanese name for the edible fungus *Grifola frondosa*, which is characterized by a large fruiting body and overlapping caps. Maitake has been used traditionally both as a food and for medicinal purposes. Polysaccharide constituents of maitake have been associated in animal studies with multiple bioactive properties. Extracts of maitake mushroom, particularly the beta-glucan polysaccharide constituent, have been associated with immune modulation in preclinical studies and are hypothesized to exert antitumor effects as a result of these immune properties. Human data are limited, and at this time there is insufficient evidence to recommend for or against the use of oral maitake for any indication.

Scientific Evidence for Common/Studied Uses	Grade*
Cancer	C
Diabetes	C
Immunostimulation	C

*Key to grades: A: Strong scientific evidence for this use; B: Good scientific evidence for this use; C: Unclear scientific evidence for this use; D: Fair scientific evidence against this use (it may not work); F: Strong scientific evidence against this use (it likely does not work). For a more detailed explanation of efficacy criteria, see "Natural Standard Evidence-Based Validated Grading Rationale" in the Introduction.

Historical or Theoretical Uses
That Lack Sufficient Evidence

- Arthritis,[1] bacterial infection,[2] hepatitis,[1,3] HIV, hypercholesterolemia,[4-6] hypertension,[7] weight loss.

Expert Opinion and Folkloric Precedent

- In Asia, maitake is used as a food, and extracts are recommended medicinally for a number of health conditions, including arthritis, hepatitis, and HIV. Recent attention has focused on possible immune and anti-tumor effects, and maitake is sometimes recommended to cancer patients.

Safety Summary

- **Likely safe:** When used as a food.
- **Possibly safe:** When used medicinally by otherwise healthy individuals, although safety and dosing are not established.
- **Possibly unsafe:** Based on animal data, maitake may lower blood sugar levels and should be used cautiously in patients with diabetes or taking hypoglycemic agents.[8-10]

DOSING/TOXICOLOGY
Standardization

- Beta-glucan (a polysaccharide constituent of maitake) contents may vary between preparations. Various fractions of maitake, such as the D-fraction, may be prepared via standardized processes, although it is not clear that different products are comparable.

Dosing: Adult (18 Years and Older)
Oral

- **Capsules/tablets/liquid extract:** Recommended doses have included 0.5 to 1 mg/kg/day of beta-glucan from maitake, taken in divided doses. Human study is limited, and safe/effective doses have not been established.
- **Raw mushroom:** Safe/effective doses have not been established.

Pediatric Dosing (Younger Than 18 Years)

- Insufficient evidence to recommend.

Toxicology

- Insufficient available evidence.

ADVERSE EFFECTS/PRECAUTIONS/CONTRAINDICATIONS
Allergy

- Insufficient available evidence.

Adverse Effects/Postmarket Surveillance

- **General:** Maitake has not been systematically assessed in humans with regular or high-dose use, and effects are largely unknown. Safety in low doses is often assumed based on traditional use as a food.
- **Cardiovascular:** Chronic oral use of maitake mushrooms in rats for 8 to 10 weeks was associated with reduced blood pressure.[6,7] Evidence in humans is lacking.
- **Endocrine:** Animal research suggests hypoglycemic properties of oral maitake,[9-11] although human data are limited in this area.[12]

Precautions/Warnings/Contraindications

- Use cautiously in patients at risk for hypotension or on antihypertensive agents.
- Use cautiously in patients with diabetes or hypoglycemia.

Pregnancy and Lactation

- Not recommended, due to lack of sufficient data.

INTERACTIONS
Maitake/Drug Interactions

- **Hypoglycemic agents:** Animal research suggests hypoglycemic properties of oral maitake,[9-11] although human data are limited in this area.[12]
- **Antihypertensive agents:** Animal studies have reported reduced blood pressure with chronic oral use of maitake mushrooms (8 to 10 weeks).[6,7] Human reports and/or interactions with antihypertensive agents have not been documented in the available literature.

Maitake/Herb/Supplement Interactions

- **Hypoglycemic herbs and supplements:** Animal research suggests hypoglycemic properties of oral maitake,[9-11] although human data are limited in this area.[12]
- **Hypotensive herbs and supplements:** Animal studies have reported reduced blood pressure with chronic oral use of maitake mushrooms (8 to 10 weeks).[6,7] Human reports and/or interactions with antihypertensive agents have not been documented in the available literature.

Maitake/Food Interactions

- Insufficient available evidence.

Maitake/Lab Interactions

- Insufficient available evidence.

MECHANISM OF ACTION
Pharmacology

- **Immune and antitumor effects:** In preclinical studies, the D-fraction of maitake, a beta-glucan extract, has been associated with activation of cellular immunity (specifically helper T cells), decreased activation of B cells; increased production of interferon-gamma, interleukin-12 p70, and interleukin-18; and suppression of interleukin-4.[13,14] Multiple antitumor mechanisms have been proposed, based on results of *in vitro* and animal research, including induction of nitric oxide synthase by maitake D-fraction,[14,15] enhanced production of tumor necrosis factor by macrophages (induced by the beta-glucan "grifolan" or gel-forming [1→3]-beta-D-glucan),[16-18] anti-angiogenesis with increased vascular endothelial growth factor (VEGF) levels induced by the D-fraction,[19] oxidative damage and induced apoptosis by beta-glucan,[20] increased Kupffer cell activity against neoplastic cells stimulated by a branched type gel-forming (1→3)-beta-D-glucan,[21] enhanced lymphocyte activity,[22] and alternative complement pathway activation.[23] *In vitro* antitumor effects of maitake polysaccharide fractions have been demonstrated.[24]

Pharmacodynamics/Kinetics

- Limited data are available. In mice, beta-glucans from maitake are distributed to the liver and spleen with a prolonged half-life.[25]

HISTORY

- The name *maitake* stems from the Japanese word *mai*, meaning "dance," and *take*, meaning "mushroom." This edible fungus is characterized by a large fruiting body and overlapping caps. It has been used traditionally both as a food and for medicinal purposes. Various fractions of the mushroom have been isolated in Japan during the past 40 years with the aim of isolating beta-glucans with potent medicinal properties. These include the D-fraction, and more recently the MD-fraction.

REVIEW OF THE EVIDENCE: TABLE

- No studies qualify for inclusion in the evidence table.

REVIEW OF THE EVIDENCE: DISCUSSION
Cancer
Summary

- Maitake extracts have been demonstrated in animal studies to stimulate immune function and potentially to prompt host-mediated anti-tumor activity.[8,26] However, systematic human data are lacking in this area. Therefore, a recommendation cannot be made either for or against the use of maitake for cancer treatment or prevention.

Human Evidence

- Kodama et al. reported the results of a case series in human patients with various types of cancer at a variety of stages.[57] A combination of whole maitake powder and the MD-fraction of maitake mushroom (containing beta-1,6 glucan) was administered to subjects and was associated with tumor regression or symptomatic improvement in 58% of liver cancer patients, 69% of breast cancer patients, and 63% of lung cancer patients. A <20% improvement was observed for leukemia, stomach, and brain tumors. However, baseline patient characteristics and history of disease and therapy were not universally clear. Although compelling, the lack of controls diminishes the clinical applicability of these results.

Preclinical Evidence

- Multiple anti-tumor mechanisms have been proposed based on results of *in vitro* and animal research, including induction of nitric oxide synthase by maitake D-fraction,[14,15] enhanced production of tumor necrosis factor by macrophages (induced by the beta-glucan "grifolan" or gel-forming [1→3]-beta-D-glucan),[16-18] anti-angiogenesis with increased vascular endothelial growth factor (VEGF) levels induced by D-fraction,[19] oxidative damage and induced apoptosis by beta-glucan,[20] increased Kupffer cell activity against neoplastic cells stimulated by a branched type gel-forming (1→3,)-beta-D-glucan,[21] enhanced lymphocyte activity,[22] and alternative complement pathway activation.[23] *In vitro* antitumor effects of maitake polysaccharide fractions have been demonstrated.[24]

Diabetes
Summary

- Animal research suggests possible hypoglycemic properties of oral maitake extracts. Reliable human data are lacking. Without additional evidence, a recommendation cannot be made either for or against the use of maitake in the management of diabetes or hypoglycemia.

Evidence

- Multiple animal studies have demonstrated hypoglycemic effects of maitake mushroom extracts. In insulin-resistant mice, a water-soluble maitake extract ("Fraction X") has been associated with enhanced peripheral insulin sensitivity.[11] Decreased blood glucose levels and glucosuria and elevated serum insulin levels have been found with dietary maitake extract in experimentally diabetic mice.[9,10] Human evidence is limited in this area.[12]

Immunostimulation
Summary

- Animal research suggests possible immunomodulatory properties of oral maitake extracts. Reliable human data are lacking. Without additional evidence, a recommendation cannot be made either for or against the use of maitake as an immune stimulant.

Evidence

- In preclinical studies, the D-fraction of maitake, a beta-glucan extract, has been associated with activation of cellular immunity (specifically helper T cells), decreased activation of B cells; increased production of interferon-gamma, interleukin-12 p70, and interleukin-18; but suppression of interleukin-4.[13,14] Studies of antitumor effects have implicated maitake extracts in the enhancement of lymphocyte and macrophage activity.

References

1. Shigesue K, Kodama N, Nanba H. Effects of maitake (*Grifola frondosa*) polysaccharide on collagen-induced arthritis in mice. Jpn J Pharmacol 2000; 84(3):293-300.
2. Kodama N, Yamada M, Nanba H. Addition of Maitake D-fraction reduces the effective dosage of vancomycin for the treatment of *Listeria*-infected mice. Jpn J Pharmacol 2001;87(4):327-332.
3. Kubo K, Nanba H. The effect of maitake mushrooms on liver and serum lipids. Altern Ther Health Med 1996;2(5):62-66.
4. Fukushima M, Ohashi T, Fujiwara Y, et al. Cholesterol-lowering effects of maitake (*Grifola frondosa*) fiber, shiitake (*Lentinus edodes*) fiber, and enokitake (*Flammulina velutipes*) fiber in rats. Exp Biol Med (Maywood) 2001;226(8):758-765.
5. Kubo K, Nanba H. Anti-hyperliposis effect of maitake fruit body (*Grifola frondosa*). I. Biol Pharm Bull 1997;20(7):781-785.
6. Kabir Y, Yamaguchi M, Kimura S. Effect of shiitake (*Lentinus edodes*) and maitake (*Grifola frondosa*) mushrooms on blood pressure and plasma lipids of spontaneously hypertensive rats. J Nutr Sci Vitaminol (Tokyo) 1987; 33(5):341-346.
7. Kabir Y, Kimura S. Dietary mushrooms reduce blood pressure in spontaneously hypertensive rats (SHR). J Nutr Sci Vitaminol (Tokyo) 1989; 35(1):91-94.
8. Adachi K, Nanba H, Kuroda H. Potentiation of host-mediated antitumor activity in mice by beta-glucan obtained from *Grifola frondosa* (maitake). Chem Pharm Bull (Tokyo) 1987;35(1):262-270.
9. Kubo K, Aoki H, Nanba H. Anti-diabetic activity present in the fruit body of *Grifola frondosa* (Maitake). I. Biol Pharm Bull 1994;17(8):1106-1110.
10. Horio H, Ohtsuru M. Maitake (*Grifola frondosa*) improve glucose tolerance of experimental diabetic rats. J Nutr Sci Vitaminol (Tokyo) 2001;47(1):57-63.
11. Manohar V, Talpur NA, Echard BW, et al. Effects of a water-soluble extract of maitake mushroom on circulating glucose/insulin concentrations in KK mice. Diabetes Obes Metab 2002;4(1):43-48.
12. Konno S, Tortorelis DG, Fullerton SA, et al. A possible hypoglycaemic effect of maitake mushroom on Type 2 diabetic patients. Diabet Med 2001; 18(12):1010.
13. Inoue A, Kodama N, Nanba H. Effect of maitake (*Grifola frondosa*) D-fraction on the control of the T lymph node Th-1/Th-2 proportion. Biol Pharm Bull 2002;25(4):536-540.
14. Ohno N, Egawa Y, Hashimoto T, et al. Effect of beta-glucans on the nitric oxide synthesis by peritoneal macrophage in mice. Biol Pharm Bull 1996; 19(4):608-612.
15. Sanzen I, Imanishi N, Takamatsu N, et al. Nitric oxide-mediated antitumor activity induced by the extract from *Grifola frondosa* (Maitake mushroom) in a macrophage cell line, RAW264.7. J Exp Clin Cancer Res 2001;20(4): 591-597.
16. Ishibashi K, Miura NN, Adachi Y, et al. Relationship between solubility of grifolan, a fungal 1,3-beta-D-glucan, and production of tumor necrosis factor by macrophages *in vitro*. Biosci Biotechnol Biochem 2001;65(9): 1993-2000.
17. Okazaki M, Adachi Y, Ohno N, et al. Structure-activity relationship of (1→3)-beta-D-glucans in the induction of cytokine production from macrophages, *in vitro*. Biol Pharm Bull 1995;18(10):1320-1327.
18. Adachi Y, Okazaki M, Ohno N, et al. Enhancement of cytokine production by macrophages stimulated with (1→3)-beta-D-glucan, grifolan (GRN), isolated from *Grifola frondosa*. Biol Pharm Bull 1994;17(12):1554-1560.
19. Matsui K, Kodama N, Nanba H. Effects of maitake (*Grifola frondosa*) D-Fraction on the carcinoma angiogenesis. Cancer Lett 2001;172(2):193-198.
20. Fullerton SA, Samadi AA, Tortorelis DG, et al. Induction of apoptosis in human prostatic cancer cells with beta-glucan (Maitake mushroom polysaccharide). Mol Urol 2000;4(1):7-13.
21. Adachi Y, Ohno N, Yadomae T. Activation of murine Kupffer cells by administration with gel-forming (1→3)-beta-D-glucan from *Grifola frondosa*. Biol Pharm Bull 1998;21(3):278-283.
22. Kurashige S, Akuzawa Y, Endo F. Effects of Lentinus edodes, *Grifola frondosa* and *Pleurotus ostreatus* administration on cancer outbreak, and activities of macrophages and lymphocytes in mice treated with a carcinogen, N-butyl-N-butanolnitrosoamine. Immunopharmacol Immunotoxicol 1997; 19(2):175-183.
23. Suzuki I, Hashimoto K, Oikawa S, et al. Antitumor and immunomodulating activities of a beta-glucan obtained from liquid-cultured *Grifola frondosa*. Chem Pharm Bull (Tokyo) 1989;37(2):410-413.
24. Suzuki I, Itani T, Ohno N, et al. Antitumor activity of a polysaccharide fraction extracted from cultured fruiting bodies of *Grifola frondosa*. J Pharmacobiodyn 1984;7(7):492-500.
25. Miura NN, Ohno N, Aketagawa J, et al. Blood clearance of (1→3)-beta-D-glucan in MRL lpr/lpr mice. FEMS Immunol Med Microbiol 1996;13(1): 51-57.
26. Li X, Rong J, Wu M, et al. [Anti-tumor effect of polysaccharide from *Grifola frondosa* and its influence on immunological function]. Zhong Yao Cai 2003;26(1):31-32.
27. Kodama N, Komuta K, Nanba H. Can maitake MD-fraction aid cancer patients? Altern Med Rev 2002;7(3):236-239.

M

Marshmallow
(*Althaea officinalis* L.)

SYNONYMS/COMMON NAMES/RELATED SUBSTANCES

- Althaea leaf, althaea root, *Althaea officinalis* L. var robusta, *Althaeae folium*, althaeae radi, althaea radix, althea, althea leaf, althea root, altheia, apothekerstockmalve, bismalva, buonvischio, eibischwurzel, guimauve, gul hatem, herba malvae, hitm, kitmi, mallards, Malvaceae, malvacioni, malve, malvavisco, mortification root, racine de guimauve, sweet weed, wymote, witte malve.
- *Note:* Not to be confused with mallow leaf, mallow flower, or confectionery marshmallows; although confectionery marshmallows were once made from the *Althaea officinalis* plant, they now primarily contain sugar.

CLINICAL BOTTOM LINE
Background

- Both the leaf and root of marshmallow (*Althaea officinalis*) are used in commercial preparations. Herbal formulations are made from either the dried root (unpeeled or peeled) or the leaf. The actual mucilaginous content of the commercial product may vary according to the time of collection.
- No clinical trials assessing marshmallow monotherapy have been conducted for any indication. Therapeutic applications of marshmallow are supported principally by traditional use, phytochemical investigation, and preclinical research. Limited human evidence is available studying the efficacy of marshmallow-containing combination products for dermatologic conditions.
- Marshmallow may interfere with the absorption of oral medications, although this is clinically unproven. Therefore, ingestion of marshmallow several hours before or after other medicinal agents may be warranted.
- Marshmallow is generally regarded as safe, and literature review reveals no documented adverse case-reports. However, the potential for marshmallow to elicit allergic reactions or hypoglycemia has been noted anecdotally.

Scientific Evidence for Common/Studied Uses	Grade*
Skin inflammatory conditions (eczema, psoriasis)	C

*Key to grades: *A:* Strong scientific evidence for this use; *B:* Good scientific evidence for this use; *C:* Unclear scientific evidence for this use; *D:* Fair scientific evidence against this use (it may not work); *F:* Strong scientific evidence against this use (it likely does not work). For a more detailed explanation of efficacy criteria, see "Natural Standard Evidence-Based Validated Grading Rationale" in the Introduction.

Historical or Theoretical Uses
That Lack Sufficient Evidence

- Abscesses (topical), antidote to poisons, aphrodisiac, arthritis, bee stings, bronchitis, boils (topical), bruises (topical), burns (topical), cancer,[1] chilblains (erythema of the extremities with cold exposure), colitis, congestion, constipation, cough, Crohn's disease, cystitis, demulcent, dermatitis (topical), diarrhea, diuretic, diverticulitis, cough, duodenal ulcer, emollient, enteritis, evaluation of functional disturbances of the esophagus,[2-4] expectorant, gastroenteritis, inflammation, ileitis, immunostimulant, impotence, indigestion, inflammation, insect bites, irritable bowel syndrome, laxative, minor wounds, mouthwash, mucilage, muscular pain, pap smear (abnormal), peptic ulcer disease, polyuria, skin ulcers (topical), soothing agent, sore throat, sprains, toothache, ulcerative colitis, urethritis, urinary irritation, urinary tract infection, urolithiasis, varicose ulcers (topical), vomiting, vulnerary (wound healing), whooping cough.

Expert Opinion and Folkloric Precedent

- The British Herbal compendium reports marshmallow's actions as a demulcent (soothing to irritation) and topically as an emollient and vulnerary (wound healing). Its internal use has also been indicated for gastroenteritis, peptic and duodenal ulcers, and ulcerative colitis. Marshmallow has been used as a mouthwash and gargle for inflammation of the oropharynx, and as a poultice, cream, and ointment for furunculosis, eczema, and dermatitis.
- The expert panel, the German Commission E, reports that marshmallow leaf and root alleviate local irritation, inhibit mucociliary activity, and stimulate phagocytosis. The Commission E has approved marshmallow for treating irritation of oral and pharyngeal mucosa, mild inflammation of the gastric mucosa, and dry cough.
- The German Standard License has approved marshmallow root tea for soothing of irritation due to mucosal inflammation of the mouth and pharynx, upper respiratory tract, and gastrointestinal tract.
- Marshmallow has been permitted as a flavoring in the United States and in Europe. In Germany, marshmallow root and leaf are both licensed as standard medicinal teas. The root is sold as a component of couth tea and cough syrups.
- Modern herbalists recommend marshmallow for relieving digestion and respiratory problems such as cough, colds, and asthma.

Safety Summary

- **Likely safe:** When used in amounts commonly found in foods. Although systematic safety trials have not been performed, marshmallow is generally considered safe and is approved for use in foods, based on historical use.
- **Possibly safe:** When used orally or topically in recommended doses for medicinal purposes.
- **Possibly unsafe:** When used in doses above recommended range. When used in pregnancy or lactation. When used in pediatric patients. When used in diabetic patients or patients at risk for hypoglycemia.

DOSING/TOXICOLOGY
General

- Dosing regimens are based on traditional health practice patterns, expert opinion and clinical anecdote; there are no available reliable human trials demonstrating safety or efficacy for any specific doses of marshmallow. With natural products, formulations and preparation methods may vary from manufacturer to manufacturer, and from batch to batch of a specific product made by a single manufacturer. Because often the active components of a product are not known, standardization may not be possible, and the clinical effects of different brands may not be comparable.

Standardization

- Pharmacopoeia-grade marshmallow must have an "index swelling" of no less than 12 and pass botanical identification by macroscopic and microscopic authentication. The British Pharmacopoeia requires marshmallow leaf to be harvested before the flowering period, pass identification by thin-layer chromatography, and pass confirmation with additional qualitative standards, including water-soluble extraction of not less than 15%.

Dosing: Adult (18 Years and Older)
Oral

- **Leaf:** 5 g of leaf or equivalent preparation daily.
- **Root:** 6 g of root or equivalent preparation daily.
- *Note:* Use cautiously in patients taking other oral medicinal agents, as marshmallow may interfere with absorption.

Topical

- **Marshmallow topical preparation:** 5 to 10 g of marshmallow root in ointment or cream base or 5% powdered marshmallow leaf; applied three times daily.
- **Gargle (for oral and pharyngeal irritation):** 2 g of marshmallow in 1 cup of cold water; soak for 2 hours, then gargle.

Dosing: Pediatric (Younger Than 18 Years)

- Not recommended because of insufficient available evidence.

Toxicology

- Based on anecdotal reports, marshmallow is generally safe, with possible rare allergic potential. Systematic study of toxicology has not been conducted.

ADVERSE EFFECTS/PRECAUTIONS/CONTRAINDICATIONS
Allergy

- Known allergy/hypersensitivity to marshmallow (*Althaea officinalis*). Allergic reactions have been reported anecdotally.

Adverse Effects/Postmarket Surveillance

- **General:** Marshmallow is generally regarded as being safe in healthy individuals at recommended doses, based on historical use, although systematic study has not been conducted. Anecdotal reports have noted the possibility of rare allergic reactions as well as hypoglycemia. Because studies have not evaluated the safety of marshmallow, recommended doses and duration in humans have not been established.
- **Dermatologic:** Anecdotal reports have noted the possibility of allergic reactions with marshmallow; however, no reports or studies are found in the available literature.
- **Endocrine:** Marshmallow may possess hypoglycemic effects, although human data are not available.[5]

Precautions/Warnings/Contraindications

- Use cautiously in patients taking hypoglycemic medications, as marshmallow has been reported to elicit hypoglycemic effects.[5]
- Use cautiously in patients taking other oral medicinal agents, as marshmallow may interfere with absorption.

Pregnancy and Lactation

- Insufficient available data.

INTERACTIONS
Marshmallow/Drug Interactions

- **Oral drugs:** Theoretically, the fiber in marshmallow may impair absorption of oral drugs (anecdotal).
- **Hypoglycemic drugs:** Marshmallow may increase the effects of hypoglycemic agents, based on reported hypoglycemic effects in animal research.[5]
- **Topical steroids:** Marshmallow may increase the topical anti-inflammatory effects of steroids, based on clinical anecdote and theory.[6]

Marshmallow/Herb/Supplement Interactions

- **Hypoglycemic herbs and supplements:** Marshmallow may increase the effects of hypoglycemic agents, based on reported hypoglycemic effects in animal research.[5]
- **Oral agents:** Theoretically, the fiber in marshmallow may impair absorption of oral drugs (anecdotal).

Marshmallow/Food Interactions

- Insufficient available data.

Marshmallow/Lab Interactions

- **Glucose:** Marshmallow may lower blood glucose levels, based on animal research.[5]

MECHANISM OF ACTION
Pharmacology

- **Constituents:** Marshmallow root preparations consist of peeled or unpeeled dried root of *Althaea officinalis* L. and contain mucilage polysaccharides (6.2% to 11.6%) including galacturonorhamnans, arabinans, glucaris, arabinogalactans; carbohydrates (25-35%); flavanoids; glycosides; sugars (10% sucrose); amines (up to 12% asparagines); fat (1.7%); calcium oxalate; coumarins; phenolic acid[7]; and sterols. Purified homogeneous mucilage of marshmallow is composed of L-rhamsose, D-galactose, galacturonnic acid, and D-glucuronic acid in molar ratio of 3:2:3:3.[5] Scopoletin, quercitin, kaempferol, chlorgenic acid, caffeic acid, and p-coumaric acid are also present in the roots. Marshmallow is high in aluminum, iron, magnesium, selenium, and tin, and contains substantial amounts of calcium. It is also high in pectin, which may lower blood glucose concentrations. The root contains 25% to 35% of the mucilage; however, the content of purified mucilage is much lower. Asparagine, sugar, and tannin have also been identified in the root. The mucilage content of the root, leaves, and flowers is highest in the late fall and winter (approximately 11%) and lowest in the spring and summer (5% to 6%). Xylose, glucan, arabinogalactan, and an acidic polysaccharide containing 2-O-alpha-D-galacturonopyranosyl-l-rhamnose[9] are also present in the hydrolysate of leaf and flower mucilages. Extracts from hybrid plants have been found to be more mucilaginous with a different sugar composition compared to native plants.[9]
- **Antitussive/mucociliary effects:** Mucilaginous herbs such as marshmallow root may inhibit coughing by forming a protective coating on the mucosal lining of the respiratory tract, shielding it from irritants.[10,11] Marshmallow reduces the transport velocity of isolated ciliary epithelia and may protect mucus layers in the hypopharynx, exerting spasmolytic, antisecretory, and bactericidal properties.[10] Antitussive activity has been demonstrated by oral doses of marshmallow root extract and a marshmallow polysaccharide (100 mg/kg and 50 mg/kg, respectively) in cats, when compared to a non-narcotic cough suppressant. A polysaccharide dose of

M

50 mg/kg was equally effective as "Syrupus Althaeae" in a dose of 1000 mg/kg.[12] The extract was less effective than marshmallow polysaccharide.[13] Demulcent properties of marshmallow may be due to reduction of local irritation that causes gastritis.

- **Antimicrobial effects:** Marshmallow given intraperitoneally to rats at a dose of 10 mg/kg exhibits phagocytic activity, suppresses mucociliary action, and stimulates phagocytosis. It also exhibits antimicrobial activity against *Pseudomonas aeruginosa*, *Proteus vulgaris*, and *Staphylococcus aureus*.[10,14]

- **Hypoglycemic effects:** At doses of 10 mg/kg, 30 mg/kg and 100 mg/kg, marshmallow reduces plasma glucose levels to 74%, 81%, and 65% of prior values, respectively, after 7 hours in rats.[5]

- **Dermatologic effects:** Combinations of marshmallow preparations with steroids have been used in the management of dermatologic conditions, and the plant appears to possess anti-inflammatory activity that potentates the effect of topical steroids.[6,15] *In vitro*, anti-inflammatory effect of an ointment containing marshmallow extract and dexamethasone (0.05%) was superior to that of the individual ingredients in the alleviation of chemically induced rabbit ear irritation.[16] Marshmallow extract *in vivo* stimulates phagocytosis and the release of cytokines from monocytes, including interleukin-6 and tumor necrosis factor.[17]

Pharmacodynamics/Kinetics

- Marshmallow mucilage is not altered in the digestive tract until it reaches the colon, where it may be partially or completely digested via bacterial action.[13]

HISTORY

- Marshmallow (*Althaea officinalis*) is a perennial herb that is native throughout damp areas of Europe and western Asia. Marshmallow is naturalized in North America in salt marshes, from Massachusetts to Virginia, and is now cultivated from Western Europe to Russia. Marshmallow has been used in traditional European medicine for more than 2000 years, and its therapeutic use was first recorded in the 9th century. It was widely used in Greek medicine, and later its use spread to Arabian medicine. The emperor Charlemagne ordered marshmallow cultivation in monasteries.

- *Althaea officinalis* grows to 5 feet in salt marshes and moist regions. The yellow roots are tapered, long, and thick, with tough exteriors. The short leaves are round with an irregularly toothed margin. The entire plant is filled with mucilage. The plant resembles hollyhock (*Althaea rosea*). Its genus name, "althaea," comes from the Greek word *altho*, which means "to cure." Its order name, Malvaceae, is derived from the Greek word *malake*, meaning "soft". The modern common name comes from the Anglo-Saxon word *merscmealwe*, in which *mersc* means "marsh" and *mealwe* translates to "mallow."

- In the United States, marshmallow is used as a component of dietary supplements with antitussive and demulcent properties. Marshmallow root and extract were formerly official entries in the United States Pharmacopeia and the National Formulary.

- In Germany, marshmallow is used in a standard medicinal tea. The root is also used as a component of some cough preparations. Marshmallow root has been recognized as a source of mucilage, which is used to treat topical wounds, sore throats, chapped skin, and stomach ailments. The mucilage is incorporated into ointments and also added to food in small quantities to provide bulk and texture.

- Marshmallow has been used as part of rituals to treat impotence and as an aphrodisiac. Seeds collected under a full moon are made into an oil and used on the genitals. An amulet made of leaf and root has been kept under the genitals and used for the same purpose. Marshmallow has been used in rituals for the dead and has been planted over grave sites.

REVIEW OF THE EVIDENCE: TABLE

- No studies qualify for inclusion in the evidence table.

REVIEW OF THE EVIDENCE: DISCUSSION
Skin Inflammatory Conditions (Eczema, Psoriasis)
Summary

- Marshmallow extracts have been used traditionally as topical anti-inflammatory agents. Animal research has demonstrated some anti-inflammatory activity. Human research is limited in this area, and safety, dosing, and comparative efficacy have not been systematically evaluated.

Evidence

- In 1986, Huriez and Fagez conducted a case series study including 51 patients with inflammatory skin conditions, to assess efficacy of Pommade Dexalta, which is a combination of dexamethasone acetate (0.05 mg), fluid extract of marshmallow (20 g), Vaseline (5 g), and lanolin anhydrated q.s.p (100 g).[6] Subjects received Dexalta once daily for 3 to 60 days (mean, 20 days). Although the authors reported improvements in the Dexalta therapy group vs. placebo, the results cannot be extrapolated to marshmallow monotherapy. Methods, results, and statistical analysis were not well described.

- In 1966, Beaune and Balea conducted an experimental study to assess the anti-inflammatory properties of marshmallow alone and in combination with dexamethasone in rabbits.[16] The efficacy of three ointments was compared: marshmallow extract (20%), dexamethasone acetate (0.5%), and a combination of marshmallow and dexamethasone. All three ointments contained lanolin and Vaseline as excipients. All preparations demonstrated anti-inflammatory effects in response to irritants (tetrahydrofurfuric alcohol and ultraviolet rays), with the most effective therapy being the combination product. Marshmallow was reported as being superior to dexamethasone monotherapy. Although these data suggest that marshmallow may possess anti-inflammatory properties that are additive to those of topical steroids, measurement techniques and statistical methods were not adequately described. Further evaluation, in humans, is warranted in this area.

References

1. Kobayashi A, Hachiya A, Ohuchi A, et al. Inhibitory mechanism of an extract of *Althaea officinalis* L. on endothelin-1–induced melanocyte activation. Biol Pharm Bull 2002;25(2):229-234.
2. Keren S, Argaman E. [Marshmallow for investigating functional disturbances of the esophageal body]. Harefuah 1992;123(5-6):161-165.
3. Keren S, Argaman E, Golan M. Solid swallowing versus water swallowing: manometric study of dysphagia. Dig Dis Sci 1992;37(4):603-608.
4. Robertson CS, Smart H, Amar SS, et al. Oesophageal transit of marshmallow after the Angelchik procedure. Br J Surg 1989;76(3):245-247.
5. Tomoda M, Shimizu N, Oshima Y, et al. Hypoglycemic activity of twenty plant mucilages and three modified products. Planta Med 1987;53(1):8-12.
6. Huriez C, Fagez C. [An association of marshmallow-dexamethasone: the pommade Dexalta]. Lille Med 1968;13(2):121-123.
7. Gudej J. Flavonoids, phenolic acids and coumarins from the roots of *Althaea officinalis*. Planta Med 1991;57:284-285.
8. Franz G. Die Schleimpolysaccharide von *Althaea officinalis* und *Malva sylvestris*. Planta Med 1966;14:90-110.
9. Franz G, Chladek M. [Comparative studies on the composition of crude

mucus from crossbred descendants of *Althaea officinalis* L. and *Althaea armeniaca* Ten]. Pharmazie 1973;28(2):128-129.

10. Muller-Limmroth W, Frohlich HH. [Effect of various phytotherapeutic expectorants on mucociliary transport]. Fortschr Med 1980;98(3):95-101.

11. Meyer E. Behandlung akuter und chronischer Bronchitiden mit Heilpflanzen. Therapiewoche 1956;6:537-540.

12. Nosal'ova G, Strapkova A, Kardosova A, et al. [Antitussive action of extracts and polysaccharides of marsh mallow (*Althea officinalis* L., var. robusta)]. Pharmazie 1992;47(3):224-226.

13. Bone K. Marshmallow soothes cough. Br J Phytother 1993;3(2):93.

14. Recio MC, et al. Antimicrobial activity of selected plants employed in the Spanish Mediterranean area, Part II. Phytother Res 1989;3:77-80.

15. Piovano PB, Mazzocchi S. [Clinical trial of a steroid derivative (9-alpha-fluoro-prednisolone-21- acetate) in association with aqueous extract of althea in the dermatological field]. G Ital Dermatol Minerva Dermatol 1970; 45(4):279-286.

16. Beaune A, Balea T. [Anti-inflammatory experimental properties of marshmallow: its potentiating action on the local effects of corticoids]. Therapie 1966;21(2):341-347.

17. Scheffer J, König W. Einfluss von Radix althaeae und Flores chamomillae Extrakten auf Entzündungsreaktionen humaner neutrophiler Granulozyten, Monozyten und Rattenmastzellen. Abstracts of 3rd Phytotherapie-Kongress 1991; Abstract P9.

Melatonin

SYNONYMS/COMMON NAMES/RELATED SUBSTANCES

- 5-Methoxy-N-acetyltryptamine, acetamide, BMS-214778, luzindole, mel, MEL, melatonine, MLT, N-acetyl-5-methoxytryptamine, N-2-(5-methoxyindol-3-ethyl)-acetamide.
- **Brand names:** Accurate Release; Appleheart Melatonin; Mel; Melatonin-BioDynamax; Melatonin Controlled Release; Melatonin-Metabolic Response Modifier; Melatonin–New Hope Health Products; Melatonin Olympian Labs; Melatonin-Optimum Nutrition; Melatonin Tablets; Melatonin Time Release.
- **Combination products:** Melatonex (vitamin B_6); Melatonin Forte (*Piper methysticum*, kavalactones, valerian); Melatonin PM Complex (vitamin B_6, vitamin B_2, vitamin B_3); Melatonin spray (γ-aminobutyric acid, pyridoxal-5-phosphate); Super Snooze with Melatonin (valerian root, hops, scullcap, chamomile, passion flower).

CLINICAL BOTTOM LINE
Background

- Melatonin is a neurohormone produced in the brain by the pineal gland from the amino acid tryptophan. The synthesis and release of melatonin are stimulated by darkness and suppressed by light, suggesting the involvement of melatonin in circadian rhythm and regulation of diverse body functions. Levels of melatonin in the blood are highest prior to bedtime.
- Synthetic melatonin supplements have been used for a variety of medical conditions, most notably for disorders related to sleep.
- Melatonin possesses antioxidant activity,[1-9] and many of its proposed therapeutic or preventive uses are based on this property.
- New drugs that block the effects of melatonin are in development, such as BMS-214778 and luzindole, and may have uses in various disorders.[10-12]

Scientific Evidence for Common/Studied Uses	Grade*
Jet lag	A
Delayed sleep phase syndrome (DSPS)	B
Insomnia in the elderly	B
Sleep disturbances in children with neuropsychiatric disorders	B
Sleep enhancement in healthy people	B
Alzheimer's disease (sleep disorders)	C
Antioxidant (free radical scavenging)	C
Attention deficit hyperactivity disorder (ADHD)	C
Benzodiazepine tapering	C
Bipolar disorder (sleep disturbances)	C

Cancer treatment	C
Chemotherapy side effects	C
Circadian rhythm entraining (in blind persons)	C
Depression (sleep disturbances)	C
Glaucoma	C
Headache prevention	C
High blood pressure (hypertension)	C
HIV / AIDS	C
Insomnia of unknown origin in the non-elderly	C
Parkinson's disease	C
Periodic limb movement disorder	C
Preoperative sedation / anxiolysis	C
REM sleep behavior disorder	C
Rett's syndrome	C
Schizophrenia (sleep disorders)	C
Seasonal affective disorder (SAD)	C
Seizure disorder (children)	C
Sleep disturbances due to pineal region brain damage	C
Smoking cessation	C
Stroke	C
Tardive dyskinesia	C
Thrombocytopenia (low platelets)	C
Ultraviolet light skin damage protection	C
Work shift sleep disorder	C

*Key to grades: *A:* Strong scientific evidence for this use; *B:* Good scientific evidence for this use; *C:* Unclear scientific evidence for this use; *D:* Fair scientific evidence against this use (it may not work); *F:* Strong scientific evidence against this use (it likely does not work). For a more detailed explanation of efficacy criteria, see "Natural Standard Evidence-Based Validated Grading Rationale" in the Introduction.

Historical or Theoretical Indications That Lack Sufficient Evidence

- Acetaminophen toxicity,[13] acute respiratory distress syndrome (ARDS),[14] aging, aluminum toxicity, Alzheimer's disease, amikacin-induced kidney damage,[15] analgesia,[16] anxiety,[17] asthma, autoimmune demyelination,[12] beta-blocker sleep disturbance,[18,19] cachexia, cancer prevention,[20] cardiac syndrome X, cataracts,[438] cholestatic liver injury,[21] cocaine withdrawal,[22] cognitive enhancement, colic,[23] colitis,[24] contraception, coronary artery disease, craniopharyngioma,[25] critical illness/intensive care unit (ICU) sleep disturbance, cyclosporin-induced kidney toxicity,[26,27] depression, diabetes,[28] dopaminergic supersensitivity,[29] edema, endometrial cancer,[30] erectile dysfunction, fertility,[31] fibromyalgia, fibrous dysplasia,[32] food preservation,[8] idiopathic scoliosis ,[33] itching, intestinal motility disorders, lead toxicity, gastroesophageal reflux disease (GERD), gentamicin-induced kidney damage, glaucoma, heart attack prevention,[34,35] hormone-dependent uterine disorders,[309] hyperpigmentation, immunostimulant, interstitial cystitis, irritable bowel syndrome,[23] Langerhans cell histiocytosis,[369] lead toxicity,[37] Machado-Joseph disease,[38] McCune-Albright syndrome,[32] melatonin deficiency, memory enhancement, multiple sclerosis, myocardial injury,[34] myometrial functioning,[39] nephrotoxicity induced by chemotherapy,[40-42] neurodegenerative disorders, neuro-fibromatous scoliosis,[32] nitrate tolerance,[43] noise-induced hearing loss, normalization of gait,[44] obstructive jaundice,[45] oral facial movements (induced by reserpine or age),[31] pancreatitis, phenylketonuria (PKU),[46] polycystic ovarian syndrome (PCOS),[47] postmenopausal osteoporosis, post-operative adjunct, postoperative delirium,[48] prevention of post–lung transplant ischemia—reperfusion injury, prolificay,[31] pulmonary fibrosis,[49] rheumatoid arthritis, sarcoidosis, sedation, seizure prevention,[16] sexual activity enhancement, schistosomiasis,[50] shock,[51,52] Smith-Magenis syndrome,[53] spinal-cord injury,[54] sudden infant death syndrome (SIDS) prevention, tachycardia, tinnitus, testicular damage,[55] toxic kidney damage, toxic liver damage, toluene neurotoxicity,[56] traumatic brain injury,[57] tuberculosis,[58] tuberous sclerosis, ulcerative colitis,[59,60] Venezuelan equine encephalomyelitis virus,[61] Wilson's disease,[62] withdrawal from narcotics, wound healing.[63]

Expert Opinion and Folkloric Precedent

- Melatonin is widely recommended for various sleep disorders and for prevention of jet lag. In addition, it is used in conditions believed to be associated with low levels of endogenous melatonin, such as aging, sleep disorders in children, and affective disorders.

Safety Summary

- **Likely safe:** When used orally for up to 2 years at a dose of 5 mg daily.[64]
- **Possibly safe:** When used in doses up to 40 mg for short periods of time.
- **Possibly unsafe:** Case reports raise concerns about risks of blood clotting abnormalities (particularly in patients taking warfarin), increased risk of seizure, and disorientation with overdose.
- **Likely unsafe:** Melatonin supplementation should be avoided in women who are pregnant or attempting to become pregnant, based on possible hormonal effects, including alterations of pituitary-ovarian function and potential inhibition of ovulation [65] or uterine contractions.[66] High levels of melatonin during pregnancy may increase the risk of developmental disorders.[67]

DOSING/TOXICOLOGY
General

- Recommended doses are based on those most commonly used in available trials, and/or on historical practice. However, with natural products, the optimal doses needed to balance efficacy and safety often have not been determined. Formulations and preparation methods may vary from manufacturer to manufacturer, and from batch to batch of a specific product made by a single manufacturer. Because often the active components of a product are not known, standardization may not be possible, and the clinical effects of different brands may not be comparable.

Standardization

- There is no widely accepted standardization for melatonin. Experts note that many brands contain impurities that cannot be characterized, as well as dissimilar amounts of actual hormone. In 2002, ConsumerLab.com evaluated 18 melatonin-containing supplements (15 quick-release and 3 time-release products), of which 12 were melatonin-only products. It was reported that 16 of the 18 products contained between 100% and 135% of the claimed amount of melatonin, one rapid-release product contained only 83% of the claimed amount of melatonin, and another rapid-release product contained a small amount of lead (slightly more than 0.5 µg per daily recommended serving size). Among the 12 melatonin-only products that "passed" these standards are Nature's Bounty Melatonin 1-mg and 3-mg tablets; Puritan's Pride Inspired by Nature Melatonin 3-mg tablets; and Twinlab Melatonin Caps, Highest Quality, Quick-Acting 3-mg tablets. Further information is available at www.ConsumerLab.com.

Dosing: Adult (18 Years and Older)

- **Alzheimer's disease (sleep disturbances):** Studies have evaluated 0.5 mg of melatonin taken nightly by mouth one hour prior to sleep.
- **Bipolar disorder (sleep disturbances):** Studies have evaluated 10 mg of melatonin taken nightly by mouth.
- **Cancer:** Various doses of melatonin have been studied in patients with cancer, usually given in addition to other standard treatments such as chemotherapy, radiation therapy, or immune therapy. Oral doses have ranged between 10 and 50 mg taken nightly, with the most common dose being 20 mg nightly. Intramuscular injections of 20 mg of melatonin have also been studied. In studies of patients with melanoma, melatonin preparations have been applied to the skin. Patients are advised to discuss cancer treatment plans with an oncologist before considering use of melatonin either alone or with other therapies. Safety and effectiveness are not proven, and melatonin should not be used instead of more proven therapies.
- **Circadian rhythm entraining (in blind persons):** 5 to 10 mg of melatonin taken by mouth, administered in the evening, has been studied in blind patients to set the circadian rhythm to a 24-hour schedule.
- **Critical illness/ICU sleep disturbance:** Studies have evaluated 3 mg of melatonin taken nightly by mouth.
- **Delayed sleep phase syndrome:** Studies have evaluated 5 mg of melatonin given by mouth 5 hours prior to bedtime.
- **Depression (sleep disturbances):** Studies have evaluated 5 mg of melatonin taken nightly by mouth.
- **Headache prevention:** Studies have evaluated regular use of 5 to 10 mg of melatonin taken nightly by mouth.
- **Hypertension:** Studies have evaluated 1 to 3 mg of melatonin taken daily by mouth for short periods of time. Intranasal melatonin (1% solution in ethanol) at a dose of 2 mg daily for one week has also been studied.
- **Insomnia in the elderly:** Studies have evaluated melatonin taken by mouth 30 to 120 minutes prior to bedtime for insomnia in the elderly. Low doses (0.1 to 0.3 mg taken

M

nightly) appear to be equally effective as higher doses (3 to 5 mg nightly).

- **Insomnia of unknown origin in the non-elderly:** Doses ranging from 1 to 5 mg taken by mouth shortly before bedtime have been studied.
- **Jet lag:** Melatonin is usually started on the day of travel (close to the target bedtime at the destination) and then taken every 24 hours for several days. Various doses have been used and studied, including low doses between 0.1 and 0.5 mg,[68] a more common dose of 5 mg,[68-72] and a higher dose of 8 mg.[73] Overall, 0.5 mg appears to be slightly less effective than 5 mg for improvement of sleep quality and latency,[74] although this area remains controversial and other research suggests no differences.[73,75] Slow-release melatonin may not be as effective as standard (quick-release) formulations.[68] If the dose is taken too early in the day, it may actually result in excessive daytime sleepiness and greater difficulty adapting to the destination time zone.
- **Schizophrenia (sleep disturbances):** Studies have evaluated 2 mg of controlled-release melatonin taken by mouth for 3 weeks.
- **Seasonal affective disorder:** Studies have evaluated 0.25 to 5 mg of melatonin daily by mouth.
- **Sleep enhancement in healthy people:** Various doses of melatonin taken by mouth 30 to 60 minutes before bedtime have been studied and reported to have beneficial effects, including doses of 0.1, 0.3, 1, 3, 5, and 6 mg. Studies report that 0.1 to 0.3 mg may produce melatonin levels in the body within the normal physiologic range of nighttime melatonin and may be sufficient. Research suggests that quick-release melatonin may be more effective than sustained-release formulations.
- **Other:** Uses for other conditions have had limited study and unclear effectiveness or safety. Use of melatonin for these conditions should be discussed with a primary healthcare provider and should not be substituted for more proven therapies.

Dosing: Pediatric (Younger Than 18 Years)

- **General:** There is limited study of melatonin supplements in children, and safety is not established. Use of melatonin should be discussed with the child's physician prior to starting treatment.
- **Circadian rhythm entraining in blind children:** Studies have evaluated 2.5 to 10 mg of melatonin taken nightly at the desired bedtime.
- **Seizure disorder in children:** Studies have evaluated 5 to 10 mg of melatonin taken nightly. Research is limited in this area, and there are other reports that melatonin may actually increase the risk of seizure or lower seizure threshold. Therefore, caution is advised, and use of melatonin should be discussed with the child's physician.
- **Sleep disturbances in children with neuropsychiatric disorders (mental retardation, autism, psychiatric disorders):** Studies have evaluated 0.5 to 10 mg of melatonin taken nightly for reduced sleep latency and increased sleep duration. Quick-release melatonin may be most useful for sleep induction, and the slow-release formulation for sleep maintenance.

Toxicology

- The LD_{50} in mice has been reported to be greater than 800 mg/kg; in clinical trials, toxicity appears to be minimal[76] and includes mild effects such as diarrhea, headache, and abdominal cramps. A case of melatonin overdose was reported with ingestion of over 24 mg for relaxation and sleep prior to surgery, inducing symptoms of lethargy and disorientation.[77]

ADVERSE EFFECTS/PRECAUTIONS/CONTRAINDICATIONS
Allergy

- There are rare reports of allergic skin reactions after taking melatonin by mouth.[78,79] Melatonin has been linked to a case of autoimmune hepatitis.[80,81]

Adverse Effects

- **General:** Based on available studies and clinical use, melatonin is generally regarded as safe in recommended doses for short-term use. Available trials report that overall adverse effects are not significantly more common with melatonin than with placebo.[68,74,82] However, case reports raise concerns about risks of blood clotting abnormalities (particularly in patients taking warfarin), increased risk of seizure, and disorientation with overdose.
- **Neurologic (general):** Commonly reported adverse effects include fatigue, dizziness, headache, irritability, and sleepiness,[68,81,83,84] although these effects may occur due to jet-lag and not to melatonin itself. Fatigue may particularly occur with morning use or high doses (greater than 50 mg),[85] and irregular sleep-wake cycles may occur.[86] Disorientation, confusion, sleepwalking, and vivid dreams and nightmares have also been noted, with effects often resolving after cessation of melatonin.[74,77,87-89] Due to risk of daytime sleepiness, caution should be taken by those driving or operating heavy machinery.[77,83,85,87,90] Headache has been reported.[89,91] Ataxia (difficulties with walking and balance) may occur following overdose.[89]
- **Neurologic (seizure risk):** It has been suggested that melatonin may lower seizure threshold and increase the risk of seizure, particularly in children with severe neurologic disorders, as reported in 4 out of 6 children in one study[92] and in an adult in whom symptoms recurred when melatonin was given a second time.[89] However, multiple other studies actually report reduced incidence of seizure with regular melatonin use.[93-98] This remains an area of controversy.[99] Patients with seizure disorder taking melatonin should be monitored closely by a healthcare professional.
- **Psychiatric:** Mood changes have been reported, including giddiness and dysphoria (sadness).[100] Psychotic symptoms have been reported in at least two cases, including hallucinations and paranoia, possibly due to overdose.[74,101] Patients with underlying major depression or psychotic disorders taking melatonin should be monitored closely by a healthcare professional.
- **Hematologic (blood clotting abnormalities):** There are at least six reported cases of alterations in prothrombin time (a measurement of blood clotting ability) in patients taking both melatonin and the blood-thinning medication warfarin (Coumadin).[89] These cases have noted decreases in prothrombin time (PT), which would tend to decrease the effects of warfarin and increase the risk of blood clots. However, blood clots have not been noted in these patients. Rather, minor bleeding was noted in two of these cases (nosebleed and internal eye bleed), which may have been due to the blood-thinning effects of warfarin alone without a relationship to use of melatonin, or possibly to an interaction between melatonin and warfarin. It is not known if melatonin has effects on blood clotting in people who are not taking warfarin. Based on these reports, melatonin

should be avoided in patients using warfarin, and possibly in patients taking other blood-thinning medications or with clotting disorders.[102]

- **Cardiovascular:** Melatonin may cause drops in blood pressure, as observed in animals [103] and in preliminary human research.[104-109] Whether these reductions in blood pressure are clinically relevant is not clear. Caution is advised in patients taking medications that may also lower blood pressure. Based on preliminary evidence, increases in cholesterol levels may occur. Preliminary research suggests that regular use of melatonin may increase atherosclerotic plaque buildup in humans [110] and animals.[111-113] Caution is therefore advised in patients with high cholesterol levels, with atherosclerosis, or at risk for cardiovascular disease. There are several poorly described reports of abnormal heart rhythms, fast heart rate, and chest pain, although in most cases patients were taking other drugs that could account for these symptoms.[74,89]

- **Endocrine (blood sugar elevations):** Elevated blood sugar levels (hyperglycemia) have been reported in patients with type 1 diabetes (insulin-dependent diabetes),[79,114] and low doses of melatonin have reduced glucose tolerance and insulin sensitivity.[115] Caution is advised in patients with diabetes or hypoglycemia and in those taking drugs, herbs, or supplements that affect blood sugar. Serum glucose levels may need to be monitored by a healthcare professional, and medication adjustments may be necessary.

- **Endocrine (hormonal effects):** Hormonal effects are reported, including decreases or increases in levels of luteinizing hormone,[116-120] progesterone,[121] estradiol, thyroid hormone (T_4 and T_3), growth hormone, prolactin,[90] cortisol, oxytocin, and vasopressin, although there are other reports of no significant hormonal effects.[123-126] Variations may occur based on underlying patient characteristics. Gynecomastia (increased breast size) has been reported in men, as well as decreased sperm count (both of which resolved with cessation of melatonin).[102] Decreased sperm motility has been reported in rats [127] and humans.[128]

- **Gastrointestinal:** Mild gastrointestinal distress commonly occurs, including nausea, vomiting, and cramping.[79] Melatonin has been linked to a case of autoimmune hepatitis[80] and to triggering of Crohn's disease symptoms.[129]

- **Ocular (glaucoma):** It has been theorized that due to effects on photoreceptor renewal in the eye, high doses of melatonin may increase intraocular pressure and the risk of glaucoma, age-related maculopathy and myopia, and retinal damage. However, there is preliminary evidence that melatonin may actually decrease intraocular pressure in the eye, and it has been suggested as a possible therapy for glaucoma.[130,131] Patients with glaucoma taking melatonin should be monitored by a healthcare professional.

INTERACTIONS
Melatonin/Drug Interactions

- **Fluvoxamine and other cytochrome P450 (CYP) 1A2 drugs:** Melatonin is broken down (metabolized) in the body by the liver enzyme CYP1A2 (with a small contribution from CYP2C19).[132] As a result, drugs that alter the activity of these enzymes may increase or decrease the effects of melatonin supplements. For example, the drug fluvoxamine, when given with melatonin, reduces the activity of CYP1A2, thereby increasing blood levels of melatonin and theoretically increasing the effects or side effects of melatonin.[133-135] Other drugs that may increase melatonin levels (by inhibiting CYP1A2) include amiodarone, anastrozole, cimetidine, ciprofloxacin, citalopram, clarithromycin, diethyldithiocarbamate, diltiazem, enoxacin, erythromycin, ethinyl estradiol, fluoroquinolones, fluoxetine (high-dose), furafylline, interferon, isoniazid, ketoconazole, levofloxacin, methoxsalen, mexiletine, mibefradil, norfloxacin, paroxetine (high-dose), ritonavir, sertraline (mild), tacrine, tricyclic antidepressants (tertiary), ticlopidine, and zileuton. There is a case of psychotic symptoms in a patient taking both melatonin and the antidepressant drug fluoxetine, which may be due to this interaction.[101] Drugs that may reduce melatonin levels (by inducing CYP1A2) include carbamazepine, insulin, 3-methyl cholanthrene, modafinil, nafcillin, nicotine, omeprazole, phenobarbital, phenytoin, primidone, rifampin, and ritonavir.

- **Zolpidem and other sedative drugs:** Increased daytime drowsiness is reported when melatonin is used at the same time as the prescription sleep-aid zolpidem (Ambien), although it is not clear that effects are greater than with the use of zolpidem alone.[82] In theory, based on possible risk of daytime sleepiness,[77,83,85,87,90] melatonin may increase the amount of drowsiness caused by some other drugs, for example benzodiazepines such as lorazepam (Ativan) and diazepam (Valium), barbiturates such as phenobarbital, narcotics such as codeine, some antidepressants, and alcohol. Caution is advised while driving or operating machinery.

- **Warfarin and other anticoagulants:** Based on preliminary evidence, melatonin should be avoided in patients taking the blood-thinning medication warfarin (Coumadin), and possibly in patients using other blood-thinners (anticoagulants) such as aspirin and heparin.[102] There are at least six reported cases of alterations in prothrombin time (a measurement of blood clotting ability) in patients taking both melatonin and warfarin.[89] These cases have noted decreases in prothrombin time (PT), which would tend to decrease the effects of warfarin and increase the risk of blood clots. However, blood clots have not been noted in these patients. Rather, minor bleeding was noted in two of these cases (nosebleed and internal eye bleed), which may have been due to the blood-thinning effects of warfarin alone without a relationship to use of melatonin, or possibly to an interaction between melatonin and warfarin.

- **Natural melatonin levels:** Multiple drugs are reported to lower natural levels of melatonin in the body. It is not clear that there are any health hazards of lowered melatonin levels or if replacing melatonin with supplements is beneficial. Examples of drugs that may reduce production or secretion of melatonin include nonsteroidal anti-inflammatory drugs (NSAIDs) such as ibuprofen (Motrin, Advil) and naproxen (Naprosyn, Aleve),[136,137] beta-blocker blood pressure medications such as atenolol (Tenormin) and metoprolol (Lopressor, Toprol),[138] and medications that reduce levels of vitamin B_6 in the body (such as oral contraceptives, hormone replacement therapy, loop diuretics, hydralazine, and theophylline).[139-142] Other agents that may alter synthesis or release of melatonin include diazepam,[140,141] vitamin B_{12},[143] verapamil,[144] temazepam,[145] and somatostatin.[146]

- **Anti-seizure drugs:** Based on preliminary evidence, melatonin should be avoided in patients taking antiseizure medications. It has been suggested that melatonin may lower seizure threshold and increase the risk of seizure, particularly in children with severe neurologic disorders, as reported in 4 out of 6 children in one study[92] and in an adult in whom symptoms recurred when melatonin was given a second time.[89] However, multiple other studies actually report reduced incidence of seizure with regular melatonin use.[93-98]

This remains an area of controversy.[99] Patients with seizure disorder taking melatonin should be monitored closely by a healthcare professional.

- **Blood pressure medications (antihypertensives):** Melatonin may cause drops in blood pressure, as observed in animals [103] and in preliminary human research.[104,106-109] It is not known if melatonin causes further drops in blood pressure when taken with antihypertensive drugs. In animals, melatonin reduces the effects of the alpha-blocker drugs clonidine and methoxamine.[103] In contrast, in humans, blood pressure increases have been observed when 5 mg of melatonin is taken at the same time as the calcium-channel blocker nifedipine.[133,147]

- **Diabetes medications:** Elevated blood sugar levels (hyperglycemia) have been reported in patients with type 1 diabetes (insulin-dependent diabetes),[79,114] and low doses of melatonin have reduced glucose tolerance and insulin sensitivity.[115] Caution is advised in patients taking drugs for diabetes by mouth or insulin. Serum glucose levels may need to be monitored by a healthcare professional, and medication adjustments may be necessary.

- **Caffeine:** It is not clear if caffeine alters the effects of melatonin supplements in humans. Caffeine is reported to raise natural melatonin levels in the body,[148] possibly due to effects on the liver enzyme cytochrome P450 1A2 (CYP1A2).[149] However, caffeine may also alter circadian rhythms in the body, with effects on melatonin secretion.[149]

- **Succinylcholine:** Based on laboratory study, melatonin may increase the neuromuscular-blocking effect of the muscle relaxant succinylcholine, but not vecuronium.[150]

- **Methamphetamine:** Based on animal research, melatonin may increase the adverse effects of methamphetamine on the nervous system.[151]

- **Haloperidol (Haldol) (positive interaction):** Preliminary reports suggest that melatonin may aid in reversing symptoms of tardive dyskinesia associated with haloperidol use.[152-158]

- **Hormone replacement therapy (HRT):** HRT is reported to cause a decrease in daily melatonin secretion without disturbing circadian rhythm.[159,160] Clinical implications are not clear.

- **Isoniazid (positive interaction):** Based on preliminary evidence, melatonin may increase the effects of isoniazid against *Mycobacterium tuberculosis*.[58]

Melatonin/Herb/Supplement Interactions

- **Sedative herbs:** Melatonin may increase daytime sleepiness or sedation when taken with herbs or supplements that may cause sedation. Examples of such agents include 5-HTP, ashwagandha root, calamus, calendula, California poppy, capsicum, celery, cough, elecampane, German chamomile, goldenseal, hops, kava, lemon balm, sage, sassafras, shepherd's purse, Siberian ginseng, scullcap, stinging nettle, valerian, wild carrot, wild lettuce, and yerba mansa.

- **Hypoglycemic agents:** Elevated blood sugar levels (hyperglycemia) have been reported in patients with type 1 diabetes (insulin-dependent diabetes),[79,114] and low doses of melatonin have reduced glucose tolerance and insulin sensitivity.[115] Caution is advised when using herbs or supplements that may also raise blood sugar levels, such as arginine, cocoa, DHEA, and ephedra (when combined with caffeine).

- **Anticoagulant agents:** Based on preliminary evidence of an interaction with the blood-thinning drug warfarin, and isolated reports of minor bleeding, melatonin may increase

the risk of bleeding when taken with herbs and supplements that are believed to increase the risk of bleeding. Multiple cases of bleeding have been reported with the use of *Ginkgo biloba*, and fewer cases with garlic and saw palmetto. Numerous other agents may theoretically increase the risk of bleeding, although this has not been proven in most cases. Some examples include alfalfa, American ginseng, angelica, anise, *Arnica montana*, asafetida, aspen bark, bilberry, birch, black cohosh, bladderwrack, bogbean, boldo, borage seed oil, bromelain, capsicum, cat's claw, celery, chamomile, chaparral, clove, coleus, cordyceps, danshen, devil's claw, dong quai, EPA (eicosapentaenoic acid, found in fish oils), evening primrose oil, fenugreek, feverfew, fish oil, flaxseed/ flax powder (not a concern with flaxseed oil), ginger, grapefruit juice, grapeseed, green tea, guggul, gymnestra, horse chestnut, horseradish, licorice root, lovage root, male fern, meadowsweet, nordihydroguaiaretic acid (NDGA), omega-3 fatty acids, onion, papain, *Panax ginseng*, parsley, passion flower, poplar, prickly ash, propolis, quassia, red clover, reishi, rue, Siberian ginseng, sweet birch, sweet clover, turmeric, vitamin E, white willow, wild carrot, wild lettuce, willow, wintergreen, and yucca.

- **Chasteberry (*Vitex agnus-castus*):** Chasteberry may increase natural secretion of melatonin in the body, based on preliminary research.[161]

- **Folate:** Severe folate deficiency may reduce the body's natural levels of melatonin, based on preliminary study.[162]

- **DHEA (Dehydroepiandrosterone):** In mice, DHEA and melatonin have been noted to stimulate immune function, with slight additive effects when used together.[163] Effects of this combination in humans are not clear.

- *Echinacea purpurea*: In mice, a combination of echinacea and melatonin has been noted to slow the maturation of some types of immune cells, which may reduce immune function.[164] Effects of this combination in humans are not clear.

- **Caffeine:** It is not clear if caffeine alters the effects of melatonin supplements in humans. Caffeine is reported to raise natural melatonin levels in the body,[148] possibly due to effects on the liver enzyme cytochrome P450 1A2 (CYP1A2).[149] However, caffeine may also alter circadian rhythms in the body, with effects on melatonin secretion.[149]

Melatonin/Magnetic Field Interactions

- It has been theorized that chronic exposure to magnetic fields or recurrent cellular telephone use may alter melatonin levels and circadian rhythms. However, several studies suggest that this is not the case.[165-168] Melatonin was seen to reduce the effects of lipid peroxidation less effectively than vitamin E in rats exposed to static magnetic fields under laboratory conditions.[169]

Melatonin/Lab Interactions

- **Hormone levels:** Hormonal effects are reported, including decreases or increases in levels of luteinizing hormone,[116-120] progesterone,[121] estradiol, thyroid hormone (T_4 and T_3),[122] growth hormone, prolactin,[90] cortisol, oxytocin and vasopressin, although there are other reports of no significant hormonal effects.[123-126] Variations may occur based on underlying patient characteristics.

- **Glucose levels:** Elevated blood sugar levels (hyperglycemia) have been reported in patients with type 1 diabetes (insulin-dependent diabetes),[79,114] and low doses of melatonin have reduced glucose tolerance and insulin sensitivity.[115]

- **Cholesterol:** Melatonin may elicit decreases in free serum cholesterol levels.[111]

MECHANISM OF ACTION
Pharmacology

- **Endogenous melatonin:** Melatonin is synthesized from tryptophan in the pineal gland,[170] with regulation of day-night changes in synthesis by serotonin *N*-acetyltransferase.[171] Some synthesis takes place additionally in the retina, gastrointestinal tract, bone marrow, and bile.[172-174] The formation and release of melatonin are stimulated by darkness and inhibited by light,[175-177] without significant differences between polarized and nonpolarized light.[178,179] The primary melatonin-controlled events take place in the rods rather than in the cones of retina.[179] This response to light may remain in blind subjects, despite apparently complete loss of visual function.[180,181]
- Since β_1-adrenoreceptor antagonists almost completely inhibit the normal nighttime rise in melatonin, it is thought that human pineal adrenoreceptors are β_1-subtype.[138,182-186] Similar arguments indicate the involvement of α_1-adrenoreceptors in stimulation of melatonin synthesis,[187] whereas α_2-adrenoreceptors presumably operate as down-regulators.[88,189] As such, the production of melatonin is considered to be regulated by the sympathetic nervous system and its neurotransmitter norepinephrine. With the onset of darkness, norepinephrine release is followed by stimulation of postsynaptic pineal adrenoreceptors and enhancement of melatonin synthesis.[170,190] The involvement of norepinephrine is supported by an increase in nighttime plasma melatonin in humans treated with an inhibitor of norepinephrine uptake.[191,192] Activation of the sympathetic nervous system (SNS) appears to accelerate melatonin synthesis.[193-195] Animal studies suggest that endogenous melatonin is involved in the suppression of SNS activity, with possible negative feedback inhibition.[196] Melatonin reduces circulating norepinephrine in young individuals and in post-menopausal women receiving estradiol replacement, but not in menopausal women.[197]
- Melatonin secretion occurs at a constant rate in both young and older men and women.[198] Circadian melatonin rhythm appears at the end of the neonatal period and persists thereafter,[199,200] despite functioning vision.
- In humans, the daytime melatonin plasma level is less than 40 pmol/L. In the middle of the night, the concentration increases to approximately 260 pmol/L.[170] In some species, these values may reach a 50-fold difference.[201] Both high-and low-affinity binding sites have been identified in several brain regions (superchiasmatic nuclei of the hypothalamus, thalamus, and pituitary gland), retina, gut, ovaries, blood vessels, lymphocytes, and platelets.[170,202-204] A recently discovered class of melatonin-binding sites, called orphan receptors, presumably mediate the ability of melatonin to regulate gene expression.[201,205]
- Suppression of nocturnal melatonin secretion with a β_1-adrenoreceptor antagonist increases total wake time and decreases rapid eye movement (REM) and slow wave sleep.[18] These effects are reversed if melatonin is given after the antagonist. In humans, a pacemaker located in the suprachiasmatic nucleus of the hypothalamus controls the circadian rhythm of melatonin production. By binding to the receptors in the nucleus, melatonin may alter a phase of pacemaker (i.e., reset the biological clock).[206-212] The suprachiasmatic nuclei are the target sites for the effect of exogenous melatonin on the amplitude of the endogenous melatonin rhythm.[213]
- The lack of light signal in blind persons leads to various unusual free-running melatonin secretory patterns.[214-216] Low-dose melatonin has been noted to be more effective entraining free-running blind people due to the potential of excess hormone spilling into the wrong zone of the phase-response curve.[217] Free-running patterns are also observed after pineal gland damage[218] or under special working regimens.[219,220] The nocturnal onset of melatonin secretion strongly correlates with a steep rise in sleep propensity and precedes it by approximately 2 hours.[221] The specific events taking place during this interval remain obscure. It is possible that melatonin does not actively induce sleep but switches off a wakefulness-generated mechanism that opposes a sleep-inducing mechanism,[221] the alerting process being dependent on the suprachiasmatic nucleus.[207]
- The following factors can modulate the synthesis and release of melatonin: nonsteroidal anti-inflammatory drugs (NSAIDs),[137] diazepam,[140,141] vitamin B_{12},[143] γ-aminobutyric acid (GABA),[222,223] ethanol,[224] micronutrient accumulation and depletion,[225] gonadotropin-releasing hormone, gonadotropins/gonadal steroids,[226,227] estrogen plus progesterone,[142] testosterone,[226] duration of gestation,[228] prenatal growth restriction,[229] interleukin-2,[230] cancer,[230] posture,[231] balance,[232] phenelzine,[233] thorazine,[234] sleep deprivation,[194,235] hypercalcemia/verapamil,[144] temazepam, zopiclone,[145] levodopa-related motor complications,[236] modafinil,[235] *Agnus castus*,[161] desipramine,[237] prazosin,[188] intravenous L-tryptophan,[174] and exercise.[238] No effect is seen with somatostatin,[146] oral administration of 5-hydoxytryptophan,[239] exposure to pulsating magnetic fields,[166] nifedipine,[240] midazolam, sodium thiopental,[241] electroconvulsive therapy, TRH-injection, L-dopa, or bromoergocryptine.[242,243]
- Disturbances in the circadian rhythm of melatonin (and declines in nighttime melatonin) have been associated with aging.[170,244-250]
- **Exogenous melatonin:** A physiologic dose of orally administered melatonin shifts circadian rhythms in humans according to a phase-response curve (PRC) that is nearly opposite in phase to the PRCs for light exposure: melatonin delays circadian rhythms when administered in the morning and advances them when administered in the afternoon or early evening.[251]
- Multiple studies performed to date on the functions of endogenous melatonin have utilized exogenous melatonin, often at high doses. However, the most reliable data are obtained at low doses of exogenous melatonin, at which plasma levels are within a physiologic range.[202,252] It is not entirely clear what relationships exist between melatonin secretion and pharmacologic effects observed at higher concentrations.[253]
- While measuring endogenous melatonin, some authors have not found a link between melatonin secretion and the sleep-waking cycle in humans.[254] It has been suggested by some that natural sleep is largely determined by a functioning circadian system without melatonin involvement.[212,245,255,256]
- **Hypnotic properties:** Melatonin, administered either day or night in doses beyond the physiologic range, appears to elicit a hypnotic effect. Even very low doses can cause sleep when ingested before endogenous melatonin onset,[87,252,257,258] although some studies have failed to confirm this finding.[259] Melatonin seems to potentiate the effects of γ-aminobutyric acid (GABA) and benzodiazepines, and quality of sleep may

be improved by a combination of melatonin and benzodiazepines.[260] Melatonin may interact directly with the GABA-benzodiazepine-chloride ion channel,[145,261] but not with the benzodiazepine receptor.[262]

- **Phase-shifting properties:** Exogenous melatonin is able to shift circadian rhythms as well as endogenous melatonin secretion and core body temperature. Light appears to be a stronger regulator of circadian rhythm than melatonin itself.[177,251,263-268] The time of administration of melatonin is of critical importance, because it may cause both phase-delay and phase-advance. For phase-delay, melatonin should be administered in the early morning; for phase-advance, melatonin should be administered 1 to 2 hours before 2100 hours.[251]

- **Suppressing core body temperature:** Ingestion of 1.6 mg of melatonin is reported to result in approximately a 0.4° C decrease in body temperature in humans.[269-272] The mechanism of this phenomenon is not known.

- **Decreasing cognitive performance:** Although vigilance, reaction time, and tasks in humans undergo circadian variations, they do not seem to correlate with endogenous melatonin levels.[87,273] Exogenous melatonin may cause decrements in performance, including a slowing of choice-reaction time [274,275] and learning.[253] Some studies have failed to confirm a decrement in performance,[276] including a study of high-dose melatonin (50 mg) in elderly persons (mean age, 84.5 years).[277] Animal research suggests a possible role of the GABAergic system.[278]

- **Immune effects:** Activation of melatonin receptors is associated with the release of cytokines by type 1 T-helper cells (Th$_1$), including γ-interferon (γ-IFN) and IL-2, as well as novel opioid cytokines.[279] There is indirect evidence that melatonin may amplify the immunostimulatory effect of interleukin-2, as measured by an increase in the number of T lymphocytes, natural killer cells, and eosinophils in cancer patients.[280-284] Melatonin may act directly on cell proliferation by binding to high affinity receptors on spleen cells that stimulate the production of IL-2 and IL-1 beta.[285] Inhibition of the circadian synthesis of melatonin has been associated with reversible immunosuppression [286] and elicits T-cell autoimmunity in mice.[12,287] Melatonin has been reported to promote neutrophil apoptosis in patients receiving hepatectomy, involving ischemia and reperfusion of the liver.[35,288-290]

- **Antiproliferative properties:** At pharmacologic concentrations, melatonin exhibits cytotoxic activity in cancer cells.[291,292] At both physiologic and pharmacologic concentrations, melatonin acts as a differentiating agent in some cancer cells and lowers their invasive and metastatic capabilities through alterations in adhesion molecules and maintenance of gap junctional intercellular communication. In other cancer cell types, melatonin, either alone or in combination with other agents, induces apoptotic cell death. Biochemical and molecular mechanisms of melatonin's oncostatic action may include regulation of estrogen receptor expression and transactivation, calcium/calmodulin activity, protein kinase C activity, cytoskeletal architecture and function, intracellular pH, melatonin receptor-mediated signal transduction cascades, and fatty acid transport and metabolism.[291] As a chemoprotective agent, daily administration of melatonin for 6 months is reported to induce a protective effect against the formation of mammary tumors in rat models.[293]

- Nuclear signaling appears to play a central role in the function of melatonin.[294] At physiologic circulating concentrations, melatonin may inhibit cancer cell proliferation via cell cycle–specific effects identified *in vitro*.[291,292,295,296] Women with endometrial cancer have been found to have melatonin plasma levels six times lower than tumor-free controls. It is not clear if this is causative or adaptive, although a melatonin antiproliferative activity is hypothesized.[297-299] Pinealectomy is reported to enhance tumor growth and metastasis in animals.[300] In addition, increased neoplastic growth has been noted in some animal models (Morris hepatoma 7288 CTC in rats), when animals are maintained in a constant weak light (0.2 lux), thereby inducing inhibition of melatonin synthesis.[301] MT1 (high-affinity melatonin receptor subtype) receptors have been detected in normal and malignant breast epithelium, with high receptor levels occurring more frequently in tumor cells ($p < 0.001$), and tumors with moderate or strong reactivity more likely to be high nuclear grade ($p < 0.045$). These findings are proposed to have implications for the use of melatonin in breast cancer therapy.[302]

- An oncostatic effect of melatonin (cessation of cell cycle progression) has been reported in human androgen-independent DU-145 prostate cancer cells, due to involvement of nuclear rather than membrane melatonin receptors.[303] MCF-7 human breast cancer cultured cells have been reported to be melatonin-sensitive as well as estrogen receptor-positive and estrogen-responsive,[304] although this finding was not confirmed in a subsequent study.[305] Inhibition of cell proliferation may be mediated either through G-protein coupled membrane receptors, or via retinoid orphan receptors with involvement of the calcium-signaling pathway.[306] Downregulation of the receptor level indicates the possibility of an estrogen-responsive mechanism. This notion is supported by melatonin-induced stimulation of expression of the growth-inhibitory factor, TGF-beta.[304] However, other investigators have failed to reproduce the oncostatic effect on MCF-7 cells or ZR-75-1 and T-47D cell lines.[307] Melanoma M2R cells also respond to melatonin.[308] It has also been suggested that melatonin-related growth inhibition of breast cancer cells may be related to enhanced TGF-beta(1) secretion.[309]

- Melatonin is reported to elicit an increase in estrogen receptor activity in breast tumors.[234] Low plasma melatonin concentrations are associated with a greater amounts of estrogen or progesterone receptors on primary tumors.[310]

- **Antioxidant properties:** *In vitro*, melatonin has been observed to act as a direct free radical scavenger with the ability to detoxify both reactive oxygen and reactive nitrogen species.[311,312] *In vivo*, it reduces oxidative damage under conditions in which excessive free radical generation is believed to be involved.[313,314] This activity has been observed in various models of ischemia and reperfusion injury,[13,35,288-290,315-332] as well as in nerve tissues including brain, spinal cord, optic nerve, and spinal-cord white matter,[333] although in a rat model, melatonin was not effective in attenuating alcohol-induced loss of Purkinje cells.[334] Nonetheless, due to its high lipophilicity, melatonin is likely able to reach most tissues.[335]

- In preclinical studies, melatonin protects against toxicity related to oxidative damage, such as alloxan-induced pancreatic toxicity,[336] 6-hydroxydopamine damage to neuronal PC12 cells, kainic acid injury,[337-339] homocysteine-mediated oxidative stress,[110,340,341] iron-induced oxidative injury,[35,288-290] radiation-induced damage of various cell lines,[342-346] ultraviolet light–induced damage,[347,348] and copper-induced LDL oxidation.[349] Melatonin has been reported as being a more efficient antioxidant than glutathione,[350] vitamin C,[351,352] or vitamin E.[3,335,353-356] Synergy has been observed with other antioxidants.[5,357]

- Some data suggest that melatonin as a free radical scavenger can inhibit the microsomal production of hydrogen peroxide in rats treated with aflatoxin,[358] although more recent research reports that melatonin does not directly scavenge hydrogen peroxide.[359] Other conflicting evidence also exists: exogenous melatonin administered to rats via intraperitoneal injection increased photoreceptor susceptibility to light-induced damage; pinealectomy has been shown to protect photoreceptors, whereas subsequent melatonin injection has increased destruction.[360]

- **Bone effects:** Through free radical scavenging and anti-oxidant properties, melatonin may impair osteoclast activity and bone resorption.[201,361,.362]

- **Hormonal effects:** Exogenous melatonin enhances the stimulatory effect of hypothalamic gonadotropin-releasing hormone on pituitary luteinizing hormone in women.[118-120,363] This response to melatonin becomes distorted in patients with menstrual abnormalities,[195,364] is absent in postmenopausal women,[356,366] and is not observed in men,[125,367,368] in whom only a decrease in basal luteinizing hormone level is noted.[116,369,370] It has been proposed that administering melatonin to aging women may lead to a recovery of pituitary and thyroid function.[371] Melatonin decreases progesterone and estradiol plasma levels in healthy women[65] and enhances stimulatory effect of chorionic gonadotropin on progesterone production in cell culture.[372]

- Melatonin enhances basal levels of growth hormone and its stimulation by hypothalamic releasing hormone or exercise.[373-377] This result may be mediated via the serotonin pathway[378-380] or through naloxone-sensitive opioid-mediation.[381,382] However, this effect has not been confirmed in other studies.[126,383] Exogenous melatonin has been reported to generate dopamine circadian rhythms in mice.[384]

- Both endogenous[385] and exogenous melatonin appear to elevate plasma concentrations of prolactin without affecting the temporal pattern of its pulsatile secretion.[124,386-389]

- Melatonin does not affect basal levels of cortisol in young men.[389,390] Cortisol increases are reported in aged but not young women.[121]

- In rats, melatonin significantly affects vasopressin secretion.[391] In humans, melatonin may not directly alter basal and angiotensin-2 stimulated arginine-vasopressin levels.[392]

- Melatonin appears to reduce glucose tolerance and insulin sensitivity[115,393] and may increase insulin levels through direct effects on the pancreas.[394]

- Melatonin is also involved in the control of testosterone secretion.[395]

- **Anti-inflammatory properties:** Melatonin has been reported to decrease upregulation of proinflammatory cytokines.[396] Other anti-inflammatory effects may be related to inhibition of nitric oxide (NO) and methylenedioxyamphetamine (MDA) production, or increase of glutathione levels.[397,398] Use in inflammatory conditions has been proposed.[399]

- **Gastric protection:** Protective effects of melatonin have been observed in models of stress-induced gastric lesions and indomethacin-mediated gastric damage,[400] possibly due to effects on prostaglandins.[401,402] Melatonin has been reported as more effective than ranitidine but less effective than omeprazole in preventing "stress ulcer."[403,404] Melatonin significantly decreases the extent of ethanol-induced macroscopic injury.[397,398]

- **Anticonvulsant/proconvulsant properties:** Both anti-convulsant[98,405,406] and proconvulsant[99] properties have been associated with melatonin in preclinical studies. In animals, intraventricular injection of anti-melatonin antibody elicits transitory epileptiform abnormalities in the electro-encephalogram.[407] Increases in anticonvulsant effects of valproate have been observed in mice.[98,405] Proposed mechanisms of action include altered brain GABAergic neurotransmission, interactions with benzodiazepine brain receptors, tryptophan metabolite activity, free-radical scavenger activity, or modulation of brain amino acids and NO production.[99,406]

- **Opioid tolerance:** In animals, melatonin acutely reverses and prevents tolerance and dependence to morphine,[408,409] and reduces the incidence of naloxone-induced withdrawal.[409]

- **Hypotensive properties:** In humans, melatonin, even in a dose of 1 mg, has been observed to reduce blood pressure and decrease catecholamine levels after 90 minutes in human subjects, possibly via direct effects on the hypothalamus, through antioxidant activity, by decreasing catecholamine levels, or by relaxing smooth muscle in the aorta wall.[410] Dose-dependent relaxation of precontracted rat aorta and reduction of contractile response to α-adrenergic but not β-adrenergic agonists have been observed.[103] In healthy humans, melatonin is reported to decrease pulsatility index and systolic and diastolic blood pressure, blunt noradrenergic activation,[104,106,107] and increase cardiac vagal tone.[108] In healthy postmenopausal women, hypotensive action has been observed only during hormone replacement therapy.[109] Reductions in intraocular pressure have been observed[130] without changes in rate of aqueous humor flow.[131]

- **Potential therapeutic uses of melatonin:** The following are conditions in which changes in circulating or excreted melatonin have been found, indicating a possible target for pharmacological intervention (however, it is not clear if altered melatonin levels are causative, resultant, or adaptive in these cases): hypothalamic amenorrhea (increased in plasma),[411,412] ischemic stroke (impaired nocturnal excretion),[413,414] seasonal affective disorder (phase delay, reduced melatonin production, hypersensitivity to light),[415-417] primary insomnia (low plasma melatonin),[418-420] major depressive disorder (low nocturnal melatonin),[421-423] premenstrual depression (chronobiological abnormalities of melatonin secretion),[424] eating disorders (low level, enhanced circadian rhythm),[425,426] hepatic encephalopathy (increased in plasma),[427] adolescent idiopathic scoliosis (increased in plasma),[33] migraine (impaired pineal function; feverfew contains melatonin and is beneficial),[243,428-431] postoperative complications in older patients (impaired secretion rhythm),[432] sudden infant death syndrome (decreased in plasma),[433-435] glaucoma,[436] mania (decreased melatonin production),[437] coronary artery disease (impaired nocturnal secretion),[438-442] multiple sclerosis (decreased in plasma),[443,444] sleep disorder in elderly patients,[445-448] delayed sleep phase syndrome (abnormally delayed phase of circadian rhythms),[449] disturbance of sleep in blind children (delays in nocturnal secretion),[450] and intestinal motility disorders.[17]

Pharmacodynamics/Kinetics

- **Half-life:** The physiologic half-life of melatonin is approximately 30 to 60 minutes, although nutritional supplements do not appear to mimic the physiologic release of melatonin, as dissolution testing has ranged from 4 to 12 hours,[451] with controlled-release formulations available.[452] When administered in gelatin capsules, melatonin reaches peak levels after 60 to 150 minutes (350 to 10,000 times higher than nighttime concentration).[453,454] Melatonin secretion increases after the onset of darkness, peaks in the middle of the night (between 2 and 4 AM), and then gradually decreases.[170] Pharmacologic effects appear to depend on the time of administration. The time delay between administration and maximal effect varies linearly from 220 minutes at noon to 60 minutes at 9 PM.[190]

- **Bioavailability:** The calculated oral bioavailability of melatonin is 0.03 to 0.06 after a 2.5-mg dose, 0.03 to 0.76 after an 80-mg dose, and 0.09 after a 100-mg dose.[455] The poor bioavailability of melatonin may be due to the hepatic first-pass effect (melatonin is converted to its metabolite before entering the systemic circulation) and varies from 10% to 56%.[456] Bioavailability testing of 80 mg of oral melatonin in humans found peak serum melatonin levels (ranging from 350 to 10,000 times those occurring at night) were observed 60 to 150 minutes after administration and were maintained for approximately 1.5 hours.[454] Melatonin can be delivered transdermally in humans[457] or transmucosally to mimic physiological activity.[458] Melatonin can be monitored by its serum metabolite 6-sulphatoxymelatonin by radio-immunoassay[242,459] and in saliva,[460,461] although melatonin concentrations measured in saliva do not consistently reflect absolute concentrations in blood.[460] Contrary to the belief

that melatonin is highly hydrophobic, melatonin has been shown to be soluble in a purely aqueous medium up to 5 mM.[462] Melatonin easily passes the blood-brain barrier.[463]

- **Metabolism/elimination:** Melatonin is primarily inactivated by 6-hydroxylation within the liver, followed by conjugation and excretion as the sulfate or glucuronide. First-pass hepatic metabolism is extensive (up to 60% of oral dose).[455] In patients with liver cirrhosis, melatonin levels are elevated compared to controls.[464,465] Up to 85% is excreted in urine. Elimination half-life values have been observed to range from approximately 30 to 50 minutes.[456,466,467]

HISTORY

- In the early 1900s, physicians came to believe that the pineal gland was involved in the endocrine system. Melatonin was discovered in 1958, and its popularity grew dramatically in the United States following reports in 1995 of its ability to promote sleep and alleviate jet lag.
- Synthetic melatonin is sold in the United States as a food supplement; small amounts are found in foods such as bananas and rice. Some authors suggest that this categorization interferes with standardization and quality improvement of melatonin.

Review of the Evidence: Melatonin

Condition Treated*	Study Design	Author, Year	N[†]	SS[†]	Study Quality[‡]	Magnitude of Benefit	ARR[†]	NNT[†]	Comments
Improvement of normal sleep	Systematic review	Avery[503] 1998	143	NA	NA	Medium	NA	NA	Reviewed 7 trials.
Improvement of normal sleep	RCT	Atkinson[508] 2001	12	No	3	NA	NA	NA	Melatonin, 5 mg.
Improvement of normal sleep	RCT	Attenburrow[418] 1996	15	Yes	4	Medium	NA	NA	Melatonin, 0.3 mg or 1 mg; unclear blinding and randomization.
Improvement of normal sleep	RCT	Cajochen[252] 1996	8	Yes	4	Medium	NA	NA	Melatonin, 5.0 mg.
Improvement of normal sleep	RCT	Dollins[506] 1994	20	Yes	4	Medium	NA	NA	Melatonin, 0.1-10 mg; unclear blinding.
Improvement of normal sleep	RCT	Gilbert[509] 1999	20	Yes	4	Medium	NA	NA	Melatonin, 5 mg; unclear blinding and randomization.
Improvement of normal sleep	RCT	James[259] 1987	10	No	3	NA	NA	NA	Melatonin, 1 mg or 5 mg; unclear blinding and randomization.
Improvement of normal sleep	RCT	Nave[510] 1995	12	Yes	4	Large	NA	NA	Melatonin, 3 mg or 6 mg; unclear blinding and randomization.
Improvement of normal sleep	RCT	Satomura[511] 2001	7	Yes	4	Medium	NA	NA	Melatonin, 1, 3, or 6 mg; single-blinded; unclear randomization.
Improvement of normal sleep	RCT	Waldhouser 1990	20	Yes	4	Medium	NA	NA	Unclear randomization.
Improvement of normal sleep	RCT	Wyatt[521] 1999	19	Yes	4	Medium	NA	NA	Melatonin, 0.3 or 0.5 mg.
Improvement of normal sleep	RCT	Zhdanova[504] 1995	6	Yes	4	Medium	NA	NA	Melatonin, 0.3 or 1 mg.
Improvement of normal sleep	RCT	Zhdanova[505] 1996	12	Yes	4	Large	NA	NA	Melatonin, 0.3 or 1 mg.
Improvement of normal sleep	Crossover RCT	Hughes	8	No	3	Medium	NA	NA	Melatonin, 1, 10, or 40 mg or placebo.
Jet lag	Review	Herxheimer[74] 2002	692	NA	NA	Medium	NA	NA	8 randomized trials.

Review of the Evidence: Melatonin—*cont'd*

Condition Treated*	Study Design	Author, Year	N[†]	SS[†]	Study Quality[‡]	Magnitude of Benefit	ARR[†]	NNT[†]	Comments
Jet lag	RCT	Arendt[69] 1986	17	Yes	4	Medium	NA	NA	Melatonin, 5 mg.
Jet lag	RCT	Claustrat[73] 1992	30	Yes	4	Medium	NA	NA	Melatonin, 8 mg; unclear blinding and randomization.
Jet lag	RCT	Petrie[71] 1993	52	No	3	Medium	NA	NA	Melatonin, 5 mg.
Jet lag	RCT	Suhner[68] 1998	320	Yes	3	Large	NA	NA	Melatonin, 5 mg FR or 2 mg CR. Placebo.
Jet lag	RCT	Spitzer[469] 1999	257	No	3	None	NA	NA	Melatonin, 5 or 0.5 mg or placebo.
Entraining circadian rhythm in blind people	RCT	Lockley[591] 2000	7	Yes	3	Medium	NA	NA	Melatonin, 5 mg; single-blinded; unclear randomization; no statistical analysis.
Entraining circadian rhythm in blind people	RCT	Sack[589] 1991	5	Yes	4	Medium	NA	NA	Melatonin, 5 mg.
Delayed sleep phase syndrome	RCT	Dagan[470] 1998	61	Yes	4	Medium	NA	NA	Melatonin, 5 mg; positive effect in 97% of cases.
Delayed sleep phase syndrome	RCT	Dahlitz[471] 1991	8	Yes	4	Medium	NA	NA	Melatonin, 5 mg.
Delayed sleep phase syndrome	RCT	Nagtegaal 1998	30	Yes	4	Medium	NA	NA	Melatonin, 5 mg.
Delayed sleep phase syndrome	RCT	Yang[473] 2001	10	Yes	4	Medium	NA	NA	Melatonin, 6 mg.
Delayed sleep phase syndrome	RCT	Kayumov[474] 2001	20	Yes	4	Medium	NA	NA	Melatonin, 5 mg.
Delayed sleep phase syndrome	RCT	Wirz-Justice 2002	9	No	3	None	NA	NA	Melatonin, 5 mg.
Insomnia (unknown origin)	Review	Morera[615] 2000	101	NA	NA	Medium	NA	NA	Reviewed 8 trials.
Insomnia (unknown origin)	RCT	Andrade[617] 2001	33	Yes	4	Medium	NA	NA	Melatonin, average dose 5.4 mg.
Insomnia (unknown origin)	RCT	Ellis[91] 1996	15	No	4	NA	NA	NA	Melatonin, 5 mg.
Insomnia (unknown origin)	RCT	James[618] 1990	10	No	4	NA	NA	NA	Melatonin, 5 mg.
Insomnia (primary)	Crossover RCT	Almeida Montes[616] 2003	10	No	3	None	NA	NA	Melatonin, 0.3 or 1 mg.
Sleep disturbances (children)	Review	Jan[475] 1999	468	NA	NA	NA	NA	NA	Analysis over 1991-1998.
Sleep disturbances (children)	RCT	Camfield[476] 1996	6	No	4	NA	NA	NA	Melatonin, 0.5 and 1 mg.
Sleep disturbances (children)	RCT	Dodge[477] 2001	20	Yes	4	Medium	NA	NA	Unclear randomization.
Sleep disturbances (children)	RCT	Smits[478] 2001	40	Yes	4	Medium	NA	NA	Melatonin, 5 mg.
Sleep disturbances (children)	Crossover RCT	Jan 2000	42	No	3	Small	NA	NA	Melatonin, average dose 5.7 mg.
Sleep disturbances (children)	Retrospective study	Ivanenko 2003	32	Yes	NA	Large	NA	NA	Melatonin, average dose 2 mg.
Sleep disturbance (elderly)	RCT	Haimov[445,494] 1995	8	Yes	4	Medium	NA	NA	Melatonin, 1 mg.

M

Continued

Review of the Evidence: Melatonin—*cont'd*

Condition Treated*	Study Design	Author, Year	N[†]	SS[†]	Study Quality[‡]	Magnitude of Benefit	ARR[†]	NNT[†]	Comments
Sleep disturbance (elderly)	RCT	Dawson 1998	12	No	4	NA	NA	NA	Melatonin, 0.5 mg.
Sleep disturbance (elderly)	RCT	Haimov[445,494] 1995	8	Yes	4	Medium	NA	NA	Melatonin, 1 mg.
Sleep disturbance (elderly)	Crossover RCT	Baskett[501]	40	No	3	Small	NA	NA	Melatonin, 5 mg.
AIDS	Phase II pilot study	Lissoni[995]	11	Yes	NA	Medium	NA	NA	Melatonin, 40 mg plus IL-2.
Cancer	RCT	Italian study group[534] 1999	386	No	5	NA	NA	NA	Melatonin, 20 mg; combination of several therapies.
Cancer	RCT	Lissoni 1996	30	Yes	4	Medium	NA	NA	Melatonin, 20 mg; melanoma.
Cancer	Review	Lamson[536] 1999	680	NA	NA	Medium	NA	NA	14 trials.
Cancer	RCT	Lissoni 2001	30	Yes	4	Medium	NA	NA	Melatonin, 20 mg.
Cancer	RCT	Lissoni 1992	63	Yes	4	Medium	NA	NA	Melatonin, 10 mg; non–small cell lung cancer.
Cancer	RCT	Barni[561] 1996	108	Yes	NA	Medium	NA	NA	Melatonin, 20 mg; no placebo.
Cancer (adjunct to chemotherapy)	RCT	Ghielmini[532] 1999	20	No	5	NA	NA	NA	Melatonin, 40 mg; advanced lung cancer.
Cancer (adjunct to chemotherapy)	RCT	Lissoni 1997	80	Yes	4	Medium	NA	NA	Melatonin, 20 mg.
Cancer (adjunct to chemotherapy)	RCT	Lissoni 1999	250	Yes	4	Medium	NA	NA	Melatonin, 20 mg; breast cancer, lung cancer, GI tumors; head and neck tumors.
Cancer (adjunct to chemotherapy)	RCT	Lissoni 1997	70	Yes	4	Medium	NA	NA	Chemotherapy plus melatonin, 20 mg; non–small cell lung cancer.
Cancer (adjunct to chemotherapy)	RCT	Cerea[529] 2003	30	Yes	1	Small	NA	NA	Chemotherapy plus melatonin, 20 mg; colorectal cancer.
Cancer (adjunct to IL-2)	RCT	Barni[566] 1995	50	Yes	4	Medium	NA	NA	Melatonin, 40 mg, plus IL-2; metastatic colorectal cancer.
Cancer (adjunct to IL2)	RCT	Brivio[567] 1995	20	Yes	4	Medium	NA	NA	IL-2 plus melatonin, 40 mg; GI tumors.
Cancer (adjunct to IL-2)	RCT	Lissoni 1990	5	Yes	4	Medium	NA	NA	IL-2 alone or IL-2 plus melatonin, 10 mg; metastatic renal cancer.
Cancer (adjunct to IL-2)	RCT	Lissoni 1994	80	Yes	4	Medium	NA	NA	IL-2 plus melatonin, 40 mg; solid tumors.
Cancer (adjunct to IL-2)	RCT	Lissoni 1995	100	Yes	4	Medium	NA	NA	IL-2 plus melatonin, 40 mg; metastatic solid tumors.
Cancer (adjunct to IL-2)	RCT	Lissoni 1995	30	Yes	NA	Medium	NA	NA	Melatonin, 40 mg, plus IL-2; GI tumors; no placebo.
Cancer (adjunct to IL-2)	RCT	Lissoni 1996	116	Yes	NA	Medium	NA	NA	Melatonin, 40 mg, plus IL-2 and TNF; advanced solid tumors; no placebo.
Cancer (adjunct to radiotherapy)	RCT	Lissoni 1996	30	Yes	4	Medium	NA	NA	Melatonin. 20 mg, plus radiotherapy; glioblastoma.
Cancer (adjunct to supportive therapy)	RCT	Lissoni 1994	50	Yes	4	Medium	NA	NA	Supportive care plus melatonin, 20 mg; unresectable brain metastases.
Cancer (adjunct to supportive therapy)	RCT	Lissoni 1996	86	Yes	4	Medium	NA	NA	Melatonin, 20 mg daily; metastatic solid tumors.

Review of the Evidence: Melatonin—*cont'd*

Condition Treated*	Study Design	Author, Year	N[†]	SS[†]	Study Quality[‡]	Magnitude of Benefit	ARR[†]	NNT[†]	Comments
Cancer (adjunct to TNF therapy)	RCT	Braczkowski[585] 1995	14	Yes	4	Medium	NA	NA	Melatonin, 40 mg; metastatic solid tumors.
Cancer (adjunct to TNF therapy)	RCT	Lissoni 1996	116	Yes	NA	Medium	NA	NA	Melatonin, 40 mg, plus TNF; advanced solid tumors; no placebo.
Depression	Open-label trial	Dalton[603] 2000	9	NA	NA	Small	NA	NA	Melatonin, 5 mg SR, plus antidepressant therapy.
Epilepsy in children	Case report	Brueske[93] 1981	1	NA	NA	NA	NA	NA	Melatonin intravenous infusion, 3.4 mg/kg.
Epilepsy in children	Case series	Fauteck[94] 1999	Not known	Yes	NA	Medium	NA	NA	Melatonin, 5-10 mg, in children.
Epilepsy in children	Case series	Jan[95] 1999	3	NA	NA	Medium	NA	NA	Melatonin, 3-5 mg, in children.
Epilepsy in children	Case report	Molina-Carballo[96] 1997	1	NA	NA	NA	NA	NA	Combination melatonin (dose unknown).
Epilepsy in children	Case series	Peled 2001	6	NA	NA	NA	NA	NA	Melatonin, 3 mg.
Headache	Review	Gagnier[606] 2001	30	NA	NA	NA	NA	NA	1 randomized trial.
Headache	RCT	Leone[608] 1996	20	Yes	4	Medium	NA	NA	Melatonin, 10 mg.
Hypertension	RCT	Birau[613] 1981	20	Yes	4	Medium	NA	NA	Intranasal melatonin, 2 mg daily.
Hypertension	RCT	Cagnacci 1997	12	Yes	5	Medium	NA	NA	Melatonin, 1 mg.
Hypertension	RCT	Cagnacci[197] 2000	31	Yes	5	Medium	NA	NA	Melatonin, 1 mg.
Parkinsonism	RCT	Papavasiliou[84] 1972	11	No	3	NA	NA	NA	Melatonin, 100 or 300 mg, maximal dose 6.6 g daily; single-blinded.
Periodic limb disorder	Case series	Kunz[623] 2001	9	Yes	3	Medium	NA	NA	Melatonin, 3 mg.
Pineal region damage	Case report	Etzioni[117] 1996	1	NA	NA	NA	NA	NA	Melatonin, 3 mg.
Pineal region damage	Case report	Lehmann[638] 1996	1	NA	NA	NA	NA	NA	Melatonin, 3 mg.
Pineal region damage	Case report	Siebler[639] 1998	1	NA	NA	NA	NA	NA	Melatonin, 5 mg.
Preoperative anxiolysis and sedation	RCT	Naguib 1999	75	Yes	4	Medium	NA	NA	Melatonin, 5mg.
Preoperative anxiolysis and sedation	RCT	Naguib[624] 1999	75	Yes	4	Medium	NA	NA	Melatonin, 5 mg.
Preoperative anxiolysis and sedation	RCT	Naguib[627] 2000	84	Yes	4	Medium	NA	NA	Melatonin, 0.05-0.1 or 0.2 mg/kg.
REM sleep behavior disorder	Case series	Takeuchi[628] 2001	15	Yes	3	Medium	NA	NA	Melatonin, 3 mg or 6-9 mg.
Rett syndrome	RCT	McArthur[630] 1998	9	Yes	NA	NA	NA	NA	Melatonin, 2.5 to 7.5 mg.
Seasonal affective disorder	Review	Avery[503] 1998	22	NA	NA	NA	NA	NA	Small sample.
Seasonal affective disorder	RCT	Wirz-Justice[635] 1990	17	No	5	NA	NA	NA	Melatonin, 5 mg daily; small sample.

M

Continued

Review of the Evidence: Melatonin—*cont'd*

Condition Treated*	Study Design	Author, Year	N[†]	SS[†]	Study Quality[‡]	Magnitude of Benefit	ARR[†]	NNT[†]	Comments
Seasonal affective disorder	RCT	Leppamaki[633] 2003	58	Yes	1	NA	NA	NA	Melatonin, 2 mg SR; unclear blinding.
Sleep disorder (Alzheimer's disease)	RCT	Singer[515] 1997	7	No	4	NA	NA	NA	Melatonin, 0.5 mg.
Sleep disorder (Alzheimer's disease)	RCT	Serfaty 2000	44	No	3	None	NA	NA	Melatonin, 6 mg.
Sleep disturbance (bipolar disorder)	RCT	Leibenluft[527] 1997	5	No	4	NA	NA	NA	Melatonin, 10 mg.
Sleep disturbance (depression)	RCT	Dolberg[602] 1998	19	Yes	4	Medium	NA	NA	Melatonin, 5 mg, plus fluoxetine vs. placebo plus fluoxetine.
Sleep disturbance (schizophrenia)	Crossover RCT	Shamir 2000	19	Yes	5	Medium	NA	NA	Melatonin, 2 mg.
Sleep disturbance (schizophrenia)	Crossover RCT	Shamir 2000	14	Yes	5	Medium	NA	NA	Melatonin, 2 mg; improved alertness test.
Suppression of UV-induced erythema	RCT	Bangha[649] 1996	20	Yes	5	Large	NA	NA	Melatonin, 0.05%, 0.1%, or 0.5% in gel.
Suppression of UV light-induced erythema	RCT	Dreher[650] 1998	15	Yes	4	Large	NA	NA	Melatonin plus ascorbic acid plus alpha-tocopherol.
Suppression of UV-induced erythema	RCT	Fischer[651] 1999	20	Yes	5	Large	NA	NA	Melatonin, 0.6 mg/cm² of skin.
Tardive dyskinesia	Crossover RCT	Shamir[158] 2000	19	No	5	NA	NA	NA	Melatonin, 2 mg.
Tardive dyskinesia	Crossover RCT	Shamir[158] 2000	19	No	5	NA	NA	NA	Melatonin, 2 mg.
Tardive dyskinesia	Crossover RCT	Shamir 2001	22	No	3	NA	NA	NA	Melatonin, 10 mg.
Thrombocytopenia	Case series	Lissoni 1996	14	Yes	NA	Medium	NA	NA	Melatonin, 20 mg.
Thrombocytopenia	Case reports	Todisco[648] 2002	3	No	NA	Medium	NA	NA	Idiopathic thrombocytopenic purpura.
Withdrawal	RCT	Garfinkel[523] 1999	34	Yes	3	Small	NA	NA	Melatonin, 2 mg; controlled release (circadin).
Work-shift sleep disorder	Review	Chase[653] 1997	53	NA	NA	Medium	NA	NA	Two trials discussed.
Work-shift sleep disorder	RCT	Dawson[502] 1995	36	No	4	NA	NA	NA	Melatonin, 2 mg.
Work-shift sleep disorder	RCT	Folkard[654] 1993	17	Yes	4	Medium	NA	NA	Melatonin, 5 mg; unclear method of randomization.
Work-shift sleep disorder	Crossover RCT	Jorgensen[657] 1998	18	No	2	Medium	NA	NA	Melatonin, 10 mg, sublingual.
Work-shift sleep disorder	Crossover RCT	Wright[659] 1998	15	Yes	3	None	NA	NA	Melatonin, 5 mg.
Work-shift sleep disorder	Crossover RCT	Sharkey 2001	21	No	3	Small	NA	NA	Melatonin, 1.8 mg.
Neonatal sepsis	Case series	Gitto 2001	20	Yes	NA	Small	NA	NA	Melatonin, 20 mg.
Sedation prior to MRI	Case series	Johnson 2002	40	No	NA	Medium	NA	NA	Melatonin, 10 mg.

*Primary or secondary outcome.
[†]*N*, Number of patients; *SS*, statistically significant; *ARR*, absolute risk reduction; *NNT*, the number of patients who need to undergo a specific intervention in order to observe an outcome in one individual.
[‡]0-2 = poor; 3-4 = good; 5 = excellent.
GI, Gastrointestinal; *IL-2*, interleukin-2; *MRI*, magnetic resonance imaging; *NA*, not applicable; *RCT*, randomized, controlled trial; *TNF*, tumor necrosis factor.
For an explanation of each category in this table, please see Table 3 in the Introduction.

REVIEW OF THE EVIDENCE: DISCUSSION

Jet Lag
Summary

- Several randomized, placebo-controlled human trials suggest that melatonin taken by mouth, started on the day of travel (close to the target bedtime at the destination) and continued for several days reduces the number of days required to establish a normal sleep pattern, diminishes the time it takes to fall asleep ("sleep latency"), improves alertness, and reduces daytime fatigue.[68-70,82,468] Effects may be greatest when traveling eastward and when crossing more than four time zones (results may be less impressive for westward travel or crossing of fewer time zones).[72,468] Combination with prescription sleep aids such as zolpidem (Ambien) may add to these effects, although side effects such as morning sleepiness may occur.[82]
- Although these results are compelling, the majority of studies have had methodological problems with their designs and reporting, and some trials have not found benefits.[75,469] Overall, the scientific evidence does suggest benefits of melatonin in up to half the people who take it for jet lag (number needed to treat = 2).[69,73,74] Further, well-designed trials are necessary to confirm these findings, to determine optimal dosing, and to evaluate use in combination with prescription sleep aids.
- Preliminary research reports that starting melatonin on the day of travel, rather than prior to travel, may yield superior results. Higher doses (such as 5 mg nightly) may be slightly more effective than lower doses (for example, 0.1 to 0.5 mg nightly) for improvement of sleep quality and latency,[74] although this area remains controversial, with some studies suggesting no differences.[73,75] Slow-release melatonin may not be as effective as standard (quick-release) formulations.[68] If the dose is taken too early in the day, it may actually result in excessive daytime sleepiness and greater difficulty adapting to the destination time zone.

Delayed Sleep Phase Syndrome
Summary

- Delayed sleep phase syndrome (DSPS) is a condition that results in delayed sleep onset, despite normal sleep architecture and sleep duration. Several small, controlled studies and case series in healthy volunteers and in patients with DSPS have used 5 to 6 mg of melatonin, with reported improvements in sleep latency.[470-474] Although these results are promising, additional research with large, well-designed controlled studies is needed before a stronger recommendation can be made.

Sleep Disturbances in Children with Neuropsychiatric Disorders
Summary

- There are multiple controlled trials and several case reports of melatonin use in children with various neuropsychiatric disorders, including mental retardation, autism, psychiatric disorders, visual impairment, and epilepsy.[475-493] Studies have demonstrated reduced time to fall asleep (sleep latency) and increased sleep duration. Oral doses of melatonin have ranged between 2.5 and 10 mg administered at the desired bedtime. Well-designed, controlled trials in select patient populations are needed before a stronger or more specific recommendation can be made.

Insomnia in the Elderly
Summary

- Several human studies report that melatonin taken by mouth 30 to 120 minutes prior to bedtime decreases the amount of time it takes to fall asleep (sleep latency) in elderly individuals with insomnia.[123,445,494-500] It is not clear if melatonin increases the length of time that people are able to stay asleep. Low doses (0.1 to 0.3 mg taken nightly) appear to be equally effective as higher doses (3 to 5 mg nightly). However, most studies have not been of high quality in their designs, and some research has found limited or no benefits.[501,502] The majority of trials have been brief in duration (several days), and long-term effects are not known.
- Although the evidence overall does suggest short-term benefits, additional study is needed before a strong recommendation can be made. It is not known how melatonin compares to standard therapies used for insomnia, including benzodiazepines such as diazepam (Valium) and lorazepam (Ativan) and other sleep aids such as zolpidem (Ambien).

Sleep Enhancement in Healthy People
Summary

- Multiple human studies have measured the effects of melatonin supplements on sleep in healthy individuals.[252,257-259,503-514] A wide range of doses has been used, including "low-dose" melatonin (0.1 to 1.0 mg), or doses between 5 and 10 mg, often taken by mouth 30 to 60 minutes prior to sleep time. Most trials have been small, brief in duration (often single-dose studies), and have not been rigorously designed or reported (inadequate blinding and randomization). However, the weight of scientific evidence does suggest that melatonin decreases the time it takes to fall asleep (sleep latency), increases the feeling of "sleepiness," and may increase the duration of sleep. Better quality research is needed in this area. It is not known how melatonin compares to standard therapies used for insomnia, including benzodiazepines such as diazepam (Valium) and lorazepam (Ativan) and other sleep aids such as zolpidem (Ambien).

Alzheimer's Disease (Sleep Disorders)
Summary

- There is limited study of melatonin for improving sleep disorders associated with Alzheimer's disease (including nighttime agitation and poor sleep quality in patients with dementia).[515-517] It has been reported that natural melatonin levels are altered in people with Alzheimer's disease,[518-521] although it remains unclear if supplementation with melatonin is beneficial. Further research is needed in this area before a firm conclusion can be reached.

Antioxidant (Free Radical Scavenging)
Summary

- There are well over 100 laboratory and animal studies of the antioxidant (free radical scavenging) properties of melatonin.[1-9] As a result, melatonin has been proposed as a supplement to prevent or treat many conditions that are associated with oxidative damage. However, there are no well-designed trials in humans that have demonstrated benefits of melatonin as an antioxidant for any health problem.

Attention Deficit Hyperactivity Disorder (ADHD)
Summary

- There is limited research on the use of melatonin in children with ADHD.[522] A clear conclusion cannot be made at this time.

Benzodiazepine Tapering
Summary

- A small amount of research has examined the use of melatonin to assist with tapering or cessation of benzodiazepines such as diazepam (Valium) and lorazepam (Ativan).[523-526] Although preliminary results are promising, due to weaknesses in the design and reporting of this research, further study is necessary before a firm conclusion can be reached.

Bipolar Disorder (Sleep Disturbances)
Summary

- There is limited study of melatonin given to patients with sleep disturbances associated with bipolar disorder (such as insomnia and irregular sleep patterns).[527,528] No clear benefits have been reported. Further research is needed in this area before a clear conclusion can be reached.

Cancer Treatment
Summary

- There are several early-phase and controlled human trials of melatonin in patients with various advanced stage malignancies, including brain, breast, colorectal, gastric, liver, lung, pancreatic, and testicular cancers, as well as lymphoma, melanoma, renal cell carcinoma, and soft-tissue sarcoma.[529-557] Many of these studies have been conducted by the same research group.

- In this research, melatonin has been combined with other types of treatment, including radiation therapy,[547] chemotherapies (such as cisplatin, etoposide, or irinotecan),[532,550,553,558-562] hormonal treatments (such as tamoxifen),[280,546,563] and immune therapies such as interferon,[564] interleukin-2,[542,565-583] and tumor necrosis factor.[574,584,585] Most of these trials have been published by the same research group and have involved giving melatonin orally, intravenously, or injected into muscle. Results have been mixed, with some patients stabilizing and others progressing. There are some promising reported results, including small significant improvements in the survival of patients with non–small cell lung cancer given oral melatonin with chemotherapy (cisplatin and etoposide). However, the design and results of this research are not sufficient to provide definitive evidence in favor of safe and effective use of melatonin in cancer patients. High-quality follow-up trials are necessary to confirm these preliminary results.

- It has been proposed that melatonin may benefit cancer patients through antioxidant, immune-enhancing, hormonal, anti-inflammatory, antiangiogenic, apoptotic, or direct cytotoxic (cancer cell-killing) effects, and there are many ongoing laboratory and animal studies in these areas. Some experts believe that antioxidants can improve the effectiveness of chemotherapy drugs and reduce side effects, whereas others suggest that antioxidants may actually interfere with the effectiveness of chemotherapies.

- Currently, no clear conclusion can be drawn in this area. There is not enough definitive scientific evidence to discern if melatonin is beneficial against any type of cancer, whether it increases (or decreases) the effectiveness of other cancer therapies, or if it safely reduces chemotherapy side effects.

Chemotherapy Side Effects
Summary

- Several human trials have examined the effects of melatonin on side effects associated with various cancer chemotherapies (such as carboplatin, cisplatin, daunorubicin, doxorubicin, epirubicin, etoposide, 5-fluorouracil, gemcitabine, and mitoxantrone).[532,544,548,550,553,558-562] Most of these studies have been published by the same research group, and involve giving melatonin through the veins or injected into muscle. Studies have included patients with advanced lung, breast, gastrointestinal, prostate, and head and neck cancers, as well as lymphoma. Promising early results include reductions in nerve injury (neuropathy), mouth sores (stomatitis), wasting (cachexia), and platelet count (thrombocytopenia) when melatonin is used with various chemotherapy agents. Animal studies note reduced severity of heart damage from anthracycline drugs [40-42,586,587] and of lung damage from bleomycin.[49,588]

- Some researchers attribute these reported benefits to antioxidant properties of melatonin. Overall, it remains controversial whether antioxidants increase effectiveness and reduce side effects of chemotherapies or whether antioxidants actually reduce effectiveness of chemotherapies.

- Increased platelet counts after melatonin use have been observed in patients with decreased platelet counts due to cancer therapies (several studies reported by the same author),[553,555,560-562,569,570] and stimulation of platelet production (thrombopoiesis) has been suggested but not clearly demonstrated.

- Although these early reported benefits are promising, high-quality, controlled trials are necessary before a clear conclusion can be reached in this area. It remains unclear if melatonin safely reduces side effects of various chemotherapies without altering effectiveness.

Circadian Rhythm Entraining (in Blind Persons)
Summary

- In blind individuals, light and dark stimuli are not received by the eye to trigger melatonin release and the onset of sleep. In these patients, natural melatonin levels peak at a different hour every night, to the point where individuals may sleep during the day and awake at night. This is commonly referred to as "free-running" circadian rhythm. There are multiple published small case series and case reports in the literature, yet limited controlled trials to date in this population.[88,589-561] Present studies and individual cases suggest that melatonin, administered in the evening, may correct circadian rhythm. Large, well-designed controlled trials are needed before a stronger recommendation can be made.

Depression (Sleep Disturbances)
Summary

- Depression can be associated with neuroendocrine and sleep abnormalities, such as reduced time before dream sleep (REM latency). Melatonin has been suggested for the improvement of sleep patterns in patients with depression, although research is limited in this area.[602-605] Further studies are needed before a clear conclusion can be reached.

Glaucoma
Summary

- It has been theorized that due to effects on photoreceptor renewal in the eye, high doses of melatonin may increase intraocular pressure and the risk of glaucoma, age-related maculopathy and myopia,[79] and retinal damage.[102] However, there is preliminary evidence that melatonin may actually decrease intraocular pressure in the eye, and it has been suggested as a possible therapy for glaucoma.[130,131] Additional study is necessary in this area. Patients with glaucoma taking melatonin should be monitored by a healthcare professional.

Headache Prevention
Summary

- Several small studies have examined the possible role of melatonin in preventing various forms of headache, including migraine, cluster, and tension-type headaches (in people who suffer from regular headaches).[428,606-608] Limited initial research suggests possible benefits in all three types of headache, although well-designed, controlled studies are needed before a firm conclusion can be drawn.

High Blood Pressure (Hypertension)
Summary

- Several controlled studies in patients with high blood pressure report small reductions in diastolic and systolic blood pressures when taking melatonin by mouth or inhaled through the nose (intranasally).[609-613] Most trials have been small and not well designed or reported. Better-designed research is necessary before a firm conclusion can be reached.

HIV/AIDS
Summary

- There is a lack of well-designed scientific evidence to recommend for or against the use of melatonin as a treatment for AIDS.[614] Melatonin should not be used in place of more proven therapies, and patients with HIV/AIDS are advised to be treated under the supervision of a medical doctor.

Insomnia (of Unknown Origin in the Non-elderly)
Summary

- There are several small, controlled human trials and pilot research of melatonin taken by mouth in people with insomnia.[91,605-621] Results have been inconsistent, with some studies reporting benefits on sleep latency and subjective sleep quality, and other research finding no benefits. Most studies have been small and not rigorously designed or reported. Better research is needed before a firm conclusion can be drawn.
- Notably, several studies in elderly individuals with insomnia provide preliminary evidence of benefits on sleep latency (discussed above).[126,445,494-500,502]

Parkinson's Disease
Summary

- Because of very limited study to date, a recommendation cannot be made for or against the use of melatonin in parkinsonism[84] or Parkinson's disease.[236,463,622] Better-designed research is needed before a firm conclusion can be reached in this area.

Periodic Limb Movement Disorder
Summary

- There is very limited study to date for the use of melatonin as a treatment in periodic limb movement disorder.[623] Better-designed research is needed before a recommendation can be made in this area.

Preoperative Sedation/Anxiolysis
Summary

- A small number of controlled studies has compared melatonin with placebo and standard drugs (benzodiazepines) for sedation and anxiety reduction (anxiolysis) prior to general anesthesia for surgery.[624-627] Results are promising, with similar results reported for melatonin as for benzodiazepines such as midazolam (Versed) and superiority to placebo. There are also promising reports using melatonin for sedation/anxiolysis prior to magnetic resonance imaging (MRI). However, due to weaknesses in the design and reporting of the available research, better studies are needed before a clear conclusion can be drawn.
- Melatonin has been suggested as a treatment for delirium following surgery, although there is little evidence in this area.[48]

REM Sleep Behavior Disorder
Summary

- Limited case reports describe benefits in patients with rapid eye movement (REM) sleep behavior disorder who receive melatonin.[628,629] However, better research is needed before a clear conclusion can be drawn.

Rett's Syndrome
Summary

- Rett's syndrome is a presumed genetic disorder that affects female children, characterized by decelerated head growth and global developmental regression. There is limited study of the possible role of melatonin in improving sleep disturbance associated with Rett's syndrome.[64,630] Further research is needed before a recommendation can be made in this area.

Schizophrenia (Sleep Disorders)
Summary

- There is limited study of melatonin for improving sleep latency (time to fall asleep) in patients with schizophrenia.[631,632] Further research is needed in this area before a clear conclusion can be reached.

Seasonal Affective Disorder (SAD)
Summary

- There are several small, brief studies of melatonin in patients with SAD.[503,633-636] This research is not well designed or reported, and further study is necessary before a clear conclusion can be reached.

Seizure Disorder (Children)
Summary

- The role of melatonin in seizure disorder is controversial. There are several reported cases of children with intractable seizures or neurologic damage who improved with regular nighttime melatonin administration.[93-98] Limited animal research also suggests possible antiseizure effects.[337,637] However, there has also been a report that melatonin may actually lower seizure threshold and increase the risk of seizures.[92] Better evidence is needed in this area before a clear conclusion can be drawn regarding the safety or effectiveness of melatonin in seizure disorder.

Sleep Disturbances Due to Pineal Region Brain Damage
Summary

- Several published cases report improvements in sleep patterns in young people with damage to the pineal gland area of the brain due to tumors or surgery.[117,638,639] Because of the rarity of such disorders, controlled trials may not be possible. Consideration of melatonin in such patients should be under the direction of a qualified healthcare professional.

M

Smoking Cessation
Summary

- A small amount of research has examined the use of melatonin to reduce symptoms associated with smoking cessation, such as anxiousness, restlessness, irritability, and cigarette craving. Although preliminary results are promising, because of weaknesses in the design and reporting of this research, further study is necessary before a firm conclusion can be reached.

Stroke
Summary

- It has been proposed that melatonin may reduce the amount of neurologic damage patients experience after stroke, based on antioxidant properties[315,316,319,640-644] In addition, melatonin levels may be altered in people immediately after stroke,[413,645] and it has thus been suggested that melatonin supplementation may be beneficial, although this has not been shown in humans. At this time, the effects of melatonin supplements immediately after stroke are not clear.

Tardive Dyskinesia
Summary

- Tardive dyskinesia (TD) is a serious potential side effect of antipsychotic medications, characterized by involuntary muscle movements. Limited small studies of melatonin use in patients with TD report mixed findings.[152-154,156-158,646] Additional research is necessary before a clear conclusion can be drawn.[152]

Thrombocytopenia (Low Platelet Counts)
Summary

- Increased platelet counts after melatonin use have been observed in patients with decreased platelets due to cancer therapies (several studies reported by the same author).[553,555,560-562,569,570] Stimulation of platelet production (thrombopoiesis) has been suggested but not clearly demonstrated. Additional research is necessary in this area before a clear conclusion can be drawn. Cases of idiopathic thrombocytopenic purpura (ITP) treated with melatonin have been reported.[647,648]

Ultraviolet (UV) Light Skin Damage Protection
Summary

- Several small, randomized trials have examined the use of melatonin in protecting human skin against UV light skin damage.[649-652] It has been proposed that antioxidant properties of melatonin may be protective. Although this preliminary research reports reductions in erythema (skin redness) with the use of melatonin, further study is necessary before a clear conclusion can be drawn about clinical effectiveness in humans.

Work Shift Sleep Disorder
Summary

- There are several studies of melatonin use in people who work irregular shifts, such as emergency room personnel.[653-659] Results are mixed, with some studies finding no significant benefits and others reporting benefits in sleep quality compared to placebo. Because most published trials are small, with incomplete reporting of design or results, additional research is necessary before a clear conclusion can be drawn.

FORMULARY: BRANDS USED IN CLINICAL TRIALS/ THIRD-PARTY TESTING
Brands Used in Clinical Trials

- Melatonin (Penn Pharmaceuticals Ltd, USA)[481]; Crystalline Melatonin (Sigma Chemical Co., St. Louis, MO)[660]; Melatonin (Regis Chemical Co., Morton Grove, IL)[634]; Circadin (Neurim Pharmaceuticals Ltd, Tel Aviv, Israel).[523]

Third Party Testing

- In 2002, ConsumerLab.com evaluated 18 melatonin-containing supplements (15 quick-release and 3 time-release products), of which 12 were melatonin-only products. It was reported that 16 of the 18 products contained between 100% and 135% of the claimed amount of melatonin, one quick-release product contained only 83% of the claimed amount of melatonin, and another quick-release product contained a small amount of lead (slightly more than 0.5 mg per daily recommended serving size). Among the 12 melatonin-only products that "passed" these standards are: Nature's Bounty Melatonin 1-mg and 3-mg tablets, Puritan's Pride Inspired by Nature Melatonin 3-mg tablets, and Penn Pharmaceuticals Ltd Twinlab Melatonin Caps, Highest Quality, Quick Acting 3-mg tablets. Further information is available at www.ConsumerLab.com.

References

1. Reiter RJ, Tan DX, Manchester LC, et al. Melatonin reduces oxidant damage and promotes mitochondrial respiration: implications for aging. Ann N Y Acad Sci 2002;959:238-250.
2. Reiter RJ, Tan DX. Melatonin: an antioxidant in edible plants. Ann N Y Acad Sci 2002;957:341-344.
3. Mayo JC, Tan DX, Sainz RM, et al. Protection against oxidative protein damage induced by metal-catalyzed reaction or alkylperoxyl radicals: comparative effects of melatonin and other antioxidants. Biochim Biophys Acta 2003;1620(1-3):139-150.
4. Sainz RM, Mayo JC, Tan DX, et al. Antioxidant activity of melatonin in Chinese hamster ovarian cells: changes in cellular proliferation and differentiation. Biochem Biophys Res Commun 2003;302(3):625-634.
5. Tan DX, Hardeland R, Manchester LC, et al. Mechanistic and comparative studies of melatonin and classic antioxidants in terms of their interactions with the ABTS cation radical. J Pineal Res 2003;34(4):249-259.
6. Pieri C, Moroni M, Marcheselli F, et al. Melatonin is an efficient antioxidant. Arch Gerontol Geriatr 1995;20:159-165.
7. Reiter RJ, Tan DX, Acuña-Castroviejo D, et al. Melatonin: mechanisms and actions as an antioxidant. Curr Top Biophys 2000;24:171-183.
8. Gulcin I, Buyukokuroglu ME, Oktay M, et al. On the in vitro antioxidative properties of melatonin. J Pineal Res 2002;33(3):167-171.
9. Gulcin I, Buyukokuroglu ME, Kufrevioglu OI. Metal chelating and hydrogen peroxide scavenging effects of melatonin. J Pineal Res 2003;34(4):278-281.
10. Vachharajani NN, Yeleswaram K, Boulton DW. Preclinical pharmacokinetics and metabolism of BMS-214778, a novel melatonin receptor agonist. J Pharm Sci 2003;92(4):760-772.
11. Zhou MO, Jiao S, Liu Z, et al. Luzindole, a melatonin receptor antagonist, inhibits the transient outward K+ current in rat cerebellar granule cells. Brain Res 2003;970(1-2):169-177.
12. Constantinescu CS, Hilliard B, Ventura E, et al. Luzindole, a melatonin receptor antagonist, suppresses experimental autoimmune encephalomyelitis. Pathobiology 1997;65(4):190-194.
13. Sener G, Schirli AO, Ayanoglu-Dulger G. Protective effects of melatonin, vitamin E and N-acetylcysteine against acetaminophen toxicity in mice: a comparative study. J Pineal Res 2003;35(1):61-68.
14. Shiu SY, Reiter RJ, Tan DX, et al. Urgent search for safe and effective treatments of severe acute respiratory syndrome: is melatonin a promising candidate drug? J Pineal Res 2003;35(1):69-70.
15. Parlakpinar H, Ozer MK, Sahna E, et al. Amikacin-induced acute renal injury in rats: protective role of melatonin. J Pineal Res 2003;35(2):85-90.
16. Acuna-Castroviejo D, Escames G, Macias M, et al. Cell protective role of melatonin in the brain. J Pineal Res 1995;19(2):57-63.
17. Delagrange P, Atkinson J, Boutin JA, et al. Therapeutic perspectives for melatonin agonists and antagonists. J Neuroendocrinol 2003;15(4):442-448.
18. van den Heuvel CJ, Reid KJ, Dawson D. Effect of atenolol on nocturnal sleep and temperature in young men: reversal by pharmacological doses of melatonin. Physiol Behav 1997;61(6):795-802.

19. Mayeda A, Mannon S, Hofstetter J, et al. Effects of indirect light and propranolol on melatonin levels in normal human subjects. Psychiatry Res 1998;81(1):9-17.
20. Anisimov VN, Alimova IN, Baturin DA, et al. The effect of melatonin treatment regimen on mammary adenocarcinoma development in HER-2/neu transgenic mice. Int J Cancer 2003;103(3):300-305.
21. Ohta Y, Kongo M, Kishikawa T. Melatonin exerts a therapeutic effect on cholestatic liver injury in rats with bile duct ligation. J Pineal Res 2003; 34(2):119-126.
22. Zhdanova IV, Geiger DA, Schwagerl AL, et al. Melatonin promotes sleep in three species of diurnal nonhuman primates. Physiol Behav 2002;75(4):523-529.
23. Bubenik GA. Gastrointestinal melatonin: localization, function, and clinical relevance. Dig Dis Sci 2002;47(10):2336-2348.
24. Dong WG, Mei Q, Yu JP, et al. Effects of melatonin on the expression of iNOS and COX-2 in rat models of colitis. World J Gastroenterol 2003; 9(6):1307-1311.
25. Muller HL, Handwerker G, Wollny B, et al. Melatonin secretion and increased daytime sleepiness in childhood craniopharyngioma patients. J Clin Endocrinol Metab 2002;87(8):3993-3996.
26. Esrefoglu M, Kurus M, Sahna E. The beneficial effect of melatonin on chronic cyclosporin A nephrotoxicity in rats. J Int Med Res 2003;31(1): 42-44.
27. Longoni B, Migliori M, Ferretti A, et al. Melatonin prevents cyclosporine-induced nephrotoxicity in isolated and perfused rat kidney. Free Radic Res 2002;36(3):357-363.
28. Aksoy N, Vural H, Sabuncu T, et al. Effects of melatonin on oxidative-antioxidative status of tissues in streptozotocin-induced diabetic rats. Cell Biochem Funct 2003;21(2):121-125.
29. Abilio VC, Vera JA, Jr., Ferreira LS, et al. Effects of melatonin on behavioral dopaminergic supersensitivity. Life Sci 2003;72(26):3003-3015.
30. Kobayashi Y, Itoh MT, Kondo H, et al. Melatonin binding sites in estrogen receptor-positive cells derived from human endometrial cancer. J Pineal Res 2003;35(2):71-74.
31. Abilio VC, Vera JA, Jr., Ferreira LS, et al. Effects of melatonin on orofacial movements in rats. Psychopharmacology (Berl) 2002;161(4):340-347.
32. Abdel-Wanis ME, Tsuchiya H. Melatonin deficiency and fibrous dysplasia: might a relation exist? Med Hypotheses 2002;59(5):552-554.
33. Machida M, Dubousset J, Imamura Y, et al. Melatonin. A possible role in pathogenesis of adolescent idiopathic scoliosis. Spine 1996;21(10): 1147-1152.
34. Acikel M, Buyukokuroglu ME, Aksoy H, et al. Protective effects of melatonin against myocardial injury induced by isoproterenol in rats. J Pineal Res 2003;35(2):75-79.
35. Chen Z, Chua CC, Gao J, et al. Protective effect of melatonin on myocardial infarction. Am J Physiol Heart Circ Physiol 2003;284(5): H1618-H1624.
36. Imashuku S, Morimoto Y, Morimoto A, et al. Pineal dysfunction (low melatonin production) as a cause of sudden death in a long-term survivor of Langerhans cell histiocytosis? Med Pediatr Oncol 2003;41(2):151-153.
37. El Sokkary GH, Kamel ES, Reiter RJ. Prophylactic effect of melatonin in reducing lead-induced neurotoxicity in the rat. Cell Mol Biol Lett 2003; 8(2):461-470.
38. Takei A, Okawa M, Sasaki H, et al. [Effective melatonin therapy in a case of Machado-Joseph disease with insomnia]. Rinsho Shinkeigaku 2000; 40(7):736-740.
39. Schlabritz-Loutsevitch N, Hellner N, Middendorf R, et al. The human myometrium as a target for melatonin. J Clin Endocrinol Metab 2003; 88(2):908-913.
40. Dziegiel P, Suder E, Surowiak P, et al. Role of exogenous melatonin in reducing the nephrotoxic effect of daunorubicin and doxorubicin in the rat. J Pineal Res 2002;33(2):95-100.
41. Dziegiel P, Jethon Z, Suder E, et al. Role of exogenous melatonin in reducing the cardiotoxic effect of daunorubicin and doxorubicin in the rat. Exp Toxicol Pathol 2002;53(6):433-439.
42. Dziegiel P, Surowiak P, Rabczynski J, et al. Effect of melatonin on cytotoxic effects of daunorubicin on myocardium and on transplantable Morris hepatoma in rats. Pol J Pathol 2002;53(4):201-204.
43. O'Rourke ST, Hammad H, Delagrange P, et al. Melatonin inhibits nitrate tolerance in isolated coronary arteries. Br J Pharmacol 2003;139(7): 1326-1332.
44. Bloom CM, Anch AM, Dyche JS. Behavioral effects of chronic melatonin and pregnenolone injections in a myelin mutant rat (taiep). J Gen Psychol 2002;129(3):226-237.
45. Bulbuller N, Akkus MA, Cetinkaya Z, et al. Effects of melatonin and lactulose on the liver and kidneys in rats with obstructive jaundice. Pediatr Surg Int 2002;18(8):677-680.
46. Martinez-Cruz F, Pozo D, Osuna C, et al. Oxidative stress induced by phenylketonuria in the rat: Prevention by melatonin, vitamin E, and vitamin C. J Neurosci Res 2002;69(4):550-558.
47. Cagnacci A, Volpe A. A role for melatonin in PCOS? Fertil Steril 2002; 77(5):1089.
48. Hanania M, Kitain E. Melatonin for treatment and prevention of postoperative delirium. Anesth Analg 2002;94(2):338-9, table.
49. Arslan SO, Zerin M, Vural H, et al. The effect of melatonin on bleomycin-induced pulmonary fibrosis in rats. J Pineal Res 2002;32(1):21-25.
50. El Sokkary GH, Omar HM, Hassanein AF, et al. Melatonin reduces oxidative damage and increases survival of mice infected with Schistosoma mansoni. Free Radic Biol Med 2002;32(4):319-332.
51. Cuzzocrea S, Reiter RJ. Pharmacological action of melatonin in shock, inflammation and ischemia/reperfusion injury. Eur J Pharmacol 2001; 426(1-2):1-10.
52. Maestroni GJ. Melatonin as a therapeutic agent in experimental endotoxic shock. J Pineal Res 1996;20(2):84-89.
53. De Leersnyder H, Bresson JL, de Blois MC, et al. Beta 1-adrenergic antagonists and melatonin reset the clock and restore sleep in a circadian disorder, Smith-Magenis syndrome. J Med Genet 2003;40(1):74-78.
54. Topsakal C, Kilic N, Ozveren F, et al. Effects of prostaglandin E1, melatonin, and oxytetracycline on lipid peroxidation, antioxidant defense system, paraoxonase (PON1) activities, and homocysteine levels in an animal model of spinal cord injury. Spine 2003;28(15):1643-1652.
55. Semercioz A, Onur R, Ogras S, et al. Effects of melatonin on testicular tissue nitric oxide level and antioxidant enzyme activities in experimentally induced left varicocele. Neuroendocrinol Lett 2003;24(1-2):86-90.
56. Baydas G, Reiter RJ, Nedzvetskii VS, et al. Melatonin protects the central nervous system of rats against toluene-containing thinner intoxication by reducing reactive gliosis. Toxicol Lett 2003;137(3):169-174.
57. Chung SY, Han SH. Melatonin attenuates kainic acid-induced hippocampal neurodegeneration and oxidative stress through microglial inhibition. J Pineal Res 2003;34(2):95-102.
58. Wiid I, Hoal-van Helden E, Hon D, et al. Potentiation of isoniazid activity against Mycobacterium tuberculosis by melatonin. Antimicrob Agents Chemother 1999;43(4):975-977.
59. Jan JE, Freeman RD. Re: Mann—melatonin for ulcerative colitis? Am J Gastroenterol 2003;98(6):1446.
60. Mann S. Melatonin for ulcerative colitis? Am J Gastroenterol 2003;98(1): 232-233.
61. Bonilla E, Valero N, Chacin-Bonilla L, et al. Melatonin increases interleukin-1beta and decreases tumor necrosis factor alpha in the brain of mice infected with the Venezuelan equine encephalomyelitis virus. Neurochem Res 2003;28(5):681-686.
62. Parmar P, Limson J, Nyokong T, et al. Melatonin protects against copper-mediated free radical damage. J Pineal Res 2002;32(4):237-242.
63. Basak PY, Agalar F, Gultekin F, et al. The effect of thermal injury and melatonin on incisional wound healing. Ulus Travma Derg 2003;9(2): 96-101.
64. Miyamoto A, Oki J, Takahashi S, et al. Serum melatonin kinetics and long-term melatonin treatment for sleep disorders in Rett syndrome. Brain Dev 1999;21(1):59-62.
65. Voordouw BC, Euser R, Verdonk RE, et al. Melatonin and melatonin-progestin combinations alter pituitary-ovarian function in women and can inhibit ovulation. J Clin Endocrinol Metab 1992;74(1):108-117.
66. Abd-Allah AR, El Sayed eS, Abdel-Wahab MH, et al. Effect of melatonin on estrogen and progesterone receptors in relation to uterine contraction in rats. Pharmacol Res 2003;47(4):349-354.
67. Ciesla W. Low ACTH and high melatonin concentrations in amniotic fluid as hormonal markers of high risk of fetal abnormalities. Preliminary studies. Prenat Diagn 1998;18(9):980-983.
68. Suhner A, Schlagenhauf P, Johnson R, et al. Comparative study to determine the optimal melatonin dosage form for the alleviation of jet lag. Chronobiol Int 1998;15(6):655-666.
69. Arendt J, Aldhous M, Marks V. Alleviation of jet lag by melatonin: preliminary results of controlled double blind trial. Br Med J (Clin Res Ed) 1986;292(6529):1170.
70. Arendt J, Aldhous M. Further evaluation of the treatment of jet-lag by melatonin: a double-blind crossover study. Annu Rev Chronopharmacol 1988;5:53-55.
71. Petrie K, Dawson AG, Thompson L, et al. A double-blind trial of melatonin as a treatment for jet lag in international cabin crew. Biol Psychiatry 1993;33(7):526-530.
72. Petrie K, Conaglen JV, Thompson L, et al. Effect of melatonin on jet lag after long haul flights. BMJ 1989;298(6675):705-707.
73. Claustrat B, Brun J, David M, et al. Melatonin and jet lag: confirmatory result using a simplified protocol. Biol Psychiatry 1992;32(8):705-711.
74. Herxheimer A, Petrie KJ. Melatonin for the prevention and treatment of jet lag. Cochrane Database Syst Rev 2002;(2):CD001520.
75. Spitzer RL, Terman M, Malt U, et al. Failure of melatonin to affect jet lag in a randomized double blind trial. Abstracts Meet Soc Light Treatm Biolog Rhythms 1997;9:1.
76. de Lourdes M, Seabra V, Bignotto M, et al. Randomized, double-blind clinical trial, controlled with placebo, of the toxicology of chronic melatonin treatment. J Pineal Res 2000;29(4):193-200.
77. Holliman BJ, Chyka PA. Problems in assessment of acute melatonin overdose. South Med J 1997;90(4):451-453.
78. Bardazzi F, Placucci F, Neri I, et al. Fixed drug eruption due to melatonin. Acta Derm Venereol 1997;78:69-70.
79. Guardiola-Lemaitre B. Toxicology of melatonin. J Biol Rhythms 1997; 12(6):697-706.

M

80. Hong YG, Riegler JL. Is melatonin associated with the development of autoimmune hepatitis? J Clin Gastroenterol 1997;25(1):376-378.

81. Morera AL, Henry M, de L, V. [Safety in melatonin use]. Actas Esp Psiquiatr 2001;29(5):334-337.

82. Suhner A, Schlagenhauf P, Hoefer I, et al. Efficacy and tolerability of melatonin and zolpidem for the alleviation of jet-lag. 6th Conference of the International Society of Travel Medicine, Montreal. 1999: abs G03.

83. Arendt J. Safety of melatonin in long-term use (?). J Biol Rhythms 1997; 12(6):673-681.

84. Papavasiliou PS, Cotzias GC, Duby SE, et al. Melatonin and parkinsonism. JAMA 1972;221(1):88-89.

85. Nickelsen T, Demisch L, Demisch K, et al. Influence of subchronic intake of melatonin at various times of the day on fatigue and hormonal levels: a placebo-controlled, double-blind trial. J Pineal Res 1989;6(4):325-334.

86. Middleton BA, Stone BM, Arendt J. Melatonin and fragmented sleep patterns. Lancet 1996;348(9026):551-552.

87. Dollins AB, Lynch HJ, Wurtman RJ, et al. Effect of pharmacological daytime doses of melatonin on human mood and performance. Psychopharmacology (Berl) 1993;112(4):490-496.

88. Arendt J, Aldhous M, Wright J. Synchronisation of a disturbed sleep-wake cycle in a blind man by melatonin treatment. Lancet 1988;1(8588):772-773.

89. U.S.Food and Drug Administration. Special Nutritionals Adverse Events Monitoring System: registered case reports.

90. Arendt J, Borbely AA, Franey C, et al. The effects of chronic, small doses of melatonin given in the late afternoon on fatigue in man: a preliminary study. Neurosci Lett 1984;45(3):317-321.

91. Ellis CM, Lemmens G, Parkes JD. Melatonin and insomnia. J Sleep Res 1996;5(1):61-65.

92. Sheldon SH. Pro-convulsant effects of oral melatonin in neurologically disabled children. Lancet 1998;351(9111):1254.

93. Brueske V, Allen J, Kepic T, et al. Melatonin inhibition of seizure activity in man [abstract]. Electroencephalog Clin Neurophysiol 1981;51:20P.

94. Fauteck J, Schmidt H, Lerchl A, et al. Melatonin in epilepsy: first results of replacement therapy and first clinical results. Biol Signals Recept 1999; 8(1-2):105-110.

95. Jan JE, Connolly MB, Hamilton D, et al. Melatonin treatment of non-epileptic myoclonus in children. Dev Med Child Neurol 1999;41(4): 255-259.

96. Molina-Carballo A, Munoz-Hoyos A, Reiter RJ, et al. Utility of high doses of melatonin as adjunctive anticonvulsant therapy in a child with severe myoclonic epilepsy: two years' experience. J Pineal Res 1997;23(2):97-105.

97. Rufo-Campos M. [Melatonin and epilepsy]. Rev Neurol 2002; 35(Suppl 1):S51-S58.

98. Siddiqui MA, Nazmi AS, Karim S, et al. Effect of melatonin and valproate in epilepsy and depression. Indian J Pharmacol 2001;33:378-381.

99. Munoz-Hoyos A, Sanchez-Forte M, Molina-Carballo A, et al. Melatonin's role as an anticonvulsant and neuronal protector: experimental and clinical evidence. J Child Neurol 1998;13(10):501-509.

100. Carman JS, Post RM, Buswell R, et al. Negative effects of melatonin on depression. Am J Psychiatry 1976;133(10):1181-1186.

101. Force RW, Hansen L, Bedell M. Psychotic episode after melatonin. Ann Pharmacother 1997;31(11):1408.

102. Lamberg L. Melatonin potentially useful but safety, efficacy remain uncertain. JAMA 1996;276(13):1011-1014.

103. Weekley LB. Melatonin-induced relaxation of rat aorta: interaction with adrenergic agonists. J Pineal Res 1991;11(1):28-34.

104. Cagnacci A, Arangino S, Angiolucci M, et al. Influences of melatonin administration on the circulation of women. Am J Physiol 1998; 274(2 Pt 2):R335-R338.

105. Harris AS, Burgess HJ, Dawson D. The effects of day-time exogenous melatonin administration on cardiac autonomic activity. J Pineal Res 2001;31(3):199-205.

106. Arangino S, Cagnacci A, Angiolucci M, et al. Effects of melatonin on vascular reactivity, catecholamine levels, and blood pressure in healthy men. Am J Cardiol 1999;83(9):1417-1419.

107. Kitajima T, Kanbayashi T, Saitoh Y, et al. The effects of oral melatonin on the autonomic function in healthy subjects. Psychiatry Clin Neurosci 2001; 55(3):299-300.

108. Nishiyama K, Yasue H, Moriyama Y, et al. Acute effects of melatonin administration on cardiovascular autonomic regulation in healthy men. Am Heart J 2001;141(5):E9.

109. Cagnacci A, Arangino S, Angiolucci M, et al. Effect of exogenous melatonin on vascular reactivity and nitric oxide in postmenopausal women: role of hormone replacement therapy. Clin Endocrinol (Oxf) 2001;54(2):261-266.

110. Wakatsuki A, Okatani Y, Ikenoue N, et al. Effects of short-term melatonin administration on lipoprotein metabolism in normolipidemic postmenopausal women. Maturitas 2001;38(2):171-177.

111. Esquifino A, Agrasal C, Velazquez E, et al. Effect of melatonin on serum cholesterol and phospholipid levels, and on prolactin, thyroid-stimulating hormone and thyroid hormone levels, in hyperprolactinemic rats. Life Sci 1997;61(11):1051-1058.

112. Pita ML, Hoyos M, Martin-Lacave I, et al. Long-term melatonin administration increases polyunsaturated fatty acid percentage in plasma lipids of hypercholesterolemic rats. J Pineal Res 2002;32(3):179-186.

113. Tailleux A, Torpier G, Bonnefont-Rousselot D, et al. Daily melatonin supplementation in mice increases atherosclerosis in proximal aorta. Biochem Biophys Res Commun 2002;293(3):1114-1123.

114. Rasmussen DD, Boldt BM, Wilkinson CW, et al. Daily melatonin administration at middle age suppresses male rat visceral fat, plasma leptin, and plasma insulin to youthful levels. Endocrinology 1999;140(2):1009-1012.

115. Cagnacci A, Arangino S, Renzi A, et al. Influence of melatonin administration on glucose tolerance and insulin sensitivity of postmenopausal women. Clin Endocrinol (Oxf) 2001;54(3):339-346.

116. Luboshitzky R, Shen-Orr Z, Shochat T, et al. Melatonin administered in the afternoon decreases next-day luteinizing hormone levels in men: lack of antagonism by flumazenil. J Mol Neurosci 1999;12(1):75-80.

117. Etzioni A, Luboshitzky R, Tiosano D, et al. Melatonin replacement corrects sleep disturbances in a child with pineal tumor. Neurology 1996; 46(1):261-263.

118. Cagnacci A, Paoletti AM, Soldani R, et al. Melatonin enhances the luteinizing hormone and follicle-stimulating hormone responses to gonadotropin-releasing hormone in the follicular, but not in the luteal, menstrual phase. J Clin Endocrinol Metab 1995;80(4):1095-1099.

119. Cagnacci A, Soldani R, Yen SS. Exogenous melatonin enhances luteinizing hormone levels of women in the follicular but not in the luteal menstrual phase. Fertil Steril 1995;63(5):996-999.

120. Cagnacci A, Elliott JA, Yen SS. Amplification of pulsatile LH secretion by exogenous melatonin in women. J Clin Endocrinol Metab 1991;73(1): 210-212.

121. Cagnacci A, Soldani R, Yen SS. Melatonin enhances cortisol levels in aged but not young women. Eur J Endocrinol 1995;133(6):691-695.

122. Lewinski A, Karbownik M. Review. Melatonin and the thyroid gland. Neuroendocrinol Lett 2002;23 Suppl 1:73-78.

123. Siegrist C, Benedetti C, Orlando A, et al. Lack of changes in serum prolactin, FSH, TSH, and estradiol after melatonin treatment in doses that improve sleep and reduce benzodiazepine consumption in sleep-disturbed, middle-aged, and elderly patients. J Pineal Res 2001;30(1):34-42.

124. Terzolo M, Revelli A, Guidetti D, et al. Evening administration of melatonin enhances the pulsatile secretion of prolactin but not of LH and TSH in normally cycling women. Clin Endocrinol (Oxf) 1993;39(2): 185-191.

125. Weinberg U, Weitzman ED, Fukushima DK, et al. Melatonin does not suppress the pituitary luteinizing hormone response to luteinizing hormone-releasing hormone in men. J Clin Endocrinol Metab 1980; 51(1):161-162.

126. Weinberg U, Weitzman ED, Horowitz ZD, et al. Lack of an effect of melatonin on the basal and L-dopa stimulated growth hormone secretion in men. J Neural Transm 1981;52(1-2):117-121.

127. Gwayi N, Bernard RT. The effects of melatonin on sperm motility *in vitro* in Wistar rats. Andrologia 2002;34(6):391-396.

128. Luboshitzky R, Shen-Orr Z, Nave R, et al. Melatonin administration alters semen quality in healthy men. J Androl 2002;23(4):572-578.

129. Calvo JR, Guerrero JM, Osuna C, et al. Melatonin triggers Crohn's disease symptoms. J Pineal Res 2002;32(4):277-278.

130. Samples JR, Krause G, Lewy AJ. Effect of melatonin on intraocular pressure. Curr Eye Res 1988;7(7):649-653.

131. Viggiano SR, Koskela TK, Klee GG, et al. The effect of melatonin on aqueous humor flow in humans during the day. Ophthalmology 1994; 101(2):326-331.

132. Yeleswaram K, Vachharajani N, Santone K. Involvement of cytochrome P-450 isozymes in melatonin metabolism and clinical implications. J Pineal Res 1999;26(3):190-191.

133. Scott GN, Elmer GW. Update on natural product–drug interactions. Am J Health Syst Pharm 2002;59(4):339-347.

134. von Bahr C, Ursing C, Yasui N, et al. Fluvoxamine but not citalopram increases serum melatonin in healthy subjects—an indication that cytochrome P450 CYP1A2 and CYP2C19 hydroxylate melatonin. Eur J Clin Pharmacol 2000;56(2):123-127.

135. Hartter S, Wang X, Weigmann H, et al. Differential effects of fluvoxamine and other antidepressants on the biotransformation of melatonin. J Clin Psychopharmacol 2001;21(2):167-174.

136. Lapwood KR, Bhagat L, Simpson MP. Analgesic effects on endogenous melatonin secretion. J Pineal Res 1997;22(1):20-25.

137. Murphy PJ, Myers BL, Badia P. Nonsteroidal anti-inflammatory drugs alter body temperature and suppress melatonin in humans. Physiol Behav 1996; 59(1):133-139.

138. Stoschitzky K, Sakotnik A, Lercher P, et al. Influence of beta-blockers on melatonin release. Eur J Clin Pharmacol 1999;55(2):111-115.

139. Munoz-Hoyos A, Amoros-Rodriguez I, Molina-Carballo A, et al. Pineal response after pyridoxine test in children. J Neural Transm Gen Sect 1996; 103(7):833-842.

140. Djeridane Y, Touitou Y. Chronic diazepam administration differentially affects melatonin synthesis in rat pineal and Harderian glands. Psychopharmacology (Berl) 2001;154(4):403-407.

141. Wakabayashi H, Shimada K, Satoh T. Effects of diazepam administration on melatonin synthesis in the rat pineal gland *in vivo*. Chem Pharm Bull (Tokyo) 1991;39(10):2674-2676.

142. Ozaki Y, Wurtman RJ, Alonso R, et al. Melatonin secretion decreases

during the proestrous stage of the rat estrous cycle. Proc Natl Acad Sci U S A 1978;75(1):531-534.

143. Honma K, Kohsaka M, Fukuda N, et al. Effects of vitamin B$_{12}$ on plasma melatonin rhythm in humans: increased light sensitivity phase-advances the circadian clock? Experientia 1992;48(8):716-720.

144. Wikner J, Wetterberg L, Rojdmark S. Does hypercalcaemia or calcium antagonism affect human melatonin secretion or renal excretion? Eur J Clin Invest 1997;27(5):374-379.

145. Norman TR, Piccolo J, Voudouris N, et al. The effect of single oral doses of zopiclone on nocturnal melatonin secretion in healthy male volunteers. Prog Neuropsychopharmacol Biol Psychiatry 2001;25(4):825-833.

146. Wikner J, Wetterberg L, Rojdmark S. The role of somatostatin (octreotide) in the regulation of melatonin secretion in healthy volunteers and in patients with primary hypothyroidism. J Endocrinol Invest 1999;22(7): 527-534.

147. Lusardi P, Piazza E, Fogari R. Cardiovascular effects of melatonin in hypertensive patients well controlled by nifedipine: a 24-hour study. Br J Clin Pharmacol 2000;49(5):423-427.

148. Ursing C, Wikner J, Brismar K, et al. Caffeine raises the serum melatonin level in healthy subjects: an indication of melatonin metabolism by cytochrome P450(CYP)1A2. J Endocrinol Invest 2003;26(5):403-406.

149. Wright KP, Jr., Badia P, Myers BL, et al. Caffeine and light effects on nighttime melatonin and temperature levels in sleep-deprived humans. Brain Res 1997;747(1):78-84.

150. Uchida K, Aoki T, Satoh H, et al. [Effects of melatonin on muscle contractility and neuromuscular blockade produced by muscle relaxants]. Masui 1997;46(2):205-212.

151. Gibb JW, Bush L, Hanson GR. Exacerbation of methamphetamine-induced neurochemical deficits by melatonin. J Pharmacol Exp Ther 1997; 283(2):630-635.

152. Nelson LA, McGuire JM, Hausafus SN. Melatonin for the treatment of tardive dyskinesia. Ann Pharmacother 2003;37(7-8):1128-1131.

153. Naidu PS, Singh A, Kaur P, et al. Possible mechanism of action in melatonin attenuation of haloperidol-induced orofacial dyskinesia. Pharmacol Biochem Behav 2003;74(3):641-648.

154. Naidu PS, Singh A, Kulkarni SK. Effect of Withania somnifera root extract on haloperidol-induced orofacial dyskinesia: possible mechanisms of action. J Med Food 2003;6(2):107-114.

155. Bhattacharya SK, Bhattacharya D, Sairam K, et al. Effect of Withania somnifera glycowithanolides on a rat model of tardive dyskinesia. Phytomedicine 2002;9(2):167-170.

156. Shamir E, Barak Y, Shalman I, et al. Melatonin treatment for tardive dyskinesia: a double-blind, placebo-controlled, crossover study. Arch Gen Psychiatry 2001;58(11):1049-1052.

157. Shamir EZ, Barak Y, Shalman I, et al. Melatonin treatment for tardive dyskinesia: a double-blind, placebo-controlled, cross-over study. Annu Meet Am Psychiatric Assoc, May 5-10 2001;

158. Shamir E, Barak Y, Plopsky I, et al. Is melatonin treatment effective for tardive dyskinesia? J Clin Psychiatry 2000;61(8):556-558.

159. Kos-Kudla B, Ostrowska Z, Kozlowski A, et al. Circadian rhythm of melatonin in patients with colorectal carcinoma. Neuroendocrinol Lett 2002;23(3):239-242.

160. Kos-Kudla B, Ostrowska Z, Marek B, et al. Circadian rhythm of melatonin in postmenopausal asthmatic women with hormone replacement therapy. Neuroendocrinol Lett 2002;23(3):243-248.

161. Dericks-Tan JS, Schwinn P, Hildt C. Dose-dependent stimulation of melatonin secretion after administration of agnus castus. Exp Clin Endocrinol Diabetes 2003;111(1):44-46.

162. Fournier I, Ploye F, Cottet-Emard JM, et al. Folate deficiency alters melatonin secretion in rats. J Nutr 2002;132(9):2781-2784.

163. Inserra P, Zhang Z, Ardestani SK, et al. Modulation of cytokine production by dehydroepiandrosterone (DHEA) plus melatonin (MLT) supplementation of old mice. Proc Soc Exp Biol Med 1998;218(1):76-82.

164. Currier NL, Sicotte M, Miller SC. Deleterious effects of Echinacea purpurea and melatonin on myeloid cells in mouse spleen and bone marrow. J Leukoc Biol 2001;70(2):274-276.

165. Touitou Y, Lambrozo J, Camus F, et al. Magnetic fields and the melatonin hypothesis: a study of workers chronically exposed to 50-Hz magnetic fields. Am J Physiol Regul Integr Comp Physiol 2003;284(6): R1529-R1535.

166. Karasek M, Czernicki J, Woldanska-Okonska M, et al. Chronic exposure to 25-80-microT, 200-Hz magnetic field does not influence serum melatonin concentrations in patients with low back pain. J Pineal Res 2000;29(2): 81-85.

167. Karasek M, Lerchl A. Melatonin and magnetic fields. Neuroendocrinol Lett 2002;23 Suppl 1:84-87.

168. Jarupat S, Kawabata A, Tokura H, et al. Effects of the 1900 MHz electromagnetic field emitted from cellular phone on nocturnal melatonin secretion. J Physiol Anthropol Appl Human Sci 2003;22(1):61-63.

169. Jajte J, Zmyslony M, Rajkowska E. [Protective effect of melatonin and vitamin E against prooxidative action of iron ions and static magnetic field]. Med Pr 2003;54(1):23-28.

170. Brzezinski A. Melatonin in humans. N Engl J Med 1997;336(3):186-195.

171. Iuvone PM, Brown AD, Haque R, et al. Retinal melatonin production: role of proteasomal proteolysis in circadian and photic control of arylalkylamine N-acetyltransferase. Invest Ophthalmol Vis Sci 2002; 43(2):564-572.

172. Kvetnoy IM, Ingel IE, Kvetnaia TV, et al. Gastrointestinal melatonin: cellular identification and biological role. Neuroendocrinol Lett 2002; 23(2):121-132.

173. Reiter RJ, Rollag MD, Panke ES, et al. Melatonin: reproductive effects. J Neural Transm Suppl 1978;(13):209-223.

174. Hajak G, Huether G, Blanke J, et al. The influence of intravenous L-tryptophan on plasma melatonin and sleep in men. Pharmacopsychiatry 1991;24(1):17-20.

175. ewy AJ, Wehr TA, Goodwin FK, et al. Light suppresses melatonin secretion in humans. Science 1980;210(4475):1267-1269.

176. Regelson W, Pierpaoli W. Melatonin: a rediscovered antitumor hormone? Its relation to surface receptors; sex steroid metabolism, immunologic response, and chronobiologic factors in tumor growth and therapy. Cancer Invest 1987;5(4):379-385.

177. Cagnacci A, Soldani R, Yen SS. Contemporaneous melatonin administration modifies the circadian response to nocturnal bright light stimuli. Am J Physiol 1997;272(2 Pt 2):R482-R486.

178. Brainard GC, Rollag MD, Hanifin JP, et al. The effect of polarized versus nonpolarized light on melatonin regulation in humans. Photochem Photobiol 2000;71(6):766-770.

179. Rea MS, Bullough JD, Figueiro MG. Human melatonin suppression by light: a case for scotopic efficiency. Neurosci Lett 2001;299(1-2):45-48.

180. Czeisler CA, Shanahan TL, Klerman EB, et al. Suppression of melatonin secretion in some blind patients by exposure to bright light. N Engl J Med 1995;332(1):6-11.

181. Hatonen T, Laakso ML, Heiskala H, et al. Bright light suppresses melatonin in blind patients with neuronal ceroid-lipofuscinoses. Neurology 1998;50(5):1445-1450.

182. Cowen PJ, Fraser S, Sammons R, et al. Atenolol reduces plasma melatonin concentration in man. Br J Clin Pharmacol 1983;15(5):579-581.

183. Brismar K, Hylander B, Eliasson K, et al. Melatonin secretion related to side-effects of beta-blockers from the central nervous system. Acta Med Scand 1988;223(6):525-530.

184. Hanssen T, Heyden T, Sundberg I, et al. Effect of propranolol on serum-melatonin. Lancet 1977;2(8032):309-310.

185. Cowen PJ, Bevan JS, Gosden B, et al. Treatment with beta-adrenoceptor blockers reduces plasma melatonin concentration. Br J Clin Pharmacol 1985;19(2):258-260.

186. Munoz-Hoyos A, Hubber E, Escames G, et al. Effect of propranolol plus exercise on melatonin and growth hormone levels in children with growth delay. J Pineal Res 2001;30(2):75-81.

187. Palazidou E, Franey C, Arendt J, et al. Evidence for a functional role of alpha-1 adrenoceptors in the regulation of melatonin secretion in man. Psychoneuroendocrinology 1989;14(1-2):131-135.

188. Palazidou E, Papadopoulos A, Sitsen A, et al. An alpha 2 adrenoceptor antagonist, Org 3770, enhances nocturnal melatonin secretion in man. Psychopharmacology (Berl) 1989;97(1):115-117.

189. Lewy AJ, Siever LJ, Uhde TW, et al. Clonidine reduces plasma melatonin levels. J Pharm Pharmacol 1986;38(7):555-556.

190. Birdsall TC. The biological effects and clinical uses of the pineal hormone melatonin. Altern Med Rev 1996;1(2):94-102.

191. Palazidou E, Skene D, Arendt J, et al. The acute and chronic effects of (+) and (−) oxaprotiline upon melatonin secretion in normal subjects. Psychol Med 1992;22(1):61-67.

192. Monteleone P, Orazzo C, Natale M, et al. Lack of effect of short-term fluoxetine administration on nighttime plasma melatonin levels in healthy subjects. Biol Psychiatry 1994;35(2):139-142.

193. Wurtman RJ, Ozaki Y. Physiological control of melatonin synthesis and secretion: mechanisms, generating rhythms in melatonin, methoxytryptophol, and arginine vasotocin levels and effects on the pineal of endogenous catecholamines, the estrous cycle, and environmental lighting. J Neural Transm Suppl 1978;(13):59-70.

194. Goh VH, Tong TY, Lim CL, et al. Effects of one night of sleep deprivation on hormone profiles and performance efficiency. Mil Med 2001;166(5): 427-431.

195. Laughlin GA, Loucks AB, Yen SS. Marked augmentation of nocturnal melatonin secretion in amenorrheic athletes, but not in cycling athletes: unaltered by opioidergic or dopaminergic blockade. J Clin Endocrinol Metab 1991;73(6):1321-1326.

196. Brugger P, Marktl W, Herold M. Impaired nocturnal secretion of melatonin in coronary heart disease. Lancet 1995;345(8962):1408.

197. Cagnacci A, Arangino S, Angiolucci M, et al. Different circulatory response to melatonin in postmenopausal women without and with hormone replacement therapy. J Pineal Res 2000;29(3):152-158.

198. Fourtillan JB, Brisson AM, Fourtillan M, et al. Melatonin secretion occurs at a constant rate in both young and older men and women. Am J Physiol Endocrinol Metab 2001;280(1):E11-E22.

199. Ardura J, Gutierrez R, Andres J, et al. Emergence and evolution of the circadian rhythm of melatonin in children. Horm Res 2003;59(2):66-72.

200. Sandyk R. Melatonin and maturation of REM sleep. Int J Neurosci 1992; 63(1-2):105-114.

M

201. Roth JA, Kim BG, Lin WL, et al. Melatonin promotes osteoblast differentiation and bone formation. J Biol Chem 1999;274(31):22041-22047.

202. Zhdanova IV, Raz DJ. Effects of melatonin ingestion on cAMP and cGMP levels in human plasma. J Endocrinol 1999;163(3):457-462.

203. Cardinali DP, Del Zar MM, Vacas MI. The effects of melatonin in human platelets. Acta Physiol Pharmacol Ther Latinoam 1993;43(1-2):1-13.

204. Vacas MI, Cardinali DP. Diurnal changes in melatonin binding sites of hamster and rat brains. Correlations with neuroendocrine responsiveness to melatonin. Neurosci Lett 1979;15(2-3):259-263.

205. Becker-Andre M, Wiesenberg I, Schaeren-Wiemers N, et al. Pineal gland hormone melatonin binds and activates an orphan of the nuclear receptor superfamily. J Biol Chem 1994;269(46):28531-28534.

206. Short RV. Melatonin. BMJ 1993;307(6910):952-953.

207. Sack RL, Hughes RJ, Edgar DM, et al. Sleep-promoting effects of melatonin: at what dose, in whom, under what conditions, and by what mechanisms? Sleep 1997;20(10):908-915.

208. Zhdanova IV, Lynch HJ, Wurtman RJ. Melatonin: a sleep-promoting hormone. Sleep 1997;20(10):899-907.

209. Matsumoto M, Sack RL, Blood ML, et al. The amplitude of endogenous melatonin production is not affected by melatonin treatment in humans. J Pineal Res 1997;22(1):42-44.

210. Cavallo A. The pineal gland in human beings: relevance to pediatrics. J Pediatr 1993;123(6):843-851.

211. Monti JM, Cardinali DP. A critical assessment of the melatonin effect on sleep in humans. Biol Signals Recept 2000;9(6):328-339.

212. Reiter RJ. The melatonin message: duration versus coincidence hypotheses. Life Sci 1987;40(22):2119-2131.

213. Bothorel B, Barassin S, Saboureau M, et al. In the rat, exogenous melatonin increases the amplitude of pineal melatonin secretion by a direct action on the circadian clock. Eur J Neurosci 2002;16(6):1090-1098.

214. Lewy AJ, Newsome DA. Different types of melatonin circadian secretory rhythms in some blind subjects. J Clin Endocrinol Metab 1983;56(6):1103-1107.

215. Nakagawa H, Sack RL, Lewy AJ. Sleep propensity free-runs with the temperature, melatonin and cortisol rhythms in a totally blind person. Sleep 1992;15(4):330-336.

216. Lockley S, Tabandeh H, Skene D, et al. Day-time naps and melatonin in blind people. Lancet 1995;346(8988):1491.

217. Lewy AJ, Emens JS, Sack RL, et al. Low, but not high, doses of melatonin entrained a free-running blind person with a long circadian period. Chronobiol Int 2002;19(3):649-658.

218. Oren DA, Turner EH, Wehr TA. Abnormal circadian rhythms of plasma melatonin and body temperature in the delayed sleep phase syndrome. J Neurol Neurosurg Psychiatry 1995;58(3):379.

219. Waldhauser F, Vierhapper H, Pirich K. Abnormal circadian melatonin secretion in night-shift workers. N Engl J Med 1986;315(25):1614.

220. Harma M, Laitinen J, Partinen M, et al. The effect of four-day round trip flights over 10 time zones on the circadian variation of salivary melatonin and cortisol in airline flight attendants. Ergonomics 1994;37(9):1479-1489.

221. Shochat T, Haimov I, Lavie P. Melatonin—the key to the gate of sleep. Ann Med 1998;30(1):109-114.

222. Monteleone P, Tortorella A, Borriello R, et al. Suppression of nocturnal plasma melatonin levels by evening administration of sodium valproate in healthy humans. Biol Psychiatry 1997;41(3):336-341.

223. Monteleone P, Forziati D, Orazzo C, et al. Preliminary observations on the suppression of nocturnal plasma melatonin levels by short-term administration of diazepam in humans. J Pineal Res 1989;6(3):253-258.

224. Ekman AC, Leppaluoto J, Huttunen P, et al. Ethanol inhibits melatonin secretion in healthy volunteers in a dose-dependent randomized double blind cross-over study. J Clin Endocrinol Metab 1993;77(3):780-783.

225. Johnson S. Micronutrient accumulation and depletion in schizophrenia, epilepsy, autism and Parkinson's disease? Med Hypotheses 2001;56(5):641-645.

226. Luboshitzky R, Lavi S, Thuma I, et al. Testosterone treatment alters melatonin concentrations in male patients with gonadotropin-releasing hormone deficiency. J Clin Endocrinol Metab 1996;81(2):770-774.

227. Luboshitzky R, Wagner O, Lavi S, et al. Abnormal melatonin secretion in hypogonadal men: the effect of testosterone treatment. Clin Endocrinol (Oxf) 1997;47(4):463-469.

228. Nakamura Y, Tamura H, Kashida S, et al. Changes of serum melatonin level and its relationship to feto-placental unit during pregnancy. J Pineal Res 2001;30(1):29-33.

229. Kennaway DJ, Flanagan DE, Moore VM, et al. The impact of fetal size and length of gestation on 6- sulphatoxymelatonin excretion in adult life. J Pineal Res 2001;30(3):188-192.

230. Viviani S, Bidoli P, Spinazze S, et al. Normalization of the light/dark rhythm of melatonin after prolonged subcutaneous administration of interleukin-2 in advanced small cell lung cancer patients. J Pineal Res 1992;12(3):114-117.

231. Deacon S, Arendt J. Posture influences melatonin concentrations in plasma and saliva in humans. Neurosci Lett 1994;167(1-2):191-194.

232. Fraschini F, Cesarani A, Alpini D, et al. Melatonin influences human balance. Biol Signals Recept 1999;8(1-2):111-119.

233. Stewart JW, Halbreich U. Plasma melatonin levels in depressed patients before and after treatment with antidepressant medication. Biol Psychiatry 1989;25(1):33-38.

234. Danforth DN, Jr., Tamarkin L, Lippman ME. Melatonin increases oestrogen receptor binding activity of human breast cancer cells. Nature 1983;305(5932):323-325.

235. Brun J, Chamba G, Khalfallah Y, et al. Effect of modafinil on plasma melatonin, cortisol and growth hormone rhythms, rectal temperature and performance in healthy subjects during a 36 h sleep deprivation. J Sleep Res 1998;7(2):105-114.

236. Bordet R, Devos D, Brique S, et al. Study of circadian melatonin secretion pattern at different stages of Parkinson's disease. Clin Neuropharmacol 2003;26(2):65-72.

237. Franey C, Aldhous M, Burton S, et al. Acute treatment with desipramine stimulates melatonin and 6-sulphatoxy melatonin production in man. Br J Clin Pharmacol 1986;22(1):73-79.

238. Buxton OM, Lee CW, L'Hermite-Baleriaux M, et al. Exercise elicits phase shifts and acute alterations of melatonin that vary with circadian phase. Am J Physiol Regul Integr Comp Physiol 2003;284(3):R714-R724.

239. Cavallo A, Richards GE, Meyer WJ, III, et al. Evaluation of 5-hydroxytryptophan administration as a test of pineal function in humans. Horm Res 1987;27(2):69-73.

240. Kancheva R, Zofkova I, Hill M, et al. Lack of melatonin response to acute administration of nifedipine and diltiazem in healthy men. Physiol Res 2000;49 Suppl 1:S119-S124.

241. Munoz-Hoyos A, Heredia F, Moreno F, et al. Evaluation of plasma levels of melatonin after midazolam or sodium thiopental anesthesia in children. J Pineal Res 2002;32(4):253-256.

242. Wetterberg L, Eriksson O, Friberg Y, et al. A simplified radioimmunoassay for melatonin and its application to biological fluids. Preliminary observations on the half-life of plasma melatonin in man. Clin Chim Acta 1978;86(2):169-177.

243. Wetterberg L. Melatonin in humans: physiological and clinical studies. J Neural Transm Suppl 1978;(13):289-310.

244. Cugini P, Touitou Y, Bogdan A, et al. Is melatonin circadian rhythm a physiological feature associated with healthy longevity? A study of long-living subjects and their progeny. Chronobiol Int 2001;18(1):99-107.

245. Kripke DF, Elliot JA, Youngstedt SD, et al. Melatonin: marvel or marker? Ann Med 1998;30(1):81-87.

246. Pepping J. Melatonin. Am J Health Syst Pharm 1999;56(24):2520, 2523-2524, 2527.

247. Sack RL, Lewy AJ, Erb DL, et al. Human melatonin production decreases with age. J Pineal Res 1986;3(4):379-388.

248. Nathan PJ, Burrows GD, Norman TR. The effect of age and pre-light melatonin concentration on the melatonin sensitivity to dim light. Int Clin Psychopharmacol 1999;14(3):189-192.

249. Zeitzer JM, Daniels JE, Duffy JF, et al. Do plasma melatonin concentrations decline with age? Am J Med 1999;107(5):432-436.

250. Mishima K, Tozawa T, Satoh K, et al. Melatonin secretion rhythm disorders in patients with senile dementia of Alzheimer's type with disturbed sleep-waking. Biol Psychiatry 1999;45(4):417-421.

251. Lewy AJ, Ahmed S, Jackson JM, et al. Melatonin shifts human circadian rhythms according to a phase-response curve. Chronobiol Int 1992;9(5):380-392.

252. Cajochen C, Krauchi K, von Arx MA, et al. Daytime melatonin administration enhances sleepiness and theta/alpha activity in the waking EEG. Neurosci Lett 1996;207(3):209-213.

253. Lieberman HR. Behavior, sleep and melatonin. J Neural Transm Suppl 1986;21:233-241.

254. Claustrat B, Brun J, Garry P, et al. A once-repeated study of nocturnal plasma melatonin patterns and sleep recordings in six normal young men. J Pineal Res 1986;3(4):301-310.

255. Youngstedt SD, Kripke DF, Elliott JA. Melatonin excretion is not related to sleep in the elderly. J Pineal Res 1998;24(3):142-145.

256. Rommel T, Demisch L. Influence of chronic beta-adrenoreceptor blocker treatment on melatonin secretion and sleep quality in patients with essential hypertension. J Neural Transm Gen Sect 1994;95(1):39-48.

257. Tzischinsky O, Lavie P. Melatonin possesses time-dependent hypnotic effects. Sleep 1994;17(7):638-645.

258. Waldhauser F, Saletu B, Trinchard-Lugan I. Sleep laboratory investigations on hypnotic properties of melatonin. Psychopharmacology (Berl) 1990;100(2):222-226.

259. James SP, Mendelson WB, Sack DA, et al. The effect of melatonin on normal sleep. Neuropsychopharmacology 1987;1(1):41-44.

260. Ferini-Strambi L, Zucconi M, Biella G, et al. Effect of melatonin on sleep microstructure: preliminary results in healthy subjects. Sleep 1993;16(8):744-747.

261. Wang F, Li J, Wu C, et al. The GABA(A) receptor mediates the hypnotic activity of melatonin in rats. Pharmacol Biochem Behav 2003;74(3):573-578.

262. Nave R, Herer P, Haimov I, et al. Hypnotic and hypothermic effects of melatonin on daytime sleep in humans: lack of antagonism by flumazenil. Neurosci Lett 1996;214(2-3):123-126.

263. Krauchi K, Cajochen C, Mori D, et al. Early evening melatonin and

S-20098 advance circadian phase and nocturnal regulation of core body temperature. Am J Physiol 1997;272(4 Pt 2):R1178-R1188.

264. Hatonen T, Alila A, Laakso ML. Exogenous melatonin fails to counteract the light-induced phase delay of human melatonin rhythm. Brain Res 1996;710(1-2):125-130.

265. Deacon S, Arendt J. Melatonin-induced temperature suppression and its acute phase-shifting effects correlate in a dose-dependent manner in humans. Brain Res 1995;688(1-2):77-85.

266. Steinlechner S. Melatonin as a chronobiotic: PROS and CONS. Acta Neurobiol Exp (Warsz) 1996;56(1):363-372.

267. Lewy AJ, Sack RL. Exogenous melatonin's phase-shifting effects on the endogenous melatonin profile in sighted humans: a brief review and critique of the literature. J Biol Rhythms 1997;12(6):588-594.

268. Zaidan R, Geoffriau M, Brun J, et al. Melatonin is able to influence its secretion in humans: description of a phase-response curve. Neuroendocrinology 1994;60(1):105-112.

269. Cagnacci A, Elliott JA, Yen SS. Melatonin: a major regulator of the circadian rhythm of core temperature in humans. J Clin Endocrinol Metab 1992;75(2):447-452.

270. Deacon S, English J, Arendt J. Acute phase-shifting effects of melatonin associated with suppression of core body temperature in humans. Neurosci Lett 1994;178(1):32-34.

271. Slotten HA, Krekling S. Does melatonin have an effect on cognitive performance? Psychoneuroendocrinology 1996;21(8):673-680.

272. Dawson D, Gibbon S, Singh P. The hypothermic effect of melatonin on core body temperature: is more better? J Pineal Res 1996;20(4):192-197.

273. Dollins AB, Lynch HJ, Wurtman RJ, et al. Effects of illumination on human nocturnal serum melatonin levels and performance. Physiol Behav 1993;53(1):153-160.

274. Lieberman HR, Waldhauser F, Garfield G, et al. Effects of melatonin on human mood and performance. Brain Res 1984;323(2):201-207.

275. Graw P, Werth E, Krauchi K, et al. Early morning melatonin administration impairs psychomotor vigilance. Behav Brain Res 2001;121(1-2):167-172.

276. Jean-Louis G, Zizi F, Von Gizycki H, et al. Acute effects of melatonin therapy on behavior, mood, and cognition [abstract]. Sleep Res 1997;26:108.

278. Singer C, Wild K, Sack R, et al. High dose melatonin is well tolerated by the elderly [abstract]. Sleep Research 1994;23:86.

278. Feng Y, Zhang LX, Chao DM. [Role of melatonin in spatial learning and memory in rats and its mechanism]. Sheng Li Xue Bao 2002;54(1):65-70.

279. Maestroni GJ. The immunotherapeutic potential of melatonin. Expert Opin Investig Drugs 2001;10(3):467-476.

280. Lissoni P, Barni S, Meregalli S, et al. Modulation of cancer endocrine therapy by melatonin: a phase II study of tamoxifen plus melatonin in metastatic breast cancer patients progressing under tamoxifen alone. Br J Cancer 1995;71(4):854-856.

281. Lissoni P, Ardizzoia A, Tisi E, et al. Amplification of eosinophilia by melatonin during the immunotherapy of cancer with interleukin-2. J Biol Regul Homeost Agents 1993;7(1):34-36.

282. Lissoni P, Barni S, Ardizzoia A, et al. Immunological effects of a single evening subcutaneous injection of low-dose interleukin-2 in association with the pineal hormone melatonin in advanced cancer patients. J Biol Regul Homeost Agents 1992;6(4):132-136.

283. Maestroni GJ. The immunoneuroendocrine role of melatonin. J Pineal Res 1993;14(1):1-10.

284. Lissoni P, Barni S, Tancini G, et al. A study of the mechanisms involved in the immunostimulatory action of the pineal hormone in cancer patients. Oncology 1993;50(6):399-402.

285. Arias J, Melean E, Valero N, et al. [Effect of melatonin on lymphocyte proliferation and production of interleukin-2 (IL-2) and interleukin-1 beta (IL-1 beta) in mice splenocytes]. Invest Clin 2003;44(1):41-50.

286. Maestroni GJ, Conti A, Pierpaoli W. Role of the pineal gland in immunity. Circadian synthesis and release of melatonin modulates the antibody response and antagonizes the immunosuppressive effect of corticosterone. J Neuroimmunol 1986;13(1):19-30.

287. Poon AM, Liu ZM, Pang CS, et al. Evidence for a direct action of melatonin on the immune system. Biol Signals 1994;3(2):107-117.

288. Chen G, Huo Y, Tan DX, et al. Melatonin in Chinese medicinal herbs. Life Sci 2003;73(1):19-26.

289. Chen JC, Ng CJ, Chiu TF, et al. Altered neutrophil apoptosis activity is reversed by melatonin in liver ischemia-reperfusion. J Pineal Res 2003;34(4):260-264.

290. Chen KB, Lin AM, Chiu TH. Oxidative injury to the locus coeruleus of rat brain: neuroprotection by melatonin. J Pineal Res 2003;35(2):109-117.

291. Blask DE, Sauer LA, Dauchy RT. Melatonin as a chronobiotic/anticancer agent: cellular, biochemical, and molecular mechanisms of action and their implications for circadian-based cancer therapy. Curr Top Med Chem 2002;2(2):113-132.

292. Blask DE, Dauchy RT, Sauer LA, et al. Light during darkness, melatonin suppression and cancer progression. Neuroendocrinol Lett 2002;23(Suppl 2):52-56.

293. Jonage-Canonico MB, Lenoir V, Martin A, et al. Long term inhibition by estradiol or progesterone of melatonin secretion after administration of a mammary carcinogen, the dimethyl benz(a)anthracene, in Sprague-Dawley female rat; inhibitory effect of melatonin on mammary carcinogenesis. Breast Cancer Res Treat 2003;79(3):365-377.

294. Karasek M, Gruszka A, Lawnicka H, et al. Melatonin inhibits growth of diethylstilbestrol-induced prolactin-secreting pituitary tumor in vitro: possible involvement of nuclear RZR/ROR receptors. J Pineal Res 2003;34(4):294-296.

295. Blask DE, Hill SM. Effects of melatonin on cancer: studies on MCF-7 human breast cancer cells in culture. J Neural Transm Suppl 1986;21:433-449.

296. Blask DE, Hill SM, Pelletier DB, et al. Melatonin: an anticancer hormone of the pineal gland. In Reiter RJ, Pang SF (eds): Advances in Pineal Research. London, John Libbey, 1989, pp 259-263.

297. Bartsch H, Buchberger A, Franz H, et al. Effect of melatonin and pineal extracts on human ovarian and mammary tumor cells in a chemosensitivity assay. Life Sci 2000;67(24):2953-2960.

298. Grin W, Grunberger W. A significant correlation between melatonin deficiency and endometrial cancer. Gynecol Obstet Invest 1998;45(1):62-65.

299. Karasek M, Kowalski AJ, Zylinska K. Serum melatonin circadian profile in women suffering from the genital tract cancers. Neuroendocrinol Lett 2000;21(2):109-113.

300. Cos S, Sanchez-Barcelo EJ. Melatonin and mammary pathological growth. Front Neuroendocrinol 2000;21(2):133-170.

301. Dauchy RT, Sauer LA, Blask DE, et al. Light contamination during the dark phase in "photoperiodically controlled" animal rooms: effect on tumor growth and metabolism in rats. Lab Anim Sci 1997;47(5):511-518.

302. Dillon DC, Easley SE, Asch BB, et al. Differential expression of high-affinity melatonin receptors (MT1) in normal and malignant human breast tissue. Am J Clin Pathol 2002;118(3):451-458.

303. Marelli MM, Limonta P, Maggi R, et al. Growth-inhibitory activity of melatonin on human androgen-independent DU 145 prostate cancer cells. Prostate 2000;45(3):238-244.

304. Molis TM, Spriggs LL, Jupiter Y, et al. Melatonin modulation of estrogen-regulated proteins, growth factors, and proto-oncogenes in human breast cancer. J Pineal Res 1995;18(2):93-103.

305. Granzotto M, Rapozzi V, Decorti G, et al. Effects of melatonin on doxorubicin cytotoxicity in sensitive and pleiotropically resistant tumor cells. J Pineal Res 2001;31(3):206-213.

306. Dai J, Ram PT, Yuan L, et al. Transcriptional repression of RORalpha activity in human breast cancer cells by melatonin. Mol Cell Endocrinol 2001;176(1-2):111-120.

307. L'Hermite-Baleriaux M, de Launoit Y. Is melatonin really an in vitro inhibitor of human breast cancer cell proliferation? In Vitro Cell Dev Biol 1992;28A(9-10):583-584.

308. Bubis M, Zisapel N. Modulation by melatonin of protein secretion from melanoma cells: is cAMP involved? Mol Cell Endocrinol 1995;112(2):169-175.

309. Bizzarri M, Cucina A, Valente MG, et al. Melatonin and vitamin D_3 increase TGF-beta1 release and induce growth inhibition in breast cancer cell cultures. J Surg Res 2003;110(2):332-337.

310. Danforth DN, Jr., Tamarkin L, Mulvihill JJ, et al. Plasma melatonin and the hormone-dependency of human breast cancer. J Clin Oncol 1985;3(7):941-948.

311. Acuna CD, Escames G, Carazo A, et al. Melatonin, mitochondrial homeostasis and mitochondrial-related diseases. Curr Top Med Chem 2002;2(2):133-151.

312. Allegra M, Gentile C, Tesoriere L, et al. Protective effect of melatonin against cytotoxic actions of malondialdehyde: an in vitro study on human erythrocytes. J Pineal Res 2002;32(3):187-193.

313. Reiter RJ, Acuna-Castroviejo D, Tan DX, et al. Free radical-mediated molecular damage. Mechanisms for the protective actions of melatonin in the central nervous system. Ann N Y Acad Sci 2001;939:200-215.

314. Reiter RJ, Tan DX, Manchester LC. Biochemical reactivity of melatonin with reactive oxygen and nitrogen species: a review of the evidence. Cell Biochem Biophys 2001;34(2):237-256.

315. Pei Z, Pang SF, Cheung RT. Administration of melatonin after onset of ischemia reduces the volume of cerebral infarction in a rat middle cerebral artery occlusion stroke model. Stroke 2003;34(3):770-775.

316. Pei Z, Fung PC, Cheung RT. Melatonin reduces nitric oxide level during ischemia but not blood-brain barrier breakdown during reperfusion in a rat middle cerebral artery occlusion stroke model. J Pineal Res 2003;34(2):110-118.

317. Pei Z, Cheung RT. Melatonin protects SHSY5Y neuronal cells but not cultured astrocytes from ischemia due to oxygen and glucose deprivation. J Pineal Res 2003;34(3):194-201.

318. Cheung RT. The utility of melatonin in reducing cerebral damage resulting from ischemia and reperfusion. J Pineal Res 2003;34(3):153-160.

319. Reiter RJ, Sainz RM, Lopez-Burillo S, et al. Melatonin ameliorates neurologic damage and neurophysiologic deficits in experimental models of stroke. Ann N Y Acad Sci 2003;993:35-47.

320. Reiter RJ, Tan DX. Melatonin: a novel protective agent against oxidative injury of the ischemic/reperfused heart. Cardiovasc Res 2003;58(1):10-19.

321. Reiter RJ. Melatonin: clinical relevance. Best Pract Res Clin Endocrinol Metab 2003;17(2):273-285.

322. Reiter RJ, Tan DX. What constitutes a physiological concentration of melatonin? J Pineal Res 2003;34(1):79-80.

323. Sahna E, Parlakpinar H, Ozturk F, et al. The protective effects of physiological and pharmacological concentrations of melatonin on renal ischemia-reperfusion injury in rats. Urol Res 2003;31(3):188-193.

324. Sahna E, Acet A, Ozer MK, et al. Myocardial ischemia-reperfusion in rats: reduction of infarct size by either supplemental physiological or pharmacological doses of melatonin. J Pineal Res 2002;33(4):234-238.

325. Sahna E, Olmez E, Acet A. Effects of physiological and pharmacological concentrations of melatonin on ischemia-reperfusion arrhythmias in rats: can the incidence of sudden cardiac death be reduced? J Pineal Res 2002; 32(3):194-198.

326. Sener G, Tosun O, Sehirli AO, et al. Melatonin and N-acetylcysteine have beneficial effects during hepatic ischemia and reperfusion. Life Sci 2003;72(24):2707-2718.

327. Sener G, Sehirli AO, Paskaloglu K, et al. Melatonin treatment protects against ischemia/reperfusion-induced functional and biochemical changes in rat urinary bladder. J Pineal Res 2003;34(3):226-230.

328. Celebi S, Dilsiz N, Yilmaz T, et al. Effects of melatonin, vitamin E and octreotide on lipid peroxidation during ischemia-reperfusion in the guinea pig retina. Eur J Ophthalmol 2002;12(2):77-83.

329. Li XJ, Zhang LM, Gu J, et al. Melatonin decreases production of hydroxyl radical during cerebral ischemia-reperfusion. Zhongguo Yao Li Xue Bao 1997;18(5):394-396.

330. Lee YM, Chen HR, Hsiao G, et al. Protective effects of melatonin on myocardial ischemia/reperfusion injury in vivo. J Pineal Res 2002;33(2): 72-80.

331. Zhang J, Guo JD, Xing SH, et al. [The protective effects of melatonin on global cerebral ischemia-reperfusion injury in gerbils]. Yao Xue Xue Bao 2002;37(5):329-333.

332. Zhang Z, Yu CX. [Effect of melatonin on learning and memory impairment induced by aluminum chloride and its mechanism]. Yao Xue Xue Bao 2002;37(9):682-686.

333. Kaptanoglu E, Palaoglu S, Demirpence E, et al. Different responsiveness of central nervous system tissues to oxidative conditions and to the antioxidant effect of melatonin. J Pineal Res 2003;34(1):32-35.

334. Edwards RB, Manzana EJ, Chen WJ. Melatonin (an antioxidant) does not ameliorate alcohol-induced Purkinje cell loss in the developing cerebellum. Alcohol Clin Exp Res 2002;26(7):1003-1009.

335. Reiter RJ, Poeggeler B, Tan D, et al. Antioxidant capacity of melatonin: a novel action not requiring a receptor. Neuroendocrinol Lett 1993; 15(1+2):103-116.

336. Pierrefiche G, Topall G, Courboin G, et al. Antioxidant activity of melatonin in mice. Res Commun Chem Pathol Pharmacol 1993;80(2): 211-223.

337. Mohanan PV, Yamamoto HA. Preventive effect of melatonin against brain mitochondria DNA damage, lipid peroxidation and seizures induced by kainic acid. Toxicol Lett 2002;129(1-2):99-105.

338. Mayo JC, Sainz RM, Uria H, et al. Inhibition of cell proliferation: a mechanism likely to mediate the prevention of neuronal cell death by melatonin. J Pineal Res 1998;25(1):12-18.

339. Manev H, Uz T. Oral melatonin in neurologically disabled children. Lancet 1998;351(9120):1963.

340. Okatani Y, Wakatsuki A, Reiter RJ. Melatonin counteracts potentiation by homocysteine of KCl-induced vasoconstriction in human umbilical artery: relation to calcium influx. Biochem Biophys Res Commun 2001;280(3): 940-944.

341. Wakatsuki A, Okatani Y, Ikenoue N, et al. Melatonin protects against oxidized low-density lipoprotein-induced inhibition of nitric oxide production in human umbilical artery. J Pineal Res 2001;31(3):281-288.

342. Koc M, Taysi S, Emin BM, et al. The effect of melatonin against oxidative damage during total-body irradiation in rats. Radiat Res 2003;160(2): 251-255.

343. Koc M, Buyukokuroglu ME, Taysi S. The effect of melatonin on peripheral blood cells during total body irradiation in rats. Biol Pharm Bull 2002;25(5):656-657.

344. Kim BC, Shon BS, Ryoo YW, et al. Melatonin reduces X-ray irradiation-induced oxidative damages in cultured human skin fibroblasts. J Dermatol Sci 2001;26(3):194-200.

345. Vijayalaxmi, Reiter RJ, Meltz ML. Melatonin protects human blood lymphocytes from radiation-induced chromosome damage. Mutat Res 1995;346(1):23-31.

346. Taysi S, Koc M, Buyukokuroglu ME, et al. Melatonin reduces lipid peroxidation and nitric oxide during irradiation-induced oxidative injury in the rat liver. J Pineal Res 2003;34(3):173-177.

347. Fischer TW, Scholz G, Knoll B, et al. Melatonin reduces UV-induced reactive oxygen species in a dose- dependent manner in IL-3-stimulated leukocytes. J Pineal Res 2001;31(1):39-45.

348. Fischer TW, Scholz G, Knoll B, et al. Melatonin suppresses reactive oxygen species in UV-irradiated leukocytes more than vitamin C and trolox. Skin Pharmacol Appl Skin Physiol 2002;15(5):367-373.

349. Bonnefont-Rousselot D, Cheve G, Gozzo A, et al. Melatonin related compounds inhibit lipid peroxidation during copper or free radical-induced LDL oxidation. J Pineal Res 2002;33(2):109-117.

350. Lopez-Burillo S, Tan DX, Mayo JC, et al. Melatonin, xanthurenic acid, resveratrol, EGCG, vitamin C and alpha-lipoic acid differentially reduce oxidative DNA damage induced by Fenton reagents: a study of their individual and synergistic actions. J Pineal Res 2003;34(4):269-277.

351. Montilla-Lopez P, Munoz-Agueda MC, Feijoo LM, et al. Comparison of melatonin versus vitamin C on oxidative stress and antioxidant enzyme activity in Alzheimer's disease induced by okadaic acid in neuroblastoma cells. Eur J Pharmacol 2002;451(3):237-243.

352. Pappolla MA, Simovich MJ, Bryant-Thomas T, et al. The neuroprotective activities of melatonin against the Alzheimer beta- protein are not mediated by melatonin membrane receptors. J Pineal Res 2002;32(3):135-142.

353. Reiter RJ, Melchiorri D, Sewerynek E, et al. A review of the evidence supporting melatonin's role as an antioxidant. J Pineal Res 1995;18(1):1-11.

354. Pieri C, Marra M, Moroni F, et al. Melatonin: a peroxyl radical scavenger more effective than vitamin E. Life Sci 1994;55(15):L271-L276.

355. Hardeland R, Reiter RJ, Poeggeler B, et al. The significance of the metabolism of the neurohormone melatonin: antioxidative protection and formation of bioactive substances. Neurosci Biobehav Rev 1993;17(3): 347-357.

356. Mayo JC, Tan DX, Sainz RM, et al. Oxidative damage to catalase induced by peroxyl radicals: functional protection by melatonin and other antioxidants. Free Radic Res 2003;37(5):543-553.

357. Tan DX, Manchester LC, Hardeland R, et al. Melatonin: a hormone, a tissue factor, an autocoid, a paracoid, and an antioxidant vitamin. J Pineal Res 2003;34(1):75-78.

358. Awney HA, Attih AM, Habib SL, et al. Effect of melatonin on the production of microsomal hydrogen peroxide and cytochrome P-450 content in rat treated with aflatoxin B(1). Toxicology 2002;172(2):143-148.

359. Fowler G, Daroszewska M, Ingold KU. Melatonin does not "directly scavenge hydrogen peroxide": demise of another myth. Free Radic Biol Med 2003;34(1):77-83.

360. Wiechmann AF, O'Steen WK. Melatonin increases photoreceptor susceptibility to light-induced damage. Invest Ophthalmol Vis Sci 1992; 33(6):1894-1902.

361. Cardinali DP, Ladizesky MG, Boggio V, et al. Melatonin effects on bone: experimental facts and clinical perspectives. J Pineal Res 2003;34(2):81-87.

362. Koyama H, Nakade O, Takada Y, et al. Melatonin at pharmacologic doses increases bone mass by suppressing resorption through down-regulation of the RANKL-mediated osteoclast formation and activation. J Bone Miner Res 2002;17(7):1219-1229.

363. de Leiva A, Tortosa F, Peinado MA, et al. Episodic nyctohemeral secretion of melatonin in adult humans: lack of relation with LH pulsatile pattern. Acta Endocrinol (Copenh) 1990;122(1):76-82.

364. Ferrari E, Foppa S, Bossolo PA, et al. Melatonin and pituitary-gonadal function in disorders of eating behavior. J Pineal Res 1989;7(2):115-124.

365. Fideleff H, Aparicio NJ, Guitelman A, et al. Effect of melatonin on the basal and stimulated gonadotropin levels in normal men and post-menopausal women. J Clin Endocrinol Metab 1976;42(6):1014-1017.

366. Aleem FA, Weitzman ED, Weinberg U. Suppression of basal luteinizing hormone concentrations by melatonin in postmenopausal women. Fertil Steril 1984;42(6):923-925.

367. Strassman RJ, Qualls CR, Lisansky EJ, et al. Sleep deprivation reduces LH secretion in men independently of melatonin. Acta Endocrinol (Copenh) 1991;124(6):646-651.

368. Paccotti P, Terzolo M, Torta M, et al. Acute administration of melatonin at two opposite circadian stages does not change responses to gonadotropin releasing hormone, thyrotropin releasing hormone and ACTH in healthy adult males. J Endocrinol Invest 1987;10(5):471-477.

369. Luboshitzky R, Levi M, Shen-Orr Z, et al. Long-term melatonin administration does not alter pituitary-gonadal hormone secretion in normal men. Hum Reprod 2000;15(1):60-65.

370. Nordlund JJ, Lerner AB. The effects of oral melatonin on skin color and on the release of pituitary hormones. J Clin Endocrinol Metab 1977; 45(4):768-774.

371. Bellipanni G, Bianchi P, Pierpaoli W, et al. Effects of melatonin in perimenopausal and menopausal women: a randomized and placebo controlled study. Exp Gerontol 2001;36(2):297-310.

372. Brzezinski A, Fibich T, Cohen M, et al. Effects of melatonin on progesterone production by human granulosa lutein cells in culture. Fertil Steril 1992;58(3):526-529.

373. Meeking DR, Wallace JD, Cuneo RC, et al. Exercise-induced GH secretion is enhanced by the oral ingestion of melatonin in healthy adult male subjects. Eur J Endocrinol 1999;141(1):22-26.

374. Valcavi R, Zini M, Maestroni GJ, et al. Melatonin stimulates growth hormone secretion through pathways other than the growth hormone-releasing hormone. Clin Endocrinol (Oxf) 1993;39(2):193-199.

375. Valcavi R, Dieguez C, Azzarito C, et al. Effect of oral administration of melatonin on GH responses to GRF 1-44 in normal subjects. Clin Endocrinol (Oxf) 1987;26(4):453-458.

376. Smythe GA, Lazarus L. Growth hormone responses to melatonin in man. Science 1974;184(144):1373-1374.

377. Forsling ML, Wheeler MJ, Williams AJ. The effect of melatonin administration on pituitary hormone secretion in man. Clin Endocrinol (Oxf) 1999;51(5):637-642.

378. Vriend J, Sheppard MS, Borer KT. Melatonin increases serum growth hormone and insulin-like growth factor I (IGF-I) levels in male Syrian hamsters via hypothalamic neurotransmitters. Growth Dev Aging 1990;54(4):165-171.

379. Smythe GA, Lazarus L. Growth hormone regulation by melatonin and serotonin. Nature 1973;244(5413):230-231.

380. Smythe GA, Lazarus L. Suppression of human growth hormone secretion by melatonin and cyproheptadine. J Clin Invest 1974;54(1):116-121.

381. Coiro V, Volpi R, Capretti L, et al. Different effects of naloxone on the growth hormone response to melatonin and pyridostigmine in normal men. Metabolism 1998;47(7):814-816.

382. Esposti D, Lissoni P, Mauri R, et al. The pineal gland-opioid system relation: melatonin-naloxone interactions in regulating GH and LH releases in man. J Endocrinol Invest 1988;11(2):103-106.

383. Wright J, Aldhous M, Franey C, et al. The effects of exogenous melatonin on endocrine function in man. Clin Endocrinol (Oxf) 1986;24(4):375-382.

384. Doyle SE, Grace MS, McIvor W, et al. Circadian rhythms of dopamine in mouse retina: the role of melatonin. Vis Neurosci 2002;19(5):593-601.

385. Okatani Y, Sagara Y. Role of melatonin in nocturnal prolactin secretion in women with normoprolactinemia and mild hyperprolactinemia. Am J Obstet Gynecol 1993;168(3 Pt 1):854-861.

386. Ninomiya T, Iwatani N, Tomoda A, et al. Effects of exogenous melatonin on pituitary hormones in humans. Clin Physiol 2001;21(3):292-299.

387. Waldhauser F, Lieberman HR, Lynch HJ, et al. A pharmacological dose of melatonin increases PRL levels in males without altering those of GH, LH, FSH, TSH, testosterone or cortisol. Neuroendocrinology 1987;46(2):125-130.

388. Petterborg LJ, Thalen BE, Kjellman BF, et al. Effect of melatonin replacement on serum hormone rhythms in a patient lacking endogenous melatonin. Brain Res Bull 1991;27:181-185.

389. Kostoglou-Athanassiou I, Treacher DF, Wheeler MJ, et al. Melatonin administration and pituitary hormone secretion. Clin Endocrinol (Oxf) 1998;48(1):31-37.

390. McIntyre IM, Norman TR, Burrows GD, et al. Alterations to plasma melatonin and cortisol after evening alprazolam administration in humans. Chronobiol Int 1993;10(3):205-213.

391. Bojanowska E, Forsling ML. The effects of melatonin on vasopressin secretion in vivo: interactions with acetylcholine and prostaglandins. Brain Res Bull 1997;42(6):457-461.

392. Chiodera P, Volpi R, Capretti L, et al. Effect of melatonin on arginine vasopressin secretion stimulated by physical exercise or angiotensin II in normal men. Neuropeptides 1998;32(2):125-129.

393. Chiodera P, Volpi R, Capretti L, et al. Melatonin inhibits oxytocin response to insulin-induced hypoglycemia, but not to angiotensin II in normal men. J Neural Transm 1998;105(2-3):173-180.

394. Fabis M, Pruszynska E, Mackowiak P. In vivo and in situ action of melatonin on insulin secretion and some metabolic implications in the rat. Pancreas 2002;25(2):166-169.

395. Valenti S, Giusti M. Melatonin participates in the control of testosterone secretion from rat testis: an overview of our experience. Ann N Y Acad Sci 2002;966:284-289.

396. Reiter RJ, Calvo JR, Karbownik M, et al. Melatonin and its relation to the immune system and inflammation. Ann N Y Acad Sci 2000;917:376-386.

397. Bilici D, Akpinar E, Kiziltunc A. Protective effect of melatonin in carrageenan-induced acute local inflammation. Pharmacol Res 2002;46(2):133-139.

398. Bilici D, Suleyman H, Banoglu ZN, et al. Melatonin prevents ethanol-induced gastric mucosal damage possibly due to its antioxidant effect. Dig Dis Sci 2002;47(4):856-861.

399. Cuzzocrea S, Reiter RJ. Pharmacological actions of melatonin in acute and chronic inflammation. Curr Top Med Chem 2002;2(2):153-165.

400. Singh P, Bhargava VK, Garg SK. Effect of melatonin and beta-carotene on indomethacin induced gastric mucosal injury. Indian J Physiol Pharmacol 2002;46(2):229-234.

401. Cabeza J, Alarcon-de-la-Lastra C, Jimenez D, et al. Melatonin modulates the effects of gastric injury in rats: role of prostaglandins and nitric oxide. Neurosignals 2003;12(2):71-77.

402. Sjoblom M, Jedstedt G, Flemstrom G. Peripheral melatonin mediates neural stimulation of duodenal mucosal bicarbonate secretion. J Clin Invest 2001;108(4):625-633.

403. Bandyopadhyay D, Biswas K, Bhattacharyya M, et al. Gastric toxicity and mucosal ulceration induced by oxygen-derived reactive species: protection by melatonin. Curr Mol Med 2001;1(4):501-513.

404. Bandyopadhyay D, Biswas K, Bandyopadhyay U, et al. Melatonin protects against stress-induced gastric lesions by scavenging the hydroxyl radical. J Pineal Res 2000;29(3):143-151.

405. Sanchez-Forte M, Moreno-Madrid F, Munoz-Hoyos A, et al. Efecto de la melatonina como anticonvulsivante y protector neuronal. Revista de Neurologia 1997;25:1229-1234.

406. Bikjdaouene L, Escames G, Leon J, et al. Changes in brain amino acids and nitric oxide after melatonin administration in rats with pentylenetetrazole-induced seizures. J Pineal Res 2003;35(1):54-60.

407. Fariello RG, Bubenik GA, Brown GM, et al. Epileptogenic action of intraventricularly injected antimelatonin antibody. Neurology 1977;27(6):567-570.

408. Zhou YH, Huo ZY, Qiu XC. [Inhibitory effect of melatonin on morphine withdrawal syndromes and the content of NO in plasma and brain tissue in morphine dependent mice]. Yao Xue Xue Bao 2002;37(3):175-177.

409. Raghavendra V, Kulkarni SK. Reversal of morphine tolerance and dependence by melatonin: possible role of central and peripheral benzodiazepine receptors. Brain Res 1999;834(1-2):178-181.

410. Sewerynek E. Melatonin and the cardiovascular system. Neuroendocrinol Lett 2002;23(Suppl 1):79-83.

411. Brzezinski A, Lynch HJ, Seibel MM, et al. The circadian rhythm of plasma melatonin during the normal menstrual cycle and in amenorrheic women. J Clin Endocrinol Metab 1988;66(5):891-895.

412. Berga SL, Mortola JF, Yen SS. Amplification of nocturnal melatonin secretion in women with functional hypothalamic amenorrhea. J Clin Endocrinol Metab 1988;66(1):242-244.

413. Fiorina P, Lattuada G, Ponari O, et al. Impaired nocturnal melatonin excretion and changes of immunological status in ischaemic stroke patients. Lancet 1996;347(9002):692-693.

414. Kondoh T, Uneyama H, Nishino H, et al. Melatonin reduces cerebral edema formation caused by transient forebrain ischemia in rats. Life Sci 2002;72(4-5):583-590.

415. McIntyre IM, Norman TR, Burrows GD, et al. Melatonin supersensitivity to dim light in seasonal affective disorder. Lancet 1990;335(8687):488.

416. Danilenko KV, Putilov AA, Russkikh GS, et al. Diurnal and seasonal variations of melatonin and serotonin in women with seasonal affective disorder. Arctic Med Res 1994;53(3):137-145.

417. Childs PA, Rodin I, Martin NJ, et al. Effect of fluoxetine on melatonin in patients with seasonal affective disorder and matched controls. Br J Psychiatry 1995;166(2):196-198.

418. Attenburrow ME, Cowen PJ, Sharpley AL. Low dose melatonin improves sleep in healthy middle-aged subjects. Psychopharmacology (Berl) 1996;126(2):179-181.

419. Rosenthal NE, Sack DA, Jacobsen FM, et al. Melatonin in seasonal affective disorder and phototherapy. J Neural Transm Suppl 1986;21:257-267.

420. Winton F, Corn T, Huson LW, et al. Effects of light treatment upon mood and melatonin in patients with seasonal affective disorder. Psychol Med 1989;19(3):585-590.

421. Claustrat B, Chazot G, Brun J, et al. A chronobiological study of melatonin and cortisol secretion in depressed subjects: plasma melatonin, a biochemical marker in major depression. Biol Psychiatry 1984;19(8):1215-1228.

422. Beck-Friis J, Kjellman BF, Aperia B, et al. Serum melatonin in relation to clinical variables in patients with major depressive disorder and a hypothesis of a low melatonin syndrome. Acta Psychiatr Scand 1985;71(4):319-330.

423. Brown R, Kocsis JH, Caroff S, et al. Differences in nocturnal melatonin secretion between melancholic depressed patients and control subjects. Am J Psychiatry 1985;142(7):811-816.

424. Parry BL, Berga SL, Kripke DF, et al. Altered waveform of plasma nocturnal melatonin secretion in premenstrual depression. Arch Gen Psychiatry 1990;47(12):1139-1146.

425. Papezova H, Yamamotova A, Nedvidkova J. Pain modulation role of melatonin in eating disorders. Eur Psychiatry 2001;16(1):68-70.

426. Tortosa F, Puig-Domingo M, Peinado MA, et al. Enhanced circadian rhythm of melatonin in anorexia nervosa. Acta Endocrinol (Copenh) 1989;120(5):574-578.

427. Wu W, Zhang G, Wang Y, et al. [The change of serum melatonin and diagnosis value in hepatic encephalopathy]. Zhonghua Gan Zang Bing Za Zhi 2000;8(5):272-273.

428. Claustrat B, Brun J, Geoffriau M, et al. Nocturnal plasma melatonin profile and melatonin kinetics during infusion in status migrainosus. Cephalalgia 1997;17(4):511-517.

429. Murialdo G, Fonzi S, Costelli P, et al. Urinary melatonin excretion throughout the ovarian cycle in menstrually related migraine. Cephalalgia 1994;14(3):205-209.

430. Salvesen R, Bekkelund SI. Migraine, as compared to other headaches, is worse during midnight-sun summer than during polar night. A questionnaire study in an Arctic population. Headache 2000;40(10):824-829.

431. Murch SJ, Simmons CB, Saxena PK. Melatonin in feverfew and other medicinal plants. Lancet 1997;350(9091):1598-1599.

432. Leardi S, Tavone E, Cianca G, et al. [The role of melatonin in the immediate postoperative period in elderly patients]. Minerva Chir 2000;55(11):745-750.

433. Sparks DL, Hunsaker JC, III. The pineal gland in sudden infant death syndrome: preliminary observations. J Pineal Res 1988;5(1):111-118.

434. Sturner WQ, Lynch HJ, Deng MH, et al. Melatonin concentrations in the sudden infant death syndrome. Forensic Sci Int 1990;45(1-2):171-180.

435. Maurizi CP. Could exogenous melatonin prevent sudden infant death syndrome? Med Hypotheses 1997;49(5):425-427.

436. Head K. Natural therapies for ocular disorders, part two: cataracts and glaucoma. Altern Med Rev 2001;6(2):141-166.

437. Maurizi CP. A preliminary understanding of mania: roles for melatonin, vasotocin and rapid-eye-movement sleep. Med Hypotheses 2000;54(1):26-29.

438. Nagtegaal E, Smits M, Swart W, et al. Melatonin secretion and coronary heart disease. Lancet 1995;346(8985):1299.

439. Baydas G, Canatan H, Turkoglu A. Comparative analysis of the protective effects of melatonin and vitamin E on streptozocin-induced diabetes mellitus. J Pineal Res 2002;32(4):225-230.

440. Baydas G, Nedzvetsky VS, Nerush PA, et al. A novel role for melatonin: regulation of the expression of cell adhesion molecules in the rat hippocampus and cortex. Neurosci Lett 2002;326(2):109-112.

441. Baydas G, Yilmaz O, Celik S, et al. Effects of certain micronutrients and melatonin on plasma lipid, lipid peroxidation, and homocysteine levels in rats. Arch Med Res 2002;33(6):515-519.

442. Baydas G, Gursu MF, Cikim G, et al. Homocysteine levels are increased due to lack of melatonin in pinealectomized rats: is there a link between melatonin and homocysteine? J Pineal Res 2002;32(1):63-64.

443. Sandyk R, Awerbuch GI. Relationship of nocturnal melatonin levels to duration and course of multiple sclerosis. Int J Neurosci 1994;75(3-4):229-237.

444. Sandyk R. Diurnal variations in vision and relations to circadian melatonin secretion in multiple sclerosis. Int J Neurosci 1995;83(1-2):1-6.

445. Haimov I, Lavie P, Laudon M, et al. Melatonin replacement therapy of elderly insomniacs. Sleep 1995;18(7):598-603.

446. Haimov I, Laudon M, Zisapel N, et al. Sleep disorders and melatonin rhythms in elderly people. BMJ 1994;309(6948):167.

447. Zisapel N. The use of melatonin for the treatment of insomnia. Biol Signals Recept 1999;8(1-2):84-89.

448. Baskett JJ, Cockrem JF, Todd MA. Melatonin levels in hospitalized elderly patients: a comparison with community based volunteers. Age Ageing 1991;20(6):430-434.

449. Nagtegaal E, Peeters T, Swart W, et al. Correlation between concentrations of melatonin in saliva and serum in patients with delayed sleep phase syndrome. Ther Drug Monit 1998;20(2):181-183.

450. Tzischinsky O, Skene D, Epstein R, et al. Circadian rhythms in 6-sulphatoxymelatonin and nocturnal sleep in blind children. Chronobiol Int 1991;8(3):168-175.

451. Hahm H, Kujawa J, Augsburger L. Comparison of melatonin products against USP's nutritional supplements standards and other criteria. J Am Pharm Assoc (Wash) 1999;39(1):27-31.

452. Shah J, Langmuir V, Gupta SK. Feasibility and functionality of OROS melatonin in healthy subjects. J Clin Pharmacol 1999;39(6):606-612.

453. Waldhauser F, Weiszenbacher G, Frisch H, et al. Fall in nocturnal serum melatonin during prepuberty and pubescence. Lancet 1984;1(8373):362-365.

454. Waldhauser F, Waldhauser M, Lieberman HR, et al. Bioavailability of oral melatonin in humans. Neuroendocrinology 1984;39(4):307-313.

455. Lane EA, Moss HB. Pharmacokinetics of melatonin in man: first pass hepatic metabolism. J Clin Endocrinol Metab 1985;61(6):1214-1216.

456. Di WL, Kadva A, Johnston A, et al. Variable bioavailability of oral melatonin. N Engl J Med 1997;336(14):1028-1029.

457. Lee BJ, Parrott KA, Ayres JW, et al. Preliminary evaluation of transdermal delivery of melatonin in human subjects. Res Commun Mol Pathol Pharmacol 1994;85(3):337-346.

458. Benes L, Claustrat B, Horriere F, et al. Transmucosal, oral controlled-release, and transdermal drug administration in human subjects: a crossover study with melatonin. J Pharm Sci 1997;86(10):1115-1119.

459. Bojkowski CJ, Arendt J, Shih MC, et al. Melatonin secretion in humans assessed by measuring its metabolite, 6- sulfatoxymelatonin. Clin Chem 1987;33(8):1343-1348.

460. Laakso ML, Porkka-Heiskanen T, Alila A, et al. Correlation between salivary and serum melatonin: dependence on serum melatonin levels. J Pineal Res 1990;9(1):39-50.

461. Nowak R, McMillen IC, Redman J, et al. The correlation between serum and salivary melatonin concentrations and urinary 6-hydroxymelatonin sulphate excretion rates: two non-invasive techniques for monitoring human circadian rhythmicity. Clin Endocrinol (Oxf) 1987;27(4):445-452.

462. Shida CS, Castrucci AM, Lamy-Freund MT. High melatonin solubility in aqueous medium. J Pineal Res 1994;16(4):198-201.

463. Antolin I, Mayo JC, Sainz RM, et al. Protective effect of melatonin in a chronic experimental model of Parkinson's disease. Brain Res 2002;943(2):163-173.

464. Steindl PE, Ferenci P, Marktl W. Impaired hepatic catabolism of melatonin in cirrhosis. Ann Intern Med 1997;127(6):494.

465. Iguchi H, Kato K, Ibayashi H. Age-dependent reduction in serum melatonin concentrations in healthy human subjects. J Clin Endocrinol Metab 1982;55(1):27-29.

466. Aldhous M, Franey C, Wright J, et al. Plasma concentrations of melatonin in man following oral absorption of different preparations. Br J Clin Pharmacol 1985;19(4):517-521.

467. Cavallo A, Ritschel WA. Pharmacokinetics of melatonin in human sexual maturation. J Clin Endocrinol Metab 1996;81(5):1882-1886.

468. Nickelsen T, Lang A, Bergau L. The effect of 6-, 9- and 11-hour time shifts on circadian rhythms: adaptation of sleep parameters and hormonal patterns following the intake of melatonin or placebo. In Arendt J, Pevet P (eds): Advances in Pineal Research. London, John Libbey, 1991, pp 303-306.

469. Spitzer RL, Terman M, Williams JB, et al. Jet lag: clinical features, validation of a new syndrome-specific scale, and lack of response to melatonin in a randomized, double-blind trial. Am J Psychiatry 1999;156(9):1392-1396.

470. Dagan Y, Yovel I, Hallis D, et al. Evaluating the role of melatonin in the long-term treatment of delayed sleep phase syndrome (DSPS). Chronobiol Int 1998;15(2):181-190.

471. Dahlitz M, Alvarez B, Vignau J, et al. Delayed sleep phase syndrome response to melatonin. Lancet 1991;337(8750):1121-1124.

472. Nagtegaal JE, Kerkhof GA, Smits MG, et al. Delayed sleep phase syndrome: A placebo-controlled cross-over study on the effects of melatonin administered five hours before the individual dim light melatonin onset. J Sleep Res 1998;7(2):135-143.

473. Yang CM, Spielman AJ, D'Ambrosio P, et al. A single dose of melatonin prevents the phase delay associated with a delayed weekend sleep pattern. Sleep 2001;24(3):272-281.

474. Kayumov L, Brown G, Jindal R, et al. A randomized, double-blind, placebo-controlled crossover study of the effect of exogenous melatonin on delayed sleep phase syndrome. Psychosom Med 2001;63(1):40-48.

475. Jan JE, Freeman RD, Fast DK. Melatonin treatment of sleep-wake cycle disorders in children and adolescents. Dev Med Child Neurol 1999;41(7):491-500.

476. Camfield P, Gordon K, Dooley J, et al. Melatonin appears ineffective in children with intellectual deficits and fragmented sleep: six "N of 1" trials. J Child Neurol 1996;11(4):341-343.

477. Dodge NN, Wilson GA. Melatonin for treatment of sleep disorders in children with developmental disabilities. J Child Neurol 2001;16(8):581-584.

478. Smits MG, Nagtegaal EE, van der HJ, et al. Melatonin for chronic sleep onset insomnia in children: a randomized placebo-controlled trial. J Child Neurol 2001;16(2):86-92.

479. Jan JE, Hamilton D, Seward N, et al. Clinical trials of controlled-release melatonin in children with sleep- wake cycle disorders. J Pineal Res 2000;29(1):34-39.

480. Gordon K, Camfield P, Dooley J, et al. Dramatically successful treatment of severe sleep disturbance in developmentally handicapped children with melatonin [abstract]. Ann Neurol 1993;34:504.

481. O'Callaghan FJ, Clarke AA, Hancock E, et al. Use of melatonin to treat sleep disorders in tuberous sclerosis. Dev Med Child Neurol 1999;41(2):123-126.

482. Hung JC, Appleton RE, Nunn AJ, et al. The use of melatonin in the treatment of sleep disturbances in children with neurological or behavioural disorders. J Ped Pharm Practice 1998;3(5):250-256.

483. Jan JE, Espezel H, Appleton RE. The treatment of sleep disorders with melatonin. Dev Med Child Neurol 1994;36(2):97-107.

484. Jan JE, O'Donnell ME. Use of melatonin in the treatment of paediatric sleep disorders. J Pineal Res 1996;21(4):193-199.

485. Jan MM. Melatonin for the treatment of handicapped children with severe sleep disorders. Pediatr Neurol 2000;23(3):229-232.

486. Masters KJ. Melatonin for sleep problems. J Am Acad Child Adolesc Psychiatry 1996;35(6):704.

487. Pillar G, Shahar E, Peled N, et al. Melatonin improves sleep-wake patterns in psychomotor retarded children. Pediatr Neurol 2000;23(3):225-228.

488. Ross C, Morris B, Whitehouse W. Melatonin treatment of sleep-wake cycle disorders in children and adolescents. Dev Med Child Neurol 1999;41(12):850.

489. Schmitt-Mechelke TH, Steinlin M, Bolthauser E. [Melatonin for the treatment of insomnia in neuropediatric patients] (abstract). Schweiz Med Wochenschr 1997;127(Suppl 87):9.

490. Tanaka H, Araki A, Ito J, et al. Improvement of hypertonus after treatment for sleep disturbances in three patients with severe brain damage. Brain Dev 1997;19(4):240-244.

491. Zhdanova IV, Wurtman RJ, Wagstaff J. Effects of a low dose of melatonin on sleep in children with Angelman syndrome. J Pediatr Endocrinol Metab 1999;12(1):57-67.

492. Hayashi E. Effect of melatonin on sleep-wake rhythm: the sleep diary of an autistic male. Psychiatry Clin Neurosci 2000;54(3):383-384.

493. Paavonen EJ, Nieminen-Von Wendt T, Vanhala R, et al. Effectiveness of melatonin in the treatment of sleep disturbances in children with Asperger disorder. J Child Adolesc Psychopharmacol 2003;13(1):83-95.

494. Haimov I, Lavie P. Potential of melatonin replacement therapy in older patients with sleep disorders. Drugs Aging 1995;7(2):75-78.

495. Garfinkel D, Laudon M, Nof D, et al. Improvement of sleep quality in elderly people by controlled-release melatonin. Lancet 1995;346(8974):541-544.

496. Garfinkel D, Laudon M, Zisapel N. Improvement of sleep quality by controlled-release melatonin in benzodiazepine-treated elderly insomniacs. Arch Gerontol Geriat 1997;24:223-231.

497. Hughes RJ, Sack RL, Lewy AJ. The role of melatonin and circadian phase in age-related sleep- maintenance insomnia: assessment in a clinical trial of melatonin replacement. Sleep 1998;21(1):52-68.

495. Jean-Louis G, von Gizycki H, Zizi F. Melatonin effects on sleep, mood, and cognition in elderly with mild cognitive impairment. J Pineal Res 1998;25(3):177-183.

M

499. Zhdanova IV, Wurtman RJ, Regan MM, et al. Melatonin treatment for age-related insomnia. J Clin Endocrinol Metab 2001;86(10):4727-4730.

500. Wurtman RJ, Zhdanova I. Improvement of sleep quality by melatonin. Lancet 1995;346(8988):1491.

501. Baskett JJ, Broad JB, Wood PC, et al. Does melatonin improve sleep in older people? A randomised crossover trial. Age Ageing 2003;32(2):164-170.

502. Dawson D, Rogers NL, van den Heuvel CJ, et al. Effect of sustained nocturnal transbuccal melatonin administration on sleep and temperature in elderly insomniacs. J Biol Rhythms 1998;13(6):532-538.

503. Avery D, Lenz M, Landis C. Guidelines for prescribing melatonin. Ann Med 1998;30(1):122-130.

504. Zhdanova IV, Wurtman RJ, Lynch HJ, et al. Sleep-inducing effects of low doses of melatonin ingested in the evening. Clin Pharmacol Ther 1995;57(5):552-558.

505. Zhdanova IV, Wurtman RJ, Morabito C, et al. Effects of low oral doses of melatonin, given 2-4 hours before habitual bedtime, on sleep in normal young humans. Sleep 1996;19(5):423-431.

506. Dollins AB, Zhdanova IV, Wurtman RJ, et al. Effect of inducing nocturnal serum melatonin concentrations in daytime on sleep, mood, body temperature, and performance. Proc Natl Acad Sci U S A 1994;91(5):1824-1828.

507. Attenburrow ME, Dowling BA, Sharpley AL, et al. Case-control study of evening melatonin concentration in primary insomnia. BMJ 1996;312(7041):1263-1264.

508. Atkinson G, Buckley P, Edwards B, et al. Are there hangover-effects on physical performance when melatonin is ingested by athletes before nocturnal sleep? Int J Sports Med 2001;22(3):232-234.

509. Gilbert SS, van den Heuvel CJ, Dawson D. Daytime melatonin and temazepam in young adult humans: equivalent effects on sleep latency and body temperatures. J Physiol 1999;514 (Pt 3):905-914.

510. Nave R, Peled R, Lavie P. Melatonin improves evening napping. Eur J Pharmacol 1995;275(2):213-216.

511. Satomura T, Sakamoto T, Shirakawa S, et al. Hypnotic action of melatonin during daytime administration and its comparison with triazolam. Psychiatry Clin Neurosci 2001;55(3):303-304.

521. Wyatt JK, Dijk D, Ritz-De Cecco A, et al. Circadian phase-dependent hypnotic effect of exogenous melatonin [abstract]. Sleep 1999;22(Suppl):S4-S5.

513. Hughes RJ, Badia P. Sleep-promoting and hypothermic effects of daytime melatonin administration in humans. Sleep 1997;20(2):124-131.

514. Vollrath L, Semm P, Gammel G. Sleep induction by intranasal application of melatonin. Adv Biosci 1981;29:327-329.

515. Singer CM, Moffit MT, Colling ED, et al. Low dose melatonin administration and nocturnal activity levels in patients with Alzheimer's disease [abstract]. Sleep Res 1997;26:752.

516. Cardinali DP, Brusco LI, Liberczuk C. The use of melatonin in Alzheimer's disease. Neuroendocrinol Lett 2002;23(Suppl 1):20-23.

517. Brusco LI, Marquez M, Cardinali DP. Monozygotic twins with Alzheimer's disease treated with melatonin: Case report. J Pineal Res 1998;25(4):260-263.

518. Skene DJ, Swaab DF. Melatonin rhythmicity: effect of age and Alzheimer's disease. Exp Gerontol 2003;38(1-2):199-206.

519. Zhou JN, Liu RY, Kamphorst W, et al. Early neuropathological Alzheimer's changes in aged individuals are accompanied by decreased cerebrospinal fluid melatonin levels. J Pineal Res 2003;35(2):125-130.

520. Savaskan E, Olivieri G, Meier F, et al. Increased melatonin 1a-receptor immunoreactivity in the hippocampus of Alzheimer's disease patients. J Pineal Res 2002;32(1):59-62.

521. Savaskan E, Olivieri G, Brydon L, et al. Cerebrovascular melatonin MT1-receptor alterations in patients with Alzheimer's disease. Neurosci Lett 2001;308(1):9-12.

522. Tjon Pian Gi CV, Broeren JP, Starreveld JS, et al. Melatonin for treatment of sleeping disorders in children with attention deficit/hyperactivity disorder: a preliminary open label study. Eur J Pediatr 2003;162(7-8):554-555.

523. Garfinkel D, Zisapel N, Wainstein J, et al. Facilitation of benzodiazepine discontinuation by melatonin: a new clinical approach. Arch Intern Med 1999;159(20):2456-2460.

524. Cardinali DP, Gvozdenovich E, Kaplan MR. A double blind-placebo controlled study on melatonin efficacy to reduce anxiolytic benzodiazepine use in the elderly. Neuroendocrinol Lett 2002;23(1):55-60.

525. Rasmussen P. A role of phytotherapy treatment of benzodiazepine and opiate drug withdrawal. Eur J Herbal Med 1997;3(1):11-21.

526. Dagan Y, Zisapel N, Nof D, et al. Rapid reversal of tolerance to benzodiazepine hypnotics by treatment with oral melatonin: a case report. Eur Neuropsychopharmacol 1997;7(2):157-160.

527. Leibenluft E, Feldman-Naim S, Turner EH, et al. Effects of exogenous melatonin administration and withdrawal in five patients with rapid-cycling bipolar disorder. J Clin Psychiatry 1997;58(9):383-388.

528. Robertson JM, Tanguay PE. Case study: the use of melatonin in a boy with refractory bipolar disorder. J Am Acad Child Adolesc Psychiatry 1997;36(6):822-825.

529. Cerea G, Vaghi M, Ardizzoia A, et al. Biomodulation of cancer chemo-

therapy for metastatic colorectal cancer: a randomized study of weekly low-dose irinotecan alone versus irinotecan plus the oncostatic pineal hormone melatonin in metastatic colorectal cancer patients progressing on 5-fluorouracil-containing combinations. Anticancer Res 2003;23(2C):1951-1954.

530. Lissoni P, Chilelli M, Villa S, et al. Five years survival in metastatic non-small cell lung cancer patients treated with chemotherapy alone or chemotherapy and melatonin: a randomized trial. J Pineal Res 2003;35(1):12-15.

531. Lissoni P, Vaghi M, Ardizzoia A, et al. A phase II study of chemo-neuroimmunotherapy with platinum, subcutaneous low-dose interleukin-2 and the pineal neurohormone melatonin (P.I.M.) as a second-line therapy in metastatic melanoma patients progressing on dacarbazine plus interferon-alpha. In Vivo 2002;16(2):93-96.

532. Ghielmini M, Pagani O, de Jong J, et al. Double-blind randomized study on the myeloprotective effect of melatonin in combination with carboplatin and etoposide in advanced lung cancer. Br J Cancer 1999;80(7):1058-1061.

533. Gonzalez R, Sanchez A, Ferguson JA, et al. Melatonin therapy of advanced human malignant melanoma. Melanoma Res 1991;1(4):237-243.

534. Italian Study Group for the Di Bella Multitherapy Trials. Evaluation of an unconventional cancer treatment (the Di Bella multitherapy): results of phase II trials in Italy. Italian Study Group for the Di Bella Multitherapy Trials. BMJ 1999;318(7178):224-228.

535. Barni S, Lissoni P, Paolorossi F, et al. A study of the pineal hormone melatonin as a second line therapy in metastatic colorectal cancer resistant to fluorouracil plus folates. Tumori 1990;76(1):58-60.

536. Lamson DW, Brignall MS. Antioxidants in cancer therapy; their actions and interactions with oncologic therapies. Altern Med Rev 1999;4(5):304-329.

537. Lissoni P, Barni S, Tancini G, et al. Clinical study of melatonin in untreatable advanced cancer patients. Tumori 1987;73(5):475-480.

538. Lissoni P, Barni S, Crispino S, et al. Endocrine and immune effects of melatonin therapy in metastatic cancer patients. Eur J Cancer Clin Oncol 1989;25(5):789-795.

539. Lissoni P, Barni S, Cattaneo G, et al. Clinical results with the pineal hormone melatonin in advanced cancer resistant to standard antitumor therapies. Oncology 1991;48(6):448-450.

540. Lissoni P, Barni S, Ardizzoia A, et al. Randomized study with the pineal hormone melatonin versus supportive care alone in advanced nonsmall cell lung cancer resistant to a first- line chemotherapy containing cisplatin. Oncology 1992;49(5):336-339.

541. Lissoni P, Tisi E, Barni S, et al. Biological and clinical results of a neuroimmunotherapy with interleukin-2 and the pineal hormone melatonin as a first line treatment in advanced non-small cell lung cancer. Br J Cancer 1992;66(1):155-158.

542. Lissoni P, Barni S, Tancini G, et al. A randomised study with subcutaneous low-dose interleukin 2 alone vs interleukin 2 plus the pineal neurohormone melatonin in advanced solid neoplasms other than renal cancer and melanoma. Br J Cancer 1994;69(1):196-199.

543. Lissoni P, Meregalli S, Fossati V, et al. A randomized study of immunotherapy with low-dose subcutaneous interleukin-2 plus melatonin vs chemotherapy with cisplatin and etoposide as first-line therapy for advanced non-small cell lung cancer. Tumori 1994;80(6):464-467.

544. Lissoni P, Barni S, Ardizzoia A, et al. A randomized study with the pineal hormone melatonin versus supportive care alone in patients with brain metastases due to solid neoplasms. Cancer 1994;73(3):699-701.

545. Lissoni P, Barni S, Tancini G, et al. Pineal-opioid system interactions in the control of immunoinflammatory responses. Ann N Y Acad Sci 1994;741:191-196.

546. Lissoni P, Paolorossi F, Tancini G, et al. A phase II study of tamoxifen plus melatonin in metastatic solid tumour patients. Br J Cancer 1996;74(9):1466-1468.

547. Lissoni P, Meregalli S, Nosetto L, et al. Increased survival time in brain glioblastomas by a radioneuroendocrine strategy with radiotherapy plus melatonin compared to radiotherapy alone. Oncology 1996;53(1):43-46.

548. Lissoni P, Paolorossi F, Tancini G, et al. Is there a role for melatonin in the treatment of neoplastic cachexia? Eur J Cancer 1996;32A(8):1340-1343.

549. Lissoni P, Brivio O, Brivio F, et al. Adjuvant therapy with the pineal hormone melatonin in patients with lymph node relapse due to malignant melanoma. J Pineal Res 1996;21(4):239-242.

550. Lissoni P, Paolorossi F, Ardizzoia A, et al. A randomized study of chemotherapy with cisplatin plus etoposide versus chemoendocrine therapy with cisplatin, etoposide and the pineal hormone melatonin as a first-line treatment of advanced non-small cell lung cancer patients in a poor clinical state. J Pineal Res 1997;23(1):15-19.

551. Lissoni P, Rovelli F, Meregalli S, et al. Melatonin as a new possible anti-inflammatory agent. J Biol Regul Homeost Agents 1997;11(4):157-159.

552. Lissoni P, Giani L, Zerbini S, et al. Biotherapy with the pineal immunomodulating hormone melatonin versus melatonin plus aloe vera in untreatable advanced solid neoplasms. Nat Immun 1998;16(1):27-33.

553. Lissoni P, Tancini G, Paolorossi F, et al. Chemoneuroendocrine therapy of metastatic breast cancer with persistent thrombocytopenia with weekly low-dose epirubicin plus melatonin: a phase II study. J Pineal Res 1999;26(3):169-173.

554. Lissoni P, Rovelli F, Malugani F, et al. Anti-angiogenic activity of melatonin in advanced cancer patients. Neuroendocrinol Lett 2001;22(1): 45-47.

555. Lissoni P, Bucovec R, Bonfanti A, et al. Thrombopoietic properties of 5-methoxytryptamine plus melatonin versus melatonin alone in the treatment of cancer-related thrombocytopenia. J Pineal Res 2001;30(2): 123-126.

556. Neri B, de L, V, Gemelli MT, et al. Melatonin as biological response modifier in cancer patients. Anticancer Res 1998;18(2B):1329-1332.

557. Todisco M, Casaccia P, Rossi N. Cyclophosphamide plus somatostatin, bromocriptin, retinoids, melatonin and ACTH in the treatment of low-grade non-Hodgkin's lymphomas at advanced stage: results of a phase II trial. Cancer Biother Radiopharm 2001;16(2):171-177.

558. Lissoni P, Barni S, Mandala M, et al. Decreased toxicity and increased efficacy of cancer chemotherapy using the pineal hormone melatonin in metastatic solid tumour patients with poor clinical status. Eur J Cancer 1999;35(12):1688-1692.

559. Lissoni P, Tancini G, Barni S, et al. Treatment of cancer chemotherapy-induced toxicity with the pineal hormone melatonin. Support Care Cancer 1997;5(2):126-129.

560. Lissoni P, Cazzaniga M, Tancini G, et al. Reversal of clinical resistance to LHRH analogue in metastatic prostate cancer by the pineal hormone melatonin: efficacy of LHRH analogue plus melatonin in patients progressing on LHRH analogue alone. Eur Urol 1997;31(2):178-181.

561. Barni S, Lissoni P, Paolorossi F, et al. Prevention of chemotherapy-induced thrombocytopenia by the pineal hormone melatonin (MLT) [abstract]. Proc Annu Meet Am Soc Clin Oncol 1996;15:528.

562. Viviani S, Negretti E, Orazi A, et al. Preliminary studies on melatonin in the treatment of myelodysplastic syndromes following cancer chemotherapy. J Pineal Res 1990;8(4):347-354.

563. Lissoni P, Ardizzoia A, Barni S, et al. A randomized study of tamoxifen alone versus tamoxifen plus melatonin in estrogen receptor-negative heavily pretreated metastatic breast cancer patients. Oncology Reports 1995;2:871-873.

564. Neri B, Fiorelli C, Moroni F, et al. Modulation of human lymphoblastoid interferon activity by melatonin in metastatic renal cell carcinoma. A phase II study. Cancer 1994;73(12):3015-3019.

565. Lissoni P, Barni S, Ardizzoia A, et al. Immunotherapy with low-dose interleukin-2 in association with melatonin as salvage therapy for metastatic soft tissue sarcomas. Oncology Reports 1997;4:157-159.

566. Barni S, Lissoni P, Cazzaniga M, et al. A randomized study of low-dose subcutaneous interleukin-2 plus melatonin versus supportive care alone in metastatic colorectal cancer patients progressing under 5-fluorouracil and folates. Oncology 1995;52(3):243-245.

567. Brivio F, Lissoni P, Fumagalli L, et al. Preoperative neuroimmunotherapy with subcutaneous low-dose interleukin-2 and melatonin in patients with gastrointestinal tumors: its efficacy in preventing surgery-induced lymphocytopenia. Oncology Reports 1995;2:597-599.

568. Bregani ER, Lissoni P, Rossini F, et al. Prevention of interleukin-2-induced thrombocytopenia during the immunotherapy of cancer by a concomitant administration of the pineal hormone melatonin. Recenti Prog Med 1995;86(6):231-233.

569. Lissoni P, Barni S, Brivio F, et al. A biological study on the efficacy of low-dose subcutaneous interleukin- 2 plus melatonin in the treatment of cancer-related thrombocytopenia. Oncology 1995;52(5):360-362.

570. Lissoni P, Barni S, Brivio F, et al. Treatment of cancer-related thrombocytopenia by low-dose subcutaneous interleukin-2 plus the pineal hormone melatonin: a biological phase II study. J Biol Regul Homeost Agents 1995;9(2):52-54.

571. Lissoni P, Brivio F, Barni S, et al. Neuroimmunotherapy of human cancer with interleukin-2 and the neurohormone melatonin: its efficacy in preventing hypotension. Anticancer Res 1990;10(6):1759-1761.

572. Lissoni P, Barni S, Fossati V, et al. A randomized study of neuro-immunotherapy with low-dose subcutaneous interleukin-2 plus melatonin compared to supportive care alone in patients with untreatable metastatic solid tumour. Support Care Cancer 1995;3(3):194-197.

573. Lissoni P, Brivio F, Brivio O, et al. Immune effects of preoperative immunotherapy with high-dose subcutaneous interleukin-2 versus neuroimmunotherapy with low-dose interleukin-2 plus the neurohormone melatonin in gastrointestinal tract tumor patients. J Biol Regul Homeost Agents 1995;9(1):31-33.

574. Lissoni P, Pittalis S, Ardizzoia A, et al. Prevention of cytokine-induced hypotension in cancer patients by the pineal hormone melatonin. Support Care Cancer 1996;4(4):313-316.

575. Aldeghi R, Lissoni P, Barni S, et al. Low-dose interleukin-2 subcutaneous immunotherapy in association with the pineal hormone melatonin as a first-line therapy in locally advanced or metastatic hepatocellular carcinoma. Eur J Cancer 1994;30A(2):167-170.

576. Barni S, Lissoni P, Cazzaniga M, et al. Neuroimmunotherapy with subcutaneous low-dose interleukin-2 and the pineal hormone melatonin as a second-line treatment in metastatic colorectal carcinoma. Tumori 1992; 78(6):383-387.

577. Lissoni P, Barni S, Ardizzoia A, et al. Cancer immunotherapy with low-dose interleukin-2 subcutaneous administration: potential efficacy in most solid tumor histotypes by a concomitant treatment with the pineal hormone melatonin. J Biol Regul Homeost Agents 1993;7(4):121-125.

578. Lissoni P, Barni S, Rovelli F, et al. Neuroimmunotherapy of advanced solid neoplasms with single evening subcutaneous injection of low-dose interleukin-2 and melatonin: preliminary results. Eur J Cancer 1993; 29A(2):185-189.

579. Lissoni P, Brivio F, Ardizzoia A, et al. Subcutaneous therapy with low-dose interleukin-2 plus the neurohormone melatonin in metastatic gastric cancer patients with low performance status. Tumori 1993;79(6):401-404.

580. Lissoni P, Barni S, Tancini G, et al. Immunotherapy with subcutaneous low-dose interleukin-2 and the pineal indole melatonin as a new effective therapy in advanced cancers of the digestive tract. Br J Cancer 1993; 67(6):1404-1407.

581. Lissoni P, Barni S, Cazzaniga M, et al. Efficacy of the concomitant administration of the pineal hormone melatonin in cancer immunotherapy with low-dose IL-2 in patients with advanced solid tumors who had progressed on IL-2 alone. Oncology 1994;51(4):344-347.

582. Lissoni P, Barni S, Tancini G, et al. Immunoendocrine therapy with low-dose subcutaneous interleukin-2 plus melatonin of locally advanced or metastatic endocrine tumors. Oncology 1995;52(2):163-166.

583. Lissoni P, Fumagalli L, Paolorossi F, et al. Anticancer neuroimmuno-modulation by pineal hormones other than melatonin: preliminary phase II study of the pineal indole 5-methoxytryptophol in association with low-dose IL-2 and melatonin. J Biol Regul Homeost Agents 1997;11(3): 119-122.

584. Brackowski R, Zubelewicz B, Romanowski W, et al. Preliminary study on modulation of the biological effects of tumor necrosis factor-alpha in advanced cancer patients by the pineal hormone melatonin. J Biol Regul Homeost Agents 1994;8(3):77-80.

585. Braczkowski R, Zubelewicz B, Romanowski W, et al. Modulation of tumor necrosis factor-alpha (TNF-alpha) toxicity by the pineal hormone melatonin (MLT) in metastatic solid tumor patients. Ann N Y Acad Sci 1995;768:334-336.

586. Kocak G, Erbil KM, Ozdemir I, et al. The protective effect of melatonin on adriamycin-induced acute cardiac injury. Can J Cardiol 2003;19(5): 535-541.

587. Morishima I, Matsui H, Mukawa H, et al. Melatonin, a pineal hormone with antioxidant property, protects against adriamycin cardiomyopathy in rats. Life Sci 1998;63(7):511-521.

588. Reiter RJ, Tan DX, Sainz RM, et al. Melatonin: reducing the toxicity and increasing the efficacy of drugs. J Pharm Pharmacol 2002;54(10): 1299-1321.

589. Sack RL, Lewy AJ, Blood ML, et al. Melatonin administration to blind people: phase advances and entrainment. J Biol Rhythms 1991;6(3):249-261.

590. Sack RL, Brandes RW, Kendall AR, et al. Entrainment of free-running circadian rhythms by melatonin in blind people. N Engl J Med 2000; 343(15):1070-1077.

591. Lockley SW, Skene DJ, James K, et al. Melatonin administration can entrain the free-running circadian system of blind subjects. J Endocrinol 2000;164(1):R1-R6.

592. Palm L, Blennow G, Wetterberg L. Long-term melatonin treatment in blind children and young adults with circadian sleep-wake disturbances. Dev Med Child Neurol 1997;39(5):319-325.

593. Sack RL, Lewy AJ. Melatonin as a chronobiotic: treatment of circadian desynchrony in night workers and the blind. J Biol Rhythms 1997;12(6): 595-603.

594. Espezel H, Jan JE, O'Donnell ME, et al. The use of melatonin to treat sleep-wake-rhythm disorders in children who are visually impaired. J V is Impair Blind 1996;90:34-50.

595. Rivkees SA. Arrhythmicity in a child with septo-optic dysplasia and establishment of sleep-wake cyclicity with melatonin. J Pediatr 2001; 139(3):463-465.

596. Pillar G, Etzioni A, Shahar E, et al. Melatonin treatment in an institutionalised child with psychomotor retardation and an irregular sleep-wake pattern. Arch Dis Child 1998;79(1):63-64.

597. McArthur AJ, Lewy AJ, Sack RL. Non-24-hour sleep-wake syndrome in a sighted man: circadian rhythm studies and efficacy of melatonin treatment. Sleep 1996;19(7):544-553.

598. Lapierre O, Dumont M. Melatonin treatment of a non-24-hour sleep-wake cycle in a blind retarded child. Biol Psychiatry 1995;38(2):119-122.

599. Tzischinsky O, Pal I, Epstein R, et al. The importance of timing in melatonin administration in a blind man. J Pineal Res 1992;12(3): 105-108.

600. Palm L, Blennow G, Wetterberg L. Correction of non-24-hour sleep/wake cycle by melatonin in a blind retarded boy. Ann Neurol 1991;29(3): 336-339.

601. Folkard S, Arendt J, Aldhous M, et al. Melatonin stabilises sleep onset time in a blind man without entrainment of cortisol or temperature rhythms. Neurosci Lett 1990;113(2):193-198.

602. Dolberg OT, Hirschmann S, Grunhaus L. Melatonin for the treatment of sleep disturbances in major depressive disorder. Am J Psychiatry 1998;155(8):1119-1121.

603. Dalton EJ, Rotondi D, Levitan RD, et al. Use of slow-release melatonin in treatment-resistant depression. J Psychiatry Neurosci 2000;25(1):48-52.

M

604. deVries MW, Peeters FP. Melatonin as a therapeutic agent in the treatment of sleep disturbance in depression. J Nerv Ment Dis 1997;185(3):201-202.

605. Kripke DF, Youngstedt SD, Rex KM, et al. Melatonin excretion with affect disorders over age 60. Psychiatry Res 2003;118(1):47-54.

606. Gagnier JJ. The therapeutic potential of melatonin in migraines and other headache types. Altern Med Rev 2001;6(4):383-389.

607. Nagtegaal JE, Smits MG, Swart AC, et al. Melatonin-responsive headache in delayed sleep phase syndrome: preliminary observations. Headache 1998;38(4):303-307.

608. Leone M, D'Amico D, Moschiano F, et al. Melatonin versus placebo in the prophylaxis of cluster headache: a double-blind pilot study with parallel groups. Cephalalgia 1996;16(7):494-496.

609. Zaslavskaia RM, Komarov FI, Shakirova AN, et al. [Effect of moxonidine monotherapy and in combination with melatonin on hemodynamic parameters in patients with arterial hypertension]. Klin Med (Mosk) 2000; 78(4):41-44.

610. Zaslavskaia RM, Biiasilov NS, Akhmetov KZ, et al. [Capozide-50 alone and in combination with melatonin in therapy of hypertension]. Klin Med (Mosk) 2000;78(11):39-41.

611. Zaslavskaia RM, Shakirova AN, Komarov FI, et al. [Effects of melatonin alone and in combination with aceten on chronostructure of diurnal hemodynamic rhythms in patients with hypertension stage II]. Ter Arkh 1999;71(12):21-24.

612. Cagnacci A, Arangino S, Angiolucci M, et al. Potentially beneficial cardio-vascular effects of melatonin administration in women. J Pineal Res 1997; 22(1):16-19.

613. Birau N, Peterssen U, Meyer C, et al. Hypotensive effect of melatonin in essential hypertension. IRCS Med Sci 1981;9:905-906.

614. Lissoni P, Vigore L, Rescaldani R, et al. Neuroimmunotherapy with low-dose subcutaneous interleukin-2 plus melatonin in AIDS patients with CD4 cell number below 200/mm³: a biological phase-II study. J Biol Regul Homeost Agents 1995;9(4):155-158.

615. Morera AL, Henry M, Villaverde-Ruiz ML, et al. [Efficiency of melatonin in the treatment of insomnia]. Actas Esp Psiquiatr 2000;28(5):325-329.

616. Almeida Montes LG, Ontiveros Uribe MP, Cortes SJ, et al. Treatment of primary insomnia with melatonin: a double-blind, placebo-controlled, crossover study. J Psychiatry Neurosci 2003;28(3):191-196.

617. Andrade C, Srihari BS, Reddy KP, et al. Melatonin in medically ill patients with insomnia: a double-blind, placebo-controlled study. J Clin Psychiatry 2001;62(1):41-45.

618. James SP, Sack DA, Rosenthal NE, et al. Melatonin administration in insomnia. Neuropsychopharmacology 1990;3(1):19-23.

619. MacFarlane JG, Cleghorn JM, Brown GM, et al. The effects of exogenous melatonin on the total sleep time and daytime alertness of chronic insomniacs: a preliminary study. Biol Psychiatry 1991;30(4):371-376.

620. Rogers NL, Phan O, Kennaway DJ, et al. Effect of daytime oral melatonin administration on neurobehavioral performance in humans. J Pineal Res 1998;25(1):47-53.

621. Brusco LI, Fainstein I, Marquez M, et al. Effect of melatonin in selected populations of sleep-disturbed patients. Biol Signals Recept 1999;8(1-2): 126-131.

622. Shaw KM, Stern GM, Sandler M. Melatonin and parkinsonism [abstract]. Lancet 1973;1(7797):271.

623. Kunz D, Bes F. Exogenous melatonin in periodic limb movement disorder: an open clinical trial and a hypothesis. Sleep 2001;24(2):183-187.

624. Naguib M, Samarkandi AH. Premedication with melatonin: a double-blind, placebo-controlled comparison with midazolam. Br J Anaesth 1999; 82(6):875-880.

625. Naguib M, Schmid PG, III, Baker MT. The electroencephalographic effects of IV anesthetic doses of melatonin: comparative studies with thiopental and propofol. Anesth Analg 2003;97(1):238-43, table.

626. Naguib M, Hammond DL, Schmid PG, III, et al. Pharmacological effects of intravenous melatonin: comparative studies with thiopental and propofol. Br J Anaesth 2003;90(4):504-507.

627. Naguib M, Samarkandi AH. The comparative dose-response effects of melatonin and midazolam for premedication of adult patients: a double-blinded, placebo-controlled study. Anesth Analg 2000;91(2):473-479.

628. Takeuchi N, Uchimura N, Hashizume Y, et al. Melatonin therapy for REM sleep behavior disorder. Psychiatry Clin Neurosci 2001;55(3):267-269.

629. Kunz D, Bes F. Melatonin effects in a patient with severe REM sleep behavior disorder: case report and theoretical considerations. Neuropsychobiology 1997;36(4):211-214.

630. McArthur AJ, Budden SS. Sleep dysfunction in Rett syndrome: a trial of exogenous melatonin treatment. Dev Med Child Neurol 1998;40(3): 186-192.

631. Shamir E, Laudon M, Barak Y, et al. Melatonin improves sleep quality of patients with chronic schizophrenia. J Clin Psychiatry 2000;61(5):373-377.

632. Shamir E, Rotenberg VS, Laudon M, et al. First-night effect of melatonin treatment in patients with chronic schizophrenia. J Clin Psychopharmacol 2000;20(6):691-694.

633. Leppamaki S, Partonen T, Vakkuri O, et al. Effect of controlled-release melatonin on sleep quality, mood, and quality of life in subjects with seasonal or weather-associated changes in mood and behaviour. Eur Neuropsychopharmacol 2003;13(3):137-145.

634. Lewy AJ, Bauer VK, Cutler NL, et al. Melatonin treatment of winter depression: a pilot study. Psychiatry Res 1998;77(1):57-61.

635. Wirz-Justice A, Graw P, Krauchi K, et al. Morning or night-time melatonin is ineffective in seasonal affective disorder. J Psychiatr Res 1990;24(2): 129-137.

636. Sherer MA, Weingartner H, James SP, et al. Effects of melatonin on performance testing in patients with seasonal affective disorder. Neurosci Lett 1985;58(3):277-282.

637. Srivastava AK, Gupta SK, Jain S, et al. Effect of melatonin and phenytoin on an intracortical ferric chloride model of posttraumatic seizures in rats. Methods Find Exp Clin Pharmacol 2002;24(3):145-149.

638. Lehmann ED, Cockerell OC, Rudge P. Somnolence associated with melatonin deficiency after pinealectomy. Lancet 1996;347(8997):323.

639. Siebler M, Steinmetz H, Freund HJ. Therapeutic entrainment of circadian rhythm disorder by melatonin in a non-blind patient. J Neurol 1998; 245(6-7):327-328.

640. Chaudhary G, Sharma U, Jagannathan NR, et al. Evaluation of *Withania somnifera* in a middle cerebral artery occlusion model of stroke in rats. Clin Exp Pharmacol Physiol 2003;30(5-6):399-404.

641. Gupta YK, Chaudhary G, Sinha K. Enhanced protection by melatonin and meloxicam combination in a middle cerebral artery occlusion model of acute ischemic stroke in rat. Can J Physiol Pharmacol 2002;80(3):210-217.

642. Pei Z, Pang SF, Cheung RT. Pretreatment with melatonin reduces volume of cerebral infarction in a rat middle cerebral artery occlusion stroke model. J Pineal Res 2002;32(3):168-172.

643. Pei Z, Ho HT, Cheung RT. Pre-treatment with melatonin reduces volume of cerebral infarction in a permanent middle cerebral artery occlusion stroke model in the rat. Neurosci Lett 2002;318(3):141-144.

644. Adams JD, Jr., Yang J, Mishra LC, et al. Effects of ashwagandha in a rat model of stroke. Altern Ther Health Med 2002;8(5):18-19.

645. Beloosesky Y, Grinblat J, Laudon M, et al. Melatonin rhythms in stroke patients. Neurosci Lett 2002;319(2):103-106.

646. Bhattacharya SK, Bhattacharya D, Sairam K, et al. Effect of Withania somnifera glycowithanolides on a rat model of tardive dyskinesia. Phytomedicine 2002;9(2):167-170.

647. Todisco M, Casaccia P, Rossi N. Severe bleeding symptoms in refractory idiopathic thrombocytopenic purpura: a case successfully treated with melatonin. Am J Ther 2003;10(2):135-136.

648. Todisco M, Rossi N. Melatonin for refractory idiopathic thrombocytopenic purpura: a report of 3 cases. Am J Ther 2002;9(6):524-526.

649. Bangha E, Elsner P, Kistler GS. Suppression of UV-induced erythema by topical treatment with melatonin (N-acetyl-5-methoxytryptamine). A dose response study. Arch Dermatol Res 1996;288(9):522-526.

650. Dreher F, Gabard B, Schwindt DA, et al. Topical melatonin in combination with vitamins E and C protects skin from ultraviolet-induced erythema: a human study *in vivo*. Br J Dermatol 1998;139(2):332-339.

651. Fischer T, Bangha E, Elsner P, et al. Suppression of UV-induced erythema by topical treatment with melatonin. Influence of the application time point. Biol Signals Recept 1999;8(1-2):132-135.

652. Bangha E, Elsner P, Kistler GS. Suppression of UV-induced erythema by topical treatment with melatonin (N-acetyl-5-methoxytryptamine). Influence of the application time point. Dermatology 1997;195(3): 248-252.

653. Chase JE, Gidal BE. Melatonin: therapeutic use in sleep disorders. Ann Pharmacother 1997;31(10):1218-1226.

654. Folkard S, Arendt J, Clark M. Can melatonin improve shift workers' tolerance of the night shift? Some preliminary findings. Chronobiol Int 1993;10(5):315-320.

655. Dawson D, Encel N, Lushington K. Improving adaptation to simulated night shift: timed exposure to bright light versus daytime melatonin administration. Sleep 1995;18(1):11-21.

656. James M, Tremea MO, Jones JS, et al. Can melatonin improve adaptation to night shift? Am J Emerg Med 1998;16(4):367-370.

657. Jorgensen KM, Witting MD. Does exogenous melatonin improve day sleep or night alertness in emergency physicians working night shifts? Ann Emerg Med 1998;31(6):699-704.

658. Jockovich M, Cosentino D, Cosentino L, et al. Effect of exogenous melatonin on mood and sleep efficiency in emergency medicine residents working night shifts. Acad Emerg Med 2000;7(8):955-958.

659. Wright SW, Lawrence LM, Wrenn KD, et al. Randomized clinical trial of melatonin after night-shift work: efficacy and neuropsychologic effects. Ann Emerg Med 1998;32(3 Pt 1):334-340.

660. Mallo C, Zaidan R, Galy G, et al. Pharmacokinetics of melatonin in man after intravenous infusion and bolus injection. Eur J Clin Pharmacol 1990;38(3):297-301.

Milk Thistle
(*Silybum marianum*)

SYNONYMS/COMMON NAMES/RELATED SUBSTANCES

- Bull thistle, cardo blanco, cardui mariae fructus, cardui mariae herba, *Cardum marianum* L., *Carduus marianus* L., chardon-Marie, emetic root, frauendistel, fructus silybi mariae, fruit de chardon Marie, heal thistle, holy thistle, isosilibinin, kanger, kocakavkas, kuub, lady's thistle, Marian thistle, mariana mariana, Mariendistel, Marienkrörner, Mary thistle, mild thistle, milk ipecac, pig leaves, royal thistle, shui fei ji, silidianin, silybi mariae fructus, silybin, silybinin, silychristin, silymarin, snake milk, sow thistle, St. Mary's thistle, Venue thistle, variegated thistle, wild artichoke.

CLINICAL BOTTOM LINE
Background

- Milk thistle (*Silybum marianum*) has been used medicinally for over 2000 years, principally for the treatment of hepatic and biliary disorders. A flavonoid complex called silymarin can be extracted from the seeds of milk thistle and is believed to be the biologically active component. The terms *milk thistle* and *silymarin* are often used interchangeably.
- Milk thistle products are popular in Europe and the United States for the management of various types of liver disease. Although numerous clinical trials have been conducted, most studies have suffered from methodological weaknesses, including heterogeneous patient populations, inadequate blinding and randomization, small sample sizes, large dropout rates, and concomitant alcohol use. Nonetheless, there is preliminary evidence that silymarin may reduce serum transaminase levels, improve liver histology, and improve survival in patients with cirrhosis or chronic hepatitis. There is insufficient evidence regarding the efficacy of milk thistle in the management of *Amanita phalloides* mushroom toxicity or drug/toxin-induced liver damage.
- An exploratory meta-analysis was conducted on 16 placebo-controlled trials identified in a high-quality systematic review prepared for the Agency for Healthcare Research and Quality (AHRQ).[1,2] The analysis focused on serologic outcomes (transaminases, bilirubin, albumin, prothrombin time) and Child's classification of cirrhosis. Although most results favored the use of milk thistle, the majority of effect sizes were small or not statistically significant. Notably, this report concluded that the clinical efficacy of milk thistle for liver disease has not been clearly established.
- Milk thistle is generally considered to be safe. Adverse reactions appear to be mild when used within the recommended dosage parameters, with occasional gastrointestinal symptoms, and rare cases of anaphylaxis.

Scientific Evidence for Common/Studied Uses	Grade*
Cirrhosis	B
Hepatitis (chronic)	B
Acute viral hepatitis	C
Amanita phalloides mushroom toxicity	C
Cancer prevention	C
Diabetes mellitus (associated with cirrhosis)	C
Drug/toxin-induced hepatotoxicity	C
Hyperlipidemia	C

*Key to grades: *A:* Strong scientific evidence for this use; *B:* Good scientific evidence for this use; *C:* Unclear scientific evidence for this use; *D:* Fair scientific evidence against this use (it may not work); *F:* Strong scientific evidence against this use (it likely does not work). For a more detailed explanation of efficacy criteria, see "Natural Standard Evidence-Based Validated Grading Rationale" in the Introduction.

Historical or Theoretical Indications That Lack Sufficient Evidence

- Amiodarone toxicity, antioxidant,[3,4] asthma, bladder cancer,[5] bleeding, breast cancer, bronchitis, bubonic plague (*Yersinia pestis*), cancer,[5-9] cough, cholelithiasis, demulcent for pleurisy, depression, diabetic neuropathy,[10] dyspepsia,[11] edema, gallstones, gynecologic cancers,[12] hepatitis C virus (HCV)-mediated fibrogenesis, hemorrhage, hemorrhoids, immunomodulator jaundice,[13] lactation stimulation, liver cancer, liver-cleansing agent, malaria, menstrual disorders, nephrotoxicity protection, neuroprotection,[14] peritonitis, plague, primary biliary cirrhosis,[15] prostate cancer,[8,9] psoriasis, radiation sickness, radiation toxicity,[16] skin cancer,[17] snakebite, solar ultraviolet protection,[18] splenic disorders, sunscreen, uterine complaints, varicose veins.

Expert Opinion and Folkloric Precedent

- Milk thistle has been used as a medicinal agent for over 2000 years, principally for disorders of the liver and gallbladder. In Europe, milk thistle is primarily used to prevent or treat liver diseases, including hepatitis, cirrhosis, gallstones, jaundice and toxin-induced liver damage.
- Milk thistle has been recommended to improve lactation in nursing mothers, although there is insufficient evidence in this area. This traditional use may be due to the white veins on the plant's spiked green leaves, which are fabled to carry the milk of the Virgin Mary.

Safety Summary

- **Likely safe:** When taken in recommended doses for up to 4 to 6 years, by patients who are not pregnant, not taking drugs metabolized by cytochrome P450, and not using hypoglycemic agents.
- **Possibly unsafe:** When taken in doses greater than recommended, or for an extended duration (>4 to 6 years). There is insufficient evidence to support the use of milk thistle during pregnancy or nursing. Silymarin has been reported to decrease fasting plasma glucose levels in patients with insulin-dependent diabetes associated with cirrhosis.[19] There is recent preclinical evidence of inhibition of cytochrome P450 3A4 and 2C9, although this has not been proven in humans.[20,21] Patients should be made aware of the existing treatment options for their specific conditions, particularly

treatments with demonstrated efficacy. For example, although milk thistle may be efficacious in the treatment of chronic viral hepatitis, there are prescription drug regimens that have been shown to be effective in multiple clinical trials, and these should be considered.

DOSING/TOXICOLOGY
General

- Recommended doses are based on those most commonly used in available trials, or on historical practice. However, with natural products, the optimal doses needed to balance efficacy and safety often have not been determined. Formulations and preparation methods may vary from manufacturer to manufacturer, and from batch to batch of a specific product made by a single manufacturer. Because often the active components of a product are not known, standardization may not be possible, and the clinical effects of different brands may not be comparable.

Standardization

- Milk thistle capsules, tincture and powder are often standardized to contain 70% to 80% silymarin. Silymarin is a mixture of three flavonolignans: silybin, silidianin, and silychristin. Despite standardization, different preparations and brands may have varying bioavailability.
- One of the most studied and used milk thistle products, Legalon (Madeus, Germany), is prepared via extraction with ethyl acetate, although other manufacturers utilize ethyl alcohol extraction.
- Silipide (IdB 1016) is a complex of silybin and phosphatidylcholine designed to improve oral absorption of silymarin, with demonstrated greater bioavailability (up to 10-fold).[22] Dosing is expressed in silybin equivalents.
- One study analyzing stability of milk thistle tincture found a shelf life of approximately 3 months.

Dosing: Adult (18 Years and Older)
Oral

- **Cirrhosis:** Silymarin (Legalon), 280 to 420 mg per day in two or three divided doses.[23-27] Up to 450 mg daily in three divided doses has been studied.[28]
- **Hepatitis (chronic):** Silipide (IdB 1016), 160 to 480 mg per day in silybin equivalents,[29-31] or silymarin (Legalon), 420 mg daily in three divided doses.[32] Silipide is a complex of silybin and phosphatidylcholine designed to improve oral absorption of silymarin, with demonstrated greater bioavailability.
- **Hepatitis (acute, viral):** Silymarin, 420 mg daily in three divided doses.[32-36]
- **Drug/toxin-induced hepatotoxicity:** Silymarin (Legalon), 280 to 420 mg daily in three divided doses.[37-41] Up to 800 mg daily has been studied.[42]
- **Hyperlipidemia:** Silymarin, 420 mg per day, has been studied.[43,44]
- **Diabetes mellitus associated with cirrhosis (insulin-dependent):** Silymarin (Legalon), 230 to 600 mg per day, has been studied.[19,45,46] Efficacy and safety have not been established.

Intravenous

- *Amanita phalloides* **mushroom poisoning:** Silibinin, 20 to 50 mg/kg in 500 mL 5% dextrose solution, given every 6 hours, over 24 hours.[47-49] Efficacy and safety have not been established.

Tea

- Due to milk thistle's poor water solubility, tea preparations are not recommended medicinally.

Dosing: Pediatric (Younger Than 18 Years)

- Insufficient evidence to recommend.

Toxicology

- Animal and human studies have reported low toxicity of silymarin at therapeutic doses. At higher doses (1500 mg per day), a mild laxative effect has been reported, possibly due to increased bile secretion and flow. Silipide (silybinin equivalent), 360 mg three times a day for three weeks, has been given to normal volunteers without toxicity.[60]
- LD_{50} values have been reported in dogs and rabbits at 300 mg/kg and in rodents at 900 to 1000 mg/kg.[50]
- In cultured hepatocytes, a cytotoxic effect was observed after addition of silymarin or silybin to the culture medium.[51]

ADVERSE EFFECTS/PRECAUTIONS/CONTRAINDICATIONS

M

Allergy

- Known allergy/hypersensitivity to a member of the aster (Compositea/Asteraceae) family or to daisies, artichokes, common thistle, kiwi or any of milk thistle's constituents (silibinin, silychistin, silydianin, silymonin, siliandrin).
- **Anaphylaxis:** Hypersensitivity/anaphylactic reactions associated with milk thistle ingestion have been published in case reports. Anaphylactic shock, characterized by laryngeal edema, bronchospasm, facial edema, and hypotension was observed in a 55-year-old patient with kiwi fruit allergy, following consumption of a tea containing milk thistle.[52] Hypersensitivity to milk thistle was later confirmed by skin test. In a different case, ingestion of the milk thistle product Carsil was associated with laryngeal edema and fever.[53] Diaphoresis, nausea, abdominal pain, and presyncope occurred after ingestion of a single dose of the milk thistle product Vegicaps; the reaction occurred again with repeat dosing.[54] Contact with milk thistle seeds resulted in rhinitis and conjunctivitis in one case.[55]
- **Urticaria:** In a study of silymarin for alcoholic cirrhosis, three patients reported pruritus and urticaria.[8] A Russian report described possible urticaria associated with milk thistle use.[53]

Adverse Effects

- **Summary:** In clinical trials and traditional use, oral milk thistle has generally been reported as well tolerated in recommended doses for up to 6 years. Most reported adverse reactions have been mild, including occasional gastrointestinal distress, pruritus, and headache. Because many subjects in trials are liver disease patients, it is not clear if adverse effects are due to milk thistle or to underlying liver disease; rates of adverse effects are often similar to those with placebo. Anaphylactic reactions have been reported.
- **Dermatologic:** Occasional pruritus has been reported in several trials of milk thistle, with incidence similar to control groups.[27,28,56] It is not clear if these symptoms were due to underlying liver disease. Urticaria and eczema have also been reported.[28,53,57]
- **Neurologic:** Headache has been reported in subjects receiving milk thistle in clinical trials, but with a similar incidence observed in placebo/control patients.[27,28,58] Irritability and fatigue have been reported rarely in trials.[41,57]
- **Gastrointestinal:** Infrequent, mild gastrointestinal symptoms have been reported in several studies, including nausea,

heartburn, diarrhea, epigastric pain, abdominal discomfort, dyspepsia, flatulence, and loss of appetite.[24,30,31,41,56-61] It is not clear if these symptoms were due to milk thistle or to underlying liver disease. In a trial of silymarin (140 mg three times a day) for patients with primary biliary cirrhosis, two patients discontinued use because of diarrhea or abdominal pain.[15] Nausea and epigastric discomfort caused two patients to drop out of a trial of silymarin for liver cirrhosis.[24] There is one report of a 57-year-old woman with sweating, nausea, colicky abdominal pain, diarrhea, vomiting, weakness and collapse after ingesting milk thistle; symptoms subsided after 24 to 48 hours without medical treatment, and recurred with re-challenge.[62] Another case report describes hepatotoxicity in a 69-year-old woman taking a combination herbal product containing milk thistle, horse chestnut, milfoil, celandine, sweet clover, and dandelion root. Liver function returned to normal after discontinuation of the supplement.[63]

- **Musculoskeletal:** In a study of silymarin for alcoholic cirrhosis, three patients reported arthralgias.[28]
- **Genitourinary:** One case of impotence in a pilot clinical trial of silymarin for alcoholic cirrhosis has been reported.[64]
- **Endocrine (hypoglycemia):** Silymarin has been reported to decrease fasting plasma glucose, hemoglobin A1c (HbA1c), and fasting insulin levels in patients with insulin-dependent diabetes associated with cirrhosis.[19]

Precautions/Warnings/Contraindications

- Use cautiously in patients taking medications metabolized by the hepatic cytochrome P450 system, due to *in vitro* inhibition of enzymes CYP 3A4 and CYP 2C9.[20]
- Use caution in patients with diabetes or taking hypoglycemic agents, based on reported hypoglycemic effects of milk thistle in a group of patients with insulin-dependent diabetes associated with cirrhosis.[19]
- Avoid in patients with known allergy to members of the aster (Compositea/Asteraceae) family, daisies, artichokes, common thistle, kiwi, or any of milk thistle's constituents (silybinin, silychristin, silydianin, silymarin, silymonin, siliandrin, isosilybinan).

Pregnancy and Lactation

- There is insufficient evidence to support the use of milk thistle during pregnancy or when nursing. However, there has been historical use of milk thistle during lactation, and milk thistle has been recommended by herbalists to improve lactation in nursing mothers (this traditional use may be due to the white veins on the plant's spiked green leaves, which are fabled to carry the milk of the Virgin Mary).
- Reyes at al. report that silymarin has been used safely to treat mothers for as long as 3 weeks with intrahepatic cholestasis of pregnancy.[65] Giannola conducted a 60-day trial of silymarin (400 mg daily) in pregnant women and adults with "minor liver insufficiencies," with improvement in blood chemistries and subjective symptoms.[66] Although milk thistle appears to have been well tolerated in these studies, systematic research has not been conducted.

INTERACTIONS

Milk Thistle/Drug Interactions

- **Cytochrome P450 (CYP) metabolized agents:** There is equivocal data from animal studies, *in vivo*, and *in vitro* studies to suggest inhibition of the CYP system by milk thistle, and effects in humans are unknown. There is recent evidence of inhibition of CYP3A4 and CYP2C9.[20,21] There-

fore, increased concentrations of concomitant medications (substrates) may occur.

- **Glucuronidated agents:** In theory, silymarin may decrease the clearance of glucuronidated agents such as lorazepam (Ativan), lamotrigine (Lamictal), and entacapone (Comtan).[21]
- **Insulin, oral hypoglycemic agents:** Silymarin has been reported to decrease fasting plasma glucose, hemoglobin A1c (HbA1c), and fasting insulin levels in patients with insulin-dependent diabetes associated with cirrhosis.[19] Concomitant use with other hypoglycemic agents may require dose adjustments.
- **Alcohol (ethanol)** (*positive interaction*): Milk thistle may reduce hepatotoxicity associated with ethanol ingestion. In rats, the flavonolignans silybin (silibinin), silydianin, and silychristin have been found to exert hepatocyte membrane–stabilizing and antioxidant effects.[67]
- **Indinavir (Crixivan):** Milk thistle does not appear to affect the metabolism of indinavir in healthy volunteers.[68] Although preclinical research suggested that milk thistle might inhibit CYP3A4 and potentially increase indinavir levels,[21] milk thistle does not appear to affect the pharmacokinetics of indinavir in humans.
- **Estrogens:** In theory, silymarin may increase the clearance of estrogen by inhibiting beta-glucuronidase.[69]
- **Chemotherapy (platinums, anthracyclines)** (*positive interaction*): There is preclinical data that silibinin may increase the efficacy of platinum compounds (cisplatin, carboplatin) on human PCA cells[70]; doxorubicin effects may also be increased.[71]

Milk Thistle/Herb/Supplement Interactions

- **Cytochrome P450 (CYP) metabolized herbs and supplements:** There is equivocal data from animal , *in vivo*, and *in vitro* studies to suggest inhibition of the CYP system by milk thistle, and effects in humans are unknown. There is recent evidence of inhibition of CYP3A4 and CYP2C9.[20,21] Therefore, increased concentrations of concomitant medications (substrates) may occur.
- **Hypoglycemic herbs and supplements:** Silymarin has been reported to decrease fasting plasma glucose, hemoglobin A1c (HbA1c), and fasting insulin levels in patients with insulin-dependent diabetes associated with cirrhosis.[19] Concomitant use with other hypoglycemic agents may require dose adjustments.
- **Vitamin E** (*positive interaction*): Silymarin and vitamin E have been reported to prevent amiodarone toxicity in animal studies.

Milk Thistle/Food Interactions

- Insufficient available evidence.

Milk Thistle/Lab Interactions

- **Serum glucose levels:** Silymarin has been reported to decrease fasting plasma glucose, hemoglobin A1c (HbA1c), and fasting insulin levels in patients with insulin-dependent diabetes associated with cirrhosis.[19]

MECHANISM OF ACTION

Pharmacology

- **Constituents:** Silymarin, a flavonoid complex that can be extracted from the seeds of milk thistle, is composed of three isomers. Silymarin is typically extracted with 95% ethanol, yielding a bright yellow fluid, although one of the most studied and used milk thistle products, Legalon (Madaus,

Germany), is prepared via extraction with ethyl acetate. A standard milk thistle extract contains 70% silymarin, a mixture of the flavonolignans (silydianin, silychristine) and silibinin, which is the most biologically active constituent according to *in vitro* assays. Other constituents, including dehydrosilybin, desoxysilydianin, and silybinomer, have also been isolated.

- **Antioxidant and hepatic effects:** Antioxidant or free radical–antagonizing actions have been cited as a likely mechanism of action of milk thistle; however, other suggested effects include increased protein synthesis, decreased tumor promotor activity, stabilized immunologic response, protection against cellular radiation damage, and alteration and increased stability of cellular membranes. Hepatoprotective properties of milk thistle have been attributed to antioxidant properties. Flavonoids present in milk thistle, such as silymarin and silybin, have been shown to act as antioxidants and free radical scavengers.[72-80] Silymarin abolishes hepatotoxicity of microcystin-LR (a toxin from the alga *Microcystis aeruginosa*) in rats and mice, possibly due to prevention of oxidation of protein-thiol groups.[81] Silymarin may also exert an antioxidant effect on human platelets and provides antioxidant protection against liver toxicity in iron-overloaded rats.[82] In human subjects with alcoholic cirrhosis, levels of erythrocyte/lymphocyte superoxide dismutase are raised in the presence of silymarin[83]
- There have been numerous other proposed hepatoprotective mechanisms of milk thistle. *In vitro* and animal studies have demonstrated protective effects of silymarin, particularly silybin, against hepatotoxins as diverse as acetaminophen, alcohol, carbon tetrachloride, tetrachlormethane, thallium, toluene, and xylene.[84-92] The antidote effects of silymarin against *Amanita phalloides*, observed in preliminary clinical and animal studies,[47,48,93-96] have been attributed to inhibition of binding to hepatocyte membranes. A membrane-stabilizing effect of silymarin has been demonstrated in rat hepatocytes.[97] The protection of silymarin on rat livers from D-galactosamine toxicity has been attributed to an activation of enzymes involved in the UDP-glucuronic acid biosynthesis pathways, involved in detoxification of phenols and other toxic substances.[98]
- Silibinin has also been shown to have a regenerating effect on the livers of hepatectomized rats, increasing DNA synthesis by 23% to 25%.[91-101] A similar effect was observed in cells exposed to various nephrotoxic agents.[102] Silybin stimulated DNA polymerase, increasing the synthesis of ribosomal RNA and stimulating liver cell regeneration; it also stabilized cellular membranes and increased the glutathione content of the liver.[67,103-105] Malignant cell lines, specifically HeLA and Burkitt lymphoma cells, were not stimulated by this compound.[99,100]
- **Renal effects:** Renal protective effects have also been evaluated. In rats, silybin prevented cisplatin-induced glomerular and tubular nephrotoxicity as measured by BUN, creatinine, fibronectin, and histologic changes in renal tubules.[106,107] In rats, 2 weeks of treatment with silybin did not prevent cyclosporine-induced decreases in glomerular filtration rate or increases in serum creatinine but did prevent cyclosporin-induced lipid peroxidation.[108] Several animal studies suggest renal protective effects of silymarin against cyclosporin and chemotherapeutic agents such as cisplatin and ifosfamide.[106-108] These possible results of the stimulatory effect of silymarin on kidney cells were demonstrated *in vitro* studies.[102]

- **Lipid peroxidation:** In human mesangial cell cultures, silybin inhibited the formation of malondialdehyde, a product of lipid peroxidation.[109] Silybin has also been found to inhibit peroxidation of low-density lipoproteins (LDL) *in vitro*,[110] and in human mesangial cells.[109] Silybin administered to rats for 2 weeks was found to inhibit cyclosporin-induced lipid peroxidation.[108] In human and rat lung/liver microsomes, silybin protects against chemical induced lipid peroxidation [111,112] and cell damage.[113]
- **Cholesterol synthesis:** Early animal experimentation with silybin demonstrated decreased cholesterol synthesis[114] and reduced biliary excretion of cholesterol salts by 60% to 70%, while leaving biliary flow rates unchanged.[44] In perfused livers from rats fed a high-cholesterol diet, silymarin normalized the clearance of low-density lipoproteins,[115] providing significant protection against dietary induced hypercholesterolemia.[115] Other animal studies using high cholesterol diets have reported anti-atherosclerotic effects.[116]
- **Cancer/chemoprotection:** Researchers from the University of Texas Cancer Center have proposed that silymarin mediates suppression of a nuclear transcription factor via regulation of genes involved in inflammation and carcinogenesis.[6] Ongoing research on the anti- carcinogenic effects of silymarin and silibinin in human breast, cervical, and prostate cancer cells report significant inhibition of cell and DNA growth; growth of human breast and prostate carcinoma cells was almost completely inhibited by silymarin (75 to 100 µg/mL of medium), whereas cyclin-dependent kinase inhibitor Cip1/p21 expression drastically increased, resulting in G1 arrest.[3,4,117,118] In human leukocytes, silymarin has been found to protect against DNA damage caused by hydrogen peroxide. In a mouse skin model, topically applied silymarin dramatically reduced UVB and chemically induced carcinogenesis, an effect possibly attributable to strong antioxidant properties of silymarin.[17,18] Almost complete abortion of chemically induced tumor promotion in rats by silymarin was accompanied by inhibition of the hypothetical endogenous tumor promoter TNFα.[7] Hydrolysis of glucuronides may expose the intestinal mucosa to carcinogens, and inhibition of β-glucuronidase by silymarin, as demonstrated in rats,[119] may play a preventive role against intestinal carcinogenesis. Silymarin has been demonstrated to protect against chemically induced bladder carcinogenesis in mice[5] and to inhibit mitogenic signaling pathways involved in proliferation of androgen-independent and androgen-dependent prostate cancer cells.[8,9]
- **Leukocyte effects:** Silymarin exerted no significant effects on unstimulated polymorphonuclear (PMN) cell motility and phagocytic and chemotactic activities. However, when PMN cells were stimulated, silymarin inhibited myeloperoxidase release. Incubation of PMN cells with silybin prevented the action of the leukocyte motility inhibitor, fMLP.[120,121] Silymarin inhibited leukotriene production and had an antifibrotic effect.[122] In healthy volunteers, silybin enhanced leukocyte motility.[121] Silybin may selectively inhibit Kupffer cell leukotriene and free radical formation and may inhibit nitric oxide production.[77,123]
- **Glucose effects:** In rats, silymarin was observed to play a protective role and spare the pancreas from damage in experimentally induced diabetes mellitus.[124] In rats pretreated with cyclosporin, silybin did not affect glucose levels; silybin and cyclosporin were found to have an additive inhibitory effect on insulin secretion.[125] Silymarin has been reported to decrease fasting plasma glucose, hemoglobin A1c (HbA1c),

M

and fasting insulin levels in patients with insulin-dependent diabetes associated with cirrhosis.[19]

- **Other effects:** Silibinin has been found to inhibit 5-lipoxygenase products by Kupffer cells *in vitro*.[123]

Pharmacodynamics/Kinetics

- **Bioavailability:** Onset for oral activity (hepatoprotection) has been measured at 3 to 4 hours,[126] with peak silipide levels in cholecystectomy patients at approximately 4 hours.[126] In another study, peak plasma concentrations of free silybin were measured after 2 to 3 hours, with a half-life 2 hours thereafter.[127] Bioavailability of orally administered silybin ranges from 23% to 47% and appears to be higher when administered in a softgel capsule.[128] Due to milk thistle's poor water solubility, tea preparations are not recommended medicinally. A phosphatidylcholine-silybin complex called Silipide (IdB 1016) has been developed to improve bio-availability by up to 10-fold.[22] Dosing is expressed in silybin equivalents. Most IdB 1016 in the circulation is in con-jugated form. The half-life is reported as less than 4 hours. Less than 3% of free or conjugated form is recovered in the urine.

- **Cytochrome P450 (CYP) effects:** There is equivocal data from animal studies and from *in vivo* and *in vitro* studies to suggest an interaction with the CYP system, in particular inhibition of enzymes CYP3A4 and CYP2C9. Silymarin has been found to increase the hepatic mixed function oxidation system in rats, whereas elimination half-life of aminopyrine in a small human sample was not affected.[129] Miguez et al. did not find evidence of involvement of CYP2E1 in the hepatoprotective mechanism of silymarin.[51] More recently, the major flavonoid of milk thistle, silibinin, had little *in vitro* effect on CYP2E1, CYP2C19, CYP1A2, and CYP2A6. Although silibinin was found to be a minor competitive inhibitor of dextromethorphan metabolism (CYP2D6) *in vitro*, the net effect did not increase with higher silibinin concentrations. Therefore, the authors did not believe this to be clinically important.[51] Clear inhibition was reported for CYP2C9. Contradictory results were observed for CYP3A4 substrates; mixed activation (low silibinin concen-tration) and minor inhibition (high silibinin concentration) of erythromycin, compared to pronounced noncompetitive inhibition of denitronifedipine.[20] In another study, Venkataramanan et al. demonstrated significant reduction in activity of CYP3A4 by 0.1 and 0.25 mM of silymarin. Silymarin (0.5 mM) also significantly decreased mitochondrial respiration as determined by MTT reduction in human hepatocytes.[21]

- **P-glycoprotein binding:** The resulting isoprenoid dehydro-silybins from the flavonolignan silybin have been shown to display high *in vitro* affinity for direct binding to P-glycoprotein.[130]

- **Elimination:** The elimination half-life is generally less than 4 hours with silymarin and silybinin.[22]

- **Excretion:** Less than 10% was found excreted in the urine, and 20% to 40% was recovered in the bile as glucuronide and sulfate conjugate.[131] Approximately 5% of a dose was excreted in the urine as total silybinin, representing a renal clearance of about 30 mL/minute.[132]

HISTORY

- Milk thistle (*Silybum marianum*) has been used medicinally for over 2000 years, principally in the treatment of liver and gallbladder disorders. Early records indicate use by the Greek healer Dioscorides, who used the tea of milk thistle to treat the bites of certain poisonous snakes. Other early healers, including Pliny the Elder, believed that milk thistle aided in clearing bile from the body. Documentation of the use of milk thistle in Europe for hepatobiliary disorders can be found since that time.

- In the 1800s, eclectic physicians used milk thistle in the treatment of various maladies, including liver, menstrual, and vascular conditions. Herbalists used milk thistle to treat hepatic, biliary, and menstrual disorders during the early 20th century. The early United States Pharmacopoeia listed a tincture of milk thistle. Scientific interest began to focus on milk thistle in the 1970s, particularly regarding possible antioxidant and hepatoprotective properties.

- Milk thistle plants have been used as food in salads and baked goods and as animal feed.

- The word *silibum* refers to all edible thistles, and *marianum* refers to the white veins on the plant's spiked green leaves, which are fabled to carry the milk of the Virgin Mary. This legend is also the derivation of the word *milk* in milk thistle.

- Milk thistle is native to Europe and was introduced into North America by early colonists. Milk thistle is found throughout the eastern United States, California, and South America. The mature plant grows up to 6 feet high and has a large, bright purple flower and an abundance of stout spines.

REVIEW OF THE EVIDENCE: DISCUSSION
Cirrhosis
Summary

- Multiple randomized, double-blind, placebo-controlled trials have been conducted in Europe to evaluate the effects of milk thistle on alcoholic and non-alcoholic cirrhosis. Studies have examined both short-term and longer-term (4 to 5 years) outcomes, including mortality. Overall, this research has reported milk thistle to lower serum transaminase levels and to improve survival. However, methodological weaknesses in study design and reporting limit interpretation and clinical applicability. Confounding factors, such as alcohol consump-tion, have not been well controlled, and inclusion criteria, such as diagnostic criteria for liver diseases, have not been well defined. A high-quality systematic review and meta-analysis prepared for the Agency for Healthcare Research and Quality (AHRQ) concluded that the clinical efficacy of milk thistle for liver disease has not been clearly established. Although the existing evidence does suggest benefits of milk thistle, most effect sizes are small or not statistically significant when data are pooled. A high-quality, long-term, controlled trial using serologic, histologic, and survival out-comes is necessary before a strong recommendation can be made.

Systematic Review

- Lawrence et al. conducted a high-quality systematic review of studies on the efficacy of milk thistle in liver disease of various etiologies, prepared for the Agency for Healthcare Research and Quality (AHRQ).[1,2] The review identified 16 randomized, placebo-controlled trials (14 blinded), and 17 non-placebo trials. The majority of studies used the silymarin product Legalon, with doses varying between 240 and 800 mg daily. Duration of treatment ranged from 1 week to 6 years. Etiologies of liver disease were heterogeneous, including chronic alcoholic liver disease (6 trials), viral hepatitis (3 trials; acute and chronic), cirrhosis of the liver (4 trials; alcoholic and non-alcoholic), and hepatotoxins

Review of the Evidence: Milk Thistle

Condition Treated*	Study Design	Author, Year	N[†]	SS[†]	Study Quality[‡]	Magnitude of Benefit	ARR[†]	NNT[†]	Comments
Liver disease (mixed etiologies)	Systematic review and meta-analysis	Lawrence[1] 2001; Jacobs[2] 2002	16 trials	NA	NA	NA	NA	NA	16 placebo-controlled & 17 non–placebo-controlled trials identified; meta-analysis of placebo controlled trials reported reductions in transaminases, but most effects sizes were small or not significant.
Cirrhosis (alcoholic)	RCT, double-blind	Pares[28] 1998	200	No	5	NA	NA	NA	2 years of 150 mg of silymarin three times daily with no better survival than placebo; may have been confounded by concomitant alcohol or hepatitis C.
Cirrhosis (mixed etiologies, with and without hepatitis)	RCT	Ferenci[89] 1989	170	Yes	5	Medium	20%	5	420 mg of silymarin daily; 41 months mean observation; better survival in silymarin group, particularly in Child's class A (mild) cirrhosis, and alcoholic cirrhosis.
Cirrhosis (alcoholic)	RCT	Lucena[137] 2002	60	Mixed	4	Small	NA	NA	6 months of 450 mg of silymarin (MZ-80) daily associated with significant reduction in lipid peroxidation, increase in glutathione, but no changes in transaminases.
Cirrhosis (alcoholic and non-alcoholic)	Before and after comparison	Benda[23] 1980	172	Unclear	4	Medium	NA	NA	4 years of 420 mg of silymarin daily reported to improve survival, but unclear statistical analysis.
Cirrhosis (alcoholic)	Before and after comparison	Lang[26,136] 1988, 1990	40	Yes	3	Medium	NA	NA	1 month of 420 mg of silymarin daily improved transaminases vs. placebo.
Chronic alcoholic liver disease (hepatitis and cirrhosis)	RCT, double-blind	Bunout[27] 1992	72	No	3	None	NA	NA	15 months of 280 mg of daily silymarin; no difference in LFTs or mortality seen; 17% dropout; possibly confounded by concomitant alcohol use.
Chronic alcoholic liver disease (hepatitis and cirrhosis)	RCT, double-blind	Feher[25] 1989	36	Yes	3	Small	NA	NA	6 months of 420 mg of silymarin daily improved transaminases, bilirubin, and histology vs. placebo.
Chronic alcoholic liver disease (hepatitis and cirrhosis)	RCT, double-blind	Salmi[39] 1982	106	Yes	3	Small	NA	NA	4 weeks of 420 mg silymarin daily improved transaminases and histology vs. baseline; baseline characteristics dissimilar between groups.
Alcoholic hepatitis (50% with cirrhosis)	RCT	Trinchet[133] 1989	116	No	5	None	NA	NA	3 months of 420 mg of silymarin daily; no differences in transaminases between silymarin and placebo.
Chronic liver disease (hepatitis and cirrhosis)	RCT, non-blinded	Tanasescu[135] 1988	180	No	1	Small	NA	NA	Non-significant improvements in transaminases with 40 days of 210 mg of silymarin daily vs. placebo.
Chronic liver disease (hepatitis and cirrhosis)	Comparison trial, unclear blinding, unclear randomization	De Martiis[138] 1980	45	Unclear	0	Small	NA	NA	90 days of silymarin associated with non-significant improvement in bilirubin; methodologically weak study.
Alcoholic liver disease (including cirrhosis)	Controlled study, not-randomized, non-blinded	Fintelmann[134] 1970	50	Unclear	0	Small	NA	NA	42 days of 420 mg of silymarin associated with reduced AST vs. placebo, but no improvement in ALT or alkaline phosphatase.

M

Continued

Review of the Evidence: Milk Thistle—*cont'd*

Condition Treated*	Study Design	Author, Year	N[†]	SS[†]	Study Quality[‡]	Magnitude of Benefit	ARR[†]	NNT[†]	Comments
Cirrhosis	Before and after comparison	Lirussi[140] 1995	27	Yes	0	Medium	NA	NA	6 months of 140 mg of silymarin three times/day associated with decreased transaminases from baseline; control group received ursodeoxycholic acid, but no between-group comparison was conducted.
Hepatitis (chronic viral)	RCT, non-blinded	Buzzelli[29] 1993	20	Yes	3	Medium	NA	NA	7 days of 240 mg of silibin (Silipide) improved transaminases in inpatients vs. placebo; lack of blinding may introduce bias.
Hepatitis (chronic viral)	Controlled, double-blind (2 studies described in one paper)	Kiesewetter[32] 1977	45 & 15	Mixed	3	Small	NA	NA	3-12 months of 420 mg of silymarin associated with significant improvements in histology; non-significant improvements in transaminases; large dropout (47% and 20%, respectively).
Hepatitis (chronic)	RCT	Marcelli[30] 1992	65	Yes	3	Medium	NA	NA	3 months of 240 mg of Silipide (IdB1016) associated with decreased transaminases vs. placebo; baseline characteristics dissimilar between groups; blinding and randomization not adequately described.
Hepatitis (chronic)	Phase II (dosing) study, randomized, non-blinded	Vailati[31] 1993	60	Yes	2	Small	NA	NA	2-week study of Silipide; dose-response effect on ALT and GGT seen with 160 mg, 240 mg, and 360 mg of daily silibin.
Hepatitis (acute viral)	Placebo-controlled, unclear blinding, unclear randomization	Magliulo[33] 1978	59	Mixed	2	Large	32%	4	3-week study of 420 mg of silymarin daily associated with lower transaminases after 5 and 21 days; methodologically weak study.
Hepatitis (acute viral)	Randomized, placebo-controlled, non-blinded	Bode[34] 1977	151	No	2	NA	NA	NA	5-35 days of 420 mg of silymarin daily associated with no serologic difference from placebo; no power calculation conducted; methodologically weak study.
Hepatitis (acute viral)	Comparison study, unclear blinding, unclear randomization	Tkacz[149] 1983	87	No	1	None	NA	NA	3 weeks of Silimarol plus vitamins B & C; no difference from cocarboxylase plus vitamins B and C; no placebo group; methodologically weak study.
Hepatitis (acute viral)	Comparison study, unclear blinding, unclear randomization	Saba[35] 1979	38	Yes	0	Small	NA	NA	420 mg of silymarin daily compared to choline plus methionine; methodologically weak study.
Hepatitis (acute)	Comparison study, unclear blinding, unclear randomization	Cavalieri[36] 1974	40	Mixed	0	Small	NA	NA	420 mg of silymarin daily compared to multi-agent therapy (including steroids); significant reduction in transaminases after 2 weeks, but not after 3 weeks; methodologically weak study.
Hepatotoxicity, (multiple etiologies)	Controlled trial, unclear blinding, unclear randomization	Schopen[139] 1970	72	Unclear	0	Small	NA	NA	45 days of 210-420 mg of silymarin daily associated with non-significant improvements in transaminases; poorly described methods and results.
Toxin-induced liver damage	RCT, double-blind	Fintelmann[151] 1980	66	Yes	3	Medium	NA	NA	28 days of silymarin associated with significantly faster recovery of transaminases vs. placebo; poorly described methods and results.

Review of the Evidence: Milk Thistle—cont'd

Condition Treated*	Study Design	Author, Year	N[†]	SS[†]	Study Quality[‡]	Magnitude of Benefit	ARR[†]	NNT[†]	Comments
Toxin-induced liver damage	Cohort	Szilard[38] 1988	49	Mixed	0	Medium	NA	NA	30 days of 420 mg of silymarin daily associated with significant improvements in transaminases; methodologically weak study.
Toxin-induced liver damage	Controlled trial, non-randomized, non-blinded	Boari[37] 1981	55	Yes	0	Medium	NA	NA	15-20 days of 420 mg of silymarin daily associated with significant improvements in transaminases vs. vitamin B; poorly described methods and results.
Drug-induced liver damage (prophylaxis)	RCT	Allain[41] 1999	217	No	2	None	NA	NA	12 weeks of silymarin did not protect against Tacrine-induced hepatotoxicity in Alzheimer's patients.
Drug-induced liver damage (prophylaxis)	RCT, non-blinded	Magula[152] 1996	29	Yes	2	Large	NA	NA	8 weeks of combination silymarin + Fumaria associated with protection against antituberculosis drug–induced toxicity.
Drug-induced liver damage	RCT, double-blind	Palasciano[42] 1994	60	No	2	Small	NA	NA	90 days of 900 mg of silymarin daily associated with non-significant improvements in transaminases.
Toxic liver damage	RCT, unclear blinding	Schopen[139] 1970	72	No	0	None	NA	NA	Improvements observed in transaminases; limited by lack of control group.
Type 2 diabetes and cirrhosis	Randomized, non-blinded, no placebo arm	Velussi[19,45] 1993, 1997	60	Yes	1	Small	NA	NA	12 months of 600 mg of silymarin daily associated with reduced fasting glucose levels and insulin requirements vs. no treatment; methodologically weak study.

*Primary or secondary outcome.
[†]N, Number of patients; SS, statistically significant; ARR, absolute risk reduction; NNT, the number of patients who need to undergo a specific intervention in order to observe an outcome in one individual.
[‡]0-2 = poor; 3-4 = good; 5 = excellent.
ALT, Alanine aminotransferase; AST, aspartate aminotransferase; GGT, gamma-glutamyl transferase; NA, not applicable; RCT, randomized, controlled trial.
For an explanation of each category in this table, please see Table 3 in the Introduction.

M

(3 trials). An exploratory meta-analysis was conducted on the placebo-controlled trials, focusing on serologic outcomes (transaminases, bilirubin, albumin, prothrombin time) and Child's classification of cirrhosis. Although most results favored the use of milk thistle, most effect sizes were small or not statistically significant. When subgroup analysis was conducted on studies of liver disease of specific etiologies, similar results were seen (nonspecific trends toward benefits of milk thistle). Regarding cirrhosis specifically, the review noted two randomized, blinded, placebo-controlled trials of alcoholic cirrhosis,[26,28] two trials of mixed alcoholic and non-alcoholic cirrhosis,[23,24] and five studies that included patients with mixed types of liver disease, including cirrhosis.[25,27,133-135] These studies are discussed below in detail, in addition to several case studies.

Controlled Trials (Alcoholic Cirrhosis)

- Pares et al. conducted a 2-year, multi-center, randomized, placebo-controlled, double-blind trial in 200 patients with alcoholic cirrhosis.[28] Inclusion of subjects was based on histologically proven cirrhosis and a history of alcohol abuse; subjects were excluded if they had other known causes of cirrhosis (e.g., autoimmune, hepatitis B virus), a history of steroid treatment, or limited life-expectancy. The primary outcome measured was survival, and secondary outcomes included serologic measures of liver disease progression. Patients were randomized to receive 150 mg three times daily of silymarin (Legalon) or placebo. The two groups had similar baseline characteristics. The 2-year study period was completed by 55% of silymarin patients and 70% of placebo patients. Survival rate and complications due to cirrhosis were similar in both groups; mean 5-year survival rate was 0.71 ± 0.06 for silymarin compared to 0.76 ± 0.05 for placebo. Clinical and laboratory tests were not significantly different between groups. These results suggest a lack of mortality benefit of silymarin. However, a number of confounding variables, such as alcohol consumption and coexistence of hepatitis C, were not consistently controlled. In addition, the number of studied subjects may have been significant for defined power in these studies, yet too small to yield any conclusion regarding survival.

- Ferenci et al. conducted a randomized, controlled, double-blind trial in 170 patients with cirrhosis of various etiologies (54% alcoholic, 46% non-alcoholic) and mixed severities (52% Child's class A cirrhosis, 40% Child's class B, 7% Child's class C).[24] Subjects were randomized to receive silymarin (Legalon) (420 mg) daily or placebo for a treatment period of at least 2 years. The two groups had similar baseline characteristics. The mean observation time was 41 months. There were 24 dropouts (14%), and 61 deaths (36%) during the observation period. A significant survival benefit was noted in silymarin patients vs. placebo, with 4-year reported survival rates of 58% (±9%) and 39% (±9%), respectively. Subgroup analysis revealed that survival benefits were statistically significant in patients with alcoholic liver disease or Child's class A (mild) cirrhosis. However, it is not clear that this study was sufficiently large to allow for statistically significant subgroup analysis, despite the high mortality rate. Nonetheless, this study suggests possible utility of silymarin in the least severe cases of cirrhosis due to alcohol consumption.

- Benda et al. conducted a 4-year, randomized, controlled, double-blind trial in 172 patients with biopsy-proven cirrhosis (mixed alcoholic and non-alcoholic).[23] Exclusion criteria were poor compliance, recent steroid therapy, primary biliary cirrhosis, and Wilson's disease. Subjects were administered 140 mg of silymarin (Legalon) three times daily or placebo. Randomization and blinding procedures were properly conducted. The authors reported better survival in the silymarin group, although clear statistical analysis was not provided (a Kruskal-Wallis test was described). In addition, there was incomplete reporting of baseline patient characteristics, and it is not apparent that between-group comparisons were conducted. Without additional details of statistical analysis, these results are of limited utility.

- A 1-month, randomized, double-blind trial was conducted by Lang et al. in 40 patients with alcoholic cirrhosis.[26,131] Inclusion criteria included chronic alcohol intake and biopsy-proven cirrhosis; exclusion criteria were hemodynamic instability, end-organ failure, or diabetes (one fourth of patients had superimposed hepatitis). Subjects received silymarin (Legalon, Aica-P (amino-imidazole-carboxamide-phosphate, 600 mg daily) or placebo for 1 month. This trial appears to have been published twice (1988 and 1990), reporting two different silymarin doses: 140 mg twice per day and 140 mg three times per day. After one month, significant improvements in transaminases were seen in the silymarin and Aica-P groups compared to baseline values, whereas the placebo group did not demonstrate significant improvements from baseline. However, it is not evident that the groups were directly compared to each other. The authors noted that silymarin therapy was associated with increases in lectin-induced lymphoblast transformation, decreases in the percentage of OKT8+ cells, and suppression of lymphocytotoxicity, which they equated with immuno-modulatory properties of silymarin. Although the findings are suggestive, weaknesses of this trial include the short duration and incomplete reporting of blinding or randomization procedures.

- Lucena et al. conducted a 6-month randomized, placebo-controlled trial in 60 patients with alcoholic cirrhosis.[137] A silymarin preparation called MZ-80 was evaluated, which has been found in rat studies to reduce hepatic lipid peroxidation and increase glutathione activity.[80] Subjects were randomized to receive 150 mg of MZ-80 three times daily or placebo. After 6 months, small significant increases in glutathione and decreases in lipid peroxidation were observed, but there were no significant changes in transaminase levels.

Controlled Trials (Chronic Alcoholic Liver Disease)

- Bunout et al. conducted a randomized, controlled, double-blind trial in 72 patients with chronic alcoholic liver disease (cirrhosis and hepatitis).[27] Subjects were included who had a history of alcohol abuse, jaundice, ascites, hyper-bilirubinemia (>2 mg/dL), prothrombin time >75, hypo-albuminemia (<3), or encephalopathy. Patients with heart failure or renal failure were excluded. Subjects received either 280 mg daily of silymarin (Legalon) or placebo, for an average follow-up of 15 months. The authors reported no differences between groups in terms of mortality (5 deaths in each group), transaminases, bilirubin levels, or prothrombin time. Weaknesses of this study include the possible con-founding effects of concomitant alcohol use (58% of milk thistle patients and 65% of placebo patients), 17% dropout, mixed types of liver disease, and poor descriptions of randomization or blinding procedures.

- Feher et al. conducted a randomized, double-blind trial in 36 patients with chronic alcoholic liver disease (hepatitis and cirrhosis).[25] Inclusion and exclusion criteria were not clearly described but appear to include chronic alcohol abuse and lack of prior steroid therapy. Subjects received either 420 mg of silymarin (Legalon) daily or placebo for 6 months. Improvements were observed in the silymarin group in serum bilirubin, transaminases (AST, ALT), and gamma-glutamyl transferase (GGT) levels, which were significant compared to baseline and compared to the placebo group. Histologic improvements were also noted in the silymarin group, although the significance of these changes is not clear. Weaknesses of this trial include the heterogeneity of included patients and poor description of methods and statistical analysis.

- Salmi and Sarna conducted a 4-week, randomized, controlled, double-blind trial in 106 patients with alcohol-induced liver disease and elevated liver enzymes.[39] Selection criteria were not clearly specified. Subjects were randomized to 420 mg of silymarin (Legalon) daily or placebo. The authors report that significant decreases in transaminases and histologic improvements occurred in the silymarin group compared to placebo, and non-significant improvements in bilirubin levels occurred. Although these results are promising, subjects were dissimilar at baseline (transaminase levels were lower in the placebo group), and blinding and randomization procedures may not have been appropriate, allowing for the possible introduction of bias or confounding.

- Trinchet et al. conducted a 3-month randomized, double-blind trial in 116 subjects with histologically proven alcoholic hepatitis, of whom 50% had cirrhosis.[133] Patients were excluded who were encephalopathic, thrombocytopenic, or coagulopathic or who had hepatocellular cancer or another end-stage disease. Subjects were randomized to receive 420 mg of silymarin (Legalon) daily or placebo. Transaminase levels significantly improved in both the silymarin and placebo groups during the trial, attributed to abstinence from alcohol use. No significant changes were noted in other serologic markers (prothrombin time, bilirubin) or in histology. These negative results are compelling, although they may have been confounded by the changes in alcohol consumption before and after the trial started, which could affect outcomes measures such as transaminase levels and histology and could mask more subtle effects mediated by silymarin. Blinding, randomization, and statistical analysis were well described.

- Tanasescu et al. conducted a low-quality, randomized, controlled trial in 180 patients with chronic liver disease of different etiologies (cirrhosis and hepatitis).[135] Subjects were administered 210 mg of silymarin (Silymarin-A, manufactured in Romania) daily or placebo for 40 days. Improvements were reported in transaminases, bilirubin, and prothrombin time. However, it is not clear that results were statistically significant. In addition, randomization and blinding were not adequate. Therefore, these results cannot be considered reliable.

- De Martiis et al. conducted a poorly described comparison trial in patients with chronic hepatitis or cirrhosis.[138] Silymarin was compared to "traditional therapy" in 45 patients over a 90-day period. Although improvements in bilirubin were reported, statistical significance was not clear. Blinding and randomization were not described.
- In an early (1970) study, Fintelmann compared treatment with 420 mg of silymarin (Legalon) daily vs. placebo of 50 patients with alcoholic liver disease (including fatty liver and cirrhosis).[134] After 42 days, an improvement in serum aspartate aminotransferase (AST) was reported, although statistical significance for the overall group was not clear. There were no significant differences in alanine aminotransferase (ALT) or alkaline phosphatase levels. Neither a randomization process nor blinding was described in this study, and baseline patient characteristics were not clear. Therefore, these results cannot be considered clinically relevant.
- Schopen and Lange conducted a poorly described randomized trial in 72 patients with chronic liver disease of multiple etiologies, including alcoholic and toxin-induced.[139] Subjects were randomized to receive either "conventional" liver-protecting agents, or 210 to 420 mg of silymarin daily. After a mean treatment duration of 45 days, non-significant improvements in transaminases were reported. Blinding was not described.
- Lirussi et al. observed a decrease in serum AST and ALT in 27 patients with active cirrhosis of the liver during a 6-month treatment period with 140 mg of silymarin (Legalon) three times/day.[140] Although this trial was presented as crossover study, with the alternative treatment being ursodeoxycholic acid, it lacked a formal comparison between treatment groups. It is therefore classifiable as a before-and-after study, without clearly significant between-group differences.
- Deak et al. conducted a double-blind study in 36 patients with histologically proven chronic alcoholic liver disease.[141] Subjects were treated for 6 months with 140 mg of silymarin (Legalon) or placebo and were "encouraged" to reduce alcohol intake. Silymarin patients experienced significant improvement in certain immune functions: significantly enhanced proliferative activity of leukocytes and normalized T-cell and CD8-cell percentages.

Uncontrolled Trials

- Several case series have reported improvements in serum transaminase levels and histology in cirrhosis patients treated with oral milk thistle preparations. Although these results are compelling, the lack of control groups in these studies does not allow for a distinction to be made between therapeutic effects and the natural history of disease. In addition, bias and confounding may be introduced.
- In a 1971 case series of 67 patients with chronic liver diseases (primarily fatty degeneration of the liver), improvement of liver enzyme, clinical, and histological parameters was observed after 6 months of oral treatment with 350 mg of silymarin three times daily.[142]
- In an early open trial, Reutter administered silymarin to 11 patients with cirrhosis, following a 14-day placebo run-in.[143] Improvements in histologic findings, including regression of inflammatory changes and lesions, were observed. Alkaline

phosphatase, serum glutamic-oxaloacetic transaminase (GOT), bilirubin, and alpha-globulin levels decreased, whereas serum albumin and triglyceride levels increased.

- In a large open, uncontrolled trial, Albrecht et al. investigated the efficacy of milk thistle fruit extract in 2637 cases of toxic liver damage.[58] Outpatients with a clinical diagnosis of toxic liver damage (diagnostic criteria not clearly described), including cirrhosis, were treated for 8 weeks with varying doses (70 to 140 mg once to three times daily) of milk thistle (Legalon) Efficacy was assessed by laboratory parameters (liver enzymes), clinical examination (liver size and consistency), and patient and physician rating. Between 80% and 90% of patients and physicians rated efficacy at least "satisfactory." On average, liver enzymes decreased to approximately half their initial values. Liver size and consistency improved in 30% to 50% of the study subjects. Despite the apparent size of the effect, it is difficult to evaluate efficacy in the absence of a control group.

Chronic Hepatitis (Viral and Alcoholic)
Summary

- Several trials have examined milk thistle as a treatment for chronic hepatitis of viral or alcoholic origin. Most studies have produced statistically significant results in favor of milk thistle in improving liver function tests, with more consistent positive results for viral hepatitis. However, methodological weaknesses in study design and reporting limit interpretation and clinical applicability. A high-quality systematic review and meta-analysis prepared for the Agency for Healthcare Research and Quality (AHRQ) concluded that the clinical efficacy of milk thistle for liver disease has not been clearly established.[1,2] Although the existing evidence does suggest benefits of milk thistle, most effect sizes are small or not statistically significant when data are pooled. A high-quality, long-term, controlled trial using serologic, histologic, and survival outcomes is necessary before a strong recommendation can be made.

Chronic Viral Hepatitis

- Buzzelli et al. conducted a randomized, placebo-controlled trial in 20 inpatients with chronic hepatitis C virus and/or chronic hepatitis B virus infections.[29] Diagnoses were made either histologically or serologically. Patients with portal hypertension, ascites, hepatocellular carcinoma, or drug addiction were excluded. Subjects were randomized to receive either 240 mg of silybin (Silipide [IdB1016]) taken twice daily or placebo. (Silipide is a complex of silybin and phosphatidylcholine designed to improve oral absorption of silymarin.) After 7 days, significant reductions were found in transaminase levels in the Silipide group compared to baseline ($p < 0.01$) and to placebo ($p < 0.05$). Bilirubin levels were not significantly altered. This trial was not adequately blinded, which increases the risk of introducing bias.
- Kiesewetter et al. reported two controlled, double-blind trials in a single publication.[32] Patients (n = 45 and n = 15) with chronic viral hepatitis were assigned to receive 420 mg of silymarin (Legalon) in three divided daily doses or placebo, for a follow-up period ranging from 3 to 12 months. In the first study, randomization was described, while it was not clear in the description of the second trial. The dropout rate was 47% in the first trial and 20% in the second trial. An intention-to-treat analysis was not carried out. In both studies, statistically significant improvements in histology were noted in the silymarin groups, whereas non-significant

improvements in transaminase levels were observed. These two studies are limited by poor descriptions of baseline patient characteristics and statistical analyses.

Chronic Hepatitis (Etiology Unknown)

- Marcelli et al. examined the use of Silipide for chronic persistent hepatitis [30] Sixty-five patients with biopsy-proven hepatitis and liver enzymes 1.5 times greater than normal were randomized to receive placebo or 240 mg of Silipide (IdB1016) daily. After 90 days of therapy, the authors observed significant reductions in ALT and AST in the Silipide group vs. placebo. However, transaminase levels were higher in the Silipide group at baseline. Blinding and randomization were not adequately described.

- De Martiis et al. conducted a poor-quality comparison trial in patients with chronic hepatitis or cirrhosis.[138] Silymarin was compared to "traditional therapy" in 45 patients over a 90-day period. Although improvements in bilirubin were reported, statistical significance was not clear. Blinding and randomization were not described.

Alcoholic Hepatitis

- Trinchet et al. conducted a three-month randomized, double-blind trial in 116 subjects with histologically proven alcoholic hepatitis, of whom 50% had cirrhosis.[133] Patients were excluded who were encephalopathic, thrombocytopenic, or coagulopathic or who had hepatocellular cancer or another end-stage disease. Subjects were randomized to receive 420 mg of silymarin (Legalon) daily or placebo. Transaminase levels significantly improved in both the silymarin and placebo group during the trial, attributed to abstinence from alcohol use. No significant changes were noted in other serologic markers (prothrombin time, bilirubin) or in histology. These negative results are compelling, although they may have been confounded by the changes in alcohol consumption before and after the trial started, which could affect outcomes measures such as transaminases and histology and could mask more subtle effects mediated by silymarin. Blinding, randomization, and statistical analysis were well described.

- Tanasescu et al. conducted a low-quality, randomized, controlled trial in 180 patients with chronic liver disease of different etiologies (cirrhosis and hepatitis).[135] Subjects were administered 210 mg of daily silymarin (Silymarin-A, manufactured in Romania) or placebo for 40 days. Improvements were reported in transaminases, bilirubin, and prothrombin time. However, it is not clear that results were statistically significant. In addition, randomization and blinding were not adequate. Therefore, these results cannot be considered reliable.

Dosing

- Vailati et al. published a phase II randomized, non-blinded study to compare doses of Silipide in the treatment of chronic viral and alcoholic hepatitis.[31] Sixty patients with biopsy-proven chronic hepatitis and liver enzymes 1.5 times greater than normal were randomized to one of three daily doses of Silipide (based on silybin content): 160 mg silybin, 240 mg silybin, or 360 mg silybin, or control. After two weeks of therapy, the authors found that decreases in aspartase aminotransferase (AST) levels reached significance in all three dosage groups ($p < 0.001$), whereas decrease in alanine aminotransferase (ALT) levels reached significance in the two higher dosage groups ($p < 0.001$). Significant dose-response

effects on AST and gammaglutamyl transpeptidase (GGT) were detected via MANOVA analysis ($p < 0.05$).

- A poor-quality study was conducted to determine the effects of 800 µg of misoprostol per day in patients with hepatitis B infections, in comparison to 210 mg of silymarin per day or no treatment.[144] Fifty-two male patients were randomly assigned to one of the three groups. After 6 months, multiple benefits were associated with misoprostol, but results were not completely reported for silymarin (transaminases, bilirubin, alkaline phosphatase). This study is of limited use in the analysis of the efficacy of silymarin (milk thistle). Blinding and randomization were not clearly described. A different poor-quality study was conducted to evaluate the efficacy of ursodeoxycholic acid (UDCA) and silymarin in the treatment of hepatitis B infection.[145] No clear advantage of silymarin was demonstrated. Methods and results were not clearly reported.

Uncontrolled Trials

- Case series have reported improvements in serum transaminase levels and histology in hepatitis patients treated with oral milk thistle preparations. Although these results are compelling, the lack of control groups in these studies does not allow for a distinction to be made between therapeutic effects and the natural history of disease. In addition, bias and confounding may be introduced.

- In a case series of eight patients with chronic hepatitis B virus and/or hepatitis C virus infections, mean alanine aminotransferase (ALT) and aspartate aminotransferase (AST) levels were observed to significantly decrease following 2 months of treatment with 120 mg silybin per day.[146] A case series was reported in which three patients with cirrhosis of the liver due to hepatitis C virus were treated with a three-agent regimen including silymarin, alpha lipoic acid, and selenium.[147] Large reductions in ALT, alpha-feto protein (AFP), and viral load were described. However, the possible effects of silymarin cannot be separated from those of the other agents, and the results of such a small sample without controls are of limited utility.

- A case series was conducted in 17 children (ages 6 to 12 years) with acute viral hepatitis.[148] Over a 10- to 30-day period, 12 mg/kg/day of silymarin (n = 10) or 12 mg/kg/day of silymarin plus 5 mg/kg/day of S-adenosylmethionine (SAMe) was administered. Small improvements in liver function tests were reported, although statistical significance was not noted. No adverse effects of therapy were reported.

Acute Viral Hepatitis
Summary

- Several low-quality studies have examined the use of milk thistle for acute viral hepatitis. Although beneficial serologic outcomes have been reported, due to methodological weaknesses these results are not conclusive. There is insufficient evidence to recommend for or against milk thistle for the treatment of acute viral hepatitis.

Evidence

- Magliulo et al. conducted a placebo-controlled trial in 59 patients with acute hepatitis A or B.[33] Subjects were randomized to receive either 140 mg of silymarin three times daily or placebo for 21 to 28 days. The authors report that by the fifth treatment day, serum transaminase and bilirubin levels were reduced in the silymarin group compared to placebo. After 3 weeks, significantly lower aspartase aminotransferase (AST) and bilirubin levels were seen in the silymarin group vs. placebo, with a non-significant trend toward lower alanine aminotransferase (ALT) levels. No difference was detected in alkaline phosphatase levels or hepatitis B surface antigen seroconversion. Although this trial was described as being double-blinded, blinding and randomization were not described. Therefore, bias or confounding may have affected the results.

- Bode et al. conducted a low-quality controlled trial in 151 patients with acute viral hepatitis.[34] Subjects were randomized to receive 140 mg of silymarin (Legalon) three times daily or no treatment for 5 to 35 days. However, randomization was not properly conducted. There were 100 patients in the no-treatment group and 51 in the silymarin group. Over a 5-week period, measurements were made every 5 to 7 days of serum transaminase, bilirubin, and alkaline phosphatase levels and prothrombin time. No differences in these values were detected between groups, and there was no significant difference in terms of time to normalized transaminase levels between groups. This study was not blinded, allowing for the possible introduction of bias.

- Tkacz and Dworniak conducted a controlled study in 87 patients with acute viral hepatitis.[149] Subjects were assigned to receive either the milk thistle product Sylimarol plus vitamins B and C, or cocarboxylase (thiamine diphosphate) plus vitamins B and C. This study was not blinded, and randomization was not clearly described. After 3 weeks, no significant differences were noted in transaminase levels or length of hospital stay between groups, although patients' general condition was reported to improve earlier and more rapidly based on subjective measures. The lack of a placebo group and unclear reporting of methods or results limits the usefulness of this study.

- Saba et al. conducted a poor-quality comparison study in 38 patients with acute viral hepatitis.[35] Subjects were randomized to receive either 420 mg of silymarin daily or choline plus methionine and a multivitamin for an unclear period of time. Although significant improvements in aspartase aminotransferase (AST) and bilirubin levels were reported, methods, statistical analysis, and results were not clearly documented. Blinding was not reported. Due to weaknesses in design and reporting, this study cannot be considered clinically relevant.

- Cavalieri conducted a comparison study in 40 patients with acute hepatitis of various etiologies.[36] Causes were not clear in all cases but included infectious cases. Subjects were assigned to receive either 420 mg of silymarin (Legalon) daily in three divided doses or a "traditional regimen" consisting of 12 parts, including steroids and multiple vitamins. After 2 weeks of therapy, significant improvements were noted in transaminase and bilirubin levels and prothrombin time; however, after 3 and 4 weeks, these improvements were not statistically significant. Randomization and blinding were not clearly reported in this study, nor was statistical analysis.

Amanita phalloides Mushroom Toxicity
Summary

- For several decades, milk thistle has been reported anecdotally to be beneficial in the management of *Amanita phalloides* mushroom poisoning. However, most research cited in the literature has consisted of animal studies, human case reports, case series, or retrospective analyses.[47-49] The quality of reports has been limited by confounding factors and lack of controls or prospective design. However, a number of authoritative natural medicine texts support the use of milk thistle in the treatment of *Amanita phalloides* mushroom poisoning based on traditional precedent and expert opinion. At this time, there is insufficient evidence to recommend for or against milk thistle for the treatment of *Amanita phalloides* mushroom toxicity.

Evidence

- In several case reports/case series, intravenous infusion of 20 to 50 mg/kg up to 4 times a day has been used to treat patients with reported *Amanita phalloides* mushroom poisoning.[47-49] In some cases, oral silymarin followed intravenous administration. Patients have been reported to recover dramatically, based on liver function tests. However, without controls for comparison, these results cannot be distinguished from the possible natural course of illness.

- In one study, 252 patients with acute *Amanita phalloides* ingestion were treated with oral silymarin, with reported marked improvement in survival.[48] This study compared these results to historical controls and did not utilize a prospective, parallel control group. There was inadequate description of baseline patient characteristics, the course of liver failure, and additional supportive treatment measures.

Cancer Prevention
Summary

- There is ongoing research on the antiarcinogenic effects of silymarin and silibinin in human breast, cervical, and prostate cancer cells, with reports that silibinin may inhibit cell growth and DNA replication.[117,118] Investigators at M.D. Anderson Cancer Center have proposed that silymarin suppresses a nuclear transcription factor, thus regulating genes involved in inflammation and carcinogenesis.[6] Due to a lack of human clinical trials, there is insufficient evidence to recommend milk thistle for the treatment of cancer.

Evidence

- There is a case report of spontaneous regression of hepatocellular cancer in a 52-year-old man with biopsy-proven unresectable hepatocellular carcinoma, which resolved "spontaneously" following self-medication with 450 mg of silymarin daily.[150]

Drug/Toxin-Induced Hepatotoxicity
Summary

- Milk thistle has been used for treatment of or prophylaxis against liver damage induced by toxins and drugs. Numerous human trials have reported promising results, although most studies have been poorly designed and reported. There is currently insufficient evidence to recommend for or against this use of milk thistle.

Toxin-Induced Liver Disease

- In a double-blind trial of patients with laboratory and clinical evidence of acute toxic liver damage, 66 subjects were randomized to receive milk thistle extract (Legalon) (unclear dose) or placebo for up to 28 days.[151] Significantly faster mean improvements in alanine aminotransferase (ALT) levels ("normalization") were reported in the milk thistle group, whereas non-significant differences in rate of improvement of bilirubin were noted. Although promising, these results are limited by inadequate description of baseline patient characteristics, inclusion criteria, blinding procedures, and statistical analysis.

- Szilard et al. conducted a cohort study in 49 non-alcoholic patients with abnormal liver function tests and/or hematologic values, presumably due to chronic exposure to organic solvent vapors (toluene, xylene).[38] Thirty of the 49 workers were treated orally with silymarin (420 mg daily) for 1 month, and no treatment was administered to the remaining 19 subjects. The authors reported significant improvements in liver function tests and platelet counts in the silymarin patients, with non-significant mean improvements in leukocyte counts. Due to lack of blinding or randomization, unclear baseline patient characteristics, and short study duration, the clinical utility of these results is limited.

- Boari et al. conducted a controlled, non-randomized, non-blinded study in 55 patients with reported occupational toxic liver damage, possibly due to paint and solvent exposure.[37] Baseline patient characteristics and inclusion criteria were not described. Subjects were treated for 15 to 20 days with either silymarin (420 mg daily) or "placebo" (vitamin B). Significant improvements in transaminase levels were reported in the silymarin group, without significant changes in the control group. Although the findings are suggestive, the methodological weaknesses of this study limit the clinical relevance of the results.

Drug-Induced Liver Disease

- Allain et al. investigated the use of silymarin (420 mg daily) to prevent Tacrine-induced liver toxicity in 217 patients with Alzheimer's dementia.[41] Patients with a history of liver disease were excluded. Subjects were randomized to receive either silymarin or placebo over a 3-month period, during which transaminase levels were monitored. In an intention-to-treat analysis, no significant differences in liver function tests were detected after 12 or 15 weeks. Despite this lack of serologic benefit, the authors suggested that silymarin may subjectively improve adverse effects and clinical tolerance of Tacrine, without a negative impact on cognitive performance. Further evidence is warranted before a recommendation can be made.

- Magula conducted an 8-week controlled study in 29 patients with normal baseline liver function tests who were undergoing antituberculosis drug therapy.[152] Subjects were randomized in a non-blinded fashion to prophylactically receive silymarin plus *Fumaria officinalis* alkaloids (in addition to antituberculosis drugs) or antituberculosis drugs alone over an 8-week period. The authors reported a significant 28% decrease in the risk of developing "liver injury" and a decreased risk of transaminitis in the silymarin/*Fumaria* group vs. the no-additional-therapy group. However, due to lack of blinding, use of a combination therapy, and unclear descriptions of outcomes measures or statistical analytic techniques, this study is of limited clinical value.

- Palasciano et al. conducted a randomized, double-blind, placebo-controlled trial in 60 women with liver disease presumed to be due to long-term therapy with antipsychotic medications (phenothiazine and/or butyrophenones).[42] Subjects with transaminitis (twice normal values) were included, and notably some patients were hepatitis B antibody positive. Exclusion criteria were alcohol/drug abuse, autoimmune hepatitis, Wilson's disease, hemochromatosis, concurrent therapy with another hepatotoxic drug, diabetes, and pregnancy. Over a 90-day period, 800 mg of silymarin daily plus/minus antipsychotic medications, or placebo without antipsychotic medications was administered. Non-significant improvements in transaminases were observed in both the milk thistle and no-drug groups. It is not clear if this study was adequately powered to detect between-group differences, and the results are not clinically helpful.

- Schopen and Lange conducted a poorly described randomized trial in 72 patients with chronic liver disease of multiple etiologies, including alcoholic and toxin-induced injury (5 patients with chronic barbiturate use, 2 with aflatoxin, 1 with mercury ingestion, and 8 "poison-induced").[139] Subjects were randomized to receive either "conventional" liver-protecting agents or 210 to 420 mg of silymarin daily. After a mean treatment duration of 45 days, non-significant improvements in transaminases were reported. Blinding was not described.

Uncontrolled Trials

- Several case series have reported improvements in serum transaminase levels, histology, and symptoms (pruritus, nausea) in patients with toxin- or drug-induced liver damage following treatment with oral milk thistle. Although these results are compelling, the lack of control groups in these studies does not allow for a distinction to be made between therapeutic effects and the natural history of the disease. In addition, bias and confounding may be introduced.

- Saba et al. reported improved transaminases in 19 patients with liver damage (presumed to be due to psychoactive medications), following treatment with milk thistle.[153] Following 3 months of silymarin treatment, 67 outpatients with "toxic-metabolic" liver damage, chronic persistent hepatitis, and cholangitis with pericholangitis were deemed "cured," based on significant reductions in serum transaminases and on liver biopsy results.[142] In a 1973 uncontrolled study in 2000 patients with toxic liver damage of various etiologies, serum levels of hepatic enzymes were reportedly reduced following milk thistle treatment.[154] Nausea and pruritus improved in 83% of patients. In a surveillance study, 200 to 400 mg of daily "St. Mary's thistle extract" (corresponding to 140 to 280 mg of silymarin daily) was administered over a 5-week period to 108 patients with alcohol-related liver damage.[40] Eighty-five percent of patients "responded" to treatment with reductions in transaminases and procollagen-III-peptide levels (a fibrosis activity marker).

- In a large open, uncontrolled trial, Albrecht et al. investigated the efficacy of milk thistle fruit extract in 2637 cases of toxic liver damage.[58] Outpatients with a clinical diagnosis of toxic liver damage (diagnostic criteria not clearly described), including cirrhosis, were treated for 8 weeks with varying doses (70 to 140 mg once to three times daily) of milk thistle (Legalon). Efficacy was assessed by laboratory parameters (liver enzymes), clinical examination (liver size and consistency), and patient and physician rating. Between 80% and 90% of patients and physicians rated efficacy at least "satisfactory." On average, liver enzyme levels decreased to approximately half their initial values. Liver size and consistency improved in 30% to 50% of the study subjects. Despite the apparent size of the effect, it is difficult to evaluate efficacy in the absence of a control group.

Hyperlipidemia
Summary

- There is preliminary evidence from *in vitro* and animal studies suggesting a lipid-lowering effect of milk thistle, via regulation of liver lipid metabolism and inhibition of cholesterol synthesis.[114,115] However, preliminary human studies are limited by small sample sizes, and they have not consistently found benefits.[43,44] Therefore, there is insufficient evidence to recommend for or against milk thistle for the treatment of hyperlipidemia.

Evidence

- In an open clinical study, 14 hyperlipidemic outpatients were treated with 420 mg daily of silymarin (Legalon).[43] After 7 months, non-significant small decreases in both total cholesterol and high-density lipoproteins (HDLs) were observed.
- In a study of 15 cholecystectomy patients, those who received silymarin (420 mg daily for 1 month) experienced a significant decrease in biliary cholesterol concentration compared to those treated with placebo, suggesting decreased hepatic cholesterol synthesis.[44]

Diabetes Mellitus (Associated with Cirrhosis)
Summary

- Preliminary evidence from animal studies has suggested a possible role of milk thistle in the management of diabetes.[124,125] Limited human data are available, and existing studies have focused on the treatment of type 2 diabetes associated with alcoholic cirrhosis. Improved glycemic control has been reported, but due to methodological weaknesses in the available studies, a firm conclusion cannot be drawn.

Evidence

- Velussi et al. conducted a year-long controlled trial in 60 patients with alcoholic cirrhosis and type 2 diabetes (insulin resistance), who were stable on insulin therapy.[19,45] Subjects were randomized to receive either 200 mg of silymarin (Legalon) three times daily or no treatment. Silymarin therapy was associated with significant decreases in fasting glucose levels, mean daily blood glucose levels, glycosuria, and insulin requirements. Although the findings are suggestive, the lack of placebo arm or blinding limits the clinical usefulness of these results.
- In a small, uncontrolled trial of 14 type 2 diabetic patients, silybin (230 mg daily) taken daily for 4 weeks was associated with a significant reduction in red blood cell (RBC) sorbitol compared to baseline; however, fasting blood glucose levels were not affected.[46]

FORMULARY: BRANDS USED IN CLINICAL TRIALS
Brands Used in Statistically Significant Clinical Trials

- Thisylin: Nature's Way, USA.
- Legalon: IBI Lorezini, Italy[19]; and Madaus, Germany.
- IdB1016: Inverni della Beffa, Italy.[29]

References

1. Lawrence V, Jacobs B, Dennehy C, et al. Report on milk thistle: effects on liver disease and cirrhosis and clinical adverse effects. Evidence Report/Technology Assessment No. 21 (Contract 290-97-0012 to the San Antonio Evidence-based Practice Center, based at the University of Texas Health Science Center at San Antonio, and The Veterans Evidence-based Research, Dissemination, and Implementation Center, a Veterans Affairs Services Research and Development Center of Excellence). AHRQ Publication No. 01-E025. Rockville, MD: Agency for Healthcare Research and Quality. October 2000.
2. Jacobs BP, Dennehy C, Ramirez G, et al. Milk thistle for the treatment of liver disease: a systematic review and meta-analysis. Am J Med 2002; 113(6):506-515.
3. Zi X, Feyes DK, Agarwal R. Anticarcinogenic effect of a flavonoid antioxidant, silymarin, in human breast cancer cells MDA-MB 468: induction of G1 arrest through an increase in Cip1/p21 concomitant with a decrease in kinase activity of cyclin-dependent kinases and associated cyclins. Clin Cancer Res 1998;4(4):1055-1064.
4. Zi X, Grasso AW, Kung HJ, et al. A flavonoid antioxidant, silymarin, inhibits activation of erbB1 signaling and induces cyclin-dependent kinase inhibitors, G1 arrest, and anticarcinogenic effects in human prostate carcinoma DU145 cells. Cancer Res 1998;58(9):1920-1929.
5. Vinh PQ, Sugie S, Tanaka T, et al. Chemopreventive effects of a flavonoid antioxidant silymarin on n-butyl- n-(4-hydroxybutyl)nitrosamine-induced urinary bladder carcinogenesis in male ICR mice. Jpn J Cancer Res 2002; 93(1):42-49.
6. Manna SK, Mukhopadhyay A, Van NT, et al. Silymarin suppresses TNF-induced activation of NF-kappa B, c-Jun N- terminal kinase, and apoptosis. J Immunol 1999;163(12):6800-6809.
7. Zi X, Mukhtar H, Agarwal R. Novel cancer chemopreventive effects of a flavonoid antioxidant silymarin: inhibition of mRNA expression of an endogenous tumor promoter TNF alpha. Biochem Biophys Res Commun 1997;239(1):334-339.
8. Bhatia N, Agarwal R. Detrimental effect of cancer preventive phytochemicals silymarin, genistein and epigallocatechin 3-gallate on epigenetic events in human prostate carcinoma DU145 cells. Prostate 2001;46(2):98-107.
9. Zhu W, Zhang JS, Young CY. Silymarin inhibits function of the androgen receptor by reducing nuclear localization of the receptor in the human prostate cancer cell line LNCaP. Carcinogenesis 2001;22(9):1399-1403.
10. Gorio A, Donadoni ML, Finco C, et al. Alterations of protein mono-ADP-ribosylation and diabetic neuropathy: a novel pharmacological approach. Eur J Pharmacol 1996;311(1):21-28.
11. Madisch A, Melderis H, Mayr G, et al. [A plant extract and its modified preparation in functional dyspepsia. Results of a double-blind placebo controlled comparative study]. Z Gastroenterol 2001;39(7):511-517.
12. Scambia G, De Vincenzo R, Ranelletti FO, et al. Antiproliferative effect of silybin on gynaecological malignancies: synergism with cisplatin and doxorubicin. Eur J Cancer 1996;32A(5):877-882.
13. Wilasrusmee C, Kittur S, Shah G, et al. Immunostimulatory effect of Silybum marianum (milk thistle) extract. Med Sci Monit 2002;8(11): BR439-BR443.
14. Kittur S, Wilasrusmee S, Pedersen WA, et al. Neurotrophic and neuroprotective effects of milk thistle (Silybum marianum) on neurons in culture. J Mol Neurosci 2002;18(3):265-269.
15. Angulo P, Patel T, Jorgensen RA, et al. Silymarin in the treatment of patients with primary biliary cirrhosis with a suboptimal response to ursodeoxycholic acid. Hepatology 2000;32(5):897-900.
16. Hakova H, Misurova E, Kropacova K. The effect of silymarin on concentration and total content of nucleic acids in tissues of continuously irradiated rats. Vet Med (Praha) 1996;41(4):113-119.
17. Lahiri-Chatterjee M, Katiyar SK, Mohan RR, et al. A flavonoid antioxidant, silymarin, affords exceptionally high protection against tumor promotion in the SENCAR mouse skin tumorigenesis model. Cancer Res 1999;59(3): 622-632.
18. Katiyar SK, Korman NJ, Mukhtar H, et al. Protective effects of silymarin against photocarcinogenesis in a mouse skin model. J Natl Cancer Inst 1997;89(8):556-566.
19. Velussi M, Cernigoi AM, De Monte A, et al. Long-term (12 months) treatment with an anti-oxidant drug (silymarin) is effective on hyperinsulinemia, exogenous insulin need and malondialdehyde levels in cirrhotic diabetic patients. J Hepatol 1997;26(4):871-879.
20. Beckmann-Knopp S, Rietbrock S, Weyhenmeyer R, et al. Inhibitory effects of silibinin on cytochrome P-450 enzymes in human liver microsomes. Pharmacol Toxicol 2000;86(6):250-256.
21. Venkataramanan R, Ramachandran V, Komoroski BJ, et al. Milk thistle, a herbal supplement, decreases the activity of CYP3A4 and uridine diphosphoglucuronosyl transferase in human hepatocyte cultures. Drug Metab Dispos 2000;28(11):1270-1273.
22. Barzaghi N, Crema F, Gatti G, et al. Pharmacokinetic studies on IdB 1016, a silybin- phosphatidylcholine complex, in healthy human subjects. Eur J Drug Metab Pharmacokinet 1990;15(4):333-338.
23. Benda L, Dittrich H, Ferenzi P, et al. [The influence of therapy with silymarin on the survival rate of patients with liver cirrhosis (author's transl)]. Wien Klin Wochenschr 1980;92(19):678-683.
24. Ferenci P, Dragosics B, Dittrich H, et al. Randomized controlled trial of silymarin treatment in patients with cirrhosis of the liver. J Hepatol 1989; 9(1):105-113.
25. Feher J, Deak G, Muzes G, et al. [Liver-protective action of silymarin therapy in chronic alcoholic liver diseases]. Orv Hetil 1989;130(51): 2723-2727.
26. Lang I, Nekam K, Gonzalez-Cabello R, et al. Hepatoprotective and immunological effects of antioxidant drugs. Tokai J Exp Clin Med 1990; 15(2-3):123-127.
27. Bunout D, Hirsch S, Petermann M, et al. [Controlled study of the effect of silymarin on alcoholic liver disease]. Rev Med Chil 1992;120(12): 1370-1375.
28. Pares A, Planas R, Torres M, et al. Effects of silymarin in alcoholic patients with cirrhosis of the liver: results of a controlled, double-blind, randomized and multicenter trial. J Hepatol 1998;28(4):615-621.
29. Buzzelli G, Moscarella S, Giusti A, et al. A pilot study on the liver protective effect of silybinphosphatidylcholine complex (IdB1016) in

chronic active hepatitis. Int J Clin Pharmacol Ther Toxicol 1993;31(9): 456-460.

30. Marcelli R, Bizzoni P, Conte D, et al. Randomized controlled study of the efficacy and tolerability of a short course of IdB 1016 in the treatment of chronic persistent hepatitis. Eur Bull Drug Res 1992;1(3):131-135.

31. Vailati A, Aristia L, Sozze E, et al. Randomized open study of the dose-effect relationship of a short course of IdB 1016 in patients with viral or alcoholic hepatitis. Fitoterapia 1993;64(3):219-228.

32. Kiesewetter E, Leodolter I, Thaler H. [Results of two double-blind studies on the effect of silymarine in chronic hepatitis (author's transl)]. Leber Magen Darm 1977;7(5):318-323.

33. Magliulo E, Gagliardi B, Fiori GP. [Results of a double blind study on the effect of silymarin in the treatment of acute viral hepatitis, carried out at two medical centres (author's transl)]. Med Klin 1978;73(28-29): 1060-1065.

34. Bode JC, Schmidt U, Durr HK. [Silymarin for the treatment of acute viral hepatitis? Report of a controlled trial (author's transl)]. Med Klin 1977; 72(12):513-518.

35. Saba P, Mignani E, Pagliai, et al. Efficacy of silymarin treatment of acute virus hepatitis. Epatologia 1979;25:277-281.

36. Cavalieri S. A controlled clinical trial of Legalon in 40 patients. Gazz Med Ital 1974;133:628-635.

37. Boari C, Montanari FM, Galletti GP, et al. [Toxic occupational liver diseases. Therapeutic effects of silymarin]. Minerva Med 1981;72(40): 2679-2688.

38. Szilard S, Szentgyorgyi D, Demeter I. Protective effect of Legalon in workers exposed to organic solvents. Acta Med Hung 1988;45(2): 249-256.

39. Salmi HA, Sarna S. Effect of silymarin on chemical, functional, and morphological alterations of the liver. A double-blind controlled study. Scand J Gastroenterol 1982;17(4):517-521.

40. Held C. [Therapy of toxic hepatopathies: Mary's thistle extract lowers the fibrosis activity]. Therapiewoche 1993;43:2002-2009.

41. Allain H, Schuck S, Lebreton S, et al. Aminotransferase levels and silymarin in de novo tacrine-treated patients with Alzheimer's disease. Dement Geriatr Cogn Disord 1999;10(3):181-185.

42. Palasciano G, Portincasa P, Palmieri V, et al. The effect of silymarin on plasma levels of malon-dialdehyde in patients receiving long-term treatment with psychotropic drugs. Curr Ther Res 1994;55(5):537-545.

43. Somogyi A, Ecsedi GG, Blazovics A, et al. Short term treatment of type II hyperlipoproteinaemia with silymarin. Acta Med Hung 1989;46(4): 289-295.

44. Nassuato G, Iemmolo RM, Strazzabosco M, et al. Effect of Silibinin on biliary lipid composition. Experimental and clinical study. J Hepatol 1991; 12(3):290-295.

45. Velussi M, Cernigoi AM, Viezzoli L, et al. Silymarin reduces hyper-insulinemia, malondialdehyde levels, and daily insulin need in cirrhotic diabetic patients. Curr Ther Res 1993;53(5):533-545.

46. Zhang JQ, Mao XM, Zhou YP. [Effects of silybin on red blood cell sorbitol and nerve conduction velocity in diabetic patients]. Zhongguo Zhong Xi Yi Jie He Za Zhi 1993;13(12):725-6, 708.

47. Floersheim GL, Weber O, Tschumi P, et al. [Clinical death-cap (Amanita phalloides) poisoning: prognostic factors and therapeutic measures. Analysis of 205 cases]. Schweiz Med Wochenschr 1982;112(34):1164-1177.

48. Hruby K, Csomos G, Thaler H. Silbinin in the treatment of deathcap fungus poisoning. Forum 1984;6:23-26.

49. Carducci R, Armellino MF, Volpe C, et al. [Silibinin and acute poisoning with Amanita phalloides]. Minerva Anestesiol 1996;62(5):187-193.

50. Desplaces A, Choppin J, Vogel G, et al. The effects of silymarin on experimental phalloidine poisoning. Arzneimittelforschung 1975;25(1): 89-96.

51. Miguez MP, Anundi I, Sainz-Pardo LA, et al. Hepatoprotective mechanism of silymarin: no evidence for involvement of cytochrome P450 2E1. Chem Biol Interact 1994;91(1):51-63.

52. Geier J, Fuchs T, Wahl R. [Anaphylactic shock due to an extract of Silybum marianum in a patient with immediate-type allergy to kiwi fruit]. Allergologie 1990;13(10):387-388.

53. Mironets VI, Krasovskaia EA, Polishchuk II. [A case of urticaria during Carsil treatment]. Vrach Delo 1990;7:86-87.

54. Adverse Drug Reactions Advisory Committee. An adverse reaction to the herbal medication milk thistle (Silybum marianum). Med J Aust 1999; 170(5):218-219.

55. Wollemann G, Seifert HU, Borelli S. Berufsbedingte Rhinokonjunktivitis auf Mariendistelsamen (Silybum marianum L.). Allergologie 1987;10: 505-507.

56. Grungreiff K, Albrecht M, Strenge-Hesse A. Benefit of medicinal liver therapy in general practice. Med Welt 1995;46:222-227.

57. Frerick F, Kuhn U, Strenge-Hesse A. Silymarin—ein Phytopharmakon zur Behandlung toxischen Leberschaden: Anwendungsbeobachtung bei 2169 Patienten. Kassenarzt 1990;33:36-41.

58. Albrecht M, Frerick H, Kuhn U, et al. Die Therapie toxischer Leberschaden mit Legalon. Z Klin Med 1992;47(2):87-92.

59. Studlar M. Die Behandlung chronischer Leberkrankungen mit Silymarin und B-Vitaminen. Therapiewoche 1985;35:3375-3378.

60. Marena C, Lampertico M. Preliminary clinical development of silipide: a new complex of silybin in toxic liver disorders. Planta Med 1991;57(2): A124-A125.

61. Schuppan D, Strosser W, Burkard G, et al. Influence of Legalon(TM) 140 on the metabolism of collagen in patients with chronic liver disease— Review by measurement of PIIINP-values. Zeitschrift fur Allgemeinmedizin 1998;74:577-584.

62. Anonymous. Adverse reaction: milk thistle-associated toxicity. Nurse Drug Alert 1999;23(7):51.

63. De Smet PA, Van den Eertwegh AJ, Lesterhuis W, et al. Hepatotoxicity associated with herbal tablets. BMJ 1996;313(7049):92.

64. Andrade RJ, Lucena MI, De la Cruz JP, et al. Effects of silymarin on the oxidative stress in patients with alcoholic liver cirrhosis. Results from a controlled, double blind, randomized pilot clinical trial. Hepatology 1998;28(4):629a.

65. Reyes H, Simon FR. Intrahepatic cholestasis of pregnancy: An estrogen-related disease. Sem Liver Dis 1993;13:289-301.

66. Giannola C, Buogo F, Forestiere G, et al. [A two-center study on the effects of silymarin in pregnant women and adult patients with so-called minor hepatic insufficiency]. Clin Ter 1985;114(2):129-135.

67. Valenzuela A, Lagos C, Schmidt K, et al. Silymarin protection against hepatic lipid peroxidation induced by acute ethanol intoxication in the rat. Biochem Pharmacol 1985;34(12):2209-2212.

68. DiCenzo R, Shelton M, Jordan K, et al. Coadministration of milk thistle and indinavir in healthy subjects. Pharmacotherapy 2003;23(7):866-870.

69. Mulrow C, Lawrence V, Jacobs B, et al. Milk thistle: effects on liver disease and cirrhosis and clinical adverse effects. Evidence Rep/Technol Assess No.21 2000

70. Dhanalakshmi S, Agarwal P, Glode LM, et al. Silibinin sensitizes human prostate carcinoma DU145 cells to cisplatin- and carboplatin-induced growth inhibition and apoptotic death. Int J Cancer 2003;106(5):699-705.

71. Tyagi AK, Singh RP, Agarwal C, et al. Silibinin strongly synergizes human prostate carcinoma DU145 cells to doxorubicin-induced growth Inhibition, G2-M arrest, and apoptosis. Clin Cancer Res 2002;8(11): 3512-3519.

72. Hikino H, Kiso Y, Wagner H, et al. Antihepatotoxic actions of flavonolignans from Silybum marianum fruits. Planta Med 1984;50(3): 248-250.

73. Mira ML, Azevedo MS, Manso C. The neutralization of hydroxyl radical by silibin, sorbinil and bendazac. Free Radical Res Commun 1987;4(125): 129.

74. Muzes G, Deak G, Lang I. Silymarin (Legalon) kezeles hatasa idult alkoholos majbetegek antioxidans vedorendszerere es a lipid peroxidaciora (kettos vak protokoll). Orvosi Hetilap 1990;131:863-866.

75. Altorjay I, Dalmi L, Sari B, et al. The effect of silibinin (Legalon) on the free radical scavenger mechanisms of human erythrocytes in vitro. Acta Physiol Hung 1992;80(1-4):375-380.

76. Comoglio A, Tomasi A, Malandrino S, et al. Scavenging effect of silipide, a new silybin-phospholipid complex, on ethanol-derived free radicals. Biochem Pharmacol 1995;50(8):1313-1316.

77. Dehmlow C, Murawski N, de Groot H. Scavenging of reactive oxygen species and inhibition of arachidonic acid metabolism by silibinin in human cells. Life Sci 1996;58(18):1591-1600.

78. Batakov EA. [Effect of Silybum marianum oil and legalon on lipid peroxidation and liver antioxidant systems in rats intoxicated with carbon tetrachloride]. Eksp Klin Farmakol 2001;64(4):53-55.

79. Mullen K, Dasarathy S. Potential new therapies for alcoholic liver disease. Clin Liver Dis 1998;2(4):853-874.

80. Gonzalez-Correa JA, de la Cruz JP, Gordillo J, et al. Effects of silymarin MZ-80 on hepatic oxidative stress in rats with biliary obstruction. Pharmacology 2002;64(1):18-27.

81. Mereish KA, Bunner DL, Ragland DR, et al. Protection against microcystin-LR-induced hepatotoxicity by Silymarin: biochemistry, histopathology, and lethality. Pharm Res 1991;8(2):273-277.

82. Pietrangelo A, Borella F, Casalgrandi G, et al. Antioxidant activity of silybin in vivo during long-term iron overload in rats. Gastroenterology 1995; 109(6):1941-1949.

83. Feher J, Lang I, Nekam K, et al. Effect of free radical scavengers on superoxide dismutase (SOD) enzyme in patients with alcoholic cirrhosis. Acta Med Hung 1988;45(3-4):265-276.

84. Tuchweber B, Trost W, Salas M, et al. Prevention of praseodymium-induced hepatotoxicity by silybin. Toxicol Appl Pharmacol 1976;38(3): 559-570.

85. Tuchweber B, Sieck R, Trost W. Prevention of silybin of phalloidin-induced acute hepatoxicity. Toxicol Appl Pharmacol 1979;51(2):265-275.

86. Campos R, Garrido A, Guerra R, et al. Silybin dihemisuccinate protects against glutathione depletion and lipid peroxidation induced by acetaminophen on rat liver. Planta Med 1989;55:417-419.

87. Skakun N, Moseichuk I. [Clinical pharmacology of Legalon]. Vrach Delo 1988;5:5-10.

88. Mourelle M, Favari L, Amezcua JL. Protection against thallium hepatotoxicity by silymarin. J Appl Toxicol 1988;8(5):351-354.

89. Mourelle M, Muriel P, Favari L, et al. Prevention of CCL4-induced liver cirrhosis by silymarin. Fundam Clin Pharmacol 1989;3(3):183-191.

90. Muriel P, Mourelle M. Prevention by silymarin of membrane alterations in acute CCl4 liver damage. J Appl Toxicol 1990;10(4):275-279.

91. Muriel P, Garciapina T, Perez-Alvarez V, et al. Silymarin protects against paracetamol-induced lipid peroxidation and liver damage. J Appl Toxicol 1992;12(6):439-442.

92. Shear NH, Malkiewicz IM, Klein D, et al. Acetaminophen-induced toxicity to human epidermoid cell line A431 and hepatoblastoma cell line Hep G2, in vitro, is diminished by silymarin. Skin Pharmacol 1995;8(6):279-291.

93. Vogel G, Temme I. [Curative antagonism of phalloidin induced liver damage with silymarin as a model of an antihepatotoxic therapy]. Arzneimittelforschung 1969;19(4):613-615.

94. Floersheim GL, Eberhard M, Tschumi P, et al. Effects of penicillin and silymarin on liver enzymes and blood clotting factors in dogs given a boiled preparation of Amanita phalloides. Toxicol Appl Pharmacol 1978;46(2):455-462.

95. Trost W, Halbach G. Anti-phalloidine and anti-alpha-amanitine action of silybin in comparison with compounds similar to structural parts of silybin. Experientia 1978;34(8):1051-1052.

96. Vogel G, Tuchweber B, Trost W, et al. Protection by silibinin against Amanita phalloides intoxication in beagles. Toxicol Appl Pharmacol 1984;73(3):355-362.

97. Ramellini G, Meldolesi J. Liver protection by silymarin: in vitro effect on dissociated rat hepatocytes. Arzneimittelforschung 1976;26(1):69-73.

98. Tyutyulkova N, Tuneva S, Gorantcheva U, et al. Hepatoprotective effect of silymarin (carsil) on liver of D-galactosamine treated rats. Biochemical and morphological investigations. Methods Find Exp Clin Pharmacol 1981;3(2):71-77.

99. Sonnenbichler J, Zetl I. Biochemical effects of the flavonolignane silibinin on RNA, protein and DNA synthesis in rat livers. Prog Clin Biol Res 1986;213:319-331.

100. Sonnenbichler J, Goldberg M, Hane L, et al. Stimulatory effect of Silibinin on the DNA synthesis in partially hepatectomized rat livers: non-response in hepatoma and other malign cell lines. Biochem Pharmacol 1986;35(3):538-541.

101. Sonnenbichler J, Zetl I. Stimulating influence of a flavonolignane derivative on proliferation, RNA synthesis and protein synthesis in liver cells. In Okoliczanyi L, Csomos G, Crepaldi G, et al, (eds). Assessment and Management of Hepatobiliary Disease. Berlin, Springer-Verlag, 1987, pp 265-272.

102. Sonnenbichler J, Scalera F, Sonnenbichler I, et al. Stimulatory effects of silibinin and silicristin from the milk thistle Silybum marianum on kidney cells. J Pharmacol Exp Ther 1999;290(3):1375-1383.

103. Fiebrich F, Koch H. Silymarin, an inhibitor of prostaglandin synthetase. Experientia 1979;35(12):1550-1552.

104. Fiebrich F, Koch H. Silymarin, an inhibitor of lipoxygenase. Experientia 1979;35(12):1548-1560.

105. Valenzuela A, Aspillaga M, Vial S, et al. Selectivity of silymarin on the increase of the glutathione content in different tissues of the rat. Planta Med 1989;55(5):420-422.

106. Bokemeyer C, Fels LM, Dunn T, et al. Silibinin protects against cisplatin-induced nephrotoxicity without compromising cisplatin or ifosfamide anti-tumour activity. Br J Cancer 1996;74(12):2036-2041.

107. Gaedeke J, Fels LM, Bokemeyer C, et al. Cisplatin nephrotoxicity and protection by silibinin. Nephrol Dial Transplant 1996;11(1):55-62.

108. Zima T, Kamenikova L, Janebova M, et al. The effect of silibinin on experimental cyclosporine nephrotoxicity. Ren Fail 1998;20(3):471-479.

109. Wenzel S, Stolte H, Soose M. Effects of silibinin and antioxidants on high glucose-induced alterations of fibronectin turnover in human mesangial cell cultures. J Pharmacol Exp Ther 1996;279(3):1520-1526.

110. Locher R, Suter PM, Weyhenmeyer R, et al. Inhibitory action of silibinin on low density lipoprotein oxidation. Arzneimittelforschung 1998;48(3):236-239.

111. Basaga H, Poli G, Tekkaya C, et al. Free radical scavenging and antioxidative properties of 'silibin' complexes on microsomal lipid peroxidation. Cell Biochem Funct 1997;15(1):27-33.

112. Carini R, Comoglio A, Albano E, et al. Lipid peroxidation and irreversible damage in the rat hepatocyte model. Protection by the silybin-phospholipid complex IdB 1016. Biochem Pharmacol 1992;43(10):2111-2115.

113. Bosisio E, Benelli C, Pirola O. Effect of the flavanolignans of Silybum marianum L. on lipid peroxidation in rat liver microsomes and freshly isolated hepatocytes. Pharmacol Res 1992;25(2):147-154.

114. Schriewer H, Rauen HM. [The effect of silybin dihemisuccinate on cholesterol biosynthesis in rat liver homogenates (author's transl)]. Arzneimittelforschung 1977;27(9):1691-1694.

115. Skottova N, Krecman V. Silymarin as a potential hypocholesterolaemic drug. Physiol Res 1998;47(1):1-7.

116. Bialecka M. [The effect of bioflavonoids and lecithin on the course of experimental atherosclerosis in rabbits]. Ann Acad Med Stetin 1997;43:41-56.

117. Bhatia N, Zhao J, Wolf DM, et al. Inhibition of human carcinoma cell growth and DNA synthesis by silibinin, an active constituent of milk thistle: comparison with silymarin. Cancer Lett 1999;147(1-2):77-84.

118. Zi X, Agarwal R. Silibinin decreases prostate-specific antigen with cell growth inhibition via G1 arrest, leading to differentiation of prostate

119. Kim DH, Jin YH, Park JB, et al. Silymarin and its components are inhibitors of beta-glucuronidase. Biol Pharm Bull 1994;17(3):443-445.

120. Minonzio F, Venegoni E, Ongari AM, et al. Modulation of human polymorphonuclear leukocyte function by the flavonoid silybin. Int J Tissue React 1988;10(4):223-231.

121. Kalmar L, Kadar J, Somogyi A, et al. Silibinin (Legalon-70) enhances the motility of human neutrophils immobilized by formyl-tripeptide, calcium ionophore, lymphokine and by normal human serum. Agents Actions 1990;29(3-4):239-246.

122. Leng-Peschlow E, Strenge-Hesse A. [The milk thistle (Silybum marianum) and silymarin in liver therapy]. Z Phytother 1991;12:162-174.

123. Dehmlow C, Erhard J, de Groot H. Inhibition of Kupffer cell functions as an explanation for the hepatoprotective properties of silibinin. Hepatology 1996;23(4):749-754.

124. Soto CP, Perez BL, Favari LP, et al. Prevention of alloxan-induced diabetes mellitus in the rat by silymarin. Comp Biochem Physiol C Pharmacol Toxicol Endocrinol 1998;119(2):125-129.

125. von Schonfeld J, Weisbrod B, Muller MK. Silibinin, a plant extract with antioxidant and membrane stabilizing properties, protects exocrine pancreas from cyclosporin A toxicity. Cell Mol Life Sci 1997;53(11-12):917-920.

126. Schandalik R, Gatti G, Perucca E. Pharmacokinetics of silybin in bile following administration of silipide and silymarin in cholecystectomy patients. Arzneimittelforschung 1992;42(7):964-968.

127. Gatti G, Perucca E. Plasma concentrations of free and conjugated silybin after oral intake of a silybin-phosphatidylcholine complex (silipide) in healthy volunteers. Int J Clin Pharmacol Ther 1994;32(11):614-617.

128. Savio D, Harrasser PC, Basso G. Softgel capsule technology as an enhancer device for the absorption of natural principles in humans. A bioavailability cross-over randomised study on silybin. Arzneimittelforschung 1998;48(11):1104-1106.

129. Leber HW, Knauff S. Influence of silymarin on drug metabolizing enzymes in rat and man. Arzneimittelforschung 1976;26(8):1603-1605.

130. Maitrejean M, Comte G, Barron D, et al. The flavanolignan silybin and its hemisynthetic derivatives, a novel series of potential modulators of P-glycoprotein. Bioorg Med Chem Lett 2000;10(2):157-160.

131. Flory PJ, Krug G, Lorenz D, et al. [Studies on elimination of silymarin in cholecystectomized patients. I. Biliary and renal elimination after a single oral dose]. Planta Med 1980;38(3):227-237.

132. Weyhenmeyer R, Mascher H, Birkmayer J. Study on dose-linearity of the pharmacokinetics of silibinin diastereomers using a new stereospecific assay. Int J Clin Pharmacol Ther Toxicol 1992;30(4):134-138.

133. Trinchet J, Coste T, Levy V, et al. [A randomized double blind trial of silymarin in 116 patients with alcoholic hepatitis]. Gastoenterol Clin Biol 1989;13(2):120-124.

134. Fintelmann V. Zur Therapie der Fettleber mit Silymarin. Therapiewoche 1970;20:1055-2064.

135. Tanasescu C, Petrea S, Baldescu R, et al. Use of the Romanian product Silimarina in the treatment of chronic liver diseases. Med Interne 1988;26(4):311-322.

136. Lang I, Deak G, Nekam K, et al. Hepatoprotective and immunomodulatory effects of antioxidant therapy. Acta Med Hung 1988;45(3-4):287-295.

137. Lucena MI, Andrade RJ, de la Cruz JP, et al. Effects of silymarin MZ-80 on oxidative stress in patients with alcoholic cirrhosis. Results of a randomized, double-blind, placebo-controlled clinical study. Int J Clin Pharmacol Ther 2002;40(1):2-8.

138. De Martiis M, Fontana M, Assogna G, et al. [Milk thistle (Silybum marianum) derivatives in the therapy of chronic hepatopathies]. Clin Ter 1980;94(3):283-315.

139. Schopen RD, Lange OK. [Therapy of hepatoses. Therapeutic use of Silymarin]. Med Welt 1970;15:691-698.

140. Lirussi F, Nassuato G, Orlando R, et al. Treatment of active cirrhosis with ursodeoxycholic acid and a free radical scavenger: A two year prospective study. Med Sci Ress 1995;23:31-33.

141. Deak G, Muzes G, Lang I, et al. [Immunomodulator effect of silymarin therapy in chronic alcoholic liver diseases]. Orv Hetil 1990;131(24):1291-1296.

142. Poser G. [Experience in the treatment of chronic hepatopathies with silymarin]. Arzneimittelforschung 1971;21(8):1209-1212.

143. Reutter FW, Haase W. [Clinical experience with silymarin in the treatment of chronic liver disease(author's transl)]. Schweiz Rundsch Med Prax 1975;64(36):1145-1151.

144. Flisiak R, Prokopowicz D. Effect of misoprostol on the course of viral hepatitis B. Hepatogastroenterology 1997;44(17):1419-1425.

145. Lirussi F, Okolicsanyi L. Cytoprotection in the nineties: experience with ursodeoxycholic acid and silymarin in chronic liver disease. Acta Physiol Hung 1992;80(1-4):363-367.

146. Moscarella S, Giusti A, Marra F, et al. Therapeutic and antilipoperoxidant effects of silybin-phosphatidylcholine complex in chronic liver disease: preliminary results. Curr Ther Res 1993;53(1):98-102.

147. Berkson BM. A conservative triple antioxidant approach to the treatment of hepatitis C. Combination of alpha lipoic acid (thioctic acid), silymarin, and selenium: three case histories. Med Klin 1999;94 Suppl 3:84-89.

carcinoma cells: implications for prostate cancer intervention. Proc Natl Acad Sci U S A 1999;96(13):7490-7495.

M

148. Musso A, Giacchino M, Vietti M, et al. [The use of silymarin and SAMe in the treatment of acute infective hepatitis in childhood]. Minerva Pediatr 1980;32(17):1057-1067.
149. Tkacz B, Dworniak D. [Sylimarol in the treatment of acute viral hepatitis]. Wiadomosci Lekarskie 1983;36(8):613-616.
150. Grossmann M, Hoermann R, Weiss M, et al. Spontaneous regression of hepatocellular carcinoma. Am J Gastroenterol 1995;90(9):1500-1503.
151. Fintelmann V, Albert A. Nachweis der therapeutischen Wirksamkeit von Legalon bei toxischen Lebererkrankungen im Doppelblindversuch. Therapiewoche 1980;30:5589-5594.
152. Magula D, Galisova Z, Iliev N, et al. [Effect of silymarin and Fumaria alkaloids in the prophylaxis of drug-induced liver injury during antituberculotic treatment]. Studia Pneumolog Phtiseol Cech 1996;56(5):206-209.
153. Saba P, Galeone F, Salvadorini F, et al. [Therapeutic effects of Silymarin in chronic liver diseases due to psychodrugs]. Gazz Med Ital 1976;135:236-251.
154. Fintelmann V. [Postoperative behavior of serum cholinesterase and other liver enzymes]. Med Klin 1973;68(24):809-815.

Niacin

SYNONYMS/COMMON NAMES/RELATED SUBSTANCES

- Anti-blacktongue factor, antipellagra factor, B-complex vitamin, benicot, Efacin, Endur-Acin, Enduramide, Hexopal, inositol hexaniacinate, inositol hexanicotinate, Niac, niacinamide, Niacor, Niaspan, Nicalex, nicamid, Nicamin, Nico-400, Nicobid, Nicolar, Nicotinex, nicosedine, Nico-Span, nicotinamide, nicotinic acid, nicotinic acid amide, nicotinic amide, nicotylamidum, Papulex, pellagra-preventing factor, 3-pyridinecarboxamide, Slo-Niacin, Tega-Span, Tri-B3, vitamin B_3, Wampocap.

CLINICAL BOTTOM LINE
Background

- Vitamin B_3 is composed of niacin (nicotinic acid) and its amide, niacinamide, and can be found in many foods, including yeast, meat, fish, milk, eggs, green vegetables, and cereal grains. Dietary tryptophan is also converted to niacin after ingestion. Vitamin B_3 is frequently found in combination with other B vitamins including thiamine, riboflavin, pantothenic acid, pyridoxine, cyanocobalamin, and folic acid.
- Niacin (not niacinamide) has been demonstrated through numerous clinical trials to be a relatively safe, inexpensive, and effective treatment for hyperlipidemia. Niacin elicits significant increases in high-density lipoproteins (HDLs) by up to 30% at doses ranging from 1 to 1.5 g daily, with greater effects than with other drugs (including hydroxy-methyl-glutarate–coenzyme A [HMG CoA] reductase inhibitors). Niacin also causes mild reductions in low-density lipoproteins (LDLs) by 5% to 20%, with stronger effects occurring at higher doses (3 to 4.5 g daily). Additional decreases in LDL levels can be achieved by combining niacin with an HMG-CoA reductase inhibitor or bile acid sequestrant.
- Preliminary evidence suggests that niacin therapy may reduce the incidence of atherosclerosis and secondary cardiovascular events. Niacin has been demonstrated to decrease lipoprotein(a) and fibrinogen levels, both of which have been associated with a decreased risk of coronary artery disease. However, niacin therapy has also been found to increase plasma homocysteine levels by up to 55%, possibly negating any positive effects on serum lipids and increasing the risk of adverse cardiac events.
- The Food and Drug Administration has approved niacin for use in treating vitamin B_3 deficiency (pellagra), which may be characterized by dermatitis, dementia, and diarrhea.
- Niacinamide (not niacin) has been investigated for the prevention and delay of onset of type 1 diabetes mellitus, possibly mediated through the protection and preservation of pancreatic islet beta cell function. Initial human research has been equivocal. Preliminary evidence suggests potential for niacinamide as a treatment for osteoarthritis.
- Inositol hexanicotinate, an ester of niacin and inositol, has also been shown through preliminary studies to share some beneficial effects with niacin, without causing the adverse effects associated with niacin administration.[1,2]

Scientific Evidence for Common/Studied Uses	Grade*
Hypercholesterolemia (niacin)	A
Pellagra (niacin)	A
Atherosclerosis (niacin)	B
Cardiovascular disease secondary prevention (niacin)	B
Diabetes mellitus type 1: preservation of pancreatic islet beta cell function (niacinamide)	C
Diabetes mellitus type 1: prevention (niacinamide)	C
Osteoarthritis (niacinamide)	C

*Key to grades: A: Strong scientific evidence for this use; B: Good scientific evidence for this use; C: Unclear scientific evidence for this use; D: Fair scientific evidence against this use (it may not work); F: Strong scientific evidence against this use (it likely does not work). For a more detailed explanation of efficacy criteria, see "Natural Standard Evidence-Based Validated Grading Rationale" in the Introduction.

Historial or Theoretical Uses That Lack Sufficient Evidence

- Acne vulgaris,[2,3] alcohol dependence,[4] anemia,[5] annular granuloma, anti-aging,[6] anxiety, arthritis,[7] Bell's palsy,[8] blood vessel spasm, bone marrow suppression, bullous pemphigoid, bursitis, cancer prevention,[9] cataract prevention,[10] central nervous system (CNS) disorders, chemotherapy-induced bone marrow suppression,[11] chloroquine-induced pruritus,[12] choleric diarrhea,[13-15] chronic diarrhea/hypokalemia (related to pancreatic islet beta cell dysplasia),[16] circulation improvement, confusion, depression,[17] dermatitis herpetiformis,[2] diabetes mellitus (type 1) treatment,[18] diabetes mellitus (type 2),[19] diagnostic test for schizophrenia,[20-27] dermatitis herpetiformis, digestion improvement, drug-induced hallucinations, dysmenorrhea,[28] edema, encephalopathy, erythema diutinum, erythema induratum, exfoliative glossitis, fetal loss,[29] glucose intolerance, granuloma annulare,[30] heart attack prevention, hearing loss,[31] helminthic infectrions,[32] hepatic encephalopathy,[33] human immunodeficiency virus (HIV) infection,[34-37] hyperkinesis, hyperlipoproteinemia, hypertension,[38] hypertriglyceridemia,[39] hypoglycemia,[40] hypothyroidism, impaired glucose tolerance, insomnia, intermittent claudication,[41-43] ischemia-reperfusion injury prevention,[44] kava-induced dermopathy,[45] leprosy, liver disease, low blood sugar, memory enhancement,[46] memory loss, Meniere's syndrome (endolymphatic hydrops),[47-49] migraine headache,[50] motion sickness, multiple sclerosis,[51] myocardial infarction prevention,[52,53] necrobiosis lipoidica,[54,55] nuclear cataract prevention,[56] orgasm improvement, peripheral vascular disease, photosensitivity, pregnancy, pregnancy complications, premenstrual headache prevention, premenstrual syndrome,[57] prostate cancer,[58] psoriasis,[2] psychosis, polymorphous light eruption,[59] Raynaud's phenomenon,[2,60-62] schizophrenia,[63-73] scleroderma,[2] sedative,[74] seizure,[74] skin disorders, sleep deprivation–induced dermatitis,[75] smoking cessation, tardive dyskinesia, taste disturbances, tinnitus,[76] tuberculosis, tumor detection,[77] ulcers,[78] vascular spasm, vertigo, vertical HIV transmission prevention.[79]

Expert Opinion and Folkloric Precedent

- Niacin deficiency, or pellagra, was common in the early 20th century. This syndrome affects the gastrointestinal tract, skin, and CNS and is characterized by dermatitis, dementia, and diarrhea. Pellagra is now virtually eliminated in the United States as a result of niacin fortification of foods, except in chronic alcoholism.

- Strong clinical data exist to support the safety and efficacy of niacin, alone or in combination with other medications, for the treatment of hypercholesterolemia and possibly the prevention of cardiovascular events and disease. Its use in the treatment of schizophrenia and osteoarthritis has also been explored, with few positive results.

Safety Summary

- **Likely safe:** When niacin is used orally in recommended doses under the supervision of a qualified health care provider. Periodic monitoring of liver function tests is recommended (every 3 months initially).[80-102] Homocysteine levels should also be monitored. The side effects profile of niacin at therapeutic doses may limit patient compliance, and 50% of subjects in some studies have discontinued use. Most patients experience initial flushing (>80%), which is likely prostaglandin-mediated. Doses are usually started low and gradually increased, to minimize facial flushing. Concomitant nonsteroidal anti-inflammatory drugs (NSAIDs) are often recommended to reduce flushing; antihistamines may also be effective. The flushing response often spontaneously diminishes after 1 to 2 weeks of therapy. Gastrointestinal distress may also occur, and taking niacin with food may decrease stomach upset and the risk of peptic ulcer. Immediate-release (crystalline) niacin may be preferable to sustained-release formulations, owing to reports of superior HDL effects and a lower incidence of hepatotoxicity and gastrointestinal side effects. Some sustained-release products, such as Niaspan, may be associated with a lower incidence of flushing than that noted for immediate-release niacin.

- **Possibly unsafe:** When used in higher than recommended doses without supervision of a qualified healthcare provider or when taken by persons with diabetes mellitus not monitored by a qualified healthcare provider. Niacin has been shown to raise serum glucose levels and may interfere with glycemic control.[80,81,90,92,100,103-113] Caution is also warranted in patients with gout. Niacin has been shown to increase plasma uric acid levels and may cause gout exacerbation.[80,81,103,105-109,112-122] Niacin may also be unsafe in patients with peptic ulcer disease and has been reported to induce or reactivate peptic ulcer disease at therapeutic doses.[82,123] There are concerns about the use of lipid-lowering agents in children, and close medical monitoring is merited in children with dyslipidemias.

- **Likely unsafe:** When used in patients with hepatic disease or dysfunction. Niacin has been implicated as a cause of hepatotoxicity.[80,83-88,91,93,95-99,101,102,124-129]

DOSING/TOXICOLOGY
General

- Recommended doses are based on those most commonly used in available trials, or on historical practice. However,

with natural products, the optimal doses needed to balance efficacy and safety often have not been determined. Formulations and preparation methods may vary from manufacturer to manufacturer, and from batch to batch of a specific product made by a single manufacturer. Because often the active components of a product are not known, standardization may not be possible, and the clinical effects of different brands may not be comparable.

Dosing: Adult (18 Years and Older)
Oral

- **Dietary intake:** The dietary reference intake established by the Food and Nutrition Board for niacin (in the form of niacin equivalents, 1 mg of niacin = 60 mg of tryptophan) ranges from 16 to 18 mg daily for adults, with an upper intake level set at 35 mg daily.[130]

- **Hypercholesterolemia:** Clinical trials have most commonly administered immediate-release (crystalline) niacin at doses of 500 to 3000 mg daily. Dosing may be initiated at 100 mg three times daily and increased gradually to an average of 1000 mg three times daily, as tolerated.[82,105,118,131-146] Significant increases in high-density lipoproteins (HDLs) by up to 30% may occur at doses ranging from 1 to 1.5 g daily.[109,122,140,147-150] Mild reductions in low-density lipoprotein (LDL) levels may occur at these doses, with stronger effects (up to 20%) occurring at higher doses (3 to 4.5 g daily).[109,149,150] or when used in combination with an HMG-CoA reductase inhibitor or bile acid sequestrant. The maximum recommended daily dose is 3 g, although a number of clinical trials have used 4.5 to 6 g daily.[81,106,113,131,151] Extended- or sustained-release niacin may be initiated at a dose of 500 mg daily (or nightly), titrated up to 1 to 2 g daily.

- **Atherosclerosis:** Niacin in doses of 1 to 4 g daily has been reported effective in the treatment of atherosclerosis.[115,152,153]

- **Cardiovascular disease:** Niacin at a dosage of 3 g daily has been evaluated in the treatment of cardiovascular disease.[53,154-156]

- **Pellagra:** The available evidence regarding dosing of niacin in the treatment of pellagra specifies dosing in the range of 50 mg to 1 g daily.[157-159]

- **Diabetes mellitus (type 1)—preservation of pancreatic islet beta cell function:** Niacinamide has been used for the preservation of pancreatic islet beta cell function in patients with newly diagnosed diabetes mellitus (type 1) at doses of 200 mg, up to 3 g daily.[160-166]

- *Notes on niacin dosing:* Taking niacin with food may decrease stomach upset and the risk of peptic ulcer.[125] Doses are usually started low and gradually increased, to decrease the adverse effect of facial flushing.[125,167,168] Concomitant NSAIDs are often recommended during the first 1 to 2 weeks to reduce flushing (likely prostaglandin-mediated): aspirin (325 mg), ibuprofen (200 mg), naproxen, and indomethacin have been shown to significantly reduce the incidence of flushing.[24,94,125,169,170-181] Use of an antihistamine 15 minutes prior to a niacin dose may also suppress cutaneous flushing.[114,182] The flushing response often spontaneously diminishes after 1 to 2 weeks of therapy. Extended-release niacin products tend to cause less flushing than immediate-release (crystalline) formulations but may be associated with an increased incidence of gastrointestinal upset, "transaminitis" (elevated liver enzymes [aminotransferases/transaminases]), and hepatitis.[91,93,96,129,138,167,183-186] Not all niacin products are equivalent, and patients switching from one product to another have reported an increase in adverse effects.[187]

Dosing: Pediatric (Younger Than 18 Years)

- *Note:* There are insufficient safety data available to recommend niacin in children in amounts greater than found in foods for any indication.
- **Diabetes mellitus (type 1) prevention:** Niacinamide has been used in children at daily doses of 150 to 300 mg per year of the child's age (maximum dose of 3 g daily), or 25 mg/kg daily, for the prevention of type 1 diabetes mellitus in "high-risk" individuals, with no reported serious adverse events.[188-190] However, safety has not been established.

Toxicology

- Animal studies have found the median lethal dose (LD_{50}) for niacin to be 4500 mg/kg in mice and 3500 mg/kg in both rats and guinea pigs.[191] The LD_{50} for niacinamide (niacinamide) subcutaneous injection was found to be 1.68 g/kg in rats, while that for niacin was found to be 5 g/kg, and the LD_{50} for orally administered niacin in mice and rats was found to be between 5 and 7 mg/kg.[192,193]
- Numerous case reports have been published concerning the development of hepatotoxicity, with manifestations ranging from elevated aminotransferase levels to jaundice, ascites, and hepatitis, after niacin therapy.[80,83-88,91,93,95-99,101,102,124-129]
- Two case reports have been published detailing the development of lactic acidosis after ingestion of sustained-release niacin, one involving concurrent ethanol ingestion.[194,195]

ADVERSE EFFECTS/PRECAUTIONS/CONTRAINDICATIONS
Allergy

- Known allergy/hypersensitivity to niacin or niacinamide or to any of their constituents is a contraindication.
- A case report has been published detailing the development of anaphylactic shock in a 32-year-old man taking prescribed niacin, 150 mg three times daily.[196]
- Anaphylactic shock necessitating the administration of epinephrine has been described in two women after receiving intravenous niacin subsequent to sensitization with oral niacin.[197]
- A 65-year-old man developed shock after the intravenous infusion of niacin, which was reversed with intramuscular epinephrine.[198]

Adverse Effects/Postmarket Surveillance

- **General:** Niacin therapy is associated with a high incidence of initial minor adverse events, including cutaneous flushing, pruritus, and gastrointestinal upset; however, these effects often diminish after 1 to 2 weeks of continued use.[81,103,108,115,132,138,151,199-206] A retrospective cohort study performed by the Department of Epidemiology and Biostatistics at the Harvard School of Public Health found that, in practice, the 1-year probability of niacin discontinuation due to adverse effects was 26.3%.[207] Another study found a withdrawal rate of up to 50% with niacin therapy.[208] More serious adverse effects have included the development of hepatotoxicity, activation of peptic ulcer disease, and the elevation of serum glucose and uric acid concentrations. Niacinamide is generally not associated with adverse events.[209] Only one clinical trial has implicated niacinamide as the cause of increased glucose intolerance.[210] Slow-release niacin products have been shown in comparative trials to be associated with a lower incidence of flushing than that with conventional niacin preparations.[186,211,212] However, some investigators have found that sustained-release niacin simply delays the appearance of cutaneous flushing and accentuates gastrointestinal/hepatic adverse effects.[103,213,214]
- **Dermatologic:** A majority of the subjects taking niacin experience cutaneous flushing and warm sensation (>80%), especially of the face, neck, and ears, on initial ingestion and with dose escalation. This flushing and cutaneous warmth usually are mild in severity but have been reported intolerable enough to cause withdrawal of up to 50% of participants in clinical trials.[81,82,100,107-109,113,115,124,131-135,138,151,154,199-206,208,215-223] Dry skin, pruritus, and cutaneous itching also are commonly experienced with niacin administration.[81,82,109,113,124,126,127,133,135,154,199,200,217,219,220,222,224,225] Concomitant NSAIDs are often recommended to reduce the incidence of flushing (likely prostaglandin-mediated): aspirin (325 mg), ibuprofen (200 mg), naproxen, and indomethacin have been shown to significantly reduce the incidence of flushing experienced after niacin administration.[24,94,125,169,170-181] Use of an antihistamine 15 minutes prior to a niacin dose may also suppress cutaneous flushing.[114,182] The flushing response often spontaneously diminishes after 1 to 2 weeks of therapy.
- **Neurologic/CNS:** Headache has been reported by a number of subjects participating in clinical trials Two 65-year-old men taking niacin for the treatment of dyslipidemias reported the development of severe dental and gingival pain after 5 months of therapy, which was relieved by the discontinuation of niacin.[226]
- **Gastrointestinal (general):** Dyspepsia, nausea, vomiting, and diarrhea are common complaints on the initiation of niacin therapy in clinical trials.[81,82,100,107,124,131,154,199,200,217-221,223] This discomfort is usually mild and subsides with continued use. The development or activation of peptic ulcer disease has also been reported in persons receiving niacin therapy.[82,123] In one subject taking 3 to 6 g of niacin daily as part of a 1961 prospective cohort study, an esophageal hiatal hernia developed during treatment that resolved on reduction of the niacin dose.[81]
- **Gastrointestinal (hepatic):** Niacin administration has been reported to cause significant but reversible elevation of serum transaminase concentrations in clinical trials.[81,82,89,92,93,99,100,102,103,105,107,108,112,113,115,118,120,121,124,126-128,185,200,217-222]

  Numerous case reports detail the development of hepatotoxicity, with manifestations including jaundice, hepatitis, ascites, and fulminant hepatic failure, after niacin administration. Periodic monitoring of liver function tests, especially transaminase values, is recommended.[80-102]
- **Endocrine (glucose levels):** Niacin can cause significant increases in blood glucose concentrations, glucose intolerance, and insulin resistance, necessitating monitoring of niacin therapy, especially in diabetic patients, as insulin or hypoglycemic medications may require dosing alterations.[40,80,81,90,92,100,103,104,107-110,113,116,117,124,126,135,200,202,224,227-229]

  Niacinamide was shown to cause a significant 23.6% increase in insulin resistance in a group of eight subjects at high risk for the development of diabetes mellitus (type 1).[210]
- **Endocrine (urate levels):** Elevated serum uric acid levels have been observed with niacin therapy.[80-82,103,105-109,112-122,126,135,168,200] The development of gout has been reported in some patients as a result of hyperuricemia following high doses of niacin.[82,114,119,154,168,223]
- **Endocrine (thyroid effects):** Hypothyroidism and its associated alterations in thyroid hormone and binding globulin tests have been observed with niacin therapy, including:

decreased total serum thyroxine, increased triiodothyronine, decreased thyroxine-binding globulin levels, and increased triiodothyronine uptake.[103,199,230-233]

- **Renal:** One case report has been published detailing the development of lactic acidosis after ingestion of sustained-release niacin.[194] A second case report details the development of lactic acidosis in a 44-year-old man on niacin therapy for hypercholesterolemia after the ingestion of a large quantity of wine.[195] Glycosuria and ketonuria were observed in five subjects receiving 1.5 g of niacin three times daily.[117] Glycosuria and impaired glucose tolerance have also been described in three patients taking 4 g of niacin daily for hypercholesterolemia.[229]

- **Hematologic:** There are three published case reports of patients who developed a reversible coagulopathy while taking sustained-release niacin.[234] O'Brien et al. reported the development of leukopenia in two patients taking niacin for the treatment of hypercholesterolemia.[232] Mild eosinophilia was observed in six of seven subjects given sustained-release niacin (1 g three times daily) for a period of 2 weeks.[235] Thrombocytopenia has been observed in clinical trials of niacin therapy.[132,135,232] Treatment with niacin has been shown to cause a significant decrease in plasma fibrinogen levels.[236,237]

- **Musculoskeletal:** Two cases of niacin-induced myopathy have been reported in a 67-year-old man and 87-year-old woman taking 1500 mg and 1000 mg, respectively, of niacin three times daily.[238] Litin et al. reported the development of myopathy in three patients taking niacin for the treatment of hypercholesterolemia.[239] Elevated creatine kinase levels have been reported in subjects taking niacin.[113,135,219,223]

Precautions/Warnings/Contraindications

- Use niacin cautiously in patients with peptic ulcer disease.[82,114,123,240]
- Use cautiously in patients with diabetes mellitus, as niacin may cause insulin resistance, hyperglycemia, and hyperinsulinemia.[40,80,81,90,92,100,103,104,107-110,113,116,117,124,126,135,200,202,224,227-229,240,241]
- Use niacin cautiously in patients with gout. Niacin therapy has been shown to increase serum uric acid levels.[80-82,103,105-109,112-122,126,135,168,200]
- Avoid in patients with hypersensitivity to niacin or niacinamide or to any of their components.
- Avoid in patients with hepatic dysfunction or liver disease. Niacin has been observed to cause elevations in liver enzymes.[81,82,89,92,93,99,100,102,103,105,107,108,112,113,115,118,120,121,124,126-128,185,200,217-222]
- Periodic monitoring of liver function tests, especially transaminase values, is recommended (every 3 months initially).[80-102]
- Periodic monitoring of homocysteine levels may be warranted.[242]

Pregnancy and Lactation

- Not recommended owing to lack of sufficient data.

INTERACTIONS
Niacin and Niacinamide/Drug Interactions

- **Antibiotics:** Antibiotics can lead to a decreased production of B vitamins through the destruction of normal gastrointestinal flora.
- **Anticonvulsants:** Concurrent administration of niacinamide with diazepam, carbamazepine, and sodium valproate has

been shown to potentiate their anticonvulsant action in animals.[243]

- **Aspirin/nonsteroidal anti-inflammatory drugs (NSAIDs):** Concurrent use of aspirin or other NSAIDs with niacin can reduce the tingling, itching, flushing, and warmth associated with oral niacin administration.[24,94,125,169-181]
- **Benzodiazepines:** Niacinamide has been shown to increase the solubility of diazepam *in vitro*, which may or may not affect the toxicity or efficacy of diazepam and possibly other benzodiazepines.[244]
- **Bile acid sequestrants:** Concomitant use of bile acid sequestrants and niacin may result in enhanced lipid-lowering effects; however, cholestyramine and colestipol may reduce niacin absorption and alter adverse effects.[115,223,245-256] A case report has been published detailing the development of myopathy in a 63-year-old woman concurrently receiving colestipol and niacin therapy.[239]
- **Clofibrate:** Concomitant administration of clofibrate and niacin has resulted in significant reductions in serum cholesterol and triglyceride levels, so the two may have additive effects when taken together.[52,53,156,257]
- **Estrogens, oral contraceptives:** Niacinamide has been shown to increase the solubility of 17β-estradiol *in vitro*, which may affect the toxicity or efficacy of 17β-estradiol and possibly other estrogens.[244] Oral contraceptives may stimulate tryptophan oxygenase, thereby increasing the amount of tryptophan that is converted into niacin; as a result, lower doses of niacin may be needed to achieve a specific clinical effect.[254,258]
- **Anticoagulant/antiplatelet agents:** In theory, niacin therapy may increase risk of bleeding. There are three published case reports of patients who developed a reversible coagulopathy while taking sustained-release niacin.[234] In addition, thrombocytopenia has been observed in clinical trials of niacin therapy.[132,135,232]
- **Ethanol:** Niacin and ethanol administered concomitantly may increase the risk of hepatotoxicity.[195] Niacin-induced flushing may be magnified by concomitant ingestion of alcohol.[259]
- **Ganglionic-blocking drugs:** Niacin theoretically may cause a potentiation of the hypotensive effects of ganglionic-blocking drugs if administered concurrently.
- **Gemfibrozil:** Concomitant administration of niacin and gemfibrozil may result in enhanced cholesterol-lowering effects of each agent.[146,246,257] A case report has been published detailing the development of myopathy in a 64-year-old woman concurrently receiving gemfibrozil and niacin.[239]
- **Griseofulvin:** Niacinamide has been shown to increase the solubility of griseofulvin *in vitro*, which may affect the toxicity or efficacy of griseofulvin *in vivo*.[244]
- **HMG-CoA reductase inhibitors (statins):** Concomitant administration of niacin and HMG-CoA reductase inhibitors may have additive effects on the reduction of serum cholesterol levels.[141,201,205,220,223,260-268] Concomitant administration of niacin and HMG-CoA reductase inhibitors may increase the risk of adverse effects, namely, myopathy and rhabdomyolysis, and patients should be monitored closely.[219,269-271] Both niacin and HMG-CoA reductase inhibitors may elevate values on liver function tests or result in hepatotoxicity, and transaminase levels should be monitored.
- **Hypertension agents:** Niacinamide may lower blood pressure values.
- **Insulin, oral hypoglycemic agents:** Niacin has been shown to increase blood glucose levels, which may necessitate dosing

adjustments for hypoglycemic agents.[40,80,81,90,92,100,103,104,107-110,113,116,117,124,126,135,200,202,224,228,229,240,241] The concomitant administration of niacinamide and insulin has been shown to lead to a reduction in insulin requirements in children newly diagnosed with type 1 diabetes mellitus.[161,163,164] However, niacinamide at a dose of 1.2 g/m^2 for 7 days caused no significant differences from baseline in insulin sensitivity, glucose disappearance rate, or acute insulin response to glucose in nine adult volunteers.[272]

- **Isoniazid:** Isoniazid inhibits the conversion of tryptophan to niacin and may induce pellagra in poorly nourished patients.[254,273,274]
- **Neomycin:** Concomitant use of neomycin and niacin may result in additive effects on the lowering of lipoprotein(a), low-density lipoprotein (LDL), and total cholesterol levels.[136,275]
- **Nicotine:** The risk of flushing and dizziness may be increased when nicotine products are used with niacin (theoretical).
- **Pantothenic acid:** The results of one crossover study in adolescents found that supplementation with pantothenic acid increased urinary secretion of niacin, which may have implications for the concomitant use of the two B-complex vitamins.[276]
- **Probucol:** Concomitant administration of niacin and probucol results in enhanced cholesterol-lowering effects, which may allow lower doses of each medication to be used.[277]
- **Progestins:** Niacinamide has been shown to increase the solubility of progesterone *in vitro*, which may affect the toxicity or efficacy of progesterone *in vivo*.[244]
- **Pyrazinamide:** The administration of a diet rich in pyrazinamide has been shown to significantly increase the metabolism of tryptophan to niacin in rats, which may have implications for the concurrent use of niacin and pyrazinamide in humans.[278]
- **Testosterone:** Niacinamide has been shown to increase the solubility of testosterone *in vitro*, which may affect the toxicity or efficacy of testosterone *in vivo*.[244]
- **Thyroid agents:** Decreases in total serum thyroxine and free thyroxine levels and increases in triiodothyronine uptake ratios have been reported after niacin therapy.[103,199,230-233]

Niacin and Niacinamide/Herb/Supplement Interactions

- **Antioxidants:** Antioxidants may blunt the' beneficial effects of niacin on cholesterol levels and heart disease, possibly by interfering with its effects on proteins involved in the formation of high-density lipoproteins (HDLs).[279-281] In a 2001 study, arteriographic measurements of coronary atherosclerotic plaques were conducted after 3 years of treatment with one of four regimens: a combination of niacin plus simvastatin; niacin plus simvastatin plus a mixed antioxidant regimen; antioxidants alone; or placebo.[260] Niacin plus simvastatin was significantly superior to placebo (average stenosis progression by 0.4% and 3.6%, respectively). However, the addition of antioxidants to this regimen *reduced* this benefit to 0.7%, suggesting possible interference by antioxidants. Critics have suggested that this study may not have been adequately powered to detect between-group differences, and these results may thus be meaningless.[282] However, in other research, concomitant administration of niacin and vitamin A, along with vitamin E, has been shown to have more marked effects on plasma cholesterol levels than those noted with niacin alone.[283] Vitamin E in combination with colestipol and niacin has also been associated with added benefits on delaying progression of coronary

atherosclerotic lesions.[284] The question of these potential interactions remains unresolved.

- **Estrogenic herbs and supplements:** Interactions may theoretically occur between estrogens and niacin or niacinamide, but it is not clear if these interactions also may occur with herbs or supplements with phytoestrogenic constituents (chemical components that possess estrogen receptor agonist or antagonist properties, or exert estrogen-like effects clinically, but may not be structurally similar to estrogens). Niacinamide has been shown to increase the solubility of 17β-estradiol *in vitro*, which may affect the toxicity or efficacy of 17β-estradiol and possibly other estrogens.[244] Oral contraceptive drugs may stimulate tryptophan oxygenase, thereby increasing the amount of tryptophan that is converted into niacin; as a result, lower doses of niacin may be necessary to achieve a specific clinical effect.[254,258]
- **Grapeseed proanthocyanidin:** Concomitant administration of chromium polynicotinate (niacin-bound chromium) and grapeseed proanthocyanidin has been shown to result in greater improvements in the lipid profile of hypercholesterolemic subjects than with either agent alone, suggesting an additive effect.[285]
- **Hepatotoxic agents:** Theoretically, concomitant use of niacin/niacinamide and other herbs that elevate transaminases or elicit hepatotoxicity may have additive hepatotoxic effects with niacin. Examples are borage, chaparral (*Larrea tridentate* Coville), kava (*Piper methysticum* G. Forst), valerian (*Valeriana officinalis* L.), and uva ursi (*Arctostaphylos uva-ursi* Spreng).
- **Hypoglycemic/hyperglycemic herbs and supplements:** Niacin has been shown to increase blood glucose levels.[40,80,81,90,92,100,103,104,107-110,113,116,117,124,126,135,200,202,224,228,229,240,241]
- **Anticoagulant/antiplatelet herbs and supplements:** In theory, niacin therapy may increase risk of bleeding. There are three published case reports of patients who developed a reversible coagulopathy while taking sustained-release niacin.[234] In addition, thrombocytopenia has been observed in clinical trials of niacin therapy.[132,135,232]
- **Herbs and supplements with progestin-like properties:** Niacinamide has been shown to increase the solubility of progesterone *in vitro*, which may affect the toxicity or efficacy of progesterone *in vivo*.[244]
- **Salicylate-containing herbs:** Concurrent use of aspirin has been shown to reduce the tingling, itching, flushing, and warmth associated with oral niacin administration,[24,94,125,169-181] an effect that may also result from use of salicylate-containing herbs. However, levels of salicylates in herbs may vary or be too low to achieve desired clinical effects.
- **Sitosterols:** Concomitant administration of niacin and a 20% suspension of β-sitosterol and dihydro-β-sitosterol resulted in an additive decrease in plasma cholesterol, as compared with each agent alone.[199]
- **Thyroid active agents:** Decreases in total serum thyroxine and free thyroxine levels and increases in triiodothyronine uptake ratios have been reported after niacin therapy.[103,199,230-233]
- **Vitamin E, vitamin A:** Concomitant administration of vitamin E and niacin,[286] or of these two agents plus vitamin A,[283] may have additive effects on the lowering of serum cholesterol levels. However, a number of studies have demonstrated no benefits of antioxidants (vitamin E) on cardiovascular outcomes.[287-290] In addition, it has been suggested that antioxidants may blunt the beneficial effects of niacin on cholesterol levels and heart disease, possibly by interfering

N

with its effects on proteins involved in the formation of high-density lipoproteins (HDLs).[279-281]

- **Vitamin E:** Concomitant administration of niacin and vitamin E, along with vitamin A, has been shown to have more marked effects on lowering plasma cholesterol than those noted with niacin alone.[283] Concomitant administration of vitamin E and niacin may have additive effects on the lowering of serum cholesterol.[286]
- **Zinc sulfate:** Oral administration of zinc sulfate to alcoholics with pellagra has been shown to increase the urinary excretion of niacin metabolites, suggesting its ability to affect the metabolism of tryptophan to niacin, having possible implications for the concurrent administration of zinc and niacin.[291]
- **Vitamin A:** Niacin in combination with vitamin A is suggested to ameliorate dysgeusia (loss of taste/metallic taste).[292]

Niacin and Niacinamide/Food Interactions

- **Hot beverages:** Hot beverages, when ingested concomitantly with niacin, can magnify niacin-induced flushing.[259]

Niacin and Niacinamide/Lab Interactions

- **Creatine kinase:** Niacin therapy has been associated with increases in creatine kinase levels.[113,135,219,223]
- **Fibrinogen levels:** Treatment with niacin has been shown to cause a significant decrease in plasma fibrinogen levels.[237,237]
- **Glucose:** Niacin has been shown to increase blood glucose levels.[40,80,81,90,92,100,103,104,107-110,113,116,117,124,126,135,200,202,224,228,229,293]
- **Homocysteine levels:** Concomitant administration of colestipol and niacin therapy as part of the Cholesterol Lowering Atherosclerosis Study (CLAS) resulted in increased homocysteine levels, which may also be attributable to niacin therapy alone.[249] An analysis of 52 participants in the Arterial Disease Multiple Intervention Trial (ADMIT) also showed niacin therapy to cause a 55% increase in plasma homocysteine levels from baseline ($p = 0.001$).[242]
- **Liver function tests:** Niacin and niacinamide administration can increase serum bilirubin, alanine aminotransferase, aspartate aminotransferase, and lactate dehydrogenase concentrations.[81,82,89,92,93,99,100,102,103,105,107,108,112,113,115,118,120,121,124,126-128,185,200,217-222]
- **Plasma uric acid:** Niacin therapy has been shown to increase plasma uric acid levels, possibly by competing with uric acid for excretion.[80-82,103,105-109,112-122,126,135,168,200]
- **Prothrombin time:** Niacin therapy can lead to clotting factor synthesis deficiency and coagulopathy, which may result in prolonged prothrombin times.[234]
- **Thyroid function tests:** Decreases in total serum thyroxine and free thyroxine levels and increases in triiodothyronine uptake ratios have been reported after niacin therapy.[103,199,230-233]

MECHANISM OF ACTION

Pharmacology

- **Metabolism:** Niacin is metabolized to form niacinamide adenine dinucleotide (NAD), niacinamide adenine dinucleotide phosphate (NADP), and nicotinuric acid, coenzymes necessary for cell function.[209,259,294-296]
- **Cholesterol effects:** Treatment with niacin results in significant increases in high-density lipoproteins (HDLs) by up to 30%, at doses ranging from 1 to 1.5 g daily.[109,122,140,147-150] Multiple mechanisms have been suggested on the basis of results of clinical research, including delayed clearance of

HDL and decreased cholesterol transfer from HDL to very-low-density lipoprotein (VLDL).

- Niacin has also been associated with reductions in low-density lipoprotein (LDL) levels by 5% to 20%, with stronger effects generally occurring at higher doses than required for raising HDL levels (up to 3 to 4.5 g daily).[109,149,150] Suggested mechanisms include decreased hepatic synthesis of VLDL, the precursor of LDL, which may occur as a result of niacin-induced reductions in free fatty acids (FFAs) mobilized from peripheral adipose tissues and lower plasma FFA concentrations.[104,297-305] Reductions in hepatic cholesterol synthesis have also been demonstrated in human studies.[111,150,298] Niacin exerts additive effects on LDL lowering when used concomitantly with HMG-CoA reductase inhibitors or bile acid sequestrants.
- Niacin therapy has been found to change the composition of LDL and VLDL fractions toward potentially less atherogenic particles, poorer in cholesteryl esters, as shown through density-gradient ultracentrifugation of blood samples from eight subjects with primary hypertriglyceridemia before and after 6 weeks of niacin.[306] Treatment with niacin has also been shown through a randomized, controlled trial to cause a significant conversion of LDL subclass patterns.[307] Treatment with daily oral niacin has been shown to significantly decrease serum concentrations of apolipoproteins C-I, C-II, C-III, and E, which correlated with a reduction in VLDL triglyceride levels.[308,309] An early study of niacin administration in five healthy adults demonstrated a reduction in the amount of lipids transferred by VLDL and LDL associated with the administration of 3 g of niacin daily and a significant reduction in plasma cholesterol by 15%.[149] Niacin 3 g daily was also found to lower serum levels of chylomicrons, VLDL, and LDL, with the most pronounced effects in patients with severe hyperlipoproteinemia.[310] Niacin (1 g three times daily) for 5 weeks significantly decreased the triglyceride content of VLDL and significantly decreased the transport of VLDL triglycerides, by 21%.[150] Treatment with niacin has also been shown to decrease serum triglyceride levels by reducing the size of VLDL particles.[308]
- Niacin has been found to decrease the plasma concentration of nonesterified fatty acids.[104,297,300,301-305] The continuous infusion of 2 g of niacin over 11 hours at night resulted in significant decreases in plasma triglyceride levels not seen when the same infusion was administered during the day.[311]
- Plasma concentrations of lipoprotein(a) and apolipoproteins are also affected by niacin administration. At a dose of 4 g daily for 6 weeks, niacin significantly decreased lipoprotein(a) levels by 38% in 31 patients with hyperlipidemia.[312] Combination treatment with niacin and colestipol for 1 year, as part of a randomized, controlled trial, was shown to increase removal or decrease synthesis of apolipoprotein B.[245] Niacin therapy (1 g three times daily), when added to neomycin (2 g daily), led to a significant decrease in lipoprotein(a) levels.[275] The administration of 1 g of niacin three times daily has been shown to cause a significant 36.4% decrease in plasma lipoprotein(a) levels.[313] Concomitant administration of niacin and simvastatin has been shown to increase lipoprotein(a) independently of phospholipid transfer protein.[279]
- Niacin has been shown to increase lipoprotein lipase activity of adipose tissue in an animal study.[314] *In vitro* study has shown niacin to increase apoprotein A-I levels in culture medium without increasing the *de novo* synthesis of apoprotein A-I; rather, it reduces HDL protein uptake and HDL

apoprotein A-I uptake by hepatic cells.[315] The subcutaneous administration of a single 250-mg/kg dose of niacin in rats inhibited normal fasting epinephrine and norepinephrine and also theophylline-induced FFA release.[316]

- By contrast, in a 1959 study, niacinamide was reported to have no effect on serum cholesterol or lipid levels in a crossover trial in 50 human subjects.[317]
- In an analysis of blood samples from hypercholesterolemic patients who received 1000 to 2000 mg of niacin or placebo for 12 weeks, niacin was found to increase HDL cholesterol and decrease LDL as well as VLDL in a dose-dependent manner relative to placebo; to increase large HDL particles (H5 and H4, corresponding to the HDL[2ab] fraction) without having a net effect on small HDL particles (H3, H2, and H1, corresponding to the HDL[3abc] fraction); and to decrease smaller, denser LDL particles (L1 and L2) and increase the larger, more buoyant L3 subclass.[318] The inhibitory effect of niacin on VLDL was evident on the larger particles (V6, V5, V4, and V3 subclasses) rather than on the smaller ones (V2 and V1). These results suggest that niacin extended release produces a beneficial effect on lipoprotein subclasses, specifically decreasing the more atherogenic small, dense LDL particles and enhancing the cardioprotective large HDL particles.
- **Cardiovascular effects:** Niacin treatment has been shown to significantly decrease fibrinogen levels in subjects with peripheral artery disease after 1 year of therapy, which may produce favorable cardiovascular outcomes.[155,237] A significant decrease in prothrombin F1.2 has also been observed.[155] Niacin significantly inhibited beta-oxidation during pre-ischemia and reperfusion, prevented the degradation of membrane phospholipids, reduced free fatty acid accumulation, and stimulated glycolysis in arrested-reperfused pig hearts.[319] Animal experiments suggest that niacin administration causes a decrease in serum cholesterol and prevents experimentally induced atherosclerosis.[320] Niacin oral treatment has also been associated with an increase in exogenous glucose utilization by cardiac tissue, as seen in five healthy volunteers.[321]
- **Flushing/vasodilation:** Niacin administration initially causes cutaneous flushing in most subjects (>80%). Multiple explanations have been postulated, primarily regarding the release of prostaglandins and local vasodilation. Niacin inhibits the formation of thromboxane A_2 in rat platelets, while increasing the synthesis of prostaglandins PGE_2 and $PGE_{2\alpha}$ and inhibiting collagen-induced platelet aggregation.[322] *In vitro* and *in vivo* research has demonstrated niacin-induced flush to be caused by an increase in the formation of prostaglandins and the subsequent formation of cyclic adenosine monophosphate (cAMP).[169,170] In humans, the administration of oral niacin has been shown to increase the release of PGD_2, prostacyclins, $PGF_{2\alpha}$, and 6-keto-$PGF_{1\alpha}$, which initially does not persist with continued treatment, as shown through urinary analysis in eight women taking rapidly increasing oral doses of niacin.[323-325] Niacin administration to seven healthy fasting volunteers led to increased forearm blood flow, which was inhibited by the administration of indomethacin, suggesting a role of prostaglandins in this phenomenon.[179] The cutaneous flushing was found to be due not to a change in metabolic rate but rather to local vasodilatory action in the skin.[326] The tolerance to flushing observed in subjects after continued use of niacin appears to be due to a reduction in the release of PGD_2 with continued niacin administration.[327]

- **Antioxidant:** Niacinamide has been shown to decrease recombinant interleukin-1β–induced nitrite production in dose-dependent fashion *in vitro*, possibly through the inhibition of the inducible form of nitric oxide synthase.[328] The addition of niacinamide has been shown to inhibit the release of reactive oxygen intermediates from a xanthine oxidase/hypoxanthine system *in vitro*, protecting rat pancreatic islet beta cells from oxidative damage.[329]
- **Pancreatic islet beta cell protection:** Niacinamide has been reported in numerous *in vitro* and animal studies to have significant protective effects on pancreatic islet beta cell function, suggesting a role in the prevention or delay of onset of diabetes mellitus (type 1). An intravenous injection of niacinamide (7.5 mM/kg) immediately prior to a dose of alloxan (known to cause diabetes mellitus in rats) prevented the development of diabetes in 68% of the animals studied.[330] Niacin (2.5 mM/kg) had similar protective effects when administered 1 hour prior to the alloxan dose. Similar protection has been seen with the intraperitoneal injection of 500 mg/kg of niacinamide 15 minutes prior to a dose of streptozotocin (known to induce diabetes).[331] Other studies have shown intraperitoneal niacinamide to protect mouse pancreatic islet beta cells from streptozotocin-induced damage responsible for the development of diabetes, possibly through an increase in NAD levels.[332] At a concentration of 20 mM, niacinamide inhibited cytokine-induced expression of major histocompatibility complex (MHC) class II molecules on mouse pancreatic islet beta cells.[333] Niacinamide administered by injection at a dosage of 500 mg/kg also increased the cell replication rate of transplanted pancreatic islet beta cells in mice.[334] Niacinamide has been reported to decrease beta cell inflammation[335] and to significantly increase C-peptide release in subjects with diabetes mellitus (type 2).[19,162,336] Niacinamide has been shown to partially reverse the inhibition of glucose-induced insulin release of pancreatic islet beta cells caused by interleukin-1β *in vitro*.[337] It has been found that niacinamide inhibits poly(ADP-ribose) polymerase; *in vitro* studies examining the effect of niacinamide on single-strand DNA breaks caused by streptozotocin and alloxan have found that niacinamide increases the number of single-strand breaks induced by streptozotocin, consistent with the inhibition of poly(ADP-ribose) synthetase; niacinamide also reduces the number of single-strand DNA breaks induced by alloxan, consistent with the scavenging of hydroxyl free radicals induced by alloxan.[338,339] Niacinamide has been shown to induce beta cell differentiation in porcine islet-like cell clusters *in vitro*, leading to an increased number of insulin-positive cells.[340] Niacinamide was shown to block nitric oxide toxicity on beta cells *in vitro*.[341] Niacinamide inhibits ADP-ribosylation and prevents beta cell lysis due to nitric oxide toxicity.[342] The addition of niacinamide has been shown to inhibit the release of reactive oxygen intermediates from a xanthine oxidase/hypoxanthine system *in vitro*, protecting rat pancreatic islet beta cells from oxidative damage.[329]
- **Other effects:** Niacin has demonstrated inhibition of lipolysis *in vitro*.[343] Niacin has been shown to inhibit stimulated adenyl cyclase activity *in vitro* and to prevent the accumulation of ^{3}H-labeled cAMP in fat cells.[343] Intravenous niacin administration caused a significant increase in plasma cortisol and glucagons levels in eight healthy male volunteers.[344] *In vitro*, niacinamide displayed low-potency inhibition of the ^{3}H-diazepam binding site.[74] Niacin, at doses of 50 mg daily, causes a significant increase in lymphocyte NAD$^+$ levels, as

shown through a randomized, controlled study in 21 healthy smoking men.[345] Niacin was found to produce insulin resistance at a dose of 2 g daily in a group of 11 healthy male volunteers after 2 weeks of therapy.[277]

Pharmacodynamics/Kinetics

- **Absorption:** Esters of niacin, pentaerythritoltetranicotinate and meso-inositol hexanicotinate, are readily absorbed from the gastric mucosa, causing a significant increase in serum niacin levels 4 hours after ingestion, as shown in rats, dogs, and humans.[346,347]
- **Bioavailability:** The bioavailability of unchanged niacin from a single 500-mg dose was 1% from two slow-release formulations and 25% from a rapid-release formulation tested in a randomized crossover study in seven healthy volunteers.[213]
- **Distribution:** A 1-g single oral dose of niacin was shown to result in peak plasma levels at 60 minutes after ingestion and decrease to normal at 6 hours after ingestion.[300,348] Niacinamide is reported to have a plasma half-life of up to 9 hours; peak plasma levels are attained within 10 minutes of niacinamide ingestion, and metabolites of niacinamide are detected in the urine after 30 minutes.[209]
- **Metabolism:** Niacin is metabolized to form niacinamide-adenine dinucleotide (NAD) and nicotinuric acid; NAD is then catabolized to release niacinamide. NAD is a coenzyme involved in tissue respiration and is required for DNA synthesis and for the activity of poly(ADP-ribose) polymerase.[259,294-296,349] Niacinamide degradation has been determined to follow a third-order rate equation *in vitro*.[350]
- **Elimination:** Niacin and niacinamide and their metabolites are renally excreted. Urinary excretion of trigonelline, methyl niacinamide, niacin, niacinamide 2-pyridone, and nicotinuric acid was shown to peak within the first 7 hours of niacinamide or niacin administration in three healthy volunteers, with excretion of methyl niacinamide, niacinamide 2-pyridone, and niacinamide being greater after ingestion of 1 g of niacinamide and excretion of niacin and trigonelline being greater after ingestion of 1 g of niacin.[351,352] Regular niacin preparations result in higher 24-hour urinary concentrations of nicotinuric acid, the metabolite of niacin excreted in the urine, than those noted with controlled-release preparations.[353] A study of urinary excretion after both immediate- and sustained-release niacin found that the renal excretion of nicotinuric acid is four times greater with the ingestion of immediate-release niacin than with ingestion of sustained-release niacin, suggesting a difference in metabolism for these compounds.
- **Other:** Animal study has found that continuous duodenal infusion of niacin has significantly greater lipid-lowering effects than those noted for either oral or continuous infusion of equivalent doses, suggesting that the site of action of niacin may be located presystemically.[354]

HISTORY

- Niacin was reported in 1955 to have applications for the treatment of hyperlipidemic states; subsequently, a landmark study was conducted from 1966 to 1975, the Coronary Drug Project.[154,355,356] Since that time, there have been multiple controlled trials of niacin alone and in combination with other medications for hyperlipidemia. Both immediate-release and sustained-release forms have been investigated.
- Niacinamide, a derivative of niacin, was reportedly isolated in the early 1930s through hematologic study of coenzymes in horses. Investigations into the application of niacinamide

for arthritis began in the 1940s and 1950s by a Connecticut physician, who reported improved joint flexibility in several hundred patients. Although the use of niacinamide for this indication has not proven fruitful, there is promising clinical evidence that niacinamide may be useful for the prevention of diabetes mellitus (type 1) and the preservation of pancreatic islet beta cell function in newly diagnosed diabetics.

REVIEW OF THE EVIDENCE: DISCUSSION
Hypercholesterolemia (Niacin)
Summary

- Multiple trials have found that niacin (not niacinamide) administration causes significant decreases in serum cholesterol.[81,82,112,216,224,246,317,357-362] Treatment with immediate-release (crystalline) niacin results in significant increases in high-density lipoproteins (HDLs) by up to 30%, at doses ranging from 1 to 1.5 g daily, and appears to have greater effects on HDL levels than those achieved with other therapies including HMG-CoA reductase inhibitors (statins).[109,122,140,147-150] Niacin also causes reductions in low-density lipoprotein (LDL) levels by 5% to 20%, with stronger effects occurring at doses higher than required for raising HDL (up to 3 to 4.5 g daily).[109,149,150] Sustained-release formulations may elicit effects on HDL levels at 500 mg daily, and on LDL levels at 1000 mg daily. According to the American Heart Association and the National Cholesterol Education Program (NCEP) Adult Treatment Panel II (ATP II) recommendations for cholesterol management, niacin can be included in the first line of treatment for elevated LDL cholesterol.[363] The American Society of Health-System Pharmacists (ASHP) supports the use of niacin for the treatment of dyslipidemias in adults, if done under the direct supervision of a healthcare professional.[167] Despite its high associated incidence of mild adverse events, available evidence supports the use of niacin in the treatment of hypercholesterolemia as a monotherapy, and additional decreases in LDL levels may be achieved by combining niacin with an HMG-CoA reductase inhibitor or bile acid sequestrant. Immediate-release niacin may be preferable to sustained-release formulations, owing to reports of superior HDL effects and a lower incidence of hepatotoxicity, hyperglycemia, and gastrointestinal side effects.[91,93,96,129,138,167,183-186] Some sustained-release products, such as Niaspan, may be associated with a lower incidence of flushing than that with immediate-release niacin.[107,118,138,139,220] Notably, niacin therapy has also been shown to increase plasma homocysteine levels by up to 55% from baseline, possibly negating any positive effects on serum lipids and increasing the risk of adverse cardiac events.[242,249]

Systematic Review

- A systematic review conducted by Schectman et al. identified three clinical trials involving niacin monotherapy (two were dosing studies) and three clinical trials comparing and/or combining niacin with an HMG-CoA reductase inhibitor (pravastatin, fluvastatin, lovastatin), through a MEDLINE search of literature published between 1975 and 1995.[364] Results from the three niacin monotherapy trials indicated that niacin in doses of 500 mg to 3 g daily is effective at decreasing LDL cholesterol and increasing HDL cholesterol levels.[138,185,222] The authors also concluded that niacin and HMG-CoA reductase inhibitors demonstrate an additive effect equal to the sum of their individual effects on LDL cholesterol levels.[219,263,267]

Review of the Evidence: Niacin

Condition Treated*	Study Design	Author, Year	N[†]	SS[†]	Study Quality[‡]	Magnitude of Benefit	ARR[†]	NNT[†]	Comments
Hypercholesterolemia	Systematic review	Schectman[364] 1996	6 studies	NA	NA	Large	NA	NA	3 trials of niacin monotherapy demonstrated efficacy; 3 trials combining niacin with statins found additive effects.
Hypercholesterolemia (monotherapy)	RCT	Elam[105] 2000	468	Yes	5	Large	NA	NA	3 g of niacin daily associated with significant increase in HDL and decrease in LDL and triglyceride levels vs. placebo.
Hypercholesterolemia (monotherapy)	RCT	Morgan[212,365] 1996, 1998	122	Yes	4	Large	NA	NA	Niaspan 1 g vs. 2 g vs. placebo. Niaspan lowered LDL and increased HDL levels at both doses vs. placebo, with few adverse effects.
Hypercholesterolemia (monotherapy)	RCT	Keenan[222] 1991	201	Yes	4	Large	NA	NA	1.5 g of niacin daily associated with significant increases in serum HDL vs. placebo. Greater effects in older patients (ages 50-70 years), but small subgroup sample sizes.
Hypercholesterolemia (monotherapy)	RCT	Goldberg[108] 2000	132	Yes	3	Large	NA	NA	Niaspan (up to 3 g/day) for 25 weeks associated with significant improvement in plasma lipids vs. placebo.
Hypercholesterolemia (monotherapy)	RCT, crossover	Aronov[217] 1996	89	Yes	3	Medium	NA	NA	Wax-matrix sustained-release niacin (1.5-2 g/day vs. placebo). Niacin associated with significant decreases in TC and LDL.
Hypercholesterolemia (monotherapy)	RCT	Grundy[371] 2002	143	Yes	2	Small	NA	NA	Niacin significantly improved HDL and triglyceride levels vs. placebo over 16 weeks.
Hypercholesterolemia (combination therapy)	RCT	Davignon[219] 1994	158	Yes	4	Large	NA	NA	Niacin plus pravastatin was superior to either agent alone in raising HDL and lowering LDL. Pravastatin monotherapy lowered LDL levels better than niacin.
Hypercholesterolemia (combination therapy)	RCT	Vacek[267] 1995	25	Yes	4	Large	NA	NA	Niacin plus lovastatin was superior to either agent alone in lowering TC and LDL.
Hypercholesterolemia	RCT, open-label, multicenter	Capuzzi[387] 2003	270	Yes	3	Medium	NA	NA	Rosuvastatin alone superior to extended-release niacin for LDL reduction and better tolerated. Additive effect of niacin for HDL lowering.
Hypercholesterolemia	RCT, comparison study	Bays[372] 2003	315	Yes	3	Small	NA	NA	Combination of niacin/lovastatin equal or superior to other statins. But no lovastatin monotherapy arm, so true additive effects of niacin are unclear.
Hypercholesterolemia	RCT	Hunninghake[373] 2003	237	Yes	3	Medium	NA	NA	Combination of niacin/statin more effective than niacin monotherapy or statin monotherapy for improving LDL, HDL, and triglycerides.
Hypercholesterolemia (dosing study)	Randomized dosing trial, no placebo	Knopp[138] 1985	71	Yes	4	Large	NA	NA	Immediate-release and sustained-release niacin both associated with significant reductions in LDL and TC. More gastrointestinal adverse effects seen with sustained-release niacin.
Hypercholesterolemia (dosing study)	Randomized dosing trial, placebo-controlled	Goldberg[107] 1998	131	Yes	3	Large	NA	NA	Dose escalation study of sustained-release niacin found HDL increases at 500 mg daily and LDL decreases at 1000 mg daily.

N

Continued

Review of the Evidence: Niacin—*cont'd*

Condition Treated*	Study Design	Author, Year	N[†]	SS[†]	Study Quality[‡]	Magnitude of Benefit	ARR[†]	NNT[†]	Comments
Hypercholesterolemia (dosing study)	Randomized dosing trial, no placebo	McKenney[185] 1994	46	Yes	3	Large	NA	NA	Sustained-release niacin associated with superior LDL reductions, inferior HDL increases, less flushing, and greater hepatotoxicity compared with immediate-release niacin.
Atherosclerosis (monotherapy)	RCT	Blankenhorn[247-249,379] 1987 (2 studies), 1991, 1993	162	Yes	3	Medium	NA	NA	Niacin plus colestipol combination therapy associated with significant increase in HDL, decrease in LDL, decrease in disease progression, and increased perceptible improvement vs. placebo.
Atherosclerosis (monotherapy)	RCT	Brown[115,186] 1990, 1997	146	Yes	3	Small	NA	NA	Niacin (4 g daily) plus colestipol (30 g daily) vs. lovastatin (40 mg daily) plus colestipol (30 g daily) vs. placebo. Drug treatment groups yielded significant reductions in disease progression vs. placebo.
Atherosclerosis (combination therapy)	RCT	Brown[260] 2001	160	Yes	3	Large	NA	NA	Subgroup analysis of larger study. Combination niacin plus simvastatin associated with greater HDL increases than in controls.
Atherosclerosis, cardiovascular disease (combination therapy)	RCT	Personius[380] 1998	143	Yes	3	Large	NA	NA	Fewer cardiovascular events seen with combination of niacin, cholestyramine, and gemfibrozil than with cholestyramine alone.
Cardiovascular disease	Systematic review	Bucher[385] 1999	59 studies; 2 studies on niacin	No	NA	None	NA	NA	Review of mortality and all cholesterol-lowering treatments. Included two trials of niacin therapy. Pooled results showed a nonsignificant risk ratio of 0.95 for cardiac mortality, 0.96 for all-cause mortality, and 0.9 for noncardiac mortality.
Cardiovascular disease (monotherapy)	RCT	Anonymous[154] 1975 Canner[353] 1986 Berge[356] 1991	8341 1119 in niacin group	Yes	4	Medium	NA	NA	Coronary Drug Project: 1119 subjects randomized to niacin 3 g daily. At 15 years, significant decrease in mortality seen with niacin.
Cardiovascular disease, hypercholesterolemia (monotherapy)	RCT	Schoch[100] 1968	570	Yes	3	Large	NA	NA	4 g of niacin daily over 5 years associated with 20% decrease in TC, and no significant effect on mortality.
Cardiovascular disease (combination therapy)	RCT	Rosenhamer[156] 1980	555	No	2	Large	NA	NA	Niacin plus clofibrate plus cardiac diet compared with diet alone. Drug therapy yielded nonsignificant 19% reduction in cardiac deaths after 5 years. 79% dropout rate.
Type 1 diabetes mellitus: preservation of beta cell function	Meta-analysis	Pozzilli[336] 1996	10 studies; 211 subjects	Yes	NA	Medium	NA	NA	Significantly higher baseline C-peptide levels in niacinamide-treated patients than in controls at 1 year.
Type 1 diabetes mellitus: preservation of beta cell function	RCT	Vague[166] 1989	26	Yes	3	Medium	NA	NA	Niacinamide treatment resulted in significant increase in C-peptide levels and decrease in HbA$_{1c}$ levels vs. placebo.
Type 1 diabetes mellitus: preservation of beta cell function	RCT	Lewis[394] 1992	49	No	2	None	NA	NA	No changes in insulin requirements or HbA$_{1c}$ or C-peptide levels after 1 year of niacinamide therapy vs. placebo. Study may not have been adequately powered.

Review of the Evidence: Niacin—cont'd

Condition Treated*	Study Design	Author, Year	N[†]	SS[†]	Study Quality[‡]	Magnitude of Benefit	ARR[†]	NNT[†]	Comments
Type 1 diabetes mellitus: preservation of beta cell function	RCT	Ilkova[393] 1991	25	No	2	None	NA	NA	No changes in insulin requirements or HbA$_{1c}$ or C-peptide levels after 1 year of niacinamide therapy vs. placebo. Study may not have been adequately powered.
Type 1 diabetes mellitus: preservation of beta cell function	RCT	Chase[160] 1990	35	No	2	None	NA	NA	No changes in HbA$_{1c}$ or C-peptide levels after 1 year of niacinamide therapy vs. placebo. Study may not have been adequately powered to detect between-group differences.
Type 1 diabetes mellitus: preservation of beta cell function	RCT	Pozzilli[397] 1995	56	No	1	Small	NA	NA	Nonsignificant reduction in insulin requirements after 1 year of niacinamide vs. placebo.
Type 1 diabetes mellitus: preservation of beta cell function	RCT, nonblinded	Pozzilli[396] 1994	90	Yes	1	Large	15%	7	Clinical remission reported in 15% of patients with type 1 diabetes treated with niacinamide vs. no treatment.
Type 1 diabetes mellitus: preservation of beta cell function	RCT	Taboga[398] 1994	21	No	1	None	NA	NA	Niacinamide plus insulin yielded no changes in insulin requirements vs. insulin therapy alone.
Type 1 diabetes mellitus: preservation of beta cell function	RCT	Mendola[395] 1989	20	Yes	1	Small	NA	NA	Niacinamide treatment resulted in significant increase in C-peptide levels.
Type 1 diabetes mellitus: preservation of beta cell function	RCT	Vague[165] 1987	16	Yes	1	Small	30%	4	Niacinamide caused significantly more remissions than with placebo in newly diagnosed DM (type 1).
Type 1 diabetes mellitus: preservation of beta cell function	Controlled trial, nonrandomized, nonblinded	Pozzilli[162,164] 1989, 1988	35	Yes	0	Small	NA	NA	Niacinamide treatment resulted in significant increase in C-peptide levels.
Type 1 diabetes mellitus: prevention	RCT	Lampeter[189] 1998	68	No	4	None	NA	NA	Niacinamide (1.2 g/m^2 daily) failed to prevent the development of diabetes (type 1) in children at risk.
Type 1 diabetes mellitus: prevention	Cohort	Elliott[188] 1991	22	Yes	0	Small	NA	NA	Niacinamide versus no treatment in children with beta cell antibodies and first-degree relatives with diabetes (type 1). Only 1 child in niacinamide group developed diabetes, vs. all in control group.
OA	RCT	Jonas[408] 1996	72	Yes	4	Small	NA	NA	Pilot study of niacinamide in OA. Significant improvement in global arthritis impact.

*Primary or secondary outcome.
[†]N, Number of patients; SS, statistically significant; ARR, absolute risk reduction; NNT, the number of patients who need to undergo a specific intervention in order to observe an outcome in one individual.
[‡]0-2 = poor; 3-4 = good; 5 = excellent.
HbA$_{1c}$, Glycosylated hemoglobin; HDL, high-density lipoprotein; LDL, low-density lipoprotein; NA, not applicable; OA, osteoarthritis; RCT, randomized, controlled trial; TC, total cholesterol.
For an explanation of each category in this table, please see Table 3 in the Introduction.

Niacin Monotherapy Trials

- Elam randomized 468 patients, including 125 with diabetes, to receive either niacin (3 g daily) or placebo for a period of up to 60 weeks as part of the Arterial Disease Multiple Intervention Trial (ADMIT).[105] Results showed that those patients randomized to receive niacin experienced a significant 29% increase in serum HDL levels and a significant decrease in triglycerides (23% to 28%) and LDL levels (8% to 9%) as compared with the placebo group. The results of this well-designed clinical trial suggest that niacin therapy is safe and effective for use in the treatment of hyper-

cholesterolemia, including that in patients with diabetes mellitus.

- Keenan et al. randomized 201 adults (20 to 70 years of age) to receive treatment with placebo, the American Heart Association Step I Diet (AHA-I), niacin 1 g daily (Enduracin), niacin 1.25 g daily, niacin 1.5 g daily, or niacin 2 g daily in double-blind fashion.[222] Lipid profiles analyzed at baseline and at the end of treatment showed niacin at daily doses of 1.5 to 2 g to cause a significant decrease in total cholesterol and LDL cholesterol levels, as compared with placebo and diet control, and subjects taking 1.5 g of niacin daily experienced significant increases in plasma HDL cholesterol. A subsequent subgroup analysis found that older patients, 50 to 70 years of age, experienced greater improvements in their lipid profiles than those observed in younger patients. This study suffers from unclear description of methodology and small sample sizes in each of the niacin subgroups.

- Aronov et al. randomized 89 hypercholesterolemic subjects (total cholesterol >225 mg/dL) to receive 6 months of treatment with wax-matrix sustained-release niacin (1500 mg daily), niacin (2 g daily), or placebo for 2 months each in a crossover design to assess the efficacy of sustained-release niacin in lowering serum cholesterol.[217] Outcome measures included total cholesterol, serum triglycerides, HDL, LDL, and lipoprotein(a) levels. Results demonstrated significant improvements from baseline in total cholesterol and LDL levels when subjects were taking niacin vs. placebo (total cholesterol 6% to 16% improvement, LDL 6% to 21% improvement, $p < 0.001$), with the higher dosage (2 g daily) associated with more substantial improvements. During the 2-month placebo phase, levels were not significantly different from baseline. Four subjects withdrew from the study because of adverse effects. Although the results of this study indicate that niacin causes significant improvements in serum total cholesterol and LDL levels, it did not measure long-term outcomes.

- A total of 132 subjects meeting the National Cholesterol Education Program criteria for elevated baseline LDL cholesterol and risk factors for coronary heart disease were randomized to receive either sustained-release niacin (Niaspan) (in doses titrated up to 3 g daily) or placebo for a period of 25 weeks.[108] LDL and apolipoprotein B levels were assessed at baseline, and every 4 weeks for the study duration, using validated enzymatic methods and the Friedewald equation. Results showed that LDL levels were significantly decreased in the niacin group at doses of 500 mg to 3 g daily (3% to 21% decrease in LDL; $p < 0.05$ for all doses), and apolipoprotein B levels similarly decreased (2% to 20%; $p < 0.05$ for all doses). Eight subjects withdrew because of adverse effects; significant elevations in aspartate aminotransferase levels and serum uric acid were seen in the niacin group as compared with the placebo group. Overall, this was a well-designed study, adequately powered to find at least an 8% difference in LDL levels between study groups.

- Morgan et al. randomized 122 subjects with LDL levels above 160 mg/dL to receive treatment with sustained-release niacin (Niaspan) in a daily dose of either 1 g or 2 g or placebo for a period of 12 weeks in double-blind fashion.[212,365] Results of serum fasting lipid and lipoprotein concentration tests showed Niaspan to significantly decrease LDL levels (by 6% with the 1-g dose; by 14% with the 2-g dose) and increase HDL levels (17% with 1 g; 23% with 2 g) as compared with placebo. At a dose of 2 g daily, Niaspan also caused a significant decrease in serum lipoprotein(a) and triglyceride concentrations. Niaspan was well tolerated, with flushing reported as the most common adverse event by 83% and 88% of subjects, respectively, in the 1-g and 2-g Niaspan groups. This was a well-designed study, and its results suggest that sustained-release niacin is safe and effective in the treatment of hypercholesterolemia.

- In an early secondary prevention trial, the U.S. Veterans Administration Cardiology Drug-Lipid Study, 570 men who had suffered transmural infarction during the previous year were randomized to receive treatment with estrogen, niacin, dextrothyroxine, or placebo, alone and in combination, for 5 years in double-blind fashion.[100] Follow-up evaluations, during which serum cholesterol levels were recorded, were conducted every month for the first 2 years and then every 2 months for the remainder of the study. After a mean follow-up period of 38 months, a mean 20% decrease in cholesterol was seen in subjects taking 4 g of niacin daily, and a 7% decrease was seen in the dextrothyroxine group. There were no significant differences observed between groups in mortality rates or recurrence of myocardial infarction. Discontinuation of niacin therapy due to adverse effects occurred in 32% of subjects. The results of this early study provided good preliminary evidence for the use of niacin to lower serum cholesterol levels in patients with previous myocardial infarction but did not support its use to prevent death.

- Lavie et al. treated coronary artery disease in 36 consecutive men with controlled-release niacin (Slo-Niacin), initiating therapy with 500 mg twice daily and increasing as tolerated to a maximum of 3 g daily, for 3 months.[152] Lipid profiles, fasting blood sugar, and aspartate transaminase values were monitored at baseline and after 3 months of niacin treatment. Results showed niacin treatment to elicit a significant 11% reduction in total cholesterol, 20% reduction in LDL cholesterol and 30% increase in HDL cholesterol levels at 3 months in subjects with low HDL cholesterol levels at baseline. In subjects with hypertriglyceridemia at baseline, a significant 23% reduction in triglycerides, 41% increase in HDL cholesterol, and 35% reduction in LDL cholesterol were observed, with results being significant between the two subgroups analyzed. The short study duration and small subgroup sizes limit the impact of these results.

- Niacin monotherapy has also been evaluated in multiple studies of lesser methodologic quality. Retrospective studies have correlated niacin therapy with significant decreases in total cholesterol levels[90,218,268,277] and plasma LDL levels, as well as increases in plasma HDL levels.[90,92,218,268,366,367] A number of prospective observational studies have also found niacin to effectively lower total plasma cholesterol and increase plasma HDL levels.[81,82,106,118,122,124,131-134,137,139,140,142,144,145,202,368]

- Numerous comparison/equivalence trials involving niacin therapy can also be found in the published literature. Niacin has been reported to result in significantly greater increases in plasma HDL than those achieved with other available treatments for hypercholesterolemia, including safflower oil, sitosterol, gemfibrozil, and the statins (pravastatin, lovastatin, atorvastatin).[109,113,135,141,143,146,151,262,266,366,369,370]

- Grundy et al. conducted a randomized, double-blind, placebo-controlled trial in 148 patients with type 2 diabetes and dyslipidemia.[371] Subjects were assigned to receive niacin 1000 mg or 1500 mg or placebo daily by mouth, over a 16-week period. Notably, 69 patients (47%) were also taking statins. The authors reported significant increases in HDL with both niacin doses vs. placebo (+19%, +24%, and 0%, respectively; $p < 0.05$). Significant reductions in triglyceride levels were also seen (−13%, −28%, and 0%, respectively; $p < 0.05$). No large, significant change in hemoglobin A_{1c} (HbA_{1c}) levels was observed. Four patients discontinued participation because of flushing (including one receiving placebo). Rates of adverse events other than flushing were similar for the niacin and the placebo groups. No hepatotoxic effects or myopathy was observed.

Combination Therapy Trials

- Davignon et al. randomized 158 patients with hyper-cholesterolemia to receive niacin (Nicobid, 500 mg twice daily), pravastatin (40 mg at bedtime), pravastatin (40 mg at bedtime) plus niacin (Nicobid, 500 mg twice daily), or placebo in double-blind fashion.[219] After a period of 6 weeks, niacin significantly lowered plasma LDL levels as compared with placebo; pravastatin significantly lowered LDL levels as compared with placebo and niacin alone; and combination therapy with pravastatin and niacin had the greatest effect on LDL levels. HDL cholesterol levels were significantly higher in all treatment groups than in the placebo group, with no significant differences between groups, and niacin had no significant effects on serum triglyceride levels, whereas pravastatin and combination treatment produced marked decreases in triglycerides. The results of this study demonstrate the effectiveness of niacin in decreasing plasma LDL and increasing HDL levels and also demonstrate the superiority of therapy with pravastatin alone or in combination with niacin in treating hypercholesterolemia.

- Vacek et al. found that in 25 hypercholesterolemic patients randomized to receive treatment with placebo, niacin and placebo, lovastatin and placebo, and niacin and lovastatin, each administered in sequential order for 3 months each and separated by 2 months of placebo treatment, the combination of lovastatin and niacin resulted in significantly greater differences in total cholesterol (27% decrease) and LDL (37% decrease) than were noted with either placebo or each agent alone.[267] However, lovastatin alone also resulted in significant decreases in total cholesterol (17%) and LDL (25%) levels, and niacin alone caused a significant decrease in LDL (11%) levels, both as compared with baseline and placebo.

- Jacobson et al. evaluated the efficacy and safety of combination therapy with fluvastatin and niacin and found that the two agents administered together result in significantly greater effects on LDL cholesterol and lipoprotein(a) levels, without added toxicity.[201,263,264]

- Bays et al. conducted a randomized, controlled trial to compare a once-daily regimen of extended-release niacin plus lovastatin, in a fixed-dose combination, with standard doses of atorvastatin or simvastatin, with a special emphasis on relative starting doses.[372] This study was conducted over a 16-week period in 315 subjects with elevated LDL and decreased HDL (defined as LDL >159 mg/dL without coronary artery disease or >129 mg/dL with coronary artery disease, and HDL <45 mg/dL in men and <50 mg/dL in women). Patients were randomized to receive starting doses of either niacin 1000 mg plus lovastatin 40 mg, or atorvastatin 10 mg, or simvastatin 20 mg. The authors reported that after 8 weeks, both niacin plus lovastatin and atorvastatin lowered mean LDL levels by 38%; after 12 weeks, niacin plus lovastatin lowered LDL by 42%, vs. 34% with simvastatin ($p < 0.001$). In addition, niacin plus lovastatin increased HDL significantly more than did atorvastatin or simvastatin in all compared doses ($p < 0.001$). Niacin plus lovastatin also provided significant improvements in triglycerides, lipoprotein(a), apolipoprotein A-1, apolipoprotein B, and HDL subfractions. No significant differences were seen between study groups in elevated liver enzymes. No drug-induced myopathy was observed. Six percent of niacin patients withdrew because of flushing. The authors concluded that niacin plus lovastatin was comparable to atorvastatin 10 mg and more effective than simvastatin 20 mg in reducing LDL and was more effective in increasing HDL than either atorvastatin or simvastatin. However, because there was no lovastatin monotherapy arm, the true additive benefits of niacin with lovastatin are not clear.

- Hunninghake et al. conducted a randomized, controlled, double-blind, multicenter trial in 237 patients with type IIA or IIB hyperlipidemia to assess the effects of pharmacotherapy on lipid levels.[373] Subjects were assigned to receive one of four escalating-dose treatment regimens: extended-release niacin 1000 mg plus lovastatin 20 mg; niacin 2000 mg plus lovastatin 40 mg; niacin 2000 mg monotherapy; or lovastatin 40 mg monotherapy. After 28 weeks of treatment, the authors reported that the combination therapies were significantly superior to either monotherapy for improving levels of LDL, HDL, and triglycerides, with a dose-response effect. The 2000 mg/40 mg dose achieved greater mean reductions in LDL (−42%) than were noted for the 1000 mg/20 mg dose (−28%, $p < 0.001$), for lovastatin 40 mg (−32%, $p < 0.05$), or for niacin 2000 mg (−14%, $p < 0.05$). The 2000 mg/40 mg dose was significantly more effective in increasing HDL levels (+30%) than the 1000 mg/20 mg dose (+21%, $p = 0.016$). The decrease in triglycerides was greater with 2000 mg/40 mg (−43%) than with 1000 mg/20 mg (−26%, $p = 0.009$). All three niacin-containing regimens were more effective than lovastatin monotherapy in reducing lipoprotein (a) levels. Flushing caused 12 patients (11%) receiving niacin plus lovastatin and 1 patient receiving lovastatin alone to withdraw. No drug-related myopathy was noted. One patient each in the 2000 mg/40 mg group and the lovastatin 40 mg group experienced reversible elevations in liver transaminases.

- In several studies of lesser methodologic quality, niacin has been evaluated in combination with HMG-CoA reductase inhibitors (statins) including pravastatin, lovastatin, and atorvastatin. These combinations have been associated with significantly greater decreases in total cholesterol, triglycerides, and LDL levels than those achieved with niacin or statin monotherapy,[205,220,266,268,374] and with significantly greater increases in plasma HDL levels than with statin monotherapy.[205,220,262,266,268] The FDA has approved a combination tablet containing lovastatin (10 mg) and niacin (500 mg) for the treatment of hypercholesterolemia based on the results of an open-label study that found the combination tablet to be effective at decreasing LDL, triglyceride, and lipoprotein(a) levels, and at increasing HDL levels, with few adverse effects.[265] Additional observational studies have evaluated the use of niacin in combination with other agents, including colestipol, etofibrate, neomycin, probucol, and gemfibrozil. These studies have reported that the addition of niacin therapy results in significant improvements in plasma cholesterol and lipid profiles not seen with either agent alone.[136,146,220,223,245,251,255,277,375] One trial of a combination treatment found no added effect with the use of two agents and involved the addition of oat bran to niacin therapy.[221]

Dosing Trials

- Knopp et al. randomized 71 subjects with hyper-cholesterolemia to receive treatment with unmodified niacin (Nicolar, 1500 mg daily increased to 3 g daily after 1 month) or time-release niacin (Nicobid, 1500 mg daily increased to 3 g daily after 1 month) for a total study period of 6 months in double-blind fashion.[138] Lipid profiles were evaluated at baseline and after 6 months of treatment according to Lipid Research Clinic Program methodology; at 6 months, both the unmodified niacin and the sustained-release niacin resulted in decreases in LDL and total cholesterol (total cholesterol 15.1% vs. 11.5%; LDL 21.1% vs. 12.8%, respectively). Patients receiving sustained-release niacin experienced significantly more gastrointestinal adverse effects than were noted by patients using unmodified niacin.

- A dose escalation study assessing the efficacy of extended-release niacin randomized 131 subjects with primary hypercholesterolemia to receive either Niaspan (initiated at 500 mg daily and increased at 500-mg intervals every 4 weeks to a maximum of 3 g daily) or placebo for a period of 26 weeks.[107] At doses ≥1 g daily, LDL levels significantly decreased; HDL levels significantly increased at doses ≥500 mg daily; and significant decreases in apolipoprotein B were seen at doses ≥1.5 g daily. Adverse effects caused 30% of the subjects in the niacin group to withdraw from the study, including flushing, nausea, vomiting, diarrhea, and rash.

- McKenney et al. randomized 46 subjects with serum LDL >160 mg/dL to receive either immediate-release (crystalline) niacin or sustained-release niacin in a dose escalation study.[185] Subjects received each dose (500 mg, 1 g, 1.5 g, 2 g, or 3 g) twice daily for a period of 6 weeks. Blood cholesterol levels were monitored at the end of weeks 4 and 6 of each study period using Centers for Disease Control and Prevention Lipid Standardization Program requirements; the occurrence of adverse effects was determined at the end of each study period. Results showed greater reductions in total cholesterol and LDL with sustained-release niacin than with immediate-release niacin at doses ≥1.5 g daily. Immediate-release niacin caused significantly greater increases in HDL cholesterol than those noted with sustained-release niacin at all doses. Subjects taking sustained-release niacin reported less flushing than those taking immediate-release niacin; however, sustained-release niacin was also associated with a significant increase in blood glucose levels and liver aminotransferase and alkaline phosphatase levels as compared with baseline, both of which were not seen in the immediate-release niacin group. Withdrawal from the study was necessary in 78% of those taking sustained-release niacin prior to completing the 3-g daily study period, because of hepatotoxicity. This study lacked a placebo group. The significant adverse effects and manifestations of toxicity seen in the sustained-release group call into question the use of sustained-release products.

Pellagra (Niacin)
Summary

- Niacin (vitamin B_3, nicotinic acid) and niacinamide have been FDA approved for the treatment of niacin deficiency. Pellagra is a nutritional disease that develops because of a dietary deficiency of vitamin B_3 or of its amino acid precursor, tryptophan. Symptoms of pellagra include dermatitis, diarrhea, and dementia/depression. The disease may afflict individuals with chronic alcohol dependence. There are drugs such as isoniazid and medical conditions such as diabetes, liver cirrhosis, and pregnancy that may predispose the affected person to the development of pellagra. Although a majority of the evidence in this area is more than 60 years old, this is a well-established indication with a clearly defined mechanism of action.

Evidence

- An observational study followed the response to therapy of 173 subjects with pellagra given niacin (50 to 1000 mg daily) and reported that resolution of symptoms occurred within a week of initiating treatment.[159] Case reports from the 1930s detail clinical improvement with decrease in symptoms of pellagra following niacin therapy. Four patients with pellagra who received 500 mg of niacin showed clinical improvement within 48 hours of beginning therapy.[157] A 42-year-old patient with pellagra recovered after the administration of niacin (60 mg daily) for a period of 12 days.[158]

- A more recent case-control epidemiologic study reexamined the etiologic basis of pellagra.[376] In Mozambican refugee camps in Malawi, 126 pairs of patients with pellagra (characterized by dermatitis, diarrhea, and dementia) and their matched controls were observed. The authors reported that the individuals with pellagra were less likely than the controls to have consumed a source of niacin in the 6 months preceding the onset of pellagra (odds ratio 0.08; 95% CI 0.01 to 0.59).

Atherosclerosis (Niacin)
Summary

- Aggressive antilipidemic therapy has been shown in numerous trials to benefit patients with atherosclerosis by slowing or even reversing the progression of disease.[377] The effectiveness of niacin in lowering cholesterol has already been demonstrated in numerous clinical trials. Niacin has also been shown to decrease plasma lipoprotein(a) levels, which have been associated with the development of atherosclerosis.[378] However, niacin therapy has also been shown to increase plasma homocysteine levels by up to 55% from baseline, possibly negating any positive effects niacin has on the lipid profile, as high levels of homocysteine have been associated with an increased risk of arterial occlusive disease.[242,249] The evidence from available clinical trials supports the use of niacin in combination with other agents (but not for monotherapy) in patients with atherosclerosis to decrease cholesterol and to slow progression of atherosclerotic plaque formation. Further research is needed to confirm the use of niacin alone in effectively reducing the size of atherosclerotic plaques and preventing death from cardiac causes.

Evidence

- The Cholesterol Lowering Atherosclerosis Study (CLAS) was a randomized, placebo-controlled trial of niacin plus colestipol in the treatment of atherosclerosis in 162 nonsmoking men (40 to 59 years of age) with progressive atherosclerosis and prior coronary bypass surgery.[247-249,253,379] Subjects were randomized to receive treatment with niacin (average 4.2 g daily) plus colestipol (average 30.1 g daily) plus controlled diet or to placebo plus controlled diet therapy. Angiography of the carotid, coronary, and carotid arteries was performed at baseline and at 2 years of treatment to assess the effects of drug therapy on the progression of atherosclerosis.[247,248] Results showed a significant 43% reduction in plasma LDL; a significant 37% increase in HDL; a reduction in the number of lesions demonstrating progression per subject ($p < 0.03$); reduction in the number of subjects with adverse changes in their coronary bypass grafts ($p < 0.03$); and a significantly greater number of individuals with a perceptible improvement in overall coronary status ($p < 0.002$) in the treatment group vs. the controls.[248] Additional results of the CLAS trial have also shown therapy with colestipol plus niacin to significantly reduce carotid artery intimal thickness at 1, 2, and 4 years, as determined by coronary artery ultrasound study, compared with placebo.[253,379] Subsequent analysis found a significant decrease in the rate of progression of atherosclerosis in the femoral artery in the treatment group vs. the control group ($p < 0.04$).[249] The results of this well-designed trial suggest that colestipol and niacin are useful in treating atherosclerosis; however, the benefit of either drug alone cannot be determined, as they were studied only in combination.

- Brown et al. randomized 146 men (<62 years of age) with apolipoprotein B levels >125 mg/dL and a family history of vascular disease to receive lovastatin (20 mg twice daily) plus colestipol (10 g three times daily); niacin (1 g four times daily) plus colestipol (10 g three times daily); or placebo, for a period of 2.5 years, as part of the Familial Atherosclerosis Treatment Study (FATS).[115] Subjects underwent monthly follow-up evaluations for 1 year and bimonthly evaluations for the remainder of the 2.5-year study, at which times plasma LDL, HDL, cholesterol, triglycerides, and apolipoprotein B were measured. Twenty-five subjects withdrew from the study prior to completion, five because of intolerance of niacin. Niacin plus colestipol therapy resulted in significant improvements from baseline in total cholesterol, LDL, HDL, triglycerides, and apolipoprotein B ($p < 0.001$ for all values), with a 32% decrease in plasma LDL and a 43% increase in plasma HDL, vs. 7% and 5%, respectively, in the placebo group, and 46% and 15% in the lovastatin plus colestipol group. Progression of disease was lower in the drug treatment groups (21% lower with lovastatin plus colestipol and 25% lower with niacin plus colestipol), and regression was significantly more frequent with drug treatment ($p < 0.005$). The results of this well-designed trial suggest that niacin in combination therapies may have a place in the management of atherosclerosis; however, conclusions regarding niacin for monotherapy cannot be extrapolated.

- A subsequent analysis utilized 31 consecutive patients from the FATS trial and randomized them to receive treatment with niacin (500 mg four times daily), lovastatin (20 mg twice daily), and colestipol (10 g three times daily) for an additional 12 months, followed by 8 months each of conventional niacin and sustained-release niacin in combination with the other two agents.[186] Triple therapy resulted in a 57% decrease in plasma LDL and a 27% increase in HDL, with 83% of those taking controlled-release niacin reaching the target of LDL ≤100 mg/dL, vs. 52% of those taking regular niacin ($p < 0.01$).

- As part of the HDL-Atherosclerosis Treatment Study (HATS), Brown et al. randomized 160 adults with coronary heart disease (defined as previous myocardial infarction, coronary interventions or angina) and low HDL cholesterol levels to receive placebo, antioxidant vitamins, simvastatin plus niacin, or simvastatin plus niacin plus antioxidant vitamins.[260] The simvastatin-niacin combinations resulted in marked increases in HDL cholesterol, whereas the antioxidant vitamin and placebo groups experienced no change in HDL levels.

- The Armed Forces Regression Study (AFREGS) randomized 143 subjects with low HDL levels to receive treatment with gemfibrozil, niacin and cholestyramine, or cholestyramine and placebo for a period of 2.5 years in double-blind fashion.[380] Results showed that treatment with the three-drug regimen led to significantly fewer cardiac events and less progression of coronary stenosis than noted for treatment with placebo and cholestyramine.

- Hecht et al. studied the effects of statins alone or in combination with niacin on coronary plaque progression in 182 consecutive patients.[381-383]

- Sacks et al. randomized 79 patients with coronary disease and normal cholesterol levels to receive placebo or treatment with pravastatin (40 mg daily), niacin (1.5 to 3 g daily), cholestyramine (8 to 16 g daily), and gemfibrozil (600 to 1200 mg daily), added in sequential order as needed to reach the goal of total cholesterol ≤4.1 mmol/L, for an average of 35 weeks.[153] A total of 38 subjects received niacin therapy. Significant reductions in total cholesterol (28%), LDL cholesterol (41%), triglycerides (26%), and apolipoprotein B (31%) and increase in HDL cholesterol (13%) were observed between treatment and placebo groups ($p < 0.001$). The application of these results to niacin therapy is limited by the lack of a niacin-only treatment group, inadequate blinding, and significant differences between the groups at baseline.

Cardiovascular Disease: Secondary Prevention (Niacin)
Summary

- In view of the wealth of evidence demonstrating efficacy of niacin in improving serum cholesterol (a risk factor and surrogate marker for coronary artery disease), it is possible that its use in patients with cardiovascular disease could decrease the incidence of coronary events and prevent the progression of atherosclerosis. Niacin therapy has been shown to decrease lipoprotein(a) levels[275,312,384] and fibrinogen levels;[155] reductions in both have been associated with a decreased risk of coronary artery disease. Numerous human trials have evaluated the use of niacin, alone and in combination with other agents, for the prevention of cardiovascular disease and death from cardiac events. Overall, the results appear to favor the use of niacin therapy, particularly in combination with other cholesterol-lowering agents, in secondary prevention of adverse cardiac outcomes. However, results have not uniformly supported this conclusion, and further research is warranted.

Systematic Review

- A systematic review of the effects of cholesterol-lowering interventions on major mortality outcomes identified 59 randomized, controlled trials held from 1966 through 1996, via searches of MEDLINE and EMBASE.[385] Two trials were identified that involved niacin therapy and mortality.[100,154] Pooled results of these two studies yielded a risk ratio of 0.95 for coronary heart disease mortality, 0.96 for total mortality, and 0.99 for non–coronary heart disease mortality. However, none of these reductions was statistically significant.

Niacin Monotherapy Trials

- The Coronary Drug Project was a double-blind, randomized, controlled trial conducted to assess the efficacy of lipid-lowering drugs vs. placebo in the long-term therapy of coronary heart disease, and subsequent reduction in total mortality, in men with previous myocardial infarction (MI).[154] It was conducted in 53 clinical centers and included results from more than 8000 subjects (ages 30 to 64 years), 1119 of whom were randomized to receive niacin (3 g daily) for 54 to 74 months. Subjects were examined every 4 months during follow-up visits, and once yearly, compliance, serum cholesterol, and liver function tests were assessed. After 5 years, 10.7% of subjects in the niacin group had withdrawn from the study because of adverse effects. At that time, results showed no significant difference between niacin and placebo in all-cause mortality rates (21.2% and 20.9%, respectively); the 5-year rates of death due to coronary heart disease were almost identical for niacin and placebo (15.9%

vs. 16.2%). However, there was a statistically significant reduction in nonfatal, recurrent MI. The preliminary results from this large-scale, well-designed trial suggest that niacin may be useful in the secondary prevention of recurrent MI (8.9% incidence in the niacin group vs. 12.2% in the placebo group) but do not support the use of niacin to decrease mortality in patients with coronary heart disease. Subsequently, reports have been published on the long-term results of the Coronary Drug Project after 15 years of follow-up and have shown a significant 11% reduction in number of deaths in the niacin group compared with the placebo group ($p < 0.0004$).[355,356]

- In an early (1968) secondary prevention trial, the U.S. Veterans Administration Cardiology Drug-Lipid Study, 570 men who had suffered transmural infarction during the previous year were randomized to receive treatment with estrogen, niacin, dextrothyroxine, or placebo, alone and in combination, for 5 years in double-blind fashion.[100] Follow-up evaluations, during which serum cholesterol levels were recorded, were conducted every month for the first 2 years and then every 2 months for the remainder of the study. After a mean follow-up period of 38 months, a mean 20% decrease in cholesterol was seen in subjects taking 4 g of niacin daily, and a 7% decrease was observed in the dextrothyroxine group. There were no significant differences observed between groups in mortality rates or recurrence of myocardial infarction. Discontinuation of niacin therapy due to adverse effects occurred in 32% of subjects. The results of this well-designed study provided good preliminary evidence for the use of niacin to lower serum cholesterol levels in patients with previous myocardial infarction but did not support its use to prevent death.

- The Arterial Disease Multiple Intervention Trial (ADMIT), a multicenter randomized, controlled trial, was conducted to determine the efficacy of secondary prevention measures, including warfarin, niacin, and antioxidant therapy, on coagulation parameters in patients with peripheral arterial disease.[155] Eighty subjects with peripheral arterial disease were randomized to receive low-dose warfarin, niacin, anti-oxidant vitamin, or corresponding placebo for a 1-year period. Fibrinogen levels, prothrombin F1.2, and von Willebrand factor levels were measured at baseline and at 12 months to determine the effect, if any, of the treatments. After 1 year of taking 1500 mg niacin twice daily, subjects experienced a significant 14% decrease in fibrinogen levels and 60% decrease in prothrombin F1.2 levels, as compared with placebo, suggesting the ability of niacin to modify abnormal coagulation factors in peripheral arterial disease.

- In an open-label study, Vega et al. administered 1 g of extended release niacin or 40 mg of lovastatin, simvastatin, or pravastatin sodium daily to assess effects on plasma levels of 24S-hydroxycholesterol and apolipoprotein E in patients with Alzheimer's disease.[386] After 6 weeks of therapy, the authors obtained fasting serum samples and reported that niacin significantly reduced levels of 24S-hydroxycholesterol by 10% and of LDL cholesterol by 18.1%, whereas statins reduced 24S-hydroxycholesterol by 21.4% and of LDL cholesterol by 34.9%. Although between-group comparisons were not conducted, the differences in results are large enough that significant differences likely would be found in favor of statins.

Combination Therapy Trials

- Rosenhamer et al. randomized 555 subjects having suffered a previous myocardial infarction to receive treatment either with niacin (up to 3 g daily) plus clofibrate (2 g daily) plus controlled diet, or with diet alone.[156] Among the 116 subjects completing 5 years in the study, total cholesterol levels fell 14% and triglyceride levels decreased 19% in the drug treatment group, and ischemic heart disease deaths were fewer in the drug treatment group as compared with the controls. However, these differences were not statistically significant.

- The Armed Forces Regression Study (AFREGS) randomized 143 subjects with low HDL levels to receive treatment with gemfibrozil, niacin and cholestyramine, or cholestyramine and placebo for a period of 2.5 years in a double-blind fashion.[380] Results showed that treatment with the three-drug regimen led to significantly fewer cardiac events and less progression of coronary stenosis than noted for treatment with placebo and cholestyramine.

- Carlson et al. randomized myocardial infarction survivors to receive either clofibrate (1 g twice daily) plus niacin (1 g three times daily) or no treatment over a 5-year period.[53] The treatment group experienced a 60% reduction in ischemic heart disease mortality as compared with the control group, and this reduction in mortality was associated with a significant reduction in serum cholesterol and triglyceride concentrations.

- Capuzzi et al. conducted a randomized, open-label, multi-center trial to assess the efficacy and safety of the statin drug rosuvastatin and extended-release niacin, alone and in combination, in 270 patients with atherogenic dyslipidemia.[387] Adult subjects with fasting total cholesterol levels >199 mg/dL, triglycerides 200 to 800 mg/dL, apolipoprotein B >109 mg/dL, and HDL cholesterol <45 mg/dL were randomized to one of four treatment groups over a 24-week period: rosuvastatin 10 to 40 mg; extended-release niacin 0.5 to 2 g; rosuvastatin 40 mg plus niacin 0.5 to 1 g; or rosuvastatin 10 mg plus niacin 0.5 to 2 g. Percent changes from baseline in LDL, non-HDL cholesterol, and other lipid measurements were determined by analysis of variance, with statistical testing performed separately between the rosuvastatin monotherapy group and each remaining treatment group. The authors reported that rosuvastatin 40 mg reduced LDL and non-HDL cholesterol significantly more than either niacin 2 g or rosuvastatin 10 mg/niacin 2 g (−48% versus −0.1% and −36% for LDL cholesterol, and −49% versus −11% and −38% for non-HDL cholesterol, respectively; $p < 0.01$ for all comparisons). No significant reduction in LDL or non-HDL cholesterol was observed with the combination of rosuvastatin 40 mg plus niacin 1.0 g (−42% and −47%). Triglyceride reductions ranged from −21% (niacin monotherapy) to −39% (rosuvastatin 40 mg plus niacin 1 g), but no observed differences were statistically significant. Compared with rosuvastatin alone, rosuvastatin 10 mg plus niacin 2 g produced significantly greater increases in HDL (11% versus 24%; $p < 0.001$). Rosuvastatin alone was better tolerated than either niacin alone or the combination of rosuvastatin plus niacin.

- Morgan et al. conducted an analysis of blood samples collected from 60 hypercholesterolemic patients in a previous randomized trial, in order to measure the effects of extended-release niacin on lipoprotein subclasses using a proton nuclear magnetic resonance imaging method.[318] Paired plasma samples collected at baseline and after 12 weeks of treatment with daily niacin 1000 mg or 2000 mg or placebo were available for analysis. The authors reported that niacin increased HDL cholesterol and decreased LDL, as well as VLDL, in a dose-dependent manner relative to placebo.

Niacin increased large HDL particles (H5 and H4, corresponding to the HDL[2ab] fraction) without having a net effect on small HDL particles (H3, H2, and H1, corresponding to the HDL[3abc] fraction). Niacin also decreased smaller, denser LDL particles (L1 and L2) and increased the larger, more buoyant L3 subclass. The inhibitory effect of niacin on VLDL was evident on the larger particles (V6, V5, V4, and V3 subclasses) rather than on the smaller ones (V2 and V1). These results suggest that niacin ER produces a beneficial effect on lipoprotein subclasses, specifically decreasing the more atherogenic small, dense LDL particles and enhancing the cardioprotective large HDL particles.

Type 1 Diabetes Mellitus: Preservation of Pancreatic Islet Beta Cell Function (Niacinamide)

Summary

- Niacinamide, not niacin, has been shown to exert a protective effect on pancreatic islet beta cell function in animal studies.[388-390] It has been postulated that beta cell death occurs through activation of poly(ADP-ribose) polymerase (PARP) as an adaptive response to minimize oxidative damage to DNA, which results in the depletion of cellular NAD^+ and subsequent cell death.[391] It may follow that supplementation with niacinamide, which repletes cellular NAD^+ levels, would prevent cell death and preserve beta cell function. However, the available human data on the use of niacinamide to preserve pancreatic islet beta cell function do not unanimously support the use of niacinamide for this indication. A single meta-analysis and additional trials have found that niacinamide supplementation increases C-peptide levels, lowers hemoglobin A_{1c} (HbA_{1c}) (i.e., glycosylated hemoglobin) levels, and leads to a reduction in required insulin doses. However, not all results have been significant, most studies have been small without adequate randomization or blinding, and several small (possibly underpowered) trials have yielded negative results. Further research is warranted to determine the effect niacinamide has in delaying the onset of insulin dependence in type 1 diabetes mellitus.

Meta-analysis

- A meta-analysis conducted by Pozzilli et al. identified 10 randomized, controlled trials in patients with recent-onset diabetes mellitus (type 1) that utilized niacinamide treatment through a questionnaire sent to all principal investigators of published trials and abstracts involving niacinamide.[336] The authors concluded that after 1 year of treatment, baseline C-peptide levels were significantly increased in subjects receiving niacinamide as compared with controls.[160,162,392-398] However, only five of the identified studies were placebo controlled, and the methodology of the included trials varied widely.

- Pozzilli et al. randomized 56 subjects (5 to 35 years old) with newly diagnosed diabetes mellitus (type 1) to receive either niacinamide (25 mg/kg daily) plus insulin or placebo plus insulin in a 1-year, double-blind, randomized, controlled trial.[397] Glycosylated hemoglobin (HbA_{1c}) and stimulated C-peptide levels were monitored every 3 months. At the end of 1 year, all subjects experienced a significant reduction in insulin dosage from baseline, with no difference between groups. Stimulated C-peptide levels were significantly increased in the niacinamide group as compared with the placebo group, but only in subjects older than 15 years of age. The results of this trial do not suggest that niacinamide is effective in improving pancreatic islet beta cell function

in newly diagnosed diabetics (type 1). The significant differences seen between niacinamide and placebo when only subjects older than 15 were analyzed appear promising but are limited by the small subgroup size.

Niacinamide Monotherapy: Positive Evidence

- Twenty subjects, newly diagnosed with diabetes mellitus (type 1) were randomized to receive treatment with niacinamide (1 g daily) or placebo, in single-blind fashion, for a period of 45 days.[395] Pancreatic islet beta cell function was assessed by a validated glucagon-stimulated C-peptide test at baseline and on days 15, 45, 180, and 365 after the start of treatment. At 45 days of therapy, both groups experienced an increase in C-peptide levels, with a significantly greater stimulated C-peptide response in the niacinamide group ($p < 0.01$). Any increase in C-peptide response ceased after drug treatment was discontinued at 45 days. Although the results of this study appear to show that niacinamide is effective at preserving beta cell function, methodologic flaws, including inadequate blinding, small sample size, and short duration, limit application of the results in clinical practice.

- In an open controlled trial in 35 patients with newly diagnosed diabetes mellitus (type 1), niacinamide (200 mg daily) plus insulin therapy resulted in a greater percentage of partial and total remissions at 12 months than that noted for insulin alone.[162,164] Subjects taking niacinamide also experienced a significant increase in stimulated plasma C-peptide levels as compared with the control group receiving insulin alone.

- Pozzilli et al. randomized 90 patients with newly diagnosed insulin-dependent diabetes to receive either nicotinamide (25 mg/kg daily), cyclosporine (5 mg/kg daily) plus nicotinamide, or no treatment.[396] After 1 year of treatment, clinical remission was obtained in 15% of the nicotinamide subjects, 8% of the subjects receiving nicotinamide and cyclosporine, and none of the control group subjects, with the nicotinamide subjects sustaining remission significantly longer than in the other groups (7 ± 3 [SD] months). Although suggestive of the nicotinamide's effectiveness in preserving beta cell function in newly diagnosed diabetics, this study suffered from inadequate blinding and a small sample size.

- Vague et al. randomized 26 subjects with diabetes mellitus (type 1), controlled on insulin therapy for up to 5 years prior to study inclusion, to receive either placebo or niacinamide (3 g daily) for 9 months in a double-blind, randomized, controlled trial.[166] Insulin dose, HbA_{1c} levels, and C-peptide levels were measured at baseline and at 6 and at 9 months. Results showed that in the placebo group, HbA_{1c} levels rose significantly from baseline, whereas the subjects receiving niacinamide demonstrated significantly lower HbA_{1c} levels than those in the placebo group. There was also a significant difference between groups in fasting and stimulated C-peptide levels, with a significant decline seen in the placebo group. Treatment with niacinamide was well tolerated.

- Vague et al. conducted a randomized, controlled trial in which 16 subjects with newly diagnosed diabetes mellitus (type 1) were consecutively assigned to receive niacinamide (3 grams daily) or placebo, in addition to their insulin dose, for a period of 6 months.[165] The primary outcome measure was clinical remission, defined as discontinuance of insulin therapy. Insulin was discontinued in 6 of 7 (85%) patients in the niacinamide group and in 5 of 9 subjects (55%) in the placebo group; three of the niacinamide group patients are reported to have maintained remission for over 2 years. The results of this study appear promising for the use of niacinamide to induce remission in newly diagnosed diabetes mellitus (type 1). However, these results are limited by the study's small sample size and inadequate randomization.

Niacinamide Monotherapy: Negative Evidence

- Chase et al. conducted a double-blind randomized, controlled trial in 35 children (ages 6 to 18 years) newly diagnosed with diabetes mellitus (type 1) to assess the efficacy of niacinamide (100 mg per year of age daily; maximum of 1.5 g daily) in preserving pancreatic islet beta cell function.[160] After 1 year in the study, no difference was found between niacinamide and placebo in subjects' required insulin dose, HbA_{1c} levels, or C-peptide plasma levels, suggesting that neither placebo nor niacinamide significantly preserved islet beta cell function in diabetes mellitus (type 1). However, this study may not have been adequately powered to detect between-group differences.

- Ilkova et al. conducted a randomized, double-blind, controlled trial of niacinamide (25 mg/kg daily) vs. placebo for 6 months in 25 subjects newly diagnosed with diabetes mellitus (type 1).[393] Results showed no significant differences between niacinamide and placebo in daily insulin requirement or blood glucose, C-peptide, or HbA_{1c} levels. This study may not have been adequately powered to detect between-group differences.

- A double-blind, randomized, controlled trial in 49 subjects with newly diagnosed diabetes mellitus (type 1) and on insulin therapy, assigned subjects to receive treatment with either placebo or niacinamide (40 mg/kg daily) for a period of 6 months, to assess the efficacy of niacinamide at inducing complete remission (defined as the discontinuation of insulin therapy).[394] Insulin use and C-peptide and HbA_{1c} levels were monitored at baseline and at 3 and 6 months after treatment initiation. Results at 6 months showed no significant protective effect of niacinamide on islet beta cell function or on sustained remission induction.

- The IMDIAB VI study was a multicenter randomized trial of two niacinamide doses (25 mg/kg or 50 mg/kg daily) in the treatment of newly diagnosed diabetes mellitus (type 1) in 74 patients (mean age 13 years).[399] Subjects were continued on insulin therapy for the duration of the trial with instructions on how to alter insulin therapy in response to blood glucose levels. Results showed no significant differences between the two treatment groups in basal C-peptide secretion, HbA_{1c} levels, the attainment of remission (one patient in each group), or adverse events. While this study was adequately powered and well-designed, it was not appropriately blinded. In addition, there is no mention of significant differences from baseline in the niacinamide treatment groups.

- Taboga et al. randomized 21 subjects newly diagnosed with diabetes mellitus (type 1) to receive insulin and niacinamide (3 g daily) or insulin alone for 1 year.[398] No significant differences were found between the groups in bimonthly insulin requirements, HbA_{1c} levels, or glucagon-stimulated C-peptide responses.

- A comparative trial of niacinamide (25 mg/kg daily) vs. vitamin E (15 mg/kg daily), vs. niacinamide plus vitamin E together with insulin therapy, was conducted for 1 year in patients with newly diagnosed diabetes mellitus (type 1).

The study found a slight increase in stimulated C-peptide levels from baseline in both groups, with no significant differences between the two groups.[400]

Combination Therapy Trials

- Ninety patients, newly diagnosed with diabetes mellitus (type 1), were randomized to receive one of three therapy regimens: cyclosporine (5 mg/kg daily) plus niacinamide (25 mg/kg daily) plus insulin, nicotinamide plus insulin, or insulin only for a period of 1 year.[163] Outcome measures included stimulated C-peptide levels, glycosylated HbA_{1c} levels, and clinical remission. The percentage of subjects achieving clinical remission at 1 year was significantly greater and longer in the niacinamide plus insulin group than in the other groups. C-peptide and glycosylated HbA_{1c} levels were not significantly different between the groups. This study suffers from a small sample size and inadequate blinding procedures. The results cannot be extrapolated to niacinamide monotherapy.

- Vialettes et al. studied the combination of cyclosporine and niacinamide and its effectiveness at inducing remission in subjects newly diagnosed with diabetes mellitus (type 1).[401] Results showed clinical remission to be achieved in 34% of patients at 6 months and 17% at 9 months, with continued remission at 1 year in only 9% of subjects. These results were compared retrospectively with those of the Cyclosporine Diabetes France trial and showed greater efficacy than that of placebo or cyclosporine alone at inducing remission. However, the results of this pilot study can only be considered preliminary.

- In a double-blind, controlled trial, 46 children (ages 1 to 17 years) newly diagnosed with diabetes mellitus (type 1) were randomized to receive either placebo or an antioxidant tablet (containing niacinamide, vitamin C, vitamin E, beta-carotene, and selenium) for a period of 2 years.[402] Subjects received concurrent insulin therapy as needed, and HbA_{1c} and C-peptide levels were monitored over the course of the study. Results showed no significant differences between antioxidant tablet and placebo in insulin dosing, HbA_{1c} levels, or C-peptide levels.

- A study in 48 children with newly diagnosed diabetes (type 1), niacinamide (200 to 600 mg daily) and insulin therapy together resulted in significantly lower mean postprandial glucose and HbA_{1c} levels, lower insulin requirements, and longer remission duration than with insulin alone.[161]

Type 1 Diabetes Mellitus: Prevention (Niacinamide)
Summary

- Animal research has found that niacinamide (not niacin) delays the development of diabetes mellitus (type 1).[295,335,390,403,404] Niacinamide has been shown to have no effect on insulin secretion or glucose kinetics, unlike niacin, which increases insulin resistance.[405] Given the proposed development of diabetes mellitus (type 1) through pancreatic islet beta cell destruction, caused partly by depletion of niacinamide adenine dinucleotide (NAD), activation of poly(ADP-ribose) polymerase (PARP), and free radical damage, and niacinamide's ability to protect against these stimuli, it has been postulated that niacinamide may play a role in the prevention of type 1 diabetes mellitus in "high-risk" individuals (defined as those with afflicted first-degree relatives with or without the presence of beta cell antibodies).[406] Initial human studies have not been uniformly positive and most have not been adequately randomized, blinded, or powered to draw strong conclusions regarding the use of niacinamide to prevent type 1 diabetes mellitus.

Positive Evidence

- Elliott et al. found that a 1% solution of niacinamide supplied to spontaneously diabetic insulin-dependent albino mice delayed the development of diabetes mellitus when given ≤250 days after birth.[335] This finding led Elliott et al. to investigate the use of niacinamide in children prone to developing diabetes mellitus (type 1). They assigned children (younger than 16 years of age) with first-degree relatives afflicted with diabetes mellitus (type 1) and a beta cell antibody level of ≥80 IU to either observation or treatment with niacinamide 150 to 300 mg per year of age daily (maximum dose of 3 g daily) to assess the effect of niacinamide on the development of diabetes mellitus (type 1).[188] After 2 years of follow-up, diabetes mellitus (type 1) had developed in 7 of 8 untreated children, whereas it developed in none of the children receiving niacinamide supplementation. After 2 years, diabetes mellitus (type 1) developed in only one child who received niacinamide, suggesting that niacinamide may have a role in the prevention of diabetes mellitus (type 1) in children with first-degree relatives with the disease. Although these results are promising, the lack of randomization or blinding and the small sample size limit their clinical usefulness.
- In a methodologically weak investigation, Manna et al. gave niacinamide (25 mg/kg daily) to six subjects with a "high risk" of developing diabetes mellitus (type 1) for a mean duration of 8.6 months and compared the results of glucose-stimulated insulin secretion tests from these patients with the results from seven high-risk subjects who received no treatment.[190] Results showed that subjects taking niacinamide had significantly increased insulin secretion at 8 months as compared with baseline, whereas the untreated subjects experienced decreased insulin secretion as compared with baseline, with a significant difference between the two groups ($p = 0.048$).

Negative Evidence

- The Deutsche Niacinamide Intervention Study randomized 65 children (ages 3 to 12 years) at risk for the development of type 1 diabetes mellitus (based on the presence of pancreatic islet beta cell antibodies and siblings with the disease) to receive oral niacinamide (1.2 g/m^2 daily) or placebo for a period of 3 years.[189] Follow-up evaluations were conducted every 6 months for the duration of the study and included determination of fasting blood glucose and HbA_{1c} levels and clinical diagnosis to detect type 1 diabetes mellitus. At the second interim analysis, the study was terminated owing to the development of diabetes mellitus (type 1) in 11 subjects randomized to receive niacinamide treatment. The results of this well-designed and adequately powered study suggest possible inefficacy of niacinamide in preventing the development of diabetes mellitus (type 1).
- In a small case series, Herskowitz et al. identified three patients at "high risk" for the development of diabetes mellitus (type 1) and started them on oral niacinamide therapy (1 g per 23 kg of body weight, in three divided doses daily).[407] Clinical diabetes mellitus (type 1) developed in all three subjects within the predicted 3-year period despite treatment.

Osteoarthritis (Niacinamide)
Summary

- Results of preliminary human research suggest that niacinamide may be useful in the treatment of osteoarthritis. However, further trials and replication of initial study results are necessary to ascertain the usefulness of niacinamide in this area.[408]

Evidence

- In a 12-week, randomized, double-blind, placebo-controlled trial comprising 72 patients with osteoarthritis, niacinamide (3 g daily) was shown to significantly decrease global arthritis impact (by 29%), improve flexibility, reduce inflammation (22% decrease in erythrocyte sedimentation rate), and reduce the use of concomitant anti-inflammatory medications.[408] Niacinamide was well tolerated, with no withdrawals due to study medication. This was a well-designed preliminary study, and further randomized, controlled trial data are needed to confirm these results and determine the place of niacinamide in osteoarthritis treatment.

FORMULARY: BRANDS USED IN CLINICAL TRIALS/ THIRD-PARTY TESTING
Brands Used in Statistically Significant Clinical Trials

- Nicangin[310]; Niaspan[107,108,118,132,135,139,212,268,365]; Enduracin[122]; Slo-Niacin[90]; Nicolar[138]; Nicobid.[138,139]

Brands Shown to Contain Claimed Ingredients Through Third-Party Testing

- Nature's Bounty Flush Free Niacin Inositol Hexanicotinate 500 mg Dietary Supplement.

References

1. Head KA. Inositol hexaniacinate: a safer alternative to niacin. Altern Med Rev 1996;1(3):176-184.
2. Welsh AL, Ede M. Inositol hexanicotinate for improved nicotinic acid therapy. Int Record Med 1961;174:9-15.
3. Shalita AR, Smith JG, Parish LC, et al. Topical nicotinamide compared with clindamycin gel in the treatment of inflammatory acne vulgaris. Int J Dermatol 1995;34(6):434-437.
4. Smith RF. A five year field trial of massive nicotinic acid therapy of alcoholics in Michigan. J Orthomol Psych 1974;3:327-331.
5. Makola D, Ash DM, Tatala SR, et al. A micronutrient-fortified beverage prevents iron deficiency, reduces anemia and improves the hemoglobin concentration of pregnant Tanzanian women. J Nutr 2003;133(5): 1339-1346.
6. Kaufman W. The use of vitamin therapy to reverse certain concomitants of aging. J Am Geriatr Soc 1955;3:927-936.
7. Hoffer A. Treatment of arthritis by nicotinic acid and nicotinamide. Can Med Assoc J 1959;81:235-239.
8. Kime CE. Bell's palsy: a new syndrome associated with treatment by nicotinic acid. Arch Otolaryngol 1958;68:28-32.
9. Jacobson EL, Dame AJ, Pyrek JS, et al. Evaluating the role of niacin in human carcinogenesis. Biochimie 1995;77(5):394-398.
10. Cumming RG, Mitchell P, Smith W. Diet and cataract: the Blue Mountains Eye Study. Ophthalmology 2000;107(3):450-456.
11. Boyonoski AC, Gallacher LM, Simon MM, et al. Niacin deficiency in rats increases the severity of ethylnitrosourea- induced anemia and leukopenia. J Nutr 2000;130(5):1102-1107.
12. Ajayi AA, Akinleye AO, Udoh SJ, et al. The effects of prednisolone and niacin on chloroquine-induced pruritus in malaria. Eur J Clin Pharmacol 1991;41(4):383-385.
13. Rabbani GH, Butler T, Bardhan PK, et al. Reduction of fluid-loss in cholera by nicotinic acid: a randomised controlled trial. Lancet 1983; 2(8365-66):1439-1442.
14. Turjman N, Gotterer GS, Hendrix TR. Prevention and reversal of cholera enterotoxin effects in rabbit jejunum by nicotinic acid. J Clin Invest 1978; 61:1155-1160.
15. Turjman N, Cardamone A, Gotterer GS, et al. Effect of nicotinic acid on cholera-induced fluid movement and unidirectional sodium fluxes in rabbit jejunum. Johns Hopkins Med J 1980;147:209-211.
16. Kidd GS, Donowitz M, O'Dorsio T, et al. Mild chronic watery diarrhea-

hypokalemia syndrome associated with pancreatic islet cell hyperplasia. Elevated plasma and tissue levels of gastric inhibitory polypeptide and successful management with nicotinic acid. Am J Med 1979;66:883-888.

17. Chouinard G, Young SN, Annable L, et al. Tryptophan-nicotinamide, imipramine and their combination in depression. A controlled study. Acta Psychiatr Scand 1979;59(4):395-414.

18. Gonzalez-Clemente JM, Munoz A, Fernandez-Usac E, et al. Desferrioxamine and nicotinamide in newly diagnosed type 1 diabetic patients: a randomized double blind placebo controlled trial. Diabetologia 1992;35:A202.

19. Polo V, Saibene A, Pontiroli AE. Nicotinamide improves insulin secretion and metabolic control in lean type 2 diabetic patients with secondary failure to sulphonylureas. Acta Diabetologia 1998;35(1):61-64.

20. Fielder P, Wolkin A, Rotrosen J. Niacin-induced flush as a measure of prostaglandin activity in alcoholics and schizophrenics. Biol Psychiatr 1986;21:1347-1350.

21. Glen AI, Cooper SJ, Rybakowski J, et al. Membrane fatty acids, niacin flushing and clinical parameters. Prostaglandins Leukot Essent Fatty Acids 1996;55(1-2):9-15.

22. Horrobin DF. Schizophrenia: a biochemical disorder? Biomedicine 1980; 32(2):54-55.

23. Hudson CJ, Lin A, Cogan S, et al. The niacin challenge test: clinical manifestation of altered transmembrane signal transduction in schizophrenia? Biol Psychiatry 1997;41(5):507-513.

24. Kunin RA. The action of aspirin in preventing the niacin flush and its relevance to the antischizophrenic action of megadose niacin. J Orthomol Psychiatry 1976;5(2):89-100.

25. Rybakowski J, Weterle R. Niacin test in schizophrenia and affective illness. Biol Psychiatry 1991;29(8):834-836.

26. Ward PE, Sutherland J, Glen EM, et al. Niacin skin flush in schizophrenia: a preliminary report. Schizophr Res 1998;29(3):269-274.

27. Wilson DW, Douglass AB. Niacin skin flush is not diagnostic of schizophrenia. Biol Psychiatry 1986;21(10):974-977.

28. Hudgins. Vitamin P, C and niacin for dysmenorrhea therapy. West J Surg and Gyn 1954;62:610-611.

29. Christian P, West KP, Khatry SK, et al. Effects of maternal micronutrient supplementation on fetal loss and infant mortality: a cluster-randomized trial in Nepal. Am J Clin Nutr 2003;78(6):1194-1202.

30. Ma A, Medenica M. Response of generalized granuloma annulare to high-dose niacinamide. Arch Dermatol 1983;119(10):836-839.

31. Selfridge G. Nicotinic acid and the eighth nerve: a preliminary report. Ann Otol Rhin Laryng 1939;48:39-53.

32. Olsen A, Thiong'o FW, Ouma JH, et al. Effects of multimicronutrient supplementation on helminth reinfection: a randomized, controlled trial in Kenyan schoolchildren. Trans R Soc Trop Med Hyg 2003;97(1):109-114.

33. Jolliffe N. Nicotinic acid deficiency encephalopathy. JAMA 1940;114: 307-312.

34. Murray MF, Srinivasan A. Nicotinamide inhibits HIV-1 in both acute and chronic in vitro infection. Biochem Biophys Res Commun 1995;210(3): 954-959.

35. Murray MF, Nghiem M, Srinivasan A. HIV infection decreases intracellular nicotinamide adenine dinucleotide [NAD]. Biochem Biophys Res Commun 1995;212(1):126-131.

36. Murray MF. Niacin as a potential AIDS preventive factor. Med Hypotheses 1999;53(5):375-379.

37. Tang AM, Graham NM, Saah AJ. Effects of micronutrient intake on survival in human immunodeficiency virus type 1 infection. Am J Epidemiol 1996;143(12):1244-1256.

38. Gadegbeku CA, Dhandayuthapani A, Shrayyef MZ, et al. Hemodynamic effects of nicotinic acid infusion in normotensive and hypertensive subjects. Am J Hypertens 2003;16(1):67-71.

39. Carlson LA, Froberg S, Oro L. A case of massive hypertriglyceridemia corrected by nicotinic acid or nicotinamide therapy. Atherosclerosis 1972;16(3):359-368.

40. Hannan F, Davoren P. Use of nicotinic acid in the management of recurrent hypoglycemic episodes in diabetes. Diabetes Care 2001;24(7): 1301.

41. Kiff RS, Quick CR. Does inositol nicotinate (Hexopal) influence intermittent claudication? A controlled trial. Br J Clin Pract 1988;42(4): 141-145.

42. O'Hara J. A double-blind placebo-controlled study of Hexopal in the treatment of intermittent claudication. J Int Med Res 1985;13(6): 322-327.

43. O'Hara J, Jolly PN, Nicol CG. The therapeutic efficacy of inositol nicotinate (Hexopal) in intermittent claudication: a controlled trial. Br J Clin Pract 1988;42(9):377-383.

44. Trueblood NA, Ramasamy R, Wang LF, et al. Niacin protects the isolated heart from ischemia-reperfusion injury. Am J Physiol Heart Circ Physiol 2000;279(2):H764-H771.

45. Ruze P. Kava-induced dermopathy: a niacin deficiency? Lancet 1990; 335(8703):1442-1445.

46. Arwert LI, Deijen JB, Drent ML. Effects of an oral mixture containing glycine, glutamine and niacin on memory, GH and IGF-I secretion in middle-aged and elderly subjects. Nutr Neurosci 2003;6(5):269-275.

47. Atkinson M. Observations on the etiology and treatment of Meniere's syndrome. JAMA 1941;116:1753-1760.

48. Harris HE, Moore PM. The use of nicotinic acid and thiamin chloride in the treatment of Meniere's syndrome. Med Clin North Amer 1940; 24(March):533-542.

49. Hultcrantz E, Hillerdal M, Angelborg C. Effect of nicotinic acid on cochlear blood flow. Arch Otorhinolaryngol 1982;234:279-283.

50. Gedye A. Hypothesized treatment for migraines using low doses of tryptophan, niacin, calcium, caffeine, and acetylsalicylic acid. Med Hypotheses 2001;56(1):91-94.

51. Moore MT. Treatment of multiple sclerosis with nicotinic acid and vitamin B_1. Arch Intern Med 1940;65:1-20.

52. Carlson LA, Danielson M, Ekberg I, et al. Reduction of myocardial reinfarction by the combined treatment with clofibrate and nicotinic acid. Atherosclerosis 1977;28(1):81-86.

53. Carlson LA, Rosenhamer G. Reduction of mortality in the Stockholm Ischaemic Heart Disease Secondary Prevention Study by combined treatment with clofibrate and nicotinic acid. Acta Med Scand 1988;223(5): 405-418.

54. Handfield-Jones S, Jones SK, Peachey RD. Nicotinamide treatment in diabetes. Br J Dermatol 1987;116(2):277.

55. Handfield-Jones S, Jones S, Peachey R. High dose nicotinamide in the treatment of necrobiosis lipoidica. Br J Dermatol 1988;118(5):693-696.

56. Sperduto RD, Hu TS, Milton RC, et al. The Linxian cataract studies. Two nutrition intervention trials. Arch Ophthalmol 1993;111(9):1246-1253.

57. Head KA. Premenstrual syndrome: nutritional and alternative approaches. Altern Med Rev 1997;2(1):12-25.

58. Mills PK, Beeson WL, Phillips RL, et al. Cohort study of diet, lifestyle, and prostate cancer in Adventist men. Cancer 1989;64(3):598-604.

59. Neumann R, Rappold E, Pohl-Markl H. Treatment of polymorphous light eruption with nicotinamide: a pilot study. Br J Dermatol 1986;115(1):77-80.

60. Aylward M. Hexopal in Raynaud's disease. J Int Med Res 1979;7(6): 484-491.

61. Ring EF, Bacon PA. Quantitative thermographic assessment of inositol nicotinate therapy in Raynaud's phenomena. J Int Med Res 1977;5(4): 217-222.

62. Sunderland GT, Belch JJ, Sturrock RD, et al. A double blind randomised placebo controlled trial of hexopal in primary Raynaud's disease. Clin Rheumatol 1988;7(1):46-49.

63. Ban TA. Canadian niacin study. Schizophr Bull 1971;4:6-7.

64. Denson R. Nicotinamide in the treatment of schizophrenia. Dis Nerv Syst 1962;23:167-172.

65. Greenbaum GH. An evaluation of niacinamide in the treatment of childhood schizophrenia. Am J Psychiatry 1970;127(1):89-92.

66. Hoffer A, Osmond H, Callbeck M, et al. Treatment of schizophrenia with nicotinic acid and nicotinamide. J Clin Exp Psychopath 1957;18:131-158.

67. Hoffer A, Osmond H. Treatment of schizophrenia with nicotinic acid: a 10-year follow-up. Acta Psychiat Scand 1964;40:171-189.

68. Hoffer A. Megavitamin B-3 therapy for schizophrenia. Can Psychiatr Assoc J 1971;16(6):499-504.

69. Hoffer A. The effect of nicotinic acid on the frequency and duration of re-hospitalization of schizophrenic patients; a controlled comparison study. Int J Neuropsychiatry 1966;2(3):234-240.

70. Meltzer H, Shader R, Grinspoon L. The behavioral effects of nicotinamide adenine dinucleotide in chronic schizophrenia. Psychopharmacologia 1969;15(2):144-152.

71. O'Reilly PO. Nicotinic acid therapy and the chronic schizophrenic. Dis Nerv System 1955;16(3):67-72.

72. Osmond H, Hoffer A. Massive niacin treatment in schizophrenia: review of a nine year study. Lancet 1962;1:316-320.

73. Ramsay RA, Ban TA, Lehmann HE, et al. Nicotinic acid as an adjuvant therapy in newly admitted schizophrenic patients. Can Med Assoc J 1970; 102:939-942.

74. Mohler H, Polc P, Cumin R, et al. Nicotinamide is a brain constituent with benzodiazepine-like actions. Nature 1979;278(5704):563-565.

75. Reimund E. Sleep deprivation–induced dermatitis: further support of nicotinic acid depletion in sleep deprivation. Med Hypotheses 1991;36(4): 371-373.

76. Hulshof JH, Vermeij P. The effect of nicotinamide on tinnitus: a double-blind controlled study. Clin Otolaryngol 1987;12(3):211-214.

77. Nakagawa K, Miyazaka M, Okui K, et al. N1-methylnicotinamide level in the blood after nicotinamide loading as further evidence for malignant tumor burden. Jpn J Cancer Res 1991;82:277-1283.

78. van der KA, Aarts NJ. Thermographical follow-up during treatment of chronic ulcerations with iontophoresis with xanthinol nicotinate. Bibl Radiol 1975;(6):203-209.

79. Fawzi WW, Msamanga GI, Spiegelman D, et al. Rationale and design of the Tanzania Vitamin and HIV Infection Trial. Control Clin Trials 1999; 20(1):75-90.

80. Baggenstoss AH, Christensen NA, Berge KG, et al. Fine structural changes in the liver in hypercholesteremic patients receiving long-term nicotinic acid therapy. Mayo Clin Proc 1967;42(7):385-399.

81. Berge KG, Achor RW, Christensen NA, et al. Hypercholesteremia and nicotinic acid: a long term study. Am J Med 1961;31:24-36.

82. Charmon RC, Matthews LB, Braeuler C. Nicotinic acid in the treatment of hypercholesterolemia: a long-term study. Angiology 1972;23:29-35.

83. Clementz GL, Holmes AW. Nicotinic acid–induced fulminant hepatic failure. J Clin Gastroenterol 1987;9(5):582-584.

84. Coppola A, Brady PG, Nord HJ. Niacin-induced hepatotoxicity: unusual presentations. South Med J 1994;87:30-32.

85. Dalton TA, Berry RS. Hepatotoxicity associated with sustained-release niacin. Am J Med 1992;93(1):102-104.

86. Etchason JA, Miller TD, Squires RW, et al. Niacin-induced hepatitis: a potential side effect with low-dose time-release niacin. Mayo Clin Proc 1991;66(1):23-28.

87. Ferenchick G, Rovner D. Case report: hepatitis and hematemesis complicating nicotinic acid use. Am J Med Sci 1989;298:191-193.

88. Fischer DJ, Knight LL, Vestal RE. Fulminant hepatic failure following low-dose sustained-release niacin therapy in hospital. West J Med 1991;155(4):410-412.

89. Goldstein MR. Potential problems with the widespread use of niacin. Am J Med 1988;85(6):881.

90. Gray DR, Morgan T, Chretien SD, et al. Efficacy and safety of controlled-release niacin in dyslipoproteinemic veterans. Ann Intern Med 1994;121(4):252-258.

91. Henkin Y, Johnson KC, Segrest JP. Rechallenge with crystalline niacin after drug-induced hepatitis from sustained-release niacin. JAMA 1990;264(2):241-243.

92. Henkin Y, Oberman A, Hurst DC, et al. Niacin revisited: clinical observations on an important but underutilized drug. Am J Med 1991;91(3):239-246.

93. Hodis HN. Acute hepatic failure associated with the use of low-dose sustained-release niacin. JAMA 1990;264:181.

94. Kohn RM, Montes M. Hepatic fibrosis following long acting nicotinic acid therapy: a case report. Am J Med Sci 1969;258:94-99.

95. Lawrence SP. Transient focal hepatic defects related to sustained-release niacin. J Clin Gastroenterol 1993;16:234-236.

96. Mullin GE, Greenson JK, Mitchell MC. Fulminant hepatic failure after ingestion of sustained-release nicotinic acid. Ann Intern Med 1989;111(3):253-255.

97. Pardue WO. Severe liver dysfunction during nicotinic acid therapy. JAMA 1961;175(2):137-138.

98. Patterson DJ, Dew EW, Gyorkey F, et al. Niacin hepatitis. South Med J 1983;76(2):239-241.

99. Rivin AU. Jaundice occurring during nicotinic acid therapy for hypercholesterolemia. JAMA 1959;170:2088-2089.

100. Schoch HK. The US Veterans Administration cadiology drug-lipid study: an interim report. Adv Exper Med Biol 1968;4:405-420.

101. Sugarmen AA, Clark CG. Jaundice following the administration of niacin. JAMA 1974;228:202.

102. Winter SL, Boyer JL. Hepatic toxicity from large doses of vitamin B₃ (nicotinamide). N Engl J Med 1973;289:1180-1182.

103. Berge KG. Side effects of nicotinic acid in treatment of hypercholesterolemia. Geriatrics 1961;16:416-422.

104. Carlson LA, Havel RJ, Ekelund LG, et al. Effect of nicotinic acid on the turnover rate and oxydation of the free fatty acids of plasma in man during exercise. Metabolism 1963;12(9):837-845.

105. Elam MB, Hunninghake DB, Davis KB, et al. Effect of niacin on lipid and lipoprotein levels and glycemic control in patients with diabetes and peripheral arterial disease: the ADMIT study: A randomized trial. Arterial Disease Multiple Intervention Trial. JAMA 2000;284(10):1263-1270.

106. Garg A, Grundy SM. Nicotinic acid as therapy for dyslipidemia in non-insulin-dependent diabetes mellitus. JAMA 1990;264(6):723-726.

107. Goldberg AC. Clinical trial experience with extended-release niacin (Niaspan): dose-escalation study. Am J Cardiol 1998;82(12A):35U-38U.

108. Goldberg A, Alagona P, Jr., Capuzzi DM, et al. Multiple-dose efficacy and safety of an extended-release form of niacin in the management of hyperlipidemia. Am J Cardiol 2000;85(9):1100-1105.

109. Illingworth DR, Stein EA, Mitchel YB, et al. Comparative effects of lovastatin and niacin in primary hypercholesterolemia. A prospective trial. Arch Intern Med 1994;154(14):1586-1595.

110. Miettinen TA, Taskinen MR, Pelkonen R, et al. Glucose tolerance and plasma insulin in man during acute and chronic administration of nicotinic acid. Acta Med Scand 1969;186(4):247-253.

111. Parsons WB. Reduction in hepatic synthesis of cholesterol from C14-acetate in hypercholesterolemic patients by nicotinic acid. Circulation 1961;90(suppl 1):1099-1100.

112. Parsons WB. Treatment of hypercholesterolemia by nicotinic acid: progress report, with review of studies regarding mechanism of action. Arch Int Med 1961;107:639-652.

113. Vega GL, Grundy SM. Lipoprotein responses to treatment with lovastatin, gemfibrozil, and nicotinic acid in normolipidemic patients with hypoalphalipoproteinemia. Arch Intern Med 1994;154(1):73-82.

114. Alhadeff L, Gualtieri CT, Lipton M. Toxic effects of water-soluble vitamins. Nutr Rev 1984;42(2):33-40.

115. Brown G, Albers JJ, Fischer LD, et al. Regression of coronary artery disease as a result of intensive lipid-lowering therapy in men with high levels of apolipoprotein B. N Engl J Med 1990;323(18):1289-1298.

116. Gaut ZN, Solomon HM, Miller ON. Influence of antilipemic doses of nicotinic acid on carbohydrate tolerance and plasma insulin levels in man. Diabetes 1970;19:385.

117. Gaut ZN, Pocelinko R, Solomon HM, et al. Oral glucose tolerance, plasma insulin, and uric acid excretion in man during chronic administration of nicotinic acid. Metabolism 1971;20(11):1031-1035.

118. Knopp RH, Alagona P, Davidson M, et al. Equivalent efficacy of a time-release form of niacin (Niaspan) given once-a-night versus plain niacin in the management of hyperlipidemia. Metabolism 1998;47(9):1097-1104.

119. Lisi DM. Niacin and hyperuricemia: how often does it occur and how often are patients started on hypouricemic agents. Int Pharm Abstracts 1999;36(21):2223.

120. Olsson AG, Oro L, Rossner S. Clinical and metabolic effects of pentaerythritol tetranicotinate (Perycit) and a comparison with plain nicotinic acid. Atherosclerosis 1974;19(1):61-73.

121. Parsons WB. Studies of nicotinic acid use in hypercholesterolemia. Arch Intern Med 1961;107:653-667.

122. Wahlberg G, Walldius G, Olsson AG, et al. Effects of nicotinic acid on serum cholesterol concentrations of high density lipoprotein subfractions HDL2 and HDL3 in hyperlipoproteinaemia. J Intern Med 1990;228(2):151-157.

123. Parsons WB. Activation of peptic ulcer by nicotinic acid: report of five cases. JAMA 1960;173:92-96.

124. Alderman JD, Pasternak RC, Sacks FM, et al. Effect of a modified, well-tolerated niacin regimen on serum total cholesterol, high density lipoprotein cholesterol and the cholesterol to high density lipoprotein ratio. Am J Cardiol 1989;64(12):725-729.

125. Brown WV. Niacin for lipid disorders. Indications, effectiveness, and safety. Postgrad Med 1995;98(2):185-189.

126. Christensen NA, Achor RW, Berge KG, et al. Nicotinic acid treatment of hypercholesterolemia, comparison of plain and sustained action preparations and report of two cases of jaundice. JAMA 1961;177:546-550.

127. Colwell L. Adverse drug reactions: hepatotoxicity and flushing with niacin therapy in a patient with hyperlipidemia. J Pharm Practice 1994;7:V-VI.

128. Einstein N, Baker A, Galper J, et al. Jaundice due to nicotinic acid therapy. Am J Dig Dis 1975;20(3):282-286.

129. Han JJ. Nicotinic acid–induced hepatotoxicity: potentially serious adverse effect with sustained-release niacin. Int Pharm Abstracts 1995;32:2325.

130. Yates AA, Schlicker SA, Suitor CW. Dietary reference intakes: the new basis for recommendations for calcium and related nutrients, B vitamins, and choline. J Am Diet Assoc 1998;98(6):699-706.

131. Achor RWP, Berge KG, Barker NW, et al. Treatment of hypercholesterolemia with nicotinic acid. Circulation 1958;17:497-504.

132. Capuzzi DM, Guyton JR, Morgan JM, et al. Efficacy and safety of an extended-release niacin (Niaspan): a long-term study. Am J Cardiol 1998;82(12A):74U-81U.

133. Chazin BJ. Effect of nicotinic acid on blood cholesterol. Geriatrics 1960;15(6):423-429.

134. Chojnowska-Jezierska J, Adamska-Dyniewska H. Efficacy and safety of one-year treatment with slow-release nicotinic acid. Monitoring of drug concentration in serum. Int J Clin Pharmacol Ther 1998;36(6):326-332.

135. Guyton JR, Blazing MA, Hagar J, et al. Extended-release niacin vs gemfibrozil for the treatment of low levels of high-density lipoprotein cholesterol. Niaspan-Gemfibrozil Study Group. Arch Intern Med 2000;160(8):1177-1184.

136. Hoeg JM, Maher MB, Bou E, et al. Normalization of plasma lipoprotein concentrations in patients with type II hyperlipoproteinemia by combined use of neomycin and niacin. Circulation 1984;70(6):1004-1011.

137. King JM, Crouse JR, Terry JG, et al. Evaluation of effects of unmodified niacin on fasting and postprandial plasma lipids in normolipidemic men with hypoalphalipoproteinemia. Am J Med 1994;97(4):323-331.

138. Knopp RH, Ginsberg J, Albers JJ, et al. Contrasting effects of unmodified and time-release forms of niacin on lipoproteins in hyperlipidemic subjects: clues to mechanism of action of niacin. Metabolism 1985;34(7):642-650.

139. Knopp RH. Clinical profiles of plain versus sustained-release niacin (Niaspan) and the physiologic rationale for nighttime dosing. Am J Cardiol 1998;82(12A):24U-28U.

140. Martin-Jadraque R, Tato F, Mostaza JM, et al. Effectiveness of low-dose crystalline nicotinic acid in men with low high-density lipoprotein cholesterol levels. Arch Intern Med 1996;156(10):1081-1088.

141. McKenney JM, McCormick LS, Weiss S, et al. A randomized trial of the effects of atorvastatin and niacin in patients with combined hyperlipidemia or isolated hypertriglyceridemia. Collaborative Atorvastatin Study Group. Am J Med 1998;104(2):137-143.

142. Morato Hernandez ML, Ichazo Cerro MS, Alvarado Vega AG, et al. [Efficacy and safety of immediate-release niacin in patients with ischemic cardiopathy. Experience of the Instituto Nacional de Cardiologia "Ignacio Chavez"]. Arch Inst Cardiol Mex 2000;70(4):367-376.

143. Mostaza JM, Schulz I, Vega GL, et al. Comparison of pravastatin with crystalline nicotinic acid monotherapy in treatment of combined hyperlipidemia. Am J Cardiol 1997;79(9):1298-1301.

144. Schectman G, Hiatt J, Hartz A. Evaluation of the effectiveness of lipid-lowering therapy (bile acid sequestrants, niacin, psyllium and lovastatin) for treating hypercholesterolemia in veterans. Am J Cardiol 1993;71(10):759-765.

N

145. Yovos JG, Patel ST, Falko JM, et al. Effects of nicotinic acid therapy on plasma lipoproteins and very low density lipoprotein apoprotein C subspecies in hyperlipoproteinemia. J Clin Endocrinol Metab 1982;54(6): 1210-1215.

146. Zema MJ. Gemfibrozil, nicotinic acid and combination therapy in patients with isolated hypoalphalipoproteinemia: a randomized, open-label, crossover study. J Am Coll Cardiol 2000;35(3):640-646.

147. Johansson J, Carlson LA. The effects of nicotinic acid treatment on high density lipoprotein particle size subclass levels in hyperlipidaemic subjects. Atherosclerosis 1990;83(2-3):207-216.

148. Patsch JR, Yeshurun D, Jackson RL, et al. Effects of clofibrate, nicotinic acid and diet on the properties of the plasma lipoproteins in a subject with type III hyperlipoproteinemia. Am J Med 1977;63(6):1001-1009.

149. Shepherd J, Packard CJ, Patsch JR, et al. Effects of nicotinic acid therapy on plasma high density lipoprotein subfraction distribution and composition and on apolipoprotein A metabolism. J Clin Invest 1979;63(5):858-867.

150. Grundy SM, Mok HY, Zech L, et al. Influence of nicotinic acid on metabolism of cholesterol and triglycerides in man. J Lipid Res 1981; 22(1):24-36.

151. Berge KG, Achor RWP, Barker NW, et al. Comparison of the treatment of hypercholesterolemia with nicotinic acid, sitosterol, and safflower oil. Am Heart J 1959;58:849-853.

152. Lavie CJ, Mailander L, Milani RV. Marked benefit with sustained-release niacin therapy in patients with "isolated" very low levels of high-density lipoprotein cholesterol and coronary artery disease. Am J Cardiol 1992; 69(12):1083-1085.

153. Sacks FM, Pasternak RC, Gibson CM, et al. Effect on coronary atherosclerosis of decrease in plasma cholesterol concentrations in normocholesterolaemic patients. Harvard Atherosclerosis Reversibility Project (HARP) Group. Lancet 1994;344(8931):1182-1186.

154. Anonymous. Clofibrate and niacin in coronary heart disease. JAMA 1975;231(4):360-381.

155. Chesney CM, Elam MB, Herd JA, et al. Effect of niacin, warfarin, and antioxidant therapy on coagulation parameters in patients with peripheral arterial disease in the Arterial Disease Multiple Intervention Trial (ADMIT). Am Heart J 2000;140(4):631-636.

156. Rosenhamer G, Carlson LA. Effect of combined clofibrate–nicotinic acid treatment in ischemic heart disease. Atherosclerosis 1980;37(1):129-142.

157. Fouts PJ, Helmer OM, Lepkovsky S, et al. Treatment of human pellagra with nicotinic acid. Proc Soc Exp Biol Med 1937;37:405-407.

158. Smith DT, Ruffin JM, Smith SG. Pellagra successfully treated with nicotinic acid: a case report. JAMA 1937;109:2054-2055.

159. Spies TD, Grant JM, Stone RE, et al. Recent observations on the treatment of six hundred pellagrins with special emphasis on the use of nicotinic acid in prophylaxis. South Med J 1938;31(12):1231.

160. Chase HP, Butler-Simon N, Garg S, et al. A trial of nicotinamide in newly diagnosed patients with type 1 (insulin-dependent) diabetes mellitus. Diabetologia 1990;33:444-446.

161. Paskova M, Ikao I, Trozova D, et al. Nicotinamide treatment in children with newly diagnosed type 1 diabetes mellitus. Diabetologia 1992;35:A203.

162. Pozzilli P, Visalli N, Ghirlanda G, et al. Nicotinamide increases C-peptide secretion in patients with recent onset type 1 diabetes. Diabet Med 1989; 6(7):568-572.

163. Pozzilli P. The IMDIAB I multicentre study in newly diagnosed insulin dependent diabetic patients: final results. Diabetologia 1991;34(suppl 2): A29.

164. Pozzilli P, Visalli N, Ghirlanda G, et al. Nicotinamide therapy in patients with newly-diagnosed type 1 (insulin-dependent) diabetes. Diabetologia 1988;31:533A.

165. Vague P, Vialettes B, Lassmann-Vague V, et al. Nicotinamide may extend remission phase in insulin-dependent diabetes. Lancet 1987;1(8533): 619-620.

166. Vague P, Picq R, Bernal M, et al. Effect of nicotinamide treatment on the residual insulin secretion in type 1 (insulin-dependent) diabetic patients. Diabetologia 1989;32(5):316-321.

167. Anonymous. ASHP Therapeutic Position Statement on the safe use of niacin in the management of dyslipidemias. American Society of Health-System Pharmacists. Am J Health Syst Pharm 1997;54(24):2815-2819.

168. Carlson LA. The broad spectrum hypolipidaemic drug nicotinic acid. J Drug Dev 1990;3(suppl 1):223-226.

169. Andersson R, Svedmyr N, Aberg G. Studies on the mechanism of flush induced by nicotinic acid. Acta Pharmacol et Toxicol 1974;35(suppl 1):17.

170. Andersson RG, Aberg G, Brattsand R, et al. Studies on the mechanism of flush induced by nicotinic acid. Acta Pharmacol Toxicol (Copenh) 1977; 41(1):1-10.

171. Ding RW, Kolbe K, Merz B, et al. Pharmacokinetics of nicotinic acid–salicylic acid interaction. Clin Pharmacol Ther 1989;46(6):642-647.

172. Dunn RT, Ford MA, Rindone JP, et al. Low dose aspirin and ibuprofen reduce the cutaneous reactions following niacin administration. Am J Therapeut 1995;2:478-480.

173. Jay RH, Dickson AC, Betteridge DJ. Effects of aspirin upon the flushing reaction induced by niceritrol. Br J Clin Pharmacol 1990;29(1):120-122.

174. Jungnickel PW, Maloley PA, Vander Tuin EL, et al. Effect of two aspirin

175. Whelan AM, Price SO, Fowler SF, et al. The effect of aspirin on niacin-induced cutaneous reactions. J Fam Pract 1992;34(2):165-168.

176. Wilkin JK, Wilkin O, Kapp R, et al. Aspirin blocks nicotinic acid–induced flushing. Clin Pharmacol Ther 1982;31:478-482.

177. Wilkin JK, Fortner G, Reinhardt LA, et al. Prostaglandins and nicotinate-provoked increase in cutaneous blood flow. Clin Pharmacol Ther 1985; 38(3):273-277.

178. Eklund B, Kaijser L, Nowak J, et al. Prostaglandins contribute to the vasodilation induced by nicotinic acid. Prostaglandins 1979;17(6): 821-830.

179. Kaijser L, Eklund B, Olsson AG, et al. Dissociation of the effects of nicotinic acid on vasodilatation and lipolysis by a prostaglandin synthesis inhibitor, indomethacin, in man. Med Biol 1979;57(2):114-117.

180. Phillips WS, Lightman SL. Is cutaneous flushing prostaglandin mediated? Lancet 1981;1(8223):754-756.

181. Svedmyr N, Heggelund A, Aberg G. Influence of indomethacin on flush induced by nicotinic acid in man. Acta Pharmacol Toxicol 1977;41: 397-400.

182. Hoffer A. Niacin reaction. J Fam Pract 1992;34(6):677, 680-677, 681.

183. Knapp TR, Middleton RK. Adverse effects of sustained-release niacin. DICP 1991;25(3):253-254.

184. Knopp RH. Niacin and hepatic failure. Ann Intern Med 1989;111(9):769.

185. McKenney JM, Proctor JD, Harris S, et al. A comparison of the efficacy and toxic effects of sustained- vs immediate-release niacin in hypercholesterolemic patients. JAMA 1994;271(9):672-677.

186. Brown BG, Bardsley J, Poulin D, et al. Moderate dose, three-drug therapy with niacin, lovastatin, and colestipol to reduce low-density lipoprotein cholesterol <100 mg/dl in patients with hyperlipidemia and coronary artery disease. Am J Cardiol 1997;80(2):111-115.

187. Frost PH. All niacin is not the same. Ann Intern Med 1991;114(12):1065.

188. Elliott RB, Chase HP. Prevention or delay of type 1 (insulin-dependent) diabetes mellitus in children using nicotinamide. Diabetologia 1991;34(5): 362-365.

189. Lampeter EF, Klinghammer A, Scherbaum WA, et al. The Deutsche Nicotinamide Intervention Study: an attempt to prevent type 1 diabetes. DENIS Group. Diabetes 1998;47(6):980-984.

190. Manna R, Migliore A, Martini LS, et al. Nicotinamide treatment in subjects at high risk of developing IDDM improves insulin secretion. Br J Clin Pract 1991;46:177-179.

191. Chen KK, Rose CL, Robbins EB. Toxicity of nicotinic acid. Proc Soc Exp Biol Med 1938;38:241-245.

192. Brazda FG, Coulson RA. Toxicity of nicotinic acid and some of its derivatives. Proc Soc Exp Biol Med 1946;62:19-20.

193. Unna K. Studies on the toxicity and pharmacology of nicotinic acid. J Pharmacol Exp Ther 1939;65:95-103.

194. Earthman TP, Odom L, Mullins CA. Lactic acidosis associated with high-dose niacin therapy. South Med J 1991;84(4):496-497.

195. Schwab RA, Bachhuber BH. Delirium and lactic acidosis caused by ethanol and niacin coingestion. Am J Emerg Med 1991;9(4):363-365.

196. Fineberg SK. Anaphylactic shock due to nicotinic acid. N Y State J Med 1948;48:635-636.

197. Pelner L. Anaphylaxis to the injections of nicotinic acid (niacin); successful treatment with epinephrine. Ann Intern Med 1947;26:290-294.

198. Powers BR. Circulatory collapse following intravenous administration of nicotinic acid (niacin). Ann Intern Med 1948;29:558-560.

199. Berge KG, Achor RWP, Barker NW, et al. Comparison of nicotinic acid, sitosterol and safflower oil in treatment of hypercholesterolemia. Circulation 1958;28:490.

200. Gibbons LW, Gonzalez V, Gordon N, et al. The prevalence of side effects with regular and sustained-release nicotinic acid. Am J Med 1995;99(4): 378-385.

201. Jacobson TA, Amorosa LF. Combination therapy with fluvastatin and niacin in hypercholesterolemia: a preliminary report on safety. Am J Cardiol 1994;73(14):25D-29D.

202. Luria MH. Effect of low-dose niacin on high-density lipoprotein cholesterol and total cholesterol/high-density lipoprotein cholesterol ratio. Arch Intern Med 1988;148(11):2493-2495.

203. Mosher LR. Nicotinic acid side effects and toxicity: a review. Am J Psychiatry 1970;126(9):1290-1296.

204. O'Kane MJ, Trinick TR, Tynan MB, et al. A comparison of acipimox and nicotinic acid in type 2b hyperlipidaemia. Br J Clin Pharmacol 1992;33: 451-453.

205. O'Keefe JH, Jr., Harris WS, Nelson J, et al. Effects of pravastatin with niacin or magnesium on lipid levels and postprandial lipemia. Am J Cardiol 1995;76(7):480-484.

206. Tornvall P, Walldius G. A comparison between nicotinic acid and acipimox in hypertriglyceridaemia—effects on serum lipids, lipoproteins, glucose tolerance and tolerability. J Intern Med 1991;230(5):415-421.

207. Andrade SE, Walker AM, Gottlieb LK, et al. Discontinuation of antihyperlipidemic drugs—do rates reported in clinical trials reflect rates in primary care settings? N Engl J Med 1995;332:1125-1131.

208. Rindone JP, Arriola OG. Experience with crystalline niacin as the preferred

drug for dyslipidemia in a specialty clinic. Pharmacotherapy 1997;17(6): 1296-1299.

209. Pozzilli P, Andreani D. The potential role of nicotinamide in the secondary prevention of IDDM. Diabetes Metabolism Reviews 1993;9(3):219-230.

210. Greenbaum CJ, Kahn SE, Palmer JP. Nicotinamide's effects on glucose metabolism in subjects at risk for IDDM. Diabetes 1996;45(11): 1631-1634.

211. Chojnowska-Jezierska J, Adamska-Dyniewska H. [Prolonged treatment with slow release nicotinic acid in patients with type II hyperlipidemia]. Pol Arch Med Wewn 1997;98(11):391-399.

212. Morgan JM, Capuzzi DM, Guyton JR, et al. Treatment effect of Niaspan, a controlled-release niacin, in patients with hypercholesterolemia: a placebo-controlled trial. J Cardiovasc Pharmacol Ther 1996;1(3):195-202.

213. Neuvonen PJ, Roivas L, Laine K, et al. The bioavailability of sustained release nicotinic acid formulations. Br J Clin Pharmacol 1991;32:473-476.

214. Rader JI, Calvert RJ, Hathcock JN. Hepatic toxicity of unmodified and time-release preparations of niacin. Am J Med 1992;92(1):77-81.

215. Aberg G, Svedmyr N. Thermographic registration of flush. Arzneimittelforschung 1971;21(6):795-796.

216. Altschul R, Hoffer A, Stephen JD. Influence of nicotinic acid on serum cholesterol in man. Arch Biochem 1955;54:558-559.

217. Aronov DM, Keenan JM, Akhmedzhanov NM, et al. Clinical trial of wax-matrix sustained-release niacin in a Russian population with hyper-cholesterolemia. Arch Fam Med 1996;5(10):567-575.

218. Colletti RB, Neufeld EJ, Roff NK, et al. Niacin treatment of hyper-cholesterolemia in children. Pediatrics 1993;92(1):78-82.

219. Davignon J, Roederer G, Montigny M, et al. Comparative efficacy and safety of pravastatin, nicotinic acid and the two combined in patients with hypercholesterolemia. Am J Cardiol 1994;73(5):339-345.

220. Guyton JR, Goldberg AC, Kreisberg RA, et al. Effectiveness of once-nightly dosing of extended-release niacin alone and in combination for hypercholesterolemia. Am J Cardiol 1998;82(6):737-743.

221. Keenan JM, Wenz JB, Ripsin CM, et al. A clinical trial of oat bran and niacin in the treatment of hyperlipidemia. J Fam Pract 1992;34:313-319.

222. Keenan JM, Fontaine PL, Wenz JB, et al. Niacin revisited. A randomized, controlled trial of wax-matrix sustained-release niacin in hyper-cholesterolemia. Arch Intern Med 1991;151(7):1424-1432.

223. Malloy MJ, Kane JP, Kunitake ST, et al. Complementarity of colestipol, niacin, and lovastatin in treatment of severe familial hypercholesterolemia. Ann Intern Med 1987;107(5):616-623.

224. Mahl M, Lange K. A long term study of the effect of nicotinic acid medication on hypercholesterolemia. Am J Med Sc 1963;65:673.

225. Ruiter M, Meyler L. Skin changes after therapeutic administration of nicotinic acid in large doses. Dermatologica 1960;120:139-144.

226. Leighton RF, Gordon NF, Small GS, et al. Dental and gingival pain as side effects of niacin therapy. Chest 1998;114(5):1472-1474.

227. Kahn SE, Beard JC, Schwartz MW, et al. Increased beta-cell secretory capacity as mechanism for islet adaptation to nicotinic acid–induced insulin resistance. Diabetes 1989;38(5):562-568.

228. Molnar GD, Berge KG, Rosevear JW, et al. The effect of nicotinic acid in diabetes mellitus. Metabolism 1964;13(2):181-190.

229. Pollack H. Nicotinic acid and diabetes. Diabetes 1962;11(2):144.

230. Cashin-Hemphill L, Spencer CA, Nicoloff JT, et al. Alterations in serum thyroid hormonal indices with colestipol-niacin therapy. Ann Intern Med 1987;107(3):324-329.

231. Drinka PJ. Alterations in thyroid and hepatic function tests associated with preparations of sustained-release niacin. Mayo Clin Proc 1992;67(12):1206.

232. O'Brien T, Silverberg JD, Nguyen TT. Nicotinic acid-induced toxicity associated with cytopenia and decreased levels of thyroxine-binding globulin. Mayo Clin Proc 1992;67(5):465-468.

233. Shakir KM, Kroll S, Aprill BS, et al. Nicotinic acid decreases serum thyroid hormone levels while maintaining a euthyroid state. Mayo Clin Proc 1995; 70(6):556-558.

234. Dearing BD, Lavie CJ, Lohmann TP, et al. Niacin-induced clotting factor synthesis deficiency with coagulopathy. Arch Intern Med 1992;152(4): 861-863.

235. O'Reilly PO, Callbeck MJ, Hoffer A. Sustained-release nicotinic acid (Nicospan): effect on (1) cholesterol levels and (2) leukocytes. Canad Med Assn J 1959;80:359-362.

236. Johansson JO, Egberg N, Asplund-Carlson A, et al. Nicotinic acid treatment shifts the fibrinolytic balance favourably and decreases plasma fibrinogen in hypertriglyceridaemic men. J Cardiovasc Risk 1997;4(3): 165-171.

237. Philipp CS, Cisar LA, Saidi P, et al. Effect of niacin supplementation on fibrinogen levels in patients with peripheral vascular disease. Am J Cardiol 1998;82(5):697-9, A9.

238. Gharavi AG, Diamond JA, Smith DA, et al. Niacin-induced myopathy. Am J Cardiol 1994;74(8):841-842.

239. Litin SC, Anderson CF. Nicotinic acid–associated myopathy: a report of three cases. Am J Med 1989;86(4):481-483.

240. Schuna AA. Safe use of niacin. Am J Health Syst Pharm 1997;54(24):2803.

241. American Diabetes Association. Consensus statement: detection and management of lipid disorders in diabetics. Diabetes Care 1996; 19(suppl 1):S96-S102.

242. Garg R, Malinow M, Pettinger M, et al. Niacin treatment increases plasma homocyst(e)ine levels. Am Heart J 1999;138(6 Pt 1):1082-1087.

243. Kryzhanovskii GN, Shandra AA. [Effect of diazepam, carbamazepine, sodium valproate and their combinations with vitamin preparations on epileptic activity]. Biull Eksp Biol Med 1985;100(11):545-547.

244. Rasool AA, Hussain AA, Dittert LW. Solubility enhancement of some water-insoluble drugs in the presence of nicotinamide and related compounds. J Pharm Sci 1991;80(4):387-393.

245. Alaupovic P, Blankenhorn DH, Nessim SA, et al. The effect of niacin, colestipol, and low fat diet on apolipoproteins in normolipemic men with coronary bypass. Arteriosclerosis Council Abstracts 2001;1:415a.

246. Andrews TC, Whitney EJ, Green G, et al. Effect of gemfibrozil +/− niacin +/− cholestyramine on endothelial function in patients with serum low-density lipoprotein cholesterol levels <160 mg/dl and high-density lipoprotein cholesterol levels <40 mg/dl. Am J Cardiol 1997;80(7): 831-835.

247. Blankenhorn DH, Johnson RL, Nessim SA, et al. The Cholesterol Lowering Atherosclerosis Study (CLAS): design, methods and baseline results. Controlled Clin Trials 1987;8:356-387.

248. Blankenhorn DH, Nessim SA, Johnson RL, et al. Beneficial effects of combined colestipol-niacin therapy on coronary atherosclerosis and coronary venous bypass grafts. JAMA 1987;257(23):3233-3240.

249. Blankenhorn DH, Malinow MR, Mack WJ. Colestipol plus niacin therapy elevates plasma homocysteine levels. Coron Art Dis 1991;2(3):357-360.

250. Crouse JR III. New developments in the use of niacin for treatment of hyperlipidemia: new considerations in the use of an old drug. Coron Artery Dis 1996;7(4):321-326.

251. Illingworth DR, Phillipson BE, Rapp JH, et al. Colestipol plus nicotinic acid in treatment of heterozygous familial hypercholesterolaemia. Lancet 1981;1(8215):296-298.

252. Kuo PT, Kostis JB, Moreyra AE, et al. Familial type II hyperlipoproteinemia with coronary heart disease: effect of diet-colestipol-nicotinic acid treatment. Chest 1981;79(3):286-291.

253. Mack WJ, Selzer RH, Hodis HN, et al. One-year reduction and longitudinal analysis of carotid intima-media thickness associated with colestipol/niacin therapy. Stroke 1993;24(12):1779-1783.

254. Matsui MS, Rozovski SJ. Drug-nutrient interaction. Clin Ther 1982;4(6): 423-440.

255. Nessim SA, Chin HP, Alaupovic P, et al. Combined therapy of niacin, colestipol, and fat-controlled diet in men with coronary bypass. Effect on blood lipids and apolipoproteins. Arteriosclerosis 1983;3(6):568-573.

256. Superko HR, Williams PT, Alderman EL. Differential effect on HDL of niacin and resin in LDL subclass pattern A and B subjects. Circulation 1993;88:2072A.

257. Sprecher DL. Raising high-density lipoprotein cholesterol with niacin and fibrates: a comparative review. Am J Cardiol 2000;86(12A):46L-50L.

258. Leklem JE, Brown RR, Rose DP, et al. Metabolism of tryptophan and niacin in oral contraceptives users receiving controlled intakes of vitamin B6. Am J Clin Nutr 1975;28(2):146-156.

259. Figge HL, Figge J, Souney PF, et al. Nicotinic acid: a review of its clinical use in the treatment of lipid disorders. Pharmacotherapy 1988;8(5):287-294.

260. Brown BG, Zhao XQ, Chait A, et al. Simvastatin and niacin, antioxidant vitamins, or the combination for the prevention of coronary disease. N Engl J Med 2001;345(22):1583-1592.

261. Capuzzi DM, Morgan JM, Brusco OA, Jr., et al. Niacin dosing: relationship to benefits and adverse effects. Curr Atheroscler Rep 2000; 2(1):64-71.

262. Gardner SF, Schneider EF, Granberry MC, et al. Combination therapy with low-dose lovastatin and niacin is as effective as higher-dose lovastatin. Pharmacotherapy 1996;16(3):419-423.

263. Jacobson TA, Chin MM, Fromell GJ, et al. Fluvastatin with and without niacin for hypercholesterolemia. Am J Cardiol 1994;74(2):149-154.

264. Jacobson TA, Jokubaitis LA, Amorosa LF. Fluvastatin and niacin in hyper-cholesterolemia: a preliminary report on gender differences in efficacy. Am J Med 1994;96(6A):64S-68S.

265. Kashyap ML, Evans R, Simmons PD, et al. New combination niacin/statin formulation shows pronounced effects on major lipoproteins and is well tolerated. J Am Coll Cardiol 2000;35(suppl A):326.

266. Tsalamandris C, Panagiotopoulos S, Sinha A, et al. Complementary effects of pravastatin and nicotinic acid in the treatment of combined hyperlipidaemia in diabetic and non-diabetic patients. J Cardiovasc Risk 1994;1(3):231-239.

267. Vacek JL, Dittmeier G, Chiarelli T, et al. Comparison of lovastatin (20 mg) and nicotinic acid (1.2 g) with either drug alone for type II hyper-lipoproteinemia. Am J Cardiol 1995;76(3):182-184.

268. Wolfe ML, Vartanian SF, Ross JL, et al. Safety and effectiveness of Niaspan when added sequentially to a statin for treatment of dyslipidemia. Am J Cardiol 2001;87(4):476-9, A7.

269. Cooke HM. Lovastatin- and niacin-induced rhabdomyolysis. Hosp Pharm 1994;29:33-34, 46.

270. Garnett WR. Interactions with hydroxymethylglutaryl-coenzyme A reductase inhibitors. Am J Health Syst Pharm 1995;52(15):1639-1645.

271. Reaven P, Witztum JL. Lovastatin, nicotinic acid, and rhabdomyolysis. Ann Intern Med 1988;109(7):597-598.

272. Paul TL, Hramiak IM, Mahon JL, et al. Nicotinamide and insulin sensitivity. Diabetologia 1993;36(4):369.

273. Darvay A, Basarab T, McGregor JM, et al. Isoniazid induced pellagra despite pyridoxine supplementation. Clin Exp Dermatol 1999;24(3):167-169.

274. Ishii N, Nishihara Y. Pellagra encephalopathy among tuberculous patients: its relation to isoniazid therapy. J Neurol Neurosurg Psychiatry 1985; 48(7):628-634.

275. Gurakar A, Hoeg JM, Kostner G, et al. Levels of lipoprotein Lp(a) decline with neomycin and niacin treatment. Atherosclerosis 1985;57(2-3):293-301.

276. Clarke JF, Kies C. Niacin nutritional status of adolescent humans fed high-dosage, pantothenic acid supplements. Nutrit Reports Int 1985;31(6):1271-1279.

277. Cohen L, Morgan J. Effectiveness of individualized long-term therapy with niacin and probucol in reduction of serum cholesterol. J Fam Pract 1988; 26(2):145-150.

278. Shibata K, Fukuwatari T, Sugimoto E. Effects of dietary pyrazinamide, an antituberculosis agent, on the metabolism of tryptophan to niacin and of tryptophan to serotonin in rats. Biosci Biotechnol Biochem 2001;65(6):1339-1346.

279. Cheung MC, Wolfbauer G, Kennedy H, et al. Plasma phospholipid transfer protein activity in patients with low HDL and cardiovascular disease treated with simvastatin and niacin. Biochim Biophys Acta 2001;1537(2):117-124.

280. Cheung MC, Zhao XQ, Chait A, et al. Antioxidant supplements block the response of HDL to simvastatin-niacin therapy in patients with coronary artery disease and low HDL. Arterioscler Thromb Vasc Biol 2001;21(8):1320-1326.

281. Freedman JE. Antioxidant versus lipid-altering therapy—some answers, more questions. N Engl J Med 2001;345(22):1636-1637.

282. Biondi-Zoccai GG, Abbate A. Antioxidant vitamins and coronary disease. N Engl J Med 2002;346(14):1092-1093.

283. Odetti P, Cheli V, Carta G, et al. Effect of nicotinic acid associated with retinol and tocopherols on plasma lipids in hyperlipoproteinaemic patients. Pharmatherapeutica 1984;4(1):21-24.

284. Hodis HN, Mack WJ, LaBree L, et al. Serial coronary angiographic evidence that antioxidant vitamin intake reduces progression of coronary artery atherosclerosis. JAMA 1995;273(23):1849-1854.

285. Preuss HG, Wallerstedt D, Talpur N, et al. Effects of niacin-bound chromium and grape seed proanthocyanidin extract on the lipid profile of hypercholesterolemic subjects: a pilot study. J Med 2000;31(5-6):227-246.

286. Azen SP, Qian D, Mack WJ, et al. Effect of supplementary antioxidant vitamin intake on carotid arterial wall intima-media thickness in a controlled clinical trial of cholesterol lowering. Circulation 1996;94(10):2369-2372.

287. Yusuf S, Dagenais G, Pogue J, et al. Vitamin E supplementation and cardiovascular events in high-risk patients. The Heart Outcomes Prevention Evaluation Study Investigators. N Engl J Med 2000;342(3):154-160.

288. Jialal I, Devaraj S. Vitamin E supplementation and cardiovascular events in high-risk patients. N Engl J Med 2000;342(25):1917-1918.

289. De Caterina R. [Low-dose aspirin and vitamin E in people at cardiovascular risk: a randomized trial in general practice]. Ital Heart J 2001;2(6 Suppl):681-684.

290. de Gaetano G. Low-dose aspirin and vitamin E in people at cardiovascular risk: a randomised trial in general practice. Collaborative Group of the Primary Prevention Project. Lancet 2001;357(9250):89-95.

291. Vannucchi H, Moreno FS. Interaction of niacin and zinc metabolism in patients with alcoholic pellagra. Am J Clin Nutr 1989;50(2):364-369.

292. Arcavi L, Shahar A. [Drug related taste disturbances: emphasis on the elderly]. Harefuah 2003;142(6):446-50, 485, 484.

293. Lammers W, Siderins P, Gaarewstroom JH. The effect of nicotinic acid on the blood sugar level. Acta Physiol Pharmacol Neerl 1950;1:193-197.

294. Hageman GJ, Stierum RH. Niacin, poly(ADP-ribose) polymerase-1 and genomic stability. Mutat Res 2001;475(1-2):45-56.

295. Mandrup-Poulsen T, Reimers JI, Andersen HU, et al. Nicotinamide treatment in the prevention of insulin-dependent diabetes mellitus. Diabetes Metab Rev 1993;9(4):295-309.

296. Stern RH, Freeman D, Spence JD. Differences in metabolism of time-release and unmodified nicotinic acid: explanation of the differences in hypolipidemic action. Metabolism 1992;41:879-881.

297. Carlson LA, Oro L, Ostman J. Effect of nicotinic acid on plasma lipids in patients with hyperlipoproteinemia during the first week of treatment. J Atheroscler Res 1968;8(4):667-677.

298. Kudchodkar BJ, Sodhi HS, Horlick L, et al. Mechanisms of hypolipidemic action of nicotinic acid. Clin Pharmacol Ther 1978;24(3):354-373.

299. Miettinen TA. Effect of nicotinic acid on the fecal excretion of neutral sterols and bile acids. In Gey KF, Carlson LA (eds): Effect of Nicotinic Acid and Its Derivatives. Bern, Huber, 1971, pp. 677-686.

300. Carlson LA, Oro L, Ostman J. Effect of a single dose of nicotinic acid on plasma lipids in patients with hyperlipoproteinemia. Acta Med Scand 1968;183(5):457-465.

301. Carlson LA, Oro L. The effect of nicotinic acid on the plasma free fatty acids: demonstration of a metabolic type of sympathicolysis. Acta Med Scand 1962;172:641-645.

302. Carlson LA, Oro L. Persistence of the inhibitory effect of nicotinic acid on catecholamine-stimulated lipid mobilization during prolonged treatment with nicotinic acid. J Atheroscler Res 1965;5:436-439.

303. Irie M, Sakuma M, Tsushima T, et al. Effect of nicotinic acid administration on plasma growth hormone concentrations. Proc Soc Exp Biol Med 1967;126:708-711.

304. Pinter EJ, Pattee CJ. Biphasic nature of blood glucose and free fatty acid changes following intravenous nicotinic acid in man. J Clin Endocrinol Metab 1967;27(3):440-443.

305. Svedmyr N, Harthon L, Lundholm L. The relationship between the plasma concentration of free nicotinic acid and some of its pharmacologic effects in man. Clin Pharmacol Ther 1969;10(4):559-570.

306. Tornvall P, Hamsten A, Johansson J, et al. Normalisation of the composition of very low density lipoprotein in hypertriglyceridemia by nicotinic acid. Atherosclerosis 1990;84(2-3):219-227.

307. Superko HR, KOS Investigators. Effect of nicotinic acid on LDL subclass patterns. Circulation 1994;90(suppl 1):I-504.

308. Carlson LA, Wahlberg G. Relative increase in apolipoprotein CII content of VLDL and chylomicrons in a case with massive type V hyperlipoproteinaemia by nicotinic acid treatment. Atherosclerosis 1978;31(1):77-84.

309. Wahlberg G, Holmquist L, Walldius G, et al. Effects of nicotinic acid on concentrations of serum apolipoproteins B, C-I, C-II, C-III and E in hyperlipidemic patients. Acta Med Scand 1988;224(4):319-327.

310. Carlson LA, Oro L. Effect of treatment with nicotinic acid for one month on serum lipids in patients with different types of hyperlipidemia. Atherosclerosis 1973;18(1):1-9.

311. Schlierf G, Hess G. Inhibition of carbohydrate-induced hypertriglyceridemia by nicotinic acid. Artery 1977;3(2):174-179.

312. Carlson LA, Hamsten A, Asplund A. Pronounced lowering of serum levels of lipoprotein Lp(a) in hyperlipidaemic subjects treated with nicotinic acid. J Intern Med 1989;226(4):271-276.

313. Seed M, O'Connor B, Perombelon N, et al. The effect of nicotinic acid and acipimox on lipoprotein(a) concentration and turnover. Atherosclerosis 1993;101(1):61-68.

314. Nikkila EA, Pykalisto O. Induction of adipose tissue lipoprotein lipase by nicotinic acid. Biochim Biophys Acta 1968;152(2):421-423.

315. Jin FY, Kamanna VS, Kashyap ML. Niacin decreases removal of high-density lipoprotein apolipoprotein A-I but not cholesterol ester by Hep G2 cells. Implication for reverse cholesterol transport. Arterioscler Thromb Vasc Biol 1997;17(10):2020-2028.

316. Dalton CO, Mallon KJ, Marchaus C. Observations on the cholesterol-lowering mechanism of nicotinc acid and nicotinyl alcohol tartrate. J Atheroscler Res 1967;8:265-276.

317. Parsons WB, Flinn JH. Reduction of serum cholesterol levels and beta-lipoprotein cholesterol levels by nicotinic acid. Arch Int Med 1959; 103:783-790.

318. Morgan JM, Capuzzi DM, Baksh RI, et al. Effects of extended-release niacin on lipoprotein subclass distribution. Am J Cardiol 2003;91(12):1432-1436.

319. Datta S, Das DK, Engelman RM, et al. Enhanced myocardial preservation by nicotinic acid, an antilipolytic compound: mechanism of action. Basic Res Cardiol 1989;84(1):63-76.

320. Altschul VR. Die beeinflussung des blutcholesterinspiegels und der experimentellen atherosklerose durch nikotinsaur. Zstchr Kreislaufforsch 1956;45:573-576.

321. Stone CK, Holden JE, Stanley W, et al. Effect of nicotinic acid on exogenous myocardial glucose utilization. J Nucl Med 1995;36(6):996-1002.

322. Vincent JE, Zijlstra FJ. Nicotinic acid inhibits thromboxane synthesis in platelets. Prostaglandins 1978;15(4):629-636.

323. Morrow JD, Awad JA, Oates JA, et al. Identification of skin as a major site of prostaglandin D2 release following oral administration of niacin in humans. J Invest Dermatol 1992;98(5):812-815.

324. Morrow JD, Parsons WG, III, Roberts LJ. Release of markedly increased quantities of prostaglandin D2 *in vivo* in humans following the administration of nicotinic acid. Prostaglandins 1989;38(2):263-274.

325. Olsson AG, Carlson LA, Anggard E, et al. Prostacyclin production augmented in the short term by nicotinic acid. Lancet 1983;2(8349):565-566.

326. Goldsmith GA, Cordill S. The vasodilating effects of nicotinic acid (relation to metabolic rate and body temperature). Am J Med Sci 1943;205:204-208.

327. Stern RH, Spence JD, Freeman DJ, et al. Tolerance to nicotinic acid flushing. Clin Pharmacol Ther 1991;50(1):66-70.

328. Cetkovic-Cvrlje M, Sandler S, Eizirik DL. Nicotinamide and dexamethasone inhibit interleukin-1-induced nitric oxide production by RINm5F cells without decreasing messenger ribonucleic acid expression for nitric oxide synthase. Endocrinology 1993;133(4):1739-1743.

329. Burkart V, Koike T, Brenner HH, et al. Oxygen radicals generated by the enzyme xanthine oxidase lyse rat pancreatic islet cells *in vitro*. Diabetologia 1992;35(11):1028-1034.

330. Lazarow A, Liambies J, Tausch AJ. Protection against diabetes with nicotinamide. J Lab Clin Med 1950;36:249-258.

331. Lazarus SS, Shapiro SH. Influence of nicotinamide and pyridine

nucleotides on streptozotocin and alloxan-induced pancreatic B cell cytotoxicity. Diabetes 1973;22(7):499-506.

332. Schein PS, Cooney DA, Vernon ML. The use of nicotinamide to modify the toxicity of streptozotocin diabetes without loss of antitumor activity. Cancer Res 1967;27(12):2324-2332.

333. Yamada K, Miyajima E, Nonaka K. Inhibition of cytokine-induced MHC class II but not class I molecule expression on mouse islet cells by niacinamide and 3-aminobenzamide. Diabetes 1990;39(9):1125-1130.

334. Sandler S, Andersson A. Stimulation of cell replication in transplanted pancreatic islets by nicotinamide treatment. Transplantation 1988;46(1): 30-31.

335. Elliott RB, Pilcher CC, Stewart A, et al. The use of nicotinamide in the prevention of type 1 diabetes. Ann N Y Acad Sci 1993;696:333-341.

336. Pozzilli P, Browne PD, Kolb H. Meta-analysis of nicotinamide treatment in patients with recent-onset IDDM. The Nicotinamide Trialists. Diabetes Care 1996;19(12):1357-1363.

337. Buscema M, Vinci C, Gatta C, et al. Nicotinamide partially reverses the interleukin-1 beta inhibition of glucose-induced insulin release in pancreatic islets. Metabolism 1992;41(3):296-300.

338. Banasik M, Komura H, Shimoyama M. Specific inhibitors of poly (ADP-ribose) synthetase and mono (ADP-ribosyl) transferase. J Biol Chem 1992; 267:1569-1575.

339. LeDoux SP, Hall CR, Forbes PM, et al. Mechanisms of nicotinamide and thymidine protection from alloxan and streptozocin toxicity. Diabetes 1988;37(8):1015-1019.

340. Korsgren O, Andersson A, Sandler S. Pretreatment of fetal porcine pancreas in culture with nicotinamide accelerates reversal of diabetes after transplantation to nude mice. Surgery 1993;113(2):205-214.

341. Kallamann B, Burkart U, Krancke KD, et al. Toxicity of chemically generated nitric oxide towards pancreatic islet cells can be prevented by nicotinamide. Life Sci 1992;51:671-678.

342. Radons J, Heller B, Burkle A, et al. Nitric oxide toxicity in islet cells involves poly(ADP-ribose) polymerase activation and concomitant NAD$^+$ depletion. Biochem Biophys Res Commun 1994;199(3):1270-1277.

343. Skidmore IF, Kritschevsky D, Schonhofer P. Influence of nicotinic acid and nicotinic acid homologs on lipolysis, phosphodiesterase activity, adenyl-cyclase activity and cyclic AMP synthesis in fat cells. In Gey KF, Carlson LA (eds): Effect of Nicotinic Acid and Its Derivatives. Bern, Huber, 1971, pp. 371-377.

344. Quabbe HJ, Luyckx AS, L'age M, et al. Growth hormone, cortisol, and glucagon concentrations during plasma free fatty acid depression: different effects of nicotinic acid and an adenosine derivative (BM 11.189). J Clin Endocrinol Metab 1983;57(2):410-414.

345. Hageman GJ, Stierum RH, van Herwijnen MH, et al. Nicotinic acid supplementation: effects on niacin status, cytogenetic damage, and poly(ADP-ribosylation) in lymphocytes of smokers. Nutr Cancer 1998; 32(2):113-120.

346. Harthon JG, Sigroth K, Sjobom AR. Ein Beitrag zur Klarung der Resorption des Hexanicotinsaureesters des Meso-inosits im Organismus. Arzneimittelforschung 1964;14:126-128.

347. Harthon L, Brattsand R. Enzymatic hydrolysis of pentaerythritol-tetranicotinate and meso- inositolhexanicotinate in blood and tissues. Arzneimittelforschung 1979;29(12):1859-1862.

348. Miller ON, Hamilton JG, Goldsmith GA. Investigation of the mechanism of action of nicotinic acid on serum lipid levels in man. Am J Clin Nutr 1960;8:480-490.

349. Okamoto H, Ishikawa A, Yoshitake Y, et al. Diurnal variations in human urinary excretion of nicotinamide catabolites: effects of stress on the metabolism of nicotinamide. Am J Clin Nutr 2003;77(2):406-410.

350. Du J, Hoag SW. The influence of excipients on the stability of the moisture sensitive drugs aspirin and niacinamide: comparison of tablets containing lactose monohydrate with tablets containing anhydrous lactose. Pharm Dev Technol 2001;6(2):159-166.

351. Humphrey JH, McKee RW, Swendseid ME. Niacin metabolites in urine following administration of nicotinic acid or nicotinamide to humans. Fed Proc 1984;43:485.

352. Mrochek JE, Jolley RL, Young DS, et al. Metabolic response of humans to ingestion of nicotinic acid and nicotinamide. Clin Chem 1976;22(11): 1821-1827.

353. Figge HL, Figge J, Souney PF, et al. Comparison of excretion of nicotinuric acid after ingestion of two controlled release nicotinic acid preparations in man. J Clin Pharmacol 1988;28:1136-1140.

354. Lomnicky Y, Friedman M, Luria MH, et al. The effect of the mode of administration on the hypolipidaemic activity of niacin: continuous gastrointestinal administration of low-dose niacin improves lipid-lowering efficacy in experimentally-induced hyperlipidaemic rats. J Pharm Pharmacol 1998;50(11):1233-1239.

355. Canner PL, Berge KG, Wenger NK, et al. Fifteen year mortality in Coronary Drug Project patients: long-term benefit with niacin. J Am Coll Cardiol 1986;8(6):1245-1255.

356. Berge KG, Canner PL. Coronary drug project: experience with niacin. Coronary Drug Project Research Group. Eur J Clin Pharmacol 1991; 40(suppl 1):S49-S51.

357. Altschul R, Hoffer A. The effect of nicotinic acid upon serum cholesterol

and upon basal metabolic rate of young adults. Arch Biochem 1958; 73:420-424.

358. Galbraith PA, Pevry WF, Beamish RE. Effect of nicotinic acid on serum lipids in normal and atherosclerotic subjects. Lancet 1959;1:222-223.

359. Gurian H, Adlersberg D. Effect of large doses of nicotinic acid on circulating lipids and carbohydrate tolerance. Am J M Sc 1959;237:12-22.

360. Packard CJ, Stewart JM, Third JL, et al. Effects of nicotinic acid therapy on high-density lipoprotein metabolism in type II and type IV hyper-lipoproteinaemia. Biochim Biophys Acta 1980;618(1):53-62.

361. Parsons WB, Achor RW, Berge KG, et al. Changes in concentration of blood lipids following prolonged administration of large doses of nicotinic acid to persons with hypercholesterolemia: Preliminary observations. Proc Staff Meet Mayo Clin 1956;31(13):377-390.

362. Parsons WB, Flinn JH. Reduction in elevated blood cholesterol levels by large doses of nicotinic acid. JAMA 1957;165(3):234-238.

363. Anonymous. Summary of the second report of the National Cholesterol Education Program (NCEP) Expert Panel on Detection, Evaluation, and Treatment of High Blood Cholesterol in Adults (Adult Treatment Panel II). JAMA 1993;269(23):3015-3023.

364. Schectman G, Hiatt J. Dose-response characteristics of cholesterol-lowering drug therapies: implications for treatment. Ann Intern Med 1996;125(12):990-1000.

365. Morgan JM, Capuzzi DM, Guyton JR. A new extended-release niacin (Niaspan): efficacy, tolerability, and safety in hypercholesterolemic patients. Am J Cardiol 1998;82(12A):29U-34U.

366. O'Connor PJ, Rush WA, Trence DL. Relative effectiveness of niacin and lovastatin for treatment of dyslipidemias in a health maintenance organization. J Fam Pract 1997;44(5):462-467.

367. Squires RW, Allison TG, Gau GT, et al. Low-dose, time-release nicotinic acid: effects in selected patients with low concentrations of high-density lipoprotein cholesterol. Mayo Clin Proc 1992;67(9):855-860.

368. Achor RWP, Berge KG. Treatment of hypercholesteremia with large oral doses of nicotinic acid: further investigations. Med Clin North America 1958;42:871-880.

369. Lal SM, Hewett JE, Petroski GF, et al. Effects of nicotinic acid and lovastatin in renal transplant patients: a prospective, randomized, open-labeled crossover trial. Am J Kidney Dis 1995;25(4):616-622.

370. Stein EA, Zupkis RV, Mitchel YB, et al. The lovastatin-niacin trial: effects on lipoproteins. Arterioscler Thrombosis 1991;11(5):1458a.

371. Grundy SM, Vega GL, McGovern ME, et al. Efficacy, safety, and tolerability of once-daily niacin for the treatment of dyslipidemia associated with type 2 diabetes: results of the assessment of diabetes control and evaluation of the efficacy of Niaspan trial. Arch Intern Med 2002; 162(14):1568-1576.

372. Bays HE, Dujovne CA, McGovern ME, et al. Comparison of once-daily, niacin extended-release/lovastatin with standard doses of atorvastatin and simvastatin (the ADvicor Versus Other Cholesterol-Modulating Agents Trial Evaluation [ADVOCATE]). Am J Cardiol 2003;91(6):667-672.

373. Hunninghake DB, McGovern ME, Koren M, et al. A dose-ranging study of a new, once-daily, dual-component drug product containing niacin extended-release and lovastatin. Clin Cardiol 2003;26(3):112-118.

374. Gardner SF, Marx MA, White LM, et al. Combination of low-dose niacin and pravastatin improves the lipid profile in diabetic patients without compromising glycemic control. Ann Pharmacother 1997;31(6):677-682.

375. Sposito AC, Caramelli B, Serrano CV, Jr., et al. Effect of niacin and etofibrate association on subjects with coronary artery disease and serum high-density lipoprotein cholesterol <35 mg/dl. Am J Cardiol 1999; 83(1):98-100.

376. Malfait P, Moren A, Dillon JC, et al. An outbreak of pellagra related to changes in dietary niacin among Mozambican refugees in Malawi. Int J Epidemiol 1993;22(3):504-511.

377. Gotto AM, Jr. Lipid risk factors and the regression of atherosclerosis. Am J Cardiol 1995;76(2):3A-7A.

378. Spinler SA, Cziraky MJ. Lipoprotein(A): physiologic function, association with atherosclerosis, and effects of lipid-lowering drug therapy. Ann Pharmacother 1994;28(3):343-351.

379. Blankenhorn DH, Selzer RH, Crawford DW, et al. Beneficial effects of colestipol-niacin therapy on the common carotid artery. Two- and four-year reduction of intima-media thickness measured by ultrasound. Circulation 1993;88(1):20-28.

380. Personius BE, Brown BG, Gotto AM Jr, et al. Effects of increasing HDL-C, lowering triglyceride and lowering LDL-C on "fixed" atherosclerotic coronary artery disease: AFREGS (the Armed Forces Regression study). Circulation 1998;98(suppl I):I-450-I-451.

381. Hecht HS, Harman SM. Relation of aggressiveness of lipid-lowering treatment to changes in calcified plaque burden by electron beam tomography. Am J Cardiol 2003;92(3):334-336.

382. Hecht HS, Harman SM. Comparison of effectiveness of statin monotherapy versus statin and niacin combination therapy in primary prevention and effects on calcified plaque burden. Am J Cardiol 2003; 91(3):348-351.

383. Hecht HS, Harman SM. Comparison of the effects of atorvastatin versus simvastatin on subclinical atherosclerosis in primary preventionas determined by electronbeam tomography. Am J Cardiol 2003;91(1):42-45.

384. Lepre F, Campbell B, Crane S, et al. Low-dose sustained release nicotinic acid (Tri-B3) and lipoprotein (a). Am J Cardiol 1992;70:133.

385. Bucher HC, Griffith LE, Guyatt GH. Systematic review on the risk and benefit of different cholesterol- lowering interventions. Arterioscler Thromb Vasc Biol 1999;19(2):187-195.

386. Vega GL, Weiner MF, Lipton AM, et al. Reduction in levels of 24S-hydroxycholesterol by statin treatment in patients with Alzheimer disease. Arch Neurol 2003;60(4):510-515.

387. Capuzzi DM, Morgan JM, Weiss RJ, et al. Beneficial effects of rosuvastatin alone and in combination with extended-release niacin in patients with a combined hyperlipidemia and low high-density lipoprotein cholesterol levels. Am J Cardiol 2003;91(11):1304-1310.

388. Nomikos IN, Prowse SJ, Carotenuto P, et al. Combined treatment with nicotinamide and desferrioxamine prevents islet allograft destruction in NOD mice. Diabetes 1986;35(11):1302-1304.

389. Varsanyi-Nagy M, Dadufalza V, Buckingham B, et al. Protective effect of nicotinamide on preservation of mouse islet function and morphology. Diabetologia 1992;35(suppl):A129.

390. Yamada K, Nonaka K, Hanafusa T, et al. Preventive and therapeutic effects of large-dose nicotinamide injections on diabetes associated with insulitis. An observation in nonobese diabetic (NOD) mice. Diabetes 1982; 31(9):749-753.

391. Heller B, Wang ZQ, Wagner EF, et al. Inactivation of the poly(ADP-ribose) polymerase gene affects oxygen radical and nitric oxide toxicity in islet cells. J Biol Chem 1995;270(19):11176-11180.

392. Guastamacchia E, Ciampolillo A, Lollino G, et al. Effetto della terapia con nicotinamide sull'induzione della durata della remissione clinica in diabetici di tipo 1 all'esordio sottoposti a terapia insulinica ottimizzata mediante microinfusore. Il Diabete 1992;4(suppl 1):210.

393. Ilkova H, Gorpe U, Kadioglu P, et al. Nicotinamide in type 1 diabetes mellitus of recent onset: a double blind placebo controlled trial. Diabetologia 1991;34(suppl 2):179.

394. Lewis CM, Canafax DM, Sprafka JM, et al. Double-blind randomized trial of nicotinamide on early-onset diabetes. Diabetes Care 1992;15(1):121-123.

395. Mendola G, Casamitjana R, Gomis R. Effect of nicotinamide therapy upon beta-cell function in newly diagnosed type 1 (insulin-dependent) diabetic patients. Diabetologia 1989;32:160-162.

396. Pozzilli P. Randomized trial comparing nicotinamide and nicotinamide plus cyclosporin in recent onset insulin-dependent diabetes. Diabet Med 1994;11:98-104.

397. Pozzilli P, Visalli N, Signore A, et al. Double blind trial of nicotinamide in recent-onset IDDM (the IMDIAB III study). Diabetologia 1995;38(7):848-852.

398. Taboga C, Tonutti L, Noacco C. Residual B cell activity and insulin requirements in insulin-dependent diabetic patients treated from the beginning with high doses of nicotinamide. A two-year follow-up. Recenti Prog Med 1994;85(11):513-516.

399. Visalli N, Cavallo MG, Signore A, et al. A multi-centre randomized trial of two different doses of nicotinamide in patients with recent-onset type 1 diabetes (the IMDIAB VI). Diabetes Metab Res Rev 1999;15(3):181-185.

400. Pozzilli P, Visalli N, Cavallo MG, et al. Vitamin E and nicotinamide have similar effects in maintaining residual beta cell function in recent onset insulin-dependent diabetes (the IMDIAB IV study). Eur J Endocrinol 1997;137(3):234-239.

401. Vialettes B, Picq R, du RM, et al. A preliminary multicentre study of the treatment of recently diagnosed type 1 diabetes by combination nicotinamide-cyclosporin therapy. Diabet Med 1990;7(8):731-735.

402. Ludvigsson J, Samuelsson U, Johansson C, et al. Treatment with anti-oxidants at onset of type 1 diabetes in children: a randomized, double-blind placebo-controlled study. Diabetes Metab Res Rev 2001;17(2):131-136.

403. Rossini AA, Mordes JP, Gallina DL, et al. Hormonal and environmental factors in the pathogenesis of BB rat diabetes. Metabolism 1983; 32(7 Suppl 1):33-36.

404. Sarri Y, Mendola J, Ferrer J, et al. Preventive effects of nicotinamide administration on spontaneous diabetes of BB rats. Med Sci Res 1989; 17:987-988.

405. Bingley PJ, Caldas G, Bonfanti R, et al. Nicotinamide and insulin secretion in normal subjects. Diabetologia 1993;36(7):675-677.

406. Gale EAM. Molecular mechanisms of beta cell destruction in IDDM. The role of nicotinamide. Hormone Res 1996;45(suppl 1):40-43.

407. Herskowitz RD, Jackson RA, Soeldner JS, et al. Pilot trial to prevent type I diabetes: progression to overt IDDM despite oral nicotinamide. J Autoimmun 1989;2(5):733-737.

408. Jonas WB, Rapoza CP, Blair WF. The effect of niacinamide on osteoarthritis: a pilot study. Inflamm Res 1996;45(7):330-334.

Oleander
(*Nerium oleander, Thevetia peruviana*)

SYNONYMS/COMMON NAMES/RELATED SUBSTANCES

- Adelfa, adynerin, ahouai (Antilles), ahousin, Anvirzel, *Apocyanaceae* (family), ashwahan, ashwamarak (Sanskrit), be-still nuts (Hawaii), boissaisi (Haiti), cardenolides, cardiac glycosides, cascaveleira (Brazil), *Cerbera thevetia* (India), cerebrine, cerebrose, common oleander, corrigen, de-hydroadynerigen, digitoxigenin, exile, folinerin, horse poison, joro-joro (Dutch Guiana), karier, karavira, kohilphin, kokilpal (India), laurier blane (Haiti), laurier bol, laurier desjundins, laurier rose, lorier bol, lucky seed (Jamaica), neriantin, neridiginoside, neridlenone A, neriifolin, neriine, nerin, nerioside, neritaloside, *Nerium indicum*, *Nerium odorum*, nerizoside, NOAG-II, odoroside H, oleanderblatter, oleandri folium, oleandrigenin, oleandrin, oleandrinogen, oleandroside, olinerin, peruvoside, pila kaner (India), pink oleander, rosa francesa, rosagenin, rosebay, rose laurel, rosen lorbeer, ruvoside, soland, strospeside, *Thevetia nerifolia*, *Thevetia neriifolia*, thevetin A, thevetin B, thevetine, L-thevetose, thevetoxin, triterpenes, white oleander, yee tho (Thailand), yellow oleander.

CLINICAL BOTTOM LINE
Background

- The term *oleander* refers to two common plant species, *Nerium oleander* (common oleander) and *Thevetia peruviana* (yellow oleander), which grow in temperate climates throughout the world. Both species contain cardiac glycosides with digoxin-like effects, and both species are toxic, with well-described reports of fatal ingestion. Recent evidence suggests that the use of activated charcoal may be beneficial in cases of oleander toxicity or overdose;[1-3] otherwise it is often suggested to manage toxicity similarly to other cardiac glycosides such as digoxin/digitoxin.
- Traditional uses of oleander have included treatment of swelling, leprosy, eye diseases, and skin disorders. Oleander has been used as an abortifacient and as a known instrument of homicide, and it gained popularity as an agent used in suicide attempts in Sri Lanka in the 1980s. The "cardiotonic" effects of oleander were investigated in the 1930s, but this use was largely abandoned because of significant gastro-intestinal toxicity and a perceived narrow therapeutic–to-toxic window. Oleander extracts have been used in China to treat neurologic and psychiatric disorders.
- The anti-cancer effects of oleander extracts are being investigated largely in *in vitro* cell line models. Human clinical cancer trials have not yet been performed.

Scientific Evidence for Common/Studied Uses	Grade*
Cancer	C
Congestive heart failure	C

*Key to grades: *A:* Strong scientific evidence for this use; *B:* Good scientific evidence for this use; *C:* Unclear scientific evidence for this use; *D:* Fair scientific evidence against this use (it may not work); *F:* Strong scientific evidence against this use (it likely does not work). For a more detailed explanation of efficacy criteria, see "Natural Standard Evidence-Based Validated Grading Rationale" in the Introduction.

- Because of lack of efficacy data and high toxicity potential, oleander is generally not recommended for any indication.

Historical or Theoretical Uses That Lack Sufficient Evidence

- Abortifacient, alcoholism, anorexia, anthelmintic, antifertility,[4] asthma, bacterial infections, cachexia, cardiotonic, cathartic, corns, diuretic, dysmenorrhea, emetic, epilepsy, eye diseases, hemorrhoids, indigestion, inflammation, insecticide, leprosy, malaria, menstrual stimulant, neurologic disorders, parasiticide, psychiatric disorders, rat poison, ringworm, sinus problems, snake bite, skin diseases, skin eruptions, swelling, venereal disease, warts, weight gain.

Expert Opinion and Folkloric Precedent

- Oleander has been used since the mid-16th century as an insecticide and rat poison and was given a Sanskrit name meaning "horse poison." It appears to have been used as a suicidal agent for nearly as long and has been implicated in homicide attempts. Two components of oleander, rosagenin and cerebroside, appear to have strychnine-like effects. The German expert panel, the Commission E, has listed oleander with other herbs that are "unapproved" and possess documented or suspected risk. However, the German Commission E has approved use of a combination product containing oleander for "mild, limited heart action" and "circulatory instability" (Miroton, which includes pheasant's eye extract, lily of the valley, squill, and oleander).
- Haitian folk healers use oleander extracts for a variety of indi-cations. A recent case report describes a woman of Haitian descent living in Florida who consulted a local Haitian healer to improve her appetite and gain weight. She was given a potion of oleander leaf extract orally and rectally and became severely ill and eventually died, despite aggressive resuscitative efforts. In South China, oleander is used to treat a variety of neurologic and psychiatric illnesses. Use of oleander extracts to treat congestive heart failure persists in parts of the world, particularly in China and Russia.
- The use of oleander is generally not recommended because of its significant toxicity potential.

Safety Summary

- **Likely unsafe:** All parts of the oleander plant, including flowers, leaves, and nectar, are considered toxic. Deaths have occurred as a result of ingestion of all forms of oleander. As little as 1 seed of the yellow oleander fruit has been reported to cause death in a child, and the ingestion of 4 to 8 seeds may be fatal in an adult. Any degree of ingestion, such as eating meat prepared on oleander skewers, can potentially be fatal. Preparations of oleandrin exist in other countries, most notably China, as therapies for heart failure and are available in 100-µg tablets. Little, if any, reliable safety data exist concerning this particular preparation and dosage.[5] Fatal ingestions have also resulted from ingestion of tea prepared from oleander leaves, inhaling smoke from burning oleander, and ingestion of minute amounts of oleander leaves, fruits, flowers or stems.
- A fatal ingestion occurred when oleander leaves mistaken for eucalyptus leaves were prepared as a tea and ingested.[6]

DOSING/TOXICOLOGY
General

- Recommended doses are based on those most commonly used in available trials, or on historical practice. However, with natural products, the optimal doses needed to balance efficacy and safety often have not been determined. Formulations and preparation methods may vary from manufacturer to manufacturer, and from batch to batch of a specific product made by a single manufacturer. Because often the active components of a product are not known, standardization may not be possible, and the clinical effects of different brands may not be comparable.

Standardization

- There is no widely accepted standardization practice for the preparation of oleander. Wild oleander should not be ingested, and "folk medicine" applications cannot be supported because of oleander's known toxicity. Medicinal uses of oleander extracts as anticancer agents are being investigated, and further information may follow as clinical trials ensue.

Dosing: Adult (18 Years and Older)
Oral

- **Congestive heart failure:** Peruvoside, a cardiac glycoside obtained from yellow oleander kernels was tested in an oral dose of 1.8 to 3.2 mg loading dose with a mean daily maintenance dose of 0.6 mg per day.[7,8] This preparation does not appear to be available commercially.
- **Cancer:** *In vitro* studies of human tumor cell line preparations are ongoing. Human doses cannot be reported until reliable human clinical trial data are available.

Dosing: Pediatric (Younger Than 18 Years)

- Not recommended, due to risk of significant toxicity.

Toxicology

- **Background:** Ingestion of 2 to 3 leaves of *Nerium oleander* (common oleander) has been fatal in sheep. Fruits of *Thevetia peruviana* (yellow oleander) are thought to be even more toxic to mammals, including humans. Yellow oleander contains thevetins A and B, neriifolin, thevetoxin, peruvoside, and ruvoside. The thevetins and thevetoxin are cardiac glycosides with direct digoxin-like effects. The thevetins are bitter to taste and constitute 0.6% of the weight of the yellow oleander fruit seed. The fruit and leaves of yellow oleander contain an irritating astringent that produces a burning sensation in the mouth, tingling in the tongue, dryness in the mouth and throat, and emesis (thought to be protective). *N. oleander*, or common oleander, contains oleandrin, digitoxigenin, neriine, and folinerin, the antibiotic oleandromycin, and the strychnine-like toxin rosagenin. Oleandrin forms colorless, odorless, aqueous crystals, which are very bitter. It has a digoxin-like action and is slowly eliminated from the body. Extracts from *N. oleander* have been used as potent rat poison and insecticide and fish poison and are toxic to mammals including humans. A single leaf of common oleander may be lethal to children and ingestion of the leaves, flowers, or bark of *N. oleander* produces nausea, vomiting, colic, drowsiness, ataxia, mydriasis, bloody diarrhea, arrhythmia, and unconsciousness. Death may occur within 30 hours. The mechanism of action appears to be largely through cardiac glycoside action, via inhibition of the sodium-potassium ATPase, an increase in intracellular

sodium, and a decrease in intracellular potassium, producing negative chronotropic and other digoxin-like effects. In healthy hearts, high-grade heart block may ensue, whereas in diseased hearts, ventricular tachycardia and ventricular fibrillation may develop.

- In rats, oleander leaves have been associated with weight loss and death.[9] In sheep, single oral doses of 0.25 g/kg of dried *Nerium oleander* leaves has caused restlessness, chewing movements, dyspnea, bloating, malcoordination, limb paresis, and death 4-24 hours after dosing.[10] A daily oral dose of 0.06 g/kg of dried *N. oleander* leaves caused less severe signs, although death occurred between days 3 and 14. Hepatotoxicity, anemia, leukopenia, and widespread hemorrhage were noted in these animals.
- **Case reports:** A 1970s Australian series reported 13 children admitted after oleander ingestion at the median age of 2 years.[11] Six children showed signs and symptoms of poisoning, and two of these children had cardiac toxicity. Deaths did not occur. Another series compiled from the Jafna District in Sri Lanka, where yellow oleander seed ingestion had become popular for suicide, reported 170 cases between 1983 and 1985.[12] The number of seeds ingested varied from one-half to 20. The common presenting symptoms were vomiting, giddiness, and diarrhea. Other symptoms included abdominal pain, numbness of the mouth and tongue, and palpitations. Electrocardiographic (ECG) changes were present in 62%, with the majority showing atrioventricular block or other bradycardias. Ventricular ectopy in this population of predominantly young adults was rare. Seven of 170 cases of ingestion were fatal, and the authors commented that ingestion of ≥8 seeds of *Thevetia peruviana* (yellow oleander) is potentially fatal.
- A review of 13 cases of yellow oleander seed ingestion from India concluded that all patients who ingested more than 2 seeds manifested gastrointestinal and cardiovascular toxic effects and that those ingesting fewer than 4 seeds but presenting within 4 hours of ingestion generally recovered.[13] The cause of death in all patients who did expire was listed as cardiogenic shock. Another series from India reviewed four cases of intentional yellow oleander seed ingestion (as suicide attempts), with all the patients consuming 4 to 6 seeds. All patients were febrile on presentation and developed abdominal pain, vomiting, loose stools, weakness, drowsiness, icterus, and hyperbilirubinemia. All patients recovered.[14]
- In 1993, there were 2388 toxic exposures to plant glycosides reported in the United States, with *Nerium oleander* ingestion accounting for approximately 25% of cases.[15]
- **Management:** Recent evidence suggests that the use of activated charcoal may be beneficial in cases of oleander toxicity or overdose;[1-3,16] otherwise it is often suggested to manage toxicity similarly to other cardiac glycosides such as digoxin/digitoxin.

ADVERSE EFFECTS/PRECAUTIONS/ CONTRAINDICATIONS
Allergy

- Known allergy/hypersensitivity to oleander.
- Contact dermatitis may result from skin contact with the sap of freshly cut oleander leaves.[17-19]

Adverse Effects/Postmarket Surveillance

- **General:** Oleander is generally regarded as being unsafe for internal use. Any benefits of therapy may not outweigh the risk of toxicity. Generalized effects of oleander ingestion may include irritation of contacted membranes, buccal erythema, nausea, vomiting, diaphoresis, abdominal pain, diarrhea, headache, altered mental status, visual disturbances, mydriasis, cardiovascular toxicity, and risk of death.[17]

- **Dermatologic:** Contact dermatitis may result from skin contact with the sap of freshly cut oleander leaves.[17-19]
- **Neurologic/CNS:** Malaise is often reported with significant oleander ingestion.[5,20] Mydriasis, peripheral neuritis, and weakness have also been reported.[6] After ingesting yellow oleander seeds, a 28-year-old man became unconscious, not responding to deep painful stimuli.[21] The patient died despite lavage and symptomatic treatment. A 1-year old boy was noted to have lethargy, pallor, and irritability as a result of oleander ingestion.[22] The child had deterioration of consciousness and experienced seizure-like activity, for which lorazepam and phenytoin were administered. A 12-year-old boy developed hypertonia, neck stiffness, constricted pupils, and flexor plantar response when he ingested yellow oleander seeds.[23] In another report, after maternal ingestion of oleander, the heart rate of the fetus dropped to 110/minute.[24] After birth (weight 2.8 kg), the neonate experienced left-sided seizures at 40 hours and generalized convulsions at 70 hours. The infant's condition improved after symptomatic treatment. Anecdotal reports have noted the development of vertigo, headache, and stupor.
- **Ocular/otic:** Mydriasis may occur with toxicity (anecdotal). There is a report of dimness of vision and tinnitus after ingesting a water extract from oleander leaves.[25]
- **Psychiatric:** Depression has been reported anecdotally.
- **Pulmonary/respiratory:** Tachypnea has been reported anecdotally.
- **Cardiovascular:** Oleander ingestion has been associated with atrioventricular (AV) block, including complete heart block, bradycardia, ventricular ectopy, and significant ST-T wave electrocardiographic (ECG) abnormalities.[12,26] In a study evaluating cardiovascular effects of oleander in 300 patients, Bose et al. found that 52% (156) were asymptomatic, and 12% (36) experienced palpitations.[27] ECG findings showed that 46% (138) of patients experienced arrhythmias, with 49.27% (68) being sinus bradycardia. Ischemic changes were found in 39.33% (118) of patients. Among 14 deaths that occurred, all had subendocardial and perivascular hemorrhage with focal myocardial edema.[27] An intravenous dose of 4.25 mg/kg of Thevetin (an extract of *Thevetia peruviana*) was studied in 14 heart failure patients, and resulted in ST-segment changes, T-wave changes, extrasystoles, and fatal ventricular tachycardia.[28] The cardiac index of 6 of these patients increased from a mean of 2.8 L/minute to 3.7 L/minute, and the right and left heart-filling pressures decreased 25% to 35%, with the left ventricular stroke work index increasing 162%. Decreases in pulse rate ranged from 2 to 40 beats per minute.[28] Other studies have also reported bradycardia as a result of oleander ingestion.[7,8,29] As the result of a suicide attempt, a 25-year-old man experienced asymptomatic bradycardia that persisted for 4 days after ingestion of yellow oleander seeds, despite emesis and gastric lavage.[21] A 28-year-old woman who ingested yellow oleander flowers experienced sinus bradycardia with ST segment depression that lasted for 3 days.[21] After ingesting yellow oleander seeds, a 28-year-old man developed irregular heartbeats with a pulse of 30. The patient died despite lavage and symptomatic treatment.[21] Another case report documents exposure to yellow oleander by a 3-year-old girl leading to complete heart block and cardiac arrest. The child died despite intravenous atropine treatment.[30] Terminal negative ST dips in the ECG of a woman who had ingested 15 leaves of an oleander bush have been documented.[31] Another patient with oleander ingestion experienced brady and tachyarrhythmias and an elevated digoxin concentration of 4.44 ng/L.[32] Hypotension has also been reported with oleander ingestion.[33]

- **Gastrointestinal:** Anorexia, nausea, vomiting, and diarrhea have been reported following ingestion of oleander or its components.[5,7,34] In a study evaluating cardiovascular effects of oleander in 300 patients, Bose et al. found that 52% (156) were asymptomatic, and 30.66% (92) experienced vomiting.[27] In a suicide attempt, a 25-year-old man experienced vomiting, epigastric pain, and altered sensorium 6 to 8 hours following ingestion of yellow oleander seeds. The patient recovered 4 days after emesis and gastric lavage.[21] In another case, a 28-year-old woman who ingested yellow oleander flowers experienced abdominal pain, diarrhea, and emesis but recovered with gastric lavage.[21] Another patient developed vomiting, faintness, dimness of vision, tinnitus, and diaphoresis after ingesting water extract from oleander leaves.[25] Two patients developed jaundice, increased bilirubin, and hepato-splenomegaly after oleander ingestion.[14] Other possible adverse effects include cramping, peripheral neuritis, weakness, and burning and/or pain in the oral cavity (anecdotal).
- **Renal:** Cases of jaundice and renal failure have been reported in the literature.[14,35] In one report, four cases of renal toxicity were associated with oleander ingestion. All patients developed yellow-colored conjunctivae, deeply colored urine, scanty urination (less than 300 mL/day), and mild fever. Serum bilirubin, creatinine, and blood urea were all found to be elevated.[14]
- **Electrolyte abnormalities:** Hyperkalemia generally occurs due to inhibition of the sodium-potassium ATPase pump. Digoxin is usually detectable by radioimmunoassay, because of the cross-reactivity of cardiac glycosides contained in oleander with digoxin assays. One study suggested that cross reactivity of cardiac glycosides contained in oleander was more abundant and predictable with digitoxin assays than with digoxin measurements.[20,26,36-39] Oleandrigenin, a principal cardiac glycoside component of *Nerium oleander*, has been specifically identified by high-performance liquid chromotography.[22] In one case report, after exposure to oleander tea, a 33-year-old woman was noted to have a serum potassium concentration of 6.7 mEq/L and a serum creatinine of 2.3 mg/L, both of which returned to normal after supportive treatment.[40]

Precautions/Warnings/Contraindications

- Oral oleander ingestion cannot be recommended, particularly in its unprocessed "natural form," as an herbal remedy. The therapeutic-to-toxic window appears to be extremely narrow.
- Medicinal preparations of oleander lack sufficient human data on utility and have been associated with significant toxicity. Other oral cardiac glycosides such as digoxin and digitoxin may have more predictable effects.[41]
- Studies regarding the antitumor effects of oleander extracts are in the preclinical phase, and such use cannot currently be recommended.[42-44]

Pregnancy and Lactation

- Human use of oleander in its unprocessed or medicinal forms is not recommended because of the risk of toxicity. Prepartum or postpartum use cannot be recommended.

- Folkloric use of oleander as an abortifacient is not supported by scientific research. There is a case report of a mother who consumed 2 yellow oleander seed kernels 12 hours before giving birth.[24] The intention of this ingestion is unclear. The fetus, while still *in utero*, developed evidence of cardiac glycoside toxicity, with a moderate decrease in fetal heart rate immediately pre- and postpartum. At 40 hours postpartum, the baby suffered left-sided seizures, followed by generalized seizures at 70 hours. Laboratory studies were normal and the child eventually recovered uneventfully and was doing well 3 years later. It has been hypothesized that maternal/fetal transmission of lipid-soluble thevetin, the chief cardiac glycoside in yellow oleander, may have occurred.

INTERACTIONS
Oleander/Drug Interactions

- **Cardiac glycosides (digoxin, digitoxin):** Both *Nerium oleander* (common oleander) and *Tevetius peruviana* (yellow oleander) are rich in cardiac glycosides, and the cardiac glycoside effects would possibly be additive (and potential toxicity augmented) when ingested by patients also receiving digoxin. In a review of oleander ingestion by children in Australia in the 1970s, of the two children exhibiting significant cardiac toxicity following oleander ingestion, one was a young girl already receiving digoxin for congenital heart disease.[11] Both peruvoside and oleandrin (present in oleander) have similar structures to digoxin and produce similar effects in the body .[45]
- **Drugs that interact with digoxin:** The cardiac glycoside digoxin has numerous documented drug interactions. Theoretically, the same agents may interact with oleander, although this has not been systematically evaluated. Both peruvoside and oleandrin (present in oleander) have similar structures to digoxin and produce similar effects in the body.[45]
- **Anti-arrhythmic agents:** The cardiac glycoside content of oleander elicits significant atrioventricular (AV) nodal blocking effects and lowers the threshold for ventricular arrhythmia. Any co-administered antiarrhythmic agent with similar properties may have additive and potentially adverse effects.
- **Laxatives:** Due to potassium depletion caused by some laxatives, the risk of cardiac toxicity may be increased with concomitant use (theoretical).
- **Potassium-depleting diuretics:** In theory, due to potassium depletion caused by some diuretics, the risk of cardiac toxicity from oleander may be increased with concurrent use.

Oleander/Herb/Supplement Interactions

- **Cardiac glycoside–containing herbs:** A number of other plant species have been found to contain cardiac glycosides or demonstrate cardiac glycoside activity. Ingestion of these species concomitantly with oleander may augment effects and toxicity.[26,46,47]
- **Diuretic herbs and supplements:** In theory, due to potassium depletion caused by some diuretics, the risk of cardiac toxicity due to oleander may be increased with concurrent use.
- **Laxative herbs and supplements:** In theory, due to potassium depletion caused by some laxative agents, the risk of cardiac toxicity may be increased with combination use.
- **Licorice:** In theory, due to potassium depletion, the risk of cardiac toxicity may be increased with combination use.

- **Calcium:** In theory, combination use of calcium supplements with oleander may result in an increased risk of cardiac toxicity.

Oleander/Food Interactions

- Insufficient available evidence.

Oleander/Lab Interactions

- **Digoxin and digitoxin assays:** Several studies address the cross-reactivity of the cardiac glycosides contained in common and yellow oleander with digoxin and digitoxin assays. In general, cardiac glycosides contained within oleander have been shown to react with fluorescence polarization assays for digoxin, but not digoxin chemiluminescent assays. Cardiac glycosides contained in oleander have demonstrated high cross-reactivity with digitoxin fluorescence polarization immunoassays, but not with monoclonal chemiluminescent assays for digitoxin. The cross-reactivity of oleandrin, a major cardiac glycoside component of common oleander, varies with different digoxin assays. In general, the presence of cardiac glycosides can be confirmed in a qualitative sense with digoxin assays, but quantitation is not possible due to unstable binding of oleander containing cardiac glycosides with digoxin assays. Quantitation does appear to be potentially possible with selected digitoxin fluorescence polarization assays. The existence of oleandrigenin, an additional cardiac glycoside present in common oleander, has been confirmed by high performance liquid chromatography analysis of an oleander ingestion victim.[20,22,26,36-38,48-51]
- **Urine output:** Four patients with oleander-induced renal toxicity developed scant urination (less than 300 mL/day).[14]
- **Serum potassium:** Hyperkalemia may result from oleander ingestion, due to inhibition of the sodium-potassium intracellular ATPase pump. In one study, higher serum potassium levels at presentation following oleander ingestion were associated with greater risk of mortality.[6,19,39,40,51-55]
- **Serum phosphate:** A case report cites severe hypophosphatemia in a 24-year-old man who had ingested six ground leaves of *Nerium oleander*. This hypophosphatemia was refractory to initial treatment but improved almost immediately upon administration of digoxin Fab antibodies.[15]
- **Creatinine:** In one case-report, after exposure to oleander tea, a 33-year-old woman had a serum potassium concentration of 6.7 mEq/L and a serum creatinine of 2/L, both of which returned to normal after supportive treatment.[40] In four cases of oleander-induced renal toxicity, creatinine was found to be elevated.[14]
- **Blood urea:** In four cases of oleander-induced renal toxicity, blood urea was found to be elevated.[14]
- **Bilirubin:** In four cases of oleander-induced renal toxicity, bilirubin was found to be elevated.[14]

MECHANISM OF ACTION
Pharmacology

- **Cardiac glycosides:** Both common oleander (*Nerium oleander*) and yellow oleander (*Thevetia peruviana*) contain cardiac glycosides with actions and mechanisms of action very similar to those of ouabain and digoxin. *N. oleander* contains oleandrin, digitoxigenin, neriin, and folinerin. Yellow oleander contains thevetin A, thevetin B, nerifolin, thevetoxin, peruvoside, and ruvoside. The pharmacologic mode of action of the cardiac glycosides is via inhibition of the sodium-potassium ATPase pump, resulting in elevation of intracellular levels of calcium and sodium with decreased intracellular/increased extracellular potassium levels. The intracellular accumulation of calcium appears to provide the basis for increased myocardial contractility.[43]

- **Anti-proliferative properties:** Oleandrin and oleandrigenin also possess cytotoxic properties. The inhibition of the sodium-potassium ATPase exchange pump, with resulting increased intracellular calcium, is thought to cause a release of mitochondrial cytochrome C, activation of the caspase cascade, and PARP (poly[adenosine diphosphatase–ribose]polymerase) cleavage. Oleandrin also blocks activation of nuclear factor-Kβ that may also contribute to its anti-tumor effects. FGF-2 is a cellular protein involving cell differentiation and growth and tumor formation and is exported from the cell via alpha subunit binding to the sodium-potassium ATPase pump. Thus, the inhibition of the sodium-potassium ATPase pump could potentially decrease FGF-2 release from the cell.[43,56]

- **CNS effects:** Four cardiac glycosides isolated from *Nerium oleander* (nerizoside, delta-dehydroadynerigen, neritaloside, odoroside) have all demonstrated central nervous system depressant activity in mice. An extract of yellow oleander, cerebrin, also is thought to have strychnine-like actions.[14,57] Rosagenin is a component of oleander also thought to have strychnine-like actions.[11]

- **Antibacterial properties:** Oleandromycin isolated from *Nerium oleander* possesses *in vitro* antibiotic properties.[11]

Pharmacodynamics/Kinetics

- Oleandrin is highly protein bound.[38] The biological half-life of oleandrin was calculated as 44 hours in one case study of a 17-year-old female.[41]

- Oleandrin, like digoxin, is not eliminated via hemodialysis. Cases of severe oleander toxicity have been treated with digoxin antibody fragments. The elimination half-life of the Fab antibody segments is reported to be 16 hours. Administration of activated charcoal is thought to play a possible role in preventing oleander absorption following ingestion and in enhancing elimination.[5,14-16,22,26,36,48,50,54,58] Chelating agents have been used as potential remedies to counter oleander toxicity but have been largely abandoned in favor of the more modern and effective digoxin antibody preparations.[59,60]

HISTORY

- *Thevetia peruviana*, also known as *Thevetia nerifolia*, and its extract has reportedly been used in India since approximately 1000 BC in the treatment of various skin diseases. It later became known as a horse poison and began to be recognized as toxic in Europe in the 16th century.

- A "cardiotonic" activity of *T. peruviana* was discovered by Devray in 1863, and the toxic–to-therapeutic ratio was subsequently found to be very high.

- *Nerium oleander* is indigenous to the Indian subcontinent, subtropical Asia, Mediterranean regions, and temperate areas of the United States. It has long been used therapeutically in treatment of swelling, leprosy, and eye and skin diseases. It has also been used to treat venereal disease and persists as a common folk medicine in some countries, including Haiti. There are reports that *N. oleander* has been used as an arrow poison in Africa, and others have attributed snakebite-healing properties to common oleander.

REVIEW OF THE EVIDENCE: DISCUSSION
Congestive Heart Failure
Summary

- Extracts of *Thevetia peruviana* (also known as *Thevetia nerifolia*) and *Nerium oleander* have been observed to possess cardiac glycoside properties since the mid-1900s. Human clinical studies began in the 1930s but have largely been abandoned because of the significant gastrointestinal toxicity of thevetin and peruvoside preparations. These glycosides have been staples of congestive heart failure therapy in China and Russia for decades, but data supporting use are scant, and no high-quality comparative studies to other, better-tolerated cardiac glycoside preparations appear to exist. Notably, cardiac glycosides have not been shown to improve mortality in patients with congestive heart failure, although well-tolerated and widely used drugs such as digoxin have been demonstrated to alleviate symptoms and reduce frequency of hospitalization.

Evidence

- In a 1930 case series, Middleton et al. studied Thevetin, an extract of *T. peruviana*, in 40 patients with decompensated

Review of the Evidence: Oleander

Condition Treated*	Study Design	Author, Year	N[†]	SS[†]	Study Quality[‡]	Magnitude of Benefit	ARR[†]	NNT[†]	Comments
Congestive heart failure	Case series	Middleton[29] 1936	40	Unclear	NA	Moderate	NA	NA	Thevetin, an extract of *Thevetia peruviana*, as therapy.
Congestive heart failure	Case series	Bhatia[7] 1970	28	Yes	NA	Large	NA	NA	Peruvoside intravenous and oral therapy; likely duplicate publication of Bhatia[8] (1971).
Congestive heart failure	Case series	Bhatia[8] 1971	27	Yes	NA	Moderate	NA	NA	Peruvoside as therapy; likely duplicate publication of Bhatia[7] (1970).
Congestive heart failure	Case series	Storz[61] 1967	27	Unclear	NA	Moderate	NA	NA	Corrign, *N. oleander* extract, as therapy.
Congestive heart failure	Case series	Arnold[28] 1935	32	Unclear	NA	Large	NA	NA	Thevetin intravenous and oral therapy.

*Primary or secondary outcome.
[†]N, Number of patients; SS, statistically significant; ARR, absolute risk reduction; NNT, the number of patients who need to undergo a specific intervention in order to observe an outcome in one individual.
[‡]0-2 = poor; 3-4 = good; 5 = excellent.
NA, Not applicable; N. oleander, Nerium oleander.
For an explanation of each category in this table, please see Table 3 in the Introduction.

congestive heart failure.[29] Dosages ranged from 1.25 mg to 4 mg per day given orally. Twenty-seven of the 40 patients were reported to demonstrate "circulatory improvements." Reported effects included slowing of heart rate, relief of dyspnea, decrease in venous pressure, diuresis, reduced edema, and increased "vital capacity." Two of the patients who responded were deemed to be "intolerant" to digoxin administration. Sixteen patients experienced gastrointestinal side effects, with cramps and diarrhea being the most common, followed by anorexia, nausea, and vomiting. Eleven of these 16 were able to continue the drug, but often only after a brief hiatus or a reduction in dosage. No statistical analysis was reported, and outcomes were based on subjective clinical judgment.

- In 1935, Arnold et al. published a case series in which 23 subjects with congestive heart failure received intravenous or oral Thevetin.[28] Fourteen subjects received intravenous dosing, in most cases 4.25 mg/kg. This administration elicited a decrease in heart rate ranging from 2 to 40 beats per minute (observed in patients both in normal sinus rhythm and in atrial fibrillation). Two patients developed extrasystoles, and most subjects experienced ST segment changes similar to those seen with digoxin therapy. Three patients experienced relief of dyspnea as well as diuresis, although this was based on subjective reporting. Nine patients received initial oral doses of 0.45 to 1.7 mg/kg. With a single dose, four of these subjects experienced decreased heart rate, and two demonstrated ST segment changes. With dose escalation to a maximum of 8.5 mg/kg per day, all but one patient experienced subjective improvements in symptoms of congestive heart failure. However, a nodal rhythm was induced in one patient, and fatal ventricular tachycardia occurred in one patient. Nausea and vomiting occurred frequently when the drug was administered orally. This preliminary investigation did not establish a safe or efficacious dose in humans.

- In 1967, Storz published a brief review of oral use of a commercial product known as Corrigen (developed in Germany) containing N. oleander extract.[61] The paper lacks detail and was published in summary form. The loading dose used was 2 mg on the first day, with a subsequent daily dose of 1.2 mg. Seven of 27 patients (25%) did not tolerate the medication well. The author concluded that Corrigen possesses similar hemodynamic effects to digoxin, but that the toxic dose is approximately 140% of the therapeutic dose. Further details of methods or results were not provided.

- In 1970 and 1971, Bhatia et al. published two case series possibly containing multiple overlapping patients, with the first series commenting on peruvoside use in 28 patients, and the second commenting on the use of that agent in 27 patients (likely duplicate publications).[7,8] The design of the studies was similar, with 6 patients receiving intravenous injections of peruvoside 0.015 mg/kg over 4 minutes, and an additional 21 (or 22) patients receiving oral dosing. Those receiving intravenous medication also underwent invasive hemodynamic monitoring. In those patients, statistically significant alterations in several hemodynamic parameters were demonstrated with peruvoside administration. Mean heart rate decreased by 36%, and patients showed an increase in cardiac index at 30 minutes (range 10% to 132%). Overall, the mean cardiac index improved from 2.8 to 3.7 L/minute. Significant reductions in right atrial, left atrial, and mean pulmonary artery pressures were noted in the range of 25%

to 40%, with the left ventricular "stroke work index" increasing by 162%. In the larger group treated with oral therapy (mean loading dose 2.4 mg and maintenance dose 0.6 mg daily), those patients in atrial fibrillation exhibited a 40% decrease in mean heart rate while those in sinus rhythm showed a 20% decrease in heart rate. Twenty of the 28 patients in the oral treatment group demonstrated improvement in symptoms of congestive heart failure with reduction of dyspnea. Of the 10 subjects not demonstrating clinical improvement, 1 died of an acute myocardial infarction, 1 died of ongoing severe mitral regurgitation, 4 were lost to follow-up, and 4 demonstrated no clinical improvement. Significant gastrointestinal side effects were reported in 10 patients, including anorexia, nausea, vomiting, and diarrhea. Cardiac arrhythmias occurred in 9 subjects, with 1 patient demonstrating first-degree atrioventricular (AV) block, 1 demonstrating intermittent third-degree AV block, and others experiencing ventricular or atrial extrasystoles. All of the cardiac dysrhythmias were reversible with withdrawal of therapy. This uncontrolled study demonstrates the narrow therapeutic index of this preparation.

Cancer
Summary

- Extracts of *Nerium oleander* are under investigation for their antitumor effects. Anecdotal evidence had emerged from long-term use of the cardiac glycosides in *N. oleander* for treatment of cardiac illnesses that suggests beneficial side effects in patients with leiomyosarcoma, Ewing's sarcoma, prostate cancer, and breast cancer.[62] *N. oleander* extracts appear promising in *in vitro* studies against a variety of human tumor cell lines. Studies of human use from clinical cancer trials are not yet available.

Evidence

- Oleandrin, the principal glycoside component of *N. oleander*, has been shown *in vitro* to have significant dose- and time-dependent cytotoxic effects on transitional cell carcinoma cell lines, with 77% to 88% cell proliferation inhibition demonstrated.[56] This effect appears to be independent of the antigen and receptor status or grade of the cell line. The cytotoxic effects occur after even brief exposure (1 to 2 hours). This effect of oleandrin is thought to be through inhibition of activation of necrosis factors-Kβ and AP-1 and their associated kinases, which may provide a molecular basis for the ability of oleandrin to suppress inflammation and perhaps tumorigenesis. Oleandrin has also been studied and shown to have an antitumor effect in other cell lines such as human histiocytic lymphoma and human ovarian, epithelial, and T cells.

- A commercial product known as Anvirzel, consisting of oleandrin, oleandrinogen, and polysaccharides, has also demonstrated antitumor effects.[42] It has been shown to induce apoptosis in metastatic human prostatic adenocarcinoma cell lines independently of androgen receptor or prostate-specific antigen pathways. This apparently occurs through an early-sustained calcium increase intracellularly, via the inhibition of the sodium-potassium ATPase pump. Such treatment has also been shown to cause arrest in the G2-M phase of the cell cycle. Activation of caspase is thought to be an intermediary mechanism in apoptosis.[62] Another study showed both Anvirzel and oleandrin to be cytotoxic to human prostate cancer cells but incapable of killing murine melanoma cells at

100-fold higher drug concentrations. An oral cancer cell line of canine origin, however, showed intermediate susceptibility to cell killing by Anvirzel and oleandrin.

- An additional proposed mechanism for the anti-tumor effects of cardiac glycosides is preventing export of the protein FGF-2 from cells via inhibition of the sodium-potassium ATPase pump.[43] FGF-2 is usually exported from the cell via binding to the alpha subunit of the sodium-potassium ATPase pump and is involved in cell differentiation growth and tumor formation. Oleandrin, oleandrigenin (an additional component of Anvirzel), and the combination product Anvirzel itself were all tested against two prostate cancer cell lines studied because of their high-level expression of transmembrane sodium-potassium ATPase and high secretion levels of FGF-2. In both cell lines, oleandrin was potent in achieving growth inhibition, more so than the less water-soluble aglycone oleandrigenin. Anvirzel was slightly less potent than either of the pure isolates but did demonstrate significant growth inhibition. Nontoxic concentrations of all three substances were then chosen for further growth inhibition experiments, and all achieved similar reductions in FGF-2 expression in both cell lines studied. It is thought that Anvirzel may be superior to either pure cardiac glycoside isolate, as it may inhibit cell line growth without cardiac effects.

- An additional report indicates that Anvirzel appears to also contain polysaccharides that contain positive immuno-modulatory as well as cytotoxic properties.[44]

FORMULARY: BRANDS USED IN CLINICAL TRIALS
Brands Used in Statistically Significant Clinical Trials

- Anvirzel (Ozelle Pharmaceuticals Incorporated, USA).[42-44,62]
- Corrigen (Beiersdorf AG, Germany).[61]

References

1. Dasgupta A, Cao S, Wells A. Activated charcoal is effective but equilibrium dialysis is ineffective in removing oleander leaf extract and oleandrin from human serum: monitoring the effect by measuring apparent digoxin concentration. Ther Drug Monit 2003;25(3):323-330.
2. de Silva HA, Fonseka MM, Pathmeswaran A, et al. Multiple-dose activated charcoal for treatment of yellow oleander poisoning: a single-blind, randomised, placebo-controlled trial. Lancet 2003;361(9373):1935-1938.
3. Juurlink DN, Sivilotti ML. Multidose activated charcoal for yellow oleander poisoning. Lancet 2003;362(9383):581.
4. Jeong SE, Lee Y, Hwang JH, et al. Effects of the sap of the common oleander Nerium indicum (Apocyanaceae) on male fertility and spermatogenesis in the Oriental tobacco budworm Helicoverpa assulta (Lepidoptera, Noctuidae). J Exp Biol 2001;204(Pt 22):3935-3942.
5. Blum LM, Rieders F. Oleandrin distribution in a fatality from rectal and oral Nerium oleander extract administration. J Anal Toxicol 1987;11(5):219-221.
6. Haynes BE, Bessen HA, Wightman WD. Oleander tea: herbal draught of death. Ann Emerg Med 1985;14(4):350-353.
7. Bhatia ML, Manchanda SC, Roy SB. Haemodynamic studies with peruvoside in human congestive heart failure. Br Med J 1970;3(725):740-743.
8. Bhatia ML, Manchanda SS, Gupta SP, et al. Clinical and haemodynamic studies with peruvoside (Cd. 421) in congestive heart failure. Indian Heart J 1971;23(2):159-163.
9. Al Yahya MA, Al Farhan AH, Adam SE. Preliminary toxicity study on the individual and combined effects of Citrullus colocynthis and Nerium oleander in rats. Fitoterapia 2000;71(4):385-391.
10. Ada SE, Al Yahya MA, Al Farhan AH. Acute toxicity of various oral doses of dried Nerium oleander leaves in sheep. Am J Chin Med 2001;29(3-4):525-532.
11. Shaw D, Pearn J. Oleander poisoning. Med J Aust 1979;2(5):267-269.
12. Saravanapavananthan N, Ganeshamoorthy J. Yellow oleander poisoning—a study of 170 cases. Forensic Sci Int 1988;36(3-4):247-250.
13. Saraswat DK, Garg PK, Saraswat M. Rare poisoning with cerbera thevetia (yellow oleander). Review of 13 cases of suicidal attempt. J Assoc Physicians India 1992;40(9):628-629.
14. Samal KK, Sahu HK, Kar MK, et al. Yellow oleander (cerbera thevetia) poisoning with jaundice and renal failure. J Assoc Physicians India 1989;37(3):232-233.
15. Safadi R, Levy I, Amitai Y, et al. Beneficial effect of digoxin-specific Fab antibody fragments in oleander intoxication. Arch Intern Med 1995;155(19):2121-2125.
16. Eddleston M, Warrell DA. Management of acute yellow oleander poisoning. QJM 1999;92(9):483-485.
17. Langford SD, Boor PJ. Oleander toxicity: an examination of human and animal toxic exposures. Toxicology 1996;109(1):1-13.
18. Apted J. Oleander Dermatitis. Contact Dermatitis 1983;9(4):321.
19. Dorsey CS. Plant dermatitis in California. Calif Med 1962;96(6):412-413.
20. Dasgupta A, Hart AP. Rapid detection of oleander poisoning using fluorescence polarization immunoassay for digitoxin. Effect of treatment with digoxin-specific Fab antibody fragment (ovine). Am J Clin Pathol 1997;108(4):411-416.
21. Ahlawat SK, Agarwal AK, Wadhwa S. Rare poisoning with cerebra thevetia (yellow oleander): a report of three cases. Trop Doct 1994;24(1):37-38.
22. Gupta A, Joshi P, Jortani SA. A case of nondigitalis cardiac glycoside toxicity. Ther Drug Monit 1997;19(6):711-714.
23. Kakrani AL, Rajput CS, Khandare SK, et al. Yellow oleander seed poisoning with cardiotoxicity. A case report. Indian Heart J 1981;33(1):31-33.
24. Thilagar S, Thirumalaikolundusubramanian P, Gopalakrishnan S, et al. Possible yellow oleander toxicity in a neonate. Indian Pediatr 1986;23(5):393.
25. Kaojarern S, Sukhupunyarak S, Mokkhavesa C. Oleander Yee tho poisoning. J Med Assoc Thai 1986;69(2):108-112.
26. Brewster D. Herbal poisoning: a case report of a fatal yellow oleander poisoning from the Solomon Islands. Ann Trop Paediatr 1986;6(4):289-291.
27. Bose TK, Basu RK, Biswas B, et al. Cardiovascular effects of yellow oleander ingestion. J Indian Med Assoc 1999;97(10):407-410.
28. Arnold HL, Middleton WS, Chen KK. The action of thevetin, a cardiac glucoside, and its clinical application. Amer Heart J 1935;189:193-206.
29. Middleton W, Chen K. Clinical results from oral administration of thevetin, a cardiac glycoside. Amer Heart J 1936;11:75-88.
30. Ansford AJ, Morris H. Fatal oleander poisoning. Med J Aust 1981;1(7):360-361.
31. Goerre S, Frohli P. [A case from practice (261). Poisoning with digitoxin-like glycosides following eating of oleander leaves]. Schweiz Rundsch Med Prax 1993;82(4):121-122.
32. Mesa MD, Anguita M, Lopez-Granados A, et al. [Digitalis poisoning from medicinal herbs. Two different mechanisms of production]. Rev Esp Cardiol 1991;44(5):347-350.
33. Misra A. Poisoning from Thevetia nerifolia (yellow oleander). Postgrad Med J 1990;66(776):492.
34. Mallick BK. Cardiotoxicity in yellow oleander seed poisoning. J Indian Med Assoc 1984;82(8):296-297.
35. Samal KK. Yellow oleander poisoning with jaundice and renal failure. J Assoc Physicians India 1990;38(10):821-822.
36. Carranza EM, Rodriguez JG, Marquez Moreno MD, et al. [Digitalis poisoning by the leaves of Nerium oleander (common oleander)]. Revista Clin Espan 1995;195(7):516.
37. Cheung K, Hinds JA, Duffy P. Detection of poisoning by plant-origin cardiac glycoside with the Abbott TDx analyzer. Clin Chem 1989;35(2):295-297.
38. Datta P, Dasgupta A. Interference of oleandrin and oleandrigenin in digitoxin immunoassays: minimal cross reactivity with a new monoclonal chemiluminescent assay and high cross reactivity with the fluorescence polarization assay. Ther Drug Monit 1997;19(4):465-469.
39. Eddleston M. Patterns and problems of deliberate self-poisoning in the developing world. QJM 2000;93(11):715-731.
40. Nishioka S, Resende ES. Transitory complete atrioventricular block associated to ingestion of Nerium oleander. Rev Assoc Med Bras 1995;41(1):60-62.
41. Durakovic Z, Durakovic A, Durakovic S. Oleander poisoning treated by resin haemoperfusion. J Indian Med Assoc 1996;94(4):149-150.
42. Pathak S, Multani AS, Narayan S, et al. Anvirzel, an extract of Nerium oleander, induces cell death in human but not murine cancer cells. Anticancer Drugs 2000;11(6):455-463.
43. Smith JA, Madden T, Vijjeswarapu M, et al. Inhibition of export of fibroblast growth factor-2 (FGF-2) from the prostate cancer cell lines PC3 and DU145 by anvirzel and its cardiac glycoside component, oleandrin(1). Biochem Pharmacol 2001;62(4):469-472.
44. Wang X, Plomley JB, Newman RA, et al. LC/MS/MS analyses of an oleander extract for cancer treatment. Anal Chem 2000;72(15):3547-3552.
45. Begum S, Siddiqui BS, Sultana R, et al. Bio-active cardenolides from the leaves of Nerium oleander. Phytochemistry 1999;50(3):435-438.
46. Mashour NH, Lin GI, Frishman WH. Herbal medicine for the treatment of cardiovascular disease: clinical considerations. Arch Intern Med 1998;158(20):2225-2234.
47. Radford DJ, Gillies AD, Hinds JA, et al. Naturally occurring cardiac glycosides. Med J Aust 1986;144(10):540-544.
48. Clark RF, Selden BS, Curry SC. Digoxin-specific Fab fragments in the treatment of oleander toxicity in a canine model. Ann Emerg Med 1991;20(10):1073-1077.
49. Jortani SA, Helm RA, Valdes R, Jr. Inhibition of Na,K-ATPase by oleandrin

and oleandrigenin, and their detection by digoxin immunoassays. Clin Chem 1996;42(10):1654-1658.

50. Lim DC, Hegewald K, Dandamudi N. A suicide attempt with an oleander cocktail. Chest 1999;116(4):405S-406S.

51. Osterloh J, Herold S, Pond S. Oleander interference in the digoxin radioimmunoassay in a fatal ingestion. JAMA 1982;247(11):1596-1597.

52. Driggers DA, Solbrig R, Steiner JF, et al. Acute oleander poisoning. A suicide attempt in a geriatric patient. West J Med 1989;151(6):660-662.

53. Eddleston M, Ariaratnam CA, Sjostrom L, et al. Acute yellow oleander (*Thevetia peruviana*) poisoning: cardiac arrhythmias, electrolyte disturbances, and serum cardiac glycoside concentrations on presentation to hospital. Heart 2000;83(3):301-306.

54. Eddleston M, Rajapakse S, Rajakanthan, et al. Anti-digoxin Fab fragments in cardiotoxicity induced by ingestion of yellow oleander: a randomised controlled trial. Lancet 2000;355(9208):967-972.

55. Monzani V, Rovellini A, Schinco G, et al. Acute oleander poisoning after a self-prepared tisane. J Toxicol Clin Toxicol 1997;35(6):667-668.

56. Manna SK, Sah NK, Newman RA, et al. Oleandrin suppresses activation of nuclear transcription factor-kappaB, activator protein-1, and c-Jun NH2-terminal kinase. Cancer Res 2000;60(14):3838-3847.

57. Siddiqui BS, Sultana R, Begum S, et al. Cardenolides from the methanolic extract of *Nerium oleander* leaves possessing central nervous system depressant activity in mice. J Nat Prod 1997;60(6):540-544.

58. Wenger TL, Butler VP, Jr., Haber E, et al. Treatment of 63 severely digitalis-toxic patients with digoxin-specific antibody fragments. J Am Coll Cardiol 1985;5(5 Suppl A):118A-123A.

59. Burton LE, Picchioni AL, Chin L. Dipotassium edetate as an antidote in poisoning from oleander and its chief glycoside, oleandrin. Arch Int Pharmacodyn Ther 1965;158(1):202-211.

60. Eliot RS, Blount SG. Calcium, chelates, and digitalis. A clinical study. Amer Heart J 1961;62(1):7-21.

61. Storz H. [On the effect of the oleander glycoside Corrigen (Oleandrin). Clinical studies]. Med Welt 1967;28:1650-1655.

62. McConkey DJ, Lin Y, Nutt LK, et al. Cardiac glycosides stimulate Ca2+ increases and apoptosis in androgen-independent, metastatic human prostate adenocarcinoma cells. Cancer Res 2000;60(14):3807-3812.

Passion Flower
(*Passiflora incarnata* L.)

SYNONYMS/COMMON NAMES/RELATED SUBSTANCES

- Apricot vine, banana passion fruit (*Passiflora mollissima*), Calmanervin (combination product), Compoz (combination product), corona de cristo, EUP, Euphytose (combination product), fleischfarbige, fleur de la passion, flor de passion, granadilla, grenadille, Jamaican honeysuckle (*Passiflora laurifolia*), madre selva, maypops, Naturest, passiflora, passionflower, passion vine, passionsblume, purple passion flower, Sedacalm, water lemon, wild passion flower.

CLINICAL BOTTOM LINE
Background

- The dried aerial parts of *Passiflora incarnata* have historically been used as a sedative and hypnotic (for insomnia), and for "nervous" gastrointestinal complaints. However, there is no clear, controlled clinical evidence supporting any therapeutic use in humans. Preclinical studies provide preliminary support for a benzodiazepine-like calming action.
- Evidence for significant adverse effects is equally inconclusive and is complicated by the variety of poorly classified, potentially active constituents in different *Passiflora* species.
- Passion fruit (*Passiflora edulis* Sims), a related species, is used as a food flavoring.

Scientific Evidence for Common/Studied Uses	Grade*
Congestive heart failure (exercise capacity)	C
Sedation (agitation, anxiety, insomnia)	C

*Key to grades: A: Strong scientific evidence for this use; B: Good scientific evidence for this use; C: Unclear scientific evidence for this use; D: Fair scientific evidence against this use (it may not work); F: Strong scientific evidence against this use (it likely does not work). For a more detailed explanation of efficacy criteria, see "Natural Standard Evidence-Based Validated Grading Rationale" in the Introduction.

Historical or Theoretical Indications That Lack Sufficient Evidence

- Alcohol withdrawal,[1-3] analgesia, anticonvulsant, antispasmodic, aphrodisiac,[4] asthma,[5] antibacterial, antipseudomonal, attention deficit hyperactivity disorder (ADHD), burns (topical), cancer, chronic pain, generalized seizures, hemorrhoids, hypertension, neuralgia, pain, perimenopausal symptoms (hot flashes),[6] gastrointestinal discomfort ("nervous stomach"), tension, wrinkle prevention (topical).

Strength of Expert Opinion and Historic/Folkloric Precedent

- In the Americas, the region of the flower's origin, some Native American groups have traditionally used the plant as a mild sedative.
- In Europe, where it has been used since the 16th century, passion flower has traditionally been used to treat medical conditions with emotional or psychological etiologies (for example, gastrointestinal upset caused by anxiety or "worry").

Passion flower has also been used for restlessness or painful conditions associated with restlessness. In modern times, some practitioners recommend passion flower for insomnia, anxiety, cardiovascular diseases (giving it the label of a "cardiotonic"), bronchial asthma, pediatric excitability and attention deficit hyperactivity disorder (ADHD), and topically for treating burns and inflamed hemorrhoids.
- Passion flower is most commonly used in combination with other herbal products such as hawthorn (*Crategeus* species) and valerian (*Valeriana officinalis* L.), with similar purported clinical applications, making the evaluation of its efficacy difficult.

Safety Summary

- **Likely safe:** Considered by experts generally to be safe when used as a food additive/flavoring and when taken by otherwise healthy individuals in recommended doses for a short duration. Reported adverse reactions may be due to adulterants in some products, but testing for purity of products is not routinely done.
- **Possibly unsafe:** Caution should be taken during pregnancy, based on animal studies showing uterine stimulation,[7] as well as for patients using monoamine oxidase inhibitors (MAOIs), based on theoretical additive effects.[8]
- **Likely unsafe:** When raw passiflora fruit (*Passiflora adenopoda*) is consumed, because of possible cyanide constituents; deaths were reported in children in Costa Rica in the 1970s.[9] Cyanide has not been isolated from *Passiflora incarnata*, however.

DOSING/TOXICOLOGY
General

- Recommended dosing regimens are based on traditional health practice patterns, expert opinion or anecdote. There are no available reliable human trials demonstrating safety or efficacy for any specific doses of passion flower. Doses are partially based on recommendations of the European Scientific Cooperative on Phytotherapy. In general, with natural products, the optimal doses needed to balance efficacy and safety often have not been determined. Formulations and preparation methods may vary from manufacturer to manufacturer, and from batch to batch of a specific product made by a single manufacturer. Because often the active components of a product are not known, standardization may not be possible, and the clinical effects of different brands may not be comparable.

Standardization

- Standardized products are not widely available. Flavonoids have been used for standardization in some commercial products. Passion flower is often found in combination products containing other herbs. Standardization is problematic given the large number of compounds that may play a role in the clinical activity of passion flower.

Dosing: Adult (18 Years and Older)
Oral

- **Dried herb:** 0.5 to 2 g, three to four times/day.

- **Tincture:** 1 to 4 mL (1:8) three to four times/day.
- **Tea:** Made from 4 to 8 g of dried herb, taken daily.

Intravenous
- **Infusion:** 2.5 g three to four times/day have been used, although there are no reliable safety or efficacy data.

Dosing: Pediatric (Younger Than 18 Years)
- Insufficient available evidence.
- Many experts recommend that children aged 3 to 12 years be given this herb under medical supervision only, with dosing proportional to adult doses (calculated by body weight: assume adult doses are for a 60-kg individual and divide by the child's weight to determine the correct dosage).

Toxicology
- Products implicated in case reports of toxicity have rarely been tested, and many experts believe that toxicities may be due to adulterants, rather than to passion flower itself. This issue has been explored at length by the British Committee on Safety of Medicine (CSM).
- Nausea, profuse vomiting, drowsiness, and episodes of non-sustained ventricular tachycardia (NSVT) are noted in a case report of a 34-year-old female self-medicating with the passion flower product Sedacalm for anxiety. Her condition resolved within a week of hospitalization following discontinuation of passion flower and several days of supportive care. She had taken 3 tablets (equivalent to 1500 mg of passion flower) for 1 day, followed by 2 tablets (1000 mg of passion flower) on a second day prior to hospitalization.[10]
- Five cases of individuals becoming temporarily "mentally impaired" from ingestion of a combination herbal product containing passion flower are discussed in a Norwegian case report.[11]
- Idiosyncratic hypersensitivity reaction characterized by urticaria and cutaneous vasculitis has been reported in a 77-year-old man with rheumatoid arthritis taking the passion flower extract product Naturest.[12]
- In mice, the reported LD_{50} of maltol and ethyl maltol isolated from *Passiflora incarnata* are 820 and 910 mg/kg, respectively,[13] but these values are derived from a study with a very small sample size and may not be reliable.
- Children in Costa Rica who died from eating passiflora fruit (*Passiflora adenopoda*) reportedly suffered from cyanide poisoning derived from a cyanogenic B-glycoside in the fruit, although documentation is unclear.[9] Notably, in available studies cyanogenic alkaloids have not been isolated from *P. incarnata* to date.

ADVERSE EFFECTS/PRECAUTIONS/CONTRAINDICATIONS
Allergy
- **Cutaneous vasculitis:** An idiosyncratic hypersensitivity reaction characterized by urticaria and cutaneous vasculitis has been reported in a 77-year-old man with rheumatoid arthritis taking the passion flower extract product Naturest.[12]
- **Allergic asthma:** Occupational asthma and rhinitis were reported in an individual preparing passion flower products. Western blot analysis confirmed IgG and IgE antibodies in the patient's serum against a protein present in *Passiflora alata*, a species not generally relevant to clinical practice.[14]

Adverse Effects
- **General:** Passion flower is generally considered by experts to be a safe herb, with few adverse events reported. Products implicated in case reports have rarely been tested, and adverse effects may be due to adulterants rather than to passion flower itself.
- **Neurologic/CNS:** Drowsiness or sedation may be expected, based on a reported mechanism of benzodiazepine receptor affinity in animals.[15-17] There are scant human data in this area, although passion flower has been used traditionally for hundreds of years as a sedative or hypnotic.
- **Gastrointestinal:** Nausea and profuse vomiting have been reported in a single patient taking a passion flower product (Sedacalm) (1500 mg for 1 day followed by 1000 mg on the second day, prior to onset).[10] This condition resolved after 1 week of supportive care.
- **Cardiovascular:** Reversible ventricular tachycardia has been reported in a single patient taking a passion flower product (Sedacalm) (1500 mg for 1 day followed by 1000 mg on the second day, prior to onset). She recovered following passion flower discontinuation and supportive hospital care for several days.[10]

Precautions/Warnings/Contraindications
- Recommend caution in patients taking sedative medications such as benzodiazepines, due to theoretical synergistic effects.
- Recommend caution in patients taking monoamine oxidase inhibitors (MAOIs), due to theoretical additive effects.
- The ability to drive or operate machinery may be impaired by the purported sedative effects of passion flower.

Pregnancy and Lactation
- Constituents found in some species of *Passiflora*, such as harman and harmaline, were reported to stimulate the uterus in several animal studies during the early 1930s.[7] These effects have not been investigated in recent available studies. Whether passion flower contains the cyanogenic glycoside gynocardin remains controversial among experts.[18] Passion flower should thus be avoided in pregnancy until additional data are available.

INTERACTIONS
Passion Flower/Drug Interactions
- **Monoamine oxidase inhibitors (MAOIs), tricyclic antidepressants (TCAs), selective serotonin receptor antagonists (SSRIs):** Harmala alkaloids, which possess MAOI activity, reportedly are found in small amounts in some species of *Passiflora*.[13] Passion flower may therefore theoretically potentiate the activity of MAOIs. In combination with other antidepressants, sedation or hypotension could theoretically be precipitated. However, levels of these alkaloids may be too low to be clinically relevant.[8]
- **Sedative drugs (including benzodiazepines, barbiturates, opiates, and ethanol):** In theory, potentiation of the central nervous system depressant effects of alcohol or other sedative-hypnotic drugs may occur with concomitant use of passion flower, based on animal data demonstrating a central benzodiazepine ligand isolated from *Passionflora coerulea*.[15-17] Prolongation of barbiturate-induced sleep time (hexobarbital, pentobarbital) in mice and rats given passion flower has been demonstrated and has been interpreted by authors as suggesting interference with barbiturate metabolism.[13,19]
- **Anticoagulant/antiplatelet drugs:** Passionflower contains coumarin [13] and therefore may increase bleeding risk (theoretical). Literature review reveals no reported cases of clinically significant bleeding in humans.

Passion Flower/Herb/Supplement Interactions

- **Kava:** Potentiation of the sedative effects of kava extracts by passion flower has been reported in mice.[20]
- **Sedating herbs and supplements:** Passion flower has been demonstrated in animal studies to have affinity for benzodiazepine receptors and theoretically may act as a sedative agent.
- **Herbs and supplements with monoamine oxidase inhibitor (MAOI) activity:** Harmala alkaloids, which possess MAOI activity, are reportedly found in small amounts in some species of *Passiflora*.[13] Passion flower could therefore theoretically potentiate the activity of MAOI agents. However, levels of these alkaloids may be too low to be clinically relevant.
- **Anticoagulant/antiplatelet agents:** Passion flower contains coumarin[13] and therefore may increase bleeding risk (theoretical). Literature review reveals no reported cases of clinically significant bleeding in humans.
- **Caffeine:** Small amount of alkaloids with monoamine oxidase inhibitor activity are found in some species of passion flower. Taken concomitantly with caffeine, hypertension may result. However, alkaloid levels may be too low to be clinically relevant.[8]

Passion Flower/Food Interactions

- **Tyramine or tryptophan-containing foods:** Harmala alkaloids, which possess monoamine oxidase inhibitor activity, are reportedly found in small amounts in some species of *Passiflora*.[8] Passion flower could therefore theoretically interact with tyramine or tryptophan-containing foods, including red wine, cheeses, and aged foods, causing reactions including hypertensive urgency. However, alkaloid levels may be too low to be clinically relevant.

Passion Flower/Lab Interactions

- **International normalized ratio (INR):** Passion flower contains coumarin[13] and theoretically may increase INR. However, literature review reveals no studies of passion flower and coagulation factors in humans.

MECHANISM OF ACTION
Pharmacology

- Among the 400 or more species of *Passiflora*, there are many substances with potential pharmacologic activity, although not all have been identified or isolated from *P. incarnata*. The principal constituents are up to 2.5% flavonoids, including vitexin, isovitexin, coumarin, apigenin, umbeliferone, and maltol. Harmala alkaloids, including harman, harmaline, harmine, and harmalol, have been reported but may be in subtherapeutic quantities. Cyanogenic glycosides have been isolated from some species of *Passiflora* but have not been reported in *P. incarnata*.[13,21-23]
- Chrysin, a flavonoid found in *P. coerulea*, has demonstrated antianxiety effects and anticonvulsant effects (against pentylenetetrazol) in mice given a benzodiazepine receptor antagonist.[15-17] Chrysin and other flavonoids also altered the *in vitro* binding of ligands to the benzodiazepine receptor.[17] These results suggest an effect mediated by benzodiazepine receptors, which would support the claimed antianxiety and sedative effects of passion flower extracts.
- An aqueous *Passiflora* extract (400 gm/kg) has produced weak effects on a mouse model of antianxiety activity, not antagonized by a benzodiazepine receptor antagonist.[24] Extracts are also reported to produce sedation and potentiate pentobarbital-induced sleep.[20,24]

- Harmala alkaloids reportedly have monoamine oxidase inhibitor properties[8] and calcium channel blocking activity in vascular and intestinal smooth muscle.[25]
- An ethanolic extract of *Passiflora incarnata* elevated the nociceptive (pain) threshold and reduced activity in rats.[19] However, studies of several individual alkaloids failed to demonstrate analgesic effects in rats.[16]
- There is an unpublished report of antimuscarinic activity, which, if confirmed, could provide a basis for reported use as a gastrointestinal antispasmodic.
- Antibacterial and antifungal activity have been found in extracts of several species of *Passiflora* but have not been reported in *Passiflora incarnata*.[26,27]
- A compound, 4-hydroxy-2-cyclopentanone, isolated from *Passiflora tetrandra*, has been found to exert cytotoxic effects on P388 murine leukemia cells ($IC_{50} < 1$ μg/ml), but this evidence is preliminary.[26]
- Although maltol has been shown to have physiologic properties, the fact that it may be produced through heat extraction processes rather than existing in the plant itself makes its clinical relevance questionable.[28]

Pharmacodynamics/Kinetics

- Insufficient available data.

HISTORY

- Passion flower has traditionally been used by Native South Americans as a mild sedative. It was brought to Europe from Peru in 1569 by Spanish explorers, who named the plant for the symbolic connections between its appearance and that of "Christ's passion," with the plant's five anthers resembling the stigmata and its fringe-like crown resembling the crown of thorns. It has been used by European homeopaths for sleep disturbances, restless agitation, and cramps. Many species of *Passiflora* produce edible fruits.

REVIEW OF THE EVIDENCE: DISCUSSION
Sedation (Agitation, Anxiety, Insomnia)
Summary

- Passion flower is often recommended for restlessness or agitation. However, there are no well-conducted human clinical trials of passion flower for these indications. Preliminary supportive evidence stems from animal studies, methodologically weak trials, and examinations of herb combinations such as Euphytose (available in Europe). Well-designed, adequately powered human trials of single agents vs. placebo or standard of care, as well as safety data, are necessary before a recommendation can be made either for or against this use.

Preclinical Evidence

- Several animal and *in vitro* studies of passion flower have demonstrated potential sedative/calming effects mediated by the benzodiazepine receptor, which may predict potential clinical value as a sedative in humans.[15-17]

Human Evidence

- A double-blind, placebo-controlled trial of 182 patients with adjustment disorder and anxious mood was conducted using the combination product Euphytose, which contains six extracts (*Crataegus*, *Ballota*, *Passiflora*, and *Valeriana*, purported to have mild sedative effects, as well as cola and *Paullinia*, purported to act as stimulants).[29] After 28 days, mean scores on the Hamilton anxiety score (HAMA) scale

P

Review of the Evidence: Passion Flower

Condition Treated*	Study Design	Author, Year	N[†]	SS[†]	Study Quality[‡]	Magnitude of Benefit	ARR[†]	NNT[†]	Comments
Anxiety	RCT	Bourin[29] 1997	182	Yes	4	Medium	17.6%	6	Outcome measure: HAMA score; study combined 6 herbs.
Congestive heart failure (exercise capacity)	RCT	Von Eiff[34] 1994	40	Yes	5	Small	NA	NA	Study combined passion flower and hawthorn.

*Primary or secondary outcome.
[†]N, Number of patients; SS, statistically significant; ARR, absolute risk reduction; NNT, the number of patients who need to undergo a specific intervention in order to observe an outcome in one individual.
[‡]0-2 = poor; 3-4 = good; 5 = excellent.
HAMA, Hamilton anxiety score; NA, not applicable; RCT, randomized, controlled trial.
For an explanation of each category in this table, please see Table 3 in the Introduction.

had dropped in both groups, but more so in the Euphytose group, with 49.2% of patients below a HAMA score of 10, vs. 25.3% in the placebo group. Results were statistically significant. Although this was a well-designed study, the description of methodology was limited. The use of a combination product makes these results impossible to extrapolate to passion flower as a monotherapy. Safety data for Euphytose are limited.

- A randomized, double-blind trial compared the effects of a single dose of the "sedative" herbal combination Valverde (contains passion flower and valerian) to the benzodiazepine bromazepam (3 mg) and to placebo in 20 healthy males.[30] No effects were observed on several indicators of sedation/alertness. However, the small number of subjects, unclear outcomes measures, and lack of a power calculation make these results difficult to interpret. In addition, because a combination product was used the amounts of passion flower present may not be comparable to monopreparations.

- Two additional publications of poor design examined combination products, including a study of the product Compoz over a 2-week period, which found no benefit over placebo for sedation,[31] and a report using the combination product Calmanervin for preoperative sedation with inconclusive results.[32] Because of the use of combination products and weak design, these results are not relevant to the use of passion flower monotherapy in clinical practice.

- A 2001 comparison of methanol extracts of *Passiflora incarnata* vs. *Passiflora edulis* for anxiety concluded that 125 mg of *P. incarnata* had "significant" anxiolytic activity, whereas *P. edulis* had none. However, scant details of design and methodology were provided, and results are thus difficult to interpret.[33]

Congestive Heart Failure (Exercise Capacity)
Summary

- There is insufficient available evidence to recommend either for or against passion flower for the treatment of exercise capacity or dyspnea in patients with congestive heart failure (CHF). Although this indication has been studied in one trial of a passion flower–hawthorn combination product, it is not a typical clinical use of passion flower. Effects may have been attributable to hawthorn, which is commonly used in Europe for CHF and which has been shown in several initial randomized trials to possibly be beneficial in heart failure.

Evidence

- Von Eiff et al. examined the effect of an extract containing both passion flower (140 mg) and hawthorn on the exercise capacity of 46 patients ages 53 to 86 years with congestive heart failure (CHF) and chronic dyspnea on exertion (DOE).[34] Patients with cardiovascular disease or obstructive pulmonary disease were excluded. The design was a monocenter, placebo-controlled, double-blind trial, stratified according to patients' pre-screened exercise capacities, and conducted for 6 weeks. Six patients were withdrawn because of design flaws (N for analysis was 21 in the placebo group, 19 in the drug group). Outcome measures were physical exercise capacity measured by distance walked in 6 minutes and a bicycle ergometer test. Exercise capacity in the walking test significantly increased in the passion flower–hawthorn group after 6 weeks vs. placebo ($p < 0.05$, two tailed). However, maximum exercise capacity as measured by the bicycle ergometer test was increased in both groups, with no statistically significant difference between the extract and placebo. The results suggest that the extract may have had an effect on functional physical activity in elderly patients with CHF. Of note, a small but statistically significant decrease was observed in the extract group in mean blood pressure during exercise and in total cholesterol levels. However, the effect of either plant product alone was not determined.

FORMULARY: BRANDS USED IN CLINICAL TRIALS
Brands Used in Statistically Significant Clinical Trials

- Euphytose, a European combination containing *Crataegus*, *Ballota*, *Passiflora*, *Valeriana*, cola, and *Paullinia* has been shown effective for anxiety in one trial.[29]

References

1. Dhawan K, Kumar S, Sharma A. Suppression of alcohol-cessation–oriented hyper-anxiety by the benzoflavone moiety of *Passiflora incarnata* Linneaus in mice. J Ethnopharmacol 2002;81(2):239-244.
2. Dhawan K. Drug/substance reversal effects of a novel tri-substituted benzoflavone moiety (BZF) isolated from *Passiflora incarnata* Linn.—a brief perspective. Addict Biol 2003;8(4):379-386.
3. Dhawan K, Dhawan S, Chhabra S. Attenuation of benzodiazepine dependence in mice by a tri-substituted benzoflavone moiety of *Passiflora incarnata* Linnaeus: a non-habit forming anxiolytic. J Pharm Pharm Sci 2003;6(2):215-222.
4. Dhawan K, Kumar S, Sharma A. Aphrodisiac activity of methanol extract of leaves of *Passiflora incarnata* Linn in mice. Phytother Res 2003;17(4):401-403.
5. Dhawan K, Kumar S, Sharma A. Antiasthmatic activity of the methanol extract of leaves of *Passiflora incarnata*. Phytother Res 2003;17(7):821-822.
6. Israel D, Youngkin EQ. Herbal therapies for perimenopausal and menopausal complaints. Pharmacotherapy 1997;17(5):970-984.
7. Farnsworth NR, Bingel AS, Cordell GA, et al. Potential value of plants as sources of new antifertility agents I. J Pharm Sci 1975;64(4):535-598.
8. Rommelspacher H, May T, Salewski B. Harman (1-methyl-beta-carboline) is a natural inhibitor of monoamine oxidase type A in rats. Eur J Pharmacol 1994;252(1):51-59.
9. Saenz JA, Nassar M. Toxic effect of the fruit of *Passiflora adenopoda* D.C.

on humans: phytochemical determination. Rev Biol Trop 1972;20(1): 137-140.

10. Fisher AA, Purcell P, Le Couteur DG. Toxicity of *Passiflora incarnata* L. J Toxicol Clin Toxicol 2000;38(1):63-66.

11. Solbakken AM, Rorbakken G, Gundersen T. [Nature medicine as intoxicant]. Tidsskr.Nor Laegeforen. 1997;117(8):1140-1141.

12. Smith GW, Chalmers TM, Nuki G. Vasculitis associated with herbal preparation containing *Passiflora* extract. Br J Rheumatol 1993;32(1):87-88.

13. Aoyagi N, Kimura R, Murata T. Studies on *passiflora incarnata* dry extract. I. Isolation of maltol and pharmacological action of maltol and ethyl maltol. Chem Pharm Bull (Tokyo) 1974;22(5):1008-1013.

14. Giavina-Bianchi PF, Jr., Castro FF, Machado ML, et al. Occupational respiratory allergic disease induced by *Passiflora alata* and *Rhamnus purshiana*. Ann Allergy Asthma Immunol 1997;79(5):449-454.

15. Wolfman C, Viola H, Paladini A, et al. Possible anxiolytic effects of chrysin, a central benzodiazepine receptor ligand isolated from *Passiflora coerulea*. Pharmacol Biochem Behav 1994;47(1):1-4.

16. Salgueiro JB, Ardenghi P, Dias M, et al. Anxiolytic natural and synthetic flavonoid ligands of the central benzodiazepine receptor have no effect on memory tasks in rats. Pharmacol Biochem Behav 1997;58(4):887-891.

17. Medina JH, Paladini AC, Wolfman C, et al. Chrysin (5,7-di-OH-flavone), a naturally-occurring ligand for benzodiazepine receptors, with anticonvulsant properties. Biochem Pharmacol 1990;40(10):2227-2231.

18. Spencer KC, Seigler DS. Gynocardin from *Passiflora*. Planta Med 1984; 50(4):356-357.

19. Speroni E, Minghetti A. Neuropharmacological activity of extracts from *Passiflora incarnata*. Planta Med 1988;54(6):488-491.

20. Capasso A, Pinto A. Experimental investigations of the synergistic-sedative effect of passiflora and kava. Acta Therapeutica 1995;21:127-140.

21. Menghini A, Mancini LA. TLC determination of flavonoid accumulation in clonal populations of *Passiflora incarnata* L. Pharmacol Res Commun 1988;20(Suppl 5):113-116.

22. Quercia V, Turchetto L, Pierini V, et al. Identification and determination of vitexin and isovitexin in *Passiflora incarnata* extracts. J Chromatogr 1978; 161:396-402.

23. Spencer KC, Seigler DS. Cyanogenesis of Passiflora edulis. J Agric Food Chem 1983;31(4):794-796.

24. Soulimani R, Younos C, Jarmouni S, et al. Behavioural effects of *Passiflora incarnata* L. and its indole alkaloid and flavonoid derivatives and maltol in the mouse. J Ethnopharmacol 1997;57(1):11-20.

25. Karaki H, Kishimoto T, Ozaki H, et al. Inhibition of calcium channels by harmaline and other harmala alkaloids in vascular and intestinal smooth muscles. Br J Pharmacol 1986;89(2):367-375.

26. Perry NB, Albertson GD, Blunt JW, et al. 4-Hydroxy-2-cyclopentenone: an anti-*Pseudomonas* and cytotoxic component from *Passiflora tetrandra*. Planta Med 1991;57(2):129-131.

27. Birner J, Nicolls JM. Passicol, an antibacterial and antifungal agent produced by *Passiflora* plant species: preparation and physicochemical characteristics. Antimicrob Agents Chemother 1973;3(1):105-109.

28. Congura M. Isolement et identification de deux glycosyl-luteolines mono-C-substituees et de la diglucosyl-6-8-luteoline di-C-substituee dans les tiges feuillees de *Passiflora incarnata* L. Helvitica Chimica Acta 1986;69: 251-253.

29. Bourin M, Bougerol T, Guitton B, et al. A combination of plant extracts in the treatment of outpatients with adjustment disorder with anxious mood: controlled study versus placebo. Fundam Clin Pharmacol 1997;11(2): 127-132.

30. Gerhard U, Hobi V, Kocher R, et al. [Acute sedative effect of a herbal relaxation tablet as ompared to that of bromazepam]. Schweiz Rundsch. Med Prax. 1991;80(52):1481-1486.

31. Rickels K, Hesbacher PT. Over-the-counter daytime sedatives. A controlled study. JAMA 1973;223(1):29-33.

32. Yaniv R, Segal E, Trau H, et al. Natural premedication for mast cell proliferative disorders. J Ethnopharmacol 1995;46(1):71-72.

33. Dhawan K, Kumar S, Sharma A. Comparative biological activity study on *Passiflora incarnata* and *P. edulis*. Fitoterapia 2001;72(6):698-702.

34. Von Eiff M, Brunner H, Haegeli A, et al. Hawthorn/passion flower extract and improvement in physical exercise capacity of patients with dyspnoea Class II of the NYHA functional classifications. Acta Therapeutica 1994; 20:47-66.

P

SYNONYMS/COMMON NAMES/RELATED SUBSTANCES

- *Chrysanthemum morifolium* (chrysanthemum, mum, chu-hua); *Ganoderma lucidum* (reishi mushroom, ling zhi); *Glycyrrhiza glabra* (licorice); *Isatis indigotica* Fort (da qing ye, dyer's wood); *Panax pseudo-ginseng* (san qi); *Rabdosia rubescens* (rubescens, dong ling cao); *Scutellaria baicalensis* (scullcap, huang-chin); *Serenoa repens* (saw palmetto).
- Not to be confused with SPES (a different product), or with copycat products marketed with similar names.

CLINICAL BOTTOM LINE
Background

- PC-SPES is an herbal combination product that was produced and marketed until early 2002 by BotanicLab, Inc. for the treatment of prostate cancer. The initials *PC* stand for "prostate cancer," and *spes* is Latin for "hope."
- Based on a Chinese herbal formula, the ingredients of PC-SPES were officially listed as including *Serenoa repens* (saw palmetto) and seven other herbs: *Chrysanthemum morifolium* (chrysanthemum, mum, chu-hua); *Ganoderma lucidum* (reishi mushroom, ling zhi); *Glycyrrhiza glabra* (licorice); *Isatis indigotica* Fort (da qing ye, dyer's wood); *Panax pseudo-ginseng* (san qi); *Rabdosia rubescens* (rubescens, dong ling cao); and *Scutellaria baicalensis* (scullcap, huang-chin).
- In low-quality studies, PC-SPES was observed to reduce serum prostate-specific antigen (PSA) levels, reduce evidence of metastatic disease, diminish pain, and improve quality of life in patients with prostate cancer. This evidence was viewed as promising by major cancer centers in the United States.
- However, in early 2002, the FDA Safety Information and Adverse Event Reporting Program issued a warning to consumers to avoid using PC-SPES, based on findings that the product contained the anticoagulant ("blood thinner") warfarin. Bleeding disorders had previously been reported with PC-SPES. The manufacturer voluntarily recalled the product. Samples of PC-SPES were later found to contain variable amounts of the nonsteroidal anti-inflammatory drug indomethacin, the synthetic estrogen diethylstilbestrol (DES), and the estrogen ethinyl estradiol.
- A study published in the September 2002 issue of the *Journal of the National Cancer Institute* analyzed lots of PC-SPES manufactured between 1996 and 2001 (Sovak, 2002). This evaluation found variable ingredients in PC-SPES between lots, with higher levels of indomethacin and DES after 1999. These post-1999 samples were found to have much greater estrogenic properties compared to earlier samples, and to possess a higher level of activity against prostate cell lines in laboratory tests. After 2001, greater amounts of the natural constituents licochalcone A and baicalin, as well as warfarin, were found in samples. These results suggest that PC-SPES produced at different times may not be equivalent or comparable, and that the "anti-cancer" effects of PC-SPES may have been due to undeclared prescription drug ingredients.
- Several other BotanicLab products have also been found to contain undeclared prescription drugs. It is not clear if

these adulterants were present in raw materials obtained by BotanicLab from other sources or were added later in the manufacturing process.

- Since BotanicLab closed its doors, several products with similar names have been introduced on the market, but none has been evaluated scientifically to the same extent as PC-SPES. The National Center for Complementary and Alternative Medicine (NCCAM) has expressed willingness to support future research on formulations that are true to the claimed ingredients and proven not to be contaminated.

Uses Based on Scientific Evidence	Grade*
Prostate cancer Uncontrolled human studies of PC-SPES have reported improvements in patients with both androgen-dependent and androgen-independent prostate cancer (de la Taille, 2000; DiPaola, 1998; Oh, 2001; Pfeifer, 2000; Small, 2000). Overall, these studies found prostate-specific antigen (PSA) levels to fall by greater than 50% in most patients, improvements in bone scans and x-rays, reductions in pain scores, and improvements in quality of life. In a 2002 preliminary report (conference abstract) of a comparison between PC-SPES and diethylstilbestrol (DES) in patients with androgen-independent metastatic prostate cancer, patients treated with PC-SPES had a greater reduction in PSA levels (Small, 2002). However, the later finding that undeclared amounts of DES are present in some PC-SPES samples clouds these results. Various explanations for the effectiveness of PC-SPES were initially proposed. Estrogen-like effects were reported prior to 1998. These may be due to herbs with estrogen-like effects or to undeclared estrogenic drugs. The constituent baicalin, a flavone found in *Scutellaria baicalensis*, was found in laboratory experiments to inhibit the enzymes 12-lipoxygenase, 5-alpha-reductase, and aromatase. In addition, PC-SPES extracts were reported to cause cell death (apoptosis) or to slow the growth of cancer cell lines. The recent finding that different lots of PC-SPES produced between 1996 and 2001 contained different ingredients from each other has raised questions about whether studies of PC-SPES can be compared with each other. The discovery of undeclared prescription drug ingredients, including the nonsteroidal anti-inflammatory drug indomethacin, the synthetic estrogen diethylstilbestrol (DES), the estrogen ethinyl estradiol, and the anticoagulant warfarin, make it unclear if these constituents may have caused the observed clinical effects. Because of these complicated circumstances, and the fact that PC-SPES has never been compared to placebo or standard cancer treatments in a well-reported study, the question of effectiveness remains unclear.	C

Due to known and theoretical safety concerns, samples of PC-SPES that may be in the possession of patients should not be used.

*Key to grades: A: Strong scientific evidence for this use; B: Good scientific evidence for this use; C: Unclear scientific evidence for this use; D: Fair scientific evidence against this use (it may not work); F: Strong scientific evidence against this use (it likely does not work). For a more detailed explanation of efficacy criteria, see "Natural Standard Evidence-Based Validated Grading Rationale" in the Introduction.

Historical or Theoretical Indications That Lack Sufficient Evidence

Benign prostatic hypertrophy, breast cancer, breast enlargement, cancer prevention, leukemia, lymphoma, melanoma, "prostate health."

DOSING/TOXICOLOGY

The following doses are based on scientific research, publications, traditional use, or expert opinion. Many herbs and supplements have not been thoroughly tested, and safety and effectiveness may not be proven. Brands may be made differently, with variable ingredients even within the same brand. The doses shown may not apply to all products. It is important to always read product labels and discuss doses with a qualified healthcare provider before therapy is started.

Adult Dosing (18 Years and Older)

- Based on known safety concerns associated with PC-SPES, no dosing regimen is recommended. Samples of PC-SPES that may be in the possession of patients should not be used.

SAFETY

The U.S. Food and Drug Administration does not strictly regulate herbs and supplements. There is no guarantee of strength, purity, or safety of products, and effects may vary. It is important to always read product labels. People who have a medical condition, or are taking other drugs, herbs, or supplements, you should consult a qualified healthcare provider before starting a new therapy. A healthcare provider should be contacted immediately about any side effects.

Allergies

- In one human study, allergic reactions were reported in 2% of patients, and treatment was stopped in one case because of throat swelling and shortness of breath. It is not clear which ingredient in PC-SPES might have been responsible. Products containing herbs similar to PC-SPES should be avoided by people with allergies to any of the included herbs.

Side Effects and Warnings

- PC-SPES has been recalled and should not be used. Undeclared prescription drug ingredients have been found in samples of PC-SPES, including indomethacin, diethylstilbestrol (DES), ethinyl estradiol, and warfarin.
- PC-SPES may increase the risk of blood clots. Several cases of blood clots, including life-threatening clots to the lungs, have been reported with PC-SPES use. In contrast, cases of bleeding have also been reported. These are theorized to be due to undeclared amounts of the prescription drug warfarin in some samples of PC-SPES, or to the presence of the PC-SPES ingredient saw palmetto which is associated with one report of bleeding. This would add to the risk of

bleeding in patients with bleeding disorders or taking drugs that may increase the risk of bleeding. The bleeding disorder disseminated intravascular coagulation (DIC), that can include clotting, bleeding, or both, has also been reported.
- PC-SPES has also been associated with erectile dysfunction, loss of libido, hot flashes, breast/nipple tenderness, breast enlargement, water retention (edema), and leg cramps.
- Adverse effects associated with undeclared prescription drug ingredients in PC-SPES are possible, such as gastrointestinal distress from indomethacin.

Pregnancy and Breastfeeding

- PC-SPES has not been evaluated during pregnancy or breast-feeding and should be avoided. Estrogenic effects may be harmful. The undeclared prescription drug diethylstilbestrol (DES), discovered in some samples of PC-SPES, may increase the risk of reproductive tract abnormalities in daughters born to women taking this drug.

INTERACTIONS

Most herbs and supplements have not been thoroughly tested for interactions with other herbs, supplements, drugs, or foods. The interactions listed here are based on reports in scientific publications, laboratory experiments, or traditional use. It is important to always read product labels. People who have a medical condition, or are taking other drugs, herbs, or supplements, should consult a qualified healthcare provider before starting a new therapy.

Interactions with Drugs

- Based on reported cases of bleeding and inclusion of undeclared amounts of the prescription blood-thinner warfarin in some samples, PC-SPES may increase the risk of bleeding when taken with drugs that increase the risk of bleeding. Some examples include aspirin, anticoagulants ("blood thinners") such as warfarin (Coumadin) and heparin, antiplatelet drugs such as clopidogrel (Plavix), and non-steroidal anti-inflammatory drugs such as ibuprofen (Motrin, Advil) and naproxen (Naprosyn, Aleve). In contrast, PC-SPES has also been associated with an increased risk of blood clots, which may be due to estrogen-like effects. This would work against the action of blood-thinning medications.
- Based on the proposed anti-androgenic mechanism of action of saw palmetto, a major ingredient of PC-SPES, additive effects may occur with anti-androgen drugs such as the 5α-reductase inhibitor finasteride (Proscar); the androgen receptor antagonists bicalutamide (Casodex), flutamide (Eulexin), and nilutamide (Nilandron); and the GnRH antagonists leuprolide (Lupron), goserelin (Zoladex), and histrelin (Supprelin). Similarly, this therapy may decrease the effectiveness of therapeutic androgens such as testosterone (Androderm, Testoderm), methyltestosterone (Android, Testred, Virilon), fluoxymesterone (Halotestin), nandrolone decanoate (Deca-Dubrolin), and stanozolol (Winstrol).
- PC-SPES may add to the estrogenic effects of other drugs, based on estrogen-like effects reported in studies and on the presence of undeclared amounts of prescription estrogen drugs in some samples of PC-SPES.

Interactions with Herbs and Dietary Supplements

- Based on reported cases of bleeding and inclusion of undeclared amounts of the prescription blood-thinner warfarin in some samples, PC-SPES may increase the risk of bleeding when taken with herbs and supplements that are believed to increase the risk of bleeding. Multiple cases of bleeding have been reported with the use of *Ginkgo biloba*, and fewer cases with garlic and saw palmetto. Numerous other agents may theoretically increase the risk of bleeding, although this has not been proven in most cases. Some examples include alfalfa, American ginseng, angelica, anise, *Arnica montana*, asafetida, aspen bark, bilberry, birch, black cohosh, bladderwrack, bogbean, boldo, borage seed oil, bromelain, capsicum, cat's claw, celery, chamomile, chaparral, clove, coleus, cordyceps, danshen, devil's claw, dong quai, EPA (eicosapentaenoic acid, found in deep-sea fish oils), evening primrose oil, fenugreek, feverfew, fish oil, flaxseed/flax powder (not a concern with flaxseed oil), ginger, grapefruit juice, grape seed, green tea, guggul, gymnestra, horse chestnut, horseradish, licorice root, lovage root, male fern, meadowsweet, nordihydroguaiaretic acid (NDGA), onion, papain, *Panax ginseng*, parsley, passionflower, poplar, prickly ash, propolis, quassia, red clover, reishi, rue, Siberian ginseng, sweet birch, sweet clover, turmeric, vitamin E, white willow, wild carrot, wild lettuce, willow, wintergreen, yucca. In contrast, PC-SPES has also been associated with an increased risk of blood clots, which may be due to estrogen-like effects. This would work against the action of blood-thinning agents.

- PC-SPES may add to the estrogenic effects of other agents, based on estrogen-like effects reported in studies and on the presence of undeclared amounts of prescription estrogen drugs in some samples. Possible examples include alfalfa, black cohosh, bloodroot, burdock, hops, kudzu, licorice, pomegranate, red clover, soy, thyme, white horehoumd, and yucca.

Selected References

Natural Standard developed the preceding evidence-based information based on a systematic review of more than 75 articles. For comprehensive information about alternative and complementary therapies on the professional level, go to www.naturalstandard.com. Selected references are listed here.

Burton TM. Prostate cancer herbs gone for good. Wall Street Journal 2002 (May 21):D4.

Cheema P, El Mefty O, Jazieh AR. Intraoperative haemorrhage associated with the use of extract of Saw Palmetto herb: a case report and review of literature. J Intern Med 2001;250(2):167-169.

Darzynkiewicz Z, Traganos F, Wu JM, et al. Chinese herbal mixture PC SPES in treatment of prostate cancer. Int J Oncol 2000;17:729-736.

Davis NB, Nahlik L, Vogelzang NJ. Does PC-SPES interact with warfarin? J Urol 2002;167:1793.

de la Taille A, Buttyan R, Hayek O, et al. Herbal therapy PC-SPES: in vitro effects and evaluation of its efficacy in 69 patients with prostate cancer. J Urol 2000;164(4):1229-1234.

de la Taille A, Hayek OR, Buttyan R, et al. Effects of a phytotherapeutic agent, PC-SPES, on prostate cancer: a preliminary investigation on human cell lines and patients. BJU Int 1999;84:845-850.

Di Silverio F, D'Eramo G, Lubrano C, et al. Evidence that *Serenoa repens* extract displays an antiestrogenic activity in prostatic tissue of benign prostatic hypertrophy patients. Eur Urol 1992;21(4):309-314.

DiPaola RS, Zhang H, Lambert GH, et al. Clinical and biologic activity of an estrogenic herbal combination (PC-SPES) in prostate cancer. N Engl J Med 1998;339(12):785-791.

Duncan GG. Re: Does PC-SPES interact with warfarin? J Urol 2003;169(1):294-295.

Elghamry MI, Hansel R. Activity and isolated phytoestrogen of shrub palmetto fruits (*Serenoa repens* Small), a new estrogenic plant. Experientia 1969;25(8):828-829.

Food and Drug Administration. MedWatch. 2002 Safety information summaries. PC SPES, SPES (BotanicLab). http://www.fda.gov/medwatch/SAFETY/2002/safety02.htm#spes.

Geliebter J, Mittelman A, Tiwari RK. PC-SPES and prostate cancer. J Nutr 2001;131:164S-166S.

Halicka HD, Ardelt B, Juan G, et al. Apoptosis and cell cycle effects induced by extracts of the Chinese herbal preparation PC SPES. Int J Oncol 1997;11:437-448.

Hsieh T, Chen SS, Wang X, et al. Regulation of androgen receptor (AR) and prostate specific antigen (PSA) expression in the androgen-responsive human prostate LNCaP cells by ethanolic extracts of the Chinese herbal preparation, PC-SPES. Biochem Mol Biol Int 1997;42:535-544.

Hsieh TC, Ng C, Chang CC, et al. Induction of apoptosis and down-regulation of bcl-6 in mutu I cells treated with ethanolic extracts of the Chinese herbal supplement PC-SPES. Int J Oncol 1998;13:1199-1202.

Ikezoe T, Chen S, Saito T, et al. PC-SPES decreases proliferation and induces differentiation and apoptosis of human acute myeloid leukemia cells. Int J Oncol 2003;23(4):1203-1211.

Ikezoe T, Chen SS, Heber D, et al. Baicalin is a major component of PC-SPES which inhibits the proliferation of human cancer cells via apoptosis and cell cycle arrest. Prostate 2001;49:285-292.

Ikezoe T, Chen SS, Yang Y, et al. PC-SPES: Molecular mechanism to induce apoptosis and down-regulate expression of PSA in LNCaP human prostate cancer cells. Int J Oncol 2003;23(5):1461-1470.

Ikezoe T, Yang Y, Heber D, et al. PC-SPES: a potent inhibitor of nuclear factor-kappaB rescues mice from lipopolysaccharide-induced septic shock. Mol Pharmacol 2003;64(6):1521-1529.

Kao GD, Devine P. Use of complementary health practices by prostate carcinoma patients undergoing radiation therapy. Cancer 2000;88:615-619.

Kao YC, Zhou C, Sherman M, et al. Molecular basis of the inhibition of human aromatase (estrogen synthetase) by flavone and isoflavone phytoestrogens: a site-directed mutagenesis study. Environ Health Perspect 1998;106:85-92.

Kitahara S, Umeda H, Yano H. Effects of intravenous administration of high dose diethylstilbestrol diphosphate on serum hormonal levels in patients with hormone-refractory prostate cancer. Endocr J 1999;46:659-64.

Ko R, Wilson RD, Loscutoff S. PC-SPES. Urology 2003;61(6):1292.

Kubota T, Hisatake J, Hisatake Y, et al. PC-SPES: a unique inhibitor of proliferation of prostate cancer cells *in vitro* and *in vivo*. Prostate 2000;42:163-171.

Lippert MC, McClain R, Boyd JC, et al. Alternative medicine use in patients with localized prostate carcinoma treated with curative intent. Cancer 1999;86:2642-2648.

Lock M, Loblaw DA, Choo R, et al. Disseminated intravascular coagulation and PC-SPES: a case report and literature review. Can J Urol 2001;8:1326-1329.

Lu X, Guo J, Hsieh TC. PC-SPES inhibits cell proliferation by modulating p21, cyclins D, E and B and multiple cell cycle-related genes in prostate cancer cells. Cell Cycle 2003;2(1):59-63.

Malkowicz SB. The role of diethylstilbestrol in the treatment of prostate cancer. Urology 2001;58:108-113.

National Center for Complementary and Alternative Medicine (NCCAM). Recall of PC SPES and SPES Dietary Supplements. http://nccam.nih.gov/health/alerts/spes/.

Oh WK, George DJ, Hackmann K, et al. Activity of the herbal combination, PC-SPES, in the treatment of patients with androgen-independent prostate cancer. Urology 2001;57(1):122-126.

Oh WK, George DJ, Kantoff PW. Rapid rise of serum prostate specific antigen levels after discontinuation of the herbal therapy PC-SPES in patients with advanced prostate carcinoma: report of four cases. Cancer 2002;94(3):686-689.

Pfeifer BL, Pirani JF, Hamann SR, et al. PC-SPES, a dietary supplement for the treatment of hormone-refractory prostate cancer. BJU Int 2000;85:481-485.

Pirani JF. The effects of phytotherapeutic agents on prostate cancer: an overview of recent clinical trials of PC SPES. Urology 2001;58:36-38.

Reynolds T. Contamination of PC-SPES remains a mystery. J Natl Cancer Inst 2002;94(17):1266-1268.

Robertson CN, Roberson KM, Padilla GM, et al. Induction of apoptosis by diethylstilbestrol in hormone-insensitive prostate cancer cells. J Natl Cancer Inst 1996;88:908-917.

Rosenbaum E, Wygoda M, Gips M, et al. Diethylstilbestrol is an active agent in prostatic cancer patients after failure to complete androgen blockade (abstract 1372). Proc ASCO 2000:19.

Schwarz RE, Donohue CA, Sadava D, et al. Pancreatic cancer in vitro toxicity mediated by Chinese herbs SPES and PC-SPES: implications for monotherapy and combination treatment. Cancer Lett 2003;189(1):59-68.

Small EJ, Frohlich MW, Bok R, et al. Prospective trial of the herbal supplement PC-SPES in patients with progressive prostate cancer. J Clin Oncol 2000;18(21):3595-3603.

Small EJ, Kantoff P, Weinberg VK, et al. A prospective multicenter randomized trial of the herbal supplement, PC-SPES vs. diethylstilbestrol (DES) in patients with advanced, androgen independent prostate cancer (AiPCa). Proc ASCO 2002;21:178a.

Sovak M, Seligson AL, Konas M, et al. Herbal composition PC-SPES for management of prostate cancer: identification of active principles. J Natl Cancer Inst 2002;94:1275-1281.

Stepanov VN, Siniakova LA, Sarrazin B, et al. Efficacy and tolerability of the lipidosterolic extract of *Serenoa repens* (Permixon) in benign prostatic hyperplasia: a double-blind comparison of two dosage regimens. Adv Ther 1999;16(5):231-241.

Tiwari RK, Geliebter J, Garikapaty VP, et al. Anti-tumor effects of PC-SPES, an herbal formulation in prostate cancer. Int J Oncol 1999;14:713-719.

Wadsworth T, Poonyagariyagorn H, Sullivan E, et al. In vivo effect of PC-SPES on prostate growth and hepatic CYP3A expression in rats. J Pharmacol Exp Ther 2003;306(1):187-194.

Wang L. Study finds additional evidence for contamination of herbal supplement for prostate cancer. J Natl Cancer Inst 2002;94(17):1259.

Weinrobe MC, Montgomery B. Acquired bleeding diathesis in a patient taking PC-SPES. N Engl J Med 2001;345:1213-1214.

White, J. (2002). PC-SPES—A lesson for future dietary supplement research. J Natl Cancer Inst 2002;94(17):1261-1262.

Wu J, Chen D, Zhang R. Study on the bioavailability of baicalin-phospholipid complex by using HPLC. Biomed Chromatogr 1999;13:493-495.

Yip I, Cudiamat M, Chim D. PC-SPES for treatment of prostate cancer: herbal medicine. Curr Urol Rep 2003;4(3):253-257.

P

Pennyroyal

American Pennyroyal (*Hedeoma pulegioides* L.), European Pennyroyal (*Mentha pulegium* L.)

SYNONYMS/COMMON NAMES/RELATED SUBSTANCES

- Aloe herbal horse spray, brotherwort, chasse-puces, churchwort, *Cunila pulegioides*, dictamne de Virginie, fleabane, flea mint, fretillet, *Hedeoma phlebitides,* herbal horsespray, herbe aux puces, herbe de Saint-Laurent, Labiatae, la menthe pouliot, Lamiaceae, lurk-in-the-ditch, *Melissa pulegioides*, mentha pouillot, Miracle Coat spray-on dog shampoo, mock pennyroyal, mosquito plant, Old World pennyroyal, pennyroyal essential oil, petit baume, piliolerial, poley, pouliot royal, pudding herb, pudding grass, pulegium, pulegium oil, pulegium vulgare, pulioll-royall, pulegium regium, run-by-the-ground, squaw balm, squawmint, stinking balm, tickweed.

CLINICAL BOTTOM LINE
Background

- The essential oil of pennyroyal is considered toxic. Death has been reported after consumption of half an ounce (15 mL) of the oil. A characteristic noted in most cases of pennyroyal overdose is a strong minty smell on the patient's breath. The active metabolite menthofuran can be detected by gas chromatography in urine, blood, and other tissues. Overdose management includes oral decontamination by lavage, and/or administration of activated charcoal.
- The similarity of the pathogenesis of pennyroyal-induced hepatic necrosis to that produced by acetaminophen suggests a possible role for *N*-acetylcysteine (NAC) in the management of pennyroyal overdose. However, this application has not been confirmed by animal or human studies.
- Anecdotal evidence and one case report suggest that the essential oil of pennyroyal may function as an abortifacient and emmenagogue (menstrual flow stimulant). However, it may do so at lethal or near-lethal doses, making this action unpredictable and dangerous. Future research to determine the safety and efficacy of the less toxic aerial parts of the pennyroyal plant on the menstrual cycle are needed before a recommendation can be made.

Scientific Evidence for Common Studied Uses	Grade*
Abortifacient (uterine contraction stimulant)	C
Emmenagogue (menstrual flow stimulant)	C

*Key to grades: A: Strong scientific evidence for this use; B: Good scientific evidence for this use; C: Unclear scientific evidence for this use; D: Fair scientific evidence against this use (it may not work); F: Strong scientific evidence against this use (it likely does not work). For a more detailed explanation of efficacy criteria, see "Natural Standard Evidence-Based Validated Grading Rationale" in the Introduction.

Historical or Theoretical Uses
That Lack Sufficient Evidence

- Acne, antiseptic, antispasmodic, anxiolytic, bowel disorders, carminative, chest congestion, colds, colic, cough, cramps, diaphoretic, digestion, diuretic, dizziness, dysentery, fever, flatulence, flavoring agent, flea control, flu, fornication, fragrance (detergents, perfumes, soaps), gallbladder disorders, gout, hallucinations, headache, hysterical affections, immortality, indigestion, insect repellent, intestinal disorders, itchy eyes, joint problems, kidney disease, leprosy, liver disease, marks from bruises and burns, menstrual irregularities (stimulant, regulator), mouth sores, nosebleeds, pneumonia, potpourri, pregnancy, premenstrual syndrome, prepare uterus for labor, purifier (water, blood), refrigerant, respiratory ailments, rubefacient, sedative, skin ailments (itching, burning), snake bites (venomous), stimulant, stomach pain, stomach spasms, sunstroke, syncope, toothache, uterine fibroids, whooping cough.

Expert Opinion and Folkloric Precedent

- Traditionally, pennyroyal is considered to be an emmenagogue (menstrual stimulant) and an abortifacient. Although pennyroyal oil historically has been used to induce abortions, it typically does so at lethal or near-lethal doses, making this action unpredictable, dangerous, and not recommended. A tea made from pennyroyal leaves, alone or in combination with other herbs, has been used to stimulate or regulate menstruation, although safety and efficacy is unknown.
- The raw, crushed aerial plant material or tincture is sometimes mixed into an externally applied skin cream and used as an insect repellent (mosquitoes, ticks). Diluted pennyroyal oil has also been used externally for this purpose.
- Pennyroyal oil was granted GRAS (generally regarded as safe) status by Federal Emergency Management Agency (FEMA) in 1965 and was approved by the U.S. Food and Drug Administration (FDA) for food use in small amounts. In 1970, The Council of Europe included pennyroyal oil on the list of flavoring substances temporarily admitted for use, with a possible limitation on levels of specific constituents in the final product, such as pulegone.[1]

Safety Summary

- **Possibly safe:** When the aerial parts are combined with other herbs and consumed as a tea by healthy adults for short periods of time (<1 week),[2] or when the aerial parts of the plant are consumed for a short duration using small doses as a tea or topical diluted oil. The Council of Europe lists pennyroyal as a natural source of food flavoring. Pennyroyal oil was granted GRAS (generally regarded as safe) status by the Federal Emergency Management Agency (FEMA) in 1965 and has been approved by the U.S. Food and Drug Administration (FDA) for food use in small amounts.
- **Possibly unsafe:** When the aerial parts are consumed as a tea, alone or in combination with other herbs, for longer than 1 week.
- **Likely unsafe:** The repeated use of alcoholic extracts of pennyroyal over a period of 2 weeks is likely unsafe. The use of any form of pennyroyal is likely unsafe in pregnant and nursing women, children, and patients with kidney disease.[3] The essential oil of pennyroyal is considered to be highly toxic. Tea made from leaves of the plant may be toxic to children.

DOSING/TOXICOLOGY

General

- No safe dosage for pennyroyal has been clinically established. Dosing of tea made from the leaf is based on historical practice. The essential oil is a highly concentrated form of the herb and the effect of 2 tablespoons of pennyroyal oil is approximately equal to 75 gallons of strong tea. Preparation of products may vary from manufacturer to manufacturer, and from batch to batch of a specific product made by a single manufacturer.

Standardization

- American pennyroyal (*Hedeoma pulegioides*) may contain up to 2% volatile oil, and European pennyroyal (*Mentha pulegium*) may contain up to 1% volatile oil. Both oils are reported to contain 85-92% of the pennyroyal constituent pulegone.

Dosing: Adult (18 Years and Older)
Oral

- *Note:* No safe dose of pennyroyal has been clinically established.
- **Extract (1:2):** Doses of 20 to 40 mL per week of pennyroyal have been used but may be toxic.
- **Oil:** Doses of 0.5 to 3 drops of pennyroyal oil have been used but may be toxic.
- **Tincture:** Doses of 30 to 60 drops of pennyroyal twice daily or 1 to 2 mL three times a day, of unclear concentration, have been used but may be toxic.
- **Tea/infusion:** Based on traditional usage, 1 or 2 cups of tea per day made from 1 to 2 teaspoons of dried leaves per cup of boiling water, steeped for 10 to 15 minutes, have been used. Pennyroyal tincture in tea water at doses of 0.25 to 0.5 teaspoonfuls (1.25 to 2.5 mL) up to twice daily, for treating cough, congestion, and upset stomach, has been used but may be toxic.

Topical

- Crushed plant material has been rubbed on the body as an insect repellent. Use of pennyroyal tincture mixed with skin cream and rubbed on the body has also been reported. Systemic absorption and toxicity may occur, and has been reported in animals.[4]
- Pennyroyal has been used as an herbal flea collar for animals by hanging a bag of pennyroyal from a regular collar or using a pennyroyal garland.

Dosing: Pediatric (Younger Than 18 Years)

- Pennyroyal should not be given to children due to the risk of toxicity and death.

Toxicology

- In animals, pennyroyal has been associated with hepatic, lung, and cerebral toxicity following oral or topical application. Doses greater than 10 mL of pennyroyal may be associated with fatality.

Animal Studies

- Pennyroyal leaf may contain 1.0% to 2.0% essential oil consisting of 80.0% to 94.0% pulegone, a constituent that acts as a liver toxin when administered to rats in high doses. Rats given high doses of pulegone, up to 160 mg/kg body weight/day, developed encephalopathy in 28 days. Microscopic dose-related cystlike spaces were found in white matter of the cerebellum. Demyelination could not be demonstrated using staining procedures.[5]
- In rats, the oral LD_{50} of pennyroyal has been found to be 0.4 g/kg, whereas topical application on rabbits has an LD_{50} value of 4.2 g/kg.[1] The LD_{90} value for Swiss albino mice given intraperitoneal pulegone was found to be 480 mg/kg.[6] Moorthy et al. determined the LD_{50} value of pulegone in rats to be 245 mg/kg at 24 hours.[7] Pulegone was given to rats in various doses (0, 20, 80, and 160 mg) to observe toxicity. The 80-mg and 160-mg doses produced atonia, decreased terminal body weight, and elicited histopathologic changes in liver and cerebellum white matter.[8]
- Pennyroyal oil given to mice at doses of 400 mg/kg and higher caused acute hepatic and lung damage.[9] Cellular necrosis was localized to the centrilobular regions of liver, which was visualized by microscopy 24 hours after dosing, and to the bronchiolar epithelial cells of the lung. The centrilobular liver necrosis was observed to follow a dose-response pattern. Administration of 300 mg/kg of pulegone in mice resulted in severe liver necrosis and an increase in serum glutamic pyruvic transaminase two days after administration.[10] A study that administered 400 mg/kg of pulegone to rats once daily for 5 days resulted in decreases in the levels of liver microsomal cytochrome P450, with a loss in microsomal heme.[7] The authors observed hepatotoxic effects of pulegone to be both dose- and time-dependent. They also observed an increase in serum glutamic pyruvic transaminase and a decrease in glucose-6-phosphatase. Madyastha and Raj suggest that the toxicity associated with pulegone may be due to the formation of the toxic metabolite p-cresol *in vitro*, which has been shown to cause severe toxicity in both liver and lung tissue.[11]

Overdose and Management

- Signs and symptoms associated with pennyroyal oil toxicity may include nausea, vomiting, profuse sweating, chills, fever, headache, tinnitus, dizziness, hypotension, difficulty in swallowing, extreme thirst, diarrhea, rapid pulse, muscle spasms, restlessness, drowsiness, fatigue, tremor and excessive talkativeness, hallucinations, mania, convulsions, and coma.[3,12-18]
- Symptoms of pennyroyal overdose may mimic those of acetaminophen overdose, and the use of *N*-acetylcysteine treatment may prove beneficial. Doses of *N*-acetylcysteine that have been used include a loading dose of 140 mg/kg, followed by 70 mg/kg every 4 hours. There is a case report of a 22-month-old child ingesting an unknown amount of pennyroyal oil from a 30-mL bottle who arrived at the emergency room with altered heart rate and blood pressure and respiration rates.[19] The emergency room physician began gastric lavage within 30 minutes of ingestion, followed by administration of activated charcoal (1 g/kg of body weight) and sorbitol (2 mL/kg). Immediately after receiving this treatment the child was given oral *N*-acetylcysteine (190 mg/kg), followed by 70 mg/kg every 4 hours for a total of 17 doses. The child had three serum levels drawn for analyses that were positive for menthofuran, a metabolite of pennyroyal, with quantitative levels of 40 ng/mL. The child recovered and was discharged to home in good health.[19] In contrast, results from one animal study concluded that *N*-acetylcysteine did not afford a significant survival benefit in pennyroyal oil toxicity.[6]
- A 28-year-old woman ingested 1 ounce of an unknown pennyroyal oil concentration and 2 cups of an unknown

P

amount of black cohosh (*Cimicifuga racemosa*) tea to induce an abortion. She presented to the emergency room after vomiting, with nausea and diaphoresis.[20] The patient had normal vital signs and blood chemistries. She was administered an unspecified amount of activated charcoal and sorbitol. Within 10 hours of ingestion, the patient was admitted to the intensive care unit, where *N*-acetylcysteine therapy was begun. The patient subsequently recovered.

- A dog that was treated topically for fleas became listless within 1 hour of pennyroyal application. The animal experienced diarrhea, hemoptysis, and epistaxis within 30 hours of application, and upon arrival for emergency care developed seizures and died. The topical dose estimated to have caused death was 2000 mg of pennyroyal oil/kg (1600 mg of pulegone/kg).[4]

Human Case Reports

- A woman died after consuming an alcohol extract of pennyroyal herb over a 2-week period in an attempt to induce abortion.[3,21] Postmortem evaluation revealed that she had an ectopic pregnancy, and the most notable pathologic abnormalities were found in the liver. The patient demonstrated hepatic cell necrosis, elevated liver enzymes, and degenerative changes involving the proximal tubules of the kidney.
- An 8-week-old infant died from multiple organ failure 14 hours after consuming approximately 120 mL of a mint tea brewed from a homegrown mint plant.[13] Botanical analysis revealed that the mint plant contained pennyroyal oil. The autopsy results showed hepatocellular necrosis, edematous hemorrhagic kidneys with focal acute tubular necrosis, left adrenal hemorrhage, bilateral lung consolidation with diffuse alveolar damage and hemorrhage, and diffuse cerebral edema with acute ischemic necrosis. The same publication documented a case of poisoning in a 6-month-old boy who ingested approximately 90 mL of tea brewed from a homegrown mint plant containing pennyroyal, taken three times a week for 3 months, administered to soothe and reduce colic.[13] A serum sample contained 25 ng/mL of pulegone and 41 ng/mL of menthofuran. The child developed elevated liver enzymes, had generalized tonic-clonic seizures, and was cyanotic at the time of hospitalization. On the fourth day of hospitalization, the child developed increased intracranial pressure with episodes of bradycardia and hypertension. The child recovered and was discharged 2 months later.
- There is a case report of cardiopulmonary arrest and death in an 18-year-old woman following ingestion of 1 ounce of pennyroyal oil.[22] Postmortem findings included petechiae in multiple organs, bilateral pulmonary congestion, and massive centrilobular hepatic necrosis.
- There is a 1904 case report of acute poisoning in a pregnant woman after taking one-half ounce of pennyroyal oil, resulting in fetal death.[23] The woman experienced facial swelling, purpura, contracted pupils, and flaccid extremities. She was resuscitated following gastric lavage. Further details are limited.

ADVERSE EFFECTS/PRECAUTIONS/CONTRAINDICATIONS
Allergy

- Known allergy/hypersensitivity to pennyroyal or to its constituents, including pulegone.

Adverse Effects

- **General:** Pennyroyal herb and volatile oils have been associated with multiple reports of toxicity and adverse effects (when used orally or topically), including severe abdominal pain, diarrhea, vomiting, convulsions, loss of consciousness, and death.[3,12,13,22] The volatile oils in pennyroyal may irritate the genitourinary tract, exert vascular effects, and stimulate abortion. Typically, the first symptoms of poisoning, from either pennyroyal oil or pennyroyal leaves, occur in the gastrointestinal tract and are often apparent soon after ingestion.
- **Dermatologic:** Contact dermatitis and urticarial rash have been reported when pennyroyal essential oil is used undiluted on the skin. An 18-year-old female patient was seen in the emergency room 2 hours after ingestion of 1 ounce of pennyroyal; she presented with normal vital signs, generalized urticarial rash, and diffuse pain on palpation.[18,22] One case of bluish mottles appearing on the face from internal use has been reported.[23]
- **Neurologic/CNS:** Ingestion of pennyroyal oil has led to loss of consciousness, coma, confusion, dizziness, malaise, rigors, fever, lethargy, agitation, paresthesia, convulsions/seizures, shock, and death.[3,12,13,15,18] There have been reports that pennyroyal can cause vertigo and delirium after oral ingestion.[3] There is a case report in which a 24-year-old woman ingested pennyroyal extract and black cohosh (*Cimicifuga racemosa*) root over 2 weeks, followed by a large acute ingestion, and experienced anoxic encephalopathy and hemorrhagic shock.[3,21] A 20-year-old female who ingested 1 teaspoon of pennyroyal oil and one-half teaspoon of ergot fluid extract experienced respiratory depression, mydriasis, generalized seizures, and coma.[3,24] The autopsy results of an 8-week-old boy who had ingested pennyroyal showed hepatocellular necrosis, edematous hemorrhagic kidneys with focal acute tubular necrosis, left adrenal hemorrhage, and bilateral lung consolidation with diffuse alveolar damage and hemorrhage, diffuse cerebral edema with acute ischemic necrosis, and isolated vacuolation of the midbrain.[13] A case report of a 6-month-old boy who was receiving approximately 90 mL of tea containing pennyroyal three times a week since he was 3 months old presented with severe epileptic encephalopathy and spastic rigidity.[13] A 23-year-old female ingested 3 tablets of an unknown amount of pennyroyal three to four times daily for approximately 4 days before being admitted to a hospital with convulsions.[15] The patient underwent electroencephalography 7 days after ingestion that showed epileptic characteristics, which resolved 4 weeks later.
- **Ocular/optic:** Anderson et al. report that pennyroyal may cause miotic or mydriatic pupils.[3] A case of pennyroyal ingestion was associated with dilated pupils and auditory and visual hallucinations.[16]
- **Psychiatric:** There is one case report of auditory and visual hallucinations associated with pennyroyal ingestion.[16] A 23-year-old woman was reported to experience a psychotic episode after ingesting an unknown dose of pennyroyal and "Widow Welch's Female Pills," a mixture of ferrous sulfate, sulphur, licorice, and turmeric.[15]
- **Cardiovascular:** Pennyroyal ingestion has been associated with hypertension, bradycardia, and cardiac arrest. A 24-year-old woman who ingested an unknown dose of pennyroyal and black cohosh (*Cimicifuga racemosa*) root over a 2-week period followed by a large acute ingestion experienced cardiopulmonary arrest.[3,21] An 1887 case report of a 40-year-old woman who ingested 30 mL of essence of pennyroyal (1 ounce of pennyroyal oil to 7 ounces of alcohol) experienced retching, coma, diaphoresis, irregular cardiac rhythm,

and "weakened pulse."[3,17] In an 1893 case report, bradycardia, hypotension, and a "weak pulse" were observed.[16]

- **Hematologic:** There are anecdotal reports that pennyroyal may lead to hemolytic anemia or disseminated intravascular coagulation. An 18-year-old female who ingested two one-half ounce bottles of pennyroyal experienced epistaxis, vaginal bleeding, excessive bleeding at venipuncture sites, and scleral hemorrhages.[22]
- **Pulmonary:** An autopsy from an overdose in one case report showed bilateral pulmonary edema and extensive consolidation.[22]
- **Gastrointestinal (general):** Early symptoms of poisoning from pennyroyal oil or leaves involve the gastrointestinal tract. Nausea, vomiting, and abdominal pain have been reported in most cases. Abdominal cramping or burning of the throat is also common in overdose.[12,22] An 18-year-old female who ingested 30 mL of pennyroyal oil experienced hematemesis, abdominal pain, and nausea.[3] A 23-year-old female who ingested 15 mL of pennyroyal oil began vomiting immediately and died 8 days after ingestion. Postmortem findings showed stomach and ileum abnormalities.[3] Numerous case studies have reported that patients present with halitosis and/or a strong peppermint-like odor.[14,25]
- **Gastrointestinal (hepatic):** Pennyroyal may lead to hepatic failure and centrilobular necrosis. An autopsy from an overdose found massive hepatic necrosis.[22] Chemical hepatitis has been reported and is often detectable within 24 hours of ingestion.[22] Pulegone, a constituent of pennyroyal, has caused increased transaminases in humans [13] and increased plasma alkaline phosphatase and liver weight in rats after 28 days (160 mg/kg).[26]
- **Renal:** Pennyroyal oil is excreted via the kidneys, and renal damage has been reported as a secondary complication in two cases of pennyroyal oil overdose.[22] Pennyroyal ingestion has been associated with metabolic acidosis.[13] There is one case report of death in a 12-week-old boy after being administered acetaminophen, a brompheniramine/ phenylpropanolamine cold remedy, and four ounces of pennyroyal tea.[27] The child died from liver failure, metabolic acidosis, and renal dysfunction. The autopsy results of an 8-week-old infant who ingested pennyroyal showed hepatocellular necrosis, edematous hemorrhagic kidneys with acute tubular necrosis, left adrenal hemorrhage, bilateral lung consolidation with diffuse alveolar damage and hemorrhage, and diffuse cerebral edema with acute ischemic necrosis.[13] A 24-year-old female who ingested 2 unknown doses of pennyroyal within 12 hours presented with oliguria; postmortem findings showed proximal tubule degeneration.[3] Pennyroyal has been associated with hematuria.
- **Endocrine:** Two pediatric patients admitted to a hospital with pennyroyal toxicity presented with hypoglycemia.[13]
- **Genitourinary:** There are anecdotal reports that pennyroyal possesses abortifacient effects, and there is a case report of pennyroyal oil association with an aborted fetus 4 days following ingestion.[23] There are anecdotal reports that large amounts of pennyroyal may be irritating to the urinary tract. Pennyroyal has been used historically as an emmenagogue (menstrual stimulant) and may elicit menstrual bleeding.

Precautions/Warnings/Contraindications

- Use cautiously in all forms, orally and topically, in all patients, because of the risk of toxicity and death.
- Avoid in children because of the risk of toxicity and death.
- Avoid in pregnant women because of the risk of abortion.

- Avoid in nursing women, based on theoretical potential for pennyroyal constituents to be transferred to infants through breast milk.
- Avoid in patients with kidney disease, as pennyroyal oil is excreted via the kidneys and has been associated with renal damage.
- If an essential oil is to be used topically, it should first be diluted in a carrier oil such as almond oil, olive oil, or safflower oil. The dilution ratio may depend upon the type of essential oil, the patient, and the desired therapeutic outcome. A 2% dilution is sometimes used when formulating whole body oil or lotions, and a 1% dilution is sometimes used for children and older patients. However, safety and efficacy are unproven, and topical preparations have been associated with systemic toxicity.

Pregnancy and Lactation

- The volatile oil of pennyroyal is traditionally considered to be an abortifacient,[28] and pennyroyal is not recommended in pregnant women because of the risk of uterine contractions, stimulation of menstruation, and abortion. There is a case report of pennyroyal oil association with an aborted fetus 4 days following ingestion,[23] although pennyroyal leaf combined with other herbs in a tea had no effect on pregnancy outcome in a different case report.[2]
- Pennyroyal is not recommended for nursing women, based on a theoretical risk of transfer of harmful constituents through breast milk.

INTERACTIONS
Pennyroyal/Drug Interactions

- **Acetaminophen (Tylenol):** The toxicity of pennyroyal theoretically may be increased when combined with acetaminophen. Acetaminophen may induce hepatotoxicity when glutathione stores are depleted, and data suggest that pennyroyal may also deplete hepatic glutathione stores.[29,30] The similarity of the pathogenesis of pennyroyal-induced hepatic necrosis to that produced by acetaminophen, supported by case reports, suggests a possible role for N-acetylcysteine (NAC) in treatment of pennyroyal or mixed pennyroyal-acetaminophen toxicity. However, one animal study found that NAC did not afford a significant survival benefit in pennyroyal oil toxicity.[6]
- **Antihistamines:** Pulegone, a constituent of pennyroyal, has been shown to exert antihistamine effects on guinea-pig ileum.[31]
- **Cytochrome P450 (CYP)–metabolized drugs:** Based on the suggested inhibition of the CYP system by pennyroyal, concomitant use with drugs metabolized by the CYP system may increase serum levels of those drugs. Similarly, pennyroyal levels may be affected by agents altering the CYP system. In vivo and in vitro studies suggest that the pennyroyal constituent pulegone diminishes the function of rat liver CYP in an irreversible, time-dependent fashion.[32] In vitro and in vivo research suggests that the pulegone metabolite menthofuran is a potent inhibitor of human liver CYP2A6[33] and may account for a significant degree of pennyroyal's hepatotoxic effects.[34,35] Pulegone and menthofuran may deplete cellular glutathione levels, leaving hepatocytes vulnerable to free radical damage.[36]
- **Oral hypoglycemic drugs, insulin:** Theoretically, pennyroyal may enhance the effects of hypoglycemic agents. There are two case reports of hypoglycemia in pediatric patients after ingesting pennyroyal.[13]

P

- **Hepatotoxic drugs:** Ingestion of pennyroyal may lead to hepatic failure and centrilobular necrosis, and may potentiate the effects of other hepatotoxic agents. An autopsy from an overdose found massive hepatic necrosis.[22] Chemical hepatitis has been reported and is often detectable within 24 hours of ingestion of pennyroyal.[22] Pulegone, a constituent of pennyroyal, has caused increased transaminases in humans [13] and increased plasma alkaline phosphatase and liver weight in rats after 28 days (160 mg/kg).[26]

Pennyroyal/Herb/Supplement Interactions

- **Black cohosh:** Pennyroyal and black cohosh (*Cimicifuga racemosa*) are sometimes taken together to induce abortion, although the use of these herbs together cannot be recommended because of the possibility of increased toxicity and death. There is a case report of a 24-year-old woman who took 48% to 56% pennyroyal herb in an alcohol base and an unknown amount of black cohosh root for 2 weeks in an attempt to induce abortion.[3] Following a single subsequent dose of this combination, the patient died within 48 hours.
- **Blue cohosh:** Pennyroyal and blue cohosh (*Caulophyllum thalictroides*) have traditionally been taken together to normalize the menstrual cycle in women and may act synergistically to increase menstrual flow. This use has not been scientifically investigated. Notably, blue cohosh may act as a vasoconstrictor and has been associated with multiple adverse outcomes.
- **Iron supplements:** Pennyroyal has been found to inhibit the absorption of iron in meals by up to 75%.[37]
- **Licorice:** In a 1961 case report, a 23-year-old woman, 6 weeks pregnant, was noted to experience a severe psychotic episode and seizures after ingesting an unknown dose of pennyroyal three to four times daily and "Widow Welch's Female Pills," a combination of ferrous sulfate, sulfur, licorice (*Glycyrrhiza glabra*), and turmeric (*Curcuma longa*).[15] The patient recovered 2 days following hospital admission, without recurrence, and delivered a healthy child.
- **Turmeric:** In a 1961 case report, a 23-year-old woman, 6 weeks pregnant, was noted to experience a severe psychotic episode and seizures after ingesting an unknown dose of pennyroyal three to four times daily and "Widow Welch's Female Pills," a combination of ferrous sulfate, sulfur, licorice (*Glycyrrhiza glabra*), and turmeric (*Curcuma longa*).[15] The patient recovered 2 days following hospital admission, without recurrence, and delivered a healthy child.
- **Cytochrome P450 (CYP)–metabolized agents:** Based on the suggested inhibition of the CYP system by pennyroyal, concomitant use with drugs metabolized by the CYP system may increase serum levels of those drugs. Similarly, pennyroyal levels may be affected by agents altering the CYP system. *In vivo* and *in vitro* studies suggest that the pennyroyal constituent pulegone diminishes the function of rat liver CYP in an irreversible, time-dependent fashion.[32] *In vitro* and *in vivo* research suggests that the pulegone metabolite menthofuran is a potent inhibitor of human liver CYP2A6[33] and may account for a significant degree of pennyroyal's hepatotoxic effects.[34,35] Pulegone and menthofuran may deplete cellular glutathione levels, leaving hepatocytes vulnerable to free radical damage.[36]
- **Hypoglycemic herbs and supplements:** Theoretically, pennyroyal may enhance the effects of hypoglycemic agents. The available scientific literature reports two cases of hypoglycemia in pediatric patients after ingesting pennyroyal.[13]

- **Hepatotoxic herbs and supplements:** The use of pennyroyal may lead to hepatic failure and centrilobular necrosis and may potentiate the effects of other hepatotoxic agents. An autopsy from an overdose found massive hepatic necrosis.[22] Chemical hepatitis has been reported and is often detectable within 24 hours of ingestion of pennyroyal.[22] Pulegone, a constituent of pennyroyal, has caused increased transaminases in humans [13] and increased plasma alkaline phosphatase and liver weight in rats after 28 days (160 mg/kg).[26]

Pennyroyal/Food Interactions

- Insufficient available evidence.

Pennyroyal/Lab Interactions

- **Liver function tests (LFTs):** Hepatic toxicity due to the pennyroyal constituent pulegone has been associated with elevations in transaminases in rats[26] and humans.[13,22]

MECHANISM OF ACTION
Pharmacology

- **Constituents:** Constituents of the aerial parts of pennyroyal which are highly concentrated in the essential oil include hedeomal, tannins, alpha-pinene, beta-pinene, limonene, 3-octanone, p-cymene, 3-octylacetate, 3-octanol, 1-octen-3-ol, 3-methylcyclohexanone, menthone, piperitenone, and paraffins.
- **Hepatic effects:** Pulegone, the constituent terpene of the volatile oil of pennyroyal, has been shown to be toxic to the urinary tract and kidneys.[32] Menthofuran is a mammalian metabolite of pulegone and may account for some of the hepatotoxic effects.[34,35] Pulegone and menthofuran may deplete cellular glutathione levels, leaving hepatocytes vulnerable to free radical damage.[36]

Pharmacodynamics/Kinetics

- The toxic properties of the pennyroyal constituent pulegone appear to follow first-order kinetics.[32] In rats given a 150-mg/kg intraperitoneal injection of pulegone, a terminal half-life of $2.08 + 0.29$ and a C_{max} of $7.02 + 1.15$ µg/mL was found.[38]
- Pennyroyal oil is reported to be excreted by the kidneys following oral ingestion.[39]
- *In vivo* and *in vitro* studies suggest that the pennyroyal constituent pulegone diminishes the function of rat liver cytochrome P450 (CYP) in an irreversible, time-dependent fashion.[32] *In vitro* and *in vivo* research suggests that the pulegone metabolite menthofuran is a potent inhibitor of human liver CYP2A6,[33] and may account for a significant degree of pennyroyal's hepatotoxic effects.[34,35] Pulegone and menthofuran may deplete cellular glutathione levels, leaving hepatocytes vulnerable to free radical damage.[36]

HISTORY

- Use of pennyroyal to induce abortions dates back to ancient Rome at the time of Pliny the Elder. In the Middle Ages, pennyroyal was dubbed *puliol royale*, or "royal thyme." Later, the French classified it as a mint, naming it *la menthe pouliot*. Its antiseptic properties were believed to be so strong, that it could purify water. The name *pulegium* derives from the Latin "flea," because of the herb's historic use to repel fleas either by topical application or by burning bunches of hanging plants. Today, both the oil and the herb are common ingredients in pet flea collars and powders used for keeping dogs and cats free of fleas. There are several plants of varying genus and species that may be dubbed "pennyroyal."

- Pennyroyal was highly prized by Europeans, and the pilgrims brought it to America. A popular stuffing, "pudding grass," was made from pennyroyal, pepper, and honey.
- The British Pharmaceutical Codex removed pennyroyal from its list in 1934, but it remains easily obtainable by the public.[40]

REVIEW OF THE EVIDENCE: TABLE

- No studies qualify for inclusion in the evidence table.

REVIEW OF THE EVIDENCE: DISCUSSION

Abortifacient (Uterine Contraction Stimulant)

Summary

- Pennyroyal oil has been used traditionally as an abortifacient, although efficacy is documented only in case reports. The use of pennyroyal is potentially dangerous, with published reports of morbidity and death.

Case Reports

- In a 1904 case report, acute pennyroyal oil toxicity (from one-half ounce of pennyroyal oil) was associated with the expulsion of a dead fetus 4 days following ingestion.[23] The face of the mother was swollen with purpura and contracted pupils, her extremities were flaccid, and respirations were diminished. The mother survived following gastric lavage and supportive measures.
- In a 1955 case report, a 24-year-old woman, 3 months pregnant, ingested two bottles of an unknown amount of pennyroyal with the intention of inducing an abortion. Several hours after ingestion, the patient aborted her fetus. The case was complicated by heavy bleeding, rash, nausea, vomiting, abdominal pain, and diarrhea.[40]
- In a 1961 case report, a 23-year-old woman, 6 weeks pregnant, was noted to experience a severe psychotic episode and seizures after ingesting an unknown dose of pennyroyal three to four times daily and "Widow Welch's Female Pills," a combination of ferrous sulfate, sulfur, licorice (*Glycyrrhiza glabra*), and turmeric (*Curcuma longa*).[15] The patient recovered 2 days following hospital admission, without recurrence, and delivered a healthy child.
- There is a 1985 case report of a pregnancy that remained unaffected by ingestion of pennyroyal tea. In a postpartum interview, a 24-year-old Amish woman noted that she drank herbal "PNC" tea during her pregnancy. PNC contains pennyroyal, red raspberry, lobelia, blue cohosh, black cohosh, and blessed thistle. Following a normal full-term pregnancy, she delivered a healthy child with mild hyperbilirubinemia that resolved without complication.[2] It is not clear what the concentration of pennyroyal was in this tea preparation.

Emmenagogue (Menstrual Flow Stimulant)

Summary

- Pennyroyal oil has been used traditionally as an emmenagogue. The available scientific literature does not support the efficacy of pennyroyal for this indication. Furthermore, this use is potentially dangerous, and there are case reports of morbidity and death. Future research of the effect of the aerial parts of the plant on the menstrual cycle, alone or in combination with other herbs, may provide useful information. In one review of plants with potential value as antifertility agents, the volatile oil of pennyroyal is listed as an emmenagogue, based on traditional information.[28]

Evidence

- There is a 1996 case report of a 24-year-old woman who drank 2 glasses of pennyroyal tea with the intention of inducing menses.[3] She noted that she prepared the tea by steeping 2 teaspoons of pennyroyal leaves in 1 pint of hot water for 5 to 10 minutes. Within 15 minutes of ingestion, she experienced mild abdominal pain. She again drank the tea 13 hours later, allowing the tea to steep for 20 minutes, and experienced nausea and severe abdominal cramping which lasted for 4 days, following which time menses began. She reported no residual symptoms. Causality is not clear.
- A 1983 case report describes a 20-year-old woman who took pennyroyal leaves and oil to induce menses.[12] She intermittently drank a tea (one teaspoon of leaves per cup of water) approximately three times per day, for 1 week. She then ingested 1 dose of the leaves packed in a gelatin capsule. She experienced some menstrual spotting later that day. She then took 2 more capsules, and 2 days later ingested 15 mL of pennyroyal oil. Within two hours of taking the pennyroyal oil, she experienced a feeling of euphoria, vomited, and lost consciousness. She was admitted to an intensive care unit, received supportive treatment, and recovered fully.

References

1. Opdyke DL. Pennyroyal oil eurafrican. Food Cosmet Toxicol 1974;12:949-950.
2. Black DR. Pregnancy unaffected by pennyroyal usage. J Am Osteopath Assoc 1985;85(5):282.
3. Anderson IB, Mullen WH, Meeker JE, et al. Pennyroyal toxicity: measurement of toxic metabolite levels in two cases and review of the literature. Ann Intern Med 1996;124(8):726-734.
4. Sudekum M, Poppenga RH, Raju N, et al. Pennyroyal oil toxicosis in a dog. J Am Vet Med Assoc 1992;200(6):817-818.
5. Olsen P, Thorup I. Neurotoxicity in rats dosed with peppermint oil and pulegone. Arch Toxicol 1984;Suppl 7:408-409.
6. Giorgi DF, Lobel D, Morasco R, et al. N-acetylcysteine for pennyroyal oil toxicity. Vet Human Toxicol 1994;36(4):358.
7. Moorthy B, Madyastha P, Madyastha KM. Hepatotoxicity of pulegone in rats: its effects on microsomal enzymes, in vivo. Toxicology 1989;55(3):327-337.
8. Thorup I, Wurtzen G, Carstensen J, et al. Short term toxicity study in rats dosed with pulegone and menthol. Toxicol Lett 1983;19(3):207-210.
9. Gordon WP, Forte AJ, McMurtry RJ, et al. Hepatotoxicity and pulmonary toxicity of pennyroyal oil and its constituent terpenes in the mouse. Toxicol Appl Pharmacol 1982;65(3):413-424.
10. Mizutani T, Nomura H, Nakanishi K, et al. Effects of drug metabolism modifiers on pulegone-induced hepatotoxicity in mice. Res Commun Chem Pathol Pharmacol 1987;58(1):75-83.
11. Madyastha KM, Raj CP. Biotransformations of R-(+)-pulegone and menthofuran in vitro: chemical basis for toxicity. Biochem Biophys Res Commun 1990;173(3):1086-1092.
12. Buechel DW, Haverlah VC, Gardner ME. Pennyroyal oil ingestion: report of a case. J Am Osteopath Assoc 1983;82(10):793-794.
13. Bakerink JA, Gospe SM, Jr., Dimand RJ, et al. Multiple organ failure after ingestion of pennyroyal oil from herbal tea in two infants. Pediatrics 1996;98(5):944-947.
14. Braithwaite PF. A case of poisoning by pennyroyal: recovery. Br Med J 1906;2:865.
15. Early DF. Pennyroyal: a rare cause of epilepsy. Lancet 1961;580-581.
16. Flynn EF. Poisoning by essence of pennyroyal. Br Med J 1893;2:1270.
17. Girling J. Poisoning by pennyroyal. Br Med J 1887;1:1214.
18. Anonymous. Fatality and illness associated with consumption of pennyroyal oil — Colorado. Morbid Mortal Week Rep 1978;27(51):511-513.
19. Mullen W, Anderson I, Oishii S, et al. Accidental pennyroyal oil ingestion in a toddler with the first human serum metabolite detection. Vet Human Toxicol 1994;36(4):342.
20. McCormick M, Manoguerra A. Toxicity of pennyroyal oil: a case report and review abstract]. Vet Human Toxicol 1988;30(4):347.
21. Anderson IB, Nelson SD, Blanc PD. Pennyroyal metabolites in human poisoning. Ann Intern Med 1997;126(3):250-251.

P

22. Sullivan JB, Jr., Rumack BH, Thomas H, Jr., et al. Pennyroyal oil poisoning and hepatotoxicity. JAMA 1979;242(26):2873-2874.

23. Runnalls HB. Report of a case of acute poisoning by oil of pennyroyal. Med Sentinel 1904;12:325.

24. Wingate UO. A case of poisoning by the oil of hedeoma (pennyroyal). Boston Med Surg J 1889;120:536.

25. Jones C. A case of poisoning by pennyroyal. Brit Med J 1913;746.

26. Molck AM, Poulsen M, Tindgard LS, et al. Lack of histological cerebellar changes in Wistar rats given pulegone for 28 days. Comparison of immersion and perfusion tissue fixation. Toxicol Lett 1998;95(2):117-122.

27. Mack RB. "Boldly they rode . . . into the mouth of hell". Pennyroyal oil toxicity. N C Med J 1997;58(6):456-457.

28. Farnsworth NR, Bingel AS, Cordell GA, et al. Potential value of plants as sources of new antifertility agents I. J Pharm Sci 1975;64(4):535-598.

29. Rumack BH. Acetaminophen overdose in young children. Treatment and effects of alcohol and other additional ingestants in 417 cases. Am J Dis Child 1984;138(5):428-433.

30. Lich-Lai MW, Sarnaik AP, Newton JF, et al. Metabolism and pharmacokinetics of acetaminophen in a severely poisoned young child. J Pediatr 1984;105(1):125-128.

31. Ortiz de Urbina AV, Martin ML, Montero MJ, et al. Antihistaminic activity of pulegone on the guinea-pig ileum. J Pharm Pharmacol 1990;42(4): 295-296.

32. Madyastha P, Moorthy B, Vaidyanathan CS, et al. *In vivo* and *in vitro* destruction of rat liver cytochrome P-450 by a monoterpene ketone, pulegone. Biochem Biophysl Res Comm 1985;128(2):921-927.

33. Khojasteh-Bakht SC, Koenigs LL, Peter RM, et al. (R)-(+)-Menthofuran is a potent, mechanism-based inactivator of human liver cytochrome P450 2A6. Drug Metab Dispos 1998;26(7):701-704.

34. Gordon WP, Huitric AC, Seth CL, et al. The metabolism of the abortifacient terpene, (R)-(+)-pulegone, to a proximate toxin, menthofuran. Drug Metab Dispos 1987;15(5):589-594.

35. Thomassen D, Pearson PG, Slattery JT, et al. Partial characterization of biliary metabolites of pulegone by tandem mass spectrometry. Detection of glucuronide, glutathione, and glutathionyl glucuronide conjugates. Drug Metab Dispos 1991;19(5):997-1003.

36. Thomassen D, Slattery JT, Nelson SD. Menthofuran-dependent and independent aspects of pulegone hepatotoxicity: roles of glutathione. J Pharmacol Exp Ther 1990;253(2):567-572.

37. Hurrell RF, Reddy M, Cook JD. Inhibition of non-haem iron absorption in man by polyphenolic-containing beverages. Br J Nutr 1999;81(4):289-295.

38. Thomassen D, Slattery JT, Nelson SD. Contribution of menthofuran to the hepatotoxicity of pulegone: assessment based on matched area under the curve and on matched time course. J Pharmacol Exp Ther 1988;244(3): 825-829.

39. Briggs CJ. Pennyroyal: A traditional medicinal herb with toxic potential. Canad Pharm J 1989;122:369-372.

40. Vallance M. Pennyroyal poisoning. A fatal case. Lancet 1955;850-853.

Peppermint
(*Mentha x piperita* L.)

SYNONYMS/COMMON NAMES/RELATED SUBSTANCES

- Balm mint, black peppermint, brandy mint, curled mint, feullis de menthe, Japanese peppermint, katzenkraut (German), lamb mint, *Mentha arvensis* L. var *piperascens*, menta prima (Italian), Menthae piperitae aetheroleum (peppermint oil), *Mentha piperita* var *officinalis*, Menthae piperitae folium (peppermint leaf), menthe anglaise, menthe poivre, menthe poivree, *Mentha piperita* var *vulgaris*, Our Lady's mint, pebermynte (Danish), pfefferminz (German), porminzen, schmecker, spearmint (*Mentha spicata* L.), water mint (*Mentha aquatica*), white peppermint, WS 1340.
- **Essential oil constituents:** Cineol, isomenthone, liminene, menthofuran, menthol, menthone, menthyl acetate, terpenoids.
- **Leaf constituents:** Caffeic acid, chlorogenic acid, luteolin, hesperidin, rutin, "volatile" oil.
- **Selected brand names:** Ben-Gay, Colpermin, China Maze, Cholaktol, Citaethol, Enteroplant (contains peppermint and caraway oil), Kiminto, Mentacur, Mentholatum, Mintec, Rhuli Gel, Robitussin cough drops, SX Mentha, Vicks VapoRub.
- **Combination products:** Absorbine Jr., Iberogast, Listerine.
- *Note: Mentha* x *villosa* L. is a different species of mint with a similar appearance, used primarily as a flavoring agent.

CLINICAL BOTTOM LINE
Background

- Peppermint is a perennial flowering plant that grows throughout Europe and North America. Peppermint is widely cultivated for its fragrant oil, which is obtained through steam distillation of the fresh above-ground parts of the plant. Peppermint oil has been used historically for numerous health conditions, including common cold symptoms, cramps, headache, indigestion, joint pain, and nausea. Peppermint leaf has been used for stomach/intestinal disorders and for gallbladder disease.
- Mint plants such as peppermint and spearmint have a long history of medicinal use, dating back to ancient Egypt, Greece, and Rome. The scientific name for peppermint (*Mentha* x *piperita*) is derived from the name *Mintha*, a Greek mythological nymph who transformed herself into the plant, and from the Latin *piper*, meaning "pepper." Peppermint is believed to be a cross (hybrid) between spearmint and water mint that arose naturally.
- Peppermint oil is available in bulk herb oil, enteric-coated capsules, soft gelatin capsules, and liquid form. In small doses such as in tea or chewing gum, peppermint is generally believed to be safe in healthy, non-pregnant, non-allergic adults. The United States is a principal producer of peppermint, and the largest markets for peppermint oil are manufacturers of chewing gum, toothpaste, mouthwash, and pharmaceuticals.

Uses Based on Scientific Evidence	Grade*
Antispasmodic (gastric spasm) One study reports that peppermint oil solution administered intraluminally can be used as an antispasmodic agent with superior efficacy and fewer side effects than hyoscine-*N*-butylbromide administered by intramuscular injection during upper endoscopy.	
Indigestion (non-ulcer dyspepsia) Several human trials examined the effects of peppermint oil or a combination of peppermint/caraway oil on dyspepsia. Overall, these studies have not been well designed or reported, and it remains unclear if peppermint oil is beneficial for this condition.	C
Irritable bowel syndrome (IBS) There are several human trials of peppermint oil for the relief of IBS symptoms such as abdominal pain, bloating, diarrhea, and gas. Results have been mixed, with some studies reporting benefits, and others finding lack of effect. Overall, these trials have been small and not well designed or reported. Better scientific studies are necessary before a firm conclusion can be drawn.	C
Nasal congestion Menthol, a constituent of peppermint oil, is sometimes included in inhaled preparations for nasal congestion, including "rubs" that are applied to the skin and inhaled. Early research suggests that the nose breathing may be improved, although it is not clear if there are true benefits on breathing or nasal congestion. High-quality research is lacking in this area.	C
Nausea Due to limited human study, there is not enough evidence to recommend for or against the use of peppermint oil in the treatment of nausea. Further research is needed before a recommendation can be made.	C
Tension headache Application of diluted peppermint oil to the forehead and temples has been tested in people with headache. Studies have not been well conducted, and it is not clear if this is an effective treatment.	C
Urinary tract infection There is limited study of peppermint tea added to other therapies for urinary tract infections. It is not clear if this is an effective treatment, and it is not recommended to rely on peppermint tea alone to treat this condition.	C

*Key to grades: *A:* Strong scientific evidence for this use; *B:* Good scientific evidence for this use; *C:* Unclear scientific evidence for this use; *D:* Fair scientific evidence against this use (it may not work); *F:* Strong scientific evidence against this use (it likely does not work). For a more detailed explanation of efficacy criteria, see "Natural Standard Evidence-Based Validated Grading Rationale" in the Introduction.

P

611

Historical or Theoretical Indications That Lack Sufficient Evidence

Antacid, anorexia, antiviral, arthritis, asthma, bile duct disorders, bronchial spasm, cancer, chickenpox, cholelithiasis (gallstones), colonic spasm (during colonoscopy or barium enema), common cold, cough, cramps, dysmenorrhea (menstrual pain), enteritis, fever, fibromyositis, gallbladder disorders, gas (flatulence), gastrointestinal disorders, gastritis, gonorrhea, head lice (*Pediculus humanus capitis*), ileus (postoperative), inflammation of oral mucosa, influenza, intestinal colic, laryngeal spasm, local anesthetic, morning sickness, motility disorders, mouthwash, musculoskeletal pain, myalgia (muscle pain), neuralgia (nerve pain), postherpetic neuralgia, pruritus (itching), rheumatic pain, sun block, tendonitis, toothache, tuberculosis, urticaria (hives).

DOSING/TOXICOLOGY

The following below doses are based on scientific research, publications, traditional use, or expert opinion. Many herbs and supplements have not been thoroughly tested, and safety and effectiveness may not be proven. Brands may be made differently, with variable ingredients even within the same brand. The doses shown may not apply to all products. It is important to always read product labels and discuss doses with a qualified healthcare provider before therapy is started.

Adults (18 Years and Older)

- **Peppermint oil:** Peppermint oil should be used cautiously, as doses of the constituent menthol over 1 gram per kilogram of body weight may be deadly. For intestinal/digestion disorders, doses of 0.2 to 0.4 ml of peppermint oil in enteric-coated capsules, dilute preparations, or suspensions taken three times daily by mouth have been used or studied. Lozenges containing 2 to 10 mg of peppermint oil have been used. 10% peppermint oil (in methanol) has been applied to the skin (forehead and temples) multiple times per day for headache relief. Some sources recommend using peppermint oil preparations on the skin no more than 3 to 4 times per day, although reliable safety information is limited in this area. For inhalation, 3 to 4 drops of oil added to 150 ml of hot water and inhaled up to three times per day or 1% to 5% essential oil as a nasal ointment has been used to relieve congestion. Enteric coated peppermint oil capsules may be better tolerated than other dosage forms.
- **Peppermint leaf:** There is limited study of the safety/effectiveness of peppermint leaf preparations, and doses are based on traditional use or anecdote. As an infusion, 3 to 6 g of peppermint leaf has been used daily. Doses of other liquid preparations depend on concentration, for example, 2 to 3 ml of tincture (1:5 in 45% ethanol) three times daily, or 1 ml of spirits (10% oil and 1% leaf extract, mixed with water) has been taken. Various doses of dried herb extract have been noted traditionally, ranging from 0.8 g daily up to 4 g taken three times daily, although safety is not clear.

Children (Younger Than 18 Years)

- There is not enough scientific information available to recommend the safe use of peppermint leaf or oil in children.

SAFETY

The U.S. Food and Drug Administration does not strictly regulate herbs and supplements. There is no guarantee of strength, purity, or safety of products, and effects may vary. It is important to always read product labels. People who have a medical condition, or are taking other drugs, herbs, or supplements, should consult a qualified healthcare provider before starting a new therapy. A healthcare provider should be contacted immediately about any side effects.

Allergies

- Allergic/hypersensitivity reactions may occur from using peppermint or menthol by mouth or on the skin, including throat closing (laryngeal spasm), breathing problems (bronchial constriction/asthma symptoms), and skin rash/hives/contact dermatitis. People with known allergy/hypersensitivity to peppermint leaf or oil should avoid peppermint products.

Side Effects and Warnings

- Peppermint is generally regarded as being safe in non-allergic adults when taken in small doses, for example as tea.
- Peppermint oil may be safe in small doses, although multiple adverse effects are possible. When used on the skin, peppermint oil has been associated with allergic/hypersensitivity reactions, skin rash/hives/contact dermatitis, mouth ulcers/sores, and eye irritation. Peppermint oil taken by mouth may cause headache, dizziness, heartburn, anal burning, slow heart rate, or muscle tremor. Mouth sores may occur with peppermint oil-containing mouthwashes. There is report of asthma symptoms related to a mint-flavored toothpaste. Very large doses of peppermint oil taken by mouth in animals have resulted in muscle weakness, brain damage, and seizure. Peppermint oil should be used cautiously by people with G6PD deficiency (based on reports of jaundice in babies exposed to menthol) or gallbladder disease (gallstones, bile duct obstruction). Enteric-coated tablets have been recommended in those with hiatal hernia or heartburn/gastroesophageal reflux disease (GERD), over other dosage forms. Use in infants or children is discouraged because of potential toxicity, including when inhaled, taken by mouth, or used on the skin around the facial area.
- Menthol, a constituent of peppermint oil that is included in mouthwashes, toothpastes, mentholated cigarettes, and decongestant "rubs" or lozenges, has been associated with multiple adverse effects. Although small amounts may be safe in non-allergic adults, doses over 1 gram per kilogram of body weight may be deadly in humans, and toxic doses can be absorbed through the skin (and may be increased with local application of heat, such as with a heating pad). Serious breathing difficulties or triggering of asthma symptoms may occur with menthol use near the nose or on the chest. Mouth sores have been associated with use of mint-flavored toothpaste, mouthwash, or mentholated cigarettes. Mentholated cigarettes have been linked with skin bruising (purpura), although the exact cause has not been proven. Use on the skin of menthol or methyl salicylate (also a peppermint oil constituent) has rarely been associated with rash, severe skin damage (necrosis), or kidney damage (interstitial nephritis). Inhalation of large doses of menthol may lead to dizziness, confusion, muscle weakness, nausea, or double vision. High doses of menthol have caused brain damage in animal studies.

Pregnancy and Breastfeeding

- Peppermint oil and menthol should be avoided during pregnancy and breastfeeding because of insufficient information and potential for toxicity.

INTERACTIONS

Most herbs and supplements have not been thoroughly tested for interactions with other herbs, supplements, drugs, or foods. The interactions listed here are based on reports in scientific publications, laboratory experiments, or traditional use. It is important to always read product labels. People who have a medical condition, or are taking other drugs, herbs, or supplements, should consult a qualified healthcare provider before starting a new therapy.

Interactions with Drugs

- There is a preliminary report that taking peppermint oil by mouth may increase blood levels of the drugs felodipine (Plendil) and simvastatin (Zocor). In rats, peppermint oil increases levels of cyclosporine in the blood, although effects in humans are not clear. Based on rat research, peppermint oil used on the skin with 5-fluorouracil (5-FU) may increase the rate of absorption of 5-FU.

- Based on laboratory studies, peppermint oil may interfere with the way the body processes certain drugs using the liver's cytochrome P450 enzyme system. As a result, the levels of these drugs may be increased in the blood and may cause increased effects or potentially serious adverse reactions. People who are using any medications should always read the package insert and consult their healthcare provider or pharmacist about possible interactions.

Interactions with Herbs and Supplements

- Based on laboratory studies, peppermint oil may interfere with the way the body processes certain herbs or supplements using the liver's cytochrome P450 enzyme system. As a result, the levels of other herbs or supplements to be too high in the blood. It may also alter the effects that other herbs or supplements possibly have on the P450 system, such as bloodroot, cat's claw, chamomile, chaparral, chasteberry, damiana, *Echinacea angustifolia*, goldenseal, grapefruit juice, licorice, oregano, red clover, St. John's wort, wild cherry, and yucca. People who are using any medications should always read the package insert and consult their healthcare provider and pharmacist about possible interactions.

Selected References

Natural Standard developed the preceding evidence-based information based on a systematic review of more than 140 articles. For comprehensive information about alternative and complementary therapies on the professional level, go to www.naturalstandard.com. Selected references are listed here.

Abdullah D, Ping QN, Liu GJ. Enhancing effect of essential oils on the penetration of 5-fluorouracil through rat skin. Yao Xue Xue Bao (Acta Pharmaceutica Sinica) 1996;31(3):214-221.

Barnick CG, Cardozo LD. The treatment of abdominal distension and dyspepsia with enteric coated peppermint oil following routine gynaecological intraperitoneal surgery. J Obstet Gynecol 1990;10(5):423-424.

Bell GD, Richmond CR, Somerville KW. Peppermint oil capsules (Colpermin) for the irritable bowel syndrome: a pharmacokinetic study. Br J Clin Pharmacol 1983;16:228P-229P.

Camarasa G, Alomar A. Menthol dermatitis from cigarettes. Contact Derm 1978;4:169-170.

Carling L, Svedberg L, Hultsen S. Short term treatment of the irritable bowel syndrome: a placebo-controlled trial of peppermint oil against hyoscyamine. Opuscula Med 1989;34:55-57.

Chrisman BR. Menthol and dermatitis. Arch Dermatol 1976;114:286.

Davies SJ, Harding LM, Baranowski AP. A novel treatment of postherpetic neuralgia using peppermint oil. Clin J Pain 2002;18(3):200-202.

Dew MJ, Evans BK, Rhodes J. Peppermint oil for the irritable bowel syndrome: a multicentre trial. Br J Clin Pract 1984;38(11-12):394-398.

Dresser GK, Wacher V, Ramtoola Z, et al. Peppermint oil increases the oral bioavailability of felodipine and simvastatin. Amer Soc Clin Pharmacol Ther Ann Meeting, March 24-27, 2002;TPII-95.

Dresser GK, Wacher V, Wong S, et al. Evaluation of peppermint oil and ascorbyl palmitate as inhibitors of cytochrome P4503A4 activity in vitro and in vivo. Clin Pharmacol Ther 2002;72(3):247-255.

Ebbinghaus K D. A 'tea' containing various plant products as adjuvant to chemotherapy of urinary tract infections. Therapiewoche 1985;35:2041-2051.

Evans BK, Levine DF, Mayberry JF, et al. Multicentre trial of peppermint oil capsules in irritable bowel syndrome. Scand J Gastroenterol 1982;17:503.

Feng XZ. [Effect of peppermint oil hot compresses in preventing abdominal distension in postoperative gynecological patients.] Zhonghua Hu Li Za Zhi 1997;32(10):577-578.

Freise J, Kohler S. [Peppermint oil-caraway oil fixed combination in non-ulcer dyspepsia—comparison of the effects of enteric preparations.] Pharmazie 1999;54(3):210-215.

Gobel H, Fresenius J, Heinze A, et al. [Effectiveness of Oleum menthae piperitae and paracetamol in therapy of headache of the tension type.] Nervenarzt 1996; 67(8):672-681.

Gobel H, Schmidt G, Soyka D. Effect of peppermint and eucalyptus oil preparations on neurophysiological and experimental algesimetric headache parameters. Cephalalgia 1994;14(3):228-234.

Goerg KJ, Spilker T. Effect of peppermint oil and caraway oil on gastrointestinal motility in healthy volunteers: a pharmacodynamic study using simultaneous determination of gastric and gall-bladder emptying and orocaecal transit time. Aliment Pharmacol Ther 2003;17(3):445-451.

Heng MC. Local necrosis and interstitial nephritis due to topical methyl salicylate and menthol. Cutis 1987;39(5):442-444.

Hiki N, Kurosaka H, Tatsutomi Y, et al. Peppermint oil reduces gastric spasm during upper endoscopy: a randomized, double-blind, double-dummy controlled trial. Gastrointest Endosc 2003;57(4):475-482.

Holtman G, Gschossmann J, Buenger L, et al. Effects of a fixed peppermint oil caraway oil combination (FPCO) on symptoms of functional dyspepsia accentuated by pain or discomfort. Digestive Disease Week 2002

Kawane H. Menthol and aspirin-induced asthma. Respir Med 1996;90(4):247.

Kline RM, Kline JJ, Di Palma J, et al. Enteric-coated, pH-dependent peppermint oil capsules for the treatment of irritable bowel syndrome in children. J Pediatr 2001;138(1):125-128.

Lawson MJ, Knight RE, Tran K, et al. Failure of enteric-coated peppermint oil in the irritable bowel syndrome: a randomized, double-blind crossover study. J Gastroenterol Hepatol 1988;3(3):235-238.

Lech Y, Olesen KM, Hey H, et al. [Treatment of irritable bowel syndrome with peppermint oil. A double- blind study with a placebo.] Ugeskr Laeger 1988; 150(40):2388-2389.

Leicester RJ, Hunt RH. Peppermint oil to reduce colonic spasm during endoscopy. Lancet 1982;2(8305):989.

Liu JH, Chen GH, Yeh HZ, et al. Enteric-coated peppermint-oil capsules in the treatment of irritable bowel syndrome: a prospective, randomized trial. J Gastroenterol 1997;32(6):765-768.

Madisch A, Heydenreich CJ, Wieland V, et al. Treatment of functional dyspepsia with a fixed peppermint oil and caraway oil combination preparation as compared to cisapride. A multicenter, reference-controlled double-blind equivalence study. Arzneimittelforschung 1999;49(11):925-932.

Mascher H, Kikuta Ch, Schiel H. [Pharmacokinetics of carvone and menthol after administration of peppermint oil and caraway oil containing enteric formulation.] [Article in German.] Wien Med Wochenschr 2002;152(15-16):432-436.

May B, Kohler S, Schneider B. Efficacy and tolerability of a fixed combination of peppermint oil and caraway oil in patients suffering from functional dyspepsia. Aliment Pharmacol Ther 2000;14(12):1671-1677.

May B, Kuntz HD, Kieser M, et al. Efficacy of a fixed peppermint oil/caraway oil combination in non-ulcer dyspepsia. Arzneimittelforschung 1996;46(12): 1149-1153.

McGowan EM. Menthol urticaria. Arch Dermatol 1966;94:62-63.

Micklefield GH, Greving I, May B. Effects of peppermint oil and caraway oil on gastroduodenal motility. Phytother Res 2000;14(1):20-23.

Moghadam BK, Gier R, Thurlow T. Extensive oral mucosal ulcerations caused by misuse of a commercial mouthwash. Cutis 1999;64(2):131-134.

Morice AH, Marshall AE, Higgins KS, et al. Effect of inhaled menthol on citric acid induced cough in normal subjects. Thorax 1994;49(10):1024-1026.

Morton CA, Garioch J, Todd P, et al. Contact sensitivity to menthol and peppermint in patients with intra-oral symptoms. Contact Dermatitis 1995;32(5): 281-284.

Nash P, Gould SR, Bernardo DE. Peppermint oil does not relieve the pain of irritable bowel syndrome. Br J Clin Pract 1986;40(7):292-293.

Nicolay K. [Double blind trial of metoclopramide and Iberogast in functional gastroenteropathy.] Gastro-Entero-Hepatologie 1984;4:24-38.

Papa CM, Shelly WB. Menthol hypersensitivity. JAMA 1964;189:546-548.

Pittler MH, Ernst E. Peppermint oil for irritable bowel syndrome: a critical review and meta-analysis. Am J Gastroenterol 1998;93(7):1131-1135.

Rees WD, Evans BK, Rhodes J. Treating irritable bowel syndrome with peppermint oil. Br Med J 1979;2(6194):835-836.

Rhodes J, Evans BK, Rees WD. Peppermint oil in enteric coated capsules for the treatment of irritable bowel syndrome: a double blind controlled trial. Hepato-Gastroenterol 1980;27(Suppl):252.

Shkurupii VA, Kazarinova NV, Ogirenko AP, et al. [Efficiency of the use of peppermint (Mentha piperita L) essential oil inhalations in the combined multi-drug therapy for pulmonary tuberculosis.] [Article in Russian.] Probl Tuberk 2002;(4):36-9.Sparks MJ, O'Sullivan P, Herrington AA, et al. Does peppermint oil relieve spasm during barium enema? Br J Radiol 1995;68(812): 841-843.

P

Subiza J, Subiza JL, Valdivieso R, et al. Toothpaste flavor-induced asthma. J Allergy Clin Immunol 1992;90(6 Pt 1):1004-1006.

Tamaoki J, Chiyotani A, Sakai A, et al. Effect of menthol vapour on airway hyperresponsiveness in patients with mild asthma. Respir Med 1995;89(7):503-504.

Tate S. Peppermint oil: a treatment for postoperative nausea. J Adv Nurs 1997;26(3):543-549.

Veal L. The potential effectiveness of essential oils as a treatment for headlice, *Pediculus humanus capitis.* Complement Ther Nurs Midwifery 1996;2(4):97-101.

Weston CF. Anal burning and peppermint oil. Postgrad Med J 1987;63(742):717.

Wilkinson SM, Beck MH. Allergic contact dermatitis from menthol in peppermint. Contact Dermatitis 1994;30(1):42-43.

Wolf E. Peppermint oil and caraway oil for the irritable stomach. Pharmazeutische Zeitung 2001;146(27):29-30.

Wyllie JP, Alexander FW. Nasal instillation of 'Olbas Oil' in an infant. Arch Dis Child 1994;70(4):357-358.

Polypodium Leucotomos
(Ferns)

SYNONYMS/COMMON NAMES/RELATED SUBSTANCES

- Anapsos, calaguala, ferns, samambaia, Polypodiaceae, *Polypodium cambricum*, *Polypodium decumanum*, *Polypodium leucotomos extract*, *Polypodium vulgare*.

CLINICAL BOTTOM LINE
Background

- Extracts of fern species (family Polypodiaceae) have been used traditionally for numerous indications, most commonly in South America and Europe.
- The South American species *Polypodium leucotomos* L. is commonly known as "calaguala." Extracts of this species, called "anapsos," have been marketed and used as a treatment for multiple indications. Although *in vitro* and animal studies have reported anti-inflammatory, cytokine-suppressing, and leukotriene inhibitory properties, the small number of available human trials have not demonstrated efficacy for any specific indication.

Scientific Evidence for Common/Studied Uses	Grade*
Atopic dermatitis	C
Dementia	C
Psoriasis	C

*Key to grades: A: Strong scientific evidence for this use; B: Good scientific evidence for this use; C: Unclear scientific evidence for this use; D: Fair scientific evidence against this use (it may not work); F: Strong scientific evidence against this use (it likely does not work). For a more detailed explanation of efficacy criteria, see "Natural Standard Evidence-Based Validated Grading Rationale" in the Introduction.

Historical or Theoretical Uses
That Lack Sufficient Evidence

- Asthma, autoimmune diseases, cancer, diuretic, fever, hypertension, immunostimulant, inflammation, pertussis, rheumatic diseases, sunburn protection, upper respiratory tract infection, vitiligo.[1]

Expert Opinion and Folkloric Precedent

- Traditionally, fern species (family Polypodiaceae) have been used medicinally for numerous indications, most commonly in South America and Europe. In Brazil, the species *Polypodium decumanum*, commonly referred to as "samambaia," has been used orally to treat joint disorders, cough, upper respiratory infections, and cancer. In Europe, the fern species *Polypodium vulgare* has been used as an oral therapy to treat upper respiratory tract infections. There is limited scientific evidence regarding the safety or efficacy of these uses.
- *Polypodium leucotomos* is a South American fern species and is commonly known as "calaguala." Extracts of this species, referred to as "anapsos," have been marketed and used as a treatment for psoriasis, arthritis, cancer, dermatitis, and pertussis and as an immunosuppressant, immunostimulant, and antimicrobial agent.

Safety Summary

- **Possibly safe:** Limited safety data are available for extracts of *Polypodium leucotomos*. Few adverse effects have been reported in the small number of available human studies. A different species of fern, *Polypodium vulgare*, has been associated with central nervous system (CNS) depressant effects, positive inotropic and chronotropic effects in frog hearts, and hypotension and tachycardia in dogs (possibly due to beta-agonist activity).[2]

DOSING/TOXICOLOGY
General

- Recommended doses are based on those most commonly used in available trials, or on historical practice. However, with natural products, the optimal doses needed to balance efficacy and safety often have not been determined. Formulations and preparation methods may vary from manufacturer to manufacturer, and from batch to batch of a specific product made by a single manufacturer. Because often the active components of a product are not known, standardization may not be possible, and the clinical effects of different brands may not be comparable.

Standardization

- There is no widely accepted standardization for the preparation of *Polypodium leucotomos* extract.

Dosing: Adult (18 Years and Older)
Oral

- **Psoriasis:** 120 mg/day of anapsos (*Polypodium leucotomos* extract) has been administered for short periods of time.[3]
- **Dementia:** 360 mg/day of anapsos (*Polypodium leucotomos* extract), administered for 4 weeks in a poor-quality case series, was reported as more efficacious than a 720-mg daily dose (or placebo).[4]

Topical

- No clear dosing has been reported or established.

Dosing: Pediatric (Younger Than 18 Years)
- Insufficient evidence to recommend.

Toxicology
- Insufficient available evidence.

ADVERSE EFFECTS/PRECAUTIONS/CONTRAINDICATIONS
Allergy

- Pruritis of unclear etiology was reported in one patient in a case series of 495 subjects.[5]
- Patients with allergies to ferns (family Polypodiaceae) should avoid *Polypodium vulgare*.

Adverse Effects/Postmarket Surveillance

- **Dermatologic:** Pruritis of unclear etiology was reported in one patient in a case series of 495 subjects.[5]
- **Neurologic/CNS:** A pharmacodynamic study of a different fern species, *Polypodium vulgare*, reported CNS depressant effects.[2]

P

- **Cardiovascular:** A pharmacodynamic study of a different fern species, *Polypodium vulgare*, reported positive inotropic and chronotropic effects in frog hearts, and hypotension and tachycardia in dogs, possibly due to beta-agonist activity.[2]
- **Gastrointestinal:** Gastrointestinal discomfort was reported in one patient in a case series of 495 subjects.[5]

Precautions/Warnings/Contraindications

- Avoid driving and use of heavy machinery when taking *Polypodium leucotomos* extract, based on theoretical CNS depressant effects.
- Use cautiously in patients with cardiac disease or taking blood pressure medications, based on theoretical beta-agonist properties.

Pregnancy and Lactation

- Not recommended because of lack of sufficient data.

INTERACTIONS
Polypodium leucotomos Extract/Drug Interactions

- **Blood pressure medications:** A pharmacodynamic study of a different fern species, *Polypodium vulgare*, reported hypotension and tachycardia in dogs, possibly due to beta-agonist activity.[2] In theory, the hypotensive effects of other drugs may be potentiated.
- **Cardiac drugs (beta-blockers, calcium channel blockers, cardiac glycosides, inotropes):** A pharmacodynamic study of a different fern species, *Polypodium vulgare*, reported positive inotropic and chronotropic effects in frog hearts, and hypotension and tachycardia in dogs, possibly due to beta-agonist activity.[2] In theory, the effects of other cardiac drugs may be affected.
- **Sedatives, CNS depressants:** A pharmacodynamic study of a different fern species, *Polypodium vulgare*, reported CNS depressant effects.[2] In theory, the effects of CNS depressants may be potentiated.

Polypodium leucotomos Extract/Herb/Supplement Interactions

- **Hypotensive herbs:** A pharmacodynamic study of a different fern species, *Polypodium vulgare*, reported hypotension and tachycardia in dogs, possibly due to beta-agonist activity.[2] In theory, the hypotensive effects of other agents may be potentiated.
- **Cardiac glycoside herbs:** A pharmacodynamic study of a different fern species, *Polypodium vulgare*, reported positive inotropic and chronotropic effects in frog hearts, and hypotension and tachycardia in dogs, possibly due to beta-agonist activity.[2] In theory, the effects of other cardioactive agents may be affected.
- **Sedative herbs and supplements:** A pharmacodynamic study of a different fern species, *Polypodium vulgare*, reported CNS depressant effects.[2] In theory, the effects of CNS depressants may be potentiated.

Polypodium leucotomos Extract/Food Interactions

- Insufficient available evidence.

Polypodium leucotomos Extract/Lab Interactions

- Insufficient available evidence.

MECHANISM OF ACTION
Pharmacology

- *In vitro* and animal research on *Polypodium leucotomos* extract (anapsos) has reported free radical scavenging activity,[6,7] inhibition of cytokine production (interleukin-2, interferon-gamma, tumor necrosis factor-alpha),[8-10] stimulation of interleukin-1 secretion,[11] inhibition of platelet-activating factor activity,[12,13] inhibition of leukotriene B_4 formation,[14] suppression of T-lymphocyte proliferation,[11,15] antimicrobial activity,[16] and inhibition of ultraviolet light–induced skin damage.[17-19]

Pharmacodynamics/Kinetics

- Insufficient available evidence.

HISTORY

- There are more than 8000 species of ferns globally, most of which are in the family Polypodiaceae. Multiple species are used medicinally, including the South American *Polypodium decumanum*, commonly referred to as "samambaia," and *Polypodium vulgare*, used in Europe for respiratory tract infections.
- Recent research has focused on the anti-inflammatory effects of *Polypodium leucotomos* extract (anapsos), and its possible use in the management of psoriasis. Anapsos is sometimes marketed as an immune system modulator.

REVIEW OF THE EVIDENCE: DISCUSSION
Psoriasis
Summary

- Extracts of *Polypodium leucotomos* (anapsos) have been used medicinally in Europe and South America for the treatment of psoriasis since the 1970s. Preclinical studies have suggested anti-inflammatory properties and ultraviolet light skin protection (associated with topical use). A small number of poor quality human studies have reported beneficial effects of oral anapsos for the "whitening" of skin lesions in psoriasis. However, there is currently insufficient evidence demonstrating the efficacy of *Polypodium leucotomos* for this indication.

Evidence

- In a poor-quality 1982 placebo-controlled study, 37 patients with psoriasis were assigned to receive either 120 mg of daily oral anapsos or placebo.[3] In the anapsos group, 86% of patients experienced partial or total "whitening" of lesions. Statistical analysis and comparison to placebo were not reported, intention-to-treat analysis was not conducted, and outcomes measures were not clearly described. Therefore, the results are of limited clinical usefulness.
- In a poorly reported 1983 case series of 495 patients with psoriasis treated with *Polypodium leucotomos* extract for a mean period of 6 months (119 dropouts), skin "whitening" was reported in 70% of subjects.[5] Statistical analysis was not reported. In a brief published letter, "repigmentation" of vitiligo lesions was reportedly associated with *Polypodium leucotomos* extract.[1] In another letter, reduction of inflammation in psoriatic arthritis was reported.[20] Similar positive results have been reported in additional studies but are of limited clinical utility because of methodological weaknesses.[21-24]

Atopic Dermatitis
Summary

- *Polypodium leucotomos* extract (anapsos) has been suggested as a treatment for atopic dermatitis. *In vitro* and animal studies have reported anti-inflammatory, cytokine-suppressing, and leukotriene inhibitory properties of *Polypodium leucotomos*. However, there is insufficient human evidence supporting the use of *Polypodium leucotomos* for this indication.

Review of the Evidence: Polypodium Leucotomos

Condition Treated*	Study Design	Author, Year	N†	SS†	Study Quality‡	Magnitude of Benefit	ARR†	NNT†	Comments
Psoriasis	Controlled study, non-blinded, non-randomized	Del Pino[3] 1982	37	Unclear	0	Large	NA	NA	Skin "whitening" reported in 86% of *P. leucotomos* subjects; inadequate statistical analysis.
Atopic dermatitis	Comparison study, non-blinded, non-randomized	Jimenez[25] 1987	76	Unclear	0	Large	NA	NA	*P. leucotomos* extract compared to antihistamines, with improvement in both groups; subjective outcome measures used, no power calculation, inadequate statistical analysis.
Dementia (vascular and Alzheimer's)	Before-and-after	Alvarez[4] 2000	45	Yes	2	Small	NA	NA	Improved cognition on ADAScog scale with 360 mg/day of *P. leucotomos* extract vs. placebo, but no improvement with 720 mg /day.

*Primary or secondary outcome.
†*N*, Number of patients; *SS*, statistically significant; *ARR*, absolute risk reduction; *NNT*, the number of patients who need to undergo a specific intervention in order to observe an outcome in one individual.
‡0-2 = poor; 3-4 = good; 5 = excellent.
ADAScog, Alzheimer's disease assessment scale—cognitive-; *NA*, not applicable.
For an explanation of each category in this table, please see Table 3 in the Introduction.

P

Evidence

- In a poorly reported 1987 non-blinded comparison study, 76 patients with atopic dermatitis were treated with either oral anapsos or antihistamines for an unclear duration.[25] Reduction of inflammation was reported in both groups, with subjective superiority of anapsos therapy. No statistical analysis was provided. Serologic evaluation of lymphocytes revealed decreased T8 (suppressor) cells and increased T4 (helper) cells in subjects using anapsos. The lack of placebo group, statistical analysis, validated measurement scale, and blinding limits the clinical usefulness of these results.

Dementia
Summary

- There are insufficient human data to recommend for or against the use of *Polypodium leucotomos* extract (anapsos) in the management of dementia.

Evidence

- Anapsos was studied as a therapy for dementia in a randomized, placebo controlled, double-blind study in 45 patients.[4] Subjects carried a diagnosis of vascular or Alzheimer's dementia. Patients were randomized to receive either anapsos (360 mg), anapsos (720 mg), or placebo daily. After 4 weeks of therapy, significant improvements in cognition on the ADAScog (Alzheimer's disease assessment scale—cognitive) were noted in the 360-mg anapsos group, whereas improvements were not seen in the placebo and 720-mg anapsis groups. Although results were compared to baseline values in each group, it is not clear that results were compared between groups, making this possibly a "before and after" study rather than a controlled trial. In addition, blinding was not adequately described, allowing for the possible introduction of bias.

References

1. Mohammad A. Vitiligo repigmentation with Anapsos (*Polypodium leucotomos*). Int J Dermatol 1989;28(7):479.
2. Mannan A, Khan RA, Asif M. Pharmacodynamic studies on *Polypodium*
vulgare (Linn.). Indian J Exp Biol 1989;27(6):556-560.
3. Del Pino GJ, De Sambricio GF, Colomo GC. [Comparative study between 120 mg. of anapsos and a placebo in 37 psoriasis patients]. Med Cutan Ibero Lat Am 1982;10(3):203-208.
4. Alvarez XA, Pichel V, Perez P, et al. Double-blind, randomized, placebo-controlled pilot study with anapsos in senile dementia: effects on cognition, brain bioelectrical activity and cerebral hemodynamics. Methods Find Exp Clin Pharmacol 2000;22(7):585-594.
5. Pineiro AB. [2 years personal experience in anapsos treatment of psoriasis in various clinical forms]. Med Cutan Ibero Lat Am 1983;11(1):65-72.
6. Gomes AJ, Lunardi CN, Gonzalez S, et al. The antioxidant action of *Polypodium leucotomos* extract and kojic acid: reactions with reactive oxygen species. Braz J Med Biol Res 2001;34(11):1487-1494.
7. Fernandez-Novoa L, Alvarez XA, Sempere JM, et al. Effects of anapsos on the activity of the enzyme Cu-Zn-superoxide dismutase in an animal model of neuronal degeneration. Methods Find Exp Clin Pharmacol 1997;19(2):99-106.
8. Nogal-Ruiz JJ, Gomez-Barrio A, Escario JA, et al. Modulation by *Polypodium leucotomos* extract of cytokine patterns in experimental trichomoniasis model. Parasite 2003;10(1):73-78.
9. Gonzalez S, Alcaraz MV, Cuevas J, et al. An extract of the fern *Polypodium leucotomos* (Difur) modulates Th1/Th2 cytokines balance *in vitro* and appears to exhibit anti-angiogenic activities *in vivo*: pathogenic relationships and therapeutic implications. Anticancer Res 2000;20(3A):1567-1575.
10. Sempere JM, Rodrigo C, Campos A, et al. Effect of Anapsos (*Polypodium leucotomos* extract) on *in vitro* production of cytokines. Br J Clin Pharmacol 1997;43(1):85-89.
11. Bernd A, Theilig C, Ramirez-Bosca A, et al. Comparison of extract from *Polypodium leucotomos* with further fractions regarding their immuno-modulating activities [published abstract]. Presented at the International Symposium on the Impact of Cancer Biotechnology on Diagnostic and Prognostic Indicators, Nice, France, October 26-28, 1996.
12. Vasange M, Rolfsen W, Bohlin L. A sulphonoglycolipid from the fern *Polypodium decumanum* and its effect on the platelet activating-factor receptor in human neutrophils. J Pharm Pharmacol 1997;49(5):562-566.
13. Tuominen M, Bohlin L, Rolfsen W. Effects of Calaguala and an active principle, adenosine, on platelet activating factor. Planta Med 1992;58(4): 306-310.
14. Vasange-Tuominen M, Perera-Ivarsson P, Shen J, et al. The fern *Polypodium decumanum*, used in the treatment of psoriasis, and its fatty acid constituents as inhibitors of leukotriene B₄ formation. Prostaglandins Leukot Essent Fatty Acids 1994;50(5):279-284.
15. Rayward J, Villarrubia VG, Guillen C, et al. An extract of the fern *Polypodium leucotomos* inhibits human peripheral blood mononuclear cells proliferation *in vitro*. Int J Immunopharmacol 1997;19(1):9-14.
16. Dea-Ayuela M, Rodero M, Rodriguez-Bueno R, et al. Modulation by Anapsos (*Polypodium* leucotomos extract) of the antibody responses against the nematode parasite *Trichinella spiralis*. Phytother Res 1999;13(7):566-570.
17. Alcaraz MV, Pathak MA, Rius F, et al. An extract of *Polypodium leucotomos* appears to minimize certain photoaging changes in a hairless albino mouse animal model. A pilot study. Photodermatol Photoimmunol Photomed 1999;15(3-4):120-126.

18. Gonzalez S, Pathak MA, Cuevas J, et al. Topical or oral administration with an extract of Polypodium leucotomos prevents acute sunburn and psoralen-induced phototoxic reactions as well as depletion of Langerhans cells in human skin. Photodermatol Photoimmunol Photomed 1997;13(1-2):50-60.

19. Gonzalez S, Pathak MA. Inhibition of ultraviolet-induced formation of reactive oxygen species, lipid peroxidation, erythema and skin photo-sensitization by *Polypodium leucotomos*. Photodermatol Photoimmunol Photomed 1996;12(2):45-56.

20. Navarro-Blasco FJ, Sempere JM. Modification of the inflammatory activity of psoriatic arthritis in patients treated with extract of *Polipodium leucotomos* (Anapsos). Br J Rheumatol 1998;37(8):912.

21. Capella Perez MC, Castells RA. [Double-blind study using "anapsos" 120 mg. in the treatment of psoriasis]. Actas Dermosifiliogr 1981;72(9-10): 487-494.

22. Mercadal PO, Maesci CF. [Preliminary communication on the treatment of psoriasis with anapsos]. Actas Dermosifiliogr 1981;72(1-2):65-68.

23. Padilla H, Lainez H, Pacheco J. A new agent (hydrophilic fraction of *Polypodium leucotomis*) for management of psoriasis. Int J Derm 1974; 13:276-282.

24. Del P, De S, Colomo G. Comparison of *Polypodium leucotomis* extract with placebo in 37 cases of psoriasis. Med Cutan Iber Lat Am 1982;10:203-208.

25. Jimenez D, Naranjo R, Doblare E, et al. Anapsos, an antipsoriatic drug, in atopic dermatitis. Allergol Immunopathol (Madr) 1987;15(4):185-189.

Propolis
(Bee propolis)

SYNONYMS/COMMON NAMES/RELATED SUBSTANCES

- Bee glue, bee propolis, bee putty, bienenharz, hive dross, propolisina, propolis balsam, propolis resin, propolis wax, Russian penicillin.

CLINICAL BOTTOM LINE
Background

- Propolis is a natural resin created by bees, used in the construction of hives. Propolis is produced from the buds of conifer and poplar trees, in combination with beeswax and other bee secretions. Historically, propolis was used in Greece to treat abscesses, by the Assyrians to heal wounds and tumors, and by the Egyptians for mummification. Today, propolis is commonly found in chewing gum, cosmetics, creams, lozenges, and ointments.
- Propolis has shown promise in dentistry for dental caries, as a natural sealant and enamel hardener.[1-3] Effectiveness of propolis against herpes simplex virus types 1 and 2[4-6] and parasitic infections[5-7] has been demonstrated in preliminary studies. However, properly controlled, randomized human trials are lacking, and further evidence is warranted in order to establish the therapeutic efficacy of propolis for any indication.
- Numerous case reports have demonstrated propolis to be a potent allergen and sensitizing agent, and therefore it should be used cautiously in hypersensitive individuals. Toxicity with propolis is rare, although there are multiple case reports of contact dermatitis, erythema, eczema, vesiculitis, and pruritus.

Scientific Evidence for Common/Studied Use	Grade*
Acute cervicitis	C
Burns	C
Dental analgesia	C
Dental plaque and gingivitis (mouthwash)	C
Dental wound healing	C
Genital herpes simplex virus (HSV) infection	C
Infections (bacterial, parasitic)	C
Legg-Calve-Perthes disease, avascular hip necrosis	C
Postherpetic corneal complications	C
Rheumatic diseases	C
Rhinopharyngitis prevention (children)	C

*Key to grades: *A:* Strong scientific evidence for this use; *B:* Good scientific evidence for this use; *C:* Unclear scientific evidence for this use; *D:* Fair scientific evidence against this use (it may not work); *F:* Strong scientific evidence against this use (it likely does not work). For a more detailed explanation of efficacy criteria, see "Natural Standard Evidence-Based Validated Grading Rationale" in the Introduction.

Historical or Theoretical Indications That Lack Sufficient Evidence

- Acne, anticoagulant, antimycotic, antioxidant,[8-14] cancer,[8-15] Crohn's disease,[19] corneal regeneration,[20] dermatitis, diverticulitis, duodenal ulcers, eczema, eye infections, fungal infections,[21] HIV,[22] hypotension, immunostimulation, laryngitis, nasopharyngeal carcinoma, osteoporosis, pruritus, psoriasis, rheumatoid arthritis, skin rejuvenant, spasmolytic, thyroid disease,[23] tuberculosis, ulcerative colitis,[19] viral infections,[24] wound healing.[25]

Expert Opinion and Historic Precedent

- The history of propolis in traditional medicine is a testament to its versatility. It has been used for inflammation, as a mouthwash, and as a skin rejuvenant. Propolis is thought by some experts to possess antibacterial and antiviral properties. Some believe that it stimulates the immune system, thereby raising the body's natural resistance to infection.

Safety Summary

- **Likely safe:** Propolis is generally considered safe when used orally as a mouth rinse,[26] and when used by children as a nasal spray for rhinopharyngitis in recommended doses.[24]
- **Possibly safe:** Repeated topical application of propolis to the skin may lead to the development of sensitivity.[27-32]

DOSING/TOXICOLOGY
General

- Recommended doses are based on those most commonly used in available trials, or on historical practice. However, with natural products, the optimal doses needed to balance efficacy and safety often have not been determined. Formulations and preparation methods may vary from manufacturer to manufacturer, and from batch to batch of a specific product made by a single manufacturer. Because often the active components of a product are not known, standardization may not be possible, and the clinical effects of different brands may not be comparable.

Standardization

- There is no widely accepted method of standardization for propolis preparations.

Dosing: Adult (18 Years and Older)
Oral

- **Antibacterial:** Two 250-mg propolis capsules, three times daily for 3 days.[33]
- **Giardiasis:** 20% to 30% propolis extract for 5 days (specific milligram dosing not established).[5]

Mouthwash

- **Dental plaque:** Swish 10 mL of 0.2% to 10% propolis ethanol extract mouthwash in mouth for 60 to 90 seconds, then spit out; use once or twice daily.[26,34]

Topical

- **Genital herpes simplex infection:** 3% propolis ointment (made from 75% to 85% concentrated propolis extract), four times daily for 10 days, or, in cases of cervical or vaginal lesions, apply the same amount of ointment to the tip of a tampon and insert vaginally four times daily for 10 days.[6]

- **Acute cervicitis:** 5% ointment/cream of propolis applied in the form of vaginal dressings daily for 10 days.[7]

Intra-articular Injection

- **Legg-Calve-Perthes disease/avascular necrosis of the hip (postoperative):** Intra-articular injection of aqueous propolis extract (2 mL), every 14 days for up to 7 months.[25] Efficacy and safety have not been adequately evaluated, and dosing should only be under the supervision of an appropriately licensed healthcare professional.

Dosing: Pediatric (Younger Than 18 Years)
Nasal spray

- **Rhinopharyngitis:** 0.5-mL propolis nasal spray (Nivcrisol), once weekly for 5 months.[24]

Oral

- **Giardiasis:** 10% ethanol extract of propolis has been used to treat giardiasis in children over 5 days (specific milligram dose not established).[5]

Toxicology

- Toxicity data for propolis are limited, and because of variability in extraction levels, safety or toxicity of one preparation may not be applicable to other preparations. Preliminary studies have found propolis to be relatively nontoxic, with a no-effect level (NOEL) of 1400 mg/kg body weight/day in mice.[36]
- The LD_{50} in mice of raw unprocessed propolis has been reported as 2050 to 7340 mg, or for an ether extract as 700 mg/kg at 19 hours.[36]
- Anecdotally, treatment of skin reactions to propolis may consist of washing with soap and water, and supportive therapy. Topical corticosteroids and diphenhydramine (Benadryl) may be used to treat propolis-induced dermatitis.

ADVERSE EFFECTS/PRECAUTIONS/CONTRAINDICATIONS
Allergy

- Known allergy/hypersensitivity to propolis, *Populus nigra* L. (black poplar), poplar bud,[27,28,30,31,37] bee stings, bee products (including honey),[38,39] and Balsam of Peru.
- Propolis is a known sensitizing agent. Several case reports of edema, erythema, eczema, and swelling and other forms of allergic reactions as the result of repeated topical use have emphasized the need for caution when using propolis.[30-32,40-45]
- There have been numerous reports that have analyzed the constituents of propolis and balsam of Peru and found them to contain at least eight active components in common (benzyl benzoate, benzyl cinnamate, benzyl alcohol, benzoic acid, cinnamic acid, caffeic acid, cinnamic alcohol, and vanillin).[29,46,47] One study reported patch testing with a 10% alcoholic solution of propolis of 605 patients, of which 25 experienced allergic reactions (4.2%). Sixteen of the 25 patients with a positive reaction reported using propolis previously. Thirteen patients exhibited a simultaneous positive patch test for balsam of Peru.[48,49]

Adverse Effects/Postmarket Surveillance

- **General:** Although there have been several case reports of allergic reactions to propolis,[28,29,40,41,50] its use is generally believed to be well tolerated, with few adverse reactions reported.

- **Dermatologic:** Case reports have noted burning, cheilitis, perioral eczema,[51] contact dermatitis,[32,42,52-54] hyperkeratotic dermatitis,[55-59] erythematous vesicular lesions,[60] itching, swelling, and vesiculitis with topical application of propolis.[55,61-64] A 31-year-old woman with a history of relapsing psoriasis for a decade reported red vesicular dermatitis around psoriatic patches after 1-month use of two topical propolis products.[61] In another case, a 53-year-old man treated a nasal abrasion with 20% propolis and developed an erythematous nodule, fever, and lymphadenopathy.[50]
- **Neurologic/CNS:** A case of fever associated with an allergic response to propolis has been reported.[50]
- **Gastrointestinal:** Case reports of mucositis and stomatitis have been cited after the use of propolis lozenges or oral ingestion of propolis extract.[41,65]

Precautions/Warnings/Contraindications

- Use cautiously in patients who are allergic to bee stings or bee products (including honey), conifers, or poplars.[27-29,66]
- Use cautiously in patients who are allergic to Balsam of Peru, due to potential cross reactivity.[30,31]
- Use cautiously in allergic asthmatics, due to the possible presence of allergens in propolis.

Pregnancy and Lactation

- Insufficient available data to evaluate safety.

INTERACTIONS
Propolis/Drug Interactions

- Insufficient available data.
- **General:** Some tinctures contain high concentrations of ethanol, and may lead to vomiting if used concomitantly with disulfiram (Antabuse) or metronidazole (Flagyl).

Propolis/Herb/Supplement Interactions

- **Balsam of Peru:** Balsam of Peru and propolis are both known to result in allergic sensitization in some individuals, and they have eight known compounds in common: benzyl benzoate, benzyl cinnamate, benzyl alcohol, benzoic acid, cinnamic acid, caffeic acid, cinnamic alcohol, and vanillin.[29] Allergic sensitization may be more prominent in those using both products concurrently.[28,29,46,49,66]

Propolis/Food Interactions

- Insufficient available data.

Propolis/Lab Interactions

- Insufficient available data.

MECHANISM OF ACTION
Pharmacology

- **Antimicrobial properties:** Propolis contains flavonoids, including pinocembrin, galangin, pinobanksin, and pinobanksin-3-acetate, which are thought to be responsible for antimicrobial effects. Propolis extracts that contain the constituents pinocembrin and galangin have been shown to inhibit the growth of *Streptococcus mutans*, an organism that causes dental caries. *In vitro* studies have shown propolis to inhibit bacterial growth by disrupting the cell wall, the cytoplasmic membrane, and the cytoplasm, causing a partial bacteriolysis and inhibition of cellular protein synthesis.[67,68] Other *in vitro* experiments have demonstrated activity against gram-positive bacteria.[69-74] However, in an experiment designed to measure induction of resistance, Scheller et al.

found that out of 62 strains of *Staphylococcus aureus* isolated from various sources, approximately 90% showed either initial reduced sensitivity or complete resistance to propolis, regardless of the concentration of the ethanol extract of propolis used.[73] The *in vitro* antiviral activity of propolis has been attributed to a synergistic action of both flavonoid and flavanol components in propolis. Studies evaluating the efficacy of isolated constituents have demonstrated minimal effectiveness compared to the natural compound.[75]

- **Anti-inflammatory and antioxidant properties:** There is preliminary *in vitro* and *in vivo* evidence that propolis suppresses the lipoxygenase pathway of arachidonic acid metabolism and decreases the synthesis of prostaglandins and leukotrienes involved in inflammation.[76,77] Propolis has also demonstrated free radical–scavenging properties, and to a lesser extent, activity against the generation of superoxides.[8,78,79] Propolis may inhibit cellular apoptosis via effects on glutathione (GSH) and TNF-kappa B in macrophages.[10,80] Anticomplement activities of lysine complexes of propolis' phenolic constituents have been demonstrated *in vitro*.[81] In a prospective, open human trial in 10 healthy subjects, Propolis XNP (500 mg over 13 days) did not significantly alter plasma cytokine levels.[82]

- **Antineoplastic properties:** *In vitro* cytotoxicity against human fibrosarcoma, human lung carcinoma, and murine colon carcinoma cells has been demonstrated by propolis, and attributed to its benzofuran derivatives.[15,16,83,84] Other constituents such as artepillin C and diethyl ether have demonstrated cytostatic activity against myeloid cell lines.[17,85] Significant results have been seen against T-cell lines.[17] The propolis constituent galangin has been found to possess anti-genotoxic activity *in vitro*.[78]

- **Epithelial repair:** Applied topically, propolis has been reported to accelerate epithelial repair after tooth extraction in animal models.[86]

- **Osteoporosis:** Propolis has been reported to contain trace amounts of ipriflavone, an isoflavone with purported efficacy in the prevention of osteoporosis. However, it is not clear if the presence of ipriflavone in propolis is of clinical significance.

Pharmacodynamics/Kinetics

- Literature review reveals scant evidence regarding the absorption, distribution, metabolism, or elimination of propolis either topically or orally. The flavonoids, many of which are found in propolis, are known to exhibit a wide range of solubility. In natural propolis, flavonoids exist as glycosides.

- Animal studies have found that byproducts of flavonoid metabolism do not accumulate in the body and are renally excreted.[87]

HISTORY

- Propolis literally translates from the Greek words *pro* (before) and *polis* (the city), referring to its use by bees to reduce the size of hive entrances. In ancient Egypt, propolis was used in the mummification process to embalm the dead.

- Traditionally, propolis has been used for a variety of ailments. It was listed as an official drug in the London pharmacopoeia during the 17th century. Propolis has been applied topically to accelerate wound healing,[25] and as an antibacterial, particularly against gram-positive infections. Proponents of propolis believe that it stimulates the immune system, thereby raising the body's natural resistance to infection. Today, it is used in a variety of products, including toothpaste as a purported means of hardening tooth enamel.

REVIEW OF THE EVIDENCE: DISCUSSION
Acute Cervicitis
Summary

- Literature review reveals scant human studies of topical propolis for cervicitis. One poor-quality trial reported a small benefit of propolis vs. control. However, without additional human trial evidence or comparison to standard of care, the evidence cannot be considered compelling in favor (or against) this use of propolis.

Evidence

- Santana et al. conducted a randomized, double-blind, controlled study to evaluate the effects of a 5% propolis ointment/cream for the treatment of acute cervicitis.[7] Forty female patients diagnosed with cervicitis (age >20) were instructed to apply either vaginal dressings using 5% propolis daily or Lugol's (iodine) dressings for the same time period. After 10 days, no patient from the study group presented with further symptoms, and all vaginal smear cultures were negative. Total epithelization of the cervix within 10 days of treatment was achieved in 90% of the treatment group. Although this represented a small advantage vs. control, this study was poorly reported, with incomplete description of methods or statistical analysis and possible inadequate blinding.

Dental Plaque and Gingivitis (Mouthwash)
Summary

- Propolis mouthwash has been evaluated for a variety of dental applications, including prevention of plaque formation. The scientific basis for this use is the proposed antibacterial activity of propolis.[69-74,88] Propolis is believed to be particularly effective against *Streptococcus mutans*, a gram-positive bacteria which is highly colonized in the mouth, and is chiefly responsible for the fermentation of carbohydrates and formation of dental carries and plaque. Although preliminary studies have reported reduction in oral bacterial counts and short-term reduction of plaque formation associated with propolis rinsing, these experiments have been methodologically weak and inadequately blinded. Without additional properly conducted trials in this area, the evidence cannot be considered conclusive. In the United States, propolis is not a common ingredient in toothpastes.

Evidence

- A double-blind, parallel study evaluated plaque growth in 42 subjects receiving a propolis mouthwash (10% extract in ethanol), chlorhexidine, or placebo.[26] Three weeks and 1 week prior to treatment, subjects underwent teeth cleaning and polishing. Then, during a 5-day treatment period, subjects were instructed to rinse in the morning and evening for 1 minute and to refrain from using any other oral hygiene measures until final examination. Plaque growth was evaluated at six sites (mesio-, mid-, and distobuccal; mesio-, mid-, and distolingual), using the established plaque index of Silness and Loe. Although no significant difference in plaque regrowth was found between the propolis and other mouth rinses, there was a non-significant 14% reduction in plaque formation between the active and placebo groups. Since no power calculation was conducted, it is not clear that this study was of sufficient size to detect statistically significant differences between groups, and therefore the results are of unclear clinical relevance.

P

Review of the Evidence: Propolis

Condition Treated*	Study Design	Author, Year	N[†]	SS[†]	Study Quality[‡]	Magnitude of Benefit	ARR[†]	NNT[†]	Comments
Acute cervicitis	RCT, double-blind	Santana[7] 1995	40	Yes	2	Small	NA	NA	Poor description of methods and statistical analysis.
Dental plaque (mouthwash)	RCT, double-blind	Murray[26] 1997	42	No	3	None	NA	NA	14% reduction in plaque with active mouth rinses compared to placebo.
Dental plaque (mouthwash)	Controlled, double-blind	Schmidt[89] 1980	100	No	2	Small	NA	NA	Sample not randomized.
Dental plaque (toothpaste)	Controlled, double-blind	Poppe[92] 1986	103	No	1	None	NA	NA	No beneficial effects demonstrated; sample not randomized.
Oral bacteria (mouthwash)	Uncontrolled (observational)	Steinberg[34] 1996	10	Yes	NA	Small	NA	NA	Demonstrated short bactericidal effect.
Dental analgesia	Case series	Mahmoud[93] 1999	26	Yes	NA	Small	NA	NA	Subjective, non-validated questionnaire used; poor description of methods.
Dental surgical wound healing	Controlled	Magro-Filho[94] 1994	27	No	0	Small	NA	NA	Non-randomized, possible inadequate power; methodologically weak trial.
Genital HSV infection	Equivalence trial, placebo-controlled, single-blind	Vynograd[6] 2000	90	Yes	2	Medium	NA	NA	Topical propolis shown superior to topical acyclovir and placebo; possible bias due to lack of subject blinding.
Rheumatic diseases	Controlled, single-blind	Siro[100] 1996	190	Yes	2	Small	NA	NA	Poor reporting of methods and statistical analysis.
Infections (bacterial)	Case series	Brumfitt[33] 1990	3	NA	NA	Small	NA	NA	Reduced urine gram-positive bacteria; of unclear clinical significance.
Infections (giardiasis)	RCT	Miyares[5], 1988	138	Yes	1	Medium	NA	NA	Higher concentration of propolis more efficacious. Poor description of methods.
Legg-Calve-Perthes disease	Equivalence trial	Przybylski[35] 1985	54	No	1	Small	NA	NA	Inadequate comparison between groups; methodologically weak trial.
Postherpetic corneal complications (keratitis)	Controlled	Maichuk[101] 1995	55	Yes	1	Small	NA	NA	Methodologically weak trial.
Rhinopharyngitis	Case-control	Crisan[24] 1995	94	No	1	Small	NA	NA	No benefit seen with propolis; methodologically weak trial.
Rhinopharyngitis	Controlled	Szmeja[102] 1989	50	No	1	Small	NA	NA	Methodologically weak trial.

*Primary or secondary outcome.
[†]N, Number of patients; SS, statistically significant; ARR, absolute risk reduction; NNT, the number of patients who need to undergo a specific intervention in order to observe an outcome in one individual.
[‡]0-2 = poor; 3-4 = good; 5 = excellent.
HSV, Herpes simplex virus; NA, not applicable; RCT, randomized, controlled trial.
For an explanation of each category in this table, please see Table 3 in the Introduction.

- Steinberg et al. conducted a small, uncontrolled study in 10 volunteers to evaluate the bactericidal and bacteriostatic properties of propolis.[34] Subjects were instructed to swish a 0.2% propolis solution in their mouth for 90 seconds. Swabs of oral bacteria were collected and analyzed prior to the experiment, and then at 10 and 60 minutes following treatment. It was found that 10 minutes after swishing, total mean bacterial counts were reduced from baseline by 38%, and S. mutans counts were reduced by 42%. Sixty minutes after swishing, mean reduction in bacterial counts was maintained, although a slight increase in S. mutans counts was observed ($p < 0.05$). Although these results are promising, this study utilized a "surrogate" end point (bacterial counts) rather than a "hard" end point (plaque formation or dental caries). In addition, because of the short duration of the study and the possibility of S. mutans resistance formation,[73] the long-term clinical relevance of this case series remains unclear.

- In an early non-randomized, double-blind, placebo-controlled trial, the effects of a mouth rinse containing propolis were assessed in 100 individuals.[89] Although the study reported some positive effects on the Silness and Loe plaque index after 4 weeks of treatment, the statistical significance of results was not clear, and baseline patient characteristics, blinding, and outcomes measurement were not adequately reported.

- In a small preliminary human study, the efficacy of a therapeutic form of propolis called Propolan was evaluated for gingivitis and oral ulcerations.[90] Although an improvement was reported, the study population, methods, and analysis were not well described, and the results cannot be considered conclusive. In a poorly described study, use of propolis was reported to be beneficial in 460 cases of local oral infections, including abscesses, phlegmons, and wound infections.[91] Although the findings are suggestive, due to unclear description of methodology or analysis, results are of limited clinical utility. In a non-randomized, inadequately blinded trial of 103 subjects, dental plaque was evaluated during the use of propolis toothpaste vs. control.[92] No differences were observed between groups, although results cannot be considered definitive, due to methodological weaknesses.

Dental Analgesia and Dental Wound Healing
Summary

- It has been suggested that based on the purported properties of propolis as a sealant, analgesic, antibiotic, and inducer of bone regeneration, it may be a useful agent in the treatment of dental caries, periodontitis, and chronic dental pain. Although there is preliminary supportive evidence from preclinical studies and small case series, adequate human data are lacking, and no firm conclusions can be drawn based on the available evidence.

Dental Analgesia

- In a case series, Mahmoud et al. investigated the use of propolis as a desensitizing agent in 26 subjects with reported dental hypersensitivity for a period of 4 weeks.[93] Cervical dental sensitivity (CDS) was assessed after 1 and 4 weeks by cold air stimulation and subjective reporting of pain. The findings between baseline and after 4 weeks were statistically significant, and 85% of patients reported being "highly satisfied." However, there were no controls, and improvement of subjects' pain may have been due to the natural history of the disorder rather than to propolis. A non-validated questionnaire was used, and statistical methods were not adequately described. Results cannot be considered conclusive.

Dental Sealant/Filler

- Propolis has been found effective both *in vitro* and in animal studies for dentinal tubule occlusion.[1,2] It has been proposed that propolis be added to filler for root canal surgery. One poorly described study reported beneficial effects of propolis in patients with severe and chronic forms of periodontitis, based on clinical and x-ray exams.[3] Further experimentation in this area is warranted before a firm conclusion can be drawn.

Dental Wound Healing

- Preclinical experiments suggest a possible role for propolis in the healing of wounds.[25,76] Magro-Filho and Carvalho investigated whether dental wound repair in 27 sulcoplasty patients would be enhanced with a 5% propolis aqueous alcohol solution.[94] Two thirds of the patients were instructed to use either a propolis solution or a 5% aqueous alcohol solution and rinse five times/day for 1 week after surgery. The remainder of patients did not use a mouth rinse. Post-surgical inflammation was found to be "moderate" in the propolis group after 7 days, compared to "intense" in the other groups. Quantitative analysis of exfoliative cytology showed that mouth-rinsing with 5% propolis solution enhanced epithelialization of intra-buccal surgical wounds. Although these results are promising, the lack of randomization, blinding, or use of an adequately validated measurement instrument limit the usefulness of results.

Genital Herpes Simplex Virus (HSV) Infection
Summary

- A limited number of *in vitro* studies have demonstrated effectiveness of propolis and its constituents against herpes simplex virus types 1 and 2, rotavirus, coronavirus and adenovirus.[4,75,95,96] No specific active constituent has been identified. Preliminary results from methodologically weak human trials suggest some degree of efficacy of topical propolis for resolving the lesions associated with genital herpes virus infections. However, without further study and comparisons both to placebo and standard of care, no firm conclusions can be drawn.

Evidence

- Vynograd et al. conducted a randomized, single-blind (masked investigator), controlled trial in 90 patients with recurrent genital HSV type 2.[6] Thirty patients were randomized to each group receiving one of three ointments: 3% propolis, 5% acyclovir, or placebo. Patients were instructed to apply the ointment four times daily, starting in the blister phase. In women with vaginal or cervical lesions, a tampon with the appropriate ointment was inserted four times daily. Patients were examined on the 3rd, 7th, and 10th day of treatment for symptoms and number and size of genital lesions. End points included resolution of symptoms and/or lesions. On the 10th day, it was found that 24 of the 30 individuals in the propolis group had healed. In the acyclovir group, only 14 of 30 had healed, and in the placebo group 12 of 30 had healed. The healing process appeared to be faster in the propolis group: on day 3, 15 propolis patients had crusted lesions, compared to 8 in the acyclovir group and 3 in the placebo group. Improvements were statistically significant. However, lack of subject blinding may have biased results. In addition, standard of care is more commonly oral (acyclovir or other anti-herpes agents) rather than topical, and thus any trial of propolis for this indication should be compared to an oral formulation. Because herpes is a chronic, relapsing infection, long-term effects should be considered.
- Anecdotal reports and other small methodologically weak investigations have proposed efficacy, although these sources of evidence have been inconclusive.[97]

Infections (Bacterial, Parasitic)
Summary

- *In vitro* studies testing the antimicrobial efficacy of propolis have reported mixed results.[98] Preliminary human data suggest possible efficacy against urinary gram-positive bacteria (but not gram-negative bacteria) and gastrointestinal *Giardia*, although no definitive studies have been conducted.

Bacterial Infections

- Metzner et al. tested the antibacterial effects of various antibiotics, including streptomycin, oxytetracycline, chloramphenicol, nystatin, griseofulvin, and sulfamerazine, vs. 25 constituents of propolis.[67] None of the propolis constituents was found to be as potent as the antibiotics against any of the bacterial strains (*Bacillus subtilis*, *Staphylococcus aureus*, *Candida albicans*, *Trichophyton mentagrophytes*). Brumfitt et al. evaluated the antimicrobial action of propolis in the urine of three human subjects.[33] Over the course of 3 days, subjects took two 250-mg capsules of propolis three times daily. Each subject produced 10 specimens of urine. Weak inhibitory activity was reported in three specimens against some gram-positive bacteria, although no activity was found against gram-negative bacteria. Without controls or a larger sample size, the clinical significance of these results is uncertain.

Parasitic Infections

• Higashi and de Castro conducted an *in vitro* study to evaluate the sensitivity of *Trypanosoma cruzi* to propolis.[99] The study found a dose-dependent inhibition of parasite proliferation when propolis was added directly to *T. cruzi* suspensions at concentrations of 12.5 to 200 μg/mL. Miyares et al. conducted an equivalence trial comparing various strengths of a propolis extract (10% in children; 20% and 30% in adults) to tinidazole (an imidazole derivative), for the treatment of giardiasis in 138 patients.[5] Diagnosis was confirmed via duodenal aspiration in children and duodenoscopy in adults. Propolis was found to possess a statistically significant concentration-dependent beneficial effect, with the 30% concentration having a higher efficacy than tinidazole (60% versus 40%, respectively). However, it is not clear if this study was adequately blinded or randomized, and results therefore may have been biased. Additional study is merited in this area.

Rheumatic Diseases
Summary

• Based on anti-inflammatory properties observed *in vitro*, propolis has been proposed as a possible agent in the treatment of rheumatic and other inflammatory diseases. Although there are promising results from one poorly described human trial, there is currently insufficient evidence to recommend either for or against this use of propolis.

Evidence

• Siro et al. conducted a single-blind, controlled trial in 190 patients with rheumatic diseases.[100] There were two arms in this study, using different routes of administration: topical administration and iontophoresis. Topical treatment consisted of purified propolis, propolis with "anti-inflammatory trace elements," or placebo. Iontophoresis treatment involved propolis saturated with trace metal elements, poplar bud ointment saturated with trace metal elements, or placebo. All groups treated showed moderate significant improvement in inflammatory end points compared to placebo, and no adverse effects were observed. However, reporting of methods, statistical analysis, and outcomes is limited. Additional study is warranted in this area.

Legg-Calve-Perthes Disease, Avascular Necrosis
Summary

• Intra-articular injection of propolis has been studied in one methodologically weak experiment following hip replacement surgery. There is inconclusive safety or efficacy evidence in this area.

Evidence

• Przyblski et al. studied 54 patients who had undergone hip replacement surgery for avascular necrosis of the femoral head.[35] In 22 patients, aqueous extracts (2 mL) of propolis were injected (intra-articular) every 14 days (13 subjects received 5 to 8 total injections, and nine received 10 to 14 injections). The remaining patients were given "other forms" of treatment. Although the study concluded that treatment with propolis injection enriched patient outcomes, results cannot be considered conclusive because of lack of clear outcomes measurements and statistical analysis.

Postherpetic Corneal Complications
Summary

• Propolis has been found to exhibit antiviral and anti-inflammatory properties *in vitro* and has been proposed as a promoter of "corneal regeneration."[20] Literature review reveals one methodologically weak study of topical propolis for the treatment of corneal complications of varicella zoster. This study reported accelerated corneal epithelialization and improved visual acuity, although as an isolated report it cannot be considered definitive.

Evidence

• In a controlled trial of 35 patients with postherpetic trophic keratitis and 20 patients with postherpetic nebula, Maichuk et al. studied the use of propolis.[101] Propolis films were placed behind the lower eyelids at bedtime over a course of 10 to 15 days. The treated group was observed to have accelerated corneal epithelialization; epitheliopathy and micropoint edema of the cornea resolved. Mean recovery time was significantly reduced from 14.1 to 7.6 days in the propolis group compared to control ($p = 0.001$). On average, the visual acuity of propolis patients increased from 0.112 to 0.27. Although promising, the results of this isolated study (which did not adequately blind, randomize, or describe methods) cannot be considered definitive. Further trials are warranted in this area.

Rhinopharyngitis Prevention (Children)
Summary

• Currently, there is insufficient human evidence to recommend for or against the use of propolis for rhinopharyngeal infections.

Evidence

• Crisan et al. conducted a controlled clinical trial evaluating rhinopharyngitis symptoms in preschool children (mean age, 6 years) and school-age children (mean age, 9 years) over a 5-month period.[24] Subjects were administered 0.5 mL weekly of either a propolis nasal spray (Nivcrisol) or a salt solution. Baseline nasopharyngeal samples were obtained and cultured (viral, bacterial, fungal) for each child, followed by monthly cultures during treatment. The children were evaluated for nasal catarrh, pharyngeal congestion, conjunctival mucosa congestion, fever, duration/severity of infection, and treatment tolerance. There was no significant difference in bacterial or viral pharyngeal flora scores in either group over the course of 5 months. Symptoms were reported to be significantly less severe in the treated groups compared to placebo, although this was not a consistent finding over the course of treatment in either arm. As a result, the conclusions of this study are unclear. Methodological weaknesses of this trial include lack of blinding of investigators, dissimilar baseline characteristics of subjects (age), and lack of use of a validated measurement instrument.

• Szmeja et al. conducted a case-control trial evaluating symptoms in 50 patients with rhinovirus infections who were given propolis vs. placebo.[102] Of the patients treated with propolis, 5 experienced symptom relief on day 1, 16 on day 2, and 3 on day 3. In comparison, mean recovery time in the placebo group was 4.8 days (mean duration was 2.5 times shorter in the treatment group). Although the results are promising, the inherent difficulties of case control trials, such as the presence of possible confounders or bias, limit the clinical applicability of this study.

Burns
Summary

• Preliminary research reports that propolis may have a beneficial effect on the healing of partial thickness burn wounds.[103]

FORMULARY: BRANDS USED IN CLINICAL TRIALS
Brands Used in Clinical Trials (Efficacy Not Proven)

• Nivcrisol nasal spray (Propolis Immuntinktur)

References

1. Almas K, Mahmoud A, Dahlan A. A comparative study of propolis and saline application on human dentin. A SEM study. Indian J Dent Res 2001; 12(1): 21-27.
2. Ikeno K, Ikeno T, Miyazawa C. Effects of propolis on dental caries in rats. Caries Res 1991;25(5):347-351.
3. Kosenko SV, Kosovich TI. [The treatment of periodontitis with prolonged-action propolis preparations (clinical x-ray research)]. Stomatologiia (Mosk) 1990;69(2):27-29.
4. Amoros M, Lurton E, Boustie J, et al. Comparison of the anti-herpes simplex virus activities of propolis and 3-methyl-but-2-enyl caffeate. J Nat Prod 1994;57(5):644-647.
5. Miyares C, Hollands I, Castaneda C, et al. [Clinical trial with a preparation based on propolis "propolisina" in human giardiasis]. Acta Gastroenterol Latinoam 1988;18(3):195-201.
6. Vynograd N, Vynograd I, Sosnowski Z. A comparative multi-centre study of the efficacy of propolis, acyclovir and placebo in the treatment of genital herpes (HSV). Phytomedicine 2000;7(1):1-6.
7. Santana PE, Lugones BM, Perez SO, et al. [Vaginal parasites and acute cervicitis: local treatment with propolis. Preliminary report]. Rev Cubana Enferm 1995;11(1):51-56.
8. Scheller S, Wilczok T, Imielski S, et al. Free radical scavenging by ethanol extract of propolis. Int J Radiat Biol 1990;57(3):461-465.
9. Ichikawa H, Satoh K, Tobe T, et al. Free radical scavenging activity of propolis. Redox Rep 2002;7(5):347-350.
10. Pascual C, Gonzalez R, Torricella RG. Scavenging action of propolis extract against oxygen radicals. J Ethnopharmacol 1994;41(1-2):9-13.
11. Nakanishi I, Uto Y, Ohkubo K, et al. Efficient radical scavenging ability of artepillin C, a major component of Brazilian propolis, and the mechanism. Org Biomol Chem 2003;1(9):1452-1454.
12. Russo A, Longo R, Vanella A. Antioxidant activity of propolis: role of caffeic acid phenethyl ester and galangin. Fitoterapia 2002;73(Suppl 1): S21-S29.
13. Hegazi AG, Abd El Hady FK. Egyptian propolis: 3. Antioxidant, antimicrobial activities and chemical composition of propolis from reclaimed lands. Z Naturforsch [C] 2002;57(3-4):395-402.
14. Kwon YS, Park DH, Shin EJ, et al. Antioxidant propolis attenuates kainate-induced neurotoxicity via adenosine A(1) receptor modulation in the rat. Neurosci Lett 2004;355(3):231-235.
15. Banskota AH, Tezuka Y, Midorikawa K, et al. Two novel cytotoxic benzofuran derivatives from Brazilian propolis. J Nat Prod 2000;63(9): 1277-1279.
16. Banskota AH, Tezuka Y, Adnyana IK, et al. Cytotoxic, hepatoprotective and free radical scavenging effects of propolis from Brazil, Peru, the Netherlands and China. J Ethnopharmacol 2000;72(1-2):239-246.
17. Kimoto T, Aga M, Hino K, et al. Apoptosis of human leukemia cells induced by Artepillin C, an active ingredient of Brazilian propolis. Anticancer Res 2001;21(1A):221-228.
18. Banskota AH, Nagaoka T, Sumioka LY, et al. Antiproliferative activity of the Netherlands propolis and its active principles in cancer cell lines. J Ethnopharmacol 2002;80(1):67-73.
19. Dano P, Moller EH, Jarnum S. [Effect of the natural product propolis on ulcerative colitis and Crohn's disease]. Ugeskr Laeger 1979;141(28): 1888-1890.
20. Bezuglyi BS. [Effect of the Propomix preparation on corneal regeneration]. Oftalmol Zh 1980;35(1):48-52.
21. D'Auria FD, Tecca M, Scazzocchio F, et al. Effect of propolis on virulence factors of Candida albicans. J Chemother 2003;15(5):454-460.
22. Harish Z, Rubinstein A, Golodner M, et al. Suppression of HIV-1 replication by propolis and its immunoregulatory effect. Drugs Exp Clin Res 1997; 23(2):89-96.
23. Mihailescu NN, Gorgos C, Palos E, et al. Contributions to the study and treatment of some thyroidal diseases with Propolis H (Romanian). The First Symposium on Apitherapy 1974;128-132.
24. Crisan I, Zaharia CN, Popovici F, et al. Natural propolis extract NIVCRISOL in the treatment of acute and chronic rhinopharyngitis in children. Rom J Virol 1995;46(3-4):115-133.
25. Hartwich A, Legutko J, Wszolek J. [Propolis: its properties and administration to patients treated for some surgical diseases]. Przegl Lek 2000;57(4): 191-194.
26. Murray MC, Worthington HV, Blinkhorn AS. A study to investigate the effect of a propolis-containing mouthrinse on the inhibition of de novo plaque formation. J Clin Periodontol 1997;24(11):796-798.
27. Bousquet J, Menardo JL, Michel FB. Allergy in beekeepers. Allergol Immunopathol (Madr) 1982;10(5):395-398.
28. Hausen BM, Wollenweber E, Senff H, et al. Propolis allergy. (II). The sensitizing properties of 1,1-dimethylallyl caffeic acid ester. Contact Dermatitis 1987;17(3):171-177.
29. Hausen BM, Wollenweber E. Propolis allergy. (III). Sensitization studies with minor constituents. Contact Dermatitis 1988;19(4):296-303.
30. Petersen HO. Hypersensitivity to propolis. Contact Dermatitis 1977;3(5): 278-279.
31. Petersen HO. [Allergy to propolis in patients with eczema]. Ugeskr Laeger 1977;139(39):2331-2333.
32. Trevisan G, Kokelj F. Contact dermatitis from propolis: role of gastrointestinal absorption. Contact Dermatitis 1987;16(1):48.
33. Brumfitt W, Hamilton-Miller JM, Franklin I. Antibiotic activity of natural products: 1. Propolis. Microbios 1990;62(250):19-22.
34. Steinberg D, Kaine G, Gedalia I. Antibacterial effect of propolis and honey on oral bacteria. Am J Dent 1996;9(6):236-239.
35. Przybylski J, Scheller S. [Early results in the treatment of Legg-Calve-Perthes disease using intra-articular injections of aqueous propolis extract]. Z Orthop Ihre Grenzgeb 1985;123(2):163-167.
36. Burdock GA. Review of the biological properties and toxicity of bee propolis (propolis). Food Chem Toxicol 1998;36(4):347-363.
37. Monti M, Berti E, Carminati G, et al. Occupational and cosmetic dermatitis from propolis. Contact Dermatitis 1983;9(2):163.
38. Machackova J. Contact dermatitis to propolis. Contact Dermatitis 1985; 13(1):43-44.
39. Valsecchi R, Cainelli T. Dermatitis from propolis. Contact Dermatitis 1984; 11(5):317.
40. Junghans V, Geier J, Fuchs T. Allergy to propolis caused by beeswax-containing ointment. Am J Contact Dermat 2002;13(2):87.
41. Bellegrandi S, D'Offizi G, Ansotegui IJ, et al. Propolis allergy in an HIV-positive patient. J Am Acad Dermatol 1996;35(4):644.
42. Schuler TM, Frosch PJ. [Propolis-induced contact allergy]. Hautarzt 1988;39(3):139-142.
43. Tumova L, Pasavova D. [Allergic contact dermatitis caused by propolis]. Ceska Slov Farm 2000;49(6):285-287.
44. Wanscher B. Contact dermatitis from propolis. Br J Dermatol 1976;94(4): 451-455.
45. Young E. Sensitivity to propolis. Contact Dermatitis 1987;16(1):49-50.
46. Ginanneschi M, Acciai MC, Sertoli A, et al. Propolis allergy: synthesis and patch testing of gamma,gamma-dimethylallyl caffeic acid ester and its o-methyl derivatives. Contact Dermatitis 1989;21(4):267-269.
47. Hegyi E, Suchy V, Nagy M. [Propolis allergy]. Hautarzt 1990;41(12): 675-679.
48. Machackova J. The incidence of allergy to propolis in 605 consecutive patients patch tested in Prague. Contact Dermatitis 1988;18(4):210-212.
49. Rudzki E, Grzywa Z. Dermatitis from propolis. Contact Dermatitis 1983; 9(1):40-45.
50. Teraki Y, Shiohara T. Propolis-induced granulomatous contact dermatitis accompanied by marked lymphadenopathy. Br J Dermatol 2001;144(6): 1277-1278.
51. Kokelj F, Trevisan G. Contact dermatitis from propolis. Contact Dermatitis 1983;9(6):518.
52. Kleinhans D. Airborne contact dermatitis due to propolis. Contact Dermatitis 1987;17(3):187-188.
53. Thomas P, Korting HC, Przybilla B. Propolis-induced allergic contact dermatitis mimicking pemphigus vulgaris. Arch Dermatol 1998;134(4): 511-513.
54. Tosti A, Caponeri GM, Bardazzi F, et al. Propolis contact dermatitis. Contact Dermatitis 1985;12(4):227-228.
55. Ayala F, Lembo G, Nappa P, et al. Contact dermatitis from propolis. Contact Dermatitis 1985;12(3):181-182.
56. Downs AM, Sansom JE. Occupational contact dermatitis due to propolis. Contact Dermatitis 1998;38(6):359-360.
57. Pincelli C, Motolese A, Pincelli L. Contact dermatitis from propolis. Contact Dermatitis 1984;11(1):49.
58. Raton JA, Aguirre A, Diaz-Perez JL. Contact dermatitis from propolis. Contact Dermatitis 1990;22(3):183-184.
59. Rudzki E, Grzywa Z, Pomorski Z. New data on dermatitis from propolis. Contact Dermatitis 1985;13(3):198-199.
60. Silvani S, Spettoli E, Stacul F, et al. Contact dermatitis in psoriasis due to propolis. Contact Dermatitis 1997;37(1):48-49.

P

61. Angelini G, Vena GA, Meneghini CL. Psoriasis and contact allergy to propolis. Contact Dermatitis 1987;17(4):251-253.

62. Cirasino L, Pisati A, Fasani F. Contact dermatitis from propolis. Contact Dermatitis 1987;16(2):110-111.

63. Garcia M. Allergic contact dermatitis from beeswax nipple-protective. Contact Dermatitis 1995;33:440-441.

64. Nakamura T. Sensitivity to propolis in Japan. Contact Dermatitis 1988; 18(5):313.

65. Hay KD, Greig DE. Propolis allergy: a cause of oral mucositis with ulceration. Oral Surg Oral Med Oral Pathol 1990;70(5):584-586.

66. Hausen BM, Wollenweber E, Senff H, et al. Propolis allergy. (I). Origin, properties, usage and literature review. Contact Dermatitis 1987;17(3): 163-170.

67. Metzner J, Bekemeier H, Paintz M, et al. [On the antimicrobial activity of propolis and propolis constituents (author's transl)]. Pharmazie 1979; 34(2):97-102.

68. Takaisi-Kikuni NB, Schilcher H. Electron microscopic and micro-calorimetric investigations of the possible mechanism of the antibacterial action of a defined propolis provenance. Planta Med 1994;60(3):222-227.

69. Bankova V, Marcucci MC, Simova S, et al. Antibacterial diterpenic acids from Brazilian propolis. Z Naturforsch [C] 1996;51(5-6):277-280.

70. Bosio K, Avanzini C, D'Avolio A, et al. *In vitro* activity of propolis against *Streptococcus pyogenes*. Lett Appl Microbiol 2000;31(2):174-177.

71. Grange JM, Davey RW. Antibacterial properties of propolis (bee glue). J R Soc Med 1990;83(3):159-160.

72. Park YK, Koo MH, Abreu JA, et al. Antimicrobial activity of propolis on oral microorganisms. Curr Microbiol 1998;36(1):24-28.

73. Scheller S, Tustanowski J, Kurylo B, et al. Biological properties and clinical application of propolis. III. Investigation of the sensitivity of *Staphylococci* isolated from pathological cases to ethanol extract of propolis (EEP). Attempts on inducing resistance in laboratory Staphylococcus strain to EEP. Arzneimittelforschung 1977;27(7):1395.

74. Sforcin JM, Fernandes A, Jr., et al. Seasonal effect on Brazilian propolis antibacterial activity. J Ethnopharmacol 2000;73(1-2):243-249.

75. Amoros M, Simoes CM, Girre L, et al. Synergistic effect of flavones and flavonols against herpes simplex virus type 1 in cell culture. Comparison with the antiviral activity of propolis. J Nat Prod 1992;55(12):1732-1740.

76. Volpert R, Elstner EF. Interactions of different extracts of propolis with leukocytes and leukocytic enzymes. Arzneimittelforschung 1996;46(1): 47-51.

77. Mirzoeva OK, Calder PC. The effect of propolis and its components on eicosanoid production during the inflammatory response. Prostaglandins Leukot Essent Fatty Acids 1996;55(6):441-449.

78. Heo MY, Sohn SJ, Au WW. Anti-genotoxicity of galangin as a cancer chemopreventive agent candidate. Mutat Res 2001;488(2):135-150.

79. Scheller S, Gazda G, Krol W, et al. The ability of ethanolic extract of propolis (EEP) to protect mice against gamma irradiation. Z Naturforsch [C] 1989; 44(11-12):1049-1052.

80. Claus R, Kinscherf R, Gehrke C, et al. Antiapoptotic effects of propolis extract and propol on human macrophages exposed to minimally modified low density lipoprotein. Arzneimittelforschung 2000;50(4):373-379.

81. Georgieva P, Ivanovska N, Bankova V, et al. Anticomplement activity of lysine complexes of propolis phenolic constituents and their synthetic analogs. Z Naturforsch [C.] 1997;52(1-2):60-64.

82. Bratter C, Tregel M, Liebenthal C, et al. [Prophylactic effectiveness of propolis for immunostimulation: a clinical pilot study]. Forsch Komplementarmed 1999;6(5):256-260.

83. Banskota AH, Tezuka Y, Prasain JK, et al. Chemical constituents of Brazilian propolis and their cytotoxic activities. J Nat Prod 1998;61(7): 896-900.

84. Hirota M, Matsuno T, Fujiwara T, et al. Enhanced cytotoxicity in a Z-photoisomer of a benzopyran derivative of propolis. J Nat Prod 2000; 63(3):366-370.

85. Hladon B, Bylka W, Ellnain-Wojtaszek M, et al. In vitro studies on the cytostatic activity of propolis extracts. Arzneimittelforschung 1980;30(11): 1847-1848.

86. Filho OM, de Carvalho AC. Application of propolis to dental sockets and skin wounds. J Nihon Univ Sch Dent 1990;32(1):4-13.

87. Havsteen B. Flavonoids, a class of natural products of high pharmacological potency. Biochem Pharmacol 1983;32(7):1141-1148.

88. Eley BM. Antibacterial agents in the control of supragingival plaque—a review. Br Dent J 1999;186(6):286-296.

89. Schmidt H, Hampel CM, Schmidt G, et al. [Double-blind trial of the effect of a propolis-containing mouthwash on inflamed and healthy gingiva]. Stomatol DDR 1980;30(7):491-497.

90. Martinez SG, Gou GA, Ona TR, et al. [Preliminary study of the effects of propolis in the treatment of chronic gingivitis and oral ulceration]. Rev Cubana Estomatol 1988;25(3):36-44.

91. Tsarev NI, Petrik EV, Aleksandrova VI. [Use of propolis in the treatment of local suppurative infection]. Vestn Khir Im I I Grek 1985;134(5): 119-122.

92. Poppe B, Michaelis H. [Results of a twice-yearly controlled oral hygiene activity using a propolis-containing toothpaste (double-blind study)]. Stomatol DDR 1986;36(4):195-203.

93. Mahmoud AS, Almas K, Dahlan AA. The effect of propolis on dentinal hypersensitivity and level of satisfaction among patients from a university hospital Riyadh, Saudi Arabia. Indian J Dent Res 1999;10(4):130-137.

94. Magro-Filho O, de Carvalho AC. Topical effect of propolis in the repair of sulcoplasties by the modified Kazanjian technique. Cytological and clinical evaluation. J Nihon Univ Sch Dent 1994;36(2):102-111.

95. Debiaggi M, Tateo F, Pagani L, et al. Effects of propolis flavonoids on virus infectivity and replication. Microbiologica 1990;13(3):207-213.

96. Dumitrescu M, Crisan I, Esanu V. [The mechanism of the antiherpetic action of an aqueous propolis extract. II. The action of the lectins of an aqueous propolis extract]. Rev RoumVirol 1993;44(1-2):49-54.

97. Feiks FK. Topical application of propolis tincture in the treatment of herpes zoster. Third International Symposium on Apitherapy 1978;109-111.

98. Focht J, Hansen SH, Nielsen JV, et al. Bactericidal effect of propolis in vitro against agents causing upper respiratory tract infections. Arzneimittelforschung 1993;43(8):921-923.

99. Higashi KO, de Castro SL. Propolis extracts are effective against *Trypanosoma cruzi* and have an impact on its interaction with host cells. J Ethnopharmacol 1994;43(2):149-155.

100. Siro B, Szelekovszky S, Lakatos B, et al. [Local treatment of rheumatic diseases with propolis compounds]. Orv Hetil 1996;137(25):1365-1370.

101. Maichuk IF, Orlovskaia LE, Andreev VP. [The use of ocular drug films of propolis in the sequelae of ophthalmic herpes]. Voen Med Zh 1995;12: 36-9, 80.

102. Szmeja Z, Kulczynski B, Sosnowski Z, et al. [Therapeutic value of flavonoids in Rhinovirus infections]. Otolaryngol Pol 1989;43(3):180-184.

103. Gregory SR, Piccolo N, Piccolo MT, et al. Comparison of propolis skin cream to silver sulfadiazine: a naturopathic alternative to antibiotics in treatment of minor burns. J Altern Complement Med 2002;8(1):77-83.

Psyllium
(Plantago ovata, Plantago isphagula)

SYNONYMS/COMMON NAMES/RELATED SUBSTANCES

- Bran Buds cereal, Effersyllium, Fiberall, flea seed, Fybogel, Heartwise cereal, Hydrocil, I-so-gel, ispaghula, ispaghula husk, ispaghula seed, Konsyl, Lunelax, Metamucil, Minolest, Natural Vegetable Laxative, Perdiem, *Plantago arenaria*, *Plantago psyllium*, Prodiem Plain, psyllion, psyllios, psyllium husk, psyllium seed, Regulan, Serutan, Vi-Siblin, Yerba Prima Psyllium hush powder.

CLINICAL BOTTOM LINE

Background

- Psyllium, also referred to as *ispaghula*, is derived from the husks of the seeds of *Plantago ovata*. Psyllium contains a high level of soluble dietary fiber and is the chief ingredient in many commonly used bulk laxatives, including products such as Metamucil and Serutan.
- Psyllium has been studied as a "non-systemic" cholesterol-lowering agent, with generally modest effects seen on total cholesterol and high-density lipoprotein levels. Several psyllium-containing cereals such as Heartwise and Bran Buds have appeared in the United States marketplace during the last 15 years, and have been touted for their potential lipid-lowering and "heart health promoting" effects.
- Allergic reactions, including anaphylaxis, have been reported, particularly in healthcare workers with previous experience preparing psyllium-containing bulk laxatives. Obstruction of the gastrointestinal tract by such laxatives has also been reported, particularly in patients with prior bowel surgeries or anatomic abnormalities, or when mixed with inadequate amounts of water.

Uses Based on Scientific Evidence	Grade*
High cholesterol Psyllium is well studied as a lipid-lowering agent with generally modest reductions seen in blood levels of total cholesterol and low-density lipoprotein ("bad cholesterol"). Effects have been observed following 8 weeks of regular use. Psyllium does not appear to have significant effects on high-density lipoprotein ("good cholesterol") or triglyceride levels. Because only small reductions have been observed, people with high cholesterol should discuss the use of more potent agents with their healthcare provider. Effects have been observed in adults and children, although long-term safety in children is not established.	A
Constipation Psyllium has long been used as a chief ingredient in "bulk laxatives." Studies exploring the mechanisms of the laxative effects of psyllium are somewhat conflicting, but have generally revealed an increase in stool weight, an increase in bowel movements per day, and a decrease in total gut transit time.	B
Diarrhea Psyllium has been studied for the treatment of diarrhea, particularly in patients undergoing tube feeding. It has also been studied in addition to Orlistat therapy in hopes of decreasing gastrointestinal effects (diarrhea and oily discharge) of this weight loss agent. An effective stool bulking effect has generally been found in scientific studies.	B
Fat excretion in stool Early research shows that dietary psyllium and chitosan supplementation may help to increase the excretion of fat in the stool.	C
Hyperglycemia (high blood sugar levels) Several studies have examined the administration of psyllium with meals or just prior to meals in order to measure effects on blood sugar levels. Measurements have been done immediately after meals and throughout the day. Effects of regular (chronic) psyllium use have also been investigated. In general, no immediate (acute) changes in blood sugar levels have been reported. Long-term effects have been inconsistent across studies, although modest reductions have been reported in some research. Better evidence is necessary before a firm conclusion can be drawn.	C
Inflammatory bowel disease There is limited and unclear evidence regarding the use of psyllium in patients with inflammatory bowel disease.	C
Irritable bowel syndrome Psyllium preparations have been studied for more than 20 years in the treatment of irritable bowel syndrome symptoms. Results of these trials have been conflicting. Better research is necessary before a firm conclusion can be reached.	C

*Key to grades: *A*: Strong scientific evidence for this use; *B*: Good scientific evidence for this use; *C*: Unclear scientific evidence for this use; *D*: Fair scientific evidence against this use (it may not work); *F*: Strong scientific evidence against this use (it likely does not work). For a more detailed explanation of efficacy criteria, see "Natural Standard Evidence-Based Validated Grading Rationale" in the Introduction.

Historical or Theoretical Indications That Lack Sufficient Evidence
Abscesses, anti-parasitic, atherosclerosis, bleeding hemorrhoids, boils, bronchitis, Crohn's disease, colon cancer prevention, cystitis, demulcent, diverticular disease, duodenal ulcer, dysentery, excessive menstrual bleeding, fecal (stool) incontinence, gallstones, hearing damage, high blood pressure, incontinence, leishmaniasis, obesity, poison ivy rash, primary biliary cirrhosis, psoriasis, radiation-induced colitis/diarrhea, sclerosing cholangitis, stomach ulcer, urethritis, wound healing (used on the skin).

P

DOSING/TOXICOLOGY

The following doses are based on scientific research, publications, traditional use, or expert opinion. Many herbs and supplements have not been thoroughly tested, and safety and effectiveness may not be proven. Brands may be made differently, with variable ingredients even within the same brand. The doses shown may not apply to all products. It is important to always read product labels and discuss doses with a qualified healthcare provider before therapy is started.

Standardization

- Standardization involves measuring the amounts of certain chemicals in products to try to make different preparations similar to each other. It is not always known if the chemicals being measured are the "active" ingredients.
- Psyllium products may contain husks of *Plantago ovata* seeds or the seeds themselves, with the husks being more commonly used. Amounts of psyllium in products are generally reported as total grams. Seed preparations contain approximately 47% soluble fiber by weight, while husk preparations generally contain 67 to 71% soluble fiber and 85% total fiber by weight.

Adults (18 Years and Older)

- **Dietary amounts:** Recommendations for dietary fiber intake for adults fall within the range of 20 to 35 g per day, or 10 to 13 g per 1,000 kilocalories ingested. However, popular U.S. foods are not high in dietary fiber, and common serving sizes of grains, fruits, and vegetables contain only 1 to 3 g of dietary fiber. The usual intake of dietary fiber in the U.S. remains lower than these recommended levels, averaging only 14 to 15 g daily.
- **General:** It is important to take laxatives such as psyllium with sufficient amounts of water or liquid in order to reduce the risk of bowel obstruction.
- **Cholesterol lowering:** A wide range of doses of psyllium has been studied, from 3.4 to 45 g per day, taken daily by mouth in two or three divided doses. Studies using psyllium-enriched cereals or other food products have administered preparations providing between 3 and 12 g of soluble fiber daily. Psyllium husk preparations have generally been used in cholesterol-lowering studies, although seed preparations have also been used.
- **Constipation:** Doses ranging from 7 to 30 g by mouth daily in single or divided doses have been used in studies.
- **Diarrhea:** Doses ranging from 7.5 to 30 g by mouth daily in single or divided doses have been used in studies.
- **Blood sugar lowering:** Doses ranging from 2.2 to 45 g by mouth daily in divided doses, often administered just prior to meals, have been used in studies. Blood sugar levels should be monitored by a qualified healthcare professional.
- **Inflammatory bowel disease:** 7 g by mouth daily in divided doses has been used in studies, although effects are not clearly established.
- **Irritable bowel syndrome:** Doses ranging from 6 to 30 g by mouth daily have been used in studies, although effects are not clearly established.

Children (Younger Than 18 Years)

- **High cholesterol:** 6 to 7 g by mouth daily of psyllium-enriched cereal has been studied, although more research is needed to establish benefits and long-term safety.
- **Diarrhea:** 3 to 4 g by mouth daily has been studied, although more research is needed to establish benefits and long-term safety.
- **Inflammatory bowel disease:** 16 g by mouth daily has been studied, although effects are not clearly established. More

research is needed to establish potential benefits and long-term safety.

SAFETY

The U.S. Food and Drug Administration does not strictly regulate herbs and supplements. There is no guarantee of strength, purity, or safety of products, and effects may vary. It is important to always read product labels. People who have a medical condition, or are taking other drugs, herbs, or supplements, should consult a qualified healthcare provider before starting a new therapy. A healthcare provider should be contacted immediately about any side effects.

Allergies

- Serious allergic reactions, including anaphylaxis, difficulty breathing/wheezing, skin rash, and hives, have been reported after ingestion of psyllium products. Less severe hypersensitivity reactions have also been noted. Cross-sensitivity may occur in people with allergy to English plantain pollen (*Plantago lanceolata*), grass pollen, or melon. Plantain allergy may be associated with latex sensitivity, although it is not clear if this applies to psyllium as well. Workers in the healthcare and pharmaceutical industries can become sensitized and develop allergic respiratory (breathing) symptoms due to handling bulk laxatives containing psyllium powder. Occupational asthma associated with psyllium exposure has been observed. Reactions may also occur from breathing in the dust or from skin contact.

Side Effects and Warnings

- Psyllium-containing laxatives, cereals, and other products are generally believed to be safe. Important exceptions include those with repeated psyllium exposure (such as healthcare workers frequently handling bulk laxatives who are at risk for hypersensitivity reactions), and patients with significant pre-existing bowel abnormalities (such as gastrointestinal strictures or impaired motility) or prior bowel surgery.
- Obstruction of the gastrointestinal tract has been noted in numerous case reports of patients taking psyllium-containing laxatives, particularly in individuals with previous bowel surgery or problems, and/or when the laxatives are mixed with inadequate amounts of water.
- Gastrointestinal side effects are generally mild and have not prompted discontinuation of psyllium in most clinical trials. Flatulence (gas), bloating, diarrhea, and constipation have been reported, and all were less frequent when compared to wheat bran therapy in one study. Since many patients in studies of psyllium have pre-existing bowel concerns, it is difficult to discern which symptoms are caused by psyllium specifically. Esophageal obstruction has been reported in a patient with Parkinson's disease.
- Due to potential reductions in blood sugar levels caused by psyllium, blood glucose levels in diabetic patients should be closely monitored.

Pregnancy and Breastfeeding

- Psyllium-containing laxatives are considered class C-2 drugs in pregnancy, meaning that they appear to be safe in all three trimesters, although studies in pregnant humans and animals have not been done. Psyllium-containing products are considered class 1 (apparently safe) during breastfeeding.

INTERACTIONS

Most herbs and supplements have not been thoroughly tested for interactions with other herbs, supplements, drugs, or foods. The interactions listed here are based on reports in scientific publications, laboratory experiments, or traditional use. It is important to always read product labels. People who have a medical condition, or are taking other drugs, herbs, or supplements, should consult a qualified healthcare provider before starting a new therapy.

Interactions with Drugs

- Psyllium-containing products may delay gastric emptying time and reduce absorption of some drugs. For example, lithium, potassium-sparing diuretics such as spironolactone (Aldactone), carbamazepine, salicylates such as aspirin, tetracyclines, and nitrofurantoin may have decreased absorption when taken with psyllium. Digoxin (Lanoxin) levels may also be affected. It is advised that drugs be taken at separate administration times from psyllium to minimize potential interactions (for example, 1 hour before or a few hours after taking psyllium).
- Although no effect on warfarin (Coumadin) levels with co-administration of psyllium was reported in one study, administration of these agents should be separated until better research is available.
- Because of potential reductions in blood sugar levels caused by psyllium, requirements for insulin or other diabetes drugs in diabetic patients may be reduced. Blood glucose levels should be closely monitored, and dosing adjustments may be necessary.

Interactions with Herbs and Dietary Supplements

- Psyllium-containing products may delay gastric emptying time and reduce absorption of some herbs, supplements, vitamins, or minerals. For example, long-term use of psyllium can reduce absorption of iron, zinc, copper, magnesium and vitamin B_{12}. Absorption of calcium may also be affected. Other agents should be taken 1 hour before or a few hours after psyllium to avoid potential interactions.
- Psyllium and chitosan taken together may increase fat excretion in the stool.

Interactions with Foods

- Psyllium-containing products may delay gastric emptying time and reduce absorption of dietary carbohydrates. Long-term use of psyllium with meals may reduce nutrient absorption, requiring vitamin or mineral supplementation. However, in a review of eight human trials, the use of blond psyllium husk for up to 6 months did not alter vitamin or mineral status.

Selected References

Natural Standard developed the preceding evidence-based information based on a systematic review of more than 275 scientific articles. For comprehensive information about alternative and complementary therapies on the professional level, go to www.naturalstandard.com. Selected references are listed here.

Abraham ZD, Mehta T. Three-week psyllium-husk supplementation: effect on plasma cholesterol concentrations, fecal steroid excretion, and carbohydrate absorption in men. Am J Clin Nutr 1988;47(1):67-74.

Anderson JW, Allgood LD, Lawrence A, et al. Cholesterol-lowering effects of psyllium intake adjunctive to diet therapy in men and women with hypercholesterolemia: meta-analysis of 8 controlled trials. Am J Clin Nutr 2000; 71(2):472-479.

Anderson JW, Allgood LD, Turner J, et al. Effects of psyllium on glucose and serum lipid responses in men with type 2 diabetes and hypercholesterolemia. Am J Clin Nutr 1999;70(4):466-473.

Anderson JW, Davidson MH, Blonde L, et al. Long-term cholesterol-lowering effects of psyllium as an adjunct to diet therapy in the treatment of hypercholesterolemia. Am J Clin Nutr 2000;71(6):1433-1438.

Anderson JW, Floore TL, Geil PB, et al. Hypocholesterolemic effects of different bulk-forming hydrophilic fibers as adjuncts to dietary therapy in mild to moderate hypercholesterolemia. Arch Intern Med 1991;151(8):1597-1602.

Arthurs Y, Fielding JF. Double blind trial of ispaghula/poloxamer in the irritable bowel syndrome. Ir Med J 1983;76(5):253.

Ashraf W, Park F, Lof J, et al. Effects of psyllium therapy on stool characteristics,

colon transit and anorectal function in chronic idiopathic constipation. Aliment Pharmacol Ther 1995;9(6):639-647.

Ashraf W, Park F, Lof J, et al. Effects of psyllium therapy on stool characteristics, colon transit and anorectal function in chronic idiopathic constipation. Aliment Pharmacol Ther 1995;9(6):639-647.

Belknap D, Davidson LJ, Smith CR. The effects of psyllium hydrophilic mucilloid on diarrhea in enterally fed patients. Heart Lung 1997;26(3):229-237.

Barroso Aranda J, Contreras F, Bagchi D, Preuss HG. Efficacy of a novel chitosan formulation on fecal fat excretion: a double-blind, crossover, placebo-controlled study. J Med 2002;33(1-4):209-225.

Bhatnagar D. Should pediatric patients with hyperlipidemia receive drug therapy? Paediatr Drugs 2002;4(4):223-230.

Bianchi M, Capurso L. Effects of guar gum, ispaghula and microcrystalline cellulose on abdominal symptoms, gastric emptying, orocaecal transit time and gas production in healthy volunteers. Dig Liver Dis 2002;34(Suppl 2): S129-S133.

Burton R, Manninen V. Influence of a psyllium-based fibre preparation on faecal and serum parameters. Acta Med Scand Suppl 1982;668:91-94.

Campbell S. Dietary fibre supplementation with psyllium or gum arabic reduced incontinent stools and improved stool consistency in community living adults. Evid Based Nurs 2002;5(2):56.

Cavaliere H, Floriano I, Medeiros-Neto G. Gastrointestinal side effects of Orlistat may be prevented by concomitant prescription of natural fibers (psyllium mucilloid). Int J Obes Relat Metab Disord 2001;25(7):1095-1099.

Chan EK, Schroeder DJ. Psyllium in hypercholesterolemia. Ann Pharmacother 1995;29(6):625-628.

Chapman ND, Grillage MG, Mazumder R, et al. A comparison of mebeverine with high-fibre dietary advice and mebeverine plus ispaghula in the treatment of irritable bowel syndrome: an open, prospectively randomised, parallel group study. Br J Clin Pract 1990;44(11):461-466.

Cherbut C, Bruley d, V, Schnee M, et al. Involvement of small intestinal motility in blood glucose response to dietary fibre in man. Br J Nutr 1994;71(5): 675-685.

Davidson MH, Dugan LD, Burns JH, et al. A psyllium-enriched cereal for the treatment of hypercholesterolemia in children: a controlled, double-blind, crossover study. Am J Clin Nutr 1996;63(1):96-102.

Davidson MH, Maki KC, Kong JC, et al. Long-term effects of consuming foods containing psyllium seed husk on serum lipids in subjects with hypercholesterolemia. Am J Clin Nutr 1998;67(3):367-376.

Dennison BA, Levine DM. Randomized, double-blind, placebo-controlled, two-period crossover clinical trial of psyllium fiber in children with hypercholesterolemia. J Pediatr 1993;123(1):24-29.

Dettmar PW, Sykes J. A multi-centre, general practice comparison of ispaghula husk with lactulose and other laxatives in the treatment of simple constipation. Curr Med Res Opin 1998;14(4):227-233.

Doerfler OC, Ruppert-Kohlmayr AJ, Reittner P, Hinterleitner T, Petritsch W, Szolar DH. Helical CT of the small bowel with an alternative oral contrast material in patients with Crohn's disease. Abdom Imaging 2003;28(3):313-318.

Eherer AJ, Santa Ana CA, Porter J, Fordtran JS. Effect of psyllium, calcium polycarbophil, and wheat bran on secretory diarrhea induced by phenolphthalein. Gastroenterology 1993;104(4):1007-1012.

Everson GT, Daggy BP, McKinley C, Story JA. Effects of psyllium hydrophilic mucilloid on LDL-cholesterol and bile acid synthesis in hypercholesterolemic men. J Lipid Res 1992; 33(8):1183-1192.

Fernandez-Banares F, Hinojosa J, Sanchez-Lombrana JL, et al. Randomised clinical trial of Plantago ovata efficacy as compared to mesalazine in maintaining remission in ulcerative colitis. Gastroenterology 1997;112:A971.

Frape DL, Jones AM. Chronic and postprandial responses of plasma insulin, glucose and lipids in volunteers given dietary fibre supplements. Br J Nutr 1995;73(5):733-751.

Frati Munari AC, Benitez PW, Raul Ariza AC, et al. Lowering glycemic index of food by acarbose and Plantago psyllium mucilage. Arch Med Res 1998; 29(2):137-141.

Frost GS, Brynes AE, Dhillo WS, Bloom SR, McBurney MI. The effects of fiber enrichment of pasta and fat content on gastric emptying, GLP-1, glucose, and insulin responses to a meal. Eur J Clin Nutr 2003;57(2):293-298.

Gaw A. A new reality: achieving cholesterol-lowering goals in clinical practice. Atheroscler Suppl 2002;2(4):5-8; discussion, 8-11.

Gelissen IC, Brodie B, Eastwood MA. Effect of Plantago ovata (psyllium) husk and seeds on sterol metabolism: studies in normal and ileostomy subjects. Am J Clin Nutr 1994;59(2):395-400.

Gupta RR, Agrawal CG, Singh GP, et al. Lipid-lowering efficacy of psyllium hydrophilic mucilloid in non-insulin dependent diabetes mellitus with hyperlipidaemia. Indian J Med Res 1994;100:237-241.

Hallert C, Kaldma M, Petersson BG. Ispaghula husk may relieve gastrointestinal symptoms in ulcerative colitis in remission. Scand J Gastroenterol 1991;26(7): 747-750.

Heather DJ, Howell L, Montana M, et al. Effect of a bulk-forming cathartic on diarrhea in tube-fed patients. Heart Lung 1991;20(4):409-413.

Hermansen K, Dinesen B, Hoie LH, Morgenstern E, Gruenwald J. Effects of soy and other natural products on LDL:HDL ratio and other lipid parameters: a literature review. Adv Ther 2003;20(1):50-78.

Hotz J, Plein K. [Effectiveness of plantago seed husks in comparison with wheat brain on stool frequency and manifestations of irritable colon syndrome with constipation.] Med Klin 1994;89(12):645-651.

P

Hunsaker DM, Hunsaker JC 3rd. Therapy-related cafe coronary deaths: two case reports of rare asphyxial deaths in patients under supervised care. Am J Forensic Med Pathol 2002;23(2):149-154.

Jenkins DJ, Kendall CW, Vuksan V, Vidgen E, Parker T, Faulkner D, Mehling CC,

Garsetti M, Testolin G, Cunnane SC, Ryan MA, Corey PN. Soluble fiber intake at a dose approved by the US Food and Drug Administration for a claim of health benefits: serum lipid risk factors for cardiovascular disease assessed in a randomized controlled crossover trial. Am J Clin Nutr 2002;75(5):834-839.

Juarranz M, Calle-Puron ME, Gonzalez-Navarro A, et al. Physical exercise, use of *Plantago ovata* and aspirin, and reduced risk of colon cancer. Eur J Cancer Prev 2002;11(5):465-472.

Kanauchi O, Mitsuyama K, Araki Y, Andoh A. Modification of intestinal flora in the treatment of inflammatory bowel disease. Curr Pharm Des 2003;9(4):333-346.

Korula J. Dietary fiber supplementation with psyllium or gum arabic reduced fecal incontinence in community-living adults. ACP J Club 2002;136(1):23. Comment in: Nurs Res 2001;50(4):203-213.

Kris-Etherton PM, Taylor DS, Smiciklas-Wright H, Mitchell DC, Bekhuis TC, Olson BH, Slonim AB. High-soluble-fiber foods in conjunction with a telephone-based, personalized behavior change support service result in favorable changes in lipids and lifestyles after 7 weeks. J Am Diet Assoc 2002;102(4):503-10. Comment in: J Am Diet Assoc 2002;102(12):1751.

Kumar A, Kumar N, Vij JC, et al. Optimum dosage of ispaghula husk in patients with irritable bowel syndrome: Correlation of symptom relief with whole gut transit time and stool weight. Gut 1987;28(2):150-155.

Longstreth GF, Fox DD, Youkeles L, et al. Psyllium therapy in the irritable bowel syndrome. A double-blind trial. Ann Intern Med 1981;95(1):53-56.

Maciejko JJ, Brazg R, Shah A, et al. Psyllium for the reduction of cholestyramine-associated gastrointestinal symptoms in the treatment of primary hypercholesterolemia. Arch Fam Med 1994;3(11):955-960.

MacMahon M, Carless J. Ispaghula husk in the treatment of hypercholesterolaemia: a double-blind controlled study. J Cardiovasc Risk 1998;5(3):167-172.

Marlett JA, Fischer MH. A poorly fermented gel from psyllium seed husk increases excreta moisture and bile Acid excretion in rats. J Nutr 2002;132(9):2638-2643.

Marlett JA, Li BU, Patrow CJ, et al. Comparative laxation of psyllium with and without senna in an ambulatory constipated population. Am J Gastroenterol 1987;82(4):333-337.

McRorie JW, Daggy BP, More JG, et al. Psyllium is superior to docusate sodium for treatment of chronic constipation. Aliment Pharmacol Ther 1998;12(5):491-497.

Murphy J, Stacey D, Crook J, Thompson B, Panetta D. Testing control of radiation-induced diarrhea with a psyllium bulking agent: a pilot study. Can Oncol Nurs J 2000;10(3):96-100.

Olson BH, Anderson SM, Becker MP, et al. Psyllium-enriched cereals lower blood total cholesterol and LDL cholesterol, but not HDL cholesterol, in hypercholesterolemic adults: results of a meta-analysis. J Nutr 1997;127(10):1973-1980.

Rai J, Singh J. Ispaghula husk. J Assoc Physicians India 2002;50:576-578.

Reid R, Fodor G, Lydon-Hassen K, D'Angelo MS, McCrea J, Bowlby M, Difrancesco L. Dietary counselling for dyslipidemia in primary care: results of a randomized trial. Can J Diet Pract Res. 2002;63(4):169-75.

Rodriguez-Moran M, Guerrero-Romero F, Lazcano-Burciaga G. Lipid- and glucose-lowering efficacy of Plantago Psyllium in type II diabetes. J Diabetes Complications 1998;12(5):273-278.

Romero AL, West KL, Zern T, Fernandez ML. The seeds from *Plantago ovata* lower plasma lipids by altering hepatic and bile acid metabolism in guinea pigs. J Nutr 2002;132(6):1194-1198.

Roy S, Freake HC, Fernandez ML. Gender and hormonal status affect the regulation of hepatic cholesterol 7-alpha-hydroxylase activity and mRNA abundance by dietary soluble fiber in the guinea pig. Atherosclerosis 2002;163(1):29-37.

Sierra M, Garcia JJ, Fernandez N, et al. Therapeutic effects of psyllium in type 2 diabetic patients. Eur J Clin Nutr 2002;56(9):830-842.

Spence JD, Huff MW, Heidenheim P, et al. Combination therapy with colestipol and psyllium mucilloid in patients with hyperlipidemia. Ann Intern Med 1995;123(7):493-499. Ref ID: 97

van Rosendaal GM, Shaffer EA, Edwards AL et al. Issues raised by psyllium meta-analysis. Am J Clin Nutr 2001; 73(3):653-654.

Voderholzer WA, Schatke W, Muhldorfer BE, et al. Clinical response to dietary fiber treatment of chronic constipation. Am J Gastroenterol 1997;92(1):95-98.

Westerhof W, Das PK, Middelkoop E, et al. Mucopolysaccharides from psyllium involved in wound healing. Drugs Exp Clin Res. 2001;27(5-6):165-75.

Williams CL, Bollella M, Spark A, et al. Soluble fiber enhances the hypocholesterolemic effect of the step I diet in childhood. J Am Coll Nutr 1995;14(3):251-257.

Zaman V, Manzoor SM, Zaki M, et al. The presence of antiamoebic constituents in psyllium husk. Phytother Res 2002;16(1):78-79.

Pycnogenol
(*Pinus pinaster* ssp. atlantica)

SYNONYMS/COMMON NAMES/RELATED SUBSTANCES

- Cocklebut, condensed tannins, French maritime pine bark extract, leucoanthocyanidins, *Pinus pinaster*, *Pinus maritime*, oligomeric proanthocyanidin complexes (OPCs), Pinaceae, proanthocyanidins, pygenol, stickwort.

CLINICAL BOTTOM LINE

Background

- Pycnogenol is the patented trade name for a water extract of the bark of the French maritime pine (*Pinus pinaster* ssp. *atlantica*), which is grown in coastal southwest France. Pycnogenol contains oligomeric proanthocyanidins (OPCs) as well as several other bioflavonoids: catechin, epicatechin, phenolic fruit acids (such as ferulic acid and caffeic acid), and taxifolin.
- There has been some confusion in the U.S. market regarding OPC products containing Pycnogenol or grape seed extract (GSE), because one of the generic terms for chemical constituents ("pycnogenols") is the same as the patented trade name (Pycnogenol). Some GSE products were formerly erroneously labeled and marketed in the U.S. as containing "pycnogenols." Although GSE and Pycnogenol do contain similar chemical constituents (primarily in the OPC fraction), the chemical, pharmacologic, and clinical literature on the two products is distinct. The term Pycnogenol should therefore only be used to refer to this specific proprietary pine bark extract. Scientific literature regarding this product should not be referenced as a basis for the safety or effectiveness of GSE.

Uses Based on Scientific Evidence	Grade*
Chronic venous insufficiency Chronic venous insufficiency (CVI) is a syndrome that includes leg swelling, varicose veins, pain, itching, skin changes, and skin ulcers. The term is more commonly used in Europe than in the United States. Pycnogenol used in people with chronic venous insufficiency is reported to reduce edema and pain. Pycnogenol may also be used in the management of other CVI symptoms.	B
ADHD (attention deficient hyperactivity disorder) Preliminary research comparing Pycnogenol vs. placebo in adults with ADHD reported improved concentration with both agents. After release of this study, Enfamol Nutraceuticals Inc. (maker of Efalex and Efalex Focus) and J&R Research (maker of Pycnogenol) settled a suit with the Federal Trade Commission (FTC) agreeing to no longer advertise these supplements as treatments for ADHD. The companies were not required to pay fines. FTC officials stated they are particularly concerned about dietary supplements with unproven claims being marketed for children. Further research is necessary in this area before a firm conclusion can be reached.	C
Antioxidant Due to conflicting study results, it is unclear if Pycnogenol has significant antioxidant effects in humans. Further research is necessary.	C
Asthma (chronic therapy) Pycnogenol is reported to reduce leukotriene levels in humans, suggesting possible benefits in the chronic management of asthma. Although these data are promising, well-designed controlled study is needed before a firm conclusion can be reached.	C
Erectile dysfunction Pycnogenol, in combination with L-arginine, may cause an improvement in sexual function in men with erectile dysfunction. It is not known what effect each of the individual compounds may have directly on this condition. Further research is needed.	C
Gingival bleeding/plaque Chewing gum containing 5 mg of Pycnogenol is reported to minimize gingival bleeding and plaque formation. Further research is needed to confirm these results.	C
High cholesterol One human trial reports Pycnogenol to significantly reduce low-density lipoprotein (LDL/"bad cholesterol") levels and increased high-density lipoprotein (HDL/"good cholesterol") levels. Other studies have reported decreases in total cholesterol and LDL levels with no change in HDL. Because of conflicting data and methodological problems with available research, further studies are necessary before clear conclusions can be drawn.	C
Male infertility Human studies report that Pycnogenol may improve sperm quality and function in sub-fertile men. Further research is needed to confirm these results.	C
Melasma (chloasma) Melasma (or chloasma) is a common disorder of hyperpigmentation of the skin predominately affecting sun-exposed areas in women. Formation of tan or brown patches/spots may occur. Pycnogenol has been reported to decrease the darkened area and the pigment intensity of melasma and improve symptoms of fatigue, constipation, body pains, and anxiety. Further well-designed research is needed before a clear recommendation can be made.	C
Platelet aggregation One human study reports reduced platelet aggregation in smokers. Further research is needed before a clear conclusion can be reached.	C
Retinopathy Several studies report benefits of Pycnogenol in the treatment and prevention of retinopathy, including	C

P

Continued

slowing the progression of retinopathy in diabetics. Reported mechanisms include improvement of capillary resistance and reduction of leakage into the retina. Improvement of visual acuity has also been reported. Better-quality research is needed before a firm conclusion can be reached.

Sunburn Pycnogenol, taken orally, may reduce erythema (redness of the skin) caused by solar ultraviolet light. Further study is needed before a recommendation can be made.	C
Systemic lupus erythematosus (SLE) Preliminary human and non-human data suggest that Pycnogenol may be useful as a second-line therapy to reduce inflammatory features of SLE. Further research is needed before a recommendation can be made.	C

*Key to grades: *A:* Strong scientific evidence for this use; *B:* Good scientific evidence for this use; *C:* Unclear scientific evidence for this use; *D:* Fair scientific evidence against this use (it may not work); *F:* Strong scientific evidence against this use (it likely does not work). For a more detailed explanation of efficacy criteria, see "Natural Standard Evidence-Based Validated Grading Rationale" in the Introduction.

Historical or Theoretical Indications That Lack Sufficient Evidence

ACE-inhibitor activity, Alzheimer's disease, antihistamine, antiparasitic, atherosclerosis, autoimmune disorders, bone marrow production, cancer prevention, cancer treatment, cardiovascular disease, cerebral ischemia, chemotherapy side effects, exercise capacity, fat burning, G6PD deficiency, gout prevention (xanthine oxidase and dehydrogenase inhibitor), hemorrhoids, high blood pressure, hypoglycemic agent, immune enhancement, immune suppression, inflammation, inhibition of TNF-alpha, increased human growth hormone, lung cancer, premenstrual syndrome, macular degeneration, myocardial ischemia/reperfusion injury, night vision, pelvic pain, neurodegenerative diseases, prevention of fat formation, psoriasis, retinal protection, rheumatoid arthritis, sickle cell anemia, skin disorders, skin aging, vasorelaxant.

DOSING/TOXICOLOGY

The following doses are based on scientific research, publications, traditional use, or expert opinion. Many herbs and supplements have not been thoroughly tested, and safety and effectiveness may not be proven. Brands may be made differently, with variable ingredients even within the same brand. The doses shown may not apply to all products. It is important to always read product labels and discuss doses with a qualified healthcare provider before therapy is started.

Standardization

- Standardization involves measuring the amounts of certain chemicals in products to try to make different preparations similar to each other. It is not always known if the chemicals being measured are the "active" ingredients. Pycnogenol is a proprietary patented formula.

Adults (18 Years and Older)

- *Note:* Pycnogenol appears to be absorbed into the bloodstream in about 20 minutes. Once absorbed, therapeutic effects are purported to last for approximately 72 hours,

followed by excretion in the urine. Because of its astringent taste and occasional minor stomach discomfort, it may be best to take Pycnogenol with or after meals.

- **Antioxidant/cholesterol reduction:** 150-360 mg/day for 4 to 6 weeks has been used.
- **Antiparasitic:** 30 mg/kg/day has been used.
- **Chronic venous insufficiency (CVI):** 100-360 mg/day in divided doses for 1 to 2 months has been used.
- **Asthma chronic therapy):** 1 mg/lb/day (maximum 200 mg/day) for up to 4 weeks has been used.
- **Erectile dysfunction:** A regimen combining Pycnogenol and L-arginine that has been used involves 1.7 g of L-arginine/day during month #1; 1.7 g of L-arginine/day and 40 mg of Pycnogenol 2 times/day during month #2; and 1.7 g of L-arginine/day and 40 mg of Pycnogenol 3 times/day during month #3.
- **Sunburn:** 1.10 mg/kg/day for 4 weeks, followed by 1.66 mg/kg/day for 4 weeks has been used.
- **Gum health (gingival bleeding/plaque):** 5 mg Pycnogenol in chewing gum for 14 days has been used.
- **Male infertility:** 200 mg/day of Pycnogenol for 90 days has been used.
- **Platelet aggregation reduction:** 100 to 200 mg/day has been used.
- **Melasma (chloasma):** 25-mg tablet with meals 3 times a day (75 mg/day) for 30 days has been used.
- **Retinopathy:** 50 mg taken three times a day for 2 months has been used.

Children (Younger Than 18 Years)

- Due to insufficient data, pycnogenol is not recommended for use by children.

SAFETY

The U.S. Food and Drug Administration does not strictly regulate herbs and supplements. There is no guarantee of strength, purity, or safety of products, and effects may vary. It is important to always read product labels. People who have a medical condition, or are taking other drugs, herbs, or supplements, should consult a qualified healthcare provider before starting a new therapy. A healthcare provider should be contacted immediately about any side effects.

Allergies

- Individuals should not take Pycnogenol if allergic to it or any of its components.

Side Effects and Warnings

- Pycnogenol is generally reported as being well tolerated. Low acute and chronic toxicity with mild unwanted effects may occur in a small percentage of patients following oral administration. Because of Pycnogenol's astringent taste and occasional minor stomach discomfort, it may be best to take Pycnogenol with or after meals. To date, no serious adverse effects have been reported in the available scientific literature, although systematic study of safety is not available.
- In theory, Pycnogenol may alter blood sugar levels. Caution is advised in patients with diabetes or hypoglycemia, and in those taking drugs, herbs, or supplements that affect blood sugar. Serum glucose levels may need to be monitored by a healthcare provider, and medication adjustments may be necessary.
- In theory, Pycnogenol may increase the risk of bleeding. Caution is advised in patients with bleeding disorders or taking drugs that may increase the risk of bleeding. Dosing adjustments may be necessary.

Pregnancy and Breastfeeding

- Pycnogenol is not recommended during pregnancy or breastfeeding because of lack of scientific evidence.

INTERACTIONS

Most herbs and supplements have not been thoroughly tested for inter-actions with other herbs, supplements, drugs, or foods. The interactions listed here are based on reports in scientific publications, laboratory experiments, or traditional use. It is important to always read product labels. People who have a medical condition, or are taking other drugs, herbs, or supplements, should consult a qualified healthcare provider before starting a new therapy.

Interactions with Drugs

- Based on mechanism of action, there are potential inter-actions with other antihypertensive medications, specifically angiotensin-converting enzyme inhibitors (ACE-I) such as benazepril (Lotensin), captopril (Capoten), enalapril (Vasotec), fosinopril (Monopril), lisinopril (Prinivil), moexipril (Univasc), perindopril (Aceon), quinapril (Accupril), ramipril (Altace), trandolapril (Mavik), and angiotensin-converting enzyme receptor blockers such as losartan (Cozaar), irbesartan (Avapro), candesartan, cilexetil (Atacand), and valsartan (Diovan).
- Based on mechanism of action, Pycnogenol may lower blood sugar levels. Caution is advised when using medications that may also lower blood sugar levels. Patients taking drugs for diabetes by mouth (such as metformin, glyburide, glipizide) or insulin should be monitored closely by a qualified healthcare provider. Medication adjustments may be necessary.
- Based on mechanism of action, Pycnogenol may increase the risk of bleeding when taken with drugs that increase the risk of bleeding. Some examples include aspirin, anticoagulants ("blood thinners") such as warfarin (Coumadin) and heparin, antiplatelet drugs such as clopidogrel (Plavix), and nonsteroidal anti-inflammatory drugs such as ibuprofen (Motrin, Advil) and naproxen (Naprosyn, Aleve).
- Because of proposed immunomodulating activity, Pycnogenol may interfere with immunosuppressant or immunostimulant drugs.
- In theory, Pycnogenol and antioxidants may have additive effects.

Interactions with Herbs and Dietary Supplements

- Although data have yet to confirm this claim, it has been proposed that Pycnogenol may increase vitamin C levels.
- Based on mechanism of action, Pycnogenol may lower blood sugar levels. Caution is advised when using herbs or supple-ments that may also lower blood sugar levels. Blood glucose levels may require monitoring, and doses may need adjust-ment. Possible examples include *Aloe vera*, American ginseng, bilberry, bitter melon, burdock, dandelion, devil's claw, fenugreek, fish oil, gymnema, horse chestnut seed extract (HCSE), maitake mushroom, marshmallow, melatonin, milk thistle, *Panax ginseng*, rosemary, shark cartilage, Siberian ginseng, stinging nettle, and white horehound.
- In theory, Pycnogenol may increase the risk of bleeding when taken with herbs and supplements that are believed to increase the risk of bleeding. Multiple cases of bleeding have been reported with the use of *Ginkgo biloba*, and fewer cases with garlic and saw palmetto. Numerous other agents may theoretically increase the risk of bleeding, although this has not been proven in most cases. Some examples include alfalfa, American ginseng, angelica, anise, *Arnica montana*, asafetida, aspen bark, bilberry, birch, black cohosh, bladderwrack, bogbean, boldo, borage seed oil, bromelain, capsicum, cat's claw, celery, chamomile, chaparral, clove, coleus, cordyceps, danshen, devil's claw, dong quai, EPA (eicosapentaenoic acid, found in fish oils), evening primrose oil, fenugreek, feverfew, fish oil, flaxseed/flax powder (not a concern with flaxseed oil), ginger, grapefruit juice, grape seed, green tea, guggul, gymnestra, horse chestnut, horse-radish, licorice root, lovage root, male fern, meadowsweet, nordihydroguaiaretic acid (NDGA), omega-3 fatty acids, onion, papain, *Panax ginseng*, parsley, passion flower, poplar, prickly ash, propolis, quassia, red clover, reishi, rue, Siberian ginseng, sweet birch, sweet clover, turmeric, vitamin E, white willow, wild carrot, wild lettuce, willow, wintergreen, and yucca.
- In theory, Pycnogenol may interact with herbs and supple-ments that affect blood pressure. Potential hypotensive herbs include aconite/monkshood, arnica, baneberry, betel nut, bilberry, black cohosh, bryony, calendula, California poppy, coleus, curcumin, eucalyptol, eucalyptus oil, flaxseed/flaxseed oil, garlic, ginger, ginkgo, goldenseal, green hellebore, hawthorn, Indian tobacco, jaborandi, mistletoe, night-blooming cereus, oleander, pasque flower, periwinkle, pleurisy root, *Polypodium vulgare*, shepherd's purse, Texas milkweed, turmeric, wild cherry. Potential hypertensive herbs include American ginseng, arnica, bayberry, betel nut, blue cohosh, broom, cayenne, cola, coltsfoot, ephedra/ma huang, ginger, licorice, and yerba mate.
- Because of proposed immunomodulating activity, Pycnogenol may interfere with immunosuppressant or immunostimulant herbs and supplements.
- In theory, Pycnogenol and other antioxidants may have additive effects.

Selected References

Natural Standard developed the preceding evidence-based information based on a systematic review of more than 70 scientific articles. For comprehensive information about alternative and complementary therapies on the professional level, go to www.naturalstandard.com. Selected references are listed here.

Araghi-Niknam M, Hosseini S, Larson D, et al. Pine bark extract reduces platelet aggregation. Integr Med 2000;2(2):73-77.

Arcangeli P. Pycnogenol in chronic venous insufficiency. Fitoterapia 2000;71(3): 236-244.

Bito T, Roy S, Sen CK, Packer L. Pine bark extract pycnogenol downregulates IFN-gamma-induced adhesion of T cells to human keratinocytes by inhibiting inducible ICAM-1 expression. Free Radic Biol Med 2000;28(2):219-227.

Bors W, Michel C, Stettmaier K. Electron paramagnetic resonance studies of radical species of proanthocyanidins and gallant esters. Arch Biochem Biophys 2000;374(2):347-355.

Buz'Zard AR, Peng Q, Lau BH. Kyolic and Pycnogenol increase human growth hormone secretion in genetically-engineered keratinocytes. Growth Horm IGF Res 2002;12(1):34-40.

Cheshier JE, Ardestani-Kaboudanian S, Liang B, et al. Immunomodulation by pycnogenol in retrovirus-infected or ethanol-fed mice. Life Sci 1996;58(5):PL 87-96.

Chida M, Suzuki K, Nakanishi-Ueda T, et al. *In vitro* testing of antioxidants and biochemical end-points in bovine retinal tissue. Ophthalmic Res 1999; 31(6):407-415.

Cho KJ, Yun CH, Packer L, Chung AS. Inhibition mechanisms of bioflavonoids extracted from the bark of *Pinus maritime* on the expression of proinflammatory cytokines. Ann N Y Acad Sci 2001;928:141-156.

Cho KJ, Yun CH, Yoon DY, et al. Effect of bioflavonoids extracted from the bark of *Pinus maritime* on proinflammatory cytokine interleukin-1 production in lipopolysaccharide-stimulated RAW 264.7. Toxicol Appl Pharmacol 2000; 168(1):64-71.

Devaraj S, Vega-Lopez S, Kaul S, et al. Supplementation with a pine bark extract rich in polyphenols increases plasma antioxidant capacity and alters the plasma lipoprotein profile. Lipids 2002;37(10):931-934.

Feng WH, Wei HL, Liu GT. Effect of PYCNOGENOL on the toxicity of heart, bone marrow and immune organs as induced by antitumor drugs. Phytomedicine 2002;9(5):414-418.

Fitzpatrick DF, Bing B, Rohdewald P. Endothelium-dependent vascular effects of Pycnogenol. J Cardiovasc Pharmacol 1998;32(4):509-515.

P

Hasegawa N. Inhibition of lipogenesis by pycnogenol. Phytother Res 2000; 14(6):472-473.

Hasegawa N. Stimulation of lipolysis by pycnogenol. Phytother Res 1999; 13(7):619-620.

Horakova L, Licht A, Sandig G, et al. Standardized extracts of flavonoids increase the viability of PC12 cells treated with hydrogen peroxide: effects on oxidative injury. Arch Toxicol 2003;77(1):22-29.

Hosseini S, Pishnamazi S, Sadrzadeh SM, et al. Pycnogenol in the management of Asthma. J Med Food 2001;4(4):201-209.

Huynh HT, Teel RW. Effects of intragastrically administered Pycnogenol on NNK metabolism in F344 rats. Anticancer Res 1999;19(3A):2095-2099.

Huynh HT, Teel RW. Effects of pycnogenol on the microsomal metabolism of the tobacco-specific nitrosamine NNK as a function of age. Cancer Lett 1998; 132(1-2):135-139.

Huynh HT, Teel RW. Selective induction of apoptosis in human mammary cancer cells (MCF-7) by pycnogenol. Anticancer Res 2000;20(4):2417-2420.

Kim HC, Healey JM. Effects of pine bark extract administered to immuno-suppressed adult mice infected with *Cryptosporidium parvum*. Am J Chin Med 2001;29(3-4):469-475.

Kim J, Chehade J, Pinnas JL, Mooradian AD. Effect of select antioxidants on malodialdehyde modification of proteins. Nutrition 2000;16(11-12): 1079-1081.

Kimbrough C, Chun M, dela Roca G, Lau BH. pycnogenol chewing gum minimizes gingival bleeding and plaque formation. Phytomedicine 2002; 9(5):410-413.

Kobayashi MS, Han D, Packer L. Antioxidants and herbal extracts protect HT-4 neuronal cells against glutamate-induced cytotoxicity. Free Radic Res 2000; 32(2):115-124.

Koch R. Comparative study of Venostasin and Pycnogenol in chronic venous insufficiency. Phytother Res 2002;16(Suppl 1):S1-S5.

Liu F, Lau BH, Peng Q, Shah V. Pycnogenol protects vascular endothelial cells from beta-amyloid-inducted injury. Biol Pharm Bull 2000;23(6):735-737.

Liu FJ, Zhang YX, Lau BH. Pycnogenol enhances immune and haemopoietic functions in senescence-accelerated mice. Cell Mol Life Sci 1998;54(10): 1168-1172.

Macrides TA, Shihata A, Kalafatis N, Wright PF. A comparison of the hydroxyl radical scavenging properties of the shark bile steroid 5 beta-scymnol and plant pycnogenols. Biochem Mol Biol Int 1997;42(6):1249-1260.

Maritim A, Dene BA, Sanders RA, Watkins JB 3rd. Effects of pycnogenol treatment on oxidative stree in streptozotocin-induced diabetic rats. J Biochem Mol Toxicol 2003;17(3):193-199.

Masquelier J. Flavonoids and pycnogenols. Int J Vitam Nutr Res 1979;49: 307-11.

Moini H, Guo Q, Packe L. Xanthine oxidase and xanthine dehydrogenase inhibition by the procyanidin-rich French maritime pine bark extract, pycnogenol: a protein binding effect. Adv Exp Med Biol 2002;505:141-149.

Moini H, Guo Q, Packer L. Enzyme inhibition and protein-binding action of procyanidin-rich French maritime pine bark extract, pycnogenol: effect on xanthine oxidase. J Agric Food Chem 2000;48(11):5630-5639.

Nelson A, Lau B, Ide N, Rong Y. Pycnogenol inhibits macrophage oxidative burst, lipoprotein oxidation, and hydroxyl radical induced DNA damage. Drug Devel Industr Pharm 1998; 24:139-44.

Ni Z, Mu Y, Gulati O. Treatment of melasma with Pycnogenol. Phytother Res 2002;16(6):567-571.

Noda Y, Anzai K, Mori A, Kohno M, et al. Hydroxyl and superoxide anion radical scavenging activities of natural source antioxidants using the computerized JES-FR30 ESR spectrometer system. Biochem Mol Biol Int 1997;42(1):35-44.

Ohnishi ST, Ohnishi T, Ogunmola GB. Sickle cell anemia: a potential nutritional approach for a molecular disease. Nutrition 2000;16(5):330-338.

Packer L, Rimbach G, Virgili F. Antioxidant activity and biologic properties of a procyanidin-rich extract from pine (*Pinus maritime*) bark, pycnogenol. Free Radic Biol Med 1999;27(5-6):704-724.

Park YC, Rimbach G, Saliou C, et al. Activity of monomeric , dimeric, and trimeric flavonoids on NO production, TNF-alpha secretion, and NF-kappaB-dependent gene expression in RAW 264.7 macrophages. FEBS Lett 2000; 465(2-3):93-97.

Peng Q, Wei Z, Lau BH. Pycnogenol inhibits tumor necrosis factor-alpha-induced nuclear factor kappa B activation and adhesion molecule expression in human vascular endothelial cells. Cell Mol Life Sci 2000;57(5):834-841.

Peng QL, Buz'Zard AR, Lau BH. Pycnogenol protects neurons from amyloid-beta peptide-induced apoptosis. Brain Res Mol Brain Res 2002;104(1):55-65.

Petrassi C, Mastromarino A, Spartera C. pycnogenol in chronic venous insufficiency. Phytomedicine 2000;7(5):383-388.

Putter M. Grotemeyer KH, Wurthwein G, et al. Inhibition of smoking-induced platelet aggregation by aspirin and Pycnogenol. Thromb Res 1999;95(4): 155-161.

Rihn B, Saliou C, Bottin MC, et al. From ancient remedies to modern therapeutics: pine bark uses in skin disorders revisited. Phytother Res 2001;15(1):76-78.

Rohdewald P. A review of the French maritime pine bark extract (Pycnogenol), a herbal medication with a diverse clinical pharmacology. Int J Clin Pharmacol Ther 2002;40(4):158-168.

Rong Y, Li L, Shah V, Lau BH. Pycnogenol protects vascular endothelial cells from t-butyl hydroperoxide induced oxidant injury. Biotechnol Ther 1994-95;5(3-4):117-126.

Roseff SJ. Improvement of sperm quality and function with French maritime pine tree bark extract. J Reprod Med 2002;47(10):821-824.

Saliou C, Rimbach G, Moini H, et al. Solar ultraviolet-induced erythema in human skin and nuclear factor-kappa-B-dependent gene expression in keratinocytes are modulated by a French maritime pine bark extract. Free Radic Biol Med 2001;30(2):154-160.

Schonlau F, Rohdewald P. Pycnogenol for diabetic retinopathy. A review. Int Ophthalmol 2001;24(3):161-171.

Sharma SC, Sharma S, Gulati OP. Pycnogenol inhibits the release of histamine from mast cells. Phytother Res 2003;17(1):66-69.

Sharma SC, Sharma S, Gulati OP. Pycnogenol prevents haemolytic injury in G6PD deficient human erythrocytes. Phytother Res 2003;17(6):671-674.

Silliman K, Parry J, Kirk LL, Prior RL. Pycnogenol does not impact the antioxidant or vitamin C status of health young adults. J Am Diet Assoc 2003; 103(1):67-72.

Spadea L, Balestrazzi E. Treatment of vascular retinopathies with Pycnogenol. Phytother Res 2001;15(3):219-223.

Stanislavov R, Nikolova V. Treatment of erectile dysfunction with pycnogenol and L-arginine. J Sex Marital Ther 2003;29(3):207-213.

Stefanescu M, Matach C, Onu A, et al. Pycnogenol efficacy in the treatment of systemic lupus erythematosus. Phytother Res 2001;15(8):698-704.

Suarez-Almazor ME, Kendall CJ, Dorgan M. Surfing the Net – information on the World Wide Web for persons with arthritis: patient empowerment or patient deceit? J Rheumatol 2001;28(1):185-191.

Tenebaum S, Paull JC, Sparrow EP. An experimental comparison of Pycnogenol and methylphenidate in adults with Attention-Deficit/Hyperactivity Disorder (ADHD). J Atten Disord 2002;6(2):49-60.

van Jaarsveld H, Kuyl JM, Schulenburg DH, Wiid NM. Effect of flavonoids on the outcome of myocaridial mitochondrial ischemia/reperfusion injury. Res Commun Mol Pathol Pharmacol 1996;91(1):65-75.

Veurink G, Liu D, Taddei K, et al. Reduction of inclusion body pathology in ApoE-deficient mice fed a combination of antioxidants. Free Radic Biol Med 2003;34(8):1070-1077.

Virgili F, Kim D, Packer L. Procyanidins extracted from pine bark protect alpha-tocopherol in ECV 304 endothelial cells challenged by activated RAW 264.7 macrophages: role of nitric oxide and peroxynitrite. FEBS Lett 1998;431(3): 315-318.

Virgili F, Kobuchi H, Packer L. Procyanidins extracted from *Pinus maritime* (Pycnogenol): scavengers of free radical species and modulators of nitrogen monoxide metabolism in activated murine RAW 264.7 macrophages. Free Radic Biol Med 1998;24(7-8):1120-1129.

Wang MY, Su C. Cancer preventive effect of Morinda *citrifolia* (Noni). Ann N Y Acad Sci 2001;952:161-168.

Watson, R. (1999). Reduction of cardiovascular disease risk factors by French Maritime Pine Bark Extract. Cardiovascular Reviews and Reports, XX(VI): 326-329.

Wei Z, Peng Q, Lau B. Pycnogenol enhances endothelial cell antioxidant defenses. Redox Report 1997;3:219-24.

Pygeum
(Pygeum africanum, Prunus africana)

SYNONYMS/COMMON NAMES/RELATED SUBSTANCES

- African plum tree, African prune tree, African *Pygeum africanum* extract, alumty, iluo, kirah, natal tree, *Pigeum africanum*, Pigenil, Pronitol, Provol, prunier d'afrique, *Pygeum africana*, Rosaceae, Tadenan, V1326, vla, wotangue.

CLINICAL BOTTOM LINE
Background

- The *Pygeum africanum* (African plum) tree is a tall evergreen of the family Rosaceae found in central and southern Africa. Its bark has been used medicinally for thousands of years. Traditional African healers have used the bark to treat bladder and micturition (urination) disorders, particularly symptoms associated with benign prostatic hypertrophy (BPH). Historically, the bark was powdered and used to make a tea, which was taken by mouth for these conditions.
- The African plum tree has become endangered due to the demand for its bark to process *P. africanum* extract.
- The majority of trials conducted since the 1970s report improvements in BPH symptoms with the administration of *P. africanum* bark extract, including frequency of nocturia (nighttime urination), urinary flow rate, and residual urine volume. This research has led some credibility to the common use of this agent in Europe for BPH. The herb is less commonly used in the United States, where prescription drugs or the herb saw palmetto is more commonly used.

Scientific Evidence for Common/Studied Uses	Grade*
Benign prostatic hypertrophy (BPH) symptoms	B

*Key to grades: A: Strong scientific evidence for this use; B: Good scientific evidence for this use; C: Unclear scientific evidence for this use; D: Fair scientific evidence against this use (it may not work); F: Strong scientific evidence against this use (it likely does not work). For a more detailed explanation of efficacy criteria, see "Natural Standard Evidence-Based Validated Grading Rationale" in the Introduction.

Historical or Theoretical Indications
That Lack Sufficient Evidence

- Aphrodisiac, bladder sphincter disorders, fever, impotence, inflammation, kidney disease, malaria, male baldness, partial bladder outlet obstruction, prostate cancer, prostatic adenoma, prostatitis, psychosis, sexual performance, stomach upset, urinary tract health.

Expert Opinion and Historic/Folkloric Precedent

- Traditional African healers used the bark of *P. africanum* to treat bladder and micturition disorders consistent with symptomatic benign prostatic hypertrophy (BPH). Other uses included inflammation, kidney disease, malaria, stomachache, fever, and as an aphrodisiac.[1]
- The majority of trials conducted since the 1970s report improvement in BPH symptoms, including frequency of nocturia, urinary flow rate, and residual urine volume, with the administration of *P. africanum* extract, lending credibility to its popular use in Europe.

Safety Summary

- **Likely safe:** When used orally in otherwise healthy men for the treatment of mild to moderate symptomatic benign prostatic hypertrophy (PBH) in doses of 100 mg per day for up to 1 year.[2,3]
- **Possibly unsafe:** When used in doses greater than recommended or with long-term use; when used orally during pregnancy or lactation; when used in pediatric patients.
- *Note:* The formulation of *P. africanum* most commonly used in clinical trials is Tadenan. No long-term studies have been conducted on the effects of *P. africanum* extract. BPH is not a self-diagnosed or self-limiting disease, and it is recommended that patients use *P. africanum* extract under the supervision of a licensed healthcare professional.

DOSING/TOXICOLOGY
General

- *Note:* Recommended doses are based on those most commonly used in available trials, or on historical practice. However, with natural products, the optimal doses needed to balance efficacy and safety often have not been determined. Formulations and preparation methods may vary from manufacturer to manufacturer, and from batch to batch of a specific product made by a single manufacturer. Because often the active components of a product are not known, standardization may not be possible, and the clinical effects of different brands may not be comparable.

Standardization

- The active component(s) of *Pygeum africanum* bark extract has not been identified. Tadenan (Laboratoires DEBAT, Garches, France), the most popular and commonly studied brand in Europe, is a lipophilic extract of *P. africanum* standardized to 13% total sterols. Other guidelines specify standardization to 14% triterpenes with 0.5% n-docosanol.[4] One capsule of Tadenan contains 50 mg of standardized extract.
- Other studied brands include Pigenil (Inverni della Beffa, Milan, Italy), Harzol (Hoyer, Germany), and Prostatonin (Pharmaton SA, Lugano, Switzerland). Some brands contain other herbs in addition to pygeum.
- Safety of use of pygeum beyond 12 months has not been reliably studied.

Dosing: Adults (18 Years and Older)

- **Capsules:** For treating benign prostatic hypertrophy, 75- to 200-mg capsules of standardized pygeum extract taken daily by mouth either as a single dose or divided into two equal doses have been used and studied.[2,3]

Dosing: Pediatric (Younger Than 18 Years)

- There is not sufficient scientific information to recommend pygeum for use in children.

Toxicology

- *Pygeum africanum* extract in a dosage of 50-100 mg/kg per day for 52 days in rats had no toxic effect on blood chemistry or on testes, prostate, adrenal, and kidney function.[5] An *in vitro* study evaluating the effect of *P. africanum* extract on fibroblast proliferation in rat prostatic cells observed the recovery of prostatic cell growth after 24-hour incubation with the extract and found *P. africanum* to be cytostatic.[6]

ADVERSE EFFECTS/PRECAUTIONS/CONTRAINDICATIONS
Allergies
- People with known allergies to pygeum should avoid this herb.

Side Effects and Warnings
- **General:** Pygeum has been well tolerated in most studies, with adverse effects similar to placebo.[7-9] However, safety of pygeum has not been extensively or systematically studied; safety of use beyond 12 months has not been reliably studied.
- **Gastrointestinal:** Some people may experience abdominal discomfort, including diarrhea, constipation, stomach pain, and nausea. Stomach upset is usually mild and does not typically cause people to stop using pygeum.[10,11]
- **Genitourinary:** *P. africanum* extract appears to inhibit human prostatic 5 alpha-reductase (IC$_{50}$ 63,000 ng/mL), but much less powerfully than the prescription drug finasteride (IC$_{50}$ 1.0 ng/mL).[12] In theory, prostate-specific antigen (PSA) serum values may be reduced with the use of 5 alpha-reductase inhibitors, masking otherwise elevated levels. Patients with prostate cancer should discuss the use of any 5 alpha-reductase inhibitor (drug or herb such as pygeum and saw palmetto) with their oncologist or urologist.

Precautions/Warnings/Contraindications
- Use caution in patients taking 5 alpha-reductase inhibitors such as finasteride (Proscar) or saw palmetto.

Pregnancy and Lactation
- Pygeum cannot be recommended during pregnancy or lactation because of a lack of scientific information and possible hormonal effects.

INTERACTIONS
Interactions with Drugs
- **5 alpha-reductase inhibitors:** 5 alpha-reductase inhibitors such as terazosin (Hytrin) and finasteride (Proscar) are commonly used to treat symptoms of prostate enlargement and may increase the effects of pygeum, although this is not well studied. Pygeum extract appears to inhibit human prostatic 5 alpha-reductase (IC$_{50}$, 63,000 ng/mL), but much less powerfully than finasteride (IC$_{50}$, 1.0 ng/mL).[12] In theory, prostate specific-antigen (PSA) values in serum may be reduced with the use of 5 alpha-reductase inhibitors, masking otherwise elevated levels. Patients with prostate cancer should discuss the use of any 5 alpha-reductase inhibitor (drug or herb such as pygeum and saw palmetto) with their oncologist or urologist.
- **Hormonal therapies:** In theory, pygeum may interact with estrogen or other hormones.[13,14]

Interactions with Herbs and Dietary Supplements
- **Saw palmetto (*Serenoa repens*), stinging nettle (*Urtica dioica*):** Pygeum may result in increased effects on the prostate if used with saw palmetto (*Serenoa repens*) or stinging nettle (*Urtica dioica*).[15] Combination products are available containing both stinging nettle and pygeum.
- **Estrogenic herbs:** Pygeum may interact with herbs/supplements containing chemicals with estrogen-like constituents ("phytoestrogens"). Possible examples include alfalfa, black cohosh, bloodroot, burdock, hops, kudzu, licorice, pomegranate, red clover, soy, thyme, white horehound, and yucca.

MECHANISM OF ACTION
Pharmacology
- **General:** Multiple mechanisms have been proposed for the genitourinary effects of pygeum, including 5 alpha-reductase inhibition, estrogenic effects, and anti-inflammatory properties.
- **Genitourinary effects:** *Pygeum africanum* extract appears to inhibit human prostatic 5 alpha-reductase (IC$_{50}$, 63,000 ng/mL), but much less powerfully than finasteride (IC$_{50}$, 1.0 ng/mL).[12] Reduction of urethral obstruction and improvement of bladder function have been observed.[16] Most studies of *P. africanum* extract have addressed outcomes related to the obstructive component. In rats, pygeum inhibits dihydrotestosterone-induced prostate hyperplasia[17] by a mechanism that appears unrelated to androgen receptor blockade.[12] In rats and men, *P. africanum* extract has been found to stimulate secretory activity of the prostate and seminal vesicles.[5,18] Reduction of contractile dysfunction of the bladder caused by partial outlet obstruction has been observed with pre-treatment of rabbits with *P. africanum* extract (Tadenan, 1 to 100 mg/kg/day).[19]
- **Anti-inflammatory effects:** *In vitro* studies report that *P. africanum* extract inhibits production of 5-lipoxygenase metabolites at concentrations of 3 µg/mL when dissolved in DMSO, and 10 µg/mL when dissolved in NaOH/HCl ($p<0.01$).[20,21] *P. africanum* inhibits fibroblast proliferation induced by epidermal growth factor (EGF; IC$_{50}$ = 4.5 µg/mL), insulin-like growth factor type I (IGF-I; IC$_{50}$ = 7.7 µg/mL), and basic fibroblast growth factor (bFGF; IC$_{50}$ = 12.6 µg/mL) *in vitro*.[6]
- **Hormonal properties:** *P. africanum* extract appears to possess phytoestrogenic properties.[14]

Pharmacodynamics/Kinetics
- Insufficient evidence available.

HISTORY
- The bark of *Pygeum africanum* (the African plum tree) has been used medicinally for thousands of years. Traditional African healers used the bark to treat bladder and micturition (urination) disorders, particularly symptoms associated with benign prostatic hypertrophy (BPH). Other uses included inflammation, kidney disease, malaria, stomachache, fever, and as an aphrodisiac.[1] Historically, the bark was powdered and used to make a tea, which was taken by mouth for these conditions.
- Since the 1960s, *P. africanum* extract has been used in Western clinical practice, especially in France and Italy, where most clinical trials evaluating efficacy in benign prostatic hypertrophy (BPH) have been conducted.
- The African plum tree is a tall evergreen of the family Rosaceae, found in central and southern Africa. It has become endangered due to the demand for its bark to process *P. africanum* extract for medicinal use.

REVIEW OF THE EVIDENCE: DISCUSSION
Benign prostatic hypertrophy (BPH) symptoms
Summary
- Pygeum (*Pygeum africanum* bark extract) has been observed to moderately improve urinary symptoms associated with enlargement of the prostate gland or prostate inflammation.

Review of the Evidence: Pygeum

Condition Treated*	Study Design	Author, Year	N[†]	SS[†]	Study Quality[‡]	Magnitude of Benefit	ARR[†]	NNT[†]	Comments
BPH	Systematic review and meta-analysis	Wilt[8] 2002	1562 (18 trials)	Yes	NA	Moderate	NA	NA	Mean study duration, 64 days (30-122 days); moderately large improvement in combined outcome of urologic symptoms and flow; men using pygeum were 2.1 times as likely to report improvement in overall symptoms. Nocturia reduced 19%; residual urine volume reduced 24%; peak urinary flow increased 23%. No studies compared pygeum to alpha-adrenergic blockers or 5 alpha-reductase inhibitors.
BPH	Systematic review; meta-analysis	Ishani[9] 2000	18 studies	Yes	NA	Small-moderate	NA	NA	No common outcome or dosage among studies.
BPH	Systematic review	Andro[7] 1995	12 studies	NA	NA	Small-moderate	NA	NA	No meta-analysis; unclear inclusion/exclusion criteria.
BPH	RCT, double-blind, placebo-controlled	Barlet[10] 1990	263	Yes	4	Large	35%	3	Superior design compared to other available studies; efficacy reported for multiple urological endpoints.
BPH	RCT, double-blind, placebo- controlled	Bassi[4] 1987	40	Yes	2	Small	69% for urgency (varies by symptom)	2	Efficacy in terms of urologic symptoms and urinary flow.
BPH	RCT	Blitz[22] 1985	57	Yes	1	Medium	33	3	Randomization and blinding methods not described; statistical significance for symptom improvement.
BPH	RCT, double-blind, placebo controlled	Bongi[23] 1972	50	Yes	3	Large	76%	2	Early study reporting functional and morphologic benefits.
BPH	Uncontrolled, open trial	Breza[24] 1998	85	Yes	1	Small	NA	NA	No control group, no blinding; no randomization.
BPH	8-week randomized, double-blind comparison trial, followed by 40-week open-phase trial	Chatelain[3] 1999	209 in trial 1; 174 in trial 2	No	3	NA	NA	NA	50 mg twice daily vs. 100 mg daily of pygeum; both doses reported as equally efficacious and safe.
BPH	RCT, double-blind, placebo-controlled	Donkervoort[25] 1977	20	No	4	None	NA	NA	Small study; higher dose used than other trials (620 mg/day).
BPH	RCT, double-blind, placebo-controlled	Dufour[26] 1984	120	Yes	2	NA	29%	4	Improvement in symptoms reported.
BPH	Comparison trial	Dutkiewicz[27] 1996	89	Yes	3	Negative (inferior)	23%	4	4 months of Cernilton (cernitin pollen extract) (n = 51) vs. Tadenan (n = 38); significant subjective improvement reported in 78% of patients vs. 55% of Tadenan patients.
BPH	RCT, placebo-controlled	Frasseto[28] 1986	20	Yes	1	Large	NA	NA	Reported efficacy in reducing symptoms; poor study design.
BPH	Randomized, double-blind, placebo-controlled equivalence trial (vs. anti-inflammatory therapy)	Gagliardi[29] 1983	40	Yes	3-5	Large	NA	NA	Relative efficacy in comparison with anti-inflammatory treatment.

Continued

Review of the Evidence: Pygeum—*cont'd*

Condition Treated*	Study Design	Author, Year	N[†]	SS[†]	Study Quality[‡]	Magnitude of Benefit	ARR[†]	NNT[†]	Comments
BPH	Randomized, double-blind, dosing trial	Krzeski[15] 1993	134	No	4	None	NA	NA	Both study arms improved compared to baseline, but the two dosages were found equivalent.
BPH	RCT, double-blind, placebo-controlled	Mandressi[31] 1983	60	Yes	3	Large	NA	NA	Comparison of saw palmetto vs. *P. africanum* extract vs. placebo.
BPH	RCT, double-blind, placebo-controlled	Maver[32] 1972	60	Yes	3	Large	NA	NA	No adverse effects reported.
BPH	Crossover trial	Mehrsai[33] 1997	26	NA	1	NA	NA	NA	Favorable effects on symptoms of BPH, but no statistical comparison presented; not blinded.
BPH	Randomized, comparative study	Pavone-Macaluso 1997	128	No	1	None	−25%	−4	Active control group used, with no proven efficacy in treating BPH.
BPH	Double-blind study	Ranno[33] 1986	39	No	2	Large	NA	NA	Not randomized; methodologically weak.
BPH	RCT, double-blind, placebo-controlled	Rigatti[35] 1983	39	Yes	3	Large	NA	NA	Methodologically weak.

*Primary or secondary outcome.
[†]*N*, Number of patients; *SS*, statistically significant; *ARR*, absolute risk reduction; *NNT*, the number of patients who need to undergo a specific intervention in order to observe an outcome in one individual.
[‡]0-2 = poor; 3-4 = good; 5 = excellent.
BPH, Benign prostatic hypertrophy; *NA*, not applicable; *RCT*, randomized, controlled trial.
For an explanation of each category in this table, please see Table 3 in the Introduction.

Numerous controlled trials in humans[2-4,7,10,11,15,19,22-36] and studies that combine the results of other research (meta-analyses,[7-9] report that pygeum significantly reduces the number of nighttime urinary episodes (nocturia), urinary hesitancy, urinary frequency, and dysuria (pain with urination) in men who experience mild to moderate symptoms. However, pygeum does not appear to reduce the size of the prostate gland or reverse the process of BPH. It is unclear how pygeum compares to the effectiveness or safety of other medical therapies, such as prescription drugs (e.g., alpha-adrenergic blockers and 5 alpha-reductase inhibitors), surgical approaches, or other herbs/supplements (e.g., saw palmetto). Although many of the available studies are not well designed or reported, the weight of scientific evidence supports the benefits of pygeum. Better research would strengthen the scientific support for this therapy, and there is ongoing study in this area. It is recommended that patients with BPH speak with their healthcare provider about the various available treatment options.

Evidence

• Most studies have used the European brand Tadenan. The mechanism of action of pygeum remains unclear. Early research reports reductions in urethral obstruction and improved bladder function.[16,17,19,37,38] Laboratory studies report inhibition of enzymes including 5-lipoxygenase[20] and 5 alpha-reductase,[12] by a mechanism similar to the prescription drug finasteride. Stimulation of secretory activity of the prostate and seminal vesicles is reported in rats and humans,[5,18] and some estrogen-like properties are noted[14] as well as anti-inflammatory properties.[6]

• In 2002, Wilt et al. conducted a systematic review and meta-analysis to investigate the evidence surrounding the use of pygeum in the treatment of BPH.[8] The authors searched for trials in multiple databases, including MEDLINE, Embase, the Cochrane Library, and Phytodok, by checking bibliographies, and by contacting relevant manufacturers and researchers. Trials were eligible if they were randomized, included men with BPH, compared preparations of *Pygeum africanum* (alone or in combination) with placebo or other BPH medications, and if they included clinical outcomes such as urologic symptom scales, symptoms, or urodynamic measurements. The main outcome measure for adverse effects was the number of men reporting adverse effects. A total of 18 randomized controlled trials involving 1562 men met inclusion criteria and were analyzed. Only one of the studies reported a method of treatment allocation concealment, although 17 were double-blinded. There were no studies comparing *Pygeum africanum* to standard pharmacologic interventions such as alpha-adrenergic blockers and 5 alpha-reductase inhibitors. The mean study duration was 64 days (range, 30 to 122 days). According to the authors, most studies did not report results in a method that permitted meta-analysis. Compared to men receiving placebo, pygeum provided a moderately large improvement in the combined outcome of urologic symptoms and flow measures as assessed by an effect size defined by the difference of the mean change for each outcome divided by the pooled standard deviation for each outcome (−0.8 SD [95% CI, −1.4, −0.3]; n = 6 studies). Men using pygeum were more than twice as likely to report an improvement in overall symptoms (RR = 2.1; 95% CI, 1.4, 3.1). Nocturia was reduced by 19%, residual urine volume by 24%, and peak urine flow was increased by 23%. Adverse effects due to pygeum were mild and comparable to placebo. The overall dropout rate was 12% and was similar for pygeum (13%), placebo (11%), and other controls (8%). Although the authors concluded that standardized preparations of pygeum may be a useful treatment option for men with lower urinary symptoms consistent with BPH, they noted that further research is necessary, as the reviewed studies overall were small in size, short in duration, used varied doses/preparations, and rarely reported outcomes using standardized validated measures of efficacy.

- In 2000, Ishani et al. conducted a systematic review and meta-analysis of 18 randomized controlled trials that evaluated the efficacy of pygeum extract in the treatment of symptomatic BPH.[9] Out of 31 randomized trials with a duration of 30 days or greater, 18 matched the inclusion criteria for this analysis. All 18 trials were conducted in Europe and included a total of 1562 subjects. Ten trials compared *P. africanum* to placebo,[4,10,22,23,25,26,28,32,34,36] 2 trials evaluated *P. africanum* versus an anti-inflammatory drug,[29,35] 1 study compared *P. africanum* to both placebo and *P. africanum* plus medroxyprogesterone,[30] 1 trial compared once-daily versus twice-daily dosing of *P. africanum*,[3] 2 trials compared *P. africanum* combined with another herbal vs. placebo,[31,39] 1 trial compared *P. africanum* to another herbal agent,[27] and 1 trial compared two different doses of *P. africanum* plus *Urtica dioica*.[15] The doses of *P. africanum* extract used in trials varied from 75 mg to 200 mg daily. The data were pooled using two methods: First, for summarizing trials with various outcome measures, treatment effect size for continuous variables was assessed by dividing the difference of the mean change for each outcome by the pooled standard deviation for that outcome. Second, effect size was estimated using the most clinically important outcome per study, according to the following preference scale: symptom score > nocturia > peak urine flow > residual urine volume. The summary effect size (difference in mean outcome divided by the pooled standard deviation for that outcome) was then assessed using the following key: 0.8 = large effect, 0.5 = moderate effect, 0.2 = small effect. Among 474 men from 6 trials comparing *P. africanum* to placebo, summary effect size was calculated to be −0.8 (95% CI, −1.4 to −0.3), which suggests a large, statistically significant improvement in symptomatic BPH with *P. africanum* compared to placebo. Furthermore, men taking *P. africanum* were 2.1 (95% CI, 1.4 to 3.4) times more likely to experience an overall improvement of symptoms than those taking placebo, and they also experienced a 19% reduction in nocturia compared to those taking placebo (weighted mean difference of −0.9). The latter two results, however, were not statistically significant (95% CI, −2.0 to 0.1). Peak urine flow, as analyzed from 4 trials (363 subjects), was significantly increased by 23% compared to placebo (95% CI, 0.3 to 4.7). For none of the effect measures, in none of the analyzed studies, was control treatment superior to *P. africanum* extract. Only 1 study did not find a difference between both treatments in terms of overall improvement. No studies compared pygeum to conventional treatments for BPH such as 5 alpha-reductase inhibitors and alpha-adrenergic blockers (or saw palmetto).

- In 1995, Andro and Riffuad performed a systematic review of 12 blinded, placebo-controlled trials assessing the efficacy of pygeum in the treatment of BPH.[7] The authors concluded that pygeum extract is a safe and effective treatment for mild to moderate BPH. All included studies[4,10,22,23,25,26,28,30,32,34,36] were also included in the Ishani analysis.[9]

FORMULARY: BRANDS USED IN CLINICAL TRIALS
Brands Used in Statistically Significant Clinical Trials

- Tadenan (Laboratoires DEBAT, Garches, France)[10,22,23,25,26,28,30,34,36]; Pigenil (Inverni della Beffa, Milan, Italy)[4]; Harzol (Hoyer, Germany) [11]; Prostatonin (a combination product containing 300 mg of *Urtica dioica* extract and 25 mg of *P. africanum* extract) (Pharmaton SA, Lugano, Switzerland).[15]

U.S. Equivalents of Most Commonly Recommended European Brands

- Provol (Upsher-Smith); Nature's Way Standardized Pygeum (standardized to 13% sterols); Solaray African Pygeum Bark Extract (standardized to 13% sterols); VitaHealthy Pygeum Bark Extract (standardized to 3 mg phytosterols).

References

1. McQueen CE, Bryant PJ. Pygeum. Am J Health Syst Pharm 2001;58(2):120-123.
2. Brackman F, Autet W. Once and twice daily dosage regimens of *Pygeum africanum* extract (PA): a double-blind study in patients with benign prostatic hyperplasia (BPH) [abstract]. J Urology 1999;161(4S):361.
3. Chatelain C, Autet W, Brackman F. Comparison of once and twice daily dosage forms of *Pygeum africanum* extract in patients with benign prostatic hyperplasia: a randomized, double-blind study, with long-term open label extension. Urology 1999;54(4):473-478.
4. Bassi P, Artibani W, De L, V, et al. [Standardized extract of *Pygeum africanum* in the treatment of benign prostatic hypertrophy. Controlled clinical study versus placebo]. Minerva Urol Nefrol 1987;39(1):45-50.
5. Thieblot L, Grizard G, Boucher D. [Effect of V 1326 (active principle of *Pygeum africanum* bark extract) on hypophyseo-genito-adrenal axis in rats]. Therapie 1977;32(1):99-110.
6. Yablonsky F, Nicolas V, Riffaud JP, et al. Antiproliferative effect of *Pygeum africanum* extract on rat prostatic fibroblasts. J Urol 1997;157(6):2381-2387.
7. Andro M, Riffaud J. *Pygeum africanum* extract for the treatment of patients with benign prostatic hyperplasia: a review of 25 years of published experience. Curr Ther Res 1995;56(8):796-817.
8. Wilt T, Ishani A, Mac DR, et al. *Pygeum africanum* for benign prostatic hyperplasia (Cochrane Review). Cochrane Database Syst Rev 2002;(1):CD001044.
9. Ishani A, MacDonald R, Nelson D, et al. *Pygeum africanum* for the treatment of patients with benign prostatic hyperplasia: a systematic review and quantitative meta-analysis. Am J Med 2000;109(8):654-664.
10. Barlet A, Albrecht J, Aubert A, et al. [Efficacy of *Pygeum africanum* extract in the medical therapy of urination disorders due to benign prostatic hyperplasia: evaluation of objective and subjective parameters. A placebo-controlled double-blind multicenter study]. Wien Klin Wochenschr 1990;102(22):667-673.
11. Berges RR, Windeler J, Trampisch HJ, et al. Randomised, placebo-controlled, double-blind clinical trial of beta-sitosterol in patients with benign prostatic hyperplasia. Beta-sitosterol Study Group. Lancet 1995;345(8964):1529-1532.
12. Rhodes L, Primka RL, Berman C, et al. Comparison of finasteride (Proscar), a 5 alpha reductase inhibitor, and various commercial plant extracts in in vitro and in vivo 5 alpha reductase inhibition. Prostate 1993;22(1):43-51.
13. Mathe G, Hallard M, Bourut CH, et al. A *Pygeum africanum* extract with so-called phyto-estrogenic action markedly reduces the volume of true and large prostatic hypertrophy. Biomed Pharmacother 1995;49(7-8):341-343.
14. Mathe G, Orbach-Arbouys S, Bizi E, et al. The so-called phyto-estrogenic action of *Pygeum africanum* extract. Biomed Pharmacother 1995;49(7-8):339-340.
15. Krzeski T, Kazon M, Borkowski A, et al. Combined extracts of *Urtica dioica* and *Pygeum africanum* in the treatment of benign prostatic hyperplasia: double-blind comparison of two doses. Clin Ther 1993;15(6):1011-1020.
16. Levin RM, Das AK. A scientific basis for the therapeutic effects of *Pygeum africanum* and *Serenoa repens*. Urol Res 2000;28(3):201-209.
17. Choo M, Constantinou CE, Bellamy F. Beneficial effects of *Pygeum africanum* extract (PA) on dihydrotestosterone (DHT) induced modifications of micturition and prostate growth in rat [abstract]. J Urology 1999;161(4S):229.
18. Clavert A, Cranz C, Riffaud JP, et al. [Effects of an extract of the bark of *Pygeum africanum* (V.1326) on prostatic secretions in the rat and in man]. Ann Urol (Paris) 1986;20(5):341-343.

P

19. Levin RM, Riffaud JP, Bellamy F, et al. Protective effect of Tadenan on bladder function secondary to partial outlet obstruction. J Urol 1996; 155(4):1466-1470.

20. Paubert-Braquet M, Cave A, Hocquemiller R, et al. Effect of *Pygeum africanum* extract on A23187-stimulated production of lipoxygenase metabolites from human polymorphonuclear cells. J Lipid Mediat Cell Signal 1994;9(3):285-290.

21. Paubert-Braquet M, Monboisse JC, Servant-Saez N, et al. Inhibition of bFGF and EGF-induced proliferation of 3T3 fibroblasts by extract of *Pygeum africanum* (Tadenan). Biomed Pharmacother 1994;48(Suppl 1): 43-47.

22. Blitz M, Garbit JL, Masson JC, et al. [Controlled study on the effect of a medical treatment on subjects consulting for the first time for prostatic adenoma]. Lyon Mediterr Med 1985;21:11.

23. Bongi G. [Tadenan in the treatment of prostatic adenoma. Anatomo-clinical study]. Minerva Urol 1972;24(4):129-139.

24. Breza J, Dzurny O, Borowka A, et al. Efficacy and acceptability of tadenan (*Pygeum africanum* extract) in the treatment of benign prostatic hyperplasia (BPH): a multicentre trial in central Europe. Curr Med Res Opin 1998; 14(3):127-139.

25. Donkervoort T, Sterling A, van Ness J, et al. A clinical and urodynamic study of tadenan in the treatment of benign prostatic hypertrophy. Eur Urol 1977;3(4):218-225.

26. Dufour B, Choquenet C, Revol M, et al. [Controlled study of the effects of *Pygeum africanum* extract on the functional symptoms of prostatic adenoma]. Ann Urol (Paris) 1984;18(3):193-195.

27. Dutkiewicz S. Usefulness of Cernilton in the treatment of benign prostatic hyperplasia. Int Urol Nephrol 1996;28(1):49-53.

28. Frasseto G, Bertoglio S, Mancuso S, et al. [Study of the efficacy and tolerability of Tadenan 50 in patients with prostatic hypertrophy]. Progresso Medico 1986;42:49-53.

29. Gagliardi V, Apicella F, Pino P, et al. Terapia medica dell'ipertrofia prostatica. Sperimentazione clinica controllata. Arch Ital Urol Nefrol Andrologia 1983;55:51-59.

30. Giacobini S, von Heland M, de Natale G, et al. Valutazione clinica e morfo-funzionale del trattamento a doppio cieco con placebo, Tadenan 50 e Tadenan 50 associato a Farlutal nei pazienti con ipertrofia prostatica benigna. Antologia Medica Italiana 1986;6:1-10.

31. Mandressi A, Tarallo U, Maggioni A, et al. Terapia medica dell'adenoma prostatico: confronto della efficacia dell'estratto di *Serenoa repens* (Permixon) versus l'estratto di *Pigeum africanum* e placebo. Valutazione in doppio cieco. Urologia 1983;50(4):752-757.

32. Maver A. [Medical treatment of fibroadenomatous hypertrophy of the prostate with a new plant substance]. Minerva Med 1972;63(37):2126-2136.

33. Mehrsai AR, Pourmand G, Taheri M. Evaluation of the clinical and urodynamic effects of *Pygeum africanum* (Tadenan) in the treatment of benign prostatic hyperplasia (BPH) [abstract]. Br J Urol 1997;80(suppl 2): 227.

34. Ranno S, Minaldi G, Viscusi G, et al. [Efficacy and tolerability in the treatment of prostatic adenoma with Tadenan 50]. Progresso Medico 1986; 42:165-169.

35. Rigatti P, Zennaro F, Fraschini O, et al. L'impegio del Tadenan nell'adenoma prostatico. Ricerca clinica controllata. Atti della Accademia Medica Lombarda 1983;38:1-4.

36. Rizzo M. Terapia medica dell'adenoma della prostata: valutazione clinica comparativa tra estratto di *Pygeum africanum* ad alte dosi e placebo. Farmacia Terapia 1985;2:105-110.

37. Choo MS, Bellamy F, Constantinou CE. Functional evaluation of Tadenan on micturition and experimental prostate growth induced with exogenous dihydrotestosterone. Urology 2000;55(2):292-298.

38. Yoshimura Y, Yamaguchi O, Bellamy F, et al. Effect of *Pygeum africanum* tadenan on micturition and prostate growth of the rat secondary to coadministered treatment and post-treatment with dihydrotestosterone. Urology 2003;61(2):474-478.

39. Barth H. Non hormonal treatment of benign prostatic hypertrophy. Clinical evaluation of the active extract of *Pygeum africanum*. Proc Symp Benign Prostat Hypertrophy 1981;1:45-48.

Red Clover
(*Trifolium pratense*)

SYNONYMS/COMMON NAMES/RELATED SUBSTANCES

- Ackerklee, beebread, cow clover, genistein, isoflavone, meadow clover, phytoestrogen, Promensil, purple clover, rotklee, Rimostil, trefoil, trefle des pres, Trinovin, wild clover.

CLINICAL BOTTOM LINE
Background

- Red clover is a legume that, like soy, contains phytoestrogens (plant-based compounds structurally similar to estradiol, capable of binding to estrogen receptors as an agonist or antagonist). Red clover was traditionally used to treat asthma, pertussis, cancer, and gout. In modern times, isoflavone extracts of red clover are most often used to treat menopausal symptoms, as an alternative hormone replacement therapy, for hyperlipidemia, and to prevent osteoporosis.
- At this time, there are no high-quality human trials supporting the efficacy of red clover for any indication.[1] Soy protein, another source of isoflavones, has been reported to significantly reduce serum lipid levels, but this benefit has not been demonstrated for red clover and may be due to the presence of other constituents in soy (saponins, pectins, essential fatty acids).

Scientific Evidence for Common/Studied Uses	Grade*
Benign prostatic hypertrophy (BPH)	C
Hormone replacement therapy (HRT)	C
Hypercholesterolemia	C
Menopausal signs and symptoms	C
Osteoporosis	C
Prostate cancer	C

*Key to grades: *A:* Strong scientific evidence for this use; *B:* Good scientific evidence for this use; *C:* Unclear scientific evidence for this use; *D:* Fair scientific evidence against this use (it may not work); *F:* Strong scientific evidence against this use (it likely does not work). For a more detailed explanation of efficacy criteria, see "Natural Standard Evidence-Based Validated Grading Rationale" in the Introduction.

Historical or Theoretical Indications That Lack Sufficient Evidence

- Acne, AIDS, antibacterial, antioxidant,[2] antispasmodic, appetite suppressant, arthritis, asthma, "blood purification," bronchitis, burns, cancer prevention (antitumor), canker sores, cough, chronic skin diseases (topical), diuretic, eczema (topical), gout, hypertension,[3] indigestion, mastalgia,[4] premenstrual syndrome, psoriasis (topical), sexually transmitted diseases (STDs), skin ulcers/sores (topical), sore eyes, tuberculosis, venereal diseases, whooping cough (pertussis).

Expert Opinion and Folkloric Precedent

- Chinese and Russian folk healers have used red clover to treat respiratory problems such as asthma and bronchitis. Native American healers recommended red clover for pertussis and cancer.
- Some experts believe that topical red clover accelerates wound healing and alleviates psoriasis. Recently, it has been speculated that red clover may have beneficial effects on bone metabolism, serum lipid levels, and arterial compliance, due to its phytoestrogen properties. Red clover is often recommended for these indications, although there is a paucity of scientific evidence.

Safety Summary

- **Likely safe:** When used in recommended doses as a supplement for the relief of menopausal symptoms and as an adjunctive preventive therapy for osteoporosis.[5-7] Small trials have not noted significant adverse effects after one year of red clover isoflavone therapy.[8,9]
- **Possibly safe:** Caution should be taken by patients on hormone replacement therapy (HRT) or oral contraceptives (OCPs), as red clover binds to intracellular estrogen receptors and may enhance estrogenic effects.[10]
- **Possibly unsafe:** Red clover, which contains coumarin, may alter platelet aggregation and therefore may theoretically be unsafe in persons with bleeding disorders/coagulopathies or taking anticoagulants. Caution should be exercised in patients with or at risk for breast cancer/estrogen receptor–positive neoplasia, because of the variable estrogen receptor–binding properties of red clover (may have estrogen agonist or antagonist properties, with unclear long-term effects). In theory, estrogenic activity unopposed by progesterone may lead to endometrial hyperplasia and ultimately may increase risk of uterine (endometrial) cancer, although short-term studies (less than 6 months) have found no visible changes on ultrasound.[11,12] It remains unclear if phytoestrogens such as red clover affect these risks, and further research is warranted in these areas.

DOSING/TOXICOLOGY
General

- Recommended doses are based on those most commonly used in available trials, or on historical practice. However, with natural products, the optimal doses needed to balance efficacy and safety often have not been determined. Formulations and preparation methods may vary from manufacturer to manufacturer, and from batch to batch of a specific product made by a single manufacturer. Because often the active components of a product are not known, standardization may not be possible, and the clinical effects of different brands may not be comparable.

Standardization

- Isoflavones are isolated from red clover via alcohol extraction. The brand of red clover isoflavone extract used in most trials, and which is most commonly available commercially, is Promensil (Novogen). Each tablet is standardized to contain 40 mg of isoflavones: 4 mg of genistein, 3.5 mg of daidzein, 24.5 mg of biochanin A, and 8.0 mg of formononetin (present as hydrolyzed aglycones).

R

- Methods used to identify constituents of red clover include high-performance liquid chromatography (HPLC)[13] and, more recently, polymerase chain reaction (PCR) techniques.[14]

Dosing: Adult (18 Years and Older)
Oral

- *Note:* Recommended doses are based on those most commonly used in available trials.
- **Hormone replacement:** 40 to 80 mg of red clover isoflavones/day (Promensil).[7,11,12,15,16]
- **Hypercholesterolemia:** 28.5, 57, or 85.5 mg of red clover isoflavones/day (Rimostil)[5] or 80 mg of red clover isoflavones/day (Promensil).[17]
- **Osteoporosis:** 40 mg of red clover isoflavones/day (Promensil).[5]
- **Menopausal symptoms:** 40, 80, or 160 mg of red clover isoflavones/day (Promensil).[6,11]
- **Benign prostatic hypertrophy:** 40 mg of red clover isoflavones/day (Trinovin).[18]

Dosing: Pediatric (Younger Than 18 Years)

- Insufficient available evidence to recommend.

Toxicology

- Insufficient human data available. In grazing animals, red clover has been noted anecdotally to be associated with cachexia, bloating, and abortion.

ADVERSE EFFECTS/PRECAUTIONS/CONTRAINDICATIONS
Allergy

- Known allergy/hypersensitivity to red clover (scant data are available).

Adverse Effects

- **General:** The small number of human studies using isoflavone extracts of red clover have all reported good tolerance.[5,7,19] Trials have not noted significant adverse effects after up to 1 year of red clover isoflavone therapy.[8,9]
- **Endocrine:** Red clover isoflavones possess varying affinity for estradiol receptors and are capable of acting as both agonists and antagonists.[20] Weight gain and breast tenderness may theoretically occur, based on the known estrogenic properties of red clover, although a human study of 93 postmenopausal women did not report these adverse effects.[19] Isoflavones may affect levels of gonadotropin-releasing hormone (GrH), follicle-stimulating hormone (FSH), and luteinizing hormone (LH) via hormonal feedback mechanisms.[10] However, in a randomized trial of 205 women receiving Promensil (40 mg of red clover isoflavones/tablet) or placebo daily for 1 year, no significant differences in FSH or LH levels were detected between groups, and no differences in breast density were found (women with a history of breast cancer were excluded).[9] Case control studies of soy (also a source of isoflavones) have reported a decreased risk of breast cancer, and high levels of urinary isoflavones have been associated with decreased risk of breast cancer, although results may not be generalizable to red clover.[21]
- **Genitourinary:** As a phytoestrogen, red clover possesses estrogen receptor agonist and antagonist properties. In theory, menstrual changes and endometrial hyperplasia may occur due to estrogenic activity unopposed by progesterone, which may increase the risk of uterine (endometrial) cancer. However, preliminary short-term (less than 6 months) studies have found no increases in endometrial thickness on ultrasound examination.[11,12] It remains unclear if phytoestrogens such as red clover affect these risks. Patients with endometrial hyperplasia should be evaluated by a qualified healthcare professional and may require an endometrial biopsy. Discontinuation of red clover should be considered, and/or addition of a progesterone product or phytoprogesterone such as chasteberry (*Vitex agnus-castus*), bloodroot (*Sanguinaria canadensis*), oregano, damiana (*Turnera* spp), or yucca.
- **Hematologic:** Red clover contains coumarin and coumarin-like compounds and additionally may alter platelet aggregation, theoretically increasing the risk of bleeding. However, literature review reveals no human reports of bleeding.

Precautions/Warnings/Contraindications

- Use cautiously in patients with bleeding disorders or taking nonsteroidal anti-inflammatory drugs (NSAIDs), anticoagulants, or antiplatelet medications: Red clover contains coumarin and may alter platelet aggregation and theoretically may increase risk of bleeding. Human data are scant in this area.
- Use cautiously in patients taking hormone replacement therapy (HRT) or oral contraceptives (OCP). Red clover binds to intracellular estrogen receptors and may enhance estrogenic effects.[10]
- Avoid use in patients with or at risk for breast cancer, estrogen receptor–positive neoplasia, or endometrial hyperplasia: Red clover binds to intracellular estrogen receptors and may enhance estrogenic effects.[10]

Pregnancy and Lactation

- Red clover often is not recommended during pregnancy and lactation because of its estrogenic activity.[10]
- One small rat study found that maternal exposure to subcutaneous genistein (an isoflavone) increases the incidence of mammary tumors in offspring, mimicking the effects of *in utero* estrogenic exposures.[22]
- Red clover has been implicated as a cause of infertility and abortion in grazing livestock.

INTERACTIONS
Red Clover/Drug Interactions

- **Agents metabolized via cytochrome P450 (CYP) 3A4:** There is *in vitro* evidence that red clover may inhibit CYP3A4 enzyme. Agents metabolized by this enzyme may potentially accumulate when taken concomitantly.
- **Anticoagulant/antiplatelet agents, nonsteroidal anti-inflammatory drugs (NSAIDS):** Red clover contains coumarin and coumarin-like compounds, which theoretically may have additive or synergistic effects when taken with anticoagulants or antiplatelet agents.
- **Hormone replacement therapy (HRT), oral contraceptives (OCPs), tamoxifen, raloxifene:** Red clover isoflavones possess varying affinity for estradiol receptors (estradiol-β and estradiol-α) and are capable of acting as both agonists and antagonists.[20] Preliminary evidence suggests a preferential binding to estrogen receptor β, which is found in the vasculature, brain, bone, and heart, as opposed to estrogen receptor α, which is found in the ovaries, breast, uterus, and adrenal glands. Concomitant use of red clover may enhance or inhibit the estrogenic effects of hormonal therapies. Isoflavones may affect levels of gonadotropin-releasing hormone (GrRH), follicle-stimulating hormone (FSH), and luteinizing hormone (LH) via hormonal feedback mechanisms.[10]

Red Clover/Herb/Supplement Interactions

- **Agents metabolized via cytochrome P450 (CYP) 3A4:** There is *in vitro* evidence that red clover may inhibit CYP3A4 enzyme. Therefore, there may be the potential for agents metabolized by this enzyme to accumulate.
- **Anticoagulant/antiplatelet agents:** Red clover contains coumarin and coumarin-like compounds, which theoretically may have additive or synergistic effects when taken with anticoagulants or antiplatelet agents.
- **Phytoestrogens/estrogenic agents:** Red clover isoflavones possess varying affinity for estradiol receptors (estradiol-α and estradiol-β), and are capable of acting as both agonists and antagonists.[20] Preliminary evidence suggests a preferential binding to estrogen receptor β, which is found in the vasculature, brain, bone, and heart, as opposed to estrogen receptor α, which is found in the ovaries, breast, uterus, and adrenal glands. Concomitant use of red clover may enhance or inhibit the estrogenic effects of other phytoestrogens, such as alfalfa (*Medicago sativa*), black cohosh (*Cimicifuga racemosa*), bloodroot (*Sanguinaria canadensis*), hops (*Humulus lupulus*), kudzu (*Pueraria lobata*), licorice (*Glycyrrhiza glabra*), pomegranate (*Punica granatum*), soybean (*Glycine max*), thyme (*Thymus vulgaris*), and yucca.

Red Clover/Food Interactions

- Red clover has been on the FDA's GRAS (generally recognized as safe) list and is included in many beverages and teas. It is believed that the amounts found in these beverages are too small to be of clinical relevance.

Red Clover/Lab Interactions

- **International normalized ratio (INR):** Red clover contains coumarin and coumarin-like compounds that may increase bleeding time, thereby raising the INR (theoretical).
- **Hormonal levels:** In theory, because of their estrogenic properties, isoflavones may affect levels of gonadotropin-releasing hormone (GrH), follicle-stimulating hormone (FSH), and luteinizing hormone (LH) via hormonal feedback mechanisms.[10] However, in a randomized trial of 205 women receiving Promensil (40 mg of red clover isoflavones/tablet) or placebo daily for 1 year, no significant differences in FSH or LH levels were detected between groups.[9]

MECHANISM OF ACTION
Pharmacology

- **Estrogenic properties:** Although red clover has been found to contain over 125 chemical compounds, the isoflavone component of the plant is thought to be responsible for the majority of its therapeutic applications. Isoflavones, like those found in red clover, are considered to be phytoestrogens, which are plant compounds that are structurally similar to estradiol and are capable of binding to estradiol receptors. Isoflavones have a varying affinity for estradiol receptors (estradiol-α and estradiol-β), and are capable of acting as both agonists and antagonists.[20] There is some evidence that suggests a preferential binding to estrogen receptor β, which is found in the vasculature, brain, bone, and heart, as opposed to estrogen receptor α, which is found in the ovaries, breast, uterus, and adrenal glands.
- As an estrogen agonist, red clover may lead to the inhibition of gonadotropin-releasing hormone (GrH), follicle-stimulating hormone (FSH), and luteinizing hormone (LH) secretion via negative feedback.[10] However, the clinical significance of this activity in humans has not been determined. The constituent isoflavones biochanin A and genistein have

been reported to have relatively high levels of estrogenic activity. Daidzein appears to be less active.[23] However, biochanin A, formononetin, genistein, and daidzein do not possess observable progestational or androgenic effects[23] and, in fact, have been proposed to possess anti-androgen properties.[24] Red clover has demonstrated estrogenic activity via the induction of alkaline phosphatase activity and upregulation of progesterone receptor mRNA,[25] with physiologic effects observed in animal research.[26]

- **Antiproliferative properties:** Biochanin A and genistein have been shown to inhibit cell proliferation *in vitro* (apoptosis is believed to be the primary mechanism of action, based on demonstrated DNA fragmentation).[27-29] Genistein inhibits cell proliferation via inhibition of tyrosine kinases and DNA topoisomerases I and II.[20] It has been speculated that genistein's cytotoxicity may be the result of disruption of transcriptional processes.[30] Coumestrol is a phytoestrogen found in high quantities in red clover. *In vitro*, coumestrol has been shown to exhibit both mutagenic and clastogenic (chromosome-breaking) properties in cultured human lymphoblastoid cells.[31] Anti-androgenic properties have also been proposed as possibly beneficial in cases of prostatic hypertrophy or prostate cancer.[24]
- **Antioxidant properties:** Red clover's purported antioxidant properties have been attributed to the isoflavone genistein. Genistein inhibits the formation of hydrogen peroxide and superoxide anion, and scavenges hydrogen peroxide *in vitro*. Daidzein also appears to possess antioxidant properties, although to a lesser extent.[28]

Pharmacodynamics/Kinetics

- Red clover differs from the phytoestrogen soy in that the principal isoflavones in red clover are biochanin A and formononetin, whereas those in soy consist solely of genistein and diadzein. However, biochanin A and formononetin are metabolized extensively *in vivo* to genistein and daidzein, respectively.[19] Daidzein is further broken down to form the estrogenic metabolite equol and the less estrogenic *O*-desmethylangolensin (*O*-DMA).[32] Metabolism and absorption (which may be influenced by food) are highly variable.[32]
- Genistein, daidzein, and equol have been detected in human urine, plasma, saliva, breast aspirate, and prostatic fluid.[20]
- The plasma half-life of daidzein and genistein is approximately 7.9 hours in adults; peak plasma concentrations occur 6 to 8 hours after oral administration of the pure compound.[33]
- Although isoflavones are structurally related to estrogen, they have a variable affinity for the estradiol-binding site and may act as either agonists or antagonists.[20]

HISTORY

- Historically, red clover has played a role in medicine, agriculture, and religion. Chinese and Russian folk healers used it to treat respiratory conditions such as asthma and bronchitis. In the Middle Ages, it was considered a charm against witchcraft. Red clover serves as a grazing food for many animals and has been implicated as a cause of infertility in livestock. Some believe that topical red clover can accelerate wound healing and alleviate psoriasis.

REVIEW OF THE EVIDENCE: DISCUSSION
Menopausal Signs and Symptoms
Summary

- Isoflavones, such as those present in red clover, are believed by many experts to reduce signs and symptoms of meno-

Review of the Evidence: Red Clover

Condition Treated*	Study Design	Author, Year	N[†]	SS[†]	Study Quality[‡]	Magnitude of Benefit	ARR[†]	NNT[†]	Comments
Menopausal symptoms	RCT, placebo-controlled, crossover, single-blind	Baber[11] 1999	51	No	2	None	NA	NA	No benefit of Promensil vs. placebo, but no power calculation; sample may have been too small to detect benefit.
Menopausal symptoms	RCT	Knight[6] 1999	37	No	2	NA	NA	NA	No benefit of Promensil vs. placebo; isoflavone ingestion in placebo group may have confounded results; no power calculation.
Menopausal symptoms	RCT, double-blind	Jeri[16] 1999	30	Yes	2	Large	53%	2	Significant reduction in hot flash frequency vs. placebo; conference abstract only (poorly reported).
Menopausal symptoms	RCT, double-blind	Van de Weijer[15,34] 2001, 2002	30	Yes	2	Mixed	NA	NA	44% decrease in median number of hot flashes, but unclear statistical significance vs. placebo; no change in subjective symptom severity; conference abstract only.
Menopausal symptoms	Case series	Nachtigall[12] 1999	23	Yes	NA	Large	NA	NA	Improvement in hot flashes and night sweats, but lack of controls limits usefulness of results.
Menopausal symptoms	Case series	Abernathy[35] 2001	33	Yes	NA	Mixed	NA	NA	44% reduction in hot flash frequency, but no change in subjective symptoms; lack of controls limits usefulness of results.
Arteriovascular resistance	RCT	Nestel[7] 1999	26	No	2	NA	NA	NA	Inappropriate randomization; data collection from 16 participants only.
Bone density and lipid metabolism	Case series (dose escalation study)	Clifton-Bligh[5] 2001	46	Yes	0	NA	NA	NA	Rimostil superior to placebo; no control group or dietary log to rule out increases in isoflavone-enriched foods.
Bone mineral density	RCT, double-blind	Atkinson[8] 2000	107	Yes	2	Mixed	NA	NA	Improvement with Promensil in pre- and perimenopausal, but not in postmenopausal women; conference abstract only with limited details.
Bone mineral density	Case series (dose escalation study)	Baber[11] 1999	50	Yes	2	Small	NA	NA	Improved bone density in some forearm areas with Promensil vs. placebo (3%); conference abstract only; 8 dropouts.
Hypercholesterolemia	RCT, double-blind	Howes[19] 2000	93	No	3	NA	NA	NA	Small study with high dropout rate: 18 dropouts.
Hypercholesterolemia	RCT, double-blind	Blakesmith[41] 2003	25	No	2	None	NA	NA	86 mg of isoflavones/day; small study in healthy premenopausal women; increased urinary isoflavones without changes in LDLs or HDLs; may have been underpowered.
Hypercholesterolemia	RCT, single-blind, crossover	Samman[17] 1999	21	Yes	1	None	NA	NA	86 mg of isoflavones/day no better than placebo; 33% dropout and no power calculation.
BPH	Case series	Gerber[42] 2000	29	Yes	NA	NA	NA	NA	Trinovin decreased BPH symptoms; Abstract only; study funded by manufacturer.

*Primary or secondary outcome.
[†] N, Number of patients; SS, statistically significant; ARR, absolute risk reduction; NNT, the number of patients who need to undergo a specific intervention in order to observe an outcome in one individual.
[‡] 0-2 = poor; 3-4 = good; 5 = excellent.
BPH, Benign prostatic hypertrophy; HDLs, high-density lipoproteins; LDLs, low-density lipoproteins; NA, not applicable; RCT, randomized, controlled trial.
For an explanation of each category in this table, please see Table 3 in the Introduction.

pause (such as hot flashes). Although the isoflavones present in red clover have been demonstrated to possess estrogenic properties in pre-clinical studies, there is currently insufficient evidence demonstrating efficacy or safety in humans. Trials have been methodologically weak and short in duration (≤12 weeks of treatment), which may not be sufficient to assess efficacy for menopausal symptoms, which tend to wax and wane over longer periods of time. Nonetheless, red clover products remain popular.

Randomized Trials

- Baber et al. conducted a randomized, placebo-controlled, crossover study in 51 menopausal women.[11] After a 1-week assessment period, subjects received either 40 mg of red clover isoflavones (Promensil) or placebo daily. After 12 weeks, all patients received placebo for 1 month, then crossed over to the alternative arm for a further 14 weeks of treatment. Subjects maintained symptom diaries that were evaluated at the start and end of treatment. Biochemical profiles, complete blood counts, vaginal swabs, and vaginal ultrasound scans were performed, as well as isoflavone levels (determined by 24-hour urine collection). The study found no significant differences in hot flashes, flushing, or other physiologic parameters between the Promensil and placebo groups. Treatment was well tolerated, and no adverse effects were reported. The study used a validated self-reporting instrument to measure results. However, there were several methodological weaknesses in this trial. Because the natural progression of hot flashes and related symptoms is characterized by a waxing and waning progression with time, the trial may have been too short to adequately measure a response; a 1- to 2- year course would be more appropriate. The study was not investigator-blinded, which may have introduced bias. No power calculation was conducted, and given the small sample size and negative result, it is conceivable that a larger study group may have been necessary to detect important clinical benefits. In addition, many subjects in the placebo groups displayed higher urinary isoflavone levels at the end of the trial compared to baseline, raising questions about possible dietary confounders or misclassification. Due to the crossover design of this study, a carryover effect in the group receiving isoflavones initially may have brought results closer to a null effect.
- A randomized, placebo-controlled study by Knight et al. examined menopausal symptoms in 37 postmenopausal women having at least three hot flashes per day (age range, 40 to 65 years; amenorrheic for ≥6 months).[6] Subjects were given 40 or 160 mg daily of isoflavones from red clover (Promensil), or placebo. After 12 weeks of therapy, no statistically significant difference in alleviation of symptoms was observed between the 40-mg, 160-mg, and placebo groups (reduction in hot flashes of 29%, 34%, and 29%, respectively). A small and insignificant increase in urinary isoflavones was noted in the placebo group, which may have been due to other dietary phytoestrogen consumption (alfalfa taken by one subject, possibly skewing the mean).
- A randomized, double-blind, placebo-controlled trial was reported by Jeri et al. as an abstract only at the 9th International Menopause Society World Congress on the Menopause (1999).[16] In this study, 30 postmenopausal Peruvian women were given 40 mg of red clover isoflavones (Promensil) or placebo for 4 months. The authors reported significant reductions in hot flash frequency in 73% of red clover patients vs. 20% in placebo, and a 47% reduction in

hot flash severity ($p < 0.001$). However, details of blinding, randomization, measurements, and statistical analysis were limited. Without further details provided, the results cannot be adequately analyzed or considered conclusive.
- In an abstract presented at the North American Menopause Society's 12th Annual Meeting (2001)[15] and subsequently published in the journal Maturitas,[34] van de Weijer and Barentsen reported the results of a randomized, double-blind, placebo-controlled study of 80 mg of red clover isoflavones/day (Promensil) in 30 menopausal women (ages 49 to 65 years). After 12 weeks of treatment, the authors reported a 44% decrease in the median frequency of hot flashes vs. no change in placebo, although it is not entirely clear how this calculation was made, and it is not apparent that there was a statistically significant difference between groups. No significant differences between groups were found in the patient-reported "Greene score" of symptom severity. Of some interest, an inverse relationship between urine isoflavone levels and hot flashes was found. This poorly reported study did not provide adequate description of methodology and calculations, had a large dropout (20%), and was not an intention-to-treat analysis (subjects were excluded from analysis after enrollment). Therefore, the results cannot be considered conclusive.

Case Series

- In a case series presented at the 9th International Menopause Society World Congress on the Menopause (1999),[12] Nachtigall et al. administered 40 mg of red clover isoflavones/day (Promensil) to 23 menopausal women (mean age, 53 years), who experienced ≥5 hot flashes/day and were not taking hormonal therapy. Subjects reported their own menopausal symptoms using a 4-point scoring system ("Greene score"). After 2 months of treatment, a statistically significant 56% reduction in hot flash frequency, 43% reduction in hot flash severity, and 52% reduction in night sweat severity were reported. Transvaginal ultrasound revealed no changes in endometrial thickness. Although these results are suggestive, the design flaws inherent to case series make the results impossible to extrapolate to clinical practice. These flaws include lack of controls in the setting of a condition that waxes and wanes; lack of blinding which may introduce bias; short duration; and small sample size.
- In an abstract presented at the British Menopause Society (2001), Abernathy et al. reported a case series in 33 postmenopausal women (ages 40 to 65 years).[35] Subjects received 40 mg of red clover isoflavones/day (Promensil) for 12 weeks, at which time a statistically significant 58.5% decrease in frequency of hot flashes was found. A non-significant reduction in the patient-reported "Greene score" of symptom severity was found. Although suggestive, this abstract lacked any description of methods or statistical analysis and as a case series has the same limitations as described for Nachtigall et al. above.

Hormone Replacement Therapy (HRT)
Summary

- High-quality controlled clinical trials supporting the use of red clover isoflavones as an alternative to conventional HRT are lacking. *In vitro* estrogenic responses have been observed with the isoflavones genistein and daidzein and their respective precursors biochanin A and formononetin, as well as with the steroid-like phytochemical coumestrol. However, human data are limited. Specific doses that would be equivalent to ethinyl estradiol or conjugated equine estrogens have not been established.[32] Evidence that isoflavones may possess similar benefits to those purported for estrogens (reduction of cardiovascular disease, positive effects on lipid profiles, vascular benefits) has not been demonstrated, and in fact such effects remain controversial for estrogens in general.[19,36,37]

Evidence

- Nestel et al. conducted a randomized, double-blind, controlled study in 26 postmenopausal women.[7] After a 3-week run-in period in which all subjects received placebo, the women were randomized to placebo or Promensil (each tablet standardized to 40 mg of isoflavones derived from red clover). Treatment was divided into three 5-week phases: 40 or 80 mg of isoflavones daily or placebo. Dietary education and instruction were provided prior to and throughout treatment. Isoflavone excretion was measured via 24-hour urinary collection. The study found that arterial compliance significantly increased dose-dependently in the isoflavone group compared to placebo. This small study had several methodological flaws. Subjects were inappropriately randomized (every fifth subject was allocated to receive placebo), and complete data were collected only from 60% of treated subjects entered in the study. These design weaknesses make it difficult to draw any conclusions from this trial.

Osteoporosis
Summary

- It is unclear to what extent bone loss is affected by dietary isoflavones such as those present in red clover. Most studies investigating isoflavones and bone metabolism have used soy products, which have a higher concentration of the isoflavones genistein and daidzein than red clover, and contain other potentially active ingredients (saponins, pectins, essential fatty acids). Therefore, at this time there is insufficient evidence to recommend for or against red clover as a treatment for osteoporosis.

Evidence

- Clifton-Bligh et al. conducted a case series in 46 postmenopausal women in order to determine the effect of red clover isoflavones on bone and lipid metabolism.[5] After a single-blind placebo phase, subjects received 28.5, 57, or 85.5 mg of a red clover isoflavone tablet (Rimostil) daily for 6 months. Bone mineral density (BMD) of the proximal radius and ulna significantly increased 4.1% over this period in subjects taking 57 mg of Rimostil. Subjects taking 85.5 mg had a 3% increase in BMD. Although these results are encouraging, this study was methodologically flawed. There was no control group or dietary log to rule out increases in isoflavone-containing foods. In addition, the changes in BMD were large and rapid, raising the question of concomitant therapy with agents known to be highly active (such as bisphosphonates) or inaccurate measurements. These results can be interpreted only as preliminary suggestive evidence.
- In a conference abstract by Atkinson et al., preliminary data from a controlled study giving 40 mg daily of red clover isoflavones (Promensil) or placebo for 1 year to 107 pre-, peri-, and postmenopausal women found no significant overall effect on spine and hip bone mineral density.[8] Subgroup analysis suggested that spine bone mineral density decreased less with isoflavones in the pre- and peri-menopausal groups, but there was no benefit over placebo for post-

menopausal women. Details of randomization, blinding, and statistical analysis were not provided. The authors proposed a potential benefit in pre- and perimenopausal women, but in light of the limited reporting in this publication and inconclusive supportive evidence elsewhere, these results cannot be considered definitive.

- In a conference abstract describing a dose escalation study by Baber et al., the red clover isoflavone preparation P081, prepared by the makers of Promensil, was given to 50 postmenopausal women.[11] Subjects were randomized to 25, 50, or 75 mg for 6 months, after which time high-density lipoprotein (HDL) levels increased and low-density lipoprotein (LDL) levels decreased significantly in all groups. However, lack of placebo and incomplete description of methodology or statistical analysis limit the clinical applicability of these results.

Hypercholesterolemia
Summary

- Because estrogens have been reported to decrease low-density lipoproteins (LDLs) and increase high-density lipoproteins (HDLs), some effort has been undertaken to discern the effects of red clover isoflavones, which appear to possess estrogenic activity, on lipid metabolism. To date, the available evidence of red clover's effects on lipid levels in humans remains inconclusive; although most available research in humans reports no clinically significant effects, because of the small sample sizes used and other methodological weaknesses, a firm conclusion cannot be reached.[7,36,38] Notably, soy protein, another source of isoflavones, has been reported to reduce serum lipid levels by up to 10%. However, soy proteins contain higher levels of the isoflavones genistein and daidzein than red clover, and contain other potentially active ingredients (saponins, pectins, essential fatty acids). Preliminary evidence suggests that soy protein is superior to isolated red clover isoflavones for reduction of serum lipid levels.

Negative Evidence

- Howes et al. conducted a randomized, controlled, double-blind trial to assess the effect of dietary isoflavone supplementation on lipid levels in 93 postmenopausal women with elevated total cholesterol levels (5.0 to 9.0 mmol/L).[19] Isoflavones from red clover were extracted to formulate a tablet containing approximately 26 mg of biochanin A, 16 mg of formononetin, 0.5 mg of daidzein, and 1 mg of genistein. Baseline lipid levels and urine analysis for isoflavones were performed after all subjects received placebo for the first 3 to 4 weeks. After the run-in period, subjects were randomly assigned to receive placebo or isoflavone therapy, 1 tablet daily for 5 weeks followed by 2 tablets daily for 5 weeks. At the end of each treatment period, fasting blood was collected on two consecutive days for lipid analysis, as was a 24-hour urine collection for the measurement of urinary excretion of isoflavones. The trial found no significant changes in total cholesterol, LDL-cholesterol, HDL-cholesterol or plasma triglycerides during supplementation with either dose of isoflavone. (Of note, this trial specifically examined the effects of isoflavones derived from red clover vs. soy protein fortified with isoflavones (reported elsewhere to reduce serum lipid levels[39,40]). Soy isoflavones were found to reduce serum lipids, compared with a lack of effect of red clover. However, 18 initial subjects (19.3%) did not complete the trial, and the study design and methods were not well described. Because of the small size and poor methodological quality, this study does not rule out a beneficial effect of red clover isoflavones on lipids.

- Samman et al. conducted a single-blind, randomized, controlled trial in 21 healthy women (ages 18 to 45 years, presumably premenopausal).[17] A red clover isoflavone preparation similar to Promensil containing 86 mg of isoflavones/day or placebo was given to subjects for 2 months prior to crossover. No significant differences were noted in HDLs, LDLs, oxidation, total cholesterol, or triglycerides. However, 33% of subjects dropped out, and there was no adequate description of those who left or reasons for leaving, and no power calculation was conducted. It is therefore conceivable that the small sample size and significant attrition rate could have masked potential true benefits of red clover isoflavones. The evidence remains inconclusive.

- Blakesmith et al. report the results of a randomized, controlled trial in 25 healthy premenopausal women.[41] An isoflavone preparation from red clover (86 mg/day) was administered to 12 subjects for three menstrual cycles, and placebo was given to the remaining women for four cycles. Although urinary isoflavones increased 15-fold in the red clover group, no significant mean changes were observed in LDL, HDL, insulin, or glucose concentrations compared to the placebo group. Although suggestive, the small sample size raises the question of whether this study was adequately powered to detect between-group differences.

Positive Evidence

- Clifton-Bligh et al. conducted a study in 46 postmenopausal women in order to determine the effects of red clover isoflavones on lipid and bone metabolism.[5] After a single-blind placebo phase, subjects received 28.5, 57, or 85.5 mg of a red clover isoflavone tablet (Rimostil) daily for 6 months. The study found that HDL levels significantly increased, regardless of dose, and apolipoprotein B levels significantly decreased. Although these results are encouraging, this study was methodologically flawed. Patients served as their own controls, and there was no dietary log or urine analysis to rule out increases in isoflavone-enriched food intake or increases due to other lifestyle changes. These results can be interpreted only as preliminary, particularly in light of prior negative evidence described above.[19,41]

Benign Prostatic Hypertrophy
Summary

- There is inconclusive evidence in support of the use of red clover or isoflavones for benign prostatic hypertrophy (BPH). Proposed mechanisms include anti-androgenic properties[24] or estrogenic effects.

Evidence

- Gerber presented an abstract at The Endocrine Society's 82nd Annual Meeting (2000) which outlined a case series of red clover isoflavones used for BPH symptomatology.[42] This study consisted of 29 men who acted as their own historical "controls," reportedly taking either 1 or 2 500 mg tablet(s) (Trinovin), standardized to 40 mg of red clover isoflavones per tablet. In this study, 3 months of treatment significantly decreased mean nocturia frequency (29%, $p < 0.0003$), increased urinary flow rates (9.8%, $p < 0.15$), improved quality of life score (15%, $p < 0.01$), and decreased the International Prostate Symptom Score (IPSS) (22.65%, $p < 0.002$). Prostate specific antigen (PSA) values, blood biochemistry, and hematology were not altered from baseline, and prostate size was not altered. The abstract did not disclose the estimated prostate volumes for the study participants upon enrollment (an important variable in the assessment of disease severity and projected response to therapy). Although these results are suggestive, BPH is a chronic condition meriting a long-term study of outcomes, comparison to standard of care, and adequate reporting of methodology. Notably, this study was funded by an unrestricted educational grant from Novogen, Inc., the manufacturer of Trinovin.

Prostate Cancer
Summary

- Red clover contains isoflavones, a class of phytoestrogen. Certain isoflavones have been shown in vitro to possess antineoplastic properties related to the suppression of angiogenesis, inhibition of tyrosine kinase activity, cellular antiproliferation, antiandrogen effects,[24] and partial antagonism of estrogen receptors.[20,28,29] The effects of isoflavones have been examined in human cancer cell lines, including prostate and breast cancer cells.[43-36] However, there is no convincing clinical evidence that red clover exerts similar effects in humans.

Evidence

- A patient scheduled for radical suprapubic prostatectomy took 4 40-mg red clover isoflavone tablets (Promensil) for 7 days before surgery. After excision, histologic changes analyzed in the prostatectomy specimen, particularly apoptosis, were interpreted as suggestive of androgen deprivation.[18] As a case report, this study is suggestive, but is not a basis for therapeutic recommendation.

FORMULARY: BRANDS USED IN CLINICAL TRIALS
Brands Used in Statistically Significant Clinical Trials

- Promensil (Novogen Laboratories: Sydney, Australia); Rimostil (Novogen Laboratories); Trinovin (Novogen Laboratories).

References

1. Nelsen J, Ulbricht C, Barrette EP, et al. Red clover (*Trifolium pratense*) monograph: a clinical decision support tool. J Herbal Pharmacother 2002; 2(3):49-72.
2. Campbell MJ, Woodside JV, Honour JW, et al. Effect of red clover-derived isoflavone supplementation on insulin-like growth factor, lipid and antioxidant status in healthy female volunteers: a pilot study. Eur J Clin Nutr 2004;58(1):173-179.
3. Howes JB, Tran D, Brillante D, et al. Effects of dietary supplementation with isoflavones from red clover on ambulatory blood pressure and endothelial function in postmenopausal type 2 diabetes. Diabetes Obes Metab 2003;5(5):325-332.
4. Ingram D, Sanders K, Kolybaba M, et al. Case-control study of phyto-oestrogens and breast cancer. Lancet 1997;350(9083):990-994.
5. Clifton-Bligh PB, Baber RJ, Fulcher GR, et al. The effect of isoflavones extracted from red clover (Rimostil) on lipid and bone metabolism. Menopause 2001;8(4):259-265.
6. Knight DC. The effect of Promensil, an isoflavone extract, on menopausal symptoms. Climacteric 1999;2:79-84.
7. Nestel PJ, Pomeroy S, Kay S, et al. Isoflavones from red clover improve systemic arterial compliance but not plasma lipids in menopausal women. J Clin Endocrinol Metab 1999;84(3):895-898.
8. Atkinson C, Compston JE, Robins SP, et al. The effects of isoflavone phytoestrogens on bone: preliminary results from a large randomized controlled trial. Endocr Soc Annu Meet Program 2000;82:196.
9. Atkinson C, Warren RM, Dowsett M, et al. Effects of isoflavones on breast density, oestradiol, and gonadotrophins: a double blind randomised placebo controlled trial. poster presented at: Endoc Soc 83rd Annu Meet (2000).
10. Zava DT, Dollbaum CM, Blen M. Estrogen and progestin bioactivity of foods, herbs, and spices. Proc Soc Exp Biol Med 1998;217(3):369-378.
11. Baber R, Clifton Bligh P, Fulcher G, et al. The effect of an isoflavone extract

(po81) on serum lipids, forearm bone density and endometrial thickness in postmenopausal women [abstract]. Proc North Am Menopause Soc (New York, 1999).

12. Nachtigall LB, La Grega L, Lee WW, et al. The effects of isoflavones derived from red clover on vasomotor symptoms and endometrial thickness. 9th Int Menopause Soc World Congress Menopause 1999;331-336.

13. Krenn L, Unterrieder I, Ruprechter R. Quantification of isoflavones in red clover by high-performance liquid chromatography. J Chromatogr B Analyt Technol Biomed Life Sci 2002;777(1-2):123-128.

14. Leroy A, Potter E, Woo HH, et al. Characterization and identification of alfalfa and red clover dietary supplements using a PCR-based method. J Agric Food Chem 2002;50(18):5063-5069.

15. Van De Weijer, Barentsen R. Isoflavones from red clover (Promensil®) significantly reduce hot flashes compared with placebo [abstract]. Poster presented at North Am Menopause Soc 12th Annu Meet (2001).

16. Jeri AR. The effect of isoflavone phytoestrogens in relieving hot flushes in peruvian postmenopausal women [abstract]. 9th Int Menopause Soc World Congress Menopause (1999).

17. Samman S, Lyons Wall PM, Chan GS, et al. The effect of supplementation with isoflavones on plasma lipids and oxidisability of low density lipoprotein in premenopausal women. Atherosclerosis 1999;147(2):277-283.

18. Stephens FO. Phytoestrogens and prostate cancer: possible preventive role. Med J Aust 1997;167(3):138-140.

19. Howes JB, Sullivan D, Lai N, et al. The effects of dietary supplementation with isoflavones from red clover on the lipoprotein profiles of postmenopausal women with mild to moderate hypercholesterolaemia. Atherosclerosis 2000;152(1):143-147.

20. Umland EM, Cauffield JS, Kirk JK, et al. Phytoestrogens as therapeutic alternatives to traditional hormone replacement in postmenopausal women. Pharmacotherapy 2000;20(8):981-990.

21. Messina M, Barnes S, Setchell KD. Phyto-oestrogens and breast cancer. Lancet 1997;350(9083):971-972.

22. Hilakivi-Clarke L, Cho E, Onojafe I, et al. Maternal exposure to genistein during pregnancy increases carcinogen-induced mammary tumorigenesis in female rat offspring. Oncol Rep 1999;6(5):1089-1095.

23. Zand RS, Jenkins DJ, Diamandis EP. Steroid hormone activity of flavonoids and related compounds. Breast Cancer Res Treat 2000;62(1):35-49.

24. Jarred RA, Mcpherson SJ, Jones ME, et al. Anti-androgenic action by red clover-derived dietary isoflavones reduces non-malignant prostate enlargement in aromatase knockout (ArKo) mice. Prostate 2003;56(1):54-64.

25. Liu J, Burdette JE, Xu H, et al. Evaluation of estrogenic activity of plant extracts for the potential treatment of menopausal symptoms. J Agric Food Chem 2001;49(5):2472-2479.

26. Burdette JE, Liu J, Lantvit D, et al. *Trifolium pratense* (red clover) exhibits estrogenic effects *in vivo* in ovariectomized Sprague-Dawley rats. J Nutr 2002;132(1):27-30.

27. Jarred RA, Keikha M, Dowling C, et al. Induction of apoptosis in low to moderate-grade human prostate carcinoma by red clover-derived dietary isoflavones. Cancer Epidemiol Biomarkers Prev 2002;11(12):1689-1696.

28. Knight DC, Eden JA. A review of the clinical effects of phytoestrogens. Obstet Gynecol 1996;87(5 Pt 2):897-904.

29. Yanagihara K, Ito A, Toge T, et al. Antiproliferative effects of isoflavones on human cancer cell lines established from the gastrointestinal tract. Cancer Res 1993;53(23):5815-5821.

30. Barnes S, Kim H, Darley-Usmar V, et al. Beyond eralpha and erbeta: estrogen receptor binding is only part of the isoflavone story. J Nutr 2000;130(3):656S-657S.

31. Domon OE, Mcgarrity LJ, Bishop M, et al. Evaluation of the genotoxicity of the phytoestrogen, coumestrol, in Ahh- 1 Tk(+/-) human lymphoblastoid cells. Mutat Res 2001;474(1-2):129-137.

32. Setchell KD, Cassidy A. Dietary Isoflavones: Biological effects and relevance to human health. J Nutr 1999;129(3):758S-767S.

33. Setchell KD. Phytoestrogens: the biochemistry, physiology, and implications for human health of soy isoflavones. Am J Clin Nutr 1998;68(6 Suppl):1333S-1346S.

34. Van De Weijer PH, Barentsen R. Isoflavones from red clover (Promensil) significantly reduce menopausal hot flush symptoms compared with placebo. Maturitas 2002;42(3):187-193.

35. Abernethy K, Brockie J, Suffling K, et al. An open study of the effects of a 40-mg isoflavone food supplement (derived from red clover), on menopausal symptoms [abstract]. Br Menopause Soc (2001).

36. Simons LA, Von Konigsmark M, Simons J, et al. Phytoestrogens do not influence lipoprotein levels or endothelial function in healthy, post-menopausal women. Am J Cardiol 2000;85(11):1297-1301.

37. Finking G, Wohlfrom M, Lenz C, et al. The phytoestrogens genistein and daidzein, and 17 beta-estradiol inhibit development of neointima in aortas from male and female rabbits *in vitro* after injury. Coron Artery Dis 1999;10(8):607-615.

38. Hodgson JM, Puddey IB, Beilin LJ, et al. Supplementation with isoflavonoid phytoestrogens does not alter serum lipid concentrations: a randomized controlled trial in humans. J Nutr 1998;128(4):728-732.

39. Anderson JW, Johnstone BM, Cook-Newell ME. Meta-analysis of the effects of soy protein intake on serum lipids. N Engl J Med 1995; 333(5):276-282.

40. Lovati MR, Manzoni C, Canavesi A, Et Al. Soybean protein diet increases low density lipoprotein receptor activity in mononuclear cells from hypercholesterolemic patients. J Clin Invest 1987;80(5):1498-1502.

41. Blakesmith SJ, Lyons-Wall PM, George C, et al. Effects of supplementation with purified red clover (*Trifolium pratense*) isoflavones on plasma lipids and insulin resistance in healthy premenopausal women. Br J Nutr 2003;89(4):467-474.

42. Gerber G, Lowe FC, Spigekman S. The use of a standardized extract of red clover isoflavones for the alleviation of BPH Symptoms [abstract]. Endocr Soc 82nd Annu Meet 2000;82:2359.

43. Le Bail JC, Champavier Y, Chulia AJ, et al. Effects of phytoestrogens on aromatase, 3 beta and 17 beta-hydroxysteroid dehydrogenase activities and human breast cancer cells. Life Sci 2000;66(14):1281-1291.

44. Peterson G, Barnes S. Genistein and biochanin a inhibit the growth of human prostate cancer cells but not epidermal growth factor receptor tyrosine autophosphorylation. Prostate 1993;22(4):335-345.

45. Peterson G, Barnes S. Genistein inhibition of the growth of human breast cancer cells: independence from estrogen receptors and the multi-drug resistance gene. Biochem Biophys Res Commun 1991;179(1):661-667.

46. Barnes S. Effect of genistein on in vitro and in vivo models of cancer. J Nutr 1995;125(3 Suppl):777S-783S.

Red Yeast
(Monascus purpureus)

SYNONYMS/COMMON NAMES/RELATED SUBSTANCES

- Angkak, beni-koji, hong qu, hung-chu, monascus, red koji, red leaven, red rice, red rice yeast, red yeast, went, Xuezhikang, Zhitai.

CLINICAL BOTTOM LINE
Background

- Red yeast rice (RYR) is the product of yeast (*Monascus purpureus*) grown on rice and serves as a dietary staple in some Asian countries. It contains several compounds collectively known as "monacolins," substances known to inhibit cholesterol synthesis. One of these, monacolin K, is a potent inhibitor of HMG-CoA reductase and is also known as mevinolin and lovastatin (Mevacor).
- Red yeast rice extract (RYRE) has been sold as a natural cholesterol-lowering agent in over-the-counter supplements such as Cholestin. However, there has been legal and industrial dispute as to whether RYR is a drug or a dietary supplement, involving the manufacturer of Cholestin (Pharmanex, Inc.), the U.S. Food and Drug Administration (FDA), and the pharmaceutical industry (particularly producers of HMG-CoA reductase inhibitor prescription drugs, or "statins").
- The use of RYR in China was first documented during the Tang Dynasty in 800 AD. A detailed description of its manufacture is found in the ancient Chinese pharmacopoeia, Ben Cao Gang Mu-Dan Shi Bu Yi, published during the Ming Dynasty (1368 to 1644). In this text, RYR is proposed to be a mild aid for gastric problems (indigestion, diarrhea), blood circulation, and spleen and stomach health. RYR in a dried, powdered form is called Zhitai. When extracted with alcohol it is called Xuezhikang.
- According to the Pharmanex Web site (accessed in September 2003), new and improved Cholestin contains policosanol, a natural product from the wax of honey bees (*Apis mellifera*). It no longer contains any red yeast. Policosanols are potent inhibitors of cholesterol synthesis and have been well studied in clinical trials in Cuba and South America.

Uses Based on Scientific Evidence	Grade*
High cholesterol Since the 1970s, human studies have reported that red yeast lowers blood levels of total cholesterol, low-density lipoprotein (LDL) ("bad cholesterol"), and triglyceride. In March 2001, a U.S. District Court ruled that the RYRE product Cholestin contains the same chemical as the prescription cholesterol-lowering drug lovastatin (Mevacor) and therefore cannot be sold without a prescription. Lovastatin, like other statin drugs, has been shown in multiple well-designed controlled trials to reduce total cholesterol and LDL levels. Cholestin has since been reformulated to contain different ingredients (such as policosanol). Other products containing RYRE can still be purchased, mostly over the Internet. However, these products may not be	A

standardized, and effects are not predictable. For lowering cholesterol, there is better evidence for using prescription drugs such as lovastatin.

*Key to grades: *A:* Strong scientific evidence for this use; *B:* Good scientific evidence for this use; *C:* Unclear scientific evidence for this use; *D:* Fair scientific evidence against this use (it may not work); *F:* Strong scientific evidence against this use (it likely does not work). For a more detailed explanation of efficacy criteria, see "Natural Standard Evidence-Based Validated Grading Rationale" in the Introduction.

Uses Based on Tradition, Theory, or Limited Scientific Evidence

Anthrax, blood circulation problems, bruised muscles, bruises, colic in children, diarrhea, dysentery (bloody diarrhea), hangover, high blood pressure, indigestion, postpartum problems, spleen problems, stomach problems, wounds.

DOSING

The following doses are based on scientific research, publications, traditional use, or expert opinion. Many herbs and supplements have not been thoroughly tested, and their safety and effectiveness may not be proven. Brands may be made differently, with variable ingredients even within the same brand. The doses shown may not apply to all products. It is important to always read product labels and discuss doses with a qualified healthcare provider before therapy is started.

Adults (18 Years and Older)

- *Capsules:* 1200 mg of concentrated red yeast powder two times per day by mouth with food has been used.

Children (Younger Than 18 Years)

- There is not enough scientific evidence to recommend red yeast for children.

SAFETY

The U.S. Food and Drug Administration does not strictly regulate herbs and supplements. There is no guarantee of strength, purity, or safety of products, and effects may vary. It is important to always read product labels. People who have a medical condition, or are taking other drugs, herbs, or supplements, should consult a qualified healthcare provider before starting a new therapy. A healthcare provider should be consulted immediately about any side effects.

Allergies

- There is one report of anaphylaxis (a severe allergic reaction) in a butcher who touched meat containing red yeast.

Side Effects and Warnings

- There is limited evidence about the side effects of red yeast. Mild headache and abdominal discomfort can occur. Side effects may be similar to those for the prescription drug lovastatin (Mevacor). Heartburn, gas, bloating, muscle pain, dizziness, and kidney problems are possible. People with liver disease should not use red yeast products.
- In theory, red yeast may increase the risk of bleeding. Caution is advised in patients with bleeding disorders or

R

taking drugs that may increase the risk of bleeding. Dosing adjustments may be necessary.

Pregnancy and Breastfeeding

- Prescription drugs with component chemicals similar to red yeast cannot be used during pregnancy. Therefore, it is strongly recommended that pregnant or breastfeeding women not take red yeast.

INTERACTIONS

Most herbs and supplements have not been thoroughly tested for interactions with other herbs, supplements, drugs, or foods. The interactions listed here are based on reports in scientific publications, laboratory experiments, or traditional use. It is important to always read product labels. People who have a medical condition, or are taking other drugs, herbs, or supplements, should consult a qualified healthcare provider before starting a new therapy.

Interactions with Drugs

- There are not many studies of the interactions of red yeast rice extract with drugs. However, because RYRE contains the same chemicals as the prescription drug lovastatin, the interactions may be the same. Alcohol and other drugs that may be toxic to the liver should be avoided with use of RYRE. Taking cyclosporine, ranitidine (Zantac), and certain antibiotics with red yeast rice extract may increase the risk of muscle breakdown or kidney damage.
- Certain drugs may interfere with how the body uses the liver's cytochrome P450 enzyme system to process red yeast. Inhibitors of cytochrome P450 may increase the chance of muscle and kidney damage if taken with red yeast. People using any medications should always read the package insert and consult their healthcare provider and pharmacist about possible interactions.
- In theory, red yeast may increase the risk of bleeding when taken with drugs that increase the risk of bleeding. Some examples are aspirin, anticoagulants (blood thinners) such as warfarin (Coumadin) and heparin, antiplatelet drugs such as clopidogrel (Plavix), and nonsteroidal anti-inflammatory drugs such as ibuprofen (Motrin, Advil) and naproxen (Naprosyn, Aleve).
- Red yeast may produce gamma-aminobutyric acid (GABA) and therefore can have additive effects when taken with drugs that affect GABA such as neurontin (Gabapentin).

Interactions with Herbs and Dietary Supplements

- Red yeast may interact with products that cause liver damage or are broken down in the liver. Grapefruit juice may increase the blood levels of red yeast. Milk thistle, St. John's wort, niacin, and vitamin A may interact with RYRE. Coenzyme Q levels may be lowered by RYRE.
- Certain herbs and supplements may interfere with how the body uses the liver's cytochrome P450 enzyme system to process red yeast. Inhibitors of cytochrome P450 may increase the chance of muscle and kidney damage if taken with red yeast. Examples are bloodroot, cat's claw, chamomile, chaparral, chasteberry, damiana, *Echinacea angustifolia*,

goldenseal, grapefruit juice, licorice, oregano, red clover, St. John's wort, wild cherry, and yucca. People who are using any other herbs or supplements should always read the package insert and consult their healthcare provider and pharmacist about possible interactions.

- In theory, red yeast may increase the risk of bleeding when taken with herbs and supplements that are believed to increase the risk of bleeding. Multiple cases of bleeding have been reported with the use of *Ginkgo biloba*, and fewer cases with garlic and saw palmetto. Numerous other agents may theoretically increase the risk of bleeding, although this has not been proven in most cases. Some examples include alfalfa, American ginseng, angelica, anise, *Arnica montana*, asafetida, aspen bark, bilberry, birch, black cohosh, bladderwrack, bogbean, boldo, borage seed oil, bromelain, capsicum, cat's claw, celery, chamomile, chaparral, clove, coleus, cordyceps, danshen, devil's claw, dong quai, EPA (eicosapentaenoic acid, found in fish oils), evening primrose oil, fenugreek, feverfew, fish oil, flaxseed/flax powder (not a concern with flaxseed oil), ginger, grapefruit juice, grapeseed, green tea, guggul, gymnestra, horse chestnut, horseradish, licorice root, lovage root, male fern, meadowsweet, nordihydroguaiaretic acid (NDGA), omega-3 fatty acids, onion, *Panax ginseng*, papain, parsley, passionflower, poplar, prickly ash, propolis, quassia, red clover, reishi, rue, Siberian ginseng, sweet birch, sweet clover, turmeric, vitamin E, white willow, wild carrot, wild lettuce, willow, wintergreen, and yucca.

Selected References

Natural Standard developed the preceding evidence-based information based on a systematic review of more than 160 articles. For comprehensive information about alternative and complementary therapies on the professional level, go to www.naturalstandard.com. Selected references are listed here.

Bonovich K, Colfer H, Petoskey MI, et al. A multi-center, self-controlled study of Cholestin in subjects with elevated cholesterol. J Invest Med 1999; 47(2):54A.

Gavagan T. Cardiovascular disease. Prim Care 2002 Jun;29(2):323-338, vi.

Heber D, Yip I, Ashley JM, et al. Cholesterol-lowering effects of a proprietary Chinese red-yeast-rice dietary supplement. Am J Clin Nutr 1999;69(2): 231-236.

Heber D. Dietary supplement or drug? The case for cholestin [letter]. Am J Clin Nutr 1999;70(1):106-108.

Hsieh PS, Tai YH. Aqueous extract of *Monascus purpureus* M9011 prevents and reverses fructose-induced hypertension in rats. J Agric Food Chem 2003 Jul 2;51(14):3945-3950.

Liu L, Zhao SP, Cheng YC, Li YL. Xuezhikang decreases serum lipoprotein(a) and C-reactive protein concentrations in patients with coronary heart disease. Clin Chem 2003 Aug;49(8):1347-1352.

Su YC, Wang JJ, Lin TT, Pan TM. Production of the secondary metabolites gamma-aminobutyric acid and monacolin K by *Monascus*. J Ind Microbiol Biotechnol 2003 Jan;30(1):41-46. Epub 2003 Jan 03.

Thompson Coon JS, Ernst E. Herbs for serum cholesterol reduction: a systematic view. J Fam Pract 2003 Jun;52(6):468-478.

Wang J, Lu Z, Chi J, et al. Multicenter clinical trial of the serum lipid-lowering effects of a *Monascus purpureus* (red yeast) rice preparation from traditional Chinese medicine. Curr Ther Res 1997;58(12):964-978.

Wei W, Li C, Wang Y, et al. Hypolipidemic and anti-atherogenic effects of long-term Cholestin (*Monascus purpureus*–fermented rice, red yeast rice) in cholesterol fed rabbits. J Nutr Biochem 2003 Jun;14(6):314-318.

Wei J, Yang H, Zhang C, et al. A comparative study of xuezhikang and mevalotin in treatment of essential hyperlipidemia. Chin J New Drugs 1997;6:265-268.

Saw Palmetto
(Serenoa repens [Bartram] Small)*

SYNONYMS/COMMON NAMES/RELATED SUBSTANCES

- American dwarf palm tree, Arecaceae, cabbage palm, dwarf palm, Elusan Prostate, IDS 89, LSESR, PA 109, Palmae, palmetto scrub, palmier de l' Amerique du Nord, palmier nain, Permixon, Prostagutt, Prostaserine, sabal, *Sabal serrulata*, *Sabal serrulata* (Michx.) Nutall ex. T. Schultes & Schultes, sabalfruchte, sabal fructus, savpalme, saw palmetto berryserenoa, *Serenoa serrulata*, *Serenoa serrulata* Hook F., SG 291, Strogen, WS 1473, zwegpalme.

CLINICAL BOTTOM LINE
Background

- Saw palmetto (*Serenoa repens*) is used popularly in Europe for the management of symptoms associated with benign prostatic hypertrophy (BPH). Although not considered a standard of medical care in the United States, it is the most popular phytotherapy for this indication.
- Numerous controlled trials have reported saw palmetto to be superior to placebo and possibly equivalent to the anti-androgenic agent finasteride/Proscar (with fewer adverse effects) for the alleviation of nocturia, improvement of urinary flow, reduction of postvoid residual bladder volume, and improvement of quality of life (but possibly not measurable reduction in prostate size). However, the majority of studies have been brief (1 to 6 months), included small sample sizes, and have not employed standardized outcomes measurements such as the International Prostate Symptom Score (IPSS). Nonetheless, the weight of available evidence favors the efficacy of saw palmetto for this indication; despite the heterogeneity of study designs and reporting of results, two pooled analyses have suggested modest benefits of saw palmetto.[1-3] One trial reported superiority of a European alpha-1 blocker (alfuzosin) over saw palmetto, although methodological weaknesses limit the clinical significance of this result.[4] Most available studies have assessed the standardized saw palmetto product Permixon.
- Saw palmetto has been used in the management of other genitourinary problems, including low sperm count and lack of libido, as well as for androgenic alopecia. Additional indications have been suggested, including cancer, diabetes, bronchitis, inflammation, and migraine headache. However, there is currently insufficient evidence to recommend for or against these uses.
- Multiple mechanisms of action have been proposed, and saw palmetto appears to possess 5-α-reductase inhibitory activity (thereby preventing the conversion of testosterone to dihydrotestosterone). Hormonal/estrogenic effects have also been reported, as well as direct inhibitory effects on androgen receptors and anti-inflammatory properties.

Scientific Evidence for Common/Studied Uses	Grade*
Benign prostatic hypertrophy (BPH)	A
Androgenetic alopecia (topical)	C
Hypotonic neurogenic bladder	C
Category III prostatitis/chronic pelvic pain syndrome (CP/CPPS)	D

*Key to grades: *A:* Strong scientific evidence for this use; *B:* Good scientific evidence for this use; *C:* Unclear scientific evidence for this use; *D:* Fair scientific evidence against this use (it may not work); *F:* Strong scientific evidence against this use (it likely does not work). For a more detailed explanation of efficacy criteria, see "Natural Standard Evidence-Based Validated Grading Rationale" in the Introduction.

Historical or Theoretical Uses That Lack Sufficient Evidence

- Acne,[5] anti-androgen, antiestrogen, antiexudative, anti-inflammatory, aphrodisiac, asthma, bladder inflammation, breast augmentation, breast reduction,[6] bronchitis, cancer, catarrh, cough, cystitis, diabetes, diarrhea, digestive aid, diuretic, dysentery, dysmenorrhea, estrogenic agent, excess hair growth, expectorant, genitourinary tract disorders, hirsutism,[7] hormone imbalances (estrogen or testosterone), hypertension,[8] immunostimulant, impotence, indigestion, inflammation, lactation stimulation, laryngitis, libido, male tonic, menstrual pain, migraine headache, muscle and intestinal spasms, ovarian cysts, pelvic congestive syndrome, polycystic ovarian syndrome, postnasal drip, prostate cancer, reproductive organ problems, salpingitis, sedation, sexual vigor, sore throat, spasmolytic, sperm production, testicular atrophy, upper respiratory tract infection, urethritis,[9] urinary antiseptic, uterine disorders, vaginal disorders.

Expert Opinion and Folkloric Precedent

- Extracts of the fruit of saw palmetto were traditionally used by Native Americans indigenous to the southeastern United States for urinary complaints and as an expectorant and anti-septic. In the 19th century, it was used by naturopaths to treat a wide range of genitourinary or endocrine-related conditions, including enhancement of breast size, sperm production, and sexual vigor.
- Saw palmetto has been studied extensively for the treatment of benign prostatic hypertrophy (BPH) and has been approved by the German expert panel, the Commission E, for the treatment of mild to moderate BPH (stage I-II). In Italy, herbal therapy represents approximately half of treatment for BPH, whereas in Germany and Austria, it is a first-line treatment.[1]
- In the United States, the herb has not become part of standard medical care, although saw palmetto is the most commonly used non-prescription therapy for lower urinary tract symptoms in BPH.[10]

Safety Summary

- **Likely safe:** When saw palmetto is used orally in recommended doses in otherwise healthy adults for up to 3 to 5 years[11,12]; the most common complaints are gastrointestinal. Anecdotally, lipidosterolic extract of *Serenoa repens* (LSESR) may be a better tolerated formulation.

- **Possibly unsafe:** May be unsafe in patients with bleeding disorders, in those taking medications or herbs/supplements that may increase the risk of bleeding, or prior to some surgical/dental procedures, based on a report of cerebral hemorrhage[13] and a report of intra-operative bleeding [14] associated with oral saw palmetto use. Saw palmetto may be unsafe during pregnancy and lactation because of its proposed ability to inhibit the conversion of testosterone to dihydrotestosterone (DHT), which may cause abnormalities in the genitalia of the male fetus. Saw palmetto may be unsafe when used with finasteride (Proscar) or other anti-androgenic drugs (due to its proposed similar mechanism of action), when used with therapeutic androgens, or when used with hormone replacement therapy.

DOSING/TOXICOLOGY
General
- Recommended doses are based on those most commonly used in available trials, or on historical practice. However, with natural products, the optimal doses needed to balance efficacy and safety often have not been determined. Formulations and preparation methods may vary from manufacturer to manufacturer, and from batch to batch of a specific product made by a single manufacturer. Because often the active components of a product are not known, standardization may not be possible, and the clinical effects of different brands may not be comparable.

Standardization
- A standardized extract of saw palmetto containing 80% to 95% sterols and fatty acids (liposterolic content) has been recommended.
- One study examining amounts of saw palmetto contained in six commercial preparations compared to amounts stated on labels reported a –97% to +140% difference compared to label claims.[15] Half the samples (3 samples) contained less than 25% of the stated amounts .

Dosing: Adult (18 Years and Older)
Oral
- **Benign prostatic hypertrophy (BPH):** 320 mg daily in 1 dose or 2 divided doses (80% to 90% liposterolic content) has been used in multiple clinical trials and is recommended by the German expert panel of the Commission E. A 1-year dosing study in 84 subjects suggests equivalence of 160 mg twice daily and 320 mg once daily.[16] A subsequent dosing evaluation reports that 160 mg once daily may be as effective as twice daily, although the lack of a placebo group limits the clinical significance of this finding.[13]
- **Other formulations:** Saw palmetto has also been used or recommended as 1 to 2 g of ground, dried, or whole berries daily; 2 to 4 mL of tincture (1:4) three times daily; 1 to 2 mL of fluid extract of berry pulp (1:1) three times daily; or tea (2 teaspoons dried berry, simmered slowly in 24 ounces water until liquid is reduced by half), taken as 4 ounces three times daily. Teas prepared from saw palmetto berries are potentially ineffective because the purported active constituents are water insoluble.[17] Anecdotally, lipidosterolic extract of *Serenoa repens* (LSESR) may be a better-tolerated formulation.

Rectal
- **Benign prostatic hypertrophy (BPH):** Rectal administration of saw palmetto extract (640 mg once daily) was reported as being clinically equivalent to oral administration (160 mg four times daily) in a 30-day controlled trial in 40 men, although it is not clear that this sample size was large enough to assess equivalence.[18]

Dosing: Pediatric (Younger Than 18 Years)
- Insufficient available evidence to recommend.

Toxicology
- No toxic effects of saw palmetto have been reported in the available literature,[1,19] although systematic study of toxicity is lacking.
- One study of sperm motility suggested effects on sperm metabolism, while other reports by the same authors did not find adverse effects on sperm DNA, oocytes, or fertilization.[20]

ADVERSE EFFECTS/PRECAUTIONS/CONTRAINDICATIONS
Allergy
- Known allergy/hypersensitivity to saw palmetto or any of its constituents.
- In an open trial of the discontinued combination product PC-SPES, which contains saw palmetto and seven other herbs, in 70 patients with prostate cancer, 3 allergic reactions were reported. In one case, treatment was discontinued because of uvular swelling and shortness of breath.[21] It is not clear which constituent(s) might have contributed to this reaction.

Adverse Effects
- **General:** Saw palmetto appears to be well tolerated by most patients for up to 3 to 5 years; the most common complaints are gastrointestinal (anecdotally, lipidosterolic extract of *Serenoa repens* [LSESR] may be a better-tolerated formulation). There have been two case reports of clinically significant bleeding associated with saw palmetto products.[13,14] In a systematic review of 18 randomized trials (2939 male subjects) of up to 48 weeks' duration adverse effects associated with saw palmetto were reported as generally mild and comparable to placebo; erectile dysfunction and study withdrawal were less common with saw palmetto than with finasteride.[1] In a 3-year trial, tolerability of a saw palmetto extract was classified as "good" or "very good" by 98% of participating physicians and patients; a total of 46 adverse events were reported in the 315 subjects, one third of which were gastrointestinal (leading to study withdrawal by 1.8% of subjects).[11] A 5-year study in 26 patients with benign prostatic hypertrophy did not find any cases of intolerance to saw palmetto.[12]
- **Neurologic/CNS:** Rare headaches have been noted in clinical trials.[16,22,23] In a multicenter, placebo-controlled trial investigating the safety of saw palmetto (320 mg), one of 84 patients reported headache,[16] whereas headache was reported in 3 of 32 subjects receiving saw palmetto in a different controlled study.[23] Occasional reports of mild headache have been noted in other studies.[13,22] Rare reports of dizziness, insomnia, and fatigue have been documented in an open trial of 160 mg of saw palmetto extract given twice daily.[24] Dizziness requiring temporary withdrawal of saw palmetto (Permixon, 320 mg) has also been reported.[25] A case of cerebral hemorrhage occurred during a study of saw palmetto (Permixon, 320 mg) for benign prostatic hypertrophy, although there was limited additional detail regarding this event.[13]
- **Psychiatric:** In a double-blind, placebo-controlled, multicenter study of saw palmetto (Permixon, 160 mg twice

daily), one subject discontinued treatment, due to fatigue, depression, and stomach upset.[26] Causality was not clearly established.

- **Pulmonary/respiratory:** One report of "breathlessness" was made in an open multicenter trial of 160 mg of saw palmetto given twice daily.[24] Two instances of respiratory depression were reported in a study of Permixon (320 mg) for benign prostatic hypertrophy (BSP).[13] Three thromboembolic events (pulmonary emboli) were reported in a prospective trial of 70 patients with prostate cancer treated with the now discontinued combination product PC-SPES, which contains saw palmetto and seven other herbs. Causality cannot easily be determined because of the increased risk of hypercoagulable events in some types of cancer.[21] Some batches of PC-SPES were notably found to contain warfarin, which would presumably reduce the risk of clotting.

- **Cardiovascular:** Occasional occurrences of hypertension, tachycardia, angina pectoris, atrial arrhythmia, extra systole, angiopathy, myocardial infarction, and congestive heart failure have been noted in the clinical literature in association with oral saw palmetto use, although these reports have provided limited information to determine causality.[13,21,24] Infrequent hypertension has been reported in controlled trials: 3.1% of 551 subjects treated with saw palmetto (Permixon, 320 mg) compared to 2.2% of 542 subjects treated with finasteride (5 mg)[27]; 2 subjects in a controlled trial of 238 patients randomized to saw palmetto (320 mg) or placebo[28]; and 3 of 50 patients with benign prostatic hypertrophy taking Permixon (320 mg).[13] There have been case reports of aggravation of preexisting angina, myocardial infarction,[25] death following a myocardial infarction in a 80-year-old patient with a history of heart disease,[27] death due to cardiac disease,[29] and two episodes of congestive heart failure in a study of prostate cancer patients.[21] However, causality has not been clear in these cases.[25] Three thromboembolic events (pulmonary emboli) were reported in a prospective trial of 70 patients with prostate cancer treated with PC-SPES, a discontinued combination therapy which includes saw palmetto.[21] Events occurred at 2 weeks and at 7 months. Causality cannot be easily determined because of the increased risk of hypercoagulability in some types of cancer.

- **Gastrointestinal:** The most commonly reported side effects associated with saw palmetto use are gastrointestinal, including abdominal discomfort or pain, nausea, vomiting, and diarrhea; there are also rare reports of duodenal ulcer and cholestatic hepatitis. These effects may be associated with the fatty nature of the berries or liposterolic extract. One third of the 46 clinical adverse effects identified in an open multicenter trial of 315 subjects were gastrointestinal.[11] Nausea, constipation, vomiting, diarrhea, gastralgia, and halitosis (bad breath) have been noted with doses of 160 mg twice daily or 320 mg once daily of saw palmetto.[16,21,24,25,30] These adverse effects have led to study withdrawal in some cases[25] or dose reduction (in one study, 39% of 70 patients experienced diarrhea and 2 patients required dose reduction).[21] One patient in a trial investigating the tolerability of 160 to 320 mg of Permixon daily withdrew because of development of a duodenal ulcer.[13] One case report has documented protracted cholestatic hepatitis in a 65-year-old man after a 2-week trial of Prostata (zinc picolinate, pyridoxine, l-alanine, glutamic acid, *Apis mellifica* pollen, silica, hydrangea extract, *Panex ginseng*, *Serenoa serrulata*, and *Pygeum africanum*); the patient's liver enzymes remained

abnormal for >3 months after cessation of this therapy. In a controlled study, a 71-year-old patient developed acute cholecystitis while taking saw palmetto (Permixon), although this was not considered to be drug-related and did not require cessation of treatment.[27]

- **Genitourinary:** Controlled trials and open studies have reported occasional genitourinary effects associated with saw palmetto, most commonly related to sexual dysfunction. However, most enrolled patients have been previously diagnosed with prostate disorders, and causality has remained unclear. In a 6-month equivalence study of saw palmetto (Permixon, 320 mg) vs. finasteride involving 1098 patients, decreased libido (2.2%), impotence (1.5%), and urinary retention (1.3%) were reported in the Permixon group, and one patient developed prostatitis and withdrew from the study.[27] In an earlier trial, one of 33 patients taking Permixon (320 mg) reported an increase in libido after 2 weeks.[25] In a three-year, open multicenter study in 435 patients, adverse urologic outcomes were noted in 9 patients, including carcinoma of the prostate (n = 4), urinary tract infection (n = 3), impotence (n =1), and ejaculatory disorder (n = 1).[11] In an open-label trial, 1 of 18 patients taking a saw palmetto herbal blend experienced a decrease in ejaculatory volume.[29] Rare cases of testicular pain, vesical tenesmus, and urinary tract infection were reported in an open multicenter trial of saw palmetto extract.[24] In a trial of the discontinued herbal mixture PC-SPES (which includes saw palmetto and seven other herbs) in 70 patients with prostate cancer, 15 subjects reported erectile dysfunction, 19 patients developed hot flushes, and 60 experienced breast tenderness/enlargement.[21] It is not clear which constituent(s) might have contributed to this effect.

- **Oncologic (PSA levels):** In theory, PSA (prostate-specific antigen) levels may be artificially lowered by saw palmetto, based on a proposed mechanism of action of saw palmetto (inhibition of 5-α-reductase). Therefore, there may be a delay in diagnosis of prostate cancer or interference with following PSA levels during treatment or monitoring in men with known prostate cancer. In contrast, a statistically significant small increase in PSA levels has been reported in association with saw palmetto use in one study[16] that has not been observed in other studies.[27,32]

- **Hematologic:** There have been two reports of bleeding complications associated with the use of saw palmetto. In one case, severe intra-operative hemorrhage was associated with saw palmetto use, requiring premature termination of neurosurgery for meningioma in a 53-year-old male patient who had been taking saw palmetto (unknown duration) for benign prostatic hypertrophy.[14] The patient exhibited prolonged bleeding time (21 minutes), which normalized 5 days after cessation of saw palmetto therapy. In a second case, cerebral hemorrhage occurred in one patient during a study of saw palmetto (Permixon, 320 mg) for benign prostatic hypertrophy, although there was limited additional detail regarding this event.[13] Three thromboembolic events (pulmonary emboli) were reported in a prospective trial of 70 patients with prostate cancer treated with the discontinued combination product PC-SPES which contains saw palmetto. Causality cannot easily be determined because of the increased risk of hypercoagulable events in some types of cancer.[21] Notably, some batches of PC-SPES were found to contain warfarin, which would presumably reduce the risk of clotting. In early 2002, the U.S. Food and Drug Administration issued a warning regarding the presence of warfarin in PC-SPES, and the manufacturer agreed to remove the product from the market.

- **Endocrine:** Saw palmetto is purported to possess anti-androgenic properties and possibly to exert effects on estrogen receptors.[33-35] Systemic endocrine effects have not been noted, although use during pregnancy and lactation are not advised because of potential hormonal effects on the developing fetus or infant.
- **Musculoskeletal:** Rare reports of fatigue and muscle pain were noted in an open multicenter trial of saw palmetto extract.[24] Back pain was reported in 1.6% of a sample of 551 patients treated with saw palmetto (Permixon) for benign prostatic hypertrophy.[27] New or worsening leg cramps was reported in 48 patients (69% of sample) with prostate cancer during a phase II study of the discontinued herbal mixture PC-SPES, which includes saw palmetto and 7 other herbs.[21]

Precautions/Warnings/Contraindications

- Avoid in women who are or may potentially be pregnant due to theoretical risks to fetal genital development.
- Avoid during lactation.
- Use cautiously in patients with bleeding disorders, in those taking medications that may increase the risk of bleeding, or prior to some surgical/dental procedures, based on a report of cerebral hemorrhage [13] and a report of intra-operative bleeding [4] associated with oral saw palmetto use.
- Use cautiously in patients taking hormone replacement therapy or with hormone-sensitive conditions.
- Use cautiously in patients taking anti-androgens (such as finasteride/Proscar) or therapeutic androgens.
- Use cautiously in patients with gastrointestinal disorders, based on multiple reports in clinical trials of mild to moderate gastrointestinal symptoms, including nausea, diarrhea, and abdominal discomfort.
- Use cautiously in patients with hypertension, based on reports of increased blood pressure in several patients in clinical studies.[13,27,28]
- Avoid the supplement/herbal combination products PC SPES and SPES, which may contain the ingredients warfarin and alprazolam, respectively.

Pregnancy and Lactation

- Because of potential anti-androgenic activity and effects on estrogen receptors, saw palmetto extract is not indicated in women who are pregnant or lactating. Use has been discouraged during pregnancy and lactation because of saw palmetto's proposed ability to inhibit the conversion of testosterone to dihydrotestosterone (DHT), which may cause abnormalities in the genitalia of a male fetus/infant.

INTERACTIONS
Saw Palmetto/Drug Interactions

- **Anti-androgenic drugs:** Based on the proposed anti-androgenic mechanism of action of saw palmetto, additive effects may occur with anti-androgen drugs such as the 5α-reductase inhibitor finasteride (Proscar); the androgen receptor antagonists bicalutamide (Casodex), flutamide (Eulexin), and nilutamide (Nilandron); and the GnRH (gonadotropin-releasing hormone) antagonists leuprolide (Lupron), goserelin (Zoladex), and histrelin (Supprelin).
- **Androgenic drugs:** Based on the proposed anti-androgenic mechanism of action of saw palmetto, therapy may decrease the effectiveness of therapeutic androgens such as testosterone (Androderm, Testoderm), methyltestosterone (Android,

Testred, Virilon), fluoxymesterone (Halotestin), nandrolone decanoate (Deca-Dubrolin), and stanozolol (Winstrol).

- **Estrogen, hormone replacement therapy (HRT), oral contraceptive pills (OCPs):** Based on *in vitro* observations that saw palmetto may be anti-androgenic and may exert activity on estrogen receptors,[33-35] saw palmetto therapy may interfere with oral contraceptive use and hormone replacement therapy.
- **Anticoagulants, anti-platelet agents, NSAIDs:** Based on a case report of severe intraoperative hemorrhage and prolonged bleeding time[14] and a report of cerebral hemorrhage,[13] saw palmetto should be used cautiously with other agents that increase the risk of bleeding.
- **Antihypertensive agents:** Occasional cases of hypertension have been reported in controlled trials: 3.1% of a sample of 551 subjects treated with saw palmetto (Permixon, 320 mg), vs. 2.2% of 542 subjects treated with finasteride (5 mg) (statistical significance not known)[27]; 2 subjects in a controlled trial of 238 patients randomized to saw palmetto (320 mg) or placebo[28]; and 6% of 50 patients with benign prostatic hypertrophy taking saw palmetto (Permixon, 320 mg) in a controlled trial.[13] Effects of saw palmetto on blood pressure and interactions with hypotensive agents have not been systematically studied.

Saw Palmetto/Herb/Supplement Interactions

- **Anticoagulant agents:** Based on one case report of severe intraoperative hemorrhage and prolonged bleeding time[14] and a report of cerebral hemorrhage,[13] saw palmetto should be used cautiously with other agents that increase the risk of bleeding.
- **Estrogenic herbs and supplements:** Based on *in vitro* observations that saw palmetto may be anti-androgenic and may exert activity on estrogen receptors,[33-35] saw palmetto therapy may interfere with the activity of estrogenic herbs and supplements.
- **Antihypertensive agents:** Occasional cases of hypertension have been reported in controlled trials: 3.1% of a sample of 551 subjects treated with saw palmetto (Permixon, 320 mg), vs. 2.2% of 542 subjects treated with finasteride (5 mg) (statistical significance not known)[27]; 2 subjects in a controlled trial of 238 patients randomized to saw palmetto (320 mg) or placebo;[28] and 6% of 50 patients with benign prostatic hypertrophy taking saw palmetto (Permixon, 320 mg) in a controlled trial[13] Effects of saw palmetto on blood pressure and interactions with hypotensive agents have not been systematically studied.
- **Androgenic/anti-androgenic agents:** Based on the proposed anti-androgenic action of saw palmetto, therapy may decrease the effectiveness of other agents used as therapeutic androgens.

Saw Palmetto/Food Interactions

- **General:** Taking saw palmetto extract with food may decrease the gastrointestinal distress sometimes associated with saw palmetto use.
- **Tea forms:** Teas prepared from saw palmetto berries are potentially ineffective because the active constituents are water insoluble.[17]

Saw Palmetto/Lab Interactions

- **Prostate specific antigen:** In theory, PSA (prostate-specific antigen) levels may be artificially lowered by saw palmetto, based on a proposed mechanism of action of saw palmetto (inhibition of 5-α-reductase). Therefore, there may be a delay in diagnosis of prostate cancer, or interference with following PSA levels during treatment or monitoring in men with known prostate cancer. In contrast, a statistically significant small increase in PSA levels has been reported in association with saw palmetto use in one study[16] that has not been observed in other studies.[27,32]

- **Dihydrotestosterone (DHT):** A modest but significant decline in prostatic DHT levels was observed in a 6-month placebo-controlled trial involving 40 men.[36] However, conflicting evidence was reported in an open, randomized, placebo-controlled study that reported that saw palmetto (Permixon) may not reduce plasma DHT levels.[37]
- **Bleeding time:** Bleeding time is a measure not often used currently in the United States. There are two reported clinical cases of bleeding associated with saw palmetto use, including one patient who was noted to have a prolonged bleeding time (21 minutes), which normalized 5 days after cessation of saw palmetto therapy.[14] Effects of saw palmetto on more common first-line measures of coagulation such as prothrombin time (PT) or international normalized ratio (INR) are not clear.
- **Liver function tests (LFTs):** One case report documents protracted cholestatic hepatitis in a 65-year-old man after a 2-week trial of Prostata (zinc picolinate, pyridoxine, l-alanine, glutamic acid, *Apis mellifica* pollen, silica, hydrangea extract, *Panex ginseng, Serenoa serrulata,* and *Pygeum africanum*).[31] The patient was found to have elevated levels of alanine aminotransferase (ALT), aspartate aminotransferase (AST), gamma-glutamyltransferase (GGT), alkaline phosphatase, and bilirubin.

MECHANISM OF ACTION
Pharmacology

- **Hormonal effects:** Active agents within saw palmetto (*Serenoa repens, Sabal serrulata*) may be sterols and fatty acids, such as myristoleic acid.[38] The exact mechanism of action is unknown. Saw palmetto has been shown to inhibit 5-α-reductase activity on testosterone *in vitro*, thereby preventing the conversion of testosterone to dihydrotestosterone (DHT) and possibly exerting an anti-tumor effect.[39-42] However, evidence of 5-α-reductase inhibition from randomized trials is conflicting.[19,29,37,42-45] A modest but significant decline in prostatic DHT levels was observed in a 6-month placebo-controlled trial involving 40 men.[36] Di Silvero et al. noted a decrease in epidermal growth factor, which they associated with DHT suppression in prostatic tissue of patients treated with saw palmetto (Permixon).[45] However, an open, randomized, placebo-controlled study indicated that Permixon may not reduce plasma DHT levels,[37] although this study was limited by its short (1 week) duration.
- A 6-month controlled trial of saw palmetto in 41 men from whom prostate biopsy specimens were obtained revealed significant contraction of transition zone epithelium and epithelial atrophy.[46] The authors suggest that because no evidence of alteration in prostatic androgen metabolism was demonstrated, saw palmetto may suppress prostatic epithelium via a nonhormonal mechanism. Clinical observations have suggested a lack of systemic hormonal effects, including unchanged levels of testosterone, follicle-stimulating hormone, and luteinizing hormone.[47] Possible estrogenic effects of saw palmetto have been suggested to derive from β-sitosterol,[34] although subsequent evaluation reports possible inhibitory effects on estrogen receptor binding.[33]

- **Androgen receptor effects:** Saw palmetto may act to increase the metabolism and excretion of dihydrotestosterone (DHT) through inhibition of cellular and nuclear receptor binding. Saw palmetto extract has demonstrated inhibition of androgen activity via competition with DHT at the androgen receptor in several animal and human tissue culture studies.[48-61] In a placebo-controlled study of 35 patients with benign prostatic hypertrophy treated with saw palmetto 3 months prior to transvesical adenomectomy, nuclear and cytosolic concentrations of estrogen and androgen receptors were examined, and the authors suggested that inactivation of androgen receptors may occur secondary to blockade of estrogen receptors.[33] Rhodes et al. did not observe either finasteride or various formulations of saw palmetto (Permixon, Talso, Strogen Forte, Prostagutt, Tadenan, Remigeron, Bazoton, and Harzol) to inhibit DHT binding to rat prostatic androgen receptors.[39]
- **Adrenergic effects:** Despite anti–α_1-adrenoceptor activity *in vitro*,[52] no evidence for α_1-adrenoceptor antagonism of saw palmetto extract was subsequently found *in vivo*.[8]
- **Anti-proliferative effects:** An *in vitro* study of cultured fibroblasts and epithelial cells derived from prostate, epididymis, testes, skin and breast suggests that saw palmetto (Permixon) may selectively act to disrupt intracellular nuclear membranes of prostate cells, yielding increased apoptosis.[53] Antiproliferative and proapoptotic properties have been attributed to saw palmetto, based on the results of other *in vitro* studies, demonstrating inhibition of growth factor-induced hyperplasia.[54-58] In human urologic cancer cell lines, saw palmetto extract inhibited urokinase-type plasminogen activator, an enzyme implicated in tumor cell invasion.[59]
- **Anti-inflammatory effects:** Anti-inflammatory properties have been attributed to saw palmetto,[60] based on the ability to inhibit lipoxygenase and cyclooxygenase *in vitro*,[61,62] as well as the ability to inhibit mast cell accumulation *in vivo*.[63]

Pharmacodynamics/Kinetics

- Studies of the pharmacodynamics and kinetics of saw palmetto or its constituents are limited.
- One study in 12 healthy men (mean age, 24-years) measured a peak plasma concentration of 2.6 mg/L at 1.5 hours and a half-life of 19 hours following administration of 320 mg of oral saw palmetto.[64]
- De Bernardi et al. conducted an open, randomized, crossover, bioequivalence study in 12 healthy volunteers and found that the concentration-time profile (AUC, C_{max}, T_{max}) of a 320-mg capsule of saw palmetto was similar to the profile of 160 mg of saw palmetto taken twice daily.[65]
- **Cytochrome P450 (CYP) activity:** In an evaluation of the effects of saw palmetto on the activity of CYP2D6 and CYP3A4 in normal volunteers, no significant effect of multiple doses was found.[66]

HISTORY

- Historical use of saw palmetto can be traced in the Americas to the Mayans, who used it as a tonic, and to the Seminoles, who used the berries as an expectorant and antiseptic. In more recent times, saw palmetto has been studied and popularized for the treatment of benign prostatic hypertrophy and other male genitourinary conditions, such as increasing sperm production and erectile dysfunction.
- Saw palmetto was listed in the United States Pharmacopeia from 1906 to 1917, and in the National Formulary from

S

Review of the Evidence: Saw Palmetto

Condition Treated*	Study Design	Author, Year	N[†]	SS[†]	Study Quality[‡]	Magnitude of Benefit	ARR[†]	NNT[†]	Comments
BPH	Systematic review and pooled analysis	Wilt[1,2] 1998, 2000	2939 (18 trials)	Yes	NA	Medium	28%	3	Well-conducted review of trials with heterogeneous designs and outcomes measures; pooled analysis of selected studies suggests improved nocturia and IPSS (superior to placebo, equivalent to finasteride); ARR & NNT calculated for self-rated symptom scores vs. placebo.
BPH	Meta-analysis	Boyle[3] 2000	2859	Yes	NA	Medium	NA	NA	Included 13 trials of the product Permixon; unclear search strategy and selection criteria; pooled analysis found reductions in peak urinary flow rate by 2.2 mL/s and nocturia by 0.5 episodes; included trials may be too heterogeneous for reliable meta-analysis.
BPH	Randomized, placebo-controlled, double-blind trial	Willetts[67] 2003	100	No	4	None	NA	NA	320 mg of saw palmetto for 12 weeks demonstrated no significant benefits over placebo (paraffin oil); may not have been adequately powered.
BPH	Randomized, placebo-controlled, double-blind trial	Mohanty[68] 1999	75	Yes	5	Medium	41%	3	Unclear dose of saw palmetto for 8 weeks associated with improved composite symptom score and subjective improvement.
BPH	Randomized, placebo-controlled, double-blind trial	Gerber[30] 2001	85	No	4	Medium	NA	NA	160 mg twice daily of saw palmetto associated with improved IPSS but not urinary flow rate; baseline characteristics differed between groups.
BPH	Randomized, placebo-controlled, double-blind trial	Bauer[69] 1999	101	Yes	4	Large	NA	NA	160 mg twice daily of Talso for 24 weeks associated with improved IPSS and dysuria but not postvoid residual volume.
BPH	Randomized, placebo-controlled, double-blind trial	Reece Smith[25] 1986	80	No	4	NA	NA	NA	160 mg twice daily of Permixon for 12 weeks associated with no significant improvement in urinary flow rate, residual volume, or subjective symptoms.
BPH	Randomized, placebo-controlled, double-blind trial	Cukier[70] 1985	168	Yes	4	Medium	40%	3	160 mg twice daily of Permixon for 10 weeks associated with improved dysuria, residual volume, and nocturia.
BPH	Randomized, placebo-controlled, double-blind trial (published letter)	Champault[22] 1984	110	Yes	4	Large	23%	5	160 mg twice daily of PA109 for 4 weeks associated with improved nocturia, urinary flow rate, and residual volume; 15% dropout.
BPH	Randomized, placebo-controlled, double-blind trial	Boccafoschi[87] 1983	22	Yes	4	Small	NA	NA	160 mg twice daily of Permixon for 8 weeks associated with improved urinary flowrate; baseline characteristics differed between groups.
BPH	Randomized, placebo-controlled, double-blind trial	Braeckman[28] 1997	238	Yes	3	Medium	NA	NA	160 mg twice daily of Permixon for 12 weeks associated with improved urinary flow and residual volume.
BPH	Randomized, placebo-controlled, double-blind trial	Descotes[26] 1995	176	Yes	3	Medium	NA	NA	160 mg twice daily of Permixon associated with improved urinary frequency, flow rate, and dysuria. Not intention-to-treat analysis.

Review of the Evidence: Saw Palmetto—*cont'd*

Condition Treated*	Study Design	Author, Year	N†	SS†	Study Quality‡	Magnitude of Benefit	ARR†	NNT†	Comments
BPH	Randomized, placebo-controlled, double-blind trial	Löbelenz[71] 1992	60	Unclear	3	Small	NA	NA	100 mg of saw palmetto extract once daily for 6 weeks associated with improved urinary flow rate, residual volume, and frequency; statistical analysis not provided.
BPH	Randomized, placebo-controlled, double-blind trial	Mattei[72] 1990	40	Yes	2	Small	NA	NA	160 mg twice daily of Talso for 13 weeks associated with improved dysuria, residual volume, and urinary frequency.
BPH	Randomized, placebo-controlled, double-blind trial	Gabric[73] 1987	59	Yes	2	Medium	NA	NA	60 drops daily of Prostagutt for 6 weeks associated with improved urinary frequency and retention and prostate size.
BPH	Randomized, placebo-controlled, double-blind trial	Tasca[74] 1985	30	Unclear	2	Large	23%	5	PA109 daily for 8 weeks associated with improved dysuria, urinary flow rate, nocturia and urgency. Poorly described trial.
BPH	Randomized, placebo-controlled, double-blind trial	Emili[73] 1983	30	Yes	2	Large	59%	2	160 mg twice daily of Permixon for 4 weeks associated with improved nocturia, urinary flow rate, and prostate volume; poorly described trial.
BPH	Randomized, placebo-controlled trial, unclear blinding (published abstract)	Mandressi[76] 1987	60	Yes	1	Unclear	NA	NA	160 mg twice daily of saw palmetto for 8 weeks associated with reduced urinary symptoms; poorly described abstract.
BPH	Non-randomized, placebo-controlled, double-blind comparison study	Mandressi[77] 1983	60	Yes	1	Small	NA	NA	160 mg twice daily of Permixon for 8 weeks vs. pygeum or placebo associated with improved dysuria, urinary frequency, and residual volume.
BPH	Comparison study, no placebo arm	Carraro[27] 1996	1098	Yes	3	Medium	NA	NA	160 mg twice daily of Permixon vs. 5 mg of finasteride daily for 26 weeks; 38% mean decrease in symptom scores in both groups from baseline; sexual function worse with finasteride but unchanged with Permixon.
BPH	Comparison study, no placebo arm	Grasso[4] 1995	63	Yes	3	Medium	24%	4	160 mg of saw palmetto twice daily vs. alpha- inhibitor alfazosin for 3 weeks; higher response rate in alfazosin group to increased urinary flow than saw palmetto group.
BPH	Comparison study (published abstract)	Semino[77] 1992	45	No	1	None	NA	NA	Saw palmetto less efficacious than prazosin.
BPH	Comparison study	Comar[79] 1986	20	NA	1	None	NA	NA	Saw palmetto less efficacious than mepartricin.
BPH	Comparison study	Pannunzio[80] 1986	60	Yes	1	Variable	NA	NA	Saw palmetto vs. Depostat; similar improved urinary symptoms from baseline in both groups; no power calculation.
BPH	Comparison study, non-randomized	Flamm[81] 1979	74	Unclear	0	None	NA	NA	Saw palmetto vs. testosterone injections weekly; both therapies ineffective in relieving urinary symptoms; no statistical analysis.
BPH	Combination product, randomized, double-blind, placebo-controlled trial	Metzker[82] 1996	40	Yes	5	Small	NA	NA	Combination of saw palmetto (320 mg) plus stinging nettle (240 mg) (Prostagutt forte) for 24 weeks, associated with improved frequency of urination.

S

Continued

Review of the Evidence: Saw Palmetto—*cont'd*

Condition Treated*	Study Design	Author, Year	N[†]	SS[†]	Study Quality[‡]	Magnitude of Benefit	ARR[†]	NNT[†]	Comments
BPH	Combination product, randomized, double-blind, placebo-controlled trial	Carbin[83] 1990	53	Yes	5	Large	NA	NA	Combination of pumpkin seeds, saw palmetto, and *Cucurbita pepo* for 12 weeks associated with improved nocturia and subjective symptoms.
BPH	Combination product, comparison, randomized, double-blind, placebo-controlled trial	Marks[29] 2000	44	No	4	NA	NA	NA	Combination of saw palmetto, nettle, pumpkin seed oil, lemon bioflavonoid extract, and vitamin A associated with non-significant improvement in urinary symptoms.
BPH	Combination product, comparison, randomized, double-blind trial	Sökeland[84] 1997	542	No	4	None	NA	NA	Combination of saw palmetto 320 mg + stinging nettle 240 mg (Prostagutt forte) vs. finasteride 5 mg daily for 52 weeks. Similar improved flow and IPSS in both groups.
BPH	Dosing study, randomized, double-blind, no placebo arm	Stepanov[13] 1999	100	No	3	NA	NA	NA	No difference between 160 mg of Permixon taken once or twice daily for 12 weeks in urinary flow rate, IPSS, or quality of life; no power calculation.
BPH	Dosing study, randomized, single-blind, placebo-controlled	Braeckman[16] 1997	84	No	1	Large	NA	NA	No difference between Prostaserene 160mg twice daily and 320 mg once daily for 52 weeks in flow rate, IPSS, or quality of life. No power calculation. 24% dropout.
BPH	Dosing study, randomized, unblinded	Roveda[18] 1994	40	No	NA	NA	NA	NA	No difference between 160 mg of oral saw palmetto 4 times daily and 640 mg of rectal saw palmetto once daily in residual volume or IPSS; no power calculation.
CP/CPP	Prospective, randomized, open label, comparison trial	Kaplan[23] 2004	64	No	3	Inferior	NA	NA	Saw palmetto (325 mg daily) inferior to finasteride (5 mg once daily) after 1 year of treatment.
Androgenetic alopecia	Randomized, double-blind, placebo-controlled, before- and -after study	Morganti[85] 1998	24	Yes	2	Medium	NA	NA	Topical saw palmetto for 50 weeks associated with improved hair density compared to baseline; smaller improvement noted in placebo group.
Hypotonic neurogenic bladder	Combination product, placebo-controlled, non-randomized trial	Timmermans[86] 1990	30	Yes	1	Small	NA	NA	Combination of echinacea and saw palmetto (Urgenin) for 7 weeks associated with improved "bladder capacity" and residual volume; poorly described trial.

*Primary or secondary outcome.

[†]*N*, Number of patients; *SS*, statistically significant; *ARR*, absolute risk reduction; *NNT*, the number of patients who need to undergo a specific intervention in order to observe an outcome in one individual.

[‡]0-2 = poor; 3-4 = good; 5 = excellent.

BPH, Benign prostatic hypertrophy; *CP/CPP*, category III prostatitis/chronic pelvic pain; *IPSS*, International Prostate Symptom Scale; *NA*, not applicable; *RCT*, randomized, controlled trial.

For an explanation of each category in this table, please see Table 3 in the Introduction.

1926 to 1950. Saw palmetto extract is a licensed product in several European countries.

REVIEW OF THE EVIDENCE: DISCUSSION
Benign prostatic hypertrophy (BPH)
Summary

- Numerous controlled trials have reported saw palmetto to be superior to placebo and possibly equivalent to the anti-androgenic agent finasteride/Proscar (with fewer adverse effects) in the alleviation of nocturia, improvement of urinary flow, reduction of postvoid residual bladder volume, and improvement of quality of life (but possibly not measurable reduction in prostate size). However, the majority of studies have been brief (1 to 6 months), included small sample sizes, and have not employed standardized outcomes measurements such as the International Prostate Symptom Score (IPSS). Nonetheless, the weight of available evidence favors the efficacy of saw palmetto for this indication; despite the heterogeneity of study designs and reporting of results, two pooled analyses have suggested modest benefits of saw palmetto.[1-3] One trial has reported superiority of a European alpha-1 blocker alfuzosin) over saw palmetto, although methodological weaknesses limit the clinical significance of this result.[4] Most available studies have assessed the standardized saw palmetto product Permixon.

Systematic Review and Meta-analysis

- In 1998, Wilt et al. conducted a well-designed systematic review of randomized, controlled trials of saw palmetto extracts taken for a minimum of 4 weeks.[1,2] Trials were identified via searches of MEDLINE, EMBASE, Phytodok, and the Cochrane library through 1997, as well as review of relevant study bibliographies and consultation with experts and manufacturers. No limitations were placed on language of publication. Of 24 identified studies, 18 randomized, controlled trials met inclusion criteria (16 double-blind), involving a total of 2939 men (mean age, 65 years).[18,22,25-28, 70-75,77,80,82-84,87,88] The mean duration of study was 9 weeks (range, 4 to 48 weeks). Main outcomes of included studies were urologic symptom scale scores and global report of symptoms, and secondary measures were peak and mean urinary flow, residual urine volume, prostate size, and nocturia. A meta-analysis was not performed because of the variability in reporting of results; only three trials used standardized validated urologic symptom scales.[27,82,84] A random effects model was therefore used. Compared to placebo, saw palmetto was associated with a significant improvement in urinary tract symptom scale scores (weighted mean difference, -1.41 [95% CI, -2.52 to -0.30] [n = 1 study]), with an absolute improvement vs. placebo of 28%; a significant improvement in nocturia nightly events (weighted mean difference, -0.76 [95% CI, -1.22 to -0.32] [n = 10 studies]); and a significant improvement in self-rated urinary tract symptoms (risk ratio 1.72 [95% CI, 1.21 to 2.44]). Compared to finasteride, saw palmetto appeared to yield similar improvements in urinary tract symptoms measured via the International Prostate Symptom Scale (IPSS) (weighted mean difference 0.37 [95% CI, -0.45 to 0.18] [n = 2 studies]). Although the included studies were limited by short duration and inconsistent study design, the evidence suggests improvement in urinary symptoms and flow compared to placebo, and similarity to finasteride.

- In 2000, Boyle et al. performed a meta-analysis of clinical trial data available for the standardized saw palmetto extract, Permixon.[3] Permixon is a registered trademark of Pierre Fabre Medicament, Castres, France.[3] The authors examined 11 randomized clinical trials (7 placebo-controlled, 4 compared to alpha-1-blockers or finasteride) and 2 open label trials, for an aggregate patient number of 2859.[4,22,25-27,70, 74,75,77,78,87,89,90] The strategy for identifying eligible studies was not described. Trial sample sizes ranged from 22 to 592 subjects, and duration was from 3 to 26 weeks. No symptom score was consistently used, and only two trials utilized the validated International Prostate Symptom Scale (IPSS). Common end points included nocturia in all studies and peak urinary flow rate (Q_{max}) in all but two studies. Pooled data revealed Permixon (320 mg daily) to increase Q_{max} rates by 2.2 mL/s relative to placebo (95% CI, 1.2 to 3.2), and to reduce the average number of episodes of nocturia by 0.5 episodes versus placebo (95% CI, 0.48 to 0.52). The significant finding of increased urinary flow rate compared to placebo is compelling. However, reporting of results and data quality were not uniform across studies, and incomplete statistical information was available from several included trials. Few studies have reported long-term results using standardized symptom scales, and high quality trials are warranted using such end points.

Placebo-Controlled Monotherapy Trials Not Included in Wilt or Boyle Review

- In 2003, Willetts et al. reported the results of a randomized, double-blind, placebo-controlled trial of saw palmetto extract in 100 men with symptoms of BPH.[67] Included subjects were less than 80 years old, with a maximum urinary flow rate of 5 to 15 mL/s, for a voiding volume of 150 mL. Patients were assigned to receive 320 mg of saw palmetto extract or placebo (paraffin oil) over a 12-week period. Primary outcome measures included the International Prostate Symptom Score (IPSS), peak urinary flow rate, and the Rosen International Index of Erectile Function (IIEF) questionnaire. After 12 weeks, the authors reported no significant differences between the two groups in terms of IPSS, peak urinary flow rate, or IIEF. Notably, improvements from baseline occurred in both groups, and as a result, actual differences between groups (if present) may not have been detectable with a sample size of 100.

- Mohanty et al. published a randomized, double-blind, placebo-controlled trial of saw palmetto extract in 75 men with mild to moderate symptomatic (grade I-II) BPH.[68] Over an 8-week period, subjects were assigned to receive either 1 capsule twice daily of an unclear dose of saw palmetto or placebo. The primary outcome measured was a single symptom score based on a composite questionnaire that assessed urinary hesitancy, "terminal dribbling," impairment of size and force of urinary stream, interruption of urination, incomplete emptying, urgency, dysuria, clothes wetting, and straining/pushing to start urinary flow. After 8 weeks, the authors reported a significant reduction in mean symptom score in the saw palmetto group compared to the placebo group (81% reduction versus 64% reduction, respectively). In addition, a secondary outcome of "grouped response" (excellent, good, satisfactory) yielded a significant overall superiority of saw palmetto compared to placebo ($p < 0.005$), with response in 76% of the extract group compared to 35% in the placebo group. The composite outcome measure that was employed is not commonly used in research, and therefore the results may not be comparable with other studies in the same area.

- In 2001, Gerber et al. reported results of a randomized, controlled, double-blind trial to examine the efficacy of saw palmetto in 85 men with lower urinary tract symptoms.[30] Patients with an IPSS of 8 or greater at baseline were enrolled. After a 4-week placebo run-in period, subjects were randomized to placebo or saw palmetto at a dose of 160 mg twice daily for 24 weeks. Outcome parameters included IPSS, urinary flow rate, peak flow rate, quality of life score, and sexual function. The authors reported a significant decrease in mean IPSS of 4.4 points in the saw palmetto group (16.7 to 12.3), compared to a mean score reduction of 2.2 in the placebo group (15.8 to 13.6; $p = 0.038$). However, there was no significant difference between groups in urinary flow rate (1.0 mL/s and 1.4 mL/s in the saw palmetto and placebo groups, respectively; $p = 0.73$). Saw palmetto had no measurable effect on mean quality-of-life score or results of the sexual function questionnaire. Critics have noted that this study did not document a 3-point difference in symptom score between saw palmetto and placebo, as it was designed to demonstrate, and that the baseline IPSS results were dissimilar between groups.

- In 1999, Bauer et al. conducted a randomized, double-blind, placebo-controlled trial evaluating the effects of saw palmetto in 101 men with BPH.[69] Patients were randomized

S

to receive 160 mg twice daily of saw palmetto (Talso, LG 166/S; Germany) or placebo for 24 weeks. Outcome measures were measured via the IPSS including urinary obstruction, dysuria, postvoid residual volume, and quality of life. Statistically significant mean reductions in urinary obstruction (31.8%) and dysuria (38.3%) but not post-void residual volume were observed in the treatment group compared to the placebo group (5.1% and 14.8% reductions, respectively). A significant mean improvement in quality of life was also noted among those ingesting saw palmetto vs. placebo. Randomization procedures and statistical analysis were not well described.

Placebo-Controlled Monotherapy Trials Included in Wilt or Boyle Review

- Reece Smith et al. conducted a randomized, placebo-controlled, double-blind study examining the effects of saw palmetto in 80 men with BPH.[25] Subjects were randomized to receive placebo or Permixon at a dose of 160 mg twice daily for 12 weeks. Measured outcomes included urinary flow rates, residual volume, and subjective symptoms. The authors reported no significant differences between groups in any of these results. Randomization and blinding procedures were adequately documented, although inclusion criteria and statistical analysis were not clearly described. The dropout rate was 12.5%, without follow-up.

- Cukier et al. conducted a randomized, double-blind, placebo-controlled trial to investigate the effect of Permixon (160 mg twice daily) in 168 men diagnosed with uncomplicated BPH ("prostatism").[70] Treatment was administered for an average of 10 weeks. Measured outcomes included dysuria, frequency of urination, postvoid residual volume, and nocturia. The authors reported that subjects treated with Permixon experienced significant improvement vs. placebo in all outcomes.

- In a published letter, Champault et al. reported the effects of saw palmetto extract in 110 men with BPH in a randomized, double-blind, placebo-controlled trial.[88] Subjects were randomized to receive placebo or saw palmetto extract PA109 at a dose of 160 mg twice daily for 4 weeks. Outcome measures included nocturia, flow rate, and post-void residual volume. The authors reported significant mean improvement in all parameters with saw palmetto compared to the placebo group. Nocturia decreased by 46% vs. 15%, flow rate increased 51% vs. 5%, and postvoid residual volume decreased by 42% vs. −9%, respectively. Patient self-rating and physician-rating of improvement were superior in the saw palmetto group (11% and 14%, respectively) compared to placebo (0%). Because of the format of this report as a published letter, only limited details of methods and statistical analysis are available. Dropout was 15%, without clear follow-up.

- Boccafoschi et al. conducted a randomized, double-blind, placebo-controlled trial to assess the effects of saw palmetto in 22 men with symptomatic BPH.[87] Patients were randomized to receive placebo or Permixon at a dose of 160 mg twice daily for 8 weeks. Evaluated outcomes included mean urinary flow rates and residual urine volume. The authors reported a significant improvement in mean urinary flow in the saw palmetto group compared to placebo (9.6 mL/s to 13.7 mL/s vs. 10.2 mL/s to 12.2 mL/s, respectively), and in residual volume (103 mL to 55 mL vs. 66 mL to 36 mL, respectively). Notably, baseline patient characteristics were dissimilar between groups, including residual volume values.

- Braeckman et al. conducted a randomized, placebo-controlled trial in 238 men with BPH.[28] Patients were excluded who had cancer, urinary flow <5 mL/s, residual volume >60 mL, or active urinary tract infection, as well as patients who were >80 years of age or taking medications. Subjects received saw palmetto extract (Prostaserine) (160 mg twice daily) or placebo for 12 weeks. Outcome measures included urinary flow rate and residual volume. Significant improvements were reported in these parameters. Limitations include scant descriptions of blinding, randomization, and statistical analysis.

- Descotes et al. reported the results of a randomized, placebo-controlled trial to evaluate the efficacy of saw palmetto in BPH.[26] Patients with very "mild" BPH symptoms, incontinence, bladder distension, urinary flow < 5 mL/s, urinary tract infection, or cancer were excluded. After a 30-day single-blind placebo run-in period in 271 subjects, 43 were excluded from the trial because they "responded" to placebo (defined as >29% improvement in urinary flow), and 13 were excluded due to loss to follow-up. The remaining patients were randomized to receive Permixon (160 mg twice daily) or placebo for 30 days. Outcome measures included dysuria, daytime urination frequency, nocturia, and urinary flow rate. The authors reported a significant reduction in dysuria compared to placebo ($p = 0.02$), and significant improvement in daytime urination frequency ($p = 0.012$), nocturia ($p = 0.03$), and urinary flow rate ($p = 0.04$) compared to placebo. Little difference was found between saw palmetto and placebo in physician and patient global assessments. Notably, this was not an intention-to-treat analysis, and 39 subjects were excluded from the analysis because of inclusion error, protocol violation, or dropout.

- Löbelenz et al. conducted a randomized, double-blind, placebo-controlled trial examining the effects of saw palmetto extract in the treatment of 60 patients with mild to moderate BPH (stage I-II).[71] Subjects were assigned to receive 100 mg of *Sabal serrulata* extract or placebo once daily for 6 weeks. Outcome measures included urinary flow, postvoid residual volume, urinary frequency, and incontinence. The authors reported improvement in all outcomes parameters in the treatment group compared to placebo, including an increase in mean urinary flow of 0.6 mL with *Sabal serrulata* extract, as compared to 0.3 mL in the placebo group. However, statistical analysis was not clearly described, diminishing the clinical usefulness of these results.

- Mattei et al. reported the results of a randomized, double-blind, placebo-controlled trial in 40 men with uncomplicated BPH and without cancer.[72] Subjects were administered saw palmetto extract (Talso, 160 mg twice daily) or placebo for an average of 13 weeks. Measured outcomes included a dysuria symptom score, postvoid residual volume score, and urinary frequency. Small significant mean improvements in these measures were noted by the authors with saw palmetto vs. placebo. However, randomization methods were not described, and results and statistical analysis were not clearly presented.

- Gabric et al. conducted a randomized, double-blind, placebo-controlled study in 30 patients with moderate to severe BPH (stage II-III) and 29 patients with prostatitis.[73] Subjects were randomized to receive placebo or stinging nettle (*Urtica diotica*) or Prostagutt (a proprietary European saw palmetto extract preparation) at a dose of 60 drops daily for 6 weeks. The primary outcomes of prostate size, urinary retention, and urination frequency were assessed via a physician rating score. The authors reported a statistically significant improvement in outcomes for both treatment groups compared to placebo. However, the method used to evaluate prostate size, digital rectal examination, is not considered to be a highly reproducible method of assessment.

- Tasca et al. conducted a randomized, double-blind, placebo-controlled trial in 30 men with mild to moderate BPH (stage I-II).[74] Subjects were assigned to receive saw palmetto extract PA109 or placebo for 8 weeks. Outcomes measured included dysuria, urinary flow, nocturia, and urgency. Significant improvement was reported for the saw palmetto group vs. placebo, although methods, results, and statistical analysis were not clearly described.

- Emili et al. conducted a randomized, double-blind, placebo-controlled trial assessing the efficacy of saw palmetto in 30 patients with mild symptomatic BPH.[75] Subjects were randomized to receive saw palmetto (Permixon) (160 mg twice daily) or placebo for 4 weeks. Outcome measures included number of daytime urinations, prostate volume, maximum urinary flow rate, and postvoid residual volume. The authors reported that nocturia and number of daily urinations significantly improved in the saw palmetto group compared to placebo. Similarly, prostate volume decreased in 27% of saw palmetto subjects, but in no placebo subjects. Maximum urinary flow rate increased from 10.3 mL/s to 13.7 mL/s with saw palmetto vs. 9.2 mL/s to 9.4 mL/s with placebo, and postvoid residual volume decreased from 71 mL to 35 mL vs. 79 mL to 67 mL, respectively. However, methods were not clearly described and no statistical analysis was presented.

- In a brief published abstract, Mandressi et al. reported a randomized trial (blinding not reported) comparing 160 mg twice daily of saw palmetto with placebo in 60 men with symptomatic BPH.[76] After 8 weeks of therapy, reduced urinary symptoms were noted in the saw palmetto group vs. placebo. However, these results were not quantified, and methods and statistical analysis were not well described.

- Mandressi et al. reported a non-randomized, controlled trial evaluating the efficacy of saw palmetto in the treatment of 60 patients with symptomatic BPH "verified" by digital prostate examination.[77] Patients were assigned to receive saw palmetto (Permixon) (160 mg twice daily) or *Pygeum africanum* or placebo for 8 weeks. Outcome measures included symptoms of dysuria, frequency of urination, nocturia, and residual volume. The authors reported a 42% mean reduction in nocturia and a 10% improvement in residual volume in the Permixon group, compared to a 38% reduction in nocturia and no change in residual volume in the pygeum group. The placebo group experienced a 4% worsening of nocturia and residual volume. Although these results were reported to be statistically significant, statistical methods were not described.

Comparison Trials

- Carraro et al. conducted a trial comparing the effects of saw palmetto and finasteride in the treatment of 1098 men with BPH diagnosed by digital rectal examination.[27] Subjects were excluded who had prostate cancer, transaminitis, or urinary tract infection and those who were taking drugs with diuretic or anti-adrenergic properties. Patients were randomized to receive either 160 mg of Permixon twice daily or 5 mg of finasteride daily (with placebo in the evening) for 26 weeks. Outcomes assessed included IPSS, urinary flow rates, prostate volume, prostate-specific antigen (PSA), and postvoid residual volume. There were 951 completers.

In these subjects, the authors reported that a 38% decrease in mean symptom score occurred in both groups and that urinary flow improved in both groups by 36% to 39% from baseline. Sexual function was unchanged in the Permixon group but deteriorated significantly in the finasteride group ($p < 0.001$). The finasteride group experienced a greater reduction in prostate volume compared to the Permixon group (16% vs. 7%). Notably, mean PSA values fell significantly in the finasteride group ($p < 0.001$) but did not change in the Permixon group. These results suggest equivalence of the two therapies in several parameters, although the lack of a placebo arm leaves open the question of magnitude of effect.

- Grasso et al. compared the efficacy of saw palmetto extract with the alpha-1-inhibitor alfuzosin (Xatral) used in Europe for BPH, in 63 patients with BPH.[4] In this double-blind trial, subjects were randomly allocated to receive saw palmetto extract (160 mg twice daily) or alfuzosin (2.5 mg three times daily) for 3 weeks. Outcome parameters included an obstructive score, score on the Boyarsky scale of clinical symptoms, and number of therapy "responders" (defined as a >25% increase in maximum urinary flow rate). The authors reported that greater mean improvements occurred in the Boyarsky scale and in the obstructive score in the alfuzosin group vs. saw palmetto (p<0.01). There were more responders to therapy in the alfuzosin group compared to the saw palmetto group (72% vs. 48%; p = 0.06). This trial suggests superiority of alpha-1 blockers to saw palmetto in some measures of BPH, although the results are limited by the study's short duration and lack of a placebo group.

- Additional comparison studies have been conducted of lower methodological quality, including unclear descriptions of study design, outcomes, and statistical analysis. In general, these publications have not included analyses to calculate sample size adequate to make between-group comparisons.

- Semino et al. compared the effect of saw palmetto and the anti-adrenergic agent prazosin on urinary flow in 45 patients with BPH.[77] The authors reported that prazosin was "slightly more effective" than saw palmetto in controlling BPH symptoms, although there was no description of statistical analysis, randomization, or blinding in the study. No placebo group was included.

- In a small double-blind study by Comar and Di Rienzo, both saw palmetto and the purported anti-estrogenic agent mepartricin (Ipertrofan; injected subcutaneously) were found to reduce functional symptoms in 20 patients with BPH.[79] No statistical comparison of efficacy was provided, although mepartricin was reportedly associated with greater reduction in symptoms. The sample size may not have been adequate to compare groups.

- Pannunzio et al. reported a trial in 60 men comparing saw palmetto (Permixon) with hydroprogesterone caproate (Depostat, Schering AG, Berlin, Germany) with respect to several functional and subjective indicators of BPH, including prostate size and obstructive symptoms (dysuria, polyuria, nocturia).[80] Improvement was noted in each group vs. baseline, with similar results between groups. However, the lack of a placebo group or randomization, and the possibly inadequate sample size, limit the clinical significance of this study.

- In a 1979 non-randomized, open-label comparison trial, Flamm et al. compared the efficacy of saw palmetto extract with that of testosterone injections in improving several functional parameters in 74 men with BPH.[81] The authors reported that neither saw palmetto taken weekly nor testosterone injections yielded improvements vs. baseline. However, no statistical analysis was presented, and there was no placebo arm. These results are of limited clinical significance.

Combination Product Studies

- Several studies have been published examining the effects of combination therapies, including saw palmetto in the management of BPH. The quality of study designs and reporting have varied. Overall, the effects of saw palmetto monotherapy cannot be adequately assessed by trials using combination regimens, owing to the possible confounding effects of other constituents.

- Metzker et al. conducted a randomized, placebo-controlled trial to assess the efficacy of Prostagutt forte (which contains saw palmetto extract and stinging nettle extract) (Schwabe, Karlsruhe, Germany) in the treatment of 40 men with BPH.[82] After a 2-week pre-trial period when all patients received placebo, subjects were randomized to continue taking placebo or to receive Prostagutt forte at a dose of 1 capsule twice daily for 24 to 48 weeks. The initial 24 weeks were conducted under double-blind conditions. After 24 weeks, patients receiving placebo were crossed over to receive Prostagutt forte, and the trial became single-blinded. Outcome measures included urinary flow, transabdominal ultrasound, quality of life, and prostate size as measured by digital rectal examination. The authors reported significant small improvement in urine pressure, decreased urinary frequency, and improved quality of life. There was no change in prostate size, although digital rectal examination is not considered to be a highly reproducible measurement.

- Carbin et al. conducted a randomized, double-blind, three-month study in which the preparation Curbicin, made from pumpkin seeds and *Sabal serrulata*, was compared to placebo in 53 patients with BPH.[83] Urinary flow, micturition time, postvoid residual volume, frequency of micturition and subjective assessment of treatment benefit were all noted as being significantly improved in the treatment group. However, details of methods and statistical analysis were limited.

- Marks et al. conducted a randomized, placebo-controlled trial in 45 men with BPH, ages 45 to 80 years.[29] Subjects were administered a combination product that contained saw palmetto, nettle root extract, pumpkin seed oil extract, lemon bioflavonoid extract, and vitamin A, vs. placebo. End points included symptom score, urinary flow, postvoid residual volume, prostate-specific antigen (PSA), prostate volume by magnetic resonance imaging (MRI), and prostate biopsy. Both groups demonstrated improved clinical parameters, with a non-significant slight advantage in the saw palmetto group. No adverse effects were noted in either group.

- Sökeland and Albrecht compared the efficacy of Prostagutt forte vs. finasteride in a year-long randomized, double-blind, multicenter trial in 542 outpatients with mild to moderate BPH (stage I-II).[84] After a 2-week run-in placebo phase, subjects were randomly allocated to receive 2 capsules daily of Prostagutt forte (160 mg of saw palmetto extract WS 1473 and 120 mg of stinging nettle extract WS 1031 per capsule) or finasteride (5 mg) daily in a double-dummy design. The main outcome variable was change in maximum urinary flow between baseline and week 24. Secondary

outcomes included IPSS, mean urinary flow rate, urinary volume, and sonographic size of the prostate. The authors reported that maximum urinary flow increased in both groups, with a marginal, statistically insignificant greater increase in the finasteride group (2.8 mL/s vs. 2.0 mL/s). The difference was noted to be smaller than the "maximum irrelevant difference" of 1.5 mL/s, although no power calculation was presented. From weeks 24 to 48, no further changes were observed. Mean IPSS results similarly decreased in both groups from week 0 to week 48 (from 11.3 to 6.5 in the Prostagutt group, and from 11.8 to 6.2 in the finasteride group). Prostate size remained constant in the Prostagutt group but decreased in the finasteride group; this difference was not statistically significant. Adverse effects, such as reduced ejaculation volume, erectile dysfunction, and arthralgia, were more common in the finasteride group. This analysis suggests equivalence of treatments for some measures. Although no power analysis was conducted to determine optimal sample size, there was likely a sufficient number of patients to make between-group comparisons.

Dosing Studies

- In 1999, Stepanov et al. performed a randomized, double-blind, parallel-group study examining the efficacy of two different doses of saw palmetto in 100 patients with BPH.[13] Subjects were randomized to receive 160 mg of Permixon once daily or twice daily for 12 weeks. Outcome parameters included IPSS, quality of life, maximum urinary flow rate, mean urinary flow rate, and residual urine volume. The authors reported that both regimens significantly reduced IPSS and improved quality-of-life scores, maximum and mean urinary flow rates, and residual urine volumes. There were no significant differences between regimens. Incidence of adverse events was similar in both groups. Limitations of this trial include the lack of a separate placebo group and short duration.

- In 1997, Braeckman et al. conducted a multicenter, randomized, single-blind, placebo-controlled trial to assess the efficacy of two different doses of saw palmetto or placebo in 84 patients with BPH.[16] Subjects were randomized to receive 160 mg of Prostaserene twice daily, 320 mg of Prostaserene once daily, or placebo. Outcomes assessed included IPSS, quality of life scores, maximum urinary flow rate, mean urinary flow rate, and residual urinary volume. At one year, both dosage regimens produced a significant improvement in IPSS results (60%), quality of life scores (85% patient satisfaction), maximum flow rates (22%), mean flow rates (17%), and residual urinary volumes (16%). This trial is limited by the lack of double-blinding and dropout of 24%.

- In 1994, Roveda and Colombo compared the efficacy of an oral saw palmetto extract (160 mg four times daily) with a rectal formulation (640 mg daily).[18] This randomized but unblinded study was conducted for 12 weeks and measured outcomes including IPSS and postvoid residual volume. The trial included 40 men with mild to moderate BPH (stage I-II) who were older than 50 years, not taking other prostate agents, and without other major comorbidities or infection. Outcomes measured included postvoid residual volume, prostate size, and dysuria. The authors reported equivalence of the two dosing regimens, although it is not clear that the sample size was adequate to detect between-group differences. In addition, there was no placebo arm against which to measure the efficacy of the two regimens.

Case Series (Uncontrolled Studies)

- Numerous case series have been conducted largely documenting improved signs and symptoms of BPH following therapy with saw palmetto. Many have been short in duration with small sample sizes, and the lack of control groups limits clinical significance. However, useful data can be derived from several case series conducted for longer periods of time (3 to 5 years) or in >1000 subjects, suggesting possible safety and tolerance of saw palmetto.[11,91-93]

- In 1996, Bach et al. reported the results of a 3-year multicenter study in which 435 BPH stage I or II patients received 160 mg of saw palmetto (IDS 89) extract twice daily.[11] Subjects were excluded who had postvoid residual volumes of >150 mL, neurogenic bladder, prostatitis, urinary tract infection, bladder stones, prostate cancer, or hematuria. The age range of patients was 41 to 89 years. Completed data were obtained for 315 subjects (72%). Clinical "controls" were carried out prior to treatment, after 1 and 3 months, and then every 3 months until the 36th month; however, a specific description of how these control measurements were carried out was not provided. The authors found significant changes compared to baseline in several parameters, including nocturia, which improved in 73% of patients. There was an improvement in daytime frequency and feeling of incomplete emptying (54% and 76%, respectively), and 62% of patients who initially reported a feeling of incomplete emptying were symptom-free after 3 years. Residual urine volume fell by 50% after 3 years of treatment. A 6.1-mL increase in peak urinary flow was also observed. Although this study was not clearly reported, and measures and statistical analysis were not well described, the tolerability of saw palmetto over a 3-year period was documented, which is a relatively long duration in this area. Tolerance was subjectively rated as "good" or "very good" by patients and clinicians in 98% of cases. Four patients reported poor tolerance. A total of 46 adverse effects occurred in 34 patients; 30% were gastrointestinal (with 1.8% of patients withdrawing for this reason). Urologic complaints occurred in 9 subjects, impotence in 1 subject, and prostate cancer in 4 subjects. However, the lack of a placebo group hinders comparison of the incidence of adverse effects to controls.

- Romics et al. treated 42 patients with moderate to severe BPH (stage II-III) with 160 mg of saw palmetto extract twice daily (Strogen forte) for 1 year.[91] As measured by ultrasound, a continuous significant decrease was observed in postvoid residual volume (from 62.8 mL to 12.3 mL) over 12 months. The frequency of nocturia decreased in 68.4% of patients. At the endpoint, 80% of patients reported no symptoms (including hesitancy, interrupted stream, and terminal dribbling).

- In an observational study sponsored by a major European manufacturer of saw palmetto products, 2080 patients with mild to moderate BPH (Alken stages I-II) from hundreds of urologic practices were treated with a fixed combination of saw palmetto extract (WS 1473) and stinging nettle extract (WS 1031).[92] After treatment, most patients and clinicians reported "improvement" of prostatic symptoms, although this study was not well described.

- Vahlensieck et al. conducted an open 12-week study to assess the effects of saw palmetto in 1334 patients with moderate to severe BPH (stage II-III).[93] Mean postvoid residual volume was reported to decrease by approximately 50%. The treatment was subjectively reported as being effective by 83% of patients and by 87% of treating physicians. The reproducibility of these results is not clear.

- Numerous additional case series and case studies have been published, employing outcomes measures including the IPSS, urinary flow rates, prostatic volume, post-void residual volume, quality of life, and subjective sense of improvement.[12,24,32,47,94-102] Almost universally there has been reported improvement over baseline, although true efficacy is not clear in these reports because of the lack of control groups. Few adverse effects have been noted in these observational studies.

Androgenetic Alopecia (Topical)
Summary

- Saw palmetto has been proposed to possess anti-androgenic properties, and to possibly possess efficacy as a treatment for hair loss, similar to topical finasteride (Propecia). However, there is currently insufficient evidence to recommend for or against the use of topical saw palmetto for the treatment of androgenetic alopecia.

Evidence

- Morganti et al. conducted a randomized, double-blind, 3-arm, before-and-after study in 48 men and women with androgenetic alopecia (type III-IV on the Hamilton Scale).[85] Half of subjects (n = 24) were randomized to receive a topical lotion containing saw palmetto extract or an identical lotion without saw palmetto (the other half of subjects received a dietary supplement containing L-cysteine and L-methionine). The patients using topical therapies were instructed to apply the lotion twice daily for 50 weeks. Hair density was measured using a standardized instrument. In the saw palmetto group, mean hair density was noted to significantly increase by 17% after 10 weeks, and by 27% after 50 weeks (compared to baseline values). The mean increase in hair density in the placebo group was significant at 13% by week 50 compared to baseline. However, no between-group comparisons were conducted, and it is not clear if the number of patients receiving topical therapies was sufficient to make between-group comparisons. Although these preliminary results are compelling, further evidence is warranted before a firm conclusion can be drawn.

Hypotonic Neurogenic Bladder
Summary

- There is currently insufficient evidence to recommend for or against the use of saw palmetto for the management of hypotonic neurogenic bladder (also known as underactive or flaccid neurogenic bladder).

Evidence

- Timmermans et al. conducted a non-randomized, placebo-controlled trial in 30 women with hypotonic neurogenic bladder.[86] Subjects were assigned to receive placebo or 90 to 120 drops daily of the combination product Urgenin (containing 84 to 112 mg of echinacea and 78 to 104 mg of saw palmetto extract). The Urgenin group received treatment for a mean of 77 days, and the placebo arm received therapy for a mean of 52 days. No change in symptomatology was reported in the placebo patients, but a significantly improved mean "bladder capacity" and postvoid residual volume was reported in the Urgenin group. Although these results are compelling, the use of a combination product, lack of use of standardized measurement techniques, difference in treatment duration between groups, and unclear reporting of methods and statistical analysis limit the clinical significance of this trial.

Prostatitis/Chronic Pelvic Pain Syndrome
Summary

- Initial study suggests that saw palmetto is inferior to finasteride in the treatment of men diagnosed with category III prostatitis/chronic pelvic pain (CP/CPPS) over a 1-year period, without appreciable benefits.

Evidence

- Kaplan et al. conducted a randomized, open-label study in 64 men with CP/CPPS.[23] Included subjects were ages 24-58 years (mean, 43 years). All had previously received antibiotics (duration of 3 to 93 weeks); 52 (82%) had been on alpha-blocker drugs. Patients were assigned to receive finasteride (5 mg daily) or saw palmetto (325 mg daily) for 1 year. Enrollees were evaluated using the National Institutes of Health Chronic Prostatitis Symptom Index (NIH CPSI), individual domains (pain, urinary symptoms, quality of life, mean pain score), and the American Urological Association Symptom Score. Measurements of these scales were conducted at baseline and 3, 6, and 12 months. The authors reported that at 1 year, the mean total NIH CPSI score decreased from 23.9 to 18.1 in the finasteride group ($p < 0.003$), and from 24.7 to 24.6 in the saw palmetto arm ($p = 0.41$). In the finasteride arm, quality of life and pain domains were significantly improved at 1 year, although urination was not. Adverse events included headache (3 cases) in the saw palmetto group and decreased libido (2 cases) in the finasteride group.

FORMULARY: BRANDS USED IN CLINICAL TRIALS/THIRD-PARTY TESTING
Saw Palmetto Brands Used in Statistically Significant Clinical Trials

- Elusan Prostate (U.S. equivalent to Permixon [imported by Plantes & Medicines, Inc.]); Permixon 160 mg Tablet available in Europe (ASTA Medica, Pierre Fabre Medicament, Castres, France); Prostagutt; Prostagutt forte (combination preparation including saw palmetto and stinging nettle); Prostaserene; Strogen forte; Strogen (Sabal extract IDS 89).

Saw Palmetto Brands Tested by Impartial Third Party Laboratories

- **Consumer Reports (2000):** Celestial Seasoning Prostate Health Ultimate Health Blend with Saw Palmetto, Centrum Herbals Saw Palmetto, CVS Premium Quality Herbs Saw Palmetto, GNC Herbal Plus Standardized Saw Palmetto, Natrol Saw Palmetto, Nature's Herbs Power-Herbs Saw Palmetto Power 160 Std. Extract, Nutrilite Saw Palmetto, One-A-Day Prostate Health with Natural Saw Palmetto and Zinc, Pharmassure Standardized Saw Palmetto, Promalmex, Prosta Pro, Puritans' Pride Saw Palmetto with Pygeum, Quanterra Prostate Saw Palmetto, Shaklee Saw Palmetto Plus, Solaray Saw Palmetto Berry Extract 160 mg, Spring Valley Saw Palmetto Extract, Sundown Herbals Standardized Saw Palmetto Extract, Super Saw Palmetto, Your Life Saw Palmetto Standardized Herbal Extract, Walgreens Saw Palmetto Standardized Extract.

References

1. Wilt TJ, Ishani A, Stark G, et al. Saw palmetto extracts for treatment of benign prostatic hyperplasia: a systematic review. JAMA 1998;280(18):1604-1609.
2. Wilt T, Ishani A, Stark G, et al. Serenoa repens for benign prostatic hyperplasia. Cochrane Database Syst Rev 2000;(2):CD001423.
3. Boyle P, Robertson C, Lowe F, et al. Meta-analysis of clinical trials of permixon in the treatment of symptomatic benign prostatic hyperplasia. Urology 2000;55(4):533-539.
4. Grasso M, Montesano A, Buonaguidi A, et al. Comparative effects of alfuzosin versus Serenoa repens in the treatment of symptomatic benign prostatic hyperplasia. Arch Esp Urol 1995;48(1):97-103.
5. Oberpichler-Schwenk H. [Finasteride or sabal extract in acne?]. Med Monatsschr Pharm 1998;21(3):83.
6. Grant K. Top-selling herbal supplements. J Managed Primary Care 1999;5(4):357-370.
7. el Sheikh MM, Dakkak MR, Saddique A. The effect of Permixon on androgen receptors. Acta Obstet Gynecol Scand 1988;67(5):397-399.
8. Goepel M, Dinh L, Mitchell A, et al. Do saw palmetto extracts block human alpha1-adrenoceptor subtypes in vivo? Prostate 2001;46(3):226-232.
9. Gutierrez M, Garcia de Boto MJ, Cantabrana B, et al. Mechanisms involved in the spasmolytic effect of extracts from Sabal serrulata fruit on smooth muscle. Gen Pharmacol 1996;27(1):171-176.
10. Lowe FC, Fagelman E. Phytotherapy in the treatment of benign prostatic hyperplasia: an update. Urology 1999;53(4):671-678.
11. Bach D, Ebeling L. Long-term drug treatment of benign prostatic hyperplasia—results of a prospective 3-year multicenter study using Sabal extract IDS 89. Phytomed 1996;3:105-111.
12. Anonymous. Effectiveness of lipidosterol extract Serenoa repens (Permixon) in patients with prostatic hyperplasia. Urologiia 2002;(1):23-25.
13. Stepanov VN, Siniakova LA, Sarrazin B, et al. Efficacy and tolerability of the lipidosterolic extract of Serenoa repens (Permixon) in benign prostatic hyperplasia: a double-blind comparison of two dosage regimens. Adv Ther 1999;16(5):231-241.
14. Cheema P, El Mefty O, Jazieh AR. Intraoperative haemorrhage associated with the use of extract of Saw Palmetto herb: a case report and review of literature. J Intern Med 2001;250(2):167-169.
15. Feifer AH, Fleshner NE, Klotz L. Analytical accuracy and reliability of commonly used nutritional supplements in prostate disease. J Urol 2002;168(1):150-154.
16. Braeckman J, Bruhwyler J, Vandekerckhove K, et al. Efficacy and safety of the extract of Serenoa repens in the treatment of benign prostatic hyperplasia: therapeutic equivalence between twice and once daily dosage forms. Phytother Res 1997;11:558-563.
17. Klepser TB, Klepser ME. Unsafe and potentially safe herbal therapies. Am J Health Syst Pharm 1999;56(2):125-138.
18. Roveda S, Colombo P. Clinical controlled trial on therapeutical bioequivalence and tolerability of Serenoa repens oral capsules 160 mg or rectal capsules 640 mg. Arch Med Interna 1994;46(2):61-75.
19. Marks LS, Tyler VE. Saw palmetto extract: newest (and oldest) treatment alternative for men with symptomatic benign prostatic hyperplasia. Urology 1999;53(3):457-461.
20. Ondrizek RR, Chan PJ, Patton WC, et al. An alternative medicine study of herbal effects on the penetration of zona-free hamster oocytes and the integrity of sperm deoxyribonucleic acid. Fertil Steril 1999;71(3):517-522.
21. Small EJ, Frohlich MW, Bok R, et al. Prospective trial of the herbal supplement PC-SPES in patients with progressive prostate cancer. J Clin Oncol 2000;18(21):3595-3603.
22. Champault G, Patel JC, Bonnard AM. A double-blind trial of an extract of the plant Serenoa repens in benign prostatic hyperplasia. Br J Clin Pharmacol 1984;18(3):461-462.
23. Kaplan SA, Volpe MA, Te AE. A prospective, 1-year trial using saw palmetto versus finasteride in the treatment of category III prostatitis/chronic pelvic pain syndrome. J Urol 2004;171(1):284-288.
24. Braeckman J. The extract of Serenoa repens in the treatment of benign prostatic hyperplasia: a multicentre open study. Curr Thera Res 1994;55(7):776-785.
25. Reece Smith H, Memon A, Smart C, et al. The value of Permixon in benign prostatic hypertrophy. Br J Urol 1986;58(1):36-40.
26. Descotes J, Rambeaud J, Deschaseaux P, et al. Placebo-controlled evaluation of the efficacy and tolerability of Permixon in benign prostatic hyperplasia after exclusion of placebo responders. Clin Drug Invest 1995; 9(5):291-297.
27. Carraro JC, Raynaud JP, Koch G, et al. Comparison of phytotherapy (Permixon) with finasteride in the treatment of benign prostate hyperplasia: a randomized international study of 1,098 patients. Prostate 1996;29(4):231-240.
28. Braeckman J, Denis L, de Leval J, et al. A double-blind, placebo-controlled study of the plant extract Serenoa repens in the treatment of benign hyperplasia of the prostate. Eur J Clin Res 1997;9:247-259.
29. Marks LS, Partin AW, Epstein JI, et al. Effects of a saw palmetto herbal blend in men with symptomatic benign prostatic hyperplasia. J Urol 2000;163(5):1451-1456.

30. Gerber GS, Kuznetsov D, Johnson BC, et al. Randomized, double-blind, placebo-controlled trial of saw palmetto in men with lower urinary tract symptoms. Urology 2001;58(6):960-964.
31. Hamid S, Rojter S, Vierling J. Protracted cholestatic hepatitis after the use of prostata. Ann Intern Med 1997;127(2):169-170.
32. Gerber GS, Zagaja GP, Bales GT, et al. Saw palmetto (*Serenoa repens*) in men with lower urinary tract symptoms: effects on urodynamic parameters and voiding symptoms. Urology 1998;51(6):1003-1007.
33. Di Silverio F, D'Eramo G, Lubrano C, et al. Evidence that *Serenoa repens* extract displays an antiestrogenic activity in prostatic tissue of benign prostatic hypertrophy patients. Eur Urol 1992;21(4):309-314.
34. Elghamry MI, Hansel R. Activity and isolated phytoestrogen of shrub palmetto fruits (*Serenoa repens* Small), a new estrogenic plant. Experientia 1969;25(8):828-829.
35. DiPaola RS, Zhang H, Lambert GH, et al. Clinical and biologic activity of an estrogenic herbal combination (PC- SPES) in prostate cancer. N Engl J Med 1998;339(12):785-791.
36. Marks LS, Hess DL, Dorey FJ, et al. Tissue effects of saw palmetto and finasteride: use of biopsy cores for in situ quantification of prostatic androgens. Urology 2001;57(5):999-1005.
37. Strauch G, Perles P, Vergult G, et al. Comparison of finasteride (Proscar) and *Serenoa repens* (Permixon) in the inhibition of 5-alpha reductase in healthy male volunteers. Eur Urol 1994;26(3):247-252.
38. Iguchi K, Okumura N, Usui S, et al. Myristoleic acid, a cytotoxic component in the extract from *Serenoa repens*, induces apoptosis and necrosis in human prostatic LNCaP cells. Prostate 2001;47(1):59-65.
39. Rhodes L, Primka RL, Berman C, et al. Comparison of finasteride (Proscar), a 5 alpha reductase inhibitor, and various commercial plant extracts in *in vitro* and *in vivo* 5 alpha reductase inhibition. Prostate 1993; 22(1):43-51.
40. Bayne C, Donnelly F, Ross M, et al. *Serenoa repens* (Permixon): a 5 alpha-reductase types I and II inhibitor-new evidence in a coculture model of BPH. Prostate 999;40(4):232-241.
41. Iehle C, Delos S, Guirou O, et al. Human prostatic steroid 5 alpha-reductase isoforms—a comparative study of selective inhibitors. J Steroid Biochem Mol Biol 1995;54(5-6):273-279.
42. Weisser H, Tunn S, Behnke B, et al. Effects of the sabal serrulata extract IDS 89 and its subfractions on 5 alpha-reductase activity in human benign prostatic hyperplasia. Prostate 1996;28(5):300-306.
43. Buck AC. Phytotherapy for the prostate. Br J Urol 1996;78(3):325-336.
44. Di Silverio F, Sciarra A, D'Eramo G, et al. Zonal distribution of androgens and epidermal growth factor (EGF) in human BPH tissue: responsiveness to flutamide, finasteride, and *Serenoa repens* administration. Br J Urol 1997;80(Suppl 2):214.
45. Di Silverio F, Monti S, Sciarra A, et al. Effects of long-term treatment with *Serenoa repens* (Permixon) on the concentrations and regional distribution of androgens and epidermal growth factor in benign prostatic hyperplasia. Prostate 1998;37(2):77-83.
46. Epstein J, Partin A, Simon I, et al. Prostate tissue effects of saw palmetto extract in men with symptomatic BPH. J Urol 1999;161(4S):362.
47. Casarosa C, Cosci dC, Fratta M. Lack of effects of a lyposterolic extract of *Serenoa repens* on plasma levels of testosterone, follicle-stimulating hormone, and luteinizing hormone. Clin Ther 1988;10(5):585-588.
48. Briley M, Carilla E, Fauran F. Permixon, a new treatment for benign prostatic hyperplasia, acts directly at the cytosolic androgen receptor in the rat prostate. Br J Pharmacol 1983;79:327P.
49. Ravenna L, Di Silverio F, Russo MA, et al. Effects of the lipidosterolic extract of *Serenoa repens* (Permixon) on human prostatic cell lines. Prostate 1996;29(4):219-230.
50. Stenger A, Rarayre JP, Carilla E. Etude pharmacologique et biochimique de l'extrait hexanique de *Serenoa repens* B. Gaz Med Fr 1982;89:2041-2048.
51. Sultan C, Terraza A, Carilla E, et al. Anti-androgenic effects of Permixon: *In vitro* studies.: Di Silverio F, Steg A (eds): New Trends in BPH Etiopathogenesis. Rome, Acta Medica, 1988, pp 297-313.
52. Goepel M, Hecker U, Krege S, et al. Saw palmetto extracts potently and noncompetitively inhibit human alpha1-adrenoceptors *in vitro*. Prostate 1999;38(3):208-215.
53. Bayne CW, Ross M, Donnelly F, et al. The selectivity and specificity of the actions of the lipido-sterolic extract of *Serenoa repens* (Permixon) on the prostate. J Urol 2000;164(3 Pt 1):876-881.
54. Paubert-Braquet M, Richardson FO, Servent-Saez N, et al. Effect of *Serenoa repens* extract (Permixon) on estradiol/testosterone-induced experimental prostate enlargement in the rat. Pharmacol Res 1996; 34(3-4):171-179.
55. Paubert-Braquet M, Raynaud JP, Braquet PG, et al. Permixon [lipid sterolic extract of *Serenoa repens* (LSESr)] and some of its components inhibit b-FGF and EGF induced proliferation of human prostate organtypic cell lines. J Urol 1997;157(suppl):138.
56. Paubert-Braquet M, Cousse H, Raynaud JP, et al. Effect of the lipidosterolic extract of *Serenoa repens* (Permixon) and its major components on basic fibroblast growth factor-induced proliferation of cultures of human prostate biopsies. Eur Urol 1998;33(3):340-347.
57. Vacherot F, Azzouz M, Gil-Diez-De-Medina S, et al. Induction of apoptosis and inhibition of cell proliferation by the lipido-sterolic extract of *Serenoa repens* (LSEr, Permixon) in benign prostatic hyperplasia. Prostate 2000;45(3):259-266.
58. Van Coppenolle F, Le Bourhis X, Carpentier F, et al. Pharmacological effects of the lipidosterolic extract of *Serenoa repens* (Permixon) on rat prostate hyperplasia induced by hyperprolactinemia: comparison with finasteride. Prostate 2000;43(1):49-58.
59. Ishii K, Usui S, Sugimura Y, et al. Extract from *Serenoa repens* suppresses the invasion activity of human urological cancer cells by inhibiting urokinase-type plasminogen activator. Biol Pharm Bull 2001;24(2):188-190.
60. Hiermann A. [The contents of sabal fruits and testing of their anti-inflammatory effect]. Arch Pharm (Weinheim) 1989;322(2):111-114.
61. Breu W, Hagenlocher M, Redl K, et al. [Anti-inflammatory activity of sabal fruit extracts prepared with supercritical carbon dioxide. *In vitro* antagonists of cyclooxygenase and 5-lipoxygenase metabolism]. Arzneimittelforschung 1992;42(4):547-551.
62. Paubert-Braquet M, Mencia Huerta JM, Cousse H, et al. Effect of the lipidic lipidosterolic extract of *Serenoa repens* (Permixon) on the ionophore A23187-stimulated production of leukotriene B4 (LTB4) from human polymorphonuclear neutrophils. Prostaglandins Leukot Essent Fatty Acids 1997;57(3):299-304.
63. Mitropoulos D, Kiroudi A, Mitsogiannis I, et al. *In vivo* effect of the lipido-sterolic extract of *Serenoa repens* (Permixon) on mast cells accumulation and glandular epithelium trophism in the rat prostate. J Urol 1999;161(4S):362.
64. Plosker GL, Brogden RN. *Serenoa repens* (Permixon). A review of its pharmacology and therapeutic efficacy in benign prostatic hyperplasia. Drugs Aging 1996;9(5):379-395.
65. De Bernardi VM, Tripodi AS, Contos S, et al. Serenoa repens capsules: a bioequivalence study. Acta Toxicol Ther 1994;15(1):21-39.
66. Markowitz JS, Donovan JL, Devane CL, et al. Multiple doses of saw palmetto (*Serenoa repens*) did not alter cytochrome P450 2D6 and 3A4 activity in normal volunteers. Clin Pharmacol Ther 2003;74(6):536-542.
67. Willetts KE, Clements MS, Champion S, et al. *Serenoa repens* extract for benign prostate hyperplasia: a randomized controlled trial. BJU Int 2003;92(3):267-270.
68. Mohanty NK, Jha RJ, Dutt C. Randomized double-blind controlled clinical trial of *Serenoa repens* versus placebo in the management of patients with symptomatic grade I to grade II benign prostatic hyperplasia (BPH). Indian J Urol 1999;16(1):26-31.
69. Bauer HW, Casarosa C, Cosci M, et al. [Saw palmetto fruit extract for treatment of benign prostatic hyperplasia. Results of a placebo-controlled double-blind study]. MMW Fortschr Med 1999;141(25):62.
70. Cukier J, Ducassou J, Le Guillou M, et al. Permixon versus placebo; resultats d'une etude multicentrique. C R Ther Pharmacol Clin 1985; 4(25):15-21.
71. Löbelenz J. Extractum Sabal fructus bei benigner Prostatahyperplasie (BPH): Klinische Prüfung im Stadium I und II. Therapeutikon 1992; 6(1-2):34, 37.
72. Mattei FM, Capone M, Acconcia A. Medikamentose therapie der benignen prostatahyperplasie mit einem extrakt der sagepalme. TW Urol Nephrol 1990;2(5):346-350.
73. Gabric V, Miskic H. Behandlung des benignen Prostataadenoms und der chronischen Prostatitis. Placebokontrollierte randomisierte doppelblindstudie mit Prostagutt. Therapiewoche 1987;37:1775-1788.
74. Tasca A, Barulli M, Cavazzana A, et al. [Treatment of obstructive symptomatology caused by prostatic adenoma with an extract of *Serenoa repens*. Double-blind clinical study vs. placebo]. Minerva Urol Nefrol 1985;37(1):87-91.
75. Emili E, Lo Cigno M, Petrone U. Risultati clinici su un nuovo farmaco nella terapia dell'ipertrofia della prostata (Permixon). Urologia 1983; 50(5):1042-1048.
76. Mandressi A. Treatment of uncomplicated benign prostatic hypertrophy (BPH) by an extract of *Serenoa repens*: clinical results. J Endocrinol Invest 1987;10 (Suppl 2):49.
77. Mandressi A, Tarallo U, Maggioni A, et al. Terapia medica dell'adenoma prostatico: confronto della efficacia dell'estratto di *Serenoa repens* (Permixon) versus l'estratto di *Pigeum africanum* e placebo. Valutazione in doppio cieco. Urologia 1983;(4):752-757.
78. Semino A, Ortega L, Cobo G, et al. [Symptomatic treatment of benign hypertrophy of the prostate. Comparative study of prazosin and *Serenoa repens*.]. Archivos Espanoles de Urologia 1992;45(3):211-213.
79. Comar OB, Di Rienzo A. Mepartricina versus *Serenoa repens*: studio sperimentale doppio cieco su 20 casi di iperplasia prostatica benigna. Riv Ital Biol Med 1986;6(2):122-125.
80. Pannunzio E, D'Ascenzo R, Giardinetti F, et al. *Serenoa repens* vs. gestonorone caproato nel trattamento dell'ipertrofia prostatica benigna. Studio randomizzato. Urologia 1986;53(5):696-705.
81. Flamm J, Kiesswetter H, Englisch M. [An urodynamic study of patients with benign prostatic hypertrophy treated conservatively with phytotherapy or testosterone (author's transl)]. Wien Klin Wochenschr 1979;91(18):622-627.

82. Metzker H, Kieser M, Hölscher U. Wirksamkeit eines Sabal-Urtica-kombinationspraparates bei der behandlung der benignen prostatahyperplasie (BPH). Urologe 1996;36(4):292-300.

83. Carbin BE, Larsson B, Lindahl O. Treatment of benign prostatic hyperplasia with phytosterols. Br J Urol 1990;66(6):639-641.

84. Sökeland J, Albrecht J. Kombination aus Sabal und Urticaextrakt vs. finasterid bei BPH (Stad I bis II nach Alken). Urologe 1997;36(4):327-333.

85. Morganti P, Fabrizi G, James B, et al. Effect of gelatin-cystine and *Serenoa repens* extract on free radicals level and hair growth. J Appl Cosmetol 1998; 16:57-64.

86. Timmermans LM, Timmermans LG, Jr. [Determination of the activity of extracts of Echinaceae and Sabal in the treatment of idiopathic megabladder in women]. Acta Urol Belg 1990;58(2):43-59.

87. Boccafoschi C, Annoscia S. Confronto fra estratto di *Serenoa repens* e placebo mediante prova clinica controllata in pazienti con adenomatosi prostatica. Urologia 1983;50(6):1257-1268.

88. Champault G, Bonnard AM, Cauquil J, et al. [Medical treatment of prostatic adenoma. Controlled trial: PA 109 vs placebo in 110 patients]. Ann Urol (Paris) 1984;18(6):407-410.

89. Authie D, Cauquil J. Appreciation de l'efficacite de permixon en pratique quotidienne. [Appreciation of the in practice daily effectiveness of permixon]. C R Ther Pharmacol Clin 1987;5(56):4-13.

90. Foroutan F. Wirksamkeit und vertraglichkeit von permixon bei einem grosseren patientenkollektiv (592 patienten) unter praxisbedingungen. J Urol Urogynakol 1997;2:17-21.

91. Romics I, Schmitz H, Frang D. Experience in treating benign prostatic hypertrophy with *Sabal serrulata* for one year. Int Urol Nephrol 1993; 25(6):565-569.

92. Schneider HJ, Honold E, Masuhr T. [Treatment of benign prostatic hyperplasia. Results of a treatment study with the phytogenic combination of Sabal extract WS 1473 and Urtica extract WS 1031 in urologic specialty practices]. Fortschr Med 1995;113(3):37-40.

93. Vahlensieck W, Jr., Volp A, Lubos W, et al. [Benign prostatic hyperplasia—treatment with sabal fruit extract. A treatment study of 1,334 patients]. Fortschr Med 1993;111(18):323-326.

94. Medvedev AA, Siniakova LA, Zaitsev AV. [Prostaplant treatment of benign prostatic hyperplasia]. Urologiia 2000;(4):13-15.

95. Tosto A, Rovereto B, Paoletti MC, et al. Study of *Serenoa repens* in treatment of functional secondary adenoma of the prostate: consideration of 20 cases. Urologia 1985;52:536-542.

96. Greca P, Volip R. Experience with a new drug in the medical treatment of prostatic adenoma. Urologia 1985;52:532-535.

97. Carreras JO. Novel treatment with a hexane extract of *Serenoa repens* in the treatment of benign prostatic hypertrophy. Archiv Esp de Urolog 1987; 40:310-313.

98. Redecker KD. [Sabal extract WS 1473 in benign prostatic hyperplasia]. Extracta Urologica 1998;21(3):23-25.

99. Ziegler H, Holscher U. Efficacy of saw palmetto fruit special extract WS1473 in patients with Alken stage I-II benign prostatic hyperplasia—open multicentre study. Jatros Uro 1998;14(3):34-43.

100. Paoletti PP, Francalanci R, Tenti S, et al. Medical treatment of prostatic hypertrophy. Experience with *Serenoa repens* extract. Urologia 1986;53: 182-187.

101. Kondas J, Philipp V, Dioszeghy G. *Sabal serrulata* extract (Strogen forte) in the treatment of symptomatic benign prostatic hyperplasia. Int Urol Nephrol 1996;28(6):767-772.

102. Cirillo-Marucco E, Pagliarulo A, Tritto G, et al. L'estratto di *Serenoa repens* (Permixon) nel trattamento precoce dell'ipertrofia prostatica. Urologia 1983;50(6):1269-1277.

Shark Cartilage
(AE-941, Neovastat)

SYNONYMS/COMMON NAMES/RELATED SUBSTANCES

- Cartilage, haifischknorpel, Houtsmuller Diet, Neovastat, shark fin soup, *Sphyrna lewini* (hammerhead shark), *Squalus acanthias* (spiny dogfish shark), squalamine, U-955.
- *Note:* Catrix is a preparation of bovine cartilage, not shark cartilage.

CLINICAL BOTTOM LINE
Background

- With over 40 brand-name products sold in 1995 alone, shark cartilage has become one of the most commonly recognized supplements in the United States. Primarily used for cancer, its use became popular in the 1980s after several poorly conducted case series reported "miracle" cancer cures.
- Commercial shark cartilage is primarily composed of chondroitin sulfate (a type of glycosaminoglycan), which is further metabolized to glucosamine and other end products. Although chondroitin and glucosamine have been extensively studied for osteoarthritis, there is no evidence supporting the use of unprocessed shark cartilage preparations for this indication. Shark cartilage also contains an abundant supply of calcium (up to 600 to 780 mg of elemental calcium/daily dose). Manufacturers sometimes promote its use for calcium supplementation rather than for its purported antiangiogenic effects.
- Monthly expenditures on shark cartilage can be as much as $700 to $1000. Many trials of shark cartilage have been supported by manufacturers, raising questions about bias.
- There has been growing interest in the shark cartilage derivative product AE-941 (Neovastat), a matrix metalloproteinase inhibitor, which in preclinical studies has demonstrated antiangiogenic, antitumor, and anti-inflammatory properties. Several clinical trials have been conducted using AE-941, and the U.S. Food and Drug Administration granted orphan drug status to this agent in 2002.
- Research on AE-941 has rejuvenated interest in shark cartilage for malignancies, macular degeneration, psoriasis, and a range of inflammatory disorders. However, there is currently insufficient human evidence to recommend for or against shark cartilage for any indication.

Scientific Evidence for Common/Studied Uses	Grade*
Analgesia	C
Cancer (solid tumors)	C
Inflammatory joint diseases (rheumatoid arthritis, osteoarthritis)	C
Macular degeneration	C
Psoriasis	C

*Key to grades: *A:* Strong scientific evidence for this use; *B:* Good scientific evidence for this use; *C:* Unclear scientific evidence for this use; *D:* Fair scientific evidence against this use (it may not work); *F:* Strong scientific evidence against this use (it likely does not work). For a more detailed explanation of efficacy criteria, see "Natural Standard Evidence-Based Validated Grading Rationale" in the Introduction.

Historical or Theoretical Uses That Lack Sufficient Evidence

- Allergic dermatitis, ankylosing spondylitis, atherosclerosis, bacterial infections, contact dermatitis, diabetic retinopathy, diarrhea, enteritis, fungal infections, glaucoma, immunostimulant, intestinal disorders, Kaposi's sarcoma, nephrolithiasis, Reiter's syndrome, rheumatoid arthritis, sarcoidosis, scar healing, Sjögren's syndrome, skin rash, systemic lupus erythematosus, wound healing, wrinkle prevention.

Expert Opinion and Folkloric Precedent

- The medicinal use of shark cartilage began fairly recently, originating with basic science and observational studies in the 1950s.
- Early theories regarding use of shark cartilage for cancer stemmed from the belief that sharks are not afflicted by cancer. In particular, the cartilaginous skeleton of the Pacific spiny dogfish shark was thought to provide a naturally occurring substance that protects the animal from metastatic disease. However, contrary to initial reports, sharks can be afflicted with cancer.[1]
- Cartilage is often recommended by natural medicine experts for cancer, psoriasis, and inflammatory joint diseases.

Safety Summary

- **Likely safe:** When taken in recommended doses for up to 18 months.[2,3]
- **Possibly unsafe:** In pregnant women, due to known teratogenicity of other antiangiogenic agents; in children and lactating women, due to potential adverse effects of antiangiogenesis on growth; in patients perioperatively or posttrauma, due to theoretical inhibition of wound healing; in patients with myocardial ischemia and peripheral vascular disease, due to theoretical inhibition of remodeling/collateral neovascularization.[4]
- **Likely unsafe:** In patients with hypercalcemia, renal failure, or cardiac arrhythmias, due to shark cartilage's high calcium content.[5]

DOSING/TOXICOLOGY
General

- Recommended doses are based on those most commonly used in available studies, or on historical practice. Doses have not been proven safe or efficacious. With natural products, the optimal doses needed to balance efficacy and safety often have not been determined. Formulations and preparation methods may vary from manufacturer to manufacturer, and from batch to batch of a specific product made by a single manufacturer. Because often the active components of a product are not known, standardization may not be possible, and the clinical effects of different brands may not be comparable.

Standardization

- The method of preparation and purification of shark cartilage is not standardized. In general, preparation involves sterilization and grinding of dried shark (hammerhead or spiny dogfish) cartilage into a powdered form. Some manufacturing processes can denature the antiangiogenic proteins and some products have been found to contain only binding agents and fillers.[6] On analysis, of one shark cartilage extract was found to contain 99.27% water.

Dosing: Adult (18 Years and Older)

Oral

- *Note:* To maximize absorption of oral preparations, shark cartilage should be taken on an empty stomach. Acidic fruit juices (apple, grape, orange, tomato, cranberry) should be avoided for 15 to 30 minutes prior to and after dosing.[7]
- **Cancer:** 80 to 100 g/day or 1 to 1.3 g/kg/day of ground cartilage extract in 2 to 4 divided doses.[5,8] Doses of the shark cartilage derivative AE-941 (Neovastat) have ranged from 30 to 240 mL/day or 20 mg/kg twice daily in clinical trials.[2,3,9]
- **Inflammatory joint diseases:** 0.2 to 2 g/kg/day in 2 to 3 divided doses.[7]
- **Kaposi's sarcoma:** 100 g/day.[10]
- **Psoriasis:** 0.4 to 0.5 g/kg/day for 4 weeks. If skin lesions improve, reduce to 0.2 to 0.3 g/kg/day for 4 additional weeks.[11]

Rectal/Intravaginal

- Doses of 15 g/day or 0.5 to 1 g/kg/day in 2 to 3 divided doses (shark cartilage prepared as an enema) have been described in case series.[8,12] Safety and efficacy have not been demonstrated.

Topical

- **Psoriasis:** Topical creams with 5% to 30% shark cartilage are available and have been recommended by some practitioners for treatment of psoriasis as monotherapy, or with oral shark cartilage, for 4 to 6 weeks. Studies have used 5% to 10% preparations applied daily.[11,13]

Dosing: Pediatric (Younger Than 18 Years)

- Shark cartilage is not recommended in children, due to the theoretical risk of its antiangiogenic effect interfering with normal growth.
- There is a case report of a 9-year-old child with a brain tumor whose parents opted to treat with shark cartilage.[14] The child died 4 months later, following marked tumor progression.

Toxicology

- Insufficient available evidence.

ADVERSE EFFECTS/PRECAUTIONS/CONTRAINDICATIONS

Allergy

- Known allergy/hypersensitivity to shark cartilage or any of its ingredients, including chondroitin sulfate and glucosamine.
- Occupational asthma in workers exposed to shark cartilage powder/dust has been reported, including death of a 38-year-old man, possibly related to hypersensitivity with respiratory complications although it is not clear if shark cartilage or underlying severe reactive airways disease was the cause.[15]

Adverse Effects/Postmarket Surveillance

- **General:** The limited available evidence suggests that shark cartilage is well tolerated in recommended doses. An 18-month phase I (preclinical) study in 330 human subjects, reported by the makers of the shark cartilage derivative

Neovastat, did not report any major toxicities after exposure to the product for more than 4 years.[3] The most commonly reported adverse effects are mild to moderate gastrointestinal distress and nausea.
- **Dermatologic:** Inhibition of angiogenesis theoretically may inhibit wound healing and recovery from surgery or trauma.
- **Neurologic/CNS:** One occurrence of each of the following was noted in an open-label trial: altered consciousness, decreased motor strength, decreased sensation, and generalized weakness.[8] Dizziness and fatigue have also been reported anecdotally.[7]
- **Cardiovascular:** Transient hypotension was noted in one of 60 patients in an open-label study.[8] Theoretically, there is a small risk of arrhythmia in patients with known arrhythmias, because of the calcium in shark cartilage. Patients with coronary artery disease and peripheral vascular disease may depend on blood vessel collateralization, which theoretically could be inhibited by the antiangiogenic properties of shark cartilage.
- **Gastrointestinal:** In open-label and phase I/II trials, 5% to 10% of patients discontinued shark cartilage because of gastrointestinal distress (nausea, vomiting, constipation, dyspepsia), and 20% to 40% experienced milder symptoms of cramping and bloating.[5,8,16,17] Gastrointestinal upset may be due to the high calcium concentration in some shark cartilage preparations. One case report documents hepatitis (transaminitis, low-grade fever, right upper quadrant abdominal tenderness, jaundice) in an elderly male patient using shark cartilage, which resolved 6 weeks after the supplement was discontinued (the product in question was never checked for adulterants or impurities).[18] Taste alteration may occur.
- **Renal:** There is a theoretical risk of hypercalcemia in patients with renal disease because of the high calcium content in some shark cartilage preparations.
- **Endocrine:** Hyperglycemia was reported in one of 60 patients in an open-label study.[8] Shark cartilage preparations may contain up to 25% calcium, and hypercalcemia was reported in 2 of 36 prostate/breast cancer patients in an open study.[5] However, both of these patients had experienced episodes of hypercalcemia prior to initiating shark cartilage therapy.
- **Hematologic:** Inhibition of angiogenesis theoretically may inhibit wound healing and recovery from surgery or trauma.

Precautions/Warnings/Contraindications

- Use cautiously in patients with coronary artery disease and peripheral vascular disease, based on theoretical inhibition of collateral neovascularization due to the antiangiogenesis properties of shark cartilage.
- Use cautiously in patients with liver dysfunction, based on one case report of hepatitis.
- Use cautiously in patients with diabetes or glucose intolerance, based on an isolated report of hypoglycemia.
- Follow calcium levels in patients with renal insufficiency or cardiac arrhythmias because of the high calcium content in shark cartilage products.
- Consider discontinuation perioperatively and post-trauma because of the antiangiogenesis properties of shark cartilage.

Pregnancy and Lactation

- Although no specific human studies have been conducted, shark cartilage should be avoided in pregnant or lactating women because of the risk of impaired angiogenesis (other

antiangiogenic agents, such as thalidomide, are known teratogens).[4]
- Shark cartilage is contraindicated in children, due to the risk of impaired angiogenesis.[4]

INTERACTIONS
Shark Cartilage/Drug Interactions

- **Thiazide diuretics:** Shark cartilage products contain calcium (up to 25%) and may cause hypercalcemia when taken with drugs known to elevate serum calcium, such as with prolonged thiazide therapy.
- **Oral hypoglycemic agents:** One patient with type 2 diabetes mellitus and renal carcinoma was noted to develop hypoglycemia during a phase I/II study using shark cartilage.[19]
- **Interferon α and β:** Both interferon α and β possess antiangiogenic properties and may act synergistically with shark cartilage to inhibit blood vessel growth, slow wound healing, reduce inflammation, and cause birth defects.[20]
- **Thalidomide:** As an angiogenesis inhibitor, thalidomide may act synergistically with shark cartilage to inhibit blood vessel growth, slow wound healing, reduce inflammation, and cause birth defects.[20,21]
- **Experimental antiangiogenic agents:** Patients in treatment protocols involving other antiangiogenic agents should avoid shark cartilage, based on its theoretical additive or synergistic activity. Examples include Ag3340, Bay12-9566, Leflunomide, Marimastat, Anti-VEGF antibody, Carboxyaminotriazole, CGS 27023A, AGM-1470, SU5416, Vitaxin, EMD 121974, Interleukin-12, and CM 101.[20]
- **Cisplatin:** Based on one animal study, cisplatin and shark cartilage may act synergistically against tumors, although there is no human supporting evidence. Intravenous shark cartilage derivative AE-941 (Neovastat) (500 mg/kg) was given to mice using the Lewis lung carcinoma metastatic model, resulting in a statistically significant 49% reduction in lung surface metastases vs. placebo.[22] Notably, cisplatin (4 mg/kg) reduced metastases by 69% (with greater toxicity), and cisplatin plus shark cartilage reduced metastases by 87%. The authors reported reduced toxicity with AE-941 plus cisplatin vs. cisplatin alone.

Shark Cartilage/Herb/Supplement Interactions

- **Calcium supplements:** Shark cartilage preparations contain up to 25% calcium. Certain products provide 600 to 780 mg of elemental calcium per day (Cartilade, BefeFin), which may have an additive effect when taken with calcium supplements, leading to hypercalcemia.
- **Hypoglycemic herbs/supplements:** One patient with type 2 diabetes mellitus and renal carcinoma was noted to develop hypoglycemia during a phase I/II study using shark cartilage.[19]
- **Chondroitin sulfate:** Chondroitin, a popular therapy for osteoarthritis, is a constituent of shark cartilage. Concomitant use may lead to higher than expected serum levels of chondroitin, with unknown toxicity (although 3 g one-time doses of chondroitin have been observed without adverse outcomes).
- **Glucosamine sulfate:** Glucosamine, a popular therapy for osteoarthritis, in a constituent of shark cartilage. Concomitant use may lead to higher than expected serum levels of glucosamine, with unknown toxicity. Anecdotally, clinicians have reported increased insulin resistance in diabetics with high levels of glucosamine, although this has not been substantiated in clinical studies.

Shark Cartilage/Food Interactions
- **Acidic fruit juices (apple, grape, orange, tomato, cranberry):** Acidic fruit juices may reduce the absorption of shark cartilage.[7,10]

Shark Cartilage/Lab Interaction
- **Calcium levels:** Shark cartilage preparations contain up to 25% calcium. Certain products provide 600 to 780 mg of elemental calcium per day (Cartilade, BefeFin), which may elevate calcium levels.
- **Keratan sulfate:** Keratan is a protein measured in basic science research and experimentally as a marker of cartilage metabolism. A protein in shark cartilage reacts with the same antibodies as in the keratan sulfate ELISA assay, which may lead to erroneous results.[23]
- **Troponin-I:** In theory, the troponin-I in shark cartilage may cause a false-positive result in human serum troponin-I assays, a test commonly used to evaluate cardiac ischemia.[24] It is unclear, however, if the troponin-I is digested by proteolytic enzymes prior to absorption.

MECHANISM OF ACTION
Pharmacology

- Shark cartilage contains approximately 40% protein (troponin-I, tetranectin-type protein, collagenase, cartilage-derived inhibitor [CDI], tissue inhibitor of metalloproteinases), and 5% to 20% glycosaminoglycans (chondroitin sulfate-D, chondroitin-6-sulfate, keratan sulfate). The remainder is made up of calcium salts (up to 25% of some preparations) and glycoproteins (sphyrnastatin-1 and 2, galactosamines, glucosamine).[20,24]
- There have been numerous proposed anticancer mechanisms for shark cartilage, including direct toxicity against tumor cells and stimulation of the immune system. However, the mechanism for which there is the most support in basic science research is the inhibition of tumor angiogenesis.[4,25-31] As with other experimental antiangiogenic agents, it is theorized that blocking formation of new blood vessels may inhibit growth/metastasis of solid tumors. Research has isolated a variety of molecular fractions from cartilage that exhibit antiangiogenic activity.[29,32-34] Peptides and glycosaminoglycans have been examined, and constituent glycoproteins have been found to have antiangiogenic activity, with ability to inhibit tumor neorevascularization in animal models.
- A proposed biochemical basis of shark cartilage's antiangiogenic activity is blockade of vascular endothelial cell growth factor (VEGF) receptors, which in turn inhibits endothelial cell proliferation.[26,32] Shark cartilage has also been found to modify the organization of focal adhesion proteins responsible for endothelial attachment[35] and to inhibit the proteolytic enzymes that break down extracellular matrix and allow tumor invasion and metastasis (matrix metalloproteinase inhibition).[31,34,36-38] This latter mechanism is the proposed activity of the shark cartilage derivative Neovastat (AE-941), currently in clinical trials.
- The antiangiogenic properties of shark cartilage in humans have been studied. In a placebo-controlled double-blind study, 30 healthy volunteers received placebo or oral shark cartilage extract for 23 days.[39] On day 12, an inert implant was inserted subcutaneously into subjects' arms. Endothelial cell densities were measured as an indirect means of assessing angiogenesis, and were significantly lower in the cartilage group compared to placebo ($p < 0.01$).

- There has also been preliminary investigation of a reef shark protein with similarities to the human plasminogen-binding protein tetranectin (tetranectin-type protein). Tetranectin enhances activation of plasminogen and alters the balance between blood clotting and fibrinolysis. Tetranectin, which is integral to connective tissue structure, is often reduced in the serum of cancer patients.[40]
- Angiogenesis is also believed to play a role in inflammatory processes. In diseases such as rheumatoid arthritis, angiogenesis inducers outweigh the activity of angiogenesis inhibitors.[41] It has therefore been proposed that antiangiogenic agents may have potency against inflammatory conditions. In a mouse model, contact hypersensitivity, a form of inflammation, was inhibited by the shark cartilage derivative AE-941.[42]
- Ongoing research has reported that shark cartilage acts as a scavenger for reactive oxygen species,[43,44] interferes with cellular adhesion,[35] inhibits calcium channels, and possesses anti-inflammatory properties.[7]
- Chondroitin sulfate and glucosamine sulfate are also found in shark cartilage. Both of these agents have been studied in osteoarthritis. Most available chondroitin and glucosamine supplements are obtained from chitin, which is a major component of the exoskeleton in marine invertebrates. Other sources include fungi, yeast and synthetic sources. Shark cartilage itself has not been extensively studied for its role in osteoarthritis.
- The matrix metalloproteinase inhibitor AE-941 (Neovastat), in addition to reported antiangiogenic properties,[19,22,25,38,45,46] has been noted to exhibit vascular endothelial growth factor inhibition,[26] tissue plasminogen activator activity stimulation,[47] and pro-apoptotic properties.[48] Preclinical research[22,27,49] and initial human research[3,9,17,50-58] report good tolerance and potential benefits in renal cell carcinoma, with research in other tumor types including prostate and lung cancer.

Pharmacodynamics/Kinetics

- Early research suggests that constituent proteins in shark cartilage are absorbed via the intestinal tract[32] and are bioavailable.[39] However, reliable data are limited at this time.

HISTORY

- Investigations of cartilage began in the 1950s. Reportedly, this was prompted by the visit of a Canadian scientist to Columbia-Presbyterian Hospital in New York, who suggested possible medicinal uses to a group of other scientists. Some mystery surrounds this anecdote, as the scientist apparently disappeared after making the suggestion.[59]
- Prior to the 1970s, research focused primarily on mammalian (bovine) cartilage, in areas including immune stimulation, cancer, and inflammation.[59,60] It was subsequently observed that sharks contain more active cartilage per animal than calves, and that shark cartilage exhibits *in vitro* anti-inflammatory activity at a cruder stage of purification.[28] In addition, researchers had appreciated the apparent excellent lifetime health of sharks, with arguably rare affliction of cancer or disease.
- During the 1970s and 1980s, bench research demonstrated antiangiogenic and antitumor properties of shark cartilage, raising interest in the possibility of treating human cancers with shark cartilage.
- Public enthusiasm for shark cartilage as a cancer treatment increased following three controversial studies by William

Lane. Lane processed shark cartilage and conducted two trials with cancer patients in Mexico, followed by a widely cited Cuban trial of terminally ill cancer patients, showing dramatic improvements in survival (Menendez-Lopez, unpublished data, 1992). His results were highly publicized, and he was featured on the television show "60 Minutes." However, these trials were subsequently discredited.[60,61] Notably, Lane's son is president of Lane Labs, which manufactures the BeneFin brand of shark cartilage. In 1999, the U.S. Food and Drug Administration sought an injunction against the makers of BeneFin for alleged illegal promotion of the product as a cancer treatment.
- Despite the lack of convincing human data, shark cartilage remains widely used by cancer patients in the United States. Three phase III trials are in progress to obtain high-quality, scientific evidence regarding the efficacy of shark cartilage (notably, two of the studies are sponsored by product manufacturers).

REVIEW OF THE EVIDENCE: DISCUSSION
Cancer (Solid Tumors)
Summary

- Promotion of new blood vessels (angiogenesis) is necessary for tumors to grow and metastasize. Numerous synthetic and naturally derived antiangiogenic agents have been studied *in vitro*, in animals, and in early-phase human trials. Enthusiasm about shark cartilage has stemmed from preclinical evidence of its antiangiogenic properties and from several poorly described case series of patients with numerous types of end-stage malignancies. At this time, however, the evidence is not adequate to recommend either for or against shark cartilage in the treatment of any type of cancer. Despite lack of approval by the U.S. Food and Drug Administration (FDA), products containing shark cartilage have been marketed to U.S. consumers as cancer treatments. This has caused the FDA to send a warning letter to shark cartilage manufacturers prohibiting the promotion of shark cartilage as a treatment for cancer.[62] There are ongoing trials of several shark cartilage derivatives, most notably the matrix metalloproteinase inhibitor Neovastat (AE-941). Diseases under investigation include renal cell carcinoma, lung cancer, prostate cancer, and multiple myeloma.

Evidence (Shark Cartilage)

- Brem and Folkman[4] and Langer et al[31,36] conducted early basic science research on cartilage and angiogenesis inhibition. Lee and Langer reported that shark cartilage extract (incorporated into pellets) implanted alongside tumors in rabbit cornea inhibited tumor neovascularization.[28] Inhibition was 75% greater than that in controls, with statistical significance. Animal studies have demonstrated that shark cartilage inhibits angiogenesis in rats[63-65] and exhibits activity against several mouse tumor lines *in vivo*.[32,34,46,66,67] This has been demonstrated in a mouse model of lung carcinoma.[2,25] Other animal antitumor models have been less definitive, and one study showed no improvement after 25 days in squamous cell carcinoma VII (SCCVII) tumors implanted in the feet of mice.[68] A more recent report demonstrated regression of implanted mouse brain tumors after 43 days of shark cartilage, but no additive effect with the borono-phenylalanine-mediated neutron capture therapy (BNCT).[69] Intravenous shark cartilage derivative AE-941 (500 mg/kg) was given to mice using the Lewis lung carcinoma metastatic model and resulted in a statistically significant 49% reduction

Review of the Evidence: Shark Cartilage

Condition Treated*	Study Design	Author, Year	N[†]	SS[†]	Study Quality[‡]	Magnitude of Benefit	ARR[†]	NNT[†]	Comments
Cancer: suppression and quality of life	Case series	Miller[8] 1998	60	NA	NA	None	NA	NA	Phase I/II trial.
Cancer: suppression and quality of life	Case series	Riviere[3] 1998	25	NA	NA	Positive trend	NA	NA	Published abstract with limited details.
Cancer: suppression and quality of life	Case series	Leitner[5] 1998	20	NA	NA	None	NA	NA	Phase II study; 10 breast cancer, 10 prostate cancer.
Cancer: suppression and quality of life	Case series	Mathews[61] 1993	20	NA	NA	Small	NA	NA	Preliminary unpublished results only.
Cancer: suppression	Case series	Lane 1996	8	NA	NA	Large	NA	NA	5 patients reported cancer-free.
Cancer: suppression	Case series	Lane[12] 1992	8	NA	NA	Large	NA	NA	Poor documentation; no objective measurement of improvement.
Cancer: suppression	Case series	Menendez-Lopez 1992	29	NA	NA	Large	NA	NA	Unpublished data; reported improvement in 55% of subjects; results discredited by National Cancer Institute.
Prostate cancer: suppression	Case series	Wisniewski, 2000	12	NA	NA	None	NA	NA	No improvement with BeneFin; 4 patients died.
Brain tumors: suppression	Case series	Rosenbluth[16] 1999	12	NA	NA	None	NA	NA	No improvement with BeneFin over 20 weeks.
Psoriasis	Case series	Goldman[73] 1998 (principal investigator, Saunder)	49	NA	NA	Dose-dependent response	NA	NA	45% dropout rate; no response with 30-60 mL/day; best response with 240 mL/day.
Macular degeneration	Case series	Turcotte[58] 1999	10	NA	NA	Large	NA	NA	Improved visual acuity in 8 patients.

*Primary or secondary outcome.
[†] N, Number of patients; SS, statistically significant; ARR, absolute risk reduction; NNT, the number of patients who need to undergo a specific intervention in order to observe an outcome in one individual.
[‡] 0-2 = poor; 3-4 = good; 5 = excellent.
NA, Not applicable.
For an explanation of each category in this table, please see Table 3 in the Introduction.

in lung surface metastases vs. placebo.[22] Notably, in this study cisplatin (4 mg/kg) reduced metastases by 69% (with greater toxicity), and cisplatin plus shark cartilage reduced metastases by 87%.

- In humans, although shark cartilage has been shown to inhibit angiogenesis during wound healing,[39] there is only preliminary cancer trial evidence. Data presented by William Lane on the television show "60 Minutes" demonstrated dramatic benefits in a group of Cuban cancer patients treated with shark cartilage. This research, which is unpublished but available on the Lane Laboratories Inc. website (principal investigator, Menendez-Lopez, 1992), was subsequently deemed "unimpressive" by the National Cancer Institute.[61] This open-label study administered 0.5 g/kg/day of shark cartilage rectally for 16 weeks in 29 patients with advanced-stage cancers of several types (breast, ovarian, uterine, liver, throat, esophageal, bladder, gastric), and reported clinical improvement in 55% of subjects (Karnofsky Index). Despite criticism, Dr. Lane has defended the Cuban trial results and the efficacy of shark cartilage. He has cited benefit in a more recent 11-week open trial in eight end-stage cancer patients, conducted in Tijuana, Mexico. In this study, subjects with multiple types of cancer (breast, ovarian, uterine, cervical, and soft tissue sarcoma) and one patient with vaginal hemangioma were administered 30 g/day of shark cartilage (in women as one 15-g enema and one 15-g intravaginal treatment, and in the one male subject as two 15-g enemas). At the study's end, seven subjects were reported to have responded favorably by subjective criteria, and five to be tumor-free.[12] There are several problems with the documentation of this study. No objective measures of improvement are provided, numerous types of cancers are grouped together, and there is misclassification of hemangioma as a malignancy. Another source of potential bias stems from Dr. Lane's involvement in commercial endeavors, both holding a patent in this area, and having family members in control of a major shark cartilage manufacturing company (Lane Labs). This was an uncontrolled study.

- A news item in the National Cancer Institute's journal reported preliminary positive findings in a small U.S. trial. This study, originally sponsored by the Office of Alternative Medicine of the U.S. National Institutes of Health, found improved quality of life, objectively measured, in 10 of 20 patients after treatment with shark cartilage. Four of the 20 patients had a partial or complete response.[61]

- In a published abstract, Riviere (an officer of the manufacturing company Aeterna Laboratories) reported a positive "trend in favor of a dose/response effect in patients' clinical benefits" (tumor assessment, ECOG criteria, body weight, and analgesic consumption combined) in 25 patients administered 10 to 80 mg/kg/day of shark cartilage over 18 months. Details beyond this abstract are not known.[3]

- Miller conducted a 12-week phase I/II open-label, non-randomized investigation of shark cartilage in 60 adult patients with advanced cancer.[8] Cancers included bladder, brain, breast, colon, rectal, lung, non-Hodgkin's lymphoma, and prostate. Shark cartilage, 1 g/kg/day administered in divided doses, was the only agent given during the trial. The dose was increased to 1.3 g/kg/day at 6 weeks if no effect was observed. No significant anticancer activity or improvement in quality of life was found.

- In a published abstract, Leitner reported preliminary results of two phase II studies of shark cartilage monotherapy (1 g/kg/day in four divided doses) in patients with either metastatic breast cancer or metastatic prostate cancer refractory to standard treatments.[5] Of 36 patients enrolled, 10 breast cancer and 10 prostate cancer patients were evaluable at 8 weeks. Among these patients, no changes in performance status, quality of life, or pain scores were observed.

- In a published abstract, Wisniewski described a case series of 12 patients with advanced prostate cancer who were "asked" to stop hormonal therapy and begin oral treatment with BeneFin (1 g/kg/day for 10 weeks, followed by 20 g/day thereafter). No patients completed the study, which was designed to last 6 months. All patients showed signs of advancing disease during the trial, including rising prostate-specific antigen (PSA) titers. Four patients died. The ethics of stopping standard-of-care therapy in favor of an unproven treatment were not explored. Prostate cancer was also studied in an open-label trial of the shark cartilage derivative AE-941 (Neovastat), which found that 40% of patients did not experience more than a 25% increase in baseline PSA values.[17] Results are difficult to interpret because of lack of controls.

- In a phase II pilot study, 12 patients with advanced refractory brain tumors (10 glioblastomas, 1 oligoastrocytoma, 1 unspecified) were treated with 96 g/day of BefeFin taken in four divided doses.[16] Disease progression was measured at 8 and 20 weeks. At the study's conclusion, 9 patients exhibited no clinical improvement, 1 patient had withdrawn due to disease progression, and 2 had dropped out for unknown reasons.

- In a case report, Coppes described a 9-year-old girl with recurrent neuroectodermal brain tumor, whose family elected to use shark cartilage monotherapy rather than radiotherapy and conventional chemotherapy.[14] Four months later she died from tumor progression.

- Based on his claimed self-cure from malignant melanoma using a diet rich in shark cartilage powder, vitamins, and antioxidants, the Dutch internist Dr. A.J. Houtsmuller promoted consumption of the "Houtsmuller Diet" during the 1980s and 1990s. Notably, more than 60% of cancer patients in the Netherlands have used this diet. Dr. Houtsmuller later admitted he had never had melanoma, bringing disrepute to the diet regimen.[70]

- In 1995, the FDA granted Phase II study approval for the treatment of advanced prostate cancer and Kaposi's sarcoma using oral doses of 100 mg/day of shark cartilage.[10]

- AE-941 (Neovastat): There are numerous cartilage-derived angiogenesis inhibitors in ongoing human trials. The matrix metalloproteinase inhibitor AE-941 (Neovastat), manufactured by Aeterna Laboratories, has been of particular research interest and was granted orphan drug status in 2002 by the FDA.[71] In addition to reports of antiangiogenic properties,[19,22,25,38,45,46] AE-941 has been noted to exhibit vascular endothelial growth factor inhibition,[26] tissue plasminogen activator activity stimulation,[47] and pro-apoptotic properties.[48] Preclinical research[22,27,49] and initial human research[3,9,17,50-58] report good tolerance and potential benefits in renal cell carcinoma,[51,53,54,56,71] with research in other tumor types including prostate[17] and non–small-cell lung cancer,[3,19,50] multiple myeloma,[55,72] and bony metastases.[27] Human trials are also reportedly underway in Chile, Japan and China.[60]

Psoriasis

Summary

- There are insufficient human data on the use of shark cartilage in the treatment of psoriasis.

Evidence

- Dupont demonstrated that the application of the shark cartilage preparation AE-94 (Neovastat) results in reduction of skin irritation on the forearms of human subjects.[13] No difference in effect was seen between 5%, 10%, and 50% topical preparations. Results were statistically significant.

- Several early-phase clinical trials have been undertaken in patients with psoriasis.[11,13,52,57,73] Preliminary results have been reported by Daniel Saunder at Sunnybrook Health Science Center in Toronto.[73] In an open-label trial, 49 patients were given oral doses of 30, 60, 120, or 240 mL/day of an unreported concentration of shark cartilage derivative AE-941 (Neovastat), for up to 12 weeks. Of the initial subjects, 25 dropped out for unclear reasons. The remaining patients on the 30-mL and 60-mL doses exhibited no response, but the 120-mL group demonstrated a 4% to 5% improvement by objective criteria (Psoriasis Area and Severity Index [PASI] score), and the 240-mL group experienced a 26% improvement. Although results are promising, the large dropout rate and open-label nature of this study point to the need for larger, randomized studies of this indication.

Macular Degeneration

Summary

- There are insufficient human data on the use of shark cartilage in the treatment of macular degeneration.

Evidence

- A promising open-label study of shark cartilage over 24 weeks observed improved or stabilized visual acuity in 8 out of 10 patients.[58] Further data from controlled studies are required before a stronger recommendation can be made.

Analgesia

Summary

- There are insufficient human data on the use of shark cartilage as an analgesic agent.

Evidence

- Fontenele and colleagues have demonstrated anti-inflammatory and analgesic properties of shark cartilage in animal studies. The authors suggest that inhibition of nitric oxide synthesis may be involved in the mechanism of action.[74,75]

Inflammatory Joint Diseases (Rheumatoid Arthritis, Osteoarthritis)

Summary

- There are insufficient human data on the use of shark cartilage for inflammatory joint diseases.

Evidence

- Derivatives of shark cartilage, such as AE-941, have been shown in animal models to reduce inflammatory responses. Shark cartilage itself has also been demonstrated to diminish inflammation *in vitro* and in animal studies. However, no human data are available.[42,74,75]
- In rheumatoid arthritis, it is believed that the activity of angiogenesis inducers outweighs that of angiogenesis inhibitors.[41] It has therefore been proposed that shark cartilage, as an antiangiogenic agent, may have potency against inflammatory conditions. There is currently no supporting human evidence.
- Chondroitin sulfate and glucosamine sulfate have been shown to benefit patients with osteoarthritis. However, concentrations in shark cartilage preparations may be too low for clinical benefit, and shark cartilage has not been assessed for this indication.

FORMULARY: BRANDS USED IN CLINICAL TRIALS
Brands Used in Case Reports and Human Trials

- AE-941/Neovastat (Aeterna Laboratories, Canada), BeneFin (Lane Labs, USA) (clinical trial availability only); MIA Shark Powder, Sharkilage, Shark Cartilage Hydrosoluable Fraction.
- *Note:* Catrix is a preparation of bovine cartilage, not shark cartilage.

References

1. Anonymous. Sharks do get cancer, so shark cartilage unlikely to contain anticancer agent. Reuters Medical News for the Professional 1999;1-2.
2. Riviere M, Alaoui-Jamali M, Falardeau P, et al. Neovastat: an inhibitor of angiogenesis with anti-cancer activity. Proc Amer Assoc Cancer Res 1998;39:46.
3. Riviere M, Falardeau P, Latreille J, et al. Phase I/II lung cancer clinical trial results with AE-941 (Neovastat®) an inhibitor of angiogenesis. Clin Invest Med (Supplt) 1998;S14.
4. Brem H, Folkman J. Inhibition of tumor angiogenesis mediated by cartilage. J Exp Med 1975;141(2):427-439.
5. Leitner SP, Rothkopf MM, Haverstick DD, et al. Two phase II studies of oral dry shark cartilage powder (SCP) in patients with either metastatic breast or prostate cancer refractory to standard treatment. Amer Soc Clin Oncol 1998;17:A240.
6. Holt S. Shark cartilage and nutraceutical update. Alt Comp Ther 1995;1:414-416.
7. Milner M. A guide to the use of shark cartilage in the treatment of arthritis and other inflammatory joint diseases. Amer Chiropractor 1999;21:40-42.
8. Miller DR, Anderson GT, Stark JJ, et al. Phase I/II trial of the safety and efficacy of shark cartilage in the treatment of advanced cancer. J Clin Oncol 1998;16(11):3649-3655.
9. Riviere M, Latreille J, Falardeau P. AE-941 (Neovastat), an inhibitor of angiogenesis: phase I/II cancer clinical trial results. Cancer Invest 1999;17(suppl 1):16-17.
10. Hunt TJ, Connelly JF. Shark cartilage for cancer treatment. Am J Health Syst Pharm 1995;52(16):1756, 1760.
11. Wilson JL. Topical shark cartilage subdues psoriasis. Altern Comp Ther 2000;6:291.
12. Lane IW, Contreras E. High rate of bioactivity (reduction in gross tumor size) observed in advanced cancer patients treated with shark cartilage material. J Naturopath Med 1992;3(1):86-88.
13. Dupont E, Savard RE, Jourdain C, et al. Antiangiogenic properties of a novel shark cartilage extract: potential role in the treatment of psoriasis. J Cutan Med Surg 1998;2(3):146-152.
14. Coppes MJ, Anderson RA, Egeler RM, et al. Alternative therapies for the treatment of childhood cancer. N Engl J Med 1998;339(12):846-847.
15. Ortega HG, Kreiss K, Schill DP, et al. Fatal asthma from powdering shark cartilage and review of fatal occupational asthma literature. Am J Ind Med 2002;42(1):50-54.
16. Rosenbluth R, Jennis A, Cantwell S, et al. Oral shark cartilage in the treatment of patients with advanced primary brain tumors. A phase II pilot study (meeting abstract). Proc Annu Meet Am Soc Clin Oncol 1999;18:A554.
17. Saad F, Klotz L, Babaian R, et al. Phase I/II trial on AE-941 (Neovastat) in patients with metastatic refractory prostate cancer (abstract presentation). Can Urologl Assoc Annu Meet (June 24-27, 2001).
18. Ashar B, Vargo E. Shark cartilage-induced hepatitis. Ann Intern Med 1996;125(9):780-781.
19. Evans WK, Latreille J, Batist G, et al. AE-941, an inhibitor of angiogenesis: rationale for development in combination with induction chemotherapy/

radiotherapy in patients with non-small-cell lung cancer (NSCLC). Proffered Papers 1999;S250.
20. Talks KL, Harris AL. Current status of antiangiogenic factors. Br J Haematol 2000;109(3):477-489.
21. Corral LG, Kaplan G. Immunomodulation by thalidomide and thalidomide analogues. Ann Rheum Dis 1999;58 Suppl 1:I107-I113.
22. Jamali MA, Riviere P, Falardeau A, et al. Effect of AE-941 (Neovastat), an angiogenesis inhibitor, in the Lewis lung carcinoma metastatic model, efficacy, toxicity prevention and survival. Clin Invest Med 1998;(suppl):S16.
23. Moller HJ, Moller-Pedersen T, Damsgaard TE, et al. Demonstration of immunogenic keratan sulphate in commercial chondroitin 6-sulphate from shark cartilage. Implications for ELISA assays. Clin Chim Acta 1995;236(2):195-204.
24. Moses MA, Wiederschain D, Wu I, et al. Troponin I is present in human cartilage and inhibits angiogenesis. Proc Natl Acad Sci U S A 1999;96(6):2645-2650.
25. Dupont E, Falardeau P, Mousa SA, et al. Antiangiogenic and antimetastatic properties of Neovastat (AE-941), an orally active extract derived from cartilage tissue. Clin Exp Metastasis 2002;19(2):145-153.
26. Beliveau R, Gingras D, Kruger EA, et al. The antiangiogenic agent Neovastat (AE-941) inhibits vascular endothelial growth factor-mediated biological effects. Clin Cancer Res 2002;8(4):1242-1250.
27. Weber MH, Lee J, Orr FW. The effect of Neovastat (AE-941) on an experimental metastatic bone tumor model. Int J Oncol 2002;20(2):299-303.
28. Lee A, Langer R. Shark cartilage contains inhibitors of tumor angiogenesis. Science 1983;221(4616):1185-1187.
29. Moses MA, Sudhalter J, Langer R. Identification of an inhibitor of neovascularization from cartilage. Science 1990;248(4961):1408-1410.
30. Kuettner KE, Pauli BU. Inhibition of neovascularization by a cartilage factor. Ciba Found Symp 1983;100:163-173.
31. Langer R, Brem H, Falterman K, et al. Isolations of a cartilage factor that inhibits tumor neovascularization. Science 1976;193(4247):70-72.
32. McGuire TR, Kazakoff PW, Hoie EB, et al. Antiproliferative activity of shark cartilage with and without tumor necrosis factor-alpha in human umbilical vein endothelium. Pharmacotherapy 1996;16(2):237-244.
33. Oikawa T, Ashino-Fuse H, Shimamura M, et al. A novel angiogenic inhibitor derived from Japanese shark cartilage (I). Extraction and estimation of inhibitory activities toward tumor and embryonic angiogenesis. Cancer Lett 1990;51(3):181-186.
34. Sheu JR, Fu CC, Tsai ML, et al. Effect of U-995, a potent shark cartilage-derived angiogenesis inhibitor, on anti-angiogenesis and anti-tumor activities. Anticancer Res 1998;18(6A):4435-4441.
35. Chen JS, Chang CM, Wu JC, et al. Shark cartilage extract interferes with cell adhesion and induces reorganization of focal adhesions in cultured endothelial cells. J Cell Biochem 2000;78(3):417-428.
36. Langer R, Conn H, Vacanti J, et al. Control of tumor growth in animals by infusion of an angiogenesis inhibitor. Proc National Acad Sci USA 1980;77.
37. Moses MA. A cartilage-derived inhibitor of neovascularization and metalloproteinases. Clin Exp Rheumatol 1993;11(Suppl 8):S67-S69.
38. Gingras D, Renaud A, Mousseau N, et al. Matrix proteinase inhibition by AE-941, a multifunctional antiangiogenic compound. Anticancer Res 2001;21(1A):145-155.
39. Berbari P, Thibodeau A, Germain L, et al. Antiangiogenic effects of the oral administration of liquid cartilage extract in humans. J Surg Res 1999;87(1):108-113.
40. Neame PJ, Young CN, Treep JT. Primary structure of a protein isolated from reef shark (*Carcharhinus springeri*) cartilage that is similar to the mammalian C-type lectin homolog, tetranectin. Protein Sci 1992;1(1):161-168.
41. Koch AE. The role of angiogenesis in rheumatoid arthritis: recent developments. Ann Rheum Dis 2000;59(Suppl 1):i65-i71.
42. Zhuang L, Wang B, Shivji G, et al. AE-941, a novel inhibitor of angiogenesis has significant anti-inflammatory effect on contact hypersensitivity. J Invest Derm 1997;108(4):633.
43. Gomes EM, Souto PR, Felzenszwalb I. Shark-cartilage containing preparation protects cells against hydrogen peroxide induced damage and mutagenesis. Mutat Res 1996;367(4):204-208.
44. Felzenszwalb I, Pelielo de Mattos JC, Bernardo-Filho M, et al. Shark cartilage-containing preparation: protection against reactive oxygen species. Food Chem Toxicol 1998;36(12):1079-1084.
45. Dupont E, Alaoui-Jamali M, Wang T, et al. Angiostatic and antitumoral activity of AE-941 (Neovastat), a molecular fraction derived from shark cartilage. Proc Annu Meet Am Assoc Cancer Res 1997;38:227.
46. Anonymous. Angiostatic and antitumoral activity of AE-941 (Neovastat-R), a molecular fraction derived from shark cartilage (meeting abstract). Proc Annu Meet Am Assoc Cancer Res 1997;38:A1530.
47. Gingras D, Labelle D, Nyalendo C, et al. The antiangiogenic agent Neovastat (AE-941) stimulates tissue plasminogen activator activity. Invest New Drugs 2004;22(1):17-26.
48. Boivin D, Gendron S, Beaulieu E, et al. The antiangiogenic agent Neovastat (AE-941) induces endothelial cell apoptosis. Mol Cancer Ther 2002;1(10):795-802.
49. Weber MH, Lee J, Orr FW. The effect of Neovastat (AE-941) on an experimental metastatic bone tumor model. Int J Oncol 2002;20(2):299-303.
50. Latreille J, Batist G, Laberge F, et al. Phase I/II trial of the safety and

efficacy of AE-941 (Neovastat) in the treatment of non-small-cell lung cancer. Clin Lung Cancer 2003;4(4):231-236.

51. Bukowski RM. AE-941, a multifunctional antiangiogenic compound: trials in renal cell carcinoma. Expert Opin Investig Drugs 2003;12(8):1403-1411.

52. Sauder DN, Dekoven J, Champagne P, et al. Neovastat (AE-941), an inhibitor of angiogenesis: Randomized phase I/II clinical trial results in patients with plaque psoriasis. J Am Acad Dermatol 2002;47(4):535-541.

53. Batist G, Patenaude F, Champagne P, et al. Neovastat (AE-941) in refractory renal cell carcinoma patients: report of a phase II trial with two dose levels. Ann Oncol 2002;13(8):1259-1263.

54. Escudier B, Patenaude F, Bukowski R, et al. Rationale for a phase III clinical trial with AE-941 (Neovastat) in metastatic renal cell carcinoma patients refractory to immunotherapy. Ann Oncol 2000;11(Suppl 4):143-144.

55. Aeterna Laboratories Inc. Phase II study of AE-941 (Neovastat; Shark Cartilage) in patients with early relapse or refractory multiple myeloma. 2001. Information Contact Number 1-888-349-3232.

56. Aeterna Laboratories Inc. Phase III randomized study of AE-941 (Neovastat; Shark Cartilage Extract) in patients with metastatic renal cell carcinoma refractory to immunotherapy. 2001. Information Contact Number 1-888-349-3232.

57. Saunder DN. Angiogenesis antagonist as treatment for psoriasis: Phase I clinical trial results with AE-941. Am Acad Dermatol Conf, New Orleans, March 19-24, 1999.

58. Turcotte P. Phase I dose escalation study of AE-941, an antiangiogenic agent, in age-related macular degeneration patient. Retina Soc Conf, Hawaii, December 2, 1999.

59. Prudden JF. Cartilage as therapy. Adjuv Nutr Cancer Treatm Symp, Tampa, Florida, September 27-30, 1995.

60. Lane W, Milner M. A comparison of shark cartilage and bovine cartilage. Townsend Lett 1996;153:40-42.

61. Mathews J. Media feeds frenzy over shark cartilage as cancer treatment. J Natl Cancer Inst 1993;85(15):1190-1191.

62. U.S. Food and Drug Administration. FDA takes action against firm marketing unapproved drugs. FDA talk paper (December 10, 1999).

63. Davis PF, He Y, Furneaux RH, et al. Inhibition of angiogenesis by oral ingestion of powdered shark cartilage in a rat model. Microvasc Res 1997; 54(2):178-182.

64. Cataldi J, Osborne D. Effects of shark cartilage on mammary tumor neovascularization in vivo and cell proliferation in vitro (meeting abstract). FASEB J 1995;9(3):A135.

65. Gonzalez RP, Soares FS, Farias RF, et al. Demonstration of inhibitory effect of oral shark cartilage on basic fibroblast growth factor-induced angiogenesis in the rabbit cornea. Biol Pharm Bull 2001;24(2):151-154.

66. Barber R, Delahunt B, Grebe SK, et al. Oral shark cartilage does not abolish carcinogenesis but delays tumor progression in a murine model. Anticancer Res 2001;21(2A):1065-1069.

67. Shimizu-Suganuma M, Mwanatambwe M, Iida K, et al. Effect of shark cartilage on tumor growth and survival time in vivo (meeting abstract). Proc Annu Meet Am Soc Clin Oncol 1999;18:A1760.

68. Horsman MR, Alsner J, Overgaard J. The effect of shark cartilage extracts on the growth and metastatic spread of the SCCVII carcinoma. Acta Oncol 1998;37(5):441-445.

69. Morris GM, Coderre JA, Micca PL, et al. Boron neutron capture therapy of the rat 9L gliosarcoma: evaluation of the effects of shark cartilage. Br J Radiol 2000;73(868):429-434.

70. Renckens CN, van Dam FS. [The national cancer fund (Koningin Wilhelmina Fonds) and the Houtsmuller-therapy for cancer]. Ned Tijdschr Geneeskd 1999;143(27):1431-1433.

71. Anon. FDA grants orphan-drug status to Aeterna's Neovastat for kidney cancer. Expert Rev Anticancer Ther 2002;2(6):618.

72. Jagannath S, Champagne P, Hariton C, et al. Neovastat in multiple myeloma. Eur J Haematol 2003;70(4):267-268.

73. Goldman E. Shark cartilage extract tried as a novel psoriasis treatment. Skin All News 1998;29(12):14.

74. Fontenele JB, Viana GS, Xavier-Filho J, et al. Anti-inflammatory and analgesic activity of a water-soluble fraction from shark cartilage. Braz J Med Biol Res 1996;29(5):643-646.

75. Fontenele JB, Araujo GB, de Alencar JW, et al. The analgesic and anti-inflammatory effects of shark cartilage are due to a peptide molecule and are nitric oxide (NO) system dependent. Biol Pharm Bull 1997;20(11): 1151-1154.

Slippery Elm
(Ulmus rubra Muhl, *Ulmus fulva* Michx)*

SYNONYMS/COMMON NAMES/RELATED SUBSTANCES

- Indian elm, moose elm, red elm, rock elm, slippery elm, American elm, sweet elm, Ulmaceae (family), *Ulmi rubrae cortex, Ulmus fulva* Michaux, winged elm, gray elm.
- **Combination products:** Essiac, Essiac-like products such as Flor-Essence, Robert's Formula.
- *Note:* Do not confuse the inner bark of slippery elm with the whole bark. Californian slippery elm (*Fremontia californica*) has bark with similar properties and, although not botanically related, is used in a similar way.

CLINICAL BOTTOM LINE
Background

- Slippery elm inner bark has been used historically as a demulcent, emollient, nutritive, astringent, antitussive and vulnerary. It is included as one of four primary ingredients in the herbal cancer remedy Essiac and in a number of Essiac-like products such as Flor-Essence.[1-4] Although anecdotal reports suggest that this combination formulation has anti-cancer activity, there are no reliable clinical trials to prove or discount this use.
- There are no scientific studies evaluating the common uses of this herb, but because of its high mucilage content, slippery elm bark may be a safe herbal remedy to treat irritations of the skin and mucous membranes.
- Although allergic reactions after contact have been reported, there is no known toxicity with typical dosing when products made only from the inner bark are used.
- In manufacturing, slippery elm is used in some baby foods and adult nutritional products and in some oral lozenges for soothing throat pain. Avoid confusing whole bark with inner bark. Commercial lozenges containing slippery elm are preferred to the native herb when used for cough and sore throat because they provide sustained release of mucilage to the throat.

Scientific Evidence for Common/Studied Uses	Grade*
Cancer	C
Diarrhea	C
Gastrointestinal disorders	C
Sore throat	C

*Key to grades: *A:* Strong scientific evidence for this use; *B:* Good scientific evidence for this use; *C:* Unclear scientific evidence for this use; *D:* Fair scientific evidence against this use (it may not work); *F:* Strong scientific evidence against this use (it likely does not work). For a more detailed explanation of efficacy criteria, see "Natural Standard Evidence-Based Validated Grading Rationale" in the Introduction.

Historical, Common, or Theoretical Indications That Lack Sufficient Evidence

- Abortifacient, abrasions, abscesses, acidity, adrenal insufficiency, anal fissures, boils, bronchitis, burns, carbuncles, cleansing impurities from the body, cold sores, colic, colitis, congestion, constipation, convalescence, cough, Crohn's disease, cystitis, diuretic, diverticulitis, duodenal ulcer, dysentery, enteritis, fever, gastric ulcer, gastritis, gastroesophageal reflux disease, gout, gynecologic disorders, heartburn, hemorrhoids, herpes, increased stomach acid, inflammation, irritable bowel syndrome (IBS), irritated mucous membranes, lung diseases, milk intolerance, nutrition, peptic ulcer disease, pleurisy, poison ivy, respiratory disorders, rheumatic disorders, tapeworm, toothache, tuberculosis, typhoid fever, scalded skin, skin ulcer, splinters, stomach inflammation, suppuration, swollen glands, synovitis, syphilis, ulcerative colitis, urinary tract infections, vaginitis, varicose ulcers, wound healing.

Strength of Expert Opinion and Historic/Folkloric Precedent

- Native American healers have used the dried inner bark of the slippery elm tree for centuries. The bark, collected in the spring, yields thick, viscous mucilage that is primarily used to treat urinary tract inflammation, inflammation of the digestive tract, cold sores, boils, and irritated skin and mucous membranes. Poultices made from slippery elm bark were applied to bruises and black eyes and often recommended to help heal minor burns and abrasions. Ground inner bark was added to milk as a nutrient for infants and the chronically ill.[5]
- From 1820 to 1960, elm bark was listed in the U.S. Pharmacopoeia as a demulcent, emollient, and antitussive. In modern times, the powdered inner bark is included in herbal teas and throat lozenges to soothe throat irritation. It is also a common ingredient in many herbal emollients and antitussives.
- Some herbalists and naturopathic doctors recommend slippery elm bark topically to treat diaper rash and other skin lesions, and internally to treat gastritis and ulcers. It is also one of the primary ingredients in the herbal cancer remedy Essiac and a number of other Essiac-like products.

Safety Summary

- **Possibly unsafe:** Due to the potential for poor-quality products to contain elements of the whole bark, slippery elm products should be avoided during pregnancy. For general use in foods, it has been recommended by the FACC (Food Additives and Contaminants Committee) that the use of slippery elm should be prohibited as a flavoring agent. It has been listed as a natural source for food flavoring (category N3), which indicates that there is insufficient information available on the toxicity of this herb.
- **Likely unsafe:** Preparations made from the whole bark may be abortifacient and should not be taken during pregnancy.

DOSING/TOXICOLOGY
General

- Recommended doses are based on historical practice, and there are no established and universally accepted dosing regimens for slippery elm. Recommended doses vary between texts and different healing traditions. The doses listed below are based on traditional use. With natural products, the optimal doses needed to balance efficacy and safety often have not been determined. Formulations and preparation methods may vary from manufacturer to manufacturer, and from batch to batch of a specific product made by a single manufacturer. Because often the active components of a product are not known, standardization may not be possible, and the clinical effects of different brands may not be comparable.

Standardization

- There is no widely accepted standardization for slippery elm preparations. Amounts of slippery elm used in Essiac and Essiac-like products are proprietary and therefore not disclosed by the manufacturers.
- Mucilage, U.S.P. is made by digesting 6 g of bruised slippery elm in 100 cc of water and heating in a closed vessel in a water-bath for 1 hour, followed by straining.

Dosing: Adults (18 Years and Older)
Oral

- *Note:* Slippery elm could theoretically slow down or decrease absorption of other oral medications, due to hydrocolloidal fibers, although no actual interactions have been reported.
- **Decoction:** Powdered inner bark of slippery elm mixed with water (4 to 5 g [about 1 teaspoon] mixed in 500 mL of boiling water) in a 1:8 ratio. A dose range that has been used is 4 to 15 mL (1 teaspoon to 1 tablespoon) orally three times daily.
- **Liquid extract:** 5 mL (1:1 in 60% alcohol) three times daily has been used.
- **Powdered inner bark:** As a decoction (1:8), 4 to 16 mL (or 4 g in 500 mL of boiling water) three times daily has been used. For gastrointestinal upset, 7 g of slippery elm powder in 20 fluid ounces of boiling water has been used as a hot or cold infusion. For cough, 1 part powdered bark of slippery elm added to 8 parts water, or 1 teaspoon of slippery elm powder in 500 mL of water taken one to three times daily has been used.
- **Tea:** Half a teaspoon of powdered bark in 1 cup of hot water taken twice or three times daily, or 0.5 to 1 gr of the bark in 200 mL of water taken as 3 to 4 cups daily has been used. For gastrointestinal upset, 1 teaspoon of slippery elm powder in 1 cup of boiling water taken multiple times during the day has been used.
- **Capsules/tablets:** 400- to 500-mg tablets or capsules taken three or four times daily has been used, although strengths may vary due to lack of standardization. Lower doses of 200-mg capsules taken twice or three times daily have been used for bronchitis.

Topical

- Slippery elm has been used topically for wound care and inflammation. Typically, the coarse powdered inner bark is mixed with boiling water to make a paste. Various concentrations and application schedules have been used.

Dosing: Pediatric (Younger Than 18 Years)

- Traditionally it has been accepted that slippery elm can be used safely in children complaining of stomach upset and diarrhea. However, there are no safety studies conducted in this area, and therefore use in children should only be under the strict supervision of a licensed healthcare professional.

Toxicology

- It is unlikely that products made only from the inner bark of slippery elm pose any appreciable risk if taken in recommended doses. However, tannins and calcium oxalate present in low quantities may pose a risk with large doses.
- Due to the potential for poor-quality products to contain elements of the whole bark, slippery elm products should be avoided during pregnancy. For general use in foods, it has been recommended by the FACC (Food Additives and Contaminants Committee) that the use of slippery elm should be prohibited as a flavoring agent. It has been listed as a natural source for food flavoring (category N3), which indicates that there is insufficient information available on the toxicity of this herb.

ADVERSE EFFECTS/PRECAUTIONS/CONTRAINDICATIONS
Allergy

- Urticaria has been reported following contact exposure to slippery elm, confirmed via patch testing in a 39-year-old man.[6] Aeroallergic or contact sensitivity to elm tree pollen may not be uncommon, although the clinical relevance in terms of medicinal use of slippery elm inner bark is not known.

Adverse Effects/Postmarket Surveillance

- **Dermatologic:** Contact dermatitis and urticaria have been reported after exposure to slippery elm or an oleoresin contained in the slippery elm bark.
- **Genitourinary:** Based on historical accounts, whole bark of slippery elm (but not inner bark) may possess abortifacient properties.

PRECAUTIONS/WARNINGS/CONTRAINDICATIONS

- Use cautiously during pregnancy.

Pregnancy and Lactation

- Avoid during pregnancy because of the risk of contamination with slippery elm whole bark, which may have abortifacient properties.

INTERACTIONS
Slippery Elm/Drug Interactions

- **Orally taken medications:** Slippery elm could theoretically slow down or decrease absorption of other oral medications, due to hydrocolloidal fibers, although no actual interactions have been reported. Slippery elm contains tannins that could theoretically decrease absorption of nitrogen-containing substances such as alkaloids, although no actual interactions have been reported.

Slippery Elm/Herb/Supplement Interactions

- **Orally taken agents:** Slippery elm could theoretically slow down or decrease absorption of other oral medications, due to hydrocolloidal fibers, although no actual interactions have been reported.

MECHANISM OF ACTION
Pharmacology

- Constituents present in slippery elm bark include carbohydrates made up primarily of complex mucilage containing a number of sugars such as hexoses, pentoses, methylpentoses, polyuronidesgalactose, glucose, and fructose; tannins (3% to 6.5%); phytosterols; sesquiterpenes; flavonoids; and salicylic acid (0.002%).[7] Oleic and palmitic acid are the principal fatty acids.[8] The bark also contains traces of beta-carotene, tannins, calcium oxalate, cholesterol, and proanthocyanidins, as well as phytosterols (beta-sitosterol, citrostandienol, and dolichol). The amount of salicylic acid present is generally thought to be too low to be considered clinically relevant.

- The inner bark of slippery elm is rich in mucilage, consisting of insoluble polysaccharides (hexose, pentose, methylpentose) which form a viscous material following oral administration or when used topically.[8] Following hydrolysis, these polysaccharides break down to produce galactose, with traces of glucose and fructose. The fiber content is thought to reduce gastrointestinal transit time and to act as a bulk-forming laxative.

- Fatty acids and fatty acid esters similar to those present in slippery elm have been reported *in vitro* and in animal studies to possess cytostatic and pro-apoptotic activity in tumor models, as well as immunomodulation.[9,10]

- In commercially available lozenges, the presence of slippery elm may result in sustained release of mucilage to the throat, forming a soothing layer over mucous membranes.[11]

Pharmacodynamics/Kinetics

- Insufficient available data.

HISTORY

- The slippery elm is native to eastern Canada and to eastern and central United States, where it is found mostly in the Appalachian Mountains. Its name refers to the slippery consistency the inner bark assumes when it is chewed or mixed with water. This property is responsible for the name used by the Iroquois Indians, *do-hoosh-ah*, which literally means "it slips." The tree can grow from 60 to 66 feet in height and is found primarily in moist woodlands. It typically has spreading branches and an open crown with young branches that are orange and reddish brown in color. The bark is deeply fissured and the dark green leaves are 4 to 8 inches long with serrated edges. Supplies of slippery elm have dwindled, due to devastation by Dutch elm disease. Slippery elm is easily mistaken for other elms.

- Native American healers have used the dried inner bark of slippery elm tree for centuries. Bark, collected in the spring, yields thick, viscous mucilage when mixed with water and is used to treat conditions such as urinary tract inflammation, inflammation of the digestive tract, cold sores, boils, and irritated skin and mucous membranes. Poultices made from slippery elm bark were applied to bruises and black eyes and recommended to help heal minor burns and abrasions. Ground bark was added to milk and taken as a nutrient for infants and chronically ill patients.[5]

- Surgeons during the American revolution used bark poultices as their primary treatment for gunshot wounds. As with Native American healers, physicians in the 19th century also recommended slippery elm broth for infants and chronically ill individuals and as a tea for gastric ulcer and colitis.

- From 1820 to 1960, elm bark was listed in the U.S. Pharmacopoeia as a demulcent, emollient, and antitussive. In modern times, the powdered bark is included in herbal teas and throat lozenges used to soothe throat irritation. It is also an ingredient in herbal emollients and antitussives.

REVIEW OF THE EVIDENCE: TABLE

- No studies qualify for inclusion in the evidence table.

REVIEW OF THE EVIDENCE: DISCUSSION

Cancer

Summary

- Slippery elm is found as a common ingredient in a purported herbal anticancer product called Essiac and a number of

Essiac-like products. These products contain other herbs such as rhubarb, sorrel and burdock root. There is limited available human evidence regarding the efficacy or safety of Essiac and Essiac-like products.[3]

Evidence

- There are no properly conducted published human studies of Essiac for cancer. A laboratory at Memorial Sloan-Kettering Cancer Center tested Essiac on mice during the 1970s, although results were never formally published and remain controversial. Questions were raised about improper preparation of the formula. A human study was started in Canada in the late 1970s but was stopped early because of concerns about inconsistent preparation of the formula and inadequate study design. In the 1980s, the Canadian Department of National Health and Welfare collected information about 86 cancer patients treated with Essiac. Results were inconclusive (17 patients had died at the time of the study, inadequate information was available for 8 patients, "no benefits" were found in 47 patients, 5 reported reduced need for pain medications, and 1 noted subjective improvement). Most individuals also received other cancer treatments such as chemotherapy, making the effects of Essiac impossible to isolate.

- Currently, there is not enough evidence to recommend for or against the use of this herbal mixture as a therapy for any type of cancer. Different brands may contain variable ingredients, and the comparative effectiveness of these formulas is not known. None of the individual herbs used in Essiac has been tested in rigorous human cancer trials (rhubarb has shown some antitumor properties in animal experiments; slippery elm inner bark has not; sheep sorrel and burdock have been used traditionally in cancer remedies). Numerous individual patient testimonials and reports from manufacturers are available on the Internet, although these cannot be considered scientifically viable as evidence. Individuals with cancer are advised not to delay treatment with more proven therapies.

Sore Throat

Summary

- Slippery elm is commonly used to treat sore throats, most typically taken as a lozenge. While anecdotally reported to be effective, supporting evidence is largely based on traditional evidence and the fact that the mucilages contained in the herb appear to possess soothing properties. Scientific evidence is necessary in this area before a clear conclusion can be drawn.

Gastrointestinal Disorders

Summary

- Slippery elm is traditionally used to treat inflammatory conditions of the digestive tract such as gastritis, peptic ulcer disease, and enteritis. It may be taken alone or in combination with other herbs. While anecdotally reported to be effective, supporting evidence is largely based upon traditional evidence and the fact that the mucilages contained in the herb appear to possess soothing properties. Scientific evidence is necessary in this area before a clear conclusion can be drawn.

Diarrhea

Summary

- Traditionally, slippery elm has been used to treat diarrhea. Although theoretically the tannins found in the herb may decrease the water content of stool, and mucilage may act as a soothing agent applied to inflamed mucous membranes, there is no reliable scientific evidence to support this indication. Systematic research is necessary in this area before a clear conclusion can be drawn.

References

1. Ernst E, Cassileth BR. How useful are unconventional cancer treatments? Eur J Cancer 1999;35(11):1608-1613.
2. Kaegi E. Unconventional therapies for cancer: 1. Essiac. The Task Force on Alternative Therapies of the Canadian Breast Cancer Research Initiative. CMAJ 1998;158(7):897-902.
3. Karn H, Moore MJ. The use of the herbal remedy ESSIAC in an outpatient cancer population. Proc Annu Meet Am Soc Clin Oncol 1997;16:A245.
4. Locock RA. Essiac. Can Pharm J 1997;130:18-20.
5. DeHaan RL. Home remedies for pets. J Am Holistic Vet Med Assoc 1994; 12:26.
6. Czarnecki D, Nixon R, Bekhor P, et al. Delayed prolonged contact urticaria from the elm tree. Contact Dermatitis 1993;28:196-197.
7. Luo W, Ang CY, Schmitt TC, et al. Determination of salicin and related compounds in botanical dietary supplements by liquid chromatography with fluorescence detection. J AOAC Int 1998;81(4):757-762.
8. Tamayo C, Richardson MA, Diamond S, et al. The chemistry and biological activity of herbs used in Flor-Essence herbal tonic and Essiac. Phytother Res 2000;14(1):1-14.
9. Kaegi E. Unconventional therapies for cancer: 1. Essiac. The Task Force on Alternative Therapies of the Canadian Breast Cancer Research Initiative. CMAJ 1998;158(7):897-902.
10. Kato A, Ando K, Tamura G, et al. Effects of some fatty acid esters on the viability and transplantability of Ehrlich ascites tumor cells. Cancer Res 1971;31(5):501-504.
11. Gallagher R. Use of herbal preparations for intractable cough. J Pain Symptom Manage 1997;14(1):1-2.

Sorrel

(*Rumex acetosa* L., *Rumex acetosella* L.); Sinupret

SYNONYMS/COMMON NAMES/RELATED SUBSTANCES

- Acedera, acid sorrel, azeda-brava, buckler leaf, cigreto, common sorrel, cuckoo sorrow, cuckoo's meate, dock, dog-eared sorrel, field sorrel, French sorrel, garden sorrel, gowke-meat, greensauce, green sorrel, *Herba acetosa*, kemekulagi, Polygonaceae, red sorrel, red top sorrel, round leaf sorrel, *Rumex scutatus*, sheephead sorrel, sheep sorrel, sheep's sorrel, sorrel dock, sour dock, sour grass, sour sabs, sour suds, sour sauce, wiesensauerampfer, wild sorrel.
- **Combination products that include this agent:** Essiac and Essiac-like products contain a combination of herbs, often including sorrel as well as burdock root, slippery elm inner bark, and Turkish rhubarb. Sinupret and its U.S. equivalent Quanterra Sinus Defense (currently off the market) contain sorrel as well as elder flowers, gentian root, verbena, and cowslip flower.
- *Note:* Not to be confused with shamrock (*Oxalis hedysaroides*, also called redwood sorrel, sorrel, violet wood sorrel) or roselle (*Hibiscus sabdariffa*, also called Guinea sorrel, Jamaican sorrel).

CLINICAL BOTTOM LINE

Background

- Historically, sorrel has been used as a salad green, spring tonic, diarrhea remedy, and weak diuretic and to soothe irritated nasal passages. In Turkey it is utilized as a treatment for anemia and as an appetite stimulant. Sorrel is one of the main ingredients in the combination herbal cancer remedy Essiac and in the European combination herbal sinus remedy Sinupret. Despite preliminary studies and widespread use of these multi-herb formulas, scientific evidence remains indeterminate for both.
- Sorrel contains oxalate (oxalic acid), which is potentially toxic in large doses. Reports of organ damage and one report of death following ingestion of a concentrated sorrel soup have been published. Sorrel may also cause kidney stones, precipitation of drugs taken concomitantly, and malabsorption of minerals such as calcium and iron.

Scientific Evidence for Common/Studied Indications	Grade*
Antibacterial	C
Antiviral	C
Bronchitis	C
Cancer	C
Sinusitis	C

*Key to grades: *A:* Strong scientific evidence for this use; *B:* Good scientific evidence for this use; *C:* Unclear scientific evidence for this use; *D:* Fair scientific evidence against this use (it may not work); *F:* Strong scientific evidence against this use (it likely does not work). For a more detailed explanation of efficacy criteria, see "Natural Standard Evidence-Based Validated Grading Rationale" in the Introduction.

Historical or Theoretical Indications That Lack Sufficient Evidence

- Acne, anemia, appetite stimulation, astringent, boils, constipation, diarrhea, diuresis, fever, hemorrhage, infection, itching, jaundice, kidney stones, nasal inflammation, nettle rash, oral ulcers, respiratory inflammation, ringworm, scurvy, sinusitis, skin cancer, sore throat, stimulation of secretion, ulcerated bowel, wound care.

Expert Opinion and Folkloric Precedent

- In ancient Greece and Rome, sorrel was used to aid digestion and offset the effects of rich foods, because of its acidity. In use since the Middle Ages in Europe, it has traditionally been employed as a salad green and later became popular for prevention of scurvy, because of its vitamin C content.[1]
- In combination with other herbs, sorrel has been prescribed as an expectorant in bronchitis and sinusitis treatments in Germany since the 1930s as the product Sinupret, and this combination product's claims have recently been evaluated in clinical studies.[2,3]
- Although sorrel initially was thought to possess antibacterial and antiviral properties, *in vitro* studies have not been able to identify antimicrobial activity against major human pathogens.[4]

Safety Summary

- **Possibly safe:** When used as a food in limited amounts. May also be safe when taken orally as a part of combination herbal therapies, such as with gentian root, European elder flower, verbena, and cowslip flower.[2,3]
- **Likely unsafe:** When taken in large amounts; a case report described the death of a 53-year-old man after ingestion of 500 g of sorrel in soup equivalent to approximately 6 to 8 g of oxalic acid.[5] The mean lethal dose of oxalic acid for adults is estimated to be 15 to 30 g, although doses as low as 5 g have been shown to be fatal.[5,6]
- **Possibly unsafe:** Sorrel is possibly unsafe in children because of its oxalic acid content; ingestion of rhubarb leaves, another source of oxalic acid, is reported to have caused death in a 4-year-old child.[6]

DOSING/TOXICOLOGY

General

- Recommended doses are based on those most commonly used in available trials or on historical practice. However, with natural products, the optimal doses needed to balance efficacy and safety often have not been determined. Formulations and preparation methods may vary from manufacturer to manufacturer, and from batch to batch of a specific product made by a single manufacturer. Because often the active components of a product are not known, standardization may not be possible, and the clinical effects of different brands may not be comparable.

Standardization

- There is no established standardization for sorrel as a monotherapy.

S

- **Doses used in herbal combinations:** According to the manufacturer, each Sinupret tablet contains the equivalent of 18 mg of sorrel. Quanterra Sinus Defense for sinusitis prophylaxis contains 29 mg of sorrel per tablet; however, manufacture of this product was suspended in 2000, and it is now off the market. There are more than 40 different Essiac-like products available. The original formulation of Essiac consisted of burdock root, sheep sorrel, slippery elm, and Turkish rhubarb root, but it has now been modified to include other herbs as well.[1] The amount of sorrel in Essiac and Essiac-like formulas is proprietary information and likely varies from brand to brand.

Dosing: Adult (18 Years and Older)

- *Note regarding concomitant medications:* In theory, precipitation of some drugs may occur when taken concomitantly with sorrel. Therefore, separate administration is recommended.

Oral

- **Use in foods:** Sorrel is used in foods—for example, to make soup or sauces. In small doses, sorrel is likely safe. However, based on reports of significant oxalate toxicity when taken in larger doses, caution is advised, particularly in children.
- **Monotherapy doses:** Sorrel is most often used medicinally as a part of combination formulas. No specific single-agent dosing is established.
- **Tablets for sinusitis:** 1 to 2 Sinupret tablets taken three times daily for 2 weeks has been used.[3,7] Sinupret is a combination product containing sorrel, gentian root, European elder flower, verbena, and cowslip flower.
- **Tincture for sinusitis:** 50 drops of alcohol-based (19%) Sinupret tincture taken three times daily has been used.[7]
- **Tea for cancer:** 30 mL of Essiac tea taken one to three times daily on an empty stomach has been used (anecdotal). Historically, Essiac was administered by mouth or injection. The most common current use is as a tea. There are no reliable published human studies of Essiac or Essiac-like products, and safety and effectiveness have not been established scientifically for any dose. Instructions for tea preparation and dosing vary from product to product.

Dosing: Pediatric (Younger Than 18 Years)

- Insufficient evidence to recommend. In large amounts, sorrel can be unsafe in children because of its oxalic acid content (ingestion of rhubarb leaves, another source of oxalic acid, is reported to have caused death in a 4-year-old child).[6]

Toxicology

- Sorrel leaves contain 7% to 15% tannins. Plants that contain more than 10% tannins possess potential adverse effects including upset stomach, renal damage, hepatic necrosis, and increased risk of esophageal and nasal cancer.
- Sorrel leaves contain 0.3% oxalate (oxalic acid). Oxalic acid combines with calcium in plasma, forming insoluble calcium oxalate crystals that may precipitate in the kidneys, blood vessels, heart, lungs, and liver, leading to hypocalcemia and renal lesions. Oxalate crystals can damage mucosal tissue, resulting in severe irritation and possible damage.[6] The mean lethal dose of oxalic acid for adults is estimated to be 15 to 30 g, although doses as low as 5 g have been shown to be fatal.[5,6] There is a case report of fatal oxalic acid poisoning in a 53-year-old man who consumed soup containing 500 g of sorrel, equivalent to approximately 6 to 8 g of oxalic acid.

Onset of symptoms of oxalate poisoning may occur 2 to 12 hours after ingestion.[6]

ADVERSE EFFECTS/PRECAUTIONS/CONTRAINDICATIONS
Allergy

- Known allergy/hypersensitivity to *Rumex acetosella* L. or members of the Polygonaceae family. There are anecdotal reports of allergic reactions to oral products containing this herb, and hay fever symptoms may occur with sheep sorrel.[1] Exposure to sorrel pollen is a potential trigger for allergic rhinitis or bronchial asthma in hypersensitive individuals, and allergic cross-sensitivity may occur in up to 19% of people allergic to weed pollen.[8]

Adverse Effects/Postmarket Surveillance

- **General:** There is limited scientific evidence regarding the use of sorrel alone. It is likely safe when used in very small amounts in foods. However, toxicity may occur when taken in larger amounts, including damage to the kidneys, liver, and gastrointestinal tract. These outcomes are likely related to the oxalate (oxalic acid) content in sorrel. Sorrel leaves contain 0.3% oxalate.[6] There is a case report of death of a 53-year-old man after ingestion of 500 g of sorrel in soup (equivalent to approximately 6 to 8 g of oxalic acid).[5] The mean lethal dose of oxalic acid for adults is estimated to be 15 to 30 g, although doses as low as 5 g have been shown to be fatal.[5,6] Sorrel is possibly unsafe in children because of its oxalic acid content (ingestion of rhubarb leaves, another source of oxalic acid, is reported to have caused death in a 4-year-old child).[6] The combination formula Sinupret (which contains sorrel in combination with gentian root, European elder flower, verbena, and cowslip flower) anecdotally is said to be well tolerated, although infrequent gastrointestinal upset has been reported.
- **Dermatologic:** There are anecdotal reports of dermatitis following consumption of large amounts of sorrel (doses beyond the amount commonly found in foods).
- **Pulmonary/respiratory:** Environmental exposure to sorrel pollen is a potential trigger for allergic rhinitis or bronchial asthma in hypersensitive individuals, and allergic cross-sensitivity may occur in up to 19% of people allergic to weed pollen.[8] This adverse effect applies more to growers than to those using the herb medicinally.
- **Gastrointestinal:** The oxalate content in sorrel may exert corrosive effects on the digestive tract, and large amounts of sorrel may cause irritation of the esophagus/stomach, nausea, diarrhea, and colic.[6]
- **Renal:** Urolithiasis and nephrosis may result from the systemic absorption of oxalates in sorrel, and can result in kidney damage.[6] Hypocalcemia may result from ingestion of oxalate in sorrel. There are anecdotal reports of polyuria occurring with sorrel ingestion.
- **Hepatic:** Extensive liver necrosis with hepatic failure has been reported with the ingestion of large amounts of sorrel, likely due to its oxalate content.[5]

Precautions/Warnings/Contraindications

- Avoid large doses of sorrel, due to the risk of oxalate toxicity.
- Avoid in children, due to the risk of oxalate toxicity.
- Use cautiously in patients with peptic ulcer disease, due to the risk of gastrointestinal irritation.
- Use cautiously in patients with a history of oxalate kidney stones, due to the oxalate content of sorrel.

Pregnancy and Lactation

- Not recommended, due to lack of sufficient data and the potential for oxalate toxicity.
- A surveillance study of Sinupret in pregnant women reported no excess teratogenicity compared to controls not using Sinupret.[9]

INTERACTIONS
Sorrel/Drug Interactions

- **General:** In theory, precipitation of some drugs may occur when taken concomitantly with sorrel. Therefore, separate administration is recommended.
- **Alkaloid agents:** In theory, herbs with high tannin content such as sorrel should not be used in combination with alkaloid agents such as atropine, belladonna, galantamine, scopolamine, or vinblastine, due to the possibility of precipitate formation.
- **Antibiotics (positive interaction):** Concurrent use of doxycycline with Quanterra Sinus Defense or Sinupret is reported in a human trial to synergistically improve outcomes in patients with acute bacterial sinusitis.[3] Additional supporting evidence in this area is limited.
- **Diuretics:** Polyuria has been reported anecdotally with the use of sorrel, which may add to the effects of diuretics.
- **Hepatotoxic drugs:** In large amounts, ingestion of sorrel may lead to liver damage; its use should be avoided with agents that are hepatotoxic.
- **Renal toxic drugs:** In large amounts, ingestion of sorrel may lead to kidney stones or kidney damage; its use should be avoided with agents that are renotoxic.

Sorrel/Herb/Supplement Interactions

- **General:** In theory, precipitation of some herbs or supplements may occur when they are taken concomitantly with sorrel. Therefore, separate administration is recommended.
- **Alkaloid agents:** In theory, herbs with high tannin content such as sorrel should not be used in combination with alkaloid agents such as atropine, belladonna, galantamine, or scopolamine, due to the possibility of precipitate formation.
- **Diuretic herbs:** Polyuria has been reported anecdotally with the use of sorrel, which may add to the effects of diuretics.
- **Mineral absorption:** Sorrel may impair calcium, iron, and zinc absorption, due to its high oxalate content. Therefore, separate administration is recommended.
- **Hepatotoxic herbs:** In large amounts, ingestion of sorrel may lead to liver damage, and its use should be avoided with agents that are hepatotoxic.

- **Rhubarb:** Rhubarb is a source of oxalate and may add to the toxic effects of oxalate in sorrel.
- **Shamrock:** Shamrock is a source of oxalate and may add to the toxic effects of oxalate in sorrel.

Sorrel/Food Interactions

- **Minerals (calcium, iron, zinc):** Sorrel may impair absorption of calcium, iron, and zinc, due to its oxalate content. Therefore, separate administration is recommended.

MECHANISM OF ACTION
Pharmacology

- **Constituents:** Ascorbic acid, oxalates (including calcium oxalate), tannins, anthracene derivatives (anthranoids, aglycones, physcion, aloe-emodin, aloe-emodin acetate, emodin, rhein), quinoids, flavonoids, and phenylpropanoid.[10]
- All active chemical compounds have not been isolated. Sorrel leaves may contain 0.3% oxalate and 7% to 15% tannins. Oxalate crystals can damage mucosal tissues (resulting in severe irritation) and can combine with calcium to form insoluble calcium oxalate crystals, which precipitate in the kidneys, blood vessels, heart, lungs, and liver, potentially resulting in hypocalcemia and kidney damage.[5,6] Tannins, which are phenolic compounds, exert an astringent effect on mucosal tissues, causing dehydration of tissues, and reducing secretions.

Pharmacodynamics/Kinetics

- There is limited reliable information in this area. Approximately 2% to 5% of ingested oxalates are absorbed in healthy human volunteers.[6] Oral oxalates administered to animals are excreted unchanged in the urine within 24 to 36 hours after ingestion.[6]

HISTORY

- Sorrel is commonly grown in Europe and was introduced to North America, where it is now widely naturalized. The herb's name derives from the old French word *surele*, meaning "sour." Its sharp taste is due to its oxalic acid and vitamin C content.[1]
- The plant can grow over 3 feet tall. The leaves are fleshy, green, and long, with a fringed cone at the base. The leaves alternate on the reddish, grooved stems. Sorrel has greenish flowers with six stamens and three styles, as well as a paintbrush-like stigma. The fruit is a triangular brown-black nut.
- The leaves, flowers, roots, and seeds are used medicinally and for culinary purposes. Apothecaries used sorrel as a common ingredient until the 19th century.

Review of the Evidence: Sorrel

Condition Treated*	Study Design	Author, Year	N†	SS†	Study Quality‡	Magnitude of Benefit	ARR†	NNT†	Comments
Sinusitis (acute)	RCT	Neubauer 1994	160	Yes	3	Small	NA	NA	Study of a combination product sorrel.
Sinusitis	Review	Marz 1999	NA	NA	NA	NA	NA	NA	Review of data for a combination product sorrel.

*Primary or secondary outcome.
†N, Number of patients; SS, statistically significant; ARR, absolute risk reduction; NNT, the number of patients who need to undergo a specific intervention in order to observe an outcome in one individual.
‡0-2 = poor; 3-4 = good; 5 = excellent.
NA, Not applicable; RCT, randomized, controlled trial.
For an explanation of each category in this table, please see Table 3 in the Introduction.

REVIEW OF THE EVIDENCE: DISCUSSION
Cancer
Summary

- There is no reliable human evidence evaluating sorrel mono-therapy as a cancer treatment.[11,12] Sorrel is included as an ingredient in the combination herbal formula Essiac and in several Essiac-like products that are used in the management of cancer. However, there is limited reliable research on these formulas.[1,13-17] It remains unclear if there are any health benefits of Essiac or Essiac-like products.

Essiac Background

- Essiac contains a combination of herbs, including sorrel as well as burdock root (*Arctium lappa*), the inner bark of slippery elm (*Ulmus fulva*), and Turkish rhubarb (*Rheum palmatum*). The original formula was developed by the Canadian nurse Rene Caisse (1888-1978) in the 1920s ("Essiac" is Caisse spelled backward). The recipe is said to be based on a traditional Ojibwa (Native American) remedy, and Caisse administered the formula by mouth and injection to numerous cancer patients during the 1920s and 1930s. The exact ingredients and amounts in the original formulation remain a secret.

- During investigations by the Canadian government and public hearings in the late 1930s, it remained unclear if Essiac was an effective cancer treatment. Amidst controversy, Caisse closed her clinic in 1942. In the 1950s, Caisse provided samples of Essiac to Dr. Charles Brusch, founder of the Brusch Medical Center in Cambridge, Massachusetts, who administered Essiac to patients (it is unclear if Brusch was given access to the secret formula). According to some accounts, additional herbs were added to these later formulations, including blessed thistle (*Cnicus benedictus*), red clover (*Trifolium pratense*), kelp (*Laminaria digitata*), and watercress (*Nasturtium officinale*).

- A laboratory at Memorial Sloan-Kettering Cancer Center tested Essiac samples (provided by Caisse) on mice during the 1970s. This research was never formally published, and there is controversy regarding the results, with some accounts noting no benefits and others reporting significant effects (including an account by Dr. Brusch). Questions were later raised about improper preparation of the formula. Caisse subsequently refused requests by researchers at Memorial Sloan-Kettering and the U.S. National Cancer Institute for access to the formula.

- In the 1970s, Caisse provided the formula to Resperin Corporation Ltd., with the understanding that Resperin would coordinate a scientific trial in humans. Although a study was initiated, it was stopped early because of questions about improper preparation of the formula and inadequate study design. This research was never completed. Resperin Corporation Ltd., which owned the Essiac name, formally went out of business after transferring rights to the Essiac name and selling the secret formula to Essiac Products Ltd., which currently distributes products through Essiac International.

- Despite the lack of available scientific evidence, Essiac and Essiac-like products (with similar ingredients) remain popular among patients, particularly those with cancer. Essiac is most commonly taken as a tea. A survey conducted in 2000 found almost 15% of Canadian women with breast cancer to be using Essiac. It has also become popular with patients with HIV and diabetes, and with healthy individuals for its purported immune-enhancing properties, although there is no reliable scientific research in these areas.

- There are more than 40 Essiac-like products available in North America, Europe, and Australia. Flor-Essence includes the original four herbs (burdock root, sorrel, slippery elm bark, Turkish rhubarb) as well as herbs that were later added as "potentiators" (blessed thistle, red clover, kelp, watercress). Virginias Herbal E contains the four original herbs along with echinacea and black walnut. Other commercial formulations may include additional ingredients, such as cat's claw (*Uncaria tomentosa*).

Essiac Scientific Research

- There are no properly conducted published human studies of Essiac for cancer. A laboratory at Memorial Sloan-Kettering Cancer Center tested Essiac on mice during the 1970s, although results were never formally published and remain controversial. Questions were raised about improper preparation of the formula. A human study was started in Canada in the late 1970s but was stopped early due to concerns about inconsistent preparation of the formula and inadequate study design. In the 1980s, the Canadian Department of National Health and Welfare collected information about 86 cancer patients treated with Essiac. Results were inconclusive (17 patients had died at the time of the study, inadequate information was available for 8 patients, "no benefits" were found in 47 patients, 5 reported reduced need for pain medications, and 1 noted subjective improvement). Most individuals also received other cancer treatments such as chemotherapy, making the effects of Essiac impossible to isolate.

- Currently, there is not enough evidence to recommend for or against the use of this herbal mixture as a therapy for any type of cancer. Different brands may contain variable ingredients, and the comparative effectiveness of these formulas is not known. None of the individual herbs used in Essiac has been tested in rigorous human cancer trials (rhubarb has shown some antitumor properties in animal experiments; slippery elm inner bark has not; sheep sorrel and burdock have been used traditionally in cancer remedies). Numerous individual patient testimonials and reports from manufacturers are available on the Internet, although these cannot be considered scientifically viable as evidence. Individuals with cancer are advised not to delay treatment with more proven therapies.

Bronchitis
Summary

- There is no reliable human evidence evaluating sorrel mono-therapy as a treatment for bronchitis. However, it is an ingredient in the combination herbal product Sinupret, which also contains cowslip flower, European elder flower, gentian root, and verbena. This proprietary formula has been used historically in Europe for the treatment of acute bronchitis and sinusitis. Although no studies have been conducted comparing the combination product to placebo, there is initial evidence from a comparison trial of various expectorants vs. Sinupret in the treatment of acute bronchitis.[7] Additional evidence is necessary before a firm conclusion can be drawn regarding the use of sorrel or Sinupret in the management of bronchitis.

Evidence

- Ernst et al. conducted a comparison trial to evaluate the safety and efficacy of Sinupret vs. 72 commonly prescribed expectorants, chosen freely by physicians at the point of care (for example, products containing acetylcysteine, bromhexine, or carbocysteine).[7] The trial was open (non-blinded, non-randomized) and included 3187 patients with acute, uncomplicated bronchitis, ages 1 to 94 years. The product was administered for 10 days, and the primary outcome was improvement in bronchitis-related symptoms. The authors reported that results with Sinupret were superior to the mean improvement seen in the reference drugs, both in terms of efficacy and adverse effects. However, Sinupret was not compared to individual expectorants. A subgroup analysis of 535 patients with acute-on-chronic bronchitis demonstrated lower efficacy of both Sinupret and the reference expectorants. Because Sinupret was compared to multiple agents and the study was neither randomized nor blinded, the results can only be considered preliminary.

Sinusitis
Summary

- There is no reliable human evidence evaluating sorrel monotherapy as a treatment for sinusitis. However, it is an ingredient in combination formulas used for sinusitis, including Sinupret (a combination product including cowslip flower, European elder flower, gentian root, and verbena), which is available in Europe, and Quanterra Sinus Defense (the U.S. equivalent of Sinupret, not manufactured since 2000). Although there is promising early evidence for this formula in patients with sinusitis, better-quality research is necessary before a firm conclusion can be drawn regarding the use of sorrel or Sinupret in the management of sinusitis.

Evidence

- Neubauer and Marz conducted a randomized, placebo-controlled trial comparing Sinupret as an adjunct to a regimen including doxycycline and a nasal decongestant, vs. doxycycline and the decongestant alone without Sinupret.[3] Treatment was administered to 160 patients diagnosed clinically with acute sinusitis over a 14-day period. In subjects who received Sinupret (n = 81), 1 tablet was given orally three times per day. The authors reported mean improvements in response rate in the Sinupret group compared to the non-Sinupret group. No adverse effects were noted in either treatment group. However, because of limited descriptions of methods and statistical analysis, these results cannot be considered definitive.
- Marz et al. published a review of the evidence regarding the use of Sinupret for sinusitis.[2] The authors cited pre-clinical reports of secretolytic, anti-inflammatory, immuno-modulatory, and antiviral effects. They also noted human research suggesting a favorable safety profile and efficacy when Sinupret was added to antibiotics and conventional decongestant drugs.

Antiviral and Antibacterial
Summary

- There are no well-conducted published studies that demonstrate sorrel to possess activity against viruses or bacteria that are important human pathogens. In an *in vitro* study, sorrel did not demonstrate activity against herpes simplex virus-1, herpes simplex virus-2, HIV, *Bacillus subtilis*, *Escherichia coli*, *Proteus morganii*, *Pseudomonas aeruginosa*, *Proteus vulgaris*, *Serratia marcescens*, or *Staphylococcus aureus*.[4]

FORMULARY: BRANDS USED IN CLINICAL TRIALS
Brands Used In Statistically Significant Clinical Trials

- Sinupret (consisting of a combination of cowslip flower, European elder flower, gentian root, sorrel, and verbena).

U.S. Equivalents of Most Commonly Recommended European Brands

- Quanterra Sinus Defense (U.S. equivalent of Sinupret, not manufactured since 2000).

References

1. Locock RA. Herbal medicine: essiac. Can Pharm J 1997;130(Feb):18-19, 51.
2. Marz RW, Ismail C, Popp MA. [Profile and effectiveness of a phytogenic combination preparation for treatment of sinusitis]. Wien Med Wochenschr 1999;149(8-10):202-208.
3. Neubauer N, Marz RW. Placebo-controlled, randomized double-blind clinical trial with Sinupret sugar coated tablets on the basis of a therapy with antibiotics and decongestant nasal drops in acute sinusitis. Phytomedicine 1994;1:177-181.
4. Dornberger K, Lich H. [Screening for antimicrobial and presumed cancerostatic plant metabolites (author's transl)]. Pharmazie 1982;37(3):215-221.
5. Farre M, Xirgu J, Salgado A, et al. Fatal oxalic acid poisoning from sorrel soup. Lancet 1989;2(8678-8679):1524.
6. Sanz P, Reig R. Clinical and pathological findings in fatal plant oxalosis. A review. Am J Forensic Med Pathol 1992;13(4):342-345.
7. Ernst E, Marz RW, Sieder C. [Acute bronchitis: effectiveness of Sinupret. Comparative study with common expectorants in 3,187 patients]. Fortschr Med 1997;115(11):52-53.
8. Gniazdowska B, Doroszewska G, Doroszewski W. [Hypersensitivity to weed pollen allergens in the region of Bygdoszcz]. Pneumonol Alergol Pol 1993;61(7-8):367-372.
9. Ismail C, Wiesel A, Marz RW, et al. Surveillance study of Sinupret in comparison with data of the Mainz birth registry. Arch Gynecol Obstet 2003;267(4):196-201.
10. Choe S, Hwang B, Kim M, et al. Chemical components of *Rumex acetellosa* L. Korean J Pharmacog 1998;29:209-216.
11. Bhakuni DS, Bittner M, Marticorena C, et al. Screening of Chilean plants for anticancer activity. I. Lloydia. 1976;39(4):225-243.
12. Ito H. Effects of the antitumor agents from various natural sources on drug-metabolizing system, phagocytic activity and complement system in sarcoma 180-bearing mice. Jpn J Pharmacol 1986;40(3):435-443.
13. Richardson MA. Research of complementary/alternative medicine therapies in oncology: promising but challenging. J Clin Oncol 1999;17(11 Suppl):38-43.
14. Karn H, Moore MJ. The use of the herbal remedy ESSIAC in an outpatient cancer population. Proc Annu Meet Am Soc Clin Oncol 1997;16:A245.
15. US Congressional Office of Technology Assessment. Essiac. US Government Printing Office 1990.
16. Kaegi E. Unconventional therapies for cancer: 1. Essiac. The Task Force on Alternative Therapies of the Canadian Breast Cancer Research Initiative. CMAJ 1998;158(7):897-902.
17. Yamamoto A. Essiac. Can J Hosp Pharm 1988;41(3):158.

S

Soy
(Glycine max L. Merr.)

SYNONYMS/COMMON NAMES/RELATED SUBSTANCES

- Coumestrol, daidzein, edamame, frijol de soya, genistein, greater bean, haba soya, hydrolyzed soy protein, isoflavone, isoflavonoid, legume, natto, phytoestrogen, plant estrogen, shoyu, soja, sojabohne, soybean, soy fiber, soy food, soy product, soy protein, soya, soya protein, ta-tou, texturized vegetable protein.
- **Selected brands used in human clinical trials:** Abalon (Nutri Pharma ASA, Oslo, Norway); SOYSELECT (Indena SpA, Milan, Italy); Takeda (Italia Farmaceutici, SpA, Catania, Italy); Osteofix (Chiesi, Parma, Italy); Piascledine 300 (Pharmascience Laboratories, Courbevoie, France); Isomil DF (Ross Products Division, Abbott Laboratories, Columbus, Ohio); Prosobee (Mead Johnson, Evansville, Indiana); Nursoy (Wyeth Laboratories); Nursoy Ready to Feed (Wyeth Laboratories); Isomil (Ross Laboratories, Columbus, Ohio); Hyprovit (Hayes Ltd., Ashdod, Israel); TakeCare (Protein Technology International, St. Louis, Missouri); Fibrim Brand Soy Fiber (Protein Technologies International); Purina 660 (Ralston Purina Company, St. Louis, Missouri); Supro 660 (Protein Technologies International); Supro 675 (Protein Technologies International); Supro 675 IF (Protein Technologies International); Supro Plus 675HG (Protein Technologies International); Temptein (Miles Laboratories, Elkhart, Indiana).

CLINICAL BOTTOM LINE
Background

- Soy is a subtropical plant native to southeastern Asia. This member of the pea family (Fabaceae) grows from 1 to 5 feet tall and forms clusters of three to five pods, each containing two to four beans per pod. Soy has been a dietary staple in Asian countries for at least 5000 years, and during the Chou dynasty in China (1134 to 246 BC), fermentation techniques were discovered that allowed soy to be prepared in more easily digestible forms such as tempeh, miso, and tamari soy sauce. Tofu was invented in second century China.
- Soy was introduced to Europe in the 1700s, and to the United States in the 1800s. Large-scale soybean cultivation began in the United States during World War II. Currently, Midwestern U.S. growers produce approximately half of the world's supply of soybeans.
- Soy and components of soy called "isoflavones" have been studied scientifically for numerous health conditions. Isoflavones (such as genistein) are believed to have estrogen-like effects in the body and therefore are sometimes called "phytoestrogens." In laboratory studies, it is not clear if isoflavones stimulate or block the effects of estrogen, or both (acting as mixed receptor agonists/antagonists).

Uses Based on Scientific Evidence	Grade*
Dietary source of protein Soy products such as tofu are high in protein and are an acceptable source of dietary protein.	A

High cholesterol — A

Numerous human studies report that adding soy protein to the diet can moderately decrease blood levels of total cholesterol and low-density lipoprotein ("bad" cholesterol). Small reductions in triglycerides may also occur, while high-density lipoprotein ("good" cholesterol) does not seem to be significantly altered. The greatest effects seem to occur in people with elevated cholesterol levels, with benefits lasting as long as the diet is continued. Total replacement of dietary animal proteins with soy protein yields the greatest benefits. People on low-cholesterol diets experience further reductions in cholesterol levels by adding soy to the diet.

Some scientists have proposed that specific components of soybean, such as the isoflavones genistein and daidzein, may be responsible for the cholesterol-lowering properties of soy. However, this has not been clearly demonstrated in research and remains controversial. It is not known if products containing isolated soy isoflavones have the same effects as those of regular dietary intake of soy protein.

Dietary soy protein has not been proven to affect long-term cardiovascular outcomes such as heart attack or stroke.

Diarrhea (acute) in infants and young children — B

Numerous studies report that infants and young children (ages 2 to 36 months) with diarrhea who are fed soy formula experience fewer bowel movements per day and fewer days of diarrhea. This research suggests soy to have benefits over other types of formula, including cow milk–based solutions. The addition of soy fiber to soy formula may increase the effectiveness. Although many of the trials in this area are not of high quality, and some report conflicting results (lack of benefits), overall the evidence supports this use of soy. Better-quality research is needed before a strong recommendation can be made.

Parents are advised to consult a qualified healthcare provider if infants experience prolonged diarrhea, become dehydrated, demonstrate signs of infection such as fever, or have blood in the stool. A healthcare provider should be consulted for current breastfeeding recommendations, and to suggest long-term formulas with adequate nutritional value.

Menopausal hot flashes — B

Soy products containing isoflavones have been studied for the reduction of menopausal symptoms such as hot flashes. The scientific evidence is mixed in this area, with several human trials suggesting reduced number of hot flashes and decrease in other menopausal symptoms, but with more recent research reporting no benefits. Overall, the scientific evidence does suggest benefits, although better-quality studies are needed in this area in order to form a firm conclusion.

Continued

Many researchers have attributed these effects to the presence in soy of "phytoestrogens" (plant-based compounds with weak estrogen-like properties), such as isoflavones. An area of concern has been whether phytoestrogens carry the same risks as for prescription drug hormone replacement therapy (HRT), which includes estrogens. For example, HRT has been associated with increased risk for development of hormone-sensitive cancers (breast, ovarian, uterine) and of blood clots. This is an important area of concern for patients, as some women may consider soy as an alternative to HRT in order to avoid these risks. Early studies report that soy isoflavones do not cause the same thickening of the uterus lining (endometrium) as occurs with estrogen and therefore may not carry the same risks as those associated with HRT. In addition, some scientists theorize that isoflavones may actually reduce the risk of cancer by blocking estrogen effects in the body, based on laboratory studies showing isoflavones to partially block (noncompetitively inhibit) estrogen receptors. Additional research is needed in this area before a clear risk assessment can be conducted.

Breast cancer prevention   C

Several large population studies have asked women about their eating habits and have reported higher soy intake (such as dietary tofu) to be associated with a decreased risk of developing breast cancer. However, this type of research (retrospective, case-control, epidemiologic) can only be considered preliminary, because people who choose to eat soy may also partake in other lifestyle decisions that may lower the risk of cancer. These other habits, rather than soy, could theoretically be the cause of the benefits seen in these studies (for example, lower fat intake, more frequent exercise, lack of smoking). Controlled human trials are necessary before a firm conclusion can be drawn. Theoretical concerns have been raised that soy may actually *increase* the risk of breast cancer because of the presence in soy of phytoestrogens (plant-based compounds with weak estrogen-like properties), such as isoflavones. This possibility remains an area of controversy. Recently, some scientists have theorized that isoflavones may reduce the risk of cancer by blocking estrogen effects in the body, based on laboratory studies showing isoflavones to partially block (noncompetitively inhibit) estrogen receptors. In fact, early research suggests that soy isoflavones do not have the same effects on the body as those of estrogens, such as increasing the thickening of the uterus lining (endometrium). Genistein has been found in laboratory and animal studies to have other anticancer effects, such as blocking new blood vessel growth (antiangiogenesis), acting as a tyrosine kinase inhibitor (a mechanism of many new cancer treatments), or causing cancer cell death (apoptosis). Until better research is available, it remains unclear if dietary soy or soy isoflavone supplements increase or decrease the risk of developing breast cancer.

Cancer treatment   C

Genistein, an isoflavone found in soy, has been found in laboratory and animal studies to possess anticancer effects, such as blocking new blood vessel growth (antiangiogenesis), acting as a tyrosine kinase inhibitor (a mechanism of many new cancer treatments), or causing cancer cell death (apoptosis). By contrast, genistein has also been reported to *increase* the growth of pancreas tumor cells in laboratory research. None of these effects has been adequately assessed in humans.

In the past, theoretical concerns have been raised that soy may increase the risk of hormone-sensitive cancers (for example, breast, ovarian, endometrial/uterine) because of the presence in soy of phytoestrogens (plant-based compounds with weak estrogen-like properties), such as isoflavones (genistein and others). This remains an area of controversy. Recently, some scientists have suggested that isoflavones may actually reduce the risk of hormone-sensitive cancers by blocking estrogen effects in the body, based on laboratory studies showing isoflavones to partially block (non-competitively inhibit) estrogen receptors. Preliminary human research suggests that soy isoflavones do not have the same effects on the body as those of estrogens, such as increasing the thickening of the uterus lining (endometrium).

Until reliable human research is available, it remains unclear if dietary soy or soy isoflavone supplements are beneficial, harmful, or neutral in people with various types of cancer.

Cardiovascular disease   C

Dietary soy protein has not been shown to affect long-term cardiovascular outcomes such as heart attack or stroke. Research does suggest cholesterol-lowering effects of dietary soy, which in theory may reduce cardiovascular risk. Soy has also been studied for blood pressure–lowering and blood sugar–reducing properties in people with type 2 diabetes, although the evidence is not definitive in these areas. Although the addition of soy to a regimen of exercise and diet may theoretically improve cardiovascular outcomes, this has not been scientifically proven. Some studies show an association between soy food consumption and lower risk of coronary heart disease in women, but further investigation is needed.

Cognitive function   C

A recent study suggests that isoflavone supplementation in postmenopausal women may have favorable effects on cognitive function, particularly verbal memory. Further research is necessary before a firm conclusion can be drawn.

Colon cancer prevention   C

There is not enough scientific evidence to determine if dietary intake of soy affects the risk of developing colon cancer.

Crohn's disease   C

Because of limited human study, there is not enough evidence to recommend for or against the use of soy as a therapy in preventing Crohn's disease. Further research is needed before a recommendation can be made.

Continued

Cyclic breast pain

It has been theorized that the presence in soy of phytoestrogens (plant-based compounds with weak estrogen-like properties) such as isoflavones may be beneficial to premenopausal women with cyclic breast pain. However, because of limited human study, there is not enough evidence to recommend for or against the use of dietary soy protein as a therapy for this condition.

C

Diarrhea in adults

Because of limited human study, there is not enough evidence to recommend for or against the use of soy-polysaccharide/fiber in the treatment of diarrhea. Further research is needed before a recommendation can be made.

C

Endometrial cancer prevention

Theoretical concerns have been raised that soy may actually *increase* the risk of endometrial cancer because of the presence in soy of phytoestrogens (plant-based compounds with weak estrogen-like properties), such as isoflavones. This remains an area of controversy. Recently, some scientists have theorized that isoflavones may reduce the risk of cancer by blocking estrogen effects in the body, based on laboratory studies showing isoflavones to partially block (noncompetitively inhibit) estrogen receptors. In fact, early research suggests that soy isoflavones do not have the same effects on the uterus as those of estrogens, such as increasing the thickening of the endometrium (lining of the uterus). Genistein has been found in laboratory and animal studies to have other anticancer effects, such as blocking new blood vessel growth (antiangiogenesis), acting as a tyrosine kinase inhibitor (a mechanism of many new cancer treatments), or causing cancer cell death (apoptosis).

C

Gallstones (cholelithiasis)

Because of limited human study, there is not enough evidence to recommend for or against the use of soy as a therapy in cholelithiasis. Further research is needed before a recommendation can be made.

C

High blood pressure

Because of limited human study, the effects of dietary soy on blood pressure are not clear. Further research is necessary before any recommendation can be made.

C

Kidney disease (chronic renal failure, nephrotic syndrome, proteinuria)

Because of limited human study, there is not enough evidence to recommend for or against the use of soy in the treatment of kidney diseases such as nephrotic syndrome. People with kidney disease should consult their healthcare provider about recommended amounts of dietary protein and should bear in mind that soy is a high-protein food.

C

Menstrual migraine

One study of a phytoestrogen combination in the prophylactic treatment of menstrual migraines reduced the number of migraine attacks suffered. Further

C

research is needed before a recommendation can be made.

Obesity, weight reduction

Because of limited human study, there is not enough evidence to recommend for or against the use of soy for weight reduction. Further research is needed before a recommendation can be made.

C

Osteoporosis, postmenopausal bone loss

It has been theorized that the presence in soy of phytoestrogens (plant-based compounds with weak estrogen-like properties) such as isoflavones may increase bone mineral density in postmenopausal women, reducing the risk of fractures. A small number of studies in this area report benefits, particularly in the lumbar spine (lower back). However, most studies have not been well designed or reported. Until better research is available, a firm conclusion cannot be drawn. Individuals at risk for osteoporosis should consult a qualified healthcare provider about the therapeutic options for increasing bone mineral density.

C

Prostate cancer prevention

It has been theorized that the presence in soy of phytoestrogens (plant-based compounds with weak estrogen-like properties) such as isoflavones may be beneficial in the treatment of prostate cancer. In addition, the isoflavone genistein has been found in laboratory and animal studies to have anticancer effects, such as blocking new blood vessel growth (antiangiogenesis), acting as a tyrosine kinase inhibitor (a mechanism of many new cancer treatments), or causing cancer cell death (apoptosis). These mechanisms have not been clearly demonstrated to work in humans.
Preliminary research has examined the effects of dietary soy intake on prostate cancer development in humans, but results have not been conclusive. Better study is needed before a recommendation can be made.

C

Stomach cancer

Preliminary study suggests that intake of soy products may be associated with a reduced risk of death from stomach cancer. Further investigation is needed before a conclusion can be drawn.

C

Type 2 diabetes mellitus

Several small studies have examined the effects of soy products on blood sugars in people with type 2 (adult-onset) diabetes mellitus. Results are mixed, with some research reporting decreased blood glucose levels and other trials noting no effects. Overall, research in this area is not well designed or reported, and better information is needed before the effects of soy on blood sugar levels can be clearly described.

C

*Key to grades: A: Strong scientific evidence for this use; B: Good scientific evidence for this use; C: Unclear scientific evidence for this use; D: Fair scientific evidence against this use (it may not work); F: Strong scientific evidence against this use (it likely does not work). For a more detailed explanation of efficacy criteria, see "Natural Standard Evidence-Based Validated Grading Rationale" in the Introduction.

Historical or Theoretical Indications That Lack Sufficient Evidence

Anemia, anorexia, antifungal, antioxidant, antithrombotic, atherosclerosis, athletic endurance, attention deficit hyperactivity disorder (ADHD), autoimmune diseases, breast enlargement, cancer prevention (general), cystic fibrosis, diabetic neuropathy, fever, gastric cancer, gastrointestinal motility, headache, hepatitis (chronic), inflammation, insect repellent, lymphoma, memory enhancement, nosebleed (chronic), osteosarcoma, premature ovarian failure, rheumatoid arthritis, urinary tract cancer, vaginitis, vasoregulator.

DOSING/TOXICOLOGY

The following doses are based on scientific research, publications, traditional use, or expert opinion. Many herbs and supplements have not been thoroughly tested, and their safety and effectiveness may not be proven. Brands may be made differently, with variable ingredients even within the same brand. The doses shown may not apply to all products. It is important to always read product labels and discuss doses with a qualified healthcare provider before therapy is started.

Adults (18 Years and Older)

- **High cholesterol:** 30 to 50 g of soy protein taken daily by mouth has been studied in people with high cholesterol. Isoflavone content of the daily intake of soy has ranged from 60 to 80 mg per day. Cholesterol and low-density lipoprotein levels have been reduced in individuals ingesting 28 g daily of soy protein with a high isoflavone content, or with Abacor, a brand that contains 26 g of soy protein. There is limited study of soymilk (400 ml daily) in premenopausal women, with reported benefits on cholesterol levels.
- **Menopausal symptoms (hot flashes):** Isolated soy protein, such as Supro (60 g), soy flour (45 g), and a range of isoflavone products have been studied. Doses of 50 to 75 mg of isoflavones have been used in research.
- **Diarrhea:** In infants and young children (2 to 36 months of age), Hyprovit formula, Isomil formula, Nursoy formula or powder, and Prosobee formula taken by mouth have been studied. Because of potential safety concerns, a qualified healthcare provider should be consulted regarding the choice of infant formula. In adults, soy-derived diets and intake of soy polysaccharide/fiber have been studied, although benefits are not clear.
- **Cancer and cancer prevention:** Population and laboratory studies have examined levels of dietary soy intake. No specific doses can be recommended at this time.
- **Cardiovascular health:** Studies have examined regular intake of dietary soy, or 40 to 80 mg of isoflavones taken by mouth daily.
- **Osteoporosis/postmenopausal bone loss:** Isoflavones/isoflavone-rich soy (60 to 80 mg daily by mouth) and soy protein (for example, 40 g daily of Supro 675) have been studied.
- **Gallstones (cholelithiasis):** Dietary intake of soy has undergone limited study. Because of limited research in humans, no specific doses can be recommended at this time.
- **Crohn's disease:** Because of limited research in humans, no specific doses can be recommended at this time.
- **Cyclic breast pain:** A soy protein drink (17 g of soy protein per 200 ml) has undergone limited study.
- **Diabetes:** A fermented soybean-derived extract tea, various doses of soy protein (such as Abalon), and up to 7 g of soya fibers taken daily by mouth have undergone limited study in humans.
- **High blood pressure:** Soymilk (1000 ml daily for 3 months) for this indication has undergone limited study.
- **Kidney disease/chronic renal failure:** Soy-based diets have undergone limited study in people with kidney diseases such as the nephrotic syndrome. However, soy is a source of dietary protein, and low-protein diets may be more desirable in patients with kidney failure. People with kidney failure should consult a qualified healthcare provider before making any dietary changes.
- **Obesity:** A soy-derived diet has undergone limited study.

Children (Younger Than 18 Years)

- **Diarrhea:** In infants and young children (2 to 36 months of age), Hyprovit formula, Isomil formula, Nursoy formula or powder, and Prosobee formula taken by mouth have been studied. Because of potential safety concerns, a qualified healthcare provider should be consulted regarding the choice of infant formula.

SAFETY

Many complementary techniques are practiced by healthcare professionals with formal training, in accordance with the standards of national organizations. However, this is not universally the case, and adverse effects are possible. Owing to limited research, in some cases only limited safety information is available.

Allergies

- Soy can act as a food allergen similar to milk, eggs, peanuts, fish, and wheat. The prevalence of soy allergy in children with positive skin tests has been reported as high as 6%. In limited research, soy has been well tolerated by most children with immunoglobulin E (IgE)-associated cow milk allergy (CMA), although allergic cross-reactivity has occasionally been reported. Rare allergic reactions have been reported in human research, and two subjects withdrew from a cholesterol study because of suspected allergy to soy. In a study involving young adults with asthma, soy beverages were associated with an increased risk of asthma. Asthma-like breathing problems have also been associated with inhaling soybean dust.

Side Effects and Warnings

- Soy has been a dietary staple in many countries for over 5000 years and is generally not regarded as having significant long-term toxicity. Limited side effects have been reported in infants, children, and adults.
- Soy protein taken by mouth has been associated with stomach and intestinal difficulties such as bloating, nausea, and constipation. More serious intestinal side effects have been uncommonly reported in infants fed soy protein formula, including vomiting, diarrhea, growth failure, and damage to or bleeding of the intestine walls. Soy protein fed to infants recovering from acute gastroenteritis may cause persistent intestinal damage and diarrhea. People who experience intestinal irritation (colitis) from cow milk may also react to soy formula.
- Based on human case reports and animal research, decreased thyroid hormone and increased thyroid-stimulating hormone (TSH) levels may occur during the use of soy formula in

infants. This includes rare reports of goiter (enlargement in neck due to increased thyroid size). Hormone levels have become normal again after soy formula is stopped. Infants fed soy or cow milk formula may also have higher rates of atopic eczema than are seen in infants who are breastfed.

- Acute migraine headache has been reported with the use of a soy isoflavone product. Based on animal research, damage to the pancreas may theoretically occur from regularly eating raw soybeans or soy flour/protein powder made from raw, unroasted, or unfermented beans.
- The use of soy is often discouraged in patients with hormone-sensitive malignancies such as breast, ovarian, or uterine cancer, because of concerns about possible estrogen-like effects (which theoretically may stimulate tumor growth). Other hormone-sensitive conditions such as endometriosis may also theoretically be worsened. In laboratory studies, it is not clear if isoflavones stimulate or block the effects of estrogen, or both (acting as a receptor agonist/antagonist). Until additional research is available, patients with these conditions should exercise caution and consult a qualified healthcare practitioner before starting use of soy.
- It is not known if soy or soy isoflavones share the same side effects as those of estrogens, such as increased risk of blood clots. Preliminary studies suggest that soy isoflavones, unlike estrogens, do not cause the lining of the uterus (endometrium) to build up.

Pregnancy and Breastfeeding

- Soy as a part of the regular diet is traditionally considered to be safe during pregnancy and breastfeeding, although scientific research is limited in these areas. The effects of high doses of soy or soy isoflavones in humans are not clear, and therefore intake at these levels is not recommended.
- Recent study demonstrates that isoflavones, which may have estrogen-like properties, are transferred through breast milk from mothers to infants. High doses of isoflavones given to pregnant rats have resulted in tumors in female offspring, although this has not been tested in humans.
- In one human study, male infants born to women who ingested soymilk or soy products during pregnancy experienced more frequent hypospadias (a birth defect in which the urethral meatus, the opening from which urine passes, is abnormally positioned on the underside of the penis). However, other human and animal studies have examined males or females fed soy formula as infants and have not found abnormalities in infant growth, head circumference, height, or weight, or in occurrence of puberty, menstruation, or reproductive ability.
- Research in children during the first year of life has found that the substitution of soy formula for cow milk may be associated with significantly lower bone mineral density. Parents considering the use of soy formula should consult a qualified healthcare practitioner to make sure the appropriate vitamins and minerals are provided in the formula.

INTERACTIONS

Most herbs and supplements have not been thoroughly tested for interactions with other herbs, supplements, drugs, or foods. The interactions listed here are based on reports in scientific publications, laboratory experiments, or traditional use. It is important to always read product labels. People who have a medical condition, or are taking other drugs, herbs, or supplements, should consult a qualified healthcare provider before starting a new therapy.

Interactions with Drugs

- **Estrogen:** Soy contains phytoestrogens (plant-based compounds with weak estrogen-like properties) such as isoflavones. In laboratory studies, it is not clear if isoflavones stimulate or block the effects of estrogen, or both (acting as a receptor agonist/antagonist). It is not known if taking soy or soy isoflavone supplements increases or decreases the effects of estrogen on the body, such as the risk of blood clots. It is unclear if taking soy alters the effectiveness of oral contraceptives containing estrogen.
- **Selective estrogen receptor modulators, aromatase inhibitors:** It is not known what the effects of soy phytoestrogens are on the antitumor effects of selective estrogen receptor modulators (SERMs) such as tamoxifen. The effects of aromatase inhibitors such as anastrozole (Arimidex), exemestane (Aromasin), and letrozole (Femara) may be reduced. Because of the potential estrogen-like properties of soy, people receiving these drugs should consult their oncologist before taking soy in amounts greater than normally found in the diet.
- **Warfarin (Coumadin):** Soy protein may interact with warfarin, although this potential interaction is not well characterized. Patients taking warfarin should consult their healthcare provider and pharmacist before taking soy supplementation.

Interactions with Herbs and Dietary Supplements

- **Iron:** The effects of soy protein or flour on iron absorption are not clear. Studies in the 1980s reported decreases in iron absorption, although more recent research has noted no effects or increased iron absorption in people taking soy. People using iron supplements as well as soy products should consult a qualified healthcare practitioner to follow blood iron levels.
- *Panax ginseng:* Some experts believe that there may be a potential interaction between soy extract and *Panax ginseng*, although this potential interaction is not well characterized.

Interactions with Laboratory Assays

- **Calcium, phosphate:** Animal research suggests that soy may possess estrogen-like effects that affect calcium and phosphate levels. Urinary calcium excretion may be reduced. Further study is needed before a firm conclusion can be drawn.

Interactions with Foods

- **Wheat:** Based on limited human study, reduced absorption of the soy isoflavone genistein (theorized to possess phytoestrogen properties) may occur when soy is taken in combination with wheat fiber.

Selected References

Natural Standard developed the preceding evidence-based information based on a systematic review of more than 600 published articles. For comprehensive information about alternative and complementary therapies on the professional level, go to www.naturalstandard.com. Selected references are listed here.

Adams KF, Newton KM, Chen C, et al. Soy isoflavones do not modulate circulating insulin-like growth factor concentrations in an older population in an intervention trial. J Nutr 2003;133(5):1316-1319.

Albert A, Altabre C, Baro F, et al. Efficacy and safety of a phytoestrogen preparation derived from *Glycine max* (L.) Merr in climacteric symptomatology: a multicentric, open, prospective and non-randomized trial. Phytomedicine 2002;9(2):85-92.

Albertazzi P, Pansini F, Bonaccorsi G, et al. The effect of dietary soy supplementation on hot flushes. Obstet Gynecol 1998;91(1):6-11.

Alekel DL, Germain AS, Peterson CT, et al. Isoflavone-rich soy protein isolate attenuates bone loss in the lumbar spine of perimenopausal women. Am J Clin Nutr 2000;72(3):844-852.

Allen UD, McLeod K, Wang EE. Cow's milk versus soy-based formula in mild and moderate diarrhea: a randomized, controlled trial. Acta Paediatr 1994; 83(2):183-187.

Allison DB, Gadbury, G, Schwartz LG, et al. A novel soy-based meal replacement formula for weight loss among obese individuals: a randomized controlled clinical trial. Eur J Clin Nutr 2003;57(4):514-522.

Andersson C, Servetnyk Z, Roomans GM. Activation of CFTR by genistein in human airway epithelial cell lines. Biochem Biophys Res Commun 2003; 308(3):518-522.

Anderson GD, Rositio G, Mohustsy MA, et al. Drug interaction potential of soy extract and *Panax ginseng*. J Clin Pharmacol 2003;43(6):643-648.

Arjmandi BH, Khalil DA, Smith BJ, et al. Soy protein has a greater effect on bone in postmenopausal women not on hormone replacement therapy, as evidenced by reducing bone resorption and urinary calcium excretion. J Clin Endocrinol Metab 2003;88(3):1048-1054.

Atkinson C, Skor HE, Dawn Fitzgibbons E, et al. Urinary equol excretion in relation to 2-hydroxyestrone and 16alpha-hydroxyestrone concentrations: an observational study of young to middle-aged women. J Steroid Biochem Mol Biol 2003;86(1):71-77.

Bakhit RM, Klein BP, Essex-Sorlie D, et al. Intake of 25 g of soybean protein with or without soybean fiber alters plasma lipids in men with elevated cholesterol concentrations. J Nutr 1994;124(2):213-222.

Baird DA, Umbach DM, Lansdell L, et al. Dietary intervention study to assess estrogenicity of dietary soy among postmenopausal women. J Clin Endocrinol Metab 1995;80(5):1685-1690.

Baxa DM, Yoshimura FK. Genistein reduces NF-kappa B in T lymphoma cells via a caspase-mediated cleavage of I kappa B alpha. Biochem Pharmacol 2003; 66(6):1009-1018.

Beck V, Unterrieder E, Krenn L, et al. Comparison of hormonal activity (estrogen, androgen, and progestin) of standardized plant extracts for large scale use in hormone replacement therapy. J Steroid Biochem Mol Biol 2003; 84(2-3):259-26.

Blum A, Lang N, Peleg A, et al. Effects of oral soy protein on markers of inflammation in postmenopausal women with mild hypercholesteremia. Am Heart J 2003;145(2):e7.

Blum A, Lang N, Vigder F, et al. Effects of soy protein on endothelium-dependent vasodilation and lipid profile in postmenopausal women with mild hypercholesterolemia. Clin Invest Med 2003;26(1):20-26.

Blum A. Possible beneficial effects of soy protein on the vascular endothelium in postmenopausal women—future directions. Is Med Assoc J 2003;5(1):56-58.

Bos C, Metges CC, Gaudichon C, et al. Postprandial kinetics of dietary amino acids are the main determinant of their metabolism after soy or milk protein ingestion in humans. J Nutr 2003;133(5):1308-1315.

Bowey E, Adlercreutz H, Rowland I. Metabolism of isoflavones and lignans by the gut microflora: a study in germ-free and human flora associated rats. Food Chem Toxicol 2003;41(5):631-636.

Burke BE, Olson RD, Cusack BJ. Randomized, controlled trial of phytoestrogen in the prophylactic treatment of menstrual migraine. Biomed Pharmacother 2002;56(6):283-288.

Burke GL, Legault C, Anthony M, et al. Soy protein and isoflavone effects on vasomotor symptoms in peri- and postmenopausal women: the Soy Estrogen Alternative Study. Menopause 2003;10(2):147-153.

Burks AW, Vanderhoof JA, Mehra S, et al. Randomized clinical trial of soy formula with and without added fiber in antibiotic-induced diarrhea. J Pediatr 2001;139(4):578-582.

Bus AE, Worsley A. Consumers' sensory and nutritional perceptions of three types of milk. Public Health Nutr 2003;6(2):201-208.

Cambria-Kiely JA. Effect of soy milk on warfarin efficacy. Ann Pharmacother 2002;36(12):1893-1896.

Cassidy A. Potential risks and benefits of phytoestrogen-rich diets. Int J Vitam Nutr Res 2003;73(2):120-126.

Chavez M. Soybeans as an alternative to hormone replacement therapy. J Herbal Pharmacother 2002;1(1):91-99.

Chen HL, Huang YC. Fiber intake and food selection of the elderly in Taiwan. Nutrition 2003;19(4):332-336.

Chen WF, Huang MH, Tzang CH, et al. Inhibitory actions of genistein in human breast cancer (MCF-7) cells. Biochem Biophys Acta 2003;1638(2) 187-196.

Chiechi LM, Secreto G, Vimercati A, et al. The effects of a soy rich diet on serum lipids: the Menfis randomized trial. Maturitas 2002;41(2):97-104.

Choi Em, Koo SJ. Effects of soybean ethanol extract on the cell survival and oxidative stress in osteoblastic cells. Phytother Res 2003;17(6):627-632.

Chorazy PA, Himelhoch S, Hopwood NJ, et al. Persistent hypothyroidism in an infant receiving a soy formula: case report and review of the literature. Pediatrics 1995;96(1 Pt 1):148-150.

Colquhoun D, Hicks BJ, Kelly GE. Lack of effect of isoflavones on human serum lipids and lipoproteins [abstract]. Atherosclerosis 1994;109:75.

Cressey PJ, Vannoort RW. Pesticide content of infant formulae and weaning foods available in New Zealand. Food Addit Contam 2003;20(1):57-64.

Crouse JR III, Morgan T, Terry JG, et al. A randomized trial comparing the effect of casein with that of soy protein containing varying amounts of isoflavones on plasma concentrations of lipids and lipoproteins. Arch Intern Med 1999;159(17):2070-2076.

Dalais FS, Ebeling PR, Kotsopoulos D, et al. The effects of soy protein containing isoflavones on lipids and indices of bone resorption in postmenopausal women. Clin Endocrinol 2003;58(6):704-709.

Dean TS, O'Reilly J, Bowey E, et al. The effects of soybean isoflavones on plasma HDL concentrations in healthy male and female subjects [abstract]. Proc Nutr Soc 1998;57:123A.

De Lemos ML. Effects of soy phytoestrogens genistein and daidzein on breast cancer growth. Ann Pharmacother 2001;35(9):1118-1121.

Demonty I, Lamrache B, Jones PJ. Role of isoflavones in the hypocholesterolemic effect of soy. Nutr Rev 2003;61(6 Pt 1):189-203.

Dewell A, Hollenbeck CB, Bruce B. The effects of soy-derived phytoestrogens on serum lipids and lipoproteins in moderately hypercholesterolemic postmenopausal women. J Clin Endocrinol Metab 2002;87(1):118-121.

Dreon DM, Slavin JL, Phinney SD. Oral contraceptive use and increased plasma concentration of C-reactive protein. Life Sci 2003;73(10):1245-1252.

Duncan AM, Underhill KEW, Xu X, et al. Modest hormonal effects of Soy isoflavones in postmenopausal women. J Clin Endocrinol Metab 1999;84(10): 3479-3484.

Endres J, Barter S, Theodora P, et al. Soy-enhanced lunch acceptance by preschoolers. J Am Diet Assoc 2003;103(3):345-351.

Engel PA. New onset migraine associated with use of soy isoflavone supplements. Neurology 2002 Oct 22;59(8):1289-1290

Fiocchi A, Restani P, Leo G, et al. Clinical tolerance to lactose in children with cow's milk allergy. Pediatrics 2003;112(2):359-362.

Fouillet H, Gaudichon C, Bos C, et al. Contribution of plasma proteins to splanchnic and total anabolic utilization of dietary nitrogen in humans. Am J Physiol Endocrinol Metab 2003;285(1):E88-97.

Fowke JH, Chung FL, Jin F, et al. Urinary isothiocyanate levels, brassica, and human breast cancer. Cancer Res 2003;63(14):3980-3886.

Frankenfeld CL, Patterson RE, Horner NK, et al. Validation of a soy food-frequency questionnaire and evaluation of correlates of plasma isoflavone concentrations in postmenopausal women. Am J Clin Nutr 2003;77(3): 674-680.

Franke AA, Custer LJ, Tanaka Y. Isoflavones in human breast milk and other biological fluids. Am J Clin Nutr 1998;68(6 Suppl):1466S-1473S.

Fujita H, Yamagami T, Ohshima K. Long-term ingestion of a fermented soybean-derived Touchi-extract with alpha-glucosidase inhibitory activity is safe and effective in humans with borderline and mild type-2 diabetes. J Nutr 2001;131(8):2105-2108.

Garcia-Martinez MC, Hermenegildo C, Tarin JJ, et al. Phytoestrogens increase the capacity of serum to stimulate prostacyclin release in human endothelial cells. Acta Obstet Gynecol Scand 2003;82(8):715-710.

Gentile MG, Manna G, D'Amico G. Soy consumption and renal function in patients with nephrotic syndrome: clinical effects and potential mechanism. Am J Clin Nutr 1998;68(suppl):1516s.

Gentile MS, Vasu C, Green A, et al. Targeting colon cancer cells with genistein-17.1A immunoconjugate. Int J Oncol 2003;22(5):955-959.

Gianazza E, Eberini I, Arnoldi A, et al. A proteomic investigation of isolated soy proteins with variable effects in experimental and clinical studies. J Nutr 2003; 133(1):9-14.

Goodman MT, Wilkens LR, Hankin JH, et al. Association of soy and fiber consumption with the risk of endometrial cancer. Am J Epidemiol 1997; 146(4):294-306.

Greendale GA, FitzGerald G, Huang MH, et al. Dietary soy isoflavones and bone mineral density: results from the study of women's health across the nation. Am J Epidemiol 2002;155(8):746-754.

Hargraves DF, Potten CF, Harding C, et al. Two-week dietary soy supplementation has an estrogenic effect on normal premenopausal breast. J Clin Endocrinol Metab 1999;84(11):4017-4024.

Haselkorn T, Stewart SL, Horn-Ross PL. Why are thyroid cancer rates so high in Southeast Asian women living in the United States? The Bay Area Thyroid Cancer Study. Cancer Epidemiol Biomarkers Prev 2003;12(2):144-150.

Hedlund TE, Johannes WU, Miller GJ. Soy isoflavonoid equol modulates the growth of benign and malignant prostatic epithelial cells in vitro. Prostate 2003;54(1):68-78.

Hermansen K, Dinesen B, Hoie LH, et al. Effects of soy and other natural products on LDL:HDL ratio and other lipid parameters: a literature review. Adv Ther 2003;20(3):50-78.

Hermansen K, Sondergaard M, Hoie L, et al. Beneficial effects of a soy-based dietary supplement on lipid levels and cardiovascular risk markers in type 2 diabetic subjects. Diabetes Care 2001;24(2):228-233.

Hidvegi E, Arato A, Cserhati E, et al. Slight decrease in bone mineralization in cow milk-sensitive children. J Pediatr Gastroenterol Nutr 2003;36(1):44-49.

Ishikawa-Takata K, Ohta T. Relationship of lifestyle factors to bone mass in Japanese women. J Nutr Health Aging 2003;7(1):44-53.

Ingram D, Sanders K, Kolybaba M, et al. Case-control study of phyto-oestrogens and breast cancer. Lancet 1997;350(9083):990-994.

Irvine C, Fitzpatrick M, Robertson I, et al. The potential adverse effects of soybean phytoestrogens in infant feeding. N Z Med J 1995;108(1000): 208-209.

S

Jenkins DJ, Kendall CW, Marchie A., et al. Effects of a dietary portfolio of cholesterol-lowering foods vs lovastatin on serum lipids and C-reactive protein. JAMA 2003;290(4):531-533.

Jenkins DJ, Kendall CW, Marchie A, et al. Type 2 diabetes and the vegetarian diet. Am J Clin Nutr 2003;78(3 Suppl):610S-616S.

Jenkins DJ, Kendall CW, D'Costa MA, et al. Soy consumption and phytoestrogens: effect on serum prostate specific antigen when blood lipids and oxidized low-density lipoprotein are reduced in hyperlipidemic men. J Urol 2003;169(2):507-511.

Jacobsen BK, Knutsen SF, Fraser GE. Does high soy milk intake reduce prostate cancer incidence? The Adventist Health Study (United States). Cancer Causes Control 1998;9(6):553-557.

Johns P, Dowlati L, Wargo W. Determination of isoflavones in ready-to-feed soy-based infant formula. J AOAC Int 2003;86(1):72-78.

Kazi A, Daniel KG, Smith DM, et al. Inhibition of the proteasome activity, a novel mechanism associated with tumor cell apoptosis-inducing ability of genistein. Biochem Pharmacol 2003;66(6):965-976.

Knight DC, Howes JB, Eden JA, et al. Effects on menopausal symptoms and acceptability of isoflavone-containing soy powder dietary supplementation. Climacteric 2001;4(1):13-18.

Koo WW, Hammami M, Margeson DP, et al. Reduced bone mineralization in infants fed palm olein–containing formula; a randomized, double-blinded, prospective trial. Pediatrics 2003;111(5 Pt 1):1017-1023.

Kritz-Silverstein D, Von Muhlen D, Barrett-Connor E, et al. Isoflavones and cognitive function in older women: the Soy and Postmenopausal Health In Aging (SOPHIA) Study. Menopause 2003;10(3)196-202.

Kurzer MS. Phytoestrogen supplement use by women. J Nutr 2003;133(6): 1983S-1986S.

Lack G, Fox D, Northstone K, et al. Factors associated with the development of peanut allergy in childhood. N Engl J Med 2003;348(11):977-985.

LaCroix DE, Wolf WR. Determination of total fat in milk- and soy-based infant formula powder by supercritical fluid extraction. J AOAC Int 2003;86(1): 86-95.

Lampe JW. Isoflavonoid and lignan phytoestrogens as dietary biomarkers. J Nutr 2003;133(Suppl 3):956S-964S.

Laurin D, Jacques H, Moorjani S, et al. Effects of a soy-protein beverage on plasma lipoproteins in children with familial hypercholesterolemia. Am J Clin Nutr 1991;54(1):98-103.

Lombaert GA, Pellaers P, Roscoe V, et al. Mycotoxins in infant cereal foods from the Canadian retail market. Food Addit Contam 2003;20(5);494-504.

Macfarlane BJ, van der Riet WB, Bothwell TH, et al. Effect of traditional oriental soy products on iron absorption. Am J Clin Nutr 1990;51(5):873-880.

Mahady GB, Parrot J, Lee C, et al. Botanical dietary supplement use in peri- and postmenopausal women. Menopause 2003;10(1):65-72.

Maskirinec G, Robbins C, Riola B, et al. Three measures show high compliance in a soy intervention among premenopausal women. J Am Diet Assoc 2003; 103(7):861-866.

Maskarinec G, Williams AE, Carlin L. Mammographic densities in a one-year isoflavone intervention. Eur J Cancer Prev 2003;12(2):165-169.

Maskarinec G, Williams AE, Inouye JS, et al. A randomized isoflavone intervention among premenopausal women. Cancer Epidemiol Biomarkers Prev 2002;11(2):195-201.

Maubach J, Bracke ME, Heyerick A, et al. Quantative of soy-derived phytoestrogens in human breast tissue and biological fluids by high-performance liquid chromatography. J Chromatogr B Analyt Technol Biomed Life Sci 2003;784(1):137-144.

McFadyen IJ, Chetty U, Setchell KDR, et al. A randomized double blind, cross over trial of soya protein for the treatment of cyclical breast pain. Breast 2000;9:271-276.

Merz-Demlow BE, Duncan AM, Wangen KE, et al. Soy isoflavones improve plasma lipids in normocholesterolemic, premenopausal women. Am J Clin Nutr 2000;71(6):1462-1469.

Messina M, Hughes C. Efficacy of soyfoods and soybean isoflavone supplements for alleviating menopausal symptoms is positively related to initial hot flush frequency. J Med Food 2003;6(1):1-11.

Messina MJ. Emerging evidence on the role of soy in reducing prostate cancer risk. Nutr Rev 2003;61(4):117-131.

Migliaccio S, Anderon JJ. Isoflavones and skeletal health: are these molecules ready for clinical application? Osteoporos Int 2003;14(5):361-368.

Miltyk W, Craciunescu CN, Fischer L, et al. Lack of significant genotoxicity of purified soy isoflavones (genistein, daidzein, and glycitein) in 20 patients with prostate cancer. Am J Clin Nutr 2003;77(4):875-882.

Mimouni F, Campaigne B, Neylan M, et al. Bone mineralization in the first year of life in infants fed human milk, cow-milk formula, or soy-based formula. J Pediatr 1993;122(3):348-354.

Moeller Le, Peterson CT, Hanson KB, et al. Isoflavone-rich soy protein prevents loss of hip lean mass but does not prevent the shift in regional fat distribution in perimenopausal women. Menopause 2003;10(4):322-331.

Morens C, Bos C, Pueyo ME, et al. Increasing habitual protein intake accentuates differences in postprandial dietary nitrogen utilization between protein sources in humans. J Nutr 2003;133(9):2733-2740.

Nagata C, Kabuto M, Kurisu Y, et al. Decreased serum estradiol concentration associated with high dietary intake of soy products in premenopausal Japanese women. Nutr Cancer 1997;29(3):228-233.

Nagata C, Shimizu H, Takami R, et al. Association of blood pressure with intake of soy products and other food groups in Japanese men and women. Prev Med 2003;36(6):692-697.

Nagata C, Shimizu H, Takami R, et al. Soy product intake is inversely associated with serum homocysteine level in premenopausal Japanese women. J Nutr 2003;133(3):797-800.

Nagata C, Takatsuka N, Kawakami N, et al. A prospective cohort study of soy product intake and stomach cancer death. Br J Cancer 2002;87(1):31-36.

Nagata C, Takatsuka N, Kawakami N, et al. Soy product intake and hot flashes in Japanese women: results from a community-based prospective study. Am J Epidemiol 2001;153(8):790-793.

Nagata C, Takatsuka N, Kurisu Y, et al. Decreased serum total cholesterol concentration is associated with high intake of soy products in Japanese men and women. J Nutr 1998;128(2):209-213.

Nikitovic D, Tsatsakis AM, Karamanos NK, et al. The effects of genistein on the synthesis and distribution of glycosaminoglycans/proteoglycans by two osteosarcoma cell lines depends on tyrosine kinase and the estrogen receptor density. Anticancer Res 2003;23(1A):459-464.

North K, Golding J. A maternal vegetarian diet in pregnancy is associated with hypospadias. The ALSPAC Study Team. Avon Longitudinal Study of Pregnancy and Childhood. BJU Int 2000;85(1):107-113.

Nowak-Wegrzyn A, Sampson HA, Wood RA, et al. Food protein-induced enterocolitis syndrome caused by solid food proteins. Pediatrics 2003; 111(4 Pt 1):829-835.

Oerter Klein K, Janfaza M, Wong JA, et al. Estrogen bioactivity in fo-ti and other herbs used for their estrogen-like effects as determined by a recombinant cell bioassay. J Clin Endocrinol Metab. 2003;88(9): 4075-4076.

Pathak SK, Sharma RA, Mellon JK. Chemoprevention of prostate cancer by diet-derived antioxidant agents and hormonal manipulation (Review). Int J Oncol 2003;22(1):5-13.

Penotti M, Fabio E, Modena AB, et al. Effect of soy-derived isoflavones on hot flushes, endometrial thickness, and the pulsatility index of the uterine and cerebral arteries. Fertil Steril 2003;79(5):1112-1117.

Pino AM, Vallardes LE, Palma MA, et al. Dietary isoflavones affect sex hormone-binding globulin levels in postmenopausal women. J Clin Endocrinol Metab 2000;85(8):2797-2800.

Potter SM, Bakshit RM, Essex-Sorlie DL, et al. Depression of plasma cholesterol in men by consumption of baked products containing soy protein. Am J Clin Nutr 1993;58(4):501-506.

Potter SM, Baum JA, Teng H, et al. Soy protein and isoflavones: their effects on blood lipids and bone density in postmenopausal women. Am J Clin Nutr 1998;68(6 Suppl):1375S-1379S.

Puska P, Korpelainen V, Hoie LH, et al. Soy in hypercholesterolaemia: a double-blind, placebo-controlled trial. Eur J Clin Nutr 2002;56(4):352-357.

Quella SK, Loprinzi CL, Barton DL, et al. Evaluation of soy phytoestrogens for the treatment of hot flashes in breast cancer survivors: A North Central Cancer Treatment Group Trial. J Clin Oncol 2000;18(5):1068-1074.

Rajaram S. The effect of vegetarian diet, plant foods, and phytochemicals on hemostasis and thrombosis. Am J Clin Nutr 2003;78(3 Suppl):552S-558S.

Register TC, Jayo MJ, Anthony MS. Soy phytoestrogens do not prevent bone loss in postmenopausal monkeys. J Clin Endocrinol Metab 2003; 88(9): 4362-4370.

Rivas M, Garay RP, Escanero JF, et al. Soy milk lowers blood pressure in men and women with mild to moderate essential hypertension. J Nutr 2002;132(7): 1900-1902.

Rossi EA, Vendramini RC, Carlos IZ, et al. Effect of a new fermented soy milk product on serum lipid levels in normocholesterolemic adult men. Arch Latinoam Nutr 2003;53(1):47-51.

Santosham M, Goepp J, Burns B, et al. Role of a soy-based lactose-free formula in the outpatient management of diarrhea. Pediatrics 1991;87(5):619-622.

Scambia G, Mango D, Signorile PG, et al. Clinical effects of a standardized soy extract in postmenopausal women: a pilot study. Menopause 2000;7(2): 105-111.

Scheiber MD, Liu JH, Subbiah MT, et al. Dietary inclusion of whole soy foods results in significant reductions in clinical risk factors for osteoporosis and cardiovascular disease in normal postmenopausal women. Menopause 2001; 8(5):384-392.

Setchell KD, Brown NM, Desai PB, et al. Bioavailability, disposition, and dose-response effects of soy isoflavones when consumed by healthy women at physiologically typical dietary intakes. J Nutr 2003;133(4):1027-1035.

Setchell KD, Cassidy A. Dietary isoflavones: biological effects and relevance to human health. J Nutr 1999;129:758S-767S.

Setchell KD, Faughnan MS, Avades T, et al. Comparing the pharmacokinetics of daidzein and genistein with the use of ^{13}C-labeled tracers in premenopausal women. Am J Clin Nutr 2003;77(2):411-419.

Setchell KD, Lydeking-Olsen E. Dietary phytoestrogens and their effect on bone: evidence from in vitro and in vivo, human observational, and dietary intervention studies. Am J Clin Nutr 2003;78(3 Suppl):593S-609S.

Shimakawa Y, Matsubara S, Yuki N, et al. Evaluation of *Bifidobacterium breve* strain Yakult-fermented soymilk as a probiotic food. Int J Food Microbiol 2003;81(2):131-136.

Shu XO, Jin F, Dai Q, et al. Soyfood intake during adolescence and subsequent risk of breast cancer among Chinese women. Cancer Epidemiol Biomarkers Prev 2001;10(5):483-488.

Sirtori CR. Dubious benefits and potential risk of soy phyto-oestrogens. Lancet 2000;355(9206):849.

Somekawa Y, Chiguchi M, Ishibashi T, et al. Soy intake related to menopausal symptoms, serum lipids, and bone mineral density in postmenopausal Japanese women. Obstet Gynecol 2001;97(1):109-115.

Spilburg CA, Goldberg AC, McGill JB, et al. Fat-free foods supplemented with soy stanol-lecithin powder reduce cholesterol absorption and LDL cholesterol. J Am Diet Assoc 2003;103(5):577-581.

St Germain A, Peterson CT, Robinson JG, et al. Isoflavone-rich or isoflavone-poor soy protein does not reduce menopausal symptoms during 24 weeks of treatment. Menopause 2001;8(1):17-26.

Steichen JJ, Tsang RC. Bone mineralization and growth in term infants fed soy-based or cow milk-based formula. J Pediatr 1987;110(5):687-692.

Steinberg FM, Guthrie NL, Villablanca AC, et al. Soy protein with isoflavones has favorable effects on endothelial function that are independent of lipid and antioxidant effects in healthy postmenopausal women. Am J Clin Nutr 2003;78(1):123-130.

Strom BL, Schinnar R, Ziegler EE, et al. Exposure to soy-based formula in infancy and endocrinological and reproductive outcomes in young adulthood. JAMA 2001;286(7):807-814.

Strom SS, Yamamura Y, Duphorne CM, et al. Phytoestrogen intake and prostate cancer: a case-control study using a new database. Nutr Cancer 1999;33(1):20-25.

Taylor M. Alternatives to HRT: an evidence-based review. Int J Fertil Womens Med 2003;48(2):64-68.

Teede HJ, Dalais FS, Kotsopoulos D, et al. Dietary soy has both beneficial and potentially adverse cardiovascular effects: a placebo-controlled study in men and postmenopausal women. J Clin Endocrinol Metab 2001;86(7):3053-3060.

Teixeira SR, Potter SM, Weigel R, et al. Effects of feeding 4 levels of soy protein for 3 and 6 wk on blood lipids and apolipoproteins in moderately hypercholesterolemic men. Am J Clin Nutr 2000;71(5):1077-1084.

Tice JA, Ettinger B, Ensrud K, et al. Phytoestrogen supplements for the treatment of hot flashes: the Isoflavone Clover Extract (ICE) Study: a randomized controlled trial. JAMA 2003;290(2):207-214.

Tonstad S, Smerud K, Hoie L. A comparison of the effects of 2 doses of soy protein or casein on serum lipids, serum lipoproteins, and plasma total homocysteine in hypercholesterolemic subjects. Am J Clin Nutr 2002;76(1):78-84.

Tsuchida K, Mizushima S, Toba M, et al. Dietary soybeans intake and bone mineral density among 995 middle-aged women in Yokohama. J Epidemiol 1999;9(1):14-19.

Turner NJ, Thomson BM, Shaw IC. Bioactive isoflavones in functional foods: the importance of gut microflora on bioavailability. Nutr Rev 2003;61(6 Pt 1):204-213.

Uesugi T, Fukui Y, Yamori Y. Beneficial effects of soybean isoflavone supplementation on bone metabolism and serum lipids in postmenopausal Japanese women: a four-week study. J Am Coll Nutr 2002;21(2):97-102.

Upmalis DH, Lobo R, Bradley L, et al. Vasomotor symptom relief by soy isoflavone extract tablets in postmenopausal women: a multicenter, double-blind, randomized, placebo-controlled study. Menopause 2000;7(4):236-242.

Van Patten CL, Olivotto IA, Chambers GK, et al. Effect of soy phytoestrogens on hot flashes in postmenopausal women with breast cancer: A randomized, controlled clinical trial. J Clin Oncol 2002;20(6):1449-1455.

Vanderhoof JA, Murray ND, Paule CL, et al. Use of soy fiber in acute diarrhea in infants and toddlers. Clin Pediatr (Phila) 1997;36(3):135-139.

Wangen KE, Duncan AM, Xu X, et al. Soy isoflavones improve plasma lipids in normocholesterolemic and mildly hypercholesterolemic postmenopausal women. Am J Clin Nutr 2001;73(2):225-231.

Watanabe S, Uesugi S, Zhuo X, et al. Phytoestrogens and cancer prevention. Gan To Kagaku Ryoho 2003;30(7):902-908.

White LR, Petrovitch H, Ross GW, et al. Brain aging and midlife tofu consumption. J Am Coll Nutr 2000;19(2):242-255.

Whitten PL, Lewis C, Russell E, et al. Potential adverse effects of phytoestrogens. J Nutr 1995;125(3 Suppl):771S-776S.

Wietzke JA, Welsh J. Phytoestrogen regulation of a vitamin D_3 receptor promoter and 1,25-dihydroxyvitamin D_3 actions in human breast cancer cells. J Steroid Biochem Mol Biol;84(2-3):149-157.

Willett W. Lessons from dietary studies in Adventists and questions for the future. Am J Clin Nutr 2003;78(3 Suppl):539S-543S.

Wilson LC, Baek SJ, Call A, et al. Nonsteroidal anti-inflammatory drug-activated gene (NAG-1) is induced by genistein through the expression of p53 in colorectal cancer cells. Int J Cancer 2003;105(6):747-753.

Wong WW, Smith EO, Stuff JE, et al. Cholesterol-lowering effect of soy protein in normocholesterolemic and hypercholesterolemic men. Am J Clin Nutr 1998;68(6 Suppl):1385S-1389S.

Woods RK, Walters EH, Raven JM. Food and nutrient intakes and asthma risk in young adults. Am J Clin Nutr 2003;78(3):414-423.

Wu AH, Yu MC, Tseng CC, et al. Green tea and risk of breast cancer in Asian Americans. Int J Cancer 2003;106(4):574-579.

Wu AH, Ziegler RG, Horn-Ross PL, et al. Tofu and risk of breast cancer in Asian-Americans. Cancer Epidemiol Biomarkers Prev 1996;5(11):901-906.

Yamamoto S, Sobue T, Kobayashi M, et al. Soy, isoflavones, and breast cancer risk in Japan. J Natl Cancer Inst 2003;95(12):906-913.

Yimyaem P, Chongsrisawat V, Vivatvakin B, et al. Gastrointestinal manifestations of cow's milk protein allergy during the first year of life. J Med Assoc Thai 2003;86(2):116-123.

Yu L, Blackburn GL, Zhou JR. Genistein and daidzein downregulate prostate androgen-regulated transcript-1 (PART-1) gene expression induced by dihydrotestosterone in human prostate LNCaP cancer cells. J Nutr 2003;133(2):389-392.

Zhang X, Shu XO, Gao YT, et al. Soy food consumption is associated with lower risk of coronary heart disease in Chinese women. J Nutr 2003;133(9):2874-2878.

Zhang Y, Hendrich S, Murphy PA. Glucuronides are the main isoflavone metabolites in women. J Nutr 2003;133(2):399-404.

Zhao XF, Hao LY, Yin SA, et al. Effect of long term supplementation of mineral-fortified dephytinized soy milk powder on biomarkers of bone turnover in boys aged 12 to 14 years. Zhonghua Yu Fang Yi Xue Za Zhi 2003;37(1):9-11.

Zhou JR, Yu L, Zhong Y, et al. Soy phytochemicals and tea bioactive components synergistically inhibit androgen-sensitive human prostate tumors in mice. J Nutr 2003;133(2):516-521.

Zubik L, Meydani M. Bioavailability of soybean isoflavones from aglycone and glucoside forms in American women. Am J Clin Nutr 2003;77(6):1459-1465.

S

SYNONYMS/COMMON NAMES/RELATED SUBSTANCES

- AFA (*Aphanizomenon flos-aquae*), *Arthrospira platensis*, blue-green algae (BGA), cyanobacteria, dihe, klamath, *Microcystis aeruginosa*, *Microcystis wesenbergii*, Multinal, *Nostoc* spp., plant plankton, pond scum, *Spirulina fusiformis*, *Spirulina maxima*, *Spirulina platensis*, tecuitatl.
- *Note:* Non-*Spirulina* species, such as *Anabaena*, *Aphanizomenon*, and *Microcystis* species, are possibly unsafe because they are usually harvested naturally and may be subject to contamination.

CLINICAL BOTTOM LINE
Background

- The term "spirulina" refers to a large number of cyanobacteria, or blue-green algae. Both *Spirulina* and non-*Spirulina* species fall into the classification of cyanobacteria and include *Aphanizomenon* spp., *Microcystis* spp., *Nostoc* spp., and *Spirulina* spp. Most commercial products contain *Aphanizomenon flos-aquae*, *Spirulina maxima*, and/or *Spirulina platensis*, now called *Arthrospira platensis*. These algae are found in the warm, alkaline waters of the world, especially off Mexico and Central Africa. *Spirulina* species are most often grown under controlled conditions and are subject to less contamination than may occur with the non-*Spirulina* species that are harvested naturally.
- Spirulina is a rich source of nutrients, containing up to 70% protein, B-complex vitamins, phycocyanin, chlorophyll, beta-carotene, vitamin E, and numerous minerals. In fact, spirulina contains more beta-carotene than that in carrots. Spirulina has been used since ancient times as a source of nutrients and has been said to possess a variety of medical uses, including as an antioxidant, antiviral, antineoplastic, weight loss aid, and lipid-lowering agent. Preliminary data from animal studies demonstrate effectiveness for some conditions as well as safety, although human evidence is lacking. Based on available research, no recommendation can be made either for or against the use of spirulina for any indication.

Scientific Evidence for Common/Studied Uses	Grade*
Diabetes mellitus (type 2)	C
Lipid-lowering effects	C
Oral leukoplakia/cancer	C
Weight loss	C
Malnutrition	D

*Key to grades: *A:* Strong scientific evidence for this use; *B:* Good scientific evidence for this use; *C:* Unclear scientific evidence for this use; *D:* Fair scientific evidence against this use (it may not work); *F:* Strong scientific evidence against this use (it likely does not work). For a more detailed explanation of efficacy criteria, see "Natural Standard Evidence-Based Validated Grading Rationale" in the Introduction.

Historical or Theoretical Uses That Lack Sufficient Evidence

- Anaphylaxis inhibition,[1,2] anemia,[3] antifungal, anti-inflammatory,[4] antineoplastic,[5,6] antioxidant,[7,8] antiviral, anxiety, atherosclerosis,[9] attention deficit-hyperactivity disorder (ADHD), bowel health, candidal infection, cardiovascular disease, colitis,[4] cytomegalovirus, depression, digestion, energy booster, fatigue, fatty liver,[10] fibromyalgia, gastric secretory inhibition, hair loss, hepatoprotection,[10,11] herpes simplex virus type 1 (HSV-1),[12] human immunodeficiency virus type 1 (HIV-1),[12,13] hypertension, immunomodulation,[14-16] influenza, iron deficiency,[3,17,18] kidney dysfunction,[19] measles, memory improvement, mood stimulant, mumps, obstetric and gynecologic disorders, premenstrual syndrome, radiation sickness,[20] skin disorders, skin papillomas,[21] stress, ulcers, vitamin and nutrient depletion,[22] wound healing.

Expert Opinion and Folkloric Precedent

- Spirulina has been harvested from warm, alkaline lakes for thousands of years. It was a common addition to the diets of the Aztecs in Mexico and of the Kanembu people in Central Africa. Spirulina is rich in protein and other vitamins and minerals. It has been postulated that spirulina prevents cancer, lowers cholesterol, reduces body weight, and kills viruses when it is eaten regularly. Spirulina has been proposed as a high-protein food supplement to aid in treating or preventing global hunger, although human data are lacking, and this idea has not been widely accepted.

Safety Summary

- **Possibly safe:** When uncontaminated species of blue-green algae are taken orally in recommended doses.
- **Possibly unsafe:** When contaminated species of blue-green algae are taken orally. Contamination is more likely when products are harvested naturally, rather than grown in controlled environments. Notably, the blue-green algae species that are commonly harvested naturally include *Anabaena* spp., *Aphanizomenon* spp., and *Microcystis* spp.

DOSING/TOXICOLOGY
General

- Recommended doses are based on those most commonly used in available trials, or on historical practice. However, with natural products, the optimal doses needed to balance efficacy and safety often have not been determined. Formulations and preparation methods may vary from manufacturer to manufacturer, and from batch to batch of a specific product made by a single manufacturer. Because often the active components of a product are not known, standardization may not be possible, and the clinical effects of different brands may not be comparable.

Standardization

- Insufficient available data.

Dosing: Adult (18 Years and Older)
Oral

- **Hypercholesterolemia:** 1.4 g of spirulina three times daily with meals for 8 weeks.[9]
- **Diabetes mellitus (type 2):** 1 g of spirulina twice daily with meals.[23]
- **Weight loss:** 200 mg of spirulina tablets three times daily, immediately preceding meals.[24]
- **Oral leukoplakia:** 1 g of *S. fusiformis* per day for up to 1 year (used in one study).[25]

Dosing: Pediatric (Younger Than 18 Years)

- Insufficient evidence to recommend.

Toxicology
Oral

- Although reliable human toxicity studies have not been performed, when given to mice at a dose of 800 mg/kg of body weight, *S. fusiformis* was nontoxic.[26] After 13 weeks of dietary supplementation with up to 30% *S. maxima* in 40 mice, no effect on behavior, dietary intake, growth, or survival was seen.[27] A similar study in rats assessing the effect of *S. maxima* on reproductive performance and perinatal/postnatal toxicity showed no adverse effects.[28]
- Chamorro et al. found that when spirulina was fed to pregnant mice through week 19 of gestation, diets of up to 30% spirulina did not cause any toxic effects to either mother or fetus.[29] The same diet fed to both male and female rats for 13 weeks also showed no toxic effects.[30,31]

Parenteral

- Mice injected with *Microcystis aeruginosa* extract intraperitoneally became lethargic; experienced piloerection, difficulty breathing, and a decrease in peripheral circulation; and died within 1 hour.[32] The investigators found the LD_{50} in mice to be 14.4 mg of algae cells/kg of body weight in mice and 67.4 mg of cells/kg of body weight in rats.
- **Heavy metal contamination:** In an analysis of eight *S. platensis* commercial samples, Johnson et al. found that the algae contained high amounts of mercury, lead, copper, iron, manganese, and zinc.[33] High levels of these heavy metals may lead to toxicity.

ADVERSE EFFECTS/PRECAUTIONS/CONTRAINDICATIONS
Allergy

- Known allergy/hypersensitivity to spirulina or blue-green algae species, or to any of their constituents, is a contraindication.

Adverse Effects/Postmarket Surveillance

- **General:** Spirulina appears to be well tolerated in human subjects.[9,23-25] The only reported adverse effects following the ingestion of spirulina have been headache, muscle pain, facial flushing, and sweating. Contamination of blue-green algae with heavy metals is possible, especially in species that are often harvested in uncontrolled settings.
- **Neurologic/CNS:** In one study, subjects taking *S. fusiformis* 1 g daily for 1 year reported frequent headaches.[25] In a different trial, patients noted reduced concentration when taking 1 g of spirulina daily for weight loss.[24]
- **Musculoskeletal:** Subjects in one study reported occasional muscle pains while taking 1 g of *S. fusiformis* daily for 1 year.[25]

- **Gastrointestinal:** Hepatotoxicity has been reported.[34]
- **Dermatologic:** Subjects in one study occasionally reported facial flushing and sweating while taking 1 g of spirulina daily for weight loss.[24]
- **Metabolic:** The phenylalanine content in blue-green algae theoretically may exacerbate the condition phenylketonuria.

Precautions/Warnings/Contraindications

- Use cautiously in patients with phenylketonuria, as the phenylalanine content in blue-green algae theoretically may exacerbate this condition.
- Use caution with products containing the blue-green algae species *Anabaena* spp., *Aphanizomenon* spp., and *Microcystis* spp., because of the risk of contamination with heavy metals.

Pregnancy and Lactation

- There are insufficient data to safely recommend the use of spirulina in pregnancy or lactation. Chamorro et al. found that when fed to pregnant mice through week 19 of gestation, diets of up to 30% spirulina did not cause any toxic effects to either mother or fetus.[29] However, no human safety trials have been performed in pregnant or lactating women.

INTERACTIONS
Spirulina/Drug Interactions

- Insufficient available data.

Spirulina/Herb/Supplement Interactions

- **Calcium:** In a weight-loss study of 15 volunteers receiving 200-mg spirulina tablets for 4 weeks, small, statistically significant increases in serum calcium were detected.[24] Individuals had also been on a reduced-calorie diet with unclear constituents. Concomitant use with calcium supplements theoretically may increase serum levels beyond those expected.

Spirulina/Food Interactions

- **Phenylalanine-containing foods:** The phenylalanine content of blue-green algae may exacerbate the condition phenylketonuria.

Spirulina/Lab Interactions

- **Alkaline phosphatase:** In a weight-loss study of 15 volunteers receiving 200-mg spirulina tablets for 4 weeks, small, statistically significant increases in alkaline phosphatase were detected.[24] These individuals had also been on a reduced-calorie diet. Follow-up was not documented.
- **Serum calcium:** In a weight-loss study of 15 volunteers receiving 200-mg spirulina tablets for 4 weeks, small, statistically significant increases in serum calcium were detected.[24] These individuals had also been on a reduced-calorie diet with unclear constituents. Follow-up was not documented.

MECHANISM OF ACTION
Pharmacology

- **Inflammation:** Spirulina has been found *in vitro* and *in vivo* to significantly increase cyclic adenosine monophosphate (cAMP) levels in mast cells and to inhibit the production of tumor necrosis factor-alpha.[1] *S. platensis* (now *A. platensis*) was shown to inhibit immunoglobulin E (IgE)-mediated histamine release from activated mast cells in rats, preventing anaphylactic reactions after exposure with a known allergen.[2]

S

S. platensis (*A. platensis*) was demonstrated *in vitro* to stimulate macrophages, phagocytosis, and interleukin-1 production.[14] In a poorly described controlled human study, children who were exposed to radiation during the Chernobyl nuclear accident were given daily spirulina (1250 mg for ages 3 to 5 and 1750 mg for ages 5 to 7).[20] Results showed a significant decrease in serum IgE levels in the children taking spirulina, and no change in the control children.

- **Antioxidant:** *In vitro* study has demonstrated that phycocyanin, a sulfated polysaccharide pigment isolated from blue-green algae such as *Arthrospira maxima* (formerly known as *S. platensis*) scavenges free radicals and inhibits liver microsomal lipid peroxidation.[8] A study in rats with acetic acid–induced colitis found that phycocyanin significantly reduced myeloperoxidase activity, inhibited inflammatory cell infiltration of the colon, and decreased damage to the colon, compared with findings in a control group.[4] *S. fusiformis* has been shown to decrease lead-induced toxicity in mice; this effect is postulated to be due to the presence of antioxidants, beta-carotene, and superoxide dismutase enzyme.[26] Dietary 5% *S. maxima* significantly prevented the development of fatty liver in rats exposed to intraperitoneal carbon tetrachloride, compared with rats fed a regular diet.[11]
- **Anticarcinogenic:** Shklar et al. found that the application of *Spirulina-Dunaliella* algae extract to buccal pouch carcinoma in hamsters induced tumor necrosis factor-alpha production and promoted tumor regression.[6] In a similar study, animals administered oral *Spirulina-Dunaliella* algae extract three times weekly along with application of a known carcinogen to their buccal pouch were prevented from developing tumors seen in the control and other experimental groups.[5] Through a series of *in vitro* experiments, calcium spirulan, a sulfated polysaccharide from *S. platensis* (*A. platensis*), has been shown to inhibit the invasion, migration, and adhesion of tumor cells.[35]
- **Antiviral:** Hayashi et al. have isolated a sulfated polysaccharide, calcium spirulan, from *S. platensis* (*A. platensis*) and have found that it inhibits both HSV-1 and HIV-1 *in vitro* and in animals.[12] Additional research has shown a polysaccharide-containing fraction of *A. platensis* (formerly known as *S. platensis*) extract to inhibit replication of HIV-1 *in vitro*.[13]
- **Gastrointestinal:** *A. platensis* (formerly known as *S. platensis*) is made up of 60% protein.[36] *S. maxima*, when fed to adult male rats in varying concentrations, has been shown to alter the storage and utilization of vitamin A and vitamin E.[37] *S. maxima* in the diet caused an increase in the amount of fat in the feces; reduced plasma, liver, and heart alpha-tocopherol levels; and increased liver retinoid levels at low concentrations. *S. platensis* (*A. platensis*) has been shown to stimulate the *in vitro* growth of lactic acid bacteria, which may explain the use of spirulina as a digestive aid.[38] An animal study showed that gastric intubation with spirulina suspension for 15 days led to a decrease in the hepatic content of cytochrome P450 enzymes and an increase of glutathione *S*-transferase activity.[21]
- **Lipids:** Rats fed a high-fructose diet supplemented with *S. maxima* experienced significantly lower hepatic triglyceride levels, elevated hepatic phospholipid concentration, and significantly lower plasma cholesterol levels compared with findings in rats fed a high-fructose diet alone.[10] Iwata et al. also found that *S. platensis* (*A. platensis*), when added to a high-fructose diet, resulted in significant inhibition of total and high-density lipoprotein cholesterol and triglyceride

and phospholipid elevation in rats.[39] These rats exhibited an increase in the level of plasma lipoprotein lipase and hepatic triglyceride lipase activity when *S. platensis* (*A. platensis*) was added to their diet, as compared with rats fed a high-fructose diet alone.

Pharmacodynamics/Kinetics

- Insufficient available data.

HISTORY

- Spirulina has been used since the 16th century as a source of food and nutrients. The Aztecs were known to harvest and ingest "blue mud," which contained spirulina. Natives of the Sahara Desert, including the Kanembu people, also harvested spirulina from what is now known as Lake Chad and included spirulina in their diets as *dihe*. Many *in vitro* and animal studies have been performed to assess the use of spirulina as a high-protein food supplement to prevent or treat global hunger; however, data for human subjects are lacking, and this idea has not been widely accepted. Since the late 1970s, spirulina has been sold in the United States and around the world as a "health food."

REVIEW OF THE EVIDENCE: DISCUSSION

Lipid-Lowering Effects

Summary

- Animal studies have found spirulina to be effective at decreasing serum cholesterol and triglyceride levels.[9,39-41] Preliminary positive results from a small number of methodologically flawed trials suggest possible efficacy in humans.[9,23] To date, however, it remains unclear if lipid-lowering effects are seen in humans, and a recommendation cannot be made either for or against the use of spirulina for this indication.

Evidence

- Nakaya et al. conducted a study in 30 healthy male volunteers to assess the cholesterol-lowering effects of 4.2 g of oral spirulina daily.[9] Volunteers were selected because they had one or more of the following conditions: total serum cholesterol >220 mg/dL; serum triglycerides >150 mg/dL; and diastolic blood pressure >90 mm Hg. Patients were observed for 4 weeks and then assigned to one of two study groups. Both groups were instructed to take seven 200-mg spirulina tablets three times daily before meals. Group A took spirulina for an 8-week period; group B took spirulina for 4 weeks and then were observed for 4 weeks. Blood pressure and body weight were measured once weekly and serum cholesterol levels were determined every 2 weeks. Results demonstrated a significant decrease in total serum cholesterol and low-density lipoprotein (LDL) cholesterol levels. Subjects in group B experienced similar significant reductions in cholesterol levels, which returned to baseline during the 4-week observation period. Subjects reported no adverse effects. Although promising, this study can only be considered preliminary because of methodologic weaknesses, including lack of adequate blinding or randomization.
- Mani et al. observed the effects of 2 g of spirulina daily for 2 months (Multinal, New Ambadi Estate, Algal Division, Madras, India) in 15 patients with type 2 diabetes.[23] Seven additional diabetic patients served as a control group and received no spirulina supplementation. Patients were instructed to take one spirulina tablet (1 g) with lunch and dinner each day for 2 months, and to change nothing else about their lifestyle during this time (diet, exercise, medications).

Review of the Evidence: Spirulina

Condition Treated*	Study Design	Author, Year	N[†]	SS[†]	Study Quality[‡]	Magnitude of Benefit	ARR[†]	NNT[†]	Comments
Hyperlipidemia (children with nephrotic syndrome)	Before and after trial	Samuels[42] 2002	23	Mixed	1	Unclear	NA	NA	Significant decreases in triglyceride/LDL levels with medications plus spirulina compared with baseline; unclear if statistically superior to medications alone.
Hyperlipidemia	Cohort study	Nakaya[9] 1988	30	Yes	0	Small	NA	NA	Significant reduction in LDL and blood pressure from baseline in both groups; no significant change in body weight, HDL, triglycerides.
Diabetes mellitus (type 2)	Cohort study	Mani[23] 2000	15	No	0	Small	NA	NA	Control group received no intervention; significant decrease in FBS levels, triglycerides, and total cholesterol after 2 months of 200 mg of spirulina bid.
Weight loss	Double-blind, crossover study	Becker[24] 1986	16	No	3	Small	NA	NA	Brief study; no significant difference between groups (no power calculation); few adverse effects noted.
Oral leukoplakia	RCT, placebo-controlled	Mathew[25] 1995	115	Yes	2	Small	38%	3	*S. fusiformis* superior to placebo for regression of lesions; 45% relapsed after discontinuing spirulina. 24% dropout; no intention-to-treat analysis.

*Primary or secondary outcome.
[†]N, Number of patients; SS, statistically significant; ARR, absolute risk reduction; NNT, the number of patients who need to undergo a specific intervention in order to observe an outcome in one individual.
[‡]0-2 = poor; 3-4 = good; 5 = excellent.
FBS, Fasting blood sugar; HDL, high-density lipoprotein; LDL, low-density lipoprotein; NA, not applicable; RCT, randomized, controlled trial.
For an explanation of each category in this table, please see Table 3 in the Introduction.

Triglycerides, free fatty acids, and cholesterol levels were measured at baseline and at 1 and 2 months after the start of the study. The authors reported a significant decrease in serum triglycerides, free fatty acids, and total cholesterol levels after 2 months in the spirulina group, with no differences in the control group. However, these results can only be considered preliminary: The study design was incompletely described; lack of blinding or randomization increases the possibility of bias or confounding; the study was short in duration in the setting of serum values that may take several weeks to change during therapy; and magnitude of benefit and statistical analysis were not clearly reported. Additional study is warranted in this area before a firm conclusion can be drawn.

- Samuels et al. conducted a controlled trial in which 23 children with hyperlipidemia associated with nephrotic syndrome were assigned to receive a medication regimen either with or without spirulina.[42] After a 2-month period, triglycerides and LDL levels fell significantly in both groups compared with baseline. Although this decrease appeared to be greater in the spirulina group, no between-group statistical comparisons were made. Therefore, these results can only be considered preliminary.

Diabetes Mellitus (Type 2)
Summary

- Preliminary human data from a small, methodologically weak trial in patients with type 2 diabetes found beneficial effects on lipids and fasting blood sugars after 2 months of oral spirulina treatment.[23] Animal studies using spirulina have

demonstrated reductions in serum cholesterol and triglyceride levels.[9,10,39-41] Currently, there is insufficient human evidence to recommend either for or against the use of spirulina for the control of blood glucose or lipid levels in diabetics.

Evidence

- Mani et al. observed the effects of 2 g of spirulina daily for 2 months (Multinal, New Ambadi Estate Pvt. Ltd., Algal Division, Madras, India) in 15 patients with type 2 diabetes.[23] Seven additional diabetic patients served as a control group and received no spirulina supplementation. Patients were instructed to take one spirulina tablet (1 g) with lunch and dinner each day for two months, and to change nothing else about their lifestyle during this time (diet, exercise, medications). Baseline assessment included fasting blood sugar, glycated serum protein, uronic acid, triglycerides, free fatty acids, and cholesterol levels. These parameters were reevaluated at 1 and 2 months after the start of the study. The authors reported a significant decrease in fasting blood sugars, glycated serum protein, triglycerides, free fatty acids, and total cholesterol levels after 2 months in the spirulina group vs. no change in the control group. However, these results can only be considered preliminary: the study design was incompletely described; lack of blinding or randomization increased the possibility of bias or confounding; the study was short in duration in the setting of serum values that may take several weeks to change during therapy; and magnitude of benefit and statistical analysis were not clearly reported. Additional study is warranted in this area before any conclusion can be drawn.

Weight Loss
Summary

- Spirulina is a popular therapy for weight loss and is sometimes marketed as a "vitamin enriched" appetite suppressant. Preliminary research has been conducted in animals, but there is a paucity of human data. A small, methodologically flawed study from 1986 found no benefit of spirulina over placebo. At this time, the evidence does not support a recommendation either for or against the use of spirulina for weight loss.

Evidence

- Becker et al. conducted a double-blind, crossover study evaluating the effect of 200-mg spirulina tablets vs. placebo (tablets containing 200 mg of spinach powder) on weight loss in 15 volunteers.[24] These individuals had been following a dietitian-approved reduced-calorie diet for 3 months before beginning spirulina supplementation. The subjects were instructed to take 14 tablets before meals three times daily and to return every 2 weeks for a physical exam. Four weeks of treatment were followed by a 2-week washout period and then crossover to the alternate therapy. Individuals taking spirulina experienced a small, significant decrease in body weight from baseline, but there was no significant difference from findings with placebo. This suggests that either there was no benefit of spirulina, or that the study was underpowered (too small) to detect benefits. A possible confounding factor is the reduced-calorie diet that subjects were on prior to the study. The brief study period may not have been adequate to detect results. Measures of appetite were not used in this study. Because of the methodologic flaws, the results cannot be considered conclusive. Further study is warranted in light of the popularity of this indication.

Oral Leukoplakia/Cancer
Summary

- Animal studies have shown spirulina to prevent the development of 7,12-dimethylbenz[a]anthracene-induced oral tumors when fed to hamsters.[5,6] These preventive properties of spirulina may or may not extend to the development of oral cancers in humans. One methodologically weak human trial reported benefit of S. fusiformis for precancerous oral leukoplakia (of homogeneous histology) in tobacco and alcohol users. However, additional human studies are warranted before a recommendation can be made.

Evidence

- Mathew et al. randomized 115 patients with oral leukoplakia to receive either S. fusiformis 1 g daily (New Ambadi Estates, Madras, India) or placebo for a 1-year period.[25] Patients were also encouraged to discontinue the use of tobacco and alcohol products. The number, type, and size of the lesions were assessed at baseline and every 2 months during the study. Complete response to spirulina was defined as disappearance of lesions as assessed by visual inspection. At the end of 1 year, 44 subjects in the spirulina group and 43 subjects in the placebo group had completed the study. The other 24% were considered dropouts because of noncompliance after the first month and were not included in the remainder of the trial. The authors reported that a significantly larger number of subjects with homogeneous lesions in the spirulina group entered complete remission as compared with the placebo group, with a calculated absolute risk reduction of 38% and number needed to treat of 3.

Notably, 45% of those experiencing a complete remission in the spirulina group relapsed within 1 year of stopping treatment. Although these results are compelling, a number of design flaws weaken the clinical applicability of these results. The blinding protocol was not described and may have been inadequate; a majority of subjects were diagnosed with histologically homogeneous leukoplakia, which has a tendency to spontaneously regress even without treatment; benefit was not demonstrated for nonhomogeneous oral leukoplakia; and the lack of an intention-to-treat analysis limits the validity of results. Additional studies with adequate power, proper blinding and randomization, and longer duration are warranted before a firm conclusion can be drawn.

Malnutrition
Summary

- Spirulina has been studied as a food supplement in infant malnutrition. In a clinical, multicenter, randomized, controlled trial, 182 malnourished children under the age of 2 years were given spirulina as a food supplement.[43] The authors observed no added benefit of spirulina over traditional nutrition. Spirulina supplementation is often more costly and is currently not recommended for this condition.

FORMULARY: BRANDS USED IN CLINICAL TRIALS
Brands Used in Statistically Significant Clinical Trials

- Multinal (New Ambadi Estate, Madras, India).[23]

References

1. Kim HM, Lee EH, Cho HH, et al. Inhibitory effect of mast cell–mediated immediate-type allergic reactions in rats by spirulina. Biochem Pharmacol 1998;55(7):1071-1076.
2. Yang HN, Lee EH, Kim HM. *Spirulina platensis* inhibits anaphylactic reaction. Life Sci 1997;61(13):1237-1244.
3. Kapoor R, Mehta U. Iron status and growth of rats fed different dietary iron sources. Plant Foods Hum Nutr 1993;44(1):29-34.
4. Gonzalez R, Rodriguez S, Romay C, et al. Anti-inflammatory activity of phycocyanin extract in acetic acid–induced colitis in rats. Pharmacol Res 1999;39(1):1055-1059.
5. Schwartz J, Shklar G, Reid S, et al. Prevention of experimental oral cancer by extracts of *Spirulina-Dunaliella* algae. Nutr Cancer 1988;11(2):127-134.
6. Shklar G, Schwartz J. Tumor necrosis factor in experimental cancer regression with alphatocopherol, beta-carotene, canthaxanthin and algae extract. Eur J Cancer Clin Oncol 1988;24(5):839-850.
7. Miranda MS, Cintra RG, Barros SB, et al. Antioxidant activity of the microalga *Spirulina maxima*. Braz J Med Biol Res 1998;31(8):1075-1079.
8. Romay C, Armesto J, Remirez D, et al. Antioxidant and anti-inflammatory properties of C-phycocyanin from blue-green algae. Inflamm Res 1998;47(1):36-41.
9. Nakaya N, Homma Y, Goto Y. Cholesterol lowering effect of spirulina. Nutrit Rep Int 1988;37(6):1329-1337.
10. Gonzalez dR, Miranda-Zamora R, Diaz-Zagoya JC, et al. Preventive effect of *Spirulina maxima* on the fatty liver induced by a fructose-rich diet in the rat, a preliminary report. Life Sci 1993;53(1):57-61.
11. Torres-Duran PV, Miranda-Zamora R, Paredes-Carbajal MC, et al. *Spirulina maxima* prevents induction of fatty liver by carbon tetrachloride in the rat. Biochem Mol Biol Int 1998;44(4):787-793.
12. Hayashi K, Hayashi T, Kojima I. A natural sulfated polysaccharide, calcium spirulan, isolated from *Spirulina platensis*: in vitro and ex vivo evaluation of anti-herpes simplex virus and anti-human immunodeficiency virus activities. AIDS Res Hum Retroviruses 1996;12(15):1463-1471.
13. Ayehunie S, Belay A, Baba TW, et al. Inhibition of HIV-1 replication by an aqueous extract of *Spirulina platensis* (*Arthrospira platensis*). J Acquir Immune Defic Syndr Hum Retrovirol 1998;18(1):7-12.
14. Hayashi O, Katoh T, Okuwaki Y. Enhancement of antibody production in mice by dietary *Spirulina platensis*. J Nutr Sci Vitaminol (Tokyo) 1994;40(5):431-441.
15. Jensen GS, Ginsberg DI. Consumption of *Aphanizomenon flos aquae* has rapid effects on the circulation and function of immune cells in humans. J Amer Nutraceut Assoc 2000;2(3):50-58.
16. Jensen GS, Ginsberg DI, Drapeau C. Blue-green algae as an immunoenhancer and biomodulator. J Amer Nutraceut Assoc 2001;3(4):24-30.
17. Johnson PE, Shubert LE. Availability of iron to rats from *Spirulina*, a blue-green alga. Nutr Res 1986;6:85.

18. Kapoor R, Mehta U. Supplementary effect of spirulina on hematological status of rats during pregnancy and lactation. Plant Foods Hum Nutr 1998; 52(4):315-324.

19. Fukino H. Effect of spirulina (*S. platensis*) on the renal toxicity induced by inorganic mercury and cisplatin. Eisei Kagaku 1990;36:5.

20. Evets L. Means to normalize the levels of immunoglobulin E, using the food supplement spirulina. Russian Federation Committee of Patents and Trade 1994; Patent (19)(RU (11)):2005486.

21. Mittalo A, Kumar A, Rao T. Modulatory influence of *Spirulina fusiformis* on 7, 12-dimethylbenz[a]anthracene induced papillomagenesis in the skin of mice. Pharmaceut Biol 1998;36(5):341-346.

22. Kapoor R, Mehta U. Effect of supplementation of blue green alga (*Spirulina*) on outcome of pregnancy in rats. Plant Foods Hum Nutr 1993; 43(1):29-35.

23. Mani UV, Desai S, Iyer U. Studies on the long-term effect of spirulina supplementation on serum lipid profile and glycated proteins in NIDDM patients. J Nutraceut 2000;2(3):25-32.

24. Becker EW, Jakober B, Luft D, et al. Clinical and biochemical evaluations of the alga spirulina with regard to its application in the treatment of obesity. A double-blind cross-over study. Nutr Report Internat 1986;33(4):565-574.

25. Mathew B, Sankaranarayanan R, Nair PP, et al. Evaluation of chemoprevention of oral cancer with *Spirulina fusiformis*. Nutr Cancer 1995;24(2):197-202.

26. Shastri D, Kumar M, Kumar A. Modulation of lead toxicity by *Spirulina fusiformis*. Phytother Res 1999;13(3):258-260.

27. Salazar M, Martinez E, Madrigal E, et al. Subchronic toxicity study in mice fed *Spirulina maxima*. J Ethnopharmacol 1998;62(3):235-241.

28. Salazar M, Chamorro GA, Salazar S, et al. Effect of *Spirulina maxima* consumption on reproduction and peri- and postnatal development in rats. Food Chem Toxicol 1996;34(4):353-359.

29. Chamorro G, Salazar M. [Teratogenic study of *Spirulina* in mice]. Arch Latinoam Nutr 1990;40(1):86-94.

30. Chamorro GA, Herrera G, Salazar M, et al. Short-term toxicity study of *Spirulina* in F3b generation rats. J Toxicol Clin Exp 1988;8(3):163-167.

31. Chamorro GA, Herrera G, Salazar M, et al. Subchronic toxicity study in rats fed *Spirulina*. J Pharm Belg 1988;43(1):29-36.

32. Oishi S, Watanabe MF. Acute toxicity of *Microcystis aeruginosa* and its cardiovascular effects. Environ Res 1986;40(2):518-524.

33. Johnson PE, Shubert LE. Accumulation of mercury and other elements by *Spirulina* (Cyanophyceae). Nutr Rep Int 1986;34:1063-1070.

34. Iwasa M, Yamamoto M, Tanaka Y, et al. Spirulina-associated hepatotoxicity. Am J Gastroenterol 2002;97(12):3212-3213.

35. Mishima T, Murata J, Toyoshima M, et al. Inhibition of tumor invasion and metastasis by calcium spirulan (Ca-SP), a novel sulfated polysaccharide derived from a blue-green alga, *Spirulina platensis*. Clin Exp Metastasis 1998;16:541-550.

36. Narasimha DL, Venkataraman GS, Duggal SK, et al. Nutritional quality of the blue-green alga *Spirulina platensis* Geitler. J Sci Food Agric 1982;33(5):456-460.

37. Mitchell GV, Grundel E, Jenkins M, et al. Effects of graded dietary levels of *Spirulina maxima* on vitamins A and E in male rats. J Nutr 1990; 120(10):1235-1240.

38. Parada JL, Zulpa dC, Zaccaro de Mule MC, et al. Lactic acid bacteria growth promoters from *Spirulina platensis*. Int J Food Microbiol 1998; 45(3):225-228.

39. Iwata K, Inayama T, Kato T. Effects of *Spirulina platensis* on plasma lipoprotein lipase activity in fructose-induced hyperlipidemic rats. J Nutr Sci Vitaminol (Tokyo) 1990;36(2):165-171.

40. Iwata K, Inayama T, Kato T. Effects of *Spirulina platensis* on fructose-induced hyperlipidemia in rats. Nippon Eiyo Shokuryo Gakkaishi (J Jpn Soc Nutr Food Sci) 1987;40:463-467.

41. Kato T, Takemoto K, Katayama H, et al. Effects of spirulina (*Spirulina platensis*) on dietary hypercholesterolemia in rats. Nippon Eiyo Shokuryo Gakkaishi (J Jpn Soc Nutr Food Sci) 1984;37:323-332.

42. Samuels R, Mani UV, Iyer UM, et al. Hypocholesterolemic effect of spirulina in patients with hyperlipidemic nephrotic syndrome. J Med Food 2002;5(2):91-96.

43. Branger B, Cadudal JL, Delobel M, et al. [Spiruline as a food supplement in case of infant malnutrition in Burkina-Faso]. Arch Pediatr 2003;10(5): 424-431.

S

St. John's Wort
(*Hypericum perforatum* L.)

SYNONYMS/COMMON NAMES/RELATED SUBSTANCES

- Amber touch-and-heal, balm-of-warrior's wound, balsana, bassant, blutkraut, bossant, corancillo, dendlu, devil's scourge, eisenblut, flor de Sao Joa, fuga daemonum, goatweed, hartheu, heofarigo on herba de millepertius, herba hyperici, herrgottsblut, hexenkraut, hierba de San Juan, hipericao, hiperico, hipericon, Johanniskraut, klammath weed, liebeskraut, LI 160, Lord God's wonder plant, millepertius, pelicao, perforate, pinillo de oro, rosin rose, tenturotou, teufelsflucht, touch and heal, Walpurgiskraut, witcher's herb.

CLINICAL BOTTOM LINE
Background

- Extracts of *Hypericum perforatum* L. (St. John's wort) have been used traditionally for a wide range of medical conditions. The most common modern-day application for St. John's wort is in the treatment of depressive disorders.[1] Meta-analyses of small, heterogeneous studies conducted over the past two decades, and several subsequent randomized trials, have reported St. John's wort to be more effective than placebo and equally effective as tricyclic antidepressants in the short-term management of mild to moderate depression (1 to 3 months in duration). Comparisons with selective serotonin reuptake inhibitor (SSRI) antidepressants have provided equivocal data.
- Controversy has been raised by the negative results of two well-conducted trials of St. John's wort for major depression. However, one of these studies did not include a reference-agent arm (comparison only with placebo),[2] and the other reported negative results for an SSRI (sertraline) as well as for St. John's wort in a study of patients with severe (rather than mild to moderate) major depressive disorder.[3] Overall, the evidence supporting the efficacy of St. John's wort in mild to moderate major depression remains compelling, whereas the evidence for severe major depression is equivocal.
- Although this herb is generally well tolerated in clinical use, there is accumulating evidence of significant St. John's wort/drug interactions, particularly when the herb is used with medications metabolized by the cytochrome P450 system. St. John's wort is not recommended in patients with HIV infection/AIDS who are taking protease inhibitors or non-nucleoside reverse transcriptase inhibitors, in patients receiving immunosuppressive therapy (particularly with cyclosporine), and in users of oral contraceptives, warfarin, or digoxin. St. John's wort may induce mania in individuals with an underlying mood disorder and may result in the serotonin syndrome if used alone or with other serotonergic agents.

Scientific Evidence for Common/Studied Uses	Grade*
Depressive disorder (mild to moderate)	A
Anxiety disorder	C
Depressive disorder (severe)	C
Obsessive-compulsive disorder (OCD)	C
Perimenopausal symptoms	C
Premenstrual syndrome (PMS)	C
Seasonal affective disorder (SAD)	C
Human immunodeficiency virus (HIV) infection	D

*Key to grades: *A:* Strong scientific evidence for this use; *B:* Good scientific evidence for this use; *C:* Unclear scientific evidence for this use; *D:* Fair scientific evidence against this use (it may not work); *F:* Strong scientific evidence against this use (it likely does not work). For a more detailed explanation of efficacy criteria, see "Natural Standard Evidence-Based Validated Grading Rationale" in the Introduction.

Historical or Theoretical Indications That Lack Sufficient Evidence

- Abrasions (topical), alcoholism,[4,5] analgesia, anti-inflammatory,[6,7] antioxidant,[8,9] antimalarial, antiviral,[10] athletic performance,[11] bacterial skin infections (topical), bedwetting, bruises (topical), benzodiazepine withdrawal, burns (topical), cancer,[12] contusions, chronic nonspecific colitis,[13] chronic suppurative otitis,[14] dental pain,[15] diarrhea, dyspepsia, diuretic, Epstein-Barr virus infection,[16] fatigue,[17] gastroenteritis, glioma,[18] hemorrhoids, hepatoprotection,[19] herpes virus infection,[20] hypnotic,[21] influenza, menorrhagia, neuralgia, nicotine withdrawal,[22] painful polyneuropathy,[23] rheumatism, snakebite, sprains, ulcers, wound healing (topical).[24]

Expert Opinion and Folkloric Precedent

- References to the use of St. John's wort in healing can be found for the last 2000 years, dating back to the time of the early Greeks. St. John's wort has been extensively investigated for mild to moderate depression. It is a popular agent internationally, with approval by the German federal drug regulatory agency (Bundesgesundheitsamt). It is a leading treatment for depression in Germany.[25]
- There is growing popularity in the United States, accompanied by efforts to develop more rigorous scientific support.

Safety Summary

- **Likely safe:** Extensive clinical trials of limited duration (<3 months) at recommended doses support the safety and benign side effect profile of St. John's wort in individuals not taking other drugs.
- **Possibly unsafe:** When used in larger than recommended doses, or for extended duration (>3 months).
- **Likely unsafe:** When taken by individuals with HIV infection or AIDS concomitantly with protease inhibitors, or non-nucleoside reverse transcriptase inhibitors because of multiple reported interactions. When taken by individuals receiving immunosuppressive therapy, particularly cyclosporine, because of to case reports of reduced cyclosporine serum levels, and associated transplant rejection. When taken by women on concomitant oral contraceptives, because

of recent reports of unwanted pregnancies. When taken by individuals on concomitant warfarin and digoxin, because of reports of reduced efficacy or drug concentration. When used concomitantly with drugs metabolized by the P450 system (particularly CYP 3A4 and CYP 2D6).

DOSING/TOXICOLOGY
General

- Recommended doses are based on those most commonly used in available trials, or on historical practice. However, with natural products, the optimal doses needed to balance efficacy and safety often have not been determined. Formulations and preparation methods may vary from manufacturer to manufacturer, and from batch to batch of a specific product made by a single manufacturer. Because often the active components of a product are not known, standardization may not be possible, and the clinical effects of different brands may not be comparable.

Standardization

- St. John's wort products are often standardized to 0.3% hypericin extract, although there has been a movement within the manufacturing industry to standardize to hyperforin (usually 2% to 5%). Standardization of extracts may not be clinically relevant in predicting effectiveness, as the active ingredient in St. John's wort has not been definitively determined.
- Analysis of eight German St. John's wort products revealed large differences in hypericin and hyperforin content and varying degrees of interbatch variability. Therefore, the authors of the study concluded that the St. John's wort brands tested are not interchangeable for the treatment of mild to moderate depression, and that health care providers should take this into consideration when counseling patients.[26]
- An analysis of the hypericin and pseudohypericin levels in commercially available St. John's wort products using liquid chromatography reported wide variations in levels of constituents compared with label claims (0% to 109% for capsules; 31% to 80% for tablets; 0% to 119% for tinctures).[27] The levels of these constituents in most products were not within 10% of claimed levels.

Dosing: Adult (18 Years and Older)
Oral

- **Depression:** *Starting dose:* 300 mg of standardized 0.3% hypericin extract by mouth three times daily (may be standardized to 2% to 5% hyperforin as well). *Maintenance dose:* 300 to 600 mg daily may be sufficient for maintenance therapy, although this has not been extensively studied. Clinical trials have used a range of doses, including 0.17 to 2.7 mg of hypericin[28] and 900 to 1450 mg of extract daily.[2,29] A liquid form may be used as well, taken three times daily and standardized to contain equivalent amounts of hypericin or hypericin, as noted.[30-35]
- *Note:* Depression is a serious illness, and individuals should be evaluated by a physician or mental health professional before self-medicating with St. John's wort.[36]

Dosing: Pediatric (Younger Than 18 Years)

- There is insufficient available evidence to recommend the safe use of St. John's wort in children. For depression, limited clinical information exists in pediatric populations. A multicenter trial of 101 children younger than 12 years of

age used 300 to 1800 mg of extract daily, with good tolerability.[37] An open-label study in 33 children (6 to 16 years old, mean age 10.5 years) administered 900 mg daily of St. John's wort for 4 weeks, with good reported tolerance.[38]

Toxicology

- Toxicologic research using St. John's wort extract LI 160 reports a no-effect dose to be above 5000 mg/kg in mice and rats. Study of chronic toxicity in rats and dogs has found only nonspecific symptoms such as weight loss.[39] *In vivo* and *in vitro* studies have not demonstrated significant mutagenic properties of St. John's wort.[40,41] One study in genotoxicity in *Salmonella typhimurium*, suggesting that this effect was due to quercetin.[42,43]
- The United States Cosmetic Ingredient Review Expert Panel recently concluded that there are insufficient data to support the safety of St. John's wort and its constituents in cosmetic formulations.

ADVERSE EFFECTS/PRECAUTIONS/CONTRAINDICATIONS
Allergy

- Infrequent allergic skin reactions, including rash, itching, and pruritus, have been reported in clinical trials.
- In a drug monitoring study of 3250 patients, there were 17 cases of allergic reactions and 10 cases of allergy-related treatment discontinuation.[44]

Adverse Effects

- **General:** In published studies, St. John's wort has been generally well tolerated at recommended doses for up to 1 to 3 months. Most common adverse effects include gastrointestinal symptoms, skin reactions, fatigue/sedation, restlessness or anxiety, dizziness, headache, and dry mouth.[44-47] Several recent meta-analyses and a report of a clinical trial conclude that adverse event rates are comparable to those noted for placebo[2,28,48,49] and less than with standard antidepressant treatment.[28,48,50-52] Data from observational studies indicate that adverse events may occur in 1% to 3% of patients. A review of adverse events occurring during treatment with Jarsin 300/Jarsin (LI 160; daily dose of 900 mg of extract = 1.08 mg of hypericin) from 1991 to 1999, involving approximately 8 million people, documented 95 adverse event reports.[47] A European drug-monitoring study of 3250 patients (Jarsin 300 in a dose of 900 mg daily) reported an overall adverse reaction rate of 2.4%.[44] A postmarketing study of Aristoforat documented the incidence of adverse events to be 1% in 2404 ambulatory patients, over a 4- to 6-week period.[45] Plasma levels to 300 ng/mL have been tolerated.[53]
- **Dermatologic (allergy):** Infrequent allergic skin reactions, including rash, itching, and pruritus, have been reported in clinical trials. A review of adverse events occurring during treatment with Jarsin/Jarsin 300 from 1991 to 1999, involving approximately 8 million people, documented 27 adverse skin reactions.[47]
- **Dermatologic (photosensitization):** Photosensitization has been reported since the early 1900s in grazing animals consuming St. John's wort flowering plants.[54] Several cases of reversible photosensitivity to St. John's wort have been reported.[55] Itchy erythematous lesions developed on light-exposed areas of skin in one patient after taking 240 mg of hypericum extract daily for 3 years.[56] In another case, a burning, erythematous eruption occurred after 4 days of treatment with 333 mg of hypericum extract.[56,57] Lane-

Brown presented three cases of phototoxicity associated with topical and oral St. John's wort, with manifestations of erythematobullous dermatosis and facial bullae related to sun exposure in one patient, ultraviolet B (UVB) phototherapy–related follicular erythema in a second patient, and urticarial edema in a third.[58] Phase I studies of intravenous and oral hypericin in HIV-infected adults observed severe cutaneous phototoxicity in 11 of 23 subjects[59] and a variety of photosensitivity reactions in 14 of 19 subjects with hepatitis C.[10] However, Brockmöller did not find a correlation between photosensitivity and total plasma hypericum concentrations in human volunteers, after a single oral dose of 900 to 3600 mg of hypericin extract.[60] The same report noted a small but significant increase in solar and ultraviolet A (UVA) light sensitivity over 15 days of 1800 mg of hypericum extract daily. Another study did not find phototoxic potential with oral L160.[61] A more recent study found peak hypericin levels in skin blister fluid following administration of an oral dose of 1800 mg or steady-state administration (900 mg/day for 7 days) to be at least 20 times less than the estimated phototoxic concentration of 100 μg/mL.[62] An additional study found phototoxicity after irradiation with UVA and visible light only at high concentrations.[63]

- **Dermatologic (alopecia):** Persistent scalp and eyebrow hair loss has been described in a 24-year-old woman with schizophrenia treated with the antipsychotic medication olanzapine (Zyprexa), occurring 5 months following augmentation with 900 mg/day of St. John's wort.[64]
- **Neurologic/CNS (headache):** In a large controlled trial, headache occurred more frequently in the St. John's wort group than in the placebo group ($p < 0.02$): 40% vs. 26% of respective samples.[2] However, in multiple other reports, headache has been found rarely.[45-47]
- **Neurologic/CNS (neuropathy):** Isolated cases of paresthesia[46] and neuropathy have been reported. Bove described a 35-year-old woman who developed subacute toxic neuropathy after taking 500 mg/day of St. John's wort for 4 weeks.[65] The subject experienced a stinging pain on exposure to mechanical stimuli that worsened during and after exposure to sun on her face and dorsa of both hands. Her symptoms began to subside after St. John's wort was withdrawn and gradually disappeared over 2 months.
- **Psychiatric (anxiety):** Restlessness, insomnia, and anxiety have been noted; 15 psychiatric adverse events were reported in a World Health Organization database up to 1998[46]; 8 reports of anxiety occurred in a sample of 3250 subjects[66]; 5 patients reported nervousness and anxiety in a postmarketing trial comprising 2404 patients.[45]
- **Psychiatric (mania):** Possible St. John's wort–induced mania has been described in several case reports; a majority had histories of affective illness, including unipolar (major depression) and bipolar (major depression and mania or hypomania) disorder.[67-70] Barbenel described a manic episode in a 28-year-old man, following 5 weeks of simultaneous ingestion of St. John's wort and 50 mg/day of sertraline (Zoloft), an SSRI antidepressant.[71]
- **Psychiatric (serotonin syndrome):** Serotonin syndrome is characterized by rigidity, hyperthermia, delirium, confusion, autonomic instability, and coma. There is a case report of possible serotonin syndrome associated with St. John's wort, manifested by transient flushing, diaphoresis, hypertension, disorientation, dyspnea, and tremors in a 40-year-old man. The patient, who had a history of depression and SSRI-

induced mania, was not taking other medications.[64] Another report described a 33-year-old woman with mild anxiety who experienced multiple anxiety episodes with autonomic arousal (blood pressure to a maximum of 195/110 mm Hg) following three doses of St. John's wort.[72] In a telephone survey, one woman reported nausea, diaphoresis, muscle cramping, weakness, and elevated pulse and blood pressure after a single dose of combination St. John's wort, kava, and valerian.[73]
- **Psychiatric (psychosis):** Lal reported psychotic decompensation in two schizophrenic patients that was temporally associated with the consumption of St. John's wort. However, both patients had discontinued antipsychotic medication prior to relapse.[74] An additional case report described psychotic features and delirium in a 76-year-old woman with Alzheimer's dementia, associated with 3 weeks of self-medication with St. John's wort.[75]
- **Psychiatric (withdrawal):** Possible withdrawal symptoms associated with cessation of chronic St. John's wort has been reported.[76]
- **Cardiovascular:** Cases of possible serotonin syndrome have been reported with the use of St. John's wort. This syndrome is characterized by rigidity, hyperthermia, delirium, confusion, autonomic instability, and coma. A recent case report described recurrent episodes of autonomic arousal with blood pressures up to 195/110 mm Hg in a previously healthy woman after taking three doses of St. John's wort.[72] Other case reports of hypertension and tachycardia have also been described.[64,77,78] No cardiac conduction abnormalities have been found with high dose St. John's wort.[79] No difference in blood pressure or heart rate was found in a 6-week comparison of 1800 mg/day of St. John's wort and 150 mg/day of imipramine in 200 adults.[50] "Swelling" was noted in 19% of patients taking 900 to 1500 mg of St. John's wort daily for 8 weeks, vs. 8% of placebo patients and 8% of sertraline (Zoloft) patients.[3]
- **Gastrointestinal:** Infrequent dyspepsia, anorexia, diarrhea, nausea, and constipation have been reported in controlled trials.[51,80] Gastrointestinal symptoms were reported in 18 of 3250 adult subjects.[66]
- **Genitourinary:** Anorgasmia was reported in 25% of patients taking 900 to 1500 mg of St. John's wort daily for 8 weeks, vs. 16% of those taking placebo and 32% of those taking sertraline (Zoloft).[3] In addition, there are two published reports of sexual dysfunction associated with St. John's wort. A 42-year-old man with mood and anxiety disorders experienced decreased libido after ingesting St. John's wort for 9 months. Notably, the subject had subsequent recurrent depressive symptoms. His sexual libido returned when St. John's wort was discontinued and an SSRI, citalopram (Celexa), was initiated.[81] A 49-year-old man with a 10-year history of recurrent depression experienced orgasmic delay, erectile dysfunction, and inhibited sexual desire when taking the SSRI sertraline (Zoloft).[82] The SSRI was discontinued, with resolution of symptoms; however, 1 week after beginning therapy with St. John's wort, the patient experienced erectile dysfunction and orgasmic delay. Co-administration of sildenafil (Viagra), 25 to 50 mg, prior to sexual activity reversed the sexual dysfunction. Frequent urination was reported in 27% of patients taking 900 to 1500 mg of St. John's wort daily for 8 weeks, vs. 11% of those taking placebo and 21% of those taking sertraline (Zoloft).[3] Inhibition of sperm motility due to St. John's wort has been observed *in vitro*.[83]

Precautions/Warnings/Contraindications

- Avoid in patients with known allergy/hypersensitivity to St. John's wort or to any of its constituents.
- Avoid in patients with HIV infection/AIDS who are taking protease inhibitors or non-nucleoside reverse transcriptase inhibitors (NNRTIs), as suggested by the U.S. Food and Drug Administration, because of documented reductions in drug concentrations with concomitant St. John's wort.[84-86]
- Avoid in transplant recipients on cyclosporine, because of numerous reports of significant reduction in drug levels and possible organ rejection with concomitant St. John's wort.[87-99]
- Use cautiously in patients taking medications metabolized by cytochrome P450, because of reported significant interactions.[100-102] This may be of particular concern with substrates of CYP 3A4, which St. John's wort appears to acutely inhibit and chronically induce.[86,103-106]
- Use cautiously in patients with sensitive skin or those taking photosensitizing drugs, because of risk of photosensitivity, documented in case reports.[107,108]
- Use cautiously in patients taking warfarin, because of case reports of reduced efficacy with concomitant St. John's wort.[86,109]
- Use cautiously in patients on monoamine oxidase inhibitors (MAOIs) or selective serotonin reuptake inhibitors (SSRIs), because of theoretical risk of serotonin syndrome with concomitant St. John's wort.[59,64,72,77]
- Use cautiously in patients taking digoxin, because of a controlled study that demonstrated reduced drug concentration with concomitant St. John's wort.[86,110,111]
- Use cautiously in women on oral contraceptives, because of reports of altered menstrual flow, bleeding, and unwanted pregnancies with concomitant St. John's wort.[109,112]
- Use cautiously in persons with a history of mania, hypomania (as in bipolar disorder), or affective illness, because of case reports of possible St. John's wort–induced manic episodes, as has been observed with standard antidepressant medications.[67-71]

Pregnancy and Lactation

- Although case reports exist of human exposure to St. John's wort during pregnancy,[113] there are insufficient data available at this time to recommend use during pregnancy or breastfeeding.[114]
- Breast milk samples were obtained from a woman with postnatal depression, taking St. John's wort (Jarsin 300, three times daily). Only hyperforin was excreted into the breast milk at quantifiable levels. No adverse effects on mother or infant were noted.[115]
- In a small safety study, 33 breastfeeding women taking St. John's wort who reported to a teratogen/toxicology reporting service were matched with 101 breastfeeding women not taking St. John's wort.[116] The authors reported no significant differences in adverse effects or lactation duration between groups, although there were nonsignificant differences: There were 2 reports of colicky infants in the St. John's wort group vs. 1 in the group not taking St. John's wort, and 2 cases of "drowsiness" and 1 case of "lethargy" with St. John's wort vs. none reported in the matched controls. Because of the small sample size and nature of the reporting mechanism (leading to possible bias and self-selection), it remains unclear if the excess adverse events were actually attributable to St. John's wort. None of the adverse events required medical treatment.

- Administration of St. John's wort to mice before and throughout gestation did not significantly impact cognitive tasks performed by their offspring.[117]

INTERACTIONS
St. John's Wort/Drug Interactions

- **Drugs metabolized via cytochrome P450 (CYP 2C9, CYP 2D6, CYP 2E1, CYP 3A4):** Concurrent use of drugs metabolized via the CYP450 liver enzyme system may result in altered therapeutic levels of pharmacologic agents, due to induction or inhibition of enzymes by St. John's wort.[118] Human studies have reported induction of 3A/3A4 according to reduction of nifedipine concentration,[103] midazolam,[104] and in pharmacokinetic study.[105] Moore et al. have recently demonstrated that St. John's wort (hyperforin) activates a regulator (pregnane X receptor) of 3A4 transcription and thereby induces expression of 3A4 in human liver cells.[106] Although authors have reported *in vivo* and *in vitro* 2C9, 2D6, and 3A4 inhibition,[100,101] a brief, 3-day human trial did not demonstrate a similar significant effect on drugs metabolized by the 2D6 or 3A4 enzyme.[119] Bray has demonstrated induction of 3A and 2E1 in mice.[102] On review, it appears that St. John's wort inhibits CYP 3A4 acutely and then induces this enzyme with repeated administration.[86] Pharmacokinetic studies are ongoing in this area.
- **Cyclosporine (CYP 3A4):** There are numerous reports of significant reduction in cyclosporine drug levels and possible organ rejection with concomitant use of St. John's wort.[87-99] A significant drop in cyclosporine levels was observed in 30 kidney transplant recipients taking St. John's wort. Cyclosporine levels markedly increased after St. John's wort was discontinued.[90,91] There are multiple additional case reports of reduced cyclosporine serum levels in kidney transplant patients receiving concomitant St. John's wort.[92-96] A recent case report of two heart transplant patients demonstrated reductions in cyclosporine levels and acute transplant rejection with St. John's wort.[97] In addition, severe acute rejection developed 14 months after liver transplantation in a 63-year-old patient. Rejection was associated with a sudden drop in cyclosporine levels, which occurred during a 2-week period of ingesting 1800 mg/day of St. John's wort.[98] Reductions in cyclosporine levels in heart transplant patients have been described elsewhere.[99] Effects on cyclosporine levels may also be due to an induction of the drug pump P-glycoprotein.[86,96]
- **Tacrolimus (FK506, Prograf):** There are several reports of decreases in tacrolimus levels in association with St. John's wort use, likely due to effects on P450 3A4.[120-122]
- **Protease inhibitors and non-nucleoside reverse transcriptase inhibitors (NNRTIs) (CYP 3A4):** St. John's wort has been shown to decrease plasma concentrations of protease inhibitors, and non-nucleoside reverse transcriptase inhibitors, possibly due to cytochrome P450 induction. The oral clearance of the NNRTI nevirapine was significantly increased in five HIV-seropositive patients receiving nevirapine and concomitant St. John's wort.[84] An open-label study demonstrated a significant reduction in concentrations of the protease inhibitor indinavir when taken concurrently with St. John's wort by healthy volunteers.[85] Effects on these medications may also be due to an induction of the drug pump P-glycoprotein.[86] The U.S. Food and Drug Administration (FDA) issued an advisory regarding the findings of this trial on February 10, 2000.

S

- **Oral contraceptives/ethinyloestradiol/desogestrol (CYP 3A4):** There are multiple reports of reduced serum level/half-life of oral contraceptives in association with St. John's wort use, likely related to effects on P450 3A4, with alterations in hormone levels, increased breakthrough bleeding, and possible unwanted pregnancies in some cases.[112,123-126] The Medical Products Agency of Sweden received eight case reports of breakthrough bleeding and one case report of changes in menstrual flow from women who were long-time users of oral contraceptives and St. John's wort,[109] also observed in a controlled trial of healthy subjects.[124] The time period between initiation of St. John's wort and the reported event was approximately 1 week.[109] Ratz reported a case of irregular bleeding with St. John's wort and oral contraceptives.[112] In early 2002, warnings emerged following several reports, in Sweden and the United Kingdom, of unwanted pregnancies in women taking oral contraceptives and St. John's wort. Pharmacokinetic/dynamic study is ongoing in this area of concern.

- **Irinotecan (CPT-11, Camptosar):** Patients taking CPT-11 should avoid St. John's wort because of reported significant reductions in serum levels of the pharmacologically active CPT-11 metabolite SN-38. CPT-11 is a chemotherapeutic agent that is eliminated principally via cytochrome P450 3A4 oxidation. An abstract presented by Mathijssen et al. at the American Association for Cancer Research 93rd Annual Meeting reported the effects of St. John's wort in patients taking CPT-11.[127] The regimen used was intravenous CPT-11, 350 mg/m^2, once every 3 weeks. Subjects were randomized to receive either concomitant St. John's wort therapy (300 mg orally three times daily for a 21-day period starting 2 weeks prior to CPT-11) or no additional therapy. Subjects were then "crossed over." "Complete pharmacological data" were available for three subjects (median age, 60 years). The authors report that the addition of St. John's wort to CPT-11 therapy resulted in a >50% mean reduction in the area under the concentration curve (UAC) for the pharmacologically active CPT-11 metabolite SN-38, whereas the UAC for CPT-11 itself was not significantly altered.

- **Warfarin (CYP 2C9):** Seven cases of reduced effects of warfarin (lowered international normalized ratio [INR]) with concomitant St. John's wort have been reported.[109] In most cases, the patients had been stabilized on warfarin for some time prior to ingesting St. John's wort. None of the patients in these cases experienced thromboembolic events; however, the decrease in INR was thought to be clinically significant. Increases in warfarin dose or discontinuation of St. John's wort resulted in return of INR to target values. This interaction may also have been due to an induction of the drug pump P-glycoprotein.[86]

- **Selective serotonin reuptake inhibitors (SSRIs):** Concomitant St. John's wort may lead to increased adverse effects typically associated with SSRI antidepressants, including serotonin syndrome. A case series of elderly depressed patients described dizziness, nausea, vomiting, headache, anxiety, confusion, irritability, and restlessness. Symptoms were associated with addition of St. John's wort to ongoing treatment with sertraline (4 cases) and nefazodone (1 case). Symptoms resolved within 1 week after discontinuation of St. John's wort.[128] A 50-year-old woman with depression became incoherent, groggy, and lethargic after a single evening dose of 20 mg of paroxetine was added to her ongoing St. John's wort regimen of 600 mg/day'. The patient had previously tolerated paroxetine for 8 months.[129] One report appears most consistent with serotonin syndrome: A 61-year-old well woman took a single 20-mg dose of paroxetine 3 days after discontinuing St. John's wort (600 mg daily). Within 24 hours she presented to the hospital restless, diaphoretic, and hypertensive, with hyperreflexia and involuntary movements of all extremities. Her creatine kinase peaked at 1024 U/L. She was discharged 2 days later, following supportive treatment.[130] Barbenel described a manic episode in a 28-year-old man, following 5 weeks of simultaneous ingestion of St. John's wort and 50 mg/day of sertraline.[71]

- **Monoamine oxidase inhibitors (MAOIs):** Early work reported *in vitro* inhibition of monoamine oxidase (MAO) A and B by hypericin,[131] as well as other components, such as xanthon and flavonols.[132] Thiede and Walper found both MAO and catechol-*O*-methyltransferase (COMT) inhibition.[133] Other studies similarly reported weak MAOI properties *in vitro*.[134-137] Yet several of these authors, and others,[134] subsequently suggested that the concentrations causing inhibition were likely not adequate to explain antidepressant activity. Cott reported that hypericin lacked significant MAO inhibition at concentrations up to 10 μM[136] and, on the basis of other findings, such as those from one pharmacokinetic study,[138] suggested that this inhibition may not be pharmacologically relevant. Nonetheless, in theory, St. John's wort may potentiate the effects of MAOIs, theoretically leading to clinical manifestations of toxicity, such as serotonin syndrome or hypertensive crisis.[139]

- **Tricyclic antidepressant drugs (multiple CYP enzymes):** A 14-day open study in 12 depressed patients found a significant reduction in amitriptyline concentration with concurrent ingestion of St. John's wort (900 mg/day).[140,141] A number of CYP enzymes including 1A2, 2C19, 3A4, and 2D6 are involved in the metabolism of tricyclic antidepressants.[142]

- **HMG CoA reductase inhibitors (statins) (CYP 3A4):** The concentrations of simvastatin and its metabolite (but not pravastatin) were significantly lowered with concomitant use of St. John's wort.[142]

- **Anesthetic drugs:** It has been hypothesized that St. John's wort may interact with anesthetic drugs.[144] Cardiovascular collapse during anesthesia was reported in a healthy 23-year-old woman who had been taking St. John's wort daily for 6 months prior to surgery. The patient had undergone uneventful general anesthesia 2 years earlier when she was not taking St. John's wort.[145]

- **Opioids:** A case of decreased methadone levels associated with St. John's wort in a chronic methadone user has been reported.[146] Interactions with oxycodone and fentanyl have also been proposed.

- **5-Hydroxytryptamine-1 (5-HT$_1$) receptor agonists (triptans):** Interaction with various triptan medications, via enhanced serotonergic activity, is possible in theory. Examples of such drugs are naratriptan (Amerge), rizatriptan (Maxalt), sumatriptan (Imitrex), and zolmitriptan (Zomig).

- **Photosensitizing products:** Concurrent use with these numerous agents, including several antibiotics and oral contraceptives, may increase risk of photosensitization.[107] A phototoxic reaction was observed in a patient undergoing experimental treatment with delta-aminolevulinic acid for breast cancer who also had been taking St. John's wort.[108]

- **Antineoplastic drugs:** Theoretically, St. John's wort may antagonize chemotherapeutic agents that are directed against topoisomerase II alpha, such as anthracyclines or cytotoxic agents, as shown *in vitro*.[147]

- **Carbamazepine (CYP 3A4):** A 2-week open study in eight healthy volunteers did not find significant difference in carbamazepine concentrations with concomitant use of St. John's wort. This lack of effect may be due to a system already induced (autoinduction) or to increased clearance of hyperforin by carbamazepine.[148]
- **Digoxin:** A controlled study demonstrated that 10 days of treatment with hypericum extract resulted in a 25% decrease in digoxin AUC. The mechanism may be induction of the P-glycoprotein drug transporter.[86,110,111,141,149-152] Bigeminy was reported in an 80-year-old man taking both digoxin and St. John's wort.[153] Other reports also support this possible interaction.
- **Loperamide (Imodium):** Delirium and agitation were reported in one patient taking loperamide (Imodium), St. John's wort, and valerian.[154] The condition resolved rapidly with discontinuation of treatment.
- **Midazolam (Versed) (CYP 3A4):** A human study reported reductions in midazolam concentration, presumed to be due to CYP 3A4 induction.[103]
- **Nifedipine (Procardia, Adalat) (CYP 3A4):** A human study reported reductions in nifedipine concentration, presumed to be due to CYP 3A4 induction.[103]
- **Theophylline (CYP 1A2):** It remains unclear if serum levels of theophylline or its metabolites are affected by St. John's wort.[86] One report describes a 42-year-old woman who experienced lowered serum theophylline levels on concomitant ingestion of 300 mg/day of St. John's wort. The patient was on multiple other medications and smoked tobacco. Within 1 week of discontinuation of St. John's wort, her theophylline level rose from 9 to 19 µg/mL.[155] However, in a 48-hour study in 12 healthy volunteers given both agents (theophylline 400 mg and St. John's wort 300 mg), no changes were observed in blood or serum levels of theophylline or its metabolites (13U, 1U, 3X). The duration of this study may not have been sufficient to adequately assess this interaction.
- **Alcohol:** A 7-day, randomized, controlled crossover trial (n = 32) concluded that St. John's wort (900 mg/day) did not significantly interact with alcohol to impair cognitive capacities.[156]
- **Thyroid agents:** A retrospective case-control study reported elevated thyroid-stimulating hormone (TSH) levels to be associated with taking St. John's wort (odds ratio of 2.12; 95% confidence interval [CI] 0.36 to 12.36).[157] This small retrospective sample does not present a clear, significant relationship or imply causality.

St. John's Wort/Herb/Supplement Interactions

- **Selective serotonin reuptake inhibitor (SSRI) herbs and supplements:** Concomitant St. John's wort may lead to increased adverse effects typically associated with SSRI antidepressants, including serotonin syndrome. A case series of elderly depressed patients described dizziness, nausea, vomiting, headache, anxiety, confusion, irritability, and restlessness. Symptoms were associated with addition of St. John's wort to ongoing treatment with sertraline (4 cases) and nefazodone (1 case). Symptoms resolved within 1 week after discontinuation of St. John's wort.[128] A 50-year-old woman with depression became incoherent, groggy, and lethargic after a single evening dose of 20 mg of paroxetine was added to her ongoing St. John's wort regimen of 600 mg/day'. The patient had previously tolerated paroxetine for 8 months.[129] One report appears most consistent with serotonin syndrome:

A 61-year-old healthy woman took a single 20-mg dose of paroxetine 3 days after discontinuing St. John's wort (600 mg daily). Within 24 hours she presented to the hospital restless, diaphoretic, and hypertensive, with hyperreflexia and involuntary movements of all extremities. Her creatine kinase peaked at 1024 U/L. She was discharged 2 days later, following supportive treatment.[130] Barbenel described a manic episode in a 28-year-old man, following 5 weeks of simultaneous ingestion of St. John's wort and 50 mg/day of sertraline.[71]

- **Monoamine oxidase inhibitor (MAOI)-like herbs and supplements:** Early work reported *in vitro* inhibition of monoamine oxidase (MAO) A and B by hypericin,[131] as well as other components, such as xanthon and flavonols.[132] Thiede and Walper found both MAO and catechol-O-methyltransferase (COMT) inhibition.[133] Other studies similarly reported weak MAOI properties *in vitro*.[134-137] Yet several of these authors, and others,[134] subsequently suggested that the concentrations causing inhibition were likely not adequate to explain antidepressant activity. Cott reported that hypericin lacked significant MAO inhibition at concentrations up to 10 µM[136] and, on the basis of other findings, such as those from one pharmacokinetic study,[138] suggested that this inhibition may not be pharmacologically relevant. Nonetheless, in theory, St. John's wort may potentiate effects of other herbs with MAOI properties, theoretically leading to clinical manifestations of toxicity, such as serotonin syndrome or hypertensive crisis.[139]
- **Cardiac glycoside herbs and supplements:** A controlled study demonstrated that 10 days of treatment with hypericum extract resulted in a decrease of digoxin by 25%. The mechanism may be induction of the P-glycoprotein drug transporter.[110] Herbs such as foxglove and oleander contain cardiac glycosides that behave similarly to digoxin.
- **Photosensitizing herbs and supplements:** Concurrent use of St. John's wort with other photosensitizing agents may increase the risk of photosensitization[107] (for example, capsaicin). A phototoxic reaction was observed in a patient undergoing experimental treatment with delta-aminolevulinic acid for breast cancer who also had been taking St. John's wort.[108]
- **Iron:** Because of the presence of tannins in St. John's wort, iron absorption may be inhibited.[107]
- **Red yeast rice (*Monascus purpureus*) (CYP 3A4):** Red yeast contains constituents that are identical to the hydroxymethylglutaryl-coenzyme A (HMG-CoA) reductase inhibitor (statin) lovastatin. Because statins such as lovastatin are known substrates of P450 3A4, which is induced by St. John's wort, it is likely that the cholesterol-lowering effects of red yeast would be diminished by St. John's wort. Concentrations of a different statin, simvastatin, and its metabolite (but not pravastatin) were significantly lowered with concomitant St. John's wort.[143] The principal product containing red yeast that had been available in the United States, Cholestin, no longer includes lovastatin.
- **Valerian:** Delirium and agitation were reported in one patient taking valerian (*Valeriana officinalis*), St. John's wort, and loperamide (Imodium).[154] The condition resolved rapidly with discontinuation of treatment.

St. John's Wort/Food Interactions

- **Tyramine-containing foods/beverages:** Weak monoamine oxidase inhibitor (MAOI) activity of St. John's wort has been observed *in vitro*.[131-137] In keeping with warnings accompanying the use of MAOI antidepressants, consumption of tyramine-containing foods with St. John's wort may pose an increased risk of hypertensive crisis. In a telephone survey of 43 subjects who had taken St. John's wort, 39 persons reported ingesting tyramine-rich foods or products. Two persons taking 600 to 900 mg/day reported associated flushing and pounding headaches.[77]

St. John's Wort/Lab Interactions

- **Thyroid-stimulating hormone (TSH):** A retrospective case-control study reported elevated TSH levels to be associated with taking St. John's wort (odds ratio of 2.12; 95% CI, 0.36 to 12.36).[157] This small retrospective sample does not present a clear, significant relationship or imply causality.

MECHANISM OF ACTION
Pharmacology

- **Overview:** St. John's wort for medicinal use is harvested when the flowers start to open and is prepared from the flowering tops or aerial parts of the plant. Herbal preparations are then extracted with ethanol or methanol. Notably, the hyperforin, hypericin, and flavonol components may vary widely according to harvest time, plant quality, and region of origin.[158] The apparent broad mechanism of St. John's wort is not fully understood, yet biologically active constituents may include hyperforin and adhyperforin (phloroglucinols), hypericin and pseudohypericin (naphthodianthrones), flavonoids, xanthones, oligomeric procyanidins, and amino acids.[159,160] Methods for evaluation and standardization of the components are still being identified.[161,162] St. John's wort's antidepressant activity may be mediated by serotonergic (via 5-HT), noradrenergic (via norepinephrine [NE]), and dopaminergic (via dopamine [DA]) systems,[163-168] as well as via gamma-aminobutyric acid (GABA) and glutamate amino acid neurotransmitters.[136,169-171] Weak activity *in vitro* suggests a combination of multiple mechanisms,[172] several of which are presented in the following paragraphs.

- **Monoamine oxidase inhibitor (MAOI) activity:** Early work reported *in vitro* inhibition of monoamine oxidase (MAO) A and B by hypericin,[131] as well as other components, such as xanthon and flavonols.[132] Thiede and Walper found both MAO and catechol-*O*-methyltransferase (COMT) inhibition.[133] Yet these authors, with others,[134] concluded that the concentrations causing inhibition were not adequate to explain antidepressant activity. Cott reported hypericin lacked significant MAO inhibition at concentrations to $10 \mu M$[136] and, on the basis of other findings, such as those from a pharmacokinetics study,[138] suggested that this inhibition may not be pharmacologically relevant.

- **Serotonin (5-HT), norepinephrine (NE), and dopamine (DA) activities:** A more recent proposal is that activity is via inhibition of serotonin, norepinephrine, and dopamine synaptic reuptake.[164,169,173,174] Müller reported that hyperforin is likely the active component; hyperforin approximated the molar efficacy of standard tricyclic antidepressants, with uniquely similar potencies in serotonin, norepinephrine, and dopamine systems.[164] Although not definitive, efficacy in behavioral paradigms of depression (learned helplessness, behavioral despair) has correlated with hyperforin content.[175] Bhattacharya reported dose-dependent potentiation of serotonin-mediated animal behaviors, with greater effect in the hyperforin-enriched (38.8% hyperforin) CO_2 extract. By contrast, the ethanolic extract (4.5% hyperforin) potentiated

dopamine-mediated behaviors.[165] In addition, significant downregulation of B-receptor density and an increase in 5-HT$_2$ receptors have been demonstrated in animal cortex following treatment with hypericum extract.[164] The number of both 5-HT$_1$ A and 5-HT$_2$ A receptors was significantly increased by 50% over that in controls in another report.[176] In the Müller study, the effect on serotonergic receptors varied according to the extract; a methanolic extract led to a significant increase in receptor density, compared with a (nonsignificant) decrease in receptor density found with a hyperforin-enriched CO_2 extract.[164] Neuroendocrine study in healthy adults demonstrated an increase in cortisol with a 600-mg oral dose of WS5570 extract, suggesting central NE or serotonin neurotransmitter activity. The authors suggest that hyperforin plasma concentrations vary according to dose of extract and should be considered in evaluating biochemical and clinical activity.[177]

- **Other neurotransmitter biochemical effects:** The mechanism of St. John's wort activity may be different from that for standard antidepressants.[178] Monoamine inhibition may be noncompetitive, mediated via sodium channels, such as with enhancement of intracellular Na^+ concentrations.[170,171,179] Jensen has also suggested that a direct effect on known transporter sites may not be the mechanism.[180] In this study, neither hyperforin nor adhyperforin inhibited binding of a cocaine analog to the dopamine transporter. Benzodiazepine, adenosine, inositol triphosphate, GABA, *N*-methyl-D-aspartic acid (NMDA),[136] and cholinergic[181] receptor activity may also contribute to psychotropic effects. Likewise, St. John's wort has been found to affect night-time melatonin levels, modulate cytokine expression,[182] increase cortisol,[177] inhibit sigma opioid receptor activity,[181] and antagonize naloxone.[163]

- **Electroencephalogram (EEG) findings:** Electrophysiologic studies have found enhanced striatal alpha-1 activity early after oral administration, which may indicate an interaction with serotonin reuptake; later increases in delta and beta-2 activity may be a correlate with GABA binding and NMDA agonism.[183] Enhanced activation in beta-2 regions had been previously reported.[184] In a human study, alpha-1, delta, and theta activity was found to increase with St. John's wort.[185] These evaluations of EEG activity may provide more insight into neurophysiology of St. John's wort than that obtained by examinations of REM sleep.[186] However, Sharpley reported that hypericum increased latency to REM sleep, as occurs with standard antidepressants.[187,188]

- **Antiproliferative/anti-inflammatory effects:** St. John's wort was found to inhibit growth of and induce apoptosis in experimental leukemia and glioma cell lines,[18,189] as well as in mouse tumor models.[190] An immunosuppressive effect of hypericin was found *in vitro*, mediated by inhibition of arachidonic acid and interleukin-6 release and of leukotriene B$_4$ and interleukin-1α production.[182,191] Proliferation of T-lymphocytes and enhancement of the mixed endothelial cell (EC) lymphocyte reaction were seen *in vitro* and *in vivo* after topical application of St. John's wort, which may provide a rationale for the treatment of inflammatory skin disorders with St. John's wort extracts.[192] *In vitro* inhibition of free radical production has been demonstrated in cell-free and human vascular tissue.[9]

- **Antiviral effects:** A variety of *in vitro* studies have documented "antiviral properties of St. John's wort.[193-202] A photodynamic mechanism has been proposed for the mechanism of action of HIV inactivation.[199,201,203]

Pharmacodynamics/Kinetics

- **Bioavailability:** Systemic availability of hypericin and pseudohypericin after oral administration has been estimated at 14% and 21%, respectively.[204] Time to peak is 2 to 6 hours,[205] with dose-dependent half-life of various compounds ranging from 24 to 36 hours.[159] A steady state is reached after 4 days.[138] The bioavailability of hyperforin has more recently been investigated in rats and human volunteers.[53] Mean plasma concentration (C_{max}) of hyperforin was 370 ng/mL at 3 hours after oral administration of 300 mg/kg of extract (5% hyperforin) in rats. Estimates of terminal half-life and clearance were 6 hours and 70 mL/min/kg respectively. In humans given 300 mg of extract (5% hyperforin), C_{max} of hyperforin was 150 ng/mL at 3.5 hours after oral administration. An open, two-compartment model best fit the data, with a distribution half-life of 3 hours and an elimination half-life of 9 hours. With increasing doses, the pharmacokinetics were linear to 600-mg doses. Mean clearance rates significantly differed for doses of 300 mg and 1200 mg, and C_{max} and AUC values after doses of 900 to 1200 mg were lower than expected. Furthermore, despite a long elimination half-life, there was no observed accumulation of hyperforin following 900 mg of extract once daily for 8 days.[53]
- **Cytochrome P450:** St. John's wort may have multiple effects (inhibition and induction) on various enzymes of the liver cytochrome P450 system.[105] Human studies have reported induction of CYP 3A/3A4 as indicated by reduction in nifedipine[103] and midazolam[104] concentrations. Moore et al. have recently demonstrated that St. John's wort (hyperforin) activates a regulator (pregnane X receptor) of CYP 3A4 transcription and thereby induces expression of 3A4 in human liver cells.[106] Although authors have reported *in vivo* and *in vitro* 2C9, 2D6, and 3A4 inhibition,[100,101] a brief, 3-day trial did not demonstrate a similar significant effect on the 2D6 or 3A4 enzyme.[119] Bray has demonstrated induction of 3A and 2E1 in mice.[102] On review, it appears that St. John's wort inhibits CYP 3A4 acutely and then induces this enzyme with repeated administration.[86,206]
- **P-glycoprotein:** P-glycoprotein, an ATP-dependent drug transporter found in the intestinal tract, genitourinary system, and central nervous system (CNS), may be clinically relevant as well in the absorption or metabolism of St. John's wort and may be activated by St. John's wort.[86,96,151]

HISTORY

- The genus *Hypericum* occurs throughout the world and encompasses 378 known species. The crude drug is obtained from the species *Hypericum perforatum*. The common name, "St. John's wort," is apparently a reference to John the Baptist, as the plant begins to flower on approximately June 25 (the feast day of St. John the Baptist).
- Euryphon, a Greek physician in 288 BC, provides the first known reference to the medicinal value of the plant. Greek derivation of hypericum is from the words *hyper* and *eikon*, which translate to "over" and "icon," respectively, a reference to protection from evil demonic spirits ("over an apparition"). Hippocrates reportedly used the plant as a cooling and anti-inflammatory agent. In 1650, Culpepper employed St. John's wort for the treatment of wounds. In the 19th century, the Eclectic doctors employed oily preparations in the treatment of ulcers, diarrhea, "hysteria," and nervous disorders, such as depression.
- Although well known abroad, St. John's wort has only become popular more recently in the United States. By the late-1990s, industry estimates reported U.S. sales to be in the hundreds of millions of dollars.

Review of the Evidence: St. John's Wort

Condition Treated*	Study Design	Author, Year	N[†]	SS[†]	Study Quality[‡]	Magnitude of Benefit	ARR[†]	NNT[†]	Comments
Depression	Review, meta-analysis	Linde[52] 2000/2002 (1998 update)	2291	Yes	NA	Medium	33%	3	27 randomized trials included, with heterogeneous patient populations, methods, & quality. Average follow-up 5.3 weeks. NNT 4 when limited to placebo controlled trials.
Depression	Meta-analysis	Linde 1996	1757	Yes	NA	Medium	NA	NA	23 randomized trials included, with heterogeneous patient populations, methods, & quality. Superior to placebo with rate ratio 2.67 (95% CI 1.78-4.01) vs. placebo. Statistically equivalent to TCAs.
Depression	Meta-analysis	Kim[48] 1999	651	Yes	NA	Medium	35%	3	Rigorous inclusion criteria. 6 randomized trials selected: 2 vs. placebo & 4 vs. antidepressant medications. NNT 3 for placebo controlled trials.
Depression	Systematic review, meta-analysis	Whiskey[229] 2001	22 studies	Yes	NA	Medium	NA	NA	22 studies included in review, 6 in meta-analysis. St. John's wort found superior to placebo with relative risk (RR) 1.98 (95% CI 1.49-2.62) vs. placebo. Statistically equivalent to TCAs.

Continued

Review of the Evidence: St. John's Wort—*cont'd*

Condition Treated*	Study Design	Author, Year	N[†]	SS[†]	Study Quality[‡]	Magnitude of Benefit	ARR[†]	NNT[†]	Comments
Depression (severe)	RCT, double-blind	HDTS Group[3] 2002	340	Yes	5	None	NA	NA	8 weeks of LI 160 900-1500 mg daily vs. sertraline 50-100 mg daily vs. placebo. Outcome measures: HAM-D and CGI scores. Improvement in all groups without significant differences between groups. Study may have been too brief or underpowered (due to large improvements in placebo arm). Patients were diagnosed with severe (rather than mild-to-moderate) major depression.
Depression	RCT, double-blind	Kalb[241] 2001	72	Yes	5	Medium	19%	6	6 weeks of WS 5572 900 mg vs. placebo. Outcome measured: >50% HAM-D reduction. Baseline HAM-D >16.
Depression	RCT, double-blind	Shelton[239] 2001	200	No	5	None	NA	NA	8 weeks of 300 mg extract three times/day vs. placebo. No improvement in HAM-D. Baseline >20 on HAM-D. Well-designed, but no arm comparing to agent with known efficacy.
Depression	Equivalence study, double-blind	Wheatley[226] 1997	165	No	5	NA	NA	NA	6 weeks of LI 160 900 mg equal to amitriptyline on HAM-D. Baseline HAM-D >17.
Depression	RCT, double-blind	Hänsgen[224,228,242] 1996, 1994, 1993	108	Yes	5	Medium	55%	2	4 weeks of LI 160 900 mg superior to placebo on HAM-D. Baseline diagnosis of major depression (DSM-III-R). Study published initially with 72 subjects (1993, 1994), then later with 108 (1996).
Depression	Equivalence study	Harrer[219,220] 1994, 1993	102	No	5	NA	NA	NA	4 weeks of LI 160 900 mg daily equal to maprotiline 75 mg on HAM-D, CGI. Baseline diagnosis of moderate depressive episode (ICD-10).
Depression	RCT, double-blind	Hubner[221,247] 1994, 1993	39	Yes	5	Medium	23%	4	4 weeks of LI 160 900 mg vs. placebo. Baseline HAM-D > 10.
Depression	RCT, double-blind	Halama[212] 1991	50	Yes	5	Large	28%	4	4 weeks of LI 160 900 mg vs. placebo. Baseline ICD-9 diagnosed neurotic depression and adjustment disorder.
Depression	Equivalence study	Vorbach[223,250] 1994, 1993	135	No	5	NA	NA	NA	6 weeks of LI 160 900 mg daily equal to imipramine 75 mg on HAM-D, CGI. Baseline HAM-D > 19.
Depression	Equivalence study	Brenner[257] 2000	30	No	4	NA	NA	NA	6 weeks of LI 160 600-900 mg equal to sertraline 50-75 mg. Baseline DSM-IV diagnosed major depressive disorder.
Depression	Equivalence study	Schrader[51] 2000	240	No	4	NA	NA	NA	6 weeks of St. John's wort preparation ZE 117 equal to 20 mg fluoxetine on HAM-D. Baseline HAM-D >16.
Depression	Equivalence study, double-blind	Woelk[251] 2000	324	No	4	NA	NA	NA	6 weeks of St. John's wort preparation ZE 117 500 mg equal to 150 mg imipramine on HAM-D, CGI. Baseline ICD-10 diagnosed mild or moderate depressive episode.

Review of the Evidence: St. John's Wort—*cont'd*

Condition Treated*	Study Design	Author, Year	N[†]	SS[†]	Study Quality[‡]	Magnitude of Benefit	ARR[†]	NNT[†]	Comments
Depression	RCT, double-blind	Laakmann[243] 1998	147	Yes	4	Medium	NA	NA	6 weeks of WS 5573 (0.5% hyperforin) vs. WS 5572 (5%) vs. placebo. Best HAM-D improvement with 5% hyperforin. Baseline mild to moderate depression (DSM-IV).
Depression	Equivalence study	Schmidt[259] 1999	149	No	4	NA	NA	NA	6 weeks of LoHyp-57 800 mg daily equal to fluoxetine 20 mg on HAM-D. Baseline mild or moderate depressive episode (ICD-10).
Depression	Equivalence study, single-blind	Vorbach[50] 1997	209	No	4	NA	NA	NA	6 weeks of LI 160 1800 mg ~equal to 150 mg imipramine on HAM-D, CGI. Baseline HAM-D >25.
Depression	RCT, double-blind	Witte[227] 1995	97	Yes	4	Medium	25%	4	6 weeks of Psychotonin forte 100-120 mg superior to placebo on HAM-D. Baseline diagnosis of depression (ICD-9).
Depression	RCT, double-blind	Randløv[29] 2001	150	Mixed	3	Variable	NA	NA	Published abstract. 6 weeks of St. John's wort vs. placebo for moderate depression/dysthymia on HAM-D. Results variable by diagnosis or instrument used.
Depression	RCT, double-blind	Philipp[255] 1999	263	Yes	3	Small	NA	NA	8 weeks of STEI better than placebo on HAM-D and equal to imipramine. Baseline HAM-D >17.
Depression	RCT, double-blind	Schlich[34] 1987	46	Yes	3	Medium	48%	2	4 weeks of Psychotonin M drops (0.5 mg hypericin in three divided doses) superior to placebo on HAM-D (ratio 4.8; 95% CI 1.59-14.50). Baseline HAM-D >15.
Depression	RCT, double-blind	Sommer[222,244] 1994, 1993	105	Yes	3	Medium	39%	3	4 weeks of LI 160 900 mg superior to placebo on HAM-D. Baseline HAM-D >15.
Depression	RCT, double-blind	Hubner[221,247] 1994, 1993	40	Yes	3	Small	NA	NA	4 weeks of LI 160 900 mg no better than placebo in heterogeneous group.
Depression	Equivalence trial, randomized, double-blind	Bergmann[215] 1993	80	No	3	NA	NA	NA	6 weeks of Esbericum vs. amitriptyline yielded similar results on HAM-D. No placebo arm. Baseline HAM-D >15.
Depression	RCT, double-blind	Lehrl[217] 1993	50	Yes	3	Medium	NA	NA	4 weeks of LI 160 300 mg three times daily superior to placebo on HAM-D, CGI, HAM-A. Baseline depression of mixed severity.
Depression	RCT, double-blind	Quandt[33] 1993	88	Yes	3	Medium	NA	NA	4 weeks of daily Psychotonin M (90 drops = 500 mg extract in three divided doses) superior to placebo on HAM-D. Baseline HAM-D >15.
Depression	RCT, double-blind	Schmidt[156] 1993	65	Yes	3	Medium	40%	3	6 weeks of LI 160 300 mg three times/day superior to placebo on HAM-D. Baseline diagnosis of neurotic depression of adjustment disorder (ICD-9). Sponsored by manufacturer.
Depression	RCT, double-blind	Ditzler[218,260] 1994, 1992	60	Yes	3	Medium	NA	NA	8 weeks of combination product Neuropas (480 mg hypericum, passion flower, valerian, 4 other herbs) superior to placebo on CGI. Unclear inclusion criteria, poor reporting of results.

S

Continued

Review of the Evidence: St. John's Wort—cont'd

Condition Treated*	Study Design	Author, Year	N[†]	SS[†]	Study Quality[‡]	Magnitude of Benefit	ARR[†]	NNT[†]	Comments
Depression	RCT, double-blind	Osterheider[32] 1992	46	Yes	3	Medium	NA	NA	8 weeks of Psychotonin M drops three times daily (0.75 mg hypericin) superior to placebo on HAM-D. Reported intention to treat analysis, but published abstract only with limited details. Baseline moderate to severe depression.
Depression	RCT, double-blind	Schmidt[35] 1989	40	Yes	3	Medium	NA	NA	4 weeks of daily Psychotonin M (90 drops = 500 mg extract in three divided doses) superior to placebo on HAM-D. Baseline HAM-D >25.
Depression	Equivalence study, combination product	Kniebel[210] 1988	153	No	3	NA	NA	NA	6 weeks of combination St. John's wort/valerian and amitriptyline of similar efficacy on HAM-D, CGI. Baseline HAM-D >20.
Depression	Equivalence study, combination product	Steger[208] 1985	100	No	3	NA	NA	NA	6 weeks of combination St. John's wort/valerian and desipramine of similar efficacy on HAM-D, CGI. Baseline HAM-D >15.
Depression	RCT, double-blind	Harrer[30] 1991	120	Yes	2	Medium	NA	NA	6 weeks of daily Psychotonin M (90 drops = 0.75 mg hypericin) superior to placebo on HAM-D. Baseline HAM-D >20.
Depression	Equivalence study, not blinded	Kugler[31] 1990	80	No	2	NA	NA	NA	4 weeks of Psychotonin M (500 mg daily) and 6 mg bromazepam of similar efficacy on several standardized measures (DSI, STAI, SDS); no power calculation.
Depression	RCT, double-blind	Hoffmann[207] 1979	60	Yes	2	Medium	NA	NA	6 weeks of hypericum drops superior to placebo on nonstandardized depression & global questionnaires. Baseline depression of mixed severity.
Depression prevention	RCT, double-blind	Häring[225] 1996	28	No	1	None	NA	NA	LI 160 300 mg three times daily in cancer patients (heterogeneous tumors) for 3 chemotherapy cycles vs. placebo showed no differences in "reactive" depression. Published abstract only, with limited details.
Depression	RCT	Maisenbacher[261] 1992	339	Unclear	1	Large	NA	NA	6 weeks of St. John's wort reported to decrease/relieve depressive symptoms, anxiety, nervousness, exhaustion, sleep disturbances. Assessment instruments not validated. Baseline HAM-D >15.
Depression	RCT, double-blind	Reh[214] 1992	50	Yes	1	Medium	NA	NA	8 weeks of Neuroplant (500 mg extract) superior to placebo on HAM-D, CGI, HAM-A. Baseline HAM-D >15.
Depression prevention	Equivalence study, randomized, single-blind	Werth[211] 1989	30	No	1	None	NA	NA	1-2 weeks of Psychotonin M drops (500 mg extract) found equal to imipramine for prevention of depression in amputee patients on HAM-D. However, no power calculation and likely underpowered.
Depression in children	Case series	Hubner[37] 2001	74	NA	NA	NA	NA	NA	Children under 12 years; 300 to 1800 mg of LI 160 daily for 4-6 weeks.

Review of the Evidence: St. John's Wort—cont'd

Condition Treated*	Study Design	Author, Year	N[†]	SS[†]	Study Quality[‡]	Magnitude of Benefit	ARR[†]	NNT[†]	Comments
Anxiety	Equivalence trial	Panijel[262] 1985	100	Yes	3	Small	NA	NA	Sedariston (St. John's wort/valerian root) vs. diazepam.
Obsessive-compulsive disorder	Case series	Taylor[264] 2000	12	Yes	NA	Medium	NA	NA	450 mg (0.3% hypericin) twice daily for 12 weeks.
Perimenopause	RCT, double-blind, placebo-controlled	Boblitz[266] 2000	179	Yes	2	Medium	NA	NA	Published conference abstract. Fixed combination of black cohosh and St. John's wort improved Kupperman score after 6 weeks.
Perimenopause	Case series	Grube[265] 1999	111	Yes	NA	Medium	NA	NA	Kira 900 mg daily for 12 weeks.
Peri-menopause	Before and after comparison	Warnecke[209] 1986	60	NA	NA	NA	NA	NA	Hyperforat vs. diazepam 6 mg for 12 weeks.
Premenstrual syndrome	Case series	Stevinson[267] 2000	19	Yes	NA	Medium	NA	aNA	Kira 300 mg for two menstrual cycles.
SAD	RCT, single-blind	Martinez[268] 1994	20	Yes	NA	Medium	NA	NA	LI 160 900 mg plus bright or dim light for 4 weeks.
SAD	Before and after comparison	Wheatley[270] 1999	301	Yes	NA	Medium	NA	NA	Kira 900 mg vs. combination with bright light for 8 weeks.
HIV infection	Open study	Gulick[59] 1999	30	No	NA	NA	NA	NA	High attrition rate (16 of 30 subjects) due to adverse effects.

*Primary or secondary outcome.
[†]N, Number of patients; SS, statistically significant; ARR, absolute risk reduction; NNT, the number of patients who need to undergo a specific intervention in order to observe an outcome in one individual.
[‡]0-2 = poor; 3-4 = good; 5 = excellent.
HIV, Human immunodeficiency virus; NA, not applicable; RCT, randomized, controlled trial; SAD, seasonal affective disorder.
For an explanation of each category in this table, please see Table 3 in the Introduction.

S

REVIEW OF THE EVIDENCE: DISCUSSION
Depression
Summary

- St. John's wort has been reported to be more effective than placebo and equally effective as tricyclic antidepressants in the short-term management of mild to moderate depression (1 to 3 months in duration). This conclusion is supported by overlapping meta-analyses and a review of multiple trials over the last two decades, and by several more recent short-term, randomized trials. Comparisons with selective serotonin reuptake inhibitor (SSRI) antidepressants have provided limited equivalence data to date. Questions have been raised regarding the methodologic quality of available studies, which have examined heterogeneous patient populations and inconsistently used standardized symptom rating instruments. Negative results have been published in two recent well-conducted trials of St. John's wort for major depression; however, one did not include a reference-agent arm (comparison was made only with placebo), and the other yielded negative results for an SSRI as well as for St. John's wort. Therefore, these results cannot be considered conclusive. Overall, the evidence supporting the efficacy of St. John's wort for mild to moderate depression remains compelling, whereas the evidence for major depression is equivocal.

Meta-analyses

- In 1996, Linde et al.[28] published a meta-analysis of 23 randomized trials of St. John's wort in 1757 patients with mild to moderate depression.[30-35,156,207-223] Selection criteria for studies included randomization, control, use of scales for measuring clinical outcomes, and diagnosis of subjects with depression. Twenty trials were double-blind in design, and 15 were placebo controlled. Results of pooled data from 13 placebo comparison trials revealed a 55.1% response to St. John's wort, compared with a 22.3% placebo response (pooled rate ratio 2.67; 95% CI 1.78 to 4.01; absolute risk reduction 33%; number needed to treat 3). Results were similar if studies using scores on the Hamilton Rating Scale for Depression (HAM-D) or clinical global impression scales as their response outcome measure were independently analyzed (rate ratios of 2.71 and 2.54, respectively). Three studies compared St. John's wort monotherapy with tricyclic antidepressants (rate ratio 1.10; 95% CI 0.93 to 1.31), and two trials compared St. John's wort in combination with other herbals with tricyclic antidepressants (rate ratio 1.52; 95% CI 0.78 to 2.94). The studies reviewed had numerous limitations. Subjects were heterogeneous, with diagnoses including adjustment disorder, "reactive" depression, "neurotic" depression, and major depressive disorder with single or recurrent episodes. Several studies did not present criteria for diagnosis, whereas others used criteria set forth in the World Health Organization's International Statistical Classification of Diseases and Related Health Problems (ICD 9 or ICD 10) or the American Psychiatric Association's *Diagnostic and Statistical Manual of Mental Disorders*, edition 3 or revised edition 3 (DSM-III or DSM-III-R).

Trials were of limited duration (2 to 8 weeks, with one 12-week trial), and the hypericin daily dose varied greatly, ranging from 0.4 to 2.7 mg.

- Linde and Mulrow followed up with a review,[52] including an expanded meta-analysis (substantive amendment in July 1998). Standardized search and analysis methods were employed, and inclusion criteria were similar to those for the 1996 meta-analysis. In addition to the trials reported in the 1996 meta-analysis, four studies were added.[50,224-226] The 27 trials that met inclusion criteria consisted of 16 randomized controlled trials, 8 equivalence/comparison trials, and 3 studies of combination products, with a total of 2291 patients. Quantitative analysis was performed on 14 studies that compared St. John's wort monotherapy with placebo, showing benefits of St. John's wort (rate ratio 2.47; 95% CI 1.69 to 3.61). Analysis was conducted on five studies that compared St. John's wort with antidepressant medications, suggesting equivalence (pooled rate ratio 1.01; 95% CI 0.97 to 1.16). Limitations of this analysis are similar to those of the 1996 meta-analysis: heterogeneous baseline patient characteristics and dosing, small sample sizes, and study design flaws. Nonetheless, this was a well-conducted analysis with suggestive results.

- In 1999, Kim et al. published a meta-analysis of use of St. John's wort for depression.[48] The authors included double-blind, controlled studies in which St. John's wort was compared with placebo or with agents used in standard therapy in subjects with depressive disorders, as defined by ICD 10, DSM-III-R, or DSM-IV criteria. In addition, all studies used the HAM-D as the primary clinical outcome measure. The analysis comprised six randomized controlled trials, including 651 patients. Two studies compared St. John's wort with placebo,[219,227] and four compared it with tricyclic antidepressants.[215,223,226,228] Two of these trials were not included in the Linde analysis.[225,227] The study concluded that St. John's wort was 1.5 times more likely than placebo to be effective (fixed RR 1.48; 95% CI 1.03 to 1.92; absolute risk reduction 35%; number needed to treat 4) and was equivalent to short-term, low-dose tricyclic antidepressants used for treatment of mild-moderate depression (fixed RR 1.11; 95% CI 0.92 to 1.29).

- In 2001, a less rigorous meta-analysis/systematic review was conducted by Whiskey et al.[229] Analysis of 22 studies demonstrated a benefit of St. John's wort over placebo, with a relative risk of 1.98 (95% CI 1.49 to 2.62), and lack of significant difference from outcomes with antidepressant medications, largely tricyclics, with a relative risk of 1.0 (95% CI 0.90 to 1.11). Six placebo-controlled trials were identified as being of higher quality, and meta-analysis revealed slightly less benefit, with a relative risk of 1.77 (95% CI 1.16 to 2.70). Subanalysis of four higher-quality equivalence trials showed no difference from outcomes with antidepressant medications.

Systematic Reviews

- Multiple systematic reviews have been conducted. A 2000 systematic review of St. John's wort monotherapy in depression by Gaster and Holroyd[49] involved eight English-language, randomized, controlled, double-blind trials.[50,80,219,221-223,226,230] Two of these trials[50,80] were not included in the aforementioned meta-analyses. Use of St. John's wort was associated with a 23% to 55% absolute increase in response rate over that seen with placebo, yet 6% to 18% less

than that noted for tricyclic antidepressants. The results of this review were in general agreement with the Linde meta-analysis. Methodologic limitations of the studies remain apparent, including lack of intention-to-treat analysis and absence of statistical comparison between placebo and active treatment. In addition, the authors excluded non–English-language studies. Although additional systematic reviews have concluded similar efficacy of St. John's wort,[231-237] recent mixed findings may alter these conclusions.[2,238,239]

Placebo-Controlled Trials (Positive Results)

- Trials of higher methodologic quality (3 or more on the validated scale developed by Jadad et al.[240]) are discussed next.

- Kalb et al. investigated St. John's wort (WS 5572; 300 mg three times daily) compared with placebo in a 6-week, randomized, double-blind trial.[41] Adult outpatients with a DSM-IV diagnosis of major depressive disorder (single or recurrent, mild or moderate severity), and baseline 17-item HAM-D score >16 were enrolled into this study. Primary outcome was the change in HAM-D score. An early difference detected between the two groups in the intention-to-treat analysis reached statistical significance on day 28 ($p = 0.01$) and day 42 ($p < 0.001$); the HAM-D total score decreased from 19.7 (±3.4) at baseline to 8.9 (±4.3) on day 42 in the St. John's wort group and from 20.2 (±2.6) to 14.4 (±6.8) in the placebo group. In patient assessment, 73% of the St. John's wort group described themselves as much or very much less depressed, compared with 46% of the placebo group. No adverse drug reactions or clinically relevant changes in vital signs, blood count, or liver enzymes were identified.

- Schrader et al. conducted a 6-week, randomized placebo-controlled, multicenter trial in 159 patients diagnosed with mild to moderate depression (ICD-10 criteria) comparing St. John's wort (250 mg of ZE117 extract twice daily = 1 mg of hypericin daily) with placebo.[80] Response rate was defined as a >50% change from baseline in the 21-item HAM-D or a total end point score <10. According to the intention-to-treat analysis, there was a significant response difference in between groups in favor of ZE 117 ($p < 0.001$). In the treatment group, the median HAM-D changed from 20 to 10 at end point, compared with a median score of 17 at study onset and of 20 at end point in the placebo group.

- Hänsgen et al. investigated the effects of St. John's wort (LI 160; 900 mg daily in three divided doses) in 72 patients diagnosed with major depression (DSM-III-R criteria; HAM-D >15) in a 6-week double-blind, placebo-controlled trial.[219] Patients were randomized to receive either placebo or St. John's wort. After 4 weeks of therapy, those taking St. John's wort showed significant improvement in HAM-D and Clinical Global Impression (CGI) scale scores. Subjects on placebo were then switched to St. John's wort for weeks 5 and 6 of treatment and showed significant improvement after 2 weeks of St. John's wort treatment. As with other studies, this trial has been criticized for its short duration and concerns about adequate blinding. This study was previously published in Germany[242] and then republished in 1996 with a larger sample size of 108.[224] In the 1996 version, similar results were reported.

- In an early well-designed trial, Halama assessed the effects of Jarsin (LI 160; 900 mg extract = 1.08 mg of hypericin daily) on 50 psychiatric outpatients suffering from ICD-9 diagnosed neurotic depression and adjustment disorder.[212] A 4-week, randomized, double-blind, placebo-controlled trial was conducted. Patients receiving St. John's wort experienced significant improvement as measured by both the HAM-D and a list of complaints. Approximately half of treated subjects (10 of 25) responded, compared with none (0 of 25) in the placebo group. The rate ratio and accompanying 95% CI (21 and 1.3 to 3.40, respectively) were therefore high in comparison with other trials conducted.[28]

- Laakman et al. evaluated the efficacy of St. John's wort extract WS 5573 (0.5% hyperforin) vs. WS 5572 extract (5% hyperforin) and vs. placebo in 147 male and female outpatients diagnosed with mild to moderate depression according to DSM-IV criteria in a 6-week, randomized, double-blind protocol.[243] The authors used an intention-to-treat analysis to assess HAM-D scores, the main outcome measure. There was a statistically significant dose-response effect based on the hyperforin content; on day 42, the 5% hyperforin group exhibited the largest change in HAM-D score from baseline (10.3 + 4.6 points), followed by the 0.5% hyperforin group (8.5 + 6.1 points) and placebo (7.9 + 5.2 points).

- Witte et al. conducted a double-blind, placebo-controlled trial in 97 depressed patients (ICD diagnosis), comparing St. John's wort (100 to 120 mg Psychotonin forte extract) with placebo in a twice-daily regimen for 6 weeks.[227] The HAM-D score improved significantly more in the St. John's wort group than in the placebo group (79% vs. 54%). However, interpretations of the results are limited by an inadequate description of baseline group characteristics and blinding protocols.

- In a published abstract, Randlov et al. investigated the antidepressant effects of St. John's wort in a 6-week randomized, placebo-controlled, double-blind study.[29] Adult patients (n = 150) enrolled in the study met ICD-10 criteria for either mild or moderately depressive episodes or dysthymia and had a baseline 17-item HAM-D score between 10 and 17. Participants were randomized to receive St. John's wort (either 900 mg or 1450 mg of standardized extract) or placebo. Primary outcome was defined as a 50% reduction in HAM-D score or an end point score of <7. There was a significant reduction in HAM-D score and Beck Depression Inventory (BDI) (self-report scale) in all three groups compared with baseline ($p < 0.05$). A nonsignificant trend toward more frequent response as measured by HAM-D score was found in the non-dysthymic patients, compared with those with dysthymia ($p < 0.06$). This difference was significant according to patient BDI self-report ($p < 0.045$). Because this was a published abstract, specific details and numerical results were not included. Therefore, the ability to assess the quality of this study is limited.

- Sommer and Harrer assessed the effects of St. John's wort (LI 160; 900 mg) in 105 patients diagnosed with neurotic depression and brief depressive reaction (ICD-9 criteria) in a 4-week randomized, placebo-controlled trial.[222,244] Use of St. John's wort was associated with significant improvement on the HAM-D score in comparison with the placebo group at both 2-week ($p < 0.05$) and 4-week ($p < 0.01$) end points.

Placebo-Controlled Trials (Negative Results)

- Shelton et al. conducted a multicenter, randomized, double-blind, placebo-controlled trial to evaluate the efficacy of St. John's wort vs. placebo.[2,239] St. John's wort was given in a dose of 900 mg daily for at least 4 weeks, which was increased to 1200 mg for the remaining 4 weeks if there was insufficient improvement by week 4. Two hundred outpatients with DSM-IV diagnosis of major depressive disorder (single episode or recurrent, without psychotic features) of at least 4 weeks in duration, and a baseline 17-item HAM-D >20, were enrolled. Sixteen subjects had been excluded following improvement during a 1-week, single-blind placebo run-in period. The random coefficient regression model examining the main outcome measure, the rate of change of HAM-D score, found no significant treatment effect ($p = 0.16$) and no time-by-treatment interaction ($p = 0.58$) in intention-to-treat analysis. Similarly, in analysis of the completers, there was a nonsignificant difference in response rate between herb and placebo. In the intention-to-treat sample, the number of patients in the St. John's wort treatment group who reached remission (14 of 98, or 14.3%) was significantly higher than in the placebo group (5 of 102, or 4.9%); however, this was likely influenced by very low remission rates in both groups. Further analysis of less severely depressed patients (subgroup with HAM-D score <22) found no significant treatment effect as well. This study has been criticized because of the abnormally low remission rates reported in both groups,[206,245] and lack of a conventional antidepressant arm to ensure that the study was sensitive enough to detect effectiveness.[206,245,246] (In a letter to the editor, the authors defend against these criticisms.[239]) Despite its methodologic weaknesses, this was overall a well-designed study. Although its negative result stands in contrast with those of multiple prior studies of lesser quality, it is notable that this was a trial in patients with major depression, whereas numerous positive trials have administered St. John's wort in patients with mild to moderate depression.

- The Hypericum Depression Trial Study (HIDS) Group conducted a multicenter trial investigating St. John's wort in the treatment of severe major depression, in comparison with sertraline (Zoloft) and placebo.[3] A total of 340 outpatients older than 18 years were included, having met DSM-IV criteria for major depressive disorder and with HAM-D score ≥20 and CGI score ≤60. Exclusion criteria were suicidality, pregnancy, transaminitis (elevated liver enzymes), seizure disorder, alcoholism/drug abuse, thyroid disease, lack of response to two prior antidepressant medication courses, and other significant DSM-IV diagnosis. Subjects were randomized to receive the St. John's wort extract LI 160 (900 to 1500 mg sertraline (50 to 100 mg), or placebo daily for 8 weeks in a blinded fashion. Primary outcome measures included HAM-D score and CGI score. Baseline patient characteristics were similar between groups at baseline. Prior to completing 8 weeks of therapy, 95 subjects (29%) withdrew from the study, with similar numbers in each group; adequate discussion of dropouts was included. An intention-to-treat analysis was conducted. After 8 weeks of therapy, improvements in HAM-D and CGI scores were observed in all groups compared with baseline, with no significant differences between groups, except for a small significant benefit of sertraline over placebo in one of the CGI subscores (CGI-I). Mean changes in HAM-D score for St. John's wort, sertraline, and placebo were –8.68, –9.20, and –10.53 respectively. The overall effect size for sertraline on the HAM-D was 0.24, which is comparable with reported effects in trials of tricyclic antidepressants, but lower than reported for SSRI antidepressants (0.31 to 0.45). The lack of superiority of sertraline to placebo may be attributed to the short trial period and use of maximum permitted dosage of 100 mg in only 36% of this group. Similarly, 8 weeks of therapy may not be sufficient to detect full effects of St. John's wort, and maximum permitted dosage was administered to only 54% of this group. The study was powered to detect moderate effect sizes of at least 0.40, although observed effect sizes on the HAM-D were lower, resulting in a lack of statistical significance. Unfortunately, this trial does not resolve the pending questions of efficacy of St. John's wort in major depressive disorder, or its comparable value relative to SSRIs. This trial included subjects with severe major depressive disorder, whereas most evidence has supported the use of St. John's wort in mild to moderate major depression. The study may have been too brief and used doses too low to detect full therapeutic effects of St. John's wort or sertraline. In addition, it may not have been adequately powered to detect between-group differences, taking into account the potential improvements in the placebo group ("placebo effect").

- Hubner et al. enrolled 40 patients with neurotic depression and temporary depressive neurosis (ICD-9 criteria) in a randomized, placebo-controlled study of St. John's wort (LI 160; 900 mg daily).[221,247] After 4 weeks of treatment, the St. John's wort group showed significant improvement in HAM-D scores compared with those obtained in the placebo group ($p < 0.05$). Limitations of this study include its short duration, as well as its heterogeneous sample that included patients with mild and transient depressive symptoms (HAM-D score of 12 at baseline). A company that manufactures St. John's wort sponsored the study.

Comparison with Tricyclic Antidepressants

- Several well-designed trials have compared St. John's wort with tricyclic antidepressants (TCAs) and report similar efficacy.
- Wheatley compared St. John's wort (LI 160, 900 mg daily) with amitriptyline (75 mg daily) in a 6-week, multicenter randomized, controlled trial in 156 subjects with DSM-IV diagnosis of major depressive episode and a baseline 17-item HAM-D score between 17 and 24.[226] There was no significant difference ($p = 0.064$) found in the main outcome variable, the HAM-D response rate, or overall clinical impression (as assessed by the CGI scale). However, the amitriptyline group scored significantly better than the St. John's wort group on median total scores on the HAM-D and the Montgomery-Asberg rating scale for depression ($p < 0.05$). Patients taking St. John's wort reported fewer adverse effects than those in the amitriptyline group. This study has been criticized because of the low dose of amitriptyline and the lack of placebo group.
- Harrer assessed the effectiveness of St. John's wort (LI 160; 900 mg daily) vs. maprotiline (75 mg daily) over a period of 4 weeks in patients (n = 102) with a moderate depressive episode (ICD-10 criteria).[220,248,249] No significant differences between the two treatment groups were observed on the HAM-D scale (scores dropped approximately 50%), the Depression scale according to von Zerssen, or the CGI scale. The maprotiline group experienced more adverse effects than were reported in the St. John's wort group. Limitations of this study include the low dose of maprotiline, the lack of a placebo control group, and the lack of intention-to-treat analysis (86 subjects).

- Vorbach conducted a comparison of St. John's wort (LI 160; 900 mg daily) and imipramine (75 mg daily) in a randomized, blinded study of 135 patients with heterogeneous DSM-III-R diagnoses: major depressive episode, single or recurrent; dysthymia; or adjustment disorder, with depressed mood.[223,250] There was no difference found in scores on the HAM-D scale, the Depression scales according to von Zerssen, or the CGI scale. This study has been criticized because of the wide range of depressive disorders among the patients, the low dose of imipramine, and the lack of a placebo group.
- Woelk et al. conducted a 6-week, randomized, controlled trial comparing St. John's wort (ZE 117 extract; 250 mg twice daily) with imipramine (75 mg twice daily) in a sample of 324 patients with ICD-10 diagnosis of mild or moderate depressive episode (single or recurrent).[251] A higher dose of the tricyclic antidepressant was used than in previous trials. Main outcome measures included the scores on the HAM-D scale, CGI scale, and a patient global impression scale. In an intention-to-treat analysis, the authors found no significant difference between the two groups' mean global HAM-D or CGI scores. However, the imipramine-treated group scored significantly better on one subscale of the HAM-D (anxiety-somatization subscale). St. John's wort was better tolerated ($p < 0.01$) than placebo, with fewer patients who discontinued treatment because of adverse events (n = 4) compared with those on imipramine (n = 26). The authors concluded that St. John's wort and imipramine are therapeutically equivalent, but that St. John's wort is better tolerated. Criticisms of this study include rapid and nonindividualized dosing of imipramine, which may have contributed to the dropout rate; small sample size[252]; short duration[253]; lack of a placebo[253]; and the assumption that a difference of 3.5 points on the Hamilton depression scale was not clinically relevant.[254]
- Vorbach evaluated the efficacy of St. John's wort (LI 160; 1800 mg daily) vs. imipramine (150 mg daily) in the management of recurrent severe depressive episode (ICD-10 criteria).[50] This trial followed the author's earlier study utilizing lower-dose treatment.[223] All patients (n = 209) participated in a 3- to 5-day single-blind placebo wash-out phase before beginning the 6-week trial. The dose of both products was increased stepwise during the first week to reach the full study dose. The main outcome measure was the HAM-D score. Both LI 160 and imipramine significantly decreased HAM-D scores, with a decrease in mean values of 25 to 14 and 26 to 13, respectively, and were found to be equivalent based on several secondary outcome measures. However, they were not identified as equivalent based on an *a priori* defined 25% interval of deviation for HAM-D reduction. The authors concluded that they could not reject the nonequivalence hypothesis. This trial has been criticized for its short duration and failure to monitor drug plasma levels to ensure treatment adequacy.
- Philipp et al. conducted the first reported three-arm double-blind controlled comparison trial of St. John's wort extract (STEI 300; 1050 mg, 0.2% to 0.3% hypericin, 2% to 3% hyperforin), 100 mg (titrated) imipramine, and placebo.[255] The study duration was 8 weeks. All patients enrolled in the study (n = 263) were diagnosed with a single or recurrent moderate depressive episode (ICD 10 criteria) and had a minimum baseline 17-item HAM-D score >18. After 6 weeks, a greater mean reduction in HAM-D score was observed in the St. John's wort group than in the placebo group (mean

difference −3.1: 95% CI −5.4 to −1.5); mean reduction in score was equivalent in the imipramine group (mean difference −1.4; 95% CI −2.7 to −0.3). A trend toward greater efficacy of imipramine relative to placebo was found (mean difference −1.7; 95% CI −3.9 to −0.1). The differences between the two treatment groups and the placebo group were comparable at week 8, but less pronounced because of further improvement in placebo group. The study is limited by the lack of significant difference between imipramine and placebo treatments.

- Kniebel and Burchard compared a combination product of St. John's wort (300 mg) and valerian (*Valeriana officinalis*) (150 mg) with amitriptyline (75 mg or 150 mg daily) for the treatment of moderate depression (DSM-III criteria) over a 6-week treatment period.[210] In this randomized, blinded trial comprising 162 patients, progressive and significant improvements were seen in the scores of both groups on the HAM-D scale. Details of the statistical analysis were not provided. In addition, the methods used to conduct this trial were incompletely described.

- Steger compared a combination product of St. John's wort and valerian (*Valeriana officinalis*) with the tricyclic antidepressant desipramine in 100 outpatient subjects with moderate depression.[208] In the first week, 600 mg of St. John's wort plus 300 mg of valerian daily was administered, followed by 400 mg of St. John's wort plus 200 mg of valerian daily for the remaining 5 weeks. The comparison treatment was 150 mg of desipramine for 1 week, followed by 100 mg daily for 5 weeks. Results and statistical analysis of this trial were poorly reported. However, there appeared to be little difference between the treatment groups on the CGI scale. This was not an intention-to-treat analysis (93 subjects).

Comparison with Selective Serotonin Reuptake Inhibitor (SSRI) Antidepressants

- Volz & Laux completed a review of clinical trials assessing St. John's wort or fluoxetine in the management of depression.[256] They identified 16 studies of St. John's wort[30,33,50,80,212,214,215,217,224,226,227,242,243,247,248,250] and nine studies of fluoxetine. a majority of the studies with fluoxetine included patients with higher baseline HAM-D scores than were reported for the subjects in St. John's wort trials. The authors were unable to conduct a formal meta-analysis, because of the heterogeneous methodologic standards and multiple St. John's wort products used in the trials. However, the authors reported that, on average, neither the absolute nor the percent reduction in HAM-D score showed difference between St. John's wort and fluoxetine. The clinical relevance of this study is limited by the lack of direct comparison of St. John's wort with SSRIs, and by the heterogeneity of included trials.

- Brenner et al. conducted a double-blind, randomized, controlled study comparing St. John's wort (LI 160; 600 mg daily for 1 week, followed by 900 mg daily for 6 weeks) with sertraline (50 mg daily for 1 week, followed by 75 mg daily for 6 weeks). The study subjects were 30 patients with DSM-IV diagnosis of major depressive disorder, single or recurrent.[257] All patients discontinued conventional antidepressant therapy prior to commencing the trial (7 days prior for SSRIs and tricyclic antidepressants; 14 days prior for MAOIs). At the end of the 7-week trial, the HAM-D scores for patients on both therapies had significantly im-

proved ($p < 0.05$). In intention-to-treat analysis, the clinical response (>50% reduction in HAM-D score) did not differ between the two groups.

- Schrader et al. compared St. John's wort (Ze 117; 250 mg twice daily) with fluoxetine (20 mg) in a 6-week randomized double-blind, controlled trial comprising 240 patients.[51] Patients were diagnosed with mild to moderate depression according to ICD-10 criteria, with a baseline HAM-D score range of 16 to 24. Data were analyzed on an intention-to-treat basis. The mean HAM-D scores in the St. John's wort group were no different from those in the fluoxetine group. Sixty percent of St. John's wort patients experienced a 50% reduction in HAM-D score, <10 at end point, compared with 40% of fluoxetine-treated patients. In addition, those taking St. John's wort experienced fewer adverse effects. This trial is limited by its short duration and lack of placebo control.

- Schmidt et al. evaluated the efficacy of a St. John's wort extract (LoHyp-57; 800 mg daily) vs. fluoxetine (20 mg daily) in a 6-week, randomized, controlled trial comprising 149 patients with mild or moderate depressive episode (ICD-10 criteria).[258,259] The primary outcome measure in this study was the HAM-D score. In intention-to-treat analysis, the Hamilton global score decreased significantly in both treatment groups.

Evidence in Children

- Hubner and Kirste conducted an open-label, uncontrolled observational study of 74 children between the ages of 1 and 12 years with symptoms of depression and neurovegetative disturbances.[37] The children (median age, 9 years) were administered St. John's wort (LI 160) at the discretion of the individual physician for 4 to 6 weeks. Doses ranged from 300 to 1800 mg daily. Only descriptive analyses of the questionnaire data supplied by parents and physicians are available. Most symptoms appear to have decreased in a majority of the study participants. No adverse events were reported. Because of the lack of controls and incomplete reporting of this study, these results are of limited clinical relevance. An open-label study in 33 children (6 to 16 years of age; mean age, 10.5 years) used a daily dose of 900 mg of St. John's wort for 4 weeks, with good reported tolerance.[38]

Studies of Lesser Methodologic Quality

- A number of other trials have been conducted to assess the efficacy of St. John's wort for depression in humans.[30,32-35,207,209,211,214,215,217,218,225,260,261] These studies can be classified as being of lower methodologic quality, as evaluated by the validated scale developed by Jadad et al. (score ≤3).[240]

Anxiety Disorders
Summary

- Although studies of depression have reported benefit in anxiety symptom reduction, there is currently insufficient evidence to recommend St. John's wort for the primary treatment of anxiety disorders.

Evidence

- Panijel completed a randomized, double-blind trial comparing a combination herbal product, Sedariston (100 mg of St. John's wort and 50 mg of valerian), with the benzodiazepine diazepam (Valium) in moderately severe anxiety states.[262] Patients received either 1 capsule of Sedariston twice daily for 1 week, followed by 2 capsules twice daily (in 54% of the patients in an attempt to increase response), or 2 mg of diazepam twice daily for 1 week, followed by 4 mg twice daily (in 70% of the patients in an attempt to increase response). Fifty-four percent of the Sedariston group were judged to have a very good outcome, compared with 16% of those in the diazepam group ($p = 0.002$). However, the effects of the two herbs cannot be separated from each other, and this study did not adequately describe blinding or randomization.

- There is a report of three cases of generalized anxiety disorder associated with use of St. John's wort.[263]

Obsessive-Compulsive Disorder (OCD)

Summary

- Due to a lack of controlled trials, there is insufficient evidence to recommend St. John's wort in the management of obsessive-compulsive disorder (OCD). Preliminary suggestive evidence from a case series merits follow-up with a controlled trial.

Evidence

- Taylor and Kobak conducted a 12-week open-label trial to assess the effect of St. John's wort (450 mg = 0.3% hypericin twice daily) in the management of obsessive-compulsive disorder (OCD).[264] Twelve patients with a primary DSM-IV diagnosis of OCD of at least 12 months' duration were enrolled in the study. The authors reported a significant change on the Yale-Brown Obsessive-Compulsive Scale (YBOCS) after the first week of therapy (mean = 2.09 points; $p = 0.02$). At end point, five patients (42%) rated themselves much or very much improved. An equivalent assessment was reported in the clinician-rated global impression (using the CGI scale). In subgroup analysis, those patients who reported prior failure to respond to SSRI had a mean YBOCS score change of 4.3, compared with those patients without prior SSRI failure, whose mean YBOCS score change was 10.5 points ($p < 0.049$). Although these results are promising, the open and uncontrolled nature of this study allows for the possible introduction of bias or confounding. Further study is warranted in this area.

Perimenopausal Symptoms

Summary

- There is currently insufficient evidence to recommend St. John's wort in the management of perimenopausal symptoms, including depressed mood.

Evidence

- Warnecke completed an open-label trial to compare St. John's wort (Hyperforat drops; 0.4 mg of hypericin per day) with diazepam (6 mg) for the management of psychological symptoms associated with perimenopause over a 12-week period.[209] Sixty patients were enrolled. The statistical analysis of this trial was not adequately reported, although it appears that patients in both treatment groups improved slightly during the study period. These results are suggestive, but cannot be considered conclusive because of the open-label nature of this study, which allows for the introduction of bias.
- Grube et al. investigated the effects of St. John's wort (Kira; 900 mg daily) in 111 women suffering from psychological symptoms associated with perimenopause or menopause.[265] This open-label uncontrolled study lasted for 12 weeks.

Approximately three quarters of the patients participating in the study experienced improvement as evidenced by decrease in climacteric complaints on both self-rating ($p < 0.001$) and physician rating ($p < 0.001$). However, as this was a case series without controls, the results are subject to confounding.

- Boblitz et al. conducted a double-blind, randomized, placebo-controlled trial of Remifemin plus a fixed combination of St. John's wort and black cohosh (*Cimicifuga racemosa*).[266] In this study, 179 patients with complaints associated with menopause received two capsules given together once daily of either Remifemin plus or placebo. The Kupperman index for those ingesting Remifemin plus decreased from 31.4 to 18.7, compared with a decrease in the placebo group from 30.3 to 22.3 ($p < 0.001$). Psychological parameters were also significantly improved in the Remifemin plus group. However, it is not possible to separate the possible effects of St. John's wort from those of black cohosh, which in initial studies has been found independently to relieve menopausal symptoms (such as hot flashes) and to improve Kupperman scores. As a published abstract (poster presentation), this report included only limited descriptions of baseline patient characteristics and methods.

Premenstrual Syndrome

Summary

- There is currently insufficient evidence to recommend St. John's wort in the management of premenstrual syndrome (PMS). Preliminary evidence from a case series merits follow-up with a controlled trial.

Evidence

- Stevinson and Ernst completed a prospective, open-label, uncontrolled observational study to investigate whether St. John's wort (Kira; 300 mg standardized to hypericin) could relieve symptoms of PMS during a two-cycle treatment period.[267] The Hospital Anxiety and Depression Scale and modified Social Adjustment Scale scores were the outcomes used. Over two thirds of the 19 women who completed the trial demonstrated at least a 50% decrease in symptom severity.

Seasonal Affective Disorder

Summary

- Despite some promising preliminary data, there is currently insufficient evidence to recommend St. John's wort in the management of DSM-IV depressive disorder, with seasonal pattern or seasonal affective disorder (SAD).

Evidence

- One study investigated the use of St. John's wort (LI 160, 900 mg daily) plus bright white light (3000 lux) or dim light (<300 lux) for the treatment of SAD (DSM-III-R) in a single-blind, randomized trial (n = 20), 4 weeks in duration.[268] Patients experienced a significant reduction in HAM-D, yet there was no significant difference between the scores of those receiving bright light and of those receiving dim light. Limitations of this trial include the small sample size, the lack of placebo control, and the single-blind design.[268,269]
- Wheatley conducted an open-label, controlled study of St. John's wort (Kira; 3 tablets daily standardized to hypericin) alone or in combination with light therapy for the treatment

of SAD.[270] Volunteers (n = 301) completed questionnaires about the severity of their symptoms before and after an 8-week course of St. John's wort. Volunteers were also asked to indicate whether they were using light therapy during the study period (no randomization). The author found that patients' SAD symptoms significantly decreased during treatment with St. John's wort. Interpretation of these findings is limited by the lack of blinding, randomization, or placebo control, and the use of nonvalidated outcome measures.

Human Immunodeficiency Virus (HIV) Infection
Summary

- Antiviral effects noted *in vitro* have not been substantiated by the one clinical trial conducted to date. In addition, multiple reports of significant adverse effects and interactions with protease inhibitors and non-nucleoside reverse transcriptase inhibitors (NNRTIs) may preclude any use in patients with HIV infection/AIDS. Therefore, there is evidence to recommend against using St. John's wort in the treatment of patients with HIV infection/AIDS.

Evidence

- A phase I trial by Gulick et al. that included 30 patients with CD4[+] counts <350 cells/mm[3] did not find significant virologic marker or CD4[+] count improvement with hypericin (0.25 to 0.50 mg/kg given intravenously or 0.50 mg/kg orally).[59] Notably, 16 patients discontinued treatment early because of side effects, including frequent cutaneous phototoxicity.

FORMULARY: BRANDS USED IN CLINICAL TRIALS/ THIRD-PARTY TESTING
Brands Used in Statistically Significant Clinical Trials

- Hyperforat; Jarsin (LI 160; 900 mg of extract = 1.08 mg of hypericin daily) or Jarsin 300; Kira (300-mg tablets standardized to hypericin); Neuroplant (WS 5572; each capsule contains 112 to 138 mg of St. John's wort, equal to 0.5 mg of hypericin); Psychotonin forte; Psychotonin or Psychotonin M (drops: 0.4:1 in ethanol, standardized to contain 0.25 mg/mL total hypericin); Remotive (ZE 117, 250-mg tabs standardized to 0.2% hypericin).

Brands Shown to Contain Claimed Ingredients Through Reliable Third-Party Testing

- *Consumer Reports* (2000), testing for standardized dose of dianthrones: CVS Herbal Supplement St. John's wort, Mood Enhancer; GNC Herbal Plus Standardized St. John's wort; Nature Made Herbs St. John's wort; Nature's Herbs Power-Herbs St. John's-Power 0.3% (inexpensive); Nature's Resource Premium Herb St. John's wort; Nature's Way Standardized St. John's wort Extract; Nutrilite St. John's wort with Lemon Balm; Puritan's Pride St. John's wort Standardized Extract (inexpensive); Schiff St. John's wort 300 mg, Mood Support; Spring Valley St. John's wort 0.3% (Wal-Mart); Sundown Herbals St. John's wort Xtra Advanced Formula; Trader Darwin's St. John's wort Extract; YourLife St. John's wort Standardized Herbal Extract, Mood Enhancer.

References

1. Hammerness P, Basch E, Ulbricht C, et al. St John's wort: a systematic review of adverse effects and drug interactions for the consultation psychiatrist. Psychosomatics 2003;44(4):271-282.
2. Shelton RC, Keller MB, Gelenberg A, et al. Effectiveness of St John's wort in major depression: a randomized controlled trial. JAMA 2001;285(15):1978-1986.
3. Hypericum Depression Trial Study [HDTS] Group. Effect of *Hypericum perforatum* (St John's wort) in major depressive disorder: a randomized controlled trial. JAMA 2002;287(14):1807-1814.
4. Rezvani AH, Yang Y, Overstreet D, et al. *Hypericum perforatum* (St. John's wort) reduces alcohol intake in alcohol preferring rats. Alcohol Clin Exp Res 1988;22(Suppl 3):121A.
5. Wright CW, Gott M, Grayson B, et al. Correlation of hyperforin content of *Hypericum perforatum* (St. John's wort) extracts with their effects on alcohol drinking in C57BL/6J mice: a preliminary study. J Psychopharmacol 2003;17(4):403-408.
6. Tedeschi E, Menegazzi M, Margotto D, et al. Anti-Inflammatory actions of St. John's wort: inhibition of human inducible nitric-oxide synthase expression by down-regulating signal transducer and activator of transcription-1alpha (STAT-1alpha) activation. J Pharmacol Exp Ther 2003;307(1):254-261.
7. Kumar V, Singh PN, Bhattacharya SK. Anti-inflammatory and analgesic activity of Indian *Hypericum perforatum* L. Indian J Exp Biol 2001; 39(4):339-343.
8. El Sherbiny DA, Khalifa AE, Attia AS, et al. *Hypericum perforatum* extract demonstrates antioxidant properties against elevated rat brain oxidative status induced by amnestic dose of scopolamine. Pharmacol Biochem Behav 2003;76(3-4):525-533.
9. Hunt EJ, Lester CE, Lester EA, et al. Effect of St. John's wort on free radical production. Life Sci 2001;69(2):181-190.
10. Jacobson JM, Feinman L, Liebes L, et al. Pharmacokinetics, safety, and antiviral effects of hypericin, a derivative of St. John's wort plant, in patients with chronic hepatitis C virus infection. Antimicrob Agents Chemother 2001;45(2):517-524.
11. Hottenrott K, Sommer HM, Lehrl S, et al. Der Einfluss von Vitamin E und Johanniskraut-Trockenextrakt auf die Ausdauerleistungsfahigkeit von Wettkampfsportlern. Eine Placebo-Kontrollierte Doppelblindstudie eit Langstreckenlaufern und Triathleten. Dtsch Zeitschr Sportmed 1997;48:22-27.
12. Vandenbogaerde A, De Witte P. Antineoplastic properties of photosensitized hypericin (meeting). Anticancer Res 1995;15(5A):1757-1758.
13. Chakurski I, Matev M, Koichev A, et al. [Treatment of chronic colitis with an herbal combination of *Taraxacum officinale, Hipericum perforatum, Melissa officinalis, Calendula officinalis* and *Foeniculum vulgare*]. Vutr Boles 1981;20(6):51-54.
14. Shaparenko BA, Slivko AB, Bazarova OV, et al. On use of medicinal plants for treatment of patients with chronic suppurative otitis. Zh Ushn Gorl Bolezn 1979;39:48-51.
15. Albertini H. Evaluation d'un traitement homeopathique de la nevralgie dentaire. *In* Boiron J, Belon P, Hariveau E (eds): Recherche en Homeopathie. Lyon, Fondation Francaise Pour la Recheche en Homeopathie, 1986, pp. 75-77.
16. Someya H. Effect of a constituent of *Hypericum erectum* on infection and multiplication of Epstein-Barr virus. J Tokyo Med Coll 1985;43:815-826.
17. Stevinson C, Dixon M, Ernst E. Hypericum for fatigue—a pilot study. Phytomedicine 1998;5(6):443-447.
18. Couldwell WT, Gopalakrishna R, Hinton DR, et al. Hypericin: a potential antiglioma therapy. Neurosurgery 1994;35(4):705-710.
19. Ozturk Y, Aydin S, Baser KHC, et al. Hepatoprotective activity of *Hypericum perforatum* L. alcoholic extract in rodents. Phytotherapy Res 1992;6:44-46.
20. Halm I, Elõzetes Vizsgálatok A. [Preliminary investigations on the application of *Hypericum perforatum* in herpes therapy]. Gyogyszereszet 1979;23:217-218.
21. Girzu M, Carnat A, Privat A, et al. Sedative activity in mice of a hydroalcohol extract of *Hypericum perforatum* L. Phytother Res 1997;11(5):395-397.
22. Catania MA, Firenzuoli F, Crupi A, et al. *Hypericum perforatum* attenuates nicotine withdrawal signs in mice. Psychopharmacology (Berl) 2003;169(2):186-189.
23. Sindrup SH, Madsen C, Bach FW, et al. St. John's wort has no effect on pain in polyneuropathy. Pain 2001;91(3):361-365.
24. Rao SG, Udupa AL, Udupa SL, et al. *Calendula* and *Hypericum*: two homeopathic drugs promoting wound healing in rats. Fitoterapia 1991;62(6):508-510.
25. Yager J, Siegfried SL, Dimatteo TL. Use of alternative remedies by psychiatric patients: illustrative vignettes and a discussion of the issues. Am J Psychiatry 1999;156(9):1432-1438.
26. Wurglics M, Westerhoff K, Kaunzinger A, et al. Comparison of German St. John's wort products according to hyperforin and total hypericin content. J Am Pharm Assoc (Wash) 2001;41(4):560-566.
27. Draves AH, Walker SE. Analysis of the hypericin and pseudohypericin content of commercially available St John's wort preparations. Can J Clin Pharmacol 2003;10(3):114-118.
28. Linde K, Ramirez G, Mulrow CD, et al. St John's wort for depression—an

overview and meta-analysis of randomised clinical trials. BMJ 1993; 313(7052):253-258.

29. Randløv C, Thomsen C, Winther K, et al. Effects of hypericum in mild to moderately depressed outpatients—a placebo-controlled clinical trial [abstract]. Altern Ther Health Med 2001;7(3):108.

30. Harrer G, Schmidt U, Kuhn U. Depressionsbehandlung mit einem Hypericum-Extrakt. Therapiewoche Neurol Psych 1991;5:710-716.

31. Kugler J, Schmidt A, Groll S, Et Al. Untersuchungen bei Patienten mit Depressiven Zustanden im Vergleich zu Bromazepam und Placebo. Ztschr Allgemeinmed 1990;66 (Suppl):13-20.

32. Osterheider M, Schmidtke A, Beckman H. Behandlung Depressiver Syndrome mit Hypericum (Johanniskraut)—eine Placebokontrollierte Doppelblindstudie. Fortschr Neurol Psychiat 1992;60(2):210-211.

33. Quandt J, Schmidt U, Schenk N. Ambulante Behandlung Leichter und Mittelschwerer Depressiver Verstiimmungen. Der Allgemeinarzt 1993; 2:97-102.

34. Schlich D, Braukmann F, Schenk N. Behandlung Depressiver Zustandsbilder mit Hypericum. Psycho 1987;13:440-447.

35. Schmidt U, Schenk N, Schwarz I, et al. Zur Therapie Depressiver Verstimmungen. Psycho 1989;15:665-671.

36. American Psychiatric Association (APA). Fact sheet on St. John's wort. American Psychiatric Publishing Group, Washington, DC, 1998.

37. Hubner WD, Kirste T. Experience with St John's wort (Hypericum perforatum) in children under 12 years with symptoms of depression and psychovegetative disturbances. Phytother Res 2001;15(4):367-370.

38. Findling RL, Mcnamara NK, O'Riordan MA, et al. An open-label pilot study of St. John's wort in juvenile depression. J Am Acad Child Adolesc Psychiatry 2003;42(8):908-914.

39. Leuschner G. Preclinical toxicology profile of hypericum extract LI 160. Phytomedicine 1996;Supplement 1:104.

40. Okpanyi SN, Lidzba H, Scholl BC, Et Al. [Genotoxicity of a standardized hypericum extract]. Arzneimittelforschung 1990;40(8):851-855.

41. Greeson JM, Sanford B, Monti DA. St. John's wort (Hypericum perforatum): a review of the current pharmacological, toxicological, and clinical literature. Psychopharmacology (Berl) 2001;153(4):402-414.

42. Poginsky B, Westendorf J, Prosenc N, et al. Johanniskraut (Hypericum perforatum L.). Genotoxizität Bedingt durch den Quercetingehalt. Deutsche Apotheker Zeitung 1988;128:1364-1366.

43. Schimmer O, Hafele F, Kruger A. The mutagenic potencies of plant extracts containing quercetin in Salmonella typhimurium TA98 and TA100. Mutat Res 1988;206(2):201-208.

44. Woelk H, Burkard G, Grunwald J. Benefits and risks of the hypericum extract LI 160: drug monitoring study with 3250 patients. J Geriat Psychiatry Neurol 1994;7 Suppl 1:S34-S38.

45. Schakau D, Hiller K, Schultz-Zehden W, et al. Risk/benefit profile of St. John's wort extract: STEI 300 in 2404 patients with various degrees of psychiatric disturbance. Psychopharmakotherapie 1996;3:116-122.

46. Ernst E, Rand JI, Barnes J, Et Al. Adverse effects profile of the herbal antidepressant St. John's wort (Hypericum perforatum L.). Eur J Clin Pharmacol 1998;54(8):589-594.

47. Schulz V. Incidence and clinical relevance of the interactions and side effects of hypericum preparations. Phytomedicine 2001;8(2):152-160.

48. Kim HL, Streltzer J, Goebert D. St. John's wort for depression: a meta-analysis of well-defined clinical trials. J Nerv Ment Dis 1999;187(9): 532-539.

49. Gaster B, Holroyd J. St John's wort for depression: a systematic review. Arch Intern Med 2000;160(2):152-156.

50. Vorbach EU, Arnoldt KH, Hubner WD. Efficacy and tolerability of St. John's wort extract LI 160 versus imipramine in patients with severe depressive episodes according to ICD- 10. Pharmacopsychiatry 1997; 30(Suppl 2):81-85.

51. Schrader E. Equivalence of St John's wort extract (Ze 117) and fluoxetine: a randomized, controlled study in mild-moderate depression. Int Clin Psychopharmacol 2000;15(2):61-68.

52. Linde K, Mulrow CD. St John's wort for depression. Cochrane Database Syst Rev 2000;(2):CD000448.

53. Biber A, Fischer H, Romer A, et al. Oral bioavailability of hyperforin from hypericum extracts in rats and human volunteers. Pharmacopsychiatry 1998;31 Suppl 1:36-43.

54. Araya OS, Ford EJ. An investigation of the type of photosensitization caused by the ingestion of St John's wort (Hypericum perforatum) by calves. J Comp Pathol 1981;91(1):135-141.

55. Schempp CM, Winghofer B, Muller K, et al. Effect of oral administration of Hypericum perforatum extract (St. John's wort) on skin erythema and pigmentation induced by UVB, UVA, visible light and solar simulated radiation. Phytother Res 2003;17(2):141-146.

56. Golsch S, Vocks E, Rakoski J, Et Al. [Reversible increase in photosensitivity to UV-B caused by St. John's wort extract]. Hautarzt 1997;48(4): 249-252.

57. Holme SA, Roberts DL. Erythroderma associated with St John's wort. Br J Dermatol 2000;143(5):1127-1128.

58. Lane-Brown MM. Photosensitivity associated with herbal preparations of St John's wort (Hypericum perforatum). Med J Aust 2000;172(6):302.

59. Gulick RM, Mcauliffe V, Holden-Wiltse J, et al. Phase I studies of hypericin, the active compound in St. John's wort, as an antiretroviral agent in HIV-infected adults. AIDS Clinical Trials Group Protocols 150 And 258. Ann Intern Med 1999;130(6):510-514.

60. Brockmöller J, Reum T, Bauer S, et al. Hypericin and pseudohypericin: pharmacokinetics and effects on photosensitivity in humans. Pharmacopsychiatry 1997;30 Suppl 2:94-101.

61. Schempp CM, Muller K, Winghofer B, et al. Single-dose and steady-state administration of Hypericum perforatum extract (St John's wort) does not influence skin sensitivity to UV radiation, visible light, and solar-simulated radiation. Arch Dermatol 2001;137(4):512-513.

62. Schempp CM, Pelz K, Wittmer A, et al. Antibacterial activity of hyperforin from St John's wort, against multiresistant Staphylococcus aureus and gram-positive bacteria. Lancet 1999;353(9170):2129.

63. Bernd A, Ramirez-Bosca A, Kippenberger S, et al. Phototoxic effects of hypericum extract in cultures of human keratinocytes compared with those of psoralen. Photochem Photobiol 1999;2(69):218-221.

64. Parker V, Wong AH, Boon HS, Et Al. Adverse reactions to St John's wort. Can J Psychiatry 2001;46(1):77-79.

65. Bove GM. Acute neuropathy after exposure to sun in a patient treated with St John's wort. Lancet 1998;352(9134):1121-1122.

66. Woelk H, Burkard G, Grunwald J. Nutzen und Risikobewertung des Hypericum-Extraktes LI 160 auf der Basis einer Drug-Monitoring-Studie mit 3250 Patienten. Nervenheilkunde 1993;12:308-313.

67. Schneck C. St. John's wort and hypomania. J Clin Psychiatry 1998;59(12): 689.

68. Nierenberg AA, Burt T, Matthews J, et al. Mania associated with St. John's wort. Biol Psychiatry 1999;46(12):1707-1708.

69. Moses EL, Mallinger AG. St. John's wort: three cases of possible mania induction. J Clin Psychopharmacol 2000;20(1):115-117.

70. Guzelcan Y, Scholte WF, Assies J, et al. [Mania during the use of a combination preparation with St. John's wort (Hypericum perforatum)]. Ned Tijdschr Geneeskd 2001;145(40):1943-1945.

71. Barbenel DM, Yusufi B, O'Shea D, et al. Mania in a patient receiving testosterone replacement postorchidectomy taking St John's wort and sertraline. J Psychopharmacol 2000;14(1):84-86.

72. Brown TM. Acute St. John's wort toxicity. Am J Emerg Med 2000;18(2): 231-232.

73. Beckman SE, Sommi RW, Switzer J. Consumer use of St. John's wort: a survey on effectiveness, safety, and tolerability. Pharmacotherapy 2000; 20(5):568-574.

74. Lal S, Iskandar H. St. John's wort and schizophrenia. CMAJ 2000;163(3): 262-263.

75. Laird RD, Webb M. Psychotic episode during use of St John's wort. J Herbal Pharmacother 2001;1(2):81-87.

76. Dean AJ, Moses GM, Vernon JM. Suspected withdrawal syndrome after cessation of St. John's wort. Ann Pharmacother 2003;37(1):151.

77. Bachmann LM. Hypericum (St. John's wort) is just as effective as low dose imipramine. Schweizerische Rundschau Fur Medizin Praxis 2000;89(14): 597.

78. Zullino D, Borgeat F. Hypertension induced by St. John's wort—a case report. Pharmacopsychiatry 2003;36(1):32.

79. Czekalla J, Gastpar M, Hubner WD, et al. The effect of hypericum extract on cardiac conduction as seen in the electrocardiogram compared to that of imipramine. Pharmacopsychiatry 1997;30 Suppl 2:86-88.

80. Schrader E, Meier B, Brattstrom A. Hypericum treatment of mild-moderate depression in a placebo-controlled study. A prospective, double-blind, randomized, placebo-controlled, multicentre study. Human Psychopharm 1998;13:163-169.

81. Bhopal JS. St John's wort–induced sexual dysfunction. Can J Psychiatry 2001;46(5):456-457.

82. Assalian P. Sildenafil for St. John wort–induced sexual dysfunction. J Sex Marital Ther 2000;26(4):357-358.

83. Ondrizek RR, Chan PJ, Patton WC, et al. Inhibition of human sperm motility by specific herbs used in alternative medicine. J Assist Reprod Genet 1999;16(2):87-91.

84. De Maat MM, Hoetelmans RM, Math T RA, et al. Drug interaction between St John's wort and nevirapine. AIDS 2001;15(3):420-421.

85. Piscitelli SC, Burstein AH, Chaitt D, et al. Indinavir concentrations and St John's wort. Lancet 2000;355(9203):547-548.

86. Cott JM. Herb-drug interactions. CNS Spectrums: Int J Neuropsychiatr Med 2001;6:827-832.

87. Alscher DM, Klotz U. Drug interaction of herbal tea containing St. John's wort with cyclosporine. Transpl Int 2003;16(7):543-544.

88. Bauer S, Stormer E, Johne A, et al. Alterations in cyclosporin A pharmacokinetics and metabolism during treatment with St John's wort in renal transplant patients. Br J Clin Pharmacol 2003;55(2):203-211.

89. Dresser GK, Schwarz UI, Wilkinson GR, et al. Coordinate induction of both cytochrome P4503A and MDR1 by St John's wort in healthy subjects. Clin Pharmacol Ther 2003;73(1):41-50.

90. Breidenbach T, Kliem V, Burg M, et al. Profound drop of cyclosporin A whole blood trough levels caused by St. John's wort (Hypericum perforatum). Transplantation 2000;69(10):2229-2232.

91. Breidenbach T, Hoffmann MW, Becker T, et al. Drug interaction of St John's wort with cyclosporin. Lancet 2000;355(9218):1912.

92. Mai I, Kruger H, Budde K, et al. Hazardous pharmacokinetic interaction of Saint John's wort (*Hypericum perforatum*) with the immunosuppressant cyclosporin. Int J Clin Pharmacol Ther 2000;38(10):500-502.

93. Barone GW, Gurley BJ, Ketel BL, et al. Herbal supplements: a potential for drug interactions in transplant recipients. Transplantation 2001;71(2): 239-241.

94. Beer AM, Ostermann T. [St. John's wort: interaction with cyclosporine increases risk of rejection for the kidney transplant and raises daily cost of medication]. Med Klin 2001;96(8):480-483.

95. Moschella C, Jaber BL. Interaction between cyclosporine and *Hypericum perforatum* (St. John's wort) after organ transplantation. Am J Kidney Dis 2001;38(5):1105-1107.

96. Turton-Weeks S, Barone GW, Gurley BJ, et al. St. John's wort: a hidden risk for transplant patients. Prog Transplant 2001;11(2):116-120.

97. Ruschitzka F, Meier PJ, Turina M, et al. Acute heart transplant rejection due to Saint John's wort. Lancet 2000;355(9203):548-549.

98. Karliova M, Treichel U, Malago M, et al. Interaction of *Hypericum perforatum* (St. John's wort) with cyclosporin A Metabolism in a patient after liver transplantation. J Hepatol 2000;33(5):853-855.

99. Ahmed SM, Banner NR, Dubrey SW. Low cyclosporin-A level due to Saint-John's-wort in heart transplant patients. J Heart Lung Transplant 2001;20(7):795.

100. Budzinski JW, Foster BC, Vandenhoek S, et al. An *in vitro* evaluation of human cytochrome P450 3A4 inhibition by selected commercial herbal extracts and tinctures. Phytomedicine 2000;7(4):273-282.

101. Obach RS. Inhibition of human cytochrome P450 enzymes by constituents of St. John's wort, an herbal preparation used in the treatment of depression. J Pharmacol Exp Ther 2000;294(1):88-95.

102. Bray BJ, Perry NB, Menkes DB, et al. St. John's wort extract induces CYP3A and CYP2E1 in the Swiss Webster mouse. Toxicol Sci 2002; 66(1): 27-33.

103. Smith M, Lin KM, Zheng YP. PIII-89 an open trial of nifedipine-herb interactions: nifedipine with St. John's wort, ginseng or *Ginkgo biloba*. Clin Pharm Ther 2001;69:P86.

104. Wang Z, Gorski JC, Hamman MA, et al. The Effects of St John's wort (*Hypericum perforatum*) on human cytochrome P450 activity. Clin Pharmacol Ther 2001;70(4):317-326.

105. Roby CA, Anderson GD, Kantor E, et al. St John's wort: effect on CYP3A4 activity. Clin Pharmacol Ther 2000;67(5):451-457.

106. Moore LB, Goodwin B, Jones SA, et al. St. John's wort induces hepatic drug metabolism through activation of the pregnane X receptor. Proc Natl Acad Sci U S A 2000;97(13):7500-7502.

107. Miller LG. Drug interactions known or potentially associated with St. John's wort. J Herbal Pharmacother 2001;1(3):51-64.

108. Ladner DP, Klein SD, Steiner RA, et al. Synergistic toxicity of delta-aminolaevulinic acid-induced protoporphyrin IX used for photodiagnosis and *Hypericum* extract, a herbal antidepressant. Br J Dermatol 2001; 144(4):916-918.

109. Yue QY, Bergquist C, Gerden B. Safety of St John's wort (*Hypericum perforatum*). Lancet 2000;355(9203):576-577.

110. Johne A, Brockmoller J, Bauer S, et al. Pharmacokinetic interaction of digoxin with an herbal extract from St John's wort (*Hypericum perforatum*). Clin Pharmacol Ther 1999;66(4):338-345.

111. Johne A, Brockmöller J, Bauer S, et al. Interaction of St.John's wort extract with digoxin. Eur J Clin Pharmacol 1999;55:A22.

112. Ratz AE, Von Moos M, Drewe J. [St. John's wort: a pharmaceutical with potentially dangerous interactions]. Schweiz Rundsch Med Prax 2001;90(19):843-849.

113. Grush LR, Nierenberg A, Keefe B, et al. St John's wort during pregnancy. JAMA 1998;280(18):1566.

114. Goldman RD, Koren G. Taking St John's wort during pregnancy. Can Fam Physician 2003;49:29-30.

115. Klier CM, Schafer MR, Schmid-Siegel B, et al. St. John's wort (*Hypericum perforatum*)—is it safe during breastfeeding? Pharmacopsychiatry 2002; 35(1):29-30.

116. Lee A, Minhas R, Matsuda N, et al. The safety of St. John's wort (*Hypericum perforatum*) during breastfeeding. J Clin Psychiatry 2003; 64(8):966-968.

117. Rayburn WF, Gonzalez CL, Christensen HD, et al. Effect of prenatally administered hypericum (St John's wort) on growth and physical maturation of mouse offspring. Am J Obstet Gynecol 2001;184(2): 191-195.

118. Markowitz JS, Donovan JL, Devane CL, et al. Effect of St John's wort on drug metabolism by induction of cytochrome P450 3A4 enzyme. JAMA 2003;290(11):1500-1504.

119. Markowitz JS, Devane CL, Boulton DW, et al. Effect of St. John's wort (*Hypericum perforatum*) on cytochrome P-450 2D6 And 3A4 activity in healthy volunteers. Life Sci 2000;66(9):L133-L139.

120. Hebert MF, Park JM, Chen YL, et al. Effects of St. John's wort (*Hypericum perforatum*) on tacrolimus pharmacokinetics in healthy volunteers. J Clin Pharmacol 2004;44(1):89-94.

121. Mai I, Stormer E, Bauer S, et al. Impact of St John's wort treatment on the pharmacokinetics of tacrolimus and mycophenolic acid in renal transplant patients. Nephrol Dial Transplant 2003;18(4):819-822.

122. Bolley R, Zulke C, Kammerl M, et al. Tacrolimus-induced nephrotoxicity unmasked by induction of the CYP3A4 system with St John's wort. Transplantation 2002;73(6):1009.

123. Hall SD, Wang Z, Huang SM, et al. The interaction between St John's wort and an oral contraceptive. Clin Pharmacol Ther 2003;74(6): 525-535.

124. Pfrunder A, Schiesser M, Gerber S, et al. Interaction of St John's wort with low-dose oral contraceptive therapy: a randomized controlled trial. Br J Clin Pharmacol 2003;56(6):683-690.

125. Schwarz UI, Buschel B, Kirch W. Unwanted pregnancy on self-medication with St John's wort despite hormonal contraception. Br J Clin Pharmacol 2003;55(1):112-113.

126. Baede-Van Dijk PA, Van Galen E, Lekkerkerker JF. [Drug interactions of *Hypericum perforatum* (St. John's wort) are potentially hazardous]. Ned Tijdschr Geneeskd 2000;144(17):811-812.

127. Mathijssen RHJ, Verweij J, De Bruijn P, et al. Modulation of irinotecan (CPT-11) metabolism by St. John's wort in cancer patients. American Association For Cancer Research, 93rd Annual Meeting, April 6-10, 2002, San Francisco, CA, USA.

128. Lantz MS, Buchalter E, Giambanco V. St. John's wort and antidepressant drug interactions in the elderly. J Geriatr Psychiatry Neurol 1999;12(1): 7-10.

129. Gordon JB. SSRIs and St. John's wort: possible toxicity? Am Fam Physician 1998;57(5):950, 953.

130. Waksman JC, Hard K, Jolliff H, et al. Serotonin syndrome associated with the use of St. John's wort (*Hypericum perforatum*) and paroxetine. J Toxicol Clin Toxicol 2000;38(5):521.

131. Suzuki O, Katsumata Y, Oya M, et al. Inhibition of monoamine oxidase by hypericin. Planta Med 1984;50(3):272-274.

132. Demisch L, Holzl J, Gollnik B, et al. Identification of selective MAO-type-A inhibitors in *Hypericum perforatum* L. (Hyperforat). Pharmacopsychiat 1989;22:194.

133. Thiede HM, Walper A. Inhibition of MAO and COMT by hypericum extracts and hypericin. J Geriatr Psychiatry Neurol 1994;7(Suppl 1): S54-S56.

134. Bladt S, Wagner H. Inhibition of MAO by fractions and constituents of hypericum extract. J Geriatr Psychiatry Neurol 1994;7(Suppl 1): S57-S59.

135. Cott J. NCDEU Update. Natural Product formulations available in Europe for psychotropic indications. Psychopharmacol Bull 1995;31(4): 745-751.

136. Cott JM. *In vitro* receptor binding and enzyme inhibition by *Hypericum perforatum* extract. Pharmacopsychiatry 1997;30 Suppl 2:108-112.

137. Miller AL. St. John's wort (*Hypericum perforatum*): clinical effects on depression and other conditions. Alt Med Rev 1998;3(1):18-26.

138. Staffeldt B, Kerb R, Brockmoller J, et al. Pharmacokinetics of hypericin and pseudohypericin after oral intake of the *Hypericum perforatum* extract LI 160 in healthy volunteers. J Geriatr Psychiatry Neurol 1994;7 Suppl 1: S47-S53.

139. Devane CL, Nemeroff CB. 2000 guide to psychotropic drug interactions. Primary Psych 2000;7(10):40-68.

140. Roots I, Johne A, Schmider J, et al. Interaction of a herbal extract from St. John's wort with amitriptyline and its metabolites. Clin Pharm Ther 2000;67(2):159.

141. Johne A, Schmider J, Brockmoller J, et al. Decreased plasma levels of amitriptyline and its metabolites on comedication with an extract from St. John's wort (*Hypericum perforatum*). J Clin Psychopharmacol 2002; 22(1):46-54.

142. Nelson JC. Tricyclics and tetracyclics. *In* Sadock BJ, Sadock VA (eds): Comprehensive Textbook of Psychiatry. Philadelphia, Lippincott Williams & Wilkins, 2000.

143. Sugimoto K, Ohmori M, Tsuruoka S, et al. Different effects of St John's wort on the pharmacokinetics of simvastatin and pravastatin. Clin Pharmacol Ther 2001;70(6):518-524.

144. Koupparis LS. Harmless herbs: a cause for concern? Anaesthesia 2000; 55(1):101-102.

145. Irefin S, Sprung J. A possible cause of cardiovascular collapse during anesthesia: long- term use of St. John's wort. J Clin Anesth 2000;12(6): 498-499.

146. Eich-Hochli D, Oppliger R, Golay KP, et al. Methadone maintenance treatment and St. John's wort—a case report. Pharmacopsychiatry 2003;36(1):35-37.

147. Peebles KA, Baker RK, Kurz EU, et al. Catalytic inhibition of human DNA topoisomerase II alpha by hypericin, a naphthodianthrone from St. John's wort (*Hypericum perforatum*). Biochem Pharmacol 2001;62(8): 1059-1070.

148. Burstein AH, Horton RL, Dunn T, et al. Lack of effect of St John's wort on carbamazepine pharmacokinetics in healthy volunteers. Clin Pharmacol Ther 2000;68(6):605-612.

149. Perloff MD, Von Moltke LL, Stormer E, et al. Saint John's wort: an *in*

S

vitro analysis of P-glycoprotein induction due to extended exposure. Br J Pharmacol 2001;134(8):1601-1608.

150. Cheng TO. St John's wort interaction with digoxin. Arch Intern Med 2000;160(16):2548.

151. Durr D, Stieger B, Kullak-Ublick GA, et al. St John's wort induces intestinal P-glycoprotein/MDR1 and intestinal and hepatic CYP3A4. Clin Pharmacol Ther 2000;68(6):598-604.

152. Troutman MD, Thakker DR, Carson SW, et al. Activation and inhibition of P-glycoprotein (P-GP) mediated efflux of digoxin by St John's wort extract [Abstract]. AAPS Pharm Sci 2000;2(4 Suppl)

153. Andelic S. [Bigeminy—the result of interaction between digoxin and St. John's wort]. Vojnosanit Pregl 2003;60(3):361-364.

154. Khawaja IS, Marotta RF, Lippmann S. Herbal medicines as a factor in delirium. Psychiatr Serv 1999;50(7):969-970.

155. Nebel A, Schneider BJ, Baker RK, et al. Potential metabolic interaction between St. John's wort and theophylline. Ann Pharmacother 1999; 33(4):502.

156. Schmidt U, Harrer U, Kuhn W, et al. Interaction of hypericum extract with alcohol. Placebo controlled study with 32 volunteers. Nervenheilkunde 1993;12(6):314-319.

157. Ferko N, Levine MA. Evaluation of the association between St. John's wort and elevated thyroid-stimulating hormone. Pharmacotherapy 2001; 21(12):1574-1578.

158. Pietta P, Gardana C, Pietta A. Comparative evaluation of St. John's wort from different Italian regions. Farmaco 2001;56(5-7):491-496.

159. Bombardelli E, Morazzoni P. *Hypericum perforatum*. Fitoterapia 1995;66(1):43-68.

160. Nahrstedt A, Butterweck V. Biologically active and other chemical constituents of the herb of *Hypericum perforatum* L. Pharmacopsychiatry 1997;30 Suppl 2:129-134.

161. Los Reyes GC, Koda RT. Development of a simple, rapid and reproducible HPLC assay for the simultaneous determination of hypericins and stabilized hyperforin in commercial St. John's wort preparations. J Pharm Biomed Anal 2001;26(5-6):959-965.

162. Jensen AG, Hansen SH. Separation of hypericins and hyperforins in extracts of *Hypericum perforatum* L. using non-aqueous capillary electrophoresis with reversed electro-osmotic flow. J Pharm Biomed Anal 2002;27(1-2):167-176.

163. Butterweck V, Wall A, Lieflander-Wulf U, et al. Effects of the total extract and fractions of *Hypericum perforatum* in animal assays for antidepressant activity. Pharmacopsychiatry 1997;30 Suppl 2:117-124.

164. Müller WE, Rolli M, Schafer C, et al. Effects of hypericum extract (LI 160) in biochemical models of antidepressant activity. Pharmacopsychiatry 1997;30 Suppl 2:102-107.

165. Bhattacharya SK, Chakrabarti A, Chatterjee SS. Activity profiles of two hyperforin-containing *Hypericum* extracts in behavioral models. Pharmacopsychiatry 1998;31 Suppl 1:22-29.

166. Calapai G, Crupi A, Firenzuoli F, et al. Serotonin, norepinephrine and dopamine involvement in the antidepressant action of *Hypericum perforatum*. Pharmacopsychiatry 2001;34(2):45-49.

167. Di M, V, Di Giovanni G, Di Mascio M, et al. Effect of acute administration of *Hypericum perforatum*-CO_2 extract on dopamine and serotonin release in the rat central nervous system. Pharmacopsychiatry 2000;33(1):14-18.

168. Simbrey K, Winterhoff H, Butterweck V. Extracts of St. John's wort and various constituents affect beta-adrenergic binding in rat frontal cortex. Life Sci 2004;74(8):1027-1038.

169. Chatterjee SS, Bhattacharya SK, Singer A, et al. Hyperforin inhibits synaptosomal uptake of neurotransmitters *in vitro* and shows antidepressant activity *in vivo*. Pharmazie 1998;53(1):9.

170. Wonnemann M, Singer A, Muller WE. Inhibition of synaptosomal uptake of 3H-L-glutamate and 3H-GABA by hyperforin, a major constituent of St. John's wort: the role of amiloride sensitive sodium conductive pathways. Neuropsychopharmacology 2000;23(2):188-197.

171. Nathan PJ. Hypericum perforatum (St John's wort): a non-selective reuptake inhibitor? A review of the recent advances in its pharmacology. J Psychopharmacol 2001;15(1):47-54.

172. Bennett DA, Jr., Phun L, Polk JF, et al. Neuropharmacology of St. John's wort (hypericum). Ann Pharmacother 1998;32(11):1201-1208.

173. Neary JT, Bu Y. Hypericum LI 160 inhibits uptake of serotonin and norepinephrine in astrocytes. Brain Res 1999;816(2):358-363.

174. Franklin M. Sub-chronic treatment effects of an extract of *Hypericum perforatum* (St. John's wort, LI 160) on neuroendocrine responses to the 5-T2A agonist, DOI in the rat. Pharmacopsychiatry 2003;36(4):161-164.

175. Chatterjee SS, Bhattacharya SK, Wonnemann M, et al. Hyperforin as a possible antidepressant component of hypericum extracts. Life Sci 1998;63(6):499-510.

176. Teufel-Mayer R, Gleitz J. Effects of long-term administration of hypericum extracts on the affinity and density of the central serotonergic 5-HT1 A and 5-HT2 A receptors. Pharmacopsychiatry 1997;30 Suppl 2:113-116.

177. Schule C, Baghai T, Ferrera A, et al. Neuroendocrine effects of hypericum extract WS 5570 in 12 healthy male volunteers. Pharmacopsychiatry 2001; 34(Suppl 1):S127-S133.

178. Yu PH. Effect of the *Hypericum perforatum* extract on serotonin turnover in the mouse brain. Pharmacopsychiatry 2000;33(2):60-65.

179. Singer A, Wonnemann M, Muller WE. Hyperforin, a major antidepressant constituent of St. John's wort, inhibits serotonin uptake by elevating free intracellular Na^+. J Pharmacol Exp Ther 1999;290(3):1363-1368.

180. Jensen AG, Hansen SH, Nielsen EO. Adhyperforin as a contributor to the effect of *Hypericum perforatum* L. in biochemical models of antidepressant activity. Life Sci 2001;68(14):1593-1605.

181. Raffa RB. Screen of receptor and uptake-site activity of hypericin component of St. John's wort reveals sigma receptor binding. Life Sci 1998;62(16):L265-L270.

182. Thiele B, Brink I, Ploch M. Modulation of cytokine expression by hypericum extract. J Geriatr Psychiatry Neurol 1994;7(Suppl 1):S60-S62.

183. Dimpfel W, Todorova A, Vonderheid-Guth B. Pharmacodynamic properties of St. John's wort: a single blind neurophysiological study in healthy subjects comparing two commercial preparations. Eur J Med Res 1999;4(8):303-312.

184. Johnson D, Ksciuk H, Woelk H, et al. Effects of hypericum extract LI 160 compared with maprotiline on resting EEG and evoked potentials in 24 volunteers. J Geriatr Psychiatry Neurol 1994;7(Suppl 1):S44-S46.

185. Schellenberg R, Sauer S, Dimpfel W. Pharmacodynamic effects of two different hypericum extracts in healthy volunteers measured by quantitative EEG. Pharmacopsychiatry 1998;31(Suppl 1):44-53.

186. Schulz H, Jobert M. Effects of hypericum extract on the sleep EEG in older volunteers. J Geriatr Psychiatry Neurol 1994;7 Suppl 1:S39-S43.

187. Sharpley AL, Mcgavin CL, Whale R, et al. Antidepressant-like effect of *Hypericum perforatum* (St John's wort) on the sleep polysomnogram. Psychopharmacology (Berl) 1998;139(3):286-287.

188. Sharpley AL, Mcgavin Cl, Whale R, et al. *Hypericum perforatum* (St. John's wort) and depression: changes in sleep architecture in normal volunteers. XXIth Collegium Internationale Neuro-Psychopharmacologicum, Glasgow, Scotland, July 12-16, 1998.

189. Hostanska K, Reichling J, Bommer S, et al. Hyperforin a constituent of St John's wort (*Hypericum perforatum* L.) extract induces apoptosis by triggering activation of caspases and with hypericin synergistically exerts cytotoxicity towards human malignant cell lines. Eur J Pharm Biopharm 2003;56(1):121-132.

190. Di Carlo G, Nuzzo I, Capasso R, et al. Modulation of apoptosis in mice treated with echinacea and St. John's wort. Pharmacol Res 2003;48(3):273-277.

191. Panossian AG, Gabrielian E, Manvelian V, et al. Immunosuppressive effects of hypericin on stimulated human leukocytes: inhibition of the arachidonic acid release, leukotriene B4 and interleukin-1alpha production, and activation of nitric oxide formation. Phytomedicine 1996;3(1):19-28.

192. Schempp CM, Winghofer B, Ludtke R, et al. Topical application of St John's wort (*Hypericum perforatum* L.) and of its metabolite hyperforin inhibits the allostimulatory capacity of epidermal cells. Br J Dermatol 2000;142(5):979-984.

193. Meruelo D, Lavie G, Lavie D. Therapeutic agents with dramatic antiretroviral activity and little toxicity at effective doses: aromatic polycyclic diones hypericin and pseudohypericin. Proc Natl Acad Sci U S A 1988;85(14):5230-5234.

194. Lavie G, Valentine F, Levin B, et al. Studies of the mechanisms of action of the antiretroviral agents hypericin and pseudohypericin. Proc Natl Acad Sci U S A 1989;86(15):5963-5967.

195. Schinazi RF, Chu CK, Babu JR, et al. Anthraquinones as a new class of antiviral agents against human immunodeficiency virus. Antiviral Res 1990; 13(5):265-272.

196. Tang J, Colacino JM, Larsen SH, et al. Virucidal activity of hypericin against enveloped and non-enveloped DNA and RNA viruses. Antiviral Res 1990;13(6):313-325.

197. Wood S, Huffman J, Weber N, et al. Antiviral activity of naturally occurring anthraquinones and anthraquinone derivatives. Planta Med 1990;56:651-652.

198. Carpenter S, Kraus GA. Photosensitization is required for inactivation of equine infectious anemia virus by hypericin. Photochem Photobiol 1991;53(2):169-174.

199. Hudson JB, Lopez-Bazzocchi I, Towers GH. Antiviral activities of hypericin. Antiviral Res 1991;15(2):101-112.

200. Lopez-Bazzocchi I, Hudson JB, Towers GH. Antiviral activity of the photoactive plant pigment hypericin. Photochem Photobiol 1991;54(1): 95-98.

201. Degar S, Prince AM, Pascual D, et al. Inactivation of the human immunodeficiency virus by hypericin: evidence for photochemical alterations of P24 and a block in uncoating. AIDS Research And Human Retroviruses 1992; 8(11):1929-1936.

202. Cohen PA, Hudson JB, Towers GH. Antiviral activities of anthraquinones, bianthrones and hypericin derivatives from lichens. Experientia 1996; 52(3):180-183.

203. Hudson JB, Graham EA, Towers GH. Antiviral assays on phytochemicals: the influence of reaction parameters. Planta Med 1994;60(4):329-332.

204. Kerb R, Brockmoller J, Staffeldt B, et al. Single-dose and steady-state pharmacokinetics of hypericin and pseudohypericin. Antimicrob Agents Chemother 1996;40(9):2087-2093.

205. Stock S, Holzi J. Pharmakokinetics test of [^{14}C] labeled and pseudohypericin from *Hypericum perforatum* and kinetics of hypericin in man. Planta Med 1991;57(2):A61-A62.

206. Cott JM, Rosenthal N, Blumenthal M. St John's wort and major depression. JAMA 2001;286(1):42-45.

207. Hoffmann J, Kuhl ED. Therapie von Depressiven Zuständen mit Hypericin. Z Allgemeinmed 1979;55:776-782.

208. Steger W. Depressive Verstimmungen. Z Allg Med 1985;61:914-918.

209. Warnecke G. Beeinflussung Klimakterischer Depressionen. Z Allg Med 1986;62:1111-1113.

210. Kniebel R, Burchard J. Zur Therapie Depressiver Verstimmungen in der Praxis. Z Allg Med 1988;64:689-696.

211. Werth W. Psychotonin M versus Imipramin in der Chirurgie. Der Kassenarzt 1989;15:64-68.

212. Halama P. Efficacy of the hypericum extract LI160 in the treatment of 50 patients of a psychiatrist [Wirksamkeit des Johanniskrautextraktes LI 160 bei Depressiver Verstimmung Nervenheilkunde]. Nervenheilkunde 1991;10:305-307.

213. Halama P. Wirksamkeit des Johanniskrautextraktes LI 160 bei Depressiver Verstimmung. Nervenheilkunde 1991;10:250-253.

214. Reh C, Laux P, Schenk N. Hypericum-Extrakt bei Depressionen eine Wirksame alternative. Therapiewoche 1992;42:1576-1581.

215. Bergmann R, Nuessner J, Demling J. Treatment of mild to moderate depressions: a comparison between *Hypericum perforatum* and amitriptiyline. Neurologie/Psychiatrie 1993;7:235-240.

216. König CD. *Hypericum Perforatum* L. (Gemeines Johanniskraut) als Therapeutikum bei Depressiven Verstimmungszuständen—eine Alternative zu Synthetischen Arzneimitteln. University of Basel Thesis, 1993 (not available for review, cited in: Linde K, Mulrow CD. St John's wort for Depression. The Cochrane Library, Oxford, Update Software, 2002[1])

217. Lehrl S, Willemsen A, Papp R, et al. Ergebnisse von Messungen der Kognitiven Leistungsfahigkeit bei Patienten unter der Therapie mit Johanniskraut-Extrakt. Nervenheilkunde 1993;12:281-289.

218. Ditzler K, Gessner B, Schatton WFH, et al. Clinical trial on Neuropas versus placebo in patients with mild to moderate depressive symptoms: a placebo-controlled, randomised double-blind study. Comp Ther Med 1994;2:5-13.

219. Hänsgen KD, Vesper J, Ploch M. Multicenter double-blind study examining the antidepressant effectiveness of the hypericum extract LI 160. J Geriatr Psychiatry Neurol 1994;7(Suppl 1):S15-S18.

220. Harrer G, Hubner WD, Podzuweit H. Effectiveness and tolerance of the hypericum extract LI 160 compared to maprotiline: a multicenter double blind study. J Geriatr Psychiatry Neurol 1994;7(1):S24-S28.

221. Hubner WD, Lande S, Podzuweit H. Hypericum treatment of mild depression with somatic symtoms. J Geriatr Psychiatry Neurol 1994;7(1):S12-S14.

222. Sommer H, Harrer G. Placebo-controlled double-blind study examining the effectiveness of an hypericum preparation in 105 mildly depressed patients. J Geriatr Psychiatry Neurol 1994;7(Suppl 1):S9-11.

223. Vorbach EU, Hubner WD, Arnoldt KH. Effectiveness and tolerance of the hypericum extract LI 160 in comparison with imipramine: randomized double-blind study with 135 outpatients. J Geriatr Psychiatry Neurol. 1994;7(Suppl 1):S19-S23.

224. Hänsgen KD, Vesper J. Antidepressive Wirksamkeit eines Hochdosierten Hypericum-Extraktes. Munch Med Wschr 1996;138(3):29-33.

225. Haring B, Hauns B, Hermann C, et al. A double-blind, placebo-controlled pilot study of LI 160 in combination with chemotherapy in patients with solid tumors. Abstracts of the 2nd International Congress on Phytomedicine 1996;SL-88.

226. Wheatley D. LI 160, an extract of St. John's wort, versus amitriptyline in mildly to moderately depressed outpatients—a controlled 6-week clinical trial. Pharmacopsychiatry 1997;30 Suppl 2:77-80.

227. Witte B, Harrer G, Kaptan T, et al. [Treatment of depressive symptoms with a high concentration hypericum preparation. a multicenter placebo-controlled double-blind study]. Fortschr Med 1995;113(28):404-408.

228. Harrer G, Sommer H. Treatment of mild /moderate depressions with hypericum. Phytomed 1994;1:3-8.

229. Whiskey E, Werneke U, Taylor D. A systematic review and meta-analysis of Hypericum perforatum in depression: a comprehensive clinical review. Int Clin Psychopharmacol 2001;16(5):239-252.

230. Harrer G, Schulz V. Clinical investigation of the antidepressant effectiveness of hypericum. J Geriatr Psychiatry Neurol 1994;7(Suppl 1):S6-S8.

231. Ernst E. St. John's wort, an anti-depressant? a systematic, criteria-based review. Phytomed 1995;2(1):67-71.

232. Chavez ML, Chavez PI. Saint John's wort. Hospital Pharm 1997;32:1621-1632.

233. Volz HP. Controlled clinical trials of hypericum extracts in depressed patients—an overview. Pharmacopsychiatry 1997;30(Suppl 2):72-76.

234. Josey ES, Tackett RL. St. John's wort: a new alternative for depression? Int J Clin Pharmacol Ther 1999;37(3):111-119.

235. Stevinson C, Ernst E. Hypericum for depression. An update of the clinical evidence. Eur Neuropsychopharmacol 1999;9(6):501-505.

236. Nangia M, Syed W, Doraiswamy PM. Efficacy and safety of St. John's wort for the treatment of major depression. Public Health Nutr 2000;3(4A):487-494.

237. Williams JW, Jr., Mulrow CD, Chiquette E, et al. A systematic review of newer pharmacotherapies for depression in adults: evidence report summary. Ann Intern Med 2000;132(9):743-756.

238. Meltzer-Brody SE. St. John's wort: clinical status in psychiatry. CNS Spectrums: Int J Neuropsychiatr Med 2001;6:835-847.

239. Shelton R, Crits-Christoph P. St. John's wort and major depression. JAMA 2001;286(1):42-45.

240. Jadad AR, Moore RA, Carroll D, et al. Assessing the quality of reports of randomized clinical trials: is blinding necessary? Control Clin Trials 1996;17(1):1-12.

241. Kalb R, Trautmann-Sponsel RD, Kieser M. Efficacy and tolerability of hypericum extract WS 5572 versus placebo in mildly to moderately depressed patients. a randomized double-blind multicenter clinical trial. Pharmacopsychiatry 2001;34(3):96-103.

242. Hänsgen, D, Vesper J, et al. Multizentrische Dopple-Blinstudie zur Anti-depressiven Wirksamkeit des Hypercum Extraktes LI 160. Nervenheilkunde 1993;10:285-289.

243. Laakmann G, Dienel A, Kieser M. Clinical significance of hyperforin for the efficacy of hypericum extracts on depressive disorders of different severities. Phytomedicine 1998;5(6):435-442.

244. Sommer H, Harrer G. Plazebo-Kontrollierte Studie zur Wirksamkeit des Hypericum-Praparates LI 160 bei 105 Patienten mit Depression. Nervenheilkunde 1993;12(274):277.

245. Brenner R, Madhusoodanan S, Pawlowska M, et al. St John's wort and major depression. JAMA 2001;286(1):43.

246. Fomous CM, Cardellina JH. St John's wort and major depression. JAMA 2001;286(1):44-45.

247. Hubner WD, Lande S, Podzuweit H. Behandlung Larvierter Depressionen mit Johanniskraut. Nervenheilkunde 1993;12:278-280.

248. Harrer G, Hubner W-D, Podzuweit H. Wirksamkeit und Vertraglichkeit des Hypericum-Praparates LI 160 im Vergleich mit Maprotilin. Nervenheilkunde 1993;12:297-301.

249. Harrer G, Sommer H. Therapie Leichter/Mittelschwerer Depressionen mit Hypericum. Muench Med Wschr 1993;135:305-309.

250. Vorbach EU, Hubner W-D, Arnoldt K. Wirksamkeit und Vertraglichkeit der Hypericum-Extraktes LI 160 im Verleich mit Imipramin. Nervenheilkunde 1993;12:290-296.

251. Woelk H. Comparison of St John's wort and imipramine for treating depression: randomised controlled trial. BMJ 2000;321(7260):536-539.

252. Alkhenizan A. Comparison of St John's wort and imipramine: finding must be treated with caution. BMJ 2001;322(7284):493.

253. Spira JL. Comparison of St John's wort and imipramine. Study design casts doubt on value of St John's wort in treating depression. BMJ 2001;322(7284):493.

254. Volp A. Comparison of St John's wort and imipramine. Sensitivity of assay is questionable. BMJ 2001;322(7284):493-494.

255. Philipp M, Kohnen R, Hiller KO. Hypericum extract versus imipramine or placebo in patients with moderate depression: randomised multicentre study of treatment for eight weeks. BMJ 1999;319(7224):1534-1538.

256. Volz HP, Laux P. Potential treatment for subthreshold and mild depression: a comparison of St. John's wort extracts and fluoxetine. Compr Psychiatry 2000;41(2 Suppl 1):133-137.

257. Brenner R, Azbel V, Madhusoodanan S, et al. Comparison of an extract of hypericum (LI 160) and sertraline in the treatment of depression: a double-blind, randomized pilot study. Clin Ther 2000;22(4):411-419.

258. Schmidt U, Harrer G, Biller A, et al. A long-term change-over study with the St. John's wort extract Lohyp-57. An observational study of 95 patients with mild and moderate depression. Nervenheilkunde 1999;18(10):106-109.

259. Schmidt U, Harrer G, Kuhn U, et al. [Equivalence comparison of the St. John's wort extract Lohyp-57 versus fluoxetine HCl]. Zeitschr Phytother 1999;20(2):89-90.

260. Ditzler K, Schatton W. Johanniskraut bei Leichten bis Mittelschweren Depressionen-Ergebnisse einer Plazebo-Kontrollierten Doppelblindstudie. Heilkunst 1992;104:263-270.

261. Maisenbacher HJ, Kuhn U. The therapy of depressions in practice: results of a post-marketing surveillance study with herba hyperici. Natura Medica 1992;7(5):394-399.

262. Panijel M. [Treatment of moderately severe anxiety states]. Therapiewoche 1985;35(41):4659-4668.

263. Kobak KA, Taylor L, Futterer R, et al. St. John's wort in generalized anxiety disorder: three more case reports. J Clin Psychopharmacol 2003;23(5):531-532.

264. Taylor LH, Kobak KA. An open-label trial of St. John's wort (*Hypericum perforatum*) in obsessive-compulsive disorder. J Clin Psychiatry 2000;61(8):575-578.

265. Grube B, Walper A, Wheatley D. St. John's wort extract: efficacy for menopausal symptoms of psychological origin. Adv Ther 1999;16(4):177-186.

266. Boblitz N, Schrader E, Henneicke-Von Zepelin HH, et al. Benefit of a fixed drug combination containing St. John's wort and black cohosh for

climacteric patients—results of a randomised clinical trial (poster presentaion from 6th Annual Symposium on Complementary Health Care, Exeter, England, December 2-4, 1999). Focus Alt Comp Ther (FACT) 2000;5(1):85-86.

267. Stevinson C, Ernst E. A pilot study of *Hypericum perforatum* for the treatment of premenstrual syndrome. Br J Obstet Gynaecol 2000;107(7): 870-876.

268. Martinez B, Kasper S, Ruhrmann S, et al. Hypericum in the treatment of seasonal affective disorders. J Geriatr Psychiatry Neurol 1994;7 Suppl 1: S29-S33.

269. Kasper S. Treatment of seasonal affective disorder (SAD) with hypericum extract. Pharmacopsychiatry 1997;30 Suppl 2:89-93.

270. Wheatley D. Hypericum in seasonal affective disorder (SAD). Curr Med Res Opin 1999;15(1):33-37.

Sweet Almond
(Prunus amygdalus dulcis)

SYNONYMS/COMMON NAMES/RELATED SUBSTANCES

- Almendra, almendra dulce, almond oil, amande, amande douce, amandel, amendoa, amêndoa doce, amigdalo, *Amygdalus communis, Amygdala dulcis,* badam, badami, badamo, badamshirin, bedamu, bian tao, bilati badam, cno ghreugach, expressed almond oil, fixed almond oil, harilik mandlipuu, Jordan almond, lawz, lozi, mandel, mandla, mandorla, mandorla dulce, mandula, mangel, mantelli, migdal, migdala, migdalo, mindal, Prunoidae (subfamily), *Prunus communis dulcis, Prunus dulcis* var. *dulcis,* Rosaceae (family), sladkiy mindal, sötmandel, süßmandel, sweet almond oil, tatli badem, tian wei bian tao, tian xing ren, vaadaam, vadumai, zoete amandel.
- *Note:* Sweet almond should not be confused with bitter almond, which contains amygdalin and can be hydrolyzed to the toxic substance hydrocyanic acid.

CLINICAL BOTTOM LINE
Background

- The almond is closely related to the peach, apricot, and cherry (all classified as drupes). Unlike with the others, however, the outer layer of the almond is not edible. The edible portion of the almond is the seed.
- Sweet almonds are a popular nutritious food. Researchers are especially interested in their level of monounsaturated fats, as these appear to have a beneficial effect on blood lipids.
- Almond oil is widely used in lotions and cosmetics.

Scientific Evidence for Common/Studied Uses	Grade*
Hyperlipidemia (whole almonds)	B
Radiation therapy skin reaction (topical)	D

*Key to grades: *A:* Strong scientific evidence for this use; *B:* Good scientific evidence for this use; *C:* Unclear scientific evidence for this use; *D:* Fair scientific evidence against this use (it may not work); *F:* Strong scientific evidence against this use (it likely does not work). For a more detailed explanation of efficacy criteria, see "Natural Standard Evidence-Based Validated Grading Rationale" in the Introduction.

Historical or Theoretical Indications That Lack Sufficient Evidence

- Antibacterial,[1] aphrodisiac,[2] bladder cancer, breast cancer, colon cancer,[3] demulcent for chapped lips (a soothing substance extracted from an emulsion), emollient, increasing sperm count,[2] mild laxative, oropharyngeal cancers, phytoestrogen,[4] solvent for injectable drugs, uterine cancer.

Expert Opinion and Folkloric Precedent

- Almonds are generally regarded as safe for food consumption.
- When blended with water, sweet almonds produce a white mixture called "almond milk," which is recommended by some practitioners as a dairy milk substitute.

Safety Summary

- **Likely safe:** When the almond seed is consumed orally or used topically, there are no safety concerns (assuming no allergy).
- **Possibly unsafe:** Allergies to almonds are common and have resulted in severe reactions, including oral allergic syndrome (OAS), angioedema, and laryngeal edema.[5]

DOSING/TOXICOLOGY
General

- Recommended doses are based on those most commonly used in available trials, or on historical practice. However, with natural products, the optimal doses needed to balance efficacy and safety often have not been determined. Formulations and preparation methods may vary from manufacturer to manufacturer, and from batch to batch of a specific product made by a single manufacturer. Because often the active components of a product are not known, standardization may not be possible, and the clinical effects of different brands may not be comparable.

Standardization

- One study found 14% of 74 almond samples to be contaminated with aflatoxin. Diced almonds were found to contain a higher concentration of aflatoxin than that found in whole almonds. Aflatoxin, a toxin produced by several species of *Aspergillus,* is also present in small quantities in peanut products. The U.S. Department of Agriculture (USDA) is responsible for monitoring aflatoxin concentrations.[6]

Dosing: Adult (18 Years and Older)
Oral

- **Hyperlipidemia:** Whole almonds: Studies have used 100 g/day[7] and 84 g/day[8] with no reported side effects.
- **Laxative:** Sweet almond oil: Doses of up to 30 mL have been reported anecdotally.
- *Note:* Sweet almonds and sweet almond oil are therapeutically distinguished from bitter almonds or bitter almond oil, as bitter almonds can be toxic to humans.

Dosing: Pediatric (Younger Than 18 Years)

- There is insufficient evidence to recommend for or against the use of almonds in children. Based on their nutritional profile, however, almonds appear to be a healthful food.

Toxicology

- One study found 14% of 74 almond samples to be contaminated with aflatoxin, a toxin produced from several species of *Aspergillus.*[6]
- In acute toxicity tests conducted in mice, *P. amygdalus* at doses between 500 mg/kg and 3 g/kg showed no signs of toxicity. During chronic treatment, the average weight of the mice increased significantly ($p < 0.05$) compared with their initial weights. There was one incidence of alopecia and inflammation in leg joints and two instances of an "anemic appearance." The mortality rate in the *P. amygdalus* group was not significantly different from that in the control group.[2]

ADVERSE EFFECTS/PRECAUTIONS/CONTRAINDICATIONS
Allergy

- Allergies to almonds are common and have led to severe reactions, including oral allergic syndrome (OAS), angioedema, and laryngeal edema.[5]
- Hypersensitivity cross-reactions to other nuts may occur. A case report documents the development of status asthmaticus leading to death in a woman who ate a slice of cake with hazelnuts and almond icing.[9] The patient had a history of peanut allergy.

Adverse Effects

- **General:** In most reports, sweet almond is generally considered to be safe when taken orally. Few nonallergic adverse reactions have been reported in the literature. However, hypersensitivity to almonds is common and may lead to severe reactions.
- **Endocrine:** One study in rats found almonds to have a significant hypoglycemic effect.[10] Clemetson et al. reported that almonds exert estrogenic activity in rats, although subsequent samples of different varieties of almonds did not confirm this finding.[4] Theoretically, increased intake of almonds (and therefore increased intake of unsaturated fat) can lead to weight gain. However, a small randomized, controlled trial reports that consuming approximately 320 calories of almonds daily for 6 months does not lead to statistically or biologically significant average changes in body weight and does increase the consumption of unsaturated fats.[11] During chronic treatment with *P. amygdalus* in mice, the average weight of mice increased significantly compared with their initial weights.[2] However, it is not clear if this was due to the nutritional content of the almond diets.
- **Rheumatologic:** During chronic treatment with *P. amygdalus* in mice, there was one instance of alopecia and inflammation in leg joints reported.[2]
- **Other:** A human case of fat embolism following intrapenile injection of almond oil for the treatment of impotence has been reported in the literature.[12] The patient presented with hemoconcentration and fat globules in his urine. The patient recovered after oxygen therapy and hydration.

Precautions/Warnings/Contraindications

- Avoid in patients with known hypersensitivity to almonds, almond constituents, or other nuts. Cross-reactivity to other nuts may occur.

Pregnancy and Lactation

- There is insufficient evidence to recommend for or against the use of almonds in pregnant or lactating women.

INTERACTIONS
Sweet Almond/Drug Interactions

- **Hypoglycemic agents:** Theoretically, the use of almonds with hypoglycemic agents may have additive effects. A study in rats found almonds to have a significant hypoglycemic effect.[10]
- **Cholesterol-lowering agents:** Theoretically, almonds and cholesterol-lowering agents may have additive effects when taken concomitantly. Almonds have been reported to lower low-density lipoproteins (LDLs) and total cholesterol levels.[7,8,13-15]

Sweet Almond/Herb/Supplement Interactions

- **Hypoglycemic herbs and supplements:** Theoretically the use of almonds with hypoglycemic agents may have additive effects. A study in rats found almonds to have a significant hypoglycemic effect.[10]
- **Cholesterol-lowering agents:** Theoretically almonds and cholesterol-lowering agents may have additive effects when taken concomitantly. Almonds have been reported to lower LDL and total cholesterol levels.[7,8,13-15]

Sweet Almond/Food Interactions

- Insufficient evidence in the available literature.

Sweet Almond/Lab Interactions

- **Serum glucose:** Theoretically, almonds may decrease serum glucose levels. A study in rats found almonds to have a significant hypoglycemic effect.[10]
- **Serum lipid profile:** Almonds have been reported to lower LDL and total cholesterol levels.[7,8,13-15]

MECHANISM OF ACTION
Pharmacology

- Analysis of sweet almond has detected protein, emulsin, prunasin, daucosterol, and other sterols. Trace amounts of vitamins A, B complex, and E and amino acids, including glutamic acid, aspartic acid, and arginine, are also present.[16] Constituents of almond emulsin include mannosidase, glucosidase, and galactosidase, with β-D-glucosidase being the main enzymatic component.[17] Almond glycopeptidase cleaves β-aspartylglycosylamine linkages in glycopeptides.[18] Almond β-galactosidase's enzymatic activity appears to depend on its histidine and carboxyl groups.[19,20] Derivatives of L-histidine, histamine, and imidazole may possess the ability to inhibit almond α-glucosidase.[21] Isofagomine, azafagomine, and isogalactofagomine have been shown to inhibit almond β-glucosidase.[22]
- Teotia et al. conducted a study in rats in which almonds were found to have a highly significant hypoglycemic effect.[10]
- Almonds have been reported to lower LDL and total cholesterol levels.[7,8,13-15] It has been proposed that the most likely mechanism of LDL lowering is enhancement of LDL receptor activity when monounsaturated fatty acids replace saturated ones in the diet. Saturated fatty acids may suppress LDL receptors.[13]
- Clemetson et al. reported that almonds exert estrogenic activity in rats, although subsequent samples of different varieties of almonds did not confirm this finding.[4] Qureshi et al. found that almond extracts increase sperm count and sperm motility in rats, with no evidence of spermatotoxicity.[2]

Pharmacodynamics/Kinetics

- Insufficient evidence in the available literature.

HISTORY

- References to almonds are found in the Old Testament. Almonds were prized as an ingredient in breads served to the Pharaohs in Egypt and have maintained religious, ethnic, and social significance throughout history.
- The almond tree is native to Western Asia. It was brought to California from Spain in the 1700s.
- Almonds are extensively cultivated in modern times. Worldwide cultivation has expanded in recent decades, with the largest amounts of almonds being produced in California and Spain.
- The increasing popularity of almonds is largely due to their nutritional profile.[16] Almonds are available whole, as flour-like almond meal, and as almond butter or almond milk. Almond oil is often used to flavor cookies and other baked goods.

Review of the Evidence: Sweet Almond

Condition Treated*	Study Design	Author, Year	N[†]	SS[†]	Study Quality[‡]	Magnitude of Benefit	ARR[†]	NNT[†]	Comments
Hyperlipidemia	RCT	Spiller[7] 1998	45	Yes	2	Small	NA	NA	Significant reductions in total cholesterol and LDL, no change in HDL; almond-based diet superior to olive oil–based diet.
Hyperlipidemia	Case series	Abbey[8] 1994	16	Yes	1	Small	NA	NA	Significant reductions in total cholesterol and LDL with both almonds and walnuts.
Hyperlipidemia	Case series	Spiller[14] 1992	26	Yes	NA	Small	NA	NA	Significant reductions in total cholesterol and LDL, no change in HDL.
Radiation therapy skin reactions	Randomized, single-blind	Maiche[24] 1991	48	No	2	None	NA	NA	No benefits of either almond ointment or chamomile cream. No placebo group.

*Primary or secondary outcome.
[†]N, Number of patients; SS, statistically significant; ARR, absolute risk reduction; NNT, the number of patients who need to undergo a specific intervention in order to observe an outcome in one individual.
[‡]0-2 = poor; 3-4 = good; 5 = excellent.
NA, Not applicable.
For an explanation of each category in this table, please see Table 3 in the Introduction.

REVIEW OF THE EVIDENCE: DISCUSSION

Hyperlipidemia
Summary

- There is initial positive evidence from human studies to support the use of almonds in the diet to lower serum lipids. There are supporting data from animal studies.[15] Proposed mechanisms include the presence of monounsaturated fats in raw almonds, or direct effects on low-density lipoprotein (LDL) receptors.[13] Further study is warranted in this area to establish dosing guidelines and degree of benefit.

Evidence

- Spiller et al. conducted a randomized trial in 45 individuals comparing an almond-based diet with an olive oil-based diet or a dairy-based diet.[7] In the almond group, statistically significant reductions were observed for total cholesterol, LDL, and the ratio of total cholesterol to high-density lipoprotein (HDL). HDL values remained unchanged. Significant changes were not observed in the olive oil group. Total cholesterol and HDL increased significantly in the dairy-based group.
- In a prior study, Spiller et al. assessed the efficacy of 100 mg/day of almonds on LDL, HDL, and total cholesterol in 26 patients over 9 weeks.[14] Total cholesterol levels significantly decreased, LDL decreased, and HDL was unchanged.
- A case series in 16 patients studied the effects of 84 g of almonds daily for 3 weeks.[8] Results included a 7% reduction in total cholesterol and 10% reduction in LDL. Following almond consumption, subjects supplemented their diets with walnuts for 3 weeks, which led to 5% and 9% reductions in total cholesterol and LDL levels respectively.
- In a case-control study that did not specifically focus on almonds, Hu et al. examined a cohort of women from the Nurses' Health Study (n = 86,016), and concluded that frequent nut consumption (eating nuts >5 times per week) is associated with a 35% reduced risk of coronary artery disease or myocardial infarction.[23] It is unclear if almonds specifically would provide such a benefit, and without confirmation of these results by prospective controlled trials, the influence of confounders on these results cannot be ruled out. It is

also not clear if effects of nuts on lipids were associated with these effects.

Radiation Therapy Skin Reactions
Summary

- In one methodologically weak human trial, topical almond ointment had no beneficial effect on the skin of breast cancer patients receiving radiotherapy.

Evidence

- Maiche et al. conducted a single-blind study in 48 breast cancer patients receiving radiotherapy.[24] Subjects were randomized to receive either almond ointment or Kamillosan cream (chamomile-based cream), and patients served as their own controls. Neither agent was found to be effective for preventing radiation-induced skin reactions, and there were no statistically significant differences between the Kamillosan and almond ointment groups. The Kamillosan group appeared to develop skin reactions later and to a lesser extent in comparison with the almond ointment group, but this difference was not statistically significant. This was a poorly described and methodologically weak study, and no true placebo group was included to measure potential benefits. Nonetheless, it provides sufficient preliminary evidence against the efficacy of this use of almond ointment, until more convincing evidence of efficacy emerges.

References

1. Sachdev Y. A new antimicrobial agent from almond (*Prunus amygdalus*) shells. Indian J Physiol Pharmacol 1968;12(4):207-212.
2. Qureshi S, Shah AH, Tariq M, et al. Studies on herbal aphrodisiacs used in Arab systems of medicine. Am J Chin Med 1989;17(1-2):57-63.
3. Davis PA, Iwahashi CK. Whole almonds and almond fractions reduce aberrant crypt foci in a rat model of colon carcinogenesis. Cancer Lett 2001;165(1):27-33.
4. Clemetson CA, de Carlo SJ, Burney GA, et al. Estrogens in food: the almond mystery. Int J Gynaecol Obstet 1978;15(6):515-521.
5. Pasini G, Simonato B, Giannattasio M, et al. IgE binding to almond proteins in two CAP-FEIA-negative patients with allergic symptoms to almond as compared to three CAP-FEIA-false-positive subjects. Allergy 2000;55(10):955-958.
6. Schade JE, McGreevy K, King A, Jr, et al. Incidence of aflatoxin in California almonds. Appl Microbiol 1975;29(1):48-53.

7. Spiller GA, Jenkins DA, Bosello O, et al. Nuts and plasma lipids: an almond-based diet lowers LDL-C while preserving HDL-C. J Am Coll Nutr 1998; 17(3):285-290.

8. Abbey M, Noakes M, Belling GB, et al. Partial replacement of saturated fatty acids with almonds or walnuts lowers total plasma cholesterol and low-density-lipoprotein cholesterol. Am J Clin Nutr 1994;59(5):995-999.

9. Evans S, Skea D, Dolovich J. Fatal reaction to peanut antigen in almond icing. CMAJ 1988;139(3):231-232.

10. Teotia S, Singh M. Hypoglycemic effect of *Prunus amygdalus* seeds in albino rabbits. Indian J Exp Biol 1997;35(3):295-296.

11. Fraser GE, Jaceldo KB, Sabate J. Effect on body weight of a free 76 Kilojoule (320 calorie) daily supplement of almonds for six months. J Am Coll Nutr 2002;21(3):275-283.

12. Thomas P, Boussuges A, Gainnier M, et al. [Fat embolism after intrapenile injection of sweet almond oil]. Rev Mal Respir 1998;15(3):307-308.

13. Grundy SM. Monounsaturated fatty acids, plasma cholesterol, and coronary heart disease. Am J Clin Nutr 1987;45(5 Suppl):1168-1175.

14. Spiller GA, Jenkins DJ, Cragen LN, et al. Effect of a diet high in mono-unsaturated fat from almonds on plasma cholesterol and lipoproteins. J Am Coll Nutr 1992;11(2):126-130.

15. Teotia S, Singh M, Pant MC. Effect of *Prunus amygdalus* seeds on lipid profile. Indian J Physiol Pharmacol 1997;41(4):383-389.

16. Saura-Calixto FS, Bauza M, de Toda FM, et al. Amino acids, sugars, and inorganic elements in the sweet almond (*Prunus amygdalus*). J Agric Food Chem 1981;29(3):509-511.

17. Schwartz J, Sloan J, Lee YC. Mannosidase, glucosidase, and galactosidase in sweet almond emulsin. Arch Biochem Biophys 1970;137(1):122-127.

18. Nishibe H, Takahashi N. The release of carbohydrate moieties from human fibrinogen by almond glycopeptidase without alteration in fibrinogen clottability. Biochim Biophys Acta 1981;661:274-279.

19. Dey PM, Malhotra OP. Kinetic behaviour of sweet almond alpha-galactosidase. Biochim Biophys Acta 1969;185(2):402-408.

20. Dey P. Inhibition, transgalactosylation and mechanism of action of sweet almond alpha-galactosidase. Biochim Biophys Acta 1969;191:644-652.

21. Field RA, Haines AH, Chrystal EJ, et al. Histidines, histamines and imidazoles as glycosidase inhibitors. Biochem J 1991;274 (Pt 3):885-889.

22. Bulow A, Plesner IW, Bols M. Slow inhibition of almond beta-glucosidase by azasugars: determination of activation energies for slow binding. Biochim Biophys Acta 2001;1545(1-2):207-215.

23. Hu FB, Stampfer MJ, Manson JE, et al. Frequent nut consumption and risk of coronary heart disease in women: prospective cohort study. BMJ 1998;317(7169):1341-1345.

24. Maiche A. Effect of chamomile cream and almond ointment on acute radiation skin reaction. Acta Oncol 1991;30(3):395-396.

Tea Tree Oil
(Melaleuca alternifolia [Maiden & Betche] Cheel)

SYNONYMS/COMMON NAMES/RELATED SUBSTANCES

- Australian tea tree oil, breathaway, Bogaskin (veterinary formulation), Burnaid (40 mg/g of tea tree oil, 1 mg/g of triclosan), cymene, malaleuca, *Melaleuca alternifolia*, Melaleuca Alternifolia Hydrogel (burn dressing), melaleucae, melaleuca oil, oil of melaleuca, oleum, oleum melaleucae, T36-C7, tea tree oil, Tebodont, teebaum, terpinen, terpinen-4-ol, terpinenol-4, ti tree.
- *Note:* Tea tree oil should not be confused with cajeput oil, niauouli oil, kanuka oil, or manuka oil obtained from other *Melaleuca* species.

CLINICAL BOTTOM LINE
Background

- Tea tree oil is obtained by steam distillation of the leaves of *Melaleuca alternifolia*. Tea tree oil is purported to have antiseptic properties and has been used traditionally to prevent and treat infections. Although numerous *in vitro* studies have demonstrated antimicrobial properties of tea tree oil (likely attributable to the constituent terpinen-4-ol), only a small number of randomized, controlled human trials have been published. Human studies have focused on the use of topical tea tree oil for fungal infections (including onychomycosis and tinea pedis), acne, and vaginal infections. However, no definitive evidence exists for the use of tea tree oil in any of these conditions, and further study is warranted.
- Oral use of tea tree oil should be avoided, as reports of toxicity after ingestion have been published. When used topically, tea tree oil is reported to be mildly irritating and has been associated with the development of allergic contact dermatitis, which may limit its potential as a topical agent for some patients.

Scientific Evidence for Common/Studied Uses	Grade*
Acne vulgaris	C
Allergic skin reactions	C
Dandruff	C
Methicillin-resistant *Staphylococcus aureus* (MRSA) colonization	C
Onychomycosis	C
Recurrent herpes labialis infection	C
Thrush (oral candidiasis)	C
Tinea pedis (athlete's foot)	C
Vaginal infections (yeast and bacterial)	C
Plaque	D

*Key to grades: *A:* Strong scientific evidence for this use; *B:* Good scientific evidence for this use; *C:* Unclear scientific evidence for this use; *D:* Fair scientific evidence against this use (it may not work); *F:* Strong scientific evidence against this use (it likely does not work). For a more detailed explanation of efficacy criteria, see "Natural Standard Evidence-Based Validated Grading Rationale" in the Introduction.

Historical or Theoretical Indications That Lack Sufficient Evidence

- Antibacterial,[1-16] antifungal,[12,17-23] antihistamine, anti-inflammatory,[24] antioxidant, antiseptic, aphthous ulcers, body odor, boils, bronchial congestion, bruises, burns,[25,26] carbuncles, colds, contraction cessation (in labor), corns, cough, eczema, fungal skin infections, furunculosis, gingivitis, herpes simplex virus infection, immune system deficiencies, impetigo,[6,17] insect bites and stings, lice,[27] lung inflammation, mouth sores, muscle and joint distress, nasopharyngitis, nose and throat irritation, oral candidiasis,[28] periodontal disease, pharyngitis, plaque formation,[29] psoriasis, pulmonary inflammation, ringworm, root canal treatment, scabies,[30] sinus infections, skin ailments, solvent, sore throat, tonsillitis,[31] warts, wound healing.[32]

Expert Opinion and Folkloric Precedent

- The tea tree was first used medicinally by the Bundalung aborigines, who crushed the leaves and applied them to cuts and wounds. Since then, topical tea tree oil has been recommended for the treatment of multiple conditions, including acne, burns, eczema, wounds, boils, and topical fungal infections, and as an astringent. The evidence is sparse regarding the efficacy of tea tree oil in the treatment of such indications, and its use is limited by the incidence of contact dermatitis, which may occur following use.

Safety Summary

- **Likely safe:** When used topically in concentrations up to 100% in patients with no known allergy to tea tree oil, any of its constituents, or other plants in the myrtle (Myrtaceae) family.[33-39]
- **Possibly safe:** In patients who have used tea tree oil in the past, as some have become sensitized to the oil after use and are at higher risk of developing allergic contact dermatitis.[40-45]
- **Likely unsafe:** When ingested orally in any concentration,[40,42,46,47] or when used topically in patients with known allergy to tea tree oil, other members of the myrtle (Myrtaceae) family, or any of the constituents of tea tree oil.

DOSING/TOXICOLOGY
General

- Recommended doses are based on those most commonly used in available trials, or on historical practice. However, with natural products, the optimal doses needed to balance efficacy and safety often have not been determined. Formulations and preparation methods may vary from manufacturer to manufacturer, and from batch to batch of a specific product made by a single manufacturer. Because often the active components of a product are not known, standardization may not be possible, and the clinical effects of different brands may not be comparable.

Standardization

- In 1996, the International Organization for Standardization specified the component limits for 14 of the almost 100 elements that make up tea tree oil (ISO 4730 Oil of

Melaleuca—terpinen-4-ol [tea tree oil]).[48] Tea tree oil must contain terpinolene 1.5% to 5%; 1,8-cineole ≤15%; α-terpinene 5% to 13%; γ-terpinene 10% to 28%; *p*-cymene 0.5% to 12%; terpinen-4-ol ≥30%; α-terpineol 1.5% to 8%; limonene 0.5% to 4%; sabinene trace 3.5%; aromadendrene trace 7%; δ-cadinene trace 8%; globulol trace 3%; viridiflorol trace 1.5%; and α-pinene 1% to 6%.[35]

- Prior to the development of the international standard (ISO 4730), an Australian standard existed (AS2782-1985) that required tea tree oil preparations to contain >30% terpinene-4-ol and <15% 1,8-cineole.[49]
- While 100% tea tree oil is sometimes used, it is often diluted with inert dilutants.

Dosing: Adult (18 Years and Older)
Topical

- *Note:* Recommended doses are based on those most commonly used in available trials. These doses have not necessarily been proven to be effective or safe.
- **Acne:** Tea tree oil 5% gel applied to acne areas daily for up to 3 months.[33]
- **Onychomycosis:** 100% tea tree oil applied twice daily for 6 months.[34]
- **Tinea pedis:** 10% tea tree oil cream (developed by Pharmaco Pty Ltd, Sydney, Australia) applied twice daily after thoroughly washing and drying feet, or 25% to 50% tea tree oil solution applied twice daily to the affected area for up to 4 weeks.[39]
- **Burns:** It is recommended that tea tree oil products not be used on burn wounds because of the toxicity of tea tree oil to human skin cells.
- **Dandruff:** 5% tea tree oil shampoo daily for at least 4 weeks has been used.
- **Genital herpes:** 6% tea tree oil gel has been used.
- **Methicillin-resistant *Staphylococcus aureus* (MRSA) colonization:** 4% tea tree oil nasal ointment and 5% tea tree oil body wash have been used.
- **Thrush:** Alcohol-based or alcohol-free solution four times daily for 2 to 4 weeks has been used.

Oral

- Due to a number of published case reports involving toxicity after ingestion, oral use of tea tree oil is not recommended.[40,42,46,47,50] Although tea tree oil solution has been used as a mouthwash, it should not be swallowed.

Dosing: Pediatric (Younger Than 18 Years)

- Insufficient evidence to recommend.

Toxicology
Oral

- Tea tree oil has been reported to cause cutaneous allergic responses and central nervous system (CNS) depression when ingested orally.[40,42,46,47] For these reasons, it is not recommended that tea tree oil be administered orally.
- A 17-month-old child ingested <10 mL of 100% tea tree oil and within 10 minutes became drowsy and unsteady, unable to sit or stand.[46] The child was given 2 g/kg of activated charcoal and experienced persistent ataxia for a period of roughly 5 hours, after which time he recovered fully and was discharged from the hospital.
- A 60-year-old man who had taken tea tree oil orally three to four times previously ingested one-half teaspoonful of tea tree oil and developed a red rash over his entire body

and feelings of malaise 1 day later.[42] The rash dissipated after 2 days and was replaced by a petechial rash in the same areas. One week later, the patient developed marked neutropenia, which resolved after an additional 10 days.

- A 23-month-old boy ingested less than 10 mL of T36-C7, a 100% tea tree oil product marketed as an antifungal and antiseptic (36% terpinen-4-ol and 7% cineol). He became confused and was unable to walk within 30 minutes.[47] He was taken to the emergency department, where he was given activated charcoal and sorbitol via a nasogastric tube; he returned to normal within 5 hours.
- There is a report of an adult who ingested one-half cup of tea tree oil and became comatose for approximately 12 hours, followed by a period of 36 hours in which the patient was semiconscious and hallucinating.[50] For 6 weeks following the ingestion of the tea tree oil, the patient experienced abdominal pain and diarrhea.

Topical

- Reported toxicities after application of tea tree oil to the skin of cats and dogs have included ataxia, weakness, muscle tremors, CNS depression, and malcoordination.[51]
- In an animal study, Zhang et al. found that 100% tea tree oil instilled into the middle ear for 30 minutes caused a change in the compound auditory nerve action potential threshold elevation.[52] A 2% solution of tea tree oil did not cause any significant lasting threshold changes under the same conditions. Thus, it is suggested that high concentrations of tea tree oil instilled in the middle ear may cause ototoxicity to the high-frequency region of the cochlea.
- An *in vitro* study on the cytotoxic effects of tea tree oil on human fibroblast cells showed that concentrations of tea tree oil up to 30 μg/mL incubated for 1, 4, 24, and 48 hours were nontoxic. Higher concentrations incubated for longer than 4 hours caused an increase in fibroblast death.[53]

ADVERSE EFFECTS/PRECAUTIONS/CONTRAINDICATIONS
Allergy

- The use of tea tree oil should be avoided in patients with a history of allergy/hypersensitivity to tea tree oil (*M. alternifolia*), any of its constituents, or plants that are members of the myrtle (Myrtaceae) family.
- There have been numerous case reports of allergic contact dermatitis occurring after topical application of tea tree oil.[43-45,54-60] Patients have presented with symptoms ranging from mild redness to bullous, blistering rashes and erythema multiforme. All episodes have reportedly subsided within weeks of the discontinuation of tea tree oil use. Some patients have required the use of topical corticosteroids to resolve their dermatitis.[44,54,55]
- De Groot and Weyland reported the development of dermatitis in two patients, one after oral ingestion and one after inhalation of tea tree oil.[40,41]
- A 28-year-old woman using tea tree oil and lavender oil containing products developed a rash on her right hand, legs, forearms, periorbital area, axillae, groin, suprapubic area, and perianal and vulval mucosa.[45] The rash cleared completely 1 month after discontinuation of tea tree and lavender oil products and treatment with clobetasone butyrate, nystatin, and oxytetracycline cream applied to her skin lesions.
- In a patch testing study of eight tea tree oil preparations in 28 healthy human volunteers, Rubel et al. found 3 patients who experienced strong allergic contact dermatitis, characterized by edema, erythema, and itching.[58,59] These authors

concluded that allergic reactions to tea tree oil appear to be caused by sesquiterpene components.

- Fritz et al. conducted allergy testing with tea tree oil in a total of 1216 patients in 1997.[43] Of those tested, seven developed allergic contact dermatitis. All of the patients who tested positive had used tea tree oil–containing products previously.
- Knight and Hausen patch tested seven patients with allergic contact dermatitis to tea tree oil to determine which components may be responsible for the allergic reaction.[57] They found that six of the seven patients reacted to limonene, five to α-terpinene and aromadendrene, two to terpinen-4-ol, one to p-cymene, and one to α-phellandrene.
- In animal studies by Hausen et al., sensitization was increased threefold with oxidized tea tree oil over that noted with fresh tea tree oil.[61] The authors suggested that the oxidized degradation products of tea tree oil may be responsible for the development of allergic contact dermatitis.
- People with a history of allergy to tincture of benzoin or colophony (rosin) should not use tea tree oil products, because cross-reactions have been reported. There is a case report of a patient with linear IgA disease, a subepidermal blistering disorder that can be precipitated by contact with tea tree oil.[62]
- Use cautiously with allergy to eucalyptol, as many tea tree preparations contain eucalyptol.

Adverse Effects/Postmarket Surveillance

- **General:** Tea tree oil is generally believed to be well tolerated when applied topically.[33-39] The most common adverse effects associated with the use of topical tea tree oil include contact dermatitis and skin and mucous membrane irritation. Oral ingestion has been associated with numerous case reports of toxicity.
- **Dermatologic:** Both topical and oral formulations of tea tree oil have been associated with cutaneous reactions. A number of reports of contact dermatitis after the topical application of tea tree oil have been documented.[43-45,54-60] Most episodes were reported to subside after the discontinuation of tea tree oil application. A number of patients have required treatment with topical corticosteroids after discontinuation of tea tree oil products, after which skin irritation/rashes subsided within weeks.[54-56] There is a case report of a 45-year-old man who developed a severe exacerbation of his long-standing atopic dermatitis after oral ingestion of 100% tea tree oil mixed with honey.[40] Another instance of rash has been reported in a 40-year-old man with hand eczema who inhaled a hot aqueous solution of tea tree oil from under a towel to treat bronchitis. He subsequently developed an edematous dermatitis on his face, eyelids, trunk, and arms.[41] Additionally, a 60-year-old man who had taken tea tree oil orally three to four times previously ingested one-half teaspoonful of tea tree oil and developed a red rash over his entire body and feelings of malaise 1 day later.[42] The red rash dissipated after 2 days and was replaced by a petechial rash in the same areas, which resolved within 1 week. Fritz et al. conducted allergy testing with tea tree oil in a total of 1216 patients in 1997, seven of whom developed allergic contact dermatitis due to tea tree oil.[43] Note: Carson et al., in defense of tea tree oil, have pointed out that the composition of the oil in the reports by van der Valk and DeGroot did not meet the international standard (ISO 4730) for tea tree oil.[35]
- **Neurologic/CNS:** CNS depression has been associated in multiple human case reports with oral tea tree oil, and in animal studies with topical tea tree oil. A 17-month-old child ingested <10 mL of 100% tea tree oil and within 10 minutes became drowsy and unsteady, unable to sit or stand.[46] A 23-month-old boy also ingested <10 mL of T36-C7, a 100% tea tree oil product marketed as an antifungal and antiseptic (36% terpinen-4-ol and 7% cineol), and became confused and was unable to walk within 30 minutes.[47] Neurologic sequelae following dermal application of tea tree oil to cats and dogs have included ataxia, weakness, muscle tremors, depressed behavior, and malcoordination.[51] Many tea tree preparations contain large volumes of alcohol.
- **Otic:** It has been suggested that high concentrations of tea tree oil instilled in the middle ear may cause ototoxicity to the high-frequency region of the cochlea. In an animal study, Zhang et al. found that 100% tea tree oil instilled into the middle ear for 30 minutes caused a change in the compound auditory nerve action potential threshold elevation.[52] A 2% solution of tea tree oil did not cause any significant lasting threshold changes under the same conditions.
- **Gastrointestinal:** One patient was reported to experience diarrhea and abdominal pain for a period of 6 weeks after the ingestion of one-half teacup of tea tree oil.[50] There have been reports of nausea, unpleasant taste, and bad breath associated with tea tree oil use.
- **Hematologic:** Profound neutropenia developed in a 60-year-old man 1 week following ingestion of one-half teaspoonful of tea tree oil.[42] Notably, a petechial rash and malaise developed shortly after the ingestion, followed by the hematologic abnormality. All symptoms and signs resolved after an additional 10 days. The patient had taken tea tree oil orally three to four times previously with no adverse effects.

Precautions/Warnings/Contraindications

- Use topical tea tree oil cautiously in patients with previous tea tree oil use, as sensitization can occur, increasing the risk of developing allergic contact dermatitis.[40-45]
- Avoid oral tea tree oil, because of multiple reports of CNS toxicity and cutaneous allergic responses.[40,42,46,47]

Pregnancy and Lactation

- Not recommended because of a lack of sufficient data.
- Animal studies suggest caution in the use of tea tree oil during childbirth, because tea tree oil has been reported to decrease the force of spontaneous contractions, which theoretically could put the baby and the mother at risk.

INTERACTIONS
Tea Tree Oil/Drug Interactions

- **Topical drying agents/astringents:** Topical tea tree oil preparations may result in drying of the skin and may act additively with other agents such as tretinoin (Retin-A, Renova).

Tea Tree Oil/Herb/Supplement Interactions

- Insufficient available data.

Tea Tree Oil/Food Interactions

- Insufficient available data.

Tea Tree Oil/Lab Interactions

- **Neutropenia:** A 60-year-old man who had taken tea tree oil orally three to four times previously ingested one-half teaspoonful of tea tree oil; 1 day later, a red rash developed over his entire body, accompanied by feelings of malaise.[42]

The rash dissipated after 2 days and was replaced by a petechial rash in the same areas. One week later, marked neutropenia developed, which resolved after an additional 10 days.

MECHANISM OF ACTION
Pharmacology

- The tea tree is related to *Melaleuca quinquenervia* and *Melaleuca cajuputi* (trees that produce oils commonly used in aromatherapy, similar to camphor and peppermint). However, tea tree oil comes exclusively from *M. alternifolia* and should not be confused with cajeput oil, niauouli oil, kanuka oil, or manuka oil obtained from other *Melaleuca* species. Their composition is quite different, and these other species contain higher concentrations of cineole, a skin irritant that may decrease the antiseptic activity of the purported active ingredient of tea tree oil (terpinen-4-ol).

- **Antimicrobial:** Tea tree oil has been found to stimulate autolysis of bacterial cells in both the exponential and stationary growth phases, with greater activity during the exponential phase.[10] *In vitro* studies conducted by Cox et al. found that at concentrations that inhibit the growth of several bacterial species, tea tree oil also inhibits glucose-stimulated leakage of intracellular potassium.[8,9] A single *in vitro* study reported that the antibacterial activity of tea tree oil is decreased by the presence of organic matter or the surfactants Tween 20 and Tween 80.[63] Tea tree oil inhibits the *in vitro* conversion of *Candida albicans* from yeast to mycelial form.[19] Through *in vitro* studies of the antimicrobial activity of tea tree oil, it has been demonstrated that terpinen-4-ol is the component most likely responsible for its antimicrobial properties.[4]

- **Inflammation:** Hart et al. have found that tea tree oil suppresses the production of tumor necrosis factor-alpha, interleukin-1β, interleukin-10, and prostaglandin E$_2$ by activated monocytes *in vitro*.[64] Budhiraja et al. found that tea tree oil induces differentiation of myelocytes into monocytes *in vitro*.[65] Tea tree oil suppresses the production of superoxide by activated monocytes *in vitro*.[24] Terpinen-4-ol has been isolated by gas chromatography to be the most likely active anti-inflammatory constituent of tea tree oil *in vitro*.[64]

Pharmacodynamics/Kinetics

- Insufficient available data.

HISTORY

- The Bundalung aborigines traditionally used tea tree oil to treat cuts and wounds. The term "tea" was coined by early European settlers in Australia who attempted to make a beverage from the leaves. In the early 20th century, the Australian chemist A.R. Penfold described antiseptic properties of tea tree leaves. Tea tree oil was used in surgery and dentistry during the 1920s. Tea tree oil was first written about in the *Medical Journal of Australia* in 1930, when a surgeon in Sydney reported good results after using a solution of tea tree oil to clean surgical wounds. In 1933, the *British Medical Journal* also published an article about the use of tea tree oil as a disinfectant. During World War II, tea tree oil was classified as an essential for the prevention and treatment of wound infections. It was used in munitions factories in Australia and was believed to have greatly reduced the number of hand infections that developed from abrasions due to metal filings and turnings. Tea tree oil was seen as such an essential product that harvesters and farmers of tea tree oil were exempt from military service in World War II. However, the use of tea tree oil as an antiseptic fell out of favor when antibiotics were discovered.

Review of the Evidence: Tea Tree Oil

Condition Treated*	Study Design	Author, Year	N[†]	SS[†]	Study Quality[‡]	Magnitude of Benefit	ARR[†]	NNT[†]	Comments
Acne	Equivalence trial, single-blind	Bassett[33] 1990	124	Mixed	2	Small	NA	NA	No significant difference between tea tree oil and benzoyl peroxide; significant improvement from baseline in both groups; lack of placebo or power calculation limits conclusions.
MRSA colonization	Randomized, equivalence study	Caelli[36,37] 1998, 2000	20	No	2	Unclear	NA	NA	Tea tree oil nasal ointment plus body wash vs. triclosan body wash plus mupirocin nasal ointment. No difference between regimens, but no power calculation, so unclear if results indicate equivalence.
Onychomycosis	Equivalence trial, double-blind	Buck[34] 1994	117	Mixed	5	Small	NA	NA	No significant difference between groups, but no placebo or power calculation.
Onychomycosis	Equivalence trial, double-blind	Syed[38] 1999	60	Yes	4	Small	NA	NA	Placebo was not inactive; combined tea tree oil with known antifungal agent; unequal randomization.
Tinea pedis	Equivalence trial	Tong[39] 1992	120	No	3	Small	NA	NA	Similar to tolnaftate in resolving symptoms.

*Primary or secondary outcome.
[†]*N*, Number of patients; *SS*, statistically significant; *ARR*, absolute risk reduction; *NNT*, the number of patients who need to undergo a specific intervention in order to observe an outcome in one individual.
[‡]0-2 = poor; 3-4 = good; 5 = excellent.
MRSA, Methicillin-resistant *Staphylococcus aureus*; *NA*, not applicable.
For an explanation of each category in this table, please see Table 3 in the Introduction.

REVIEW OF THE EVIDENCE: DISCUSSION

Acne Vulgaris

Summary

- Tea tree oil has been suggested as a topical treatment for acne, based on its demonstrated *in vitro* antibacterial properties.[1,3,4,6-12,14,16] However, there is insufficient human evidence at this time to recommend either for or against this use of tea tree oil. One methodologically weak human trial has yielded preliminary equivocal results.[33]

Evidence

- In a single blind, randomized equivalence trial, Bassett et al. studied the effects of tea tree oil 5% gel (developed by Product Development Laboratory, Lederle Laboratories, using Ateol tea tree oil from Australian Plantations Pty Ltd.) vs. benzoyl peroxide 5% lotion in 124 patients with mild to moderate acne (mean age, 19.7 years).[33] Acne severity was assessed using the established counting technique, which measures the number and severity of lesions. After 3 months, a statistically significant decrease in the number of lesions from baseline was seen in both groups, with no significant difference between groups. These results can be interpreted in one of two ways: Either tea tree oil was in fact equivalent in efficacy to benzoyl peroxide, or there were too few subjects enrolled in the trial to adequately detect a difference between the groups (inadequately powered). The study was only single-blinded, which introduces the possibility of bias. There was no placebo group, which raises the question of whether the improvements were simply due to the natural history of the disease, which may include periodic resolution of lesions even without intervention. Notably, patients in the tea tree oil group reported fewer adverse effects—namely, less skin dryness, pruritus, stinging, and redness—than were experienced by patients in the benzoyl peroxide group ($p < 0.001$). Because of methodologic weaknesses in this trial, the results cannot be considered conclusive. Further study is warranted in this area.

Thrush (Oral Candidiasis)

Summary

- Numerous *in vitro* studies have demonstrated the ability of tea tree oil to kill fungal pathogens such as *Candida* organisms.[17-22] It has been hypothesized that tea tree oil may be efficacious as a gargle for the treatment of thrush. One human case series has reported promising early results in patients with AIDS, but at this time there is insufficient evidence to recommend either for or against this use of tea tree oil. It should be noted that tea tree oil is toxic when ingested orally and therefore should not be swallowed.

Evidence

- Jandourek et al. performed a preliminary open-label study investigating the effectiveness of tea tree oil oral solution, used four times daily for 2 to 4 weeks, in treating fluconazole-refractory oral candidiasis in 13 AIDS patients.[66] The primary outcome measure was resolution of oral lesions, as evaluated on a weekly basis. After 4 weeks, 8 of 12 evaluable patients had responded to the treatment with tea tree oil oral solution and two patients were cured. The overall clinical response rate was 67%, and the only adverse effects reported were mild to moderate oral burning when the solution contacted oral mucosa (reported by two thirds of the patients). Although these results are promising, open-label studies cannot be considered definitive, because of the possible introduction of bias and confounding. Further study is warranted in this area.

- In a case series, Vasquez et al. treated refractory oropharyngeal candidiasis in 14 patients with AIDS using Melaleuca Oral Solution M (Breathaway).[28] The regimen consisted of "swish and spit" of tablespoon of the solution four times daily. Clinical improvement measures were based on physical evaluation of the oropharynx, as well as culture data. After 4 weeks, 12 patients were evaluable. The authors reported cure in five patients, improvement in five, and lack of effect in two (nonresponders). Although these results are promising, this was not a controlled study, and therefore the results cannot clearly be attributed to tea tree oil. Further study is warranted in this area.

Methicillin-Resistant *Staphylococcus aureus* Colonization

Summary

- In multiple *in vitro* studies, tea tree oil has been shown to have antimicrobial activity against methicillin-resistant *Staphylococcus aureus* (MRSA).[3,7,13] However, there is currently insufficient human evidence to recommend either for or against this use of tea tree oil.

Evidence

- Calli et al. performed a randomized equivalence trial comparing the use of 4% tea tree oil nasal ointment and 5% tea tree oil body wash with triclosan body wash and 2% mupirocin nasal ointment for decolonization in 20 hospital inpatients carrying MRSA.[36,37] The main outcome measure was defined as the absence of MRSA at the end of a 7-day course of treatment. A nonsignificant trend toward better performance of tea tree oil than of triclosan and mupirocin was reported. This small trial may not have been adequately powered to detect significant differences between groups, and these results cannot be considered clinically relevant. Further study using both placebo and standard therapies as controls, as well as an initial power calculation, would provide a higher standard of evidence.

Onychomycosis

Summary

- Tea tree oil has been proposed as a potential topical therapeutic agent for onychomycosis, based on multiple studies demonstrating *in vitro* antifungal activity.[12,17-23] Initial human trials have been methodologically flawed, and at this time there is insufficient evidence to recommend either for or against this use of tea tree oil.

Evidence

- In a double-blind, randomized equivalence trial, Buck et al. studied the efficacy of 100% tea tree oil (Thursday Plantation Inc., Monetite, California) vs. 1% clotrimazole solution (Schering-Plough Corp., Liberty Corner, New Jersey) in the topical treatment of lower extremity onychomycosis in 117 patients.[34] Primary outcome measures after 6 months of twice-daily study drug application included clinical assessment (defined by the investigator as "full," "partial," or "no" resolution); culture results (using the validated dermatophyte infection test medium); and subjective patient assessment of improvement. A power calculation was performed by the investigators prior to the study to calculate the appropriate sample size. Four participants withdrew from the study because of adverse effects (erythema and irritation). Five additional participants were lost to follow-

T

up. At 6 months, no significant difference was found between the two treatments in clinical assessment, culture results, or subjective assessment. The percent of patients experiencing full or partial resolution of their onychomycosis at the end of 6 months in the tea tree oil and the clotrimazole groups was 60% and 61%, respectively, and these results represented significant improvements from baseline. Although this study was generally well designed, it suffers from several methodologic flaws. First, the lack of a placebo group raises questions about whether the improvements in both groups were simply due to the natural history of onychomycosis, which tends to periodically subside even without intervention. In addition, blinding was not described, and given the distinctive odor of tea tree oil, full blinding of patients may not have been possible, thus introducing bias. As a result of these weaknesses, the results of this trial can only be considered suggestive. The relevance of this study is also diminished in current times because tea tree oil was compared with a therapeutic agent that is not currently standard, topical clotrimazole. Future studies would be useful if outcomes were compared with a standard systemic therapy.

- In a double-blind, randomized equivalence trial, Skyed et al. studied the efficacy of 2% butenafine hydrochloride plus 5% tea tree oil cream vs. a "control" cream (containing an unclear amount of tea tree oil) in treating toenail onychomycosis in 60 outpatients.[38] Patients were randomized to receive either butenafine/tea tree oil cream or control; they were instructed to apply cream to their large toenail three times daily for up to 8 weeks and to return once weekly for assessment and toenail debridement if possible. Outcome was based on symptomatic and mycologic cure; clinical success was defined as 100% remission or 90% to 99% improvement in the treated toenail. Results showed cure in 80% of patients using the butenafine/tea tree oil cream, compared with 0% cure in the control group, with statistical significance. From this study, it appears that a combination butenafine/tea tree oil cream is more effective in treating toenail onychomycosis than a cream containing an unclear concentration of tea tree oil. However, these results do not have an implication for the use of tea tree oil monotherapy in the treatment of onychomycosis. Because the concentration of tea tree oil in the control cream was not reported, the absence of clinical success in the control group is not clinically relevant. The amount of tea tree oil in the control cream may have been quite low, in order to provide a scent similar to that of the test cream without including active amounts, but this remains unclear. A superior study design would include a butenafine monotherapy group, a tea tree oil monotherapy group, a standard care therapy group (for example, oral terbinafine), and a true placebo group.

Recurrent Herpes Labialis Infection
Summary
- Tea tree oil has been proposed as a potential topical therapy for genital herpes simplex virus infections based on *in vitro* findings of antiviral activity.[67] However, at this time there is insufficient human evidence to recommend either for or against this use of tea tree oil.

Evidence
- Carson et al. evaluated the efficacy of tea tree oil in 20 patients with a self-reported history of recurrent herpes labialis.[68] Subjects were randomized to receive either 6% tea tree oil in an aqueous gel base (Australian Body care Pty Ltd., Mudgeeraba, Queensland, Australia) or placebo for application to lesions five times daily. The primary outcome measures were time to re-epithelialization, time to crust formation, and duration of virus detection by polymerase chain reaction (PCR) assay. Tea tree oil therapy was well tolerated, and there was a trend toward reduced duration of positive cultures, although no statistically significant difference was found for tea tree oil vs. placebo. Because no power calculation was performed, it is possible that the sample size was too small to detect benefits. Therefore, the results are equivocal and of limited clinical relevance.

Tinea Pedis (Athlete's Foot)
Summary
- Tea tree oil has been proposed as a potential topical therapy for tinea pedis (athlete's foot), based on multiple studies demonstrating *in vitro* antifungal activity.[12,17-23] Literature review reveals a single human study with equivocal results. Therefore, at this time there is insufficient reliable human evidence to recommend either for or against this use of tea tree oil.

Evidence
- In a randomized, double-blind equivalence trial (with placebo control), Tong et al. studied the effects of 10% tea tree oil cream (developed by Pharmaco Pty Ltd, Sydney, Australia) vs. 1% tolnaftate cream (Tinaderm, Schering Pty Ltd, Sydney, Australia) and placebo in the treatment of 121 patients with tinea pedis.[39] Patients were randomized and instructed to apply the cream twice daily for 4 weeks and to return for evaluation weekly. The signs and symptoms of tinea pedis were assessed at each visit. The amounts of scaling, inflammation, itching, and burning were rated subjectively on a scale of 0 to 4, with 0 for absence of symptoms and 4 for "very severe." After 4 weeks, a skin scraping/culture was analyzed. The authors reported that 104 subjects completed the protocol (86%), and no subjects withdrew because of adverse effects. More patients in the tolnaftate group converted to negative cultures than those in the tea tree oil or placebo group (85%, 30%, and 21%, respectively; $p < 0.001$). The relatively high rate of mycologic cure in the placebo group (21%) may be explained by the increased attention to foot care, as all subjects were instructed to wash and dry their feet twice daily before the application of study cream. By contrast, patients in the tea tree oil group experienced symptomatic improvement similar to that in patients in the tolnaftate group, and superior to that in patients in the placebo group, with statistical significance. Although aspects of this study were well designed, such as randomization and controls, methodologic weaknesses included the lack of a validated scale to assess symptomatic improvement and the small sample size. These mixed results leave the question of efficacy unanswered.

Vaginal Infections (Yeast and Bacterial)
Summary
- *In vitro* studies have demonstrated tea tree oil to possess antimicrobial activity against pathogens that commonly cause vaginal infections.[12,17-23] However, the existing human evidence is methodologically weak, and the efficacy of tea tree oil for vaginal infections remains unclear.

Evidence

- In a 1962 study, Pena investigated the use of a tea tree oil solution in the treatment of 130 cases of vaginal infections (96 cases of trichomonal vaginosis, 4 cases of *Candida albicans* infection, 20 cases of nulliparous *Trichomonas vaginalis* cervicitis, and 10 cases of chronic endocervicitis).[69] A 20% solution of tea tree oil applied via saturated tampon for 24 hours was reported to cure the 10 chronic cervicitis cases after four weekly treatments, with no adverse effects. Clinical cure of the 96 cases of trichomonal vaginitis occurred after application of a tea tree oil–saturated tampon for 24 hours, followed by daily douching with 0.4% tea tree oil in 1 quart of water. Patients used a mean of 42 douches and 6 tea tree oil tampon applications during the study. A control group of 50 patients with trichomonal vaginitis received "standard" 1962 antitrichomonal suppositories and experienced no better results than those for treatment with tea tree oil. Although this evidence seemed promising, the lack of adequate blinding, randomization, or statistical analysis limited the clinical relevance of these results. Additional studies of safety and efficacy are warranted before a recommendation can be made.
- Blackwell reported the case of a 41-year-old woman with anaerobic bacterial vaginosis.[70] She refused metronidazole treatment and instead used a 5-day course of 200-mg tea tree oil vaginal pessaries in vegetable oil base. One month later, her vaginal secretions were reported as normal. It is not clear if her infection would have cleared spontaneously (without tea tree oil treatment). These results can only be considered preliminary.

FORMULARY: BRANDS USED IN CLINICAL TRIALS
Brands Used in Statistically Significant Clinical Trials

- Trials have used products from the following manufacturers: Australian Plantation Pty Ltd. (Wyrallah, New South Wales, Australia)[33]; Thursday Plantation Inc. (Montecito, California)[34]; Australian Bodycare Pty Ltd (Mudgeeraba, Queensland, Australia).[68]

References

1. Carson CF, Riley TV. The antimicrobial activity of tea tree oil. Med J Aust 1994;160(4):236.
2. Carson CF, Riley TV. Susceptibility of *Propionibacterium acnes* to the essential oil of *Melaleuca alternifolia*. Lett Appl Microbiol 1994;19(1):24-25.
3. Carson CF, Cookson BD, Farrelly HD, et al. Susceptibility of methicillin-resistant *Staphylococcus aureus* to the essential oil of *Melaleuca alternifolia*. J Antimicrob Chemother 1995;35(3):421-424.
4. Carson CF, Riley TV. Antimicrobial activity of the major components of the essential oil of *Melaleuca alternifolia*. J Appl Bacteriol 1995;78(3):264-269.
5. Carson CF, Hammer KA, Riley TV. Broth micro-dilution method for determining the susceptibility of *Escherichia coli* and *Staphylococcus aureus* to the essential oil of *Melaleuca alternifolia* (tea tree oil). Microbios 1995;82(332):181-185.
6. Carson CF, Hammer KA, Riley TV. In-vitro activity of the essential oil of *Melaleuca alternifolia* against *Streptococcus* spp. J Antimicrob Chemother 1996;37(6):1177-1178.
7. Chan CH, Loudon KW. Activity of tea tree oil on methicillin-resistant *Staphylococcus aureus* (MRSA). J Hosp Infect 1998;39(3):244-245.
8. Cox SD, Gustafson JE, Mann CM, et al. Tea tree oil causes K+ leakage and inhibits respiration in Escherichia coli. Lett Appl Microbiol 1998;26(5):355-358.
9. Cox SD, Mann CM, Markham JL, et al. The mode of antimicrobial action of the essential oil of *Melaleuca alternifolia* (tea tree oil). J Appl Microbiol 2000;88(1):170-175.
10. Gustafson JE, Liew YC, Chew S, et al. Effects of tea tree oil on *Escherichia coli*. Lett Appl Microbiol 1998;26(3):194-198.
11. Hammer KA, Carson CF, Riley TV. Susceptibility of transient and commensal skin flora to the essential oil of *Melaleuca alternifolia* (tea tree oil). Am J Infect Control 1996;24(3):186-189.
12. Kulik E, Lenkeit K, Meyer J. [Antimicrobial effects of tea tree oil (*Melaleuca*

13. *alternifolia*) on oral microorganisms]. Schweiz Monatsschr Zahnmed 2000;110(11):125-130.
13. May J, Chan CH, King A, et al. Time-kill studies of tea tree oils on clinical isolates. J Antimicrob Chemother 2000;45(5):639-643.
14. Raman A, Weir U, Bloomfield SF. Antimicrobial effects of tea-tree oil and its major components on *Staphylococcus aureus*, *Staph. epidermidis* and *Propionibacterium acnes*. Lett Appl Microbiol 1995;21(4):242-245.
15. Shapiro S, Meier A, Guggenheim B. The antimicrobial activity of essential oils and essential oil components towards oral bacteria. Oral Microbiol Immunol 1994;9(4):202-208.
16. Williams LR, Home VN, Zhang X, et al. The composition and bactericidal activity of oil of *Melaleuca alternifolia* (tea tree oil). Int J Aromather 1988;1:15-17.
17. Belaiche P. Treatment of skin infections with the essential oil of *Melaleuca alternifolia*. Phytotherapy 1985;15:15, 17.
18. Concha JM, Moore LS, Holloway WJ. Antifungal activity of *Melaleuca alternifolia* (tea-tree) oil against various pathogenic organisms. J Am Podiatr Med Assoc 1998;88(10):489-492.
19. D'Auria FD, Laino L, Strippoli V, et al. In vitro activity of tea tree oil against *Candida albicans* mycelial conversion and other pathogenic fungi. J Chemother 2001;13(4):377-383.
20. Hammer KA, Carson CF, Riley TV. In vitro susceptibility of *Malassezia furfur* to the essential oil of *Melaleuca alternifolia*. J Med Vet Mycol 1997;35(5):375-377.
21. Hammer KA, Carson CF, Riley TV. In-vitro activity of essential oils, in particular *Melaleuca alternifolia* (tea tree) oil and tea tree oil products, against *Candida* spp. J Antimicrob Chemother 1998;42(5):591-595.
22. Hammer KA, Carson CF, Riley TV. In vitro activities of ketoconazole, econazole, miconazole, and *Melaleuca alternifolia* (tea tree) oil against *Malassezia* species. Antimicrob Agents Chemother 2000;44(2):467-469.
23. Nenoff P, Haustein UF, Brandt W. Antifungal activity of the essential oil of *Melaleuca alternifolia* (tea tree oil) against pathogenic fungi in vitro. Skin Pharmacol 1996;9(6):388-394.
24. Brand C, Ferrante A, Prager RH, et al. The water-soluble components of the essential oil of *Melaleuca alternifolia* (tea tree oil) suppress the production of superoxide by human monocytes, but not neutrophils, activated in vitro. Inflamm Res 2001;50(4):213-219.
25. Faoagali J, George N, Leditschke JF. Does tea tree oil have a place in the topical treatment of burns? Burns 1997;23(4):349-351.
26. Jandera V, Hudson DA, de Wet PM, et al. Cooling the burn wound: evaluation of different modalites. Burns 2000;26(3):265-270.
27. Veal L. The potential effectiveness of essential oils as a treatment for headlice, *Pediculus humanus capitis*. Complement Ther Nurs Midwifery 1996;2(4):97-101.
28. Vazquez JA, Vaishampayan J, Arganoza MT, et al. Use of an over the counter product, Breathaway (*Melaleuca* oral solution), as an alternative agent for refractory oropharyngeal candidiasis in AIDS patients [abstract]. Int Conf AIDS 1996;11:109.
29. Arweiler NB, Donos N, Netuschil L, et al. Clinical and antibacterial effect of tea tree oil—a pilot study. Clin Oral Invest 2000;4(2):70-73.
30. Walton SF, Myerscough MR, Currie BJ. Studies in vitro on the relative efficacy of current acaricides for *Sarcoptes scabiei* var. hominis. Trans R Soc Trop Med Hyg 2000;94(1):92-96.
31. Hammer KA, Carson CF, Riley TV. In vitro susceptibilities of lactobacilli and organisms associated with bacterial vaginosis to *Melaleuca alternifolia* (tea tree) oil. Antimicrob Chemother 1999;43(1):196.
32. Sherry E, Boeck H, Warnke PH. Percutaneous treatment of chronic MRSA osteomyelitis with a novel plant- derived antiseptic. BMC Surg 2001;1(1):1.
33. Bassett IB, Pannowitz DL, Barnetson RS. A comparative study of tea-tree oil versus benzoylperoxide in the treatment of acne. Med J Aust 1990;153(8):455-458.
34. Buck DS, Nidorf DM, Addino JG. Comparison of two topical preparations for the treatment of onychomycosis: *Melaleuca alternifolia* (tea tree) oil and clotrimazole. J Fam Pract 1994;38(6):601-605.
35. Carson CF, Riley TV. Safety, efficacy and provenance of tea tree (*Melaleuca alternifolia*) oil. Contact Dermatitis 2001;45(2):65-67.
36. Caelli M, Riley T. Tea tree oil - an alternative topical decolonisation agent for adult inpatients with methicillin-resistant *Staphylococcus aureus* (MRSA)—a pilot study. J Hosp Infect 1998;40(Suppl A):9.
37. Caelli M, Porteous J, Carson CF, et al. Tea tree oil as an alternative topical decolonization agent for methicillin-resistant *Staphylococcus aureus*. J Hosp Infect 2000;46(3):236-237.
38. Syed TA, Qureshi ZA, Ali SM, et al. Treatment of toenail onychomycosis with 2% butenafine and 5% *Melaleuca alternifolia* (tea tree) oil in cream. Trop Med Int Health 1999;4(4):284-287.
39. Tong MM, Altman PM, Barnetson RS. Tea tree oil in the treatment of tinea pedis. Australas J Dermatol 1992;33(3):145-149.
40. De Groot AC, Weyland JW. Systemic contact dermatitis from tea tree oil. Contact Dermatitis 1992;27(4):279-280.
41. De Groot AC. Airborne allergic contact dermatitis from tea tree oil. Contact Dermatitis 1996;35(5):304-305.
42. Elliott C. Tea tree oil poisoning. Med J Aust 1993;159(11-12):830-831.
43. Fritz TM, Burg G, Krasovec M. [Allergic contact dermatitis to cosmetics

containing *Melaleuca alternifolia* (tea tree oil)]. Ann Dermatol Venereol 2001;128(2):123-126.

44. Selvaag E, Eriksen B, Thune P. Contact allergy due to tea tree oil and cross-sensitization to colophony. Contact Dermatitis 1994;31(2):124-125.

45. Varma S, Blackford S, Statham BN, et al. Combined contact allergy to tea tree oil and lavender oil complicating chronic vulvovaginitis. Contact Dermatitis 2000;42(5):309-310.

46. Del Beccaro MA. *Melaleuca* oil poisoning in a 17-month-old. Vet Hum Toxicol 1995;37(6):557-558.

47. Jacobs MR, Hornfeldt CS. *Melaleuca* oil poisoning. J Toxicol Clin Toxicol 1994;32(4):461-464.

48. Anonymous. Essential oils of *Melaleuca*, terpinen-4-ol type (tea tree oil). International Organization for Standardization, 1996.

49. Anonymous. Australian standard for essential oils-oil of *Melaleuca*, terpinen-4-ol type (AS 2782-1985). Standards Association of Australia, 1985.

50. Seawright A. Comment: Tea tree oil poisoning. Med J Aust 1993;159:830-831.

51. Villar D, Knight MJ, Hansen SR, et al. Toxicity of *Melaleuca* oil and related essential oils applied topically on dogs and cats. Vet Human Toxicol 1994;36(2):139-142.

52. Zhang SY, Robertson D. A study of tea tree oil ototoxicity. Audiol Neurootol 2000;5(2):64-68.

53. Soderberg TA, Johansson A, Gref R. Toxic effects of some conifer resin acids and tea tree oil on human epithelial and fibroblast cells. Toxicology 1996;107(2):99-109.

54. Apted JH. Contact dermatitis associated with the use of tea-tree oil. Australas J Dermatol 1991;32(3):177.

55. Bhushan M, Beck MH. Allergic contact dermatitis from tea tree oil in a wart paint. Contact Dermatitis 1997;36(2):117-118.

56. Khanna M, Qasem K, Sasseville D. Allergic contact dermatitis to tea tree oil with erythema multiforme–like id reaction. Am J Contact Dermat 2000;11(4):238-242.

57. Knight TE, Hausen BM. *Melaleuca* oil (tea tree oil) dermatitis. J Am Acad Dermatol 1994;30(3):423-427.

58. Rubel DM, Freeman S, Southwell IA. Tea tree oil allergy: what is the offending agent? Report of three cases of tea tree oil allergy and review of the literature. Australas J Dermatol 1998;39(4):244-247.

59. Southwell IA, Freeman S, Rubel D. Skin irritancy of tea tree oil. J Essent Oil Res 1997;9:47-52.

60. van der Valk PG, De Groot AC, Bruynzeel DP, et al. [Allergic contact eczema due to 'tea tree' oil]. Ned Tijdschr Geneeskd 1994;138(16):823-825.

61. Hausen BM, Reichling J, Harkenthal M. Degradation products of monoterpenes are the sensitizing agents in tea tree oil. Am J Contact Dermat 1999;10(2):68-77.

62. Perrett CM, Evans AV, Russell-Jones R. Tea tree oil dermatitis associated with linear IgA disease. Clin Exp Dermatol 2003;28(2):167-170.

63. Hammer KA, Carson CF, Riley TV. Influence of organic matter, cations and surfactants on the antimicrobial activity of *Melaleuca alternifolia* (tea tree) oil *in vitro*. J Appl Microbiol 1999;86(3):446-452.

64. Hart PH, Brand C, Carson CF, et al. Terpinen-4-ol, the main component of the essential oil of *Melaleuca alternifolia* (tea tree oil), suppresses inflammatory mediator production by activated human monocytes. Inflamm Res 2000;49(11):619-626.

65. Budhiraja SS, Cullum ME, Sioutis SS, et al. Biological activity of *Melaleuca alternifola* (tea tree) oil component, terpinen-4-ol, in human myelocytic cell line HL-60. J Manipulative Physiol Ther 1999;22(7):447-453.

66. Jandourek A, Vaishampayan JK, Vazquez JA. Efficacy of melaleuca oral solution for the treatment of fluconazole refractory oral candidiasis in AIDS patients. AIDS 1998;12(9):1033-1037.

67. Schnitzler P, Schon K, Reichling J. Antiviral activity of Australian tea tree oil and eucalyptus oil against herpes simplex virus in cell culture. Pharmazie 2001;56(4):343-347.

68. Carson CF, Ashton L, Dry L, et al. *Melaleuca alternifolia* (tea tree) oil gel (6%) for the treatment of recurrent herpes labialis. J Antimicrob Chemother 2001;48(3):450-451.

69. Peña EF. *Melaleuca alternifolia* oil. Its use for trichomonal vaginitis and other vaginal infections. Obstet Gynecol 1962;19(6):793-795.

70. Blackwell AL. Tea tree oil and anaerobic (bacterial) vaginosis. Lancet 1991;337(8736):300.

Thyme
(Thymus vulgaris L.)

SYNONYMS/COMMON NAMES/RELATED SUBSTANCES

- Common thyme, common garden thyme, English thyme, farigola, folia thymi, French thyme, garden thyme, gartenthymian, herba thymi, herba timi, Labiatae (family), Lamiaceae (family), mother of thyme, red thyme, rubbed thyme, serpyllium, shepherd's thyme, Spanish thyme, ten, thick leaf thyme, time, timo, thym, thyme aetheroleum, thyme oil, thymi herba, Thymian, thymol, *Thymus serpyllum*, *Thymus zygis* L., wild thyme, white thyme oil.
- *Note:* There are up to 400 subspecies of thyme; common thyme (*Thymus vulgaris*) and Spanish thyme (*Thymus zygis*) are often used interchangeably for medicinal purposes. Not to be confused with calamint (*Calamintha ascendens*, basil thyme) or with Spanish origanum oil (*Thymus capitatus*, Sicilian thyme or Spanish thyme).

CLINICAL BOTTOM LINE
Background

- Thyme has been used medicinally for thousands of years. Beyond its common culinary application, it has been recommended for a myriad of indications, based on proposed antimicrobial, antitussive, spasmolytic, and antioxidant activity. To date there are no well-defined controlled clinical trials to support thyme monotherapy for therapeutic use in humans.
- Thymol, one of the constituents of thyme, is contained in antiseptic mouthwashes, with limited clinical studies in the available literature to corroborate its efficacy as a monotherapy in dental outcomes, such as reductions in plaque formation, gingivitis, and caries.
- Although no well-defined clinical data exist, traditional health practice patterns, expert opinion, and anecdote suggest that the herb is generally well tolerated in common doses; a majority of the adverse events appear to be related to dermatologic or allergic reactions. The essential oil of thyme should not be used orally, since it has been associated with toxic reactions ranging from nausea to respiratory arrest.

Scientific Evidence for Common/Studied Uses	Grade*
Alopecia areata	C
Bronchitis, cough	C
Dental plaque	C
Inflammatory skin disorders	C
Paronychia, onycholysis, antifungal	C

*Key to grades: *A:* Strong scientific evidence for this use; *B:* Good scientific evidence for this use; *C:* Unclear scientific evidence for this use; *D:* Fair scientific evidence against this use (it may not work); *F:* Strong scientific evidence against this use (it likely does not work). For a more detailed explanation of efficacy criteria, see "Natural Standard Evidence-Based Validated Grading Rationale" in the Introduction.

Historical or Theoretical Indications
That Lack Sufficient Evidence

- Abscess, acne, appetite stimulant, antioxidant,[1-3] anxiety, arthritis, asthma, burns, cancer,[4] cellulitis, depression, colic, cystitis, dermatitis, dermatomyositis, diarrhea, diuresis, dysmenorrhea, dyspepsia, dyspnea, eczema, edema, enuresis, epilepsy, fever, flatulence, flu, gas, gastritis, gingivitis, gout, halitosis, headache, heartburn, *Helicobacter pylori* infection,[5] hookworms, indigestion, inflammation of the colon, insect bites, insomnia, intestinal parasites, laryngitis, lice, methicillin-resistant *Staphylococcus aureus* colonization (MRSA),[6] neuralgia, nightmares, obesity, pertussis, pruritus, rheumatism, roundworms, scabies, scleroderma, sinusitis, sore throat, spasms, sprains, stomach cramps, stomatitis, tonsillitis, urethritis, upper respiratory tract infection, urinary tract infection, vaginal irritation, warts, wound healing.

Expert Opinion and Folkloric Precedent

- Thyme leaf is renowned as a culinary spice and has also been used cosmetically and medicinally.
- Traditional uses of thyme include symptomatic treatment of cough and upper respiratory congestion; it continues to be one of the most commonly recommended herbs in Europe for these indications. The German expert panel Commission E has approved thyme for relief of symptoms of bronchitis, whooping cough, and catarrh (inflammation of upper respiratory tract mucous membranes).
- Topically, thymol (a major constituent of thyme) has been used for various bacterial infections. Recent studies of combination products including thymol, such as Listerine, have shown antibacterial activity when used as a mouthwash to reduce oral bacteria.
- Experts have recommended the use of thymol in treatment of actinomycosis, onycholysis (separation or loosening of a fingernail or toenail from its nail bed), and paronychia (inflammation of the tissue surrounding a fingernail or toenail) because of its antifungal properties. Anecdotal reports of successful healing date to the 1960s,[7] although there are no well-designed clinical studies to advise for human therapeutic use.

Safety Summary

- **Likely safe:** When thyme is used in amounts found in foods; thyme was granted "generally recognized as safe" (GRAS) status in the United States.
- **Possibly safe:** When thyme is used orally or topically in recommended amounts. It is often recommended not to exceed oral doses of 10 g of dried leaf containing 0.03% phenol (calculated as thymol) per day.
- **Likely unsafe:** When thyme oil is used either orally or topically in nondiluted form.

DOSING/TOXICOLOGY
General

- There is limited scientific evidence supporting any specific dose of thyme. Listed doses are based primarily on historical practice. However, with natural products, the optimal doses needed to balance efficacy and safety often have not been determined. Formulations and preparation methods may vary from manufacturer to manufacturer, and from batch to batch of a specific product made by a single manufacturer. Because often the active components of a product are not known, standardization may not be possible, and the clinical effects of different brands may not be comparable.

Standardization

- Standardized amounts of thyme oil may be found in commercial products such as topical cosmetic formulations or mouthwash.[8]
- Standardized extracts may contain 0.6% to 1.2% volatile oil and 0.5% phenol.
- Common thyme contains a greater quantity of volatile oil (0.4% to 3.4%) than that found in Spanish thyme (0.7% to 1.38%).

Dosing: Adult (18 Years and Older)
Oral

- **General:** 1 to 2 g of thyme extract taken daily in divided doses has been used.
- **Tea:** For upper respiratory tract infection/bronchitis symptoms, it has been recommended to steep 1 to 2 g of dried herb in 150 mL of boiling water for 10 minutes, strain, and drink several times daily as needed for symptom alleviation. Safety and efficacy have not been proven.
- **Liquid extract:** Traditional doses for various ailments including upper respiratory tract infection symptoms include 1 to 2 g of extract in fluid in 1 cup of water up to three times daily; 20 to 40 drops of liquid extract (1:1 weight/volume fresh leaf or 1:4 dried leaf) three times daily in juice; or 40 drops tincture (1:10 in 70% ethanol) up to three times daily. Safety and efficacy have not been proven.
- **Oil:** 2 or 3 drops of thyme oil on a sugar cube two or three times daily has been used. Safety and efficacy have not been proven, and thyme oil is considered to be highly toxic.
- **Combination with primrose root (primulae radix):** In one study, 1 tablet of Bronchipret containing 60 mg dried extract of primulae radix and 160 mg dried extract of thyme was used, although the specific number of tablets and frequency of administration were not clear.[9]

Gargle/Mouthwash

- For periodontal prophylaxis, it has been recommended to steep 5 g of dried leaf per 100 mL of boiling water for 10 minutes and strain (5% infusion). Thymol is a constituent in some combination mouthwash products such as Listerine (demonstrated to be efficacious in the reduction of oral bacteria).

Topical

- **Oil/ointment:** For alopecia areata, 2 or 3 drops of an essential oil combination (thyme, lavender, rosemary, and cedarwood added to grapeseed and jojoba oils) massaged into the scalp every night for 7 months has been studied.[10] For paronychia, 1 drop of 1% to 2% thymol in chloroform to the affected area three times daily, or 1 drop of 4% thymol in chloroform to a chronically affected area three times daily, has been used.[7] Diluted thyme oil has been applied as needed in 1% to 2% ointments for a variety of skin disorders. Safety and efficacy have not been proven, and thyme oil is considered to be highly toxic.
- **Compress:** As a compress for rheumatic diseases, bruises, and miscellaneous skin disorders, it has been recommended to steep 5 g of dried leaf per 100 mL of boiling water for 10 minutes and strain. Safety and efficacy have not been proven.

Dosing: Pediatric (Younger Than 18 Years)

- There is insufficient available evidence to recommend medicinal use of thyme in children for any indication. For periodontal prophylaxis, a combination product containing 1% chlorhexidine-thymol varnish (Cervitec) was tolerated in 110 healthy children, ages 8 to 10 years, when taken three times within 2 weeks.[11]

Toxicology

- Anecdotally, it has been suggested not to exceed oral doses of 10 g of dried leaf with 0.03% phenol (calculated as thymol) per day to prevent toxicity.
- Thyme oil is considered to be highly toxic. Signs of toxicity include nausea and, as supported by animal studies, may include tachypnea and hypotension.[12]
- The LD_{50} of the essential oil of thyme is 2.84 g/kg of body weight in rats.[13] Oral doses (0.5 to 3 g/kg of body weight) of concentrated thyme extract (equivalent to 4.3 to 26 g/kg of thyme) decreased locomotor activity and respiratory activity in mice.[14] Following 3 months of oral administration of 0.9 g of dried herb daily as an extract in 95% ethanol, mice experienced an increase in liver and testes weight; 30% of male animals and 10% of female and control animals died.[14]

ADVERSE EFFECTS/PRECAUTIONS/CONTRAINDICATIONS
Allergy

- Avoid with known allergy/hypersensitivity to members of the Lamiaceae (mint) family or to any component of thyme, or to rosemary (*Rosmarinus officinalis*).[15]
- Contact allergies to thyme or thyme oil have been reported by numerous sources, dating to the 1940s and 1950s. In a study of 100 patients with contact allergies, 5% were attributed to thyme oil as an allergen contained in wound dressings.[16] Several case reports have described allergic contact dermatitis and allergic alveolitis provoked by thyme and thymol (a main component of thyme oil).[17-19] In one case report, pruritic contact dermatitis developed following topical application of the combination antiseptic solution Listerine to a chronic paronychia of the toe; patch testing with single ingredients revealed selective allergic hypersensitivity to thymol.[20]
- Cross-reactions to birch pollen, celery, oregano, and to other species in the Lamiaceae/Labiatae (mint) family may occur. A cross-reaction was reported in a 45-year-old man allergic to thyme with a history of immunoglobulin E (IgE)-mediated rhinitis and asthma.[21] Manifestations included nausea, emesis, pruritus, angioedema, dysphagia, dysphonia, hypotension, and progressive respiratory difficulty. The subject recovered with supportive therapy including epinephrine, antihistamines, and corticosteroids, and cross-reactivity was confirmed using *in vitro* assays.

Adverse Effects

- **General:** Based on historical use and clinical anecdote, thyme flower and leaves appear to be safe in culinary and in limited medicinal use. However, caution is warranted with the use of thyme oil, which should not be taken orally and should be diluted for topical administration because of potential toxic effects.
- **Neurologic/CNS:** Headache and dizziness have been associated with oral ingestion of thyme and thyme oil. Oral ingestion of thyme oil may cause seizure and coma.

- **Ocular/otic:** Conjunctivitis has been reported in a farmer exposed to thyme dust.[19]
- **Dermatologic:** Contact dermatologic reactions have been reported in numerous sources, dating to the 1940s and 1950s. Spiewak et al. described occupational airborne contact dermatitis caused by thyme dust in farmers exposed to dried thyme.[19] Allergic contact dermatitis was reported in a 70-year-old woman six weeks after initiation of 4% thymol once daily to a chronic paronychia.[17] Topical application of Listerine antiseptic solution to a chronic parenchyma of the toe by a 43-year-old man resulted in contact dermatitis.[20] Cases of inflammation of the lips and tongue have anecdotally been attributed to thyme oil as an ingredient in toothpaste.
- **Pulmonary/respiratory:** Occupational asthma provoked by thyme and confirmed by inhalation challenge has been described in a butcher.[22] Allergic alveolitis and rhinitis due to thyme dust exposure have been reported in farmers.[18,19] High doses of thyme or thyme oil have elicited tachypnea in animals.[12] Oral ingestion of thyme oil may lead to respiratory arrest (anecdotal).
- **Cardiovascular:** Hypotension developed after ingestion of thyme seasoning in a 45-year-old man, possibly related to an allergic response.[21] Animal studies have reported both hypotension and increased cardiac contractility.[12] Anecdotal reports suggest that bradycardia may be associated with ingestion of thyme, and cardiac arrest may occur with oral intake of thyme oil.
- **Gastrointestinal:** Oral thyme and thyme oil may elicit heartburn, nausea, vomiting, diarrhea, and gastrointestinal irritation (anecdotal).
- **Endocrine:** An extract of *Thymus serpyllum*, a related species to *Thymus vulgaris*, has been shown to exert antithyrotropic effects in rats, causing decline in thyroid-stimulating hormone and prolactin.[23] Estradiol and progesterone receptor–binding activity has been demonstrated *in vivo*.[24] Endocrine effects of *T. vulgaris* in humans are unclear.
- **Genitourinary:** Oral thyme has anecdotally been reported to exacerbate inflammation associated with urinary tract infections.
- **Musculoskeletal:** Oral use of thyme or thyme oil has been associated with muscle weakness in anecdotal reports, although details are limited.

Precautions/Warnings/Contraindications

- Avoid with known allergy/hypersensitivity to members of the Lamiaceae (mint) family or to any component of thyme.
- Avoid oral ingestion or nondiluted topical application of thyme oil, because of potential toxicity.
- Avoid topical preparations in areas of skin breakdown or injury, or in atopic patients, because of multiple reports of contact dermatitis.
- Use cautiously in patients with gastrointestinal irritation or peptic ulcer disease, because of anecdotal reports of gastrointestinal irritation.
- Use cautiously in patients with thyroid disorders, because of observed antithyrotropic effects in animal research on the related species *T. serpyllum*.

Pregnancy and Lactation

- Thyme is not recommended in pregnancy or lactation, because of lack of sufficient data. A 1975 review of plants as possible new antifertility agents classified thyme as an emmenagogue and abortifacient.[25]

INTERACTIONS
Thyme/Drug Interactions

- **Thyroid replacement therapy, antithyroid agents:** An extract of *Thymus serpyllum*, a related species to *Thymus vulgaris*, has been shown to exert antithyrotropic effects in rats causing decline in thyroid-stimulating hormone and prolactin.[23] Therefore, in theory, thyme may decrease levels of thyroid hormone, although this has not been systematically studied or demonstrated in humans.
- **Estrogen, progesterone:** Thyme has demonstrated estradiol and progesterone receptor–binding activity *in vivo*,[24] although this effect has not been systematically studied or demonstrated in humans.
- **5-Fluorouracil (topical):** Topical thymol significantly enhanced percutaneous absorption of 5-fluorouracil through porcine epidermis in comparison with control.[26]

Thyme/Herb/Supplement Interactions

- **Herbs with estrogen or progesterone receptor activity:** Thyme has demonstrated estradiol and progesterone receptor–binding activity *in vivo*,[24] although this effect has not been systematically studied or demonstrated in humans.

Thyme/Food Interactions

- Insufficient available evidence.

Thyme/Lab Interactions

- **Thyroid-stimulating hormone (TSH):** TSH levels have been suppressed by administration of thyme extract in rats.[23] Effects in humans are unknown.
- **Thyroid hormones (triiodothyronine [T_3], thyroxine [T_4]):** Thyroid hormone levels have been reported to decrease after a single intravenous injection of thyme extract in rats.[23]
- **Prolactin:** Based on preclinical data, prolactin levels theoretically may be decreased with high thyme doses.[23]

MECHANISM OF ACTION
Pharmacology

- **Constituents:** The key constituents of thyme include essential oils, such as the phenols thymol and carvacrol, glycosides, flavonoids, *p*-cymene, borneol, linalool, alcohols, rosmarinic acid, saponins, tannins, and terpenoids.[19,27,28] Four acetophenone glycosides have been isolated from the butanol-soluble fraction of thyme extracts, with weak cytotoxic and antioxidant effects *in vitro*.[29]
- **Antimicrobial effects:** Antimicrobial activities of thyme and thymol have been reported *in vitro*.[8] Antibacterial efficacy has been noted against several bacterial species, including *Salmonella typhimurium*, *Staphylococcus aureus*, and *Helicobacter pylori*.[5,8,30-33] Activity against cariogenic and periodontopathogenic bacteria such as *Porphyromonas gingivalis*, *Selenomonas artemidis*, *Streptococcus sobrinus*, and *Streptococcus mutans* has been reported, possibly related to membrane perforation and rapid efflux of intracellular components.[11,34] Thymol has exhibited activity against some fungi and yeasts, including *Aspergillus parasiticus*, *Aspergillus flavus*, and *Candida albicans*), and suppresses fungal growth and aflatoxin synthesis at doses of 250 ppm *in vitro*.[8,35-38]
- **Spasmolytic/antitussive effects:** Spasmolytic and antitussive activity have historically been attributed to thymol and carvacrol.[39] In animal models, flavonoids in thyme appear to relax tracheal and ileal smooth muscle via inhibition of acetylcholine and histamine receptors, or via calcium channel

T

antagonism.[27,28,40] *In vitro*, thyme extract and volatile oil exert a relaxant effect on tracheal and ileal smooth muscle by inhibiting phasic contractions[41,42]; this effect may depend on the concentration of flavone aglycones.[40]

- **Antioxidant effects:** A biphenyl compound and a flavonoid isolated from thyme have been reported to inhibit superoxide anion production and to protect red blood cells against oxidative damage.[43] Rat and *in vitro* studies have noted antioxidant properties of thyme oil and thymol.[1,44-46]
- **Anti-inflammatory effects:** Inhibition of prostaglandin synthesis by thymol and carvacrol[47] and *in vivo* inhibition of mouse macrophages and complement activation have been reported.[48]

Pharmacodynamics/Kinetics

- There is limited available pharmacodynamic information for thyme and its constituents or derivatives. In one study of thymol and carvacrol in rats, urinary excretion of metabolites occurred rapidly; only small amounts were excreted after 24 hours.[49]

HISTORY

- Thyme has been used historically for cosmetic, culinary, and medicinal purposes. Ancient Sumerian and Egyptian cultures employed thyme for medicinal purposes and to embalm the dead. Romans burnt thyme to deter dangerous animals and used thyme to flavor cheese and alcoholic beverages. Roman soldiers bathed in thyme, as this was believed to provide vigor.
- Thyme's common name may be derived from a Greek word meaning "to fumigate," based on its use as incense, or may come from the Greek word *thymon*, meaning "courage." In medieval times, women sometimes embroidered a sprig of thyme on gifts for knights.
- In modern times, thyme oil is commonly used in manufacturing as a constituent of soaps, cosmetics, mouthwash, and toothpaste. Red thyme oil is used in perfumes.

REVIEW OF THE EVIDENCE: DISCUSSION
Alopecia Areata
Summary

- There is no available clinical evidence regarding the use of thyme as a monotherapy for hair loss. Combination preparations of essential oils including thyme have been evaluated,

without definitive results. Therefore, there is currently insufficient information to recommend for or against the use of topical thyme oil for alopecia areata.

Evidence

- In a randomized double-blind trial, 86 subjects with alopecia were assigned to massage a combination of essential oils (thyme, rosemary, lavender, and cedarwood) or a placebo oil into the scalp nightly.[10] After 7 months, it was reported that 44% of the essential oil group experienced new hair growth, compared with 15% of controls, with statistical significance. However, assessment of affected areas was performed in only 32 patients. Although this study was designed to be double-blinded, the oils were not identical in smell, and therefore differences could be discerned both by enrollees and evaluators. There was a 32% attrition rate in the control group, without follow-up of dropouts. Conceivably, if patients experiencing hair growth dropped out of the control group, this would skew results favorably toward the treatment group.

Dental Plaque
Summary

- One of thyme's main constituents, thymol, has been found *in vitro* to have activity against cariogenic and periodontopathogenic bacteria such as *Porphyromonas gingivalis*, *Selenomonas artemidis*, *Streptococcus sobrinus*, and *Streptococcus mutans* (possibly related to membrane perforation and rapid efflux of intracellular components).[11,34] Thymol is included as one of several ingredients in antiseptic mouthwashes such as Listerine. Clinical studies have reported efficacy of Listerine in decreasing plaque formation and gingivitis, although human evidence for a beneficial effect of thymol as a monotherapy mouthrinse is limited.[11,50-52]

Cervitec

- A combination product of 1% chlorhexidine and 1% thymol varnish (Cervitec) has been evaluated in the treatment of *S. mutans* in plaque and saliva in 110 schoolchildren. Subjects were assigned to receive this preparation over 2 years and were compared with those in an untreated reference group. Statistically significant reductions in bacterial colonization levels (at 1 month only) and in interdental plaque (at 1 and 3 months) were reported in treated children.[11] These results

Review of the Evidence: Thyme

Condition Treated*	Study Design	Author, Year	N†	SS†	Study Quality‡	Magnitude of Benefit	ARR†	NNT†	Comments
Alopecia areata	RCT	Hay[10] 1998	86	Yes	2	Small	NA	NA	Thyme used in a combination oil.
Bronchitis	Matched pair comparison	Ernst[9] 1997	7783	NA	NA	NA	NA	NA	Thyme used in combination with primula root (Bronchipret) vs. synthetic secretolytics.
Cough	RCT, double-blind	Knols[74] 1994	60	No	2	NA	NA	NA	Thyme compared with bromhexine.

*Primary or secondary outcome.
†*N*, Number of patients; *SS*, statistically significant; *ARR*, absolute risk reduction; *NNT*, the number of patients who need to undergo a specific intervention in order to observe an outcome in one individual.
‡0-2 = poor; 3-4 = good; 5 = excellent.
NA, Not applicable; *RCT*, randomized, controlled trial.
For an explanation of each category in this table, please see Table 3 in the Introduction.

are of limited clinical utility because of the open and uncontrolled nature of the trial and the use of a combination product.

Listerine

- Listerine antiseptic mouthrinse contains a combination of essential oils, including eucalyptol, menthol, thymol, and methyl salicylate. Broad-spectrum antibiotic properties have been demonstrated for Listerine,[53] including against *S. mutans*,[81] herpes simplex virus, and influenza A virus.[54] Listerine has been demonstrated in several randomized, double-blind trials to be efficacious in the treatment of supragingival plaque and gingivitis when used twice daily for up to 6 months.[56-59]
- Listerine mouthrinse has been reported to significantly reduce gingivitis and plaque in several additional human studies,[60-62] and to be less efficacious than Peridex (chlorhexidine) against plaque,[63-65] but less likely than Peridex to cause stains or supragingival calculus.[66] A 2001 human trial conducted by Pfizer (the manufacturer of Listerine) reported Listerine mouthrinse plus a fluoride toothpaste to be superior to Colgate Total dentifrice (toothpaste) for the reduction of plaque and gingivitis in 316 individuals with plaque after 6 months.[67]
- There is early evidence that Listerine is able to penetrate dental plaque biofilm and kill gram-positive organisms interproximally (in the area most associated with periodontitis and dental caries, heretofore thought to be cleansed primarily only via flossing).[68,69]
- Adverse effects of Listerine have included case reports of allergic contact dermatitis,[20] attributed to thymol, and cardiac asystole in an alcoholic patient who ingested a large volume of Listerine.[70] Other uses of Listerine have included the removal of orally inhaled corticosteroids following inhalation[71] and wound-dressing following periodontal surgery.[72]

Paronychia, Onycholysis, Antifungal
Summary

- *In vitro* studies suggest that thyme essential oil and thymol exert activity against a number of fungi, including *Aspergillus parasiticus* and *Aspergillus flavus*, and may completely suppress growth and aflatoxin synthesis. Topical thymol has been used traditionally in the treatment of paronychia and onycholysis. However, because of a lack of controlled clinical trials, there is insufficient evidence to recommend for or against use of thyme/thymol as a treatment for fungal infections.

Evidence

- In the 1930s, Myers reported five cases of actinomycosis successfully treated to resolution with thymol in oral doses, ranging from 1 g twice weekly up to 2 g once daily.[73] Three of the five patients received additional thymol as a 10% to 25% injection into the sinus tract. A sixth patient received local thymol injection only and subsequently died of fungemia. Adverse effects were not clearly reported, and in light of the known toxicity of thymol, and the current availability of other antifungal agents with demonstrated efficacy and more favorable therapeutic indices, thymol may not be advisable for such cases.
- Topical thymol has been used traditionally in the treatment of paronychia and onycholysis. In a 1965 review article in the *Archives of Dermatology*, Wilson suggested that one drop of 1% or 2% thymol in chloroform can be used for acute paronychia, whereas chronic cases may be treated with 4% thymol, applied three times daily.[7] The author noted personal experience treating patients over 20 years with these formulations with good results and excellent tolerance.

Bronchitis, Cough
Summary

- Thyme has traditionally been used for the treatment of respiratory conditions including cough and bronchitis. Animal studies have identified spasmolytic properties of thyme constituents. The German expert panel Commission E has approved thyme for use in bronchitis. However, because of a lack of data regarding thyme as a monotherapy for any specific respiratory indication, there is currently insufficient scientific evidence to recommend for or against use of thyme as a treatment for bronchitis or coughs.

Evidence

- Ernst et al. conducted a multicenter postmarket surveillance study comparing Bronchipret (combination of thyme and primula root) with other pharmaceutical options for acute bronchitis.[9] The study was designed as a matched-pair comparison of 7783 patients. Patients received Bronchipret, "other herbals" pooled into one treatment group (Bronchoforton—eucalyptus, peppermint, Hedelix—ivy extract, Prospan—ivy extract, Sinupret—Rad. Gentianae, Flos Primulae cum calycibus, Herba Rumicis, Flos Sambuci, Herba Verbenae, Soledum—extract of thyme) or the synthetic agents *N*-acetylcysteine (NAC) and Ambroxal. Clinical outcomes of bronchitis and adverse reactions were documented. Data were evaluated by comparing the treatment success of the test medication and three control groups using ordinal regression. The authors reported that the clinical effectiveness of Bronchipret was not less than that of the synthetic drugs. There was a trend toward better results with Bronchipret, particularly in adults. Bronchipret was associated with a favorable adverse effects profile compared with controls. The authors concluded a possible risk/benefit advantage of Bronchipret over these controls for the management of acute bronchitis. This preliminary finding may merit follow-up with a prospective controlled trial with both a placebo arm and use of a control medication with established evidence of efficacy.
- In a double-blind, randomized trial, 60 patients with productive cough resulting from an uncomplicated respiratory infection received either syrup of thyme or bromhexine for a period of 5 days.[74] Both groups made similar gains from day 0 to day 5. The authors reported no significant difference between the two groups based on self-reported symptom relief. The study concluded that bromhexine may be no better in alleviating coughing complaints than syrup of thyme. However, no power calculation was conducted prior to the study, and it is conceivable that the sample size was too small to detect significant differences between groups. Without a placebo arm, these results cannot be discriminated from the natural course of disease.

Inflammatory Skin Disorders
Summary

- Historically, thyme has been used topically for a number of dermatologic conditions. Although several case reports note possible beneficial effects, controlled trial evidence of effectiveness for treating dermatologic disorders is conflicting. Because of a lack of controlled trials, there is insufficient evidence to recommend for or against use of thyme as a treatment for inflammatory disorders of the skin.

Evidence

- Oral administration of large doses of thymol was reported to result in resolution of a case of dermatomyositis and a case of progressive scleroderma in a 1965 publication.[75]
- A case study of two sisters with vulval lichen sclerosis reported successful treatment of both patients with a topical cream containing thyme extract. There were no reported side effects.[76]
- A randomized controlled clinical trial evaluated the effects of aromatherapy with essential oils including thyme on a group of children with atopic eczema. The essential oil mixture (containing thyme, benzoin, boswellia, German chamomile, Litsea cubeba, myrrh, spike lavender, and sweet marjoram oil) was massaged into the scalp daily in conjunction with counseling by a therapist. No significant difference in improvement was detected between the treatment group (aromatherapy with massage) and the control group (massage only).[77]

FORMULARY: BRANDS USED IN CLINICAL TRIALS
Combination Products

- Listerine contains thymol, a phenolic constituent of thyme, as well as other essential oils such as eucalyptol.

References

1. Aeschbach R, Loliger J, Scott BC, et al. Antioxidant actions of thymol, carvacrol, 6-gingerol, zingerone and hydroxytyrosol. Food Chem Toxicol 1994;32(1):31-36.
2. Dapkevicius A, van Beek TA, Lelyveld GP, et al. Isolation and structure elucidation of radical scavengers from Thymus vulgaris leaves. J Nat Prod 2002;65(6):892-896.
3. Miura K, Kikuzaki H, Nakatani N. Antioxidant activity of chemical components from sage (Salvia officinalis L.) and thyme (Thymus vulgaris L.) measured by the oil stability index method. J Agric Food Chem 2002; 50(7):1845-1851.
4. Aschhoff B. Retrospective study of Ukraine treatment in 203 patients with advanced-stage tumors. Drugs Exp Clin Res 2000;26(5-6):249-252.
5. Tabak M, Armon R, Potasman I, et al. In vitro inhibition of Helicobacter pylori by extracts of thyme. J Appl Bacteriol 1996;80(6):667-672.
6. Nostro A, Blanco AR, Cannatelli MA, et al. Susceptibility of methicillin-resistant staphylococci to oregano essential oil, carvacrol and thymol. FEMS Microbiol Lett 2004;230(2):191-195.
7. Wilson JW. Paronychia and onycholysis, etiology and therapy. Arch Dermatol 1965;92(6):726-730.
8. Manou I, Bouillard L, Devleeschouwer MJ, et al. Evaluation of the preservative properties of Thymus vulgaris essential oil in topically applied formulations under a challenge test. J Appl Microbiol 1998;84(3):368-376.
9. Ernst E, Marz R, Sieder C. A controlled multi-centre study of herbal versus synthetic secretolytic drugs for acute bronchitis. Phytomedicine 1997;4: 287-293.
10. Hay IC, Jamieson M, Ormerod AD. Randomized trial of aromatherapy. Successful treatment for alopecia areata. Arch Dermatol 1998;134(11): 1349-1352.
11. Twetman S, Petersson LG. Interdental caries incidence and progression in relation to mutans streptococci suppression after chlorhexidine-thymol varnish treatments in schoolchildren. Acta Odontol Scand 1999;57(3):144-148.
12. Kagramanov KM, et al. Effect of the essential oils of some thyme growing in Azerbaidzhan on cardiovascular activity and respiration. Chem Abstr 1977; 87:145896.
13. Skramlik EV. Toxicity and toleration of volatile oils. Pharmazie 1959;14: 435-445.
14. Qureshi S, Shah AH, Al-Yahya MA, et al. Toxicity of Achillea fragrantissima and Thymus vulgaris in mice. Fitoterapia 1991;62(4):319-323.
15. Armisen M, Rodriguez V, Vidal C. Photoaggravated allergic contact dermatitis due to Rosmarinus officinalis cross-reactive with Thymus vulgaris. Contact Dermatitis 2003;48(1):52-53.
16. Le Roy R, Grosshans E, Foussereau J. [Investigation of contact allergies in 100 cases of ulcus cruris (author's transl)]. Derm Beruf Umwelt 1981; 29(6):168-170.
17. Lorenzi S, Placucci F, Vincenzi C, et al. Allergic contact dermatitis due to thymol. Contact Dermatitis 1995;33(6):439-440.
18. Mackiewicz B, Skorska C, Dutkiewicz J, et al. Allergic alveolitis due to herb dust exposure. Ann Agric Environ Med 1999;6(2):167-170.
19. Spiewak R, Skorska C, Dutkiewicz J. Occupational airborne contact dermatitis caused by thyme dust. Contact Dermatitis 2001;44(4):235-239.
20. Fisher AA. Allergic contact dermatitis due to thymol in Listerine for treatment of paronychia. Cutis 1989;43(6):531-532.
21. Benito M, Jorro G, Morales C, et al. Labiatae allergy: systemic reactions due to ingestion of oregano and thyme. Ann Allergy Asthma Immunol 1996; 76(5):416-418.
22. Lemiere C, Cartier A, Lehrer SB, et al. Occupational asthma caused by aromatic herbs. Allergy 1996;51(9):647-649.
23. Sourgens H, Winterhoff H, Gumbinger HG, et al. Antihormonal effects of plant extracts. TSH- and prolactin-suppressing properties of Lithospermum officinale and other plants. Planta Med 1982;45(2):78-86.
24. Zava DT, Dollbaum CM, Blen M. Estrogen and progestin bioactivity of foods, herbs, and spices. Proc Soc Exp Biol Med 1998;217(3):369-378.
25. Farnsworth NR, Bingel AS, Cordell GA, et al. Potential value of plants as sources of new antifertility agents I. J Pharm Sci 1975;64(4):535-598.
26. Gao S, Singh J. Mechanism of transdermal transport of 5-fluorouracil by terpenes: carvone, 1,8-cineole, and thymol. Int J Pharmaceutics 1997;154: 67-77.
27. Van den Broucke CO, Lemli JA. Action spasmolytique des flavones de differentes especes de Thymus. Plantes Med Phytother 1983;16(4):310-317.
28. Van den Broucke CO, Lemli JA. Spasmolytic activity of the flavonoids from Thymus vulgaris. Pharm Weekbl Sci 1983;5(1):9-14.
29. Wang M, Kikuzaki H, Lin CC, et al. Acetophenone glycosides from thyme (Thymus vulgaris L.). J Agric Food Chem 1999;47(5):1911-1914.
30. Ramanoelina AR, Terrom GP, Bianchini JP, et al. [Antibacterial action of essential oils extracted from Madagascar plants]. Arch Inst Pasteur Madagascar 1987;53(1):217-226.
31. Juven BJ, Kanner J, Schved F, et al. Factors that interact with the antibacterial action of thyme essential oil and its active constituents. J Appl Bacteriol 1994;76(6):626-631.
32. Agnihotri S, Vaidya AD. A novel approach to study antibacterial properties of volatile components of selected Indian medicinal herbs. Indian J Exp Biol 1996;34(7):712-715.
33. Ceyhan N, Ugur A. Investigation of in vitro antimicrobial activity of honey. Riv Biol 2001;94(2):363-371.
34. Shapiro S, Guggenheim B. The action of thymol on oral bacteria. Oral Microbiol Immunol 1995;10(4):241-246.
35. Mahmoud AL. Antifungal action and antiaflatoxigenic properties of some essential oil constituents. Lett Appl Microbiol 1994;19(2):110-113.
36. Tantaoui-Elaraki A, Beraoud L. Inhibition of growth and aflatoxin production in Aspergillus parasiticus by essential oils of selected plant materials. J Environ Pathol Toxicol Oncol 1994;13(1):67-72.
37. Arras G, Usai M. Fungitoxic activity of 12 essential oils against four postharvest citrus pathogens: chemical analysis of Thymus capitatus oil and its effect in subatmospheric pressure conditions. J Food Prot 2001;64(7): 1025-1029.
38. Inouye S, Uchida K, Yamaguchi H. In-vitro and in-vivo anti-Trichophyton activity of essential oils by vapour contact. Mycoses 2001;44(3-4):99-107.
39. Van den Broucke CO. Chemical and pharmacological investigation on Thymi herba and its liquid extracts. Planta Med 1980;39:253-254.
40. Van den Broucke CO, Lemli JA. Pharmacological and chemical investigation of thyme liquid extracts. Planta Med 1981;41(2):129-135.
41. Reiter M, Brandt W. Relaxant effects on tracheal and ileal smooth muscles of the guinea pig. Arzneimittelforschung 1985;35(1A):408-414.
42. Meister A, Bernhardt G, Christoffel V, et al. Antispasmodic activity of Thymus vulgaris extract on the isolated guinea-pig trachea: discrimination between drug and ethanol effects. Planta Med 1999;65(6):512-516.
43. Haraguchi H, Saito T, Ishikawa H, et al. Antiperoxidative components in Thymus vulgaris. Planta Med 1996;62(3):217-221.
44. Youdim KA, Deans SG. Dietary supplementation of thyme (Thymus vulgaris L.) essential oil during the lifetime of the rat: its effects on the antioxidant status in liver, kidney and heart tissues. Mech.Ageing Dev. 1999;109(3): 163-175.
45. Youdim KA, Deans SG. Effect of thyme oil and thymol dietary supplementation on the antioxidant status and fatty acid composition of the ageing rat brain. Br J Nutr 2000;83(1):87-93.
46. Takacsova M, Pribela A, Faktorova M. Study of the antioxidative effects of thyme, sage, juniper and oregano. Nahrung 1995;39(3):241-243.
47. Wagner H, Wierer M, Bauer R. [In vitro inhibition of prostaglandin biosynthesis by essential oils and phenolic compounds]. Planta Med 1986; (3):184-187.
48. Englberger W, Hadding U, Etschenberg E, et al. Rosmarinic acid: a new inhibitor of complement C3-convertase with anti- inflammatory activity. Int J Immunopharmacol 1988;10(6):729-737.
49. Austgulen LT, Solheim E, Scheline RR. Metabolism in rats of p-cymene derivatives: carvacrol and thymol. Pharmacol Toxicol 1987;61(2):98-102.
50. Baca P, Junco P, Bravo M, et al. Caries incidence in permanent first molars after discontinuation of a school-based chlorhexidine-thymol varnish program. Community Dent Oral Epidemiol 2003;31(3):179-183.
51. Baca P, Munoz MJ, Bravo M, et al. Effectiveness of chlorhexidine-thymol varnish for caries reduction in permanent first molars of 6-7-year-old children: 24-month clinical trial. Community Dent Oral Epidemiol 2002; 30(5):363-368.

52. Haukali G, Poulsen S. Effect of a varnish containing chlorhexidine and thymol (Cervitec) on approximal caries in 13- to 16-year-old schoolchildren in a low caries area. Caries Res 2003;37(3):185-189.

53. Ross NM, Charles CH, Dills SS. Long-term effects of Listerine antiseptic on dental plaque and gingivitis. J Clin Dentistry 1988;1(4):92-95.

54. Fine DH, Furgang D, Barnett ML, et al. Effect of an essential oil–containing antiseptic mouthrinse on plaque and salivary *Streptococcus mutans* levels. J Clin Periodontol 2000;27(3):157-161.

55. Dennison DK, Meredith GM, Shillitoe EJ, et al. The antiviral spectrum of Listerine antiseptic. Oral Surg Oral Med Oral Pathol Oral Radiol Endod 1995;79(4):442-448.

56. Lamster IB. The effect of Listerine antiseptic on reduction of existing plaque and gingivitis. Clin Prev Dent 1983;5:12-16.

57. Gordon JM, Lamster IB, Seiger MC. Efficacy of Listerine antiseptic in inhibiting the development of plaque and gingivitis. J Clin Periodontol 1985;12(8):697-704.

58. DePaola LG, Overholser CD, Meiller TF, et al. Chemotherapeutic inhibition of supragingival dental plaque and gingivitis development. J Clin Periodontol 1989;16(5):311-315.

59. Minah GE, DePaola LG, Overholser CD, et al. Effects of 6 months use of an antiseptic mouthrinse on supragingival dental plaque microflora. J Clin Periodontol 1989;16(6):347-352.

60. Brecx M, Brownstone E, MacDonald L, et al. Efficacy of Listerine, Meridol and chlorhexidine mouthrinses as supplements to regular tooth cleaning measures. J Clin Periodontol 1992;19(3):202-207.

61. Pitts G, Brogdon C, Hu L, et al. Mechanism of action of an antiseptic, anti-odor mouthwash. J Dent Res 1983;62(6):738-742.

62. Nelson RF, Rodasti PC, Tichnor A, et al. Comparative study of four over-the-counter mouthrinses claiming antiplaque and/or antigingivitis benefits. Clin Prev Dent 1991;13(6):30-33.

63. Maruniak J, Clark WB, Walker CB, et al. The effect of 3 mouthrinses on plaque and gingivitis development. J Clin Periodontol 1992;19(1):19-23.

64. McKenzie WT, Forgas L, Vernino AR, et al. Comparison of a 0.12% chlorhexidine mouthrinse and an essential oil mouthrinse on oral health in institutionalized, mentally handicapped adults: one-year results. J Periodontol 1992;63(3):187-193.

65. Brecx M, Netuschil L, Reichert B, et al. Efficacy of Listerine, Meridol and chlorhexidine mouthrinses on plaque, gingivitis and plaque bacteria vitality. J Clin Periodontol 1990;17(5):292-297.

66. Overholser CD, Meiller TF, DePaola LG, et al. Comparative effects of 2 chemotherapeutic mouthrinses on the development of supragingival dental plaque and gingivitis. J Clin Periodontol 1990;17(8):575-579.

67. Charles CH, Sharma NC, Galustians HJ, et al. Comparative efficacy of an antiseptic mouthrinse and an antiplaque/antigingivitis dentifrice. A six-month clinical trial. J Am Dent Assoc 2001;132(5):670-675.

68. Pan P, Barnett ML, Coelho J, et al. Determination of the in situ bactericidal activity of an essential oil mouthrinse using a vital stain method. J Clin Periodontol 2000;27(4):256-261.

69. Fine DH, Furgang D, Barnett ML. Comparative antimicrobial activities of antiseptic mouthrinses against isogenic planktonic and biofilm forms of *Actinobacillus actinomycetemcomitans*. J Clin Periodontol 2001;28(7):697-700.

70. Westermeyer RR, Terpolilli RN. Cardiac asystole after mouthwash ingestion: a case report and review of the contents. Mil Med 2001;166(9):833-835.

71. Kelloway JS, Wyatt NN, Adlis S, et al. Does using a mouthwash instead of water improve the oropharyngeal removal of inhaled Flovent (fluticasone propionate)? Allergy Asthma Proc 2001;22(6):367-371.

72. Yukna RA, Broxson AW, Mayer ET, et al. Comparison of Listerine mouthwash and periodontal dressing following periodontal flap surgery. I. Initial findings. Clin Prev Dent 1986;8(4):14-19.

73. Myers HB. Thymol therapy in actinomycosis. JAMA 1937;108(22):1875.

74. Knols G, Stal PC, Van Ree JW. Productive coughing complaints: sirupus thymi or bromhexine? A double-blind randomized study. Huisarts en Wetenschap 1994;37:392-394.

75. Buccellato G. [Dermatomyositis cured by administration of para-methyl-isopropyl-phenol (thymol)]. G Ital Dermatol Minerva Dermatol 1965;106(1):89-94.

76. Hagedorn M. [Genital vulvar lichen sclerosis in 2 siblings]. Z Hautkrankh 1989;64(9):810, 813-810, 814.

77. Anderson C, Lis-Balchin M, Kirk-Smith M. Evaluation of massage with essential oils on childhood atopic eczema. Phytother Res 2000;14(6):452-456.

T

Turmeric

(*Curcuma longa* L.)

SYNONYMS/COMMON NAMES/RELATED SUBSTANCES

- Amomoum curcuma, anlatone, curcuma, *Curcuma aromatica*, *Curcuma aromatica* Salisb., *Curcuma domestica*, *Curcuma domestica* Valet., curcuma oil, curcumae longae rhizoma, curcumin (I, II, III), diferuloylmethane, e zhu, gelbwurzel, gurkemeje, haldi, haridra, Indian saffron, Indian yellow root, jiang huang, kunir, kunyit, kurkumawurzelstock, kyoo, olena, radix zedoariae longae, rhizome de curcuma, safran des Indes, shati, turmeric root, tumerone, ukon, yellowroot, zedoary, Zingiberaceae (family), zingiberene, zitterwurzel.

CLINICAL BOTTOM LINE
Background

- The rhizome (root) of turmeric (*Curcuma longa* L.) has long been used in traditional Asian medicine to treat gastrointestinal upset, arthritic pain, and "low energy." *In vitro* and animal research has demonstrated anti-inflammatory, antioxidant, and antiproliferative properties of turmeric and its constituent curcumin. Preliminary human evidence, albeit of poor quality, suggests possible efficacy in the management of dyspepsia, hyperlipidemia, and scabies (topical therapy). However, because of methodologic weaknesses in the available studies, an evidence-based recommendation cannot be made regarding the use of turmeric or curcumin for any specific indication.

Scientific Evidence for Common/Studied Uses	Grade*
Cancer	C
Cholelithiasis prevention/cholagogue (gallbladder contraction/bile flow stimulant)	C
Dyspepsia	C
HIV	C
Hyperlipidemia	C
Inflammation	C
Osteoarthritis	C
Peptic ulcer disease	C
Rheumatoid arthritis	C
Scabies	C
Uveitis	C

*Key to grades: *A:* Strong scientific evidence for this use; *B:* Good scientific evidence for this use; *C:* Unclear scientific evidence for this use; *D:* Fair scientific evidence against this use (it may not work); *F:* Strong scientific evidence against this use (it likely does not work). For a more detailed explanation of efficacy criteria, see "Natural Standard Evidence-Based Validated Grading Rationale" in the Introduction.

Historical or Common Indications That Lack Supportive Evidence

- Abdominal bloating, Alzheimer's disease,[1] antifungal,[2] antiprotozoal,[3] antispasmodic, antivenom,[4] amenorrhea, appetite stimulant, asthma,[5] bleeding, boils, bruises, cataracts, colic, contraception, cough,[5] diabetes,[6] flatulence, diarrhea, dizziness, dysmenorrhea, enhancement of sperm count/motility, epilepsy, gonorrhea, hepatitis, hepatoprotection, hypertension, insect bites, insect repellent, jaundice, kidney disease,[7] lactation stimulant, leprosy, pain, ringworm, toxin-mediated liver damage,[8,9] urolithiasis.

Expert Opinion and Folkloric Precedent

- In traditional Indian Ayurvedic medicine, turmeric has been used to strengthen the body, tone the digestive system and the liver, dispel worms, regulate menstruation, dissolve gallstones, and relieve arthritis. Ancient Hindu texts refer to its carminative, aromatic, and stimulant properties. Mixed with slaked lime, it has been used in topical treatment for sprains and strains. In Chinese medicine, turmeric is an important herb for digestive and urinary complaints, gallstones, and menstrual pain.[10]

Safety Summary

- **Likely safe:** When used in amounts commonly found in foods.
- **Possibly safe:** When used orally or topically in medicinal amounts in healthy individuals. Turmeric appears to be nontoxic, even in large doses.[11]
- **Possibly unsafe:** Turmeric may cause gastric irritation in medicinal amounts and is inadvisable in patients with peptic ulcer disease or gastric hyperacidity disorders.
- **Likely unsafe:** In patients with bile duct obstruction or gallstones. Use cautiously in combination with immunosuppressants. Avoid in patients allergic to yellow food colorings.

DOSING/TOXICOLOGY
General

- Recommended doses are based on those most commonly used in available trials, or on historical practice. However, with natural products, the optimal doses needed to balance efficacy and safety often have not been determined. Formulations and preparation methods may vary from manufacturer to manufacturer, and from batch to batch of a specific product made by a single manufacturer. Because often the active components of a product are not known, standardization may not be possible, and the clinical effects of different brands may not be comparable.

Standardization

- Turmeric may be standardized to contain 95% curcuminoids per dose.
- The dried root of turmeric is reported to contain 3% to 5% curcumin.[12]

Dosing: Adult (18 Years and Older)
Oral

- **Dosing range:** Traditional doses range from 1.5 to 3 g of turmeric root daily in divided doses. Studies have used 750 mg to 1.5 g of turmeric daily in 3 to 4 divided doses,[13,14] with daily doses up to 8 g used for the treatment of duodenal ulcer.[15] As a tea, 1 to 1.5 g of dried root may be steeped in 150 mL of water for 15 minutes; this infusion is taken twice daily.
- **Dietary intake:** Average dietary intake in the Indian population may range between 2 and 2.5 g, corresponding to 60 to 200 mg of curcumin per day.[12,16,17]
- **Absorption:** Because of the questionable absorption of orally administered turmeric, turmeric is often formulated with bromelain to enhance absorption. A lipid base of lecithin, fish oils, or essential fatty acids may also be used to enhance absorption.

Topical

- **Scabies:** Cover affected areas once daily with a paste consisting of a 4:1 mixture of *Azadirachta indica* ADR (neem) and turmeric, for up to 15 days.[18] Treatment of scabies should be conducted under the supervision of a healthcare professional.

Dosing: Pediatric (Younger Than 18 Years)
Topical

- **Scabies:** Cover affected areas once daily with a paste consisting of a 4:1 mixture of *Azadirachta indica* ADR (neem) and turmeric, for up to 15 days.[18] Treatment of scabies should be conducted under the supervision of a healthcare professional.

Toxicology

- In mice, 100 mg/kg of turmeric has been reported to increase heart and lung weight and to decrease leukocyte count and hemoglobin level.[19] Mice have also demonstrated alopecia, central nervous system (CNS) excitation, and priapism with doses of 3 mg/kg.[19] The turmeric constituent curcumin has been reported to induce abnormalities in liver function tests in rats and may be mildly hepatotoxic in high doses.[20] Turmeric has been reported as nonmutagenic[21] and nontoxic at high doses (300 mg/kg in rats, 2.5 g/kg in monkeys).[22] The oral LD_{50} in mice is >2 g/kg.[23]

ADVERSE EFFECTS/PRECAUTIONS/CONTRAINDICATIONS
Allergy

- Allergic reactions to turmeric have been reported anecdotally. Cases of contact dermatitis have been reported following occupational exposure, with manifestations including erythema, induration, papules, vesicles, and pruritus.[24,25] One subject out of 62 in a trial reported local pruritus after topical application of a curcumin ointment to the scalp for treatment of melanoma.[26]
- Turmeric should be used cautiously in patients allergic to yellow food colorings, or to other members of the Zingiberaceae (ginger) family.

Adverse Effects

- **Dermatologic:** Cases of contact dermatitis have been reported following occupational exposure, with manifestations including erythema, induration, papules, vesicles, and pruritus.[24,25] In a trial, 1 subject out of 62 reported local pruritus after topical application of a curcumin ointment to

the scalp for treatment of melanoma.[26] In rats, high doses of turmeric (10% of diet) have caused alopecia.[27]
- **Neurologic/CNS:** Turmeric has been reported anecdotally to cause mild, transient giddiness.
- **Cardiovascular:** Transient hypotension has been noted in dogs following administration of the turmeric constituent curcumin.[28]
- **Gastrointestinal (GI upset):** Turmeric may cause gastrointestinal irritation or upset, particularly in high or prolonged doses, despite its traditional use as a treatment for gastrointestinal disorders. In one study of patients with duodenal ulcer, 6 g of daily turmeric was associated with epigastric burning in 27% of subjects, compared with 13% of those in the placebo group.[15] Dyspepsia and aggravation of peptic ulcer disease have been reported anecdotally with high doses or chronic use. Since turmeric is sometimes used for the treatment of dyspepsia or ulcers, caution may be warranted in some patients. Nausea was reported by 3 of 38 subjects (8%) taking 1 g of oral turmeric daily in a trial of turmeric for dyspepsia, compared with 3% of placebo patients; diarrhea was reported by a small number of turmeric patients, with no difference vs. placebo.[14]
- **Gastrointestinal (hepatobiliary effects):** The turmeric constituent curcumin has been reported to induce abnormalities in liver function tests in rats and may be mildly hepatotoxic in high doses.[20] In a human cohort study, 750 mg of turmeric administered twice daily for 30 days to 22 subjects did not have significant effects on indices of liver function (levels of aspartate aminotransferase or alanine aminotransferase),[13] and in a case series, 20 mg of curcumin daily for 60 days did not raise transaminases in 45 subjects.[29] Gallbladder contraction in humans has been associated with oral curcumin and occurs over a 2-hour period following administration of a single 20-mg dose.[30] Curcumin may therefore be inadvisable in patients with cholelithiasis.
- **Hematologic:** *In vitro* and animal studies report turmeric to inhibit platelet aggregation,[31-34] possibly because of effects on eicosanoids.[16,31,35-37] Therefore, turmeric may increase the risk of bleeding. Human data are limited, and there are no reports of significant bleeding in the small number of available human studies.
- **Endocrine:** Turmeric may lower serum low-density lipoproteins (LDL) and increase high-density lipoproteins (HDL); studies in rats report that turmeric may alter cholesterol metabolism by stimulating cholesterol-7α-hydroxylase activity.[38,39]
- **Immunologic:** Turmeric has been found to possess anti-inflammatory properties *in vitro* and in animals, which may be attributable to effects on cytokines,[28,40] inhibition of prostaglandins,[31] or inhibition of neutrophils.[41]

Precautions/Warnings/Contraindications

- Avoid in patients allergic to turmeric or any of its constituents (including curcumin), to yellow food colorings, or to members of the Zingiberaceae (ginger) family.
- Avoid in patients with bile duct obstruction or cholelithiasis.
- Avoid in patients with gastric or duodenal ulcers, or with gastric hyperacidity disorders.
- Use cautiously in immunosuppressed patients.

Pregnancy and Lactation

- Based on historical use, turmeric is generally considered to be safe when used as a spice in foods during pregnancy and lactation. However, turmeric is not recommended to be ingested in high doses from foods, or to be used medicinally, because of potential emmenagogue (menstrual flow stimulant) or uterine stimulant effects.

- Oral turmeric has not been found to be teratogenic in mice or rats.[42-44] In mice, turmeric has been associated with increased weight of sexual organs and increased sperm motility without spermatoxic effects.[19]

INTERACTIONS

Turmeric/Drug Interactions

- **Anticoagulants, nonsteroidal anti-inflammatory drugs (NSAIDs), antiplatelet agents:** *In vitro* and animal studies report turmeric to inhibit platelet aggregation,[31-34] possibly because of effects on eicosanoids.[16,31,35-37] Therefore, turmeric may potentiate the effects of other agents that increase bleeding risk. An observed positive effect of turmeric in rats has been the reduction of NSAID (indomethacin)-induced peptic ulcers, although at high doses turmeric may be ulcerogenic.[45,46]
- **Cytochrome P450–metabolized drugs:** In rats, curcumin is reported to be a potent inhibitor of cytochrome P450 (CYP) 1A1/1A2, a less potent inhibitor of CYP 2B1/2B2, and a weak inhibitor of CYP 2E1.[46] Inhibition of cytochrome P450 has also been demonstrated *in vitro* and in other animal studies.[47-50] Human data are lacking.
- **Lipid-lowering agents:** Turmeric has been found to decrease LDL, increase HDL, and decrease serum lipid peroxides; rat studies suggest that turmeric may produce changes in cholesterol metabolism by stimulating cholesterol-7α-hydroxylase activity.[38,39] Turmeric may potentiate the effects of lipid-lowering agents.
- **Reserpine (Serpasil):** *Positive interaction*: Turmeric root solid alcoholic extract significantly reduced the frequency of reserpine-induced gastric and duodenal ulcers in rats; however, in high doses, turmeric may be ulcerogenic.[45]
- **Doxorubicin (Adriamycin, Doxil):** *Positive interaction*: Curcumin (200 mg/kg) protects against acute doxorubicin-induced myocardial toxicity in rats.[51]

Turmeric/Herb Interactions

- **Anticoagulant herbs and supplements:** *In vitro* and animal studies report turmeric to inhibit platelet aggregation,[31-34] possibly because of effects on eicosanoids.[16,31,35-37] Therefore, turmeric may potentiate the effects of other agents that increase bleeding risk.
- **P450-metabolized herbs and supplements:** In rats, curcumin is reported to be a potent inhibitor of cytochrome P450 (CYP) 1A1/1A2, a less potent inhibitor of CYP 2B1/2B2, and a weak inhibitor of CYP 2E1.[46] Inhibition of cytochrome P450 has also been demonstrated *in vitro* and in other animal studies.[47-50] Human data are lacking.
- **Lipid-lowering agents:** Turmeric has been found to decrease LDLs and increase HDLs; rat studies suggest that turmeric may produce changes in cholesterol metabolism by stimulating cholesterol-7α-hydroxylase activity.[38,39] Turmeric may potentiate the effects of lipid-lowering agents such as fish oil, garlic, guggul, and niacin.

Turmeric/Food Interactions

- Insufficient data available.

Turmeric/Lab Interactions

- **Serum lipids:** Turmeric has been found to decrease LDL and increase HDL; rat studies suggest that turmeric may produce changes in cholesterol metabolism by stimulating cholesterol-7α-hydroxylase activity.[38,39]

MECHANISM OF ACTION
Pharmacology

- **Constituents:** Curcumin, a polyphenol compound responsible for the bright yellow color of turmeric, is believed to be the principal pharmacologic agent. In addition to curcumin, turmeric contains the curcuminoids atlantone, bisdemethoxycurcumin, demethoxycurcumin, diaryl heptanoids, and tumerone. Other constituents include sugars, resins, proteins, vitamins, and minerals (including iron and potassium).
- **Anti-inflammatory effects:** Turmeric has been associated with inhibition of tumor necrosis factor-alpha, interleukin-8, monocyte inflammatory protein-1, interleukin-1β, and monocyte chemotactic protein-1.[40] Turmeric and its constituent curcumin have been found to inhibit lipoxygenase and cyclooxygenase in rat tissues and *in vitro*,[31,35,36] as well as thromboxane B_2[32] and leukotriene B_4 formation.[36,52] In rat macrophages, curcumin inhibits the incorporation of arachidonic acid into membrane lipids, as well as prostaglandin E_2, leukotriene B_4, and leukotriene C_4, but does not affect the release of arachidonic acid.[53] Curcumin also inhibits the secretion of collagenase, elastase, and hyaluronidase. Inhibition of neutrophil function has been noted,[41] and *in vitro* research demonstrates that curcumin inhibits 5-hydroxy-eicosatetraenoic acid (5-HETE) in intact human neutrophils.[31] Turmeric has been found to block cytokine-induced transcription of leukocyte adhesion molecules ICAM-1, VCAM-1, and E-selectin[54] and appears to induce production of endogenous transforming growth factor-beta-1 (TGF-β_1) in animal wounds.[55] Curcumin downregulates transcription of genes responsible for the production of chemotactic cytokines in bone marrow stromal cells.[56] Curcumin reduces chemically induced rat paw edema[57,58] and liver inflammation.[59]
- **Antioxidant effects:** Turmeric has been reported to possess antioxidant properties *in vitro* and in animal studies.[56,60-67] Turmeric preparations have been found to scavenge free radicals (peroxides) and phenolic oxidants,[54] inhibit lipid peroxidation induced by chemical agents,[68,69] and inhibit iron-dependent lipid peroxidation in rat tissues.[35,70] *In vitro* research shows turmeric to prevent oxidative damage to DNA[71] and to be a potent scavenger of nitric acid.[64] Curcumin appears to generate a hydroxyl radical.[72] Structural features of curcuminoids that may contribute to antioxidant activity include phenolic and methoxy groups on phenyl rings and 1,3-diketones.[73] Research using aqueous extracts of turmeric suggests that curcumin is not the only antioxidant in turmeric,[74] and turmerin has been identified as a water-soluble peptide from turmeric with antioxidant properties.[75] Animal studies have reported turmeric-associated reversal of hepatonecrosis and fatty changes, with reversal of aflatoxin-induced liver damage.[9]
- **Platelet effects:** Curcumin inhibits thromboxane A_2 without affecting the synthesis of prostaglandin I_2.[76] *In vitro*, curcumin inhibits platelet aggregation induced by adenosine diphosphate (ADP), epinephrine, or collagen.[32,34] Turmeric appears to inhibit arachidonic acid incorporation into platelet phospholipids and degradation of phospholipids and cyclooxygenase.[16,37]
- **Antiproliferative effects:** Multiple preclinical studies have explored potential anticancer mechanisms of curcumin.[26,47,77-93] In a rat model, the effects of 0.2% or 0.6% dietary

curcumin were evaluated on chemically induced colon adenocarcinoma.[94] Histologic examination after 1 year revealed both preventive and therapeutic benefits in animals receiving curcumin, in comparison with findings in animals not receiving curcumin, with better response at higher doses. Histologic examination revealed evidence of apoptosis of cancer cells. In mice, 6 weeks of a 2% curcumin diet was found to decrease cellular proliferation and increase apoptosis of implanted androgen-dependent LNCaP prostate cancer cells.[83] However, *in vitro* research on the antiproliferative effects of curcumin on breast cancer cells reports no evidence of apoptosis.[95] Dietary turmeric extract given to mice (2% or 5% of diet) significantly inhibited chemically induced skin and gastric tumors.[48] A 57% reduction in the incidence of chemically induced colonic epithelial cell dysplasia was noted in mice fed a 2% curcumin diet.[96] Curcumin has been found to inhibit the formation of chemically induced aberrant crypt foci in rat colon, and to inhibit colonic mucosal tyrosine protein kinase activity.[35] *In vitro*, curcumin derivatives demonstrate antitumor effects against leukemic cells, and in test animals decrease the incidence of experimentally induced forestomach tumors by 20% and the number of skin tumors and papillomas by 68% and 57%, respectively.[47] HL-60 leukemia cells are susceptible to curcumin treatment *in vitro*.[97] Extracts of turmeric and curcumin have been found to be nonmutagenic using the Ames test, and to serve protective roles against experimental mutagenesis induced by capsaicin, chili extract, and tobacco-derived mutagens.[21] In a different animal study, however, concentrations up to 5 mM curcumin did not protect against cytotoxicity of paracetamol in freshly isolated hepatocytes, and curcumin itself was found to be mildly hepatotoxic at high doses.[20] Curcumin inhibits the growth of human epidermoid carcinoma A431 cells *in vitro*.[98] Topical application of curcumin inhibits chemically induced tumor promotion in mouse skin,[99] which may be attributable to suppression of protein kinase C activity.[100] Curcumins have also been noted *in vitro* to inhibit nitrosation of methyl urea by sodium nitrate.[101] *In vitro* research suggests that curcumin exerts activity against human breast cancer cells,[93] including hormone-dependent, hormone-independent, and multidrug-resistant cell lines,[95] which may occur via effects on aryl hydrocarbon receptors[49] or ornithine decarboxylase activity.[95] The protective role of curcumin against carcinogenesis has also been attributed to antioxidant effects.[71] In rats, curcumin is reported to be protective against radiation-induced lung fibrosis and formation of micronuclei,[102] and to protect against acute doxorubicin (Adriamycin)-induced myocardial toxicity.[51] In rat aortic smooth muscle cells, curcumin inhibited cell proliferation, arrested cell cycle progression, and induced cell apoptosis.[103] *In vitro*, curcumin has exhibited activity against human B cells immortalized by Epstein-Barr virus.[104] Antiangiogenic properties have been proposed.[83,105-107]

- **Lipid-lowering effects:** In rat models of hyperlipidemia, a diet of 0.5% curcumin for 8 weeks significantly lowered serum LDL, very-low-density lipoprotein (VLDL), total cholesterol, and triglyceride levels, possibly by enhancing the activity of hepatic cholesterol-7α-hydroxylase and increasing cholesterol catabolism.[38,39,108] The turmeric constituents demethoxycurcumin, bisdemethoxycurcumin, and acetylcurcumin appear to inhibit iron-stimulated lipid peroxidation in rat tissues and liver microsomes.[69] In a rat model of hyperlipidemia, a 50% ethanolic extract of turmeric was associated with a significant reduction in the ratio

of total cholesterol to phospholipids.[109] In rabbits fed a high-cholesterol diet, oral turmeric (1.6 to 3.2 mg/kg) was associated with lower levels of plasma cholesterol and triglycerides than in a control group, although no differences in atherogenesis were noted on histologic examination of aortas.[110] Cholesterol levels were lower in the 1.6-mg/kg group.

- **Gastroprotective effects:** Oral administration of turmeric to rats (500 mg/kg) significantly reduces the incidence of chemically induced duodenal ulcers and is associated with an increase in intestinal wall mucus and nonprotein sulfhydryl content.[45] However, early research in guinea pigs reported that various constituents of turmeric do not protect against histamine-induced gastric ulcerations.[111]

- **Gallbladder effects:** Gallbladder contraction over the 2-hour period following administration of 20 mg of curcumin has been demonstrated in humans.[30] Animal research reports that curcumin in the diet reduces the incidence of chemically induced gallstones in mice.[112]

- **Other effects:** *In vitro* research on liposomal membranes has demonstrated that curcumin forms chelates with iron.[113,114] Curcumin in low concentrations has been found to potentiate phototoxicity to the bacteria *Salmonella typhimurium* and *Escherichia coli*.[115]

Pharmacodynamics/Kinetics

- Animal research shows absorption of curcumin after oral administration to vary from 25% to 60%, with most of the absorbed flavonoid being metabolized in the intestinal mucosa and liver.[116] The remainder is excreted in the feces.[117]

- In rats, curcumin is reported to be a potent inhibitor of cytochrome P450 (CYP) 1A1/1A2, a less potent inhibitor of CYP 2B1/2B2, and a weak inhibitor of CYP 2E1.[46] Inhibition of cytochrome P450 has also been demonstrated *in vitro*.[47] Turmeric may decrease hepatocyte glutathione levels[118]; curcumin appears to induce glutathione *S*-transferase activity in mice.[119]

HISTORY

- Turmeric has been used in Asian food preparation, medicine, cosmetics, and fabric dying for more than 2000 years. Marco Polo described turmeric in his memoirs, and the herb became popular in Europe during medieval times for its coloring value and medicinal uses. Traditionally, turmeric has been used to relieve gastrointestinal upset, reduce symptoms of arthritis, and improve overall body energy. As an ingredient in foods, turmeric provides a yellow tint as well as flavoring to curry dishes. Turmeric also plays a role in some Indian religious ceremonies.

- Turmeric is produced most extensively in India but is also cultivated in other countries in Asia and Latin America.

- During the 1970s, research began to focus on the pharmacologic properties of turmeric and its constituent curcumin, particularly regarding possible anti-inflammatory and antioxidant properties.

REVIEW OF THE EVIDENCE: DISCUSSION
Cancer
Summary

- Multiple animal and *in vitro* studies report anti-mutagenic properties of curcumin, including activity against colon, skin, and breast cancer cells.[26,47,77,79-83,87-89,91,94] Numerous mechanisms have been implicated, including antioxidant activity and effects on transcription, with antiproliferative effects on cancer cells at various stages of differentiation

Review of the Evidence: Turmeric

Condition Treated*	Study Design	Author, Year	N[†]	SS[†]	Study Quality[‡]	Magnitude of Benefit	ARR[†]	NNT[†]	Comments
Cancer	Case series	Kuttan[26] 1985	111	Unclear	NA	Unclear	NA	NA	Topical curcumin associated with decreased "foul smell" and exudates of cutaneous lesions from various cancer types. Poor-quality study; unclear outcome measures; 44% dropout; no statistical analysis.
Cancer	Case series	Polasa[13] 1992	22	Yes	NA	Medium	NA	NA	Reduced urine mutagens in smokers after 15-30 days of oral turmeric, 750 mg twice daily. Results may not correlate with improved cancer outcomes.
Dyspepsia	RCT	Thamlikitkul[14] 1989	116	Yes	4	Medium	34%	3	Reduced dyspepsia symptoms with 250 mg turmeric, four times daily. Outcomes measures not clearly defined; blinding, randomization not described.
Biliary colic	Controlled trial	Niederau[120] 1999	76	Yes	3	Small	NA	NA	Combination of 45 mg turmeric and celandine decreased symptoms of colic. Randomization, blinding not described.
Gastric ulcer	Comparison trial, randomized, nonblinded	Kositchaiwat[121] 1993	50	Yes	3	Small	Negative	Negative	Antacid with aluminum hydroxide and magnesium hydroxide superior to 250 mg turmeric four times daily for healing of gastric ulcers. No placebo group.
Duodenal ulcer	RCT, double-blind	Van Dau[115] 1998	118	Unclear	3	None	NA	NA	Turmeric 6 g daily no better than placebo for duodenal ulcer healing or relief of symptoms. Statistical analysis not described.
Gallbladder contraction	RCT, crossover	Rasyid[30] 1999	12	Yes	4	Medium	NA	NA	Single dose of 20 mg curcumin associated with gallbladder contraction over 2 hours vs. gallbladder volume increase in placebo.
Hyperlipidemia	Case series	Soni[124] 1992	10	Yes	NA	Medium	NA	NA	Increased HDL and decreased total cholesterol with 500 mg of curcumin daily for 7 days. Unclear if confounders such as dietary change may have played a role.
Inflammation	RCT	Satoskar[125] 1986	40	Yes	3	Medium	NA	NA	Curcumin 400 mg daily for 5 days found more effective than placebo or phenylbutazone on measures of postoperative inflammation.
Osteoarthritis	RCT, crossover	Kulkarni[127] 1991	42	Yes	4	Large	NA	NA	Combination product used (Articulin-F); effects of turmeric alone not clear.
Rheumatoid arthritis	Comparison study, randomized, double-blind	Deodhar[128] 1980	18	Unclear	3	Equivalent	NA	NA	Curcumin 1200 mg daily and phenylbutazone equally decreased morning stiffness, joint pain vs. baseline. Unclear if benefits would be greater than with placebo; sample size likely inadequate to detect between-group differences.

Review of the Evidence: Turmeric—cont'd

Condition Treated*	Study Design	Author, Year	N†	SS†	Study Quality‡	Magnitude of Benefit	ARR†	NNT†	Comments
Scabies	Case series	Charles[18] 1992	824	Yes	NA	Large	NA	NA	Topical combination of turmeric and *Azadirachta indica* ADR (neem) highly efficacious against scabies; no control group.
HIV infection	Open-label study	Hellinger[136] 1996	40	No	NA	None	NA	NA	Published abstract only. No decrease in viral load or CD4+ count after 8 weeks of high-dose curcumin.
HIV infection	Controlled trial	Copeland[137] 1994	18	Yes	NA	Small	NA	NA	Published abstract only. Increased CD4+ count vs. control with ~2000 mg curcumin daily. Limited details provided.
Chronic anterior uveitis	Case series	Lal[138] 1999	32	Unclear	NA	Unclear	NA	NA	Improvement seen with curcumin therapy over 12 weeks. During 3-year follow-up, 47% recurrence rate and 22% vision loss. No control group, and unclear benefits of curcumin vs. no therapy or steroids. 40% dropout rate.

*Primary or secondary outcome.

†*N*, Number of patients; *SS*, statistically significant; *ARR*, absolute risk reduction; *NNT*, the number of patients who need to undergo a specific intervention in order to observe an outcome in one individual.

‡0-2 = poor; 3-4 = good; 5 = excellent.

HIV, Human immunodeficiency virus; *NA*, not applicable; *RCT*, randomized, controlled trial.

For an explanation of each category in this table, please see Table 3 in the Introduction.

or division. Human data in this area is limited to poor-quality case series, and at this time it is not clear if turmeric or curcumin is beneficial in the prevention or treatment of human cancers.

Human Evidence

- In a human case series, topical application of turmeric (as a turmeric ethanol extract or 0.5% curcumin ointment in petrolatum [Vaseline]) was assessed in 111 patients with cutaneous lesions due to cancers of various types.[88] Treatment was administered three times daily for up to 4 weeks. Outcome measures included lesion size, pain, pruritus, and "foul smell," although details were not provided of how these measurements were conducted. At the time of evaluation, 49 subjects had dropped out (44%). Descriptions of dropouts were not provided. Of the 62 evaluable patients, diagnoses were heterogeneous, including 37 oral cancers (including 5 with oral leukoplakia), 7 with breast lesions [presumably due to breast cancer], 4 with vulvar lesions, 3 with skin cancer of unspecified type, and 11 "other." The authors reported a reduction in "foul smell" of lesions in >90% of patients, a reduction in lesion pain in 50% of subjects (although concomitant analgesics were allowed during the study), decreased exudates in 70% of patients, and reduced "thickness" of lesions in 10% of patients. No statistical analysis was described, and statistical significance was not calculated. The lack of clearly defined outcome measures or use of a control group makes these results difficult to interpret.
- In a case series, Polasa et al. examined the effects of oral turmeric on the urinary excretion of mutagens in 16 otherwise healthy chronic cigarette smokers and 6 nonsmokers.[13] Over a 30-day period, subjects were administered 750 mg

of turmeric in tablet form twice daily. All subjects were maintained on a fixed-calorie vegetarian diet. In smokers, 24-hour urine collection revealed a significant 32% to 39% reduction in urinary mutagen excretion compared with baseline after 15 days (with no significant change after 30 days); no differences were noted in nonsmokers. Notably, baseline urinary mutagen levels were significantly lower in nonsmokers. Although the evidence is suggestive, the measurement of surrogate outcomes such as urinary mutagens does not clearly correlate with reduction of cancer incidence. Further evaluation that correlates turmeric use with reduced cancer incidence in comparison with a control group is merited before a firm conclusion can be made in this area.

Animal and In Vitro Evidence

- In a rat model, the effects of 0.2% or 0.6% dietary curcumin were evaluated in chemically induced colon adenocarcinoma.[94] Histological examination after 1 year revealed both preventative and therapeutic benefits of curcumin when compared with animals not receiving curcumin, with better response at higher doses. Histologic examination revealed evidence of apoptosis of cancer cells. In mice, 6 weeks of a 2% curcumin diet was found to decrease cellular proliferation and increase apoptosis of implanted androgen-dependent LNCaP prostate cancer cells.[83] However, *in vitro* research on the antiproliferative effects of curcumin on breast cancer cells reports no evidence of apoptosis.[95] Dietary turmeric extract given to mice (2% or 5% of diet) significantly inhibited chemically induced skin and gastric tumors.[48] A 57% reduction in the incidence of chemically induced colonic epithelial cell dysplasia was noted in mice fed a 2% curcumin diet.[96] Curcumin has been found to inhibit the formation of chemically induced aberrant crypt foci in rat colon and

T

to inhibit colonic mucosal tyrosine protein kinase activity.[35] Curcumin derivatives demonstrate antitumor effects against leukemic cells *in vitro* and decrease the incidence of experimentally induced forestomach tumors in test animals by 20% and the number of skin tumors and papillomas by 68% and 57%, respectively.[47] HL-60 leukemia cells are susceptible to curcumin treatment *in vitro*.[97] Extracts of turmeric and curcumin have been found to be nonmutagenic using the Ames test, and to serve protective roles against experimental mutagenesis induced by capsaicin, chili extract, and tobacco-derived mutagens.[21] In a different animal study, however, concentrations up to 5 mM curcumin did not protect against cytotoxicity of paracetamol in freshly isolated hepatocytes, and curcumin itself was found to be mildly hepatotoxic at high doses.[20] Curcumin inhibits the growth of human epidermoid carcinoma A431 cells *in vitro*.[98] Topical application of curcumin inhibits chemically induced tumor promotion in mouse skin,[99] which may be attributable to suppression of protein kinase C activity.[100] Curcumins have also been noted *in vitro* to inhibit nitrosation of methyl urea by sodium nitrate.[101] *In vitro* research suggests that curcumin exerts activity against human breast cancer cells,[93] including hormone-dependent, hormone-independent, and multidrug-resistant cell lines,[95] which may occur via effects on aryl hydrocarbon receptors[49] or ornithine decarboxylase activity.[95] The protective role of curcumin against carcinogenesis has also been attributed to antioxidant effects.[71] In rats, curcumin is reported to be protective against radiation-induced lung fibrosis and formation of micronuclei[102] and to protect against acute doxorubicin (Adriamycin)-induced myocardial toxicity.[51]

Dyspepsia
Summary

• Turmeric has been used traditionally to treat a variety of gastrointestinal disorders, particularly indigestion associated with fatty meals. Notably, turmeric may cause gastrointestinal irritation or upset, particularly in high or prolonged doses. There are limited data in the area of treating dyspepsia, although preliminary evidence suggests that turmeric may provide some symptomatic relief. Further study is warranted before an evidence-based recommendation can be made.

Evidence

• Thamlikitkul et al. in Thailand conducted a randomized, double-blind trial in 116 patients clinically diagnosed with dyspepsia.[14] Subjects were older than 12 years and were excluded if they exhibited clinical evidence of bowel obstruction, cholecystitis, pancreatitis, hepatitis, peritonitis, or pregnancy. Subjects received treatment four times daily with either turmeric capsules (250 mg of dried root powder containing 0.02 mL of volatile oil and 0.024 g of total curcuminoids), placebo (starch powder), or a herbal preparation (called "flatulence") consisting of cascara dry extract, nux vomica dry extract, asafetida tincture, capsicum powder, ginger powder, and diastase. Baseline characteristics were similar between groups. After 7 days of treatment, 71% of turmeric patients had clinically improved and 16% were cured, vs. 42% and 11%, respectively, in the placebo group and 57% and 27% in the "flatulence" group. Ten subjects (9%) dropped out, and analysis of dropouts revealed no significant baseline differences from the remaining patients. Differences between groups were statistically significant. Although these results are suggestive, the measurement

techniques used to evaluate symptomatic improvements or cures in patients were not described. Blinding and randomization procedures were not detailed and may not have been appropriate.

• Niederau et al. conducted a placebo-controlled trial in 76 patients with diagnosed "biliary dyskinesia" and chronic right upper quadrant pain (colic).[120] Subjects received either placebo or a combination product, Cholagogum F Nattermann, consisting of 45 mg of curcumin and 104 mg of celandine (*Chelidonium majus* L.). Notably, celandine is used traditionally as a treatment for gallbladder diseases such as cholelithiasis or cholecystitis; it contains multiple alkaloids and has been implicated in cases of neurotoxicity and hepatotoxicity in large or prolonged doses. After 3 weeks of therapy, a small significant reduction in colicky pain was noted in the treatment group compared with the placebo group. Secondary outcomes, including symptoms of food intolerance, nausea, and vomiting, were similar between groups. This study did not describe blinding or randomization and therefore was subject to the introduction of bias or confounding. The possible effects of turmeric and celandine cannot be separated from each other. Because of methodologic weaknesses, these results are of limited clinical value.

Peptic Ulcer Disease
Summary

• Turmeric has been used traditionally to treat a variety of gastrointestinal disorders, particularly indigestion associated with fatty meals. Notably, turmeric may cause gastrointestinal irritation or upset, particularly in high or prolonged doses. Turmeric has also been used historically to treat gastric and duodenal ulcers and was approved for the treatment of benign gastric ulcers in Thailand in 1986. In rats, oral turmeric reduces the incidence of chemically induced duodenal ulcers and is associated with an increase in intestinal wall mucus.[45] However, there is insufficient human research in this area to make an evidence-based recommendation. With the discovery of the role of *H. pylori* in duodenal and some gastric ulcers, and the demonstrated efficacy of antibiotics and proton pump inhibitors, turmeric may not be an appropriate first-line therapy. Comparisons of turmeric with proton pump inhibitors or H_2-receptor blockers have not been conducted.

Gastric Ulcer

• A comparison trial was conducted in 60 Thai patients with endoscopically proven gastric ulcers >0.5 cm in diameter.[121] Subjects were randomized to receive a 250-mg capsule of powdered turmeric root four times daily, or 30 mL of a liquid antacid containing aluminum hydroxide and magnesium hydroxide four times daily. Baseline patient characteristics were similar. After 6 weeks of therapy, endoscopy was repeated. The authors report that ulcers completely healed in 33.3% of turmeric patients, compared with 65.2% of antacid patients. Some improvement, presumably based on reduction in ulcer size, was observed in an additional 51.9% of the turmeric group and 34.8% of the antacid group. Notably, 10 patients (17%) dropped out prior to study completion. Because of the lack of placebo control in this study, it is not clear that the healing rate of gastric ulcers in the turmeric group was superior to that for no treatment; healing may be attributed to the natural history of gastric ulcers, which spontaneously heal in some patients. However, this study does suggest that this dose of turmeric is inferior to other antacid therapies. Methodologic weaknesses of this study include lack of blinding (turmeric was administered in capsule form, whereas the antacid was a liquid).

- Small case series have reported healing of peptic ulcers and decreased abdominal discomfort with the oral administration of turmeric.[122,123] Because of the lack of placebo control, clinical improvements cannot be distinguished from the natural history of disease, which resolves spontaneously in some patients.

Duodenal Ulcer

- Van Dau et al. conducted a placebo-controlled, double-blind trial in 130 Vietnamese patients with endoscopically proven duodenal ulcers >0.5 cm in diameter.[15] Subjects were randomized to receive either turmeric 6 g daily in three divided doses or placebo. Baseline patient characteristics were similar between groups. Outcome measures included endoscopic ulcer size and subjective patient responses to questions regarding severity of symptoms, using a multipoint scale to assess epigastric pain, constipation, nocturnal pain, pain with meals, nausea/vomiting, and hematemesis/melena. Details of the scoring system were not provided, and it does not appear to be a validated measurement system. An intention-to-treat analysis was not performed, and 12 subjects (9%) were excluded from final assessment because of unclear diagnoses or dropout. After 4 weeks of therapy, ulcers were found to be healed in 2% of turmeric patients and in 15% of placebo patients (significance not reported). After 8 weeks, ulcers were found to be healed in 27% of turmeric patients and in 29% of placebo patients (significance not reported). Symptoms as evaluated by the multipoint symptom scale decreased in both groups, without statistical differences. The authors concluded that turmeric is not an effective treatment for duodenal ulcer, although the critical style of the report's discussion section raise the possibility of bias. Methodologic weaknesses of this study include the lack of intention-to-treat analysis and lack of statistical analysis of the primary outcome measure. Randomization and blinding procedures were adequately described.

Cholelithiasis Prevention/Cholagogue (Gallbladder Contraction/Bile Flow Stimulant)
Summary

- Anecdotally, it has been observed that there is a low incidence of cholelithiasis in Indian populations, in which the diet typically includes large amounts of turmeric. Animal research reports that the turmeric constituent curcumin in the diet reduces the incidence of chemically induced gallstones in mice,[112] and it has been suggested that turmeric may inhibit the formation of cholesterol gallstones. Preliminary human data suggest that curcumin possesses cholagogic (gallbladder-contracting) properties. This mechanism may play a role in the prevention of gallstones. However, use of turmeric may be inadvisable in patients with active gallstones.

Evidence

- A randomized, double-blind, crossover study examined the effect of 20 mg of curcumin or placebo on gallbladder volume in 12 healthy volunteers.[30] A dose of 20 mg of curcumin or placebo was administered to subjects following a night of fasting, and gallbladder volume was measured by ultrasonography. Following a 1-week washout period, subjects received the alternate therapy. The authors report that gallbladder contraction occurred in the curcumin group 30

minutes after administration, and after 2 hours there was a mean reduction in volume by 16% ($p < 0.01$). In the placebo group, there was initial contraction similar to curcumin, but after 2 hours the mean gallbladder volume increased by 31%. Between-group differences were statistically significant. These results suggest an effect of curcumin on gallbladder function, although it is not clear what the clinical applications or long-term implications would be. In addition, because of the small sample size and unclear statistical analysis in this study, the results can only be considered preliminary.

Hyperlipidemia
Summary

- Animal studies report that oral turmeric lowers serum LDL and total cholesterol levels.[38,39,108] Preliminary evidence from small human case series suggest similar effects in humans, although in the absence of controlled trials, an evidence-based recommendation cannot be made.

Human Evidence

- In a case series, the effect of curcumin administration on serum lipids was examined in 10 healthy human volunteers.[124] Subjects received 500 mg of oral curcumin daily for 7 days. The authors noted a significant 29% increase in HDL cholesterol and a significant 12% decrease in total cholesterol. Although these findings are suggestive, it is not clear if other factors, such as change in diet, may have been implicated.
- In a poorly described case series of longer duration, healthy individuals were administered 20 mg of curcumin daily to assess effects on serum lipids.[67] After 45 days, a significant mean decrease in serum lipid peroxides was found, as determined by measuring levels of malondialdehyde (>60% decrease).
- A similar case series was conducted in 30 healthy individuals over a 60-day period.[29] A daily dose of 20 mg of curcumin was associated with a decrease in peroxidation of HDL and LDL cholesterol. Results were significantly greater in subjects with higher baseline levels.

Animal Studies

- In rat models of hyperlipidemia, a diet of 0.5% curcumin for 8 weeks significantly lowered serum LDL, VLDL, total cholesterol, and triglyceride levels, possibly by enhancing the activity of hepatic cholesterol-7α-hydroxylase and increasing cholesterol catabolism.[38,39,108] The turmeric constituents demethoxycurcumin, bisdemethoxycurcumin, and acetylcurcumin appear to inhibit iron-stimulated lipid peroxidation in rat tissues and liver microsomes.[69] In a rat model of hyperlipidemia, a 50% ethanolic extract of turmeric was associated with a significant reduction in the ratio of total cholesterol to phospholipids.[109] In rabbits fed a high-cholesterol diet, oral turmeric (1.6 to 3.2 mg/kg) was associated with lower levels of plasma cholesterol and triglycerides than those measured in a control group, although no differences in atherogenesis were noted on histologic examination of aortas.[110] Cholesterol levels were lower in the 1.6-mg/kg group.

Inflammation
Summary

- *In vitro* and animal studies have demonstrated anti-inflammatory activity of turmeric and its constituent curcumin. Multiple mechanisms have been implicated,

T

including effects on prostaglandins and cytokines. Human data are limited, and the specific mechanism of action and efficacy remain unproven.

Human Study

- In a controlled, double-blind study of 40 subjects with postoperative inflammation after hernia or hydrocele repair, 400 mg of curcumin was compared with placebo or 100 mg of phenylbutazone three times daily for 5 days.[125] Ampicillin 500 mg four times daily was given concurrently to all patients. Curcumin was found to significantly reduce edema and tenderness compared to placebo.[125] Details of outcome measurements, statistical analysis, randomization, and blinding were limited.

Animal and In Vitro Studies

- Pre-clinical studies have demonstrated multiple mechanisms that may be involved in the reduction of inflammation. Turmeric has been associated with inhibition of tumor necrosis factor-alpha, interleukin-8, monocyte inflammatory protein-1, interleukin-1β, and monocyte chemotactic protein-1.[40] Turmeric and its constituent curcumin have been found to inhibit lipoxygenase and cyclooxygenase in rat tissues and *in vitro*.[31,36,126] Inhibition of neutrophil function has been noted,[41] and *in vitro* research demonstrates that curcumin inhibits 5-hydroxy-eicosatetraenoic acid (5-HETE) in intact human neutrophils.[31] Turmeric has been found to block cytokine-induced transcription of leukocyte adhesion molecules intercellular adhesion molecule-1 (ICAM-1), vascular cell adhesion molecule-1 (VCAM-1), and E-selectin[54] and appears to induce production of endogenous TGF-beta$_1$ in animal wounds.[55] Curcumin downregulates transcription of genes responsible for the production of chemotactic cytokines in bone marrow stromal cells.[56] Curcumin reduces chemically induced rat paw edema[57,58] and liver inflammation.[59] In rat macrophages, curcumin inhibits the incorporation of arachidonic acid into membrane lipids, as well as prostaglandin E$_2$, leukotriene B$_4$, and leukotriene C$_4$, but does not affect the release of arachidonic acid.[53] Curcumin also inhibits the secretion of collagenase, elastase, and hyaluronidase.

Osteoarthritis
Summary

- Turmeric has been used historically to treat rheumatic conditions. Recent *in vitro* and animal studies have demonstrated anti-inflammatory properties of turmeric and its constituent curcumin that may play a role in the symptomatic relief of osteoarthritis. Human data are limited in this area, and no evidence-based recommendation can be made.

Evidence

- Kulkarni et al. conducted a randomized, double-blind, placebo-controlled, crossover study in 42 patients with osteoarthritis.[127] Patients were randomized to receive either the combination product Articulin-F (2 capsules three times daily) or placebo for 3 months. Each tablet of Articulin-F contains extracts of 50 mg of turmeric root, 100 mg of *Boswellia serrata*, 450 mg of *Withania somnifera* (ashwagandha), and 50 mg of zinc complex. Pain severity and disability scores were tabulated using validated instruments (Ritchie articular index, American Rheumatism Association joint score). At the study's end, treatment with

Articulin-F was found to have significantly improved the mean pain severity score ($p < 0.001$) and mean disability score ($p < 0.05$). Other parameters such as morning stiffness, grip strength, and joint score also showed improvement, but without statistical significance. The lack of significance of these results may reflect an absence of true benefit, or inadequate sample size to detect true benefits. Weaknesses of this study also include poor description of randomization and blinding methods, and unclear diagnostic criteria by which patients were judged to have osteoarthritis (unclear inclusion criteria). As a result, the patient population may not have been uniform. The mixed statistical significance of results and the isolated nature of this study leave open the question of the efficacy of Articulin-F for osteoarthritis. Because Articulin-F is a combination product, no firm conclusions can be drawn regarding turmeric specifically.

Rheumatoid Arthritis
Summary

- Turmeric has been used historically to treat rheumatic conditions. Recent *in vitro* and animal studies have demonstrated anti-inflammatory properties of turmeric and its constituent curcumin that may play a role in the symptomatic relief of rheumatoid arthritis. Human data are limited in this area, and no evidence-based recommendation can be made.

Evidence

- Deodhar et al. conducted a double-blind, crossover study in 18 patients with diagnosed rheumatoid arthritis (RA).[128,129] Subjects were randomized to receive either 1200 mg of curcumin or 300 mg of phenylbutazone daily for 2 weeks. Other anti-inflammatory medications were discontinued. Outcome measures included evaluation by a clinician of multiple parameters, including morning stiffness, walking time, fatigue time, and grip strength. In addition, erythrocyte sedimentation rate (ESR) and "articular index" were measured. An overall assessment score was assigned both by a clinician and subjectively by patients. It is not clear that any of the nonserologic measurements were based on standardized scales, and limited details were provided. After 2 weeks, both treatment groups experienced significant improvement as indicated by decrease in morning stiffness, increase in walking time, and decrease in joint swelling vs. baseline, and there was no difference between groups. Significant improvement did not occur in other measures, including ESR and articular index. Although the authors concluded that "antirheumatic" activity was exhibited by both therapies, because there was no placebo arm, it is possible that improvements were due to the natural history of RA symptoms (which may wax and wane) or to a "placebo effect." The lack of significant differences between groups may be attributable to the small sample size and inadequate power to detect differences.

Scabies
Summary

- Topical turmeric has been used historically in Ayurvedic medicine to treat chronic skin ulcers and scabies, sometimes in conjunction with leaves of the herb *Azadirachta indica* ADR (neem). Preliminary research from a large case series using this combination in patients with scabies is promising, although a controlled study is necessary before a strong recommendation can be made.

Evidence

- A case series was conducted in 824 individuals with diagnosed scabies in a rural area of India.[18] A paste was prepared for topical application to affected areas, consisting of a 4:1 mixture of neem (*Azadirachta indica* ADR) leaves and turmeric. Lesions were treated with paste daily until they disappeared, for up to 15 days. In addition to this treatment, clothing was boiled, and a scrub bath was performed on patients daily. The authors report complete resolution of lesions in 97.9% of cases within 3 to 15 days of treatment, and resolution in 95.8% of subjects with localized lesions within 3 to 5 days. These results are impressive and suggest a treatment that may be used in rural areas where access to pharmaceuticals is limited. However, it is not clear to what extent these benefits were due to the scrub baths and clothes-boiling; without a control group, the results must be considered preliminary. Because a combination preparation was used, the isolated efficacy of turmeric cannot be assessed.

HIV Infection
Summary

- *In vitro* studies suggest that curcumin may inhibit HIV-1 and HIV-2 proteases[130-133] and HIV-1 integrase.[134,135] Initial human evidence is limited, although lack of efficacy is suggested by a well-designed phase I/II trial reported as a conference abstract. At this time, there are insufficient data to make an evidence-based judgment regarding efficacy.

Human Studies

- A clinical trial, published as an abstract, was reported at the 3rd Conference on Retroviruses and Opportunistic Infections in 1996.[136] Based on the prior finding that the turmeric constituent curcumin inhibits TNF-alpha stimulation of HIV long terminal repeat (LTR) in several cell lines, this open-label study was conducted in 40 HIV-positive individuals, using either 4800 mg or 2700 mg of curcumin daily in divided doses. Curcumin was obtained from the brand Turmeric Power (Nature's Herbs, Orem, Utah). After 8 weeks of therapy, no significant changes were detected in HIV RNA copy number or CD4+ cell counts.
- In a study published as an abstract only, 18 HIV-positive patients with CD4+ cell counts between 5 and 615 were administered an average of 2000 mg of curcumin daily.[137] This regimen was reported to significantly increase CD4+ counts compared with control levels. However, this report did not include specific details of the CD4+ rise.

Uveitis
Summary

- Turmeric and its constituent curcumin have been demonstrated *in vitro* and in animals to possess anti-inflammatory and antioxidant properties. One human case series suggests a possible benefit of curcumin in the management of chronic anterior uveitis. However, because of methodologic weaknesses with this study, and lack of controlled trials in this area, no evidence-based recommendation can be made at this time.

Evidence

- A case series was performed in 53 patients with chronic anterior uveitis.[138] Subjects were administered 375 mg of curcumin derived from turmeric, three times daily. Outcome measures included decrease in uveitis signs and symptoms,

recurrence rate, and vision loss. Over the 12-week trial period, 21 patients dropped out (40%). The remaining 32 subjects were analyzed as two separate cohorts: those taking turmeric alone (n = 18) and those taking turmeric plus antituberculosis treatment for a positive purified protein derivative (PPD) reaction (n = 14). In the turmeric-only group, all patients improved during the study period, whereas in the turmeric/antituberculin group, 86% improved. Criteria for improvement were not clearly described, and statistical significance was not clear. Additional follow-up of these 32 subjects was conducted over 3 years, during which time uveitis recurred in 47% of patients and 22% lost their vision. The authors assert that these rates of recurrence and vision loss are comparable to rates observed with steroid treatment. However, without a control group, the benefits attributable to curcumin remain unclear. The 40% attrition rate without adequate description of dropouts raises questions about whether the remaining patients may have been self-selected for good outcomes, while subjects with worse outcomes dropped out.

FORMULARY: BRANDS USED IN CLINICAL TRIALS

- Turmeric Power (Nature's Herbs, Orem, Utah): not efficacious in the treatment of HIV infection.[136]

References

1. Kim DS, Park SY, Kim JK. Curcuminoids from Curcuma longa L. (Zingiberaceae) that protect PC12 rat pheochromocytoma and normal human umbilical vein endothelial cells from betaA(1-42) insult. Neurosci Lett 2001;303(1):57-61.
2. Apisariyakul A, Vanittanakom N, Buddhasukh D. Antifungal activity of turmeric oil extracted from *Curcuma longa* (Zingiberaceae). J Ethnopharmacol 1995;49(3):163-169.
3. Rasmussen HB, Christensen SB, Kvist LP, et al. A simple and efficient separation of the curcumins, the antiprotozoal constituents of *Curcuma longa*. Planta Med 2000;66(4):396-398.
4. Ferreira LA, Henriques OB, Andreoni AA, et al. Antivenom and biological effects of ar-turmerone isolated from *Curcuma longa* (Zingiberaceae). Toxicon 1992;30(10):1211-1218.
5. Li C, Li L, Luo J, et al. [Effect of turmeric volatile oil on the respiratory tract]. Zhongguo Zhong Yao Za Zhi 1998;23(10):624-5, inside.
6. Sajithlal GB, Chithra P, Chandrakasan G. Effect of curcumin on the advanced glycation and cross-linking of collagen in diabetic rats. Biochem Pharm 1998;56:1607-1614.
7. Cohly HH, Taylor A, Angel MF, et al. Effect of turmeric, turmerin and curcumin on H$_2$O$_2$-induced renal epithelial (LLC-PK1) cell injury. Free Radic Biol Med 1998;24(1):49-54.
8. Kiso Y, Suzuki Y, Watanabe N, et al. Antihepatotoxic principles of *Curcuma longa* rhizomes. Planta Med 1983;49(3):185-187.
9. Soni KB, Rajan A, Kuttan R. Reversal of aflatoxin induced liver damage by turmeric and curcumin. Cancer Lett 1992;66(2):115-121.
10. Kosuge T, Ishida H, Yamazaki H. Studies on active substances in the herbs used for oketsu ("stagnant blood") in Chinese medicine. III. On the anti-coagulative principles in curcumae rhizoma. Chem Pharm Bull (Tokyo) 1985;33(4):1499-1502.
11. Shalini VK, Srinivas L. Fuel smoke condensate induced DNA damage in human lymphocytes and protection by turmeric (*Curcuma longa*). Mol Cell Biochem 1990;95(1):21-30.
12. Govindarajan VS. Turmeric—chemistry, technology, and quality. Crit Rev Food Sci Nutr 1980;12(3):199-301.
13. Polasa K, Raghuram TC, Krishna TP, et al. Effect of turmeric on urinary mutagens in smokers. Mutagenesis 1992;7(2):107-109.
14. Thamlikitkul V, Bunyapraphatsara N, Dechatiwongse T, et al. Randomized double blind study of *Curcuma domestica* Val. for dyspepsia. J Med Assoc Thai 1989;72(11):613-620.
15. Van Dau N, Ngoc Ham N, Huy Khac D, et al. The effects of a traditional drug, turmeric (*Curcuma longa*), and placebo on the healing of duodenal ulcer. Phytomed 1998;5(1):29-34.
16. Shah BH, Nawaz Z, Pertani SA, et al. Inhibitory effect of curcumin, a food spice from turmeric, on platelet-activating factor– and arachidonic acid–mediated platelet aggregation through inhibition of thromboxane formation and Ca^{2+} signaling. Biochem Pharmacol 1999;58(7):1167-1172.
17. Commandeur JN, Vermeulen NP. Cytotoxicity and cytoprotective activities

of natural compounds. The case of curcumin. Xenobiotica 1996;26(7): 667-680.

18. Charles V, Charles SX. The use and efficacy of *Azadirachta indica* ADR ('neem') and *Curcuma longa* ('turmeric') in scabies. A pilot study. Trop Geogr Med 1992;44(1-2):178-181.

19. Qureshi S, Shah AH, Ageel AM. Toxicity studies on *Alpinia galanga* and *Curcuma longa*. Planta Med 1992;58:124-127.

20. Donatus IA, Sardjoko, Vermeulen NP. Cytotoxic and cytoprotective activities of curcumin. Effects on paracetamol-induced cytotoxicity, lipid peroxidation and glutathione depletion in rat hepatocytes. Biochem Pharmacol 1990;39(12):1869-1875.

21. Nagabhushan M, Amonkar AJ, Bhide SV. *In vitro* antimutagenicity of curcumin against environmental mutagens. Food Chem Toxicol 1987; 25(7):545-547.

22. Shankar TN, Murthy VS. Effect of turmeric (*Curcuma longa*) fractions on the growth of some intestinal and pathogenic bacteria *in vitro*. J Exper Biol 1979;17:1363-1366.

23. Srimal RC, Dhawan BN. Pharmacology of diferuloyl methane (curcumin), a non-steroidal anti-inflammatory agent. J Pharm Pharmacol 1973;25(6): 447-452.

24. Kiec-Swierczynska M, Krecisz B. Occupational allergic contact dermatitis due to curcumin food colour in a pasta factory worker. Contact Dermatitis 1998;39(1):30-31.

25. Goh CL, Ng SK. Allergic contact dermatitis to *Curcuma longa* (turmeric). Contact Dermatitis 1987;17(3):186.

26. Kuttan R, Bhanumathy P, Nirmala K, et al. Potential anticancer activity of turmeric (*Curcuma longa*). Cancer Lett 1985;29(2):197-202.

27. Patil TN, Srinivasan M. Hypocholesteremic effect of curcumin in induced hypercholesteremic rats. Indian J Exp Biol 1971;9(2):167-169.

28. Ammon HP, Wahl MA. Pharmacology of *Curcuma longa*. Planta Med 1991;57(1):1-7.

29. Bosca A, et al. Effects of the antioxidant tumeric on lipoprotein peroxides: implications for the prevention of atherosclerosis. Age 1997;20:165-168.

30. Rasyid A, Lelo A. The effect of curcumin and placebo on human gallbladder function: an ultrasound study. Aliment Pharmacol Ther 1999; 13(2):245-249.

31. Flynn DL, Rafferty MF, Boctor AM. Inhibition of 5-hydroxy-eicosatetraenoic acid (5-HETE) formation in intact human neutrophils by naturally-occurring diarylheptanoids: inhibitory activities of curcuminoids and yakuchinones. Prostaglandins Leukot Med 1986;22(3):357-360.

32. Srivastava KC, Bordia A, Verma SK. Curcumin, a major component of food spice turmeric (*Curcuma longa*) inhibits aggregation and alters eicosanoid metabolism in human blood platelets. Prostaglandins Leukot Essent Fatty Acids 1995;52(4):223-227.

33. Srivastava R, Dikshit M, Srimal RC, et al. Anti-thrombotic effect of curcumin. Thromb Res 1985;40(3):413-417.

34. Srivastava R, Puri V, Srimal RC, et al. Effect of curcumin on platelet aggregation and vascular prostacyclin synthesis. Arzneimittelforschung 1986; 36(4):715-717.

35. Rao CV, Simi B, Reddy BS. Inhibition by dietary curcumin of azoxymethane-induced ornithine decarboxylase, tyrosine protein kinase, arachidonic acid metabolism and aberrant crypt foci formation in the rat colon. Carcinogenesis 1993;14(11):2219-2225.

36. Ammon HP, Safayhi H, Mack T, et al. Mechanism of antiinflammatory actions of curcumine and boswellic acids. J Ethnopharmacol 1993;38(2-3): 113-119.

37. Srivastava KC. Extracts from two frequently consumed spices—cumin (*Cuminum cyminum*) and turmeric (*Curcuma longa*)—inhibit platelet aggregation and alter eicosanoid biosynthesis in human blood platelets. Prostaglandins Leukot Essent Fatty Acids 1989;37(1):57-64.

38. Babu PS, Srinivasan K. Hypolipidemic action of curcumin, the active principle of turmeric (*Curcuma longa*) in streptozotocin induced diabetic rats. Mol Cell Biochem 1997;166(1-2):169-175.

39. Srinivasan K, Sambaiah K. The effect of spices on cholesterol 7 alpha-hydroxylase activity and on serum and hepatic cholesterol levels in the rat. Int J Vit Nutr Res 1991;61:364-369.

40. Abe Y, Hashimoto S, Horie T. Curcumin inhibition of inflammatory cytokine production by human peripheral blood monocytes and alveolar macrophages. Pharmacol Res 1999;39(1):41-47.

41. Srivastava R. Inhibition of neutrophil response by curcumin. Agents Actions 1989;28(3-4):298-303.

42. Chandra D, Gupta SS. Anti-inflammatory and anti-arthritic activity of volatile oil of *Curcuma longa* (haldi). Indian J Med Res 1972;60(1): 138-142.

43. Garg SK. Effect of *Curcuma longa* (rhizomes) on fertility in experimental animals. Planta Med 1974;26(3):225-227.

44. Vijayalaxmi. Genetic effects of turmeric and curcumin in mice and rats. Mutat Res 1980;79(2):125-132.

45. Rafatullah S, Tariq M, Al Yahya MA, et al. Evaluation of turmeric (*Curcuma longa*) for gastric and duodenal antiulcer activity in rats. J Ethnopharmacol 1990;29(1):25-34.

46. Oetari S, Sudibyo M, Commandeur JN, et al. Effects of curcumin on cytochrome P450 and glutathione *S*-transferase activities in rat liver. Biochem Pharmacol 1996;51(1):39-45.

47. Nagabhushan M, Bhide SV. Curcumin as an inhibitor of cancer. J Am Coll Nutrit 1992;11(2):192-198.

48. Azuine MA, Bhide SV. Chemopreventive effect of turmeric against stomach and skin tumors induced by chemical carcinogens in Swiss mice. Nutr Cancer 1992;17(1):77-83.

49. Ciolino HP, Daschner PJ, Wang TT, et al. Effect of curcumin on the aryl hydrocarbon receptor and cytochrome P450 1A1 in MCF-7 human breast carcinoma cells. Biochem Pharmacol 1998;56(2):197-206.

50. Firozi PF, Aboobaker VS, Bhattacharya RK. Action of curcumin on the cytochrome P450-system catalyzing the activation of aflatoxin B1. Chem Biol Interact 1996;100(1):41-51.

51. Venkatesan N. Curcumin attenuation of acute Adriamycin myocardial toxicity in rats. Br J Pharmacol 1998;124(3):425-427.

52. Ammon HP, Anazodo MI, Safayhi H, et al. Curcumin: a potent inhibitor of leukotriene B$_4$ formation in rat peritoneal polymorphonuclear neutrophils (PMNL). Planta Med 1992;58(2):226.

53. Joe B, Lokesh BR. Effect of curcumin and capsaicin on arachidonic acid metabolism and lysosomal enzyme secretion by rat peritoneal macrophages. Lipids 1997;32(11):1173-1180.

54. Gupta B, Ghosh B. *Curcuma longa* inhibits TNF-alpha induced expression of adhesion molecules on human umbilical vein endothelial cells. Int J Immunopharmacol 1999;21(11):745-757.

55. Sidhu GS, Singh AK, Thaloor D, et al. Enhancement of wound healing by curcumin in animals. Wound Repair Regen 1998;6(2):167-177.

56. Xu YX, Pindolia KR, Janakiraman N, et al. Curcumin, a compound with anti-inflammatory and anti-oxidant properties, down-regulates chemokine expression in bone marrow stromal cells. Exp Hematol 1997;25(5): 413-422.

57. Nurfina AN, Reksohadiprodjo MS, Timmerman H, et al. Synthesis of some symmetrical curcumin derivatives and their antiinflammatory activity. Eur J Med Chem 1997;32:321-328.

58. Mukhopadhyay A, Basu N, Ghatak N, et al. Anti-inflammatory and irritant activities of curcumin analogues in rats. Agents Actions 1982;12(4): 508-515.

59. Srimal RC, Khanna NM, Dhawan BN. A preliminary report on anti-inflammatory activity of curcumin. Indian J Pharmacol 1971;3:10.

60. Iqbal M, Sharma SD, Okazaki Y, et al. Dietary supplementation of curcumin enhances antioxidant and phase II metabolizing enzymes in ddY male mice: possible role in protection against chemical carcinogenesis and toxicity. Pharmacol Toxicol 2003;92(1):33-38.

61. Balogun E, Hoque M, Gong P, et al. Curcumin activates the haem oxygenase-1 gene via regulation of Nrf2 and the antioxidant-responsive element. Biochem J 2003;371(Pt 3):887-895.

62. Braga ME, Leal PF, Carvalho JE, et al. Comparison of yield, composition, and antioxidant activity of turmeric (*Curcuma longa* L.) extracts obtained using various techniques. J Agric Food Chem 2003;51(22):6604-6611.

63. Motterlini R, Foresti R, Bassi R, et al. Curcumin, an antioxidant and anti-inflammatory agent, induces heme oxygenase-1 and protects endothelial cells against oxidative stress. Free Radic Biol Med 2000;28(8):1303-1312.

64. Sreejayan, Rao MN. Nitric oxide scavenging by curcuminoids. J Pharm Pharmacol 1997;49(1):105-107.

65. Ruby AJ, Kuttan G, Babu KD, et al. Anti-tumour and antioxidant activity of natural curcuminoids. Cancer Lett 1995;94(1):79-83.

66. Osawa T, Sugiyama Y, Inayoshi M, et al. Antioxidative activity of tetrahydrocurcuminoids. Biosci Biotechnol Biochem 1995;59(9): 1609-1612.

67. Ramirez-Bosca A, Soler A, Guiterrez MA, et al. Antioxidant curcuma extracts decrease the blood lipid peroxide levels of human subjects. Age 1995;18(4):167-169.

68. Reddy AC, Lokesh BR. Effect of dietary turmeric (*Curcuma longa*) on iron-induced lipid peroxidation in the rat liver. Food Chem Toxicol 1994; 32(3):279-283.

69. Sreejayan, Rao MN. Curcuminoids as potent inhibitors of lipid peroxidation. J Pharm Pharmacol 1994;46(12):1013-1016.

70. Sreejayan, Rao MNA. Curcumin inhibits iron-dependent lipid peroxidation. Int J Pharmaceut 1993;100:93-97.

71. Subramanian M, Sreejayan, Rao MN, et al. Diminution of singlet oxygen-induced DNA damage by curcumin and related antioxidants. Mutat Res 1994;311(2):249-255.

72. Kunchandy E, Rao MN. Effect of curcumin on hydroxyl radical generation through Fenton reaction. Int J Pharmaceut 1989;57:173-176.

73. Sreejayan N, Rao MN. Free radical scavenging activity of curcuminoids. Arzneimittelforschung 1996;46(2):169-171.

74. Shalini VK, Srinivas L. Lipid peroxide induced DNA damage: protection by turmeric (Curcuma longa). Mol Cell Biochem 1987;77(1):3-10.

75. Srinivas L, Shalini VK. DNA damage by smoke: protection by turmeric and other inhibitors of ROS. Free Radic Biol Med 1991;11(3):277-283.

76. Srivastava R, Srimal RC. Modification of certain inflammation-induced biochemical changes by curcumin. Indian J Med Res 1985;81:215-223.

77. Aggarwal BB, Kumar A, Bharti AC. Anticancer potential of curcumin: preclinical and clinical studies. Anticancer Res 2003;23(1A):363-398.

78. Bharti AC, Donato N, Singh S, et al. Curcumin (diferuloylmethane) down-regulates the constitutive activation of nuclear factor-kappa B and IkappaBalpha kinase in human multiple myeloma cells, leading to

suppression of proliferation and induction of apoptosis. Blood 2003; 101(3):1053-1062.

79. Chaudhary LR, Hruska KA. Inhibition of cell survival signal protein kinase B/Akt by curcumin in human prostate cancer cells. J Cell Biochem 2003;89(1):1-5.

80. Deeb D, Xu YX, Jiang H, et al. Curcumin (diferuloyl-methane) enhances tumor necrosis factor-related apoptosis-inducing ligand-induced apoptosis in LNCaP prostate cancer cells. Mol Cancer Ther 2003;2(1):95-103.

81. Devasena T, Rajasekaran KN, Gunasekaran G, et al. Anticarcinogenic effect of bis-1,7-(2-hydroxyphenyl)-hepta-1,6-diene-3,5-dione, a curcumin analog, on DMH-induced colon cancer model. Pharmacol Res 2003; 47(2):133-140.

82. Di GH, Li HC, Shen ZZ, et al. [Analysis of anti-proliferation of curcumin on human breast cancer cells and its mechanism]. Zhonghua Yi Xue Za Zhi 2003;83(20):1764-1768.

83. Dorai T, Cao YC, Dorai B, et al. Therapeutic potential of curcumin in human prostate cancer. III. Curcumin inhibits proliferation, induces apoptosis, and inhibits angiogenesis of LNCaP prostate cancer cells in vivo. Prostate 2001;47(4):293-303.

84. Elattar TM, Virji AS. The inhibitory effect of curcumin, genistein, quercetin and cisplatin on the growth of oral cancer cells in vitro. Anticancer Res 2000;20(3A):1733-1738.

85. Gautam SC, Xu YX, Pindolia KR, et al. Nonselective inhibition of proliferation of transformed and nontransformed cells by the anticancer agent curcumin (diferuloylmethane). Biochem Pharmacol 1998;55(8): 1333-1337.

86. Hastak K, Lubri N, Jakhi SD, et al. Effect of turmeric oil and turmeric oleoresin on cytogenetic damage in patients suffering from oral submucous fibrosis. Cancer Lett 1997;116(2):265-269.

87. Jiang MC, Yang-Yen HF, Yen JJ, et al. Curcumin induces apoptosis in immortalized NIH 3T3 and malignant cancer cell lines. Nutr Cancer 1996; 26(1):111-120.

88. Kuttan R, Sudheeran PC, Josph CD. Turmeric and curcumin as topical agents in cancer therapy. Tumori 1987;73(1):29-31.

89. Moragoda L, Jaszewski R, Majumdar AP. Curcumin induced modulation of cell cycle and apoptosis in gastric and colon cancer cells. Anticancer Res 2001;21(2A):873-878.

90. Pereira MA, Grubbs CJ, Barnes LH, et al. Effects of the phytochemicals, curcumin and quercetin, upon azoxymethane-induced colon cancer and 7,12-dimethylbenz[a]anthracene- induced mammary cancer in rats. Carcinogenesis 1996;17(6):1305-1311.

91. Rashmi R, Santhosh Kumar TR, Karunagaran D. Human colon cancer cells differ in their sensitivity to curcumin-induced apoptosis and heat shock protects them by inhibiting the release of apoptosis-inducing factor and caspases. FEBS Lett 2003;538(1-3):19-24.

92. Sharma RA, McLelland HR, Hill KA, et al. Pharmacodynamic and pharmacokinetic study of oral Curcuma extract in patients with colorectal cancer. Clin Cancer Res 2001;7(7):1894-1900.

93. Verma S, Salamone E, Goldin B. Curcumin and genistein, plant natural products, show synergistic inhibitory effects on the growth of human breast cancer MCF-7 cells induced by estrogenic pesticides. Biochem Biophys Res Commun 1997;233(3):692-696.

94. Kawamori T, Lubet R, Steele VE, et al. Chemopreventive effect of curcumin, a naturally occurring anti-inflammatory agent, during the promotion/ progression stages of colon cancer. Cancer Res 1999;59(3): 597-601.

95. Mehta K, Pantazis P, McQueen T, et al. Antiproliferative effect of curcumin (diferuloylmethane) against human breast tumor cell lines. Anticancer Drugs 1997;8(5):470-481.

96. Huang MT, Deschner EE, Newmark HL, et al. Effect of dietary curcumin and ascorbyl palmitate on azoxymethanol- induced colonic epithelial cell proliferation and focal areas of dysplasia. Cancer Lett 1992;64(2):117-121.

97. Kuo ML, Huang TS, Lin JK. Curcumin, an antioxidant and anti-tumor promoter, induces apoptosis in human leukemia cells. Biochim Biophys Acta 1996;1317(2):95-100.

98. Korutla L, Kumar R. Inhibitory effect of curcumin on epidermal growth factor receptor kinase activity in A431 cells. Biochim Biophys Acta 1994;1224(3):597-600.

99. Conney AH, Lysz T, Ferraro T, et al. Inhibitory effect of curcumin and some related dietary compounds on tumor promotion and arachidonic acid metabolism in mouse skin. Adv Enzyme Regul 1991;31:385-396.

100. Liu JY, Lin SJ, Lin JK. Inhibitory effects of curcumin on protein kinase C activity induced by 12-O-tetradecanoyl-phorbol-13-acetate in NIH 3T3 cells. Carcinogenesis 1993;14(5):857-861.

101. Nagabhushan M, Nair UJ, Amonkar AJ, et al. Curcumins as inhibitors of nitrosation in vitro. Mutat Res 1988;202(1):163-169.

102. Thresiamma KC, George J, Kuttan R. Protective effect of curcumin, ellagic acid and bixin on radiation induced toxicity. Indian J Exp Biol 1996;34(9):845-847.

103. Chen HW, Huang HC. Effect of curcumin on cell cycle progression and apoptosis in vascular smooth muscle cells. Br J Pharmacol 1998;124(6): 1029-1040.

104. Ranjan D, Siquijor A, Johnston TD, et al. The effect of curcumin on human B-cell immortalization by Epstein-Barr virus. Am Surg 1998; 64(1):47-51.

105. Robinson TP, Ehlers T, Hubbard IV RB, et al. Design, synthesis, and biological evaluation of angiogenesis inhibitors: aromatic enone and dienone analogues of curcumin. Bioorg Med Chem Lett 2003;13(1):115-117.

106. Gao C, Ding Z, Liang B, et al. [Study on the effects of curcumin on angiogenesis]. Zhong Yao Cai 2003;26(7):499-502.

107. Thaloor D, Singh AK, Sidhu GS, et al. Inhibition of angiogenic differentiation of human umbilical vein endothelial cells by curcumin. Cell Growth Differ 1998;9(4):305-312.

108. Babu PS, Srinivasan K. Influence of dietary curcumin and cholesterol on the progression of experimentally induced diabetes in albino rat. Mol Cell Biochem 1995;152(1):13-21.

109. Dixit VP, Jain P, Joshi SC. Hypolipidaemic effects of Curcuma longa L and Nardostachys jatamansi, DC in triton-induced hyperlipidaemic rats. Indian J Physiol Pharmacol 1988;32(4):299-304.

110. Ramirez-Tortosa MC, Mesa MD, Aguilera MC, et al. Oral administration of a turmeric extract inhibits LDL oxidation and has hypocholesterolemic effects in rabbits with experimental atherosclerosis. Atherosclerosis 1999;147(2):371-378.

111. Bhatia A, Singh GB, Khanna NM. Effect of curcumin, its alkali salts & Curcuma longa oil in histamine-induced gastric ulceration. Indian J Exp Biol 1964;2:158-160.

112. Hussain MS, Chandrasekhara N. Effect on curcumin on cholesterol gallstone induction in mice. Indian J Med Res 1992;96:288-291.

113. Tonnesen HH. Chemistry of curcumin and curcuminoids. Phenol Comp Food Effects Health 1992;143-153.

114. Tonnesen HH, Greenhill JV. Studies on curcumin and curcuminoids. XXII: Curcumin as a reducing agent and as a radical scavenger. Int J Pharmaceut 1992;87:79-87.

115. Tonnesen HH, de Vries H, Karlsen J, et al. Studies on curcumin and curcuminoids. IX: Investigation of the photobiological activity of curcumin using bacterial indicator systems. J Pharm Sci 1987;76(5):371-373.

116. Wahlstrom B, Blennow G. A study on the fate of curcumin in the rat. Acta Pharmacol Toxicol (Copenh) 1978;43(2):86-92.

117. Ravindranath V, Chandrasekhara N. Absorption and tissue distribution of curcumin in rats. Toxicology 1980;16(3):259-265.

118. Mathews S, Rao MNA. Interaction of curcumin with glutathione. Int J Pharmaceut 1991;76:257-259.

119. Susan M, Rao MN. Induction of glutathione S-transferase activity by curcumin in mice. Arzneimittelforschung 1992;42(7):962-964.

120. Niederau C, Gopfert E. [The effect of chelidonium- and turmeric root extract on upper abdominal pain due to functional disorders of the biliary system. Results from a placebo-controlled double-blind study]. Med Klin 1999;94(8):425-430.

121. Kositchaiwat C, Kositchaiwat S, Havanondha J. Curcuma longa Linn. in the treatment of gastric ulcer: comparison to liquid antacid: a controlled clinical trial. J Med Assoc Thai 1993;76(11):601-605.

122. Intanonta A. Treatment of abdominal pain with Curcuma longa L. Report submitted to Primary Health Care Office, Ministry of Public Health, Thailand, 1986.

123. Prucksunand C, et al. Effect of the long turmeric (Curcumina longa L.) on healing peptic ulcer: a preliminary report of 10 case studies. Thai J Pharmacol 1986;8:139-151.

124. Soni KB, Kuttan R. Effect of oral curcumin administration on serum peroxides and cholesterol levels in human volunteers. Indian J Physiol Pharmacol 1992;36(4):273-275.

125. Satoskar RR, Shah SJ, Shenoy SG. Evaluation of anti-inflammatory property of curcumin (diferuloyl methane) in patients with postoperative inflammation. Int J Clin Pharmacol Ther Toxicol 1986;24(12):651-654.

126. Rao S, Rao M. Curcumin inhibits iron-dependent lipid peroxidation. Int J Pharmaceut 1993;1993:93-97.

127. Kulkarni RR, Patki PS, Jog VP, et al. Treatment of osteoarthritis with a herbomineral formulation: a double-blind, placebo-controlled, cross-over study. J Ethnopharmacol 1991;33(1-2):91-95.

128. Deodhar SD, Sethi R, Srimal RC. Preliminary study on antirheumatic activity of curcumin (diferuloyl methane). Indian J Med Res 1980;71: 632-634.

129. Deodhar SD, Srimal R, Dhawan BN. Antirheumatic activity of curcumin. Proc World Conference on Clinical Pharmacology and Therapeutics, London, Abstract No. 0668. London, Macmillan, 1980, p. 668.

130. Barthelemy S, Vergnes L, Moynier M, et al. Curcumin and curcumin derivatives inhibit Tat-mediated transactivation of type 1 human immunodeficiency virus long terminal repeat. Res Virol 1998;149(1):43-52.

131. Li CJ, Zhang LJ, Dezube BJ, et al. Three inhibitors of type 1 human immunodeficiency virus long terminal repeat–directed gene expression and virus replication. Proc Natl Acad Sci U S A 1993;90(5):1839-1842.

132. Mazumder A, Wang S, Neamati N, et al. Antiretroviral agents as inhibitors of both human immunodeficiency virus type 1 integrase and protease. J Med Chem 1996;39(13):2472-2481.

133. Sui Z, Salto R, Li J, et al. Inhibition of the HIV-1 and HIV-2 proteases by curcumin and curcumin boron complexes. Bioorg Med Chem 1993;1(6): 415-422.

134. Mazumder A, Raghavan K, Weinstein J, et al. Inhibition of human immunodeficiency virus type-1 integrase by curcumin. Biochem Pharmacol 1995;49(8):1165-1170.

T

135. Mazumder A, Neamati N, Sunder S, et al. Curcumin analogs with altered potencies against HIV-1 integrase as probes for biochemical mechanisms of drug action. J Med Chem. 1997;40(19):3057-3063.
136. Hellinger JA, Cohen CJ, Dugan ME, et al. Phase I/II randomized, open-label study of oral curcumin safety, and antiviral effects on HIV-RT PCR in HIV⁺ individuals. 3rd Conference on Retroviruses and Opportunistic Infections, January 28–February 1, 1996, Washington, DC.
137. Copeland R. Curcumin therapy in HIV-infected patients initially increased CD-4 and CD-8 cell counts. X Int Conf AIDS 1994;10:216.
138. Lal B, Kapoor AK, Asthana OP, et al. Efficacy of curcumin in the management of chronic anterior uveitis. Phytother Res 1999;13(4):318-322.

Valerian
(*Valeriana officinalis* L.)

SYNONYMS/COMMON NAMES/RELATED SUBSTANCES

- All-heal, amantilla, balderbrackenwurzel, baldrian, baldrianwurzel, baldrion, Belgian valerian, common valerian, fragrant valerian, garden heliotrope, garden valerian, great wild valerian, herba benedicta, heliptrope, Indian valerian, Jacob's ladder, Japanese valerian, katzenwurzel, laege-baldrian, Mexican valerian, Nervex, Neurol, Orasedon, Pacific valerian, phu, phu germanicum, phu parvum, pinnis dentatis, racine de valèriane, radix valerian, red valerian, Sanox-N, Sedonium, setewale capon's tail, setwall, setwell, theriacaria, Ticalma, *Valeriana. edulis, Valeriana faurieri , Valeriana foliis pinnatis, Valeriana jatamansi, Valeriana radix, Valeriana sitchensis, Valeriana wallichii,* valerianae radix, Valerianaceae, Valerianaheel, valeriane, Valmane, vandal root.

CLINICAL BOTTOM LINE
Background

- Valerian is widely used to treat insomnia and anxiety. Preliminary data from several human trials suggest that valerian improves subjective measures of sleep quality and sleep latency. Better effects have been noted in poor sleepers. Early evidence suggests that ongoing use may be more effective than acute (single-dose) use, with progressive effects over several weeks. However, most available studies have been methodologically weak, and in most cases results have not been confirmed using objective sleep pattern data in a sleep laboratory or validated measurement scales.
- Studies report that valerian is generally well tolerated for up to 4 to 6 weeks but rarely may produce mild adverse effects (dizziness, hangover, headache). Preliminary research suggests that valerian is nonsedating in recommended doses and has little effect on reaction time, concentration, or coordination compared to benzodiazepines. However, other studies report that valerian may impair vigilance or slow the processing of complex thoughts for a few hours after use.

Scientific Evidence for Common/Studied Uses	Grade*
Insomnia	B
Anxiety	C
Sedation	D

*Key to grades: *A:* Strong scientific evidence for this use; *B:* Good scientific evidence for this use; *C:* Unclear scientific evidence for this use; *D:* Fair scientific evidence against this use (it may not work); *F:* Strong scientific evidence against this use (it likely does not work). For a more detailed explanation of efficacy criteria, see "Natural Standard Evidence-Based Validated Grading Rationale" in the Introduction.

Historical or Theoretical Indications
That Lack Sufficient Evidence

- Acne, angina pectoris, amenorrhea, anodyne (pain relief), anorexia, anticonvulsive, antiperspirant, antispasmodic, anti-viral, arthritis, asthma, bloating, bronchospasm, carminative, colic, congestive heart failure, constipation, convulsions, cough, cramping (abdominal, pelvic, menstrual), cyanosis, depression (in combination with St. John's wort [*Hypericum perforatum*]),[1-4] digestive problems, diuretic, dysmenorrhea, emmenagogue, exhaustion, fatigue, fever, flatulence, hangovers, heart disease, heartburn, hepatic disorders, HIV, hypertension, hypochondria, intestinal disorders, irritable bowel syndrome, measles, memory, menopause, migraine, mood enhancement, motor syndromes, muscle pain/spasm/tension, nausea, nervous excitability, nervous palpitation, nervous tachycardia, neuralgia, pain, peptic ulcer disease, premenstrual syndrome, restlessness, restless leg syndrome, rheumatic pain, skin disorders, spasmolytic, stress, tension headaches, urinary tract disorders, urolithiasis, vaginal yeast infections, vertigo, viral gastroenteritis, vision, withdrawal from tranquilizers.[5-7]

Expert Opinion and Folkloric Precedent

- Valerian root has a history of widespread use in North America and Europe since the mid- 1800s for the treatment of restlessness and nervous sleep disturbances and has been called the "Valium of the 19th century." Today, valerian is popular in parts of Europe as a prescription or non-prescription hypnotic and sedative. The German government expert panel, Commission E, has approved the use of valerian as a mild sedative. The American Pharmaceutical Association has given valerian a high rating for safety and efficacy in its use as a mild sedative.

Safety Summary

- **General:** Valerian root is widely reported as being safe in recommended doses for brief periods of time (4 to 6 weeks). In the United States, valerian has been categorized by the U.S. Food and Drug Administration as GRAS (generally recognized as safe). The German Commission E has approved valerian as a nonprescription agent to treat nervous restlessness and sleeping disorders. In Canada, it is approved for use as a sedative and spasmolytic.
- **Likely safe:** When used orally at recommended doses (400 to 600 mg of aqueous or aqueous-alcoholic root extract/day) by otherwise healthy adults for short- or intermediate-term use.
- **Possibly unsafe:** When preparations are used that contain high concentrations of valeprotriates and baldrinals, when taken in conjunction with CNS-depressing drugs, or when used by patients with liver dysfunction. Use cautiously if at all during the perioperative period.[8]
- **Likely unsafe:** When used in high dosages with other CNS-acting drugs. Notably, certain degradation products of valpotriates (e.g., baldrinals, homobaldrinal) have been shown to be cytotoxic and mutagenic *in vitro*[9,10]; however, they have not been demonstrated to cause birth defects in a limited body of animal studies and are poorly absorbed into the blood and easily hydrolyzed.[11-13] Because of the lack of human safety data, it is nevertheless prudent to discontinue valerian use during pregnancy and lactation.

V

DOSING/TOXICOLOGY
General

- Recommended doses are based on those most commonly used in available trials, or on historical practice. However, with natural products, the optimal doses needed to balance efficacy and safety often have not been determined. Formulations and preparation methods may vary from manufacturer to manufacturer, and from batch to batch of a specific product made by a single manufacturer. Because often the active components of a product are not known, standardization may not be possible, and the clinical effects of different brands may not be comparable.

Standardization

- Extracts are often standardized to contain 0.3% valerenic, or valeric, acid, although other chemical constituents may be responsible for valerian's pharmacologic activity. Some products are standardized to contain 0.8% valerenic acid.
- Some natural medicine texts have suggested that Mexican and Indian sources of valerian may contain excessive levels of valepotriates and thus should be avoided.
- Valerian is typically sold in combination with other herbs and supplements, such as hops (*Flores humuli*), lemon balm (*Melissa officinalis*), and 5-hydroxytryptophan (5-HTP). The safety and efficacy of such formulations has not been evaluated in most cases.

Dosing: Adult (18 Years and Older)
Oral

- **Insomnia:** Studied doses have ranged from 400 to 900 mg of an aqueous or aqueous-ethanolic extract (corresponding to 1.5 to 3 g of herb), taken 30 to 60 minutes before going to bed. The better available trials have used 600 mg daily, taken 1 hour before bedtime.[14,15] Valerian has historically been used in the form of a tea (1.5 to 3 g of root steeped for 5 to 10 minutes in 150 mL of boiling water), although this formulation has not been studied in randomized, controlled trials.
- **Sedation/anxiety:** One study evaluated the effect of 100 mg of aqueous or aqueous-ethanolic extract before a stressful event.[16] Valerian is also used traditionally as a relaxant in the form of a tea (1.5 to 3 g of root steeped for 5 to 10 minutes in 150 mL of boiling water), but this formulation has not been studied in randomized, controlled trials.

Dosing: Pediatric (Younger Than 18 Years)

- Insufficient evidence to recommend. In their 1996-1997 review, an expert panel, the European Scientific Cooperative on Phytotherapy (ESCOP), recommended against the use of valerian in children less than 3 years old.
- A 2002 pilot study evaluated the efficacy of a valerian species in five children with sleep difficulties and learning disorders and reported no serious adverse effects and possible benefits.[17]

Toxicology

- Valerian has been on the U.S. Food & Drug Administration's GRAS (generally regarded as safe) list, and no fatalities due to overdose have been reported.
- There is a case report of an overdose involving 40 to 50 capsules of valerian capsules containing 470 mg of the powdered root that resulted in gastrointestinal upset, chest tightness, tremor, and lightheadedness in an 18-year-old female.[18] Symptoms resolved within 24 hours. Severe hypotension (suspected to be due to vasodilation), hypo-

calcemia, and hypokalemia were reported in a patient who had injected an unknown quantity of a crude tap water extract of raw valerian root.[19] Symptoms from acute overdose or chronic use may include blurred vision, cardiac disturbance, excitability, headache, hypersensitivity reactions, insomnia, and nausea.
- In rats, intraperitoneal doses of an ethanol extract ranging from 400 to 600 mg/kg/day for 45 days resulted in no detrimental effects on growth, blood pressure, organ weight, and hematologic and biochemical parameters.
- Hepatotoxicity has been associated with some multi-herb preparations that include valerian.[20] The contribution of valerian itself cannot be determined from these reports, due to the potential hepatotoxicity of other ingredients (e.g., scullcap), as well as the possibility of adulteration with unlisted herbs (such as the known hepatotoxic herb germander, which is often mistakenly harvested as scullcap). Furthermore, reports on 50 cases of overdose with a combination preparation containing hyoscine, cyproheptadine, and valerian indicated the expected symptoms of cyproheptadine and hyoscine toxicity, but no signs of hepatotoxicity developed in the short or long term.[21,22]
- Cytotoxicity has been reported in cultured hepatic tumor cells incubated with valtrate and related analogs.[9]
- The LD_{50} value for valerian essential oil has been reported as 15 g/kg,[23] and for valerenic acid as 300 mg/kg given intraperitoneally in mice.[24]

ADVERSE EFFECTS/PRECAUTIONS/CONTRAINDICATIONS
Allergy

- Known allergy/hypersensitivity to valerian. No reports of allergic reactions to valerian were found in a systematic literature search.

Adverse Effects/Postmarket Surveillance

- **General:** Valerian has been reported to cause headache, excitability, insomnia, uneasiness, ataxia, and hypothermia, although the level of adverse effects reported in clinical trials has not been greater than for placebo.
- **Neurologic/CNS:** Short-term mild impairments in vigilance, concentration, and processing time for complex thoughts, as well as mild fatigue, have been reported in trials (lasting for several hours), although residual sedative effects appear to be less pronounced than those associated with benzodiazepines.[16,25-27] Preliminary evidence suggests that valerian is nonsedating in recommended doses.[25,26,28] In one trial, use of a combination product containing valerian and lemon balm (*Melissa officinalis*) did not impair performance on psychometric tests that correlate with the ability to drive or operate machinery.[29] A drug "hangover" effect has been reported in patients taking high doses of valerian extracts.[30] A "valerian withdrawal" effect has been reported with chronic high-dose use; delirium, ameliorated by benzodiazepines, was reported in a single patient undergoing withdrawal from high doses of valerian.[31] Dizziness and headache have been reported rarely in human studies.[32,33] Anecdotally, some patients may develop a "paradoxical reaction" leading to nervousness or excitability, and use for longer than 2 to 4 months may result in insomnia.
- **Cardiovascular:** Tachycardia and high-output cardiac failure were reported following withdrawal of valerian in one patient with a history of coronary artery disease who had been self-medicating with high doses "for many years."[31] Large doses have reportedly caused bradycardia (anecdotal).

- **Gastrointestinal (GI upset):** Mild, transient stomach upset as well as nausea and vomiting have been reported anecdotally. Large doses may be associated with decreased intestinal motility.
- **Gastrointestinal (hepatotoxicity):** It remains unclear if valerian is hepatotoxic. Hepatotoxicity has been associated with some multi-herb preparations that include valerian.[20] However, the contribution of valerian itself cannot be determined from these reports, due to the potential hepatotoxicity of other ingredients (e.g., scullcap), as well as the possibility of adulteration with unlisted herbs (such as the known hepatotoxic herb germander, which is often mistakenly harvested as scullcap). Furthermore, reports on 50 cases of overdose with a combination preparation containing hyoscine, cyproheptadine, and valerian indicated the expected symptoms of cyproheptadine and hyoscine toxicity, but no signs of hepatotoxicity developed in the short or long term.[21,22]

Precautions/Warnings/Contraindications

- Use cautiously in patients with liver dysfunction, due to possible risk of hepatotoxicity.
- Valerian should be used cautiously if at all during the perioperative period.[8]
- Use cautiously in patients taking other sedative agents, due to the risk of additive effects.
- Avoid the use of valerian if driving or operating heavy machinery because of the risk of sedation or reduced vigilance, although in one study use of a combination product containing valerian and lemon balm (*Melissa officinalis*) did not impair performance on psychometric tests that correlate with the ability to drive or operate machinery.[29]

Pregnancy and Lactation

- Valerian is not recommended for use in pregnant and lactating women because of theoretical concerns over the teratogenic effects of valepotriates. Valepotriates and baldrinals have been shown to be cytotoxic and mutagenic *in vitro*.[9,10] However, these substances are unstable and generally not found in commercial valerian products. In rats, a 30-day administration of a mixture of valepotriates failed to demonstrate any changes in fertility, estrous phases, or development of offspring.[12] Furthermore, valepotriates are poorly absorbed and subject to a significant first pass effect.[11,13] No teratogenic actions have been reported in the very few known cases of valerian intoxication during pregnancy.[34] Because of the lack of human safety data, it is nevertheless prudent to discontinue valerian use during pregnancy and lactation.

INTERACTIONS
Valerian/Drug Interactions

- **Sedative drugs/CNS depressants:** Valerian theoretically may potentiate the effects of CNS depressant drugs, although studies in patients taking CNS-active medications concurrently with valerian have not revealed an increased rate of adverse effects.[35] Valerian has been found to potentiate the effects of CNS depressants in rats.[36] Data from *in vitro* and animal studies suggest that valerian may prolong barbiturate-induced sleeping time.[11,24,37] Preliminary evidence suggests that valerian alone is nonsedating in recommended doses,[25,26] although short term impairment in vigilance and concentration, as well as mild fatigue, have been reported in trials; residual sedative effects appear to be less pronounced than those associated with benzodiazepines.[16,25-27]

- **Selective serotonin reuptake inhibitors (SSRIs):** A patient taking fluoxetine (Prozac) for a mood disorder (in the setting of alcohol use) reported that approximately 12 hours after taking valerian tablets, he experienced mental status changes and lost control of his left arm.[38] Other reported symptoms included agitation and obsession, which led him to self-inflict cuts on his hand. After another 12 hours, his symptoms resolved. The specific role of valerian in this isolated case is not clear.
- **Beta blockers:** In a randomized trial, a combination of 100 mg of valerian extract and 20 mg of propranolol was found to impair performance on a written concentration test more than valerian alone (which was reported to slightly improve performance).[16] However, there was no comparison with propranolol alone, so it is not clear if the effects were due to the beta blocker only or to the combination with valerian. The study itself was methodologically weak, raising questions about the validity of the results.
- **Alcohol:** Concomitant use of valerian and ethanol should be avoided because of the theoretical risk of potentiation of CNS depressant effects and a report of mental status changes in an individual using both.[39] However, in one study of a combination product containing valerian and lemon balm (*Melissa officinalis*), no potentiation was seen.[29] Other studies in patients taking CNS-active medications concurrently with valerian have not revealed an increased rate of adverse effects.[35] Valerian does not appear to alter the ethanol blood concentration curve in rats.[40]
- **Antiseizure agents:** It has been suggested anecdotally that valerian products may interact with antiseizure medications, although literature review reveals no human data to support this assertion.
- **Loperamide (Imodium):** A brief episode of acute delirium was reported in one patient during concomitant use of loperamide and valerian.[41] However, causality could not be established, as the patient was also taking St. John's wort (*Hypericum perforatum*). The condition resolved rapidly with discontinuation of treatment.
- **Disulfiram (Antabuse):** Valerian tinctures often have a high alcohol content (15% to 90%) and theoretically may elicit a disulfiram reaction.
- **Metronidazole (Flagyl):** A disulfiram reaction can occur when metronidazole and alcohol are used concomitantly. Because of the high alcohol content in some valerian tinctures, this combination theoretically may cause such a reaction.
- **Vasopressin (positive interaction):** In rabbits given vasopressin, valepotriates have been found to reduce the incidence of cardiac arrhythmias.[42] The clinical relevance in humans is not clear.

Valerian/Herb/Supplement Interactions

- **St. John's wort (*Hypericum perforatum*):** Delirium and agitation were reported in one patient taking valerian, St. John's wort, and loperamide (Imodium).[41] The condition resolved rapidly with discontinuation of treatment. In a telephone survey, one woman reported nausea, diaphoresis, muscle cramping, weakness, and elevated pulse and blood pressure after a single dose of a combination product containing St. John's wort, kava, and valerian.[43]
- **Kava (*Piper methysticum*):** In a telephone survey, one woman reported nausea, diaphoresis, muscle cramping, weakness and elevated pulse and blood pressure after a single dose of a combination product containing St. John's wort, kava, and valerian.[43]

V

- **Sedative herbs and supplements/CNS depressants:** Valerian may theoretically potentiate the effects of CNS depressant agents, although studies in patients taking CNS-active medications concurrently with valerian have not revealed an increased rate of adverse effects.[35] Valerian has been found to potentiate the effects of CNS depressants in rats.[36] Preliminary evidence suggests that valerian alone is nonsedating in recommended doses,[25,26] although short-term impairment in vigilance and concentration, as well as mild fatigue, have been reported in trials; residual sedative effects appear to be less pronounced than those associated with benzodiazepines.[16,25-27]

Valerian/Food Interactions

- Insufficient available evidence.

Valerian/Lab Interactions

- **Transaminases (alanine aminotransferase [ALT], aspartate aminotransferase [AST], gamma-glutamyltransferase [GGT]), lactate dehydrogenase (LDH), alkaline phosphatase, bilirubin:** Hepatotoxicity has been associated with some multi-herb preparations that include valerian.[20] The contribution of valerian itself cannot be determined from these reports, due to the potential hepatotoxicity of other ingredients (e.g., scullcap), as well as the possibility of adulteration with unlisted herbs (such as the known hepatotoxic herb germander, which is often mistakenly harvested as scullcap). Furthermore, reports on 50 cases of overdose with a combination preparation containing hyoscine, cyproheptadine, and valerian indicated the expected symptoms of cyproheptadine and hyoscine toxicity, but no signs of hepatotoxicity developed in the short or long term.[21,22]

MECHANISM OF ACTION
Pharmacology

- **Constituents:** Valerian root may contain as many as 150 compounds, not all of which have been thoroughly investigated. The known major constituents are the valepotriates (irioids), notably valtrate and related analogs, and volatile oils, notably kessanes, valerenal, valeranone and valerenic acid. The valeprotriates decompose to other potentially active compounds, notably baldrinal and homobaldrinal.[44-46] Valerenic acid and the valepotriates have received the most attention. The herb has a characteristic, unpleasant odor, due to isovaleric acid, and is reported to contain a "cat attractant," actinidine.
- **CNS effects:** The constituents of valerian responsible for its clinical effects have not been conclusively identified. Although pharmacologic activity has been shown for some components, the concentrations found in typical valerian extracts appear to fall short of therapeutic levels. The flavonoid glycoside linarin, flavone 6-methylapigenin, and flavanone glycoside 2S (-) hesperidin have been suggested as possessing anxiolytic or sedative properties.[47] It is possible that a combination of compounds impart clinical activity to valerian.[46,48,49] Extracts of valerian and some of its components have been shown to have effects on gamma-aminobutyric acid (GABA)–related mechanisms in the CNS, exerting potential activity at both pre- and postsynaptic sites.[50-58] Valerian extracts can alter binding at benzodiazepine receptors[48,53] and GABA-A (muscimol) receptors.[50] Extracts have been reported to increase synaptasomal GABA concentrations, possibly by enhancing GABA release and inhibiting GABA uptake.[48,53,55,57] However, other research suggests that the presence of small quantities of GABA in valerian extracts may have confounded these results by directly elevating measured GABA levels in the synaptic cleft.[50,56]
- Extracts of valerian exert anticonvulsant actions and prolong barbiturate sleep times in mice.[11,37,59,60] Evidence regarding effects on spontaneous activity in lab animals is mixed.[11,37,59] Studies suggest that some of the pharmacologic properties of the extract may be shared by valerenic acid [11,24] or homobaldrinal.[49] An ethanolic extract of Japanese valerian root [60] and α-kessyl alcohol derived from a methanol extract of *Valeriana fauriei* [4] exerted activity in a mouse model of antidepressant activity.
- **Antiproliferative effects:** Valepotriates exert cytotoxic effects on hepatoma cell lines and inhibit DNA and protein synthesis; didrovaltrate prolongs survival in mice with ascitic tumors.[9,10]

Pharmacodynamics/Kinetics

- Valepotriates are poorly absorbed and subject to a significant first-pass effect when administered orally. Degradation may occur in the presence of heat or alkaline conditions.
- Valepotriates as well as their metabolites have reportedly been found in the stomach lining, intestines, blood, liver, kidneys, heart, lungs, and brain.

HISTORY

- Valerian is an herb native to Europe and Asia and now grows in most parts of the world. The name is believed to derive from the Latin word *valere*, meaning to be healthy or strong. The root and rhizome of the plant are believed to contain its active constituents. Use of valerian as a sedative and anxiolytic has been reported for more than 2000 years; for example, in the 2nd century AD, Galen recommended valerian as a treatment for insomnia. Related species have been used in traditional Chinese and Ayurvedic medicine. Topical treatments have been used to treat skin sores and acne, and valerian has been used for other conditions such as digestive problems, flatulence, congestive heart failure, urinary tract disorders, and angina pectoris.
- Valerian extracts became popular in the United States and Europe in the mid-1800s, and continued to be used by both physicians and the lay public until it was superseded by pharmaceutical compounds such as barbiturates.
- Valerian remains popular in North America, Europe, and Japan for its presumed sedative properties. Although the active ingredients in valerian are not known, preparations are typically standardized to the content of valerenic acid.

REVIEW OF THE EVIDENCE: DISCUSSION
Insomnia (Sleep Onset and Quality)
Summary

- Preliminary data from several human trials suggest that valerian improves subjective measures of sleep quality and sleep latency, for up to 4 to 6 weeks. Better effects have been noted in poor sleepers. Preliminary evidence suggests that ongoing use may be more effective than acute (single-dose) use, with progressive effects over 4 weeks.[14] However, most available studies have been methodologically weak, and in most cases results have not been confirmed using objective sleep pattern data in a sleep laboratory or validated measurement scales. Preliminary studies of combination valerian-hops (*Flores humuli*) or valerian-St. John's wort (*Hypericum*

Review of the Evidence: Valerian

Condition Treated*	Study Design	Author, Year	N[†]	SS[†]	Study Quality[‡]	Magnitude of Benefit	ARR[†]	NNT[†]	Comments
Sleep quality	Double-blind, placebo-controlled trial	Vorbach[14] 1996	121	Yes	5	Large	NA	NA	Subjective improvement; compliance monitored.
Sleep quality	Comparison trial (no placebo arm)	Dorn[15] 2000	75	Mixed	4	NA	NA	NA	Valerian and oxazepam reported as equally effective; no placebo control group.
Sleep quality	Comparison trial (no placebo arm)	Ziegler[66] 2002	202	Mixed	4	NA	NA	NA	Valerian and oxazepam reported as equally effective; no placebo control group.
Sleep latency and quality	Double-blind, placebo controlled, crossover trial	Leathwood[62] 1982	128	Yes	3	Small	14	7	Acute effect on sleep latency in insomniacs.
Sleep quality and structure	RCT, double-blind	Donath[67] 2000	16	No	3	Small	NA	NA	Chronic but no acute effect in insomniacs; improvement of slow-wave sleep with chronic dosing.
Sleep latency and quality	Randomized, double-blind, placebo-controlled trial	Leathwood[30] 1985	8	Yes	2	Small	NA	NA	Acute effect on sleep latency in insomniacs, but sample size too small for a decisive conclusion.
Sleep quality and structure	Randomized, double-blind, placebo-controlled trial	Schulz[65] 1994	14	No	2	Small	NA	NA	Acute effect in poor sleepers; improvement of slow-wave sleep.
Sleep quality	Double-blind crossover trial	Lindahl[70] 1989	27	Yes	3	Large	NA	NA	Combination product; acute effect in patients with sleep difficulties; end point, patient self-rating; no placebo group.
Sleep latency and quality	RCT, double-blind	Balderer[64] 1985	18	Mixed	2	Small	NA	NA	Acute effect primarily on sleep latency in healthy subjects at home.
Sleep quality (patients with sleep disorders)	Double-blind, crossover trial	Gessner[63] 1984	11	Yes	2	Medium	NA	NA	Results limited by small sample size.
Sleep quality	RCT, double-blind trial	Kamm-Kohl[32] 1984	80	Yes	2	Medium	29%	3	Improvement noted in behavioral abnormalities, quality of life and sleep; baseline characteristics of groups differed.
Sleep disorders	RCT, double-blind	Jansen[71] 1977	150	Unclear	2	Medium	NA	NA	Statistical analysis and outcomes measures not clear.
Sleep quality (healthy patients; noise exposure)	RCT, double-blind;	Muller-Limroth[75] 1977	12	No	2	NA	NA	NA	Non-significant trend for drug group to facilitate sleep; drug was combination of valerian and hops (Flores humuli).
Sleep quality	Equivalence trial	Schmitz[76] 1998	46	Yes	3	Medium	NA	NA	Combination of valerian and hops (low-dose valerian); equivalence to benzodiazepines by Mann-Whitney statistic of 0.50, with lower boundary of 95% CI, 0.46.
Sleep quality	Equivalence trial, combination product	Dressing[77] 1992	20	No	1	None	NA	NA	Valerian and lemon balm (Melissa officinalis) combination vs. benzodiazepine triazolam, with no significant difference between groups; methodologically weak, possibly underpowered.
Sleep quality	RCT, double-blind	Cerny[74] 1999	98	Yes	4	NA	NA	NA	Study of combination of valerian and lemon balm (Melissa officinalis); primarily evaluated adverse effects, not efficacy.

Continued

Review of the Evidence: Valerian—cont'd

Condition Treated*	Study Design	Author, Year	N[†]	SS[†]	Study Quality[‡]	Magnitude of Benefit	ARR[†]	NNT[†]	Comments
Sleep quality	Case series	Dominguez[72] 2000	23	Yes	1	Large	NA	NA	End point, patient self-rating on subjective ordinal scale.
Sleep quality	Case series	Schmidt-Vogt[73] 1986	11,168	Yes	0	Large	NA	NA	Suggestive results limited by lack of controls.
Sleep quality	Case series	Seifert[33] 1988	1,689	Unclear	NA	Large	NA	NA	Drug monitoring study with poor description of baseline patient characteristics.
Anxiety	Equivalence trial	Panijel[83] 1985	100	Yes	3	Medium	38%	3	St. John's wort (Hypericum perforatum) plus valerian combination yielded "very good" outcome in 54% of subjects, vs. 16% with diazepam.
Anxiety	RCT, double-blind	Andreatini[78] 2002	36	No	2	None	NA	NA	Valerian, diazepam, and placebo all improved anxiety scores compared to baseline (HAM-A) but no significant differences between groups; likely underpowered to detect between-group differences.
Anxiety	RCT, double-blind	Sousa[79] 1992	80	Unclear	2	Equal	NA	NA	Valerian reported as equivalent to the benzodiazepine clobazam, but no power calculation conducted.
Anxiety	Equivalence trial	Schellenberg[82] 1994	20	Yes	1	Small	NA	NA	Similar EEG changes (and reduced anxiety) with valerian plus passion flower (Passiflora incarnata) combination and chlorpromazine, but no power calculation for between-group differences.
Anxiety	RCT	Delsignore[80] 1980	40	Unclear	0	Small	NA	NA	Results reported individually for subjects; unclear mean improvement.
Sedation	RCT, double-blind	Kuhlmann[26] 1999	102	No	3	None	NA	NA	No effects after single or repeated dosages.
Sedation, anxiety	Randomized, double-blind, placebo-controlled trial	Kohnen[16] 1988	48	NA	2	NA	NA	NA	Insufficient statistical reporting.
Sedation, anxiety	RCT, double-blind	Gerhard[25] 1996	80	Yes	2	Medium	NA	NA	No "hangover" the morning after valerian use; methodologically weak study, designed to detect adverse effects.

*Primary or secondary outcome.
[†]N, Number of patients; SS, statistically significant; ARR, absolute risk reduction; NNT, the number of patients who need to undergo a specific intervention in order to observe an outcome in one individual.
[‡]0-2 = poor; 3-4 = good; 5 = excellent.
EEG, Electroencephalographic; HAM-A, Hamilton Anxiety Scale; NA, not applicable; RCT, randomized, controlled trial.
For an explanation of each category in this table, please see Table 3 in the Introduction.

perforatum) products are promising, but have similarly been methodologically weak. Further evidence is warranted before a strong recommendation can be made.

Systematic Review
• Stevinson and Ernst conducted a well-designed systematic review of randomized, placebo-controlled, double-blind clinical trials of valerian for insomnia and concluded that the results are promising but inconclusive.[61] Nine trials (from eight reports), published between 1984 and 1996, met the selection criteria. Of these, six trials [30,62-64] examined acute effects of valerian, while three[14,32,65] examined cumulative effects. Several of the trials reported positive effects on sleep latency or quality, but all had methodological flaws. Pre-bedtime variables (e.g., caffeine, alcohol) were not fully controlled in any study. Other weaknesses in more than one study included inadequate details of randomization, inclusion/exclusion criteria, blinding methods, and validation of outcome measures.

Evidence from Randomized Trials
• Ziegler at al. conducted a randomized, controlled, double-blind, comparison study, published after the Stevinson systematic review.[66] The authors randomized 202 adult

outpatients with insomnia of mean duration of 3.5 months, to receive either 600 mg/day of valerian standardized extract LI 156 or 10 mg/day of the benzodiazepine oxazepam. Following 6 weeks of therapy, no statistically significant mean differences were detected between groups in sleep quality on the Sleep Questionnaire B (SF-B; CIPS 1996), Clinical Global Impressions (CGI) scale, or several other validated measures of sleep and fatigue. Treatment was rated as "very good" by 83% of valerian patients and by 73% of oxazepam patients. Adverse effects rated as mild or moderate occurred in 28% of valerian patients and in 36% of oxazepam patients. These results are promising, although without a placebo arm to demonstrate improvements in both the valerian and oxazepam arms compared to a control, they cannot be considered definitive. Future comparison studies would be more clinically useful if a placebo arm were included.

- Vorbach et al. reported a well-designed, 28-day multi-center, double-blind, placebo-controlled parallel group study of 121 patients with nonorganic insomnia according to ICD-10 criteria.[14] The treatment group received a dry ethanolic valerian extract (Sedonium) at a dose of 600 mg 1 hour before bedtime. The authors state that the placebo used was indistinguishable from the valerian pill by size, appearance, taste, and smell. Randomization was carried out by means of a validated random number generator. Effectiveness was judged according to the Goetelmeyer Sleep Questionnaire B, Zerssen Well-Being Scale, and CGI scale. Pretrial evaluation showed no relevant baseline differences. Four participants dropped out, and an intention-to-treat (ITT) analysis was used. Data were analyzed using a t-test for data scaled in intervals, and the Wilcoxon-Mann-Whitney Test for data with an ordinal scale. Interim results at 14 days demonstrated statistically insignificant trends in favor of valerian for most measures, although evaluation of therapeutic effectiveness by the physician on the CGI scale attained statistical significance ($p < 0.05$). At 28 days, statistically significant differences in favor of valerian were seen in all primary outcome measures. This study suggests that valerian's effects may be cumulative, with optimal effects occurring with persistent use over a period of at least 1 month.

- Dorn et al. reported a well-designed double-blind trial (n = 75) comparing a dry ethanolic valerian extract (Sedonium, 600 mg/day) with the benzodiazepine oxazepam (10 mg/ day).[15] The study was done in a population of primarily older female patients who had complained of insomnia for over 1 year. The primary outcome measure was sleep quality as defined by the SFB questionnaire. Patients took valerian or oxazepam for 28 days. Both the oxazepam and valerian groups showed significant improvement in sleep quality over baseline ($p < 0.001$), and the two groups were not statistically different from each other in their efficacy. The effect size was small for both groups (between 0.02 and 0.05), with valerian exhibiting a more favorable adverse event profile. A power calculation was not conducted, and it is not clear if the sample size was adequate to detect differences between groups. In addition, the lack of placebo and small effect sizes overall raise questions about the benefits of therapy in either group.

- Leathwood et al. (1982) conducted a double-blind, randomized trial using self-rated measures to assess sleep latency and sleep quality in 128 healthy participants.[62] Subjects received either 2 placebo capsules, 2 specially-prepared Hova capsules, prepared by grinding Hova tablets and preparing capsules containing valerian (200 mg) plus hops (*Flores*

humuli) (100 mg) in each capsule, or 2 valerian capsules (200 mg dried powder/capsule) for 1 night before bedtime. The alternate therapies were administered on the subsequent 2 nights. A questionnaire was filled out by the subjects, reflecting back on their sleep quality after each treatment. Results showed a significant improvement in subjective assessments of sleep latency (decreased time until falling asleep) with valerian monotherapy (37% of patients) and Hova (31%) vs. placebo (23%) ($p < 0.05$ for valerian, but non-significant for Hova). Subgroup analysis revealed the greatest benefit in poor sleepers and older (>40 years old) subjects. The data presented for sleep quality state that 43% of respondents reported improved sleep after taking valerian monotherapy vs. 25% for placebo ($p < 0.05$); there was no significant improvement in the Hova group. Subgroup analysis of individuals who rated themselves as good sleepers vs. poor sleepers showed that good sleepers were largely unaffected by valerian, whereas 54% of poor sleepers had improved sleep quality. Although methodologically flawed by poor description of randomization and blinding, a no-validated questionnaire, and 23% dropout, this study does suggest that the effects of valerian may be clinically insignificant in healthy patients with no reported sleep disturbances.

- Donath et al. reported a double-blind, randomized, crossover study (n = 16) after a single dose and over 14 days using 600 mg/day of a commercially prepared extract of valerian (Sedonium).[67] The test population (median age, 49 years) consisted of patients suffering from mild psychophysiologic insomnia. The primary target variable of the study was sleep efficiency, which was measured through subject self-assessment. Objective polysomnographic data were also obtained. No effects on sleep structure or subjective sleep assessment were observed with single dose administration. No significant difference in subjective assessment was observed with multiple-dose administration. There was a significant increase in slow-wave sleep (SWS) time in the treatment group over placebo (9.8 vs. 8.1%, respectively) and a significant reduction in SWS latency over placebo (21.3% vs. 13.5%; $p < 0.05$) for chronic dosing. The authors concluded that, compared with benzodiazepines, the effect of valerian is slight and delayed. However, Giedke and Breyer-Pfaff[68] criticized this study, calling it "clinically irrelevant." These authors criticized the diagnostic criteria used for psychophysiologic insomnia, disputed the lack of positive effects on any sleep parameter except for the "questionable" evaluation of SWS, and pointed out that the largest effects were found in the short-term placebo group.

- Leathwood et al. (1985) conducted a small study (n = 8) comparing nighttime motor activity, using a wrist-worn activity meter, during sleep in mild insomniacs receiving 450 mg or 900 mg of valerian root extract, or placebo.[30] The study was double-blind and utilized a repeated measure, random order design. Sleep latency was reduced from 16 minutes in the placebo group to 9 minutes in the 450-mg valerian group (significantly different at $p < 0.05$, by a one tailed t-test); the 900-mg group (11 minutes) did not differ from the 450-mg group. No difference was observed in subjective sleep quality or in total sleep time. Complete data were obtained in only 5 subjects, with one subject providing no useful information. The study size may be too small to yield results of meaningful significance or generalizability. Given the number of limitations of this study, no reliable conclusion can be made. Leathwood et al. previously conducted a small trial of valerian (400 mg) in 10 healthy, male volunteers in a sleep laboratory.[69] No effect was observed on electroencephalographic (EEG) measurements of sleep, although this study had similar methodological weaknesses.

- Schulz et al. conducted a double-blind, placebo-controlled parallel group study with an aqueous alkaline dried extract of valerian (Valdispert Forte, 405 mg three times daily).[65] Subjects (n = 14) were elderly females who were poor sleepers. Valerian or placebo was given for 8 consecutive days, and measurements were made after the first and last day. Valerian increased the percentage of slow wave sleep (SWS, S3 + S4) and K-complex density. Sleep onset time and subjective measures of sleep parameters were unaffected by the treatment. Although the authors concluded that valerian had a mild tranquilizing effect, the study is marred by the small sample size and the lack of equivalence in baseline values for the two groups.

- Lindahl et al. conducted a small, double-blind, crossover trial (n = 27) examining the effects of a standardized combination valerian preparation (Valerina Natt) containing 400 mg valerian, 160 mg of lemon balm (*Melissa officinalis*) and 375 mg of hops (*Flores humuli*) against a preparation containing an incidental amount of valerian and the same amounts of the other constituents.[70] Subjects were randomized to one therapy on the first night and then received the other on the following night. Subjects then rated their sleep quality by comparing the 2 nights on an ordinal scale the morning after the second night. It was reported that 21 (78%) subjects rated their sleep quality following the test preparation as "perfect" or "clearly better" compared to 5 (11%) controls (*p* < 0.001). No noticeable improvement was reported by 15 of the 27 subjects in the control group and 3 subjects in the valerian group. Because there is limited available information about the pharmacokinetics of valerian, it is not clear if residual effects might have been present on the second night in patients who received valerian on the first night (i.e., inadequate washout period). In addition, the clinical relevance of these results is limited by the incomplete description of methods and statistical analysis.

- In a poorly described study, Balderer and Borbely reported the effects of an aqueous extract of valerian root (confirmed to be free of valepotriates) vs. placebo on sleep in two groups of healthy, young subjects.[64] One group (n = 10) was studied at home, and the other group (n = 8) was studied in a sleep laboratory. Two doses (450 mg and 900 mg) were used in this double-blind, crossover study. In the home study group, both sleep latency and wake time after sleep onset were shown to have decreased for doses of 450 mg (non-significant) and 900 mg (*p* < 0.01). Nighttime motor activity was unchanged overall, but a small but significant decrease was observed in the last third of the night, although the clinical relevance of this finding is unclear. No statistically significant change in self-ratings of sleep was reported, but a trend toward improvement with valerian was noted. Results from the laboratory group revealed no changes in outcome parameters, including EEG measurements and sleep stages, in the valerian group.

- Kamm-Kohl et al. conducted a trial in 80 chronically ill patients with difficulty sleeping.[32] Participants were randomized to an aqueous valerian extract (Baldrian Dispert, 3 capsules twice daily) or placebo for 14 days. Primary outcome measures included the von Zerssen Emotional State Scale, the Nurse's Observation Scale for Inpatient Evaluation (NOSIE) scale, and subjective ratings of symptoms, quantified numerically (0 = "none" to 4 = "very strong"). Baseline

characteristics of the two groups were comparable except in the NOSIE scale, on which the valerian group demonstrated more severe initial symptoms. At 14 days, improvement in the valerian group was greater than that for placebo for all measures (*p* < 0.01). However, because of the lack of baseline equivalence on the NOSIE scale and the lack of description of randomization, these results cannot be considered conclusive.

- Gessner et al. conducted a randomized study with 11 healthy, young volunteers in a sleep laboratory.[63] Polygraphic measures and sleep questionnaires were recorded in subjects taking 60 mg or 120 mg of valerian (Harmonicum Much) or placebo in a random order on 3 nonconsecutive nights. Small, dose-dependent changes in EEG measurements of sleep (increases in stages 1 to 3, decreases in stage 4 and REM) were reported, with no changes in subjective measures of sleep. Maximal effects occurred after 2 to 3 hours. The clinical relevance of these results is not clear.

- Jansen et al. conducted a double-blind study to test the effects of Baldisedron (valerian) in patients with sleep disorders.[71] Patients (n = 150) received placebo or valerian. Psychological and somatic symptoms were noted to improve significantly in the valerian group. Significant improvements were observed in sleep disorders and agitation. Although the results are suggestive, this study was poorly reported with inadequate descriptions of blinding, results, and statistical analysis.

- **Evidence from case series:** Dominguez et al. conducted a case series (n = 23) in a Hispanic population receiving mental health services, generally for depression or anxiety.[72] A commercial preparation (Nature's Way) of valerian capsules (470 mg) was administered daily to patients complaining of insomnia. All study participants had been on a stable psychotropic medication regimen for at least 1 month. The authors reported that 15 out of 20 patients reported moderate to extreme improvement in subjective assessments of insomnia by week 2 of therapy (*p* = 0.005). No adverse interactions with psychotropic regimens were encountered during the study period. However, the clinical effects of the other medications are not clear, and as with other open label studies, the possible introduction of bias may influence results.

- Schmidt-Voigt et al. conducted a large, open, multi-center observational trial assessing the efficacy of valerian for sleep disorders.[73] Patients (n = 11,168) were given 450 mg of valerian over a 10-day period. Subjects were asked to keep a log of the perceived effects of the intervention. Self-rated scores suggested that valerian decreased sleep latency, restlessness, and tension in 72% of patients and improved discontinuous sleep in 76%. Although the results are suggestive, the use of subjective measurements, lack of controls, and open nature of this study allow for the possible influences of bias and confounding, which reduce the clinical usefulness of the results.

- Seifert et al. conducted a drug monitoring trial of 1689 children and adults using 3 to 9 valerian (45 mg) tablets daily for treatment for sleep disturbances and anxiety.[33] Among patients that complained of difficulty concentrating, 50% were symptom free at the end this 10-day trial. Reductions in symptoms of cardiac palpitations, depression and menopausal associated anxiety were also noted. Due to the absence of a control group, this trial may be regarded as providing general information on safety rather than an assessment of effectiveness. Even in this regard, poor description of patient baseline characteristics limits the meaningfulness of the results.

- **Evidence for combination products:** Cerny et al. conducted a 30-day randomized, placebo-controlled, double-blind trial to assess the safety of a valerian/lemon balm (*Melissa officinalis*) combination in the treatment of sleep disorders.[74] A total of 98 healthy volunteers were randomized to receive placebo (n = 32) or valerian/lemon balm (n = 66). The primary end point was assessment of the overall tolerability of the preparation on a 5-point self-rating scale, and incidence of adverse effects. The preparation was well tolerated, and adverse effects did not differ significantly between the valerian and placebo groups. A secondary end point measuring sleep quality yielded inconsistent findings. Results of informal questioning regarding sleep improvement found a small statistically significant improvement in sleep quality. However, intergroup differences on a visual analog scale of sleep quality failed to attain statistical significance. Self-ratings of general well-being did not differ between groups. Methodological weaknesses of this trial include incomplete reporting of baseline patient characteristics, randomization, and blinding. Notably, this study was not principally designed to measure efficacy, and therefore its clinical applicability is limited.
- In a double-blind trial, Müller-Limroth et al. studied the effects of a valerian/hops (*Flores humuli*) combination product on sleep disturbances.[75] Patients (n = 12) were given placebo or 4 capsules of Seda-Kneipp (60 mg of valerian plus 100 mg of hops) each night at bedtime. Results showed a trend for valerian to facilitate sleep, but results were not statistically significant. Limitations of this trial include inadequate descriptions of baseline patient characteristics, lack of randomization, and a sample size that may not have been adequate to detect beneficial effects.
- Schmitz and Jackel conducted a randomized, double-blind trial comparing a hops/valerian combination product (Hova-Filmtabletten) and benzodiazepines in 46 patients diagnosed with sleep disorders by DSM-IV (*Diagnostic and Statistical Manual of Mental Disorders, Fourth Edition*) criteria.[76] In the herb group, 2 daily capsules were given, each containing 200 mg of hops extract and 45.5 mg of valerian. After 2 weeks of therapy, the authors report that the "state of health" was observed to improve equally during therapy in both groups, with statistical significance; these benefits deteriorated 1 week after cessation of therapy. No withdrawal symptoms were reported with hops/valerian but were observed with benzodiazepines. The clinical relevance of this study is limited by the inadequate reporting of randomization, blinding procedures, and outcomes measures and by the small sample size. The effects of hops and valerian cannot be separated from each other.
- Dressing conducted a double-blind, crossover trial to assess the efficacy of the combination of valerian and lemon balm (*Melissa officinalis*) vs. the benzodiazepine triazolam (Halcion) in sleep disorders.[77] Healthy volunteers (n = 20) were randomized to 1 tablet of the combination (160 mg of valerian plus 80 mg of lemon balm) or 0.125 mg of triazolam at bedtime, in a double-dummy study design. Participants were supervised for 9 nights in a sleep laboratory. Sleep quality was analyzed according to the international criteria of Rechtschaffen and Kales. Primary outcome measures were sleep continuity, sleep architecture, and REM (rapid eye movement) sleep parameters. Statistical analysis included parametric procedures (Analysis of Variance [ANOVA], t-test) to evaluate possible statistical interference. Use of triazolam resulted in a significant improvement in most sleep

parameters. In contrast, statistically significant sleep improvement could only be demonstrated for the valerian/lemon balm group through post-hoc subgroup analysis. The dose of valerian used was lower than that in most trials of valerian monotherapy, and therefore the value of these results is limited.

Anxiety and Panic Disorder
Summary

- Valerian has been proposed as a treatment for anxiety and panic disorder, although these conditions have not been directly evaluated in controlled clinical trials. Studies have generally been of poor methodological quality, and several have used valerian in combination with other herbs, such as passion flower (*Passiflora incarnata* L.) and St. John's wort (*Hypericum perforatum*).

Evidence for Valerian Monotherapy

- Andreatini et al. conducted a randomized, controlled, double-blind trial in 36 outpatients with generalized anxiety disorder, diagnosed by DSM III-R criteria.[78] Following a 2-week washout period, subjects were randomized to receive valerian extract (mean daily dose, 81 mg), diazepam (mean daily dose, 6.5 mg), or placebo. Outcomes included change from baseline in the Hamilton Anxiety Scale (HAM-A) or State-Trait Anxiety Index (STAI-trait). Following 4 weeks of therapy, the authors reported significant improvements in the HAM-A in all three groups compared to baseline, with improvement in STAI-trait only in the diazepam group. However, there were no significant differences in mean scores between groups. This small study was likely underpowered, and therefore its results cannot be considered conclusive.
- Sousa et al. conducted a randomized, double-blind, comparison (equivalence) study in 80 adults with various anxiety diagnoses, comparing the effects of a standardized valerian extract (Valdispert, 270 mg/day) and the benzodiazepine clobazepam.[79] Levels of anxiety were measured using validated scales, including the Hamilton Anxiety Rating Scale and the Leeds anxiety questionnaire. Although the study reported equal benefits from the two therapies, it is not clear that this trial was adequately powered to detect significant between-group differences. In addition, randomization and blinding were not adequately reported.
- Delsignore et al. conducted a trial in 40 patients with mild anxiety.[80] Subjects were randomized to receive placebo or valerian at a dose of 100 mg three times daily for 21 days. Results were reported individually for each subject, with unclear mean improvement. The authors reported that, overall, the valerian group experienced statistically significant reductions in levels of anxiety vs. placebo. Although the results are suggestive, this study was poorly reported, with inadequate descriptions of randomization, blinding, and statistical analysis.
- In a double-blind trial by Kohnen et al. designed to measure sedation in adults taking valerian, level of anxiety was also measured.[16] Subjects (n = 48) were administered valerian extract (100 mg), the beta blocker propranolol (Inderal) (20 mg/tablet), a combination of valerian and propranolol (100 mg of valerian extract plus 20 mg of propranolol), or placebo. After being administered a verbal "test" in front of an audience, participants filled out a questionnaire (50-point analog scale) quantifying their feelings of "psychic strain." Subjective reports of anxiety were reduced in the valerian

V

group vs. placebo, but no statistical analysis was performed. The outcomes measure utilized was not validated, with unclear reproducibility; there was inadequate description of blinding, randomization, baseline patient characteristics, and statistical analysis. Although this study was creative in design, the results cannot be applied to clinical practice.

- In a 1969 open-label case series, 70 hospitalized patients with diverse psychosomatic diagnoses were given 150- to 300-mg daily doses of the valerian product Valmane.[27] The preparation was reported to produce mild sedative effects and to be effective in the treatment of "restlessness" and "tension." However, in the absence of a control group, these results are of limited clinical relevance.

- Glass et al. reported no difference between a single dose of valerian extract (400 mg or 800 mg) and placebo in validated measures of sedation and mood in 14 healthy volunteers (Visual Analog Scale [VAS], Tufts Benzodiazepine Scale).[81]

Evidence for Combination Products

- Schellenberg et al. conducted a trial comparing the efficacy of a valerian/passion flower (*Passiflora incarnata* L.) combination product to chlorpromazine (Thorazine) in the treatment of affective disorders.[82] Patients (n = 20) with psychosomatic and affective disorders were selected. Subjects in the valerian/passion flower group received 100 mg of valerian/6.5 mg of passion flower, or 40 mg of chlorpromazine for a duration of 6 weeks. Electroencephalographic (EEG) increases in alpha- and theta-waves were noted in both groups. However, they were observed in the valerian/passion flower group only during the first 2 weeks of use, whereas they continued for the full 6 weeks with chlorpromazine. Depression and anxiety measures were shown to be decreased in both groups. The chlorpromazine group experienced side effects such as reduced vigilance and orthostatic load that were not seen in the valerian/passion flower group. No power calculation was conducted, and it is not clear that the sample size was adequate to detect between-group differences. In addition, the correlation between EEG findings and clinical outcomes is not clear.

- Panijel conducted a randomized, double-blind trial comparing the combination herbal product Sedariston (100 mg of St. John's wort [*Hypericum perforatum*] and 50 mg of valerian root) and the benzodiazepine diazepam (Valium) in moderately severe anxiety states.[83] Patients received either 1 capsule of Sedariston twice daily for 1 week, followed by 2 capsules twice daily (in 54% of the patients in an attempt to increase response), or 2 mg of diazepam twice daily for 1 week, followed by 4 mg twice daily (in 70% of the patients in an attempt to increase response). Fifty-four percent of the Sedariston group were judged to have a very good outcome, compared with 16% of those in the diazepam group ($p = 0.002$). However, the effects of the two herbs cannot be separated from each other, and this study did not adequately describe blinding or randomization.

- A poorly designed trial investigated the effects of a valerian/kava combination in 54 healthy individuals and reported reduced physiologic indicators that the authors equated with reduced stress response, including blood pressure and heart rate.[84]

Sedation
Summary

- Although valerian has not been studied explicitly as a sedative, evidence from studies conducted for other purposes suggests that valerian may not possess significant sedative effects.

Evidence

- Kuhlmann et al. conducted a double-blind trial in 102 healthy female patients randomized to receive valerian extract (600 mg), placebo, or flunitrazepam (Rohypnol) (1 mg/tablet).[26] The trial consisted of two phases. In the first phase (phase A), study participants were randomized to receive a single dose of valerian, flunitrazepam, or placebo, followed by psychometric testing the morning after to assess the effect of these preparations on reaction time. Phase A was then followed by a 7-day washout phase, whereupon study participants were further randomized to receive 14 days of either valerian or placebo (the benzodiazepine group was not included in the chronic phase). The primary outcome measure was described as the change in median reaction time as defined by the Vienna Determination Test (VDT). Secondary criteria included alertness, two-handed coordination, and sleep quality. Following single-dose administration, reaction time was significantly lower for flunitrazepam compared to valerian or placebo. No differences between valerian and placebo were observed. The flunitrazepam group also showed a significant impairment of performance (hangover effect) compared to improvements in both the valerian and placebo groups. Alertness and coordination, however, were similar among all three groups. Following 14-day administration, effects on reaction time, alertness, and concentration were comparable between valerian and placebo. There was an insignificant trend toward improved sleep quality with valerian compared to placebo.

- Kohnen et al. conducted a randomized, double-blind study (n = 48) examining the effects of valerian extract (100 mg) on social anxiety compared to placebo, the beta blocker propranolol (20 mg/tablet), or a combination of 100 mg of valerian extract plus 20 mg of propranolol.[16] The objective of the study was to assess whether valerian affected "psychic strain" (e.g., the ability to perform mathematical calculations in a timed and/or social setting) or somatic arousal (e.g., pulse during examination period). Each subject group consisted of four people (1 from each treatment group). Subjects were required to solve a series of arithmetic calculations verbally in front of a group (90 minutes after ingestion), and were then administered a written concentration test (150 minutes after ingestion). Valerian was reported to yield a small improvement in the written concentration test, and the combination of valerian and propranolol resulted in impairment of performance. No sedative effects or increases in calculation errors were reported for valerian. However, statistical analysis was not performed, relying only on visual assessment of chart trends; the outcomes measure utilized was not validated, with unclear reproducibility; and there was inadequate description of blinding, randomization, and baseline patient characteristics.

- A controlled trial was conducted by Gerhard et al. in 80 individuals to assess the effects on vigilance/reaction time in healthy patients taking Valverde (2 capsules, each containing 150 mg of valerian extract and 150 mg of hops extract), 800 mg of valerian only (Valverde Sleeping Syrup, 10 mL), 1 mg of the benzodiazepine flunitrazepam (Rohypnol), or placebo.[25] Doses were taken before bedtime, and effects were measured the following morning. A "hangover" phenomenon was observed in 50% of benzodiazepine subjects and in 10% of the Valverde and placebo groups. Subjective measures of sleep quality were no different between groups. A substudy of 36 individuals assessed the effects of valerian or placebo 1 to 2 hours after ingestion, and the authors concluded that valerian monotherapy syrup caused a "very mild" statistically significant impairment of vigilance, whereas the valerian-hops combination caused mild slowing in the processing of complex thoughts. This study was designed to assess adverse effects rather than efficacy. The trial is limited by poor reporting of baseline patient characteristics and lack of proper randomization or blinding. In a prior low-quality trial by the same lead author, Valverde tablets were compared to 3 mg of bromazepam or placebo in 60 healthy males.[28] No sedation or effects on vigilance were detected in either treatment group throughout a series of tests, although it is not clear that any of these assessments was properly validated. Although the results suggest that valerian does not cause sedation, the lack of effect for any group raises questions about the validity of the results. Further studies are warranted in this area.

- In a 1969 open-label case series, 70 hospitalized patients with diverse psychosomatic diagnoses were given 150 to 300 mg daily doses of the valerian product Valmane.[27] The preparation was reported to produce mild sedative effects and to be effective in the treatment of "restlessness" and "tension." However, in the absence of a control group, these results are of limited clinical relevance.

FORMULARY: BRANDS USED IN CLINICAL TRIALS
Brands Used in Statistically Significant Clinical Trials

- Nature's Way Valerian (USA).[72]
- Baldisedron (Germany)[71]; Baldrian- Dispert (Germany)[32,73]; Harmonicum Much[85]; Seda-Kneipp[75]; Sedonium (Germany)[15,67]; Valdispert (Germany)[32]; Valdispert forte (Germany)[65]; Valverde[25,28]; Valverde Sleeping Syrup (Germany)[25]; Valerina Natt.[70]

References

1. Muller D, Pfeil T, von den Dreisch, V. Treating depression comorbid with anxiety—results of an open, practice-oriented study with St John's wort WS 5572 and valerian extract in high doses. Phytomedicine 2003;10(Suppl 4): 25-30.
2. Kniebel R, Burchard JM. Zur therapie depressiver verstimmungen in der praxis. Z Allg Med 1988;64:689-696.
3. Steger W. A randomised double-blind study to compare the effectiveness of a plant-based combination of metabolic substances to a synthetic anti-depressant in depressive state. Z Allg Med 1985;61:914-918.
4. Oshima Y, Matsuoka S, Ohizumi Y. Antidepressant principles of *Valeriana fauriei* roots. Chem Pharm Bull (Tokyo) 1995;43(1):169-170.
5. Andreatini R, Leite JR. Effect of valepotriates on the behavior of rats in the elevated plus maze during diazepam withdrawal. Eur J Pharmacol 1994; 260(2-3):233-235.
6. Poyares DR, Guilleminault C, Ohayon MM, et al. Can valerian improve the sleep of insomniacs after benzodiazepine withdrawal? Prog Neuropsychopharmacol Biol Psychiatry 2002;26(3):539-545.
7. Reference deleted in proofs.
8. Ang-Lee MK, Moss J, Yuan CS. Herbal medicines and perioperative care. JAMA 2001;286(2):208-216.
9. Bounthanh C, Bergmann C, Beck JP, et al. Valepotriates, a new class of cytotoxic and antitumor agents. Planta Med 1981;41(1):21-28.
10. Bounthanh C, Richert L, Beck JP, et al. The action of valepotriates on the synthesis of DNA and proteins of cultured hepatoma cells. Planta Med 1983;49(3):138-142.
11. Hiller KO, Zetler G. Neuropharmacological studies on ethanol extracts of *Valeriana officinalis* L: behavioural and anticonvulsant properties. Phytother Res 1996;10:145-151.
12. Tufik S, Fujita K, Seabra M, et al. Effects of a prolonged administration of valepotriates in rats on the mothers and their offspring. J Ethnopharmacol 1994;41(1-2):39-44.
13. Braun R, Dittmar W, Hubner GE, et al. [*In vivo* influence of valtrate/isovaltrate on hematopoiesis and metabolic liver activity in mice]. Planta Med 1984;(1):1-4.
14. Vorbach EU, Darmstadt R, Gortelmeyer, et al. Therapie von Insomnien. Psychopharmakotherapie 1996;3:109-115.
15. Dorn M. [Efficacy and tolerability of Baldrian versus oxazepam in non-organic and non-psychiatric insomniacs: a randomised, double-blind, clinical, comparative study]. Forsch Komplementarmed Klass Naturheilkd 2000; 7(2):79-84.
16. Kohnen R, Oswald WD. The effects of valerian, propranolol, and their combination on activation, performance, and mood of healthy volunteers under social stress conditions. Pharmacopsychiatry 1988;21(6):447-448.
17. Francis AJ, Dempster RJ. Effect of valerian, *Valeriana edulis*, on sleep difficulties in children with intellectual deficits: randomised trial. Phytomedicine 2002;9(4):273-279.
18. Willey LB, Mady SP, Cobaugh DJ, et al. Valerian overdose: a case report. Vet Hum Toxicol 1995;37(4):364-365.
19. Wells SR. International intravenous administration of a crude valerian root extract. NACCT 1995;33:542.
20. MacGregor FB, Abernethy VE, Dahabra S, et al. Hepatotoxicity of herbal remedies. BMJ 1989;299(6708):1156-1157.
21. Chan TY, Tang CH, Critchley JA. Poisoning due to an over-the-counter hypnotic, Sleep-Qik (hyoscine, cyproheptadine, valerian). Postgrad Med J 1995;71(834):227-228.
22. Chan TY. An assessment of the delayed effects associated with valerian overdose. Int J Clin Pharmacol Ther 1998;36(10):569.
23. Skramlik E. Uber die giftigkeit und vertaglichkeit von atherischen olen. Pharmazie 1959;14:435-445.
24. Hendriks H, Bos R, Woerdenbag HJ, et al. Central nervous depressant activity of valerenic acid in the mouse. Planta Med 1985;(1):28-31.
25. Gerhard U, Linnenbrink N, Georghiadou C, et al. Vigilanzmindernde Effekte zweier pflazlicher Schlafmittel (Effects of two plant-based sleep remedies on vigilance). Schweiz Rundsch Med Prax 1996;85(15):473-481.
26. Kuhlmann J, Berger W, Podzuweit H, et al. The influence of valerian treatment on "reaction time, alertness and concentration" in volunteers. Pharmacopsychiatry 1999;32(6):235-241.
27. Boeters VU. [On treatment of control disorders of the autonomic nervous system with valepotriaten (Valmane)]. MMW 1969;37:1873-1876.
28. Gerhard U, Hobi V, Kocher R, et al. [Acute sedating effect of a herbal tranquilizer compared to that of bromazepam]. Schweiz Rundsch Med Prax 1991;80(52):1481-1486.
29. Albrecht M, Berger W, Laux P, et al. Psychopharmaceuticals and traffic safety: the effect of Euvegal® Dragees Forte on driving ability and combination effects with alcohol. Z Allg Med 1995;71:1215-1225.
30. Leathwood PD, Chauffard F. Aqueous extract of valerian reduces latency to fall asleep in man. Planta Med 1985;(2):144-148.
31. Garges HP, Varia I, Doraiswamy PM. Cardiac complications and delirium associated with valerian root withdrawal. JAMA 1998;280(18):1566-1567.
32. Kamm-Kohl AV, Jansen W, Brockmann P. Moderne baldriantherapie gegen nervöse Störungen im Senium. Medwelt 1984;35:1450-1454.
33. Seifert T. Therapeutic effects of valerian in nervous disorders. Therapeutikon 1988;2:94-98.
34. Czeizel A, Szentesi I, Szekeres I, et al. A study of adverse effects on the progeny after intoxication during pregnancy. Arch Toxicol 1988;62(1):1-7.
35. Plushner SL. Valerian: *Valeriana officinalis*. Am J Health-Syst Pharm 2000; 57(4):328, 333, 335.
36. Miller LG. Herbal medicinals: selected clinical considerations focusing on known or potential drug-herb interactions. Arch Intern Med 1998;158(20): 2200-2211.
37. Leuschner J, Muller J, Rudmann M. Characterisation of the central nervous depressant activity of a commercially available valerian root extract. Arzneimittelforschung 1993;43(6):638-641.
38. Yager J, Siegfried SL, DiMatteo TL. Use of alternative remedies by psychiatric patients: illustrative vignettes and a discussion of the issues. Am J Psychiatry 1999;156(9):1432-1438.
39. Chen D, Klesmer J, Giovanniello A, et al. Mental status changes in an alcohol abuser taking valerian and gingko biloba. Am J Addict 2002;11(1): 75-77.
40. Mayer B, Springer E. [Psychoexperimental studies on the effect of a valepotriate combination as well as the combined effects of valtratum and alcohol]. Arzneimittelforschung 1974;24(12):2066-2070.
41. Khawaja IS, Marotta RF, Lippmann S. Herbal medicines as a factor in delirium. Psychiatr Serv 1999;50(7):969-970.
42. Petkov V. Plants and hypotensive, antiatheromatous and coronarodilatating action. Am J Chin Med 1979;7(3):197-236.
43. Beckman SE, Sommi RW, Switzer J. Consumer use of St. John's wort: a survey on effectiveness, safety, and tolerability. Pharmacotherapy 2000; 20(5):568-574.
44. Hendriks H, Bos R, Allersma DP, et al. Pharmacological screening of valerenal and some other components of essential oil of *Valeriana officinalis*. Planta Med 1981;42(1):62-68.
45. Houghton PJ. The biological activity of Valerian and related plants. J Ethnopharmacol 1988;22(2):121-142.
46. Houghton PJ. The scientific basis for the reputed activity of Valerian. J Pharm Pharmacol 1999;51(5):505-512.
47. Fernandez S, Wasowski C, Paladini AC, et al. Sedative and sleep-enhancing properties of linarin, a flavonoid-isolated from *Valeriana officinalis*. Pharmacol Biochem Behav 2004;77(2):399-404.
48. Morazzoni P, Bombardelli E. Valeriana officinalis: traditional use and recent evaluation of activity. Fitoterapia 1995;66(2):99-112.

V

49. Wagner H, Jurcic K, Schaette R. [Comparative studies on the sedative action of Valeriana extracts, valepotriates and their degradation products (author's transl)]. Planta Med 1980;38(4):358-365.

50. Cavadas C, Araujo I, Cotrim MD, et al. *In vitro* study on the interaction of *Valeriana officinalis* L. extracts and their amino acids on GABAA receptor in rat brain. Arzneimittelforschung 1995;45(7):753-755.

51. Mennini T, Bernasconi P, Bombardelli E, et al. *In vitro* study on the interaction of extracts and pure compounds from *Valeriana officinalis* roots with GABA, benzodiazepine and barbiturate receptors in rat brain. Fitoterapia 1993;64(4):291-300.

52. Nieves J, Oritz J G. Effects of valeriana officinalis extract on GABAergic transmission. J Neurochem 1997;69(Suppl 1):S128.

53. Ortiz JG, Nieves-Natal J, Chavez P. Effects of *Valeriana officinalis* extracts on [3H]flunitrazepam binding, synaptosomal [3H]GABA uptake, and hippocampal [3H]GABA release. Neurochem Res 1999;24(11):1373-1378.

54. Rodenbeck A, Simen S, Cohrs S, et al. Alterations of the sleep stage structure as a feature of GABAergic effects of a valerian-hop preparation in patients with psychophysiological insomnia. Somnologie 1998;2:26-31.

55. Santos MS, Ferreira F, Cunha AP, et al. An aqueous extract of valerian influences the transport of GABA in synaptosomes. Planta Med 1994; 60(3):278-279.

56. Santos MS, Ferreira F, Faro C, et al. The amount of GABA present in aqueous extracts of valerian is sufficient to account for [3H]GABA release in synaptosomes. Planta Med 1994;60(5):475-476.

57. Santos MS, Ferreira F, Cunha AP, et al. Synaptosomal GABA release as influenced by valerian root extract— involvement of the GABA carrier. Arch Int Pharmacodyn Ther 1994;327(2):220-231.

58. Yuan CS, Mehendale S, Xiao Y, et al. The gamma-aminobutyric acidergic effects of valerian and valerenic acid on rat brainstem neuronal activity. Anesth Analg 2004;98(2):353-8, table.

59. Capasso A. Pharmacological effects of aqueous extract from *Valeriana adscendens.* Phytother Res 1996;10:309-312.

60. Sakamoto T, Mitani Y, Nakajima K. Psychotropic effects of Japanese valerian root extract. Chem Pharm Bull (Tokyo) 1992;40(3):758-761.

61. Stevinson C, Ernst E. Valerian for insomnia: systematic review of randomized clinical trials. Sleep Med 2000;1:91-99.

62. Leathwood PD, Chauffard F, Heck E, et al. Aqueous extract of valerian root (*Valeriana officinalis* L.) improves sleep quality in man. Pharmacol Biochem Behav 1982;17(1):65-71.

63. Gessner B, Klasser M. [Studies on the effect of Harmonicum Much on sleep using polygraphic EEG recordings]. EEG EMG Z Elektroenzephalogr Elektromyogr Verwandte Geb 1984;15(1):45-51.

64. Balderer G, Borbely AA. Effect of valerian on human sleep. Psychopharmacology (Berl) 1985;87(4):406-409.

65. Schulz H, Stolz C, Muller J. The effect of valerian extract on sleep polygraphy in poor sleepers: a pilot study. Pharmacopsychiatry 1994;27(4): 147-151.

66. Ziegler G, Ploch M, Miettinen-Baumann A, et al. Efficacy and tolerability of valerian extract LI 156 compared with oxazepam in the treatment of non-organic insomnia—a randomized, double-blind, comparative clinical study. Eur J Med Res 2002;7(11):480-486.

67. Donath F, Quispe S, Diefenbach K, et al. Critical evaluation of the effect of valerian extract on sleep structure and sleep quality. Pharmacopsychiatry 2000;33(2):47-53.

68. Giedke H, Breyer-Pfaff U. Critical evaluation of the effect of valerian extract on sleep structure and sleep quality. Pharmacopsychiatry 2000;33(6):239.

69. Leathwood PD, Chauffard F. Quantifying the effects of mild sedatives. J Psychiatr Res 1982;17(2):115-122.

70. Lindahl O, Lindwall L. Double blind study of a valerian preparation. Pharmacol Biochem Behav 1989;32(4):1065-1066.

71. Jansen W. Doppelblindstudie mit Baldrisedon. Therapiewoche 1977;27: 2779-2786.

72. Dominguez RA, Bravo-Valverde RL, Kaplowitz BR, et al. Valerian as a hypnotic for Hispanic patients. Cultur Divers Ethnic Minor Psychol 2000; 6(1):84-92.

73. Schmidt-Voigt J. Die Behandlung nervöser Schlafstörungen und innerer Unruhe mit einem rein pflanzlichen Sedativum. Therapiewoche 1986; 36:663-667.

74. Cerny AS, Schmid K. Tolerability and efficacy of valerian/lemon balm in healthy volunteers; a double blind placebo controlled, multicentre study. Fitoterapia 1999;70(3):221-228.

75. Muller-Limmroth W, Ehrenstein W. [Experimental studies of the effects of Seda-Kneipp on the sleep of sleep disturbed subjects; implications for the treatment of different sleep disturbances (author's transl)]. Med Klin 1977;72(25):1119-1125.

76. Schmitz M, Jackel M. [Comparative study for assessing quality of life of patients with exogenous sleep disorders (temporary sleep onset and sleep interruption disorders) treated with a hops-valarian preparation and a benzodiazepine drug]. Wien Med Wochenschr 1998;148(13):291-298.

77. Dressing H. Valerian combination therapy vs. benzodiazepine: same efficacy in the treatment of sleeping disorders? Therapiewoche 1992;42(12):726-736.

78. Andreatini R, Sartori VA, Seabra ML, et al. Effect of valepotriates (valerian extract) in generalized anxiety disorder: a randomized placebo-controlled pilot study. Phytother Res 2002;16(7):650-654.

79. Sousa MPd, Pacheco P, Roldao V. Double-blind comparative study of the efficacy and safety of Valdispert vs. clobazepam. KaliChemi Med Res Info (Report) 1992;

80. Delsignore R, Orlando S, Costi D, et al. Placebo controlled clinical trial with valerian. Settimana Medica 1980;68(9):437-447.

81. Glass JR, Sproule BA, Herrmann N, et al. Acute pharmacological effects of temazepam, diphenhydramine, and valerian in healthy elderly subjects. J Clin Psychopharmacol 2003;23(3):260-268.

82. Schellenberg R, Schwartz A, Schellenberg V, et al. Quantitative EEG-monitoring and psychometric evaluation of the therapeutic efficacy of Biral N in psychosomatic diseases. Naturamed 1994;4:9.

83. Panijel M. [Treatment of moderately severe anxiety states]. Therapiewoche 1985;35(41):4659-4668.

84. Cropley M, Cave Z, Ellis J, et al. Effect of kava and valerian on human physiological and psychological responses to mental stress assessed under laboratory conditions. Phytother Res 2002;16(1):23-27.

85. Gessner B, Klasser M, Völp A. [Long term effect of a valerian extract (harmonicum much) in persons with sleep disorders]. Therapiewoche 1983; 33:5547-5558.

White Horehound
(*Marrubium vulgare* L.)

SYNONYMS/COMMON NAMES/RELATED SUBSTANCES

- Andorn, blanc rubi, bonhomme, bouenriblé, bull's blood, common hoarhound, eye of the star, grand bon-homme, grand-bonhomme, haran haran, herbe aux crocs, herbe vierge, hoarhound, horehound, hound-bane, houndsbane, Labiatae (family), Lamiaceae (family), llwyd y cwn, maltrasté, mapiochin, mariblé, marinclin, marrochemin, marroio, marroio-blanco, marromba, marrube, marrube blanc, marrube commun, marrube des champs, marrube officinal, marrube vulgaire, marrubii herba, marrubio, marrubium, *Marrubium vulgare*, maruil, marvel, mastranzo, mont blanc, Ricola, soldier's tea, seed of Horus, weisser andorn.
- *Note:* Not to be confused with black horehound (*Ballota nigra*) or water horehound (*Lycopus americanus*, also known as bugleweed).

CLINICAL BOTTOM LINE
Background

- Since the time of ancient Egypt, white horehound (*Marrubium vulgare* L.) has been used as an expectorant. Ayurvedic, Native American, and Australian aboriginal medicines have traditionally used white horehound to treat respiratory conditions. The U.S. Food and Drug Administration (FDA) banned horehound from cough drops in 1989 because of insufficient evidence supporting its efficacy. However, horehound is currently widely used in Europe and can be found in European-made herbal cough remedies sold in the United States (for example, Ricola). There is no well-defined clinical evidence to support this (or any other) therapeutic use of white horehound. The expert German panel Commission E has approved white horehound as a choleretic indicated for lack of appetite and dyspepsia. Again, there are no known clinical studies supporting this indication. There is promising early evidence favoring the use of white horehound as a hypoglycemic agent for diabetes mellitus and as a nonopioid pain reliever.
- There is limited evidence on tolerability or toxicity in humans. White horehound has been reported to cause hypotension, hypoglycemia, and arrhythmias in animal studies[1-3] and is not recommended in pregnancy because of possible abortifacient properties.[4]

Scientific Evidence for Common/Studied Uses	Grade*
Antispasmodic	C
Choleretic (dyspepsia, appetite stimulation)	C
Diabetes	C
Pain	C

*Key to grades: *A:* Strong scientific evidence for this use; *B:* Good scientific evidence for this use; *C:* Unclear scientific evidence for this use; *D:* Fair scientific evidence against this use (it may not work); *F:* Strong scientific evidence against this use (it likely does not work). For a more detailed explanation of efficacy criteria, see "Natural Standard Evidence-Based Validated Grading Rationale" in the Introduction.

Historical or Theoretical Uses That Lack Sufficient Evidence

- Anorexia, antihelmintic, arrhythmia, asthma, bile secretion, bloating, bronchitis, cancer, cathartic, chronic obstructive pulmonary disease (COPD), colic, congestion, constipation, cough, debility, decoction for skin conditions, diaphoretic, diarrhea, digestive aid, diuresis, dysmenorrhea, dyspepsia, emetic, expectorant, fever reduction, flatulence, food flavoring, gallbladder complaints, hepatitis, indigestion, intestinal parasites, jaundice, laxative, lung congestion, menstrual pain, morning sickness, pain, pertussis, pneumonia, rabies, respiratory spasmolytic, skin ulcers, snake poisoning, sore throat, spasms, tachycardia, tuberculosis, upper respiratory tract infections, vasodilator, vulnerary, warts, wheezing, whooping cough, wound healing.

Expert Opinion and Folkloric Precedent

- In traditional medicine, the leaves and flowers of white horehound have been used orally to treat a variety of respiratory, gastrointestinal, and menstrual conditions; as a diuretic and anthelmintic; for cancer treatment; and topically to treat skin ulcers or for wound care. Currently white horehound is widely used in Europe despite a lack of supportive clinical evidence. The German Commission E has approved white horehound as a choleretic indicated for lack of appetite and dyspepsia. Horehound is found in European-made herbal cough remedies/cough drops sold in the United States.
- In Mexico, white horehound has been used empirically for management of diabetes mellitus, with emerging data that describe the hypoglycemic effects of the plant.
- Recent evidence of antinociceptive (decreasing sensitivity to noxious stimuli) and antispasmodic properties of marrubiin, a confirmed component in white horehound tea, supports the employment of *M. vulgare* in folk medicine for the treatment of pain and spasms.

Safety Summary

- **Likely safe:** When used orally in dietary amounts found in foods. White horehound has been granted "generally recognized as safe" (GRAS) status in the United States. Safety data are based on expert opinion and anecdotal use. Reliable human studies on the tolerability or toxicity of white horehound are not available.
- **Possibly safe:** When above-ground parts of white horehound are used orally, in recommended doses, for limited duration in otherwise healthy adults.
- **Possibly unsafe:** When used in doses above the recommended range or in long-term use.
- **Likely unsafe:** When used orally during pregnancy or breastfeeding.

DOSING/TOXICOLOGY
General

- Recommended doses are based on those most commonly used in available trials, or on historical practice. However, with natural products, the optimal doses needed to balance efficacy and safety often have not been determined. Formulations and preparation methods may vary from manufacturer

W

to manufacturer, and from batch to batch of a specific product made by a single manufacturer. Because often the active components of a product are not known, standardization may not be possible, and the clinical effects of different brands may not be comparable.

Standardization

- There is no widely accepted standardization for white horehound.
- The maximum average concentration in candy has been reported as 0.073%. Crude white horehound was formerly an official remedy in the United States Pharmacopeia (USP). Strengths of extracts have been expressed in terms of flavor intensity or weight-to-weight ratio.
- Black horehound (*Ballota nigra*) may be found as an adulterant in compounds reported to contain only white horehound.

Dosing: Adult (18 Years and Older)
Oral

- **Gastrointestinal (dyspepsia, appetite stimulant):** 4.5 g per day of cut herb or 2 to 6 tablespoons of fresh plant juice, or equivalent, has been recommended by the expert German panel Commission E. Another traditional dosing suggestion is 1 to 2 g of dried herb or infusion three times daily.
- **Respiratory (cough and throat ailments):** 10 to 40 drops of extract in water up to three times a day, or lozenges dissolved in the mouth as needed (as recommended anecdotally). Ricola drops are recommended by the manufacturer at a maximum of 2 lozenges every 1 to 2 hours as needed.

Dosing: Pediatric (Younger Than 18 Years)

- Insufficient evidence to recommend.

Toxicology

- There are limited available toxicity studies in humans. The LD_{50} in rats for orally administered marrubinic acid was reported as 370 mg/kg of body weight in a 1959 study.[5] Saleh et al. found the volatile oil to be highly toxic to the flukes *Schistosoma mansoni* and *Schistosoma haematobium*.[6] Maximum average level is 0.073% reported in candy.
- Black horehound (*B. nigra*), which has indications similar to those for *M. vulgare* but is extremely bitter tasting, may sometimes be found as an adulterant in compounds reported to contain only white horehound.

ADVERSE EFFECTS/PRECAUTIONS/CONTRAINDICATIONS
Allergy

- Known allergy/hypersensitivity to members of the Lamiaceae family (mint family) or any white horehound components is a contraindication.

Adverse Effects

- **General:** White horehound is generally considered to be safe when used as a flavoring agent in foods. However, the scientific literature regarding potential clinical application consists largely of animal (not human) studies, which may or may not be indicative of human tolerability.
- **Cardiovascular:** Large doses of white horehound have caused arrhythmias in animal studies.[1] Hypotension has been reported in animals, perhaps mediated by vascular relaxant activity of *Marrubium*.[3] Theoretically, aldosterone-enhancing properties of the herb may cause hypertension, hypernatremia, and edema via its proposed mechanism of action, including loss of potassium and distal sodium reabsorption in the kidneys.

- **Dermatologic:** Skin contact with the irritant in white horehound plant juice has been reported to elicit a contact dermatitis.
- **Endocrine:** Decreases in blood glucose have been reported in hyperglycemic rabbits compared with a control (water ingestion).[2] Theoretically, aldosterone-enhancing properties of the herb may cause loss of potassium and distal sodium resorption in the kidneys.
- **Gastrointestinal:** White horehound is considered to be an emetic and cathartic in large doses and may cause diarrhea via its proposed mechanism of action on the gastrointestinal tract. White horehound may cause intestinal dilation or ileus because of its possible aldosterone-enhancing properties.
- **Musculoskeletal:** Anecdotal reports suggest white horehound may cause muscular weakness or edema via its possible aldosterone-enhancing properties.

Precautions/Warnings/Contraindications

- Avoid during pregnancy or lactation, because of emmenagogic and abortifacient effects reported in animal studies and anecdotal reports of uterine stimulant activity.
- Use cautiously in patients with diabetes mellitus, because of a report of decreased blood glucose levels in hyperglycemic animals.
- Use cautiously in patients with hypertension or hypernatremia or in patients taking diuretics, because of proposed aldosterone-enhancing properties.
- Use cautiously in patients with unstable blood pressure or hypotension, because of reported hypotension in animals.
- Use cautiously in patients with cardiac arrhythmias, because of isolated reports of arrhythmias in animals.
- Use cautiously in patients with gastrointestinal disease, such as ileus, atony, or obstruction.

Pregnancy and Lactation

- Not recommended during pregnancy, because of emmenagogic and abortifacient effects reported in animal studies.[4] In addition, anecdotal reports have noted that white horehound may stimulate uterine contractions.
- Not recommended during lactation, because of a lack of sufficient scientific study.

INTERACTIONS
White Horehound/Drug Interactions

- **Antiarrhythmics:** Large amounts of white horehound may be proarrhythmogenic and should be avoided concurrently with drugs that affect cardiac rhythm.[1]
- **Antiemetics (granisetron, ondansetron):** Theoretically, horehound may interact with serotonin receptor antagonists such as granisetron and ondansetron, as supported by *in vitro* studies suggesting that horehound may antagonize the effects of serotonin.[1]
- **Antihypertensives:** Additive hypotensive effects may occur with concomitant horehound, as supported by reports of hypotension in animals administered the plant alone.[3]
- **Antimigraine agents:** Theoretically, horehound may interact with serotonin enhancers such as ergot alkaloids (bromocriptine, dihydroergotamine, ergotamine) and triptans, as supported by *in vitro* studies suggesting that horehound may antagonize the effects of serotonin.[1]
- **Cardiac glycosides (digoxin, digitoxin):** White horehound contains glycosides and therefore theoretically could potentiate the activity of glycoside medications.
- **Diuretics:** White horehound may enhance aldosterone action and therefore may interact with diuretic medications.

- **Expectorants:** Because of possible expectorant activity of white horehound, concomitant use with other expectorants may be additive (as indicated by anecdotal reports).
- **Estrogen, oral contraceptive pills (OCPs), agents for hormone replacement therapy (HRT):** White horehound may possess phytoestrogenic chemicals that antagonize or agonize estrogen receptors, thereby altering the effects of estrogen therapies (theoretical).
- **Insulin, oral hypoglycemics:** Augmentation of the hypoglycemic effects of oral hypoglycemics may occur, as suggested by the blood glucose–lowering activity of white horehound in hyperglycemic rabbits.[2]
- **Penicillin:** Anecdotal reports suggest that white horehound may interact with the excretion of penicillin, although details and scientific data are limited.
- **Selective serotonin reuptake inhibitor (SSRI) antidepressants:** Preclinical studies with aqueous extracts of horehound suggest that white horehound may antagonize the effects of serotonin.[1] Theoretically, this antagonism may result in interaction with antidepressants that possess serotonin activity, such as SSRIs.
- **Thyroid medications:** Because of possible hypothalamic-pituitary-adrenal axis (HPA) effects of white horehound constituents, concomitant administration may interact with thyroid medications (theoretical).

White Horehound/Herb/Supplement Interactions

- **Hypotensive herbs:** Additive hypotensive effects may occur with concomitant horehound, as supported by reports of hypotension in animals administered the plant alone.[3]
- **Cardiac glycoside herbs and supplements:** White horehound contains glycosides and therefore theoretically could potentiate the activity of glycoside agents.
- **Diuretic herbs and supplements:** White horehound may enhance aldosterone action and therefore may interact with diuretics.
- **Phytoestrogenic herbs:** White horehound may possess phytoestrogenic chemicals that antagonize or agonize estrogen receptors, thereby altering the effects of other agents that act on these receptors, including herbs with estrogenic properties (theoretical).
- **Hypoglycemic herbs:** White horehound may augment the hypoglycemic effects of other agents, as suggested by the blood glucose–lowering activity of white horehound in hyperglycemic rabbits.[2]
- **Selective serotonin reuptake inhibitor (SSRI) herbs and supplements:** Preclinical studies with aqueous extracts of horehound suggest that white horehound may antagonize the effects of serotonin.[1] Theoretically, this antagonism may result in interaction with other agents that possess serotonin activity, such as herbs or supplements with SSRI properties.

White Horehound/Food Interactions
- Insufficient available evidence.

White Horehound/Lab Interactions
- **Serum glucose levels:** Hypoglycemia has been reported in animal studies in which consumption of eight plants was followed by significantly decreased hyperglycemia in rabbits.[2]
- **Serum electrolytes:** Potassium and sodium levels may be altered as a result of possible aldosterone-enhancing activity of white horehound (theoretical).
- **Serum hormone levels:** Because of possible hypothalamic-pituitary-gonadal axis (HPA) effects of white horehound constituents, various hormonal levels may be altered,

although there is limited human clinical information in this area (theoretical).

MECHANISM OF ACTION
Pharmacology
- **Constituents:** The medicinally used parts of white horehound (*Marrubium vulgare* L.) are the dried leaves and flowering tops. Processed white horehound contains 0.3% to 1% of the bitter principle marrubiin, diterpene alcohols, alkaloids, bitter lactone, flavonoids, saponin, sterols, tannins, vitamin C, and 0.06% of a volatile oil.[7-10] Marrubiin does not exist in the fresh plant but is formed from premarrubiin during processing.[11,12] Although the chemical aspects of the compound have been documented, the pharmacologically active constituents remain to be determined.
- **Analgesic/antispasmodic effects:** *In vivo* models of pain in mice report significant analgesic activity of the hydroalcoholic extract of *M. vulgare*, and antinociceptive effects as well as an anti-inflammatory effect of marrubiin.[13] A hydroalcoholic extract of *M. vulgare* has also been shown to exhibit antispasmodic and antinociceptive effects in animals.[12] The exact mechanisms remain to be determined but appear not to involve the inhibition of cyclooxygenase or opioid receptors. Nociceptive action is not reversed by naloxone.[12] An *in vitro* study of white horehound demonstrated noncompetitive, concentration-dependent antagonism of muscle contractions induced by several agonists of smooth muscle tissue.[12]
- **Cardiac effects:** Hypotensive activity has been ascribed to the herb, as supported by animal data.[3] Pharmacologically, white horehound (*M. vulgare*) may exert hypotensive action through vascular relaxation[3] or vasodilation.[15] Large amounts of horehound have been demonstrated to have proarrhythmic potential.[1]
- **Central nervous system effects:** *In vitro* research demonstrates that the aqueous extract of white horehound exhibits an antagonistic effect on serotonin.[1]
- **Expectorant effects:** Monoterpenes from the volatile oil of *M. vulgare* have exhibited expectorant activity,[15] which may stem from direct stimulation of bronchial mucosal secretions.
- **Endocrine effects:** Hypoglycemia has been reported in animal studies, in which consumption of eight plants was followed by significantly decreased hyperglycemia in rabbits compared with a control (water ingestion).[2] In anecdotal reports, horehound has been noted to possess aldosterone-enhancing properties.
- **Biliary effects:** Animal research from 1959 suggests that marrubinic acid may stimulate bile secretion.[5]

Pharmacodynamics/Kinetics
- White horehound administered to mice had a maximum duration of action for analgesia of 4 hours.[13]
- The LD_{50} for oral marrubinic acid has been reported as 370 mg/kg in an animal model.[5]

HISTORY
- White horehound is a perennial aromatic herb of the mint family, native to Eurasia and naturalized in the northeastern United States and Canada.
- Horehound has a rich history of medicinal use. Egyptian priests called this plant "seed of Horus," "bull's blood," or "eye of the star." It has been a principal ingredient in antidotes for vegetable poisons. In ancient Greece, it was used for treating rabid dog bites, and the name "horehound" may refer to its historical use as such an antidote. The Romans esteemed white horehound for its medicinal

properties, and one theory suggests that its Latin name, *Marrubium*, was derived from "Maria urbs," an ancient town of Italy. Other theories derive its name from the Hebrew for "bitter juice" and suggest that it was a bitter herb that Jews ate ceremonially during Passover.

- Horehound was an official remedy in the United States Pharmacopeia from 1820 to 1900. Horehound is currently widely used in Europe and can be found in European-made herbal cough remedies sold in the United States (for example, Ricola). In Britain, it is also brewed as Horehound Ale.

REVIEW OF THE EVIDENCE: TABLE

- No studies qualify for inclusion in the evidence table.

REVIEW OF THE EVIDENCE: DISCUSSION

Antispasmodic
Summary

- White horehound has been used traditionally as an antispasmodic in treating gastrointestinal disorders. However because of a lack of controlled trials, there is currently insufficient evidence to recommend for or against the use of white horehound for this indication.

Evidence

- A preclinical study evaluated effects of white horehound extract on smooth muscle.[14] The hydroalcoholic extract of white horehound exerted antispasmodic activity and inhibited the actions of acetylcholine, bradykinin, and histamine-induced contractions on guinea pig ileum and rat duodenum. Results demonstrated noncompetitive, concentration-dependent antagonism of smooth muscle contraction induced by several agonists.
- In a subsequent investigation, a hydroalcoholic extract of *M. vulgare* exhibited antispasmodic and antinociceptive effects in animals.[12]

Choleretic (Dyspepsia, Appetite Stimulation)
Summary

- The expert German panel Commission E has approved white horehound as a choleretic for the treatment of dyspepsia and lack of appetite. The evidence supporting this use is largely anecdotal and based on historical use, and there is currently insufficient scientific research to recommend for or against this use of white horehound.

Evidence

- In a 1959 study, the white horehound constituent marrubiin acid and its sodium salt were reported to transiently stimulate bile flow, whereas the constituent marrubiin did not do so.[5]

Diabetes
Summary

- White horehound has been used traditionally in Mexico for the management of diabetes mellitus. However, there have been no clinical trials conducted in humans to assess efficacy or safety. Recent animal data suggest possible hypoglycemic effects of white horehound, and further research may be warranted in this area.

Evidence

- In an animal study, Roman et al. compared the hypoglycemic effects of white horehound and 11 other plants with the effects of tolbutamide and water.[2] Subcutaneous injections of 50% dextrose solution were administered to rabbits to induce temporary hyperglycemia. The plant preparations, tolbutamide, and water were administered prior to the dextrose solution. The authors reported that white horehound significantly decreased hyperglycemia induced by dextrose solution when compared with water, and results with use of the herb did not differ statistically in magnitude from those with tolbutamide.

Pain
Summary

- White horehound has traditionally been used in the management of pain and spasms associated with menstruation or gastrointestinal conditions. Preliminary supportive evidence stems from limited animal research, although there are no reliable human studies of safety or efficacy in this area.

Evidence

- Mouse research has reported significant analgesic, anti-inflammatory, antinociceptive, and antispasmodic effects, with some evidence that this activity is not associated with opioid receptors.[12,13] De Jesus et al. studied mice to determine the nociceptive activity of marrubiin, a constituent of white horehound.[12] ID_{50} values (the doses that reduced chemically induced pain by 50% vs. control values) were calculated. The authors reported that ID_{50} values for formalin-induced pain were 6.6 μmol/kg for marrubiin, "inactive" for aspirin, and >94 μmol/kg for diclofenac. ID_{50} values for capsaicin-induced pain were 6.3 μmol/kg for marrubiin, 123 μmol/kg for aspirin, and 34.5 μmol/kg for diclofenac.

References

1. Cahen R. [Pharmacologic spectrum of *Marrubium vulgare* L]. C R Seances Soc Biol Fil 1970;164(7):1467-1472.
2. Roman RR, Alarcon-Aguilar F, Lara-Lemus A, et al. Hypoglycemic effect of plants used in Mexico as antidiabetics. Arch Med Res 1992;23(1):59-64.
3. El Bardai S, Lyoussi B, Wibo M, et al. Pharmacological evidence of hypotensive activity of *Marrubium vulgare* and *Foeniculum vulgare* in spontaneously hypertensive rat. Clin Exp Hypertens 2001;23(4):329-343.
4. Farnsworth NR, Bingel AS, Cordell GA, et al. Potential value of plants as sources of new antifertility agents I. J Pharm Sci 1975;64(4):535-598.
5. Krejci I, Zadina R. Die Gallentreibende Wirkung von Marrubiin und Marrabinsäure. Planta Med 1959;7:1-7.
6. Saleh MM, Glombitza KW. Volatile oil of *Marrubium vulgare* and its anti-schistosomal activity. Planta Med 1989;55:105.
7. Nicholas HJ. Isolation of marrubiin, a sterol, and a sesquiterpene from *Marrubium vulgare*. J Pharm Sci 1964;53(8):895-899.
8. Karriyev MO, Bairiyev CB, Atayeva AS. [On the curative properties and phytochemistry of *Marribum vulgare*]. Izvestiia Akademii Nauk Turkmenskoi SSR, Seriia Biol Nauk 1976;3:86-88.
9. Knoss W, Reuter B, Zapp J. Biosynthesis of the labdane diterpene marrubiin in *Marrubium vulgare* via a non-mevalonate pathway. Biochem J 1997;326 (Pt 2):449-454.
10. Takeda Y, Yanagihara K, Masuda T, et al. Labdane diterpenoids from *Marrubium globosum* ssp. *globosum*. Chem Pharm Bull (Tokyo) 2000; 48(8):1234-1235.
11. Henderson MS, McCrindle R. Premarrubiin. A diterpenoid from *Marrubium vulgare* L. J Chem Soc 1969;C:2014-2015.
12. De Jesus RA, Cechinel-Filho V, Oliveira AE, et al. Analysis of the antinociceptive properties of marrubiin isolated from *Marrubium vulgare*. Phytomedicine 2000;7(2):111-115.
13. de Souza MM, De Jesus RA, Cechinel-Filho V, et al. Analgesic profile of hydroalcoholic extract obtained from *Marrubium vulgare*. Phytomedicine 1998;5(2):103-107.
14. Schlemper V, Ribas A, Nicolau M, et al. Antispasmodic effects of hydroalcoholic extract of *Marrubium vulgare* on isolated tissues. Phytomedicine 1996;3(2):211-216.
15. Karryvev MO, Bairyev CB, Ataeva AS. Some therapeutic properties of common horehound. Chem Abstr 1977;86:2355.

Wild Yam
(Dioscorea villosa L.)

SYNONYMS/COMMON NAMES/RELATED SUBSTANCES

- Atlantic yam, barbasco, China root, colic root, devil's bones, *Dioscorea, Dioscorea barbasco, Dioscorea hypoglauca, Dioscorea macrostachya, Dioscorea opposita,* Dioscoreaceae, Dioscoreae, diosgenin, Mexican yam, natural dehydroepiandrosterone (DHEA), phytoestrogen, rheumatism root, shan yao, wild yam root, yam, yuma.
- *Note:* "Yams" sold in the supermarket are actually members of the sweet potato family and are not true yams.

CLINICAL BOTTOM LINE
Background

- It has been hypothesized that wild yam (*Dioscorea villosa* and other *Dioscorea* species) possesses dehydroepiandrosterone (DHEA)-like properties and acts as a precursor to human sex hormones such as estrogen and progesterone. Based on this proposed mechanism, extracts of the plant have been used to treat dysmenorrhea, hot flashes, and headaches associated with menopause. However, these uses are based on a misconception that wild yam contains hormones or hormonal precursors—largely because of the historical fact that progesterone, androgens, and cortisone were chemically manufactured from Mexican wild yam in the 1960s. It is unlikely that this chemical conversion to progesterone occurs in the human body. The hormonal activity of some topical wild yam preparations has been attributed to adulteration with synthetic progesterone by manufacturers, although there is limited evidence in this area.
- The effects of diosgenin, a wild yam saponin constituent, on lipid metabolism are well documented in animal models and are possibly due to impaired intestinal cholesterol absorption. However, its purported hypocholesterolemic effect in humans and the feasibility of long-term use warrant further investigation.
- There are few reported contraindications to the use of wild yam in adults. However, there are no reliable safety or toxicity studies during pregnancy, lactation, or childhood.

Scientific Evidence for Common/Studied Uses	Grade*
Hyperlipidemia	C
Menopausal symptoms	C
Hormonal properties (estrogenic, progestinic, DHEA-like)	D

*Key to grades: *A:* Strong scientific evidence for this use; *B:* Good scientific evidence for this use; *C:* Unclear scientific evidence for this use; *D:* Fair scientific evidence against this use (it may not work); *F:* Strong scientific evidence against this use (it likely does not work). For a more detailed explanation of efficacy criteria, see "Natural Standard Evidence-Based Validated Grading Rationale" in the Introduction.

Historical or Theoretical Uses
That Lack Sufficient Evidence

- Amenorrhea, antifungal,[1] anti-inflammatory, antispasmodic, asthma, biliary colic, breast enlargement, carminative (prevents flatus), childbirth, cholagogue (promotes bile flow), cramps, croup, dermatitis, diaphoresis, diverticulitis, dysmenorrhea, emetic, energy promotion, expectorant, hepatoprotection, hypoglycemia, intestinal spasm, irritable bowel syndrome, joint pain, libido enhancement, menopause, menstrual pain, morning sickness, neuralgia, osteoporosis, pelvic cramps, pancreatic enzyme inhibitor, parturition, pelvic cramps, postmenopausal vaginal dryness, premenstrual syndrome, rheumatic pain, sudorific (causes perspiration), urinary tract disorders, uterotonic.

Expert Opinion and Folkloric Precedent

- Yams were traditionally used by Native Americans to treat cough, intestinal spasm, biliary colic, and rheumatic pain. Other traditional indications included dysmenorrhea, pelvic cramps, menstrual problems, menopause, and labor/ childbirth. Large doses were used to induce vomiting. In traditional Chinese medicine, two species of yam (*Dioscorea opposita* and *Dioscorea hypoglauca*) were used for some of these conditions, and for asthma and urinary tract problems.
- Wild yam is occasionally recommended as a treatment for biliary colic, irritable bowel syndrome, diverticulitis, and intestinal inflammation/spasm. However, it is most often marketed as a natural source of estrogen, progesterone, and/ or DHEA (although wild yam does not appear to contain DHEA or to possess sex hormonal properties in its un-processed form, contrary to popular opinion). Manufacturers tout the use of wild yam products to treat menopausal symptoms, dysmenorrhea, and cramps associated with menses or childbirth. In the 1960s, Mexican wild yams were the primary source material used to synthesize progesterone, androgens, and cortisone. In areas where manufacturing resources are limited, wild yam continues to be an important steroid substrate for the pharmaceutical industry.
- Wild yam has not been used historically to treat cardio-vascular disease. However, in view of its demonstrated effects on lipid metabolism in animals, and preliminary evidence in humans, it has been suggested as an adjunctive anti-hyperlipidemic agent.[2]

Safety Summary

- **Likely safe:** Wild yam products appear to be safe when used orally or topically by healthy individuals in recommended doses.[3]
- **Possibly unsafe:** Wild yam may be unsafe in patients with sex hormone–dependent cancers (such as breast, endometrial, ovarian, and prostate cancer), because of possible steroidal effects (not supported by available scientific studies), or because of adulteration with progesterone or other hormones.

DOSING/TOXICOLOGY
General

- Recommended doses are based on those most commonly used in available trials, or on historical practice. However, with natural products, the optimal doses needed to balance efficacy and safety often have not been determined. Formulations and preparation methods may vary from manufacturer to manufacturer, and from batch to batch of a specific

W

product made by a single manufacturer. Because often the active components of a product are not known, standardization may not be possible, and the clinical effects of different brands may not be comparable.

Standardization

- Typical standardization of wild yam products is to 10% diosgenin per dose.
- Diosgenin levels vary markedly among different wild yam species.[4,5] Unless a product is standardized, consumers can expect a considerable range of diosgenin-related effects based on the source species as well as on growing, harvesting, processing, and storage conditions. Synthetic progesterone has reportedly been added to some wild yam products.

Dosing: Adult (18 Years and Older)
Oral

- **Dried root:** 2 to 4 g or 1 to 2 teaspoons daily in two or three divided doses is sometimes recommended (safety and efficacy have not been clearly demonstrated).
- **Capsules:** 250 mg of wild yam taken one to three times daily is often recommended, or 450 to 900 mg/day of dioscorea extract from wild yam (safety and efficacy have not been clearly demonstrated).
- **Liquid (1:1 in 45% alcohol):** 2 to 4 mL daily in three divided doses has been recommended anecdotally (safety and efficacy have not been clearly demonstrated).
- **Tincture:** 4 to 12 drops or 2 to 4 mL taken three to five times daily has been reported anecdotally (safety and efficacy have not been clearly demonstrated).

Topical

- **Cream:** Wild yam is available as a component of vaginal creams, although there are no universally accepted dosing standards.[6] Systemic steroidal effects of topical preparations have not been demonstrated. Adulteration with synthetic progesterone has been alleged.

Dosing: Pediatric (Younger Than 18 Years)

- Insufficient evidence to recommend. Anecdotally, pediatric doses have been weight-based in proportion to the full dose for a 70-kg (150 pound) adult. Divide the child's weight in kilograms by 70 (or weight in pounds by 150), and multiply the result times the recommended adult dose. Safety and efficacy have not been demonstrated.

Toxicology

- There is limited information available on the toxicology of wild yam. There are anecdotal reports that large doses taken by mouth may produce emesis. The precise dosage that may induce vomiting has not been specified.

ADVERSE EFFECTS/PRECAUTIONS/CONTRAINDICATIONS
Allergy

- Rubbing the skin with *Dioscorea batatas* (a related yam species to *D. villosa*) has been reported to cause allergic contact dermatitis.[7] Among workers with chronic, high-level exposure, *D. batatas* has induced occupational asthma.[8] Cross-allergenicity may occur with other *Dioscorea* species.

Adverse Effects/Postmarket Surveillance

- **Dermatologic:** Contact dermatitis has been reported after rubbing the skin with *D. batatas*, a related yam species.[7]

However, in one report, topical application of wild yam cream was well tolerated in 23 healthy women.[6]
- **Gastrointestinal:** Among seven elderly volunteers given up to 8 wild yam pills daily (standardization or dosage of diosgenin not stated), several women reported gastrointestinal upset at higher doses.[3]
- **Endocrine:** There are anecdotal reports of adulteration of wild yam topical preparations with progesterone.

Precautions/Warnings/Contraindications

- Use cautiously in patients on hormone replacement therapy, oral contraceptives, or with a history of thromboembolic disorders or stroke, because of possible estrogenic/progestinic properties (not supported by scientific studies) and reported adulteration of some wild yam preparations with synthetic progesterone.
- Avoid in pregnancy due to possible progestinic or estrogenic effects (not supported by scientific studies).
- Avoid in patients with hormone-sensitive conditions such as breast, uterine, or ovarian cancer and in patients with endometriosis or uterine fibroids, because of possible progestinic or estrogenic effects (not supported by scientific studies) and anecdotal reports of adulteration with synthetic progesterone.

Pregnancy and Lactation

- Not recommended because of a lack of sufficient data. Wild yam is believed to induce uterine contractions and therefore is frequently not recommended for use during pregnancy.[9] Wild yam is purported to possess progestinic or estrogenic effects (not supported by scientific studies), and there are anecdotal reports of adulteration with synthetic progesterone.

INTERACTIONS
Wild Yam/Drug Interactions

- **Nonsteroidal anti-inflammatory drugs (NSAIDs):** Wild yam has been found to lower serum indomethacin levels and to attenuate indomethacin-induced intestinal inflammation in rats.[10] Human data are lacking.
- **Hormone replacement therapy/oral contraceptives:** In a pilot study, a wild yam preparation was found to suppress progesterone synthesis.[11] However, clinical trial evidence is lacking, and there are anecdotal reports of adulteration with synthetic progesterone.
- **Insulin, oral hypoglycemic agents:** It is unclear to what extent serum glucose is lowered by *Dioscorea villosa* (wild yam), if at all. Although dioscoretine, a component of the related species *Dioscorea dumentorum* (bitter or African yam), has been shown to lower blood glucose in rabbits, this reaction has not been demonstrated for *D. villosa* and has not been documented in humans.[12] Nonetheless, caution is warranted.
- **Fibric acid derivatives (clofibrate [Questran], gemfibrozil [Lopid], fenofibrate [Tricor]):** *Positive interaction*: When given in combination with wild yam, clofibrate has been found to exert a greater lipid-lowering effect in animals.[13,14]
- **Cholesterol-lowering agents:** *Positive interaction*: Diosgenin, the purported active constituent of wild yam, has been found in animals to decrease intestinal cholesterol absorption and to reduce total serum cholesterol levels.[2,13,15-21] Preliminary human evidence from case studies demonstrates reductions in low-density lipoprotein (LDL) and triglycerides and

increases in high-density lipoprotein (HDL) (despite a lack of change in total serum cholesterol), and diosgenin also may potentiate the effects of other lipid-lowering agents.[2,3,13,14,22]

- **General:** Some tinctures contain high concentrations of ethanol, and may lead to vomiting if used concomitantly with disulfiram (Antabuse) or metronidazole (Flagyl).

Wild Yam/Herb/Supplement Interactions

- **Phytoestrogens/phytoprogestins:** In a pilot study, a wild yam preparation was found to suppress endogenous progesterone synthesis.[11] However, clinical trial evidence is lacking, and there are anecdotal reports of adulteration with synthetic progesterone.
- **Hypoglycemic agents:** It is unclear to what extent serum glucose is lowered by *D. villosa* (wild yam), if at all. Although dioscoretine, a component of the related species *D. dumentorum* (bitter or African yam), has been shown to lower blood glucose in rabbits, this reaction has not been demonstrated for *D. villosa* and has not been documented in humans.[12] Nonetheless, caution is warranted.
- **Hypocholesterolemic agents:** *Positive interaction*: Diosgenin, the purported active constituent of wild yam, has been found in animals to decrease intestinal cholesterol absorption and to reduce total serum cholesterol levels.[2,13-21] Preliminary human evidence from case studies demonstrates reductions in LDL and triglycerides and increases in HDL (despite a lack of change in total serum cholesterol), and diosgenin may potentiate the effects of other lipid-lowering agents.[2,3,13,14,22]
- **Vitamin C:** *Positive interaction*: Vitamin C has been shown to enhance the cholesterol-lowering effects of diosgenin and clofibrate.[21]

Wild Yam/Food Interactions

- Insufficient data available.

Wild Yam/Lab Interactions

- **Serum lipids:** Diosgenin, the purported active constituent of wild yam, has been found in animals to decrease intestinal cholesterol absorption and reduce total serum cholesterol levels.[2,13-21] Preliminary human evidence from case studies demonstrates reductions in LDL and triglycerides and increases in HDL (despite a lack of change in total serum cholesterol).[2,3,13,14,22]
- **Serum glucose:** It is unclear to what extent serum glucose is lowered by *D. villosa* (wild yam), if at all. Although dioscoretine, a component of the related species *D. dumentorum* (bitter or African yam), has been shown to lower blood glucose in rabbits, this reaction has not been demonstrated for *D. villosa* and has not been documented in humans.[12] Nonetheless, caution is warranted.

MECHANISM OF ACTION
Pharmacology

- The species considered to be yams are defined by their constituent diosgenin. This saponin is present in species originating in North America or in Asia. Medicinal species include *D. villosa, D. opposita, D. hypoglauca, D. composata, D. deltoida, D. parazeri, D. mastrostachya, D. floribunda,* and *D. barbasco.* The principal Mexican wild yam species are *D. macrostachya* and *D. barbasco.* Common names include Atlantic yam, China root, colic root, devil's bones, Mexican wild yam, rheumatism root, and yuma. African species may not have the same chemical constituents (although African

Dioscorea species possess hypoglycemic effects, hypoglycemia is not observed after administration of Mexican wild yam [*D. macrostachya, D. barbasco*]).

- *D. villosa* includes saponins (diosgenin, dioscin) and an alkaloid (dioscorin).[3,22] Diosgenin is considered the primary active ingredient in wild yam and is structurally similar to cholesterol.
- Diosgenin levels vary markedly among different yam species.[4,5] Consumers can expect a considerable range of diosgenin-related effects based on the source species as well as on techniques of growing, harvesting, and processing and storage conditions. Typical standardization of wild yam products is to 10% diosgenin per dose.
- **Hormonal properties:** Estrogenic and anti-inflammatory effects of diosgenin have been hypothesized to stem from structural similarities to estrogen precursors. However, no natural progesterones, estrogens, or other reproductive hormones are found in *Dioscorea*. Diosgenin is not converted into hormones in the human body and can be transformed into progesterone only through chemical manipulation.[3] Synthetic progesterone has reportedly been added to some wild yam products. In ovariectomized mice, 20 to 40 mg/kg of the wild yam constituent diosgenin, injected subcutaneously each day for 15 days, was found to stimulate mammary gland epithelial growth without observed progestinic effects.[23]
- **Lipid-lowering properties:** Diosgenin has been found in multiple animal studies to decrease intestinal cholesterol absorption and to reduce total serum cholesterol levels. In everted rat jejunum, diosgenin has been found to competitively inhibit cholesterol absorption.[15] Giving Wistar rats 1% diosgenin in their diets increases biliary cholesterol output between 200% to 400%.[16,17] Diosgenin has been found to reduce the total body pool of cholesterol.[18] Hypercholestoleremic rats treated with diosgenin have demonstrated decreased cholesterol absorption, increased hepatic cholesterol synthesis, and increased biliary cholesterol secretion, with no alteration in serum cholesterol.[13,14,19] Hypercholesterolemic mice fed a 1% diosgenin diet for 15 days were shown to have decreased cholesterol absorption, increased fecal excretion of cholesterol, and decreased plasma cholesterol levels.[20] Hypercholesterolemic rats fed both clofibrate and diosgenin have shown a greater decrease in LDL cholesterol than that in rats fed either compound alone; however, the combination partially reversed the elevation in HDL cholesterol seen in the diosgenin-only group.[13]
- Administering vitamin C enhanced the cholesterol—lowering effects of clofibrate and diosgenin.[21] In hypercholesterolemic monkeys, a synthetic analog of diosgenin decreased absorption of dietary cholesterol, increased biliary secretion of endogenous cholesterol, and reduced hypercholesterolemia.[2]
- In rats, oral administration of diosgenin increases cholesterol and phospholipid content in hepatocyte cell membranes while maintaining cholesterol/phospholipid molar ratios. Secretion of surfactant-like cholesterol and lipid vesicles also increases. These changes have been hypothesized to mediate protection against bile salt toxicity.[24]
- **Other properties:** Feeding rats a 0.5% diosgenin diet for 7 days almost completely prevents indomethacin-induced ulcers and lowers serum indomethacin levels.[10] In rats with cholestasis induced by estradiol-17β, diosgenin increases biliary secretion. However, estrogen-induced morphologic changes appear to be unaffected.[24] Diosgenin and dioscin have been shown to inhibit fungal growth *in vitro*.[1]

W

Pharmacodynamics/Kinetics

- After oral administration, diosgenin is metabolized in the liver and eliminated via the bile.[14]

HISTORY

- *Dioscorea villosa* (wild yam) is a perennial vine with a pale brown, cylindrical, twisted rhizome and a thin, red-brown, and woolly stem up to 12 meters long. The leaves are broad and oval. The plant has small greenish-yellow flowers. Although the purportedly active wild yam constituent diosgenin is present in both the leaves and the root, it is the root that is used medicinally. Worldwide, there are over 600 species of yam plants, of which 25 are edible. Notably, "yams" sold in the supermarket are actually members of the sweet potato family and are not true yams.
- *Dioscorea* is indigenous to North America but is now widely cultivated in tropical and subtropical regions worldwide.

REVIEW OF THE EVIDENCE: TABLE

- No studies qualify for inclusion in the evidence table

REVIEW OF THE EVIDENCE: DISCUSSION

Menopausal Symptoms

Summary

- Wild yam (*Dioscorea*) preparations are used to treat dysmenorrhea, hot flashes, and headaches associated with menopause. Manufacturers of a vaginal cream containing *Dioscorea* have claimed that the cream possesses progesterone-like effects and is a source of "natural hormones," although this claim is not supported by animal or human studies. Steroidal effects may be attributable to the presence of synthetic progesterone, which is sometimes added to commercial wild yam products. Some marketers also promote wild yam as a natural precursor of DHEA, which is unfounded in science. At this time, there is inconclusive evidence regarding the use of wild yam for menopausal symptoms.

Evidence

- Wild yam extract cream was used by 23 healthy menopausal women in a double-blind, placebo-controlled trial.[6] At the end of 3 months, there were nonsignificant mild improvements in both groups as evidenced by decreased diurnal flushing frequency, severity of non-flushing symptoms, and nocturnal sweating. Markers of menstrual status, such as serum follicle-stimulating hormone (FSH) and estradiol, were unchanged.
- In a randomized, controlled trial comprising 13 menopausal women given a combination herbal compound containing wild yam root, burdock root, licorice root, motherwort, and angelica root for 3 months (2 capsules three times a day, precise dosages of individual ingredients not described), decreases in menopausal symptoms in the active treatment group were noted but were not statistically significant.[25] The amount of wild yam present in this combination was likely lower than in recommended doses for monotherapy.

Hyperlipidemia

Summary

- Diosgenin, a constituent of wild yam, has been found in multiple animal studies to decrease intestinal cholesterol absorption and to reduce total serum cholesterol levels.[2,13-21] Limited human evidence from case studies appears promising, demonstrating reductions in low-density lipoprotein (LDL) and triglycerides and increases in high-density

lipoprotein (HDL) (despite a lack of change in total serum cholesterol). Additional data from properly randomized trials are required before a firm conclusion can be drawn. In addition, it should be noted that lipid levels serve as surrogate markers for diseases with significant morbidity and mortality, such as myocardial infarction and stroke. Convincing studies of efficacy would include these as end points, rather than serum markers.

Evidence

- In a case series, seven elderly adults who took up to 8 wild yam pills daily over a period of 6 weeks (individual doses were not stated) experienced significant decreases in serum triglycerides and phospholipids, increased serum HDL, and unchanged total serum cholesterol.[3] These findings lend support to the results of a poorly described 1970s case series in which patients with ischemic heart disease treated with *Dioscorea* were reported to show a significant decrease in serum triglycerides without a significant change in serum total cholesterol level.[22]
- Wild yam has not been used historically to treat cardiovascular disease. However, in view of its potential effects on lipid metabolism, it has been suggested as an adjunct hypocholesterolemic agent.[2]

Hormonal Properties (Estrogenic, Progestinic, DHEA-like)

Summary

- Manufacturers of vaginal creams containing *Dioscorea* (wild yam) have claimed that the preparations possess progesterone-like effects, although this claim is not supported by animal or human studies. Hormonal effects may be attributable to the presence of synthetic progesterone, which is allegedly sometimes added to commercial wild yam products. Some marketers also promote wild yam as a natural precursor of DHEA, although these claims are also not supported by science. Estrogenic effects of the wild yam constituent diosgenin have been hypothesized to stem from structural similarities to estrogen precursors. However, no natural progestins, estrogens, or other reproductive hormones are found in *Dioscorea*. Diosgenin is not converted to hormones in the human body, and can only be transformed into progesterone through chemical manipulation.[3] At this time, as supported by historical, pharmacologic, and preliminary human data, it appears that wild yam does not possess efficacy as a hormonal agent.

Evidence

- In a pilot study of women using wild yam products (*D. villosa*), it was found that progesterone synthesis was suppressed compared with controls.[26] However, no direct effect of wild yam extract on the estrogen or progesterone receptors was found. The preparation was not tested for the presence of synthetic progesterone adulterants.
- Among seven elderly volunteers given up to 8 wild yam pills daily (the dosage of diosgenin was not stated), there were no measured increases in serum DHEA.[3]
- Wild yam extract cream was used by 23 healthy menopausal women in a double-blind, placebo-controlled trial.[6] At the end of 3 months, there were no changes in FSH, glucose, estradiol, serum or salivary progesterone, weight, blood pressure, total cholesterol level, triglycerides, or high-density lipoprotein (HDL). There was mild improvement in both groups, as evidenced by decreased diurnal flushing frequency,

severity of non-flushing symptoms, and nocturnal sweating, that was found to be statistically insignificant.

References

1. Vasiukova NI, Paseshnichenko VA, Davydova MA, et al. [Fungiotoxic properties of steroid saponins from the rhizomes of deltoid dioscorea]. Prikl Biokhim Mikrobiol 1977;13(2):172-176.
2. Malinow MR, Elliott WH, McLaughlin P, et al. Effects of synthetic glycosides on steroid balance in Macaca fascicularis. J Lipid Res 1987; 28(1):1-9.
3. Araghiniknam M, Chung S, Nelson-White T, et al. Antioxidant activity of Dioscorea and dehydroepiandrosterone (DHEA) in older humans. Life Sciences 1996;59:L147-L157.
4. Datta K, Datta SK, Datta PC. Pharmacognostic evaluation of potential yams Dioscorea. Journal of Economic and Taxonomic Botany 1984;5:181-196.
5. Huai ZP, Ding ZZ, He SA, et al. [Research on correlations between climatic factors and diosgenin content in Dioscorea zingiberensis Wright]. Yao Xue Xue Bao 1989;24(9):702-706.
6. Komesaroff PA, Black CV, Cable V, et al. Effects of wild yam extract on menopausal symptoms, lipids and sex hormones in healthy menopausal women. Climacteric 2001;4(2):144-150.
7. Kubo Y, Nonaka S, Yoshida H. Allergic contact dermatitis from Dioscorea batatas Decaisne. Contact Dermatitis 1988;18(2):111-112.
8. Park HS, Kim MJ, Moon HB. Occupational asthma caused by two herb materials, Dioscorea batatas and Pinellia ternata. Clin Exp Allergy 1994; 24(6):575-581.
9. Boikova VV, Korkhov VV, Paseshnichenko VA. Contraceptive activity of deltonin isolated from Dioscorea-Deltoida wall. Rastitel'nye Resursy 1990; 26(1):85-88.
10. Yamada T, Hoshino M, Hayakawa T, et al. Dietary diosgenin attenuates subacute intestinal inflammation associated with indomethacin in rats. Am J Physiol 1997;273(2 Pt 1):G355-G364.
11. Smolinske SC. Dietary supplement-drug interactions. J Am Med Womens Assoc 1999;54(4):191-2,195.
12. Iwu MM, Okunji CO, Ohiaeri GO, et al. Hypoglycaemic activity of dioscoretine from tubers of Dioscorea dumetorum in normal and alloxan diabetic rabbits. Planta Med 1990;56(3):264-267.
13. Cayen MN, Dvornik D. Effect of diosgenin on lipid metabolism in rats. J Lipid Res 1979;20(2):162-174.
14. Cayen MN, Ferdinandi ES, Greselin E, et al. Studies on the disposition of diosgenin in rats, dogs, monkeys and man. Atherosclerosis 1979;33(1): 71-87.
15. Juarez-Oropeza MA, Diaz-Zagoya JC, Rabinowitz JL. In vivo and *in vitro* studies of hypocholesterolemic effects of diosgenin in rats. Int J Biochem 1987;19(8):679-683.
16. Ulloa N, Nervi F. Mechanism and kinetic characteristics of the uncoupling by plant steroids of biliary cholesterol from bile salt output. Biochim Biophys Acta 1985;837(2):181-189.
17. Nervi F, Bronfman M, Allalon W, et al. Regulation of biliary cholesterol secretion in the rat. Role of hepatic cholesterol esterification. J Clin Invest 1984;74(6):2226-2237.
18. Zagoya JCD, Laguna J, Guzman-Garcia J. Studies on the regulation of cholesterol metabolism by the use of structural analogue, diosgenin. Biochemical Pharmacology 1971;20:3471-3480.
19. Nervi F, Marinovic I, Rigotti A, et al. Regulation of biliary cholesterol secretion. Functional relationship between the canalicular and sinusoidal cholesterol secretory pathways in the rat. J Clin Invest 1988;82(6):1818-1825.
20. Uchida K, Takase H, Nomura Y, et al. Changes in biliary and fecal bile acids in mice after treatments with diosgenin and beta-sitosterol. J Lipid Res 1984;25(3):236-245.
21. Odumosu A. How vitamin C, clofibrate and diosgenin control cholesterol metabolism in male guinea-pigs. Int J Vitam Nutr Res Suppl 1982;23: 187-195.
22. Zakharov VN. [Hypolipemic effect of diosponine in ischemic heart disease depending on the type of hyperlipoproteinemia]. Kardiologiia 1977;17(6): 136-137.
23. Aradhana, Rao AR, Kale RK. Diosgenin—a growth stimulator of mammary gland of ovariectomized mouse. Indian J Exp Biol 1992;30(5):367-370.
24. Accatino L, Pizarro M, Solis N, et al. Effects of diosgenin, a plant-derived steroid, on bile secretion and hepatocellular cholestasis induced by estrogens in the rat. Hepatology 1998;28(1):129-140.
25. Hudson t, Standish L, Breed C, et al. Clinical and endocrinological effects of a menopausal botanical formula. J Naturopath Med 1997;7:73-77.
26. Zava DT, Dollbaum CM, Blen M. Estrogen and progestin bioactivity of foods, herbs, and spices. Proc Soc Exp Biol Med 1998;217(3):369-378.

W

Yohimbe Bark Extract

(*Pausinystalia yohimbe* Pierre ex Beille)

SYNONYMS/COMMON NAMES/RELATED SUBSTANCES

- Aphrodien, *Corynanthe johimbi*, *Corynanthe yohimbi*, corynine, johimbi, *Pausinystalia johimbe*, *Pausinystalia johimbe* (Schumann) Beille quebrachine, Rubiaceae, yohimbe bark extract, yohimbehe, yohimbehe cortex, yohimbeherinde, yohimbene, yohimbime, yohimbine, yohimbine hydrochloride.

CLINICAL BOTTOM LINE
Background

- The terms *yohimbine*, *yohimbine hydrochloride*, and *yohimbe bark extract* are related but not interchangeable. Yohimbine is an active indole alkaloid constituent found in the bark of the *Pausinystalia yohimbe* tree. Yohimbine hydrochloride is a standardized form of yohimbine that is available as a prescription drug in the United States and has been demonstrated in clinical trials to be effective in the treatment of erectile dysfunction. Yohimbine hydrochloride has also been used for the treatment of sexual side effects induced by antidepressants (selective serotonin reuptake inhibitors [SSRIs]), to treat female hyposexual disorder, as a pressor agent in autonomic failure, for xerostomia, and as a probe for noradrenergic activity.
- In contrast, there is a paucity of clinical research utilizing yohimbe bark extract, which generally contains low concentrations of yohimbine (6% indole alkaloids, of which only 10% to 15% is yohimbine), and commercial preparations may or may not share the pharmacologic and clinical effects of yohimbine hydrochloride.[1] A 1995 chemical analysis of 26 commercial yohimbe products reported that most commercial yohimbe products contain virtually no yohimbine.[1] Traditionally, yohimbe bark was used as an aphrodisiac and mild hallucinogen. However, all information related to its efficacy is folkloric, empirical, and anecdotal or extrapolated from studies of yohimbine hydrochloride.
- Most commercial sources of yohimbe bark extract do not state the level of yohimbine alkaloid content per dosage.

Therefore, use of pure pharmaceutical-derived yohimbine hydrochloride is the only method of ingesting an exact content of yohimbine.[2] Given the pronounced pharmacologic properties of yohimbine, the use of yohimbe bark products that do not give an indication of indole alkaloid content is potentially dangerous.

Historical or Theoretical Uses That Lack Sufficient Evidence

- Aphrodisiac, Alzheimer's disease,[3,4] anesthetic, angina, aphrodisiac, atherosclerosis, chest pain, clonidine overdose, cognition,[5] coronary artery disease, coughs, depression, diabetic complications, diabetic neuropathy, exhaustion, feebleness, fevers, hallucinogenic, hyperlipidemia, hypotension,[6-9] insomnia,[10] leprosy, narcolepsy,[11,12] obesity,[13-16] panic disorder,[17] Parkinson's disease,[9,18] postural hypotension, pupil dilator, schizophrenia (decreasing auditory evoked response/sensory gating),[19] syncope (neurally mediated).[20]

Expert Opinion and Folkloric Precedent

- For over a century, yohimbine has been used as a treatment for erectile dysfunction, and this remains the most popular use of this extract. It has long been thought to be an aphrodisiac and has also been smoked as a hallucinogen. Yohimbe has also been used in traditional medicine to treat hypertension, angina, and age-related cognitive disorders.
- Although yohimbe bark extract has been used in Germany for the treatment of sexual disorders, "feebleness," and "exhaustion," the expert German panel, the Commission E, does not recommend its use because of a high risk-benefit ratio.

Safety Summary

- *Note:* Because of the potential for serious side effects and interactions, the U.S. Food and Drug Administration has found yohimbine to be unsafe for over-the-counter sale. Because yohimbe bark may contain clinically significant amounts of yohimbine alkaloid, similar risks may apply. Notably, many yohimbe bark products contain only low levels of yohimbine that may not carry these risks, although most yohimbe bark products are not standardized to yohimbine content.
- **Likely safe:** When taken by adults in recommended oral doses under the direction and supervision of a qualified healthcare professional. Doses of yohimbine in clinical trials have ranged from 15 to 30 mg for 2 to 10 weeks.[21-27]
- **Possibly safe:** When used without the supervision of a qualified healthcare professional.[28-31]
- **Possibly unsafe:** In large doses, as the yohimbe constituent yohimbine has been noted to cause severe hypotension and cardiac conduction disorders.
- **Likely unsafe:** Avoid in pregnancy, as the yohimbe constituent yohimbine may potentially act as a uterine relaxant and fetal toxin. Avoid yohimbine during lactation and in children, due to reports of death in children. Yohimbine should be avoided in diabetics or patients taking agents with monoamine oxidase inhibitor (MAOI) activity because of yohimbine's MAOI activity. Use yohimbine cautiously in

Scientific Evidence for Common/Studied Uses	Grade*
Autonomic failure	C
Inhibition of platelet aggregation	C
Libido (women)	C
Male erectile dysfunction	C
Sexual side effects of selective serotonin reuptake inhibitors (SSRIs)	C
Xerostomia (psychotropic drug induced)	C

*Key to grades: *A:* Strong scientific evidence for this use; *B:* Good scientific evidence for this use; *C:* Unclear scientific evidence for this use; *D:* Fair scientific evidence against this use (it may not work); *F:* Strong scientific evidence against this use (it likely does not work). For a more detailed explanation of efficacy criteria, see "Natural Standard Evidence-Based Validated Grading Rationale" in the Introduction.

patients with cardiac disease or at risk for hypotension because of cardiovascular effects. Use yohimbine cautiously in patients with liver and kidney disease and with schizophrenia.

DOSING/TOXICOLOGY
General

- Recommended doses are based on those most commonly used in available trials, or on historical practice. However, with natural products, the optimal doses needed to balance efficacy and safety often have not been determined. Formulations and preparation methods may vary from manufacturer to manufacturer, and from batch to batch of a specific product made by a single manufacturer. Because often the active components of a product are not known, standardization may not be possible, and the clinical effects of different brands may not be comparable.

Standardization

- Standardization has not been widely established to regulate the production of yohimbe bark extract products.
- A gas chromatographic chemical analysis of 26 commercial yohimbe products conducted by Betz et al. concluded that most commercial yohimbe products contain virtually no yohimbine. Concentrations of yohimbine ranging from <0.1 to 489 parts per million (ppm) were found in the products. Nine of the 26 products contained no yohimbine, and 7 of the 26 contained trace amounts (0.1 to 1 ppm). This was compared to a standard containing 7089 ppm.[1]
- Yohimbine tablets are commonly standardized to contain 5.4 mg of yohimbine hydrochloride.

Dosing: Adult (18 Years and Older)
Oral

- *Note:* Recommended doses are based on those most commonly used in available trials for pharmaceutical standardized yohimbine hydrochloride. No clinical studies are available for administration of over-the-counter yohimbe.
- **Impotence with vascular or diabetic origin:** 16 to 18 mg of yohimbine hydrochloride daily in divided doses.
- **Erectile dysfunction (impotence):** 16 to 30 mg of yohimbine hydrochloride daily in three divided doses (e.g., 5.4 to 10 mg three times daily). More adverse effects occur with higher doses.[28,32,33]
- **Orthostatic hypotension:** 12.5 mg yohimbine hydrochloride daily (limited available evidence).
- **Antidepressant (selective serotonin reuptake inhibitors [SSRIs])-induced sexual side effects:** 18 mg of yohimbine hydrochloride daily or 15 mg of yohimbine hydrochloride daily when used with trazodone.[34]

Tea

- A tea can be prepared by simmering 5 to 10 teaspoons of shaved yohimbe bark in 1 pint of water (with a further recommendation of adding 0.5 to 1.0 g of Vitamin C to the tea, which converts the alkaloid to a more water-soluble ascorbate).[35] Safety and efficacy data are lacking.

Dosing: Pediatric (Younger Than 18 Years)

- Yohimbe is not recommended for use in children.

Toxicology

- Symptoms of toxicity from yohimbine, a constituent of yohimbe, include paralysis, severe hypotension, cardiac conduction disorders, cardiac failure, and death. These same

risks may extend to yohimbe bark extract, depending on the concentration of yohimbine present and dose ingested.
- A mouse study demonstrated no protection against yohimbine toxicity by adrafinil, whereas clonidine was shown to antagonize the yohimbine toxicity at doses of 5 and 15 mg/kg. The LD_{50} of yohimbine was calculated to be 40 mg/kg.[35-46]

ADVERSE EFFECTS/PRECAUTIONS/CONTRAINDICATIONS
Allergy

- Known allergy/hypersensitivity to yohimbe, any of its constituents, or yohimbine-containing products.

Adverse Effects/Postmarket Surveillance

- **General:** Multiple adverse effects have been associated with the use of yohimbine hydrochloride. In theory, these effects may also apply to yohimbe bark extract, which contains variable (albeit low) concentrations of yohimbine alkaloid. Evidence suggests that yohimbine is tolerated in recommended doses, and that if adverse effects become apparent, discontinuance of the product will likely discontinue the effects.
- **Dermatologic:** Rash, erythrodermic skin eruption, exanthema, and flushing have been reported with use of yohimbine.[37] In theory, these effects may also occur with the use of yohimbe bark extract. Skin flushing and piloerection have been associated with the use of yohimbe bark extract (anecdotal).
- **Neurologic/CNS:** Yohimbine has been associated with reports of general CNS and autonomic excitation, tremulousness,[38-40] head twitching, seizure threshold changes,[41] and enhanced brain norepinephrine release (increasing resting heart rate and blood pressure).[42] Yohimbine has been associated with increased and decreased locomotor activity in rats.[41] Yohimbine has also been shown to dose-dependently induce clonic seizures in mice.[43] Because yohimbine crosses the blood-brain barrier, it may elicit a centrally mediated increase in sympathetic output and peripheral presynaptic transmitter release.[44] In theory, these effects may also occur with the use of yohimbe bark extract. Anecdotal reports have noted agitation, dizziness, headache, irritability, nervousness, tremors, and insomnia with the use of yohimbe bark extract.
- **Ocular/Otic:** Mydriasis has been noted anecdotally.
- **Psychiatric:** Yohimbine is usually not recommended for use in psychiatric patients because of reports of excitation, tremor, insomnia, anxiety, irritability, the potential to trigger psychoses in predisposed patients, and possible exacerbation of post-traumatic stress disorder (PTSD).[45-53] Yohimbine may also precipitate panic attacks, anxiety, and manic episodes in predisposed patients.[42,54-61] Increased acoustic startle reflexes and fear have been noted.[62,63] In theory, these effects may also occur with the use of yohimbe bark extract.
- **Pulmonary/Respiratory:** Bronchospasm, cough, and rhinorrhea have been documented with use of yohimbine, and theoretically may also occur with yohimbe bark extract.[46,64]
- **Cardiovascular:** Small concentrations of yohimbine have been associated with hypertension, whereas higher doses may elicit hypotension.[65] Tachycardia, fluid retention, and chest discomfort have also been reported with use of yohimbine.[4,19,44,65-71] Conduction abnormalities may occur. In theory, these effects may also occur with the use of yohimbe bark extract.
- **Gastrointestinal:** Nausea, vomiting, increased lacrimal secretion (salivation), and diarrhea may occur with yohimbine

Y

use.[72-76] Yohimbine is generally avoided in patients with peptic ulcer disease. In theory, these effects may also occur with the use of yohimbe bark extract. Anorexia has been associated with the use of yohimbe bark extract (anecdotal).

- **Renal:** Use should be avoided in kidney disease because of possible antidiuretic effects of yohimbine. Renal failure and urinary frequency have been reported.[37,46,48] Dysuria has been associated anecdotally with yohimbe bark extract use.
- **Genitourinary:** Genital pain has been associated with yohimbe bark extract use (anecdotal).
- **Hematologic:** Drug-induced agranulocytosis has been noted. Yohimbine may inhibit platelet aggregation by binding to the alpha-2 adrenoceptor responsible for noradrenaline-induced platelet aggregation, and may increase risk of bleeding.[77-82]
- **Musculoskeletal:** Muscle aches have been noted.[46]
- **Rheumatologic:** A 42-year-old man developed a lupus-like syndrome after ingesting yohimbine at a dose of 5.4 mg three times daily for 1 day.[37]

Precautions/Warnings/Contraindications

- Avoid use in pregnant and lactating patients.
- Avoid use in children.
- Avoid use in patients with benign prostatic hypertrophy (BPH), as yohimbine, the active constituent of yohimbe, may exacerbate symptoms of BPH, due to its presynaptic alpha-2 blocking ability.
- Avoid use in patients with anxiety, mania, bipolar disorder, post-traumatic stress disorder, or depression, as yohimbine may cause or exacerbate anxiety or suicidality.[54,56,57,83]
- Avoid use in schizophrenic patients, as yohimbine may activate psychosis.
- Use cautiously in patients with hypertension, cardiac disease, or using hypotensive agents, as small amounts of yohimbine may increase blood pressure, whereas higher doses may elicit hypotension.[48,56]
- Use cautiously in patients with peptic ulcer disease.
- Use cautiously in patients with liver or kidney disease.[48]
- Use cautiously in patients taking hypoglycemic agents, based on unclear anecdotal reports of increased effects.

Pregnancy and Lactation

- Yohimbe should be avoided during pregnancy. Yohimbe may act as a uterine relaxant and fetal toxin.
- Yohimbe should be avoided during lactation. Deaths have been reported in children.

INTERACTIONS
Yohimbe/Drug Interactions

- **Drugs metabolized by cytochrome P450 (CYP):** Drugs that inhibit CYP3A3 or CYP3A4 may elicit increases in serum levels of yohimbine. Likewise, drugs that induce these enzymes may result in decreases in serum levels.
- **Ethanol:** Concomitant use of ethanol with yohimbine produces an additive effect of increasing severity of acute intoxication.[61] In theory, this interaction may also apply to yohimbe bark extract, which contains variable (albeit low) concentrations of yohimbine alkaloid.
- **Adrenergic or antiadrenergic drugs:** Yohimbine, an alpha-adrenergic blocker, has been reported to antagonize the effects of alpha-adrenergic drugs and may potentiate the effects of antiadrenergic agents such as clonidine and guanabenz.[5,84,85] In theory, this interaction may also apply

to yohimbe bark extract, which contains variable (albeit low) concentrations of yohimbine alkaloid.
- **Benzodiazepines:** Concomitant yohimbine administration antagonizes the effects of alprazolam on blood pressure and attenuates alprazolam induced changes in cortisol.[86]
- **Antihypertensive drugs:** Yohimbine may interfere with blood pressure control and should be used cautiously with other hypotensive agents. In theory, this interaction may also apply to yohimbe bark extract, which contains variable (albeit low) concentrations of yohimbine alkaloid. Beta blockers may possess a protective role against yohimbine toxicity.
- **Monoamine oxidase inhibitor (MAOI) antidepressants:** Due to MAOI activity of yohimbine, concomitant use may produce additive effects. In theory, this interaction may also apply to yohimbe bark extract, which contains variable (albeit low) concentrations of yohimbine alkaloid.
- **Linezolid:** Due to MAOI activity, use of linezolid with yohimbine may lead to additive effects or toxicity, and should be avoided.
- **Morphine:** Although yohimbine by itself does not appear to possess analgesic effects, yohimbine may enhance morphine analgesia, based on the results of a controlled trial.[87,88] In theory, this interaction may also apply to yohimbe bark extract, which contains variable (albeit low) concentrations of yohimbine alkaloid.
- **Opioid antagonists, naltrexone/naloxone:** Yohimbine may increase or decrease naloxone-precipitated withdrawal symptoms.[86,89,90] In theory, this interaction may also apply to yohimbe bark extract, which contains variable (albeit low) concentrations of yohimbine alkaloid.
- **Phenothiazine drugs:** Concomitant use is contraindicated because of an increased risk of alpha-2 adrenergic antagonism.
- **Physostigmine:** Concomitant use of yohimbine and physostigmine in patients with Alzheimer's disease has been associated in a pilot study with anxiety, agitation, restlessness, and chest pain.[4]
- **Sympathomimetic drugs:** Concomitant use of yohimbine is contraindicated because of an increased risk of hypertensive crisis due to yohimbine's MAOI activity.
- **Tricyclic antidepressants:** Concomitant yohimbine should be used cautiously because of potential effects on blood pressure.
- **Diabetes medications:** Anecdotally, yohimbine has been reported to increase the effects of diabetic medications, including insulin, although there is limited reliable scientific evidence in this area.
- **Antihistamines:** Use of yohimbine with antihistamines has been cautioned anecdotally, although there is limited reliable scientific evidence in this area.
- **Amphetamines:** Use of yohimbine with amphetamines has been cautioned anecdotally, although there is limited reliable scientific evidence in this area.
- **Antimuscarinic agents:** Concomitant use with antimuscarinic agents may result in transient increased risk of toxicity (anecdotal).

Yohimbe/Herb/Supplement Interactions

- **Hypotensive/hypertensive herbs and supplements:** Yohimbine may interfere with blood pressure control and should be used cautiously with other agents that affect blood pressure. In theory, these interactions may also apply to yohimbe bark extract, which contains variable (albeit low) concentrations of yohimbine alkaloid. There are anecdotal reports of a risk of hypertensive crisis when yohimbe is used concomitantly with ephedra.

- **Monoamine oxidase inhibitor (MAOI) herbs and supplements:** Due to MAOI activity of yohimbine, concomitant use may produce additive effects. In theory, this interaction may also apply to yohimbe bark extract, which contains variable (albeit low) concentrations of yohimbine alkaloid.
- **Caffeine-containing agents:** Caffeine-containing agents such as coffee, tea, cola, guarana, and mate may theoretically increase the risk of hypertensive crisis when taken with yohimbine.
- **Over-the-counter (OTC) stimulants:** OTC products containing stimulants, including caffeine, phenylephrine, phenylpropanolamine (removed from the U.S. market), may lead to additive effects when used in combination with yohimbe bark extract (anecdotal).
- **Hypoglycemic herbs and supplements:** Anecdotally, yohimbine has been reported to increase the effects of diabetic medications, including insulin, although there is limited reliable scientific evidence in this area. It is not clear if these potential effects extend to hypoglycemic herbs and supplements.
- **Goldenseal, berberine:** Berberine, an alkaloid present in goldenseal, has been shown to competitively inhibit the binding of yohimbine to cell surface receptors, which may or may not affect pharmacologic actions when the two agents are administered concurrently.[91]

Yohimbe/Food Interactions

- **Tyramine-containing foods:** Because of the monoamine oxidase inhibitor (MAOI) activity of yohimbine, tyramine-containing foods, including red wines, fermented meats, and aged cheeses, theoretically may increase the risk of hypertensive crisis when taken concomitantly with yohimbine. In theory, this interaction may also apply to yohimbe bark extract, which contains variable (albeit low) concentrations of yohimbine alkaloid.
- **Caffeine-containing foods:** Foods that increase blood pressure, such as coffee, tea, cola, or chocolate, theoretically may increase the risk of hypertensive crisis when taken concomitantly with yohimbine.

Yohimbe/Lab Interactions

- Insufficient available data.

MECHANISM OF ACTION
Pharmacology

- **Constituents:** Yohimbe bark extract contains approximately 6% indole alkaloids, of which 10% to 15% is yohimbine. A 1995 chemical analysis of 26 commercial yohimbe products reported that most commercial yohimbe products contained virtually no yohimbine.[1] The pharmacologic activity of yohimbine has been well characterized in studies, although these effects may or may not apply to yohimbe, depending on the concentration of yohimbine present.
- **Alpha-2 adrenergic antagonist effects:** Yohimbine acts as an alpha-2 adrenoceptor antagonist. It is significantly more active at presynaptic adrenoceptors than at postsynaptic receptors. This action blocks the decrease in central noradrenergic response and the reduction in peripheral sympathetic activity.[39,46,72,92-95] In 1975, Papeschi and Theiss demonstrated the dopamine antagonistic properties and serotonin-like properties of yohimbine.[96]

- Yohimbine inhibits monoamine oxidase and blocks calcium channel and peripheral serotonin receptors.
- Genital blood vessel dilation, nerve impulse transmission to genital tissue and increased reflex excitability in the sacral region of the spinal cord appear to be responsible for yohimbine's aphrodisiac activity. Yohimbine is most effective for impotence in men with organic vascular dysfunction. Yohimbine's effects on impotence are mediated through increased penile blood flow and increased central excitatory impulses to the genital tissue.[97,98]
- A clinical randomized control study demonstrated that yohimbine does not influence the function of the alpha-2 adrenoceptors on adipocytes and does not facilitate weight loss, as previously thought.[15,99]
- **Platelet aggregation inhibition:** Yohimbine has been found to inhibit epinephrine-induced platelet aggregation *ex vivo*; the lowest dose of yohimbine that significantly inhibited platelet aggregation was 8 mg.[78]
- **Norepinephrine effects:** Yohimbine acts centrally to increase sympathetic outflow, and peripherally to increase the release of norepinephrine from adrenergic nerve terminals. This increases the plasma norepinephrine, and elicits pressor effects.[20,32,40,100,101]
- **Hormonal effects:** Yohimbine was demonstrated to produce an increase in plasma prolactin levels in rats.[102] This study suggested that the increased prolactin levels were not caused by anti-dopaminergic effects, and possibly occurred through a mechanism related to prolactin-releasing factor. Yohimbine has been reported to possess mild antidiuretic effects, possibly due to stimulation of hypothalamic centers and release of pituitary hormones.
- **Insulin effects:** In a study of type 1 and type 2 diabetic rats, pretreatment with yohimbine potentiated glucose-induced insulin release in no-diabetic control rats, and an improvement of oral glucose tolerance in type 2 diabetic rats, but not in type 1 diabetic rats. Yohimbine may act via blockade of postsynaptic alpha-2 adrenoceptors to produce insulinotropic and hypoglycemic effects.[103]

Pharmacodynamics/Kinetics

- **Bioavailability:** Yohimbine's oral absorption appears to be poor, although there seems to be highly variable bioavailability. This may be the result of extensive first-pass metabolism.[104] Yohimbine displays dose-related increases in area under the curve (AUC).[104,105] There is a significant correlation between plasma norepinephrine levels and yohimbine AUC or C_{max}.[104] According to one pharmacokinetic study, a 10-mg oral dose of yohimbine produced a peak plasma concentration within 45 minutes and the half-life for plasma clearance was 0.2 to 1.1 hours. Yohimbine is fairly lipophilic and it crosses the blood-brain barrier.[106] Since alpha adrenoceptors are located in widespread locations throughout the central and peripheral nervous system, yohimbine has a variety of autonomic and psychic effects (increased noradrenaline release). As a result, yohimbine was shown to induce lipid mobilization in obese subjects.[16] In a single-dose study of yohimbine in young healthy, older healthy, and Alzheimer's patients, the authors found that the plasma disposition of yohimbine displayed large variability with no significant differences among subject groups. However, the C_{max} and AUC of the active metabolite 11-hydroxy-yohimbine were significantly lower in the older healthy subjects than in the young healthy subjects and

Y

Alzheimer's patients. They also found a strong positive correlation between cerebrospinal fluid (CSF) and plasma yohimbine concentrations and a weak positive correlation between CSF and plasma concentrations of 11-hydroxy-yohimbine.[107]

- **Elimination:** Yohimbine has an elimination half-life of less than 1 hour, whereas the active metabolite 11-hydroxy-yohimbine has a half-life of about 6 hours.[104] In a study of 32 patients, 24 displayed one-compartment elimination while 8 displayed two-compartment elimination.[104] Less than 1% of the oral dose was recovered unchanged in the urine within 24 hours.[106]

HISTORY

- Yohimbine is derived from the bark (of the trunk and branches) of an evergreen tree native to West Africa (Congo, Zaire, Cameroon, Nigeria, and Gabon). The corklike bark of the yohimbe tree contains the indole alkaloid yohimbine. The bark may be composed of approximately 6% alkaloids, of which only 10% to 15% percent is yohimbine. Yohimbine is a selective antagonist of alpha-2 receptors.
- Traditionally, yohimbe bark has been used to treat angina and hypertension and was smoked as a hallucinogen.
- Yohimbine hydrochloride is a standardized form of yohimbine that is available as a prescription drug in the United States. Yohimbine hydrochloride is used primarily for erectile dysfunction and in clinical trials as a probe for noradrenergic activity. Although erectile dysfunction is not a life-threatening condition, it may result in significant reduction in quality of life. According to the National Institutes of Health, as many as 30 million men may be affected in the United States alone.

Review of the Evidence: Yohimbe Bark Extract

Condition Treated*	Study Design	Author, Year	N[†]	SS[†]	Study Quality[‡]	Magnitude of Benefit	ARR[†]	NNT[†]	Comments
Erectile dysfunction	Meta-analysis (4 independent convergent meta-analyses)	Carey[30] 1996	874	Yes	NA	Large	NA	NA	Included 16 studies of yohimbine hydrochloride, not yohimbe bark extract; consistent improvement in erectile dysfunction compared to placebo.
Erectile dysfunction	Meta-analysis	Ernst[108] 1998	7 trials	Yes	NA	Large	NA	NA	Study of yohimbine hydrochloride, not yohimbe bark extract; benefits of yohimbine appeared to outweigh risks.
Erectile dysfunction	Meta-analysis	Yan 2000	234	Yes	3	NA	35-39%	3	Study of yohimbine hydrochloride, not yohimbe bark extract; mean age, 41 years; 5.4 mg of yohimbine t.i.d., then 10.8 mg t.i.d., with Viagra 60 minutes prior to intercourse; patients with different etiologies of erectile dysfunction. Minimal adverse effects: mild headache, flushing, tachycardia, bloating
Erectile dysfunction	RPCT, double-blind, crossover	Rowland[27] 1997	11	Yes	3	Medium	64%	2	Study of yohimbine hydrochloride, not yohimbe bark extract; mean age, 49 years; 5-10 mg of yohimbine t.i.d. for 4 weeks. Minimal adverse effects: diarrhea, frequent urination, lack of energy.
Erectile dysfunction due to organic or non-organic etiology	RPCT, double-blind	Mann[25] 1996	30	No	3	NA	20%	5	Study of yohimbine hydrochloride, not yohimbe bark extract; mean age, 43 years; 5 mg of oral yohimbine t.i.d.; small sample size. Adverse effects: sweating, agitation, anxiety, headache, tachycardia, GI disturbances
Erectile dysfunction without detectable cause	RPCT, double-blind	Vogt[26] 1997	81	No	3	NA	26%	4	Study of yohimbine hydrochloride, not yohimbe bark extract; mean age, 53 years; 10 mg of oral yohimbine t.i.d.
Organic impotence	RPCT, double-blind, partial crossover	Morales[21] 1982	100	No	3	NA	15%	7	Study of yohimbine hydrochloride, not yohimbe bark extract; mean age, 56 years; 6 mg of yohimbine capsules t.i.d.

Review of the Evidence: Yohimbe Bark Extract—*cont'd*

Condition Treated*	Study Design	Author, Year	N[†]	SS[†]	Study Quality[‡]	Magnitude of Benefit	ARR[†]	NNT[†]	Comments
Vasculogenic impotence	RCT, crossover	Knoll[48] 1996	20	No	3	NA	15%	7	Study of yohimbine hydrochloride, not yohimbe bark extract; mean age, 47 years. Adverse effects: insomnia, dyspepsia.
Psychogenic impotence	RPCT, double-blind, partial crossover	Montorsi[29] 1994	55	Yes	4	Medium	49%	2	Study of yohimbine hydrochloride, not yohimbe bark extract; mean age, 43 years; 5 mg of yohimbine t.i.d. plus 50 mg daily of trazodone vs. placebo. Adverse effects: dizziness, gastric intolerance, restlessness, agitation.)
Psychogenic impotence	RPCT, double-blind, partial crossover	Reid[22] 1987	48	Yes	3	Medium	46%	2	Study of yohimbine hydrochloride, not yohimbe bark extract; age range 18 to 70 years; 6 mg of yohimbine t.i.d. No serious adverse effects.
Erectile dysfunction	Case series	Ashton[28] 1994	8	Yes	NA	Large	NA	NA	Study of yohimbine hydrochloride, not yohimbe bark extract. Benefits of yohimbine reported to outweigh risks.
Impotence	RCT, double-blind, crossover	Mazo[114] 1984	40	NA	NA	None	NA	NA	Study of yohimbine hydrochloride, not yohimbe bark extract; 18 mg of yohimbine daily or placebo for 1 month; abstract has results of only 10 patients (remaining 30 were enrolled but had not completed trial).
Chronic erectile impotence of mixed etiology	RPCT, double-blind, crossover	Riley[23] 1989	57	Yes	4	Medium	24%	4	Study of yohimbine hydrochloride, not yohimbe bark extract; mean age, 50 years; 5.4 mg yohimbine t.i.d. Adverse effects: hypertension, rash, loss of antiepileptic action of phenytoin.
Any kind of erectile impotence	RPCT, double blind, partial crossover	Susset[24] 1989	70	No	4	NA	34%	3	Study of yohimbine hydrochloride, not yohimbe bark extract; mean age, 61 years; 5.4 mg of yohimbine tablets q.i.d. increased to 8 times daily for 4 weeks. Adverse effects: anxiety, dizziness, chills, headache, increased frequency of urination.
Sexual side effects of SSRIs	Case series	Hollander[119] 1992	6	NA	3	Small	NA	NA	Study of yohimbine hydrochloride, not yohimbe bark extract; clomipramine (5 patients) and fluoxetine (1 patient) studied; 5 of 6 patients reported improvement in sexual function; 1 patient non-compliant. Varying doses of yohimbine used.
Sexual side effects of SSRIs	Case series	Jacobsen[120] 1992	9	NA	3	Small	NA	NA	Study of yohimbine hydrochloride, not yohimbe bark extract; fluoxetine studied; 8 of 9 subjects reported complete or partial response; 5.4 mg of yohimbine t.i.d.
Autonomic failure	RCT	Jordan[124] 1998	22	Yes	4	Medium	52%	2	Study of yohimbine hydrochloride, not yohimbe bark extract; yohimbine effective in raising seated and standing blood pressure.
Xerostomia: psychotropic drug-induced	RCT, double-blind, crossover	Bagheri[122] 1997	10	Yes	3	Medium	NA	NA	Study of yohimbine hydrochloride, not yohimbe bark extract; yohimbine significantly increased salivary secretions.

Y

Continued

Review of the Evidence: Yohimbe Bark Extract—*cont'd*

Condition Treated*	Study Design	Author, Year	N[†]	SS[†]	Study Quality[‡]	Magnitude of Benefit	ARR[†]	NNT[†]	Comments
Libido (women)	RCT	Piletz[106] 1998	16	No	3	NA	NA	NA	Study of yohimbine hydrochloride, not yohimbe bark extract; mean age 41 years (range, 32-49 years). No benefit reported.
Parkinson's disease	RCT	Montastruc[125] 1981	18	Yes	2	Small	NA	NA	Study of yohimbine hydrochloride, not yohimbe bark extract; study represents preliminary data.
Erectile impotence of mixed etiology	RCT, double-blind, crossover	Kunelius[115] 1997	27	Yes	4	NA	NA	NA	Study of yohimbine hydrochloride, not yohimbe bark extract; mean age, 47 years. Adverse effects: hypertension, palpitations. Yohimbine found by authors to be no better than placebo.

*Primary or secondary outcome.
[†]*N*, Number of patients; *SS*, statistically significant; *ARR*, absolute risk reduction; *NNT*, the number of patients who need to undergo a specific intervention in order to observe an outcome in one individual.
[‡]0-2 = poor; 3-4 = good; 5 = excellent.
GI, Gastrointestinal; *NA*, not applicable; *q.i.d.*, four times daily; *RCT*, randomized, controlled trial; *SSRIs*, selective serotonin reuptake inhibitors; *t.i.d.*, three times daily.
For an explanation of each category in this table, please see Table 3 in the Introduction.

REVIEW OF THE EVIDENCE: DISCUSSION

Erectile Dysfunction

Summary

- Yohimbine is an active indole alkaloid constituent found in the bark of the *Pausinystalia yohimbe* tree. Yohimbine hydrochloride, a standardized form of yohimbine that is available as a prescription drug in the United States, has been demonstrated in multiple clinical trials to be efficacious in the management of male impotence. Although yohimbine alkaloid isolated from yohimbe bark has been used traditionally to treat male erectile dysfunction, there is no clinical evidence specifically studying these effects of yohimbe bark extract. Notably, yohimbe bark extract generally contains low concentrations of yohimbine (6% indole alkaloids, of which only 10% to 15% is yohimbine), and commercial preparations may or may not share the pharmacologic and clinical effects of yohimbine hydrochloride.[1] A 1995 chemical analysis of 26 commercial yohimbe products reported that most commercial yohimbe products contain virtually no yohimbine.[1] Therefore, although there is strong evidence to suggest the efficacy of the drug yohimbine hydrochloride for the management of certain types of erectile dysfunction, there is insufficient evidence to support the use of yohimbe bark extract for this indication. It should be noted that currently yohimbine hydrochloride is less commonly used in the United States than other drug therapies such as sildenafil (Viagra). Other options noted by the American Urologic Association include vacuum constriction devices, vasoactive drug injection therapy, and penile prosthesis implantation.

Meta-analyses of Controlled Trials of Yohimbine Hydrochloride (Not Yohimbe Bark Extract)

- Ernst and Pittler conducted a 1998 meta-analysis of randomized, controlled trials of yohimbine for erectile dysfunction.[108] Trials were located via searches of MEDLINE (1966 to 1997), Embase (1974 to 1997), and the Cochrane Library (Issue 1, 1997). Selection criteria allowed for the inclusion of seven randomized, placebo-controlled trials including a total

of 419 male patients (age range, 18 to 70 years).[21-27] Doses of yohimbine ranged from 15 to 30 mg daily for 2 to 10 weeks. All trials reported positive results, and a pooled analysis revealed an odds ratio of 3.85 (95% CI, 6.67 to 2.22). Reported adverse effects included anxiety, dizziness, increased frequency of urination, chills, headache, sweating, agitation, tachycardia, gastrointestinal disturbances, hypertension, rash, and reduced seizure threshold on phenytoin.

- An earlier evaluation was conducted in 1996 by Carey et al. and included four meta-analytic integrations of the available literature.[30] This publication reported a consistent tendency for yohimbine to enhance erectile function vs. placebo. The authors also noted several shortcomings in the studies. Other study results reported that yohimbine-containing medications enhance erectile functioning vs. placebo.[22,23,109-111]

Selected Controlled Trials of Yohimbine Hydrochloride (Not Yohimbe Bark Extract)

- Susset et al. conducted a randomized, controlled, double-blind, partial crossover study of 82 patients between the ages of 40 and 73 years.[24] Patients were included with heterogeneous causes of erectile dysfunction. Patients received 5.4 mg of yohimbine hydrochloride or placebo, with dosages increased by adding 1 tablet daily, from an initial dose of 1 tablet 4 times daily to a maximum of 2 tablets 4 times daily (maximum of 42.0 mg daily). After 4 weeks, the placebo group was crossed over to drug, and drug patients were continued as treated. Outcomes measures included vascular testing (Doppler penile segmental pressure and pulse-volume recording with plethysmography), venous outflow studies, neurologic studies, psychological testing, penile circumference changes measured by mercury strain gauge, and a Derogatis Sexual Functioning Inventory. The authors reported that 14%t of patients experienced restoration of full and sustained erections, 20% had partial response, and 65% had no improvement, with 3 patients reporting a positive placebo effect. A positive overall response was seen in 34% of patients. Younger patients (average, 4 years younger) responded better than older patients.

- A randomized, controlled, double-blind study was conducted by Mann et al. in 31 patients with erectile dysfunction of organic or nonorganic etiology.[25] Subjects were treated with 5 mg of oral yohimbine hydrochloride 3 times daily. Outcomes were measured both subjectively and via an objective scale. Improvement was reported in 60% of yohimbine patients vs. 40% of placebo patients.

- A randomized, placebo-controlled, double-blind study of the effect of yohimbine and trazodone on psychogenic impotence was studied by Montorsi et al.[29] Sixty-three patients with psychogenic impotence were administered 15 mg daily of oral yohimbine plus 50 mg daily of oral trazodone. During two 8-week treatments, assessments were made of erectile function, ejaculation, interest in sex, and sexual thoughts. Fifty-five patients were able to complete the study; 71% of completers in the yohimbine group reported positive clinical results vs. 22% in the placebo group, with clinical significance. At follow-up assessments, 58% in the yohimbine group maintained positive results at 3 months, and 56% at 6 months.

- A randomized placebo-controlled, double-blind, partial crossover study of yohimbine was conducted by Morales et al. in 100 subjects (mean age, 56 years) with psychogenic erectile dysfunction.[109] Inclusion criteria included clearly organic etiologic diagnosis, patient age between 18 and 70 years, residency within 50 km (~31 miles) of the clinic, and willingness for follow-up assessment. Patients were administered 3 dosages of yohimbine providing 18 mg daily over a period of 4 to 10 weeks. Outcome measures included urinary riboflavin marker under fluorescence slit lamp (to determine compliance), comparison of yohimbine to placebo for penile brachial index, and testosterone, luteinizing hormone, follicle-stimulating hormone, and prolactin levels. Positive effects were noted in 42.6% of patients receiving yohimbine vs. 27.6% receiving placebo.

- A randomized crossover study in 20 patients (mean age, 47 years) was conducted by Knoll et al. to evaluate yohimbine and isoxsuprine (vs. pentoxifylline) in the management of vasculogenic impotence.[48] Inclusion criteria included arterial insufficiency and cavernous venous leakage by penile duplex scanning. Patients received 5.4 mg of yohimbine plus 10 mg of isoxsuprine or 400 mg pentoxifylline orally 3 times daily. Outcome measures included penile biothesiometry, systolic peak flow velocities, sexual questionnaire, and laboratory evaluation of testosterone and prolactin levels. The study found no significant differences in response to oral regimens, and the authors reported no improvement in the pre-and post-injection cavernous arterial peak systolic flow velocities and resistance indexes. Limitations of this study included lack of a placebo group and no power calculation. It is possible that the sample size was not adequate to detect between-group differences.

- In an earlier study, Morales et al. studied oral yohimbine (6 mg taken 3 times daily) as a treatment for impotence in diabetic patients with peripheral neuropathy.[112] An incidental finding was improvement of paresthesias.

- Miller conducted a double-blind, crossover study in 22 patients, ranging from 29 to 62 years of age, complaining of impotence for 2 weeks to 5 years.[113] Subjects were assigned to receive either the yohimbine product Afrodex or placebo. The authors noted that yohimbine exerted significant positive therapeutic effects in increasing the number of erections and orgasms in impotent males. No side effects were noted.

- Mazo et al. documented, in a published abstract, a randomized, controlled, double-blind, crossover trial assessing the effects of yohimbine in the treatment of 40 patients with impotence.[114] Patients were randomized to receive placebo or yohimbine at a dose of 18 mg daily for one month. Following a 1-week washout period, patients were crossed over to receive the opposite treatment. Outcomes assessed included a sexual performance questionnaire, penile brachial index, and snap gauge testing. Results were reflective of only 10 patients who had completed the study (at the time of publishing the abstract). Of these 10 patients, 3 experienced a favorable response to yohimbine treatment. Limitations include small sample size and only brief descriptions of methods and statistical analysis.

- Kunelius et al. conducted a randomized, controlled, double-blind, crossover trial assessing the effects of yohimbine hydrochloride in the treatment of 29 patients with mixed types of impotence.[115] Patients were randomized to receive placebo or yohimbine at a dose of 36 mg daily for 25 days. After a 14-day washout, patients were crossed over to receive the opposite treatment for another 25 days. Outcome measures included erectile function, ejaculation, and interest in sex. Results, which were based on 27 patients who completed the trial, revealed no significant difference between groups in response rate: complete or partial responses were noted in 44% (n = 12) and 48% (n = 13) of patients taking yohimbine and placebo, respectively. This small, brief study may not have been adequately powered to detect between-group differences.

- Additional studies have been conducted demonstrating efficacy of yohimbine in the management of erectile dysfunction,[21,116] including 15 mg of yohimbine in combination with 50 mg of trazodone daily for the treatment of psychogenic impotence.[29] Other research has reported marginal efficacy of yohimbine.[117]

Sexual Side Effects of Selective Serotonin Reuptake Inhibitors (SSRIs)

Summary

- Yohimbine is an alkaloid constituent found in the bark of the *Pausinystalia yohimbe* tree. Yohimbine hydrochloride, a standardized form of yohimbine that is available as a prescription drug in the United States, has been shown effective in the management of erectile dysfunction and has been suggested as a potential agent to improve sexual function that has been impaired as a result of the use of SSRI antidepressants. However, there is currently limited human evidence in this area from methodologically weak studies (case series and a single-blind study). Therefore, there are insufficient scientific data to recommend for or against the use of yohimbine or yohimbe bark extract for this indication.

Evidence

- A single-blind study by Cappiello et al. reported efficacy of yohimbine as an addition to fluvoxamine in nine patients with major depression (age range, 24 to 63 years).[118] The authors reported a moderate improvement in two of the patients and a marked improvement in one patient.

- A case series conducted by Hollander and McCarley evaluated six patients who experienced sexual side effects while receiving SSRIs.[119] Five of the patients were taking clomipramine, and one was taking fluoxetine. Patients were administered varying doses of yohimbine (2.7 to 16.2 mg), taken 2 to 4 hours before they engaged in sexual activity.

Y

One patient was noncompliant, and the other five reported subjective improvement in sexual function. Reported side effects included fatigue, sweating, shakiness, insomnia, and anxiety.

- Jacobsen evaluated nine patients (two women, seven men) who reported sexual dysfunction while taking fluoxetine (20 to 40 mg daily).[120] Duration of fluoxetine treatment prior to beginning yohimbine ranged from 30 to 180 days (mean, 84 days). Each patient was administered 5.4 mg of yohimbine three times daily for a minimum of 3 weeks. Eight of the patients reported "complete response" (full restoration of sexual desire and/or function) or "partial response" (noticeable but incomplete improvement in sexual desire and/or function), and one subject reported a "poor response" (absence of improvement in sexual function).[121] Reported side effects included nausea, anxiety, insomnia, and urinary frequency.

Xerostomia (Psychotropic Drug–Induced)
Summary
- Yohimbine is an alkaloid constituent found in the bark of the *Pausinystalia yohimbe* tree. Studies have shown that acute administration of yohimbine, an alpha-2 adrenoceptor antagonist, is able to increase salivary secretion in animals and in humans. Based on these results, yohimbine has been used for the treatment of dry mouth caused by tricyclic antidepressants to increase salivary outflow. Notably, yohimbe bark extract generally contains low concentrations of yohimbine (6% indole alkaloids, of which only 10% to 15% is yohimbine), and commercial preparations may or may not share the pharmacologic and clinical effects of yohimbine.[1]

Evidence
- Bagheri et al. reported a randomized, controlled, double-blind, crossover equivalence study in 10 patients (5 men, 5 women) receiving various psychotropic drugs (clomipramine, amitriptyline, pipotiazine, loxapine, fluphenazine, topatepine) and complaining of dry mouth.[122] Patients were assigned to receive oral yohimbine (6 mg) or anetholtrithione (25 mg) three times daily. The authors reported that the yohimbine-treated group experienced a statistically significant increase in salivary volume compared to baseline, whereas no improvements were noted in the anetholtrithione group. The authors also commented that in previous experiments they had found that the sialogenic effect of yohimbine is due to the inhibition of presynaptic alpha-2 adrenoceptors located on the chorda tympani.
- Other studies have reported increased salivary secretion with yohimbine administration, both in humans[123] and in dogs (submaxillary gland secretion).[32,76]

Libido (Women)
Summary
- It has been suggested that yohimbine alkaloid, isolated from yohimbe bark, exerts no effect on male libido but may elicit increases in female libido. However, there is currently insufficient evidence demonstrating beneficial effects of yohimbine or of over-the-counter yohimbe preparations in this area.

Evidence
- Piletz et al. reported a study in which nine "hyposexual" women were placed on yohimbine (5.4 mg) orally three times daily, and seven "healthy females" were compared as controls.[106] Women in the control group were studied over two menstrual cycles, and women in the treatment group were studied over three menstrual cycles. Although women with hypoactive sexual desire had slightly lower plasma levels of the norepinephrine metabolite 3-methoxy-4-hydroxy-phenylethylene glycol (MHPG) than controls at baseline, these differences were not statistically significant. Yohimbine was observed to elicit a sustained rise in plasma MHPG levels, although there was no improvement in the subjects' sexual desire.

Autonomic Failure
Summary
- Based on its mechanism of action, it has been suggested that yohimbine alkaloid, isolated from yohimbe bark, may improve orthostatic hypotension or other manifestations of autonomic nervous system dysfunction. However, there is currently insufficient evidence demonstrating beneficial effects of yohimbine or of over-the-counter yohimbe preparations in this area.

Evidence
- Jordan et al. studied 35 patients with severe orthostatic hypotension due to multiple system atrophy or autonomic failure.[124] The authors assessed the effects on seated systolic blood pressure of placebo, phenylpropanolamine (12.5 mg and 25 mg), yohimbine (5.4 mg), indomethacin (50 mg), ibuprofen (600 mg), caffeine (250 mg), and methylphenidate (5 mg). Statistically significant increases in systolic blood pressure were observed with phenylpropanolamine (12.5 mg), yohimbine, and indomethacin compared to placebo. Notably, phenylpropanolamine has been removed from the U.S. market.
- Montastruc et al. conducted a randomized, controlled trial in 18 patients with Parkinson's disease (6 men and 12 women between the ages of 48 and 81 years).[125] Subjects received 12 mg daily of yohimbine hydrochloride as a monotherapy (n = 2), with L-dopa and inhibitors (n = 13), with bromocriptine (n = 1), or with L-dopa and inhibitors plus bromocriptine (n = 2). Treatment was administered for 1 to 6 months. The results suggested an improvement in orthostatic hypotension in the patients treated with L-dopa.
- In 1994, Biaggioni et al. reviewed the available literature regarding the use of yohimbine in the treatment of autonomic failure, and concluded that yohimbine is not only a useful tool in the study of blood pressure regulation but also may offer a therapeutic option in autonomic dysfunction.[40]

Platelet Aggregation Inhibition
Summary
- Preclinical studies report that yohimbine alkaloid, isolated from yohimbe bark, may inhibit platelet aggregation. Research in humans is limited, and it is unclear if these platelet effects are clinically significant or may be beneficial in the management of specific diseases.

Evidence
- A comparison study by Boon et al. demonstrated that yohimbine binds to the alpha-2 adrenoceptor responsible for noradrenaline-induced platelet aggregation.[77]

FORMULARY: BRANDS USED IN CLINICAL TRIALS
Brands of Yohimbine Hydrochloride (Not Yohimbe Bark Extract) Used in Clinical Trials
- Aphrodyne (Star Pharmaceuticals, Pompano Beach, FL); Dayto HimbinYocon (Pallisades Pharmaceutical, Tenafly, NJ); Afrodex (Pentax Pharmaceutical Company, Houston,

TX); Vikonon; Potensan; Yohimex; Yohimbine HCl (Sigma Chemical Co., St. Louis, MO; Watson Laboratories, Inc. Corona, CA); Goldine (Ft. Lauderdale, FL).

References

1. Betz JM, White KD, der Marderosian AH. Gas chromatographic determination of yohimbine in commercial yohimbe products. J AOAC Int 1995;78(5):1189-1194.
2. Murray M. Yohimbine vs. Muira puama in the treatment of erectile dysfunction. Am J Nat Med 1994;1(3):8.
3. Peskind ER, Wingerson D, Murray S, et al. Cerebrospinal fluid norepinephrine responses to yohimbine and clonidine in Alzheimer's disease and normal aging. Arch Gen Psychiatry 1995;52:774-782.
4. Bierer LM, Aisen PS, Davidson M, et al. A pilot study of oral physostigmine plus yohimbine in patients with Alzheimer disease. Alzheimer Dis Assoc Disord 1993;7(2):98-104.
5. Arnsten AF, Cai JX. Postsynaptic alpha-2 receptor stimulation improves memory in aged monkeys: indirect effects of yohimbine versus direct effects of clonidine. Neurobiol Aging 1993;14(6):597-603.
6. Lacomblez L, Bensimon G, Isnard F, et al. Effect of yohimbine on blood pressure in patients with depression and orthostatic hypotension induced by clomipramine. Clin Pharmacol Ther 1989;45(3):241-251.
7. Price LH, Heninger GR. Can yohimbine be used to treat orthostatic hypotension associated with the use of desipramine and other anti-depressants? What general and/or specific strategy do you recommend for treating orthostatic hypotension? J Clin Psychopharmacol 1988;8(5):384.
8. Seibyl JP, Krystal JH, Price LH, et al. Use of yohimbine to counteract nortriptyline-induced orthostatic hypotension. J Clin Psychopharmacol 1989;9(1):67-68.
9. Senard JM, Rascol O, Durrieu G, et al. Effects of yohimbine on plasma catecholamine levels in orthostatic hypotension related to Parkinson disease or multiple system atrophy. Clin Neuropharmacol 1993;16(1):70-76.
10. Gentili A, Godschalk MF, Gheorghiu D, et al. Effect of clonidine and yohimbine on sleep in healthy men: a double-blind, randomized, controlled trial. Eur J Clin Pharmacol 1996;50(6):463-465.
11. Kanno O, Clarenbach P. Effect of clonidine and yohimbine on sleep in man: polygraphic study and EEG analysis by normalized slope descriptors. Electroencephalogr Clin Neurophysiol 1985;60(6):478-484.
12. Wooten V. Yohimbine treatment in narcolepsy and idiopathic hypersomnolence [abstract]. Sleep Research 1993;22:295.
13. Des Lauriers A, Widlocher D, Allilaire JF, et al. [Treatment of orthostatic hypotension induced by tricyclic antidepressants with yohimbine (author's transl)]. Ann Med Interne (Paris) 1980;131(8):508-509.
14. Kucio C, Jonderko K, Piskorska D. Does yohimbine act as a slimming drug? Isr J Med Sci 1991;27(10):550-556.
15. Berlin I, Stalla-Bourdillon A, Thuillier Y, et al. [Lack of efficacy of yohimbine in the treatment of obesity]. J Pharmacol 1986;17(3):343-347.
16. Berlan M, Galitzky J, Riviere D, et al. Plasma catecholamine levels and lipid mobilization induced by yohimbine in obese and non-obese women. Int J Obes 1991;15(5):305-315.
17. Charney DS, Heninger GR, Breier A. Noradrenergic function in panic anxiety. Effects of yohimbine in healthy subjects and patients with agoraphobia and panic disorder. Arch Gen Psychiatry 1984;41(8):751-763.
18. Richard IH, Szegethy E, Lichter D, et al. Parkinson's disease: a preliminary study of yohimbine challenge in patients with anxiety. Clin Neuropharmacol 1999;22(3):172-175.
19. Adler LE, Hoffer L, Nagamoto HT, et al. Yohimbine impairs P50 auditory sensory gating in normal subjects. Neuropsychopharmacology 1994;10(4):249-257.
20. Mosqueda-Garcia R, Fernandez-Violante R, Tank J, et al. Yohimbine in neurally mediated syncope. Pathophysiological implications. J Clin Invest 1998;102(10):1824-1830.
21. Morales A, Surridge DH, Marshall PG, et al. Nonhormonal pharmacological treatment of organic impotence. J Urol 1982;128(1):45-47.
22. Reid K, Surridge DH, Morales A, et al. Double-blind trial of yohimbine in treatment of psychogenic impotence. Lancet 1987;2(8556):421-423.
23. Riley AJ, Goodman R, Kellett JM, et al. Double blind trial of yohimbine hydrochloride in the treatment of erection inadequacy. Sex Marital Ther 1989;4(1):17-26.
24. Susset JG, Tessier CD, Wincze J, et al. Effect of yohimbine hydrochloride on erectile impotence: a double-blind study. J Urol 1989;141(6):1360-1363.
25. Mann K, Klingler T, Noe S, et al. Effects of yohimbine on sexual experiences and nocturnal penile tumescence and rigidity in erectile dysfunction. Arch Sex Behav 1996;25(1):1-16.
26. Vogt HJ, Brandl P, Kockott G, et al. Double-blind, placebo-controlled safety and efficacy trial with yohimbine hydrochloride in the treatment of nonorganic erectile dysfunction. Int J Impot Res 1997;9(3):155-161.
27. Rowland DL, Kallan K, Slob AK. Yohimbine, erectile capacity, and sexual response in men. Arch Sex Behav 1997;26(1):49-62.
28. Ashton AK. Yohimbine in the treatment of male erectile dysfunction. Am J Psychiatry 1994;151(9):1397.
29. Montorsi F, Strambi LF, Guazzoni G, et al. Effect of yohimbine-trazodone on psychogenic impotence: a randomized, double-blind, placebo-controlled study. Urology 1994;44(5):732-736.
30. Carey MP, Johnson BT. Effectiveness of yohimbine in the treatment of erectile disorder: four meta-analytic integrations. Arch Sex Behav 1996;25(4):341-360.
31. Witt DK. Yohimbine for erectile dysfunction. J Fam Pract 1998;46(4):282-283.
32. Owen JA, Nakatsu SL, Fenemore J, et al. The pharmacokinetics of yohimbine in man. Eur J Clin Pharmacol 1987;32(6):577-582.
33. Guthrie SK, Hariharan M, Grunhaus LJ. Yohimbine bioavailability in humans. Eur J Clin Pharmacol 1990;39(4):409-411.
34. Assalian P, Margolese HC. Treatment of antidepressant-induced sexual side effects. J Sex Marital Ther 1996;22(3):218-224.
35. Buffum J. Pharmacosexology update: yohimbine and sexual function. J Psychoactive Drugs 1985;17(2):131-132.
36. Bourin M, Malinge M, Colombel MC, et al. Influence of alpha stimulants and beta blockers on yohimbine toxicity. Prog Neuropsychopharmacol Biol Psychiatry 1988;12(5):569-574.
37. Sandler B, Aronson P. Yohimbine-induced cutaneous drug eruption, progres-sive renal failure, and lupus-like syndrome. Urology 1993;41(4):343-345.
38. Charney DS, Heninger GR, Redmond DE, Jr. Yohimbine induced anxiety and increased noradrenergic function in humans: effects of diazepam and clonidine. Life Sci 1983;33(1):19-29.
39. Cameron OG, Zubieta JK, Grunhaus L, et al. Effects of yohimbine on cerebral blood flow, symptoms, and physiological functions in humans. Psychosom Med 2000;62(4):549-559.
40. Biaggioni I, Robertson RM, Robertson D. Manipulation of norepinephrine metabolism with yohimbine in the treatment of autonomic failure. J Clin Pharmacol 1994;34(5):418-423.
41. Bowes MP, Peters RH, Kernan WJ, Jr., et al. Effects of yohimbine and idazoxan on motor behaviors in male rats. Pharmacol Biochem Behav 1992;41(4):707-713.
42. Bremner JD, Innis RB, Ng CK, et al. Positron emission tomography measurement of cerebral metabolic correlates of yohimbine administration in combat-related posttraumatic stress disorder. Arch Gen Psychiatry 1997;54(3):246-254.
43. Dunn RW, Corbett R. Yohimbine-induced seizures involve NMDA and GABAergic transmission. Neuropharmacology 1992;31(4):389-395.
44. Musso NR, Vergassola C, Pende A, et al. Yohimbine effects on blood pressure and plasma catecholamines in human hypertension. Am J Hypertens 1995;8(6):565-571.
45. Shalev AY. Post-traumatic stress disorder: a biopsychological perspective. Isr J Psychiatry Relat Sci 1993;30(2):102-109.
46. Charney DS, Heninger GR, Sternberg DE. Assessment of alpha 2 adrenergic autoreceptor function in humans: effects of oral yohimbine. Life Sci 1982;30(23):2033-2041.
47. Mack RB. Taljaribu kila dawa isifal: yohimbine intoxication. N C Med J 1985;46(4):229-230.
48. Knoll LD, Benson RC, Jr., Bilhartz DL, et al. A randomized crossover study using yohimbine and isoxsuprine versus pentoxifylline in the management of vasculogenic impotence. J Urol 1996;155(1):144-146.
49. Morgan CA, III, Grillon C, Southwick SM, et al. Yohimbine facilitated acoustic startle in combat veterans with post-traumatic stress disorder. Psychopharmacology (Berl) 1995;117(4):466-471.
50. Southwick SM, Krystal JH, Bremner JD, et al. Noradrenergic and serotonergic function in posttraumatic stress disorder. Arch Gen Psychiatry 1997;54(8):749-758.
51. Rasmusson AM, Hauger RL, Morgan CA, et al. Low baseline and yohimbine-stimulated plasma neuropeptide Y (NPY) levels in combat-related PTSD. Biol Psychiatry 2000;47(6):526-539.
52. Southwick SM, Morgan CA, III, Charney DS, et al. Yohimbine use in a natural setting: effects on posttraumatic stress disorder. Biol Psychiatry 1999;46(3):442-444.
53. Becker C, Hamon M, Benoliel JJ. Prevention by 5-HT1A receptor agonists of restraint stress- and yohimbine-induced release of cholecystokinin in the frontal cortex of the freely moving rat. Neuropharmacology 1999; 38(4):525-532.
54. Albus M, Zahn TP, Breier A. Anxiogenic properties of yohimbine. I. Behavioral, physiological and biochemical measures. Eur Arch Psychiatry Clin Neurosci 1992;241(6):337-344.
55. Albus M, Zahn TP, Breier A. Anxiogenic properties of yohimbine. II. Influence of experimental set and setting. Eur Arch Psychiatry Clin Neurosci 1992;241(6):345-351.
56. Shear MK. Pathophysiology of panic: a review of pharmacologic provocative tests and naturalistic monitoring data. J Clin Psychiatry 1986; 47(6 Suppl):18-26.
57. Gurguis GN, Vitton BJ, Uhde TW. Behavioral, sympathetic and adrenocortical responses to yohimbine in panic disorder patients and normal controls. Psychiatry Res 1997;71(1):27-39.
58. Price LH, Charney DS, Heninger GR. Three cases of manic symptoms following yohimbine administration. Am J Psychiatry 1984;141(10):1267-1268.
59. Bagheri H, Picault P, Schmitt L, et al. Pharmacokinetic study of yohimbine

Y

and its pharmacodynamic effects on salivary secretion in patients treated with tricyclic antidepressants. Br J Clin Pharmacol 1994;37(1):93-96.

60. Bourin M, Malinge M, Guitton B. Provocative agents in panic disorder. Therapie 1995;50(4):301-306.

61. McDougle CJ, Krystal JH, Price LH, et al. Noradrenergic response to acute ethanol administration in healthy subjects: comparison with intravenous yohimbine. Psychopharmacology (Berl) 1995;118(2):127-135.

62. Morgan CA, III, Southwick SM, Grillon C, et al. Yohimbine-facilitated acoustic startle reflex in humans. Psychopharmacology (Berl) 1993;110(3):342-346.

63. Kehne JH, Davis M. Central noradrenergic involvement in yohimbine excitation of acoustic startle: effects of DSP4 and 6-OHDA. Brain Res 1985;330(1):31-41.

64. Landis E, Shore E. Yohimbine-induced bronchospasm. Chest 1989;96(6):1424.

65. Brodde OE, Anlauf M, Arroyo J, et al. Hypersensitivity of adrenergic receptors and blood-pressure response to oral yohimbine in orthostatic hypotension. N Engl J Med 1983;308(17):1033-1034.

66. Andrejak M, Ward M, Schmitt H. Cardiovascular effects of yohimbine in anaesthetized dogs. Eur J Pharmacol 1983;94(3-4):219-228.

67. Bolme P, Corrodi H, Fuxe K, et al. Possible involvement of central adrenaline neurons in vasomotor and respiratory control. Studies with clonidine and its interactions with piperoxane and yohimbine. Eur J Pharmacol 1974;28(1):89-94.

68. Friesen K, Palatnick W, Tenenbein M. Benign course after massive ingestion of yohimbine. J Emerg Med 1993;11(3):287-288.

69. Murburg MM, Villacres EC, Ko GN, et al. Effects of yohimbine on human sympathetic nervous system function. J Clin Endocrinol Metab 1991;73(4):861-865.

70. Kennedy SH, Gnam W, Ralevski E, et al. Melatonin responses to clonidine and yohimbine challenges. J Psychiatry Neurosci 1995;20(4):297-304.

71. Kenney WL, Zappe DH, Tankersley CG, et al. Effect of systemic yohimbine on the control of skin blood flow during local heating and dynamic exercise. Am J Physiol 1994;266(2 Pt 2):H371-H376.

72. Bagheri H, Berlan M, Montastruc JL, et al. Yohimbine and lacrimal secretion. Br J Clin Pharmacol 1990;30(1):151-152.

73. Bagheri H, Bompart G, Girolami JP, et al. Is yohimbine-induced increase in salivary secretion a kinin-dependent mechanism? Fundam Clin Pharmacol 1992;6(1):17-20.

74. Bagheri H, Schmitt L, Berlan M, et al. Effect of 3 weeks treatment with yohimbine on salivary secretion in healthy volunteers and in depressed patients treated with tricyclic antidepressants. Br J Clin Pharmacol 1992;34(6):555-558.

75. Bagheri H, Chale JJ, Guyen LN, et al. Evidence for activation of both adrenergic and cholinergic nervous pathways by yohimbine, an alpha 2-adrenoceptor antagonist. Fundam Clin Pharmacol 1995;9(3):248-254.

76. Montastruc P, Berlan M, Montastruc JL. Effects of yohimbine on submaxillary salivation in dogs. Br J Pharmacol 1989;98(1):101-104.

77. Boon NA, Elliott JM, Grahame-Smith DG, et al. A comparison of alpha 2-adrenoreceptor binding characteristics of intact human platelets identified by [3H]-yohimbine and [3H]- dihydroergocryptine. J Auton Pharmacol 1983;3(2):89-95.

78. Berlin I, Crespo-Laumonnier B, Cournot A, et al. The alpha 2-adrenergic receptor antagonist yohimbine inhibits epinephrine-induced platelet aggregation in healthy subjects. Clin Pharmacol Ther 1991;49(4):362-369.

79. Braddock L, Cowen PJ, Elliott JM, et al. Binding of yohimbine and imipramine to platelets in depressive illness. Psychol Med 1986;16(4):765-773.

80. Braddock LE, Cowen PJ, Elliott JM, et al. Changes in the binding to platelets of [3H]imipramine and [3H]yohimbine in normal subjects taking amitriptyline. Neuropharmacology 1984;23(2B):285-286.

81. Motulsky HJ, Shattil SJ, Insel PA. Characterization of alpha 2-adrenergic receptors on human platelets using [3H]yohimbine. Biochem Biophys Res Commun 1980;97(4):1562-1570.

82. Mustonen P, Savola J, Lassila R. Atipamezole, an imidazoline-type alpha(2)-adrenoceptor inhibitor, binds to human platelets and inhibits their adrenaline-induced aggregation more effectively than yohimbine. Thromb Res 2000;99(3):231-237.

83. Anonymous. Yohimbine for male sexual dysfunction. Med Lett Drugs Therapeutics 1994;36(938):115-116.

84. Roberge RJ, McGuire SP, Krenzelok EP. Yohimbine as an antidote for clonidine overdose. Am J Emerg Med 1996;14(7):678-680.

85. Roberge RJ, Kimball ET, Rossi J, et al. Clonidine and sleep apnea syndrome interaction: antagonism with yohimbine. J Emerg Med 1998;16(5):727-730.

86. Charney DS, Price LH, Heninger GR. Desipramine-yohimbine combination treatment of refractory depression. Implications for the beta-adrenergic receptor hypothesis of antidepressant action. Arch Gen Psychiatry 1986;43(12):1155-1161.

87. Gear RW, Gordon NC, Heller PH, et al. Enhancement of morphine analgesia by the alpha 2-adrenergic antagonist yohimbine. Neuroscience 1995;66(1):5-8.

88. Dwoskin LP, Neal BS, Sparber SB. Yohimbine exacerbates and clonidine

89. Rosen MI, Kosten TR, Kreek MJ. The effects of naltrexone maintenance on the response to yohimbine in healthy volunteers. Biol Psychiatry 1999;45(12):1636-1645.

90. Hameedi FA, Woods SW, Rosen MI, et al. Dose dependent effects of yohimbine on methadone maintained patients. Am J Drug Alcohol Abuse 1997;23(2):327-333.

91. Hui KK, Yu JL, Chan WF, et al. Interaction of berberine with human platelet alpha 2 adrenoceptors. Life Sci 1991;49(4):315-324.

92. Goldberg MR, Robertson D. Yohimbine: a pharmacological probe for study of the alpha 2- adrenoreceptor. Pharmacol Rev 1983;35(3):143-180.

93. Anden NE, Pauksens K, Svensson K. Selective blockade of brain alpha 2-autoreceptors by yohimbine: effects on motor activity and on turnover of noradrenaline and dopamine. J Neural Transm 1982;55(2):111-120.

94. Anonymous. Yohimbine: time for resurrection? Lancet 1986;2(8517):1194-1195.

95. Galitzky J, Taouis M, Berlan M, et al. Alpha 2-antagonist compounds and lipid mobilization: evidence for a lipid mobilizing effect of oral yohimbine in healthy male volunteers. Eur J Clin Invest 1988;18(6):587-594.

96. Papeschi R, Theiss P. The effect of yohimbine on the turnover of brain catecholamines and serotonin. Eur J Pharmacol 1975;33(1):1-12.

97. Wagner G, Saenz DT. Update on male erectile dysfunction. BMJ 1998;316(7132):678-682.

98. Balon R. The effects of anitdepressants on human sexuality: Diagnosis and management update 1999. Primary Psychology 1999;6(11):40-54.

99. Berlin I, Crespo-Laumonnier B, Turpin G, et al. The alpha-2 adrenoceptor antagonist yohimbine does not facilitate weight loss but blocks adrenaline induced platelet aggregation in obese subjects. Therapie 1989;44(4):301.

100. Grossman E, Rea RF, Hoffman A, et al. Yohimbine increases sympathetic nerve activity and norepinephrine spillover in normal volunteers. Am J Physiol 1991;260(1 Pt 2):R142-R147.

101. Dwoskin LP, Neal BS, Sparber SB. Evidence for antiserotonergic properties of yohimbine. Pharmacol Biochem Behav 1988;31(2):321-326.

102. Meltzer HY, Simonovic M, Gudelsky GA. Effect of yohimbine on rat prolactin secretion. J Pharmacol Exp Ther 1983;224(1):21-27.

103. Abdel-Zaher AO, Ahmed IT, El Koussi AD. The potential antidiabetic activity of some alpha-2 adrenoceptor antagonists. Pharmacol Res 2001;44(5):397-409.

104. Sturgill MG, Grasing KW, Rosen RC, et al. Yohimbine elimination in normal volunteers is characterized by both one- and two-compartment behavior. J Cardiovasc Pharmacol 1997;29(6):697-703.

105. Grasing K, Sturgill MG, Rosen RC, et al. Effects of yohimbine on autonomic measures are determined by individual values for area under the concentration-time curve. J Clin Pharmacol 1996;36(9):814-822.

106. Piletz JE, Segraves KB, Feng YZ, et al. Plasma MHPG response to yohimbine treatment in women with hypoactive sexual desire. J Sex Marital Ther 1998;24(1):43-54.

107. Le Corre P, Dollo G, Chevanne F, et al. Biopharmaceutics and metabolism of yohimbine in humans. Eur J Pharm Sci 1999;9(1):79-84.

108. Ernst E, Pittler MH. Yohimbine for erectile dysfunction: a systematic review and meta- analysis of randomized clinical trials. J Urol 1998;159(2):433-436.

109. Morales A, Condra M, Owen JA, et al. Is yohimbine effective in the treatment of organic impotence? Results of a controlled trial. J Urol 1987;137(6):1168-1172.

110. Sonda LP, Mazo R, Chancellor MB. The role of yohimbine for the treatment of erectile impotence. J Sex Marital Ther 1990;16(1):15-21.

111. Morales A. Yohimbine in erectile dysfunction: the facts. Int J Impot Res 2000;12 Suppl 1:S70-S74.

112. Morales A, Surridge DH, Marshall PG. Yohimbine for treatment of impotence in diabetes. N Engl J Med 1981;305(20):1221.

113. Miller WW, Jr. Afrodex in the treatment of male impotence: a double-blind cross-over study. Curr Ther Res Clin Exp 1968;10(7):354-359.

114. Mazo R, Sonda LP. A prospective double blind trial of yohimbine for erectile impotence [abstract]. 79th Annu Meeting Am Urolog Assoc, Baltimore. 1984;234/A.

115. Kunelius P, Hakkinen J, Lukkarinen O. Is high-dose yohimbine hydrochloride effective in the treatment of mixed-type impotence? A prospective, randomized, controlled double-blind crossover study. Urology 1997;49(3):441-444.

116. Melman A. The effects of yohimbine upon sexual function: a double-blind study [abstract]. 79th Annu Meeting Am Urolog Assoc, Baltimore. 1985:302/A.

117. Montague DK, Barada JH, Belker AM, et al. Clinical guidelines panel on erectile dysfunction: summary report on the treatment of organic erectile dysfunction. The American Urological Association. J Urol 1996;156(6):2007-2011.

118. Cappiello A, McDougle CJ, Malison RT, et al. Yohimbine augmentation of fluvoxamine in refractory depression: a single-blind study. Biol Psychiatry 1995;38(11):765-767.

119. Hollander E, McCarley A. Yohimbine treatment of sexual side effects induced by serotonin reuptake blockers. J Clin Psychiatry 1992;53(6):207-209.

120. Jacobsen FM. Fluoxetine-induced sexual dysfunction and an open trial of yohimbine. J Clin Psychiatry 1992;53(4):119-122.
121. Balon R. Fluoxetine-induced sexual dysfunction and yohimbine. J Clin Psychiatry 1993;54(4):161-162.
122. Bagheri H, Schmitt L, Berlan M, et al. A comparative study of the effects of yohimbine and anetholtrithione on salivary secretion in depressed patients treated with psychotropic drugs. Eur J Clin Pharmacol 1997; 52(5):339-342.

123. Chatelut E, Rispail Y, Berlan M, et al. Yohimbine increases human salivary secretion. Br J Clin Pharmacol 1989;28(3):366-368.
124. Jordan J, Shannon JR, Biaggioni I, et al. Contrasting actions of pressor agents in severe autonomic failure. Am J Med 1998;105(2):116-124.
125. Montastruc JL, Puech AJ, Clanet M, et al. [Yohimbine in treatment of Parkinson's disease. Preliminary results (author's transl)]. Nouv Presse Med 1981;10(16):1331-1332.

Y

HERBS WITH POTENTIAL HYPOGLYCEMIC OR HYPERGLYCEMIC PROPERTIES*
Possible Hypoglycemic Herbs

Based on expert opinion, anecdote, case reports, and/or preliminary trial evidence.

- Aloe vera, American ginseng (*Panax quinquefolius*), bilberry (*Vaccinium myrtillus*), bitter melon (*Momordica charantia*), burdock (*Arctium lappa*), dandelion, devil's claw, fenugreek (*Trigonella foenum-graecum*), fish oil, goldenseal (berberine), gymnema (*Gymnema sylvestre*), horse chestnut (*Aesculus hippocastanum*)/horse chestnut seed extract (HCSE), maitake mushroom (*Grifola frondosa*), marshmallow (*Althea officinalis*), melatonin, milk thistle (*Silybum marianum*), *Panax ginseng*, rosemary (*Rosmarinus officinalis*), Pycnogenol, shark cartilage, Siberian ginseng (*Eleutherococcus senticosus*), stinging nettle (*Urtica dioica*), white horehound (*Marrubium vulgare* L.).

Possible Hyperglycemic Herbs

Based on expert opinion, anecdote, case reports, and/or preliminary trial evidence.

- Arginine (L-arginine), cocoa, DHEA (dehydro-epiandrosterone), ephedra (when combined with caffeine), melatonin.

HERBS AND SUPPLEMENTS WITH POTENTIAL HEPATOTOXIC EFFECTS

Use cautiously with other possible hepatotoxic agents, consider monitoring transaminase levels.

- Ackee (*Blighia sapida*), bee pollen, birch oil (*Betula lenta*), blessed thistle (*Cnicus benedictus*)[†], borage (*Borago officinalis*), bush tea (*Crotalaria spp*)[‡], butterbur (*Petasites hybridus*), chaparral (*Larrea tridentate*), coltsfoot (*Tussilago farfara*), comfrey (*Symphytum* spp.), DHEA, *Echinacea purpurea*, *Echium* spp.[‡], germander (*Teucrium chamaedrys*), *Heliotropium* spp., horse chestnut parenteral preparations (*Aesculus hippocastanum*), Jin-bu-huan (*Lycopodium serratum*), kava (*Piper methysticum*), lobelia (*Lobelia inflata*), L-tetrahydropalmatine (THP), mate (*Ileus partaguayensis*)[‡], niacin (vitamin B₃), niacinamide, Paraguay tea (*Ilex paraguayensis*), periwinkle (*Catharanthus roseus*), *Plantago lanceolata*[†], pride of Madeira (*Echium fastuosum*)[‡], rue (*Ruta graveolus*), sassafras (*Sassafras albidum*), scullcap (Scutellaria lateriflora), *Senecio* spp./groundsel (*Senecio jacobea, Senecio spartoides, Senecio vulgaris*)[†], tansy ragwort (*Senecio jacobea*)[‡], turmeric (*Curcuma longa*), Tu-san-chi (*Gynura segetum*)[‡], uva ursi (*Arctostaphylos uva-ursi* Spreng), valerian (*Valeriana officinalis*), white chameleon (*Atractylis gummifera*).

HERBS AND SUPPLEMENTS WITH POSSIBLE HYPOTENSIVE OR HYPERTENSIVE PROPERTIES
Hypotensive Herbs

Based on expert opinion, anecdote, case reports, and/or preliminary trial evidence.

- Aconite/monkshood (*Aconitum columbianum*), alpha-linolenic acid, arnica (*Arnica montana*), baneberry (*Actaea* spp.), betel nut (*Areca catechu*), bilberry (*Vaccinium myrtillus*), black cohosh (*Cimicifuga racemosa*), bryony (*Bryonia alba*), calendula (*Calendula officinalis*), California poppy (*Eschscholtzia californica*), coleus (*Coleus forskohlii*), curcumin, Danshen (*Salvia miltiorrhiza*), eucalyptol, eucalyptus oil (*Eucalyptus globulus*), evening primrose oil (*Oenothera biennis*), fish oils, flaxseed/flaxseed oil (*Linum usitatissimum*), garlic (*Allium sativum*), ginger (*Zingiber officinale* Roscoe), *Ginkgo biloba*, goldenseal (*Hydrastis canadensis*), green hellebore (*Veratrum alba*), hawthorn (*Crataegus oxyacantha*), Indian tobacco (*Lobelia inflata*), jaborandi (*Pilocarpus jaborandi*), maitake mushroom (*Grifola frondosa*), melatonin (N-acetyl-5 methoxytryptamine), mistletoe (*Viscum album*), night blooming cereus (*Cactus grandiflorus*), oleander (*Nerium oleander, Thevetia peruviana*), omega-3 fatty acids, pasque flower (*Anemone pulsatilla*), periwinkle (*Vinca major*), pleurisy root (*Asclepias tuberosa*), *Polypodium vulgare*, shepherd's purse (*Capsella bursa-pastoris*), Texas milkweed (*Asclepias asperula*), turmeric (*Curcuma longa*), wild cherry (*Prunus serotina*).

Hypertensive Herbs

Based on anecdotal or historical reports, pre-clinical data, or human studies.

- American ginseng *(Panax quinquifolium)*, Arnica *(Arnica chamissonis, Arnica cordifolia, Arnica fulgens, Arnica latifolia, Arnica montana, Arnica sororia)*, bayberry *(Myrica cerifera)*, betel nut *(Areca catechu)*, blue cohosh *(Caulophyllum thalictroides)*, broom *(Sarothamnus scoparius)*, cayenne *(Capsicum annum)*, cola *(Cola* spp.), coltsfoot *(Tussilago farfara)*, ephedra *(Ephedra sinica)*, ginger *(Zingiber officinale* Roscoe), licorice *(Glycyrrhiza glabra)*, yerba mate *(Ilex paraguariensis)*.

HERBS WITH POTENTIAL PROGESTATIONAL OR ESTROGENIC ACTIVITY
Phytoprogestin Herbs

Contain constituents reported to exhibit progestin-like activity in basic science and/or animal studies.

- Chasteberry (*Vitex agnus-castus*), bloodroot (*Sanguinaria canadensis*), damiana (*Turnera* spp), oregano (*Oregano* spp.), yucca (*Yucca* spp.).

Phytoestrogen Herbs

Contain constituents reported to act as estrogen receptor agonists and/or to exhibit estrogenic properties in basic science studies, animal research, or human trials.

- Alfalfa *(Medicago sativa)*, black cohosh *(Cimicifuga racemosa)**, bloodroot *(Sanguinaria canadensis)*, burdock

---

*Note: This is not an all-inclusive, comprehensive list of agents that may lower serum glucose. A qualified healthcare practitioner should be consulted with specific questions or concerns regarding potential effects on blood sugar or interactions.

[†]Contains tannins and may be hepatotoxic in large quantities.

[‡]Contains pyrrolizidine alkaloids, which may account for hepatotoxicity.

---

*Estrogen and isoflavone constituents.

(*Arctium lappa*), hops (*Humulus lupulus*)[†], Kudzu (*Pueraria lobata*)[‡], licorice (*Glycyrrhiza glabra*)[†], pomegranate (*Punica granatum*)[†], red clover (*Trifolium pratense*)[‡], soy (*Glycine max*)[‡], thyme (*Thymus vulgaris*), white horehound (*Marrubium vulgare* L.), yucca (*Yucca* spp).

HERBS WITH KNOWN OR POTENTIAL DIURETIC PROPERTIES

Based on expert opinion, anecdote, case reports, and/or preliminary trial evidence.

- Artichoke (*Cynara scolymus*), celery (*Apium graveolens*), corn silk (*Zea mays*), couchgrass (*Agropyron repens*), dandelion (*Taraxacum officinale*), elder flower (*Sambucus nigra/ Sambucus canadensis*), horsetail (*Equisetum arvense*), juniper berry (*Juniperus communis*), kava (*Piper methysticum*), shepherd's purse (*Capsella bursa-pastoris*), uva ursi leaf (*Arctostaphylos uva-ursi*), yarrow flower (*Achillea millefolium*).

HERBS WITH POSSIBLE SEDATING PROPERTIES

Based on expert opinion, anecdote, case reports, and/or preliminary trial evidence):

- 5-HTP, ashwagandha root, calamus, calendula, California poppy, capsicum, catnip, celery, couch grass, danshen, dogwood, elecampane, german chamomile, goldenseal, gotu kola (*Centella asiatica*), hops, kava (believed to be hypnotic/anxiolytic without significant sedation), lavender aromatherapy, lemon balm, melatonin, sage, sassafras, scullcap, shepherd's purse, Siberian ginseng, St. John's wort, stinging nettle, valerian, wild carrot, wild lettuce, Withania root, yerba mansa.

HERBS WITH POTENTIAL CARDIAC GLYCOSIDE PROPERTIES*

Based on expert opinion, anecdote, pre-clinical data, and/or preliminary human evidence.

- Adonis (*Adonis vernalis*), *Adonis microcarpa*, balloon cotton (*Asclepias friticosa*), black hellebore root/melampode (*Helleborus niger*), black Indian hemp (*Apocynum cannabinum*), bushman's poison (*Carissa acokanthera*), cactus grandifloris (*Selenicerus grandiflorus*), convallaria (*Convallaria majalis*), eyebright (*Euphrasia* spp.), figwort (Scrophulariaceae), foxglove/digitalis (*Digitalis purpurea*), frangipani (*Plumeria rubra*), hedgemustard (*Sisymbrium officinale*), *Helleborus viridus*, hemp root/Canadian hemp root, king's crown (*Calotropis procera*), lily-of-the-valley, motherwort (*Leonurus cardiaca*), oleander leaf (*Nerium oleander* L.), pheasant's eye plant (*Adonis aestivalis*), plantain leaf (*Plantago lanceolata*), pleurisy root, psyllium husks (*Plantago psyllium*), redheaded cotton-bush (*Asclepias currassavica*), rhubarb root (*Rheum palmatum*), rubber vine (*Cryptostegia grandifolia*), sea-mango (*Cerebra manghas*), senna fruit (*Cassia senna*), squill (*Urginea maritima*), strophanthus (*Strophanthus hispidus, Strophanthus kombe*), uzara (*Xysmalobium undulatum*), wallflower (*Cheirantus*

cheiri), white horehound (*Marrubium vulgare*), wintersweet (*Carissa spectabilis*), yellow dock root (*Rumex crispus*), yellow oleander (*Thevetia peruviana*).

CYTOCHROME P450: SELECTED SUBSTRATES, INHIBITORS, AND INDUCERS

CYP 450 1A2: Substrates (Affected Herbs and Supplements)

- Melatonin (N-acetyl-5-methoxytryptamine)

CYP 450 1A2: Inducing Herbs/Foods

- Cabbage, broccoli, brussels sprouts, cauliflower, charbroiled meats, cigarette smoking.

CYP 450 1A2: Inhibiting Herbs

- Dandelion, chaparral component nordihydroguairetic acid (NDGA) inhibits cytochrome P450–mediated monoxygenase activity in rat hepatic microsomes.

CYP 450 2A6: Inhibiting Herbs

- American pennyroyal (*Hedeoma pulegioides* L.), European pennyroyal (*Mentha pulegium* L.).

CYP 450 2C19: Substrates (Affected Herbs and Supplements)

- Red yeast rice (*Monascus purpureus*): levels of lovastatin present in *Monascus purpureus* may be affected.

CYP 450 2C19: Inhibiting Herbs

- Chaparral component nordihydroguairetic acid (NDGA) inhibits cytochrome P450–mediated monoxygenase activity in rat hepatic microsomes.

CYP 450 2C9: Inhibiting Herbs

- Milk thistle (*Silybum marianum*)/silymarin, St. John's wort (*Hypericum perforatum*), which is believed to exert more prominent effects on 3A4, has also been found *in vivo* and *in vitro* to inhibit 2C9 and 2D6. The chaparral component nordihydroguairetic acid (NDGA) inhibits cytochrome P450–mediated monoxygenase activity in rat hepatic microsomes. *In vitro* inhibition of CYP 450 2C9 has also been reported for black tea, cat's claw (*Uncaria tomentosa, Uncaria guianensis*), chamomile (*Matricaria chamomilla*), clove, ginger, gotu kola, kava (weak), oregano (weak), sage, Siberian ginseng, thyme, and turmeric (weak), although interactions have not been demonstrated in humans.

CYP 450 2D6: Inhibiting Herbs

- *SSRI herbs* (in theory; see SSRI section below). St. John's wort, which is believed to exert more prominent effects on 3A4, has also been found *in vivo* and *in vitro* to inhibit 2C9 and 2D6. The chaparral component nordihydroguairetic acid (NDGA) inhibits cytochrome P450–mediated monoxygenase activity in rat hepatic microsomes. *In vitro* inhibition of CYP 450 2D6 has also been reported for black tea, cat's claw (*Uncaria tomentosa, Uncaria guianensis*), chamomile (*Matricaria chamomilla*), clove, ginger, gotu kola, kava (weak), oregano, sage, thyme, and turmeric (weak), although interactions have not been demonstrated in humans.

CYP 450 2E1: Inhibiting Herbs

- Dandelion, chaparral component nordihydroguairetic acid (NDGA) inhibits cytochrome P450–mediated monoxygenase activity in rat hepatic microsomes.

[†]Estriol, estrone, estradiol, or estrogen constituents.
[‡]Isoflavone constituents.
*This is not an all-inclusive, comprehensive list of herbs that may contain clinically relevant levels of cardiac glycosides. A qualified healthcare practitioner should be consulted for specific questions or concerns regarding potential cardiac effects or interactions of specific agents.
Note: Bufalin/Chan Su (*Secretio bufonis*) is a Chinese herbal purported aphrodisiac that has been reported to be toxic or fatal when taken with cardiac glycosides. Reliable human data are limited.

CYP 450 3A (4,5,7): Substrates (Affected Herbs)

- DHEA, eucalyptol: initial evidence suggests that 1,8-cineole (eucalyptol), a principal constituent of eucalyptus oil, and a constituent of multiple other plants including tea tree oil, has been found in laboratory studies to be a substrate of CYP 450 3A.

CYP 450 3A (4,5,7): Inducing Herbs

- St. John's wort (*Hypericum perforatum*) appears to inhibit CYP 3A4 acutely and then to induce the enzyme with repeated administration. Hops (*Humulus lupuli*) have been demonstrated *in vitro* and *in vivo* to induce P450 3A and 2B. In theory, phytoprogestins (see above section) may induce CYP 3A4, although scientific data are lacking in this area. Examples include chasteberry (*Vitex agnus-castus*), bloodroot (*Sanguinaria canadensis*), oregano (*Oregano* spp.), damiana (*Turnera* spp.), and yucca (*Yucca* spp).

CYP 450 3A (4,5,7): Inhibiting Herbs/Foods

- Cannabinoids, ginseng (*Panax* and Siberian), grapefruit juice, milk thistle (*Silybum marianum*)/silymarin (although milk thistle has been found not to affect indinavir levels), peppermint oil, St. John's wort (*Hypericum perforatum*) appears to inhibit CYP 3A4 acutely and then to induce the enzyme with repeated administration. The chaparral component nordihydroguaiaretic acid (NDGA) inhibits cytochrome P450–mediated monoxygenase activity in rat hepatic microsomes. *In vitro* inhibition of CYP 450 3A4 has also been reported for black tea, cat's claw (*Uncaria tomentosa, Uncaria guianensis*), chamomile (*Matricaria chamomilla*), clove, *Echinacea angustifolia* root, ginger, goldenseal (*Hydrastis canadensis*), gotu kola, kava (weak), licorice (*Glycyrrhiza glabra*), oregano, sage, thyme, turmeric, and wild cherry (*Trifolium pratense*), although interactions have not been demonstrated in humans. No effect on P450 3A4 has been found in a human study of saw palmetto.

SELECTIVE SEROTONIN REUPTAKE INHIBITORS (SSRI): DRUGS, HERBS, VITAMINS, SUPPLEMENTS

Herbs/Supplements with Possible SSRI Effects

Based on preliminary evidence from basic science, human case reports/trials, and/or expert opinion.

- Ephedra, evening primrose oil (*Oenothera biennis*), fenugreek, ginkgo biloba, hops, St. John's wort, tyrosine, valerian, yohimbe.

Vitamins/Minerals with Possible SSRI Effects

Based on preliminary evidence from basic science, human case reports/trials, and/or expert opinion.

- 5-HTP (5-hydroxytryptophan), adrenal extract, chromium, DHEA (dehydroepiandrosterone), DLPA (DL phenylalanine), SAMe (S-adenosylmethionine), vitamin B_6.

Homeopathic Remedies with Possible SSRI Effects

Based on preliminary evidence from basic science, human case reports/trials, and/or expert opinion.

- Aurum metcallicum, Kali bromatum, Sepia.

MONOAMINE OXIDASE INHIBITORS (MAOIs)*
MAOI Drugs*

- Isocarboxazid (Marplan), phenelzine (Nardil), tranylcypromine (Parnate).

Herbs with Possible MAOI Effects

Based on preliminary evidence from basic science, human case reports/trials, and/or expert opinion.

- California poppy (*Eschscholtzia californica*), ephedra, evening primrose oil (*Oenothera biennis*), fenugreek (*Trigonella foenum-graecum*), ginkgo biloba, hops (*Humulus lupulus*), mace (*Myristica fragrans*), St. John's wort (*Hypericum perforatum*), valerian (*Valeriana officinalis*), yohimbe bark extract.

Supplements/Vitamins with Possible MAOI Effects

Based on preliminary evidence from basic science, human case reports/trials, and/or expert opinion.

- 5-HTP (5-hydroxytryptophan), adrenal extract, chromium, DHEA (dehydroepiandrosterone), DLPA (DL phenylalanine), SAMe (S-adenosylmethionine), vitamin B_6.

Homeopathic Remedies with Possible MAOI Effects

Based on preliminary evidence from basic science, human case reports/trials, and/or expert opinion

- Aurum metcallicum, kali bromatum, sepia.

TYRAMINE/TRYPTOPHAN-CONTAINING FOODS

May induce hypertensive crisis when taken concomitantly with MAOIs.

- Anchovies, avocados, bananas, bean curd, beer (alcohol-free/reduced), caffeine (large amounts), caviar, champagne, cheeses—particularly aged, processed, or strong varieties (e.g., camembert, cheddar, stilton)—chocolate, dry sausage/salami/bologna, fava beans, figs, herring (pickled), liver (particularly chicken), meat tenderizers, papaya, protein extracts/powder, raisins, shrimp paste, sour cream, soy sauce, wine (particularly chianti), yeast extracts, yogurt.

HERBS WITH LAXATIVE/STIMULANT LAXATIVE PROPERTIES†

Based on expert opinion, anecdote, case reports, and/or preliminary trial evidence.

- Alder buckthorn, aloe dried leaf sap (*Aloe* spp.), black root, blue flag rhizome, butternut bark, dong quai, European

---

Warning: Tyramine/tryptophan-containing foods may induce hypertensive crisis when taken concomitantly with MAOIs and should be avoided by individuals taking MAOIs. These include protein foods that have been aged/preserved. Specific examples of foods include anchovies, avocados, bananas, bean curd, beer (alcohol-free/reduced), caffeine (large amounts), caviar, champagne, cheeses—particularly aged, processed, or strong varieties (e.g., camembert, cheddar, stilton)—chocolate, dry sausage/salami/bologna, fava beans, figs, herring (pickled), liver (particularly chicken), meat tenderizers, papaya, protein extracts/powder, raisins, shrimp paste, sour cream, soy sauce, wine (particularly chianti), yeast extracts, yogurt. (Note: This is not a comprehensive, all-inclusive list of foods of concern, and a nutritionist or other qualified healthcare professional should be consulted for questions regarding potential drug-food or herb/supplement-food interactions.)

Note: In general, patients taking monoamine oxidase inhibitors (MAOIs) should avoid protein foods that have been aged/preserved. This is not a comprehensive, all-inclusive list of foods of concern, and a nutritionist or other qualified healthcare professional should be consulted for questions regarding potential drug-food or herb/supplement-food interactions.
†*Note:* This informational page is not an all-inclusive, comprehensive list of laxative herbs. Other herbs and supplements may possess laxative qualities. A qualified healthcare practitioner should be consulted with specific questions or concerns regarding potential laxative effects of agents or interactions.

buckthorn, eyebright herb (*Euphrasia* spp.), cascara bark (*Rhamnus persiana*), castor oil, chasteberry (*Vitex agnus-castus*), colocynth fruit pulp, dandelion, gamboges bark exudates, horsetail (*Equisetum arvense*), jalap root, manna bark exudates, plantain leaf (*Plantago lanceolata*), podophyllum root, psyllium husks (*Plantago psyllium*), rhubarb (*Rheum palmatum*) root, senna (*Cassia senna*) fruit, wild cucumber fruit, yellow dock (*Rumex crispus*) root.

These tables are organized by specific health conditions and their related terms. Traditionally, ailments treated with herbs and supplements often are related to other illnesses, and these relationships are useful to consider. Each table is organized by level of evidence, according to the Natural Standard Evidence-Based Validated Grading Scale (see below), with therapies for which there is the best evidence graded higher on the table.

Grades reflect the level of available scientific evidence in support of the efficacy of a given therapy for a specific indication. Evidence of harm is considered separately; the grades shown apply only to evidence of benefit. Note that these tables only consider therapies that are discussed in this text, and that there are other herbs and supplements not discussed in this book that are also used for many of these conditions.

Natural Standard Evidence-Based Validated Grading Rationale

Level of Evidence Grade	Criteria
A (Strong scientific evidence)	Statistically significant evidence of benefit from >2 randomized, controlled trials (RCTs), *or* evidence from 1 RCT *and* 1 properly conducted meta-analysis, *or* evidence from multiple RCTs with a clear majority of the trials showing statistically significant evidence of benefit, *and* with supporting evidence in basic science, animal studies, or theory.
B (Good scientific evidence)	Statistically significant evidence of benefit from 1 or 2 RCTs *or* evidence of benefit from >1 properly conducted meta-analysis, *or* evidence of benefit from >1 cohort/case-controlled/non-randomized trial, *and* with supporting evidence in basic science, animal studies, or theory.
C (Unclear or conflicting scientific evidence)	Evidence of benefit from ≥1 small RCT without adequate size, power, statistical significance, or quality of design by objective criteria,* *or* conflicting evidence from multiple RCTs without a clear majority of the properly conducted trials showing evidence of benefit or ineffectiveness, *or* evidence of benefit from >1 cohort/case-controlled/non-randomized trial, *and* without supporting evidence in basic science, animal studies, or theory, *or* evidence of efficacy only from basic science, animal studies, or theory.
D (Fair negative scientific evidence)	Statistically significant negative evidence (i.e., lack of evidence of benefit) from cohort/case-controlled/non-randomized trials, *and* evidence in basic science, animal studies, or theory suggesting a lack of benefit.
F (Strong negative scientific evidence)	Statistically significant negative evidence (i.e., lack of evidence of benefit) from ≥1 properly randomized adequately powered trial of high-quality design by objective criteria.*
Lack of Evidence (Traditional/theoretical)	Unable to evaluate efficacy due to lack of adequate or available human data.

*Objective criteria are derived from validated instruments for evaluating study quality, including the 5-point scale developed by Jadad et al., in which a score below 4 is considered to indicate lesser quality methodologically (Jadad AR, Moore RA, Carroll D, et al. Assessing the quality of reports of randomized clinical trials: is blinding necessary? *Controlled Clinical Trials* 1996;17[1]:1-12).

ACNE AND RELATED CONDITIONS
Levels of Scientific Evidence for Specific Therapies

GRADE: C (Unclear or Conflicting Scientific Evidence)	
Therapy	Specific Therapeutic Use(s)
Guggul (Commifora mukul)	Acne
Tea tree oil (*Melaleuca alternifolia* [Maiden & Betche] Cheel)	Acne vulgaris

TRADITIONAL OR THEORETICAL USES THAT LACK SUFFICIENT EVIDENCE	
Therapy	Specific Therapeutic Use(s)
American pennyroyal (*Hedeoma pulegioides* L.), European pennyroyal (*Mentha pulegium* L.)	Acne

Boswellia (*Boswellia serrata* Roxb.)	Acne
Boswellia (*Boswellia serrata* Roxb.)	Pimples
Burdock (*Arctium lappa*)	Acne
Calendula (*Calendula officinalis* L.), marigold	Acne
Chamomile (*Matricaria recutita, Chamaemelum nobile*)	Acne
Dandelion (*Taraxacum officinale*)	Acne
Danshen (*Salvia miltiorrhiza*)	Acne
Echinacea (*Echinacea angustifolia* DC., *E. pallida, E. purpurea*)	Acne
Flaxseed and flaxseed oil (*Linum usitatissimum*)	Pimples
Goldenseal (*Hydrastis canadensis* L.), berberine	Acne
Hawthorn (*Crataegus laevigata, C. oxyacantha, C. monogyna, C. pentagyna*)	Acne
Lactobacillus acidophilus	Acne
Lavender (*Lavandula angustifolia* Miller)	Acne
Niacin (vitamin B_3, nicotinic acid), niacinamide, and inositol hexanicotinate	Acne
Propolis	Acne
Red clover (*Trifolium pratense*)	Acne
Saw palmetto (*Serenoa repens* [Bartram] Small)	Acne
Sorrel (*Rumex acetosa* L., *R. acetosella* L.), sinupret	Acne
Thyme (*Thymus vulgaris* L.), thymol	Acne
Valerian (*Valeriana officinalis* L.)	Acne

ADDICTION AND RELATED CONDITIONS

Levels of Scientific Evidence for Specific Therapies

GRADE: C (Unclear or Conflicting Scientific Evidence)

Therapy	Specific Therapeutic Use(s)
Globe artichoke (*Cynara scolymus* L.)	Alcohol-induced hangover
Goldenseal (*Hydrastis canadensis* L.), berberine	Narcotic concealment (urinalysis)
Melatonin	Benzodiazepine tapering
Melatonin	Smoking cessation

TRADITIONAL OR THEORETICAL USES THAT LACK SUFFICIENT EVIDENCE

Therapy	Specific therapeutic Use(s)
Betel nut (*Areca catechu* L.)	Alcoholism
Black tea (*Camellia sinensis*)	Toxin/alcohol elimination from the body
Burdock (*Arctium lappa*)	Detoxification
Chamomile (*Matricaria recutita, Chamaemelum nobile*)	Delirium tremens (DTs)

Continued

Clay	Smoking
Dandelion (*Taraxacum officinale*)	Alcohol withdrawal
Dandelion (*Taraxacum officinale*)	Smoking cessation
Essiac	Detoxification
Evening primrose oil (*Oenothera biennis* L.)	Alcoholism
Evening primrose oil (*Oenothera biennis* L.)	Hangover remedy
Ginger (*Zingiber officinale* Roscoe)	Alcohol withdrawal
Ginkgo (*Ginkgo biloba* L.)	Alcoholism
Green tea (*Camellia sinensis*)	Alcohol intoxication
Green tea (*Camellia sinensis*)	Detoxification from alcohol or toxins
Lavender (*Lavandula angustifolia* Miller)	Hangover
Licorice (*Glycyrrhiza glabra* L.) and Deglycyrrhizinated licorice (DGL)	Detoxification
Melatonin	Withdrawal from narcotics
Niacin (vitamin B_3, nicotinic acid), niacinamide, and inositol hexanicotinate	Alcohol dependence
Niacin (vitamin B_3, nicotinic acid), niacinamide, and inositol hexanicotinate	Smoking cessation
Oleander (*Nerium oleander, Thevetia peruviana*)	Alcoholism
St. John's wort (*Hypericum perforatum* L.)	Alcoholism
St. John's wort (*Hypericum perforatum* L.)	Benzodiazepine withdrawal
Valerian (*Valeriana officinalis* L.)	Hangovers

AIDS/HIV AND RELATED CONDITIONS

Levels of Scientific Evidence for Specific Therapies

GRADE: C (Unclear or Conflicting Scientific Evidence)

Therapy	Specific therapeutic Use(s)
Aloe (*Aloe vera*)	HIV
Antineoplastons	HIV
Bitter melon (*Momordica charantia* L.) and MAP30	HIV
Coenzyme Q10	HIV/AIDS
DHEA (dehydroepiandrosterone)	HIV/AIDS
Flaxseed and flaxseed oil (*Linum usitatissimum*)	HIV/AIDS
Melatonin	HIV/AIDS
Turmeric (*Curcuma longa* L.), curcumin	HIV

GRADE: D (Fair Negative Scientific Evidence)

Therapy	Specific Therapeutic Use(s)
St. John's wort (*Hypericum perforatum* L.)	HIV

TRADITIONAL OR THEORETICAL USES THAT LACK SUFFICIENT EVIDENCE

Therapy	Specific Therapeutic Use(s)
Arginine (L-arginine)	AIDS/HIV
Astragalus (*Astragalus membranaceus*)	AIDS/HIV
Bromelain	AIDS
Burdock (*Arctium lappa*)	HIV
Calendula (*Calendula officinalis* L.), marigold	HIV
Dandelion (*Taraxacum officinale*)	AIDS
Danshen (*Salvia miltiorrhiza*)	HIV
DHEA (dehydroepiandrosterone)	Lipodystrophy in HIV
Echinacea (*Echinacea angustifolia* DC., *E. pallida*, *E. purpurea*)	HIV/AIDS
Elder (*Sambucus nigra* L.)	HIV
Essiac	AIDS/HIV
Eucalyptus oil (*Eucalyptus globulus* Labillardiere, *E. fructicetorum* F. Von Mueller, *E. smithii* R.T. Baker)	AIDS
Garlic (*Allium sativum* L.)	AIDS
Garlic (*Allium sativum* L.)	HIV
Ginseng (American ginseng, Asian ginseng, Chinese ginseng, Korean red ginseng, *Panax ginseng*: *Panax* spp. including *P. ginseng* C.C. Meyer and *P. quincefolium* L., excluding *Eleutherococcus senticosus*)	HIV
Goldenseal (*Hydrastis canadensis* L.), berberine	AIDS
Green tea (*Camellia sinensis*)	HIV/AIDS
Lactobacillus acidophilus	AIDS
Lavender (*Lavandula angustifolia* Miller)	HIV
Licorice (*Glycyrrhiza glabra* L.) and deglycyrrhizinated licorice (DGL)	HIV
Lycopene	AIDS
Maitake mushroom (*Grifola frondosa*) and beta-glucan	HIV
Niacin (vitamin B3, nicotinic acid), niacinamide, and inositol hexanicotinate	HIV prevention
Omega-3 fatty acids, fish oil, alpha-linolenic acid	AIDS
Propolis	HIV
Red clover (*Trifolium pratense*)	AIDS
Spirulina	HIV

ALLERGIES AND RELATED CONDITIONS

Levels of Scientific Evidence for Specific Therapies

GRADE: B (Good Scientific Evidence)	
Therapy	Specific Therapeutic Use(s)
Bromelain	Sinusitis

Continued

GRADE: C (Unclear or Conflicting Scientific Evidence)	
Therapy	Specific Therapeutic Use(s)
Elder (*Sambucus nigra* L.)	Bacterial sinusitis
Ephedra (Ephedra sinica) ma huang	Allergic rhinitis
Eucalyptus oil (*Eucalyptus globulus* Labillardiere, *E. fructicetorum* F. Von Mueller, *E. smithii* R.T. Baker)	Decongestant/expectorant
Sorrel (Rumex acetosa L., R. acetosella L.), Sinupret	Sinusitis

TRADITIONAL OR THEORETICAL USES THAT LACK SUFFICIENT EVIDENCE	
Therapy	Specific Therapeutic Use(s)
Alfalfa (*Medicago sativa* L.)	Allergies
Alfalfa (*Medicago sativa* L.)	Hay fever
Astragalus (*Astragalus membranaceus*)	Allergies
Belladonna (*Atropa belladonna* L. or its variety *acuminata* Royle ex Lindl)	Hay fever
Bromelain	Allergic rhinitis (hay fever)
Bromelain	Food allergies
Burdock (*Arctium lappa*)	Hives
Chamomile (*Matricaria recutita, Chamaemelum nobile*)	Hay fever
Chamomile (*Matricaria recutita, Chamaemelum nobile*)	Hives
Chamomile (*Matricaria recutita, Chamaemelum nobile*)	Sinusitis
Chaparral (*Larrea tridentata* DC. Coville, *L. divaricata* Cav.), nordihydroguaiaretic acid (NDGA)	Allergies
Clove (*Eugenia aromatica*)	Antihistamine
Dandelion (*Taraxacum officinale*)	Allergies
Devil's claw (*Harpagophytum procumbens* DC.)	Allergies
DHEA (dehydroepiandrosterone)	Allergic disorders
DHEA (dehydroepiandrosterone)	Angioedema
Dong quai (*Angelica sinensis* [Oliv.] Diels), Chinese angelica	Allergy
Dong quai (*Angelica sinensis* [Oliv.] Diels), Chinese angelica	Chronic rhinitis
Dong quai (*Angelica sinensis* [Oliv.] Diels), Chinese angelica	Hay fever
Echinacea (*Echinacea angustifolia* DC., *E. pallida, E. purpurea*)	Catarrh
Elder (*Sambucus nigra* L.)	Hay fever
Ephedra (*Ephedra sinica*)/ma huang	Acute coryza (rhinitis)
Ephedra (*Ephedra sinica*)/ma huang	Decongestant
Ephedra (*Ephedra sinica*)/ma huang	Hay fever
Ephedra (*Ephedra* sinica)/ma huang	Urticaria

Eucalyptus oil (*Eucalyptus globulus* Labillardiere, *E. fructicetorum* F. Von Mueller, *E. smithii* R.T. Baker)	Runny nose
Eucalyptus oil (*Eucalyptus globulus* Labillardiere, *E. fructicetorum* F. Von Mueller, *E. smithii* R.T. Baker)	Sinusitis
Eyebright (*Euphrasia officinalis*)	Allergies
Eyebright (*Euphrasia officinalis*)	Hay fever
Eyebright (*Euphrasia officinalis*)	Rhinitis
Eyebright (*Euphrasia officinalis*)	Sinusitis
Flaxseed and flaxseed oil (*Linum usitatissimum*)	Allergic reactions
Garlic (*Allium sativum* L.)	Allergies
Ginkgo (*Ginkgo biloba* L.)	Allergies
Ginkgo (*Ginkgo biloba* L.)	Chronic rhinitis
Ginseng (American ginseng, Asian ginseng, Chinese ginseng, Korean red ginseng, *Panax ginseng*: *Panax* spp. including *P. ginseng* C.C. Meyer and *P. quincefolium* L., excluding *Eleutherococcus senticosus*)	Allergies
Globe artichoke (*Cynara scolymus* L.)	Allergies
Goldenseal (*Hydrastis canadensis* L.), berberine	Antihistamine
Goldenseal (*Hydrastis canadensis* L.), berberine	Sinusitis
Guggul (*Commifora mukul*)	Rhinitis
Lactobacillus acidophilus	Allergies
Lactobacillus acidophilus	Hives
Oleander (*Nerium oleander*, *Thevetia peruviana*)	Sinus problems
Omega-3 fatty acids, fish oil, alpha-linolenic acid	Allergies
Omega-3 fatty acids, fish oil, alpha-linolenic acid	Hay fever
Saw palmetto (*Serenoa repens* [Bartram] Small)	Catarrh
Shark cartilage	Allergic skin rashes
Sorrel (*Rumex acetosa* L., *R. acetosella* L.), Sinupret	Sinusitis
Spirulina	Anaphylaxis (severe allergic reaction) prevention
Thyme (*Thymus vulgaris* L.), thymol	Sinusitis

ALOPECIA AND RELATED CONDITIONS

Levels of Scientific Evidence for Specific Therapies

GRADE: C (Unclear or Conflicting Scientific Evidence)	
Therapy	Specific Therapeutic Use(s)
Saw palmetto (*Serenoa repens* [Bartram] Small)	Androgenetic alopecia (topical)
Thyme (Thymus vulgaris L.), thymol	Alopecia areata

Continued

TRADITIONAL OR THEORETICAL USES THAT LACK SUFFICIENT EVIDENCE

Therapy	Specific Therapeutic Use(s)
Aloe (*Aloe vera*)	Alopecia (hair loss)
Bladderwrack (*Fucus vesiculosus*)	Hair loss
Burdock (*Arctium lappa*)	Dandruff
Burdock (*Arctium lappa*)	Hair loss
Chaparral (*Larrea tridentata* DC. Coville, *L. divaricata* Cav.), nordihydroguaiaretic acid (NDGA)	Hair tonic
Coenzyme Q10	Hair loss from chemotherapy
Dandelion (*Taraxacum officinale*)	Dandruff
Elder (*Sambucus nigra* L.)	Hair dye
Fenugreek (*Trigonella foenum-graecum* L.)	Baldness
Garlic (*Allium sativum* L.)	Hair growth
Ginger (*Zingiber officinale* Roscoe)	Baldness
Goldenseal (*Hydrastis canadensis* L.), berberine	Dandruff
Gotu kola (*Centella asiatica* L.), total triterpenic fraction of *Centella asiatica* (TTFCA)	Hair growth promoter
Horsetail (*Equisetum arvense* L.)	Hair loss
Lavender (*Lavandula angustifolia* Miller)	Hair loss
Pygeum (*Prunus africana*, *Pygeum africanum*)	Male baldness
Seaweed, kelp, bladderwrack (*Fucus vesiculosus*)	Hair loss
Spirulina	Hair loss

ALZHEIMER'S DISEASE AND RELATED CONDITIONS

Levels of Scientific Evidence for Specific Therapies

GRADE: B (Good Scientific Evidence)

Therapy	Specific Therapeutic Use(s)
Ginkgo (*Ginkgo biloba* L.)	Cerebral insufficiency
Ginseng (American ginseng, Asian ginseng, Chinese ginseng, Korean red ginseng, *Panax ginseng*: *Panax* spp. including *P. ginseng* C.C. Meyer and *P. quincefolium* L., excluding *Eleutherococcus senticosus*)	Mental performance

GRADE: C (Unclear or Conflicting Scientific Evidence)

Therapy	Specific Therapeutic Use(s)
Black tea (*Camellia sinensis*)	Memory enhancement
Black tea (*Camellia sinensis*)	Mental performance/alertness
Boron	Improving cognitive function
Ginkgo (*Ginkgo biloba* L.)	Age-associated memory impairment (AAMI)

Ginkgo (*Ginkgo biloba* L.)	Memory enhancement (in healthy people)
Green tea (*Camellia sinensis*)	Memory enhancement
Green tea (*Camellia sinensis*)	Mental performance/alertness
Polypodium leucotomos extract, Anapsos	Dementia

GRADE: D (Fair Negative Scientific Evidence)	
Therapy	Specific Therapeutic Use(s)
DHEA (dehydroepiandrosterone)	Brain function and well-being in the elderly

TRADITIONAL OR THEORETICAL USES THAT LACK SUFFICIENT EVIDENCE	
Therapy	Specific Therapeutic Use(s)
Arginine (L-arginine)	Dementia
Astragalus (*Astragalus membranaceus*)	Dementia
Astragalus (*Astragalus membranaceus*)	Memory
Blessed thistle (*Cnicus benedictus* L.)	Memory improvement
Danshen (*Salvia miltiorrhiza*)	Anoxic brain injury
DHEA (dehydroepiandrosterone)	Dementia
Eyebright (*Euphrasia officinalis*)	Memory loss
Garlic (*Allium sativum* L.)	Age-related memory problems
Ginseng (American ginseng, Asian ginseng, Chinese ginseng, Korean red ginseng, *Panax ginseng. Panax* spp. including *P. ginseng* C.C. Meyer and *P. quincefolium* L., excluding *Eleutherococcus senticosus*)	Dementia
Ginseng (American ginseng, Asian ginseng, Chinese ginseng, Korean red ginseng, *Panax ginseng. Panax* spp. including *P. ginseng* C.C. Meyer and *P. quincefolium* L., excluding *Eleutherococcus senticosus*)	Improved memory and thinking after menopause
Ginseng (American ginseng, Asian ginseng, Chinese ginseng, Korean red ginseng, *Panax ginseng. Panax* spp. including *P. ginseng* C.C. Meyer and *P. quincefolium* L., excluding *Eleutherococcus senticosus*)	Senile dementia
Gotu kola (*Centella asiatica* L.), total triterpenic fraction of *Centella asiatica* (TTFCA)	Memory enhancement
Green tea (*Camellia sinensis*)	Cognitive performance enhancement
Kava (*Piper methysticum* G. Forst)	Brain damage
Lycopene	Cognitive function
Melatonin	Cognitive enhancement
Melatonin	Memory enhancement
Niacin (vitamin B_3, nicotinic acid), niacinamide, and inositol hexanicotinate	Memory loss
Omega-3 fatty acids, fish oil, alpha-linolenic acid	Memory enhancement
Soy (*Glycine max* L. Merr.)	Cognitive function
Soy (*Glycine max* L. Merr.)	Memory enhancement

Continued

Spirulina	Memory improvement
Valerian (*Valeriana officinalis* L.)	Memory
Yohimbe bark extract (*Pausinystalia yohimbe* Pierre ex Beille)	Cognition

ANEMIA AND RELATED CONDITIONS
Levels of Scientific Evidence for Specific Therapies

GRADE: C (Unclear or Conflicting Scientific Evidence)	
Therapy	Specific Therapeutic Use(s)
Antineoplastons	Sickle cell anemia/thalassemia
Betel nut (*Areca catechu* L.)	Anemia

TRADITIONAL OR THEORETICAL USES THAT LACK SUFFICIENT EVIDENCE	
Therapy	Specific Therapeutic Use(s)
Arginine (L-arginine)	Beta-hemoglobinopathies
Arginine (L-arginine)	Sickle cell anemia
Astragalus (*Astragalus membranaceus*)	Anemia
Calendula (*Calendula officinalis* L.), marigold	Anemia
Dandelion (*Taraxacum officinale*)	Anemia
Dong quai (*Angelica sinensis* [Oliv.] Diels), Chinese angelica	Anemia
Dong quai (*Angelica sinensis* [Oliv.] Diels), Chinese angelica	Hemolytic disease of the newborn
Feverfew (*Tanacetum parthenium* L. Schultz-Bip.)	Anemia
Ginseng (American ginseng, Asian ginseng, Chinese ginseng, Korean red ginseng, *Panax ginseng*: Panax spp. including *P. ginseng* C.C. Meyer and *P. quincefolium* L., excluding Eleutherococcus senticosus)	Anemia
Globe artichoke (*Cynara scolymus* L.)	Anemia
Gotu kola (*Centella asiatica* L.), total triterpenic fraction of *Centella asiatica* (TTFCA)	Anemia
Sorrel (*Rumex acetosa* L., *R. acetosella* L.), Sinupret	Anemia
Soy (*Glycine max* L. Merr.)	Anemia
Spirulina	Anemia

ANTI-AGING AND RELATED CONDITIONS
Levels of Scientific Evidence for Specific Therapies

TRADITIONAL OR THEORETICAL USES THAT LACK SUFFICIENT EVIDENCE	
Therapy	Specific Therapeutic Use(s)
Antineoplastons	Aging
Arginine (L-arginine)	Anti-aging
Astragalus (*Astragalus membranaceus*)	Aging

DHEA (dehydroepiandrosterone)	Aging
Dong quai (*Angelica sinensis* [Oliv.] Diels), Chinese angelica	Anti-aging
Ginkgo (*Ginkgo biloba* L.)	Aging
Ginseng (American ginseng, Asian ginseng, Chinese ginseng, Korean red ginseng, *Panax ginseng*: *Panax* spp. including *P. ginseng* C.C. Meyer and *P. quincefolium* L., excluding *Eleutherococcus senticosus*)	Aging
Melatonin	Aging
Niacin (Vitamin B$_3$, nicotinic acid), niacinamide, and inositol hexanicotinate	Anti-aging

ANTICOAGULATION AND RELATED CONDITIONS
Levels of Scientific Evidence for Specific Therapies

GRADE: C (Unclear or Conflicting Scientific Evidence)

Therapy	Specific Therapeutic Use(s)
Bladderwrack (*Fucus vesiculosus*)	Anticoagulant (blood thinner)
Garlic (*Allium sativum* L.)	Antiplatelet effects (blood thinning)
Seaweed, kelp, bladderwrack (*Fucus vesiculosus*)	Anticoagulant
Yohimbe bark extract (*Pausinystalia yohimbe* Pierre ex Beille)	Inhibition of platelet aggregation

TRADITIONAL OR THEORETICAL USES THAT LACK SUFFICIENT EVIDENCE

Therapy	Specific therapeutic Use(s)
Alfalfa (*Medicago sativa* L.)	Blood clotting disorders
Astragalus (*Astragalus membranaceus*)	Blood thinner
Barley (*Hordeum vulgare* L.), germinated barley foodstuff (GBF)	Blood circulation
Bromelain	Blood clot treatment
Bromelain	Platelet inhibition (blood thinner)
Calendula (*Calendula officinalis* L.), marigold	Blood vessel clots
Clove (*Eugenia aromatica*)	Blood thinner (antiplatelet agent)
Danshen (*Salvia miltiorrhiza*)	Blood clotting disorders
Danshen (*Salvia miltiorrhiza*)	Hypercoagulability
Dong quai (*Angelica sinensis* [Oliv.] Diels), Chinese angelica	Blood clots
Dong quai (*Angelica sinensis* [Oliv.] Diels), Chinese angelica	Blood flow disorders
Dong quai (*Angelica sinensis* [Oliv.] Diels), Chinese angelica	Blood stagnation
Dong quai (*Angelica sinensis* [Oliv.] Diels), Chinese angelica	Blood vessel disorders

Continued

Elder (*Sambucus nigra* L.)	Blood vessel disorders
Flaxseed and flaxseed oil (*Linum usitatissimum*)	Blood thinner
Ginger (*Zingiber officinale* Roscoe)	Blood thinner
Ginkgo (*Ginkgo biloba* L.)	Blood clots
Ginkgo (*Ginkgo biloba* L.)	Blood vessel disorders
Goldenseal (*Hydrastis canadensis* L.), berberine	Anticoagulant (blood thinner)
Goldenseal (*Hydrastis canadensis* L.), berberine	Blood circulation stimulant
Green tea (*Camellia sinensis*)	Inhibition of platelet aggregation
Horse chestnut (*Aesculus hippocastanum* L.)	Lung blood clots (pulmonary embolism)
Niacin (vitamin B_3, nicotinic acid), niacinamide, and inositol hexanicotinate	Blood circulation improvement
Omega-3 fatty acids, fish oil, alpha-linolenic acid	Anticoagulation
Propolis	Anticoagulant
Red yeast rice (*Monascus purpureus*)	Blood circulation problems

ANTIDEPRESSANT AND RELATED CONDITIONS
Levels of scientific evidence for specific therapies

GRADE: A (Strong Scientific Evidence)

Therapy	Specific Therapeutic Use(s)
St. John's wort (*Hypericum perforatum* L.)	Depressive disorder (mild to moderate)

GRADE: C (Unclear or Conflicting Scientific Evidence)

Therapy	Specific Therapeutic Use(s)
DHEA (dehydroepiandrosterone)	Depression
Evening primrose Oil (*Oenothera biennis* L.)	Postviral/chronic fatigue syndrome
Ginkgo (*Ginkgo biloba* L.)	Depression and seasonal affective disorder (SAD)
Melatonin	Bipolar disorder (sleep disturbances)
Melatonin	Depression (sleep disturbances)
Melatonin	Seasonal affective disorder (SAD)
Omega-3 fatty acids, fish oil, alpha-linolenic acid	Bipolar disorder
Omega-3 fatty acids, fish oil, alpha-linolenic acid	Depression
St. John's wort (*Hypericum perforatum* L.)	Depressive disorder (severe)
St. John's wort (*Hypericum perforatum* L.)	Seasonal affective disorder (SAD)

TRADITIONAL OR THEORETICAL USES THAT LACK SUFFICIENT EVIDENCE

Therapy	Specific Therapeutic Use(s)
Black cohosh (*Cimicifuga racemosa* L. Nutt.)	Depression
Dong quai (*Angelica sinensis* [Oliv.] Diels), Chinese angelica	Anti-aging
Ginkgo (*Ginkgo biloba* L.)	Aging
Ginseng (American ginseng, Asian ginseng, Chinese ginseng, Korean red ginseng, *Panax ginseng*: *Panax* spp. including *P. ginseng* C.C. Meyer and *P. quincefolium* L., excluding *Eleutherococcus senticosus*)	Aging
Melatonin	Aging
Niacin (vitamin B$_3$, nicotinic acid), niacinamide, and inositol hexanicotinate	Anti-aging
Ginseng (American ginseng, Asian ginseng, Chinese ginseng, Korean red ginseng, *Panax ginseng*: *Panax* spp. *including P. ginseng* C.C. Meyer and *P. quincefolium* L., excluding *Eleutherococcus senticosus*)	Antidepressant
Gotu kola (*Centella asiatica* L.), total triterpenic fraction of *Centella asiatica* (TTFCA)	Antidepressant
Gotu kola (*Centella asiatica* L), total triterpenic fraction of *Centella asiatica* (TTFCA)	Mood disorders
Hops (*Humulus lupulus* L.)	Antidepressant
Hops (*Humulus lupulus* L.)	Mood disturbances
Kava (*Piper methysticum* G. Forst)	Depression
Lavender (*Lavandula angustifolia* Miller)	Depression
Licorice (*Glycyrrhiza glabra* L.) and deglycyrrhizinated licorice (DGL)	Depression
Melatonin	Depression
Milk thistle (*Silybum marianum*), silymarin	Depression
Niacin (vitamin B$_3$, nicotinic acid), niacinamide, and inositol hexanicotinate	Depression
Spirulina	Depression
Spirulina	Mood stimulant
Thyme (*Thymus vulgaris* L.), thymol	Depression
Valerian (*Valeriana officinalis* L.)	Mood enhancement
Yohimbe bark extract (*Pausinystalia yohimbe* Pierre ex Beille)	Depression
Yohimbe bark extract (*Pausinystalia yohimbe* Pierre ex Beille)	Depression

ANTI-INFLAMMATORY AND RELATED CONDITIONS

Levels of Scientific Evidence for Specific Therapies

GRADE: B (Good Scientific Evidence)

Therapy	Specific Therapeutic Use(s)
Bromelain	Inflammation

Continued

GRADE: C (Unclear or Conflicting Scientific Evidence)	
Therapy	Specific Therapeutic Use(s)
Arginine (L-arginine)	Dental pain (ibuprofen arginate)
Black cohosh (*Cimicifuga racemosa* L. Nutt.)	Arthritis pain (rheumatoid arthritis, osteoarthritis)
Dandelion (*Taraxacum officinale*)	Anti-inflammatory
Eyebright (*Euphrasia officinalis*)	Anti-inflammatory
Propolis	Dental pain
Shark cartilage	Analgesia
Turmeric (*Curcuma longa* L.), curcumin	Inflammation
White horehound (*Marrubium vulgare*)	Pain

TRADITIONAL OR THEORETICAL USES THAT LACK SUFFICIENT EVIDENCE	
Therapy	Specific Therapeutic Use(s)
Alfalfa (*Medicago sativa* L.)	Inflammation
Arginine (L-arginine)	Pain
Astragalus (*Astragalus membranaceus*)	Myalgia (muscle pain)
Belladonna (*Atropa belladonna* L. or its variety *acuminata* Royle ex Lindl)	Anesthetic
Belladonna (*Atropa belladonna* L. or its variety *acuminata* Royle ex Lindl)	Inflammation
Belladonna (*Atropa belladonna* L. or its variety *acuminata* Royle ex Lindl)	Muscle and joint pain
Bitter almond (*Prunus amygdalus* Batch var. *amara* DC. Focke), Laetrile	Anti-inflammatory
Bitter Almond (*Prunus amygdalus* Batch var. *amara* DC. Focke), Laetrile	Local anesthetic
Bitter Almond (*Prunus amygdalus* Batch var. *amara* DC. Focke), Laetrile	Pain suppressant
Black cohosh (*Cimicifuga racemosa* L. Nutt.)	Inflammation
Black cohosh (*Cimicifuga racemosa* L. Nutt.)	Muscle pain
Black tea (*Camellia sinensis*)	Pain
Blessed thistle (*Cnicus benedictus* L.)	Inflammation
Bromelain	Pain
Bromelain	Pain (general)
Burdock (*Arctium lappa*)	Inflammation
Calendula (*Calendula officinalis* L.), marigold	Pain
Chamomile (*Matricaria recutita, Chamaemelum nobile*)	Anti-inflammatory
Chaparral (*Larrea tridentata* DC. Coville, *L. divaricata* Cav.), nordihydroguaiaretic acid (NDGA)	Anti-inflammatory
Chaparral (*Larrea tridentata* DC. Coville, *L. divaricata* Cav.), nordihydroguaiaretic acid (NDGA)	Pain

Clove (*Eugenia aromatica*)	Pain
Dandelion (*Taraxacum officinale*)	Analgesia
Devil's claw (*Harpagophytum procumbens* DC.)	Anti-inflammatory
Devil's claw (*Harpagophytum procumbens* DC.)	Muscle pain
Devil's claw (*Harpagophytum procumbens* DC.)	Pain
Dong quai (*Angelica sinensis* [Oliv.] Diels), Chinese angelica	Pain
Dong quai (*Angelica sinensis* [Oliv.] Diels), Chinese angelica	Pain from bruises
Echinacea (*Echinacea angustifolia* DC., *E. pallida*, *E. purpurea*)	Pain
Elder (*Sambucus nigra* L.)	Anti-inflammatory
Ephedra (*Ephedra sinica*)/ma huang	Anti-inflammatory
Eucalyptus oil (*Eucalyptus globulus* Labillardiere, *E. fructicetorum* F. Von Mueller, *E. smithii* R.T. Baker)	Inflammation
Eucalyptus oil (*Eucalyptus globulus* Labillardiere, *E. fructicetorum* F. Von Mueller, *E. smithii* R.T. Baker)	Muscle/joint pain (applied to the skin)
Evening primrose oil (*Oenothera biennis* L.)	Pain
Fenugreek (*Trigonella foenum-graecum* L. Leguminosae)	Inflammation
Feverfew (*Tanacetum parthenium* L. Schultz-Bip.)	Anti-inflammatory
Garlic (*Allium sativum* L.)	Dental pain
Ginger (*Zingiber officinale* Roscoe)	Pain relief
Ginseng (American ginseng, Asian ginseng, Chinese ginseng, Korean red ginseng, *Panax ginseng*: *Panax* spp. including *P. ginseng* C.C. Meyer and *P. quincefolium* L., excluding *Eleutherococcus senticosus*)	Inflammation
Ginseng (American ginseng, Asian ginseng, Chinese ginseng, Korean red ginseng, *Panax ginseng*: *Panax* spp. including *P. ginseng* C.C. Meyer and *P. quincefolium* L., excluding *Eleutherococcus senticosus*)	Pain relief
Goldenseal (*Hydrastis canadensis* L.), berberine	Anesthetic
Goldenseal (*Hydrastis canadensis* L.), berberine	Anti-inflammatory
Goldenseal (*Hydrastis canadensis* L.), berberine	Muscle pain
Goldenseal (*Hydrastis canadensis* L.), berberine	Pain
Gotu kola (*Centella asiatica* L), total triterpenic fraction of *Centella asiatica* (TTFCA)	Inflammation
Gotu kola (*Centella asiatica* L), total triterpenic fraction of *Centella asiatica* (TTFCA)	Pain
Guggul (*Commifora mukul*)	Pain
Hops (*Humulus lupulus* L.)	Anti-inflammatory
Hops (*Humulus lupulus* L.)	Pain
Kava (*Piper methysticum* G. Forst)	Anesthesia
Kava (*Piper methysticum* G. Forst)	Pain
Lavender (*Lavandula angustifolia* Miller)	Anti-inflammatory
Lavender (*Lavandula angustifolia* Miller)	Pain

Continued

Licorice (*Glycyrrhiza glabra* L.), deglycyrrhizinated licorice (DGL)	Inflammation
Marshmallow (*Althaea officinalis* L.)	Inflammation
Marshmallow (*Althaea officinalis* L.)	Muscular pain
Oleander (*Nerium oleander, Thevetia peruviana*)	Inflammation
Passionflower (*Passiflora incarnata* L.)	Chronic pain
Passionflower (*Passiflora incarnata* L.)	Pain (general)
Peppermint (*Mentha x piperita* L.)	Local anesthetic
Peppermint (*Mentha x piperita* L.)	Musculoskeletal pain
Peppermint (*Mentha x piperita* L.)	Myalgia (muscle pain)
Polypodium leucotomos extract, Anapsos	Inflammation
Pygeum (*Prunus africana, Pygeum africanum*)	Inflammation
Saw palmetto (*Serenoa repens* [Bartram] Small)	Anti-inflammatory
Slippery elm (*Ulmus rubra* Muhl., *U. fulva* Michx.)	Inflammation
Spirulina	Anti-inflammatory
St. John's wort (*Hypericum perforatum* L.)	Anti-inflammatory
St. John's wort (*Hypericum perforatum* L.)	Dental pain
St. John's wort (*Hypericum perforatum* L.)	Pain relief
Tea tree oil (*Melaleuca alternifolia* [Maiden & Betche] Cheel)	Anti-inflammatory
Tea tree oil (*Melaleuca alternifolia* [Maiden & Betche] Cheel)	Muscle and joint pain
Turmeric (*Curcuma longa* L.), curcumin	Pain
Valerian (*Valeriana officinalis* L.)	Anodyne (pain relief)
Valerian (*Valeriana officinalis* L.)	Muscle pain
Valerian (*Valeriana officinalis* L.)	Pain
White horehound (*Marrubium vulgare*)	Pain
Wild yam (*Dioscorea villosa*)	Anti-inflammatory

ANTIOXIDANT AND RELATED CONDITIONS
Levels of Scientific Evidence for Specific Therapies

GRADE: C (Unclear or Conflicting Scientific Evidence)

Therapy	Specific Therapeutic Use(s)
Bladderwrack (*Fucus vesiculosus*)	Antioxidant
Cranberry (*Vaccinium macrocarpon*)	Antioxidant
Dandelion (*Taraxacum officinale*)	Antioxidant
Globe artichoke (*Cynara scolymus* L.)	Antioxidant
Lycopene	Antioxidant
Melatonin	Antioxidant (free radical scavenging)
Seaweed, kelp, bladderwrack (*Fucus vesiculosus*)	Antioxidant

TRADITIONAL OR THEORETICAL USES THAT LACK SUFFICIENT EVIDENCE

Therapy	Specific Therapeutic Use(s)
Astragalus (*Astragalus membranaceus*)	Antioxidant
Black tea (*Camellia sinensis*)	Antioxidant
Coenzyme Q10	Antioxidant
Dandelion (*Taraxacum officinale*)	Antioxidant
Danshen (*Salvia miltiorrhiza*)	Antioxidant
Devil's claw (*Harpagophytum procumbens* DC.)	Antioxidant
Elder (*Sambucus nigra* L.)	Antioxidant
Garlic (*Allium sativum* L.)	Antioxidant
Ginger (*Zingiber officinale* Roscoe)	Antioxidant
Ginkgo (*Ginkgo biloba* L.)	Antioxidant
Green tea (*Camellia sinensis*)	Antioxidant
Horsetail (*Equisetum arvense* L.)	Antioxidant
Lavender (*Lavandula angustifolia* Miller)	Antioxidant
Licorice (*Glycyrrhiza glabra* L.), deglycyrrhizinated licorice (DGL)	Antioxidant
Propolis	Antioxidant
Red clover (*Trifolium pratense*)	Antioxidant
Spirulina	Antioxidant

ANTIPSYCHOTIC AND RELATED CONDITIONS

Levels of Scientific Evidence for Specific Therapies

GRADE: C (Unclear or Conflicting Scientific Evidence)

Therapy	Specific Therapeutic Use(s)
Betel nut (*Areca catechu* L.)	Schizophrenia
DHEA (dehydroepiandrosterone)	Schizophrenia
Melatonin	Schizophrenia (sleep disorders)
Omega-3 fatty acids, fish oil, alpha-linolenic acid	Schizophrenia

GRADE: D (Fair Negative Scientific Evidence)

Therapy	Specific Therapeutic Use(s)
Evening primrose oil (*Oenothera biennis* L.)	Schizophrenia

TRADITIONAL OR THEORETICAL USES THAT LACK SUFFICIENT EVIDENCE

Therapy	Specific Therapeutic Use(s)
American pennyroyal (*Hedeoma pulegioides* L.), European pennyroyal (*Mentha pulegium* L.)	Hallucinations
Chaparral (*Larrea tridentata* DC. Coville, *L. divaricata* Cav.), nordihydroguaiaretic acid (NDGA)	Hallucinations (including those due to LSD ingestion)

Continued

Coenzyme Q10	Psychiatric disorders
Ginkgo (*Ginkgo biloba* L.)	Schizophrenia
Ginseng (American ginseng, Asian ginseng, Chinese ginseng, Korean red ginseng, *Panax ginseng*: *Panax* spp. including *P. ginseng* C.C. Meyer and *P. quincefolium* L., excluding *Eleutherococcus senticosus*)	Psycho-asthenia
Gotu kola (*Centella asiatica* L), total triterpenic fraction of *Centella asiatica* (TTFCA)	Mental disorders
Kava (*Piper methysticum* G. Forst)	Antipsychotic
Lavender (*Lavandula angustifolia* Miller)	Psychosis
Niacin (vitamin B_3, nicotinic acid), niacinamide, and inositol hexanicotinate	Diagnostic test for schizophrenia
Niacin (vitamin B_3, nicotinic acid), niacinamide, and inositol hexanicotinate	Drug-induced hallucinations
Niacin (vitamin B_3, nicotinic acid), niacinamide, and inositol hexanicotinate	Psychosis
Niacin (vitamin B_3, nicotinic acid), niacinamide, and inositol hexanicotinate	Schizophrenia
Oleander (*Nerium oleander, Thevetia peruviana*)	Psychiatric disorders
Pygeum (*Prunus africana, Pygeum africanum*)	Psychosis
Yohimbe bark extract (*Pausinystalia yohimbe* Pierre ex Beille)	Hallucinogenic
Yohimbe bark extract (*Pausinystalia yohimbe* Pierre ex Beille)	Schizophrenia
Yohimbe bark extract (*Pausinystalia yohimbe* Pierre ex Beille)	Hallucinogenic

ANXIETY/STRESS AND RELATED CONDITIONS
Levels of Scientific Evidence for Specific Therapies

GRADE: A (Strong Scientific Evidence)

Therapy	Specific Therapeutic Use(s)
Kava (*Piper methysticum* G. Forst)	Anxiety

GRADE: B (Good Scientific Evidence)

Therapy	Specific Therapeutic Use(s)
Lavender (*Lavandula angustifolia* Miller)	Anxiety (lavender aromatherapy)

GRADE: C (Unclear or Conflicting Scientific Evidence)

Therapy	Specific Therapeutic Use(s)
Gotu kola (*Centella asiatica* L), total triterpenic fraction of *Centella asiatica* (TTFCA)	Anxiety
St. John's wort (*Hypericum perforatum* L.)	Anxiety disorder
Valerian (*Valeriana officinalis* L.)	Anxiety

TRADITIONAL OR THEORETICAL USES THAT LACK SUFFICIENT EVIDENCE

Therapy	Specific Therapeutic Use(s)
American pennyroyal (*Hedeoma pulegioides* L.), European pennyroyal (*Mentha pulegium* L.)	Anxiolytic
Belladonna (*Atropa belladonna* L. or its variety *acuminata* Royle ex Lindl)	Anxiety
Black cohosh (*Cimicifuga racemosa* L. Nutt.)	Anxiety
Black tea (*Camellia sinensis*)	Anxiety
Calendula (*Calendula officinalis* L.), marigold	Anxiety
Chamomile (*Matricaria recutita, Chamaemelum nobile*)	Anxiety
Danshen (*Salvia miltiorrhiza*)	Anxiety
DHEA (dehydroepiandrosterone)	Anxiety
DHEA (dehydroepiandrosterone)	Stress
Dong quai (*Angelica sinensis* [Oliv.] Diels), Chinese angelica	Anxiety
Dong quai (*Angelica sinensis* [Oliv.] Diels), Chinese angelica	Stress
Elder (*Sambucus nigra* L.)	Stress reduction
Eucalyptus oil (*Eucalyptus globulus* Labillardiere, *E. fructicetorum* F. Von Mueller, *E. smithii* R.T. Baker)	Aromatherapy
Garlic (*Allium sativum* L.)	Stress (anxiety)
Ginkgo (*Ginkgo biloba* L.)	Anxiety
Ginseng (American ginseng, Asian ginseng, Chinese ginseng, Korean red ginseng, *Panax ginseng*: *Panax* spp. including *P. ginseng* C.C. Meyer and *P. quincefolium* L., excluding *Eleutherococcus senticosus*)	Aggression
Ginseng (American ginseng, Asian ginseng, Chinese ginseng, Korean red ginseng, *Panax ginseng*: *Panax* spp. including *P. ginseng* C.C. Meyer and *P. quincefolium* L., excluding *Eleutherococcus senticosus*)	Anxiety
Ginseng (American ginseng, Asian ginseng, Chinese ginseng, Korean red ginseng, *Panax ginseng*: *Panax* spp. including *P. ginseng* C.C. Meyer and *P. quincefolium* L., excluding *Eleutherococcus senticosus*)	Stress
Goldenseal (*Hydrastis canadensis* L.), berberine	Anxiety
Gotu kola (*Centella asiatica* L), total triterpenic fraction of *Centella asiatica* (TTFCA)	Anxiety
Hops (*Humulus lupulus* L.)	Anxiety
Hops (*Humulus lupulus* L.)	Anxiety during menopause
Lavender (*Lavandula angustifolia* Miller)	Anxiety
Niacin (vitamin B$_3$, nicotinic acid), *Niacinamide, and Inositol hexanicotinate*	Anxiety
Omega-3 fatty acids, fish oil, alpha-linolenic acid	Panic disorder
Passionflower (*Passiflora incarnata* L.)	Tension
Spirulina	Anxiety
Thyme (*Thymus vulgaris* L.), thymol	Anxiety
Valerian (*Valeriana officinalis* L.)	Stress

ARRHYTHMIA AND RELATED CONDITIONS

Levels of Scientific Evidence for Specific Therapies

GRADE: C (Unclear or Conflicting Scientific Evidence)

Therapy	Specific Therapeutic Use(s)
Omega-3 fatty acids, fish oil, alpha-linolenic acid	Cardiac arrhythmias (abnormal heart rhythms)

TRADITIONAL OR THEORETICAL USES THAT LACK SUFFICIENT EVIDENCE

Therapy	Specific Therapeutic Use(s)
Astragalus (*Astragalus membranaceus*)	Palpitations
Black cohosh (*Cimicifuga racemosa* L. Nutt.)	Heart disease/palpitations
Clay	Heart disorders
Coenzyme Q10	Heart irregular beats
Danshen (*Salvia miltiorrhiza*)	Heart palpitations
Devil's claw (*Harpagophytum procumbens* DC.)	Irregular heartbeat
Dong quai (*Angelica sinensis* [Oliv.] Diels), Chinese angelica	Abnormal heart rhythms
Dong quai (*Angelica sinensis* [Oliv.] Diels), Chinese angelica	Palpitations
Garlic (*Allium sativum* L.)	Heart rhythm disorders
Ginkgo (*Ginkgo biloba* L.)	Cardiac rhythm abnormalities
Ginseng (American ginseng, Asian ginseng, Chinese ginseng, Korean red ginseng, *Panax ginseng*: *Panax* spp. including *P. ginseng* C.C. Meyer and *P. quincefolium* L., excluding *Eleutherococcus senticosus*)	Palpitations
Goldenseal (*Hydrastis Canadensis* L.), berberine	Abnormal heart rhythms
Valerian (*Valeriana officinalis* L.)	Nervous palpitation
Valerian (*Valeriana officinalis* L.)	Nervous tachycardia
White horehound (*Marrubium vulgare*)	Heart rate abnormalities

ASTHMA AND RELATED CONDITIONS

Levels of Scientific Evidence for Specific Therapies

GRADE: B (Good Scientific Evidence)

Therapy	Specific Therapeutic Use(s)
Boswellia (*Boswellia serrata* Roxb.)	Asthma (chronic therapy)
Ephedra (*Ephedra sinica*)/ma huang	Asthmatic bronchoconstriction

GRADE: C (Unclear or Conflicting Scientific Evidence)

Therapy	Specific Therapeutic Use(s)
Belladonna (*Atropa belladonna* L. or its variety *acuminata* Royle ex Lindl)	Airway obstruction
Black tea (*Camellia sinensis*)	Asthma

Bromelain	Chronic obstructive pulmonary disease (COPD)
Danshen (*Salvia miltiorrhiza*)	Asthmatic bronchitis
Green tea (*Camellia sinensis*)	Asthma
Lactobacillus acidophilus	Asthma
Lycopene	Asthma caused by exercise
Omega-3 fatty acids, fish oil, alpha-linolenic acid	Asthma

GRADE: D (Fair Negative Scientific Evidence)	
Therapy	Specific Therapeutic Use(s)
Evening primrose oil (*Oenothera biennis* L.)	Asthma

GRADE: F (Strong Negative Scientific Evidence)	
Therapy	Specific Therapeutic Use(s)
Arginine (L-arginine)	Asthma

TRADITIONAL OR THEORETICAL USES THAT LACK SUFFICIENT EVIDENCE	
Therapy	Specific Therapeutic Use(s)
Alfalfa (*Medicago sativa* L.)	Asthma
Aloe (*Aloe vera*)	Asthma
Astragalus (*Astragalus membranaceus*)	Asthma
Astragalus (*Astragalus membranaceus*)	Shortness of breath
Barley (*Hordeum vulgare* L.), germinated barley foodstuff (GBF)	Asthma
Belladonna (*Atropa belladonna* L. or its variety *acuminata* Royle ex Lindl)	Asthma
Betel nut (*Areca catechu* L.)	Asthma
Black cohosh (*Cimicifuga racemosa* L. Nutt.)	Asthma
Boswellia (*Boswellia serrata* Roxb.)	Chronic obstructive pulmonary disease (COPD)
Clove (*Eugenia aromatica*)	Asthma
Coenzyme Q10	Asthma
Coenzyme Q10	Breathing difficulties
Coenzyme Q10	Chronic obstructive pulmonary disease (COPD)
DHEA (dehydroepiandrosterone)	Asthma
Dong quai (*Angelica sinensis* [Oliv.] Diels), Chinese angelica	Asthma
Dong quai (*Angelica sinensis* [Oliv.] Diels), Chinese angelica	Chronic obstructive pulmonary disease (COPD)
Elder (*Sambucus nigra* L.)	Asthma
Elder (*Sambucus nigra* L.)	Respiratory distress
Ephedra (*Ephedra sinica*)/ma huang	Dyspnea
Essiac	Asthma

Continued

Eucalyptus oil (Eucalyptus globulus Labillardiere, *E. fructicetorum* F. Von Mueller, *E. smithii* R.T. Baker)	Asthma
Eucalyptus oil (*Eucalyptus globulus* Labillardiere, *E. fructicetorum* F. Von Mueller, *E. smithii* R.T. Baker)	Chronic obstructive pulmonary disease (COPD)
Eucalyptus oil (*Eucalyptus globulus* Labillardiere, *E. fructicetorum* F. Von Mueller, *E. smithii* R.T. Baker)	Emphysema
Eyebright (*Euphrasia officinalis*)	Asthma
Feverfew (*Tanacetum parthenium* L. Schultz-Bip.)	Asthma
Flaxseed and flaxseed oil (*Linum usitatissimum*)	Bronchial irritation
Garlic (*Allium sativum* L.)	Asthma
Ginger (*Zingiber officinale* Roscoe)	Asthma
Ginkgo (*Ginkgo biloba* L.)	Asthma
Ginseng (American ginseng, Asian ginseng, Chinese ginseng, Korean red ginseng, *Panax ginseng*: *Panax* spp. including *P. ginseng* C.C. Meyer and *P. quincefolium* L., excluding *Eleutherococcus senticosus*)	Asthma
Ginseng (American ginseng, Asian ginseng, Chinese ginseng, Korean red ginseng, *Panax ginseng*: *Panax* spp. including *P. ginseng* C.C. Meyer and *P. quincefolium* L., excluding *Eleutherococcus senticosus*)	Breathing difficulty
Ginseng (American ginseng, Asian ginseng, Chinese ginseng, Korean red ginseng, *Panax ginseng*: *Panax* spp. including *P. ginseng* C.C. Meyer and *P. quincefolium* L., excluding *Eleutherococcus senticosus*)	Bronchodilation
Goldenseal (*Hydrastis canadensis* L.), berberine	Asthma
Gotu kola (*Centella asiatica* L.), total triterpenic fraction of *Centella asiatica* (TTFCA)	Asthma
Guggul (*Commifora mukul*)	Asthma
Hawthorn (*Crataegus laevigata, C. oxyacantha, C. monogyna, C. pentagyna*)	Asthma
Hawthorn (*Crataegus laevigata, C. oxyacantha, C. monogyna, C. pentagyna*)	Dyspnea
Kava (*Piper methysticum* G. Forst)	Asthma
Lavender (*Lavandula angustifolia* Miller)	Asthma
Licorice (Gly*cyrrhiza glabra* L.), deglycyrrhizinated licorice (DGL)	Asthma
Melatonin	Asthma
Oleander (*Nerium oleander, Thevetia peruviana*)	Asthma
Omega-3 fatty acids, fish oil, alpha-linolenic acid	Chronic obstructive pulmonary disease
Passionflower (*Passiflora incarnata* L.)	Asthma
Peppermint (*Mentha x piperita* L.)	Asthma
Polypodium leucotomos extract, Anapsos	Asthma
Red clover (*Trifolium pratense*)	Asthma
Saw palmetto (*Serenoa repens* [Bartram] Small)	Asthma
Slippery elm (*Ulmus rubra* Muhl., *U. fulva* Michx.)	Respiratory disorders
Thyme (*Thymus vulgaris* L.), Thymol	Asthma

Thyme (*Thymus vulgaris* L.), Thymol	Dyspnea
Turmeric (*Curcuma longa* L.), curcumin	Asthma
Valerian (*Valeriana officinalis* L.)	Asthma
Valerian (*Valeriana officinalis* L.)	Bronchospasm
White horehound (*Marrubium vulgare*)	Asthma
White horehound (*Marrubium vulgare*)	Chronic obstructive pulmonary disease (COPD)
White horehound (*Marrubium vulgare*)	Wheezing
Wild yam (*Dioscorea villosa*)	Asthma

ATHEROSCLEROSIS AND RELATED CONDITIONS
Levels of Scientific Evidence for Specific Therapies

GRADE: A (Strong Scientific Evidence)

Therapy	Specific Therapeutic Use(s)
Niacin (vitamin B_3, nicotinic acid), niacinamide, and inositol hexanicotinate	High cholesterol (niacin)
Omega-3 fatty acids, fish oil, alpha-linolenic acid)	Hypertriglyceridemia (fish oil/ eicosapentaenoic acid [EPA] plus docosahexaenoic acid [DHA])
Omega-3 fatty acids, fish oil, alpha-linolenic acid	Secondary cardiovascular disease prevention (fish oil/ eicosapentaenoic acid [EPA] plus docosahexaenoic acid [DHA])
Psyllium (*Plantago ovata, P. ispaghula*)	High cholesterol
Red yeast rice (*Monascus purpureus*)	High cholesterol
Soy (*Glycine max* L. Merr.)	High cholesterol

GRADE: B (Good Scientific Evidence)

Therapy	Specific Therapeutic Use(s)
Barley (*Hordeum vulgare* L.), germinated barley foodstuff (GBF)	High cholesterol
Garlic (*Allium sativum* L.)	High cholesterol
Niacin (vitamin B_3, nicotinic acid), niacinamide, and inositol hexanicotinate	Atherosclerosis (niacin)
Niacin (vitamin B_3, nicotinic acid), niacinamide, and inositol hexanicotinate	Prevention of a second heart attack (niacin)
Omega-3 fatty acids, fish oil, alpha-linolenic acid	Primary cardiovascular disease prevention (fish intake)
Sweet Almond (*Prunus amygdalus dulcis*)	High cholesterol (whole almonds)

GRADE: C (Unclear or Conflicting Scientific Evidence)

Therapy	Specific Therapeutic Use(s)
Alfalfa (*Medicago sativa* L.)	Atherosclerosis (cholesterol plaques in heart arteries)

Continued

Alfalfa (*Medicago sativa* L.)	High cholesterol
Arginine (L-arginine)	Coronary artery disease/angina
Arginine (L-arginine)	Heart protection during coronary artery bypass grafting (CABG)
Astragalus (*Astragalus membranaceus*)	Coronary artery disease
Bilberry (*Vaccinium myrtillus*)	Atherosclerosis (hardening of the arteries) and peripheral vascular disease
Black tea (*Camellia sinensis*)	Heart attack prevention
Coenzyme Q10	Angina (chest pain from clogged heart arteries)
Coenzyme Q10	Heart attack (acute myocardial infarction)
Coenzyme Q10	Heart protection during surgery
Danshen (*Salvia miltiorrhiza*)	Cardiovascular disease/angina
DHEA (dehydroepiandrosterone)	Atherosclerosis (cholesterol plaques in the arteries)
Dong quai (*Angelica sinensis* [Oliv.] Diels), Chinese angelica	Angina pectoris/coronary artery disease
Fenugreek (*Trigonella foenum-graecum* L.)	Hyperlipidemia
Flaxseed and flaxseed oil (*Linum usitatissimum*)	Heart disease (flaxseed and flaxseed oil)
Flaxseed and flaxseed oil (*Linum usitatissimum*)	High cholesterol or triglycerides (flaxseed and flaxseed oil)
Garlic (*Allium sativum* L.)	Atherosclerosis (hardening of the arteries)
Garlic (*Allium sativum* L.)	Familial hypercholesterolemia
Garlic (*Allium sativum* L.)	Heart attack prevention in patients with known heart disease
Ginseng (American ginseng, Asian ginseng, Chinese ginseng, Korean red ginseng, *Panax ginseng*: *Panax* spp. including *P. ginseng* C.C. Meyer and *P. quincefolium* L., excluding *Eleutherococcus senticosus*)	Coronary artery (heart) disease
Globe artichoke (*Cynara scolymus* L.)	Lipid-lowering (cholesterol and triglycerides)
Green tea (*Camellia sinensis*)	Heart attack prevention
Green tea (*Camellia sinensis*)	High cholesterol
Guggul (*Commifora mukul*)	Hyperlipidemia
Gymnema (*Gymnema sylvestre* R. Br.)	High cholesterol
Hawthorn (*Crataegus laevigata, C. oxyacantha, C. monogyna, C. pentagyna*)	Coronary artery disease (angina)
Lactobacillus acidophilus	High cholesterol
Lycopene	Atherosclerosis (clogged arteries) and high cholesterol

Milk thistle (*Silybum marianum*), silymarin	Hyperlipidemia
Omega-3 fatty acids, fish oil, alpha-linolenic acid	Angina pectoris
Omega-3 fatty acids, fish oil, alpha-linolenic acid	Atherosclerosis
Omega-3 fatty acids, fish oil, alpha-linolenic acid	Prevention of graft failure after heart bypass surgery
Omega-3 fatty acids, fish oil, alpha-linolenic acid	Prevention of restenosis after percutaneous transluminal coronary angioplasty (PTCA)
Red clover (*Trifolium pratense*)	High cholesterol
Soy (*Glycine max* L. Merr.)	Cardiovascular disease
Spirulina	High cholesterol
Turmeric (*Curcuma longa* L), curcumin	High cholesterol
Wild yam *(Dioscorea villosa)*	High cholesterol

GRADE: D (Fair Negative Scientific Evidence)

Therapy	Specific Therapeutic Use(s)
Omega-3 fatty acids, fish oil, alpha-linolenic acid	Hypercholesterolemia

TRADITIONAL OR THEORETICAL USES THAT LACK SUFFICIENT EVIDENCE

Therapy	Specific Therapeutic Use(s)
Aloe (*Aloe vera*)	Heart disease prevention
Antineoplastons	Cholesterol/triglyceride abnormalities
Arginine (L-arginine)	Cardiac syndrome X
Arginine (L-arginine)	Heart attack
Arginine (L-arginine)	High cholesterol
Astragalus (*Astragalus membranaceus*)	Angina
Astragalus (*Astragalus membranaceus*)	Heart attack
Astragalus (*Astragalus membranaceus*)	High cholesterol
Bilberry (*Vaccinium myrtillus*)	Angina
Bilberry (*Vaccinium myrtillus*)	Heart disease
Bilberry (*Vaccinium myrtillus*)	High cholesterol
Black cohosh (*Cimicifuga racemosa* L. Nutt.)	Cardiac diseases
Bladderwrack (*Fucus vesiculosus*)	Atherosclerosis
Bladderwrack (*Fucus vesiculosus*)	Heart disease
Bladderwrack (*Fucus vesiculosus*)	High cholesterol
Boron	High cholesterol
Bromelain	Angina
Bromelain	Atherosclerosis (hardening of the arteries)
Bromelain	Heart disease

Continued

Calendula (*Calendula officinalis* L.), marigold	Atherosclerosis (clogged arteries)
Calendula (*Calendula officinalis* L.), marigold	Heart disease
Clay	Cardiovascular disorders
Coenzyme Q10	High cholesterol
Dandelion (*Taraxacum officinale*)	Cardiovascular disorders
Dandelion (*Taraxacum officinale*)	Clogged arteries
Dandelion (*Taraxacum officinale*)	High cholesterol
Danshen (*Salvia miltiorrhiza*)	Clogged arteries
Danshen (*Salvia miltiorrhiza*)	High cholesterol
Devil's claw (*Harpagophytum procumbens* DC.)	Atherosclerosis (clogged arteries)
Devil's claw (*Harpagophytum procumbens* DC.)	High cholesterol
DHEA (dehydroepiandrosterone)	Heart attack
DHEA (dehydroepiandrosterone)	High cholesterol
Dong quai (*Angelica sinensis* [Oliv.] Diels), Chinese angelica	Atherosclerosis
Dong quai (*Angelica sinensis* [Oliv.] Diels), Chinese angelica	High cholesterol
Evening primrose oil (*Oenothera biennis* L.)	Atherosclerosis
Evening primrose oil (*Oenothera biennis* L.)	Heart disease
Evening primrose oil (*Oenothera biennis* L.)	High cholesterol
Fenugreek (*Trigonella foenum-graecum* L.)	Atherosclerosis
Ginger (*Zingiber officinale* Roscoe)	Atherosclerosis
Ginger (*Zingiber officinale* Roscoe)	Heart disease
Ginkgo (*Ginkgo biloba* L.)	Angina
Ginkgo (*Ginkgo biloba* L.)	Atherosclerosis (clogged arteries)
Ginkgo (*Ginkgo biloba* L.)	Heart attack
Ginkgo (*Ginkgo biloba* L.)	Heart disease
Ginkgo (*Ginkgo biloba* L.)	High cholesterol
Ginseng (American ginseng, Asian ginseng, Chinese ginseng, Korean red ginseng, *Panax ginseng*: *Panax* spp. including *P. ginseng* C.C. Meyer and *P. quincefolium* L., excluding *Eleutherococcus senticosus*)	Atherosclerosis
Ginseng (American ginseng, Asian ginseng, Chinese ginseng, Korean red ginseng, *Panax ginseng*: *Panax* spp. including *P. ginseng* C.C. Meyer and *P. quincefolium* L., excluding *Eleutherococcus senticosus*)	Heart damage
Globe artichoke (*Cynara scolymus* L.)	Atherosclerosis
Goldenseal (*Hydrastis canadensis* L.), berberine	Atherosclerosis (hardening of the arteries)
Goldenseal (*Hydrastis canadensis* L.), berberine	High cholesterol
Green tea (*Camellia sinensis*)	Heart disease
Gymnema (*Gymnema Sylvestre* R. Br.)	Cardiovascular disease

Hawthorn (*Crataegus laevigata, C. oxyacantha, C. monogyna, C. pentagyna*)	Angina
Hawthorn (*Crataegus laevigata*, C. oxyacantha, *C. monogyna, C. pentagyna*)	Cardiac murmurs
Lactobacillus acidophilus	Heart disease
Licorice (*Glycyrrhiza glabra* L.), deglycyrrhizinated licorice (DGL)	High cholesterol
Lycopene	Heart disease
Maitake mushroom (*Grifola frondosa*), beta-glucan	High cholesterol
Melatonin	Cardiac syndrome X
Melatonin	Coronary artery disease
Niacin (vitamin B_3, nicotinic acid), niacinamide, and inositol hexanicotinate	Heart attack prevention
Oleander (*Nerium oleander, Thevetia peruviana*)	Heart disease
Omega-3 fatty acids, fish oil, alpha-linolenic acid	Acute myocardial infarction (heart attack)
Psyllium (*Plantago ovata, P. ispaghula*)	Atherosclerosis
Seaweed, kelp, bladderwrack (*Fucus vesiculosus*)	Atherosclerosis
Seaweed, kelp, bladderwrack (*Fucus vesiculosus*)	Fatty heart
Seaweed, kelp, bladderwrack (*Fucus vesiculosus*)	Hyperlipemia
Shark cartilage	Atherosclerosis
Soy (*Glycine max* L. Merr.)	Atherosclerosis
Spirulina	Atherosclerosis
Spirulina	Heart disease
Sweet almond (*Prunus amygdalus dulcis*)	Heart disease
Valerian (*Valeriana officinalis* L.)	Angina pectoris
Valerian (*Valeriana officinalis* L.)	Heart disease
Yohimbe bark extract (*Pausinystalia yohimbe* Pierre ex Beille)	Angina
Yohimbe bark extract (*Pausinystalia yohimbe* Pierre ex Beille)	Coronary artery disease
Yohimbe bark extract (*Pausinystalia yohimbe* Pierre ex Beille)	High cholesterol
Yohimbe bark extract (*Pausinystalia yohimbe* Pierre ex Beille)	Angina
Yohimbe bark extract (*Pausinystalia yohimbe* Pierre ex Beille)	Atherosclerosis
Yohimbe bark extract (*Pausinystalia yohimbe* Pierre ex Beille)	Chest pain
Yohimbe bark extract (*Pausinystalia yohimbe* Pierre ex Beille)	Coronary artery disease
Yohimbe bark extract (*Pausinystalia yohimbe* Pierre ex Beillee)	Hyperlipidemia

ATTENTION DEFICIT HYPERACTIVITY DISORDER (ADHD) AND RELATED CONDITIONS

Levels of Scientific Evidence for Specific Therapies

GRADE: C (Unclear or Conflicting Scientific Evidence)

Therapy	Specific Therapeutic Use(s)
Melatonin	ADHD

GRADE: D (Fair Negative Scientific Evidence)

Therapy	Specific Therapeutic Use(s)
Evening primrose oil (*Oenothera biennis* L.)	ADHD

TRADITIONAL OR THEORETICAL USES THAT LACK SUFFICIENT EVIDENCE

Therapy	Specific Therapeutic Use(s)
Black tea (*Camellia sinensis*)	Hyperactivity (children)
Ginkgo (*Ginkgo biloba* L.)	ADHD
Ginseng (American ginseng, Asian ginseng, Chinese ginseng, Korean red ginseng, *Panax ginseng*: *Panax* spp. including *P. ginseng* C.C. Meyer and *P. quincefolium* L., excluding *Eleutherococcus senticosus*)	ADHD
Omega-3 fatty acids, fish oil, alpha-linolenic acid	ADHD
Passionflower (*Passiflora incarnata* L.)	ADHD
Soy (*Glycine max* L. Merr.)	ADHD
Spirulina	ADHD

BACK PAIN AND RELATED CONDITIONS

Levels of Scientific Evidence for Specific Therapies

GRADE: C (Unclear or Conflicting Scientific Evidence)

Therapy	Specific Therapeutic Use(s)
Devil's claw (*Harpagophytum procumbens* DC.)	Low back pain

TRADITIONAL OR THEORETICAL USES THAT LACK SUFFICIENT EVIDENCE

Therapy	Specific Therapeutic Use(s)
Belladonna (*Atropa belladonna* L. or its variety *acuminata* Royle ex Lindl)	Sciatica (back and leg pain)
Black cohosh (*Cimicifuga racemosa* L. Nutt.)	Back pain
Bromelain	Back pain
Bromelain	Sciatica
Burdock (*Arctium lappa*)	Back pain
Burdock (*Arctium lappa*)	Sciatica
Chamomile (*Matricaria recutita, Chamaemelum nobile*)	Back pain
Chamomile (*Matricaria recutita, Chamaemelum nobile*)	Sciatica

Dong quai (*Angelica sinensis* [Oliv.] Diels), Chinese angelica	Back pain
Dong quai (*Angelica sinensis* [Oliv.] Diels), Chinese angelica	Sciatica
Eucalyptus oil (Eucalyptus globulus Labillardiere, *E. fructicetorum* F. Von Mueller, *E. smithii* R.T. Baker)	Back pain
Goldenseal (*Hydrastis canadensis* L.), berberine	Sciatica

BACTERIAL INFECTIONS AND RELATED CONDITIONS

Levels of Scientific Evidence for Specific Therapies

GRADE: C (Unclear or Conflicting Scientific Evidence)

Therapy	Specific Therapeutic Use(s)
Bladderwrack (*Fucus vesiculosus*)	Antibacterial/antifungal
Blessed thistle (*Cnicus benedictus* L.)	Bacterial infections
Garlic (*Allium sativum* L.)	Cryptococcal meningitis
Goldenseal (*Hydrastis canadensis* L.), berberine	Trachoma (*Chlamydia trachomatosis* eye infection)
Lavender (*Lavandula angustifolia* Miller)	Antibacterial (lavender used on the skin)
Propolis	Infections
Seaweed, kelp, bladderwrack (*Fucus vesiculosus*)	Antibacterial
Sorrel (*Rumex acetosa* L., *R. acetosella* L.), Sinupret	Antibacterial
Tea tree oil (*Melaleuca alternifolia* [Maiden & Betche] Cheel)	Methicillin-resistant *Staphylococcus aureus* (MRSA) chronic infection (colonization)

TRADITIONAL OR THEORETICAL USES THAT LACK SUFFICIENT EVIDENCE

Therapy	Specific Therapeutic Use(s)
Aloe (*Aloe vera*)	Bacterial skin infections
American pennyroyal (*Hedeoma pulegioides* L.), European pennyroyal (*Mentha pulegium* L.)	Antiseptic
Astragalus (*Astragalus membranaceus*)	Antimicrobial
Bilberry (*Vaccinium myrtillus*)	Skin infections
Bitter almond (*Prunus amygdalus* Batch var. *amara* DC. Focke),d Laetrile	Antibacterial
Blessed thistle (*Cnicus benedictus* L.)	Bubonic plague
Boron	Antiseptic
Boswellia (*Boswellia serrata* Roxb.)	Antiseptic
Bromelain	Antibiotic absorption problems in the gut
Bromelain	Infections
Burdock (*Arctium lappa*)	Bacterial infections
Calendula (*Calendula officinalis* L.), marigold	Bacterial infections

Continued

Calendula (*Calendula officinalis* L.), marigold	Cholera
Calendula (*Calendula officinalis* L.), marigold	Tuberculosis
Chamomile (*Matricaria recutita*, *Chamaemelum nobile*)	Antibacterial
Chamomile (*Matricaria recutita*, *Chamaemelum nobile*)	Skin infections
Chaparral (*Larrea tridentata* DC. Coville, *L. divaricata* Cav.), nordihydroguaiaretic acid (NDGA)	Antibacterial
Chaparral (*Larrea tridentata* DC. Coville, *L. divaricata* Cav.), nordihydroguaiaretic acid (NDGA)	Tuberculosis
Clove (*Eugenia aromatica*)	Antiseptic
Dandelion (*Taraxacum officinale*)	Antibacterial
Dong quai (*Angelica sinensis* [Oliv.] Diels), Chinese angelica	Antibacterial
Dong quai (*Angelica sinensis* [Oliv.] Diels), Chinese angelica	Antiseptic
Dong quai (*Angelica sinensis* [Oliv.] Diels), Chinese angelica	Infections
Echinacea (*Echinacea angustifolia* DC., *E. pallida*, *E. purpurea*)	Bacterial infections
Ephedra (Ephedra sinica)/ma huang	Gonorrhea
Eucalyptus oil (*Eucalyptus globulus* Labillardiere, *E. fructicetorum* F. Von Mueller, *E. smithii* R.T. Baker)	Antibacterial
Eucalyptus oil (*Eucalyptus globulus* Labillardiere, E. fructicetorum F. Von Mueller, E. smithii R.T. Baker)	Skin infections in children
Eucalyptus oil (*Eucalyptus globulus* Labillardiere, E. *fructicetorum* F. Von Mueller, *E. smithii* R.T. Baker)	Tuberculosis
Eyebright (*Euphrasia officinalis*)	Antibacterial
Fenugreek (*Trigonella foenum-graecum* L.)	Cellulitis
Fenugreek (*Trigonella foenum-graecum* L.)	Infections
Fenugreek (*Trigonella foenum-graecum* L.)	Tuberculosis
Flaxseed and flaxseed oil (*Linum usitatissimum*)	Gonorrhea
Flaxseed and flaxseed oil (*Linum usitatissimum*)	Skin infections
Garlic (*Allium sativum* L.)	Cholera
Garlic (*Allium sativum* L.)	Cryptococcal meningitis
Garlic (*Allium sativum* L.)	Tuberculosis
Ginger (*Zingiber officinale* Roscoe)	Antiseptic
Ginger (*Zingiber officinale* Roscoe)	Cholera
Ginkgo (*Ginkgo biloba* L.)	Antibacterial
Goldenseal (*Hydrastis canadensi*s L.), berberine	Antibacterial
Goldenseal (*Hydrastis canadensi*s L.), berberine	Infections
Goldenseal (*Hydrastis canadensi*s L.), berberine	Tuberculosis
Gotu kola (*Centella asiatica* L.), total triterpenic fraction of *Centella asiatica* (TTFCA)	Anti-infective
Gotu kola (*Centella asiatica* L.), total triterpenic fraction of *Centella asiatica* (TTFCA)	Cholera

Gotu kola (*Centella asiatica* L.), total triterpenic fraction of *Centella asiatica* (TTFCA)	Tuberculosis
Hawthorn (*Crataegus laevigata, C. oxyacantha, C. monogyna, C. pentagyna*)	Antibacterial
Hops (*Humulus lupulus* L.)	Antibacterial
Horsetail (*Equisetum arvense* L.)	Antibacterial
Horsetail (*Equisetum arvense* L.)	Gonorrhea
Horsetail (*Equisetum arvense* L.)	Tuberculosis
Kava (*Piper methysticum* G. Forst)	Gonorrhea
Kava (*Piper methysticum* G. Forst)	Infections
Kava (*Piper methysticum* G. Forst)	Tuberculosis
Lavender (*Lavandula angustifolia* Miller)	Antiseptic
Licorice (*Glycyrrhiza glabra* L.), deglycyrrhizinated licorice (DGL)	Antimicrobial
Licorice (*Glycyrrhiza glabra* L.), deglycyrrhizinated licorice (DGL)	Bacterial infections
Licorice (*Glycyrrhiza glabra* L.), deglycyrrhizinated licorice (DGL)	Methicillin-resistant staphylococcus aureus
Licorice (*Glycyrrhiza glabra* L.), deglycyrrhizinated licorice (DGL)	SARS
Maitake mushroom (*Grifola frondosa*), beta-glucan	Bacterial infection
Niacin (vitamin B$_3$, nicotinic acid), niacinamide, and inositol hexanicotinate	Tuberculosis
Oleander (*Nerium oleander, Thevetia peruviana*)	Bacterial infections
Omega-3 fatty acids, fish oil, alpha-linolenic acid	Bacterial infections
Passionflower (*Passiflora incarnata* L.)	Antibacterial
Peppermint (*Mentha x piperita* L.)	Gonorrhea
Propolis	Tuberculosis
Red clover (*Trifolium pratense*)	Antibacterial
Red clover (*Trifolium pratense*)	Tuberculosis
Red yeast rice (*Monascus purpureus*)	Anthrax
Shark cartilage	Bacterial infections
Slippery elm (*Ulmus rubra* Muhl., *U. fulva* Michx.)	Tuberculosis
St. John's wort (*Hypericum perforatum* L.)	Bacterial skin infections (topical)
Sweet almond (*Prunus amygdalus dulcis*)	Antibacterial
Tea tree oil (*Melaleuca alternifolia* [Maiden & Betche] Cheel)	Antibacterial
Thyme (*Thymus vulgaris* L.), thymol	Cellulitis
Turmeric (*Curcuma longa* L.), curcumin	Gonorrhea
White horehound (*Marrubium vulgare*)	Tuberculosis

BALANCE AND RELATED CONDITIONS

Levels of Scientific Evidence for Specific Therapies

GRADE: C (Unclear or Conflicting Scientific Evidence)

Therapy	Specific Therapeutic Use(s)
Coenzyme Q10	Exercise performance
DHEA (dehydroepiandrosterone)	Muscle mass/body mass
Ginseng (American ginseng, Asian ginseng, Chinese ginseng, Korean red ginseng, *Panax ginseng*: *Panax* spp. including *P. ginseng* C.C. Meyer and *P. quincefolium* L., excluding *Eleutherococcus senticosus*)	Exercise performance

GRADE: D (Fair Negative Scientific Evidence)

Therapy	Specific Therapeutic Use(s)
Boron	Bodybuilding aid (increasing testosterone)

TRADITIONAL OR THEORETICAL USES THAT LACK SUFFICIENT EVIDENCE

Therapy	Specific Therapeutic Use(s)
Arginine (L-arginine)	Enhanced athletic performance
Arginine (L-arginine)	Increased muscle mass
Barley (*Hordeum vulgare* L.), germinated barley foodstuff (GBF)	Stamina/strength enhancer
DHEA (dehydroepiandrosterone)	Performance enhancement
Ephedra (*Ephedra sinica*)/ma huang	Bodybuilding
Essiac	Energy enhancement
Ginseng (American ginseng, Asian ginseng, Chinese ginseng, Korean red ginseng, *Panax ginseng*: *Panax* spp. including *P. ginseng* C.C. Meyer and *P. quincefolium* L., excluding *Eleutherococcus senticosus*)	Physical work capacity
Ginseng (American ginseng, Asian ginseng, Chinese ginseng, Korean red ginseng, *Panax ginseng*: *Panax* spp. including *P. ginseng* C.C. Meyer and *P. quincefolium* L., excluding *Eleutherococcus senticosus*)	Rehabilitation
Gotu kola (*Centella asiatica* L.), total triterpenic fraction of *Centella asiatica* (TTFCA)	Physical exhaustion
Lavender (*Lavandula angustifolia* Miller)	Exercise recovery
Soy (*Glycine max* L. Merr.)	Athletic endurance
St. John's wort (*Hypericum perforatum* L.)	Athletic performance enhancement
Wild yam (*Dioscorea villosa*)	Energy improvement

BEDWETTING AND RELATED CONDITIONS

Levels of Scientific Evidence for Specific Therapies

GRADE: C (Unclear or Conflicting Scientific Evidence)

Therapy	Specific Therapeutic Use(s)
Cranberry (*Vaccinium macrocarpon*)	Reduction of odor from incontinence/bladder catheterization
Saw palmetto (*Serenoa repens* [Bartram] Small)	Hypotonic neurogenic bladder

TRADITIONAL OR THEORETICAL USES THAT LACK SUFFICIENT EVIDENCE

Therapy	Specific Therapeutic Use(s)
Belladonna (*Atropa belladonna* L. or its variety *acuminata* Royle ex Lindl)	Bedwetting
Calendula (*Calendula officinalis* L.), marigold	Urinary retention
Ephedra (*Ephedra sinica*)/ma huang	Enuresis
Gotu kola (*Centella asiatica* L.), total triterpenic fraction of *Centella asiatica* (TTFCA)	Urinary retention
Horsetail (*Equisetum arvense* L.)	Urinary incontinence
Kava (*Piper methysticum* G. Forst)	Urinary incontinence
St. John's wort (*Hypericum perforatum* L.)	Bedwetting
Thyme (*Thymus vulgaris* L.), thymol	Enuresis

BENIGN PROSTATIC HYPERTROPHY (BPH) AND RELATED CONDITIONS

Levels of Scientific Evidence for Specific Therapies

GRADE: A (Strong Scientific Evidence)

Therapy	Specific Therapeutic Use(s)
Saw palmetto (*Serenoa repens* [Bartram] Small)	BPH

GRADE: B (Good Scientific Evidence)

Therapy	Specific Therapeutic Use(s)
Pygeum (*Prunus africana*, *Pygeum africanum*)	BPH symptoms

GRADE: C (Unclear or Conflicting Scientific Evidence)

Therapy	Specific Therapeutic Use(s)
Red clover (*Trifolium pratense*)	Prostate enlargement (BPH)

TRADITIONAL OR THEORETICAL USES THAT LACK SUFFICIENT EVIDENCE

Therapy	Specific Therapeutic Use(s)
Alfalfa (*Medicago sativa* L.)	Prostate disorders
Astragalus (*Astragalus membranaceus*)	Prostatitis
Bladderwrack (*Fucus vesiculosus*)	BPH

Continued

Calendula (*Calendula officinalis* L.), marigold	BPH
Calendula (*Calendula officinalis* L.), marigold	Prostatitis
Dandelion (*Taraxacum officinale*)	BPH
Flaxseed and flaxseed oil (*Linum usitatissimum*)	Enlarged prostate
Goldenseal (*Hydrastis canadensis* L.), berberine	Prostatitis
Horse chestnut (*Aesculus hippocastanum* L.)	BPH
Horsetail (*Equisetum arvense* L.)	Prostate inflammation
PC-SPES	BPH
Pygeum (*Prunus africana, Pygeum africanum*)	Prostatic adenoma
Pygeum (*Prunus africana, Pygeum africanum*)	Prostatitis
Seaweed, kelp, bladderwrack (*Fucus vesiculosus*)	BPH

BLADDER DISORDERS AND RELATED CONDITIONS

Levels of Scientific Evidence for Specific Therapies

GRADE: C (Unclear or Conflicting Scientific Evidence)

Therapy	Specific Therapeutic Use(s)
Chamomile (*Matricaria recutita, Chamaemelum nobile*)	Hemorrhagic cystitis (bladder irritation with bleeding)
Saw palmetto (*Serenoa repens* [Bartram] Small)	Underactive bladder

TRADITIONAL OR THEORETICAL USES THAT LACK SUFFICIENT EVIDENCE

Therapy	Specific Therapeutic Use(s)
Alfalfa (*Medicago sativa* L.)	Bladder disorders
Bladderwrack (*Fucus vesiculosus*)	Bladder inflammatory disease
Boswellia (*Boswellia serrata* Roxb.)	Cystitis
Burdock (*Arctium lappa*)	Bladder disorders
Calendula (*Calendula officinalis* L.), marigold	Bladder irritation
Dandelion (*Taraxacum officinale*)	Bladder irritation
Flaxseed and flaxseed oil (*Linum usitatissimum*)	Bladder inflammation
Globe artichoke (*Cynara scolymus* L.)	Cystitis
Goldenseal (*Hydrastis canadensis* L.), berberine	Cystitis
Hawthorn (*Crataegus laevigata, C. oxyacantha, C. monogyna, C. pentagyna*)	Bladder disorders
Horsetail (*Equisetum arvense* L.)	Bladder disturbances
Horsetail (*Equisetum arvense* L.)	Cystic ulcers
Kava (*Piper methysticum* G. Forst)	Cystitis
Marshmallow (*Althaea officinalis* L.)	Cystitis
Marshmallow (*Althaea officinalis* L.)	Urethritis
Psyllium (*Plantago ovata, P. ispaghula*)	Cystitis

Psyllium (*Plantago ovata, P. ispaghula*)	Urethritis
Pygeum (*Prunus africana, Pygeum africanum*)	Bladder sphincter disorders
Pygeum (*Prunus africana, Pygeum africanum*)	Partial bladder outlet obstruction
Saw palmetto (*Serenoa repens* [Bartram] Small)	Cystitis
Seaweed, kelp, bladderwrack (*Fucus vesiculosus*)	Bladder inflammatory disease
Slippery elm (*Ulmus rubra* Muhl., *U. fulva* Michx.)	Cystitis
Thyme (*Thymus vulgaris* L.), thymol	Cystitis
Thyme (*Thymus vulgaris* L.), thymol	Urethritis

BLEEDING AND RELATED CONDITIONS
Levels of Scientific Evidence for Specific Therapies

TRADITIONAL OR THEORETICAL USES THAT LACK SUFFICIENT EVIDENCE

Therapy	Specific Therapeutic Use(s)
Astragalus (*Astragalus membranaceus*)	Hemorrhage (bleeding)
Blessed thistle (*Cnicus benedictus* L.)	Bleeding
Cranberry (*Vaccinium macrocarpon*)	Blood disorders
Dong quai (*Angelica sinensis* [Oliv.] Diels), Chinese angelica	Hematopoiesis (stimulation of blood cell production)
Ginger (*Zingiber officinale* Roscoe)	Bleeding
Ginseng (American ginseng, Asian ginseng, Chinese ginseng, Korean red ginseng, *Panax ginseng*: *Panax* spp. including *P. ginseng* C.C. Meyer and *P. quincefolium* L., excluding *Eleutherococcus senticosus*)	Bleeding disorders
Glucosamine	Bleeding esophageal varices (blood vessels in the esophagus)
Goldenseal (*Hydrastis canadensis* L.), berberine	Anti-heparin
Goldenseal (*Hydrastis canadensis* L.), berberine	Hemorrhage (bleeding)
Guggul (*Commifora mukul*)	Bleeding
Horsetail (*Equisetum arvense* L.)	Bleeding
Milk thistle (*Silybum marianum*), silymarin	Hemorrhage
Sorrel (*Rumex acetosa* L., *R. acetosella* L.), Sinupret	Hemorrhage
Turmeric (*Curcuma longa* L.), curcumin	Bleeding

BREAST ENLARGEMENT AND RELATED CONDITIONS
Levels of Scientific Evidence for Specific Therapies

TRADITIONAL OR THEORETICAL USES THAT LACK SUFFICIENT EVIDENCE

Therapy	Specific Therapeutic Use(s)
Dandelion (*Taraxacum officinale*)	Breast augmentation
Dong quai (*Angelica sinensis* [Oliv.] Diels), Chinese angelica	Breast enlargement

Continued

Ginseng (American ginseng, Asian ginseng, Chinese ginseng, Korean red ginseng, *Panax ginseng*: *Panax* spp. including *P. ginseng* C.C. Meyer and *P. quincefolium* L., excluding *Eleutherococcus senticosus*) Breast enlargement

PC-SPES Breast enlargement

Saw palmetto (*Serenoa repens* [Bartram] Small) Breast augmentation

Soy (*Glycine max* L. Merr.) Breast enlargement

Wild yam (*Dioscorea villosa*) Breast enlargement

BRUISES AND RELATED CONDITIONS

Levels of Scientific Evidence for Specific Therapies

TRADITIONAL OR THEORETICAL USES THAT LACK SUFFICIENT EVIDENCE

Therapy	Specific Therapeutic Use(s)
American pennyroyal (*Hedeoma pulegioides* L.), European pennyroyal (*Mentha pulegium* L.)	Bruises and burns
Bromelain	Bruises
Calendula (*Calendula officinalis* L.), Marigold	Bruises
Chaparral (*Larrea tridentata* DC. Coville, *L. divaricata* Cav.), nordihydroguaiaretic acid (NDGA)	Bruises
Dandelion (*Taraxacum officinale*)	Bruises
Danshen (*Salvia miltiorrhiza*)	Bruising
Evening primrose oil (*Oenothera biennis* L.)	Bruises (topical)
Gotu kola (*Centella asiatica* L.), total triterpenic fraction of *Centella asiatica* (TTFCA)	Bruises
Horse chestnut (*Aesculus hippocastanum* L.)	Bruising
Marshmallow (*Althaea officinalis* L.)	Bruises (topical)
Red yeast rice (*Monascus purpureus*)	Bruised muscles
Red yeast rice (*Monascus purpureus*)	Bruises
St. John's wort (*Hypericum perforatum* L.)	Bruises (topical)
Turmeric (*Curcuma longa* L.), curcumin	Bruises

BURNS AND RELATED CONDITIONS

Levels of Scientific Evidence for Specific Therapies

GRADE: C (Unclear or Conflicting Scientific Evidence)

Therapy	Specific Therapeutic Use(s)
Aloe (*Aloe vera*)	Skin burns
Arginine (L-arginine)	Burns
Danshen (*Salvia miltiorrhiza*)	Burn healing

TRADITIONAL OR THEORETICAL USES THAT LACK SUFFICIENT EVIDENCE

Therapy	Specific Therapeutic Use(s)
Bromelain	Burn and wound care
Burdock (*Arctium lappa*)	Burns
Calendula (*Calendula officinalis* L.), marigold	Burns
Chamomile (*Matricaria recutita, Chamaemelum nobile*)	Burns
DHEA (dehydroepiandrosterone)	Burns
Echinacea (*Echinacea angustifolia* DC., *E. pallida, E. purpurea*)	Burn wounds
Elder (*Sambucus nigra* L.)	Burns
Eucalyptus oil (*Eucalyptus globulus* Labillardiere, *E. fructicetorum* F. Von Mueller, *e. smithii* R.T. Baker)	Burns
Fenugreek (*Trigonella foenum-graecum* L.)	Burns
Flaxseed and flaxseed oil (*Linum usitatissimum*)	Burns (poultice)
Ginger (*Zingiber officinale* Roscoe)	Burns (applied to the skin)
Ginseng (American ginseng, Asian ginseng, Chinese ginseng, Korean red ginseng, *Panax ginseng*: *Panax* spp. including *P. ginseng* C.C. Meyer and *P. quincefolium* L., excluding *Eleutherococcus senticosus*)	Burns
Marshmallow (*Althaea officinalis* L.)	Burns (topical)
Passionflower (*Passiflora incarnata* L.)	Burns (skin)
Red clover (*Trifolium pratense*)	Burns
Slippery elm (*Ulmus rubra* Muhl., *U. fulva* Michx.)	Burns
St. John's wort (*Hypericum perforatum* L.)	Burns (topical)
Tea tree oil (*Melaleuca alternifolia* [Maiden & Betche] Cheel)	Burns
Thyme (*Thymus vulgaris* L.), thymol	Burns

CANCER/CANCER PREVENTION AND RELATED CONDITIONS

Levels of Scientific Evidence for Specific Therapies

GRADE: C (Unclear or Conflicting Scientific Evidence)

Therapy	Specific Therapeutic Use(s)
Aloe (*Aloe vera*)	Cancer prevention
Antineoplastons	Cancer
Arginine (L-arginine)	Gastrointestinal cancer surgery
Astragalus (*Astragalus membranaceus*)	Cancer
Bitter melon (*Momordica charantia* L.), MAP30	Cancer
Black tea (*Camellia sinensis*)	Cancer prevention
Bladderwrack (*Fucus vesiculosus*)	Cancer
Bromelain	Cancer

Continued

Chaparral (*Larrea tridentata* DC. Coville, *L. divaricata* Cav.), nordihydroguaiaretic acid (NDGA)	Cancer
Coenzyme Q10	Breast cancer
Cranberry (*Vaccinium macrocarpon*)	Cancer prevention
Dandelion (*Taraxacum officinale*)	Cancer
DHEA (dehydroepiandrosterone)	Cervical dysplasia
Echinacea (*Echinacea angustifolia* DC., *E. pallida*, *E. purpurea*)	Cancer
Essiac	Cancer
Evening primrose oil (*Oenothera biennis* L.)	Breast cancer
Flaxseed and flaxseed oil (*Linum usitatissimum*)	Breast cancer (flaxseed, not flaxseed oil)
Garlic (*Allium sativum* L.)	Cancer prevention
Ginseng (American ginseng, Asian ginseng, Chinese ginseng, Korean red ginseng, *Panax ginseng*: *Panax* spp. including *P. ginseng* C.C. Meyer and *P. quincefolium* L., excluding *Eleutherococcus senticosus*)	Cancer prevention
Green tea (*Camellia sinensis*)	Cancer prevention
Hoxsey formula	Cancer
Lavender (*Lavandula angustifolia* Miller)	Cancer (perillyl alcohol)
Lycopene	Breast cancer prevention
Lycopene	Cancer prevention (general)
Lycopene	Cervical cancer prevention
Lycopene	Lung cancer prevention
Lycopene	Prostate cancer prevention
Maitake mushroom (*Grifola frondosa*), beta-glucan	Cancer
Melatonin	Cancer treatment
Milk thistle (*Silybum marianum*), silymarin	Cancer prevention
Oleander (*Nerium oleander*, *Thevetia peruviana*)	Cancer
Omega-3 fatty acids, fish oil, alpha-linolenic acid	Cancer prevention
Omega-3 fatty acids, fish oil, alpha-linolenic acid	Colon cancer
PC-SPES	Prostate cancer
Red clover (*Trifolium pratense*)	Prostate cancer
Seaweed, kelp, bladderwrack (*Fucus vesiculosus*)	Cancer
Shark cartilage	Cancer (solid tumors)
Slippery elm (*Ulmus rubra* Muhl., *U. fulva* Michx.)	Cancer
Sorrel (*Rumex acetosa* L., *R. acetosella* L.), Sinupret	Cancer
Soy (*Glycine max* L. Merr.)	Breast cancer prevention
Soy (*Glycine max* L. Merr.)	Cancer treatment
Soy (*Glycine max* L. Merr.)	Colon cancer prevention
Soy (*Glycine max* L. Merr.)	Endometrial cancer prevention

Soy (*Glycine max* L. Merr.)	Prostate cancer prevention
Spirulina	Oral leukoplakia/cancer
Turmeric (*Curcuma longa* L.), curcumin	Cancer

GRADE: D (Fair Negative Scientific Evidence)	
Therapy	Specific Therapeutic Use(s)
Bitter almond (*Prunus amygdalus* Batch var. *amara* DC. Focke), Laetrile	Cancer (Laetrile)
Flaxseed and flaxseed oil (*Linum usitatissimum*)	Prostate cancer (flaxseed, not flaxseed oil)

TRADITIONAL OR THEORETICAL USES THAT LACK SUFFICIENT EVIDENCE	
Therapy	Specific Therapeutic Use(s)
Aloe (*Aloe vera*)	Untreatable tumors
American pennyroyal (*Hedeoma pulegioides* L.), European pennyroyal (*Mentha pulegium* L.)	Cancer
Antineoplastons	Acute lymphocytic leukemia
Antineoplastons	Adenocarcinoma
Antineoplastons	Astrocytoma
Antineoplastons	Basal cell epithelioma
Antineoplastons	Bladder cancer
Antineoplastons	Chronic lymphocytic leukemia
Antineoplastons	Colon cancer
Antineoplastons	Glioblastoma
Antineoplastons	Hepatocellular carcinoma
Antineoplastons	Malignant melanoma
Antineoplastons	Medulloblastoma
Antineoplastons	Metastatic synovial sarcoma
Antineoplastons	Promyelocytic leukemia
Antineoplastons	Prostate cancer
Antineoplastons	Rectal cancer
Antineoplastons	Skin cancer
Arginine (L-arginine)	Cancer
Astragalus (*Astragalus membranaceus*)	Leukemia
Astragalus (*Astragalus membranaceus*)	Lung cancer
Barley (*Hordeum vulgare* L.), germinated barley foodstuff (GBF)	Colon cancer
Bilberry (*Vaccinium myrtillus*)	Cancer
Black cohosh (*Cimicifuga racemosa* L. Nutt.)	Cervical dysplasia (abnormal pap smear)
Black tea (*Camellia sinensis*)	Melanoma
Blessed thistle (*Cnicus benedictus* L.)	Cervical dysplasia

Continued

Boron	Breast cancer
Boron	Cancer
Boron	Leukemia
Bromelain	Cancer prevention
Burdock (*Arctium lappa*)	Cancer
Calendula (*Calendula officinalis* L.), marigold	Skin cancer
Chamomile (*Matricaria recutita, Chamaemelum nobile*)	Cancer
Clay	Cancer
Coenzyme Q10	Cancer
Coenzyme Q10	Lung cancer
Cranberry (*Vaccinium macrocarpon*)	Cancer treatment
Dandelion (*Taraxacum officinale*)	Breast cancer
Dandelion (*Taraxacum officinale*)	Leukemia
Danshen (*Salvia miltiorrhiza*)	Cancer
Danshen (*Salvia miltiorrhiza*)	Leukemia
Danshen (*Salvia miltiorrhiza*)	Liver cancer
DHEA (dehydroepiandrosterone)	Bladder cancer
DHEA (dehydroepiandrosterone)	Breast cancer
DHEA (dehydroepiandrosterone)	Colon cancer
DHEA (dehydroepiandrosterone)	Pancreatic cancer
DHEA (dehydroepiandrosterone)	Prostate cancer
Dong quai (*Angelica sinensis* [Oliv.] Diels), Chinese angelica	Cancer
Dong quai (*Angelica sinensis* [Oliv.] Diels), Chinese angelica	Stomach cancer
Echinacea (*Echinacea angustifolia* DC., *E. pallida*, *E. purpurea*)	Cancer
Elder (*Sambucus nigra* L.)	Cancer
Essiac	Bladder cancer
Essiac	Breast cancer
Essiac	Colon cancer
Essiac	Endometrial cancer
Essiac	Head/neck cancers
Essiac	Leukemia
Essiac	Lip cancer
Essiac	Liver cancer (hepatocellular carcinoma)
Essiac	Lung cancer
Essiac	Lymphoma
Essiac	Multiple myeloma
Essiac	Ovarian cancer

Essiac	Pancreatic cancer
Essiac	Prostate cancer
Essiac	Stomach cancer
Essiac	Throat cancer
Essiac	Tongue cancer
Eucalyptus oil (*Eucalyptus globulus* Labillardiere, *E. fructicetorum* F. Von Mueller, *E. smithii* R.T. Baker)	Cancer prevention
Evening primrose oil (*Oenothera biennis* L.)	Cancer
Evening primrose oil (*Oenothera biennis* L.)	Melanoma
Eyebright (*Euphrasia officinalis*)	Cancer
Flaxseed and flaxseed oil (*Linum usitatissimum*)	Colon cancer
Flaxseed and flaxseed oil (*Linum usitatissimum*)	Melanoma
Ginger (*Zingiber officinale* Roscoe)	Cancer
Ginkgo (*Ginkgo biloba* L.)	Cancer
Ginseng (American ginseng, Asian ginseng, Chinese ginseng, Korean red ginseng, *Panax ginseng*: *Panax* spp. including *P.* ginseng C.C. Meyer and *P. quincefolium* L., excluding *Eleutherococcus senticosus*)	Aplastic anemia
Ginseng (American ginseng, Asian ginseng, Chinese ginseng, Korean red ginseng, *Panax ginseng*: *Panax* spp. including *P. ginseng* C.C. Meyer and *P. quincefolium* L., excluding *Eleutherococcus senticosus*)	Breast cancer
Ginseng (American ginseng, Asian ginseng, Chinese ginseng, Korean red ginseng, *Panax ginseng*: *Panax* spp. including *P. ginseng* C.C. Meyer and *P. quincefolium* L., excluding *Eleutherococcus senticosus*)	Cancer prevention
Ginseng (American ginseng, Asian ginseng, Chinese ginseng, Korean red ginseng, *Panax ginseng*: *Panax* spp. including *P. ginseng* C.C. Meyer and *P. quincefolium* L., excluding *Eleutherococcus senticosus*)	Malignant tumors
Ginseng (American ginseng, Asian ginseng, Chinese ginseng, Korean red ginseng, *Panax ginseng*: *Panax* spp. including *P. ginseng* C.C. Meyer and *P. quincefolium* L., excluding *Eleutherococcus senticosus*)	Prostate cancer
Ginseng (American ginseng, Asian ginseng, Chinese ginseng, Korean red ginseng, *Panax ginseng*: *Panax* spp. including *P. ginseng* C.C. Meyer and *P. quincefolium* L., excluding *Eleutherococcus senticosus*)	Stomach cancer
Goldenseal (*Hydrastis canadensis* L.), berberine	Cancer
Green tea (*Camellia sinensis*)	Fibrosarcoma
Green tea (*Camellia sinensis*)	Liver cancer
Green tea (*Camellia sinensis*)	Lung cancer
Green tea (*Camellia sinensis*)	Ovarian cancer
Guggul (*Commifora mukul*)	Tumors
Gymnema (*Gymnema Sylvestre* R. Br.)	Cancer
Hawthorn (*Crataegus laevigata, C. oxyacantha, C. monogyna, C. pentagyna*)	Cancer

Continued

Hops (*Humulus lupulus* L.)	Breast cancer
Hops (*Humulus lupulus* L.)	Cancer (general)
Horsetail (*Equisetum arvense* L.)	Cancer
Hoxsey formula	Breast cancer
Hoxsey formula	Cervical cancer
Hoxsey formula	Colon cancer
Hoxsey formula	Lung cancer
Hoxsey formula	Lymphoma
Hoxsey formula	Melanoma
Hoxsey formula	Mouth cancer
Hoxsey formula	Prostate cancer
Hoxsey formula	Sarcomas
Kava (*Piper methysticum* G. Forst)	Cancer
Lactobacillus acidophilus	Cancer
Lactobacillus acidophilus	Colon cancer prevention
Licorice (*Glycyrrhiza glabra* L.), deglycyrrhizinated licorice (DGL)	Aplastic anemia
Licorice (*Glycyrrhiza glabra* L.), deglycyrrhizinated l icorice (DGL)	Cancer
Licorice (*Glycyrrhiza glabra* L.), deglycyrrhizinated licorice (DGL)	Colorectal cancer
Licorice (*Glycyrrhiza glabra* L.), deglycyrrhizinated licorice (DGL)	Lung cancer
Lycopene	Bladder cancer
Lycopene	Breast cancer
Lycopene	Esophageal cancer
Lycopene	Laryngeal cancer
Lycopene	Melanoma
Lycopene	Mesothelioma
Lycopene	Ovarian cancer
Lycopene	Pancreatic cancer
Lycopene	Pharyngeal cancer
Lycopene	Skin cancer
Lycopene	Stomach cancer
Marshmallow (*Althaea officinalis* L.)	Cancer
Milk thistle (*Silybum marianum*), silymarin	Breast cancer
Milk thistle (*Silybum marianum*), silymarin	Liver cancer
Niacin (vitamin B_3, nicotinic acid), niacinamide, and inositol hexanicotinate	Cancer prevention
Niacin (vitamin B_3, nicotinic acid), niacinamide, and inositol hexanicotinate	Prostate cancer

Niacin (vitamin B$_3$, nicotinic acid), niacinamide, and inositol hexanicotinate	Tumor detection
Omega-3 fatty acids, fish oil, alpha-linolenic acid	Leukemia
Omega-3 fatty acids, fish oil, alpha-linolenic acid	Prostate cancer prevention
Passionflower (*Passiflora incarnata* L.)	Cancer
PC-SPES	Breast cancer
PC-SPES	Cancer prevention
PC-SPES	Leukemia
PC-SPES	Lymphoma
PC-SPES	Melanoma
Peppermint (*Mentha x piperita* L.)	Cancer
Polypodium leucotomos extract, Anapsos	Cancer
Propolis	Cancer
Propolis	Nasopharyngeal carcinoma
Psyllium (*Plantago ovata, P. ispaghula*)	Colon cancer prevention
Pygeum (*Prunus africana, Pygeum africanum*)	Prostate cancer
Red clover (*Trifolium pratense*)	Cancer prevention
Saw palmetto (*Serenoa repens* [Bartram] Small)	Cancer
Sorrel (*Rumex acetosa* L., *R. acetosella* L.), Sinupret	Skin cancer
Soy (*Glycine max* L. Merr.)	Cancer prevention (general)
Soy (*Glycine max* L. Merr.)	Gastric cancer
Soy (*Glycine max* L. Merr.)	Urinary tract cancer
Spirulina	Cancer prevention
St. John's wort (*Hypericum perforatum* L.)	Cancer
Sweet almond (*Prunus amygdalus dulcis*)	Bladder cancer
Sweet almond (*Prunus amygdalus dulcis*)	Breast cancer
Sweet almond (*Prunus amygdalus dulcis*)	Colon cancer
Sweet almond (*Prunus amygdalus dulcis*)	Mouth and throat cancers
White horehound (*Marrubium vulgare*)	Cancer

CARPAL TUNNEL SYNDROME AND RELATED CONDITIONS
Levels of Scientific Evidence for Specific Therapies

TRADITIONAL OR THEORETICAL USES THAT LACK SUFFICIENT EVIDENCE

Therapy	Specific Therapeutic Use(s)
Bromelain	Carpal tunnel syndrome
Chamomile (*Matricaria recutita, Chamaemelum nobile*)	Carpal tunnel syndrome
Lavender (*Lavandula angustifolia* Miller)	Carpal tunnel syndrome

CATARACTS AND RELATED CONDITIONS

Levels of Scientific Evidence for Specific Therapies

GRADE: C (Unclear or Conflicting Scientific Evidence)

Therapy	Specific Therapeutic Use(s)
Bilberry (*Vaccinium myrtillus*)	Cataracts
Danshen (*Salvia miltiorrhiza*)	Glaucoma
Ginkgo (*Ginkgo biloba* L.)	Glaucoma
Melatonin	Glaucoma

TRADITIONAL OR THEORETICAL USES THAT LACK SUFFICIENT EVIDENCE

Therapy	Specific Therapeutic Use(s)
Arginine (L-arginine)	Glaucoma
Belladonna (*Atropa belladonna* L. or its variety *acuminata* Royle ex Lindl)	Glaucoma
Betel nut (*Areca catechu* L.)	Glaucoma
Bilberry (*Vaccinium myrtillus*)	Glaucoma
Danshen (*Salvia miltiorrhiza*)	Cataracts
Dong quai (*Angelica sinensis* [Oliv.] Diels), Chinese angelica	Glaucoma
Eyebright (*Euphrasia officinalis*)	Cataracts
Green tea (*Camellia sinensis*)	Cataracts
Lycopene	Cataracts
Melatonin	Glaucoma
Niacin (vitamin B_3, nicotinic acid), niacinamide, and inositol hexanicotinate	Cataract prevention
Omega-3 fatty acids, fish oil, alpha-linolenic acid	Glaucoma
Shark cartilage	Glaucoma
Turmeric (*Curcuma longa* L.), curcumin	Cataracts

CEREBRAL INSUFFICIENCY AND RELATED CONDITIONS

Levels of Scientific Evidence for Specific Therapies

GRADE: B (Good Scientific Evidence)

Therapy	Specific Therapeutic Use(s)
Ginkgo (*Ginkgo biloba* L.)	Cerebral insufficiency
Ginseng (American ginseng, Asian ginseng, Chinese ginseng, Korean red ginseng, *Panax ginseng*: *Panax* spp. including *P. ginseng* C.C. Meyer and *P. quincefolium* L., excluding *Eleutherococcus senticosus*)	Mental performance

GRADE: C (Unclear or Conflicting Scientific Evidence)

Therapy	Specific Therapeutic Use(s)
Black tea (*Camellia sinensis*)	Memory enhancement
Black tea (*Camellia sinensis*)	Mental performance/alertness

Boron	Improving cognitive function
Ginkgo (*Ginkgo biloba* L.)	Age-associated memory impairment (AAMI)
Ginkgo (*Ginkgo biloba* L.)	Memory enhancement (in healthy people)
Green tea (*Camellia sinensis*)	Memory enhancement
Green tea (*Camellia sinensis*)	Mental performance/alertness
Polypodium leucotomos extract, Anapsos	Dementia

GRADE: D (Fair Negative Scientific Evidence)

Therapy	Specific Therapeutic Use(s)
DHEA (dehydroepiandrosterone)	Brain function and well-being in the elderly

TRADITIONAL OR THEORETICAL USES THAT LACK SUFFICIENT EVIDENCE

Therapy	Specific Therapeutic Use(s)
Arginine (L-arginine)	Dementia
Astragalus (*Astragalus membranaceus*)	Dementia
Astragalus (*Astragalus membranaceus*)	Memory
Blessed thistle (*Cnicus benedictus* L.)	Memory improvement
Danshen (*Salvia miltiorrhiza*)	Anoxic brain injury
DHEA (dehydroepiandrosterone)	Dementia
Eyebright (*Euphrasia officinalis*)	Memory loss
Garlic (*Allium sativum* L.)	Age-related memory problems
Ginseng (American ginseng, Asian ginseng, Chinese ginseng, Korean red ginseng, *Panax ginseng*: *Panax* spp. including *P. ginseng* C.C. Meyer and *P. quincefolium* L., excluding *Eleutherococcus senticosus*)	Dementia
Ginseng (American ginseng, Asian ginseng, Chinese ginseng, Korean red ginseng, *Panax ginseng*: *Panax* spp. including *P. ginseng* C.C. Meyer and *P. quincefolium* L., excluding *Eleutherococcus senticosus*)	Improved memory and thinking after menopause
Ginseng (American ginseng, Asian ginseng, Chinese ginseng, Korean red ginseng, *Panax ginseng*: *Panax* spp. including *P. ginseng* C.C. Meyer and *P. quincefolium* L., excluding *Eleutherococcus senticosus*)	Senile dementia
Gotu kola (*Centella asiatica* L.), total triterpenic fraction of *Centella asiatica* (TTFCA)	Memory enhancement
Green tea (*Camellia sinensis*)	Cognitive performance enhancement
Kava (*Piper methysticum* G. Forst)	Brain damage
Lycopene	Cognitive function
Melatonin	Cognitive enhancement
Melatonin	Memory enhancement
Niacin (vitamin B_3, nicotinic acid), niacinamide, and inositol hexanicotinate	Memory loss

Continued

Omega-3 fatty acids, fish oil, alpha-linolenic acid	Memory enhancement
Soy (*Glycine max* L. Merr.)	Cognitive function
Soy (*Glycine max* L. Merr.)	Memory enhancement
Spirulina	Memory improvement
Valerian (*Valeriana officinalis* L.)	Memory
Yohimbe bark extract (*Pausinystalia yohimbe* Pierre ex Beille)	Cognition

CEREBROVASCULAR ACCIDENT (STROKE) AND RELATED CONDITIONS
Levels of Scientific Evidence for Specific Therapies

GRADE: C (Unclear or Conflicting Scientific Evidence)	
Therapy	Specific Therapeutic Use(s)
Betel nut (*Areca catechu* L.)	Stroke recovery
Danshen (*Salvia miltiorrhiza*)	Ischemic stroke
Melatonin	Stroke
Omega-3 fatty acids, fish oil, alpha-linolenic acid	Stroke prevention

GRADE: D (Fair Negative Scientific Evidence)	
Therapy	Specific Therapeutic Use(s)
Ginkgo (*Ginkgo biloba* L.)	Stroke

TRADITIONAL OR THEORETICAL USES THAT LACK SUFFICIENT EVIDENCE	
Therapy	Specific therapeutic Use(s)
Arginine (L-arginine)	Ischemic stroke
Arginine (L-arginine)	Stroke
Astragalus (*Astragalus membranaceus*)	Stroke
Dong quai (*Angelica sinensis* [Oliv.] Diels), Chinese angelica	Stroke
Garlic (*Allium sativum* L.)	Stroke
Ginseng (American ginseng, Asian ginseng, Chinese ginseng, Korean red ginseng, *Panax ginseng*: *Panax* spp. including *P. ginseng* C.C. Meyer and *P. quincefolium* L., excluding *Eleutherococcus senticosus*)	Strokes
Green tea (*Camellia sinensis*)	Ischemia-reperfusion injury protection
Green tea (*Camellia sinensis*)	Stroke prevention
Kava (*Piper methysticum* G. Forst)	Cerebral ischemia
Lycopene	Stroke prevention
Niacin (vitamin B_3, nicotinic acid), niacinamide, and inositol hexanicotinate	Ischemia-reperfusion injury prevention

CHEMOTHERAPY SIDE EFFECTS AND RELATED CONDITIONS

Levels of Scientific Evidence for Specific Therapies

GRADE: B (Good Scientific Evidence)

Therapy	Specific Therapeutic Use(s)
Omega-3 fatty acids, fish oil, alpha-linolenic acid	Protection from cyclosporine toxicity in organ transplant patients

GRADE: C (Unclear or Conflicting Scientific Evidence)

Therapy	Specific therapeutic Use(s)
Astragalus (*Astragalus membranaceus*)	Chemotherapy side effects
Coenzyme Q10	Anthracycline chemotherapy heart toxicity
Ginkgo (*Ginkgo biloba* L.)	Chemotherapy side effects
Melatonin	Chemotherapy side effects

TRADITIONAL OR THEORETICAL USES THAT LACK SUFFICIENT EVIDENCE

Therapy	Specific Therapeutic Use(s)
Danshen (*Salvia miltiorrhiza*)	Bleomycin induced lung fibrosis
Dong quai (*Angelica sinensis* [Oliv.] Diels), Chinese angelica	Bleomycin-induced lung damage
Essiac	Chemotherapy side effects
Ginseng (American ginseng, Asian ginseng, Chinese ginseng, Korean red ginseng, *Panax ginseng*: *Panax* spp. including *P. ginseng* C.C. Meyer and *P. quincefolium* L., excluding *Eleutherococcus senticosus*)	Chemotherapy support
Omega-3 fatty acids, fish oil, alpha-linolenic acid	Anthracycline-induced cardiac toxicity
Omega-3 fatty acids, fish oil, alpha-linolenic acid	Protection from isotretinoin drug toxicity

CHOLELITHIASIS AND RELATED CONDITIONS

Levels of Scientific Evidence for Specific Therapies

GRADE: C (Unclear or Conflicting Scientific Evidence)

Therapy	Specific Therapeutic Use(s)
Globe artichoke (*Cynara scolymus* L.)	Choleretic (bile flow stimulant)
Soy (*Glycine max* L. Merr.)	Gallstones (cholelithiasis)
Turmeric (*Curcuma longa* L.), curcumin	Gallstone prevention/bile flow stimulant
White horehound (*Marrubium vulgare*)	Choleretic (dyspepsia, appetite stimulation)

Continued

TRADITIONAL OR THEORETICAL USES THAT LACK SUFFICIENT EVIDENCE	
Therapy	Specific Therapeutic Use(s)
American pennyroyal (*Hedeoma pulegioides* L.), European pennyroyal (*Mentha pulegium* L.)	Gallbladder disorders
Black cohosh (*Cimicifuga racemosa* L. Nutt.)	Gallbladder disorders
Blessed thistle (*Cnicus benedictus* L.)	Choleretic (bile flow stimulant)
Blessed thistle (*Cnicus benedictus* L.)	Gallbladder disease
Cranberry (*Vaccinium macrocarpon*)	Gallbladder stones
Dandelion (*Taraxacum officinale*)	Bile flow stimulation
Dandelion (*Taraxacum officinale*)	Gallbladder disease
Dandelion (*Taraxacum officinale*)	Gallstones
Devil's claw (*Harpagophytum procumbens* DC.)	Choleretic (bile secretion)
Dong quai (*Angelica sinensis* [Oliv.] Diels), Chinese angelica	Cholagogue
Garlic (*Allium sativum* L.)	Bile secretion problems
Garlic (*Allium sativum* L.)	Gallstones
Ginger (*Zingiber officinale* Roscoe)	Bile secretion problems
Globe artichoke (*Cynara scolymus* L.)	Cholegogue
Globe artichoke (*Cynara scolymus* L.)	Cholelithiasis
Goldenseal (*Hydrastis canadensis* L.), berberine	Bile flow stimulant
Goldenseal (*Hydrastis canadensis* L.), berberine	Gallstones
Horse chestnut (*Aesculus hippocastanum* L.)	Gallbladder infection (cholecystitis)
Horse chestnut (*Aesculus hippocastanum* L.)	Gallbladder pain (colic)
Horse chestnut (*Aesculus hippocastanum* L.)	Gall ladder stones (cholelithiasis)
Lavender (*Lavandula angustifolia* Miller)	Cholagogue
Lavender (*Lavandula angustifolia* Miller)	Choleretic
Milk thistle (*Silybum marianum*), silymarin	Cholelithiasis
Omega-3 fatty acids, fish oil, alpha-linolenic acid	Gallstones
Peppermint (*Mentha x piperita* L.)	Bile duct disorders
Peppermint (*Mentha x piperita* L.)	Cholelithiasis (gallstones)
Peppermint (*Mentha x piperita* L.)	Gallbladder disorders
Psyllium (*Plantago ovata, P. ispaghula*)	Gallstones
Turmeric (*Curcuma longa* L.), curcumin	Gallstones
White horehound (*Marrubium vulgare*)	Bile secretion
White horehound (*Marrubium vulgare*)	Gallbladder complaints
Wild yam (*Dioscorea villosa*)	Bile flow improvement
Wild yam (*Dioscorea villosa*)	Biliary colic

CHRONIC OBSTRUCTIVE PULMONARY DISEASE AND RELATED CONDITIONS

Levels of Scientific Evidence for Specific Therapies

GRADE: B (Good Scientific Evidence)

Therapy	Specific therapeutic Use(s)
Boswellia (*Boswellia serrata* Roxb.)	Asthma (chronic therapy)
Ephedra (*Ephedra sinica*)/ma huang	Asthmatic bronchoconstriction

GRADE: C (Unclear or Conflicting Scientific Evidence)

Therapy	Specific Therapeutic Use(s)
Belladonna (*Atropa belladonna* L. or its variety *acuminata* Royle ex Lindl)	Airway obstruction
Black tea (*Camellia sinensis*)	Asthma
Bromelain	Chronic obstructive pulmonary disease (COPD)
Danshen (*Salvia miltiorrhiza*)	Asthmatic bronchitis
Green tea (*Camellia sinensis*)	Asthma
Lactobacillus acidophilus	Asthma
Lycopene	Asthma caused by exercise
Omega-3 fatty acids, fish oil, alpha-linolenic acid	Asthma

GRADE: D (Fair Negative Scientific Evidence)

Therapy	Specific Therapeutic Use(s)
Evening primrose oil (*Oenothera biennis* L.)	Asthma

GRADE: F (Strong Negative Scientific Evidence)

Therapy	Specific Therapeutic Use(s)
Arginine (L-arginine)	Asthma

TRADITIONAL OR THEORETICAL USES THAT LACK SUFFICIENT EVIDENCE

Therapy	Specific Therapeutic Use(s)
Alfalfa (*Medicago sativa* L.)	Asthma
Aloe (*Aloe vera*)	Asthma
Astragalus (*Astragalus membranaceus*)	Asthma
Astragalus (*Astragalus membranaceus*)	Shortness of breath
Barley (*Hordeum vulgare* L.), germinated barley foodstuff (GBF)	Asthma
Belladonna (*Atropa belladonna* L. or its variety *acuminata* Royle ex Lindl)	Asthma
Betel nut (*Areca catechu* L.)	Asthma
Black cohosh (*Cimicifuga racemosa* L. Nutt.)	Asthma
Boswellia (*Boswellia serrata* Roxb.)	Chronic obstructive pulmonary disease (COPD)

Continued

Clove (*Eugenia aromatica*)	Asthma
Coenzyme Q10	Asthma
Coenzyme Q10	Breathing difficulties
Coenzyme Q10	Chronic obstructive pulmonary disease (COPD)
DHEA (dehydroepiandrosterone)	Asthma
Dong quai (*Angelica sinensis* [Oliv.] Diels), Chinese angelica	Asthma
Dong quai (*Angelica sinensis* [Oliv.] Diels), Chinese angelica	Chronic obstructive pulmonary disease (COPD)
Elder (*Sambucus nigra L.*)	Asthma
Elder (*Sambucus nigra* L.)	Respiratory distress
Ephedra *(Ephedra sinica)*/ma huang	Dyspnea
Essiac	Asthma
Eucalyptus oil (*Eucalyptus globulus* Labillardiere, *E. fructicetorum* F. Von Mueller, *E. smithii* R.T. Baker)	Asthma
Eucalyptus oil (*Eucalyptus globulus* Labillardiere, *E. fructicetorum* F. Von Mueller, *E. smithii* R.T. Baker)	Chronic obstructive pulmonary disease (COPD)
Eucalyptus oil (*Eucalyptus globulus* Labillardiere, *E. fructicetorum* F. Von Mueller, *E. smithii* R.T. Baker)	Emphysema
Eyebright (*Euphrasia officinalis*)	Asthma
Feverfew (*Tanacetum parthenium* L. Schultz-Bip.)	Asthma
Flaxseed and flaxseed oil (*Linum usitatissimum*)	Bronchial irritation
Garlic (*Allium sativum* L.)	Asthma
Ginger (*Zingiber officinale* Roscoe)	Asthma
Ginkgo (*Ginkgo biloba* L.)	Asthma
Ginseng (American ginseng, Asian ginseng, Chinese ginseng, Korean red ginseng, *Panax ginseng*: *Panax* spp. including *P. ginseng* C.C. Meyer and *P. quincefolium* L., excluding *Eleutherococcus senticosus*)	Asthma
Ginseng (American ginseng, Asian ginseng, Chinese ginseng, Korean red ginseng, *Panax ginseng*: *Panax* spp. including *P. ginseng* C.C. Meyer and *P. quincefolium* L., excluding *Eleutherococcus senticosus*)	Breathing difficulty
Ginseng (American ginseng, Asian ginseng, Chinese ginseng, Korean red ginseng, *Panax ginseng*: *Panax* spp. including *P. ginseng* C.C. Meyer and *P. quincefolium* L., excluding *Eleutherococcus senticosus*)	Bronchodilation
Goldenseal (*Hydrastis canadensis* L.), berberine	Asthma
Gotu kola (*Centella asiatica* L.), total triterpenic fraction of *Centella asiatica* (TTFCA)	Asthma
Guggul (*Commifora mukul*)	Asthma
Hawthorn (*Crataegus laevigata, C. oxyacantha, C. monogyna, C. pentagyna*)	Asthma
Hawthorn (*Crataegus laevigata, C. oxyacantha, C. monogyna, C. pentagyna*)	Dyspnea
Kava (*Piper methysticum* G. Forst)	Asthma

Lavender (*Lavandula angustifolia* Miller)	Asthma
Licorice (*Glycyrrhiza glabra* L.), deglycyrrhizinated licorice (DGL)	Asthma
Melatonin	Asthma
Oleander (*Nerium oleander, Thevetia peruviana*)	Asthma
Omega-3 fatty acids, fish oil, alpha-linolenic acid	Chronic obstructive pulmonary disease (COPD)
Passionflower (*Passiflora incarnata* L.)	Asthma
Peppermint (*Mentha x piperita* L.)	Asthma
Polypodium leucotomos extract, Anapsos	Asthma
Red clover (*Trifolium pratense*)	Asthma
Saw palmetto (*Serenoa repens* [Bartram] Small)	Asthma
Slippery elm (*Ulmus rubra* Muhl., *U. fulva* Michx.)	Respiratory disorders
Thyme (*Thymus vulgaris* L.), thymol	Asthma
Thyme (*Thymus vulgaris* L.), thymol	Dyspnea
Turmeric (*Curcuma longa* L.), curcumin	Asthma
Valerian (*Valeriana officinalis* L.)	Asthma
Valerian (*Valeriana officinalis* L.)	Bronchospasm
White horehound (*Marrubium vulgare*)	Asthma
White horehound (*Marrubium vulgare*)	Chronic obstructive pulmonary disease (COPD)
White horehound (*Marrubium vulgare*)	Wheezing
Wild (*Dioscorea villosa*)	Asthma

CHRONIC VENOUS INSUFFICIENCY AND RELATED CONDITIONS

Levels of Scientific Evidence for Specific Therapies

GRADE: A (Strong Scientific Evidence)	
Therapy	Specific Therapeutic Use(s)
Horse chestnut (*Aesculus hippocastanum* L.)	Chronic venous insufficiency

GRADE: B (Good Scientific Evidence)	
Therapy	Specific Therapeutic Use(s)
Gotu kola (*Centella asiatica* L.), total triterpenic fraction of *Centella asiatica* (TTFCA)	Chronic venous insufficiency/ varicose veins

GRADE: C (Unclear or Conflicting Scientific Evidence)	
Therapy	Specific Therapeutic Use(s)
Bilberry (*Vaccinium myrtillus*)	Chronic venous insufficiency
Glucosamine	Chronic venous insufficiency

Continued

TRADITIONAL OR THEORETICAL USES THAT LACK SUFFICIENT EVIDENCE

Therapy	Specific Therapeutic Use(s)
Astragalus (Astragalus membranaceus)	Edema
Barley (*Hordeum vulgare* L.), germinated barley foodstuff (GBF)	Improved blood circulation
Bilberry (*Vaccinium myrtillus*)	Poor circulation
Black cohosh (*Cimicifuga racemosa* L. Nutt.)	Edema
Black tea (*Camellia sinensis*)	Circulatory/blood flow disorders
Bladderwrack (*Fucus vesiculosus*)	Edema
Bromelain	Varicose veins
Burdock (*Arctium lappa*)	Fluid retention
Calendula (*Calendula officinalis* L.), marigold	Circulation problems
Calendula (Calendula officinalis L.), marigold	Edema
Calendula (*Calendula officinalis* L.), marigold	Varicose veins
Dandelion (*Taraxacum officinale*)	Circulation
Dandelion (*Taraxacum officinale*)	Dropsy
Danshen (*Salvia miltiorrhiza*)	Circulation
Devil's claw (*Harpagophytum procumbens* DC.)	Edema
Dong quai (*Angelica sinensis* [Oliv.] Diels), Chinese angelica	Fluid retention
Elder (*Sambucus nigra* L.)	Circulatory stimulant
Elder (*Sambucus nigra* L.)	Edema
Ephedra (*Ephedra sinica*)/ma huang	Edema
Fenugreek (*Trigonella foenum-graecum* L.)	Dropsy
Ginkgo (*Ginkgo biloba* L.)	Swelling
Globe artichoke (*Cynara scolymus* L.)	Peripheral edema
Goldenseal (*Hydrastis canadensis* L.), berberine	Circulatory stimulant
Gotu kola (*Centella asiatica* L.), total triterpenic fraction of *Centella asiatica* (TTFCA)	Vascular fragility
Green tea (*Camellia sinensis*)	Improving blood flow
Hawthorn (*Crataegus laevigata, C. oxyacantha, C. monogyna, C. pentagyna*)	Edema
Horsetail (*Equisetum arvense* L.)	Dropsy
Lavender (*Lavandula angustifolia* Miller)	Circulation problems
Lavender (*Lavandula angustifolia* Miller)	Varicose veins
Melatonin	Edema
Milk thistle (*Silybum marianum*), silymarin	Edema
Niacin (Vitamin B_3, nicotinic acid), niacinamide, and inositol hexanicotinate	Edema
Oleander (*Nerium oleander, Thevetia peruviana*)	Swelling

Polypodium leucotomos extract, Anapsos	Water retention
Seaweed, kelp, bladderwrack (*Fucus vesiculosus*)	Edema
Slippery elm (*Ulmus rubra* Muhl., *U. fulva* Michx.)	Varicose ulcers
Thyme (*Thymus vulgaris* L.), thymol	Edema
White horehound (*Marrubium vulgare*)	Water retention

CIRRHOSIS AND RELATED CONDITIONS

Levels of Scientific Evidence for Specific Therapies

GRADE: B (Good Scientific Evidence)

Therapy	Specific Therapeutic Use(s)
Milk thistle (*Silybum marianum*), silymarin	Cirrhosis
Milk thistle (*Silybum marianum*), silymarin	Hepatitis (chronic)

GRADE: C (Unclear or Conflicting Scientific Evidence)

Therapy	Specific Therapeutic Use(s)
Astragalus (*Astragalus membranaceus*)	Liver protection
Clay	Protection from aflatoxins
Dandelion (*Taraxacum officinale*)	Hepatitis B
Danshen (*Salvia miltiorrhiza*)	Liver disease (cirrhosis/chronic hepatitis B)
Eyebright (*Euphrasia officinalis*)	Hepatoprotection
Lactobacillus acidophilus	Hepatic encephalopathy (confused thinking due to liver disorders)
Licorice (*Glycyrrhiza glabra* L.), deglycyrrhizinated licorice (DGL)	Viral hepatitis
Milk thistle (*Silybum marianum*), silymarin	Acute viral hepatitis
Milk thistle (*Silybum marianum*), silymarin	*Amanita phalloides* mushroom toxicity
Milk thistle (*Silybum marianum*), silymarin	Drug/toxin-induced hepatotoxicity

TRADITIONAL OR THEORETICAL USES THAT LACK SUFFICIENT EVIDENCE

Therapy	Specific Therapeutic Use(s)
Alfalfa (*Medicago sativa* L.)	Jaundice
Aloe (*Aloe vera*)	Hepatitis
American pennyroyal (*Hedeoma pulegioides* L.), European pennyroyal (Mentha pulegium L.)	Liver disease
Arginine (L-arginine)	Ammonia toxicity
Arginine (L-arginine)	Hepatic encephalopathy
Arginine (L-arginine)	Liver disease
Astragalus (*Astragalus membranaceus*)	Chronic hepatitis

Continued

Astragalus (*Astragalus membranaceus*)	Liver disease
Bilberry (*Vaccinium myrtillus*)	Liver disease
Black cohosh (*Cimicifuga racemosa* L. Nutt.)	Liver disease
Blessed thistle (*Cnicus benedictus* L.)	Jaundice
Blessed thistle (*Cnicus benedictus* L.)	Liver disorders
Burdock (*Arctium lappa*)	Liver protection
Calendula (*Calendula officinalis* L.), marigold	Jaundice
Calendula (*Calendula officinalis* l.), marigold	Liver dysfunction
Chamomile (*Matricaria recutita*, *Chamaemelum nobile*)	Liver disorders
Coenzyme Q10	Hepatitis B
Coenzyme Q10	Liver enlargement or disease
Cranberry (*Vaccinium macrocarpon*)	Liver disorders
Dandelion (*Taraxacum officinale*)	Jaundice
Dandelion (*Taraxacum officinale*)	Liver cleansing
Dandelion (*Taraxacum officinale*)	Liver disease
Devil's claw (*Harpagophytum procumbens* DC.)	Liver and gallbladder tonic
DHEA (dehydroepiandrosterone)	Liver protection
Dong quai (*Angelica sinensis* [Oliv.] Diels), Chinese angelica	Chronic hepatitis
Dong quai (*Angelica sinensis* [Oliv.] Diels), Chinese angelica	Cirrhosis
Dong quai (*Angelica sinensis* [Oliv.] Diels), Chinese angelica	Liver protection
Elder (*Sambucus nigra* L.)	Liver disease
Eucalyptus oil (*Eucalyptus globulus* Labillardiere, *E. fructicetorum* F. Von Mueller, *E. smithii* R.T. Baker)	Liver protection
Evening primrose oil (*Oenothera biennis* L.)	Hepatitis B
Eyebright (*Euphrasia officinalis*)	Jaundice
Eyebright (*Euphrasia officinalis*)	Liver disease
Garlic (*Allium sativum* L.)	Antitoxin
Garlic (*Allium sativum* L.)	Hepatopulmonary syndrome
Garlic (*Allium sativum* L.)	Liver health
Ginger (*Zingiber officinale* Roscoe)	Liver disease
Ginkgo (*Ginkgo biloba* L.)	Hepatitis B
Ginseng (American ginseng, Asian ginseng, Chinese ginseng, Korean red ginseng, *Panax ginseng*: *Panax* spp. including *P. ginseng* C.C. Meyer and *P. quincefolium* L., excluding *Eleutherococcus senticosus*)	Hepatitis/hepatitis B infection
Ginseng (American ginseng, Asian ginseng, Chinese ginseng, Korean red ginseng, *Panax ginseng*: Panax *spp.* including *P. ginseng* C.C. Meyer and *P. quincefolium* L., excluding *Eleutherococcus senticosus*)	Liver disease
Ginseng (American ginseng, Asian ginseng, Chinese ginseng, Korean red ginseng, *Panax ginseng*: *Panax* spp. including *P. ginseng* C.C. Meyer and *P. quincefolium* L., excluding *Eleutherococcus senticosus*)	Liver health

Globe artichoke (*Cynara scolymus* L.)	Jaundice
Goldenseal (*Hydrastis canadensis* L.), berberine	Alcoholic liver disease
Goldenseal (*Hydrastis canadensis* L.), berberine	Hepatitis
Goldenseal (*Hydrastis canadensis* L.), berberine	Jaundice
Goldenseal (Hydrastis canadensis L.), berberine	Liver disorders
Gotu kola (*Centella asiatica* L.), total triterpenic fraction of *Centella asiatica* (TTFCA)	Hepatitis
Gotu kola (*Centella asiatica* L.), total triterpenic fraction of *Centella asiatica* (TTFCA)	Jaundice
Gymnema (*Gymnema Sylvestre* R. Br.)	Liver disease
Gymnema (*Gymnema Sylvestre* R. Br.)	Liver protection
Horse chestnut (*Aesculus hippocastanum* L.)	Liver congestion
Horsetail (*Equisetum arvense* L.)	Liver protection
Licorice (*Glycyrrhiza glabra* L.), deglycyrrhizinated licorice (DGL)	Liver protection
Maitake mushroom (*Grifola frondosa*), beta-glucan	Liver inflammation (hepatitis)
Melatonin	Toxic liver damage
Milk thistle (*Silybum marianum*), silymarin	Jaundice
Milk thistle (*Silybum Marianum*), silymarin	Liver-cleansing agent
Niacin (vitamin B_3, nicotinic acid), niacinamide, and inositol hexanicotinate	Liver disease
Omega-3 fatty acids, fish oil, alpha-linolenic acid	Cirrhosis

CLAUDICATION AND RELATED CONDITIONS
Levels of Scientific Evidence for Specific Therapies

GRADE: A (Strong Scientific Evidence)	
Therapy	Specific Therapeutic Use(s)
Ginkgo (*Ginkgo biloba* L.)	Claudication (painful legs from clogged arteries)

GRADE: C (Unclear or Conflicting Scientific Evidence)	
Therapy	Specific Therapeutic Use(s)
Arginine (L-arginine)	Peripheral vascular disease/claudication
Garlic (*Allium sativum* L.)	Peripheral vascular disease (blocked arteries in the legs)

TRADITIONAL OR THEORETICAL USES THAT LACK SUFFICIENT EVIDENCE	
Therapy	Specific Therapeutic Use(s)
Garlic (*Allium sativum* L.)	Claudication (leg pain due to poor blood flow)
Niacin (vitamin B_3, nicotinic acid), niacinamide, and inositol hexanicotinate	Peripheral vascular disease
Omega-3 fatty acids, fish oil, alpha-linolenic acid	Peripheral vascular disease

CONGESTIVE HEART FAILURE (CHF) AND RELATED CONDITIONS

Levels of Scientific Evidence for Specific Therapies

GRADE: A (Strong Scientific Evidence)

Therapy	Specific Therapeutic Use(s)
Hawthorn (*Crataegus laevigata*, *C. oxyacantha*, *C. monogyna*, *C. pentagyna*)	CHF

GRADE: C (Unclear or Conflicting Scientific Evidence)

Therapy	Specific Therapeutic Use(s)
Arginine (L-arginine)	Heart failure (CHF)
Astragalus (*Astragalus membranaceus*)	Heart failure
Coenzyme Q10	Cardiomyopathy (dilated, hypertrophic)
Coenzyme Q10	Heart failure
DHEA (dehydroepiandrosterone)	Heart failure
Ginseng (American ginseng, Asian ginseng, Chinese ginseng, Korean red ginseng, *Panax ginseng*: *Panax* spp. including *P. ginseng* C.C. Meyer and *P. quincefolium* L., excluding *Eleutherococcus senticosus*)	CHF
Hawthorn (*Crataegus laevigata*, *C. oxyacantha*, *C. monogyna*, *C. pentagyna*)	Functional cardiovascular disorders
Oleander (Nerium oleander, *Thevetia peruviana*)	CHF
Passionflower (*Passiflora incarnata* L.)	CHF (exercise capacity)

GRADE: D (Fair Negative Scientific Evidence)

TRADITIONAL OR THEORETICAL USES THAT LACK SUFFICIENT EVIDENCE

Therapy	Specific Therapeutic Use(s)
Dandelion (*Taraxacum officinale*)	CHF
Danshen (*Salvia miltiorrhiza*)	Left ventricular hypertrophy
Dong quai (*Angelica sinensis* [Oliv.] Diels), Chinese angelica	CHF
Ginkgo (*Ginkgo biloba* L.)	CHF
Goldenseal (*Hydrastis canadensis* L.), berberine	Heart failure
Horse chestnut (*Aesculus hippocastanum* L.)	Fluid in the lungs (pulmonary edema)
Horsetail (*Equisetum arvense* L.)	Fluid in the lungs
Omega-3 fatty acids, fish oil, alpha-linolenic acid	CHF
Passionflower (*Passiflora incarnata* L.)	CHF (exercise ability)
Valerian (*Valeriana officinalis* L.)	CHF

CONSTIPATION AND RELATED CONDITIONS

Levels of Scientific Evidence for Specific Therapies

GRADE: A (Strong Scientific Evidence)

Therapy	Specific Therapeutic Use(s)
Aloe (*Aloe vera*)	Constipation (laxative)

GRADE: B (Good Scientific Evidence)

Therapy	Specific Therapeutic Use(s)
Flaxseed and flaxseed oil (*Linum usitatissimum*)	Laxative (flaxseed, not flaxseed oil)
Psyllium (*Plantago ovata, P. ispaghula*)	Constipation

GRADE: C (Unclear or Conflicting Scientific Evidence)

Therapy	Specific therapeutic Use(s)
Barley (*Hordeum vulgare* L.), germinated barley foodstuff (GBF)	Constipation

TRADITIONAL OR THEORETICAL USES THAT LACK SUFFICIENT EVIDENCE

Therapy	Specific Therapeutic Use(s)
Astragalus (*Astragalus membranaceus*)	Laxative
Bladderwrack (*Fucus vesiculosus*)	Laxative
Bladderwrack (*Fucus vesiculosus*)	Stool softener
Burdock (*Arctium lappa*)	Laxative
Calendula (*Calendula officinalis* L.), marigold	Constipation
Chamomile (*Matricaria recutita, Chamaemelum nobile*)	Constipation
Clay	Constipation
Devil's claw (*Harpagophytum procumbens* DC.)	Constipation
Dong quai (*Angelica sinensis* [Oliv.] Diels), Chinese angelica	Constipation
Dong quai (*Angelica sinensis* [Oliv.] Diels), Chinese angelica	Laxative
Elder (*Sambucus nigra* L.)	Laxative
Fenugreek (*Trigonella foenum-graecum* L.)	Constipation
Feverfew (*Tanacetum parthenium* L. Schultz-Bip.)	Constipation
Ginger (*Zingiber officinale* Roscoe)	Laxative
Globe artichoke (*Cynara scolymus* L.)	Constipation
Goldenseal (Hydrastis Canadensis L.), Berberine	Constipation
Gymnema (*Gymnema Sylvestre* R. Br.)	Constipation
Gymnema (*Gymnema Sylvestre* R. Br.)	Laxative
Lactobacillus acidophilus	Constipation
Licorice (*Glycyrrhiza glabra* L.), deglycyrrhizinated licorice (DGL)	Constipation
Marshmallow (*Althaea officinalis* L.)	Constipation

Continued

Marshmallow (*Althaea officinalis* L.)	Laxative
Oleander (*Nerium oleander*, *Thevetia peruviana*)	Cathartic
Seaweed, kelp, bladderwrack (*Fucus vesiculosus*)	Bulk laxative
Seaweed, kelp, bladderwrack (*Fucus vesiculosus*)	Laxative
Seaweed, kelp, bladderwrack (*Fucus vesiculosus*)	Stool softener
Slippery elm (*Ulmus rubra* Muhl., *U. fulva* Michx.)	Constipation
Sorrel (*Rumex acetosa* L., *R. acetosella* L.), Sinupret	Constipation
Sweet almond (*Prunus amygdalus dulcis*)	Mild laxative
Valerian (*Valeriana officinalis* L.)	Constipation
White horehound (*Marrubium vulgare*)	Cathartic
White horehound (*Marrubium vulgare*)	Constipation
White horehound (*Marrubium vulgare*)	Laxative

CONTRACEPTIVE AND RELATED CONDITIONS

Levels of Scientific Evidence for Specific Therapies

TRADITIONAL OR THEORETICAL USES THAT LACK SUFFICIENT EVIDENCE

Therapy	Specific Therapeutic Use(s)
Blessed thistle (*Cnicus benedictus* L.)	Contraception
Kava (*Piper methysticum* G. Forst)	Contraception
Melatonin	Contraception
Oleander (*Nerium oleander*, *Thevetia peruviana*)	Anti-fertility
Turmeric (*Curcuma longa* L.), curcumin	Contraception

CORONARY ARTERY DISEASE AND RELATED CONDITIONS

Levels of Scientific Evidence for Specific Therapies

GRADE: A (Strong Scientific Evidence)

Therapy	Specific Therapeutic Use(s)
Niacin (vitamin B$_3$, nicotinic acid), niacinamide, and inositol hexanicotinate	High cholesterol (niacin)
Omega-3 fatty acids, fish oil, alpha-linolenic acid	Hypertriglyceridemia (fish oil/ eicosapentaenoic acid [EPA] plus docosahexaenoic acid [DHA])
Omega-3 fatty acids, fish oil, alpha-linolenic acid	Secondary cardiovascular disease prevention (fish oil/ eicosapentaenoic acid [EPA] plus docosahexaenoic acid [DHA])
Psyllium (*Plantago ovata*, *P. ispaghula*)	High cholesterol
Red yeast rice (*Monascus purpureus*)	High cholesterol
Soy (*Glycine max* L. Merr.)	High cholesterol

GRADE: B (Good Scientific Evidence)	
Therapy	Specific Therapeutic Use(s)
Barley (*Hordeum vulgare* L.), germinated barley foodstuff (GBF)	High cholesterol
Garlic (*Allium sativum* L.)	High cholesterol
Niacin (vitamin B$_3$, nicotinic acid), niacinamide, and inositol hexanicotinate	Atherosclerosis (niacin)
Niacin (vitamin B$_3$, nicotinic acid), niacinamide, and inositol hexanicotinate	Prevention of a second heart attack (niacin)
Omega-3 fatty acids, fish oil, alpha-linolenic acid prevention (fish intake)	Primary cardiovascular disease
Sweet almond (*Prunus amygdalus dulcis*)	High cholesterol (whole almonds)

GRADE: C (Unclear or Conflicting Scientific Evidence)	
Therapy	Specific Therapeutic Use(s)
Alfalfa (*Medicago sativa* L.)	Atherosclerosis (cholesterol plaques in heart arteries)
Alfalfa (*Medicago sativa* L.)	High cholesterol
Arginine (L-arginine)	Coronary artery disease/angina
Arginine (L-arginine)	Heart protection during coronary artery bypass grafting (CABG)
Astragalus (*Astragalus membranaceus*)	Coronary artery disease
Bilberry (*Vaccinium myrtillus*)	Atherosclerosis (hardening of the arteries) and peripheral vascular disease
Black tea (*Camellia sinensis*)	Heart attack prevention
Coenzyme Q10	Angina (chest pain from clogged heart arteries)
Coenzyme Q10	Heart attack (acute myocardial infarction)
Coenzyme Q10	Heart protection during surgery
Danshen (*Salvia miltiorrhiza*)	Cardiovascular disease/angina
DHEA (dehydroepiandrosterone)	Atherosclerosis (cholesterol plaques in the arteries)
Dong quai (*Angelica sinensis* [Oliv.] Diels), Chinese angelica	Angina pectoris/coronary artery disease
Fenugreek (*Trigonella foenum-graecum* L.)	Hyperlipidemia
Flaxseed and flaxseed oil (*Linum usitatissimum*)	Heart disease (flaxseed and flaxseed oil)
Flaxseed and flaxseed oil (*Linum usitatissimum*)	High cholesterol or triglycerides (flaxseed and flaxseed oil)
Garlic (*Allium sativum* L.)	Atherosclerosis (hardening of the arteries)

Continued

Garlic (*Allium sativum* L.)	Familial hypercholesterolemia
Garlic (*Allium sativum* L.)	Heart attack prevention in patients with known heart disease
Ginseng (American ginseng, Asian ginseng, Chinese ginseng, Korean red ginseng, *Panax ginseng*: *Panax* spp. including *P. ginseng* C.C. Meyer and *P. quincefolium* L., excluding *Eleutherococcus senticosus*)	Coronary artery (heart) disease
Globe artichoke (*Cynara scolymus* L.)	Lipid-lowering (cholesterol and triglycerides)
Green tea (*Camellia sinensis*)	Heart attack prevention
Green tea (*Camellia sinensis*)	High cholesterol
Guggul (*Commifora mukul*)	Hyperlipidemia
Gymnema (*Gymnema Sylvestre* R. Br.)	High cholesterol
Hawthorn (*Crataegus laevigata, C. oxyacantha, C. monogyna, C. pentagyna*)	Coronary artery disease (angina)
Lactobacillus acidophilus	High cholesterol
Lycopene	Atherosclerosis (clogged arteries) and high cholesterol
Milk thistle (*Silybum marianum*), silymarin	Hyperlipidemia
Omega-3 fatty acids, fish oil, alpha-linolenic acid	Angina pectoris
Omega-3 fatty acids, fish oil, alpha-linolenic acid	Atherosclerosis
Omega-3 fatty acids, fish oil, alpha-linolenic acid	Prevention of graft failure after heart bypass surgery
Omega-3 fatty acids, fish oil, alpha-linolenic acid	Prevention of restenosis after percutaneous transluminal coronary angioplasty (PTCA)
Red clover (*Trifolium pratense*)	High cholesterol
Soy (*Glycine max* L. Merr.)	Cardiovascular disease
Spirulina	High cholesterol
Turmeric (*Curcuma longa* L.), curcumin	High cholesterol
Wild yam (*Dioscorea villosa*)	High cholesterol

GRADE: D (Fair Negative Scientific Evidence)	
Therapy	Specific Therapeutic Use(s)
Omega-3 fatty acids, fish oil, alpha-linolenic acid	Hypercholesterolemia

TRADITIONAL OR THEORETICAL USES THAT LACK SUFFICIENT EVIDENCE	
Therapy	Specific therapeutic Use(s)
Aloe (*Aloe vera*)	Heart disease prevention
Antineoplastons	Cholesterol/triglyceride abnormalities
Arginine (L-arginine)	Cardiac syndrome X
Arginine (L-arginine)	Heart attack
Arginine (L-arginine)	High cholesterol

Astragalus (*Astragalus membranaceus*)	Angina
Astragalus (*Astragalus membranaceus*)	Heart attack
Astragalus (*Astragalus membranaceus*)	High cholesterol
Bilberry (*Vaccinium myrtillus*)	Angina
Bilberry (*Vaccinium myrtillus*)	Heart disease
Bilberry (*Vaccinium myrtillus*)	High cholesterol
Black cohosh (*Cimicifuga racemosa* L. Nutt.)	Cardiac diseases
Bladderwrack (*Fucus vesiculosus*)	Atherosclerosis
Bladderwrack (*Fucus vesiculosus*)	Heart disease
Bladderwrack (*Fucus vesiculosus*)	High cholesterol
Boron	High cholesterol
Bromelain	Angina
Bromelain	Atherosclerosis (hardening of the arteries)
Bromelain	Heart disease
Calendula (*Calendula officinalis* L.), marigold	Atherosclerosis (clogged arteries)
Calendula (*Calendula officinalis* L.), marigold	Heart disease
Clay	Cardiovascular disorders
Coenzyme Q10	High cholesterol
Dandelion (*Taraxacum officinale*)	Cardiovascular disorders
Dandelion (*Taraxacum officinale*)	Clogged arteries
Dandelion (*Taraxacum officinale*)	High cholesterol
Danshen (*Salvia miltiorrhiza*)	Clogged arteries
Danshen (*Salvia miltiorrhiza*)	High cholesterol
Devil's claw (*Harpagophytum procumbens* DC.)	Atherosclerosis (clogged arteries)
Devil's claw (*Harpagophytum procumbens* DC.)	High cholesterol
DHEA (dehydroepiandrosterone)	Heart attack
DHEA (dehydroepiandrosterone)	High cholesterol
Dong quai (*Angelica sinensis* [Oliv.] Diels), Chinese angelica	Atherosclerosis
Dong quai (*Angelica sinensis* [Oliv.] Diels), Chinese angelica	High cholesterol
Evening primrose oil (*Oenothera biennis* L.)	Atherosclerosis
Evening primrose oil (*Oenothera biennis* L.)	Heart disease
Evening primrose oil (*Oenothera biennis* L.)	High cholesterol
Fenugreek (*Trigonella foenum-graecum* L.)	Atherosclerosis
Ginger (*Zingiber officinale* Roscoe)	Atherosclerosis
Ginger (*Zingiber officinale* Roscoe)	Heart disease
Ginkgo (*Ginkgo biloba* L.)	Angina

Continued

Ginkgo (*Ginkgo biloba* L.)	Atherosclerosis (clogged arteries)
Ginkgo (*Ginkgo biloba* L.)	Heart attack
Ginkgo (*Ginkgo biloba* L.)	Heart disease
Ginkgo (*Ginkgo biloba* L.)	High cholesterol
Ginseng (American ginseng, Asian ginseng, Chinese ginseng, Korean red ginseng, *Panax ginseng*: *Panax* spp. including *P. ginseng* C.C. Meyer and *P. quincefolium* L., excluding *Eleutherococcus senticosus*)	Atherosclerosis
Ginseng (American ginseng, Asian ginseng, Chinese ginseng, Korean red ginseng, *Panax ginseng*: *Panax* spp. including *P. ginseng* C.C. Meyer and *P. quincefolium* L., excluding *Eleutherococcus senticosus*)	Heart damage
Globe artichoke (*Cynara scolymus* L.)	Atherosclerosis
Goldenseal (*Hydrastis canadensis* L.), berberine	Atherosclerosis (hardening of the arteries)
Goldenseal (*Hydrastis canadensis* L.), berberine	High cholesterol
Green tea (*Camellia sinensis*)	Heart disease
Gymnema (*Gymnema Sylvestre* R. Br.)	Cardiovascular disease
Hawthorn (*Crataegus laevigata, C. oxyacantha, C. monogyna, C. pentagyna*)	Angina
Hawthorn (*Crataegus laevigata, C. oxyacantha, C. monogyna, C. pentagyna*)	Cardiac murmurs
Lactobacillus acidophilus	Heart disease
Licorice (*Glycyrrhiza glabra* L.), deglycyrrhizinated licorice (DGL)	High cholesterol
Lycopene	Heart disease
Maitake mushroom (*Grifola frondosa*), beta-glucan	High cholesterol
Melatonin	Cardiac syndrome X
Melatonin	Coronary artery disease
Niacin (vitamin B_3, nicotinic acid), niacinamide, and inositol hexanicotinate	Heart attack prevention
Oleander (*Nerium oleander, Thevetia peruviana*)	Heart disease
Omega-3 fatty acids, fish oil, alpha-linolenic acid	Acute myocardial infarction (heart attack)
Psyllium (*Plantago ovata, P. ispaghula*)	Atherosclerosis
Seaweed, kelp, bladderwrack (*Fucus vesiculosus*)	Atherosclerosis
Seaweed, kelp, bladderwrack (*Fucus vesiculosus*)	Fatty heart
Seaweed, kelp, bladderwrack (*Fucus vesiculosus*)	Hyperlipemia
Shark cartilage	Atherosclerosis
Soy (*Glycine max* L. Merr.)	Atherosclerosis
Spirulina	Atherosclerosis
Spirulina	Heart disease
Sweet almond (*Prunus amygdalus dulcis*)	Heart disease
Valerian (*Valeriana officinalis* L.)	Angina pectoris

Valerian (*Valeriana officinalis* L.)	Heart disease
Yohimbe bark extract (*Pausinystalia yohimbe* Pierre ex Beille)	Angina
Yohimbe bark extract (*Pausinystalia yohimbe* Pierre ex Beille)	Coronary artery disease
Yohimbe bark extract (*Pausinystalia yohimbe* Pierre ex Beille)	High cholesterol
Yohimbe bark extract (*Pausinystalia yohimbe* Pierre ex Beille)	Angina
Yohimbe bark extract (*Pausinystalia yohimbe* Pierre ex Beille)	Atherosclerosis
Yohimbe bark extract (*Pausinystalia yohimbe* Pierre ex Beille)	Chest pain
Yohimbe bark extract (*Pausinystalia yohimbe* Pierre ex Beille)	Coronary artery disease
Yohimbe bark extract (*Pausinystalia yohimbe* Pierre ex Beille)	Hyperlipidemia

COUGH AND RELATED CONDITIONS

Levels of Scientific Evidence for Specific Therapies

GRADE: C (Unclear or Conflicting Scientific Evidence)

Therapy	Specific Therapeutic Use(s)
Eucalyptus oil (*Eucalyptus globulus* Labillardiere, *E. fructicetorum* F. Von Mueller, *E. smithii* R.T. Baker)	Decongestant-expectorant/ upper respiratory tract infection (oral/inhalation)
White horehound (*Marrubium vulgare* e)	Cough

TRADITIONAL OR THEORETICAL USES THAT LACK SUFFICIENT EVIDENCE

Therapy	Specific Therapeutic Use(s)
Alfalfa (*Medicago sativa* L.)	Cough
American pennyroyal (*Hedeoma pulegioides* L.), European pennyroyal (*Mentha pulegium* L.)	Cough
Betel nut (*Areca catechu* L.)	Cough
Bilberry (*Vaccinium myrtillus*)	Cough
Bitter almond (*Prunus amygdalus* Batch var. *amara* DC. Focke), Laetrile	Cough suppressant
Black cohosh (*Cimicifuga racemosa* L. Nutt.)	Pertussis (whooping cough)
Blessed thistle (*Cnicus benedictus* L.)	Expectorant
Boswellia (*Boswellia serrata* Roxb.)	Expectorant
Bromelain	Cough
Burdock (*Arctium lappa*)	Cough
Calendula (*Calendula officinalis* L.), marigold	Cough
Chaparral (*Larrea tridentata* DC. Coville, *L. divaricata* Cav.), nordihydroguaiaretic acid (NDGA)	Cough
Clove (*Eugenia aromatica*)	Cough
Clove (*Eugenia aromatica*)	Expectorant
Dong quai (*Angelica Sinensis* [Oliv.] Diels), Chinese angelica	Cough
Dong quai (*Angelica sinensis* [Oliv.] Diels), Chinese angelica	Expectorant

Continued

Echinacea (*Echinacea angustifolia* DC., *E. pallida*, *E. purpurea*)	Whooping cough (pertussis)
Elder (*Sambucus nigra* L.)	Cough suppressant
Ephedra (*Ephedra sinica*)/ma huang	Cough
Eucalyptus oil (*Eucalyptus globulus* Labillardiere, *E. fructicetorum* F. Von Mueller, *E. smithii* R.T. Baker)	Cough
Eucalyptus oil (*Eucalyptus globulus* Labillardiere, *E. fructicetorum* F. Von Mueller, *E. smithii* R.T. Baker)	Croup
Eucalyptus oil (*Eucalyptus globulus* Labillardiere, *E. fructicetorum* F. Von Mueller, *E. smithii* R.T. Baker)	Whooping cough
Evening primrose oil (*Oenothera biennis* L.)	Whooping cough
Eyebright (*Euphrasia officinalis*)	Cough
Eyebright (*Euphrasia officinalis*)	Expectorant
Fenugreek (*Trigonella foenum-graecum* L.)	Cough (chronic)
Flaxseed and flaxseed oil (*Linum usitatissimum*)	Antitussive
Flaxseed and flaxseed oil (*Linum usitatissimum*)	Cough
Flaxseed and flaxseed oil (*Linum usitatissimum*)	Expectorant
Garlic (*Allium sativum* L.)	Cough
Ginger (*Zingiber officinale* Roscoe)	Cough suppressant
Ginkgo (*Ginkgo biloba* L.)	Cough
Goldenseal (*Hydrastis canadensis* L.), berberine	Croup
Gymnema (*Gymnema Sylvestre* R. Br.)	Cough
Horse chestnut (*Aesculus hippocastanum* L.)	Cough
Licorice (*Glycyrrhiza glabra* L.), deglycyrrhizinated licorice (DGL)	Cough
Marshmallow (Althaea officinalis L.)	Cough
Marshmallow (*Althaea officinalis* L.)	Expectorant
Marshmallow (*Althaea officinalis* L.)	Whooping cough
Milk thistle (*Silybum marianum*), silymarin	Cough
Peppermint (*Mentha x piperita* L.)	Cough
Polypodium leucotomos extract, Anapsos	Pertussis
Red clover (*Trifolium pratense*)	Cough
Saw palmetto (*Serenoa repens* [Bartram] Small)	Cough
Saw palmetto (*Serenoa repens* [Bartram] Small)	Expectorant
Slippery elm (*Ulmus rubra* Muhl., *U. fulva* Michx.)	Cough
Tea tree oil (*Melaleuca alternifolia* [Maiden & Betche] Cheel)	Cough
Thyme (*Thymus vulgaris* L.), thymol	Pertussis
Turmeric (*Curcuma longa* L.), curcumin	Cough
Valerian (*Valeriana officinalis* L.)	Cough
White horehound (*Marrubium vulgare*)	Whooping cough
Wild yam (*Dioscorea villosa*)	Croup

Wild yam (*Dioscorea villosa*)	Expectorant
Yohimbe bark extract (*Pausinystalia yohimbe* Pierre ex Beille)	Cough
Yohimbe bark extract (*Pausinystalia yohimbe* Pierre ex Beille)	Coughs

CROHN'S DISEASE AND RELATED CONDITIONS

Levels of Scientific Evidence for Specific Therapies

GRADE: C (Unclear or Conflicting Scientific Evidence)

Therapy	Specific Therapeutic Use(s)
Barley (*Hordeum vulgare* L.), germinated barley foodstuff (GBF)	Ulcerative colitis
Betel nut (*Areca catechu* L.)	Ulcerative colitis
Boswellia (*Boswellia serrata* Roxb.)	Ulcerative colitis
Dandelion (*Taraxacum officinale*)	Colitis
Glucosamine	Inflammatory bowel disease
Licorice (*Glycyrrhiza glabra* L.), deglycyrrhizinated licorice (DGL)	Familial Mediterranean Fever (FMF)
Omega-3 fatty acids, fish oil, alpha-linolenic acid	Ulcerative colitis
Psyllium (*Plantago ovata, P. ispaghula*)	Inflammatory bowel disease

TRADITIONAL OR THEORETICAL USES THAT LACK SUFFICIENT EVIDENCE

Therapy	Specific Therapeutic Use(s)
Aloe (*Aloe vera*)	Inflammatory bowel disease
Arginine (L-arginine)	Inflammatory bowel disease
Barley (*Hordeum vulgare* L.), germinated barley foodstuff (GBF)	Inflammatory bowel disorders
Belladonna (*Atropa belladonna* L. or its variety *acuminata* Royle ex Lindl)	Colitis
Belladonna (*Atropa belladonna* L. or its variety *acuminata* Royle ex Lindl)	Ulcerative colitis
Bromelain	Colitis
Bromelain	Ulcerative colitis
Calendula (*Calendula officinalis* L.), marigold	Ulcerative colitis
DHEA (dehydroepiandrosterone)	Ulcerative colitis
Elder (*Sambucus nigra* L.)	Ulcerative colitis
Eucalyptus oil (*Eucalyptus globulus* Labillardiere, *E. fructicetorum* F. Von Mueller, *E. smithii* R.T. Baker)	Inflammatory bowel disease
Evening primrose oil (*Oenothera biennis* L.)	Ulcerative colitis
Flaxseed and flaxseed oil (*Linum usitatissimum*)	Ulcerative colitis
Ginkgo (*Ginkgo biloba* L.)	Ulcerative colitis
Ginseng (American ginseng, Asian ginseng, Chinese ginseng, Korean red ginseng, *Panax ginseng; Panax* spp. including *P. ginseng* C.C. Meyer and *P. quincefolium* L., excluding *Eleutherococcus senticosus*)	Colitis

Continued

Glucosamine	Inflammatory bowel disease
Glucosamine	Ulcerative colitis
Goldenseal (*Hydrastis canadensis* L.), berberine	Colitis
Guggul (*Commifora mukul*)	Colitis
Lactobacillus acidophilus	Colitis
Lactobacillus acidophilus	Ulcerative colitis
Licorice (*Glycyrrhiza glabra* L.), deglycyrrhizinated licorice (DGL)	Colitis
Marshmallow (*Althaea officinalis* L.)	Colitis
Marshmallow (*Althaea officinalis* L.)	Inflammation of the small intestine
Marshmallow (*Althaea officinalis* L.)	Ulcerative colitis
Melatonin	Colitis
Propolis	Ulcerative colitis
Slippery elm (*Ulmus rubra* Muhl., *U. fulva* Michx.)	Colitis
Slippery elm (*Ulmus rubra* Muhl., *U. fulva* Michx.)	Ulcerative colitis
Spirulina	Colitis
Thyme (*Thymus vulgaris* L.), thymol	Inflammation of the colon

DEEP VENOUS THROMBOSIS AND RELATED CONDITIONS

Levels of Scientific Evidence for Specific Therapies

GRADE: C (Unclear or Conflicting Scientific Evidence)

Therapy	Specific Therapeutic Use(s)
Bladderwrack (*Fucus vesiculosus*)	Anticoagulant (blood thinner)
Garlic (*Allium sativum* L.)	Antiplatelet effects (blood thinning)
Seaweed, kelp, bladderwrack (*Fucus vesiculosus*)	Anticoagulant
Yohimbe bark extract (*Pausinystalia yohimbe* Pierre ex Beille)	Inhibition of platelet aggregation

TRADITIONAL OR THEORETICAL USES THAT LACK SUFFICIENT EVIDENCE

Therapy	Specific Therapeutic Use(s)
Alfalfa (*Medicago sativa* L.)	Blood clotting disorders
Astragalus (*Astragalus membranaceus*)	Blood thinner
Barley (*Hordeum vulgare* L.), germinated barley foodstuff (GBF)	Blood circulation
Bromelain	Blood clot treatment
Bromelain	Platelet inhibition (blood thinner)
Calendula (*Calendula officinalis* L.), marigold	Blood vessel clots
Clove (*Eugenia aromatica*)	Blood thinner (antiplatelet agent)

Danshen (*Salvia miltiorrhiza*)	Blood clotting disorders
Danshen (*Salvia miltiorrhiza*)	Hypercoagulability
Dong quai (*Angelica Sinensis* [Oliv.] Diels), Chinese angelica	Blood clots
Dong quai (*Angelica sinensis* [Oliv.] Diels), Chinese angelica	Blood flow disorders
Dong quai (*Angelica sinensis* [Oliv.] Diels), Chinese angelica	Blood stagnation
Dong quai (*Angelica sinensis* [Oliv.] Diels), Chinese angelica	Blood vessel disorders
Elder (*Sambucus nigra* L.)	Blood vessel disorders
Flaxseed and flaxseed oil (*Linum usitatissimum*)	Blood thinner
Ginger (*Zingiber officinale* Roscoe)	Blood thinner
Ginkgo (*Ginkgo biloba* L.)	Blood clots
Ginkgo (*Ginkgo biloba* L.)	Blood vessel disorders
Goldenseal (*Hydrastis canadensis* L.), berberine	Anticoagulant (blood thinning)
Goldenseal (*Hydrastis canadensis* L.), berberine	Blood circulation stimulant
Green tea (*Camellia sinensis*)	Inhibition of platelet aggregation
Horse chestnut (*Aesculus hippocastanum* L.)	Lung blood clots (pulmonary embolism)
Niacin (vitamin B_3, nicotinic acid), niacinamide, and inositol hexanicotinate	Blood circulation improvement
Omega-3 fatty acids, fish oil, alpha-linolenic acid	Anticoagulation
Propolis	Anticoagulant
Red yeast rice (*Monascus purpureus*)	Blood circulation problems

DEMENTIA AND RELATED CONDITIONS

Levels of Scientific Evidence for Specific Therapies

GRADE: B (Good Scientific Evidence)

Therapy	Specific therapeutic Use(s)
Ginkgo (*Ginkgo biloba* L.)	Cerebral insufficiency
Ginseng (American ginseng, Asian ginseng, Chinese ginseng, Korean red ginseng, *Panax ginseng*: *Panax* spp. including *P. ginseng* C.C. Meyer and *P. quincefolium* L., excluding *Eleutherococcus senticosus*)	Mental performance

GRADE: C (Unclear or Conflicting Scientific Evidence)

Therapy	Specific Therapeutic Use(s)
Black tea (*Camellia sinensis*)	Memory enhancement
Black tea (*Camellia sinensis*)	Mental performance/alertness
Boron	Improving cognitive function
Ginkgo (*Ginkgo biloba* L.)	Age-associated memory impairment (AAMI)
Ginkgo (*Ginkgo biloba* L.)	Memory enhancement (in healthy people)

Continued

Green tea (*Camellia sinensis*)	Memory enhancement
Green tea (*Camellia sinensis*)	Mental performance/alertness
Polypodium leucotomos extract, Anapsos	Dementia

GRADE: D (Fair Negative Scientific Evidence)	
Therapy	Specific Therapeutic Use(s)
DHEA (dehydroepiandrosterone)	Brain function and well-being in the elderly

TRADITIONAL OR THEORETICAL USES THAT LACK SUFFICIENT EVIDENCE	
Therapy	Specific Therapeutic Use(s)
Arginine (L-arginine)	Dementia
Astragalus (*Astragalus membranaceus*)	Dementia
Astragalus (*Astragalus membranaceus*)	Memory
Blessed thistle (*Cnicus benedictus* L.)	Memory improvement
Danshen (*Salvia miltiorrhiza*)	Anoxic brain injury
DHEA (dehydroepiandrosterone)	Dementia
Eyebright (*Euphrasia officinalis*)	Memory loss
Garlic (*Allium sativum* L.)	Age-related memory problems
Ginseng (American ginseng, Asian ginseng, Chinese ginseng, Korean red ginseng, *Panax ginseng*: *Panax* spp. including *P. ginseng* C.C. Meyer and *P. quincefolium* L., excluding *Eleutherococcus senticosus*)	Dementia
Ginseng (American ginseng, Asian ginseng, Chinese ginseng, Korean red ginseng, *Panax ginseng*: *Panax* spp. including *P. ginseng* C.C. Meyer and *P. quincefolium* L., excluding *Eleutherococcus senticosus*)	Improved memory and thinking after menopause
Ginseng (American ginseng, Asian ginseng, Chinese ginseng, Korean red ginseng, *Panax ginseng*: Panax spp. including *P. ginseng* C.C. Meyer and *P. quincefolium* L., excluding *Eleutherococcus senticosus*)	Senile dementia
Gotu kola (*Centella asiatica* L.), total triterpenic fraction of *Centella asiatica* (TTFCA)	Memory enhancement
Green tea (*Camellia sinensis*)	Cognitive performance enhancement
Kava (*Piper methysticum* G. Forst)	Brain damage
Lycopene	Cognitive function
Melatonin	Cognitive enhancement
Melatonin	Memory enhancement
Niacin (vitamin B_3, nicotinic acid), niacinamide, and inositol hexanicotinate	Memory loss
Omega-3 fatty acids, fish oil, alpha-linolenic acid	Memory enhancement
Soy (*Glycine max* L. Merr.)	Cognitive function
Soy (*Glycine max* L. Merr.)	Memory enhancement
Spirulina	Memory improvement

| Valerian (*Valeriana officinalis* L.) | Memory |
| Yohimbe bark extract (*Pausinystalia yohimbe* Pierre ex Beille) | Cognition |

DENTAL CONDITIONS AND RELATED CONDITIONS

Levels of Scientific Evidence for Specific Therapies

GRADE: C (Unclear or Conflicting Scientific Evidence)

Therapy	Specific Therapeutic Use(s)
Betel nut (*Areca catechu* L.)	Dental cavities
Black tea (*Camellia sinensis*)	Dental cavity prevention
Coenzyme Q10	Gum disease (periodontitis)
Cranberry (*Vaccinium macrocarpon*)	Dental plaque
Eucalyptus oil (*Eucalyptus globulus* Labillardiere, *E. fructicetorum* F. Von Mueller, *E. smithii* R.T. Baker)	Dental plaque/gingivitis (mouthwash)
Green tea (*Camellia sinensis*)	Dental cavity prevention
Propolis	Dental plaque and gingivitis (mouthwash)
Thyme (*Thymus vulgaris* L.), thymol	Dental plaque

TRADITIONAL OR THEORETICAL USES THAT LACK SUFFICIENT EVIDENCE

Therapy	Specific Therapeutic Use(s)
Arginine (L-arginine)	Peritonitis
Astragalus (*Astragalus membranaceus*)	Denture adhesive (astragalus sap)
Bilberry (*Vaccinium myrtillus*)	Bleeding gums
Chamomile (*Matricaria recutita*, *Chamaemelum nobile*)	Gingivitis
Clove (*Eugenia aromatica*)	Cavities
Coenzyme Q10	Gingivitis
Echinacea (*Echinacea angustifolia* DC., *E. pallida*, *E. purpurea*)	Gingivitis
Goldenseal (*Hydrastis canadensis* L.), berberine	Gingivitis
Gotu kola (*Centella asiatica* L.), total triterpenic fraction of *Centella asiatica* (TTFCA)	Periodontal disease
Green tea (*Camellia sinensis*)	Bleeding of gums or tooth sockets
Green tea (*Camellia sinensis*)	Gum swelling
Guggul (*Commifora mukul*)	Gingivitis
Licorice (*Glycyrrhiza glabra* L.), deglycyrrhizinated licorice (DGL)	Dental hygiene
Licorice (*Glycyrrhiza glabra* L.), deglycyrrhizinated licorice (DGL)	Plaque
Lycopene	Periodontal disease
Milk thistle (*Silybum marianum*), silymarin	Peritonitis
Omega-3 fatty acids, fish oil, alpha-linolenic acid	Gingivitis

Continued

Tea tree oil (*Melaleuca alternifolia* [Maiden & Betche] Cheel)	Dental plaque
Tea tree oil (*Melaleuca alternifolia* [Maiden & Betche] Cheel)	Gingivitis
Tea tree oil (*Melaleuca alternifolia* [Maiden & Betche] Cheel)	Periodontal disease
Thyme (*Thymus vulgaris* L.), thymol	Gingivitis

DEPRESSION AND RELATED CONDITIONS

Levels of Scientific Evidence for Specific Therapies

GRADE: A (Strong Scientific Evidence)

Therapy	Specific Therapeutic Use(s)
St. John's wort (*Hypericum perforatum* L.)	Depressive disorder (mild to moderate)

GRADE: C (Unclear or Conflicting Scientific Evidence)

Therapy	Specific Therapeutic Use(s)
DHEA (dehydroepiandrosterone)	Depression
Evening primrose oil (*Oenothera biennis* L.)	Postviral/chronic fatigue syndrome
Ginkgo (*Ginkgo biloba* L.)	Depression and seasonal affective disorder (SAD)
Melatonin	Bipolar disorder (sleep disturbances)
Melatonin	Depression (sleep disturbances)
Melatonin	Seasonal affective disorder (SAD)
Omega-3 fatty acids, fish oil, alpha-linolenic acid	Bipolar disorder
Omega-3 fatty acids, fish oil, alpha-linolenic acid	Depression
St. John's wort (*Hypericum perforatum* L.)	Depressive disorder (severe)
St. John's wort (*Hypericum perforatum* L.)	Seasonal affective disorder (SAD)

TRADITIONAL OR THEORETICAL USES THAT LACK SUFFICIENT EVIDENCE

Therapy	Specific Therapeutic Use(s)
Black Cohosh (*Cimicifuga racemosa* L.]Nutt.)	Depression
Ephedra (*Ephedra sinica*)/ma huang	Depression
Flaxseed and flaxseed oil (*Linum usitatissimum*)	Bipolar disorder
Flaxseed and flaxseed oil (*Linum usitatissimum*)	Depression
Ginger (*Zingiber officinale* Roscoe)	Depression
Ginkgo (*Ginkgo biloba* L.)	Mood disturbances
Ginseng (American ginseng, Asian ginseng, Chinese ginseng, Korean red ginseng, *Panax ginseng*: *Panax* spp. including *P. ginseng* C.C. Meyer and *P. quincefolium* L., excluding *Eleutherococcus* senticosus)	Antidepressant
Gotu kola (*Centella asiatica* L.), total triterpenic fraction of *Centella asiatica* (TTFCA)	Antidepressant

Gotu kola (*Centella asiatica* L.), total triterpenic fraction of *Centella asiatica* (TTFCA)	Mood disorders
Hops (*Humulus lupulus* L.)	Antidepressant
Hops (*Humulus lupulus* L.)	Mood disturbances
Kava (*Piper methysticum* G. Forst)	Depression
Lavender (*Lavandula angustifolia* Miller)	Depression
Licorice (*Glycyrrhiza glabra* L.), deglycyrrhizinated licorice (DGL)	Depression
Melatonin	Depression
Milk thistle (*Silybum marianum*), silymarin	Depression
Niacin (vitamin B_3, nicotinic acid), niacinamide, and inositol hexanicotinate	Depression
Spirulina	Depression
Spirulina	Mood stimulant
Thyme (*Thymus vulgaris* L.), thymol	Depression
Valerian (*Valeriana officinalis* L.)	Mood enhancement
Yohimbe bark extract (*Pausinystalia yohimbe* Pierre ex Beille)	Depression
Yohimbe bark extract (*Pausinystalia yohimbe* Pierre ex Beille)	Depression

DIABETES MELLITUS AND RELATED CONDITIONS

Levels of Scientific Evidence for Specific Therapies

GRADE: B (Good Scientific Evidence)	
Therapy	**Specific Therapeutic Use(s)**
Bitter melon (*Momordica charantia* L.), MAP30	Diabetes (hypoglycemic agent)
Ginseng (American ginseng, Asian ginseng, Chinese ginseng, Korean red ginseng, *Panax ginseng*: Panax spp. including *P. ginseng* C.C. Meyer and *P. quincefolium* L., excluding *Eleutherococcus senticosus*)	Type 2 diabetes (adult onset)
Gymnema (*Gymnema Sylvestre* R. Br.)	Diabetes

GRADE: C (Unclear or Conflicting Scientific Evidence)	
Therapy	**Specific Therapeutic Use(s)**
Alfalfa (*Medicago sativa* L.)	Diabetes
Aloe (*Aloe vera*)	Diabetes (type 2)
Barley (*Hordeum vulgare* L.), germinated barley foodstuff (GBF)	High blood sugar/glucose intolerance
Bilberry (*Vaccinium myrtillus*)	Diabetes
Bladderwrack (*Fucus vesiculosus*)	Diabetes
Burdock (*Arctium lappa*)	Diabetes
Dandelion (*Taraxacum officinale*)	Diabetes
Evening primrose oil (*Oenothera biennis* L.)	Diabetes

Continued

Fenugreek (*Trigonella foenum-graecum* L.)	Type 1 diabetes
Fenugreek (*Trigonella foenum-graecum* L.)	Type 2 diabetes
Flaxseed and flaxseed oil (*Linum usitatissimum*)	Diabetes (flaxseed, not flaxseed oil)
Gotu kola (*Centella asiatica* L.), total triterpenic fraction of *Centella asiatica* (TTFCA)	Diabetic microangiopathy
Maitake mushroom (*Grifola frondosa*), beta-glucan	Diabetes
Milk thistle (*Silybum marianum*), silymarin	Diabetes (associated with cirrhosis)
Niacin (vitamin B$_3$, nicotinic acid), niacinamide, and inositol hexanicotinate	Type 1 Diabetes prevention (niacinamide)
Psyllium (*Plantago ovata*, *P. ispaghula*)	Hyperglycemia (high blood sugar levels)
Red clover (*Trifolium pratense*)	Diabetes
Seaweed, kelp, bladderwrack (*Fucus vesiculosus*)	Hyperglycemia (diabetes)
Soy (*Glycine max* L. Merr.)	Type 2 diabetes
Spirulina	Diabetes
White horehound (*Marrubium vulgare*)	Diabetes

GRADE: D (Fair Negative Scientific Evidence)	
Therapy	**Specific Therapeutic Use(s)**
Coenzyme Q10	Diabetes
Garlic (*Allium sativum* L.)	Diabetes
Omega-3 fatty acids, fish oil, alpha-linolenic acid	Diabetes

TRADITIONAL OR THEORETICAL USES THAT LACK SUFFICIENT EVIDENCE	
Therapy	**Specific Therapeutic Use(s)**
Arginine (L-arginine)	Diabetes
Astragalus (*Astragalus membranaceus*)	Diabetes
Chaparral (*Larrea tridentata* DC. Coville, *L. divaricata* Cav.), nordihydroguaiaretic acid (NDGA)	Diabetes
Devil's claw (*Harpagophytum procumbens* DC.)	Diabetes
DHEA (dehydroepiandrosterone)	Diabetes
Dong quai (*Angelica sinensis* [Oliv.] Diels), Chinese angelica	Diabetes
Elder (*Sambucus nigra* L.)	Diabetes
Essiac	Diabetes
Eucalyptus oil (*Eucalyptus globulus* Labillardiere, *E. fructicetorum* F. Von Mueller, *E. smithii* R.T. Baker)	Diabetes
Evening primrose oil (*Oenothera biennis* L.)	Diabetes
Ginkgo (*Ginkgo biloba* L.)	Diabetes
Goldenseal (*Hydrastis canadensis* L.), berberine	Diabetes
Green tea (*Camellia sinensis*)	Diabetes

Guggul (*Commifora mukul*)	Diabetes
Hawthorn (*Crataegus laevigata, C. oxyacantha, C. monogyna, C. pentagyna*)	Diabetes mellitus
Hops (*Humulus lupulus* L.)	Diabetes
Horsetail (*Equisetum arvense* L.)	Diabetes
Lavender (*Lavandula angustifolia* Miller)	Diabetes
Licorice (*Glycyrrhiza glabra* L.), deglycyrrhizinated licorice (DGL)	Diabetes
Lycopene	Diabetes mellitus
Niacin (vitamin B_3, nicotinic acid), niacinamide, and inositol hexanicotinate	Type 1 diabetes
Niacin (vitamin B_3, nicotinic acid), niacinamide, and inositol hexanicotinate	Type 2 diabetes
Niacin (vitamin B_3, nicotinic acid), niacinamide, and inositol hexanicotinate	Low blood sugar
Saw palmetto (*Serenoa repens* [Bartram] Small)	Diabetes
Turmeric (*Curcuma longa* L.), curcumin	Diabetes
Wild yam (*Dioscorea villosa*)	Low blood sugar

DIABETIC COMPLICATIONS AND RELATED CONDITIONS

Levels of Scientific Evidence for Specific Therapies

GRADE: C (Unclear or Conflicting Scientific Evidence)

Therapy	Specific Therapeutic Use(s)
Bilberry (*Vaccinium myrtillus*)	Retinopathy
Evening primrose oil (*Oenothera biennis* L.)	Diabetic neuropathy (nerve damage)
Gotu kola (*Centella asiatica* L.), total triterpenic fraction of *Centella asiatica* (TTFCA)	Diabetic microangiopathy

TRADITIONAL OR THEORETICAL USES THAT LACK SUFFICIENT EVIDENCE

Therapy	Specific Therapeutic Use(s)
Astragalus (*Astragalus membranaceus*)	Diabetic foot ulcers
Astragalus (*Astragalus membranaceus*)	Diabetic neuropathy
Danshen (*Salvia miltiorrhiza*)	Diabetic nerve pain
Ginkgo (*Ginkgo biloba* L.)	Diabetic eye disease
Ginkgo (*Ginkgo biloba* L.)	Diabetic nerve damage (neuropathy)
Ginseng (American ginseng, Asian ginseng, Chinese ginseng, Korean red ginseng, *Panax ginseng*: *Panax* spp. including P. ginseng C.C. Meyer and P. quincefolium L., excluding *Eleutherococcus senticosus*)	Diabetic nephropathy (kidney disease)
Milk thistle (*Silybum marianum*), silymarin	Diabetic nerve pain
Omega-3 fatty acids, fish oil, alpha-linolenic acid	Diabetic nephropathy

Continued

Omega-3 fatty acids, fish oil, alpha-linolenic acid	Diabetic neuropathy
Shark cartilage	Diabetic retinopathy
Soy (*Glycine max* L. Merr.)	Diabetic neuropathy
Yohimbe bark extract (*Pausinystalia yohimbe* Pierre ex Beille)	Diabetic complications
Yohimbe bark extract (*Pausinystalia yohimbe* Pierre ex Beille)	Diabetic neuropathy
Yohimbe bark extract (*Pausinystalia yohimbe* Pierre ex Beille)	Diabetic complications
Yohimbe bark extract (*Pausinystalia yohimbe* Pierre ex Beille)	Diabetic neuropathy

DIARRHEA AND RELATED CONDITIONS

Levels of Scientific Evidence for Specific Therapies

GRADE: B (Good Scientific Evidence)

Therapy	Specific Therapeutic Use(s)
Psyllium (*Plantago ovata*, *P. ispaghula*)	Diarrhea
Soy (*Glycine max* L. Merr.)	Diarrhea (acute) in infants and young children

GRADE: C (Unclear or Conflicting Scientific Evidence)

Therapy	Specific Therapeutic Use(s)
Bilberry (*Vaccinium myrtillus*)	Diarrhea
Chamomile (*Matricaria recutita*, *Chamaemelum nobile*)	Diarrhea in children
Clay	Fecal incontinence associated with psychiatric disorders (encopresis): clay modeling therapy in children
Goldenseal (*Hydrastis canadensis* L.), berberine	Infectious diarrhea
Lactobacillus acidophilus	Diarrhea prevention
Lactobacillus acidophilus	Diarrhea treatment (children)
Lactobacillus acidophilus	Lactose intolerance
Slippery elm (*Ulmus rubra* Muhl., *U. fulva* Michx.)	Diarrhea
Soy (*Glycine max* L. Merr.)	Diarrhea in adults

TRADITIONAL OR THEORETICAL USES THAT LACK SUFFICIENT EVIDENCE

Therapy	Specific Therapeutic Use(s)
American pennyroyal (*Hedeoma pulegioides* L.), European pennyroyal (*Mentha pulegium* L.)	Dysentery
Astragalus (*Astragalus membranaceus*)	Diarrhea
Barley (*Hordeum vulgare* L.), germinated barley foodstuff (GBF)	Diarrhea
Belladonna (*Atropa belladonna* L. or its variety *acuminata* Royle ex Lindl)	Diarrhea
Bilberry (*Vaccinium myrtillus*)	Dysentery
Black cohosh (*Cimicifuga racemosa* L. Nutt.)	Diarrhea
Black tea (*Camellia sinensis*)	Diarrhea

Blessed thistle (*Cnicus benedictus* L.)	Diarrhea
Bromelain	Diarrhea
Chaparral (*Larrea tridentata* DC. Coville, *L. divaricata* Cav.), nordihydroguaiaretic acid (NDGA)	Diarrhea
Clay	Diarrhea
Clay	Dysentery
Clove (*Eugenia aromatica*)	Diarrhea
Dandelion (*Taraxacum officinale*)	Diarrhea
Devil's Claw (*Harpagophytum procumbens* DC.)	Diarrhea
Dong quai (*Angelica sinensis* [Oliv.] Diels), Chinese angelica	Dysentery
Eucalyptus oil (*Eucalyptus globulus* Labillardiere, *E. fructicetorum* F. Von Mueller, *E. smithii* R.T. Baker)	Diarrhea
Fenugreek (*Trigonella foenum-graecum* L.)	Diarrhea
Fenugreek (*Trigonella foenum-graecum* L.)	Dysentery
Feverfew (*Tanacetum parthenium* L. Schultz-Bip.)	Diarrhea
Flaxseed and flaxseed oil (*Linum usitatissimum*)	Diarrhea
Garlic (*Allium sativum* L.)	Dysentery
Ginger (*Zingiber officinale* Roscoe)	Diarrhea
Ginkgo (*Ginkgo biloba* L.)	Dysentery (bloody diarrhea)
Ginseng (American ginseng, Asian ginseng, Chinese ginseng, Korean red ginseng, *Panax ginseng*: *Panax* spp. including *P. ginseng* C.C. Meyer and *P. quincefolium* L., excluding *Eleutherococcus senticosus*)	Dysentery
Goldenseal (*Hydrastis canadensis* L.), berberine	Diarrhea
Gotu kola (*Centella asiatica* L.), total triterpenic fraction of *Centella asiatica* (TTFCA)	Diarrhea
Gotu kola (*Centella asiatica* L.), total triterpenic fraction of *Centella asiatica* (TTFCA)	Dysentery
Green tea (*Camellia sinensis*)	Diarrhea
Hawthorn (*Crataegus laevigata, C. oxyacantha, C. monogyna, C. pentagyna*)	Diarrhea
Hawthorn (*Crataegus laevigata, C. oxyacantha, C. monogyna, C. pentagyna*)	Dysentery
Hops (*Humulus lupulus* L.)	Diarrhea caused by infection
Horse chestnut (*Aesculus hippocastanum* L.)	Diarrhea
Marshmallow (*Althaea officinalis* L.)	Diarrhea
Niacin (vitamin B_3, nicotinic acid), niacinamide, and inositol hexanicotinate	Cholera diarrhea
Niacin (vitamin B_3, nicotinic acid), niacinamide, and inositol hexanicotinate	Chronic diarrhea
Psyllium (*Plantago ovata, P. ispaghula*)	Dysentery
Psyllium (*Plantago ovata, P. ispaghula*)	Fecal (stool) incontinence
Red yeast rice (*Monascus purpureus*)	Diarrhea

Continued

Red yeast rice (*Monascus purpureus*)	Dysentery (bloody diarrhea)
Saw palmetto (*Serenoa repens* [Bartram] Small)	Dysentery
Slippery elm (*Ulmus rubra* Muhl., *U. fulva* Michx.)	Dysentery
Sorrel (*Rumex acetosa* L., *R. acetosella* L.), Sinupret	Diarrhea
St. John's wort (*Hypericum perforatum* L.)	Diarrhea
Thyme (*Thymus vulgaris* L.), thymol	Diarrhea
Turmeric (*Curcuma longa* L.), curcumin	Diarrhea
White horehound (*Marrubium vulgare*)	Diarrhea

DIURESIS AND RELATED CONDITIONS

Levels of Scientific Evidence for Specific Therapies

GRADE: B (Good Scientific Evidence)

Therapy	Specific Therapeutic Use(s)
Horsetail (*Equisetum arvense* L.)	Diuresis (increased urine)

GRADE: C (Unclear or Conflicting Scientific Evidence)

Therapy	Specific Therapeutic Use(s)
Dandelion (*Taraxacum officinale*)	Diuretic (increased urine flow)

TRADITIONAL OR THEORETICAL USES THAT LACK SUFFICIENT EVIDENCE

Therapy	Specific Therapeutic Use(s)
Alfalfa (*Medicago sativa* L.)	Diuresis (increasing urination)
American pennyroyal (*Hedeoma pulegioides* L.), European pennyroyal (*Mentha pulegium* L.)	Diuretic
Astragalus (*Astragalus membranaceus*)	Diuretic (urination stimulant)
Belladonna (*Atropa belladonna* L. or its variety *acuminata* Royle ex Lindl)	Diuretic (use as a water pill)
Betel nut (*Areca catechu* L.)	Diuretic
Black tea (*Camellia sinensis*)	Diuretic (increasing urine flow)
Blessed thistle (*Cnicus benedictus* L.)	Diuretic (increasing urine)
Boswellia (*Boswellia serrata* Roxb.)	Diuretic
Burdock (*Arctium lappa*)	Diuretic (increasing urine flow)
Calendula (*Calendula officinalis* L.), marigold	Diuretic
Chamomile (*Matricaria recutita, Chamaemelum nobile*)	Diuretic
Chaparral (*Larrea tridentata* DC. Coville, *L. divaricata* Cav.), nordihydroguaiaretic acid (NDGA)	Diuretic (increasing urine flow)
Cranberry (*Vaccinium macrocarpon*)	Diuresis (increasing urine flow)
Devil's claw (*Harpagophytum procumbens* DC.)	Diuretic
Dong quai (*Angelica sinensis* [Oliv.] Diels), Chinese angelica	Diuretic (increasing urination)
Elder (*Sambucus nigra* L.)	Diuresis (urine production)

Ephedra (*Ephedra sinica*)/ma huang	Diuretic
Garlic (*Allium sativum* L.)	Diuretic (water pill)
Ginger (*Zingiber officinale* Roscoe)	Diuresis
Ginseng (American ginseng, Asian ginseng, Chinese ginseng, Korean red ginseng, *Panax ginseng*: *Panax* spp. including *P. ginseng* C.C. Meyer and *P. quincefolium* L., excluding *Eleutherococcus senticosus*)	Diuretic (water pill)
Goldenseal (*Hydrastis canadensis* L.), berberine	Diuretic (increasing urine flow)
Gotu kola (*Centella asiatica* L.), total triterpenic fraction of *Centella asiatica* (TTFCA)	Diuretic
Green tea (*Camellia sinensis*)	Diuretic (increasing urine flow)
Green tea (*Camellia sinensis*)	Improving urine flow
Gymnema (*Gymnema Sylvestre* R. Br.)	Diuresis
Hawthorn (*Crataegus laevigata, C. oxyacantha, C. monogyna, C. pentagyna*)	Diuresis
Kava (*Piper methysticum* G. Forst)	Diuretic
Lavender (*Lavandula angustifolia* Miller)	Diuretic
Licorice (*Glycyrrhiza glabra* L.), deglycyrrhizinated licorice (DGL)	Diuretic
Marshmallow (*Althaea officinalis* L.)	Diuretic
Oleander (*Nerium oleander, Thevetia peruviana*)	Diuretic (increase urine flow)
Polypodium leucotomos extract, Anapsos	Diuretic
Red clover (*Trifolium pratense*)	Diuretic (increase urine flow)
Saw palmetto (*Serenoa repens* [Bartram] Small)	Diuretic
Slippery elm (*Ulmus rubra* Muhl., *U. fulva* Michx.)	Diuretic
Sorrel (*Rumex acetosa* L., *R. acetosella* L.), Sinupret	Diuresis
St. John's wort (*Hypericum perforatum* L.)	Diuretic (increasing urine flow)
Thyme (*Thymus vulgaris* L.), thymol	Diuresis
Valerian (*Valeriana officinalis* L.)	Diuretic
White horehound (*Marrubium vulgare*)	Diuresis

DIZZINESS AND RELATED CONDITIONS

Levels of Scientific Evidence for Specific Therapies

GRADE: C (Unclear or Conflicting Scientific Evidence)	
Therapy	Specific Therapeutic Use(s)
Ginkgo (*Ginkgo biloba* L.)	Vertigo

TRADITIONAL OR THEORETICAL USES THAT LACK SUFFICIENT EVIDENCE	
Therapy	Specific therapeutic Use(s)
American pennyroyal (*Hedeoma pulegioides* L.), European pennyroyal (*Mentha pulegium* L.)	Dizziness

Continued

Black cohosh (*Cimicifuga racemosa* L. Nutt.)	Dizziness
Calendula (*Calendula officinalis* L.), marigold	Dizziness
Echinacea (*Echinacea angustifolia* DC., *E. pallida*, *E. purpurea*)	Dizziness
Feverfew (*Tanacetum parthenium* L. Schultz-Bip.)	Dizziness
Ginkgo (*Ginkgo biloba* L.)	Dizziness
Ginseng (American ginseng, Asian ginseng, Chinese ginseng, Korean red ginseng, *Panax ginseng*: *Panax* spp. including *P. ginseng* C.C. Meyer and *P. quincefolium* L., excluding *Eleutherococcus senticosus*)	Dizziness
Horse chestnut (*Aesculus hippocastanum* L.)	Dizziness
Kava (*Piper methysticum* G. Forst)	Dizziness
Lavender (*Lavandula angustifolia* Miller)	Dizziness
Niacin (vitamin B$_3$, nicotinic acid), niacinamide, and inositol hexanicotinate	Vertigo
Turmeric (*Curcuma longa* L.), curcumin	Dizziness
Valerian (*Valeriana officinalis* L.)	Vertigo

DRUG ADDICTION AND RELATED CONDITIONS
Levels of Scientific Evidence for Specific Therapies

GRADE: C (Unclear or Conflicting Scientific Evidence)

Therapy	Specific Therapeutic Use(s)
Globe artichoke (*Cynara scolymus* L.)	Alcohol-induced hangover
Goldenseal (*Hydrastis canadensis* L.), berberine	Narcotic concealment (urinalysis)
Melatonin	Benzodiazepine tapering
Melatonin	Smoking cessation

TRADITIONAL OR THEORETICAL USES THAT LACK SUFFICIENT EVIDENCE

Therapy	Specific Therapeutic Use(s)
Betel nut (*Areca catechu* L.)	Alcoholism
Black tea (*Camellia sinensis*)	Toxin/alcohol elimination from the body
Burdock (*Arctium lappa*)	Detoxification
Chamomile (*Matricaria recutita*, *Chamaemelum nobile*)	Delirium tremens (DTs)
Clay	Smoking
Dandelion (*Taraxacum officinale*)	Alcohol withdrawal
Dandelion (*Taraxacum officinale*)	Smoking cessation
Essiac	Detoxification
Evening primrose oil (*Oenothera biennis* L.)	Alcoholism
Evening primrose oil (*Oenothera biennis* L.)	Hangover remedy
Ginger (*Zingiber officinale* Roscoe)	Alcohol withdrawal

Ginkgo (*Ginkgo biloba* L.)	Alcoholism
Green tea (*Camellia sinensis*)	Alcohol intoxication
Green tea (*Camellia sinensis*)	Detoxification from alcohol or toxins
Lavender (*Lavandula angustifolia* Miller)	Hangover
Licorice (*Glycyrrhiza glabra* L.), deglycyrrhizinated licorice (DGL)	Detoxification
Melatonin	Withdrawal from narcotics
Niacin (vitamin B_3, nicotinic acid), niacinamide, and inositol hexanicotinate	Alcohol dependence
Niacin (vitamin B_3, nicotinic acid), niacinamide, and inositol hexanicotinate	Smoking cessation
Oleander (*Nerium oleander*, *Thevetia peruviana*)	Alcoholism
St. John's wort (*Hypericum perforatum* L.)	Alcoholism
St. John's wort (*Hypericum perforatum* L.)	Benzodiazepine withdrawal
Valerian (*Valeriana officinalis* L.)	Hangover

DYSMENORRHEA AND RELATED CONDITIONS
Levels of Scientific Evidence for Specific Therapies

GRADE: B (Good Scientific Evidence)

Therapy	Specific Therapeutic Use(s)
Black cohosh (*Cimicifuga racemosa* L.]Nutt.)	Menopausal symptoms
Soy (*Glycine max* L. Merr.)	Menopausal hot flashes

GRADE: C (Unclear or Conflicting Scientific Evidence)

Therapy	Specific Therapeutic Use(s)
American pennyroyal (*Hedeoma pulegioides* L.), European pennyroyal (*Mentha pulegium* L.)	Emmenagogue (menstrual flow stimulant)
Belladonna (*Atropa belladonna* L. or its variety *acuminata* Royle ex Lindl)	Premenstrual syndrome (PMS)
Bilberry (*Vaccinium myrtillus*)	Painful menstruation (dysmenorrhea)
DHEA (dehydroepiandrosterone)	Menopausal disorders
DHEA (dehydroepiandrosterone)	Ovulation disorders
Dong quai (*Angelica sinensis* [Oliv.] Diels), Chinese angelica	Amenorrhea (lack of menstrual period)
Dong quai (*Angelica sinensis* [Oliv.] Diels), Chinese angelica	Dysmenorrhea (painful menstruation)
Flaxseed and flaxseed oil (*Linum usitatissimum*)	Menstrual breast pain (flaxseed, not flaxseed oil)
Ginkgo (*Ginkgo biloba* L.)	Premenstrual syndrome (PMS)
Ginseng (American ginseng, Asian ginseng, Chinese ginseng, Korean red ginseng, *Panax ginseng*: *Panax* spp. including *P. ginseng* C.C. Meyer and *P. quincefolium* L., excluding *Eleutherococcus senticosus*)	Menopausal symptoms

Continued

Green tea (*Camellia sinensis*)	Menopausal symptoms
Omega-3 fatty acids, fish oil, alpha-linolenic acid	Dysmenorrhea (painful menstruation)
Red clover (*Trifolium pratense*)	Hormone replacement therapy (HRT)
Red clover (*Trifolium pratense*)	Menopausal symptoms
St. John's wort (*Hypericum perforatum* L.)	Perimenopausal symptoms
St. John's wort (*Hypericum perforatum* L.)	Premenstrual syndrome (PMS)
Wild yam (*Dioscorea villosa*)	Menopausal symptoms

GRADE: D (Fair Negative Scientific Evidence)	
Therapy	Specific Therapeutic Use(s)
Belladonna (*Atropa belladonna* L. or its variety *acuminata* Royle ex Lindl)	Menopausal symptoms
Boron	Menopausal symptoms
Evening primrose oil (*Oenothera biennis* L.)	Menopause (flushing/bone metabolism)
Evening primrose oil (*Oenothera biennis* L.)	Premenstrual syndrome (PMS)
Wild yam (*Dioscorea villosa*)	Hormonal properties (to mimic estrogen, progesterone, or DHEA)

TRADITIONAL OR THEORETICAL USES THAT LACK SUFFICIENT EVIDENCE	
Therapy	Specific Therapeutic Use(s)
Alfalfa (*Medicago sativa* L.)	Estrogen replacement
Alfalfa (*Medicago sativa* L.)	Menopausal symptoms
American pennyroyal (*Hedeoma pulegioides* L.), European pennyroyal (*Mentha pulegium* L.)	Cramps
American pennyroyal (*Hedeoma pulegioides* L.), European pennyroyal (*Mentha pulegium* L.)	Premenstrual syndrome (PMS)
Astragalus (*Astragalus membranaceus*)	Menstrual disorders
Astragalus (*Astragalus membranaceus*)	Pelvic congestion syndrome
Belladonna (*Atropa belladonna* L. or its variety *acuminata* Royle ex Lindl)	Abnormal menstrual periods
Betel nut (*Areca catechu* L.)	Excessive menstrual flow
Black cohosh (*Cimicifuga racemosa* L. Nutt.)	Endometriosis
Black cohosh (*Cimicifuga racemosa* L. Nutt.)	Menstrual period problems
Black cohosh (*Cimicifuga racemosa* L. Nutt.)	Ovarian cysts
Black cohosh (*Cimicifuga racemosa* L. Nutt.)	Premenstrual syndrome (PMS)
Bladderwrack (*Fucus vesiculosus*)	Menstruation irregularities
Blessed thistle (*Cnicus benedictus* L.)	Menstrual disorders
Blessed thistle (*Cnicus benedictus* L.)	Menstrual flow stimulant
Blessed thistle (*Cnicus benedictus* L.)	Painful menstruation
Boswellia (*Boswellia serrata* Roxb.)	Amenorrhea

Boswellia (*Boswellia serrata* Roxb.)	Emmenagogue (induces menstruation)
Bromelain	Menstrual pain
Calendula (*Calendula officinalis* L.), marigold	Cramps
Calendula (*Calendula officinalis* L.), marigold	Menstrual period abnormalities
Chamomile (*Matricaria recutita*, *Chamaemelum nobile*)	Dysmenorrhea
Chamomile (*Matricaria recutita*, *Chamaemelum nobile*)	Menstrual disorders
Chaparral (*Larrea tridentata* DC. Coville, *L. divaricata* Cav.), nordihydroguaiaretic acid (NDGA)	Menstrual cramps
Clay	Menstruation difficulties
Dandelion (*Taraxacum officinale*)	Menopause
Dandelion (*Taraxacum officinale*)	Premenstrual syndrome (PMS)
Danshen (*Salvia miltiorrhiza*)	Menstrual problems
Devil's claw (*Harpagophytum procumbens* DC.)	Menopausal symptoms
Devil's claw (*Harpagophytum procumbens* DC.)	Menstrual cramps
DHEA (dehydroepiandrosterone)	Amenorrhea associated with anorexia
DHEA (dehydroepiandrosterone)	Andropause/andrenopause
DHEA (dehydroepiandrosterone)	Premenstrual syndrome (PMS)
Dong quai (*Angelica sinensis* [Oliv.] Diels), Chinese angelica	Cramps
Dong quai (*Angelica sinensis* [Oliv.] Diels), Chinese angelica	Hormonal abnormalities
Dong quai (*Angelica sinensis* [Oliv.] Diels), Chinese angelica	Menorrhagia (heavy menstrual bleeding)
Dong quai (*Angelica sinensis* [Oliv.] Diels), Chinese angelica	Menstrual cramping
Dong quai (*Angelica sinensis* [Oliv.] Diels), Chinese angelica	Ovulation abnormalities
Dong quai (*Angelica sinensis* [Oliv.] Diels), Chinese angelica	Pelvic congestion syndrome
Dong quai (*Angelica sinensis* [Oliv.] Diels), Chinese angelica	Premenstrual syndrome (PMS)
Fenugreek (*Trigonella foenum-graecum* L.)	Menopausal symptoms
Fenugreek (*Trigonella foenum-graecum* L.)	Postmenopausal vaginal dryness
Feverfew (*Tanacetum parthenium* L. Schultz-Bip.)	Menstrual cramps
Feverfew (*Tanacetum parthenium* L. Schultz-Bip.)	Promotion of menstruation
Flaxseed and flaxseed oil (*Linum usitatissimum*)	Menstrual disorders
Flaxseed and flaxseed oil (*Linum usitatissimum*)	Ovarian disorders
Garlic (*Allium sativum* L.)	Emmenagogue
Ginger (*Zingiber officinale* Roscoe)	Dysmenorrhea
Ginger (*Zingiber officinale* Roscoe)	Promotion of menstruation
Ginkgo (*Ginkgo biloba* L.)	Menstrual pain
Ginseng (American ginseng, Asian ginseng, Chinese ginseng, Korean red ginseng, *Panax ginseng*: *Panax* spp. including *P. ginseng* C.C. Meyer and *P. quincefolium* L., excluding *Eleutherococcus senticosus*)	Menopausal symptoms

Continued

Goldenseal (*Hydrastis canadensis* L.), berberine	Menstruation problems
Goldenseal (*Hydrastis canadensis* L.), berberine	Premenstrual syndrome (PMS)
Gotu kola (*Centella asiatica* L.), total triterpenic fraction of *Centella asiatica* (TTFCA)	Amenorrhea
Gotu kola (*Centella asiatica* L.), total triterpenic fraction of *Centella asiatica* (TTFCA)	Hot flashes
Gotu kola (*Centella asiatica* L.), total triterpenic fraction of *Centella asiatica* (TTFCA)	Menstrual disorders
Guggul (*Commifora mukul*)	Menstrual disorders
Hawthorn (*Crataegus laevigata, C. oxyacantha, C. monogyna, C. pentagyna*)	Amenorrhea
Hops (*Humulus lupulus* L.)	Estrogenic effects
Horse chestnut (*Aesculus hippocastanum* L.)	Menstrual pain
Horsetail (*Equisetum arvense* L.)	Menstrual pain
Kava (*Piper methysticum* G. Forst)	Menopause
Kava (*Piper methysticum* G. Forst)	Menstrual disorders
Lavender (*Lavandula angustifolia* Miller)	Menopause
Lavender (*Lavandula angustifolia* Miller)	Menstrual period problems
Licorice (*Glycyrrhiza glabra* L.), deglycyrrhizinated licorice (DGL)	Hormone regulation
Licorice (*Glycyrrhiza glabra* L.), deglycyrrhizinated licorice (DGL)	Menopausal symptoms
Melatonin	Melatonin deficiency
Milk thistle (*Silybum marianum*), silymarin	Menstrual disorders
Niacin (vitamin B_3, nicotinic acid), niacinamide, and inositol hexanicotinate	Painful menstruation
Niacin (vitamin B_3, nicotinic acid), niacinamide, and inositol hexanicotinate	Premenstrual headache prevention
Niacin (vitamin B_3, nicotinic acid), niacinamide, and inositol hexanicotinate	Premenstrual syndrome (PMS)
Oleander (*Nerium oleander, Thevetia peruviana*)	Abnormal menstruation
Oleander (*Nerium oleander, Thevetia peruviana*)	Menstrual stimulant
Omega-3 fatty acids, fish oil, alpha-linolenic acid	Menopausal symptoms
Omega-3 fatty acids, fish oil, alpha-linolenic acid	Menstrual cramps
Omega-3 fatty acids, fish oil, alpha-linolenic acid	Premenstrual syndrome (PMS)
Passionflower (*Passiflora incarnata* L.)	Menopausal symptoms (hot flashes)
Peppermint (*Mentha x piperita* L.)	Cramps
Peppermint (*Mentha x piperita* L.)	Dysmenorrhea (menstrual pain)
Psyllium (*Plantago ovata, P. ispaghula*)	Excessive menstrual bleeding
Red clover (*Trifolium pratense*)	Hot flashes
Red clover (*Trifolium pratense*)	Premenstrual syndrome (PMS)
Saw palmetto (*Serenoa repens* [Bartram] Small)	Antiandrogen

Saw palmetto (*Serenoa repens* [Bartram] Small)	Antiestrogen
Saw palmetto (*Serenoa repens* [Bartram] Small)	Dysmenorrhea
Saw palmetto (*Serenoa repens* [Bartram] Small)	Estrogenic agent
Saw palmetto (*Serenoa repens* [Bartram] Small)	Ovarian cysts
Saw palmetto (*Serenoa repens* [Bartram] Small)	Pelvic congestive syndrome
Seaweed, kelp, bladderwrack (*Fucus vesiculosus*)	Menstrual irregularities (menorrhagia)
Slippery elm (*Ulmus rubra* Muhl., *U. fulva* Michx.)	Gynecologic disorders
Spirulina	Premenstrual syndrome (PMS)
St. John's wort (*Hypericum perforatum* L.)	Menstrual pain
Sweet almond (*Prunus amygdalus dulcis*)	Plant-derived estrogen
Thyme (*Thymus vulgaris* L.), thymol	Dysmenorrhea
Turmeric (*Curcuma longa* L.), curcumin	Menstrual pain
Turmeric (*Curcuma longa* L.), curcumin	Menstrual period problems/ lack of menstrual period
Valerian (*Valeriana officinalis* L.)	Amenorrhea
Valerian (*Valeriana officinalis* L.)	Dysmenorrhea
Valerian (*Valeriana officinalis* L.)	Emmenagogue
Valerian (*Valeriana officinalis* L.)	Menopause
Valerian (*Valeriana officinalis* L.)	Premenstrual syndrome (PMS)
White horehound (*Marrubium vulgare*)	Dysmenorrhea
White horehound (*Marrubium vulgare*)	Menstrual pain
Wild yam (*Dioscorea villosa*)	Cramps
Wild yam (*Dioscorea villosa*)	Menopause
Wild yam (*Dioscorea villosa*)	Menstrual pain or irregularities
Wild yam (*Dioscorea villosa*)	Pelvic cramps
Wild yam (*Dioscorea villosa*)	Postmenopausal vaginal dryness
Wild yam (*Dioscorea villosa*)	Premenstrual syndrome (PMS)

ENERGY BOOSTER AND RELATED CONDITIONS

Levels of Scientific Evidence for Specific Therapies

GRADE: C (Unclear or Conflicting Scientific Evidence)

Therapy	Specific Therapeutic Use(s)
Betel nut (*Areca catechu* L.)	Stimulant
DHEA (dehydroepiandrosterone)	Chronic fatigue syndrome
Evening primrose oil (*Oenothera biennis* L.)	Chronic fatigue syndrome/ postviral infection symptoms
Ginseng (American ginseng, Asian ginseng, Chinese ginseng, Korean red ginseng, *Panax ginseng*: *Panax* spp. including *P. ginseng* C.C. Meyer and *P. quincefolium* L., excluding *Eleutherococcus senticosus*)	Fatigue

Continued

TRADITIONAL OR THEORETICAL USES THAT LACK SUFFICIENT EVIDENCE	
Therapy	Specific Therapeutic Use(s)
Aloe (*Aloe vera*)	Chronic fatigue syndrome
American pennyroyal (*Hedeoma pulegioides* L.), European pennyroyal (*Mentha pulegium* L.)	Stimulant
Astragalus (*Astragalus membranaceus*)	Chronic fatigue syndrome
Astragalus (*Astragalus membranaceus*)	Fatigue
Black cohosh (*Cimicifuga racemosa* L. Nutt.)	Malaise
Bladderwrack (*Fucus vesiculosus*)	Fatigue
Calendula (*Calendula officinalis* L.), marigold	Fatigue
Coenzyme Q10	Chronic fatigue syndrome
Dandelion (*Taraxacum officinale*)	Chronic fatigue syndrome
Dandelion (*Taraxacum officinale*)	Stimulant
Dong quai (*Angelica sinensis* [Oliv.] Diels), Chinese angelica	Fatigue
Ephedra (Ephedra sinica)/ma huang	Energy enhancer
Ephedra (Ephedra sinica)/ma huang	Stimulant
Essiac	Chronic fatigue syndrome
Eucalyptus oil (*Eucalyptus globulus* Labillardiere, *E. fructetorum* F. Von Mueller, *E. smithii* R.T. Baker)	Alertness
Eucalyptus oil (*Eucalyptus globulus* Labillardiere, *E. fructetorum* F. Von Mueller, *E. smithii* R.T. Baker)	Stimulant
Garlic (*Allium sativum* L.)	Fatigue
Ginger (*Zingiber officinale* Roscoe)	Stimulant
Ginkgo (*Ginkgo biloba* L.)	Fatigue
Ginseng (American ginseng, Asian ginseng, Chinese ginseng, Korean red ginseng, *Panax ginseng*: *Panax* spp. including *P. ginseng* C.C. Meyer and *P. quincefolium* L., excluding *Eleutherococcus senticosus*)	Fatigue
Goldenseal (*Hydrastis canadensis* L.), berberine	Chronic fatigue syndrome
Goldenseal (*Hydrastis canadensis* L.), berberine	Stimulant
Gotu kola (*Centella asiatica* L.), total triterpenic fraction of *Centella asiatica* (TTFCA)	Energy
Gotu kola (*Centella asiatica* L.), total triterpenic fraction of *Centella asiatica* (TTFCA)	Fatigue
Green tea (*Camellia sinensis*)	Stimulant
Lavender (*Lavandula angustifolia* Miller)	Fatigue
Licorice (*Glycyrrhiza glabra* L.), deglycyrrhizinated licorice (DGL)	Chronic fatigue syndrome
Omega-3 fatty acids, fish oil, alpha-linolenic acid	Chronic fatigue syndrome
Seaweed, kelp, bladderwrack (*Fucus vesiculosus*)	Fatigue
Spirulina	Energy booster
Spirulina	Fatigue

St. John's wort (*Hypericum perforatum* L.)   Fatigue

Valerian (*Valeriana officinalis* L.)   Fatigue

ERECTILE DYSFUNCTION AND RELATED CONDITIONS
Levels of Scientific Evidence for Specific Therapies

GRADE: C (Unclear or Conflicting Scientific Evidence)

Therapy	Specific Therapeutic Use(s)
Arginine (L-arginine)	Erectile dysfunction
Clove (*Eugenia aromatica*)	Premature ejaculation
DHEA (dehydroepiandrosterone)	Sexual function/libido/erectile dysfunction
Ephedra (*Ephedra sinica*)/ma huang	Sexual arousal
Ginkgo (*Ginkgo biloba* L.)	Decreased libido/erectile dysfunction (impotence)
Ginseng (American ginseng, Asian ginseng, Chinese ginseng, Korean red ginseng, *Panax ginseng*: *Panax* spp. including *P. ginseng* C.C. Meyer and *P. quincefolium* L., excluding *Eleutherococcus senticosus*)	Erectile dysfunction
Yohimbe bark extract (*Pausinystalia yohimbe* Pierre ex Beille)	Erectile dysfunction (male impotence)
Yohimbe bark extract (*Pausinystalia yohimbe* Pierre ex Beille)	Libido (women)
Yohimbe bark extract (*Pausinystalia yohimbe* Pierre ex Beille)	Sexual side effects of selective serotonin reuptake inhibitor (SSRI) antidepressants

TRADITIONAL OR THEORETICAL USES THAT LACK SUFFICIENT EVIDENCE

Therapy	Specific Therapeutic Use(s)
Betel nut (Areca catechu L.)	Aphrodisiac
Betel nut (*Areca catechu* L.)	Impotence
Black cohosh (*Cimicifuga racemosa* L. Nutt.)	Aphrodisiac
Burdock (*Arctium lappa*)	Aphrodisiac
Burdock (*Arctium lappa*)	Impotence
Fenugreek (*Trigonella foenum-graecum* L.)	Impotence
Garlic (*Allium sativum* L.)	Aphrodisiac
Ginger (*Zingiber officinale* Roscoe)	Aphrodisiac
Ginger (*Zingiber officinale* Roscoe)	Impotence
Ginseng (American ginseng, Asian ginseng, Chinese ginseng, Korean red ginseng, *Panax ginseng*: *Panax* spp. including *P. ginseng* C.C. Meyer and *P. quincefolium* L., excluding *Eleutherococcus senticosus*)	Aphrodisiac
Ginseng (American ginseng, Asian ginseng, Chinese ginseng, Korean red ginseng, *Panax ginseng*: *Panax* spp. including *P. ginseng* C.C. Meyer and *P. quincefolium* L., excluding *Eleutherococcus senticosus*)	Premature ejaculation

Continued

Ginseng (American ginseng, Asian ginseng,
Chinese ginseng, Korean red ginseng, *Panax ginseng*:
Panax spp. including *P. ginseng* C.C. Meyer and
P. quincefolium L., excluding *Eleutherococcus senticosus*)   Sexual arousal

Ginseng (American ginseng, Asian ginseng,
Chinese ginseng, Korean red ginseng, *Panax ginseng*:
Panax spp. including *P. ginseng* C.C. Meyer and
P. quincefolium L., excluding *Eleutherococcus senticosus*)   Sexual symptoms

Gotu kola (*Centella asiatica* L.), total triterpenic fraction
of *Centella asiatica* (TTFCA)   Aphrodisiac

Gotu kola (*Centella asiatica* L.), total triterpenic fraction
of *Centella asiatica* (TTFCA)   Libido

Gymnema (*Gymnema Sylvestre* R. Br.)   Aphrodisiac

Hops (*Humulus lupulus* L.)   Aphrodisiac

Kava (*Piper methysticum* G. Forst)   Aphrodisiac

Lavender (*Lavandula angustifolia* Miller)   Aphrodisiac

Marshmallow (*Althaea officinalis* L.)   Aphrodisiac

Marshmallow (*Althaea officinalis* L.)   Impotence

Melatonin   Erectile dysfunction

Melatonin   Sexual activity enhancement

Niacin (vitamin B_3, nicotinic acid), niacinamide,
and inositol hexanicotinate   Orgasm improvement

Pygeum (*Prunus africana*, *Pygeum africanum*)   Aphrodisiac

Pygeum (*Prunus africana*, *Pygeum africanum*)   Impotence

Pygeum (*Prunus africana*, *Pygeum africanum*)   Sexual performance

Saw palmetto (*Serenoa repens* [Bartram] Small)   Aphrodisiac

Saw palmetto (*Serenoa repens* [Bartram] Small)   Impotence

Saw palmetto (*Serenoa repens* [Bartram] Small)   Sexual vigor

Sweet almond (*Prunus amygdalus dulcis*)   Aphrodisiac

Wild yam (*Dioscorea villosa*)   Libido

Yohimbe bark extract (*Pausinystalia yohimbe* Pierre ex Beille)   Aphrodisiac

EYE DISORDERS AND RELATED CONDITIONS

Levels of Scientific Evidence for Specific Therapies

GRADE: C (Unclear or Conflicting Scientific Evidence)

Therapy	Specific Therapeutic Use(s)
Eyebright (*Euphrasia officinalis*)	Conjunctivitis
Propolis	Cornea complications from zoster infection
Turmeric (*Curcuma longa* L.), curcumin	Uveitis (eye inflammation)

TRADITIONAL OR THEORETICAL USES THAT LACK SUFFICIENT EVIDENCE

Therapy	Specific Therapeutic Use(s)
Belladonna (*Atropa belladonna* L. or its variety *acuminata* Royle ex Lindl)	Conjunctivitis
Bilberry (*Vaccinium myrtillus*)	Eye disorders
Boron	Eye cleansing
Calendula (*Calendula officinalis* L.), marigold	Conjunctivitis
Calendula (*Calendula officinalis* L.), marigold	Eye inflammation
Chamomile (*Matricaria recutita, Chamaemelum nobile*)	Eye infections
Clay	Eye disorders
Eyebright (*Euphrasia officinalis*)	Ocular compress
Eyebright (*Euphrasia officinalis*)	Ocular fatigue
Eyebright (*Euphrasia officinalis*)	Ocular rinse
Eyebright (*Euphrasia officinalis*)	Ophthalmia
Flaxseed and flaxseed oil (*Linum usitatissimum*)	Foreign body removal from the eye
Goldenseal (Hydrastis canadensis L.), berberine	Conjunctivitis
Goldenseal (*Hydrastis canadensis* L.), berberine	Eyewash
Goldenseal (*Hydrastis canadensis* L.), berberine	Keratitis (inflammation of the cornea of the eye)
Gotu kola (*Centella asiatica* L.), total triterpenic fraction of *Centella asiatica* (TTFCA)	Eye diseases
Green tea (*Camellia sinensis*)	Tired eyes
Oleander (*Nerium oleander, Thevetia peruviana*)	Eye diseases
Propolis	Eye infections/inflammation
Valerian (*Valeriana officinalis* L.)	Vision problems
Yohimbe bark extract (*Pausinystalia yohimbe* Pierre ex Beille)	Pupil dilator
Yohimbe bark extract (*Pausinystalia yohimbe* Pierre ex Beille)	Pupil dilator

FATIGUE AND RELATED CONDITIONS

Levels of Scientific Evidence for Specific Therapies

GRADE: C (Unclear or Conflicting Scientific Evidence)

Therapy	Specific Therapeutic Use(s)
Betel nut (*Areca catechu* L.)	Stimulant
DHEA (dehydroepiandrosterone)	Chronic fatigue syndrome
Evening primrose oil (*Oenothera biennis* L.)	Chronic fatigue syndrome/ post-viral infection symptoms
Ginseng (American ginseng, Asian ginseng, Chinese ginseng, Korean red ginseng, *Panax ginseng*: *Panax* spp. including *P. ginseng* C.C. Meyer and *P. quincefolium* L., excluding *Eleutherococcus senticosus*)	Fatigue

Continued

TRADITIONAL OR THEORETICAL USES THAT LACK SUFFICIENT EVIDENCE

Therapy	Specific Therapeutic Use(s)
Aloe (*Aloe vera*)	Chronic fatigue syndrome
American pennyroyal (*Hedeoma pulegioides* L.), European pennyroyal (*Mentha pulegium* L.)	Stimulant
Astragalus (*Astragalus membranaceus*)	Chronic fatigue syndrome
Astragalus (*Astragalus membranaceus*)	Fatigue
Black cohosh (*Cimicifuga racemosa* L. Nutt.)	Malaise
Bladderwrack (*Fucus vesiculosus*)	Fatigue
Calendula (*Calendula officinalis* L.), marigold	Fatigue
Coenzyme Q10	Chronic fatigue syndrome
Dandelion (*Taraxacum officinale*)	Chronic fatigue syndrome
Dandelion (*Taraxacum officinale*)	Stimulant
Dong quai (*Angelica sinensis* [Oliv.] Diels), Chinese angelica	Fatigue
Ephedra (*Ephedra sinica*)/ma huang	Energy enhancer
Ephedra (*Ephedra sinica*)/ma huang	Stimulant
Essiac	Chronic fatigue syndrome
Eucalyptus oil (*Eucalyptus globulus* Labillardiere, *E. fructicetorum* F. Von Mueller, *E. smithii* R.T. Baker)	Alertness
Eucalyptus oil (*Eucalyptus globulus* Labillardiere, *E. fructicetorum* F. Von Mueller, *E. smithii* R.T. Baker)	Stimulant
Garlic (*Allium sativum* L.)	Fatigue
Ginger (*Zingiber officinale* Roscoe)	Stimulant
Ginkgo (*Ginkgo biloba* L.)	Fatigue
Ginseng (American ginseng, Asian ginseng, Chinese ginseng, Korean red ginseng, *Panax ginseng*: *Panax* spp. including *P. ginseng* C.C. Meyer and *P. quincefolium* L., excluding *Eleutherococcus senticosus*)	Fatigue
Goldenseal (*Hydrastis canadensis* L.), berberine	Chronic fatigue syndrome
Goldenseal (*Hydrastis canadensis* L.), berberine	Stimulant
Gotu kola (*Centella asiatica* L.), total triterpenic fraction of *Centella asiatica* (TTFCA)	Energy
Gotu kola (*Centella asiatica* L.), total triterpenic fraction of *Centella asiatica* (TTFCA)	Fatigue
Green tea (*Camellia sinensis*)	Stimulant
Lavender (*Lavandula angustifolia* Miller)	Fatigue
Licorice (*Glycyrrhiza glabra* L.), deglycyrrhizinated licorice (DGL)	Chronic fatigue syndrome
Omega-3 fatty acids, fish oil, alpha-linolenic acid	Chronic fatigue syndrome
Seaweed, kelp, bladderwrack (*Fucus vesiculosus*)	Fatigue
Spirulina	Energy booster
Spirulina	Fatigue
St. John's wort (*Hypericum perforatum* L.)	Fatigue
Valerian (*Valeriana officinalis* L.)	Fatigue

FEVER AND RELATED CONDITIONS

Levels of Scientific Evidence for Specific Therapies

GRADE: C (Unclear or Conflicting Scientific Evidence)	
Therapy	Specific Therapeutic Use(s)
Clove (*Eugenia aromatica*)	Fever reduction

TRADITIONAL OR THEORETICAL USES THAT LACK SUFFICIENT EVIDENCE	
Therapy	Specific Therapeutic Use(s)
American pennyroyal (*Hedeoma pulegioides* L.), European pennyroyal (*Mentha pulegium* L.)	Diaphoretic
American pennyroyal (*Hedeoma pulegioides* L.), European pennyroyal (*Mentha pulegium* L.)	Fever
Astragalus (*Astragalus membranaceus*)	Fever
Belladonna (*Atropa belladonna* L. or its variety *acuminata* Royle ex Lindl)	Fever
Bilberry (*Vaccinium myrtillus*)	Fevers
Black cohosh (*Cimicifuga racemosa* L. Nutt.)	Fever
Blessed thistle (*Cnicus benedictus* L.)	Antipyretic
Blessed thistle (*Cnicus benedictus* L.)	Diaphoretic
Blessed thistle (*Cnicus benedictus* L.)	Fever
Burdock (*Arctium lappa*)	Fever
Calendula (*Calendula officinalis* L.), marigold	Fever
Chamomile (*Matricaria recutita*, *Chamaemelum nobile*)	Diaphoretic
Chamomile (*Matricaria recutita*, *Chamaemelum nobile*)	Fever
Clay	Fevers
Dandelion (*Taraxacum officinale*)	Fever reduction
Devil's claw (*Harpagophytum procumbens* DC.)	Fever
Elder (*Sambucus nigra* L.)	Fever
Ephedra (*Ephedra sinica*)/ma huang	Antipyretic
Ephedra (*Ephedra sinica*)/ma huang	Diaphoretic
Ephedra (*Ephedra sinica*)/ma huang	Fevers
Eucalyptus oil (*Eucalyptus globulus* Labillardiere, *E. fructicetorum* F. Von Mueller, *E. smithii* R.T. Baker)	Fever
Feverfew (*Tanacetum parthenium* L. Schultz-Bip.)	Fever
Garlic (*Allium sativum* L.)	Fever
Ginseng (American ginseng, Asian ginseng, Chinese ginseng, Korean red ginseng, *Panax ginseng*: *Panax* spp. including *P. ginseng* C.C. Meyer and *P. quincefolium* L., excluding *Eleutherococcus senticosus*)	Fever
Goldenseal (*Hydrastis canadensis* L.), berberine	Fever
Gotu kola (*Centella asiatica* L.), total triterpenic fraction of *Centella asiatica* (TTFCA)	Fever

Continued

Horse chestnut (*Aesculus hippocastanum* L.)	Fever
Horsetail (*Equisetum arvense* L.)	Fever
Lavender (*Lavandula angustifolia* Miller)	Fever
Licorice (*Glycyrrhiza glabra* L.), deglycyrrhizinated licorice (DGL)	Fever
Peppermint (*Mentha x piperita* L.)	Fever
Polypodium leucotomos extract, Anapsos	Fever
Pygeum (*Prunus africana*, *Pygeum africanum*)	Fever
Slippery elm (*Ulmus rubra* Muhl., *U. fulva* Michx.)	Fever
Sorrel (*Rumex acetosa* L., *R. acetosella* L.), Sinupret	Fever
Soy (*Glycine max* L. Merr.)	Fever
Thyme (*Thymus vulgaris* L.), thymol	Fever
Valerian (*Valeriana officinalis* L.)	Fever
White horehound (*Marrubium vulgare*)	Fever reduction
Yohimbe bark extract (*Pausinystalia yohimbe* Pierre ex Beille)	Fevers
Yohimbe bark extract (*Pausinystalia yohimbe* Pierre ex Beille)	Fevers

FIBROMYALGIA AND RELATED CONDITIONS

Levels of Scientific Evidence for Specific Therapies

TRADITIONAL OR THEORETICAL USES THAT LACK SUFFICIENT EVIDENCE

Therapy	Specific Therapeutic Use(s)
Black cohosh (*Cimicifuga racemosa* L. Nutt.)	Myalgia
Devil's claw (*Harpagophytum procumbens* DC.)	Fibromyalgia
Fenugreek (*Trigonella foenum-graecum* L.)	Myalgia
Ginseng (American ginseng, Asian ginseng, Chinese ginseng, Korean red ginseng, *Panax ginseng*: *Panax* spp. including *P. ginseng* C.C. Meyer and *P. quincefolium* L., excluding *Eleutherococcus senticosus*)	Fibromyalgia
Horse chestnut (*Aesculus hippocastanum* L.)	Nocturnal leg cramps
Melatonin	Fibromyalgia
Omega-3 fatty acids, fish oil, alpha-linolenic acid	Fibromyalgia
Peppermint (*Mentha x piperita* L.)	Fibromyositis
Spirulina	Fibromyalgia
Tea tree oil (*Melaleuca alternifolia* [Maiden & Betche] Cheel)	Muscle and joint distress

FLATULENCE AND RELATED CONDITIONS

Levels of Scientific Evidence for Specific Therapies

TRADITIONAL OR THEORETICAL USES THAT LACK SUFFICIENT EVIDENCE

Therapy	Specific Therapeutic Use(s)
American pennyroyal (*Hedeoma pulegioides* L.), European pennyroyal (*Mentha pulegium* L.)	Carminative

American pennyroyal (*Hedeoma pulegioides* L.), European pennyroyal (*Mentha pulegium* L.)	Flatulence
Betel nut (*Areca catechu* L.)	Gas
Boswellia (*Boswellia serrata* Roxb.)	Belching
Boswellia (*Boswellia serrata* Roxb.)	Carminative
Chamomile (*Matricaria recutita*, *Chamaemelum nobile*)	Gas
Chaparral (*Larrea tridentata* DC. Coville, *L. divaricata* Cav.), nordihydroguaiaretic acid (NDGA)	Gas
Clove (*Eugenia aromatica*)	Gas
Dandelion (*Taraxacum officinale*)	Gas
Devil's claw (*Harpagophytum procumbens* DC.)	Flatulence (gas)
Dong quai (*Angelica sinensis* [Oliv.] Diels), Chinese angelica	Flatulence (gas)
Fenugreek (*Trigonella foenum-graecum* L.)	Flatulence
Ginger (*Zingiber officinale* Roscoe)	Flatulence (gas)
Goldenseal (*Hydrastis canadensis* L.), berberine	Flatulence (gas)
Green tea (*Camellia sinensis*)	Flatulence
Lavender (*Lavandula angustifolia* Miller)	Gas
Peppermint (*Mentha x piperita* L.)	Gas (flatulence)
Thyme (*Thymus vulgaris* L.), thymol	Flatulence
Thyme (*Thymus vulgaris* L.), thymol	Gas
Turmeric (*Curcuma longa* L.), curcumin	Gas
Valerian (*Valeriana officinalis* L.)	Carminative
Valerian (*Valeriana officinalis* L.)	Flatulence
White horehound (*Marrubium vulgare*)	Flatulence
Wild Yam (*Dioscorea villosa*)	Flatus prevention

FLAVORING AGENT AND RELATED CONDITIONS

Levels of Scientific Evidence for Specific Therapies

TRADITIONAL OR THEORETICAL USES THAT LACK SUFFICIENT EVIDENCE

Therapy	Specific Therapeutic Use(s)
American pennyroyal (*Hedeoma pulegioides* L.), European pennyroyal (*Mentha pulegium* L.)	Flavoring agent
Clove (*Eugenia aromatica*)	Flavoring for food and cigarettes
Dandelion (*Taraxacum officinale*)	Coffee substitute
Dandelion (*Taraxacum officinale*)	Food uses
Elder (*Sambucus nigra* L.)	Flavoring
Eucalyptus oil (*Eucalyptus globulus* Labillardiere, *E. fructicetorum* F. Von Mueller, *E. smithii* R.T. Baker)	Flavoring

Continued

| Eyebright (*Euphrasia officinalis*) | Flavoring agent |
| White horehound (*Marrubium vulgare*) | Food flavoring |

FUNGAL INFECTIONS AND RELATED CONDITIONS
Levels of Scientific Evidence for Specific Therapies

GRADE: C (Unclear or Conflicting Scientific Evidence)

Therapy	Specific Therapeutic Use(s)
Garlic (*Allium sativum* L.)	Antifungal (applied to the skin)
Goldenseal (*Hydrastis canadensis* L.), berberine	Chloroquine-resistant malaria
Seaweed, kelp, bladderwrack (*Fucus vesiculosus*)	Antifungal
Tea tree oil (*Melaleuca alternifolia* [Maiden & Betche] Cheel)	Fungal nail infection (onychomycosis)
Tea tree oil (*Melaleuca alternifolia* [Maiden & Betche] Cheel)	Thrush (*Candida albicans* infection of the mouth)

TRADITIONAL OR THEORETICAL USES THAT LACK SUFFICIENT EVIDENCE

Therapy	Specific Therapeutic Use(s)
Aloe (*Aloe vera*)	Parasitic worm infections
Aloe (*Aloe vera*)	Yeast infections of the skin
Astragalus (*Astragalus membranaceus*)	Antifungal
Betel nut (*Areca catechu* L.)	Anthelminthic
Black cohosh (*Cimicifuga racemosa* L. Nutt.)	Malaria
Bladderwrack (*Fucus vesiculosus*)	Parasites
Blessed thistle (*Cnicus benedictus* L.)	Malaria
Burdock (*Arctium lappa*)	Fungal infections
Burdock (*Arctium lappa*)	Ringworm
Calendula (*Calendula officinalis* L.), marigold	Fungal infections
Chamomile (*Matricaria recutita, Chamaemelum nobile*)	Antifungal
Chamomile (*Matricaria recutita, Chamaemelum nobile*)	Fungal infections
Chamomile (*Matricaria recutita, Chamaemelum nobile*)	Malaria
Chamomile (*Matricaria recutita, Chamaemelum nobile*)	Parasites/worms
Chaparral (*Larrea tridentata* DC. Coville, *L. divaricata* Cav.), nordihydroguaiaretic acid (NDGA)	Antiparasitic
Clove (*Eugenia aromatica*)	Antifungal
Dandelion (*Taraxacum officinale*)	Antifungal
Devil's claw (*Harpagophytum procumbens* DC.)	Malaria
DHEA (dehydroepiandrosterone)	Malaria
Dong quai (*Angelica sinensis* [Oliv.] Diels), Chinese angelica	Antifungal
Dong quai (*Angelica sinensis* [Oliv.] Diels), Chinese angelica	Malaria

Echinacea (*Echinacea angustifolia* DC., *E. pallida*, *E. purpurea*)	Malaria
Eucalyptus oil (*Eucalyptus globulus* Labillardiere, *E. fructicetorum* F. Von Mueller, *E. smithii* R.T. Baker)	Antifungal
Eucalyptus oil (*Eucalyptus globulus* Labillardiere, *E. fructicetorum* F. Von Mueller, *E. smithii* R.T. Baker)	Hookworm
Eucalyptus oil (*Eucalyptus globulus* Labillardiere, *E. fructicetorum* F. Von Mueller, *E. smithii* R.T. Baker)	Parasitic infection
Eucalyptus oil (*Eucalyptus globulus* Labillardiere, *E. fructicetorum* F. Von Mueller, *E. smithii* R.T. Baker)	Ringworm
Eyebright (*Euphrasia officinalis*)	Anthelmintic
Garlic (*Allium sativum* L.)	Amoeba infections
Garlic (*Allium sativum* L.)	Malaria
Garlic (*Allium sativum* L.)	Parasites and worms
Garlic (*Allium sativum* L.)	Thrush
Ginger (*Zingiber officinale* Roscoe)	Fungal infections
Ginger (*Zingiber officinale* Roscoe)	Malaria
Ginkgo (*Ginkgo biloba* L.)	Antifungal
Ginkgo (*Ginkgo biloba* L.)	Antiparasitic
Ginkgo (*Ginkgo biloba* L.)	Filariasis
Goldenseal (*Hydrastis canadensis* L.), berberine	Antifungal
Goldenseal (*Hydrastis canadensis* L.), berberine	Thrush
Gotu kola (*Centella asiatica* L.), total triterpenic fraction of *Centella asiatica* (TTFCA)	Fungal infections
Gotu kola (*Centella asiatica* L.), total triterpenic fraction of *Centella asiatica* (TTFCA)	Malaria
Green tea (*Camellia sinensis*)	Fungal infections
Gymnema (*Gymnema Sylvestre* R. Br.)	Malaria
Hops (*Humulus lupulus* L.)	Parasites
Horsetail (*Equisetum arvense* L.)	Malaria
Kava (*Piper methysticum* G. Forst)	Antifungal
Lactobacillus acidophilus	Thrush
Lavender (*Lavandula angustifolia* Miller)	Antifungal
Lavender (*Lavandula angustifolia* Miller)	Parasites/worms
Milk thistle (*Silybum marianum*), silymarin	Malaria
Oleander (*Nerium oleander*, *Thevetia peruviana*)	Antiparasitic
Oleander (*Nerium oleander*, *Thevetia peruviana*)	Malaria
Oleander (*Nerium oleander*, *Thevetia peruviana*)	Ringworm
Omega-3 fatty acids, fish oil, alpha-linolenic acid	Malaria
Propolis	Fungal infections
Psyllium (*Plantago ovata*, *P. ispaghula*)	Antiparasitic

Continued

Pygeum (*Prunus africana*, *Pygeum africanum*)	Malaria
Seaweed, kelp, bladderwrack (*Fucus vesiculosus*)	Antiparasitic
Shark cartilage	Fungal infections
Sorrel (*Rumex acetosa* L., *R. acetosella* L.), Sinupret	Ringworm
Soy (*Glycine max* L. Merr.)	Antifungal
Spirulina	Antifungal
St. John's wort (*Hypericum perforatum* L.)	Antimalarial
Tea tree oil (*Melaleuca alternifolia* [Maiden & Betche] Cheel)	Ringworm
Turmeric (*Curcuma longa* L.), curcumin	Antifungal
Turmeric (*Curcuma longa* L.), curcumin	Parasites
Turmeric (*Curcuma longa* L.), curcumin	Ringworm
White horehound (*Marrubium vulgare*)	Anthelmintic
Wild yam (*Dioscorea villosa*)	Antifungal

GALLBLADDER DISORDERS AND RELATED CONDITIONS

Levels of Scientific Evidence for Specific Therapies

GRADE: C (Unclear or Conflicting Scientific Evidence)

Therapy	Specific Therapeutic Use(s)
Globe artichoke (*Cynara scolymus* L.)	Choleretic (bile-secretion stimulant)
Soy (*Glycine max* L. Merr.)	Gallstones (cholelithiasis)
Turmeric (*Curcuma longa* L.), curcumin	Gallstone prevention/bile flow stimulant
White horehound (*Marrubium vulgare*)	Choleretic (dyspepsia, appetite stimulation)

TRADITIONAL OR THEORETICAL USES THAT LACK SUFFICIENT EVIDENCE

Therapy	Specific Therapeutic Use(s)
American pennyroyal (*Hedeoma pulegioides* L.), European pennyroyal (*Mentha pulegium* L.)	Gallbladder disorders
Black cohosh (*Cimicifuga racemosa* L. Nutt.)	Gallbladder disorders
Blessed thistle (*Cnicus benedictus* L.)	Choleretic (bile flow stimulant)
Blessed thistle (*Cnicus benedictus* L.)	Gallbladder disease
Cranberry (*Vaccinium macrocarpon*)	Gallbladder stones
Dandelion (*Taraxacum officinale*)	Bile flow stimulation
Dandelion (*Taraxacum officinale*)	Gallbladder disease
Dandelion (*Taraxacum officinale*)	Gallstones
Devil's claw (*Harpagophytum procumbens* DC.)	Choleretic (bile secretion)
Dong quai (*Angelica sinensis* [Oliv.] Diels), Chinese angelica	Cholagogue
Garlic (*Allium sativum* L.)	Bile secretion problems

Garlic (*Allium sativum* L.)	Gallstones
Ginger (*Zingiber officinale* Roscoe)	Bile secretion problems
Globe artichoke (*Cynara scolymus* L.)	Cholegogue
Globe artichoke (*Cynara scolymus* L.)	Cholelithiasis
Goldenseal (*Hydrastis canadensis* L.), berberine	Bile flow stimulant
Goldenseal (*Hydrastis canadensis* L.), berberine	Gallstones
Horse chestnut (*Aesculus hippocastanum* L.)	Gallbladder infection (cholecystitis)
Horse chestnut (*Aesculus hippocastanum* L.)	Gallbladder pain (colic)
Horse chestnut (*Aesculus hippocastanum* L.)	Gallbladder stones (cholelithiasis)
Lavender (*Lavandula angustifolia* Miller)	Cholagogue
Lavender (*Lavandula angustifolia* Miller)	Choleretic
Milk thistle (*Silybum marianum*), silymarin	Cholelithiasis
Omega-3 fatty acids, fish oil, alpha-linolenic acid	Gallstones
Peppermint (*Mentha x piperita* L.)	Bile duct disorders
Peppermint (*Mentha x piperita* L.)	Cholelithiasis (gallstones)
Peppermint (*Mentha x piperita* L.)	Gallbladder disorders
Psyllium (*Plantago ovata, P. ispaghula*)	Gallstones
Turmeric (*Curcuma longa* L.), curcumin	Gallstones
White horehound (*Marrubium vulgare*)	Bile secretion
White horehound (*Marrubium vulgare*)	Gallbladder complaints
Wild yam (*Dioscorea villosa*)	Bile flow improvement
Wild yam (*Dioscorea villosa*)	Biliary colic

GASTROINTESTINAL DISORDERS AND RELATED CONDITIONS
Levels of Scientific Evidence for Specific Therapies

GRADE: C (Unclear or Conflicting Scientific Evidence)

Therapy	Specific Therapeutic Use(s)
Belladonna (*Atropa belladonna* L. or its variety *acuminata* Royle ex Lindl)	Irritable bowel syndrome
Chamomile (*Matricaria recutita, Chamaemelum nobile*)	Gastrointestinal conditions
Clay	Functional gastrointestinal disorders
Globe artichoke (*Cynara scolymus* L.)	Irritable bowel syndrome
Lactobacillus acidophilus	Irritable bowel syndrome
Lactobacillus acidophilus	Necrotizing enterocolitis prevention in infants
Peppermint (*Mentha x piperita* L.)	Irritable bowel syndrome

Continued

Psyllium (*Plantago ovata, P. ispaghula*)   Irritable bowel syndrome

Slippery elm (*Ulmus rubra* Muhl., *U. fulva* Michx.)   Gastrointestinal disorders

White horehound (*Marrubium vulgare*)   Intestinal disorders/ antispasmodic

TRADITIONAL OR THEORETICAL USES THAT LACK SUFFICIENT EVIDENCE	
Therapy	Specific Therapeutic Use(s)
Alfalfa (*Medicago sativa* L.)	Gastrointestinal tract disorders
Aloe (*Aloe vera*)	Bowel disorders
American pennyroyal (*Hedeoma pulegioides* L.), European pennyroyal (*Mentha pulegium* L.)	Bowel disorders
American pennyroyal (*Hedeoma pulegioides* L.), European pennyroyal (*Mentha pulegium* L.)	Colic
American pennyroyal (*Hedeoma pulegioides* L.), European pennyroyal (*Mentha pulegium* L.)	Intestinal disorders
American pennyroyal (*Hedeoma pulegioides* L.), European pennyroyal (*Mentha pulegium* L.)	Stomach pain
American pennyroyal (*Hedeoma pulegioides* L.), European pennyroyal (*Mentha pulegium* L.)	Stomach spasms
Arginine (L-arginine)	Infantile necrotizing enterocolitis
Arginine (L-arginine)	Lower esophageal sphincter relaxation
Arginine (L-arginine)	Stomach motility disorders
Astragalus (*Astragalus membranaceus*)	Gastrointestinal disorders
Barley (*Hordeum vulgare* L.), germinated barley foodstuff (GBF)	Bowel/intestinal disorders
Belladonna (*Atropa belladonna* L. or its variety *acuminata* Royle ex Lindl)	Diverticulitis
Bilberry (*Vaccinium myrtillus*)	Stomach upset
Bitter melon (*Momordica charantia* L.), MAP30	Gastrointestinal cramps
Black tea (*Camellia sinensis*)	Stomach disorders
Bladderwrack (*Fucus vesiculosus*)	Stomach upset
Bromelain	Leaky gut syndrome
Calendula (*Calendula officinalis* L.), marigold	Bowel irritation
Calendula (*Calendula officinalis* L.), marigold	Gastrointestinal tract disorders
Chamomile (*Matricaria recutita, Chamaemelum nobile*)	Abdominal bloating
Chamomile (*Matricaria recutita, Chamaemelum nobile*)	Infantile colic
Chamomile (*Matricaria recutita, Chamaemelum nobile*)	Irritable bowel syndrome
Chaparral (*Larrea tridentata* DC. Coville, *L. divaricata* Cav.), nordihydroguaiaretic acid (NDGA)	Bowel cramps
Chaparral (*Larrea tridentata* DC. Coville, *L. divaricata* Cav.), nordihydroguaiaretic acid (NDGA)	Gastrointestinal disorders
Clay	Stomach disorders
Clove (*Eugenia aromatica*)	Abdominal pain

Clove (*Eugenia aromatica*)	Colic
Cranberry (*Vaccinium macrocarpon*)	Stomach ailments
Dandelion (*Taraxacum officinale*)	Stomachache
Devil's claw (*Harpagophytum procumbens* DC.)	Gastrointestinal disorders
Dong quai (*Angelica sinensis* [Oliv.] Diels), Chinese angelica	Abdominal pain
Dong quai (*Angelica sinensis* [Oliv.] Diels), Chinese angelica	Irritable bowel syndrome
Echinacea (*Echinacea angustifolia* DC., *E. pallida*, *E. purpurea*)	Stomach upset
Elder (*Sambucus nigra* L.)	Colic
Elder (*Sambucus nigra* L.)	Gut disorders
Evening primrose oil (*Oenothera biennis* L.)	Irritable bowel syndrome
Eyebright (*Euphrasia officinalis*)	Gastric acid secretion stimulation
Fenugreek (*Trigonella foenum-graecum* L.)	Colic
Feverfew (*Tanacetum parthenium* L. Schultz-Bip.)	Abdominal pain
Flaxseed and flaxseed oil (*Linum usitatissimum*)	Abdominal pain
Flaxseed and flaxseed oil (*Linum usitatissimum*)	Diverticulitis
Flaxseed and flaxseed oil (*Linum usitatissimum*)	Irritable bowel syndrome
Flaxseed and flaxseed oil (*Linum usitatissimum*)	Laxative-induced colon damage
Flaxseed and flaxseed oil (*Linum usitatissimum*)	Stomach upset
Garlic (*Allium sativum* L.)	Stomachache
Ginger (*Zingiber officinale* Roscoe)	Colic
Ginger (*Zingiber officinale* Roscoe)	Stomachache
Ginseng (American ginseng, Asian ginseng, Chinese red ginseng, Korean red ginseng, *Panax ginseng*: *Panax* spp. including *P. ginseng* C.C. Meyer and *P. quincefolium* L., excluding *Eleutherococcus senticosus*)	Stomach upset
Goldenseal (*Hydrastis canadensis* L.), berberine	Stomachache
Green tea (*Camellia sinensis*)	Stomach disorders
Gymnema (*Gymnema Sylvestre* R. Br.)	Stomach ailments
Hawthorn (*Crataegus laevigata*, *C. oxyacantha*, *C. monogyna*, *C. pentagyna*)	Abdominal colic
Hawthorn (*Crataegus laevigata*, *C. oxyacantha*, *C. monogyna*, *C. pentagyna*)	Abdominal distention
Hawthorn (*Crataegus laevigata*, *C. oxyacantha*, *C. monogyna*, *C. pentagyna*)	Abdominal pain
Hawthorn (*Crataegus laevigata*, *C. oxyacantha*, *C. monogyna*, *C. pentagyna*)	Stomachache
Hops (*Humulus lupulus* L.)	Irritable bowel syndrome
Horsetail (*Equisetum arvense* L.)	Stomach upset
Kava (*Piper methysticum* G. Forst)	Stomach upset
Lactobacillus acidophilus	Diverticulitis

Continued

Lavender (*Lavandula angustifolia* Miller)	Colic
Licorice (*Glycyrrhiza glabra* L.), deglycyrrhizinated licorice (DGL)	Diverticulitis
Licorice (*Glycyrrhiza glabra* L.),d deglycyrrhizinated licorice (DGL)	Stomach upset
Marshmallow (*Althaea officinalis* L.)	Diverticulitis
Marshmallow (*Althaea officinalis* L.)	Irritable bowel syndrome
Melatonin	Intestinal motility disorders
Passionflower (*Passiflora incarnata* L.)	Gastrointestinal discomfort (nervous stomach)
Peppermint (*Mentha x piperita* L.)	Gastrointestinal disorders
Peppermint (*Mentha x piperita* L.)	Ileus (postoperative)
Peppermint (*Mentha x piperita* L.)	Intestinal colic
Propolis	Diverticulitis
Pygeum (*Prunus africana, Pygeum africanum*)	Stomach upset
Red yeast rice (*Monascus purpureus*)	Colic in children
Red yeast rice (*Monascus purpureus*)	Stomach problems
Shark cartilage	Intestinal disorders and inflammation
Slippery elm (*Ulmus rubra* Muhl., *U. fulva* Michx.)	Colic
Slippery elm (*Ulmus rubra* Muhl., *U. fulva* Michx.)	Diverticulitis
Slippery elm (*Ulmus rubra* Muhl., *U. fulva* Michx.)	Irritable bowel syndrome)
Sorrel (*Rumex acetosa* L., *R. acetosella* L.), Sinupret	Stimulation of secretion
Sorrel (*Rumex acetosa* L., *R. acetosella* L.), Sinupret	Ulcerated bowel
Soy (*Glycine max* L. Merr.)	Gastrointestinal motility
Spirulina	Bowel health
Thyme (*Thymus vulgaris* L.), thymol	Colic
Thyme (*Thymus vulgaris* L.), thymol	Stomach cramps
Turmeric (*Curcuma longa* L.), curcumin	Bloating
Turmeric (*Curcuma longa* L.), curcumin	Colic
Valerian (*Valeriana officinalis* L.)	Bloating
Valerian (*Valeriana officinalis* L.)	Colic
Valerian (*Valeriana officinalis* L.)	Intestinal disorders
Valerian (*Valeriana officinalis* L.)	Irritable bowel syndrome
Valerian (*Valeriana officinalis* L.)	Viral gastroenteritis
White horehound (*Marrubium vulgare*)	Bloating
White horehound (*Marrubium vulgare*)	Colic
Wild yam (*Dioscorea villosa*)	Diverticulitis
Wild yam (*Dioscorea villosa*)	Irritable bowel syndrome

GENERALIZED ANXIETY DISORDER AND RELATED CONDITIONS

Levels of Scientific Evidence for Specific Therapies

GRADE: A (Strong Scientific Evidence)

Therapy	Specific Therapeutic Use(s)
Kava (*Piper methysticum* G. Forst)	Anxiety

GRADE: B (Good Scientific Evidence)

Therapy	Specific therapeutic Use(s)
Lavender (*Lavandula angustifolia* Miller)	Anxiety (lavender aromatherapy)

GRADE: C (Unclear or Conflicting Scientific Evidence)

Therapy	Specific Therapeutic Use(s)
Gotu kola (*Centella asiatica* L.), total triterpenic fraction of *Centella asiatica* (TTFCA)	Anxiety
St. John's wort (*Hypericum perforatum* L.)	Anxiety disorder
Valerian (*Valeriana officinalis* L.)	Anxiety

TRADITIONAL OR THEORETICAL USES THAT LACK SUFFICIENT EVIDENCE

Therapy	Specific Therapeutic Use(s)
American pennyroyal (*Hedeoma pulegioides* L.), European pennyroyal (*Mentha pulegium* L.)	Anxiolytic
Belladonna (*Atropa belladonna* L. or its variety *acuminata* Royle ex Lindl)	Anxiety
Black cohosh (*Cimicifuga racemosa* L. Nutt.)	Anxiety
Black tea (*Camellia sinensis*)	Anxiety
Calendula (*Calendula officinalis* L.), marigold	Anxiety
Chamomile (*Matricaria recutita, Chamaemelum nobile*)	Anxiety
Danshen (*Salvia miltiorrhiza*)	Anxiety
DHEA (dehydroepiandrosterone)	Anxiety
DHEA (dehydroepiandrosterone)	Stress
Dong quai (*Angelica sinensis* [Oliv.] Diels), Chinese angelica	Anxiety
Dong quai (*Angelica sinensis* [Oliv.] Diels), Chinese angelica	Stress
Elder (*Sambucus nigra* L.)	Stress reduction
Eucalyptus oil (*Eucalyptus globulus* Labillardiere, *E. fructicetorum* F. Von Mueller, *E. smithii* R.T. Baker)	Aromatherapy
Garlic (*Allium sativum* L.)	Stress (anxiety)
Ginkgo (*Ginkgo biloba* L.)	Anxiety
Ginseng (American ginseng, Asian ginseng, Chinese ginseng, Korean red ginseng, *Panax ginseng*: *Panax* spp. including *P. ginseng* C.C. Meyer and *P. quincefolium* L., excluding *Eleutherococcus senticosus*)	Aggression

Continued

Ginseng (American ginseng, Asian ginseng, Chinese ginseng, Korean red ginseng, *Panax ginseng*: *Panax* spp. including *P. ginseng* C.C. Meyer and *P. quincefolium* L., excluding *Eleutherococcus senticosus*)   Anxiety

Ginseng (American ginseng, Asian ginseng, Chinese ginseng, Korean red ginseng, *Panax ginseng*: *Panax* spp. including *P. ginseng* C.C. Meyer and *P. quincefolium* L., excluding *Eleutherococcus senticosus*)   Stress

Goldenseal (*Hydrastis canadensis* L.), berberine   Anxiety

Gotu kola (*Centella asiatica* L.), total triterpenic fraction of *Centella asiatica* (TTFCA)   Anxiety

Hops (*Humulus lupulus* L.)   Anxiety

Hops (*Humulus lupulus* L.)   Anxiety during menopause

Lavender (*Lavandula angustifolia* Miller)   Anxiety

Niacin (vitamin B$_3$, nicotinic acid), niacinamide, and inositol hexanicotinate   Anxiety

Omega-3 fatty acids, fish oil, alpha-linolenic acid   Panic disorder

Passionflower (*Passiflora incarnata* L.)   Tension

Spirulina   Anxiety

Thyme (*Thymus vulgaris* L.), thymol   Anxiety

Valerian (*Valeriana officinalis* L.)   Stress

Yohimbe bark extract (*Pausinystalia yohimbe* Pierre ex Beille)   Panic disorder

GENITAL HERPES SIMPLEX VIRUS (HSV) INFECTION AND RELATED CONDITIONS

Levels of Scientific Evidence for Specific Therapies

GRADE: B (Good Scientific Evidence)

Therapy	Specific Therapeutic Use(s)
Aloe (*Aloe vera)*	Genital HSV infection

GRADE: C (Unclear or Conflicting Scientific Evidence)

Therapy	Specific Therapeutic Use(s)
Licorice (*Glycyrrhiza glabra* L.), deglycyrrhizinated licorice (DGL)	HSV infection
Propolis	Genital HSV infection
Tea tree oil (*Melaleuca alternifolia* [Maiden & Betche] Cheel)	Genital HSV infection

GRADE: D (Fair Negative Scientific Evidence)

Therapy	Specific Therapeutic Use(s)
Echinacea (*Echinacea angustifolia* DC., *E. pallida*, *E. purpurea*)	Genital HSV infection
Licorice (*Glycyrrhiza glabra* L.), deglycyrrhizinated licorice (DGL)	Genital HSV infection

TRADITIONAL OR THEORETICAL USES THAT LACK SUFFICIENT EVIDENCE

Therapy	Specific Therapeutic Use(s)
Astragalus (*Astragalus membranaceus*)	Genital HSV infection
Belladonna (*Atropa belladonna* L. or its variety *acuminata* Royle ex Lindl)	Chickenpox
Bromelain	Shingles pain/postherpetic neuralgia
Calendula (*Calendula officinalis* L.), marigold	HSV infection
Chaparral (*Larrea tridentata* DC. Coville, *L. divaricata* Cav.), nordihydroguaiaretic acid (NDGA)	Chickenpox
Clove (*Eugenia aromatica*)	HSV infection
Elder (*Sambucus nigra* L.)	HSV infection
Eucalyptus oil (*Eucalyptus globulus* Labillardiere, *E. fructicetorum* F. Von Mueller, *E. smithii* R.T. Baker)	HSV infection
Eucalyptus oil (*Eucalyptus globulus* Labillardiere, *E. fructicetorum* F. Von Mueller, *E. smithii* R.T. Baker)	Shingles
Ginseng (American ginseng, Asian ginseng, Chinese red ginseng, Korean red ginseng, *Panax ginseng*: *Panax* spp. including *P. ginseng* C.C. Meyer and *P. quincefolium* L., excluding *Eleutherococcus senticosus*)	HSV infection
Goldenseal (*Hydrastis canadensis* L.), berberine	Chickenpox
Goldenseal (*Hydrastis canadensis* L.), berberine	HSV infection
Gotu kola (*Centella asiatica* L.), total triterpenic fraction of *Centella asiatica* (TTFCA)	HSV-2 infection
Gotu kola (*Centella asiatica* L.), total triterpenic fraction of *Centella asiatica* (TTFCA)	Shingles (postherpetic neuralgia)
Peppermint (*Mentha x piperita* L.)	Chickenpox
Peppermint (*Mentha x piperita* L.)	Postherpetic neuralgia
Slippery elm (*Ulmus rubra* Muhl., *U. fulva* Michx.)	HSV infection
Spirulina	HSV-1 infection
St. John's wort (*Hypericum perforatum* L.)	HSV infection
Tea tree oil (*Melaleuca alternifolia* [Maiden & Betche] Cheel)	HSV infection

GLAUCOMA AND RELATED CONDITIONS
Levels of Scientific Evidence for Specific Therapies

GRADE: C (Unclear or Conflicting Scientific Evidence)

Therapy	Specific Therapeutic Use(s)
Bilberry (*Vaccinium myrtillus*)	Cataracts
Danshen (*Salvia miltiorrhiza*)	Glaucoma
Ginkgo (*Ginkgo biloba* L.)	Glaucoma
Melatonin	Glaucoma

Continued

TRADITIONAL OR THEORETICAL USES THAT LACK SUFFICIENT EVIDENCE	
Therapy	Specific therapeutic Use(s)
Arginine (L-arginine)	Glaucoma
Belladonna (*Atropa belladonna* L. or its variety *acuminata* Royle ex Lindl)	Glaucoma
Betel nut (*Areca catechu* L.)	Glaucoma
Bilberry (*Vaccinium myrtillus*)	Glaucoma
Danshen (*Salvia miltiorrhiza*)	Cataracts
Dong quai (*Angelica sinensis* [Oliv.] Diels), Chinese angelica	Glaucoma
Eyebright (*Euphrasia officinalis*)	Cataracts
Green tea (*Camellia sinensis*)	Cataracts
Lycopene	Cataracts
Melatonin	Glaucoma
Niacin (vitamin B_3, nicotinic acid), niacinamide, and inositol hexanicotinate	Cataract prevention
Omega-3 fatty acids, fish oil, alpha-linolenic acid	Glaucoma
Shark cartilage	Glaucoma
Turmeric (*Curcuma longa* L.), curcumin	Cataracts

GOITER AND RELATED CONDITIONS

Levels of Scientific Evidence for Specific Therapies

GRADE: C (Unclear or Conflicting Scientific Evidence)	
Therapy	Specific therapeutic Use(s)
Bladderwrack (*Fucus vesiculosus*)	Goiter (thyroid disease)

TRADITIONAL OR THEORETICAL USES THAT LACK SUFFICIENT EVIDENCE	
Therapy	Specific Therapeutic Use(s)
Essiac	Thyroid disorders
Horsetail (*Equisetum arvense* L.)	Thyroid disorders
Niacin (vitamin B_3, nicotinic acid), niacinamide, and inositol hexanicotinate	Hypothyroidism
Propolis	Thyroid disease
Seaweed, kelp, bladderwrack (*Fucus vesiculosus*)	Exophthalmos
Seaweed, kelp, bladderwrack (*Fucus vesiculosus*)	Goiter
Seaweed, kelp, bladderwrack (*Fucus vesiculosus*)	Myxedema

GOUT AND RELATED CONDITIONS

Levels of Scientific Evidence for Specific Therapies

TRADITIONAL OR THEORETICAL USES THAT LACK SUFFICIENT EVIDENCE

Therapy	Specific Therapeutic Use(s)
American pennyroyal (*Hedeoma pulegioides* L.), European pennyroyal (*Mentha pulegium* L.)	Gout
Belladonna (*Atropa belladonna* L. or its variety *acuminata* Royle ex Lindl)	Gout
Bilberry (*Vaccinium myrtillus*)	Gout
Bromelain	Gout
Burdock (*Arctium lappa*)	Gout
Calendula (*Calendula officinalis* L.), marigold	Gout
Clove (Eugenia aromatica)	Gout
Dandelion (*Taraxacum officinale*)	Gout
Devil's claw (*Harpagophytum procumbens* DC.)	Gout
Ephedra (*Ephedra sinica*)/ma huang	Gout
Fenugreek (*Trigonella foenum-graecum* L.)	Gout
Globe artichoke (*Cynara scolymus* L.)	Gout
Gymnema (*Gymnema Sylvestre* R. Br.)	Gout
Horsetail (*Equisetum arvense* L.)	Gout
Omega-3 fatty acids, fish oil, alpha-linolenic acid	Gout
Red clover (*Trifolium pratense*)	Gout
Slippery elm (*Ulmus rubra* Muhl., *U. fulva* Michx.)	Gout
Thyme (*Thymus vulgaris* L.), thymol	Gout

HAIR LOSS AND RELATED CONDITIONS

Levels of Scientific Evidence for Specific Therapies

GRADE: C (Unclear or Conflicting Scientific Evidence)

Therapy	Specific Therapeutic Use(s)
Saw palmetto (*Serenoa repens* [Bartram] Small)	Androgenetic alopecia (topical)
Thyme (*Thymus vulgaris* L.), thymol	Alopecia areata

TRADITIONAL OR THEORETICAL USES THAT LACK SUFFICIENT EVIDENCE

Therapy	Specific Therapeutic Use(s)
Aloe (*Aloe vera*)	Alopecia (hair loss)
Bladderwrack (*Fucus vesiculosus*)	Hair loss
Burdock (*Arctium lappa*)	Dandruff
Burdock (*Arctium lappa*)	Hair loss

Continued

Therapy	Specific Therapeutic Use(s)
Chaparral (*Larrea tridentata* DC. Coville, *L. divaricata* Cav.), nordihydroguaiaretic acid (NDGA)	Hair tonic
Coenzyme Q10	Hair loss
Dandelion (*Taraxacum officinale*)	Dandruff
Elder (*Sambucus nigra* L.)	Hair dye
Fenugreek (*Trigonella foenum-graecum* L.)	Baldness
Garlic (*Allium sativum* L.)	Hair growth
Ginger (*Zingiber officinale* Roscoe)	Baldness
Goldenseal (*Hydrastis canadensis* L.), berberine	Dandruff
Gotu kola (*Centella asiatica* L.), total triterpenic fraction of *Centella asiatica* (TTFCA)	Hair growth promoter
Horsetail (*Equisetum arvense* L.)	Hair loss
Lavender (*Lavandula angustifolia* Miller)	Hair loss
Pygeum (*Prunus africana, Pygeum africanum*)	Male baldness
Seaweed, kelp, bladderwrack (*Fucus vesiculosus*)	Hair loss
Spirulina	Hair loss

HALITOSIS AND RELATED CONDITIONS
Levels of Scientific Evidence for Specific Therapies

TRADITIONAL OR THEORETICAL USES THAT LACK SUFFICIENT EVIDENCE

Therapy	Specific Therapeutic Use(s)
Clove (*Eugenia aromatica*)	Bad breath
Licorice (*Glycyrrhiza glabra* L.), deglycyrrhizinated licorice (DGL)	Bad breath
Thyme (*Thymus vulgaris* L.), thymol	Halitosis

HEADACHE AND RELATED CONDITIONS
Levels of Scientific Evidence for Specific Therapies

GRADE: B (Good Scientific Evidence)

Therapy	Specific Therapeutic Use(s)
Feverfew (*Tanacetum parthenium* L. Schultz-Bip.)	Migraine headache prevention

GRADE: C (Unclear or Conflicting Scientific Evidence)

Therapy	Specific Therapeutic Use(s)
Arginine (L-arginine)	Migraine headache
Belladonna (*Atropa belladonna* L. or its variety *acuminata* Royle ex Lindl)	Headache
Eucalyptus oil (*Eucalyptus globulus* Labillardiere, *E. fructicetorum* F. Von Mueller, *E. smithii* R.T. Baker)	Headache (applied to the skin)
Melatonin	Headache prevention
Peppermint (*Mentha x piperita* L.)	Tension headache

Continued

TRADITIONAL OR THEORETICAL USES THAT LACK SUFFICIENT EVIDENCE	
Therapy	Specific Therapeutic Use(s)
American pennyroyal (*Hedeoma pulegioides* L.), European pennyroyal (*Mentha pulegium* L.)	Headache
Black cohosh (*Cimicifuga racemosa* L. Nutt.)	Headache
Black tea (*Camellia sinensis*)	Headache
Burdock (*Arctium lappa*)	Headache
Calendula (*Calendula officinalis* L.), marigold	Headache
Dandelion (*Taraxacum officinale*)	Headache
Devil's claw (*Harpagophytum procumbens* DC.)	Headache
Devil's claw (*Harpagophytum procumbens* DC.)	Migraine headache
Dong quai (*Angelica sinensis* [Oliv.] Diels), Chinese angelica	Headache
Dong quai (*Angelica sinensis* [Oliv.] Diels), Chinese angelica	Migraine headache
Echinacea (*Echinacea angustifolia* DC., *E. pallida*, *E. purpurea*)	Migraine headache
Elder (*Sambucus nigra* L.)	Headache
Elder (*Sambucus nigra* L.)	Migraine headache
Eyebright (*Euphrasia officinalis*)	Headache
Garlic (*Allium sativum* L.)	Headache
Ginger (*Zingiber officinale* Roscoe)	Headache
Ginger (*Zingiber officinale* Roscoe)	Migraine headache
Ginkgo (*Ginkgo biloba* L.)	Headache
Ginkgo (*Ginkgo biloba* L.)	Migraine headache
Ginseng (American ginseng, Asian ginseng, Chinese ginseng, Korean red ginseng, *Panax ginseng*: *Panax* spp. including *P. ginseng* C.C. Meyer and *P. quincefolium* L., excluding *Eleutherococcus senticosus*)	Headache
Ginseng (American ginseng, Asian ginseng, Chinese ginseng, Korean red ginseng, *Panax ginseng*: *Panax* spp. including *P. ginseng* C.C. Meyer and *P. quincefolium* L., excluding *Eleutherococcus senticosus*)	Migraine headache
Glucosamine	Migraine headache
Goldenseal (*Hydrastis canadensis* L.), berberine	Headache
Green tea (*Camellia sinensis*)	Headache
Kava (*Piper methysticum* G. Forst)	Migraine headache
Lavender (*Lavandula angustifolia* Miller)	Migraine headache
Lavender (*Lavandula angustifolia* Miller)	Tension headache
Niacin (vitamin B_3, nicotinic acid), niacinamide, and inositol hexanicotinate	Migraine headache
Omega-3 fatty acids, fish oil, alpha-linolenic acid	Headache
Saw palmetto (*Serenoa repens* [Bartram] Small)	Migraine headache
Soy (*Glycine max* L. Merr.)	Headache

Thyme (*Thymus vulgaris* L.), thymol	Headache
Valerian (*Valeriana officinalis* L.)	Migraine headache
Valerian (*Valeriana officinalis* L.)	Tension headaches

HEART FAILURE AND RELATED CONDITIONS

Levels of Scientific Evidence for Specific Therapies

GRADE: A (Strong Scientific Evidence)

Therapy	Specific Therapeutic Use(s)
Hawthorn (*Crataegus laevigata, C. oxyacantha, C. monogyna, C. pentagyna*)	Congestive heart failure

GRADE: C (Unclear or Conflicting Scientific Evidence)

Therapy	Specific Therapeutic Use(s)
Arginine (L-arginine)	Heart failure (congestive)
Astragalus (*Astragalus membranaceus*)	Heart failure
Coenzyme Q10	Cardiomyopathy (dilated, hypertrophic)
Coenzyme Q10	Heart failure
Dehydroepiandrosterone (DHEA)	Heart failure
Ginseng (American ginseng, Asian ginseng, Chinese ginseng, Korean red ginseng, *Panax ginseng*: *Panax* spp. including *P. ginseng* C.C. Meyer and *P. quinquefolium* L., excluding *Eleutherococcus senticosus*)	Congestive heart failure
Hawthorn (*Crataegus laevigata, C. oxyacantha, C. monogyna, C. pentagyna*)	Functional cardiovascular disorders
Oleander (*Nerium oleander, Thevetia peruviana*)	Congestive heart failure
Passionflower (*Passiflora incarnata* L.)	Congestive heart failure (exercise capacity)

GRADE: D (Fair Negative Scientific Evidence)

TRADITIONAL OR THEORETICAL USES THAT LACK SUFFICIENT EVIDENCE

Therapy	Specific Therapeutic Use(s)
Dandelion (*Taraxacum officinale*)	Congestive heart failure
Danshen (*Salvia miltiorrhiza*)	Left ventricular hypertrophy
Dong quai (*Angelica sinensis* [Oliv.] Diels), Chinese angelica	Congestive heart failure
Ginkgo (*Ginkgo biloba* L.)	Congestive heart failure
Goldenseal (*Hydrastis canadensis* L.), berberine	Heart failure
Horse chestnut (*Aesculus hippocastanum* L.)	Fluid in the lungs (pulmonary edema)
Horsetail (*Equisetum arvense* L.)	Fluid in the lungs
Omega-3 fatty acids, fish oil, alpha-linolenic acid	Congestive heart failure
Passionflower (*Passiflora incarnata* L.)	Congestive heart failure (exercise ability)
Valerian (*Valeriana officinalis* L.)	Congestive heart failure

HEARTBURN AND RELATED CONDITIONS

Levels of Scientific Evidence for Specific Therapies

GRADE: C (Unclear or Conflicting Scientific Evidence)

Therapy	Specific Therapeutic Use(s)
Bilberry (*Vaccinium myrtillus*)	Stomach ulcers (peptic ulcer disease)
Blessed thistle (*Cnicus benedictus* L.)	Indigestion and flatulence (gas)
Cranberry (*Vaccinium macrocarpon*)	Stomach ulcers caused by *Helicobacter pylori* bacteria
Globe artichoke (*Cynara scolymus* L.)	Nonulcer dyspepsia
Licorice (*Glycyrrhiza glabra* L.), deglycyrrhizinated licorice (DGL)	Bleeding stomach ulcers caused by aspirin
Licorice (*Glycyrrhiza glabra* L.), deglycyrrhizinated licorice (DGL)	Peptic ulcer disease
Peppermint (*Mentha* x *piperita* L.)	Indigestion (nonulcer dyspepsia)
Turmeric (*Curcuma longa* L.), curcumin	Dyspepsia (heartburn)
Turmeric (*Curcuma longa* L.), curcumin	Peptic ulcer disease (stomach ulcer)
White horehound (*Marrubium vulgare* L.)	Heartburn/poor appetite

GRADE: D (Fair Negative Scientific Evidence)

Therapy	Specific Therapeutic Use(s)
Garlic (*Allium sativum* L.)	Stomach ulcers caused by *Helicobacter pylori* bacteria

TRADITIONAL OR THEORETICAL USES THAT LACK SUFFICIENT EVIDENCE

Therapy	Specific Therapeutic Use(s)
Alfalfa (*Medicago sativa* L.)	Indigestion
Alfalfa (*Medicago sativa* L.)	Stomach ulcers
American pennyroyal (*Hedeoma pulegioides* L.), European pennyroyal (*Mentha pulegium* L.)	Indigestion
Arginine (L-arginine)	Stomach ulcer
Astragalus (*Astragalus membranaceus*)	Stomach ulcer
Barley (*Hordeum vulgare* L.), germinated barley foodstuff (GBF)	Gastritis
Barley (*Hordeum vulgare* L.), germinated barley foodstuff (GBF)	Gastrointestinal inflammation
Belladonna (*Atropa belladonna* L. or its variety *A. acuminata* Royle ex Lindl)	Stomach ulcers
Bilberry (*Vaccinium myrtillus*)	Dyspepsia
Bilberry (*Vaccinium myrtillus*)	Infantile dyspepsia
Bladderwrack (*Fucus vesiculosus*)	Heartburn
Bladderwrack (*Fucus vesiculosus*)	Ulcer

Continued

Boswellia (*Boswellia serrata* Roxb.)	Dyspepsia
Boswellia (*Boswellia serrata* Roxb.)	Peptic ulcer disease
Bromelain	Indigestion
Bromelain	Stomach ulcer/stomach ulcer prevention
Calendula (*Calendula officinalis* L.), marigold	Indigestion
Calendula (*Calendula officinalis* L.), marigold	Stomach ulcers
Chamomile (*Matricaria recutita, Chamaemelum nobile*)	Heartburn
Chaparral (*Larrea tridentata* DC. Coville, *L. divaricata* Cav), nordihydroguaiaretic acid (NDGA)	Heartburn
Chaparral (*Larrea tridentata* DC. Coville, *L. divaricata* Cav), nordihydroguaiaretic acid (NDGA)	Indigestion
Chaparral (*Larrea tridentata* DC. Coville, *L. divaricata* Cav), nordihydroguaiaretic acid (NDGA)	Stomach ulcer
Coenzyme Q10	Stomach ulcer
Dandelion (*Taraxacum officinale*)	Heartburn
Danshen (*Salvia miltiorrhiza*)	Gastric ulcers
Danshen (*Salvia miltiorrhiza*)	Stomach ulcers
Devil's claw (*Harpagophytum procumbens* DC.)	Dyspepsia
Devil's claw (*Harpagophytum procumbens* DC.)	Heartburn
Devil's claw (*Harpagophytum procumbens* DC.)	Indigestion
Dong quai (*Angelica sinensis* [Oliv.] Diels), Chinese angelica	Heartburn
Echinacea (*Echinacea angustifolia* DC., *E. pallida, E. purpurea*)	Dyspepsia
Evening primrose oil (*Oenothera biennis* L.)	Disorders of the stomach and intestines
Fenugreek (*Trigonella foenum-graecum* L.)	Dyspepsia
Fenugreek (*Trigonella foenum-graecum* L.)	Gastritis
Fenugreek (*Trigonella foenum-graecum* L.)	Indigestion
Flaxseed and flaxseed oil (*Linum usitatissimum*)	Enteritis
Flaxseed and flaxseed oil (*Linum usitatissimum*)	Gastritis
Garlic (*Allium sativum* L.)	Stomach acid reduction
Ginger (*Zingiber officinale* Roscoe)	Antacid
Ginger (*Zingiber officinale* Roscoe)	Dyspepsia
Ginger (*Zingiber officinale* Roscoe)	Helicobacter pylori infection
Ginger (*Zingiber officinale* Roscoe)	Stomach ulcers
Goldenseal (*Hydrastis canadensis* L.), berberine	Gastroenteritis
Goldenseal (*Hydrastis canadensis* L.), berberine	Indigestion
Goldenseal (*Hydrastis canadensis* L.), berberine	Stomach ulcers
Gotu kola (*Centella asiatica* L.) and total triterpenic fraction of *Centella asiatica* (TTFCA)	Gastritis
Green tea (*Camellia sinensis*)	Gastritis

Green tea (*Camellia sinensis*)	Helicobacter pylori infection
Hawthorn (*Crataegus laevigata, C. oxyacantha, C. monogyna, C. pentagyna*)	Dyspepsia
Hops (*Humulus lupulus* L.)	Indigestion
Horse chestnut (*Aesculus hippocastanum* L.)	Ulcers
Horsetail (*Equisetum arvense* L.)	Dyspepsia
Kava (*Piper methysticum* G. Forst)	Dyspepsia
Lactobacillus acidophilus	Heartburn
Lactobacillus acidophilus	Indigestion
Lactobacillus acidophilus	Stomach ulcer
Lavender (*Lavandula angustifolia* Miller)	Heartburn
Lavender (*Lavandula angustifolia* Miller)	Indigestion
Licorice (*Glycyrrhiza glabra* L.), deglycyrrhizinated licorice (DGL)	Gastroesophageal reflux disease
Marshmallow (*Althaea officinalis* L.)	Duodenal ulcer
Marshmallow (*Althaea officinalis* L.)	Enteritis
Marshmallow (*Althaea officinalis* L.)	Gastroenteritis
Marshmallow (*Althaea officinalis* L.)	Indigestion
Marshmallow (*Althaea officinalis* L.)	Peptic ulcer disease
Melatonin	Gastroesophageal reflux disease (GERD)
Niacin (vitamin B_3, nicotinic acid), niacinamide, inositol hexanicotinate	Stomach ulcer
Oleander (*Nerium oleander, Thevetia peruviana*)	Indigestion
Peppermint (*Mentha* x *piperita* L.)	Antacid
Peppermint (*Mentha* x *piperita* L.)	Enteritis
Peppermint (*Mentha* x *piperita* L.)	Gastritis
Propolis	Stomach ulcer
Psyllium (*Plantago ovata, P. ispaghula*)	Duodenal ulcer
Psyllium (*Plantago ovata, P. ispaghula*)	Stomach ulcer
Red clover (*Trifolium pratense*)	Indigestion
Red yeast rice (*Monascus purpureus*)	Indigestion
Saw palmetto (*Serenoa repens* [Bartram] Small)	Indigestion
Seaweed, kelp, bladderwrack (*Fucus vesiculosus*)	Dyspepsia
Seaweed, kelp, bladderwrack (*Fucus vesiculosus*)	Heartburn
Seaweed, kelp, bladderwrack (*Fucus vesiculosus*)	Ulcer
Shark cartilage	Enteritis
Slippery elm (*Ulmus rubra* Muhl. or *U. fulva* Michx.)	Duodenal ulcer
Slippery elm (*Ulmus rubra* Muhl. or *U. fulva* Michx.)	Enteritis

Continued

Slippery elm (*Ulmus rubra* Muhl. or *U. fulva* Michx.)	Gastric ulcer
Slippery elm (*Ulmus rubra* Muhl. or *U. fulva* Michx.)	Gastritis
Slippery elm (*Ulmus rubra* Muhl. or *U. fulva* Michx.)	Gastroesophageal reflux disease
Slippery elm (*Ulmus rubra* Muhl. or *U. fulva* Michx.)	Heartburn
Slippery elm (*Ulmus rubra* Muhl. or *U. fulva* Michx.)	Peptic ulcer disease
Spirulina	Stomach acid excess
Spirulina	Ulcers
St. John's wort (*Hypericum perforatum* L.)	Heartburn
St. John's wort (*Hypericum perforatum* L.)	Ulcers
Thyme (*Thymus vulgaris* L.), thymol	Dyspepsia
Thyme (*Thymus vulgaris* L.), thymol	Gastritis
Thyme (*Thymus vulgaris* L.), thymol	Heartburn
Thyme (*Thymus vulgaris* L.), thymol	Indigestion
Valerian (*Valeriana officinalis* L.)	Heartburn
Valerian (*Valeriana officinalis* L.)	Peptic ulcer disease
White horehound (*Marrubium vulgare* L.)	Indigestion

HEAVY METAL/LEAD TOXICITY AND RELATED CONDITIONS

Levels of Scientific Evidence for Specific Therapies

GRADE: C (Unclear or Conflicting Scientific Evidence)

Therapy	Specific Therapeutic Use(s)
Clay	Mercuric chloride poisoning

TRADITIONAL OR THEORETICAL USES THAT LACK SUFFICIENT EVIDENCE

Therapy	Specific Therapeutic Use(s)
Belladonna (*Atropa belladonna* L. or its variety *A. acuminata* Royle ex Lindl)	Poisoning (especially by insecticides)
Clay	Poisoning
Essiac	Blood cleanser
Essiac	Chelating agent (heavy metals)
Hoxsey formula	Elimination of toxins
Marshmallow (*Althaea officinalis* L.)	Antidote to poisons
Melatonin	Aluminum toxicity
Melatonin	Lead toxicity

HEPATITIS AND RELATED CONDITIONS

Levels of Scientific Evidence for Specific Therapies

GRADE: B (Good Scientific Evidence)

Therapy	Specific Therapeutic Use(s)
Milk thistle (*Silybum marianum*), silymarin	Cirrhosis
Milk thistle (*Silybum marianum*), silymarin	Hepatitis (chronic)

GRADE: C (Unclear or Conflicting Scientific Evidence)

Therapy	Specific Therapeutic Use(s)
Astragalus (*Astragalus membranaceus*)	Liver protection
Clay	Protection from aflatoxins
Dandelion (*Taraxacum officinale*)	Hepatitis B
Danshen (*Salvia miltiorrhiza*)	Liver disease (cirrhosis/chronic hepatitis B)
Eyebright (*Euphrasia officinalis*)	Hepatoprotection
Lactobacillus acidophilus	Hepatic encephalopathy (confused thinking due to liver disorders)
Licorice (*Glycyrrhiza glabra* L.), deglycyrrhizinated licorice (DGL)	Viral hepatitis
Milk thistle (*Silybum marianum*), silymarin	Acute viral hepatitis
Milk thistle (*Silybum marianum*), silymarin	Amanita phalloides mushroom toxicity
Milk thistle (*Silybum marianum*), silymarin	Drug/toxin-induced hepatotoxicity

TRADITIONAL OR THEORETICAL USES THAT LACK SUFFICIENT EVIDENCE

Therapy	Specific Therapeutic Use(s)
Alfalfa (*Medicago sativa* L.)	Jaundice
Aloe (*Aloe vera*)	Hepatitis
American pennyroyal (*Hedeoma pulegioides* L.), European pennyroyal (*Mentha pulegium* L.)	Liver disease
Arginine (L-arginine)	Ammonia toxicity
Arginine (L-arginine)	Hepatic encephalopathy
Arginine (L-arginine)	Liver disease
Astragalus (*Astragalus membranaceus*)	Chronic hepatitis
Astragalus (*Astragalus membranaceus*)	Liver disease
Bilberry (*Vaccinium myrtillus*)	Liver disease
Black cohosh (*Cimicifuga racemosa* L. Nutt.)	Liver disease
Blessed thistle (*Cnicus benedictus* L.)	Jaundice
Blessed thistle (*Cnicus benedictus* L.)	Liver disorders
Burdock (*Arctium lappa*)	Liver protection

Continued

Calendula (*Calendula officinalis* L.), marigold	Jaundice
Calendula (*Calendula officinalis* L.), marigold	Liver dysfunction
Chamomile (*Matricaria recutita, Chamaemelum nobile*)	Liver disorders
Coenzyme Q10	Hepatitis B
Coenzyme Q10	Liver enlargement or disease
Cranberry (*Vaccinium macrocarpon*)	Liver disorders
Dandelion (*Taraxacum officinale*)	Jaundice
Dandelion (*Taraxacum officinale*)	Liver cleansing
Dandelion (*Taraxacum officinale*)	Liver disease
Devil's claw (*Harpagophytum procumbens* DC.)	Liver and gallbladder tonic
Dehydroepiandrosterone (DHEA)	Liver protection
Dong quai (*Angelica sinensis* [Oliv.] Diels), Chinese angelica	Chronic hepatitis
Dong quai (*Angelica sinensis* [Oliv.] Diels), Chinese angelica	Cirrhosis
Dong quai (*Angelica sinensis* [Oliv.] Diels), Chinese angelica	Liver protection
Elder (*Sambucus nigra* L.)	Liver disease
Eucalyptus oil (*Eucalyptus globulus* Labillardiere, *E. fructicetorum* F. Von Mueller, *E. smithii* R.T. Baker)	Liver protection
Evening primrose oil (*Oenothera biennis* L.)	Hepatitis B
Eyebright (*Euphrasia officinalis*)	Jaundice
Eyebright (*Euphrasia officinalis*)	Liver disease
Garlic (*Allium sativum* L.)	Antitoxin
Garlic (*Allium sativum* L.)	Hepatopulmonary syndrome
Garlic (*Allium sativum* L.)	Liver health
Ginger (*Zingiber officinale* Roscoe)	Liver disease
Ginkgo (*Ginkgo biloba* L.)	Hepatitis B
Ginseng (American ginseng, Asian ginseng, Chinese ginseng, Korean red ginseng, *Panax ginseng*: *Panax* spp. including *P. ginseng* C.C. Meyer and *P. quinquefolium* L., excluding *Eleutherococcus senticosus*)	Hepatitis/hepatitis B infection
Ginseng (American ginseng, Asian ginseng, Chinese ginseng, Korean red ginseng, *Panax ginseng*: *Panax* spp. including *P. ginseng* C.C. Meyer and *P. quinquefolium* L., excluding *Eleutherococcus senticosus*)	Liver diseases
Ginseng (American ginseng, Asian ginseng, Chinese ginseng, Korean red ginseng, *Panax ginseng*: *Panax* spp. including *P. ginseng* C.C. Meyer and *P. quinquefolium* L., excluding *Eleutherococcus senticosus*)	Liver health
Globe artichoke (*Cynara scolymus* L.)	Jaundice
Goldenseal (*Hydrastis canadensis* L.), berberine	Alcoholic liver disease
Goldenseal (*Hydrastis canadensis* L.), berberine	Hepatitis
Goldenseal (*Hydrastis canadensis* L.), berberine	Jaundice
Goldenseal (*Hydrastis canadensis* L.), berberine	Liver disorders
Gotu kola (*Centella asiatica* L.), total triterpenic fraction of *Centella asiatica* (TTFCA)	Hepatitis

Gotu kola (*Centella asiatica* L.), total triterpenic fraction of *Centella asiatica* (TTFCA)	Jaundice
Gymnema (*Gymnema sylvestre* R. Br.)	Liver disease
Gymnema (*Gymnema sylvestre* R. Br.)	Liver protection
Horse chestnut (*Aesculus hippocastanum* L.)	Liver congestion
Horsetail (*Equisetum arvense* L.)	Liver protection
Licorice (*Glycyrrhiza glabra* L.), deglycyrrhizinated licorice (DGL)	Liver protection
Maitake mushroom (*Grifola frondosa*), beta-glucan	Liver inflammation (hepatitis)
Melatonin	Toxic liver damage
Milk thistle (*Silybum marianum*), silymarin	Jaundice
Milk thistle (*Silybum marianum*), silymarin	Liver cleansing agent
Niacin (vitamin B_3, nicotinic acid), niacinamide, inositol hexanicotinate	Liver disease
Omega-3 fatty acids, fish oil, alpha-linolenic acid	Cirrhosis

HERPES SIMPLEX VIRUS AND RELATED CONDITIONS

Levels of Scientific Evidence for Specific Therapies

GRADE: B (Good Scientific Evidence)

Therapy	Specific Therapeutic Use(s)
Aloe (*Aloe vera*)	Genital herpes

GRADE: C (Unclear or Conflicting Scientific Evidence)

Therapy	Specific Therapeutic Use(s)
Licorice (*Glycyrrhiza glabra* L.), deglycyrrhizinated licorice (DGL)	Herpes simplex virus
Propolis	Genital herpes simplex virus (HSV) infection
Tea tree oil (*Melaleuca alternifolia* [Maiden & Betche] Cheel)	Genital herpes

GRADE: D (Fair Negative Scientific Evidence)

Therapy	Specific Therapeutic Use(s)
Echinacea (*Echinacea angustifolia* DC., *E. pallida*, *E. purpurea*)	Genital herpes
Licorice (*Glycyrrhiza glabra* L.), deglycyrrhizinated licorice (DGL)	Genital herpes

TRADITIONAL OR THEORETICAL USES THAT LACK SUFFICIENT EVIDENCE

Therapy	Specific Therapeutic Use(s)
Astragalus (*Astragalus membranaceus*)	Genital herpes
Belladonna (*Atropa belladonna* L. or its variety *A. acuminata* Royle ex Lindl)	Chickenpox
Bromelain	Shingles pain/postherpetic neuralgia

Continued

Calendula (*Calendula officinalis* L.), marigold	Herpes simplex virus infections
Chaparral (*Larrea tridentata* DC. Coville, *L. divaricata* Cav.), nordihydroguaiaretic acid (NDGA)	Chickenpox
Clove (*Eugenia aromatica*)	Herpes simplex virus infection
Elder (*Sambucus nigra* L.)	Herpes
Eucalyptus oil (*Eucalyptus globulus* Labillardiere, *E. fructicetorum* F. Von Mueller, *E. smithii* R.T. Baker)	Herpes
Eucalyptus oil (*Eucalyptus globulus* Labillardiere, *E. fructicetorum* F. Von Mueller, *E. smithii* R.T. Baker)	Shingles
Ginseng (American ginseng, Asian ginseng, Chinese ginseng, Korean red ginseng, *Panax ginseng*: *Panax* spp. including *P. ginseng* C.C. Meyer and *P. quinquefolium* L., excluding *Eleutherococcus senticosus*)	Herpes
Goldenseal (*Hydrastis canadensis* L.), berberine	Chickenpox
Goldenseal (*Hydrastis canadensis* L.), berberine	Herpes
Gotu kola (*Centella asiatica* L.), total triterpenic fraction of *Centella asiatica* (TTFCA)	Herpes simplex virus type 2 (HSV-2) infection
Gotu kola (*Centella asiatica* L.), total triterpenic fraction of *Centella asiatica* (TTFCA)	Shingles (postherpetic neuralgia)
Peppermint (*Mentha* x *piperita* L.)	Chickenpox
Peppermint (*Mentha* x *piperita* L.)	Postherpetic neuralgia
Slippery elm (*Ulmus rubra* Muhl. or *U. fulva* Michx.)	Herpes
Spirulina	Herpes simplex virus type 1 (HSV-1) infection
St. John's wort (*Hypericum perforatum* L.)	Herpesvirus infection
Tea tree oil (*Melaleuca alternifolia* [Maiden & Betche] Cheel)	Herpes simplex virus infection

HIGH CHOLESTEROL AND RELATED CONDITIONS

Levels of Scientific Evidence for Specific Therapies

GRADE: A (Strong Scientific Evidence)	
Therapy	Specific Therapeutic Use(s)
Niacin (vitamin B_3, nicotinic acid), niacinamide, inositol hexanicotinate	High cholesterol (niacin)
Omega-3 fatty acids, fish oil, alpha-linolenic acid	Hypertriglyceridemia (fish oil/ eicosapentaenoic acid [EPA] plus docosahexaenoic acid [DHA])
Omega-3 fatty acids, fish oil, alpha-linolenic acid	Secondary cardiovascular disease prevention (fish oil/ eicosapentaenoic acid [EPA] plus docosahexaenoic acid [DHA])
Psyllium (*Plantago ovata*, *P. ispaghula*)	High cholesterol
Red yeast rice (*Monascus purpureus*)	High cholesterol
Soy (*Glycine max* L. Merr.)	High cholesterol

GRADE: B (Good Scientific Evidence)	
Therapy	**Specific Therapeutic Use(s)**
Barley (*Hordeum vulgare* L.), germinated barley foodstuff (GBF)	High cholesterol
Garlic (*Allium sativum* L.)	High cholesterol
Niacin (vitamin B_3, nicotinic acid), niacinamide, and inositol hexanicotinate	Atherosclerosis (niacin)
Niacin (vitamin B_3, nicotinic acid), niacinamide, and inositol hexanicotinate	Prevention of a second heart attack (niacin)
Omega-3 fatty acids, fish oil, alpha-linolenic acid prevention	Primary cardiovascular disease (fish intake)
Sweet almond (*Prunus amygdalus dulcis*)	High cholesterol (whole almonds)

GRADE: C (Unclear or Conflicting Scientific Evidence)	
Therapy	**Specific Therapeutic Use(s)**
Alfalfa (*Medicago sativa* L.)	Atherosclerosis (cholesterol plaques in heart arteries)
Alfalfa (*Medicago sativa* L.)	High cholesterol
Arginine (L-arginine)	Coronary artery disease/angina
Arginine (L-arginine)	Heart protection during coronary artery bypass grafting (CABG)
Astragalus (*Astragalus membranaceus*)	Coronary artery disease
Bilberry (*Vaccinium myrtillus*)	Atherosclerosis (hardening of the arteries) and peripheral vascular disease
Black tea (*Camellia sinensis*)	Heart attack prevention
Coenzyme Q10	Angina (chest pain from clogged heart arteries)
Coenzyme Q10	Heart attack (acute myocardial infarction)
Coenzyme Q10	Heart protection during surgery
Danshen (*Salvia miltiorrhiza*)	Cardiovascular disease/angina
Dehydroepiandrosterone (DHEA)	Atherosclerosis (cholesterol plaques in the arteries)
Dong quai (*Angelica sinensis* [Oliv.] Diels), Chinese angelica	Angina pectoris/coronary artery disease
Fenugreek (*Trigonella foenum-graecum* L.)	Hyperlipidemia
Flaxseed and flaxseed oil (*Linum usitatissimum*)	Heart disease (flaxseed and flaxseed oil)
Flaxseed and flaxseed oil (*Linum usitatissimum*)	High cholesterol or triglycerides (flaxseed and flaxseed oil)
Garlic (*Allium sativum* L.)	Atherosclerosis (hardening of the arteries)

Continued

Garlic (*Allium sativum* L.)	Familial hypercholesterolemia
Garlic (*Allium sativum* L.)	Heart attack prevention in patients with known heart disease
Ginseng (American ginseng, Asian ginseng, Chinese ginseng, Korean red ginseng, *Panax ginseng*: *Panax* spp. including *P. ginseng* C.C. Meyer and *P. quinquefolium* L., excluding *Eleutherococcus senticosus*)	Coronary artery (heart) disease
Globe artichoke (*Cynara scolymus* L.)	Lipid lowering (cholesterol and triglycerides)
Green tea (*Camellia sinensis*)	Heart attack prevention
Green tea (*Camellia sinensis*)	High cholesterol
Guggul (*Commifora mukul*)	Hyperlipidemia
Gymnema (*Gymnema sylvestre* R. Br.)	High cholesterol
Hawthorn (*Crataegus laevigata*, *C. oxyacantha*, *C. monogyna*, *C. pentagyna*)	Coronary artery disease (angina)
Lactobacillus acidophilus	High cholesterol
Lycopene	Atherosclerosis (clogged arteries) and high cholesterol
Milk thistle (*Silybum marianum*), silymarin	Hyperlipidemia
Omega-3 fatty acids, fish oil, alpha-linolenic acid	Angina pectoris
Omega-3 fatty acids, fish oil, alpha-linolenic acid	Atherosclerosis
Omega-3 fatty acids, fish oil, alpha-linolenic acid	Prevention of graft failure after heart bypass surgery
Omega-3 fatty acids, fish oil, alpha-linolenic acid	Prevention of restenosis after coronary angioplasty (percutaneous transluminal coronary angioplasty [PTCA])
Red clover (*Trifolium pratense*)	High cholesterol
Soy (*Glycine max* L. Merr.)	Cardiovascular disease
Spirulina	High cholesterol
Turmeric (*Curcuma longa* L.), curcumin	High cholesterol
Wild yam (*Dioscorea villosa*)	High cholesterol

GRADE: D (Fair Negative Scientific Evidence)

Therapy	Specific Therapeutic Use(s)
Omega-3 fatty acids, fish oil, alpha-linolenic acid	Hypercholesterolemia

TRADITIONAL OR THEORETICAL USES THAT LACK SUFFICIENT EVIDENCE

Therapy	Specific Therapeutic Use(s)
Aloe (*Aloe vera*)	Heart disease prevention
Antineoplastons	Cholesterol/triglyceride abnormalities
Arginine (L-arginine)	Cardiac syndrome X
Arginine (L-arginine)	Heart attack

Arginine (L-arginine)	High cholesterol
Astragalus (*Astragalus membranaceus*)	Angina
Astragalus (*Astragalus membranaceus*)	Heart attack
Astragalus (*Astragalus membranaceus*)	High cholesterol
Bilberry (*Vaccinium myrtillus*)	Angina
Bilberry (*Vaccinium myrtillus*)	Heart disease
Bilberry (*Vaccinium myrtillus*)	High cholesterol
Black cohosh (*Cimicifuga racemosa* L. Nutt.)	Cardiac diseases
Bladderwrack (*Fucus vesiculosus*)	Atherosclerosis
Bladderwrack (*Fucus vesiculosus*)	Heart disease
Bladderwrack (*Fucus vesiculosus*)	High cholesterol
Boron	High cholesterol
Bromelain	Angina
Bromelain	Atherosclerosis (hardening of the arteries)
Bromelain	Heart disease
Calendula (*Calendula officinalis* L.), marigold	Atherosclerosis (clogged arteries)
Calendula (*Calendula officinalis* L.), marigold	Heart disease
Clay	Cardiovascular disorders
Coenzyme Q10	High cholesterol
Dandelion (*Taraxacum officinale*)	Cardiovascular disorders
Dandelion (*Taraxacum officinale*)	Clogged arteries
Dandelion (*Taraxacum officinale*)	High cholesterol
Danshen (*Salvia miltiorrhiza*)	Clogged arteries
Danshen (*Salvia miltiorrhiza*)	High cholesterol
Devil's claw (*Harpagophytum procumbens* DC.)	Atherosclerosis (clogged arteries)
Devil's claw (*Harpagophytum procumbens* DC.)	High cholesterol
Dehydroepiandrosterone (DHEA)	Heart attack
Dehydroepiandrosterone (DHEA)	High cholesterol
Dong quai (*Angelica sinensis* [Oliv.] Diels), Chinese angelica	Atherosclerosis
Dong quai (*Angelica sinensis* [Oliv.] Diels), Chinese angelica	High cholesterol
Evening primrose oil (*Oenothera biennis* L.)	Atherosclerosis
Evening primrose oil (*Oenothera biennis* L.)	Heart disease
Evening primrose oil (*Oenothera biennis* L.)	High cholesterol
Fenugreek (*Trigonella foenum-graecum* L.)	Atherosclerosis
Ginger (*Zingiber officinale* Roscoe)	Atherosclerosis
Ginger (*Zingiber officinale* Roscoe)	Heart disease

Continued

Ginkgo (*Ginkgo biloba* L.)	Angina
Ginkgo (*Ginkgo biloba* L.)	Atherosclerosis (clogged arteries)
Ginkgo (*Ginkgo biloba* L.)	Heart attack
Ginkgo (*Ginkgo biloba* L.)	Heart disease
Ginkgo (*Ginkgo biloba* L.)	High cholesterol
Ginseng (American ginseng, Asian ginseng, Chinese ginseng, Korean red ginseng, *Panax ginseng*: *Panax* spp. including *P. ginseng* C.C. Meyer and *P. quinquefolium* L., excluding *Eleutherococcus senticosus*)	Atherosclerosis
Ginseng (American ginseng, Asian ginseng, Chinese ginseng, Korean red ginseng, *Panax ginseng*: *Panax* spp. including *P. ginseng* C.C. Meyer *and* *P. quinquefolium* L., excluding *Eleutherococcus senticosus*)	Heart damage
Globe artichoke (*Cynara scolymus* L.)	Atherosclerosis
Goldenseal (*Hydrastis canadensis* L.), berberine	Atherosclerosis (hardening of the arteries)
Goldenseal (*Hydrastis canadensis* L.), berberine	High cholesterol
Green tea (*Camellia sinensis*)	Heart disease
Gymnema (*Gymnema sylvestre* R. Br.)	Cardiovascular disease
Hawthorn (*Crataegus laevigata*, *C. oxyacantha*, *C. monogyna*, *C.* pentagyna)	Angina
Hawthorn (*Crataegus laevigata*, *C. oxyacantha*, *C. monogyna*, *C.* pentagyna)	Cardiac murmurs
Lactobacillus acidophilus	Heart disease
Licorice (*Glycyrrhiza glabra* L.), deglycyrrhizinated licorice (DGL)	High cholesterol
Lycopene	Heart disease
Maitake mushroom (*Grifola frondosa*), beta-glucan	High cholesterol
Melatonin	Cardiac syndrome X
Melatonin	Coronary artery disease
Niacin (vitamin B$_3$, nicotinic acid), niacinamide, inositol hexanicotinate	Heart attack prevention
Oleander (*Nerium oleander*, *Thevetia peruviana*)	Heart disease
Omega-3 fatty acids, fish oil, alpha-linolenic acid	Acute myocardial infarction (heart attack)
Psyllium (*Plantago ovata*, *P. ispaghula*)	Atherosclerosis
Seaweed, kelp, bladderwrack (*Fucus vesiculosus*)	Atherosclerosis
Seaweed, kelp, bladderwrack (*Fucus vesiculosus*)	Fatty heart
Seaweed, kelp, bladderwrack (*Fucus vesiculosus*)	Hyperlipemia
Shark cartilage	Atherosclerosis
Soy (*Glycine max* L. Merr.)	Atherosclerosis
Spirulina	Atherosclerosis
Spirulina	Heart disease
Sweet almond (*Prunus amygdalus dulcis*)	Heart disease

Valerian (*Valeriana officinalis* L.)	Angina pectoris
Valerian (*Valeriana officinalis* L.)	Heart disease
Yohimbe bark extract (*Pausinystalia yohimbe* Pierre ex Beille)	Angina
Yohimbe bark extract (*Pausinystalia yohimbe* Pierre ex Beille)	Coronary artery disease
Yohimbe bark extract (*Pausinystalia yohimbe* Pierre ex Beille)	High cholesterol
Yohimbe bark extract (*Pausinystalia yohimbe* Pierre ex Beille)	Atherosclerosis
Yohimbe bark extract (*Pausinystalia yohimbe* Pierre ex Beille)	Chest pain
Yohimbe bark extract (*Pausinystalia yohimbe* Pierre ex Beille)	Coronary artery disease
Yohimbe bark extract (*Pausinystalia yohimbe* Pierre ex Beille)	Hyperlipidemia

HUMAN IMMUNODEFICIENCY VIRUS (HIV) INFECTION/AIDS AND RELATED CONDITIONS

Levels of Scientific Evidence for Specific Therapies

GRADE: C (Unclear or Conflicting Scientific Evidence)

Therapy	Specific Therapeutic Use(s)
Aloe (*Aloe vera*)	HIV infection
Antineoplastons	HIV infection
Bitter melon (*Momordica charantia* L.), MAP30	HIV infection
Coenzyme Q10	HIV infection/AIDS
Dehydroepiandrosterone (DHEA)	HIV infection/AIDS
Flaxseed and flaxseed oil (*Linum usitatissimum*)	HIV infection/AIDS
Melatonin	HIV infection/AIDS
Turmeric (*Curcuma longa* L.), curcumin	HIV infection

GRADE: D (Fair Negative Scientific Evidence)

Therapy	Specific Therapeutic Use(s)
St. John's wort (*Hypericum perforatum* L.)	HIV infection

TRADITIONAL OR THEORETICAL USES THAT LACK SUFFICIENT EVIDENCE

Therapy	Specific Therapeutic Use(s)
Arginine (L-arginine)	AIDS/HIV infection
Astragalus (*Astragalus membranaceus*)	AIDS/HIV infection
Bromelain	AIDS
Burdock (*Arctium lappa*)	HIV infection
Calendula (*Calendula officinalis* L.), marigold	HIV infection
Dandelion (*Taraxacum officinale*)	AIDS
Danshen (*Salvia miltiorrhiza*)	HIV infection
Dehydroepiandrosterone (DHEA)	Lipodystrophy in HIV infection

Continued

Therapy	Condition
Echinacea (*Echinacea angustifolia* DC., *E. pallida*, *E. purpurea*)	HIV infection/AIDS
Elder (*Sambucus nigra* L.)	HIV infection
Essiac	AIDS/HIV infection
Eucalyptus oil (*Eucalyptus globulus* Labillardiere, *E. fructicetorum* F. Von Mueller, *E. smithii* R.T. Baker)	AIDS
Garlic (*Allium sativum* L.)	AIDS
Garlic (*Allium sativum* L.)	HIV infection
Ginseng (American ginseng, Asian ginseng, Chinese ginseng, Korean red ginseng, *Panax ginseng*: *Panax* spp. including *P. ginseng* C.C. Meyer and *P. quinquefolium* L., excluding *Eleutherococcus senticosus*)	HIV infection
Goldenseal (*Hydrastis canadensis* L.), berberine	AIDS
Green tea (*Camellia sinensis*)	HIV infection/AIDS
Lactobacillus acidophilus	AIDS
Lavender (*Lavandula angustifolia* Miller)	HIV infection
Licorice (*Glycyrrhiza glabra* L.), deglycyrrhizinated licorice (DGL)	HIV infection
Lycopene	AIDS
Maitake mushroom (*Grifola frondosa*), beta-glucan	HIV infection
Niacin (vitamin B_3, nicotinic acid), niacinamide, inositol hexanicotinate	HIV infection prevention
Omega-3 fatty acids, fish oil, alpha-linolenic acid	AIDS
Propolis	HIV infection
Red clover (*Trifolium pratense*)	AIDS
Spirulina	HIV infection

HYPERTENSION AND RELATED CONDITIONS

Levels of Scientific Evidence for Specific Therapies

GRADE: A (Strong Scientific Evidence)

Therapy	Specific therapeutic Use(s)
Omega-3 fatty acids, fish oil, alpha-linolenic acid	High blood pressure

GRADE: B (Good Scientific Evidence)

Therapy	Specific Therapeutic Use(s)
Coenzyme Q10	High blood pressure (hypertension)

GRADE: C (Unclear or Conflicting Scientific Evidence)

Therapy	Specific Therapeutic Use(s)
Arginine (L-arginine)	High blood pressure
Evening primrose oil (*Oenothera biennis* L.)	Preeclampsia/high blood pressure of pregnancy
Flaxseed and flaxseed oil (*Linum usitatissimum*)	High blood pressure (flaxseed, not flaxseed oil)

Garlic (*Allium sativum* L.)	High blood pressure
Ginseng (American ginseng, Asian ginseng, Chinese ginseng, Korean red ginseng, *Panax ginseng*: *Panax* spp. including *P. ginseng* C.C. Meyer and *P. quinquefolium* L., excluding *Eleutherococcus senticosus*)	High blood pressure
Melatonin	High blood pressure (hypertension)
Omega-3 fatty acids, fish oil, alpha-linolenic acid	Preeclampsia
Soy (*Glycine max* L. Merr.)	High blood pressure

TRADITIONAL OR THEORETICAL USES THAT LACK SUFFICIENT EVIDENCE	
Therapy	**Specific Therapeutic Use(s)**
Arginine (L-arginine)	Preeclampsia
Astragalus (*Astragalus membranaceus*)	High blood pressure
Bilberry (*Vaccinium myrtillus*)	High blood pressure
Black cohosh (*Cimicifuga racemosa* L. Nutt.)	High blood pressure
Dandelion (*Taraxacum officinale*)	High blood pressure
Danshen (*Salvia miltiorrhiza*)	Preeclampsia
Dong quai (*Angelica sinensis* [Oliv.] Diels), Chinese angelica	High blood pressure
Fenugreek (*Trigonella foenum-graecum* L.)	Hypertension
Ginger (*Zingiber officinale* Roscoe)	High blood pressure
Ginkgo (*Ginkgo biloba* L.)	High blood pressure
Ginseng (American ginseng, Asian ginseng, Chinese ginseng, Korean red ginseng, *Panax ginseng*: *Panax* spp. including *P. ginseng* C.C. Meyer and *P. quinquefolium* L., excluding *Eleutherococcus senticosus*)	High blood pressure
Goldenseal (*Hydrastis canadensis* L.), berberine	High blood pressure
Gotu kola (*Centella asiatica* L.), total triterpenic fraction of *Centella asiatica* (TTFCA)	Hypertension
Gotu kola (*Centella asiatica* L.), total triterpenic fraction of *Centella asiatica* (TTFCA)	Peripheral vasodilator
Gymnema (*Gymnema sylvestre* R. Br.)	High blood pressure
Maitake mushroom (*Grifola frondosa*), beta-glucan	High blood pressure
Niacin (vitamin B_3, nicotinic acid), niacinamide, inositol hexanicotinate	High blood pressure
Passionflower (*Passiflora incarnata* L.)	High blood pressure
Polypodium leucotomos extract, Anapsos	Hypertension
Psyllium (*Plantago ovata*, *P. ispaghula*)	High blood pressure
Red yeast rice (*Monascus purpureus*)	High blood pressure
Saw palmetto (*Serenoa repens* [Bartram] Small)	High blood pressure
Spirulina	High blood pressure
Turmeric (*Curcuma longa* L.), curcumin	High blood pressure
Valerian (*Valeriana officinalis* L.)	Hypertension

HYPOTENSION AND RELATED CONDITIONS

Levels of Scientific Evidence for Specific Therapies

GRADE: C (Unclear or Conflicting Scientific Evidence)

Therapy	Specific Therapeutic Use(s)
Dehydroepiandrosterone (DHEA)	Septicemia (serious bacterial infections in the blood)
Ephedra (*Ephedra sinica*)/ma huang	Hypotension

TRADITIONAL OR THEORETICAL USES THAT LACK SUFFICIENT EVIDENCE

Therapy	Specific Therapeutic Use(s)
Arginine (L-arginine)	Sepsis
Dong quai (*Angelica sinensis* [Oliv.] Diels), Chinese angelica	Sepsis
Echinacea (*Echinacea angustifolia* DC., *E. pallida*, *E. purpurea*)	Septicemia
Ginger (*Zingiber officinale* Roscoe)	Low blood pressure
Ginkgo (*Ginkgo biloba* L.)	Acidosis
Ginkgo (*Ginkgo biloba* L.)	Sepsis
Lavender (*Lavandula angustifolia* Miller)	Low blood pressure
Propolis	Low blood pressure
Yohimbe bark extract (*Pausinystalia yohimbe* Pierre ex Beille)	Low blood pressure

HYPOTHYROIDISM AND RELATED CONDITIONS

Levels of Scientific Evidence for Specific Therapies

GRADE: C (Unclear or Conflicting Scientific Evidence)

Therapy	Specific Therapeutic Use(s)
Bladderwrack (*Fucus vesiculosus*)	Goiter (thyroid disease)

TRADITIONAL OR THEORETICAL USES THAT LACK SUFFICIENT EVIDENCE

Therapy	Specific Therapeutic Use(s)
Essiac	Thyroid disorders
Horsetail (*Equisetum arvense* L.)	Thyroid disorders
Niacin (vitamin B_3, nicotinic acid), niacinamide, inositol hexanicotinate	Hypothyroidism
Propolis	Thyroid disease
Seaweed, kelp, bladderwrack (*Fucus vesiculosus*)	Exophthalmos
Seaweed, kelp, bladderwrack (*Fucus vesiculosus*)	Goiter
Seaweed, kelp, bladderwrack (*Fucus vesiculosus*)	Myxedema

IMMUNOMODULATION AND RELATED CONDITIONS

Levels of Scientific Evidence for Specific Therapies

GRADE: C (Unclear or Conflicting Scientific Evidence)

Therapy	Specific Therapeutic Use(s)
Astragalus (*Astragalus membranaceus*)	Immunostimulation
Astragalus (*Astragalus membranaceus*)	Low white blood cell count
Ginseng (American ginseng, Asian ginseng, Chinese ginseng, Korean red ginseng, *Panax ginseng*: *Panax* spp. including *P. ginseng* C.C. Meyer and *P. quinquefolium* L., excluding *Eleutherococcus senticosus*)	Immune system enhancement
Ginseng (American ginseng, Asian ginseng, Chinese ginseng, Korean red ginseng, *Panax ginseng*: *Panax* spp. including *P. ginseng* C.C. Meyer and *P. quinquefolium* L., excluding *Eleutherococcus senticosus*)	Low white blood cell counts
Goldenseal (*Hydrastis canadensis* L.), berberine	Immune system stimulation
Maitake mushroom (*Grifola frondosa*), beta-glucan	Immunoenhancement

GRADE: D (Fair Negative Scientific Evidence)

Therapy	Specific Therapeutic Use(s)
Dehydroepiandrosterone (DHEA)	Immune system stimulant
Lycopene	Immunostimulation

TRADITIONAL OR THEORETICAL USES THAT LACK SUFFICIENT EVIDENCE

Therapy	Specific Therapeutic Use(s)
Arginine (L-arginine)	Enhanced immune function
Arginine (L-arginine)	Immunomodulation
Black tea (*Camellia sinensis*)	Immune enhancement/ improving resistance to disease
Bromelain	Immune system regulation
Calendula (*Calendula officinalis* L.), marigold	Immune system stimulant
Chaparral (*Larrea tridentata* DC. Coville, *L. divaricata* Cav.), nordihydroguaiaretic acid (NDGA)	Immune system disorders
Coenzyme Q10	Immune system diseases
Dandelion (*Taraxacum officinale*)	Immunostimulation
Elder (*Sambucus nigra* L.)	Immunostimulant
Essiac	Immune system enhancement
Garlic (*Allium sativum* L.)	Immune system stimulation
Ginger (*Zingiber officinale* Roscoe)	Immunostimulation
Gotu kola (*Centella asiatica* L.), total triterpenic fraction of *Centella asiatica* (TTFCA)	Immunomodulator
Green tea (*Camellia sinensis*)	Improving resistance to disease
Lactobacillus acidophilus	Immune system enhancement
Marshmallow (*Althaea officinalis* L.)	Immunostimulant

Continued

Melatonin	Immunostimulant
Omega-3 fatty acids, fish oil, alpha-linolenic acid	Immunosuppression
Polypodium leucotomos extract, Anapsos	Immunostimulation
Propolis	Immunostimulation
Saw palmetto (*Serenoa repens* [Bartram] Small)	Immunostimulation
Spirulina	Immune system enhancement
Tea tree oil (*Melaleuca alternifolia* [Maiden & Betche] Cheel)	Immune system deficiencies

INCONTINENCE AND RELATED CONDITIONS

Levels of Scientific Evidence for Specific Therapies

GRADE: C (Unclear or Conflicting Scientific Evidence)

Therapy	Specific Therapeutic Use(s)
Cranberry (*Vaccinium macrocarpon*)	Reduction of odor from incontinence/bladder catheterization
Saw palmetto (*Serenoa repens* [Bartram] Small)	Hypotonic neurogenic bladder

TRADITIONAL OR THEORETICAL USES THAT LACK SUFFICIENT EVIDENCE

Therapy	Specific Therapeutic Use(s)
Belladonna (*Atropa belladonna* L. or its variety *A. acuminata* Royle ex Lindl)	Bedwetting
Calendula (*Calendula officinalis* L.), marigold	Urinary retention
Ephedra (*Ephedra sinica*)/ma huang	Enuresis
Gotu kola (*Centella asiatica* L.), total triterpenic fraction of *Centella asiatica* (TTFCA)	Urinary retention
Horsetail (*Equisetum arvense* L.)	Urinary incontinence
Kava (*Piper methysticum* G. Forst)	Urinary incontinence
St. John's wort (*Hypericum perforatum* L.)	Bedwetting
Thyme (*Thymus vulgaris* L.), thymol	Enuresis

INFERTILITY AND RELATED CONDITIONS

Levels of Scientific Evidence for Specific Therapies

GRADE: D (Fair Negative Scientific Evidence)

Therapy	Specific Therapeutic Use(s)
Arginine (L-arginine)	Infertility

TRADITIONAL OR THEORETICAL USES THAT LACK SUFFICIENT EVIDENCE

Therapy	Specific Therapeutic Use(s)
Bitter melon (*Momordica charantia* L.), MAP30	Infertility
Black cohosh (*Cimicifuga racemosa* L. Nutt.)	Infertility

Burdock (*Arctium lappa*)	Sterility
Coenzyme Q10	Infertility
Dong quai (*Angelica sinensis* [Oliv.] Diels), Chinese angelica	Infertility
Ginseng (American ginseng, Asian ginseng, Chinese ginseng, Korean red ginseng, *Panax ginseng*: *Panax* spp. including *P. ginseng* C.C. Meyer and *P. quinquefolium* L., excluding *Eleutherococcus senticosus*)	Male infertility
Lavender (*Lavandula angustifolia* Miller)	Infertility
Omega-3 fatty acids, fish oil, alpha-linolenic acid	Male infertility
Sweet almond (*Prunus amygdalus dulcis*)	Increasing sperm count

INFLAMMATION AND RELATED CONDITIONS

Levels of Scientific Evidence for Specific Therapies

GRADE: B (Good Scientific Evidence)

Therapy	Specific Therapeutic Use(s)
Bromelain	Inflammation

GRADE: C (Unclear or Conflicting Scientific Evidence)

Therapy	Specific Therapeutic Use(s)
Arginine (L-arginine)	Dental pain (ibuprofen arginate)
Black cohosh (*Cimicifuga racemosa* L. Nutt.)	Arthritis pain (rheumatoid arthritis, osteoarthritis)
Dandelion (*Taraxacum officinale*)	Anti-inflammatory
Eyebright (*Euphrasia officinalis*)	Anti-inflammatory
Propolis	Dental pain
Shark cartilage	Analgesia
Turmeric (*Curcuma longa* L.), curcumin	Inflammation
White horehound (*Marrubium vulgare* L.)	Pain

TRADITIONAL OR THEORETICAL USES THAT LACK SUFFICIENT EVIDENCE

Therapy	Specific Therapeutic Use(s)
Alfalfa (*Medicago sativa* L.)	Inflammation
Arginine (L-arginine)	Pain
Astragalus (*Astragalus membranaceus*)	Myalgia (muscle pain)
Belladonna (*Atropa belladonna* L. or its variety *A. acuminata* Royle ex Lindl)	Anesthetic
Belladonna (*Atropa belladonna* L. or its variety *A. acuminata* Royle ex Lindl)	Inflammation
Belladonna (*Atropa belladonna* L. or its variety *A. acuminata* Royle ex Lindl)	Muscle and joint pain
Bitter almond (*Prunus amygdalus* Batch var. *amara* DC. Focke), Laetrile	Anti-inflammatory

Continued

Bitter almond (*Prunus amygdalus* Batch var. *amara* DC. Focke), Laetrile	Local anesthetic
Bitter almond (*Prunus amygdalus* Batch var. *amara* DC. Focke), Laetrile	Pain suppressant
Black cohosh (*Cimicifuga racemosa* L. Nutt.)	Inflammation
Black cohosh (*Cimicifuga racemosa* L. Nutt.)	Muscle pain
Black tea (*Camellia sinensis*)	Pain
Blessed thistle (*Cnicus benedictus* L.)	Inflammation
Bromelain	Pain
Bromelain	Pain (general)
Burdock (*Arctium lappa*)	Inflammation
Calendula (*Calendula officinalis* L.), marigold	Pain
Chamomile (*Matricaria recutita, Chamaemelum nobile*)	Anti-inflammatory
Chaparral (*Larrea tridentata* DC. Coville, *L. divaricata* Cav.), nordihydroguaiaretic acid (NDGA)	Anti-inflammatory
Chaparral (*Larrea tridentata* DC. Coville, *L. divaricata* Cav.), nordihydroguaiaretic acid (NDGA)	Pain
Clove (*Eugenia aromatica*)	Pain
Dandelion (*Taraxacum officinale*)	Analgesia
Devil's claw (*Harpagophytum procumbens* DC.)	Anti-inflammatory
Devil's claw (*Harpagophytum procumbens* DC.)	Muscle pain
Devil's claw (*Harpagophytum procumbens* DC.)	Pain
Dong quai (*Angelica sinensis* [Oliv.] Diels), Chinese angelica	Pain
Dong quai (*Angelica sinensis* [Oliv.] Diels), Chinese angelica	Pain from bruises
Echinacea (*Echinacea angustifolia* DC., *E. pallida, E. purpurea*)	Pain
Elder (*Sambucus nigra* L.)	Anti-inflammatory
Ephedra (*Ephedra sinica*)/ma huang	Anti-inflammatory
Eucalyptus oil (*Eucalyptus globulus* Labillardiere, *E. fructicetorum* F. Von Mueller, *E. smithii* R.T. Baker)	Inflammation
Eucalyptus oil (*Eucalyptus globulus* Labillardiere, *E. fructicetorum* F. Von Mueller, *E. smithii* R.T. Baker)	Muscle/joint pain (applied to the skin)
Evening primrose oil (*Oenothera biennis* L.)	Pain
Fenugreek (*Trigonella foenum-graecum* L.)	Inflammation
Feverfew (*Tanacetum parthenium* L. Schultz-Bip.)	Anti-inflammatory
Garlic (*Allium sativum* L.)	Dental pain
Ginger (*Zingiber officinale* Roscoe)	Pain relief
Ginseng (American ginseng, Asian ginseng, Chinese ginseng, Korean red ginseng, *Panax ginseng: Panax* spp. including *P. ginseng* C.C. Meyer and *P. quinquefolium* L., excluding *Eleutherococcus senticosus*)	Inflammation
Ginseng (American ginseng, Asian ginseng, Chinese ginseng, Korean red ginseng, *Panax ginseng: Panax* spp. including *P. ginseng* C.C. Meyer and *P. quinquefolium* L., excluding *Eleutherococcus senticosus*)	Pain relief

Goldenseal (*Hydrastis canadensis* L.), berberine	Anesthetic
Goldenseal (*Hydrastis canadensis* L.), berberine	Anti-inflammatory
Goldenseal (*Hydrastis canadensis* L.), berberine	Muscle pain
Goldenseal (*Hydrastis canadensis* L.), berberine	Pain
Gotu kola (*Centella asiatica* L.), total triterpenic fraction of *Centella asiatica* (TTFCA)	Inflammation
Gotu kola (*Centella asiatica* L.), total triterpenic fraction of *Centella asiatica* (TTFCA)	Pain
Guggul (*Commifora mukul*)	Pain
Hops (*Humulus lupulus* L.)	Anti-inflammatory
Hops (*Humulus lupulus* L.)	Pain
Kava (*Piper methysticum* G. Forst)	Anesthesia
Kava (*Piper methysticum* G. Forst)	Pain
Lavender (*Lavandula angustifolia* Miller)	Anti-inflammatory
Lavender (*Lavandula angustifolia* Miller)	Pain
Licorice (*Glycyrrhiza glabra* L.), deglycyrrhizinated licorice (DGL)	Inflammation
Marshmallow (*Althaea officinalis* L.)	Inflammation
Marshmallow (*Althaea officinalis* L.)	Muscular pain
Oleander (*Nerium oleander*, *Thevetia peruviana*)	Inflammation
Passionflower (*Passiflora incarnata* L.)	Chronic pain
Passionflower (*Passiflora incarnata* L.)	Pain (general)
Peppermint (*Mentha* x *piperita* L.)	Local anesthetic
Peppermint (*Mentha* x *piperita* L.)	Musculoskeletal pain
Peppermint (*Mentha* x *piperita* L.)	Myalgia (muscle pain)
Polypodium leucotomos extract, Anapsos	Inflammation
Pygeum (*Prunus africana*, *Pygeum africanum*)	Inflammation
Saw palmetto (*Serenoa repens* [Bartram] Small)	Anti-inflammatory
Slippery elm (*Ulmus rubra* Muhl. or *U. fulva* Michx.)	Inflammation
Spirulina	Anti-inflammatory
St. John's wort (*Hypericum perforatum* L.)	Anti-inflammatory
St. John's wort (*Hypericum perforatum* L.)	Dental pain
St. John's wort (*Hypericum perforatum* L.)	Pain relief
Tea tree oil (*Melaleuca alternifolia* [Maiden & Betche] Cheel)	Anti-inflammatory
Tea tree oil (*Melaleuca alternifolia* [Maiden & Betche] Cheel)	Muscle and joint pain
Turmeric (*Curcuma longa* L.), curcumin	Pain
Valerian (*Valeriana officinalis* L.)	Anodyne (pain relief)
Valerian (*Valeriana officinalis* L.)	Muscle pain
Valerian (*Valeriana officinalis* L.)	Pain

Continued

White horehound (*Marrubium vulgare* L.)	Pain
Wild yam (*Dioscorea villosa*)	Anti-inflammatory
Yohimbe bark extract (*Pausinystalia yohimbe* Pierre ex Beille)	Anesthetic

INSECT BITES AND STINGS AND RELATED CONDITIONS
Levels of Scientific Evidence for Specific Therapies

GRADE: C (Unclear or Conflicting Scientific Evidence)	
Therapy	Specific Therapeutic Use(s)
Garlic (*Allium sativum* L.)	Tick repellent

TRADITIONAL OR THEORETICAL USES THAT LACK SUFFICIENT EVIDENCE	
Therapy	Specific Therapeutic Use(s)
Alfalfa (*Medicago sativa* L.)	Insect bites
American pennyroyal (*Hedeoma pulegioides* L.), European pennyroyal (*Mentha pulegium* L.)	Flea control
American pennyroyal (*Hedeoma pulegioides* L.), European pennyroyal (*Mentha pulegium* L.)	Insect repellent
Black cohosh (*Cimicifuga racemosa* L. Nutt.)	Insect repellent
Chamomile (*Matricaria recutita, Chamaemelum nobile*)	Insect bites
Echinacea (*Echinacea angustifolia* DC., *E. pallida, E. purpurea*)	Bee stings
Elder (*Sambucus nigra* L.)	Mosquito repellent
Eucalyptus oil (*Eucalyptus globulus* Labillardiere, *E. fructicetorum* F. Von Mueller, *E. smithii* R.T. Baker)	Insect repellent
Feverfew (*Tanacetum parthenium* L. Schultz-Bip.)	Insect bites
Feverfew (*Tanacetum parthenium* L. Schultz-Bip.)	Insect repellent
Ginger (*Zingiber officinale* Roscoe)	Insecticide
Lavender (*Lavandula angustifolia* Miller)	Insect repellent
Marshmallow (*Althaea officinalis* L.)	Bee stings
Marshmallow (*Althaea officinalis* L.)	Insect bites
Oleander (*Nerium oleander, Thevetia peruviana*)	Insecticide
Soy (*Glycine max* L. Merr.)	Insect repellent
Tea tree oil (*Melaleuca alternifolia* [Maiden & Betche] Cheel)	Insect bites/stings
Thyme (*Thymus vulgaris* L.), thymol	Insect bites
Turmeric (*Curcuma longa* L.), curcumin	Insect bites
Turmeric (*Curcuma longa* L.), curcumin	Insect repellent

IRRITABLE BOWEL SYNDROME AND RELATED CONDITIONS

Levels of Scientific Evidence for Specific Therapies

GRADE: C (Unclear or Conflicting Scientific Evidence)

Therapy	Specific Therapeutic Use(s)
Belladonna (*Atropa belladonna* L. or its variety *A. acuminata* Royle ex Lindl)	Irritable bowel syndrome
Chamomile (*Matricaria recutita*, *Chamaemelum nobile*)	Gastrointestinal conditions
Clay	Functional gastrointestinal disorders
Globe artichoke (*Cynara scolymus* L.)	Irritable bowel syndrome
Lactobacillus acidophilus	Irritable bowel syndrome
Lactobacillus acidophilus	Necrotizing enterocolitis prevention in infants
Peppermint (*Mentha* x *piperita* L.)	Irritable bowel syndrome
Psyllium (*Plantago ovata*, *P. ispaghula*)	Irritable bowel syndrome
Slippery elm (*Ulmus rubra* Muhl. or *U. fulva* Michx.)	Gastrointestinal disorders
White horehound (*Marrubium vulgare* L.)	Intestinal disorders/ antispasmodic

TRADITIONAL OR THEORETICAL USES THAT LACK SUFFICIENT EVIDENCE

Therapy	Specific Therapeutic Use(s)
Alfalfa (*Medicago sativa* L.)	Gastrointestinal tract disorders
Aloe (*Aloe vera*)	Bowel disorders
American pennyroyal (*Hedeoma pulegioides* L.), European pennyroyal (*Mentha pulegium* L.)	Bowel disorders
American pennyroyal (*Hedeoma pulegioides* L.), European pennyroyal (*Mentha pulegium* L.)	Colic
American pennyroyal (*Hedeoma pulegioides* L.), European pennyroyal (*Mentha pulegium* L.)	Intestinal disorders
American pennyroyal (*Hedeoma pulegioides* L.), European pennyroyal (*Mentha pulegium* L.)	Stomach pain
American pennyroyal (*Hedeoma pulegioides* L.), European pennyroyal (*Mentha pulegium* L.)	Stomach spasms
Arginine (L-arginine)	Infantile necrotizing enterocolitis
Arginine (L-arginine)	Lower esophageal sphincter relaxation
Arginine (L-arginine)	Stomach motility disorders
Astragalus (*Astragalus membranaceus*)	Gastrointestinal disorders
Barley (*Hordeum vulgare* L.), germinated barley foodstuff (GBF)	Bowel/intestinal disorders
Belladonna (*Atropa belladonna* L. or its variety *A. acuminata* Royle ex Lindl)	Diverticulitis
Bilberry (*Vaccinium myrtillus*)	Stomach upset
Bitter melon (*Momordica charantia* L.), MAP30	Gastrointestinal cramps

Continued

Black tea (*Camellia sinensis*)	Stomach disorders
Bladderwrack (*Fucus vesiculosus*)	Stomach upset
Bromelain	Leaky gut syndrome
Calendula (*Calendula officinalis* L.), marigold	Bowel irritation
Calendula (*Calendula officinalis* L.), marigold	Gastrointestinal tract disorders
Chamomile (*Matricaria recutita, Chamaemelum nobile*)	Abdominal bloating
Chamomile (*Matricaria recutita, Chamaemelum nobile*)	Infantile colic
Chamomile (*Matricaria recutita, Chamaemelum nobile*)	Irritable bowel syndrome
Chaparral (*Larrea tridentata* DC. Coville, *L. divaricata* Cav.), nordihydroguaiaretic acid (NDGA)	Bowel cramps
Chaparral (*Larrea tridentata* DC. Coville, *L. divaricata* Cav.), nordihydroguaiaretic acid (NDGA)	Gastrointestinal disorders
Clay	Stomach disorders
Clove (*Eugenia aromatica*)	Abdominal pain
Clove (*Eugenia aromatica*)	Colic
Cranberry (*Vaccinium macrocarpon*)	Stomach ailments
Dandelion (*Taraxacum officinale*)	Stomach ache
Devil's claw (*Harpagophytum procumbens* DC.)	Gastrointestinal disorders
Dong quai (*Angelica sinensis* [Oliv.] Diels), Chinese angelica	Abdominal pain
Dong quai (*Angelica sinensis* [Oliv.] Diels), Chinese angelica	Irritable bowel syndrome
Echinacea (*Echinacea angustifolia* DC., *E. pallida, E. purpurea*)	Stomach upset
Elder (*Sambucus nigra* L.)	Colic
Elder (*Sambucus nigra* L.)	Gut disorders
Evening primrose oil (*Oenothera biennis* L.)	Irritable bowel syndrome
Eyebright (*Euphrasia officinalis*)	Gastric acid secretion stimulation
Fenugreek (*Trigonella foenum-graecum* L.)	Colic
Feverfew (*Tanacetum parthenium* L. Schultz-Bip.)	Abdominal pain
Flaxseed and flaxseed oil (*Linum usitatissimum*)	Abdominal pain
Flaxseed and flaxseed oil (*Linum usitatissimum*)	Diverticulitis
Flaxseed and flaxseed oil (*Linum usitatissimum*)	Irritable bowel syndrome
Flaxseed and flaxseed oil (*Linum usitatissimum*)	Laxative-induced colon damage
Flaxseed and flaxseed oil (*Linum usitatissimum*)	Stomach upset
Garlic (*Allium sativum* L.)	Stomachache
Ginger (*Zingiber officinale* Roscoe)	Colic
Ginger (*Zingiber officinale* Roscoe)	Stomachache
Ginseng (American ginseng, Asian ginseng, Chinese ginseng, Korean red ginseng, *Panax ginseng: Panax* spp. including *P. ginseng* C.C. Meyer and *P. quinquefolium* L., excluding *Eleutherococcus senticosus*)	Stomach upset
Goldenseal (*Hydrastis canadensis* L.), berberine	Stomachache

Green tea (*Camellia sinensis*)	Stomach disorders
Gymnema (*Gymnema sylvestre* R. Br.)	Stomach ailments
Hawthorn (*Crataegus laevigata, C. oxyacantha, C. monogyna, C. pentagyna*)	Abdominal colic
Hawthorn (*Crataegus laevigata, C. oxyacantha, C. monogyna, C. pentagyna*)	Abdominal distention
Hawthorn (*Crataegus laevigata, C. oxyacantha, C. monogyna, C. pentagyna*)	Abdominal pain
Hawthorn (*Crataegus laevigata, C. oxyacantha, C. monogyna, C. pentagyna*)	Stomachache
Hops (*Humulus lupulus* L.)	Irritable bowel syndrome
Horsetail (*Equisetum arvense* L.)	Stomach upset
Kava (*Piper methysticum* G. Forst)	Stomach upset
Lactobacillus acidophilus	Diverticulitis
Lavender (*Lavandula angustifolia* Miller)	Colic
Licorice (*Glycyrrhiza glabra* L.), deglycyrrhizinated licorice (DGL)	Diverticulitis
Licorice (*Glycyrrhiza glabra* L.), deglycyrrhizinated licorice (DGL)	Stomach upset
Marshmallow (*Althaea officinalis* L.)	Diverticulitis
Marshmallow (*Althaea officinalis* L.)	Irritable bowel syndrome
Melatonin	Intestinal motility disorders
Passionflower (*Passiflora incarnata* L.)	Gastrointestinal discomfort (nervous stomach)
Peppermint (*Mentha* x *piperita* L.)	Gastrointestinal disorders
Peppermint (*Mentha* x *piperita* L.)	Ileus (postoperative)
Peppermint (*Mentha* x *piperita* L.)	Intestinal colic
Propolis	Diverticulitis
Pygeum (*Prunus africana, Pygeum africanum*)	Stomach upset
Red yeast rice (*Monascus purpureus*)	Colic in children
Red yeast rice (*Monascus purpureus*)	Stomach problems
Shark cartilage	Intestinal disorders and inflammation
Slippery elm (*Ulmus rubra* Muhl. or *U. fulva* Michx.)	Colic
Slippery elm (*Ulmus rubra* Muhl. or *U. fulva* Michx.)	Diverticulitis
Slippery elm (*Ulmus rubra* Muhl. or *U. fulva* Michx.)	Irritable bowel syndrome
Sorrel (*Rumex acetosa* L., *R. acetosella* L.), Sinupret	Stimulation of secretion
Sorrel (*Rumex acetosa* L., *R. acetosella* L.), Sinupret	Ulcerated bowel
Soy (*Glycine max* L. Merr.)	Gastrointestinal motility
Spirulina	Bowel health
Thyme (*Thymus vulgaris* L.), thymol	Colic

Continued

Thyme (*Thymus vulgaris* L.), thymol	Stomach cramps
Turmeric (*Curcuma longa* L.), curcumin	Bloating
Turmeric (*Curcuma longa* L.), curcumin	Colic
Valerian (*Valeriana officinalis* L.)	Bloating
Valerian (*Valeriana officinalis* L.)	Colic
Valerian (*Valeriana officinalis* L.)	Intestinal disorders
Valerian (*Valeriana officinalis* L.)	Irritable bowel syndrome
Valerian (*Valeriana officinalis* L.)	Viral gastroenteritis
White horehound (*Marrubium vulgare* L.)	Bloating
White horehound (*Marrubium vulgare* L.)	Colic
Wild yam (*Dioscorea villosa*)	Diverticulitis
Wild yam (*Dioscorea villosa*)	Irritable bowel syndrome

KIDNEY DISEASE AND RELATED CONDITIONS
Levels of Scientific Evidence for Specific Therapies

GRADE: C (Unclear or Conflicting Scientific Evidence)

Therapy	Specific Therapeutic Use(s)
Astragalus (*Astragalus membranaceus*)	Renal failure
Danshen (*Salvia miltiorrhiza*)	Increased rate of peritoneal dialysis
Dong quai (*Angelica sinensis* [Oliv.] Diels), Chinese angelica	Glomerulonephritis
Flaxseed and flaxseed oil (*Linum usitatissimum*)	Kidney disease/lupus nephritis (flaxseed, not flaxseed oil)
Omega-3 fatty acids, fish oil, alpha-linolenic acid	IgA nephropathy
Omega-3 fatty acids, fish oil, alpha-linolenic acid	Nephrotic syndrome
Soy (*Glycine max* L. Merr.)	Kidney disease (chronic renal failure, nephrotic syndrome, proteinuria)

GRADE: D (Fair Negative Scientific Evidence)

Therapy	Specific Therapeutic Use(s)
Arginine (L-arginine)	Cyclosporine toxicity
Arginine (L-arginine)	Kidney disease
Arginine (L-arginine)	Kidney protection during angiography

TRADITIONAL OR THEORETICAL USES THAT LACK SUFFICIENT EVIDENCE

Therapy	Specific Therapeutic Use(s)
Alfalfa (*Medicago sativa* L.)	Kidney disorders
Aloe (*Aloe vera*)	Kidney or bladder stones
American pennyroyal (*Hedeoma pulegioides* L.), European pennyroyal (*Mentha pulegium* L.)	Kidney disease

Astragalus (*Astragalus membranaceus*)	Nephritis
Bilberry (*Vaccinium myrtillus*)	Kidney disease
Bilberry (*Vaccinium myrtillus*)	Urine blood
Black cohosh (*Cimicifuga racemosa* L. Nutt.)	Kidney inflammation
Bladderwrack (*Fucus vesiculosus*)	Kidney disease
Boswellia (*Boswellia serrata* Roxb.)	Nephritis
Burdock (*Arctium lappa*)	Kidney diseases
Coenzyme Q10	Kidney failure
Dandelion (*Taraxacum officinale*)	Kidney disease
Danshen (*Salvia miltiorrhiza*)	Gentamicin toxicity
Danshen (*Salvia miltiorrhiza*)	Kidney failure
Dong quai (*Angelica sinensis* [Oliv.] Diels), Chinese angelica	Kidney disease
Elder (*Sambucus nigra* L.)	Kidney disease
Ephedra (*Ephedra sinica*)/ma huang	Nephritis
Essiac	Kidney diseases
Flaxseed and flaxseed oil (*Linum usitatissimum*)	Glomerulonephritis
Garlic (*Allium sativum* L.)	Bloody urine
Garlic (*Allium sativum* L.)	Kidney damage from antibiotics
Garlic (*Allium sativum* L.)	Kidney problems
Garlic (*Allium sativum* L.)	Nephrotic syndrome
Ginger (*Zingiber officinale* Roscoe)	Kidney disease
Ginseng (American ginseng, Asian ginseng, Chinese ginseng, Korean red ginseng, *Panax ginseng*: *Panax* spp. including *P. ginseng* C.C. Meyer and *P. quinquefolium* L., excluding *Eleutherococcus senticosus*)	Diabetic nephropathy (kidney disease)
Ginseng (American ginseng, Asian ginseng, Chinese ginseng, Korean red ginseng, *Panax ginseng*: *Panax* spp. including *P. ginseng* C.C. Meyer and *P. quinquefolium* L., excluding *Eleutherococcus senticosus*)	Kidney disease
Globe artichoke (*Cynara scolymus* L.)	Nephrosclerosis
Hawthorn (*Crataegus laevigata, C. oxyacantha, C. monogyna, C. pentagyna*)	Nephrosis
Hops (*Humulus lupulus* L.)	Kidney disorders
Horse chestnut (*Aesculus hippocastanum* L.)	Kidney diseases
Horsetail (*Equisetum arvense* L.)	Kidney disease
Kava (*Piper methysticum* G. Forst)	Kidney disorders
Licorice (*Glycyrrhiza glabra* L.), deglycyrrhizinated licorice (DGL)	Gentamicin induced kidney damage
Melatonin	Gentamicin-induced kidney damage
Melatonin	Toxic kidney damage
Milk thistle (*Silybum marianum*), silymarin	Nephrotoxicity protection

Continued

Omega-3 fatty acids, fish oil, alpha-linolenic acid	Diabetic nephropathy
Omega-3 fatty acids, fish oil, alpha-linolenic acid	Glomerulonephritis
Omega-3 fatty acids, fish oil, alpha-linolenic acid	Hepatorenal syndrome
Omega-3 fatty acids, fish oil, alpha-linolenic acid	Kidney disease prevention
Pygeum (*Prunus africana, Pygeum africanum*)	Kidney disease
Spirulina	Kidney disease
Turmeric (*Curcuma longa* L.), curcumin	Kidney disease

LABOR AND DELIVERY AND RELATED CONDITIONS
Levels of Scientific Evidence for Specific Therapies

GRADE: C (Unclear or Conflicting Scientific Evidence)

Therapy	Specific Therapeutic Use(s)
American pennyroyal (*Hedeoma pulegioides* L.), European pennyroyal (*Mentha pulegium* L.)	Abortifacient (uterine contraction stimulant)
Blessed thistle (*Cnicus benedictus* L.)	Abortifacient

TRADITIONAL OR THEORETICAL USES THAT LACK SUFFICIENT EVIDENCE

Therapy	Specific Therapeutic Use(s)
American pennyroyal (*Hedeoma pulegioides* L.), European pennyroyal (*Mentha pulegium* L.)	Pregnancy
Arginine (L-arginine)	Preterm labor contractions
Astragalus (*Astragalus membranaceus*)	Postpartum fever
Astragalus (*Astragalus membranaceus*)	Postpartum urinary retention
Black cohosh (*Cimicifuga racemosa* L. Nutt.)	Labor induction
Blessed thistle (*Cnicus benedictus* L.)	Abortifacient
Bromelain	Shortening of labor
Dandelion (*Taraxacum officinale*)	Pregnancy
Danshen (*Salvia miltiorrhiza*)	Ectopic pregnancy
Danshen (*Salvia miltiorrhiza*)	Intrauterine growth restriction/retardation
Dong quai (*Angelica sinensis* [Oliv.] Diels), Chinese angelica	Labor aid
Dong quai (*Angelica sinensis* [Oliv.] Diels), Chinese angelica	Postpartum weakness
Dong quai (*Angelica sinensis* [Oliv.] Diels), Chinese angelica	Pregnancy support
Fenugreek (*Trigonella foenum-graecum* L.)	Abortifacient
Fenugreek (*Trigonella foenum-graecum* L.)	Labor induction (uterine stimulant)
Feverfew (*Tanacetum parthenium* L. Schultz-Bip.)	Abortifacient
Feverfew (*Tanacetum parthenium* L. Schultz-Bip.)	Labor induction
Garlic (*Allium sativum* L.)	Abortion
Ginkgo (*Ginkgo biloba* L.)	Labor induction

Goldenseal (*Hydrastis canadensis* L.), berberine	Abortifacient
Goldenseal (*Hydrastis canadensis* L.), berberine	Postpartum hemorrhage
Niacin (vitamin B$_3$, nicotinic acid), niacinamide, inositol hexanicotinate	Pregnancy problems
Oleander (*Nerium oleander, Thevetia peruviana*)	Pregnancy termination
Omega-3 fatty acids, fish oil, alpha-linolenic acid	Pregnancy nutritional supplement
Omega-3 fatty acids, fish oil, alpha-linolenic acid	Premature birth prevention
Red yeast rice (*Monascus purpureus*)	Postpartum problems
Saw palmetto (*Serenoa repens* [Bartram] Small)	Postnasal drip
Slippery elm (*Ulmus rubra* Muhl. or *U. fulva* Michx.)	Abortifacient
Spirulina	Obstetric and gynecologic disorders

LACTATION STIMULATION AND RELATED CONDITIONS
Levels of Scientific Evidence for Specific Therapies

TRADITIONAL OR THEORETICAL USES THAT LACK SUFFICIENT EVIDENCE

Therapy	Specific Therapeutic Use(s)
Alfalfa (*Medicago sativa* L.)	Increasing breast milk
Blessed thistle (*Cnicus benedictus* L.)	Breast milk stimulant
Fenugreek (*Trigonella foenum-graecum* L.)	Galactagogue (lactation stimulant)
Milk thistle (*Silybum marianum*), silymarin	Lactation stimulation
Saw palmetto (*Serenoa repens* [Bartram] Small)	Lactation
Turmeric (*Curcuma longa* L.), curcumin	Lactation stimulation

LAXATIVE AND RELATED CONDITIONS
Levels of Scientific Evidence for Specific Therapies

GRADE: A (Strong Scientific Evidence)

Therapy	Specific Therapeutic Use(s)
Aloe (*Aloe vera*)	Constipation (laxative)

GRADE: B (Good Scientific Evidence)

Therapy	Specific Therapeutic Use(s)
Flaxseed and flaxseed oil (*Linum usitatissimum*)	Laxative (flaxseed, not flaxseed oil)
Psyllium (*Plantago ovata, P. ispaghula*)	Constipation

GRADE: C (Unclear or Conflicting Scientific Evidence)

Therapy	Specific Therapeutic Use(s)
Barley (*Hordeum vulgare* L.), germinated barley foodstuff (GBF)	Constipation

Continued

TRADITIONAL OR THEORETICAL USES THAT LACK SUFFICIENT EVIDENCE	
Therapy	Specific Therapeutic Use(s)
Astragalus (*Astragalus membranaceus*)	Laxative
Bladderwrack (*Fucus vesiculosus*)	Laxative
Bladderwrack (*Fucus vesiculosus*)	Stool softener
Burdock (*Arctium lappa*)	Laxative
Calendula (*Calendula officinalis* L.), marigold	Constipation
Chamomile (*Matricaria recutita, Chamaemelum nobile*)	Constipation
Clay	Constipation
Devil's claw (*Harpagophytum procumbens* DC.)	Constipation
Dong quai (*Angelica sinensis* [Oliv.] Diels), Chinese angelica	Constipation
Dong quai (*Angelica sinensis* [Oliv.] Diels), Chinese angelica	Laxative
Elder (*Sambucus nigra* L.)	Laxative
Fenugreek (*Trigonella foenum-graecum* L.)	Constipation
Feverfew (*Tanacetum parthenium* L. Schultz-Bip.)	Constipation
Ginger (*Zingiber officinale* Roscoe)	Laxative
Globe artichoke (*Cynara scolymus* L.)	Constipation
Goldenseal (*Hydrastis canadensis* L.), berberine	Constipation
Gymnema (*Gymnema sylvestre* R. Br.)	Constipation
Gymnema (*Gymnema sylvestre* R. Br.)	Laxative
Lactobacillus acidophilus	Constipation
Licorice (*Glycyrrhiza glabra* L.), deglycyrrhizinated licorice (DGL)	Constipation
Marshmallow (*Althaea officinalis* L.)	Constipation
Marshmallow (*Althaea officinalis* L.)	Laxative
Oleander (*Nerium oleander, Thevetia peruviana*)	Cathartic
Seaweed, kelp, bladderwrack (*Fucus vesiculosus*)	Bulk laxative
Seaweed, kelp, bladderwrack (*Fucus vesiculosus*)	Laxative
Seaweed, kelp, bladderwrack (*Fucus vesiculosus*)	Stool softener
Slippery elm (*Ulmus rubra* Muhl. or *U. fulva* Michx.)	Constipation
Sorrel (*Rumex acetosa* L., *R. acetosella* L.) and Sinupret	Constipation
Sweet almond (*Prunus amygdalus dulcis*)	Mild laxative
Valerian (*Valeriana officinalis* L.)	Constipation
White horehound (*Marrubium vulgare* L.)	Cathartic
White horehound (*Marrubium vulgare* L.)	Constipation
White horehound (*Marrubium vulgare* L.)	Laxative

LIVER DISEASE AND RELATED CONDITIONS

Levels of Scientific Evidence for Specific Therapies

GRADE: B (Good Scientific Evidence)

Therapy	Specific Therapeutic Use(s)
Milk thistle (*Silybum marianum*), silymarin	Cirrhosis
Milk thistle (*Silybum marianum*), silymarin	Hepatitis (chronic)

GRADE: C (Unclear or Conflicting Scientific Evidence)

Therapy	Specific Therapeutic Use(s)
Astragalus (*Astragalus membranaceus*)	Liver protection
Clay	Protection from aflatoxins
Dandelion (*Taraxacum officinale*)	Hepatitis B
Danshen (*Salvia miltiorrhiza*)	Liver disease (cirrhosis/chronic hepatitis B)
Eyebright (*Euphrasia officinalis*)	Hepatoprotection
Lactobacillus acidophilus	Hepatic encephalopathy (confused thinking due to liver disorders)
Licorice (*Glycyrrhiza glabra* L.), deglycyrrhizinated licorice (DGL)	Viral hepatitis
Milk thistle (*Silybum marianum*), silymarin	Acute viral hepatitis
Milk thistle (*Silybum marianum*), silymarin	*Amanita phalloides* mushroom toxicity
Milk thistle (*Silybum marianum*), silymarin	Drug/toxin-induced hepatotoxicity

TRADITIONAL OR THEORETICAL USES THAT LACK SUFFICIENT EVIDENCE

Therapy	Specific Therapeutic Use(s)
Alfalfa (*Medicago sativa* L.)	Jaundice
Aloe (*Aloe vera*)	Hepatitis
American pennyroyal (*Hedeoma pulegioides* L.), European pennyroyal (*Mentha pulegium* L.)	Liver disease
Arginine (L-arginine)	Ammonia toxicity
Arginine (L-arginine)	Hepatic encephalopathy
Arginine (L-arginine)	Liver disease
Astragalus (*Astragalus membranaceus*)	Chronic hepatitis
Astragalus (*Astragalus membranaceus*)	Liver disease
Bilberry (*Vaccinium myrtillus*)	Liver disease
Black cohosh (*Cimicifuga racemosa* L. Nutt.)	Liver disease
Blessed thistle (*Cnicus benedictus* L.)	Jaundice
Blessed thistle (*Cnicus benedictus* L.)	Liver disorders
Burdock (*Arctium lappa*)	Liver protection

Continued

Calendula (*Calendula officinalis* L.), marigold	Jaundice
Calendula (*Calendula officinalis* L.), marigold	Liver dysfunction
Chamomile (*Matricaria recutita, Chamaemelum nobile*)	Liver disorders
Coenzyme Q10	Hepatitis B
Coenzyme Q10	Liver enlargement or disease
Cranberry (*Vaccinium macrocarpon*)	Liver disorders
Dandelion (*Taraxacum officinale*)	Jaundice
Dandelion (*Taraxacum officinale*)	Liver cleansing
Dandelion (*Taraxacum officinale*)	Liver disease
Devil's claw (*Harpagophytum procumbens* DC.)	Liver and gallbladder tonic
Dehydroepiandrosterone (DHEA)	Liver protection
Dong quai (*Angelica sinensis* [Oliv.] Diels), Chinese angelica	Chronic hepatitis
Dong quai (*Angelica sinensis* [Oliv.] Diels), Chinese angelica	Cirrhosis
Dong quai (*Angelica sinensis* [Oliv.] Diels), Chinese angelica	Liver protection
Elder (*Sambucus nigra* L.)	Liver disease
Eucalyptus oil (*Eucalyptus globulus* Labillardiere, *E. fructicetorum* F. Von Mueller, *E. smithii* R.T. Baker)	Liver protection
Evening primrose oil (*Oenothera biennis* L.)	Hepatitis B
Eyebright (*Euphrasia officinalis*)	Jaundice
Eyebright (*Euphrasia officinalis*)	Liver disease
Garlic (*Allium sativum* L.)	Antitoxin
Garlic (*Allium sativum* L.)	Hepatopulmonary syndrome
Garlic (*Allium sativum* L.)	Liver health
Ginger (*Zingiber officinale* Roscoe)	Liver disease
Ginkgo (*Ginkgo biloba* L.)	Hepatitis B
Ginseng (American ginseng, Asian ginseng, Chinese ginseng, Korean red ginseng, *Panax ginseng*: *Panax* spp. including *P. ginseng* C.C. Meyer and *P. quinquefolium* L., excluding *Eleutherococcus senticosus*)	Hepatitis/hepatitis B virus infection
Ginseng (American ginseng, Asian ginseng, Chinese ginseng, Korean red ginseng, *Panax ginseng*: *Panax* spp. including *P. ginseng* C.C. Meyer and *P. quinquefolium* L., excluding *Eleutherococcus senticosus*)	Liver diseases
Ginseng (American ginseng, Asian ginseng, Chinese ginseng, Korean red ginseng, *Panax ginseng*: *Panax* spp. including *P. ginseng* C.C. Meyer and *P. quinquefolium* L., excluding *Eleutherococcus senticosus*)	Liver health
Globe artichoke (*Cynara scolymus* L.)	Jaundice
Goldenseal (*Hydrastis canadensis* L.), berberine	Alcoholic liver disease
Goldenseal (*Hydrastis canadensis* L.), berberine	Hepatitis
Goldenseal (*Hydrastis canadensis* L.), berberine	Jaundice
Goldenseal (*Hydrastis canadensis* L.), berberine	Liver disorders
Gotu kola (*Centella asiatica* L.), total triterpenic fraction of *Centella asiatica* (TTFCA)	Hepatitis

Gotu kola (*Centella asiatica* L.), total triterpenic fraction of *Centella asiatica* (TTFCA)	Jaundice
Gymnema (*Gymnema sylvestre* R. Br.)	Liver disease
Gymnema (*Gymnema sylvestre* R. Br.)	Liver protection
Horse chestnut (*Aesculus hippocastanum* L.)	Liver congestion
Horsetail (*Equisetum arvense* L.)	Liver protection
Licorice (*Glycyrrhiza glabra* L.), deglycyrrhizinated licorice (DGL)	Liver protection
Maitake mushroom (*Grifola frondosa*), beta-glucan	Liver inflammation (hepatitis)
Melatonin	Toxic liver damage
Milk thistle (*Silybum marianum*), silymarin	Jaundice
Milk thistle (*Silybum marianum*), silymarin	Liver cleansing agent
Niacin (vitamin B$_3$, nicotinic acid), niacinamide, inositol hexanicotinate	Liver disease
Omega-3 fatty acids, fish oil, alpha-linolenic acid	Cirrhosis

LOWER BACK PAIN AND RELATED CONDITIONS

Levels of Scientific Evidence for Specific Therapies

GRADE: C (Unclear or Conflicting Scientific Evidence)

Therapy	Specific Therapeutic Use(s)
Devil's claw (*Harpagophytum procumbens* DC.)	Low back pain

TRADITIONAL OR THEORETICAL USES THAT LACK SUFFICIENT EVIDENCE

Therapy	Specific Therapeutic Use(s)
Belladonna (*Atropa belladonna* L. or its variety *A. acuminata* Royle ex Lindl)	Sciatica (back and leg pain)
Black cohosh (*Cimicifuga racemosa* L. Nutt.)	Back pain
Bromelain	Back pain
Bromelain	Sciatica
Burdock (*Arctium lappa*)	Back pain
Burdock (*Arctium lappa*)	Sciatica
Chamomile (*Matricaria recutita, Chamaemelum nobile*)	Back pain
Chamomile (*Matricaria recutita, Chamaemelum nobile*)	Sciatica
Dong quai (*Angelica sinensis* [Oliv.] Diels), Chinese angelica	Back pain
Dong quai (*Angelica sinensis* [Oliv.] Diels), Chinese angelica	Sciatica
Eucalyptus oil (*Eucalyptus globulus* Labillardiere, *E. fructicetorum* F. Von Mueller, *e. smithii* R.T. Baker)	Back pain
Goldenseal (*Hydrastis canadensis* L.), berberine	Sciatica

LOWER EXTREMEITY EDEMA AND RELATED CONDITIONS

Levels of Scientific Evidence for Specific Therapies

GRADE: A (Strong Scientific Evidence)

Therapy	Specific Therapeutic Use(s)
Horse chestnut (*Aesculus hippocastanum* L.)	Chronic venous insufficiency

GRADE: B (Good Scientific Evidence)

Therapy	Specific Therapeutic Use(s)
Gotu kola (*Centella asiatica* L.), total triterpenic fraction of *Centella asiatica* (TTFCA)	Chronic venous insufficiency/ varicose veins

GRADE: C (Unclear or Conflicting Scientific Evidence)

Therapy	Specific Therapeutic Use(s)
Bilberry (*Vaccinium myrtillus*)	Chronic venous insufficiency
Glucosamine	Chronic venous insufficiency

TRADITIONAL OR THEORETICAL USES THAT LACK SUFFICIENT EVIDENCE

Therapy	Specific Therapeutic Use(s)
Astragalus (*Astragalus membranaceus*)	Edema
Barley (*Hordeum vulgare* L.), germinated barley foodstuff (GBF)	Improved blood circulation
Bilberry (*Vaccinium myrtillus*)	Poor circulation
Black cohosh (*Cimicifuga racemosa* L. Nutt.)	Edema
Black tea (*Camellia sinensis*)	Circulatory/blood flow disorders
Bladderwrack (*Fucus vesiculosus*)	Edema
Bromelain	Varicose veins
Burdock (*Arctium lappa*)	Fluid retention
Calendula (*Calendula officinalis* L.), marigold	Circulation problems
Calendula (*Calendula officinalis* L.), marigold	Edema
Calendula (*Calendula officinalis* L.), marigold	Varicose veins
Dandelion (*Taraxacum officinale*)	Circulation
Dandelion (*Taraxacum officinale*)	Dropsy
Danshen (*Salvia miltiorrhiza*)	Circulation
Devil's claw (*Harpagophytum procumbens* DC.)	Edema
Dong quai (*Angelica sinensis* [Oliv.] Diels), Chinese angelica	Fluid retention
Elder (*Sambucus nigra* L.)	Circulatory stimulant
Elder (*Sambucus nigra* L.)	Edema
Ephedra (*Ephedra sinica*)/ma huang	Edema
Fenugreek (*Trigonella foenum-graecum* L.)	Dropsy
Ginkgo (*Ginkgo biloba* L.)	Swelling

Globe artichoke (*Cynara scolymus* L.)	Peripheral edema
Goldenseal (*Hydrastis canadensis* L.), berberine	Circulatory stimulant
Gotu kola (*Centella asiatica* L.), total triterpenic fraction of *Centella asiatica* (TTFCA)	Vascular fragility
Green tea (*Camellia sinensis*)	Improving blood flow
Hawthorn (*Crataegus laevigata*, *C. oxyacantha*, *C. monogyna*, *C. pentagyna*)	Edema
Horsetail (*Equisetum arvense* L.)	Dropsy
Lavender (*Lavandula angustifolia* Miller)	Circulation problems
Lavender (*Lavandula angustifolia* Miller)	Varicose veins
Melatonin	Edema
Milk thistle (*Silybum marianum*), silymarin	Edema
Niacin (vitamin B_3, nicotinic acid), niacinamide, inositol hexanicotinate	Edema
Oleander (*Nerium oleander*, *Thevetia peruviana*)	Swelling
Polypodium leucotomos extract, Anapsos	Water retention
Seaweed, kelp, bladderwrack (*Fucus vesiculosus*)	Edema
Slippery elm (*Ulmus rubra* Muhl. or *U. fulva* Michx.)	Varicose ulcers
Thyme (*Thymus vulgaris* L.), thymol	Edema
White horehound (*Marrubium vulgare* L.)	Water retention

LUNG DISEASE AND RELATED CONDITIONS
Levels of Scientific Evidence for Specific Therapies

GRADE: C (Unclear or Conflicting Scientific Evidence)	
Therapy	Specific Therapeutic Use(s)

TRADITIONAL OR THEORETICAL USES THAT LACK SUFFICIENT EVIDENCE	
Therapy	Specific Therapeutic Use(s)
American pennyroyal (*Hedeoma pulegioides* L.), European pennyroyal (*Mentha pulegium* L.)	Pneumonia
Blessed thistle (*Cnicus benedictus* L.)	Pneumonitis
Bromelain	Pneumonia
Burdock (*Arctium lappa*)	Pneumonia
Coenzyme Q10	Lung disease
Danshen (*Salvia miltiorrhiza*)	Lung fibrosis
Dong quai (*Angelica sinensis* [Oliv.] Diels), Chinese angelica	Lung disease
Dong quai (*Angelica sinensis* [Oliv.] Diels), Chinese angelica	Pleurisy
Garlic (*Allium sativum* L.)	Pneumonia
Goldenseal (*Hydrastis canadensis* L.), berberine	Pneumonia

Continued

Hops (*Humulus lupulus* L.)	Lung disease (from inhalation of silica dust or asbestos)
Melatonin	Sarcoidosis
Shark cartilage	Sarcoidosis
Slippery elm (*Ulmus rubra* Muhl. or *U. fulva* Michx.)	Lung diseases
Slippery elm (*Ulmus rubra* Muhl. or *U. fulva* Michx.)	Pleurisy
Tea tree oil (*Melaleuca alternifolia* [Maiden & Betche] Cheel)	Lung inflammation
White horehound (*Marrubium vulgare* L.)	Lung congestion
White horehound (*Marrubium vulgare* L.)	Pneumonia

MACULAR DEGENERATION AND RELATED CONDITIONS

Levels of Scientific Evidence for Specific Therapies

GRADE: C (Unclear or Conflicting Scientific Evidence)

Therapy	Specific Therapeutic Use(s)
Ginkgo (*Ginkgo biloba* L.)	Macular degeneration
Lycopene	Age-related macular degeneration prevention
Shark cartilage	Macular degeneration

TRADITIONAL OR THEORETICAL USES THAT LACK SUFFICIENT EVIDENCE

Therapy	Specific Therapeutic Use(s)
Coenzyme Q10	Macular degeneration
Omega-3 fatty acids, fish oil, alpha-linolenic acid	Age-related macular degeneration

MEMORY ENHANCEMENT AND RELATED CONDITIONS

Levels of Scientific Evidence for Specific Therapies

GRADE: B (Good Scientific Evidence)

Therapy	Specific Therapeutic Use(s)
Ginkgo (*Ginkgo biloba* L.)	Cerebral insufficiency
Ginseng (American ginseng, Asian ginseng, Chinese ginseng, Korean red ginseng, *Panax ginseng*. *Panax* spp. including *P. ginseng* C.C. Meyer and *P. quinquefolium* L., excluding *Eleutherococcus senticosus*)	Mental performance

GRADE: C (Unclear or Conflicting Scientific Evidence)

Therapy	Specific Therapeutic Use(s)
Black tea (*Camellia sinensis*)	Memory enhancement
Black tea (*Camellia sinensis*)	Mental performance/alertness
Boron	Improving cognitive function
Ginkgo (*Ginkgo biloba* L.)	Age-associated memory impairment (AAMI)

Ginkgo (*Ginkgo biloba* L.)	Memory enhancement (in healthy people)
Green tea (*Camellia sinensis*)	Memory enhancement
Green tea (*Camellia sinensis*)	Mental performance/alertness
Polypodium leucotomos extract, Anapsos	Dementia

GRADE: D (Fair Negative Scientific Evidence)	
Therapy	Specific Therapeutic Use(s)
Dehydroepiandrosterone (DHEA)	Brain function and well-being in the elderly

TRADITIONAL OR THEORETICAL USES THAT LACK SUFFICIENT EVIDENCE	
Therapy	Specific Therapeutic Use(s)
Arginine (L-arginine)	Dementia
Astragalus (*Astragalus membranaceus*)	Dementia
Astragalus (*Astragalus membranaceus*)	Memory
Blessed thistle (*Cnicus benedictus* L.)	Memory improvement
Danshen (*Salvia miltiorrhiza*)	Anoxic brain injury
Dehydroepiandrosterone (DHEA)	Dementia
Eyebright (*Euphrasia officinalis*)	Memory loss
Garlic (*Allium sativum* L.)	Age-related memory problems
Ginseng (American ginseng, Asian ginseng, Chinese ginseng, Korean red ginseng, *Panax ginseng*: *Panax* spp. including *P. ginseng* C.C. Meyer and *P. quinquefolium* L., excluding *Eleutherococcus senticosus*)	Dementia
Ginseng (American ginseng, Asian ginseng, Chinese ginseng, Korean red ginseng, *Panax ginseng*: *Panax* spp. including *P. ginseng* C.C. Meyer and *P. quinquefolium* L., excluding *Eleutherococcus senticosus*)	Improved memory and thinking after menopause
Ginseng (American ginseng, Asian ginseng, Chinese ginseng, Korean red ginseng, *Panax ginseng*: *Panax* spp. including *P. ginseng* C.C. Meyer and *P. quinquefolium* L., excluding *Eleutherococcus senticosus*)	Senile dementia
Gotu kola (*Centella asiatica* L.), total triterpenic fraction of *Centella asiatica* (TTFCA)	Memory enhancement
Green tea (*Camellia sinensis*)	Cognitive performance enhancement
Kava (*Piper methysticum* G. Forst)	Brain damage
Lycopene	Cognitive function
Melatonin	Cognitive enhancement
Melatonin	Memory enhancement
Niacin (vitamin B_3, nicotinic acid), niacinamide, inositol hexanicotinate	Memory loss
Omega-3 fatty acids, fish oil, alpha-linolenic acid	Memory enhancement
Soy (*Glycine max* L. Merr.)	Cognitive function
Soy (*Glycine max* L. Merr.)	Memory enhancement

Continued

Spirulina	Memory improvement
Valerian (*Valeriana officinalis* L.)	Memory
Yohimbe bark extract (*Pausinystalia yohimbe* Pierre ex Beille)	Cognition

MENOPAUSAL SYMPTOMS AND RELATED CONDITIONS
Levels of Scientific Evidence for Specific Therapies

GRADE: B (Good Scientific Evidence)

Therapy	Specific Therapeutic Use(s)
Black cohosh (*Cimicifuga racemosa* L. Nutt.)	Menopausal symptoms
Soy (*Glycine max* L. Merr.)	Menopausal hot flashes

GRADE: C (Unclear or Conflicting Scientific Evidence)

Therapy	Specific Therapeutic Use(s)
American pennyroyal (*Hedeoma pulegioides* L.), European pennyroyal (*Mentha pulegium* L.)	Emmenagogue (menstrual flow stimulant)
Belladonna (*Atropa belladonna* L. or its variety *A. acuminata* Royle ex Lindl)	Premenstrual syndrome
Bilberry (*Vaccinium myrtillus*)	Painful menstruation (dysmenorrhea)
Dehydroepiandrosterone (DHEA)	Menopausal disorders
Dehydroepiandrosterone (DHEA)	Ovulation disorders
Dong quai (*Angelica sinensis* [Oliv.] Diels), Chinese angelica	Amenorrhea (lack of menstrual period)
Dong quai (*Angelica sinensis* [Oliv.] Diels), Chinese angelica	Dysmenorrhea (painful menstruation)
Flaxseed and flaxseed oil (*Linum usitatissimum*)	Menstrual breast pain (flaxseed, not flaxseed oil)
Ginkgo (*Ginkgo biloba* L.)	Premenstrual syndrome
Ginseng (American ginseng, Asian ginseng, Chinese ginseng, Korean red ginseng, *Panax ginseng*: *Panax* spp. including *P. ginseng* C.C. Meyer and *P. quinquefolium* L., excluding *Eleutherococcus senticosus*)	Menopausal symptoms
Green tea (*Camellia sinensis*)	Menopausal symptoms
Omega-3 fatty acids, fish oil, alpha-linolenic acid	Dysmenorrhea (painful menstruation)
Red clover (*Trifolium pratense*)	Hormone replacement therapy (HRT)
Red clover (*Trifolium pratense*)	Menopausal symptoms
St. John's wort (*Hypericum perforatum* L.)	Perimenopausal symptoms
St. John's wort (*Hypericum perforatum* L.)	Premenstrual syndrome
Wild yam (*Dioscorea villosa*)	Menopausal symptoms

GRADE: D (Fair Negative Scientific Evidence)	
Therapy	Specific Therapeutic Use(s)
Belladonna (*Atropa belladonna* L. or its variety *A. acuminata* Royle ex Lindl)	Menopausal symptoms
Boron	Menopausal symptoms
Evening primrose oil (*Oenothera biennis* L.)	Menopause (flushing/bone metabolism)
Evening primrose oil (*Oenothera biennis* L.)	Premenstrual syndrome
Wild yam (*Dioscorea villosa*)	Hormonal properties (to mimic estrogen, progesterone, or dehydroepiandrosterone [DHEA])

TRADITIONAL OR THEORETICAL USES THAT LACK SUFFICIENT EVIDENCE	
Therapy	Specific Therapeutic Use(s)
Alfalfa (*Medicago sativa* L.)	Estrogen replacement
Alfalfa (*Medicago sativa* L.)	Menopausal symptoms
American pennyroyal (*Hedeoma pulegioides* L.), European pennyroyal (*Mentha pulegium* L.)	Cramps
American pennyroyal (*Hedeoma pulegioides* L.), European pennyroyal (*Mentha pulegium* L.)	Premenstrual syndrome
Astragalus (*Astragalus membranaceus*)	Menstrual disorders
Astragalus (*Astragalus membranaceus*)	Pelvic congestion syndrome
Belladonna (*Atropa belladonna* L. or its variety *A. acuminata* Royle ex Lindl)	Abnormal menstrual periods
Betel nut (*Areca catechu* L.)	Excessive menstrual flow
Black cohosh (*Cimicifuga racemosa* L. Nutt.)	Endometriosis
Black cohosh (*Cimicifuga racemosa* L. Nutt.)	Menstrual period problems
Black cohosh (*Cimicifuga racemosa* L. Nutt.)	Ovarian cysts
Black cohosh (*Cimicifuga racemosa* L. Nutt.)	Premenstrual syndrome
Bladderwrack (*Fucus vesiculosus*)	Menstruation irregularities
Blessed thistle (*Cnicus benedictus* L.)	Menstrual disorders
Blessed thistle (*Cnicus benedictus* L.)	Menstrual flow stimulant
Blessed thistle (*Cnicus benedictus* L.)	Painful menstruation
Boswellia (*Boswellia serrata* Roxb.)	Amenorrhea
Boswellia (*Boswellia serrata* Roxb.)	Emmenagogue (inducer of menstruation)
Bromelain	Menstrual pain
Calendula (*Calendula officinalis* L.), marigold	Cramps
Calendula (*Calendula officinalis* L.), marigold	Menstrual period abnormalities
Chamomile (*Matricaria recutita, Chamaemelum nobile*)	Dysmenorrhea
Chamomile (*Matricaria recutita, Chamaemelum nobile*)	Menstrual disorders

Continued

Chaparral (*Larrea tridentata* DC. Coville, *L. divaricata* Cav.), nordihydroguaiaretic acid (NDGA)	Menstrual cramps
Clay	Menstruation difficulties
Dandelion (*Taraxacum officinale*)	Menopause
Dandelion (*Taraxacum officinale*)	Premenstrual syndrome
Danshen (*Salvia miltiorrhiza*)	Menstrual problems
Devil's claw (*Harpagophytum procumbens* DC.)	Menopausal symptoms
Devil's claw (*Harpagophytum procumbens* DC.)	Menstrual cramps
Dehydroepiandrosterone (DHEA)	Amenorrhea associated with anorexia
Dehydroepiandrosterone (DHEA)	Andropause/andrenopause
Dehydroepiandrosterone (DHEA)	Premenstrual syndrome
Dong quai (*Angelica sinensis* [Oliv.] Diels), Chinese angelica	Cramps
Dong quai (*Angelica sinensis* [Oliv.] Diels), Chinese angelica	Hormonal abnormalities
Dong quai (*Angelica sinensis* [Oliv.] Diels), Chinese angelica	Menorrhagia (heavy menstrual bleeding)
Dong quai (*Angelica sinensis* [Oliv.] Diels), Chinese angelica	Menstrual cramping
Dong quai (*Angelica sinensis* [Oliv.] Diels), Chinese angelica	Ovulation abnormalities
Dong quai (*Angelica sinensis* [Oliv.] Diels), Chinese angelica	Pelvic congestion syndrome
Dong quai (*Angelica sinensis* [Oliv.] Diels), Chinese angelica	Premenstrual syndrome
Fenugreek (*Trigonella foenum-graecum* L.)	Menopausal symptoms
Fenugreek (*Trigonella foenum-graecum* L.)	Postmenopausal vaginal dryness
Feverfew (*Tanacetum parthenium* L. Schultz-Bip.)	Menstrual cramps
Feverfew (*Tanacetum parthenium* L. Schultz-Bip.)	Promotion of menstruation
Flaxseed and flaxseed oil (*Linum usitatissimum*)	Menstrual disorders
Flaxseed and flaxseed oil (*Linum usitatissimum*)	Ovarian disorders
Garlic (*Allium sativum* L.)	Emmenagogue
Ginger (*Zingiber officinale* Roscoe)	Dysmenorrhea
Ginger (*Zingiber officinale* Roscoe)	Promotion of menstruation
Ginkgo (*Ginkgo biloba* L.)	Menstrual pain
Ginseng (American ginseng, Asian ginseng, Chinese ginseng, Korean red ginseng, *Panax ginseng*: *Panax* spp. including *P. ginseng* C.C. Meyer and *P. quinquefolium* L., excluding *Eleutherococcus senticosus*)	Menopausal symptoms
Goldenseal (*Hydrastis canadensis* L.), berberine	Menstruation problems
Goldenseal (*Hydrastis canadensis* L.), berberine	Premenstrual syndrome
Gotu kola (*Centella asiatica* L.), total triterpenic fraction of *Centella asiatica* (TTFCA)	Amenorrhea
Gotu kola (*Centella asiatica* L.), total triterpenic fraction of *Centella asiatica* (TTFCA)	Hot flashes
Gotu kola (*Centella asiatica* L.), total triterpenic fraction of *Centella asiatica* (TTFCA)	Menstrual disorders

Guggul (*Commifora mukul*)	Menstrual disorders
Hawthorn (*Crataegus laevigata*, *C. oxyacantha*, *C. monogyna*, *C. pentagyna*)	Amenorrhea
Hops (*Humulus lupulus* L.)	Estrogenic effects
Horse chestnut (*Aesculus hippocastanum* L.)	Menstrual pain
Horsetail (*Equisetum arvense* L.)	Menstrual pain
Kava (*Piper methysticum* G. Forst)	Menopause
Kava (*Piper methysticum* G. Forst)	Menstrual disorders
Lavender (*Lavandula angustifolia* Miller)	Menopause
Lavender (*Lavandula angustifolia* Miller)	Menstrual period problems
Licorice (*Glycyrrhiza glabra* L.), deglycyrrhizinated licorice (DGL)	Hormone regulation
Licorice (*Glycyrrhiza glabra* L.), deglycyrrhizinated licorice (DGL)	Menopausal symptoms
Melatonin	Melatonin deficiency
Milk thistle (*Silybum marianum*), silymarin	Menstrual disorders
Niacin (vitamin B$_3$, nicotinic acid), niacinamide, inositol hexanicotinate	Painful menstruation
Niacin (vitamin B$_3$, nicotinic acid), niacinamide, inositol hexanicotinate	Premenstrual headache prevention
Niacin (vitamin B$_3$, nicotinic acid), niacinamide, inositol hexanicotinate	Premenstrual syndrome
Oleander (*Nerium oleander*, *Thevetia peruviana*)	Abnormal menstruation
Oleander (*Nerium oleander*, *Thevetia peruviana*)	Menstrual stimulant
Omega-3 fatty acids, fish oil, alpha-linolenic acid	Menopausal symptoms
Omega-3 fatty acids, fish oil, alpha-linolenic acid	Menstrual cramps
Omega-3 fatty acids, fish oil, alpha-linolenic acid	Premenstrual syndrome
Passionflower (*Passiflora incarnata* L.)	Menopausal symptoms (hot flashes)
Peppermint (*Mentha* x *piperita* L.)	Cramps
Peppermint (*Mentha* x *piperita* L.)	Dysmenorrhea (menstrual pain)
Psyllium (*Plantago ovata*, *P. ispaghula*)	Excessive menstrual bleeding
Red clover (*Trifolium pratense*)	Hot flashes
Red clover (*Trifolium pratense*)	Premenstrual syndrome
Saw palmetto (*Serenoa repens* [Bartram] Small)	Antiandrogen
Saw palmetto (*Serenoa repens* [Bartram] Small)	Antiestrogen
Saw palmetto (*Serenoa repens* [Bartram] Small)	Dysmenorrhea
Saw palmetto (*Serenoa repens* [Bartram] Small)	Estrogenic agent
Saw palmetto (*Serenoa repens* [Bartram] Small)	Ovarian cysts
Saw palmetto (*Serenoa repens* [Bartram] Small)	Pelvic congestive syndrome
Seaweed, kelp, bladderwrack (*Fucus vesiculosus*)	Menstrual irregularities (menorrhagia)

Continued

Slippery elm (*Ulmus rubra* Muhl. or *U. fulva* Michx.)	Gynecologic disorders
Spirulina	Premenstrual syndrome
St. John's wort (*Hypericum perforatum* L.)	Menstrual pain
Sweet almond (*Prunus amygdalus dulcis*)	Plant-derived estrogen
Thyme (*Thymus vulgaris* L.), thymol	Dysmenorrhea
Turmeric (*Curcuma longa* L.), curcumin	Menstrual pain
Turmeric (*Curcuma longa* L.), curcumin	Menstrual period problems/ lack of menstrual period
Valerian (*Valeriana officinalis* L.)	Amenorrhea
Valerian (*Valeriana officinalis* L.)	Dysmenorrhea
Valerian (*Valeriana officinalis* L.)	Emmenagogue
Valerian (*Valeriana officinalis* L.)	Menopause
Valerian (*Valeriana officinalis* L.)	Premenstrual syndrome
White horehound (*Marrubium vulgare* L.)	Dysmenorrhea
White horehound (*Marrubium vulgare* L.)	Menstrual pain
Wild yam (*Dioscorea villosa*)	Cramps
Wild yam (*Dioscorea villosa*)	Menopause
Wild yam (*Dioscorea villosa*)	Menstrual pain or irregularities
Wild yam (*Dioscorea villosa*)	Pelvic cramps
Wild yam (*Dioscorea villosa*)	Postmenopausal vaginal dryness
Wild yam (*Dioscorea villosa*)	Premenstrual syndrome

METABOLIC DISORDERS AND RELATED CONDITIONS
Levels of Scientific Evidence for Specific Therapies

GRADE: A (Strong Scientific Evidence)

Therapy	Specific Therapeutic Use(s)
Arginine (L-arginine)	Inborn errors of urea synthesis

GRADE: C (Unclear or Conflicting Scientific Evidence)

Therapy	Specific Therapeutic Use(s)
Coenzyme Q10	Mitochondrial diseases, Kearns-Sayre syndrome

TRADITIONAL OR THEORETICAL USES THAT LACK SUFFICIENT EVIDENCE

Therapy	Specific Therapeutic Use(s)
Astragalus (*Astragalus membranaceus*)	Metabolic disorders
Calendula (*Calendula officinalis* L.), marigold	Metabolic disorders
Coenzyme Q10	Mitochondrial encephalopathy–lactic acidosis–stroke-like symptoms (MELAS) syndrome
Ephedra (*Ephedra sinica*)/ma huang	Metabolic enhancement

MOUTH SORES AND RELATED CONDITIONS

Levels of Scientific Evidence for Specific Therapies

GRADE: C (Unclear or Conflicting Scientific Evidence)

Therapy	Specific Therapeutic Use(s)
Aloe (*Aloe vera*)	Canker sores (aphthous stomatitis)
Chamomile (*Matricaria recutita*, *Chamaemelum nobile*)	Mucositis from cancer treatment (mouth ulcers/irritation)
Licorice (*Glycyrrhiza glabra* L.), deglycyrrhizinated licorice (DGL)	Aphthous ulcers/canker sores
Spirulina	Oral leukoplakia (precancerous mouth lesions)

TRADITIONAL OR THEORETICAL USES THAT LACK SUFFICIENT EVIDENCE

Therapy	Specific Therapeutic Use(s)
American pennyroyal (*Hedeoma pulegioides* L.), European pennyroyal (*Mentha pulegium* L.)	Mouth sores
Bilberry (*Vaccinium myrtillus*)	Oral ulcers
Burdock (*Arctium lappa*)	Canker sores
Clove (*Eugenia aromatica*)	Mouth and throat inflammation
Dandelion (*Taraxacum officinale*)	Aphthous ulcers
Fenugreek (*Trigonella foenum-graecum* L.)	Aphthous ulcers
Fenugreek (*Trigonella foenum-graecum* L.)	Chapped lips
Goldenseal (*Hydrastis canadensis* L.), berberine	Canker sores
Green tea (*Camellia sinensis*)	Oral leukoplakia
Lactobacillus acidophilus	Canker sores
Peppermint (*Mentha* x *piperita* L.)	Inflammation of oral mucosa
Red clover (*Trifolium pratense*)	Canker sores
Sorrel (*Rumex acetosa* L., *R. acetosella* L.), Sinupret	Oral ulcers
Sweet almond (*Prunus amygdalus dulcis*)	Chapped lips
Tea tree oil (*Melaleuca alternifolia* [Maiden & Betche] Cheel)	Mouth sores
Thyme (*Thymus vulgaris* L.), thymol	Stomatitis

MULTIPLE SCLEROSIS (MS) AND RELATED CONDITIONS

Levels of Scientific Evidence for Specific Therapies

GRADE: C (Unclear or Conflicting Scientific Evidence)

Therapy	Specific Therapeutic Use(s)
Evening primrose oil (*Oenothera biennis* L.)	Multiple sclerosis
Ginkgo (*Ginkgo biloba* L.)	Multiple sclerosis
Yohimbe bark extract (*Pausinystalia yohimbe* Pierre ex Beille)	Autonomic failure

Continued

TRADITIONAL OR THEORETICAL USES THAT LACK SUFFICIENT EVIDENCE	
Therapy	Specific Therapeutic Use(s)
Astragalus (*Astragalus membranaceus*)	Myasthenia gravis
Boswellia (*Boswellia serrata* Roxb.)	Multiple sclerosis
Dehydroepiandrosterone (DHEA)	Multiple sclerosis
Ephedra (*Ephedra sinica*)/ma huang	Myasthenia gravis
Evening primrose oil (*Oenothera biennis* L.)	Multiple sclerosis
Melatonin	Multiple sclerosis
Niacin (vitamin B_3, nicotinic acid), niacinamide, inositol hexanicotinate	Multiple sclerosis
Omega-3 fatty acids, fish oil, alpha-linolenic acid	Multiple sclerosis

MUSCULAR DYSTROPHY AND RELATED CONDITIONS
Levels of Scientific Evidence for Specific Therapies

GRADE: C (Unclear or Conflicting Scientific Evidence)	
Therapy	Specific Therapeutic Use(s)
Coenzyme Q10	Muscular dystrophies

TRADITIONAL OR THEORETICAL USES THAT LACK SUFFICIENT EVIDENCE	
Therapy	Specific Therapeutic Use(s)
Calendula (*Calendula officinalis* L.), marigold	Muscle wasting
Coenzyme Q10	Muscular dystrophy
Omega-3 fatty acids, fish oil, alpha-linolenic acid	Myopathy

MUSCULOSKELETAL DISORDERS AND RELATED CONDITIONS
Levels of Scientific Evidence for Specific Therapies

TRADITIONAL OR THEORETICAL USES THAT LACK SUFFICIENT EVIDENCE	
Therapy	Specific Therapeutic Use(s)
Bitter almond (*Prunus amygdalus* Batch var. *amara* DC. Focke) and Laetrile	Muscle relaxant
Black cohosh (*Cimicifuga racemosa* L. Nutt.)	Muscle spasms
Boswellia (*Boswellia serrata* Roxb.)	Bursitis
Boswellia (*Boswellia serrata* Roxb.)	Tendonitis
Bromelain	Bursitis
Bromelain	Sports or other physical injuries
Bromelain	Tendonitis
Clove (*Eugenia aromatica*)	Muscle spasm

Devil's claw (*Harpagophytum procumbens* DC.)	Tendonitis
Dong quai (*Angelica sinensis* [Oliv.] Diels), Chinese angelica	Muscle relaxant
Eucalyptus oil (*Eucalyptus globulus* Labillardiere, *E. fructicetorum* F. Von Mueller, *E. smithii* R.T. Baker)	Muscle spasm
Eucalyptus oil (*Eucalyptus globulus* Labillardiere, *E. fructicetorum* F. Von Mueller, *E. smithii* R.T. Baker)	Strains/sprains (applied to the skin)
Garlic (*Allium sativum* L.)	Muscle spasms
Goldenseal (*Hydrastis canadensis* L.), berberine	Muscle spasm
Hops (*Humulus lupulus* L.)	Muscle and joint disorders
Hops (*Humulus lupulus* L.)	Muscle spasm
Lavender (*Lavandula angustifolia* Miller)	Muscle spasm
Lavender (*Lavandula angustifolia* Miller)	Sprains
Licorice (*Glycyrrhiza glabra* L.), deglycyrrhizinated licorice (DGL)	Muscle cramps
Marshmallow (*Althaea officinalis* L.)	Sprains
Niacin (vitamin B_3, nicotinic acid), niacinamide, inositol hexanicotinate	Bursitis
Omega-3 fatty acids, fish oil, alpha-linolenic acid	Tennis elbow
Peppermint (*Mentha* x *piperita* L.)	Tendonitis
Saw palmetto (*Serenoa repens* [Bartram] Small)	Muscle or intestinal spasms
Slippery elm (*Ulmus rubra* Muhl. or *U. fulva* Michx.)	Synovitis
St. John's wort (*Hypericum perforatum* L.)	Sprains
Thyme (*Thymus vulgaris* L.), thymol	Sprains
Valerian (*Valeriana officinalis* L.)	Muscle pain/spasm/tension

NAUSEA AND RELATED CONDITIONS
Levels of Scientific Evidence for Specific Therapies

GRADE: B (Good Scientific Evidence)

Therapy	Specific Therapeutic Use(s)
Ginger (*Zingiber officinale* Roscoe)	Nausea (due to chemotherapy)
Ginger (*Zingiber officinale* Roscoe)	Nausea and vomiting of pregnancy (hyperemesis gravidarum)

GRADE: C (Unclear or Conflicting Scientific Evidence)

Therapy	Specific Therapeutic Use(s)
Ginger (*Zingiber officinale* Roscoe)	Nausea and vomiting (after surgery)
Peppermint (*Mentha* x *piperita* L.)	Nausea

Continued

TRADITIONAL OR THEORETICAL USES THAT LACK SUFFICIENT EVIDENCE

Therapy	Specific Therapeutic Use(s)
Belladonna (*Atropa belladonna* L. or its variety *A. acuminata* Royle ex Lindl)	Motion sickness
Black tea (*Camellia sinensis*)	Vomiting
Calendula (*Calendula officinalis* L.), marigold	Nausea
Chamomile (*Matricaria recutita, Chamaemelum nobile*)	Motion sickness
Chamomile (*Matricaria recutita, Chamaemelum nobile*)	Nausea
Chamomile (*Matricaria recutita, Chamaemelum nobile*)	Sea sickness
Chaparral (*Larrea tridentata* DC. Coville, *L. divaricata* Cav.), nordihydroguaiaretic acid (NDGA)	Vomiting
Clay	Vomiting
Clay	Vomiting/nausea during pregnancy
Clove (*Eugenia aromatica*)	Nausea or vomiting
Cranberry (*Vaccinium macrocarpon*)	Vomiting
Elder (*Sambucus nigra* L.)	Vomiting
Globe artichoke (*Cynara scolymus* L.)	Emesis
Lavender (*Lavandula angustifolia* Miller)	Motion sickness
Lavender (*Lavandula angustifolia* Miller)	Nausea
Lavender (*Lavandula angustifolia* Miller)	Vomiting
Marshmallow (*Althaea officinalis* L.)	Vomiting
Niacin (vitamin B_3, nicotinic acid), niacinamide, inositol hexanicotinate	Motion sickness
Oleander (*Nerium oleander, Thevetia peruviana*)	Vomiting
Valerian (*Valeriana officinalis* L.)	Nausea
White horehound (*Marrubium vulgare* L.)	Emetic
Wild yam (*Dioscorea villosa*)	Emetic

NEPHROLITHIASIS (KIDNEY STONES) AND RELATED CONDITIONS

Levels of Scientific Evidence for Specific Therapies

GRADE: C (Unclear or Conflicting Scientific Evidence)

Therapy	Specific Therapeutic Use(s)
Cranberry (*Vaccinium macrocarpon*)	Kidney stones

TRADITIONAL OR THEORETICAL USES THAT LACK SUFFICIENT EVIDENCE

Therapy	Specific Therapeutic Use(s)
Aloe (*Aloe vera*)	Urolithiasis (bladder stones)
Belladonna (*Atropa belladonna* L. or its variety *A. acuminata* Royle ex Lindl)	Kidney stones

Black tea (*Camellia sinensis*)	Kidney stone prevention
Burdock (*Arctium lappa*)	Kidney stones
Cranberry (*Vaccinium macrocarpon*)	Nephrolithiasis prevention
Evening primrose oil (*Oenothera biennis* L.)	Kidney stones
Globe artichoke (*Cynara scolymus* L.)	Nephrolithiasis
Globe artichoke (*Cynara scolymus* L.)	Urolithiasis
Glucosamine	Kidney stones
Green tea (*Camellia sinensis*)	Kidney stone prevention
Horsetail (*Equisetum arvense* L.)	Kidney stones
Marshmallow (*Althaea officinalis* L.)	Kidney stones
Omega-3 fatty acids, fish oil, alpha-linolenic acid	Kidney stones
Omega-3 fatty acids, fish oil, alpha-linolenic acid	Urolithiasis (bladder stones)
Shark cartilage	Nephrolithiasis
Sorrel (*Rumex acetosa* L., *R. acetosella* L.), Sinupret	Kidney stones
Valerian (*Valeriana officinalis* L.)	Urolithiasis

NEUROLOGIC DISORDERS AND RELATED CONDITIONS

Levels of Scientific Evidence for Specific Therapies

GRADE: C (Unclear or Conflicting Scientific Evidence)

Therapy	Specific Therapeutic Use(s)
Arginine (L-arginine)	Adrenoleukodystrophy
Belladonna (*Atropa belladonna* L. or its variety *A. acuminata* Royle ex Lindl)	Nervous system disorders
Dehydroepiandrosterone (DHEA)	Myotonic dystrophy
Dong quai (*Angelica sinensis* [Oliv.] Diels), Chinese angelica	Nerve pain
Melatonin	Periodic limb movement disorder
Yohimbe bark extract (*Pausinystalia yohimbe* Pierre ex Beille)	Nervous system dysfunction (autonomic failure)

TRADITIONAL OR THEORETICAL USES THAT LACK SUFFICIENT EVIDENCE

Therapy	Specific Therapeutic Use(s)
Belladonna (*Atropa belladonna* L. or its variety *A. acuminata* Royle ex Lindl)	Hyperkinesis (excessive motor function)
Belladonna (*Atropa belladonna* L. or its variety *A. acuminata* Royle ex Lindl)	Neuralgia
Black cohosh (*Cimicifuga racemosa* L. Nutt.)	Chorea
Black cohosh (*Cimicifuga racemosa* L. Nutt.)	Neurovegetative complaints
Black tea (*Camellia sinensis*)	Trigeminal neuralgia
Calendula (*Calendula officinalis* L.), marigold	Nervous system disorders

Continued

Chamomile (*Matricaria recutita, Chamaemelum nobile*)	Neuralgia (nerve pain)
Chaparral (*Larrea tridentata* DC. Coville, *L. divaricata* Cav.), nordihydroguaiaretic acid (NDGA)	Central nervous system disorders
Coenzyme Q10	Amyotrophic lateral sclerosis (ALS)
Coenzyme Q10	Cerebellar ataxia
Devil's claw (*Harpagophytum procumbens* DC.)	Nerve pain
Dehydroepiandrosterone (DHEA)	Movement disorders
Dong quai (*Angelica sinensis* [Oliv.] Diels), Chinese angelica	Age-related nerve damage
Dong quai (*Angelica sinensis* [Oliv.] Diels), Chinese angelica	Central nervous system disorders
Elder (*Sambucus nigra* L.)	Nerve pain
Eucalyptus oil (*Eucalyptus globulus* Labillardiere, *E. fructicetorum* F. Von Mueller, *E. smithii* R.T. Baker)	Nerve pain
Ginseng (American ginseng, Asian ginseng, Chinese ginseng, Korean red ginseng, *Panax ginseng*: *Panax* spp. including *P. ginseng* C.C. Meyer and *P. quinquefolium* L., excluding *Eleutherococcus senticosus*)	Neuralgia (pain due to nerve damage or inflammation)
Green tea (*Camellia sinensis*)	Neuroprotection
Guggul (*Commifora mukul*)	Neuralgia
Horse chestnut (*Aesculus hippocastanum* L.)	Nerve pain
Horsetail (*Equisetum arvense* L.)	Neurodermatitis
Licorice (*Glycyrrhiza glabra* L.), deglycyrrhizinated licorice (DGL)	Dropped head syndrome
Melatonin	Neurodegenerative disorders
Melatonin	Tuberous sclerosis
Niacin (vitamin B$_3$, nicotinic acid), niacinamide, inositol hexanicotinate	Central nervous system disorders
Oleander (*Nerium oleander, Thevetia peruviana*)	Neurologic disorders
Passionflower (*Passiflora incarnata* L.)	Nerve pain
Peppermint (*Mentha* x *piperita* L.)	Neuralgia (nerve pain)
St. John's wort (*Hypericum perforatum* L.)	Nerve pain
Thyme (*Thymus vulgaris* L.), thymol	Neuralgia
Valerian (*Valeriana officinalis* L.)	Nervous excitability
Valerian (*Valeriana officinalis* L.)	Neuralgia
Wild yam (*Dioscorea villosa*)	Nerve pain

NEUROPATHY AND RELATED CONDITIONS

Levels of Scientific Evidence for Specific Therapies

GRADE: C (Unclear or Conflicting Scientific Evidence)

Therapy	Specific Therapeutic Use(s)
Evening primrose oil (*Oenothera biennis* L.)	Diabetic neuropathy (nerve damage)

TRADITIONAL OR THEORETICAL USES THAT LACK SUFFICIENT EVIDENCE

Therapy	Specific Therapeutic Use(s)
Astragalus (*Astragalus membranaceus*)	Diabetic neuropathy
Belladonna (*Atropa belladonna* L. or its variety *A. acuminata* Royle ex Lindl)	Pain from nerve disorders
Danshen (*Salvia miltiorrhiza*)	Diabetic nerve pain
Ginkgo (*Ginkgo biloba* L.)	Diabetic nerve damage (neuropathy)
Milk thistle (*Silybum marianum*), silymarin	Diabetic nerve pain
Omega-3 fatty acids, fish oil, alpha-linolenic acid	Diabetic neuropathy
Omega-3 fatty acids, fish oil, alpha-linolenic acid	Neuropathy
Soy (*Glycine max* L. Merr.)	Diabetic neuropathy
Yohimbe bark extract (*Pausinystalia yohimbe* Pierre ex Beille)	Diabetic neuropathy

NOSEBLEED AND RELATED CONDITIONS

Levels of Scientific Evidence for Specific Therapies

TRADITIONAL OR THEORETICAL USES THAT LACK SUFFICIENT EVIDENCE

Therapy	Specific Therapeutic Use(s)
American pennyroyal (*Hedeoma pulegioides* L.), European pennyroyal (*Mentha pulegium* L.)	Nosebleed
Calendula (*Calendula officinalis* L.), marigold	Nosebleed
Horsetail (*Equisetum arvense* L.)	Nosebleed
Soy (*Glycine max* L. Merr.)	Nosebleed (chronic)

NUTRITIONAL DEFICIENCIES AND RELATED CONDITIONS

Levels of Scientific Evidence for Specific Therapies

GRADE: A (Strong Scientific Evidence)

Therapy	Specific Therapeutic Use(s)
Niacin (vitamin B_3, nicotinic acid), niacinamide, inositol hexanicotinate	Pellagra (niacin)
Soy (*Glycine max* L. Merr.)	Dietary source of protein

GRADE: C (Unclear or Conflicting Scientific Evidence)

Therapy	Specific Therapeutic Use(s)
Bromelain	Nutrition supplementation
Cranberry (*Vaccinium macrocarpon*)	Vitamin B_{12} absorption in people using antacids
Omega-3 fatty acids, fish oil, alpha-linolenic acid	Infant eye/brain development

Continued

GRADE: D (Fair Negative Scientific Evidence)	
Therapy	Specific Therapeutic Use(s)
Omega-3 fatty acids, fish oil, alpha-linolenic acid	Appetite/weight loss in cancer patients

TRADITIONAL OR THEORETICAL USES THAT LACK SUFFICIENT EVIDENCE	
Therapy	Specific Therapeutic Use(s)
Alfalfa (*Medicago sativa* L.)	Appetite stimulant
Alfalfa (*Medicago sativa* L.)	Nutritional support
Arginine (L-arginine)	Supplementation to a low-protein diet
Astragalus (*Astragalus membranaceus*)	Anorexia
Betel nut (*Areca catechu* L.)	Appetite stimulant
Black cohosh (*Cimicifuga racemosa* L. Nutt.)	Appetite stimulant
Bladderwrack (*Fucus vesiculosus*)	Malnutrition
Blessed thistle (*Cnicus benedictus* L.)	Anorexia
Blessed thistle (*Cnicus benedictus* L.)	Appetite stimulant
Boron	Boron deficiency
Boron	Vitamin D deficiency
Burdock (*Arctium lappa*)	Anorexia nervosa
Calendula (*Calendula officinalis* L.), marigold	Appetite stimulant
Chamomile (*Matricaria recutita*, *Chamaemelum nobile*)	Anorexia
Clay	Nutrition
Coenzyme Q10	Nutrition
Cranberry (*Vaccinium macrocarpon*)	Anorexia
Dandelion (*Taraxacum officinale*)	Appetite stimulant
Dandelion (*Taraxacum officinale*)	Nutrition
Devil's claw (*Harpagophytum procumbens* DC.)	Appetite stimulant
Devil's claw (*Harpagophytum procumbens* DC.)	Loss of appetite
Dehydroepiandrosterone (DHEA)	Malnutrition
Dong quai (*Angelica sinensis* [Oliv.] Diels), Chinese angelica	Anorexia nervosa
Dong quai (*Angelica sinensis* [Oliv.] Diels), Chinese angelica	Vitamin E deficiency
Essiac	Appetite stimulant
Essiac	Nutritional supplement
Eyebright (*Euphrasia officinalis*)	Appetite stimulant
Fenugreek (*Trigonella foenum-graecum* L.)	Appetite stimulant
Fenugreek (*Trigonella foenum-graecum* L.)	Beriberi
Fenugreek (*Trigonella foenum-graecum* L.)	Rickets
Fenugreek (*Trigonella foenum-graecum* L.)	Vitamin deficiencies

Ginger (*Zingiber officinale* Roscoe)	Diminished appetite (anorexia)
Ginseng (American ginseng, Asian ginseng, Chinese ginseng, Korean red ginseng, *Panax ginseng*: *Panax* spp. including *P. ginseng* C.C. Meyer and *P. quinquefolium* L., excluding *Eleutherococcus senticosus*)	Appetite stimulant
Goldenseal (*Hydrastis canadensis* L.), berberine	Appetite stimulant
Hawthorn (*Crataegus laevigata, C. oxyacantha, C. monogyna, C. pentagyna*)	Appetite stimulant
Hops (*Humulus lupulus* L.)	Appetite stimulant
Kava (*Piper methysticum* G. Forst)	Anorexia
Lavender (*Lavandula angustifolia* Miller)	Appetite stimulant
Melatonin	Cachexia
Oleander (*Nerium oleander, Thevetia peruviana*)	Anorexia
Peppermint (*Mentha* x *piperita* L.)	Anorexia
Seaweed, kelp, bladderwrack (*Fucus vesiculosus*)	Malnutrition
Slippery elm (*Ulmus rubra* Muhl. or *U. fulva* Michx.)	Nutrition
Sorrel (*Rumex acetosa* L., *R. acetosella* L.), Sinupret	Appetite stimulation
Soy (*Glycine max* L. Merr.)	Anorexia
Spirulina	Iron deficiency
Spirulina	Vitamin and nutrient deficiency
Thyme (*Thymus vulgaris* L.), thymol	Appetite stimulant
Turmeric (*Curcuma longa* L.), curcumin	Appetite stimulant
Valerian (*Valeriana officinalis* L.)	Anorexia
White horehound (*Marrubium vulgare* L.)	Anorexia

OBSESSIVE-COMPULSIVE DISORDER AND RELATED CONDITIONS

Levels of Scientific Evidence for Specific Therapies

GRADE: C (UNCLEAR OR CONFLICTING SCIENTIFIC EVIDENCE)

Therapy	Specific Therapeutic Use(s)
St. John's wort (*Hypericum perforatum* L.)	Obsessive-compulsive disorder (OCD)

OSTEOARTHRITIS AND RELATED CONDITIONS

Levels of Scientific Evidence for Specific Therapies

GRADE: A (Strong Scientific Evidence)

Therapy	Specific Therapeutic Use(s)
Glucosamine	Knee osteoarthritis (mild to moderate)

Continued

GRADE: B (Good Scientific Evidence)	
Therapy	Specific Therapeutic Use(s)
Devil's claw (*Harpagophytum procumbens* DC.)	Osteoarthritis
Glucosamine	Osteoarthritis (general)

GRADE: C (Unclear or Conflicting Scientific Evidence)	
Therapy	Specific Therapeutic Use(s)
Black cohosh (*Cimicifuga racemosa* L. Nutt.)	Joint pain
Boron	Osteoarthritis
Boswellia (*Boswellia serrata* Roxb.)	Osteoarthritis
Chondroitin	Osteoarthritis
Glucosamine	Temporomandibular joint (TMJ) disorders
Guggul (*Commifora mukul*)	Osteoarthritis
Niacin (vitamin B$_3$, nicotinic acid), niacinamide, inositol hexanicotinate	Osteoarthritis (niacinamide)
Turmeric (*Curcuma longa* L.), curcumin	Osteoarthritis

TRADITIONAL OR THEORETICAL USES THAT LACK SUFFICIENT EVIDENCE	
Therapy	Specific Therapeutic Use(s)
American pennyroyal (*Hedeoma pulegioides* L.), European pennyroyal (*Mentha pulegium* L.)	Joint problems
Astragalus (*Astragalus membranaceus*)	Joint pain
Betel nut (*Areca catechu* L.)	Joint pain/swelling
Black tea (*Camellia sinensis*)	Joint pain
Bromelain	Joint disease
Dandelion (*Taraxacum officinale*)	Osteoarthritis
Devil's claw (*Harpagophytum procumbens* DC.)	Hip pain
Devil's claw (*Harpagophytum procumbens* DC.)	Knee pain
Dehydroepiandrosterone (DHEA)	Joint diseases
Dong quai (*Angelica sinensis* [Oliv.] Diels), Chinese angelica	Joint pain
Elder (*Sambucus nigra* L.)	Joint swelling
Ephedra (*Ephedra sinica*), ma huang	Joint pain
Feverfew (*Tanacetum parthenium* L. Schultz-Bip.)	Joint pain
Glucosamine	Joint pain
Green tea (*Camellia sinensis*)	Joint pain
Horse chestnut (*Aesculus hippocastanum* L.)	Osteoarthritis
Kava (*Piper methysticum* G. Forst)	Joint pain and stiffness
Licorice (*Glycyrrhiza glabra* L.), deglycyrrhizinated licorice (DGL)	Osteoarthritis
Omega-3 fatty acids, fish oil, alpha-linolenic acid	Osteoarthritis

St. John's wort (*Hypericum perforatum* L.)   Joint pain

Wild yam (*Dioscorea villosa*)   Joint pain

OSTEOPOROSIS AND RELATED CONDITIONS
Levels of Scientific Evidence for Specific Therapies

GRADE: C (Unclear or Conflicting Scientific Evidence)	
Therapy	Specific Therapeutic Use(s)
Black tea (*Camellia sinensis*)	Osteoporosis prevention
Boron	Osteoporosis
Dehydroepiandrosterone (DHEA)	Bone density
Horsetail (*Equisetum arvense* L.)	Osteoporosis (weakening of the bones)
Red clover (*Trifolium pratense*)	Osteoporosis
Soy (*Glycine max* L. Merr.)	Osteoporosis/postmenopausal bone loss

TRADITIONAL OR THEORETICAL USES THAT LACK SUFFICIENT EVIDENCE	
Therapy	Specific Therapeutic Use(s)
Arginine (L-arginine)	Osteoporosis
Black cohosh (*Cimicifuga racemosa* L. Nutt.)	Bone diseases
Dehydroepiandrosterone (DHEA)	Bone diseases
Dehydroepiandrosterone (DHEA)	Bone loss associated with anorexia
Dehydroepiandrosterone (DHEA)	Osteoporosis
Dong quai (*Angelica sinensis* [Oliv.] Diels), Chinese angelica	Osteoporosis
Goldenseal (*Hydrastis canadensis* L.), berberine	Osteoporosis
Green tea (*Camellia sinensis*)	Bone density improvement
Melatonin	Postmenopausal osteoporosis
Omega-3 fatty acids, fish oil, alpha-linolenic acid	Osteoporosis
Propolis	Osteoporosis
Wild yam (*Dioscorea villosa*)	Osteoporosis

OTITIS MEDIA AND RELATED CONDITIONS
Levels of Scientific Evidence for Specific Therapies

GRADE: C (Unclear or Conflicting Scientific Evidence)	
Therapy	Specific Therapeutic Use(s)
Belladonna (*Atropa belladonna* L. or its *variety* *A. acuminata* Royle ex Lindl)	Ear infection
Calendula (*Calendula officinalis* L.), marigold	Ear infection

Continued

TRADITIONAL OR THEORETICAL USES THAT LACK SUFFICIENT EVIDENCE

Therapy	Specific Therapeutic Use(s)
Belladonna (*Atropa belladonna* L. or its variety *A. acuminata* Royle ex Lindl)	Earache
Betel nut (*Areca catechu* L.)	Ear infections
Chamomile (*Matricaria recutita, Chamaemelum nobile*)	Ear infections
Eucalyptus oil (*Eucalyptus globulus* Labillardiere, *E. fructicetorum* F. Von Mueller, *E. smithii* R.T. Baker)	Ear infections
Eyebright (*Euphrasia officinalis*)	Earache
Garlic (*Allium sativum* L.)	Earache
Goldenseal (*Hydrastis canadensis* L.), berberine	Otorrhea
Kava (*Piper methysticum* G. Forst)	Otitis

PAIN AND RELATED CONDITIONS
Levels of Scientific Evidence for Specific Therapies

GRADE: B (Good Scientific Evidence)

Therapy	Specific Therapeutic Use(s)
Bromelain	Inflammation

GRADE: C (Unclear or Conflicting Scientific Evidence)

Therapy	Specific Therapeutic Use(s)
Arginine (L-arginine)	Dental pain (ibuprofen arginate)
Black cohosh (*Cimicifuga racemosa* L. Nutt.)	Arthritis pain (rheumatoid arthritis, osteoarthritis)
Dandelion (*Taraxacum officinale*)	Anti-inflammatory
Eyebright (*Euphrasia officinalis*)	Anti-inflammatory
Propolis	Dental pain
Shark cartilage	Analgesia
Turmeric (*Curcuma longa* L.), curcumin	Inflammation
White horehound (*Marrubium vulgare* L.)	Pain

TRADITIONAL OR THEORETICAL USES THAT LACK SUFFICIENT EVIDENCE

Therapy	Specific Therapeutic Use(s)
Alfalfa (*Medicago sativa* L.)	Inflammation
Arginine (L-arginine)	Pain
Astragalus (*Astragalus membranaceus*)	Myalgia (muscle pain)
Belladonna (*Atropa belladonna* L. or its variety *A. acuminata* Royle ex Lindl)	Anesthetic
Belladonna (*Atropa belladonna* L. or its variety *A. acuminata* Royle ex Lindl)	Inflammation

Belladonna (*Atropa belladonna* L. or its variety *A. acuminata* Royle ex Lindl)	Muscle and joint pain
Bitter almond (*Prunus amygdalus* Batch var. *amara* DC. Focke), Laetrile	Anti-inflammatory
Bitter almond (*Prunus amygdalus* Batch var. *amara* DC. Focke), Laetrile	Local anesthetic
Bitter almond (*Prunus amygdalus* Batch var. *amara* DC. Focke), Laetrile	Pain suppressant
Black cohosh (*Cimicifuga racemosa* L. Nutt.)	Inflammation
Black cohosh (*Cimicifuga racemosa* L. Nutt.)	Muscle pain
Black tea (*Camellia sinensis*)	Pain
Blessed thistle (*Cnicus benedictus* L.)	Inflammation
Bromelain	Pain
Bromelain	Pain (general)
Burdock (*Arctium lappa*)	Inflammation
Calendula (*Calendula officinalis* L.), marigold	Pain
Chamomile (*Matricaria recutita, Chamaemelum nobile*)	Anti-inflammatory
Chaparral (*Larrea tridentata* DC. Coville, *L. divaricata* Cav.), nordihydroguaiaretic acid (NDGA)	Anti-inflammatory
Chaparral (*Larrea tridentata* DC. Coville, *L. divaricata* Cav.), nordihydroguaiaretic acid (NDGA)	Pain
Clove (*Eugenia aromatica*)	Pain
Dandelion (*Taraxacum officinale*)	Analgesia
Devil's claw (*Harpagophytum procumbens* DC.)	Anti-inflammatory
Devil's claw (*Harpagophytum procumbens* DC.)	Muscle pain
Devil's claw (*Harpagophytum procumbens* DC.)	Pain
Dong quai (*Angelica sinensis* [Oliv.] Diels), Chinese angelica	Pain
Dong quai (*Angelica sinensis* [Oliv.] Diels), Chinese angelica	Pain from bruises
Echinacea (*Echinacea angustifolia* DC., *E. pallida, E. purpurea*)	Pain
Elder (*Sambucus nigra* L.)	Anti-inflammatory
Ephedra (*Ephedra sinica*), ma huang	Anti-inflammatory
Eucalyptus oil (*Eucalyptus globulus* Labillardiere, *E. fructicetorum* F. Von Mueller, *E. smithii* R.T. Baker)	Inflammation
Eucalyptus oil (*Eucalyptus globulus* Labillardiere, *E. fructicetorum* F. Von Mueller, *E. smithii* R.T. Baker)	Muscle/joint pain (applied to the skin)
Evening primrose oil (*Oenothera biennis* L.)	Pain
Fenugreek (*Trigonella foenum-graecum* L.)	Inflammation
Feverfew (*Tanacetum parthenium* L. Schultz-Bip.)	Anti-inflammatory
Garlic (*Allium sativum* L.)	Dental pain
Ginger (*Zingiber officinale* Roscoe)	Pain relief

Continued

Ginseng (American ginseng, Asian ginseng, Chinese ginseng, Korean red ginseng, *Panax ginseng*: *Panax* spp. including *P. ginseng* C.C. Meyer and *P. quinquefolium* L., excluding *Eleutherococcus senticosus*)	Inflammation
Ginseng (American ginseng, Asian ginseng, Chinese ginseng, Korean red ginseng, *Panax ginseng*: *Panax* spp. including *P. ginseng* C.C. Meyer and *P. quinquefolium* L., excluding *Eleutherococcus senticosus*)	Pain relief
Goldenseal (*Hydrastis canadensis* L.), berberine	Anesthetic
Goldenseal (*Hydrastis canadensis* L.), berberine	Anti-inflammatory
Goldenseal (*Hydrastis canadensis* L.), berberine	Muscle pain
Goldenseal (*Hydrastis canadensis* L.), berberine	Pain
Gotu kola (*Centella asiatica* L.), total triterpenic fraction of *Centella asiatica* (TTFCA)	Inflammation
Gotu kola (*Centella asiatica* L.), total triterpenic fraction of *Centella asiatica* (TTFCA)	Pain
Guggul (*Commifora mukul*)	Pain
Hops (*Humulus lupulus* L.)	Anti-inflammatory
Hops (*Humulus lupulus* L.)	Pain
Kava (*Piper methysticum* G. Forst)	Anesthesia
Kava (*Piper methysticum* G. Forst)	Pain
Lavender (*Lavandula angustifolia* Miller)	Anti-inflammatory
Lavender (*Lavandula angustifolia* Miller)	Pain
Licorice (*Glycyrrhiza glabra* L.), deglycyrrhizinated licorice (DGL)	Inflammation
Marshmallow (*Althaea officinalis* L.)	Inflammation
Marshmallow (*Althaea officinalis* L.)	Muscular pain
Oleander (*Nerium oleander*, *Thevetia peruviana*)	Inflammation
Passionflower (*Passiflora incarnata* L.)	Chronic pain
Passionflower (*Passiflora incarnata* L.)	Pain (general)
Peppermint (*Mentha* x *piperita* L.)	Local anesthetic
Peppermint (*Mentha* x *piperita* L.)	Musculoskeletal pain
Peppermint (*Mentha* x *piperita* L.)	Myalgia (muscle pain)
Polypodium leucotomos extract, Anapsos	Inflammation
Pygeum (*Prunus africana*, *Pygeum africanum*)	Inflammation
Saw palmetto (*Serenoa repens* [Bartram] Small)	Anti-inflammatory
Slippery elm (*Ulmus rubra* Muhl. or *U. fulva* Michx.)	Inflammation
Spirulina	Anti-inflammatory
St. John's wort (*Hypericum perforatum* L.)	Anti-inflammatory
St. John's wort (*Hypericum perforatum* L.)	Dental pain
St. John's wort (*Hypericum perforatum* L.)	Pain relief
Tea tree oil (*Melaleuca alternifolia* [Maiden & Betche] Cheel)	Anti-inflammatory

Tea tree oil (*Melaleuca alternifolia* [Maiden & Betche] Cheel)	Muscle and joint pain
Turmeric (*Curcuma longa* L.), curcumin	Pain
Valerian (*Valeriana officinalis* L.)	Anodyne (pain relief)
Valerian (*Valeriana officinalis* L.)	Muscle pain
Valerian (*Valeriana officinalis* L.)	Pain
White horehound (*Marrubium vulgare* L.)	Pain
Wild yam (*Dioscorea villosa*)	Anti-inflammatory
Yohimbe bark extract (*Pausinystalia yohimbe* Pierre ex Beille)	Anesthetic

PEPTIC ULCER DISEASE AND RELATED CONDITIONS

Levels of Scientific Evidence for Specific Therapies

GRADE: C (Unclear or Conflicting Scientific Evidence)

Therapy	Specific Therapeutic Use(s)
Bilberry (*Vaccinium myrtillus*)	Stomach ulcers (peptic ulcer disease)
Blessed thistle (*Cnicus benedictus* L.)	Indigestion and flatulence (gas)
Cranberry (*Vaccinium macrocarpon*)	Stomach ulcers caused by Helicobacter pylori bacteria
Globe artichoke (*Cynara scolymus* L.)	Nonulcer dyspepsia
Licorice (*Glycyrrhiza glabra* L.), deglycyrrhizinated licorice (DGL)	Bleeding stomach ulcers caused by aspirin
Licorice (*Glycyrrhiza glabra* L.), deglycyrrhizinated licorice (DGL)	Peptic ulcer disease
Peppermint (*Mentha* x *piperita* L.)	Indigestion (nonulcer dyspepsia)
Turmeric (*Curcuma longa* L.), curcumin	Dyspepsia (heartburn)
Turmeric (*Curcuma longa* L.), curcumin	Peptic ulcer disease (stomach ulcer)
White horehound (*Marrubium vulgare* L.)	Heartburn/poor appetite

GRADE: D (Fair Negative Scientific Evidence)

Therapy	Specific Therapeutic Use(s)
Garlic (*Allium sativum* L.)	Stomach ulcers caused by *Helicobacter pylori* bacteria

TRADITIONAL OR THEORETICAL USES THAT LACK SUFFICIENT EVIDENCE

Therapy	Specific Therapeutic Use(s)
Alfalfa (*Medicago sativa* L.)	Indigestion
Alfalfa (*Medicago sativa* L.)	Stomach ulcers
American pennyroyal (*Hedeoma pulegioides* L.), European pennyroyal (*Mentha pulegium* L.)	Indigestion

Continued

Arginine (L-arginine)	Stomach ulcer
Astragalus (*Astragalus membranaceus*)	Stomach ulcer
Barley (*Hordeum vulgare* L.), germinated barley foodstuff (GBF)	Gastritis
Barley (*Hordeum vulgare* L.), germinated barley foodstuff (GBF)	Gastrointestinal inflammation
Belladonna (*Atropa belladonna* L. or its variety *A. acuminata* Royle ex Lindl)	Stomach ulcers
Bilberry (*Vaccinium myrtillus*)	Dyspepsia
Bilberry (*Vaccinium myrtillus*)	Infantile dyspepsia
Bladderwrack (*Fucus vesiculosus*)	Heartburn
Bladderwrack (*Fucus vesiculosus*)	Ulcer
Boswellia (*Boswellia serrata* Roxb.)	Dyspepsia
Boswellia (*Boswellia serrata* Roxb.)	Peptic ulcer disease
Bromelain	Indigestion
Bromelain	Stomach ulcer/stomach ulcer prevention
Calendula (*Calendula officinalis* L.), marigold	Indigestion
Calendula (*Calendula officinalis* L.), marigold	Stomach ulcers
Chamomile (*Matricaria recutita*, *Chamaemelum nobile*)	Heartburn
Chaparral (*Larrea tridentata* DC. Coville, *L. divaricata* Cav.), nordihydroguaiaretic acid (NDGA)	Heartburn
Chaparral (*Larrea tridentata* DC. Coville, *L. divaricata* Cav.), nordihydroguaiaretic acid (NDGA)	Indigestion
Chaparral (*Larrea tridentata* DC. Coville, *L. divaricata* Cav.), nordihydroguaiaretic acid (NDGA)	Stomach ulcer
Coenzyme Q10	Stomach ulcer
Dandelion (*Taraxacum officinale*)	Heartburn
Danshen (*Salvia miltiorrhiza*)	Gastric ulcers
Danshen (*Salvia miltiorrhiza*)	Stomach ulcers
Devil's claw (*Harpagophytum procumbens* DC.)	Dyspepsia
Devil's claw (*Harpagophytum procumbens* DC.)	Heartburn
Devil's claw (*Harpagophytum procumbens* DC.)	Indigestion
Dong quai (*Angelica sinensis* [Oliv.] Diels), Chinese angelica	Heartburn
Echinacea (*Echinacea angustifolia* DC., *E. pallida*, *E. purpurea*)	Dyspepsia
Evening primrose oil (*Oenothera biennis* L.)	Disorders of the stomach and intestines
Fenugreek (*Trigonella foenum-graecum* L.)	Dyspepsia
Fenugreek (*Trigonella foenum-graecum* L.)	Gastritis
Fenugreek (*Trigonella foenum-graecum* L.)	Indigestion
Flaxseed and flaxseed oil (*Linum usitatissimum*)	Enteritis
Flaxseed and flaxseed oil (*Linum usitatissimum*)	Gastritis

Garlic (*Allium sativum* L.)	Stomach acid reduction
Ginger (*Zingiber officinale* Roscoe)	Antacid
Ginger (*Zingiber officinale* Roscoe)	Dyspepsia
Ginger (*Zingiber officinale* Roscoe)	*Helicobacter pylori* infection
Ginger (*Zingiber officinale* Roscoe)	Stomach ulcers
Goldenseal (*Hydrastis canadensis* L.), berberine	Gastroenteritis
Goldenseal (*Hydrastis canadensis* L.), berberine	Indigestion
Goldenseal (*Hydrastis canadensis* L.), berberine	Stomach ulcers
Gotu kola (*Centella asiatica* L.), total triterpenic fraction of *Centella asiatica* (TTFCA)	Gastritis
Green tea (*Camellia sinensis*)	Gastritis
Green tea (*Camellia sinensis*)	*Helicobacter pylori* infection
Hawthorn (*Crataegus laevigata, C. oxyacantha, C. monogyna, C. pentagyna*)	Dyspepsia
Hops (*Humulus lupulus* L.)	Indigestion
Horse chestnut (*Aesculus hippocastanum* L.)	Ulcers
Horsetail (*Equisetum arvense* L.)	Dyspepsia
Kava (*Piper methysticum* G. Forst)	Dyspepsia
Lactobacillus acidophilus	Heartburn
Lactobacillus acidophilus	Indigestion
Lactobacillus acidophilus	Stomach ulcer
Lavender (*Lavandula angustifolia* Miller)	Heartburn
Lavender (*Lavandula angustifolia* Miller)	Indigestion
Licorice (*Glycyrrhiza glabra* L.), deglycyrrhizinated licorice (DGL)	Gastroesophageal reflux disease
Marshmallow (*Althaea officinalis* L.)	Duodenal ulcer
Marshmallow (*Althaea officinalis* L.)	Enteritis
Marshmallow (*Althaea officinalis* L.)	Gastroenteritis
Marshmallow (*Althaea officinalis* L.)	Indigestion
Marshmallow (*Althaea officinalis* L.)	Peptic ulcer disease
Melatonin	Gastroesophageal reflux disease
Niacin (vitamin B$_3$, nicotinic acid), niacinamide, inositol hexanicotinate	Stomach ulcer
Oleander (*Nerium oleander, Thevetia peruviana*)	Indigestion
Peppermint (*Mentha* x *piperita* L.)	Antacid
Peppermint (*Mentha* x *piperita* L.)	Enteritis
Peppermint (*Mentha* x *piperita* L.)	Gastritis
Propolis	Stomach ulcer
Psyllium (*Plantago ovata, P. ispaghula*)	Duodenal ulcer

Continued

Psyllium (*Plantago ovata, P. ispaghula*)	Stomach ulcer
Red clover (*Trifolium pratense*)	Indigestion
Red yeast rice (*Monascus purpureus*)	Indigestion
Saw palmetto (*Serenoa repens* [Bartram] Small)	Indigestion
Seaweed, kelp, bladderwrack (*Fucus vesiculosus*)	Dyspepsia
Seaweed, kelp, bladderwrack (*Fucus vesiculosus*)	Heartburn
Seaweed, kelp, bladderwrack (*Fucus vesiculosus*)	Ulcer
Shark cartilage	Enteritis
Slippery elm (*Ulmus rubra* Muhl. or *U. fulva* Michx.)	Duodenal ulcer
Slippery elm (*Ulmus rubra* Muhl. or *U. fulva* Michx.)	Enteritis
Slippery elm (*Ulmus rubra* Muhl. or *U. fulva* Michx.)	Gastric ulcer
Slippery elm (*Ulmus rubra* Muhl. or *U. fulva* Michx.)	Gastritis
Slippery elm (*Ulmus rubra* Muhl. or *U. fulva* Michx.)	Gastroesophageal reflux disease
Slippery elm (*Ulmus rubra* Muhl. or *U. fulva* Michx.)	Heartburn
Slippery elm (*Ulmus rubra* Muhl. or *U. fulva* Michx.)	Peptic ulcer disease
Spirulina	Stomach acid excess
Spirulina	Ulcers
St. John's wort (*Hypericum perforatum* L.)	Heartburn
St. John's wort (*Hypericum perforatum* L.)	Ulcers
Thyme (*Thymus vulgaris* L.), thymol	Dyspepsia
Thyme (*Thymus vulgaris* L.), thymol	Gastritis
Thyme (*Thymus vulgaris* L.), thymol	Heartburn
Thyme (*Thymus vulgaris* L.), thymol	Indigestion
Valerian (*Valeriana officinalis* L.)	Heartburn
Valerian (*Valeriana officinalis* L.)	Peptic ulcer disease
White horehound (*Marrubium vulgare* L.)	Indigestion

PERIPHERAL VASCULAR DISEASE AND RELATED CONDITIONS

Levels of Scientific Evidence for Specific Therapies

GRADE: A (Strong Scientific Evidence)	
Therapy	Specific Therapeutic Use(s)
Ginkgo (*Ginkgo biloba* L.)	Claudication (painful legs from clogged arteries)

GRADE: C (Unclear or Conflicting Scientific Evidence)	
Therapy	Specific Therapeutic Use(s)
Arginine (L-arginine)	Peripheral vascular disease/ claudication
Garlic (*Allium sativum* L.)	Peripheral vascular disease (blocked arteries in the legs)

TRADITIONAL OR THEORETICAL USES THAT LACK SUFFICIENT EVIDENCE	
Therapy	Specific Therapeutic Use(s)
Garlic (*Allium sativum* L.)	Claudication (leg pain due to poor blood flow)
Niacin (vitamin B$_3$, nicotinic acid), niacinamide, inositol hexanicotinate	Peripheral vascular disease
Omega-3 fatty acids, fish oil, alpha-linolenic acid	Peripheral vascular disease

PLAQUE/PERIODONTAL DISEASE AND RELATED CONDITIONS

Levels of Scientific Evidence for Specific Therapies

GRADE: C (Unclear or Conflicting Scientific Evidence)	
Therapy	Specific Therapeutic Use(s)
Betel nut (*Areca catechu* L.)	Dental cavities
Black tea (*Camellia sinensis*)	Dental cavity prevention
Coenzyme Q10	Gum disease (periodontitis)
Cranberry (*Vaccinium macrocarpon*)	Dental plaque
Eucalyptus oil (*Eucalyptus globulus* Labillardiere, *E. fructicetorum* F. Von Mueller, *E. smithii* R.T. Baker)	Dental plaque/gingivitis (mouthwash)
Green tea (*Camellia sinensis*)	Dental cavity prevention
Propolis	Dental plaque and gingivitis (mouthwash)
Thyme (*Thymus vulgaris* L.), thymol	Dental plaque

TRADITIONAL OR THEORETICAL USES THAT LACK SUFFICIENT EVIDENCE	
Therapy	Specific Therapeutic Use(s)
Arginine (L-arginine)	Peritonitis
Astragalus (*Astragalus membranaceus*)	Denture adhesive (astragalus sap)
Bilberry (*Vaccinium myrtillus*)	Bleeding gums
Chamomile (*Matricaria recutita, Chamaemelum nobile*)	Gingivitis
Clove (*Eugenia aromatica*)	Cavities
Coenzyme Q10	Gingivitis
Echinacea (*Echinacea angustifolia* DC., *E. pallida, E. purpurea*)	Gingivitis
Goldenseal (*Hydrastis canadensis* L.), berberine	Gingivitis
Gotu kola (*Centella asiatica* L.), total triterpenic fraction of *Centella asiatica* (TTFCA)	Periodontal disease
Green tea (*Camellia sinensis*)	Bleeding of gums or tooth sockets
Green tea (*Camellia sinensis*)	Gum swelling
Guggul (*Commifora mukul*)	Gingivitis
Licorice (*Glycyrrhiza glabra* L.), deglycyrrhizinated licorice (DGL)	Dental hygiene

Continued

Licorice (*Glycyrrhiza glabra* L.), deglycyrrhizinated licorice (DGL)	Plaque
Lycopene	Periodontal disease
Milk thistle (*Silybum marianum*), silymarin	Peritonitis
Omega-3 fatty acids, fish oil, alpha-linolenic acid	Gingivitis
Tea tree oil (*Melaleuca alternifolia* [Maiden & Betche] Cheel)	Dental plaque
Tea tree oil (*Melaleuca alternifolia* [Maiden & Betche] Cheel)	Gingivitis
Tea tree oil (*Melaleuca alternifolia* [Maiden & Betche] Cheel)	Periodontal disease
Thyme (*Thymus vulgaris* L.), thymol	Gingivitis

PNEUMONIA AND RELATED CONDITIONS
Levels of Scientific Evidence for Specific Therapies

TRADITIONAL OR THEORETICAL USES THAT LACK SUFFICIENT EVIDENCE

Therapy	Specific Therapeutic Use(s)
American pennyroyal (*Hedeoma pulegioides* L.), European pennyroyal (*Mentha pulegium* L.)	Pneumonia
Blessed thistle (*Cnicus benedictus* L.)	Pneumonitis
Bromelain	Pneumonia
Burdock (*Arctium lappa*)	Pneumonia
Coenzyme Q10	Lung disease
Danshen (*Salvia miltiorrhiza*)	Lung fibrosis
Dong quai (*Angelica sinensis* [Oliv.] Diels), Chinese angelica	Lung disease
Dong quai (*Angelica sinensis* [Oliv.] Diels), Chinese angelica	Pleurisy
Garlic (*Allium sativum* L.)	Pneumonia
Goldenseal (*Hydrastis canadensis* L.), berberine	Pneumonia
Hops (*Humulus lupulus* L.)	Lung disease (from inhalation of silica dust or asbestos)
Melatonin	Sarcoidosis
Shark cartilage	Sarcoidosis
Slippery elm (*Ulmus rubra* Muhl. or *U. fulva* Michx.)	Lung diseases
Slippery elm (*Ulmus rubra* Muhl. or *U. fulva* Michx.)	Pleurisy
Tea tree oil (*Melaleuca alternifolia* [Maiden & Betche] Cheel)	Lung inflammation
White horehound (*Marrubium vulgare* L.)	Lung congestion
White horehound (*Marrubium vulgare* L.)	Pneumonia

POISONING AND RELATED CONDITIONS
Levels of Scientific Evidence for Specific Therapies

GRADE: C (Unclear or Conflicting Scientific Evidence)

Therapy	Specific Therapeutic Use(s)
Clay	Mercuric chloride poisoning

TRADITIONAL OR THEORETICAL USES THAT LACK SUFFICIENT EVIDENCE	
Therapy	Specific Therapeutic Use(s)
Belladonna (*Atropa belladonna* L. or its variety *A. acuminata* Royle ex Lindl)	Poisoning (especially by insecticides)
Clay	Poisoning
Essiac	Blood cleanser
Essiac	Chelating agent (heavy metals)
Hoxsey formula	Elimination of toxins
Marshmallow (*Althaea officinalis* L.)	Antidote to poisons
Melatonin	Aluminum toxicity
Melatonin	Lead toxicity

POLYCYSTIC OVARY SYNDROME AND RELATED CONDITIONS

Levels of Scientific Evidence for Specific Therapies

TRADITIONAL OR THEORETICAL USES THAT LACK SUFFICIENT EVIDENCE	
Therapy	Specific Therapeutic Use(s)
Black cohosh (*Cimicifuga racemosa* L. Nutt.)	Polycystic ovary syndrome
Dehydroepiandrosterone (DHEA)	Polycystic ovary syndrome
Licorice (*Glycyrrhiza glabra* L.), deglycyrrhizinated licorice (DGL)	Polycystic ovary syndrome
Saw palmetto (*Serenoa repens* [Bartram] Small)	Polycystic ovary syndrome

PREMENSTRUAL SYNDROME AND RELATED CONDITIONS

Levels of Scientific Evidence for Specific Therapies

GRADE: B (Good Scientific Evidence)	
Therapy	Specific Therapeutic Use(s)
Black cohosh (*Cimicifuga racemosa* L. Nutt.)	Menopausal symptoms
Soy (*Glycine max* L. Merr.)	Menopausal hot flashes

GRADE: C (Unclear or Conflicting Scientific Evidence)	
Therapy	Specific Therapeutic Use(s)
American pennyroyal (*Hedeoma pulegioides* L.), European pennyroyal (*Mentha pulegium* L.)	Emmenagogue (menstrual flow stimulant)
Belladonna (*Atropa belladonna* L. or its variety *A. acuminata* Royle ex Lindl)	Premenstrual syndrome
Bilberry (*Vaccinium myrtillus*)	Painful menstruation (dysmenorrhea)
Dehydroepiandrosterone (DHEA)	Menopausal disorders
Dehydroepiandrosterone (DHEA)	Ovulation disorders
Dong quai (*Angelica sinensis* [Oliv.] Diels), Chinese angelica	Amenorrhea (lack of menstrual periods)

Continued

Dong quai (*Angelica sinensis* [Oliv.] Diels), Chinese angelica	Dysmenorrhea (painful menstruation)
Flaxseed and flaxseed oil (*Linum usitatissimum*)	Menstrual breast pain (flaxseed, not flaxseed oil)
Ginkgo (*Ginkgo biloba* L.)	Premenstrual syndrome
Ginseng (American ginseng, Asian ginseng, Chinese ginseng, Korean red ginseng, *Panax ginseng*: *Panax* spp. including *P. ginseng* C.C. Meyer and *P. quinquefolium* L., excluding *Eleutherococcus senticosus*)	Menopausal symptoms
Green tea (*Camellia sinensis*)	Menopausal symptoms
Omega-3 fatty acids, fish oil, alpha-linolenic acid	Dysmenorrhea (painful menstruation)
Red clover (*Trifolium pratense*)	Hormone replacement therapy (HRT)
Red clover (*Trifolium pratense*)	Menopausal symptoms
St. John's wort (*Hypericum perforatum* L.)	Perimenopausal symptoms
St. John's wort (*Hypericum perforatum* L.)	Premenstrual syndrome
Wild yam (*Dioscorea villosa*)	Menopausal symptoms

GRADE: D (Fair Negative Scientific Evidence)

Therapy	Specific Therapeutic Use(s)
Belladonna (*Atropa belladonna* L. or its variety *A. acuminata* Royle ex Lindl)	Menopausal symptoms
Boron	Menopausal symptoms
Evening primrose oil (*Oenothera biennis* L.)	Menopause (flushing/bone metabolism)
Evening primrose oil (*Oenothera biennis* L.)	Premenstrual syndrome
Wild yam (*Dioscorea villosa*)	Hormonal properties (to mimic estrogen, progesterone, or dehydroepiandrosterone [DHEA])

TRADITIONAL OR THEORETICAL USES THAT LACK SUFFICIENT EVIDENCE

Therapy	Specific Therapeutic Use(s)
Alfalfa (*Medicago sativa* L.)	Estrogen replacement
Alfalfa (*Medicago sativa* L.)	Menopausal symptoms
American pennyroyal (*Hedeoma pulegioides* L.), European pennyroyal (*Mentha pulegium* L.)	Cramps
American pennyroyal (*Hedeoma pulegioides* L.), European pennyroyal (*Mentha pulegium* L.)	Premenstrual syndrome
Astragalus (*Astragalus membranaceus*)	Menstrual disorders
Astragalus (*Astragalus membranaceus*)	Pelvic congestion syndrome
Belladonna (*Atropa belladonna* L. or its variety *A. acuminata* Royle ex Lindl)	Abnormal menstrual periods
Betel nut (*Areca catechu* L.)	Excessive menstrual flow
Black cohosh (*Cimicifuga racemosa* L. Nutt.)	Endometriosis

Black cohosh (*Cimicifuga racemosa* L. Nutt.)	Menstrual period problems
Black cohosh (*Cimicifuga racemosa* L. Nutt.)	Ovarian cysts
Black cohosh (*Cimicifuga racemosa* L. Nutt.)	Premenstrual syndrome
Bladderwrack (*Fucus vesiculosus*)	Menstruation irregularities
Blessed thistle (*Cnicus benedictus* L.)	Menstrual disorders
Blessed thistle (*Cnicus benedictus* L.)	Menstrual flow stimulant
Blessed thistle (*Cnicus benedictus* L.)	Painful menstruation
Boswellia (*Boswellia serrata* Roxb.)	Amenorrhea
Boswellia (*Boswellia serrata* Roxb.)	Emmenagogue (inducer of menstruation)
Bromelain	Menstrual pain
Calendula (*Calendula officinalis* L.), marigold	Cramps
Calendula (*Calendula officinalis* L.), marigold	Menstrual period abnormalities
Chamomile (*Matricaria recutita, Chamaemelum nobile*)	Dysmenorrhea
Chamomile (*Matricaria recutita, Chamaemelum nobile*)	Menstrual disorders
Chaparral (*Larrea tridentata* DC. Coville, *L. divaricata* Cav.), nordihydroguaiaretic acid (NDGA)	Menstrual cramps
Clay	Menstruation difficulties
Dandelion (*Taraxacum officinale*)	Menopause
Dandelion (*Taraxacum officinale*)	Premenstrual syndrome
Danshen (*Salvia miltiorrhiza*)	Menstrual problems
Devil's claw (*Harpagophytum procumbens* DC.)	Menopausal symptoms
Devil's claw (*Harpagophytum procumbens* DC.)	Menstrual cramps
Dehydroepiandrosterone (DHEA)	Amenorrhea associated with anorexia
Dehydroepiandrosterone (DHEA)	Andropause/andrenopause
Dehydroepiandrosterone (DHEA)	Premenstrual syndrome
Dong quai (*Angelica sinensis* [Oliv.] Diels), Chinese angelica	Cramps
Dong quai (*Angelica sinensis* [Oliv.] Diels), Chinese angelica	Hormonal abnormalities
Dong quai (*Angelica sinensis* [Oliv.] Diels), Chinese angelica	Menorrhagia (heavy menstrual bleeding)
Dong quai (*Angelica sinensis* [Oliv.] Diels), Chinese angelica	Menstrual cramping
Dong quai (*Angelica sinensis* [Oliv.] Diels), Chinese angelica	Ovulation abnormalities
Dong quai (*Angelica sinensis* [Oliv.] Diels), Chinese angelica	Pelvic congestion syndrome
Dong quai (*Angelica sinensis* [Oliv.] Diels), Chinese angelica	Premenstrual syndrome
Fenugreek (*Trigonella foenum-graecum* L.)	Menopausal symptoms
Fenugreek (*Trigonella foenum-graecum* L.)	Postmenopausal vaginal dryness
Feverfew (*Tanacetum parthenium* L. Schultz-Bip.)	Menstrual cramps
Feverfew (*Tanacetum parthenium* L. Schultz-Bip.)	Promotion of menstruation

Continued

Flaxseed and flaxseed oil (*Linum usitatissimum*)	Menstrual disorders
Flaxseed and flaxseed oil (*Linum usitatissimum*)	Ovarian disorders
Garlic (*Allium sativum* L.)	Emmenagogue
Ginger (*Zingiber officinale* Roscoe)	Dysmenorrhea
Ginger (*Zingiber officinale* Roscoe)	Promotion of menstruation
Ginkgo (*Ginkgo biloba* L.)	Menstrual pain
Ginseng (American ginseng, Asian ginseng, Chinese ginseng, Korean red ginseng, *Panax ginseng*: *Panax* spp. including *P. ginseng* C.C. Meyer and *P. quinquefolium* L., excluding *Eleutherococcus senticosus*)	Menopausal symptoms
Goldenseal (*Hydrastis canadensis* L.), berberine	Menstruation problems
Goldenseal (*Hydrastis canadensis* L.), berberine	Premenstrual syndrome
Gotu kola (*Centella asiatica* L.), total triterpenic fraction of *Centella asiatica* (TTFCA)	Amenorrhea
Gotu kola (*Centella asiatica* L.), total triterpenic fraction of *Centella asiatica* (TTFCA)	Hot flashes
Gotu kola (*Centella asiatica* L.), total triterpenic fraction of *Centella asiatica* (TTFCA)	Menstrual disorders
Guggul (*Commifora mukul*)	Menstrual disorders
Hawthorn (*Crataegus laevigata*, *C. oxyacantha*, *C. monogyna*, *C. pentagyna*)	Amenorrhea
Hops (*Humulus lupulus* L.)	Estrogenic effects
Horse chestnut (*Aesculus hippocastanum* L.)	Menstrual pain
Horsetail (*Equisetum arvense* L.)	Menstrual pain
Kava (*Piper methysticum* G. Forst)	Menopause
Kava (*Piper methysticum* G. Forst)	Menstrual disorders
Lavender (*Lavandula angustifolia* Miller)	Menopause
Lavender (*Lavandula angustifolia* Miller)	Menstrual period problems
Licorice (*Glycyrrhiza glabra* L.), deglycyrrhizinated licorice (DGL)	Hormone regulation
Licorice (*Glycyrrhiza glabra* L.), deglycyrrhizinated licorice (DGL)	Menopausal symptoms
Melatonin	Melatonin deficiency
Milk thistle (*Silybum marianum*), ,silymarin	Menstrual disorders
Niacin (vitamin B_3, nicotinic acid), niacinamide, inositol hexanicotinate	Painful menstruation
Niacin (vitamin B_3, nicotinic acid), niacinamide, inositol hexanicotinate	Premenstrual headache prevention
Niacin (vitamin B_3, nicotinic acid), niacinamide, inositol hexanicotinate	Premenstrual syndrome
Oleander (*Nerium oleander*, *Thevetia peruviana*)	Abnormal menstruation
Oleander (*Nerium oleander*, *Thevetia peruviana*)	Menstrual stimulant
Omega-3 fatty acids, fish oil, alpha-linolenic acid	Menopausal symptoms

Omega-3 fatty acids, fish oil, alpha-linolenic acid	Menstrual cramps
Omega-3 fatty acids, fish oil, alpha-linolenic acid	Premenstrual syndrome
Passionflower (*Passiflora incarnata* L.)	Menopausal symptoms (hot flashes)
Peppermint (*Mentha* x *piperita* L.)	Cramps
Peppermint (*Mentha* x *piperita* L.)	Dysmenorrhea (menstrual pain)
Psyllium (*Plantago ovata, P. ispaghula*)	Excessive menstrual bleeding
Red clover (*Trifolium pratense*)	Hot flashes
Red clover (*Trifolium pratense*)	Premenstrual syndrome
Saw palmetto (*Serenoa repens* [Bartram] Small)	Antiandrogen
Saw palmetto (*Serenoa repens* [Bartram] Small)	Antiestrogen
Saw palmetto (*Serenoa repens* [Bartram] Small)	Dysmenorrhea
Saw palmetto (*Serenoa repens* [Bartram] Small)	Estrogenic agent
Saw palmetto (*Serenoa repens* [Bartram] Small)	Ovarian cysts
Saw palmetto (*Serenoa repens* [Bartram] Small)	Pelvic congestive syndrome
Seaweed, kelp, bladderwrack (*Fucus vesiculosus*)	Menstrual irregularities (menorrhagia)
Slippery elm (*Ulmus rubra* Muhl. or *U. fulva* Michx.)	Gynecologic disorders
Spirulina	Premenstrual syndrome
St. John's wort (*Hypericum perforatum* L.)	Menstrual pain
Sweet almond (*Prunus amygdalus dulcis*)	Plant-derived estrogen
Thyme (*Thymus vulgaris* L.), thymol	Dysmenorrhea
Turmeric (*Curcuma longa* L.), curcumin	Menstrual pain
Turmeric (*Curcuma longa* L.), curcumin	Menstrual period problems/ lack of menstrual periods
Valerian (*Valeriana officinalis* L.)	Amenorrhea
Valerian (*Valeriana officinalis* L.)	Dysmenorrhea
Valerian (*Valeriana officinalis* L.)	Emmenagogue
Valerian (*Valeriana officinalis* L.)	Menopause
Valerian (*Valeriana officinalis* L.)	Premenstrual syndrome
White horehound (*Marrubium vulgare* L.)	Dysmenorrhea
White horehound (*Marrubium vulgare* L.)	Menstrual pain
Wild yam (*Dioscorea villosa*)	Cramps
Wild yam (*Dioscorea villosa*)	Menopause
Wild yam (*Dioscorea villosa*)	Menstrual pain or irregularities
Wild yam (*Dioscorea villosa*)	Pelvic cramps
Wild yam (*Dioscorea villosa*)	Postmenopausal vaginal dryness
Wild yam (*Dioscorea villosa*)	Premenstrual syndrome

PROSTATE DISORDERS AND RELATED CONDITIONS

Levels of Scientific Evidence for Specific Therapies

GRADE: A (Strong Scientific Evidence)

Therapy	Specific Therapeutic Use(s)
Saw palmetto (*Serenoa repens* [Bartram] Small)	Benign prostatic hypertrophy (BPH)

GRADE: B (Good Scientific Evidence)

Therapy	Specific Therapeutic Use(s)
Pygeum (*Prunus africana*, *Pygeum africanum*)	BPH symptoms

GRADE: C (Unclear or Conflicting Scientific Evidence)

Therapy	Specific Therapeutic Use(s)
Red clover (*Trifolium pratense*)	Prostate enlargement (BPH)

TRADITIONAL OR THEORETICAL USES THAT LACK SUFFICIENT EVIDENCE

Therapy	Specific Therapeutic Use(s)
Alfalfa (*Medicago sativa* L.)	Prostate disorders
Astragalus (*Astragalus membranaceus*)	Prostatitis
Bladderwrack (*Fucus vesiculosus*)	BPH
Calendula (*Calendula officinalis* L.), marigold	BPH
Calendula (*Calendula officinalis* L.), marigold	Prostatitis
Dandelion (*Taraxacum officinale*)	BPH
Flaxseed and flaxseed oil (*Linum usitatissimum*)	Enlarged prostate
Goldenseal (*Hydrastis canadensis* L.), berberine	Prostatitis
Horse chestnut (*Aesculus hippocastanum* L.)	BPH
Horsetail (*Equisetum arvense* L.)	Prostate inflammation
PC-SPES	BPH
Pygeum (*Prunus africana*, *Pygeum africanum*)	Prostatic adenoma
Pygeum (*Prunus africana*, *Pygeum africanum*)	Prostatitis
Seaweed, kelp, bladderwrack (*Fucus vesiculosus*)	BPH

PSYCHOSIS AND RELATED CONDITIONS

Levels of Scientific Evidence for Specific Therapies

GRADE: C (Unclear or Conflicting Scientific Evidence)

Therapy	Specific Therapeutic Use(s)
Betel nut (*Areca catechu* L.)	Schizophrenia
Dehydroepiandrosterone (DHEA)	Schizophrenia
Melatonin	Schizophrenia (sleep disorders)
Omega-3 fatty acids, fish oil, alpha-linolenic acid	Schizophrenia

GRADE: D (Fair Negative Scientific Evidence)	
Therapy	Specific Therapeutic Use(s)
Evening primrose oil (*Oenothera biennis* L.)	Schizophrenia

TRADITIONAL OR THEORETICAL USES THAT LACK SUFFICIENT EVIDENCE	
Therapy	Specific Therapeutic Use(s)
American pennyroyal (*Hedeoma pulegioides* L.), European pennyroyal (*Mentha pulegium* L.)	Hallucinations
Chaparral (*Larrea tridentata* DC. Coville, *L. divaricata* Cav.), nordihydroguaiaretic acid (NDGA)	Hallucinations (including those due to LSD ingestion)
Coenzyme Q10	Psychiatric disorders
Ginkgo (*Ginkgo biloba* L.)	Schizophrenia
Ginseng (American ginseng, Asian ginseng, Chinese ginseng, Korean red ginseng, *Panax ginseng*: *Panax* spp. including *P. ginseng* C.C. Meyer and *P. quinquefolium* L., excluding *Eleutherococcus senticosus*)	Psychoasthenia
Gotu kola (*Centella asiatica* L.), total triterpenic fraction of *Centella asiatica* (TTFCA)	Mental disorders
Kava (*Piper methysticum* G. Forst)	Antipsychotic
Lavender (*Lavandula angustifolia* Miller)	Psychosis
Niacin (vitamin B$_3$, nicotinic acid), niacinamide, inositol hexanicotinate	Diagnostic test for schizophrenia
Niacin (vitamin B$_3$, nicotinic acid), niacinamide, inositol hexanicotinate	Drug-induced hallucinations
Niacin (vitamin B$_3$, nicotinic acid), niacinamide, inositol hexanicotinate	Psychosis
Niacin (vitamin B$_3$, nicotinic acid), niacinamide, inositol hexanicotinate	Schizophrenia
Oleander (*Nerium oleander, Thevetia peruviana*)	Psychiatric disorders
Pygeum (*Prunus africana, Pygeum africanum*)	Psychosis
Yohimbe bark extract (*Pausinystalia yohimbe* Pierre ex Beille)	Hallucinogenic
Yohimbe bark extract (*Pausinystalia yohimbe* Pierre ex Beille)	Schizophrenia

PULMONARY EDEMA AND RELATED CONDITIONS

Levels of Scientific Evidence for Specific Therapies

GRADE: A (Strong Scientific Evidence)	
Therapy	Specific Therapeutic Use(s)
Hawthorn (*Crataegus laevigata, C. oxyacantha, C. monogyna, C. pentagyna*)	Congestive heart failure

GRADE: C (Unclear or Conflicting Scientific Evidence)	
Therapy	Specific Therapeutic Use(s)
Arginine (L-arginine)	Heart failure (congestive)
Astragalus (*Astragalus membranaceus*)	Heart failure

Continued

Coenzyme Q10	Cardiomyopathy (dilated, hypertrophic)
Coenzyme Q10	Heart failure
Dehydroepiandrosterone (DHEA)	Heart failure
Ginseng (American ginseng, Asian ginseng, Chinese ginseng, Korean red ginseng, *Panax ginseng*. *Panax* spp. including *P. ginseng* C.C. Meyer and *P. quinquefolium* L., excluding *Eleutherococcus senticosus*)	Congestive heart failure
Hawthorn (*Crataegus laevigata, C. oxyacantha, C. monogyna, C. pentagyna*)	Functional cardiovascular disorders
Oleander (*Nerium oleander, Thevetia peruviana*)	Congestive heart failure
Passionflower (*Passiflora incarnata* L.)	Congestive heart failure (exercise capacity)

TRADITIONAL OR THEORETICAL USES THAT LACK SUFFICIENT EVIDENCE

Therapy	Specific Therapeutic Use(s)
Dandelion (*Taraxacum officinale*)	Congestive heart failure
Danshen (*Salvia miltiorrhiza*)	Left ventricular hypertrophy
Dong quai (*Angelica sinensis* [Oliv.] Diels), Chinese angelica	Congestive heart failure
Ginkgo (*Ginkgo biloba* L.)	Congestive heart failure
Goldenseal (*Hydrastis canadensis* L.), berberine	Heart failure
Horse chestnut (*Aesculus hippocastanum* L.)	Fluid in the lungs (pulmonary edema)
Horsetail (*Equisetum arvense* L.)	Fluid in the lungs
Omega-3 fatty acids, fish oil, alpha-linolenic acid	Congestive heart failure
Passionflower (*Passiflora incarnata* L.)	Congestive heart failure (exercise ability)
Valerian (*Valeriana officinalis* L.)	Congestive heart failure

PULMONARY HYPERTENSION AND RELATED CONDITIONS

Levels of Scientific Evidence for Specific Therapies

GRADE: C (Unclear or Conflicting Scientific Evidence)

Therapy	Specific Therapeutic Use(s)
Dong quai (*Angelica sinensis* [Oliv.] Diels), Chinese angelica	Pulmonary hypertension

TRADITIONAL OR THEORETICAL USES THAT LACK SUFFICIENT EVIDENCE

Therapy	Specific Therapeutic Use(s)
Arginine (L-arginine)	Pulmonary hypertension (high blood pressure in the lungs)
Danshen (*Salvia miltiorrhiza*)	Pulmonary hypertension
Feverfew (*Tanacetum parthenium* L. Schultz-Bip.)	Blood vessel dilation (relaxation)
White horehound (*Marrubium vulgare* L.)	Vasodilator

QUALITY OF LIFE AND RELATED CONDITIONS

Levels of Scientific Evidence for Specific Therapies

GRADE: C (Unclear or Conflicting Scientific Evidence)

Therapy	Specific Therapeutic Use(s)
Chamomile (*Matricaria recutita, Chamaemelum nobile*)	Quality of life in cancer patients

TRADITIONAL OR THEORETICAL USES THAT LACK SUFFICIENT EVIDENCE

Therapy	Specific Therapeutic Use(s)
Essiac	Supportive care in advanced-cancer patients
Ginseng (American ginseng, Asian ginseng, Chinese ginseng, Korean red ginseng, *Panax ginseng*: *Panax* spp. including *P. ginseng* C.C. Meyer and *P. quinquefolium* L., excluding *Eleutherococcus senticosus*)	Qi deficiency and blood stasis syndrome in heart disease (Eastern medicine)
Ginseng (American ginseng, Asian ginseng, Chinese ginseng, Korean red ginseng, *Panax ginseng*: *Panax* spp. including *P. ginseng* C.C. Meyer and *P. quinquefolium* L., excluding *Eleutherococcus senticosus*)	Quality of life

RADIATION THERAPY SIDE EFFECTS AND RELATED CONDITIONS

Levels of Scientific Evidence for Specific Therapies

GRADE: C (Unclear or Conflicting Scientific Evidence)

Therapy	Specific Therapeutic Use(s)
Aloe (*Aloe vera*)	Radiation dermatitis
Belladonna (*Atropa belladonna* L. or its variety *A. acuminata* Royle ex Lindl)	Radiation therapy rash (radiation burn)
Echinacea (*Echinacea angustifolia* DC., *E. pallida, E. purpurea*)	Low white blood cell counts after x-ray treatment
Melatonin	Ultraviolet light skin damage protection

GRADE: D (Fair Negative Scientific Evidence)

Therapy	Specific Therapeutic Use(s)
Aloe (*Aloe vera*)	Radiation dermatitis
Sweet almond (*Prunus amygdalus dulcis*)	Radiation therapy skin reactions (used on the skin)

TRADITIONAL OR THEORETICAL USES THAT LACK SUFFICIENT EVIDENCE

Therapy	Specific Therapeutic Use(s)
Alfalfa (*Medicago sativa* L.)	Skin damage from radiation
Aloe (*Aloe vera*)	Skin protection during radiation therapy
Bladderwrack (*Fucus vesiculosus*)	Radiation protection
Danshen (*Salvia miltiorrhiza*)	Radiation-induced lung damage

Continued

Ginseng (American ginseng, Asian ginseng, Chinese ginseng, Korean red ginseng, *Panax ginseng*: *Panax* spp. including *P. ginseng* C.C. Meyer and *P. quinquefolium* L., excluding *Eleutherococcus senticosus*)   Recovery from radiation

Milk thistle (*Silybum marianum*), silymarin   Radiation sickness

Psyllium (*Plantago ovata, P. ispaghula*)   Radiation-induced colitis/diarrhea

Seaweed, kelp, bladderwrack (*Fucus vesiculosus*)   Radiation protection

Spirulina   Radiation sickness

RETINOPATHY AND RELATED CONDITIONS

Levels of Scientific Evidence for Specific Therapies

GRADE: C (Unclear or Conflicting Scientific Evidence)

Therapy	Specific Therapeutic Use(s)
Bilberry (*Vaccinium myrtillus*)	Retinopathy

TRADITIONAL OR THEORETICAL USES THAT LACK SUFFICIENT EVIDENCE

Therapy	Specific Therapeutic Use(s)
Ginkgo (*Ginkgo biloba* L.)	Diabetic eye disease
Shark cartilage	Diabetic retinopathy

RHEUMATOID ARTHRITIS AND RELATED CONDITIONS

Levels of Scientific Evidence for Specific Therapies

GRADE: B (Good Scientific Evidence)

Therapy	Specific Therapeutic Use(s)
Omega-3 fatty acids, fish oil, alpha-linolenic acid	Rheumatoid arthritis (fish oil)

GRADE: C (Unclear or Conflicting Scientific Evidence)

Therapy	Specific Therapeutic Use(s)
Boswellia (*Boswellia serrata* Roxb.)	Rheumatoid arthritis
Bromelain	Rheumatoid arthritis
Dehydroepiandrosterone (DHEA)	Systemic lupus erythematosus
Dong quai (*Angelica sinensis* [Oliv.] Diels), Chinese angelica	Arthritis
Evening primrose oil (*Oenothera biennis* L.)	Rheumatoid arthritis
Feverfew (*Tanacetum parthenium* L. Schultz-Bip.)	Rheumatoid arthritis
Ginger (*Zingiber officinale* Roscoe)	Rheumatic diseases (rheumatoid arthritis, osteoarthritis, arthralgias, muscle pain)
Glucosamine	Rheumatoid arthritis
Green tea (*Camellia sinensis*)	Arthritis
Guggul (*Commifora mukul*)	Rheumatoid arthritis

Omega-3 fatty acids, fish oil, alpha-linolenic acid	Lupus erythematosus
Propolis	Rheumatic diseases
Shark cartilage	Inflammatory joint diseases (rheumatoid arthritis, osteoarthritis)
Turmeric (*Curcuma longa* L.), curcumin	Rheumatoid arthritis

TRADITIONAL OR THEORETICAL USES THAT LACK SUFFICIENT EVIDENCE	
Therapy	Specific Therapeutic Use(s)
Alfalfa (*Medicago sativa* L.)	Rheumatoid arthritis
Aloe (*Aloe vera*)	Arthritis
Aloe (*Aloe vera*)	Lupus erythematosus
Astragalus (*Astragalus membranaceus*)	Ankylosing spondylitis
Astragalus (*Astragalus membranaceus*)	Systemic lupus erythematosus
Belladonna (*Atropa belladonna* L. or its variety *A. acuminata* Royle ex Lindl)	Arthritis
Bilberry (*Vaccinium myrtillus*)	Arthritis
Bladderwrack (*Fucus vesiculosus*)	Arthritis
Bladderwrack (*Fucus vesiculosus*)	Rheumatism
Boron	Rheumatoid arthritis
Bromelain	Autoimmune disorders
Burdock (*Arctium lappa*)	Arthritis
Burdock (*Arctium lappa*)	Rheumatoid arthritis
Chamomile (*Matricaria recutita, Chamaemelum nobile*)	Arthritis
Chaparral (*Larrea tridentata* DC. Coville, *L. divaricata* Cav.), nordihydroguaiaretic acid (NDGA)	Arthritis
Chaparral (*Larrea tridentata* DC. Coville, *L. divaricata* Cav.), nordihydroguaiaretic acid (NDGA)	Rheumatic diseases
Dandelion (*Taraxacum officinale*)	Arthritis
Dandelion (*Taraxacum officinale*)	Rheumatoid arthritis
Devil's claw (*Harpagophytum procumbens* DC.)	Rheumatoid arthritis
Dehydroepiandrosterone (DHEA)	Rheumatic diseases
Dong quai (*Angelica sinensis* [Oliv.] Diels), Chinese angelica	Chilblains
Dong quai (*Angelica sinensis* [Oliv.] Diels), Chinese angelica	Rheumatic diseases
Echinacea (*Echinacea angustifolia* DC., *E. pallida, E. purpurea*)	Rheumatism
Essiac	Arthritis
Essiac	Systemic lupus erythematosus
Eucalyptus oil (*Eucalyptus globulus* Labillardiere, *E. fructicetorum* F. Von Mueller, *E. smithii* R.T. Baker)	Arthritis
Eucalyptus oil (*Eucalyptus globulus* Labillardiere, *E. fructicetorum* F. Von Mueller, *E. smithii* R.T. Baker)	Rheumatoid arthritis (applied to the skin)

Continued

Evening primrose oil (*Oenothera biennis* L.)	Systemic lupus erythematosus
Flaxseed and flaxseed oil (*Linum usitatissimum*)	Rheumatoid arthritis
Garlic (*Allium sativum* L.)	Arthritis
Globe artichoke (*Cynara scolymus* L.)	Arthritis
Globe artichoke (*Cynara scolymus* L.)	Rheumatoid arthritis
Goldenseal (*Hydrastis canadensis* L.), berberine	Arthritis
Goldenseal (*Hydrastis canadensis* L.), berberine	Lupus
Gotu kola (*Centella asiatica* L.), total triterpenic fraction of Centella asiatica (TTFCA)	Rheumatism
Gotu kola (*Centella asiatica* L.), total triterpenic fraction of *Centella asiatica* (TTFCA)	Systemic lupus erythematosus
Gymnema (*Gymnema sylvestre* R. Br.)	Rheumatoid arthritis
Hops (*Humulus lupulus* L.)	Rheumatic disorders
Horse chestnut (*Aesculus hippocastanum* L.)	Rheumatism
Horse chestnut (*Aesculus hippocastanum* L.)	Rheumatoid arthritis
Horsetail (*Equisetum arvense* L.)	Rheumatism
Kava (*Piper methysticum* G. Forst)	Arthritis
Lavender (*Lavandula angustifolia* Miller)	Rheumatism
Licorice (*Glycyrrhiza glabra* L.), deglycyrrhizinated licorice (DGL)	Rheumatoid arthritis
Lycopene	Inflammatory conditions
Maitake mushroom (*Grifola frondosa*), beta-glucan	Arthritis
Marshmallow (*Althaea officinalis* L.)	Arthritis
Marshmallow (*Althaea officinalis* L.)	Chilblains
Melatonin	Rheumatoid arthritis
Niacin (vitamin B$_3$, nicotinic acid), niacinamide, inositol hexanicotinate	Arthritis
Omega-3 fatty acids, fish oil, alpha-linolenic acid	Dermatomyositis
Omega-3 fatty acids, fish oil, alpha-linolenic acid	Systemic lupus erythematosus
Peppermint (*Mentha* x *piperita* L.)	Arthritis
Peppermint (*Mentha* x *piperita* L.)	Rheumatic pain
Polypodium leucotomos extract, Anapsos	Autoimmune diseases
Polypodium leucotomos extract, Anapsos	Rheumatic diseases
Propolis	Rheumatoid arthritis
Red clover (*Trifolium pratense*)	Arthritis
Seaweed, kelp, bladderwrack (*Fucus vesiculosus*)	Arthritis
Seaweed, kelp, bladderwrack (*Fucus vesiculosus*)	Rheumatism
Shark cartilage	Ankylosing spondylitis
Shark cartilage	Systemic lupus erythematosus
Slippery elm (*Ulmus rubra* Muhl. or *U. fulva* Michx.)	Rheumatic disorders

Soy (*Glycine max* L. Merr.)	Autoimmune diseases
Soy (*Glycine max* L. Merr.)	Rheumatoid arthritis
St. John's wort (*Hypericum perforatum* L.)	Rheumatism
Thyme (*Thymus vulgaris* L.), thymol	Arthritis
Thyme (*Thymus vulgaris* L.), thymol	Dermatomyositis
Thyme (*Thymus vulgaris* L.), thymol	Rheumatism
Valerian (*Valeriana officinalis* L.)	Arthritis
Valerian (*Valeriana officinalis* L.)	Rheumatic pain
Wild yam (*Dioscorea villosa*)	Rheumatic pain

SCHIZOPHRENIA AND RELATED CONDITIONS

Levels of Scientific Evidence for Specific Therapies

GRADE: C (Unclear or Conflicting Scientific Evidence)

Therapy	Specific Therapeutic Use(s)
Betel nut (*Areca catechu* L.)	Schizophrenia
Dehydroepiandrosterone (DHEA)	Schizophrenia
Melatonin	Schizophrenia (sleep disorders)
Omega-3 fatty acids, fish oil, alpha-linolenic acid	Schizophrenia

GRADE: D (Fair Negative Scientific Evidence)

Therapy	Specific Therapeutic Use(s)
Evening primrose oil (*Oenothera biennis* L.)	Schizophrenia

TRADITIONAL OR THEORETICAL USES THAT LACK SUFFICIENT EVIDENCE

Therapy	Specific Therapeutic Use(s)
American pennyroyal (*Hedeoma pulegioides* L.), European pennyroyal (*Mentha pulegium* L.)	Hallucinations
Chaparral (*Larrea tridentata* DC. Coville, *L. divaricata* Cav.), nordihydroguaiaretic acid (NDGA)	Hallucinations (including those due to LSD ingestion)
Coenzyme Q10	Psychiatric disorders
Ginkgo (*Ginkgo biloba* L.)	Schizophrenia
Ginseng (American ginseng, Asian ginseng, Chinese ginseng, Korean red ginseng, *Panax ginseng*: *Panax* spp. including *P. ginseng* C.C. Meyer and *P. quinquefolium* L., excluding *Eleutherococcus senticosus*)	Psychoasthenia
Gotu kola (*Centella asiatica* L.), total triterpenic fraction of *Centella asiatica* (TTFCA)	Mental disorders
Kava (*Piper methysticum* G. Forst)	Antipsychotic
Lavender (*Lavandula angustifolia* Miller)	Psychosis
Niacin (vitamin B_3, nicotinic acid), niacinamide, inositol hexanicotinate	Diagnostic test for schizophrenia

Continued

Niacin (vitamin B₃, nicotinic acid), niacinamide, inositol hexanicotinate	Drug-induced hallucinations
Niacin (vitamin B₃, nicotinic acid), niacinamide, inositol hexanicotinate	Psychosis
Niacin (vitamin B₃, nicotinic acid), niacinamide, inositol hexanicotinate	Schizophrenia
Oleander (*Nerium oleander, Thevetia peruviana*)	Psychiatric disorders
Pygeum (*Prunus africana, Pygeum africanum*)	Psychosis
Yohimbe bark extract (*Pausinystalia yohimbe* Pierre ex Beille)	Hallucinogenic
Yohimbe bark extract (*Pausinystalia yohimbe* Pierre ex Beille)	Schizophrenia

SEASICKNESS AND RELATED CONDITIONS
Levels of Scientific Evidence for Specific Therapies

GRADE: B (Good Scientific Evidence)

Therapy	Specific Therapeutic Use(s)
Ginger (*Zingiber officinale* Roscoe)	Nausea (due to chemotherapy)
Ginger (*Zingiber officinale* Roscoe)	Nausea and vomiting of pregnancy (hyperemesis gravidarum)

GRADE: C (Unclear or Conflicting Scientific Evidence)

Therapy	Specific Therapeutic Use(s)
Ginger (*Zingiber officinale* Roscoe)	Nausea and vomiting (after surgery)
Peppermint (*Mentha* x *piperita* L.)	Nausea

TRADITIONAL OR THEORETICAL USES THAT LACK SUFFICIENT EVIDENCE

Therapy	Specific Therapeutic Use(s)
Belladonna (*Atropa belladonna* L. or its variety *A. acuminata* Royle ex Lindl)	Motion sickness
Belladonna (*Atropa belladonna* L. or its variety *A. acuminata* Royle ex Lindl)	Nausea and vomiting during pregnancy
Black tea (*Camellia sinensis*)	Vomiting
Calendula (*Calendula officinalis* L.), marigold	Nausea
Chamomile (*Matricaria recutita, Chamaemelum nobile*)	Motion sickness
Chamomile (*Matricaria recutita, Chamaemelum nobile*)	Nausea
Chamomile (*Matricaria recutita, Chamaemelum nobile*)	Sea sickness
Chaparral (*Larrea tridentata* DC. Coville, *L. divaricata* Cav.), nordihydroguaiaretic acid (NDGA)	Vomiting
Clay	Vomiting
Clay	Vomiting/nausea during pregnancy
Clove (*Eugenia aromatica*)	Nausea or vomiting

Cranberry (*Vaccinium macrocarpon*)	Vomiting
Elder (*Sambucus nigra* L.)	Vomiting
Globe artichoke (*Cynara scolymus* L.)	Emesis
Lavender (*Lavandula angustifolia* Miller)	Motion sickness
Lavender (*Lavandula angustifolia* Miller)	Nausea
Lavender (*Lavandula angustifolia* Miller)	Vomiting
Marshmallow (*Althaea officinalis* L.)	Vomiting
Niacin (vitamin B$_3$, nicotinic acid), niacinamide, inositol hexanicotinate	Motion sickness
Oleander (*Nerium oleander, Thevetia peruviana*)	Vomiting
Valerian (*Valeriana officinalis* L.)	Nausea
White horehound (*Marrubium vulgare* L.)	Emetic
Wild yam (*Dioscorea villosa*)	Emetic

SEDATION AND RELATED CONDITIONS
Levels of Scientific Evidence for Specific Therapies

GRADE: C (Unclear or Conflicting Scientific Evidence)

Therapy	Specific Therapeutic Use(s)
Chamomile (*Matricaria recutita, Chamaemelum nobile*)	Sleep aid/sedation
Hops (*Humulus lupulus* L.)	Sedation
Lavender (*Lavandula angustifolia* Miller)	Hypnotic/sleep aid (lavender)
Melatonin	Preoperative sedation/ anxiolysis
Passionflower (*Passiflora incarnata* L.)	Sedation (agitation, anxiety, insomnia)

GRADE: D (Fair Negative Scientific Evidence)

Therapy	Specific Therapeutic Use(s)
Valerian (*Valeriana officinalis* L.)	Sedation

TRADITIONAL OR THEORETICAL USES THAT LACK SUFFICIENT EVIDENCE

Therapy	Specific Therapeutic Use(s)
American pennyroyal (*Hedeoma pulegioides* L.), European pennyroyal (*Mentha pulegium* L.)	Sedative
Belladonna (*Atropa belladonna* L. or its variety *A. acuminata* Royle ex Lindl)	Sedative
Devil's claw (*Harpagophytum procumbens* DC.)	Sedative
Dong quai (*Angelica sinensis* [Oliv.] Diels), Chinese angelica	Sedative
Elder (*Sambucus nigra* L.)	Sedative
Feverfew (*Tanacetum parthenium* L. Schultz-Bip.)	Tranquilizer
Garlic (*Allium sativum* L.)	Sedative

Continued

Ginseng (American ginseng, Asian ginseng, Chinese ginseng, Korean red ginseng, *Panax ginseng*: *Panax* spp. including *P. ginseng* C.C. Meyer and *P. quinquefolium* L., excluding *Eleutherococcus senticosus*)	Sedative
Goldenseal (*Hydrastis canadensis* L.), berberine	Sedative
Melatonin	Sedation
Niacin (vitamin B$_3$, nicotinic acid), niacinamide, inositol hexanicotinate	Sedative
Saw palmetto (*Serenoa repens* [Bartram] Small)	Sedation

SEIZURE DISORDER AND RELATED CONDITIONS

Levels of Scientific Evidence for Specific Therapies

GRADE: C (Unclear or Conflicting Scientific Evidence)	
Therapy	Specific Therapeutic Use(s)
Melatonin	Seizure disorder (children)

TRADITIONAL OR THEORETICAL USES THAT LACK SUFFICIENT EVIDENCE	
Therapy	Specific Therapeutic Use(s)
Chamomile (*Matricaria recutita*, *Chamaemelum nobile*)	Convulsions
Chamomile (*Matricaria recutita*, *Chamaemelum nobile*)	Seizure disorder
Elder (*Sambucus nigra* L.)	Epilepsy
Eyebright (*Euphrasia officinalis*)	Epilepsy
Ginseng (American ginseng, Asian ginseng, Chinese ginseng, Korean red ginseng, *Panax ginseng*: *Panax* spp. *including P. ginseng* C.C. Meyer and *P. quinquefolium* L., excluding *Eleutherococcus senticosus*)	Convulsions
Gotu kola (*Centella asiatica* L.), total triterpenic fraction of *Centella asiatica* (TTFCA)	Epilepsy
Kava (*Piper methysticum* G. Forst)	Seizures
Lavender (*Lavandula angustifolia* Miller)	Anticonvulsant
Niacin (vitamin B$_3$, nicotinic acid), niacinamide, inositol hexanicotinate	Seizure
Oleander (*Nerium oleander*, *Thevetia peruviana*)	Epilepsy (seizure)
Passionflower (*Passiflora incarnata* L.)	Anticonvulsant
Passionflower (*Passiflora incarnata* L.)	Generalized seizures
Thyme (*Thymus vulgaris* L.), thymol	Epilepsy
Turmeric (*Curcuma longa* L.), curcumin	Epilepsy
Valerian (*Valeriana officinalis* L.)	Anticonvulsive
Valerian (*Valeriana officinalis* L.)	Convulsions

SEXUAL DYSFUNCTION AND RELATED CONDITIONS

Levels of Scientific Evidence for Specific Therapies

GRADE: C (Unclear or Conflicting Scientific Evidence)

Therapy	Specific Therapeutic Use(s)
Arginine (L-arginine)	Erectile dysfunction
Clove (*Eugenia aromatica*)	Premature ejaculation
Dehydroepiandrosterone (DHEA)	Sexual function/libido/erectile dysfunction
Ephedra (*Ephedra sinica*)/ma huang	Sexual arousal
Ginkgo (*Ginkgo biloba* L.)	Decreased libido and erectile dysfunction (impotence)
Ginseng (American ginseng, Asian ginseng, Chinese ginseng, Korean red ginseng, *Panax ginseng*: *Panax* spp. including *P. ginseng* C.C. Meyer and *P. quinquefolium* L., excluding *Eleutherococcus senticosus*)	Erectile dysfunction
Yohimbe bark extract (*Pausinystalia yohimbe* Pierre ex Beille)	Erectile dysfunction (male impotence)
Yohimbe bark extract (*Pausinystalia yohimbe* Pierre ex Beille)	Libido (women)
Yohimbe bark extract (*Pausinystalia yohimbe* Pierre ex Beille)	Sexual side effects of selective serotonin reuptake inhibitor (SSRI) antidepressants
Yohimbe bark extract (*Pausinystalia yohimbe* Pierre ex Beille)	Male erectile dysfunction

TRADITIONAL OR THEORETICAL USES THAT LACK SUFFICIENT EVIDENCE

Therapy	Specific Therapeutic Use(s)
Betel nut (*Areca catechu* L.)	Aphrodisiac
Betel nut (*Areca catechu* L.)	Impotence
Black cohosh (*Cimicifuga racemosa* L. Nutt.)	Aphrodisiac
Burdock (*Arctium lappa*)	Aphrodisiac
Burdock (*Arctium lappa*)	Impotence
Fenugreek (*Trigonella foenum-graecum* L.)	Impotence
Garlic (*Allium sativum* L.)	Aphrodisiac
Ginger (*Zingiber officinale* Roscoe)	Aphrodisiac
Ginger (*Zingiber officinale* Roscoe)	Impotence
Ginseng (American ginseng, Asian ginseng, Chinese ginseng, Korean red ginseng, *Panax ginseng*: *Panax* spp. including *P. ginseng* C.C. Meyer and *P. quinquefolium* L., excluding *Eleutherococcus senticosus*)	Aphrodisiac
Ginseng (American ginseng, Asian ginseng, Chinese ginseng, Korean red ginseng, *Panax ginseng*: *Panax* spp. including *P. ginseng* C.C. Meyer and *P. quinquefolium* L., excluding *Eleutherococcus senticosus*)	Premature ejaculation
Ginseng (American ginseng, Asian ginseng, Chinese ginseng, Korean red ginseng, *Panax ginseng*: *Panax* spp. including *P. ginseng* C.C. Meyer and P. *quinquefolium* L., excluding *Eleutherococcus senticosus*)	Sexual arousal

Continued

Ginseng (American ginseng, Asian ginseng, Chinese ginseng, Korean red ginseng, *Panax ginseng*: *Panax* spp. including *P. ginseng* C.C. Meyer and *P. quinquefolium* L., excluding *Eleutherococcus senticosus*)	Sexual symptoms
Gotu kola (*Centella asiatica* L.), total triterpenic fraction of *Centella asiatica* (TTFCA)	Aphrodisiac
Gotu kola (*Centella asiatica* L.), total triterpenic fraction of *Centella asiatica* (TTFCA)	Libido
Gymnema (*Gymnema sylvestre* R. Br.)	Aphrodisiac
Hops (*Humulus lupulus* L.)	Aphrodisiac
Kava (*Piper methysticum* G. Forst)	Aphrodisiac
Lavender (*Lavandula angustifolia* Miller)	Aphrodisiac
Marshmallow (*Althaea officinalis* L.)	Aphrodisiac
Marshmallow (*Althaea officinalis* L.)	Impotence
Melatonin	Erectile dysfunction
Melatonin	Sexual activity enhancement
Niacin (vitamin B_3, nicotinic acid), niacinamide, inositol hexanicotinate	Orgasm improvement
Pygeum (*Prunus africana, Pygeum africanum*)	Aphrodisiac
Pygeum (*Prunus africana, Pygeum africanum*)	Impotence
Pygeum (*Prunus africana, Pygeum africanum*)	Sexual performance
Saw palmetto (*Serenoa repens* [Bartram] Small)	Aphrodisiac
Saw palmetto (*Serenoa repens* [Bartram] Small)	Impotence
Saw palmetto (*Serenoa repens* [Bartram] Small)	Sexual vigor
Sweet almond (*Prunus amygdalus dulcis*)	Aphrodisiac
Wild yam (*Dioscorea villosa*)	Libido
Yohimbe bark extract (*Pausinystalia yohimbe* Pierre ex Beille)	Aphrodisiac

SKIN CONDITIONS/RASH AND RELATED CONDITIONS

Levels of Scientific Evidence for Specific Therapies

GRADE: B (Good Scientific Evidence)	
Therapy	Specific Therapeutic Use(s)
Aloe (*Aloe vera*)	Psoriasis vulgaris
Aloe (*Aloe vera*)	Seborrheic dermatitis (seborrhea, dandruff)
Evening primrose oil (*Oenothera biennis* L.)	Eczema (children and adults)
Evening primrose oil (*Oenothera biennis* L.)	Skin irritation (atopic dermatitis in children and adults)

GRADE: C (Unclear or Conflicting Scientific Evidence)	
Therapy	Specific Therapeutic Use(s)
Calendula (*Calendula officinalis* L.), marigold	Skin inflammation
Chamomile (*Matricaria recutita*, *Chamaemelum nobile*)	Skin conditions (eczema/radiation damage/wound healing)
Evening primrose oil (*Oenothera biennis* L.)	Scalelike dry skin (ichthyosis vulgaris)
Marshmallow (*Althaea officinalis* L.)	Inflammatory skin conditions (eczema, psoriasis)
Omega-3 fatty acids, fish oil, alpha-linolenic acid	Eczema
Omega-3 fatty acids, fish oil, alpha-linolenic acid	Psoriasis
Polypodium leucotomos extract, Anapsos	Atopic dermatitis
Polypodium leucotomos extract, Anapsos	Psoriasis
Shark cartilage	Psoriasis
Thyme (*Thymus vulgaris* L.), thymol	Inflammatory skin disorders

GRADE: D (Fair Negative Scientific Evidence)	
Therapy	Specific Therapeutic Use(s)
Boron	Psoriasis (boric acid ointment)
Evening primrose oil (*Oenothera biennis* L.)	Psoriasis

TRADITIONAL OR THEORETICAL USES THAT LACK SUFFICIENT EVIDENCE	
Therapy	Specific Therapeutic Use(s)
Belladonna (*Atropa belladonna* L. or its variety *A. acuminata* Royle ex Lindl)	Rash
Belladonna (*Atropa belladonna* L. or its variety *A. acuminata* Royle ex Lindl)	Warts
Betel nut (*Areca catechu* L.)	Dermatitis (used on the skin)
Bilberry (*Vaccinium myrtillus*)	Dermatitis
Bitter melon (*Momordica charantia* L.) and MAP30	Psoriasis
Bladderwrack (*Fucus vesiculosus*)	Eczema
Bladderwrack (*Fucus vesiculosus*)	Psoriasis
Boron	Diaper rash (avoid because of case reports of death in infants from absorbing boron through skin or when taken by mouth)
Burdock (*Arctium lappa*)	Eczema
Burdock (*Arctium lappa*)	Ichthyosis (skin disorder)
Burdock (*Arctium lappa*)	Psoriasis
Burdock (*Arctium lappa*)	Skin disorders
Burdock (*Arctium lappa*)	Skin moisturizer

Continued

Burdock (*Arctium lappa*)	Warts
Calendula (*Calendula officinalis* L.), marigold	Diaper rash
Calendula (*Calendula officinalis* L.), marigold	Eczema
Calendula (*Calendula officinalis* L.), marigold	Warts
Chamomile (*Matricaria recutita*, *Chamaemelum nobile*)	Contact dermatitis
Chamomile (*Matricaria recutita*, *Chamaemelum nobile*)	Diaper rash
Chamomile (*Matricaria recutita*, *Chamaemelum nobile*)	Impetigo
Chamomile (*Matricaria recutita*, *Chamaemelum nobile*)	Psoriasis
Chaparral (*Larrea tridentata* DC. Coville, *L. divaricata* Cav.), nordihydroguaiaretic acid (NDGA)	Skin disorders
Dandelion (*Taraxacum officinale*)	Age spots
Dandelion (*Taraxacum officinale*)	Psoriasis
Dandelion (*Taraxacum officinale*)	Skin conditions
Dandelion (*Taraxacum officinale*)	Warts
Danshen (*Salvia miltiorrhiza*)	Eczema
Danshen (*Salvia miltiorrhiza*)	Psoriasis
Dehydroepiandrosterone (DHEA)	Psoriasis
Dong quai (*Angelica sinensis* [Oliv.] Diels), Chinese angelica	Dermatitis
Dong quai (*Angelica sinensis* [Oliv.] Diels), Chinese angelica	Eczema
Dong quai (*Angelica sinensis* [Oliv.] Diels), Chinese angelica	Psoriasis
Dong quai (*Angelica sinensis* [Oliv.] Diels), Chinese angelica	Skin pigmentation disorders
Echinacea (*Echinacea angustifolia* DC., *E. pallida*, *E. purpurea*)	Eczema
Echinacea (*Echinacea angustifolia* DC., *E. pallida*, *E. purpurea*)	Psoriasis
Elder (*Sambucus nigra* L.)	Psoriasis
Evening primrose pil (*Oenothera biennis* L.)	Skin conditions due to kidney failure in dialysis patients
Eyebright (*Euphrasia officinalis*)	Skin conditions
Fenugreek (*Trigonella foenum-graecum* L.)	Dermatitis
Fenugreek (*Trigonella foenum-graecum* L.)	Eczema
Feverfew (*Tanacetum parthenium* L. Schultz-Bip.)	Rash
Flaxseed and flaxseed oil (*Linum usitatissimum*)	Eczema
Flaxseed and flaxseed oil (*Linum usitatissimum*)	Psoriasis
Flaxseed and flaxseed oil (*Linum usitatissimum*)	Skin inflammation
Garlic (*Allium sativum* L.)	Psoriasis
Garlic (*Allium sativum* L.)	Warts
Ginger (*Zingiber officinale* Roscoe)	Psoriasis (topical)
Ginkgo (*Ginkgo biloba* L.)	Dermatitis
Ginkgo (*Ginkgo biloba* L.)	Eczema
Globe artichoke (*Cynara scolymus* L.)	Eczema

Glucosamine	Psoriasis
Goldenseal (*Hydrastis canadensis* L.), berberine	Eczema
Goldenseal (*Hydrastis canadensis* L.), berberine	Impetigo
Goldenseal (*Hydrastis canadensis* L.), berberine	Psoriasis
Goldenseal (*Hydrastis canadensis* L.), berberine	Seborrhea
Gotu kola (*Centella asiatica* L.), total triterpenic fraction of *Centella asiatica* (TTFCA)	Eczema
Gotu kola (*Centella asiatica* L.), total triterpenic fraction of *Centella asiatica* (TTFCA)	Skin diseases
Guggul (*Commifora mukul*)	Psoriasis
Hops (*Humulus lupulus* L.)	Dermatitis
Horse chestnut (*Aesculus hippocastanum* L.)	Skin conditions
Lactobacillus acidophilus	Diaper rash
Licorice (*Glycyrrhiza glabra* L.), deglycyrrhizinated licorice (DGL)	Eczema
Licorice (*Glycyrrhiza glabra* L.), deglycyrrhizinated licorice (DGL)	Inflammatory skin disorders
Licorice (*Glycyrrhiza glabra* L.), deglycyrrhizinated licorice (DGL)	Skin disorders
Marshmallow (*Althaea officinalis* L.)	Dermatitis (topical)
Melatonin	Hyperpigmentation
Milk thistle (*Silybum marianum*), silymarin	Psoriasis
Niacin (vitamin B_3, nicotinic acid), niacinamide, inositol hexanicotinate	Psoriasis
Niacin (vitamin B_3, nicotinic acid), niacinamide, inositol hexanicotinate	Skin disorders
Oleander (*Nerium oleander, Thevetia peruviana*)	Corns
Oleander (*Nerium oleander, Thevetia peruviana*)	Skin diseases
Oleander (*Nerium oleander, Thevetia peruviana*)	Skin eruptions
Oleander (*Nerium oleander, Thevetia peruviana*)	Warts
Polypodium leucotomos extract, Anapsos	Vitiligo (loss of pigment in the skin)
Propolis	Dermatitis
Propolis	Eczema
Propolis	Psoriasis
Psyllium (*Plantago ovata, P. ispaghula*)	Psoriasis
Red clover (*Trifolium pratense*)	Eczema
Red clover (*Trifolium pratense*)	Psoriasis
Seaweed, kelp, bladderwrack (*Fucus vesiculosus*)	Eczema
Seaweed, kelp, bladderwrack (*Fucus vesiculosus*)	Psoriasis
Shark cartilage	Contact dermatitis

Continued

Sorrel (*Rumex acetosa* L., *R. acetosella* L.), Sinupret	Nettle rash
Spirulina	Skin disorders
Spirulina	Warts
Tea tree oil (*Melaleuca alternifolia* [Maiden & Betche] Cheel)	Corns
Tea tree oil (*Melaleuca alternifolia* [Maiden & Betche] Cheel)	Eczema
Tea tree oil (*Melaleuca alternifolia* [Maiden & Betche] Cheel)	Impetigo
Tea tree oil (*Melaleuca alternifolia* [Maiden & Betche] Cheel)	Psoriasis
Tea tree oil (*Melaleuca alternifolia* [Maiden & Betche] Cheel)	Skin ailments
Tea tree oil (*Melaleuca alternifolia* [Maiden & Betche] Cheel)	Warts
Thyme (*Thymus vulgaris* L.), thymol	Dermatitis
Thyme (*Thymus vulgaris* L.), thymol	Eczema
Thyme (*Thymus vulgaris* L.), thymol	Warts
White horehound (*Marrubium vulgare* L.)	Skin conditions
White horehound (*Marrubium vulgare* L.)	Warts
Wild yam (*Dioscorea villosa*)	Rash

SLEEP DISORDERS/INSOMNIA/JET LAG AND RELATED CONDITIONS

Levels of Scientific Evidence for Specific Therapies

GRADE: A (Strong Scientific Evidence)	
Therapy	**Specific Therapeutic Use(s)**
Melatonin	Jet lag

GRADE: B (Good Scientific Evidence)	
Therapy	**Specific Therapeutic Use(s)**
Melatonin	Delayed sleep phase syndrome (DSPS)
Melatonin	Insomnia in the elderly
Melatonin	Sleep disturbances in children with neuropsychiatric disorders
Melatonin	Sleep enhancement in healthy people
Valerian (*Valeriana officinalis* L.)	Insomnia

GRADE: C (Unclear or Conflicting Scientific Evidence)	
Therapy	**Specific Therapeutic Use(s)**
Hops (*Humulus lupulus* L.)	Insomnia/sleep quality
Lavender (*Lavandula angustifolia* Miller)	Hypnotic/sleep
Melatonin	Circadian rhythm entraining (in blind persons)
Melatonin	Insomnia (of unknown origin in the nonelderly)

Melatonin	Rapid eye movement (REM) sleep behavior disorder
Melatonin	Sleep disturbances due to pineal region brain damage
Melatonin	Work shift sleep disorder

TRADITIONAL OR THEORETICAL USES THAT LACK SUFFICIENT EVIDENCE

Therapy	Specific Therapeutic Use(s)
Astragalus (*Astragalus membranaceus*)	Insomnia
Black cohosh (*Cimicifuga racemosa* L. Nutt.)	Sleep disorders
Calendula (*Calendula officinalis* L.), marigold	Insomnia
Coenzyme Q10	Insomnia
Danshen (*Salvia miltiorrhiza*)	Sleep difficulties
Danshen (*Salvia miltiorrhiza*)	Stimulation of gamma-aminobutyric acid (GABA) release
Dehydroepiandrosterone (DHEA)	Sleep disorders
Elder (*Sambucus nigra* L.)	Insomnia
Eucalyptus oil (*Eucalyptus globulus* Labillardiere, *E. fructicetorum* F. Von Mueller, *E. smithii* R.T. Baker)	Snoring
Ginkgo (*Ginkgo biloba* L.)	Insomnia
Ginseng (American ginseng, Asian ginseng, Chinese ginseng, Korean red ginseng, *Panax ginseng*: *Panax* spp. including *P. ginseng* C.C. Meyer and *P. quinquefolium* L., excluding *Eleutherococcus senticosus*)	Insomnia
Hawthorn (*Crataegus laevigata, C. oxyacantha, C. monogyna, C. pentagyna*)	Insomnia
Kava (Piper methysticum G. Forst)	Jet lag
Niacin (vitamin B$_3$, nicotinic acid), niacinamide, inositol hexanicotinate	Insomnia
Passionflower (*Passiflora incarnata* L.)	Insomnia
St. John's wort (*Hypericum perforatum* L.)	Insomnia
Thyme (*Thymus vulgaris* L.), thymol	Insomnia
Thyme (*Thymus vulgaris* L.), thymol	Nightmares
Yohimbe bark extract (*Pausinystalia yohimbe* Pierre ex Beille)	Insomnia
Yohimbe bark extract (*Pausinystalia yohimbe* Pierre ex Beille)	Narcolepsy

SNAKE BITES AND RELATED CONDITIONS

Levels of Scientific Evidence for Specific Therapies

TRADITIONAL OR THEORETICAL USES THAT LACK SUFFICIENT EVIDENCE

Therapy	Specific Therapeutic Use(s)
American pennyroyal (*Hedeoma pulegioides* L.), European pennyroyal (*Mentha pulegium* L.)	Snake bites (venomous)

Continued

Black cohosh (*Cimicifuga racemosa* L. Nutt.)	Snake bites
Chaparral (*Larrea tridentata* DC. Coville, *L. divaricata* Cav.), nordihydroguaiaretic acid (NDGA)	Snakebite pain
Echinacea (*Echinacea angustifolia* DC., *E. pallida*, *E. purpurea*)	Snake bites
Ginger (*Zingiber officinale* Roscoe)	Poisonous snake bites
Globe artichoke (*Cynara scolymus* L.)	Snake bites
Gotu kola (*Centella asiatica* L.), total triterpenic fraction of *Centella asiatica* (TTFCA)	Antivenom
Gotu kola (*Centella asiatica* L.), total triterpenic fraction of *Centella asiatica* (TTFCA)	Snake bites
Gymnema (*Gymnema sylvestre* R. Br.)	Snake venom antidote
Milk thistle (*Silybum marianum*), silymarin	Snake bites
Oleander (*Nerium oleander*, *Thevetia peruviana*)	Snake bites
St. John's wort (*Hypericum perforatum* L.)	Snake bites

SPRAINS/STRAINS AND RELATED CONDITIONS

Levels of Scientific Evidence for Specific Therapies

TRADITIONAL OR THEORETICAL USES THAT LACK SUFFICIENT EVIDENCE

Therapy	Specific Therapeutic Use(s)
Bitter almond (*Prunus amygdalus* Batch var. *amara* DC. Focke), Laetrile	Muscle relaxant
Black cohosh (*Cimicifuga racemosa* L. Nutt.)	Muscle spasms
Boswellia (*Boswellia serrata* Roxb.)	Bursitis
Boswellia (*Boswellia serrata* Roxb.)	Tendonitis
Bromelain	Bursitis
Bromelain	Sports or other physical injuries
Bromelain	Tendonitis
Clove (*Eugenia aromatica*)	Muscle spasm
Devil's claw (*Harpagophytum procumbens* DC.)	Tendonitis
Dong quai (*Angelica sinensis* [Oliv.] Diels), Chinese angelica	Muscle relaxant
Eucalyptus oil (*Eucalyptus globulus* Labillardiere, *E. fructicetorum* F. Von Mueller, *E. smithii* R.T. Baker)	Muscle spasm
Eucalyptus oil (*Eucalyptus globulus* Labillardiere, *E. fructicetorum* F. Von Mueller, *E. smithii* R.T. Baker)	Strains/sprains (applied to the skin)
Garlic (*Allium sativum* L.)	Muscle spasms
Goldenseal (*Hydrastis canadensis* L.), berberine	Muscle spasm
Hops (*Humulus lupulus* L.)	Muscle and joint disorders
Hops (*Humulus lupulus* L.)	Muscle spasm
Lavender (*Lavandula angustifolia* Miller)	Muscle spasm
Lavender (*Lavandula angustifolia* Miller)	Sprains

Licorice (*Glycyrrhiza glabra* L.), deglycyrrhizinated licorice (DGL)	Muscle cramps
Marshmallow (*Althaea officinalis* L.)	Sprains
Niacin (vitamin B$_3$, nicotinic acid), niacinamide, inositol hexanicotinate	Bursitis
Omega-3 fatty acids, fish oil, alpha-linolenic acid	Tennis elbow
Peppermint (*Mentha* x *piperita* L.)	Tendonitis
Saw palmetto (*Serenoa repens* [Bartram] Small)	Muscle or intestinal spasms
Slippery elm (*Ulmus rubra* Muhl. or *U. fulva* Michx.)	Synovitis
St. John's wort (*Hypericum perforatum* L.)	Sprains
Thyme (*Thymus vulgaris* L.), thymol	Sprains
Valerian (*Valeriana officinalis* L.)	Muscle pain/spasm/tension

STROKE AND RELATED CONDITIONS

Levels of Scientific Evidence for Specific Therapies

GRADE: C (Unclear or Conflicting Scientific Evidence)

Therapy	Specific Therapeutic Use(s)
Betel nut (*Areca catechu* L.)	Stroke recovery
Danshen (*Salvia miltiorrhiza*)	Ischemic stroke
Melatonin	Stroke
Omega-3 fatty acids, fish oil, alpha-linolenic acid	Stroke prevention

GRADE: D (Fair Negative Scientific Evidence)

Therapy	Specific Therapeutic Use(s)
Ginkgo (*Ginkgo biloba* L.)	Stroke

TRADITIONAL OR THEORETICAL USES THAT LACK SUFFICIENT EVIDENCE

Therapy	Specific Therapeutic Use(s)
Arginine (L-arginine)	Ischemic stroke
Arginine (L-arginine)	Stroke
Astragalus (*Astragalus membranaceus*)	Stroke
Dong quai (*Angelica sinensis* [Oliv.] Diels), Chinese angelica	Stroke
Garlic (*Allium sativum* L.)	Stroke
Ginseng (American ginseng, Asian ginseng, Chinese ginseng, Korean red ginseng, *Panax ginseng*: *Panax* spp. including *P. ginseng* C.C. Meyer and *P. quinquefolium* L., excluding *Eleutherococcus senticosus*)	Strokes
Green tea (*Camellia sinensis*)	Ischemia–reperfusion injury protection
Green tea (*Camellia sinensis*)	Stroke prevention
Kava (*Piper methysticum* G. Forst)	Cerebral ischemia

Continued

Lycopene	Stroke prevention
Niacin (vitamin B$_3$, nicotinic acid), niacinamide, inositol hexanicotinate	Ischemia–reperfusion injury prevention

SUNBURN AND RELATED CONDITIONS

Levels of Scientific Evidence for Specific Therapies

GRADE: C (Unclear or Conflicting Scientific Evidence)

Therapy	Specific Therapeutic Use(s)
Green tea (*Camellia sinensis*)	Sun protection

TRADITIONAL OR THEORETICAL USES THAT LACK SUFFICIENT EVIDENCE

Therapy	Specific Therapeutic Use(s)
Aloe (*Aloe vera*)	Sunburn
American pennyroyal (*Hedeoma pulegioides* L.), European pennyroyal (*Mentha pulegium* L.)	Sunstroke
Gotu kola (*Centella asiatica* L.), total triterpenic fraction of *Centella asiatica* (TTFCA)	Sunstroke
Green tea (*Camellia sinensis*)	Sunburn
Peppermint (*Mentha* x *piperita* L.)	Sun block
Polypodium leucotomos extract, Anapsos	Sunburn protection
Propolis	Skin rejuvenant

SYSTEMIC LUPUS ERYTHEMATOSUS (LUPUS) AND RELATED CONDITIONS

Levels of Scientific Evidence for Specific Therapies

GRADE: B (Good Scientific Evidence)

Therapy	Specific Therapeutic Use(s)
Omega-3 fatty acids, fish oil, alpha-linolenic acid	Rheumatoid arthritis (fish oil)

GRADE: C (Unclear or Conflicting Scientific Evidence)

Therapy	Specific Therapeutic Use(s)
Boswellia (*Boswellia serrata* Roxb.)	Rheumatoid arthritis
Bromelain	Rheumatoid arthritis
Dehydroepiandrosterone (DHEA)	Systemic lupus erythematosus
Dong quai (*Angelica sinensis* [Oliv.] Diels), Chinese angelica	Arthritis
Evening primrose oil (*Oenothera biennis* L.)	Rheumatoid arthritis
Feverfew (*Tanacetum parthenium* L. Schultz-Bip.)	Rheumatoid arthritis
Ginger (*Zingiber officinale* Roscoe)	Rheumatic diseases (rheumatoid arthritis, osteoarthritis, arthralgias, muscle pain)
Glucosamine	Rheumatoid arthritis

Green tea (*Camellia sinensis*)	Arthritis
Guggul (*Commifora mukul*)	Rheumatoid arthritis
Omega-3 fatty acids, fish oil, alpha-linolenic acid	Lupus erythematosus
Propolis	Rheumatic diseases
Shark cartilage	Inflammatory joint diseases (rheumatoid arthritis, osteoarthritis)
Turmeric (*Curcuma longa* L.), curcumin	Rheumatoid arthritis

TRADITIONAL OR THEORETICAL USES THAT LACK SUFFICIENT EVIDENCE

Therapy	Specific Therapeutic Use(s)
Alfalfa (*Medicago sativa* L.)	Rheumatoid arthritis
Aloe (*Aloe vera*)	Arthritis
Aloe (*Aloe vera*)	Lupus erythematosus
Astragalus (*Astragalus membranaceus*)	Ankylosing spondylitis
Astragalus (*Astragalus membranaceus*)	Systemic lupus erythematosus
Belladonna (*Atropa belladonna* L. or its variety *A. acuminata* Royle ex Lindl)	Arthritis
Bilberry (*Vaccinium myrtillus*)	Arthritis
Bladderwrack (*Fucus vesiculosus*)	Arthritis
Bladderwrack (*Fucus vesiculosus*)	Rheumatism
Boron	Rheumatoid arthritis
Bromelain	Autoimmune disorders
Burdock (*Arctium lappa*)	Arthritis
Burdock (*Arctium lappa*)	Rheumatoid arthritis
Chamomile (*Matricaria recutita, Chamaemelum nobile*)	Arthritis
Chaparral (*Larrea tridentata* DC. Coville, *L. divaricata* Cav.), nordihydroguaiaretic acid (NDGA)	Arthritis
Chaparral (*Larrea tridentata* DC. Coville, *L. divaricata* Cav.), nordihydroguaiaretic acid (NDGA)	Rheumatic diseases
Dandelion (*Taraxacum officinale*)	Arthritis
Dandelion (*Taraxacum officinale*)	Rheumatoid arthritis
Devil's claw (*Harpagophytum procumbens* DC.)	Rheumatoid arthritis
Dehydroepiandrosterone (DHEA)	Rheumatic diseases
Dong quai (*Angelica sinensis* [Oliv.] Diels), Chinese angelica	Chilblains
Dong quai (*Angelica sinensis* [Oliv.] Diels), Chinese angelica	Rheumatic diseases
Echinacea (*Echinacea angustifolia* DC., *E. pallida, E. purpurea*)	Rheumatism
Essiac	Arthritis
Essiac	Systemic lupus erythematosus
Eucalyptus oil (*Eucalyptus globulus* Labillardiere, *E. fructicetorum* F. Von Mueller, *E. smithii* R.T. Baker)	Arthritis

Continued

Eucalyptus oil (*Eucalyptus globulus* Labillardiere, *E. fructicetorum* F. Von Mueller, *E. smithii* R.T. Baker)	Rheumatoid arthritis (applied to the skin)
Evening primrose oil (*Oenothera biennis* L.)	Systemic lupus erythematosus
Flaxseed and flaxseed oil (*Linum usitatissimum*)	Rheumatoid arthritis
Garlic (*Allium sativum* L.)	Arthritis
Globe artichoke (*Cynara scolymus* L.)	Arthritis
Globe artichoke (*Cynara scolymus* L.)	Rheumatoid arthritis
Goldenseal (*Hydrastis canadensis* L.), berberine	Arthritis
Goldenseal (*Hydrastis canadensis* L.), berberine	Lupus
Gotu kola (*Centella asiatica* L.), total triterpenic fraction of *Centella asiatica* (TTFCA)	Rheumatism
Gotu kola (*Centella asiatica* L.), total triterpenic fraction of *Centella asiatica* (TTFCA)	Systemic lupus erythematosus
Gymnema (*Gymnema sylvestre* R. Br.)	Rheumatoid arthritis
Hops (*Humulus lupulus* L.)	Rheumatic disorders
Horse chestnut (*Aesculus hippocastanum* L.)	Rheumatism
Horse chestnut (*Aesculus hippocastanum* L.)	Rheumatoid arthritis
Horsetail (*Equisetum arvense* L.)	Rheumatism
Kava (*Piper methysticum* G. Forst)	Arthritis
Lavender (*Lavandula angustifolia* Miller)	Rheumatism
Licorice (*Glycyrrhiza glabra* L.), deglycyrrhizinated licorice (DGL)	Rheumatoid arthritis
Lycopene	Inflammatory conditions
Maitake mushroom (*Grifola frondosa*), beta-glucan	Arthritis
Marshmallow (*Althaea officinalis* L.)	Arthritis
Marshmallow (*Althaea officinalis* L.)	Chilblains
Melatonin	Rheumatoid arthritis
Niacin (vitamin B_3, nicotinic acid), niacinamide, inositol hexanicotinate	Arthritis
Omega-3 fatty acids, fish oil, alpha-linolenic acid	Dermatomyositis
Omega-3 fatty acids, fish oil, alpha-linolenic acid	Systemic lupus erythematosus
Peppermint (*Mentha* x *piperita* L.)	Arthritis
Peppermint (*Mentha* x *piperita* L.)	Rheumatic pain
Polypodium leucotomos extract, Anapsos	Autoimmune diseases
Polypodium leucotomos extract, Anapsos	Rheumatic diseases
Propolis	Rheumatoid arthritis
Red clover (*Trifolium pratense*)	Arthritis
Seaweed, kelp, bladderwrack (*Fucus vesiculosus*)	Arthritis
Seaweed, kelp, bladderwrack (*Fucus vesiculosus*)	Rheumatism
Shark cartilage	Ankylosing spondylitis

Shark cartilage	Systemic lupus erythematosus
Slippery elm (*Ulmus rubra* Muhl. or *U. fulva* Michx.)	Rheumatic disorders
Soy (Glycine max L. Merr.)	Autoimmune diseases
Soy (*Glycine max* L. Merr.)	Rheumatoid arthritis
St. John's wort (*Hypericum perforatum* L.)	Rheumatism
Thyme (*Thymus vulgaris* L.), thymol	Arthritis
Thyme (*Thymus vulgaris* L.), thymol	Dermatomyositis
Thyme (*Thymus vulgaris* L.), thymol	Rheumatism
Valerian (*Valeriana officinalis* L.)	Arthritis
Valerian (*Valeriana officinalis* L.)	Rheumatic pain
Wild yam (*Dioscorea villosa*)	Rheumatic pain

THROMBOCYTOPENIA AND RELATED CONDITIONS

Levels of Scientific Evidence for Specific Therapies

GRADE: C (Unclear or Conflicting Scientific Evidence)

Therapy	Specific Therapeutic Use(s)
Dong quai (*Angelica sinensis* [Oliv.] Diels), Chinese angelica	Idiopathic thrombocytopenic purpura (ITP)
Melatonin	Thrombocytopenia (low platelets)

TRADITIONAL OR THEORETICAL USES THAT LACK SUFFICIENT EVIDENCE

Therapy	Specific Therapeutic Use(s)
Astragalus (*Astragalus membranaceus*)	Low platelets
Black cohosh (*Cimicifuga racemosa* L. Nutt.)	Thrombocytopenia
Dong quai (*Angelica sinensis* [Oliv.] Diels), Chinese angelica	Immune cytopenias
Goldenseal (*Hydrastis canadensis* L.), berberine	Thrombocytopenia (low platelets)

THYROID DISORDERS AND RELATED CONDITIONS

Levels of Scientific Evidence for Specific Therapies

GRADE: C (Unclear or Conflicting Scientific Evidence)

Therapy	Specific Therapeutic Use(s)
Bladderwrack (*Fucus vesiculosus*)	Goiter (thyroid disease)

TRADITIONAL OR THEORETICAL USES THAT LACK SUFFICIENT EVIDENCE

Therapy	Specific Therapeutic Use(s)
Essiac	Thyroid disorders
Horsetail (*Equisetum arvense* L.)	Thyroid disorders

Continued

Niacin (vitamin B$_3$, nicotinic acid), niacinamide, inositol hexanicotinate	Hypothyroidism
Propolis	Thyroid disease
Seaweed, kelp, bladderwrack (*Fucus vesiculosus*)	Exophthalmos
Seaweed, kelp, bladderwrack (*Fucus vesiculosus*)	Goiter
Seaweed, kelp, bladderwrack (*Fucus vesiculosus*)	Myxedema

TINNITUS AND RELATED CONDITIONS

Levels of Scientific Evidence for Specific Therapies

GRADE: C (Unclear or Conflicting Scientific Evidence)

Therapy	Specific Therapeutic Use(s)
Ginkgo (*Ginkgo biloba* L.)	Ringing in the ears (tinnitus)

TRADITIONAL OR THEORETICAL USES THAT LACK SUFFICIENT EVIDENCE

Therapy	Specific Therapeutic Use(s)
Black cohosh (*Cimicifuga racemosa* L. Nutt.)	Ringing in the ears
Calendula (*Calendula officinalis* L.), marigold	Ringing in the ears
Dong quai (*Angelica sinensis* [Oliv.] Diels), Chinese angelica	Tinnitus (ringing in the ears)
Feverfew (*Tanacetum parthenium* L. Schultz-Bip.)	Ringing in the ears
Goldenseal (*Hydrastis canadensis* L.), berberine	Tinnitis (ringing in the ears)
Horse chestnut (*Aesculus hippocastanum* L.)	Ringing in the ears (tinnitus)
Melatonin	Tinnitus
Niacin (vitamin B$_3$, nicotinic acid), niacinamide, inositol hexanicotinate	Ear ringing

ULCERATIVE COLITIS AND RELATED CONDITIONS

Levels of Scientific Evidence for Specific Therapies

GRADE: C (Unclear or Conflicting Scientific Evidence)

Therapy	Specific Therapeutic Use(s)
Barley (*Hordeum vulgare* L.), germinated barley foodstuff (GBF)	Ulcerative colitis
Betel nut (*Areca catechu* L.)	Ulcerative colitis
Boswellia (*Boswellia serrata* Roxb.)	Ulcerative colitis
Dandelion (*Taraxacum officinale*)	Colitis
Glucosamine	Inflammatory bowel disease
Licorice (*Glycyrrhiza glabra* L.), deglycyrrhizinated licorice (DGL)	Familial Mediterranean fever
Omega-3 fatty acids, fish oil, alpha-linolenic acid	Ulcerative colitis
Psyllium (*Plantago ovata, P. ispaghula*)	Inflammatory bowel disease

TRADITIONAL OR THEORETICAL USES THAT LACK SUFFICIENT EVIDENCE

Therapy	Specific Therapeutic Use(s)
Aloe (*Aloe vera*)	Inflammatory bowel disease
Arginine (L-arginine)	Inflammatory bowel disease
Barley (*Hordeum vulgare* L.), germinated barley foodstuff (GBF)	Inflammatory bowel disorders
Belladonna (*Atropa belladonna* L. or its variety *A. acuminata* Royle ex Lindl)	Colitis
Belladonna (*Atropa belladonna* L. or its variety *A. acuminata* Royle ex Lindl)	Ulcerative colitis
Bromelain	Colitis
Bromelain	Ulcerative colitis
Calendula (*Calendula officinalis* L.), marigold	Ulcerative colitis
Dehydroepiandrosterone (DHEA)	Ulcerative colitis
Elder (*Sambucas nigra* L.)	Ulcerative colitis
Eucalyptus oil (*Eucalyptus globulus* Labillardiere, *E. fructicetorum* F. Von Mueller, *E. smithii* R.T. Baker)	Inflammatory bowel disease
Evening primrose oil (*Oenothera biennis* L.)	Ulcerative colitis
Flaxseed and flaxseed oil (*Linum usitatissimum*)	Ulcerative colitis
Ginkgo (*Ginkgo biloba* L.)	Ulcerative colitis
Ginseng (American ginseng, Asian ginseng, Chinese ginseng, Korean red ginseng, *Panax ginseng*: *Panax* spp. including *P. ginseng* C.C. Meyer and *P. quinquefolium* L., excluding *Eleutherococcus senticosus*)	Colitis
Glucosamine	Inflammatory bowel disease
Glucosamine	Ulcerative colitis
Goldenseal (*Hydrastis canadensis* L.), berberine	Colitis
Guggul (*Commifora mukul*)	Colitis
Lactobacillus acidophilus	Colitis
Lactobacillus acidophilus	Ulcerative colitis
Licorice (*Glycyrrhiza glabra* L.), deglycyrrhizinated licorice (DGL)	Colitis
Marshmallow (*Althaea officinalis* L.)	Colitis
Marshmallow (*Althaea officinalis* L.)	Inflammation of the small intestine
Marshmallow (*Althaea officinalis* L.)	Ulcerative colitis
Melatonin	Colitis
Propolis	Ulcerative colitis
Slippery elm (*Ulmus rubra* Muhl. or *U. fulva* Michx.)	Colitis
Slippery elm (*Ulmus rubra* Muhl. or *U. fulva* Michx.)	Ulcerative colitis
Spirulina	Colitis
Thyme (*Thymus vulgaris* L.), thymol	Inflammation of the colon

UPPER RESPIRATORY TRACT INFECTION/BRONCHITIS/ COMMON COLD/FLU AND RELATED CONDITIONS

Levels of Scientific Evidence for Specific Therapies

GRADE: B (Good Scientific Evidence)

Therapy	Specific Therapeutic Use(s)
Echinacea (*Echinacea angustifolia* DC., *E. pallida, E. purpurea*)	Upper respiratory tract infections: treatment

GRADE: C (Unclear or Conflicting Scientific Evidence)

Therapy	Specific Therapeutic Use(s)
Astragalus (*Astragalus membranaceus*)	Upper respiratory tract infection
Chamomile (*Matricaria recutita, Chamaemelum nobile*)	Common cold
Echinacea (*Echinacea angustifolia* DC., *E. pallida, E. purpurea*)	Upper respiratory tract infections: prevention
Elder (*Sambucus nigra* L.)	Bronchitis
Elder (*Sambucus nigra* L.)	Influenza
Garlic (*Allium sativum* L.)	Upper respiratory tract infection
Goldenseal (*Hydrastis canadensis* L.), berberine	Common cold/upper respiratory tract infection
Peppermint (*Mentha* x *piperita* L.)	Nasal congestion
Propolis	Prevention of colds
Slippery elm (*Ulmus rubra* Muhl. or *U. fulva* Michx.)	Sore throat
Sorrel (*Rumex acetosa* L., *R. acetosella* L.), Sinupret	Bronchitis

TRADITIONAL OR THEORETICAL USES THAT LACK SUFFICIENT EVIDENCE

Therapy	Specific Therapeutic Use(s)
American pennyroyal (*Hedeoma pulegioides* L.), European pennyroyal (*Mentha pulegium* L.)	Chest congestion
American pennyroyal (*Hedeoma pulegioides* L.), European pennyroyal (*Mentha pulegium* L.)	Colds
American pennyroyal (*Hedeoma pulegioides* L.), European pennyroyal (*Mentha pulegium* L.)	Flu
American pennyroyal (*Hedeoma pulegioides* L.), European pennyroyal (*Mentha pulegium* L.)	Respiratory ailments
Arginine (L-arginine)	Cold prevention
Astragalus (*Astragalus membranaceus*)	Bronchitis
Barley (*Hordeum vulgare* L.), germinated barley foodstuff (GBF)	Bronchitis
Belladonna (*Atropa belladonna* L. or its variety *A. acuminata* Royle ex Lindl)	Colds
Belladonna (*Atropa belladonna* L. or its variety *A. acuminata* Royle ex Lindl)	Flu
Belladonna (*Atropa belladonna* L. or its variety *A. acuminata* Royle ex Lindl)	Sore throat

Betel nut (*Areca catechu* L.)	Respiratory stimulant
Bilberry (*Vaccinium myrtillus*)	Common cold
Bilberry (*Vaccinium myrtillus*)	Pharyngitis
Black cohosh (*Cimicifuga racemosa* L. Nutt.)	Bronchitis
Black cohosh (*Cimicifuga racemosa* L. Nutt.)	Sore throat
Black tea (*Camellia sinensis*)	Influenza
Bladderwrack (*Fucus vesiculosus*)	Sore throat
Blessed thistle (*Cnicus benedictus* L.)	Colds
Bromelain	Bronchitis
Bromelain	Common cold
Bromelain	Upper respiratory tract infection
Burdock (*Arctium lappa*)	Common cold
Burdock (*Arctium lappa*)	Respiratory infections
Burdock (*Arctium lappa*)	Tonsillitis
Calendula (*Calendula officinalis* L.), marigold	Influenza
Calendula (*Calendula officinalis* L.), marigold	Sore throat
Chaparral (*Larrea tridentata* DC. Coville, *L. divaricata* Cav.), nordihydroguaiaretic acid (NDGA)	Colds
Chaparral (*Larrea tridentata* DC. Coville, *L. divaricata* Cav.), nordihydroguaiaretic acid (NDGA)	Influenza
Chaparral (*Larrea tridentata* DC. Coville, *L. divaricata* Cav.), nordihydroguaiaretic acid (NDGA)	Respiratory tract infections
Dehydroepiandrosterone (DHEA)	Influenza
Dong quai (*Angelica sinensis* [Oliv.] Diels), Chinese angelica	Bronchitis
Dong quai (*Angelica sinensis* [Oliv.] Diels), Chinese angelica	Respiratory tract infection
Echinacea (*Echinacea angustifolia* DC., *E. pallida*, *E. purpurea*)	Tonsillitis
Elder (*Sambucus nigra* L.)	Colds
Ephedra (*Ephedra sinica*)/ma huang	Colds
Ephedra (*Ephedra sinica*)/ma huang	Flu
Ephedra (*Ephedra sinica*)/ma huang	Nasal congestion
Ephedra (*Ephedra sinica*)/ma huang	Upper respiratory tract infection
Eucalyptus oil (*Eucalyptus globulus* Labillardiere, *E. fructicetorum* F. Von Mueller, *E. smithii* R.T. Baker)	Bronchitis
Eucalyptus oil (*Eucalyptus globulus* Labillardiere, *E. fructicetorum* F. Von Mueller, *E. smithii* R.T. Baker)	Colds
Eucalyptus oil (*Eucalyptus globulus* Labillardiere, *E. fructicetorum* F. Von Mueller, *E. smithii* R.T. Baker)	Influenza
Eyebright (*Euphrasia officinalis*)	Bronchitis (chronic)
Eyebright (*Euphrasia officinalis*)	Common cold

Continued

Eyebright (*Euphrasia officinalis*)	Respiratory infections
Eyebright (*Euphrasia officinalis*)	Sore throat
Fenugreek (*Trigonella foenum-graecum* L.)	Bronchitis
Feverfew (*Tanacetum parthenium* L. Schultz-Bip.)	Colds
Flaxseed and flaxseed oil (*Linum usitatissimum*)	Sore throat
Flaxseed and flaxseed oil (*Linum usitatissimum*)	Upper respiratory tract infection
Garlic (*Allium sativum* L.)	Bronchitis
Garlic (*Allium sativum* L.)	Colds
Garlic (*Allium sativum* L.)	Influenza
Ginger (*Zingiber officinale* Roscoe)	Bronchitis
Ginger (*Zingiber officinale* Roscoe)	Colds
Ginger (*Zingiber officinale* Roscoe)	Flu
Ginkgo (*Ginkgo biloba* L.)	Bronchitis
Ginkgo (*Ginkgo biloba* L.)	Respiratory tract illnesses
Ginseng (American ginseng, Asian ginseng, Chinese ginseng, Korean red ginseng, *Panax ginseng*: *Panax* spp. including *P. ginseng* C.C. Meyer and *P. quinquefolium* L., excluding *Eleutherococcus senticosus*)	Influenza
Ginseng (American ginseng, Asian ginseng, Chinese ginseng, Korean red ginseng, *Panax ginseng*: *Panax* spp. including *P. ginseng* C.C. Meyer and *P. quinquefolium* L., excluding *Eleutherococcus senticosus*)	Upper respiratory tract infection
Goldenseal (*Hydrastis canadensis* L.), berberine	Bronchitis
Goldenseal (*Hydrastis canadensis* L.), berberine	Influenza
Goldenseal (*Hydrastis canadensis* L.), berberine	Tonsillitis
Gotu kola (*Centella asiatica* L.), total triterpenic fraction of *Centella asiatica* (TTFCA)	Bronchitis
Gotu kola (*Centella asiatica* L.), total triterpenic fraction of *Centella asiatica* (TTFCA)	Colds
Gotu kola (*Centella asiatica* L.), total triterpenic fraction of *Centella asiatica* (TTFCA)	Influenza
Gotu kola (*Centella asiatica* L.), total triterpenic fraction of *Centella asiatica* (TTFCA)	Tonsillitis
Guggul (*Commifora mukul*)	Sore throat
Hawthorn (*Crataegus laevigata, C. oxyacantha, C. monogyna, C. pentagyna*)	Sore throat
Kava (*Piper methysticum* G. Forst)	Colds
Lavender (*Lavandula angustifolia* Miller)	Bronchitis
Lavender (*Lavandula angustifolia* Miller)	Common cold
Licorice (*Glycyrrhiza glabra* L.), deglycyrrhizinated licorice (DGL)	Bronchitis
Licorice (*Glycyrrhiza glabra* L.), deglycyrrhizinated licorice (DGL)	Sore throat

Marshmallow (*Althaea officinalis* L.)	Bronchitis
Marshmallow (*Althaea officinalis* L.)	Sore throat
Milk thistle (*Silybum marianum*), silymarin	Bronchitis
Omega-3 fatty acids, fish oil, alpha-linolenic acid	Common cold
Peppermint (*Mentha* x *piperita* L.)	Bronchial spasm
Peppermint (*Mentha* x *piperita* L.)	Common cold
Peppermint (*Mentha* x *piperita* L.)	Influenza
Polypodium leucotomos extract, Anapsos	Upper respiratory tract infection
Psyllium (*Plantago ovata*, *P. ispaghula*)	Bronchitis
Red clover (*Trifolium pratense*)	Bronchitis
Saw palmetto (*Serenoa repens* [Bartram] Small)	Bronchitis
Saw palmetto (*Serenoa repens* [Bartram] Small)	Sore throat
Saw palmetto (*Serenoa repens* [Bartram] Small)	Upper respiratory tract infection
Seaweed, kelp, bladderwrack (*Fucus vesiculosus*)	Sore throat
Slippery elm (*Ulmus rubra* Muhl. or *U. fulva* Michx.)	Bronchitis
Sorrel (*Rumex acetosa* L., *R. acetosella* L.), Sinupret	Nasal inflammation
Sorrel (*Rumex acetosa* L., *R. acetosella* L.), Sinupret	Respiratory inflammation
Sorrel (*Rumex acetosa* L., *R. acetosella* L.), Sinupret	Sore throat
Spirulina	Influenza
St. John's wort (*Hypericum perforatum* L.)	Influenza
Tea tree oil (*Melaleuca alternifolia* [Maiden & Betche] Cheel)	Bronchial congestion
Tea tree oil (*Melaleuca alternifolia* [Maiden & Betche] Cheel)	Colds
Tea tree oil (*Melaleuca alternifolia* [Maiden & Betche] Cheel)	Sinus infections
Tea tree oil (*Melaleuca alternifolia* [Maiden & Betche] Cheel)	Sore throat
Tea tree oil (*Melaleuca alternifolia* [Maiden & Betche] Cheel)	Tonsillitis
Thyme (*Thymus vulgaris* L.), thymol	Flu
Thyme (*Thymus vulgaris* L.), thymol	Sore throat
Thyme (*Thymus vulgaris* L.), thymol	Tonsillitis
Thyme (*Thymus vulgaris* L.), thymol	Upper respiratory tract infection
White horehound (*Marrubium vulgare* L.)	Bronchitis
White horehound (*Marrubium vulgare* L.)	Respiratory (lung) spasms
White horehound (*Marrubium vulgare* L.)	Sore throat
White horehound (*Marrubium vulgare* L.)	Upper respiratory tract infection

URINARY INCONTINENCE AND RELATED CONDITIONS

Levels of Scientific Evidence for Specific Therapies

GRADE: C (Unclear or Conflicting Scientific Evidence)

Therapy	Specific Therapeutic Use(s)
Cranberry (*Vaccinium macrocarpon*)	Reduction of odor from incontinence/bladder catheterization
Saw palmetto (*Serenoa repens* [Bartram] Small)	Hypotonic neurogenic bladder

TRADITIONAL OR THEORETICAL USES THAT LACK SUFFICIENT EVIDENCE

Therapy	Specific Therapeutic Use(s)
Belladonna (*Atropa belladonna* L. or its variety *A. acuminata* Royle ex Lindl)	Bedwetting
Calendula (*Calendula officinalis* L.), marigold	Urinary retention
Ephedra (*Ephedra sinica*)/ma huang	Enuresis
Gotu kola (*Centella asiatica* L.), total triterpenic fraction of *Centella asiatica* (TTFCA)	Urinary retention
Horsetail (*Equisetum arvense* L.)	Urinary incontinence
Kava (*Piper methysticum* G. Forst)	Urinary incontinence
St. John's wort (*Hypericum perforatum* L.)	Bedwetting
Thyme (*Thymus vulgaris* L.), thymol	Enuresis

URINARY TRACT INFECTION AND RELATED CONDITIONS

Levels of Scientific Evidence for Specific Therapies

GRADE: B (Good Scientific Evidence)

Therapy	Specific Therapeutic Use(s)
Cranberry (*Vaccinium macrocarpon*)	Urinary tract infection prevention

GRADE: C (Unclear or Conflicting Scientific Evidence)

Therapy	Specific Therapeutic Use(s)
Bromelain	Urinary tract infection
Cranberry (*Vaccinium macrocarpon*)	Urinary tract infection treatment
Cranberry (*Vaccinium macrocarpon*)	Urine acidification
Peppermint (*Mentha* x *piperita* L.)	Urinary tract infection

GRADE: D (Fair Negative Scientific Evidence)

Therapy	Specific Therapeutic Use(s)
Cranberry (*Vaccinium macrocarpon*)	Chronic urinary tract infection prevention: children with neurogenic bladder

TRADITIONAL OR THEORETICAL USES THAT LACK SUFFICIENT EVIDENCE

Therapy	Specific Therapeutic Use(s)
Bilberry (*Vaccinium myrtillus*)	Urinary tract infections
Burdock (*Arctium lappa*)	Urinary tract infections
Chaparral (*Larrea tridentata* DC. Coville, *L. divaricata* Cav.), nordihydroguaiaretic acid (NDGA)	Urinary tract infections
Dandelion (*Taraxacum officinale*)	Urinary tract inflammation
Devil's claw (*Harpagophytum procumbens* DC.)	Urinary tract infections
Echinacea (*Echinacea angustifolia* DC., *E. pallida*, *E. purpurea*)	Urinary tract infections
Eucalyptus oil (*Eucalyptus globulus* Labillardiere, *E. fructicetorum* F. Von Mueller, *E. smithii* R.T. Baker)	Urinary tract infection
Flaxseed and flaxseed oil (*Linum usitatissimum*)	Urinary tract infection
Garlic (*Allium sativum* L.)	Urinary tract infections
Ginkgo (*Ginkgo biloba* L.)	Genitourinary disorders
Goldenseal (*Hydrastis canadensis* L.), berberine	Urinary tract disorders
Gotu kola (*Centella asiatica* L.), total triterpenic fraction of *Centella asiatica* (TTFCA)	Urinary tract infection
Horsetail (*Equisetum arvense* L.)	Urinary tract infection
Horsetail (*Equisetum arvense* L.)	Urinary tract inflammation
Kava (*Piper methysticum* G. Forst)	Urinary tract disorders
Marshmallow (*Althaea officinalis* L.)	Urinary tract infection
Saw palmetto (*Serenoa repens* [Bartram] Small)	Genitourinary tract disorders
Saw palmetto (*Serenoa repens* [Bartram] Small)	Urinary antiseptic
Slippery elm (*Ulmus rubra* Muhl. or *U. fulva* Michx.)	Urinary tract infections
Thyme (*Thymus vulgaris* L.), thymol	Urinary tract infection
Valerian (*Valeriana officinalis* L.)	Urinary tract disorders
Wild yam (*Dioscorea villosa*)	Urinary tract disorders

UTERINE DISORDERS AND RELATED CONDITIONS

Levels of Scientific Evidence for Specific Therapies

TRADITIONAL OR THEORETICAL USES THAT LACK SUFFICIENT EVIDENCE

Therapy	Specific Therapeutic Use(s)
Alfalfa (*Medicago sativa* L.)	Uterine stimulant
American pennyroyal (*Hedeoma pulegioides* L.), European pennyroyal (*Mentha pulegium* L.)	Preparation of uterus for labor
American pennyroyal (*Hedeoma pulegioides* L.), European pennyroyal (*Mentha pulegium* L.)	Uterine fibroids
Astragalus (*Astragalus membranaceus*)	Uterine bleeding
Astragalus (*Astragalus membranaceus*)	Uterine prolapse

Continued

Black cohosh (*Cimicifuga racemosa* L. Nutt.)	Uterine diseases and bleeding
Calendula (*Calendula officinalis* L.), marigold	Uterus problems
Ephedra (*Ephedra sinica*)/ma huang	Uterotonic
Eucalyptus oil (*Eucalyptus globulus* Labillardiere, *E. fructicetorum* F. Von Mueller, *E. smithii* R.T. Baker)	Urinary difficulties
Feverfew (*Tanacetum parthenium* L. Schultz-Bip.)	Uterine disorders
Goldenseal (*Hydrastis canadensis* L.), berberine	Uterus inflammation
Goldenseal (*Hydrastis canadensis* L.), berberine	Uterus stimulant
Kava (*Piper methysticum* G. Forst)	Uterus inflammation
Milk thistle (*Silybum marianum*), silymarin	Uterine complaints
Saw palmetto (*Serenoa repens* [Bartram] Small)	Uterine disorders

VERTIGO AND RELATED CONDITIONS
Levels of Scientific Evidence for Specific Therapies

GRADE: C (Unclear or Conflicting Scientific Evidence)

Therapy	Specific Therapeutic Use(s)
Ginkgo (*Ginkgo biloba* L.)	Vertigo

TRADITIONAL OR THEORETICAL USES THAT LACK SUFFICIENT EVIDENCE

Therapy	Specific Therapeutic Use(s)
American pennyroyal (*Hedeoma pulegioides* L.), European pennyroyal (*Mentha pulegium* L.)	Dizziness
Black cohosh (*Cimicifuga racemosa* L. Nutt.)	Dizziness
Calendula (*Calendula officinalis* L.), marigold	Dizziness
Echinacea (*Echinacea angustifolia* DC., *E. pallida*, *E. purpurea*)	Dizziness
Feverfew (*Tanacetum parthenium* L. Schultz-Bip.)	Dizziness
Ginkgo (*Ginkgo biloba* L.)	Dizziness
Ginseng (American ginseng, Asian ginseng, Chinese ginseng, Korean red ginseng, *Panax ginseng*: *Panax* spp. including *P. ginseng* C.C. Meyer and *P. quinquefolium* L., excluding *Eleutherococcus senticosus*)	Dizziness
Horse chestnut (*Aesculus hippocastanum* L.)	Dizziness
Kava (*Piper methysticum* G. Forst)	Dizziness
Lavender (*Lavandula angustifolia* Miller)	Dizziness
Niacin (vitamin B_3, nicotinic acid), niacinamide, inositol hexanicotinate	Vertigo
Turmeric (*Curcuma longa* L.), curcumin	Dizziness
Valerian (*Valeriana officinalis* L.)	Vertigo

VIRAL INFECTIONS AND RELATED CONDITIONS

Levels of Scientific Evidence for Specific Therapies

GRADE: C (Unclear or Conflicting Scientific Evidence)

Therapy	Specific Therapeutic Use(s)
Astragalus (*Astragalus membranaceus*)	Antiviral activity
Blessed thistle (*Cnicus benedictus* L.)	Viral infections
Cranberry (*Vaccinium macrocarpon*)	Antiviral, antifungal
Sorrel (*Rumex acetosa* L., *R. acetosella* L.), Sinupret	Antiviral

TRADITIONAL OR THEORETICAL USES THAT LACK SUFFICIENT EVIDENCE

Therapy	Specific Therapeutic Use(s)
Betel nut (*Areca catechu* L.)	Diphtheria
Calendula (*Calendula officinalis* L.), marigold	Antiviral
Chaparral (*Larrea tridentata* DC. Coville, *L. divaricata* Cav.), nordihydroguaiaretic acid (NDGA)	Antiviral
Clove (*Eugenia aromatica*)	Antiviral
Dandelion (*Taraxacum officinale*)	Antiviral
Dong quai (*Angelica sinensis* [Oliv.] Diels), Chinese angelica	Antiviral
Echinacea (*Echinacea angustifolia* DC., *E. pallida*, *E. purpurea*)	Diphtheria
Eucalyptus oil (*Eucalyptus globulus* Labillardiere, *E. fructicetorum* F. Von Mueller, *E. smithii* R.T. Baker)	Antiviral
Eyebright (*Euphrasia officinalis*)	Antiviral
Garlic (*Allium sativum* L.)	Antiviral
Garlic (*Allium sativum* L.)	Diphtheria
Ginger (*Zingiber officinale* Roscoe)	Antiviral
Goldenseal (*Hydrastis canadensis* L.), berberine	Diphtheria
Licorice (*Glycyrrhiza glabra* L.), deglycyrrhizinated licorice (DGL)	Coronavirus infection
Licorice (*Glycyrrhiza glabra* L.), deglycyrrhizinated licorice (DGL)	Epstein-Barr virus infection
Peppermint (*Mentha* x *piperita* L.)	Antiviral
Propolis	Viral infections
Spirulina	Antiviral
St. John's wort (*Hypericum perforatum* L.)	Antiviral
St. John's wort (*Hypericum perforatum* L.)	Epstein-Barr virus infectio

VISION AND RELATED CONDITIONS

Levels of Scientific Evidence for Specific Therapies

GRADE: D (Fair Negative Scientific Evidence)

Therapy	Specific Therapeutic Use(s)
Bilberry (*Vaccinium myrtillus*)	Night vision

TRADITIONAL OR THEORETICAL USES THAT LACK SUFFICIENT EVIDENCE

Therapy	Specific Therapeutic Use(s)
Betel nut (*Areca catechu* L.)	Blindness from methanol poisoning
Flaxseed and flaxseed oil (*Linum usitatissimum*)	Vision improvement
Omega-3 fatty acids, fish oil, alpha-linolenic acid	Night vision enhancement
Valerian (*Valeriana officinalis* L.)	Vision

VOMITING AND RELATED CONDITIONS

Levels of Scientific Evidence for Specific Therapies

GRADE: B (Good Scientific Evidence)

Therapy	Specific Therapeutic Use(s)
Ginger (*Zingiber officinale* Roscoe)	Nausea (due to chemotherapy)
Ginger (*Zingiber officinale* Roscoe)	Nausea and vomiting of pregnancy (hyperemesis gravidarum)

GRADE: C (Unclear or Conflicting Scientific Evidence)

Therapy	Specific Therapeutic Use(s)
Ginger (*Zingiber officinale* Roscoe)	Nausea and vomiting (after surgery)
Peppermint (*Mentha* x *piperita* L.)	Nausea

TRADITIONAL OR THEORETICAL USES THAT LACK SUFFICIENT EVIDENCE

Therapy	Specific Therapeutic Use(s)
Belladonna (*Atropa belladonna* L. or its variety *A. acuminata* Royle ex Lindl)	Motion sickness
Belladonna (*Atropa belladonna* L. or its variety *A. acuminata* Royle ex Lindl)	Nausea and vomiting during pregnancy
Black tea (*Camellia sinensis*)	Vomiting
Calendula (*Calendula officinalis* L.), marigold	Nausea
Chamomile (*Matricaria recutita, Chamaemelum nobile*)	Motion sickness
Chamomile (*Matricaria recutita, Chamaemelum nobile*)	Nausea
Chamomile (*Matricaria recutita, Chamaemelum nobile*)	Sea sickness
Chaparral (*Larrea tridentata* DC. Coville, *L. divaricata* Cav.), nordihydroguaiaretic acid (NDGA)	Vomiting

Clay	Vomiting
Clay	Vomiting/nausea during pregnancy
Clove (*Eugenia aromatica*), clove oil (eugenol)	Nausea or vomiting
Cranberry (*Vaccinium macrocarpon*)	Vomiting
Elder (*Sambucus nigra* L.)	Vomiting
Globe artichoke (*Cynara scolymus* L.)	Emesis
Lavender (*Lavandula angustifolia* Miller)	Motion sickness
Lavender (*Lavandula angustifolia* Miller)	Nausea
Lavender (*Lavandula angustifolia* Miller)	Vomiting
Marshmallow (*Althaea officinalis* L.)	Vomiting
Niacin (vitamin B_3, nicotinic acid), niacinamide, inositol hexanicotinate	Motion sickness
Oleander (*Nerium oleander, Thevetia peruviana*)	Vomiting
Valerian (*Valeriana officinalis* L.)	Nausea
White horehound (*Marrubium vulgare* L.)	Emetic
Wild yam (*Dioscorea villosa*)	Emetic

WEIGHT REDUCTION AND RELATED CONDITIONS

Levels of Scientific Evidence for Specific Therapies

GRADE: A (Strong Scientific Evidence)

Therapy	Specific Therapeutic Use(s)
Ephedra (*Ephedra sinica*)/ma huang	Weight loss

GRADE: C (Unclear or Conflicting Scientific Evidence)

Therapy	Specific Therapeutic Use(s)
Bladderwrack (*Fucus vesiculosus*)	Weight loss
Evening primrose oil (*Oenothera biennis* L.)	Obesity/weight loss
Green tea (*Camellia sinensis*)	Weight loss
Guggul (*Commifora mukul*)	Obesity
Spirulina	Weight loss

TRADITIONAL OR THEORETICAL USES THAT LACK SUFFICIENT EVIDENCE

Therapy	Specific Therapeutic Use(s)
Arginine (L-arginine)	Obesity
Astragalus (*Astragalus membranaceus*)	Weight loss
Barley (*Hordeum vulgare* L.), germinated barley foodstuff (GBF)	Appetite suppressant
Bladderwrack (*Fucus vesiculosus*)	Obesity
Bromelain	Appetite suppressant

Continued

Coenzyme Q10	Obesity
Dehydroepiandrosterone (DHEA)	Obesity
Ephedra (*Ephedra sinica*)/ma huang	Appetite suppressant
Evening primrose oil (*Oenothera biennis* L.)	Weight loss
Garlic (*Allium sativum* L.)	Obesity
Goldenseal (*Hydrastis canadensis* L.), berberine	Obesity
Guggul (*Commifora mukul*)	Obesity
Guggul (*Commifora mukul*)	Weight loss
Gymnema (*Gymnema sylvestre* R. Br.)	Obesity
Kava (*Piper methysticum* G. Forst)	Weight reduction
Licorice (*Glycyrrhiza glabra* L.), deglycyrrhizinated licorice (DGL)	Body fat reducer
Licorice (*Glycyrrhiza glabra* L.), deglycyrrhizinated licorice (DGL)	Obesity
Omega-3 fatty acids, fish oil, alpha-linolenic acid	Obesity
Psyllium (*Plantago ovata, P. ispaghula*)	Obesity
Red clover (*Trifolium pratense*)	Appetite suppressant
Seaweed, kelp, bladderwrack (*Fucus vesiculosus*)	Obesity
Thyme (*Thymus vulgaris* L.), thymol	Obesity
Yohimbe bark extract (*Pausinystalia yohimbe* Pierre ex Beille)	Obesity

WELL-BEING AND RELATED CONDITIONS

Levels of Scientific Evidence for Specific Therapies

GRADE: C (Unclear or Conflicting Scientific Evidence)	
Therapy	Specific Therapeutic Use(s)
Chamomile (*Matricaria recutita, Chamaemelum nobile*)	Quality of life in cancer patients

TRADITIONAL OR THEORETICAL USES THAT LACK SUFFICIENT EVIDENCE	
Therapy	Specific Therapeutic Use(s)
Essiac	Supportive care in advanced-cancer patients
Ginseng (American ginseng, Asian ginseng, Chinese ginseng, Korean red ginseng, *Panax ginseng*: *Panax* spp. including *P. ginseng* C.C. Meyer and *P. quinquefolium* L., excluding *Eleutherococcus senticosus*)	Qi deficiency and blood stasis syndrome in heart disease (Eastern medicine)
Ginseng (American ginseng, Asian ginseng, Chinese ginseng, Korean red ginseng, *Panax ginseng*: *Panax* spp. including *P. ginseng* C.C. Meyer and *P. quinquefolium* L., excluding *Eleutherococcus senticosus*)	Quality of life

WOUND HEALING AND RELATED CONDITIONS

Levels of Scientific Evidence for Specific Therapies

GRADE: C (Unclear or Conflicting Scientific Evidence)

Therapy	Specific Therapeutic Use(s)
Arginine (L-arginine)	Wound healing
Calendula (*Calendula officinalis* L.), marigold	Wound and burn healing
Gotu kola (*Centella asiatica* L.), total triterpenic fraction of *Centella asiatica* (TTFCA)	Wound healing

GRADE: D (Fair Negative Scientific Evidence)

Therapy	Specific Therapeutic Use(s)
Aloe (*Aloe vera*)	Infected surgical wounds

TRADITIONAL OR THEORETICAL USES THAT LACK SUFFICIENT EVIDENCE

Therapy	Specific Therapeutic Use(s)
Aloe (*Aloe vera*)	Wound healing after cosmetic dermabrasion
Astragalus (*Astragalus membranaceus*)	Diabetic foot ulcers
Blessed thistle (*Cnicus benedictus* L.)	Skin ulcers
Blessed thistle (*Cnicus benedictus* L.)	Wound healing
Boswellia (*Boswellia serrata* Roxb.)	Cicatrizant (promoting scar formation)
Burdock (*Arctium lappa*)	Sores
Chamomile (*Matricaria recutita, Chamaemelum nobile*)	Abrasions
Chamomile (*Matricaria recutita, Chamaemelum nobile*)	Bed sores
Cranberry (*Vaccinium macrocarpon*)	Wound care
Devil's claw (*Harpagophytum procumbens* DC.)	Skin ulcers (used topically)
Dehydroepiandrosterone (DHEA)	Skin graft healing
Dong quai (*Angelica sinensis* [Oliv.] Diels), Chinese angelica	Skin ulcers
Echinacea (*Echinacea angustifolia* DC., *E. pallida, E. purpurea*)	Skin ulcers
Eucalyptus oil (*Eucalyptus globulus* Labillardiere, *E. fructicetorum* F. Von Mueller, *E. smithii* R.T. Baker)	Skin ulcers
Ginkgo (*Ginkgo biloba* L.)	Skin sores (ginkgo cream)
Goldenseal (*Hydrastis canadensis* L.), berberine	Anal fissures
Guggul (*Commifora mukul*)	Sores
Hawthorn (*Crataegus laevigata, C. oxyacantha, C. monogyna, C. pentagyna*)	Skin sores
Hops (*Humulus lupulus* L.)	Skin ulcers (hops used on the skin)
Lavender (*Lavandula angustifolia* Miller)	Sores
Licorice (*Glycyrrhiza glabra* L.), deglycyrrhizinated licorice (DGL)	Graft healing

Continued

Marshmallow (*Althaea officinalis* L.)	Vulnerary
Propolis	Skin rejuvenator
Shark cartilage	Wound healing
Slippery elm (*Ulmus rubra* Muhl. or *U. fulva* Michx.)	Abrasions
Slippery elm (*Ulmus rubra* Muhl. or *U. fulva* Michx.)	Anal fissures
Slippery elm (*Ulmus rubra* Muhl. or *U. fulva* Michx.)	Skin ulcer
Spirulina	Wound healing
St. John's wort (*Hypericum perforatum* L.)	Skin scrapes
White horehound (*Marrubium vulgare* L.)	Skin ulcers
White horehound (*Marrubium vulgare* L.)	Vulnerary

Index